CURRENT THERAPY
IN EMERGENCY
MEDICINE

Current Therapy Series

CURRENT THERAPY

IN EMERGENCY

MEDICINE

MICHAEL L. CALLAHAM, M.D.

Adjunct Associate Professor of Medicine
University of California School of Medicine

Chief, Division of Emergency Medicine
Moffitt-Long Hospital
San Francisco, California

1987

B.C. DECKER INC • Toronto • Philadelphia

Publisher

B.C. Decker Inc.
3228 South Service Road
Burlington, Ontario   L7N 3H8

B.C. Decker Inc.
P.O. Box 30246
Philadelphia, Pennsylvania   19103

Sales and Distribution

United States and Possessions	**The C.V. Mosby Company** 11830 Westline Industrial Drive Saint Louis, Missouri 63146
Canada	**The C.V. Mosby Company, Ltd.** 5240 Finch Avenue East, Unit No. 1 Scarborough, Ontario M1S 4P2
United Kingdom, Europe and the Middle East	**Blackwell Scientific Publications, Ltd.** Osney Mead, Oxford OX2 OEL, England
Australia	**CBS Publishing Australia Pty. Limited** 9 Waltham Street Artarmon, N.S.W. 2064 Australia
Japan	**Igaku-Shoin Ltd.** Tokyo International P.O. Box 5063 1-28-36 Hongo, Bunkyo-ku, Tokyo 113, Japan
Asia	**CBS Publishing Asia Limited** 10/F, Inter-Continental Plaza Tsim Sha Tsui East Kowloon, Hong Kong

Current Therapy in Emergency Medicine   ISBN 0–941158–62–4

Library of Congress catalog card number: 86-71432

10 9 8 7 6 5 4 3 2 1

To those editors who came before me:

Ilya Gregorivich Bervy
John Robert Callaham
Ludmilla Ignatiev Callaham

and to Lee

SANDRA M. ABADIE, M.D.

Fellow, Department of Internal Medicine, Section of
Infectious Diseases, Ochsner Clinic and Alton Ochsner
Medical Foundation, New Orleans, Louisiana
Adult Infectious Diarrhea

EDWARD ABRAHAM, M.D.

Assistant Professor of Medicine, UCLA Medical School;
Attending Physician, Medical Intensive Care Unit, UCLA
Medical Center, Los Angeles, California
Approach to the Patient in Shock

HAROLD P. ADAMS Jr., M.D.

Professor of Neurology and Director, Division of
Cerebrovascular Diseases, Department of Neurology,
University of Iowa College of Medicine; Attending
Neurologist and Director, Acute Stroke Care and
Monitoring Unit, University of Iowa Hospitals,
Iowa City, Iowa
Cerebral Infarction and Transient Ischemic Attack

STEPHEN L. ADAMS, M.D.

Assistant Professor, Department of Medicine and
Associate Chief, Section of Emergency Medicine, Depart-
ment of Medicine, Northwestern University Medical
School; Associate Medical Director, Emergency Medical
Services, Northwestern Memorial Hospital,
Chicago, Illinois
Pleural Effusion

ALBERT ALTCHECK, M.D., F.A.C.S., F.A.C.O.G.

Associate Clinical Professor of Obstetrics, Gynecology,
and Reproductive Science, The Mount Sinai School of
Medicine; Associate Attending Obstetrician-Gynecologist,
The Mount Sinai Hospital and Director, Pediatric
Gynecology Clinic, Lenox Hill Hospital,
New York, New York
Childhood and Adolescent Gynecologic Problems

WILLIAM J. C. AMEND Jr., M.D.

Professor of Clinical Medicine and Surgery, University of
California School of Medicine; Attending Physician,
University of California Medical Center—Moffitt-Long
Hospital, San Francisco, California
Emergencies in Patients with Renal Transplants

JAMES T. AMSTERDAM, D.M.D., M.D.

Visiting Associate Professor, Medical College of
Pennsylvania, Philadelphia, Pennsylvania and Assistant
Professor of Emergency Medicine and Assistant Professor
of Surgery (Oral Surgery and Dentistry), University of
Cincinnati Medical Center; Coordinator for Medical
Operations, Center for Emergency Care, University of
Cincinnati Hospital, Cincinnati, Ohio
Infection of the Head and Neck

GAIL V. ANDERSON, M.D., F.A.C.S., F.A.C.O.G.

Professor and Chairman, Department of Emergency
Medicine and Professor of Obstetrics and Gynecology,
University of Southern California School of Medicine;
Director, Department of Emergency Medicine,
Los Angeles County—University of Southern California
Medical Center, Los Angeles, California
Ectopic Pregnancy

THOMAS E. ANDREOLI, M.D.

Edward Randall III, Professor and Chairman, Department
of Internal Medicine, University of Texas Medical
School; Chief of Medicine and Medical Director,
Texas Kidney Institute, Hermann Hospital,
Houston, Texas
Hyponatremia and Hypernatremia

HABIB ANWAR, M.D., F.A.C.I.P.

Clinical Instructor, Surgery and Urology, University of
California School of Medicine; Attending Urologist,
Mercy Hospital, Sharp Memorial Hospital,
San Diego, California
Priapism and Cutaneous Lesions of the Penis and Scrotum

CHARLES APRAHAMIAN, M.D., F.A.C.S.

Associate Professor of Surgery, Medical College of Wisconsin, Milwaukee, Wisconsin
Blunt Abdominal Trauma

PAUL S. AUERBACH, M.D.

Associate Professor of Surgery and Medicine, Vanderbilt
University School of Medicine; Director, Emergency
Services, Vanderbilt University Medical Center, and
Medical Director, Division of Emergency Medical
Services, Tennessee Department of Health and
Environment, Nashville, Tennessee
Marine Envenomation
Bee, Wasp, and Spider Envenomation

CHARLES F. BABBS, M.D., Ph.D.

Associate Research Scholar, Hillenbrand Biomedical Engineering Center, Purdue University, West Lafayette; Instructor in Family Medicine, Indiana University School of Medicine, Indianapolis, Indiana
Practical Advances in Cardiopulmonary Resuscitation

PAUL B. BAKER, M.D.

Senior Resident, Department of Emergency Medicine, University of Cincinnati Medical Center, Cincinnati, Ohio
Malaria

FREDERICK C. BALDUINI, M.D.

Assistant Professor of Orthopaedic Surgery, University of Pennsylvania School of Medicine; Orthopaedic Surgeon, Hospital of the University of Pennsylvania, Philadelphia, Pennsylvania
Musculotendinous Contusion and Rupture

SABINO T. BALUYOT, M.D., F.A.C.S.

Assistant Clinical Professor, Department of Otolaryngology–Head and Neck Surgery, University of Cincinnati Medical Center; Chairman, Department of Surgery, Deaconess Hospital and Chairman, Section of Otolaryngology–Head and Neck Surgery, Deaconess and Good Samaritan Hospitals, Cincinnati, Ohio
Foreign Bodies of the Ear, Nose, and Oropharynx

WILLIAM G. BARSAN, M.D.

Associate Professor, Department of Emergency Medicine, University of Cincinnati College of Medicine; Attending Physician, University of Cincinnati Hospital, Cincinnati, Ohio
Anaphylaxis and Serum Sickness

ALFRED V. BARTLETT III, M.D.

Assistant Professor of Pediatrics, Program in Infectious Diseases and Clinical Microbiology, University of Texas Medical School, Houston, Texas
Pediatric Diarrhea

JOHN G. BARTLETT, M.D.

Professor of Medicine, The Johns Hopkins University School of Medicine; Chief, Infectious Diseases Division, The Johns Hopkins Hospital, Baltimore, Maryland
Pulmonary Infection Caused by Aerobic Gram-Positive Cocci

DANIEL R. BENSON, M.D.

Professor, Department of Orthopaedic Surgery and Chief of the Spine Service, University of California School of Medicine, Davis, California
Thoracic and Lumbosacral Spine Injury

CAROL D. BERKOWITZ, M.D., F.A.A.P.

Adjunct Associate Professor of Pediatrics, UCLA School of Medicine, Los Angeles; Director, Pediatric Clinic and Group Practice, Harbor-UCLA Medical Center, Torrance, California
Fever in the Child

HARRY C. BISHOP, M.D.

Professor of Surgery, University of Pennsylvania School of Medicine; Surgeon, Children's Hospital of Philadelphia, Philadelphia, Pennsylvania
Pediatric Gastrointestinal Problems

BRACK A. BIVINS, M.D., F.A.C.S.

Clinical Associate Professor of Surgery, University of Michigan Medical School, Ann Arbor; Head, Division of Trauma Surgery and Director, Nutritional Support Service, Henry Ford Hospital, Detroit, Michigan
Penetrating Neck Trauma

DANIEL S. BLUMENTHAL, M.D., M.P.H.

Professor and Chairman, Department of Community Health and Preventive Medicine and Associate Professor, Department of Pediatrics, Morehouse School of Medicine; Attending Physician, Hughes Spalding Medical Center, Atlanta, Georgia
Intestinal Parasites

MAX BORTEN, M.D.

Associate Professor of Obstetrics and Gynecology, Harvard Medical School; Director, Medical Gynecology, Beth Israel Hospital, Boston, Massachusetts
Lactation Disorders and Mastitis

MARY E. BOTTONE, M.D.

Senior Resident, Division of Otolaryngology, Georgetown University School of Medicine, Washington, D.C.
Tonsillitis and Peritonsillar Abscess

HARISIOS BOUDOULAS, M.D.

Professor of Medicine, Ohio State University College of Medicine and Ohio State University Hospitals, Columbus, Ohio
Mitral Valve Prolapse

WILLIAM F. BOUZARTH, M.D., F.A.C.S.

Professor of Neurosurgery, Medical College of Pennsylvania, Philadelphia, Pennsylvania
Subarachnoid Hemorrhage

WILLIAM R. BOWIE, M.D., F.R.C.P.(C)

Associate Professor of Medicine, Division of Infectious Diseases, Department of Medicine, Vancouver General Hospital and University of British Columbia, Vancouver, British Columbia, Canada
Urethritis

MICHAEL BOWMAN, M.D., M.S.

Assistant Professor of Surgery and Medicine, University of Wisconsin School of Medicine; Chief, Section of Emergency Medicine and Director, University of Wisconsin Med Flight, University of Wisconsin Hospital and Clinics, Madison, Wisconsin
Neurologic Assessment in the Emergency Setting

MARK E. BOYD, M.D., F.R.C.S.(C)

Associate Professor of Obstetrics and Gynecology, McGill University Faculty of Medicine; Head, Division of Gynecology, Royal Victoria Hospital, Montreal, Quebec, Canada
Abnormal Uterine Bleeding

G. RICHARD BRAEN, M.D., F.A.C.E.P.

Director of Emergency Services, Brigham and Women's Hospital and Harvard Community Health Service, Boston, Massachusetts
Rape

ROBERT C. BRASCH, M.D.

Professor of Radiology and Pediatrics, University of California School of Medicine, San Francisco, California
Diagnostic Imaging in the Emergency Center

SHIMON BRAUN, M.D.

Visiting Scientist, Cardiovascular Research Institute, University of California School of Medicine and the Veterans Administration Medical Center, San Francisco, California
Pulmonary Edema

TIMOTHY J. BRAY, M.D.

Assistant Professor, Department of Orthopaedics and Chief, Orthopaedic Trauma Service, University of California School of Medicine, Davis, California
Pelvic Fracture

BARRY BRENNER, M.D.

Clinical Assistant Professor of Emergency Medicine, UCLA School of Medicine; Attending Physician, UCLA Medical Center, Los Angeles, California
Compartment Syndrome and Rhabdomyolysis

MICHAEL J. BRESLER, M.D., F.A.C.E.P.

Assistant Clinical Professor of Surgery, Stanford University School of Medicine; Associate Director, Division of Emergency Medicine, Stanford Medical Center, Stanford, California
Behavioral Emergencies

MARTIN BROTMAN, B.Sc.(Med), M.Sc., M.D.

Clinical Professor of Medicine, University of California School of Medicine; Chief, Division of Gastroenterology and Director, Division of Education, Pacific Presbyterian Medical Center, San Francisco, California
Functional Bowel Problems

CHARLES G. BROWN, M.D., F.A.C.E.P.

Assistant Professor, Ohio State University College of Medicine, Columbus, Ohio
Alcohol Intoxication and Withdrawal

DALE BROWN Jr., M.D.

Clinical Associate Professor, Baylor College of Medicine, Houston, Texas
Vulvar Disease

MICHAEL W. BROWN, M.D.

Assistant Professor of Urology, Duke University School of Medicine; Attending Urologist, Duke University Medical Center and Durham Veterans Administration Hospital, Durham, North Carolina
Prostatitis

NYDA WILLIAMS BROWN, M.D., F.A.G.P.A.

Associate Clinical Professor of Psychiatry, Emory University School of Medicine, Atlanta; Chief, Eating Disorders Service, Brawner Psychiatric Institute, Smyrna, Georgia
Starvation and Diet-Induced Emergencies

MICHAEL W. BRUNKO, M.D.

Clinical Instructor in Emergency Medicine, Department of Surgery, University of Colorado Health Sciences Center; Attending Staff, Emergency Physician, St. Anthony Hospital, Denver, Colorado
Blunt and Penetrating Chest Trauma

ROBERT W. BUCHOLZ, M.D.

Associate Professor, Division of Orthopaedic Surgery, University of Texas Southwestern Medical School, Dallas, Texas
Bursitis and Tendonitis

JURIS BUNKIS, M.D., F.A.C.S.

Assistant Clinical Professor of Surgery, University of California School of Medicine, San Francisco; Private Practice, Hayward, California
Wound Management

JOHN R. BURNS, M.D.

Associate Professor, Division of Urology, University of Alabama School of Medicine; Attending Physician, Veterans Administration Hospital, Birmingham, Alabama
Renal Stones and Urinary Obstruction

CHRISTOPHER R. BURROW, M.D.

Assistant Professor of Medicine, The Johns Hopkins University School of Medicine; Medical Director, Dialysis, The Johns Hopkins Hospital, Baltimore, Maryland
Hypertensive Crisis

EDWIN C. CADMAN, M.D.

Professor of Medicine and Director, Cancer Research Institute, Chief, Hematology and Oncology and Vice-Chairman, Department of Medicine, University of California School of Medicine, San Francisco, California
Oncologic Emergencies

RENE CAILLIET, M.D.

Clinical Professor, Department of Physical Medicine Rehabilitation, University of Southern California School of Medicine, Los Angeles, California
Shoulder Pain

MICHAEL L. CALLAHAM, M.D.

Adjunct Associate Professor of Medicine, University of California School of Medicine; Chief, Division of Emergency Medicine, Moffitt-Long Hospital, San Francisco, California
Human and Animal Bites
Cyclic Antidepressant Overdose

JOHN V. CARBONE, M.D.

Professor of Medicine, University of California School of Medicine; Attending Physician, Moffitt-Long Hospital, San Francisco, California
Inflammatory Bowel Disease

JOHN J. CARONNA, M.D.

Professor of Clinical Neurology, Cornell University Medical College; Attending Neurologist, The New York Hospital—Cornell Medical Center, New York, New York
The Comatose Patient

MARSHALL W. CARPENTER, B.S., M.D.

Assistant Professor, Department of Obstetrics and Gynecology, Brown University Program in Medicine; Associate Director, Division of Maternal-Fetal Medicine, Women and Infants Hospital of Rhode Island, Providence, Rhode Island
Abdominal Pain and Vaginal Bleeding in Late Pregnancy

RALPH R. CAVALIERI, M.D.

Professor of Medicine and Radiology, University of California School of Medicine; Chief, Nuclear Medicine, Veterans Administration Medical Center, San Francisco, California
Thyroid Disorders

JOHN P. CELLO, M.D.

Associate Professor of Medicine, University of California School of Medicine; Chief, Division of Gastroenterology, San Francisco General Hospital, San Francisco, California
Upper Gastrointestinal Bleeding

HENRY F. CHAMBERS, M.D.

Assistant Professor, Department of Medicine, University of California School of Medicine and San Francisco General Hospital, San Francisco, California
Infection in the Parenteral Drug User

THOMAS A. CHAPEL, M.D.

Clinical Professor, Wayne State University School of Medicine, Detroit, Michigan
Mucous Membrane Disease

KANU CHATTERJEE, M.B., F.R.C.P.

Professor of Medicine, Lucie Stern Professor of Cardiology, University of California School of Medicine; Associate Chief, Division of Cardiology and Director, Cardiac Care Unit, Moffit-Long Hospital, San Francisco, California
Congestive Heart Failure

MELVIN D. CHEITLIN, M.D., F.A.C.C.

Professor of Medicine, University of California School of Medicine; Associate Chief of Cardiology, San Francisco General Hospital, San Francisco, California
Myocardial Contusion

NEIL S. CHERNIACK, M.D.

Professor of Medicine, Case Western Reserve University School of Medicine; Chief, Pulmonary Division, University Hospitals and Cleveland Veterans Administration Medical Center, Cleveland, Ohio
Chronic Obstructive Pulmonary Disease

ROBERT CHUONG, D.M.D., M.D.

Assistant Professor, Oral and Maxillofacial Surgery, Harvard School of Dental Medicine; Assistant Surgeon, Brigham and Women's Hospital, Boston, Massachusetts
Maxillofacial Skeletal Fracture

PAUL M. COLOMBANI, M.D.

Assistant Professor of Surgery and Pediatrics, The Johns Hopkins University School of Medicine; Attending Pediatric Surgeon, The Johns Hopkins Hospital, Baltimore, Maryland
The Pediatric Trauma Patient

FERNANDO I. COLON-FIGUEROA, M.D.

Surgical Resident, Mount Carmel Medical Center, Columbus, Ohio
Tetanus

DAVID M. CONTRERAS, M.D.

Department of Orthopaedic Surgery, University of California School of Medicine; Chief Resident, San Francisco General Hospital, San Francisco, California
Hand Infections

MARY ANN COOPER, M.D., F.A.C.E.P.

Associate Professor and Research Director, Department of Surgery, Division of Emergency Medicine, University of Illinois College of Medicine; Staff, Emergency Department, Mercy Hospital Medical Center, Chicago, Illinois
Electrical Injury
Lightning Injury

LAURENCE CORASH, M.D.

Professor, Laboratory Medicine, University of California School of Medicine; Chief, Hematology Section, Clinical Laboratories, University of California Hospitals and Clinics, San Francisco, California
Hemorrhagic Coagulopathy

RICHARD A. CRASS, M.D.

Associate Professor of Surgery and Chief, Division of General Surgery, The Oregon Health Sciences University School of Medicine, Portland, Oregon
Biliary Tract Disease

ALVIN H. CRAWFORD, M.D., F.A.C.S.

Professor of Orthopaedic Surgery and Pediatrics, University of Cincinnati College of Medicine; Director of Orthopaedic Surgery, Childrens Hospital Medical Center, Cincinnati, Ohio
Orthopaedic Injury in Children

RICHARD A. CURRIE, M.D., C.M., F.A.C.S.

Associate Professor of Surgery, The Johns Hopkins University School of Medicine, Baltimore; Chief of Surgery, Patuxent Medical Group, Columbia, Maryland
Breast Disorders

JOHN R. CUTLER, M.D.

Instructor, Department of Neurology, University of California School of Medicine, San Francisco, California
Headache and Facial Pain

ROBERT H. DAILEY, M.D.

Clinical Professor of Medicine, University of California School of Medicine, San Francisco; Chief, Emergency Medicine, Highland Hospital, Oakland, California
Grand Mal (Major Motor) Seizures
Venous Access

DANIEL F. DANZL, M.D., F.A.C.E.P.

Associate Professor of Emergency Medicine, University of Louisville School of Medicine, Louisville, Kentucky
Principles of Airway Management

STEVEN J. DAVIDSON, M.D., F.A.C.E.P.

Associate Professor of Emergency Medicine, Medical College of Pennsylvania, Philadelphia, Pennsylvania
Approach to Acute Abdominal Pain

MICHAEL E. DeBAKEY, M.D.

Olga Keith Wiess Professor of Surgery and Chairman of the Department of Surgery, Baylor College of Medicine, Houston, Texas
Dissecting Aneurysm of the Aorta

KATHLEEN DELANEY, M.D.

Clinical Instructor in Medicine, New York University School of Medicine; Attending Physician, Bellevue Emergency Department, New York, New York
Metabolic Acidosis and Alkalosis

DAVID R. DEMARTINI, M.D.

Assistant Clinical Professor, Department of Ophthalmology, Pacific Medical Center, San Francisco; Vice-Chairman, Department of Ophthalmology, Highland General Hospital, Oakland, California
Corneal Abrasion and Burn
Acute Eye Inflammation

THOMAS A. DEUTSCH, M.D.

Assistant Professor and Program Director, Department of Ophthalmology, Rush Medical College; Assistant Attending, Department of Ophthalmology, Rush-Presbyterian-St. Luke's Medical Center, Chicago, Illinois
Eye and Orbit Trauma

RONALD A. DIECKMANN, M.D., M.P.H., F.A.A.P., F.A.C.E.P.

Assistant Clinical Professor, Pediatrics and Medicine, University of California School of Medicine; Attending Physician, Emergency Department, San Francisco General Hospital, San Francisco, California
Seizures in Children

DENNIS A. DIEDERICH, M.D.

Professor of Medicine, Department of Medicine, Division of Nephrology, University of Kansas Medical Center, Kansas City, Kansas
Acute Renal Failure

RALPH J. DiLIBERO, M.D., F.A.A.O.S.

Staff, Southern California Permanente Medical Group, Department of Orthopaedic Surgery and Sports Medicine, Kaiser Foundation Hospital, Hollywood, California
Fractures Not Requiring Orthopaedic Consultation

ALAN R. DIMICK, M.D., F.A.C.S.

Associate Professor of Surgery, University of Alabama School of Medicine; Director, Burn Center, University of Alabama Hospital and Children's Hospital, Birmingham, Alabama
Thermal and Chemical Burns

JAMES R. DINGFELDER, M.D.

Clinical Instructor, Obstetrics and Gynecology, Duke University School of Medicine; Attending Physician, Durham County General Hospital, Durham, North Carolina
Vaginal Trauma and Foreign Bodies

LYNNETTE A. DOAN, M.D., F.A.C.E.P.

Assistant Professor of Emergency Medicine, University of Chicago; Associate Chairman, Department of Emergency Medicine, University of Chicago Medical Center, Chicago, Illinois
Hematuria

HILLARY DON, M.D.

Associate Professor, Department of Anesthesia, University of California School of Medicine; Attending Staff, Department of Anesthesia, Veterans Administration Medical Center, San Francisco, California
Oxygen Therapy

MICHAEL V. DRAKE, M.D.

Assistant Professor, Department of Ophthalmology and Chief, Eye Clinic, University of California School of Medicine; Attending Surgeon, San Francisco General Hospital and Veterans Administration Hospital, San Francisco, California
Approach to Ocular Emergencies

STEVEN C. DRONEN, M.D.

Assistant Professor and Coordinator, Emergency Medicine Residency Program, University of Cincinnati College of Medicine; Attending Physician, Emergency Medicine Department, University Hospital, Cincinnati, Ohio
Monitoring in the Emergency Department
Malaria

DENIS S. DRUMMOND, M.D.

Professor of Orthopaedic Surgery, The Hospital of the University of Pennsylvania; Chairman, Department of Orthopaedic Surgery, The Children's Hospital of Philadelphia, Philadelphia, Pennsylvania
Acute Back Pain in Physically Active Individuals

HERBERT L. DuPONT, M.D.

Professor and Director, Program in Infectious Diseases and Clinical Microbiology, The University of Texas Medical School; Attending Physician, Hermann Hospital, Houston, Texas
Prophylaxis for Travelers

LAWRENCE DURBAN, M.D.

Chief Resident in Surgery, Cornell University Medical College; Attending Staff, The New York Hospital, New York, New York
Penetrating Cardiac Trauma

RAPHAEL B. DURFEE, M.D.

Professor of Reproductive Medicine, University of California School of Medicine; Clinical Professor, UCSD Medical Center, San Diego, California
Spontaneous Abortion and Bleeding in Early Pregnancy

STEPHEN H. EMBURY, M.D.

Associate Professor of Medicine, University of California School of Medicine; Chief, Adult Hematology Division, San Francisco General Hospital, San Francisco, California
Sickle Cell Anemia

KENNETH ENG, M.D.

Professor of Surgery, New York University School of Medicine, New York, New York
Appendicitis and Diverticulitis

G. THOMAS EVANS Jr., M.D.

Clinical Assistant Professor of Medicine, University of California Medical Center, San Francisco and Assistant Chief of Emergency Medicine, Valley Medical Center, Fresno, California
The Patient with S-T and T Wave Changes on Electrocardiography

EVAN R. FARMER, M.D.

Associate Professor of Dermatology, The Johns Hopkins University School of Medicine, Baltimore, Maryland
Approach to Skin Disease

BARRY M. FARR, M.D., M.Sc.

Assistant Professor of Medicine, University of Virginia School of Medicine; Attending Physician, University of Virginia Hospital, Charlottesville, Virginia
The Common Cold

JOHN M. FIELD, M.D.

Assistant Professor of Medicine and Surgery, Director of Clinical Cardiology and Director, Emergency Medical Services, Penn State University School of Medicine, Hershey Medical Center, Hershey, Pennsylvania
Valvular Heart Disease

MICHAEL L. FISCHMAN, M.D., M.P.H.

Clinical Instructor in Medicine, Division of Occupational Medicine, Department of Medicine, University of California School of Medicine, San Francisco; Consulting Practice in Occupational Medicine and Toxicology, Hughes, Lewis, Fischman and Associates, Oakland, California
Exposure to Chemicals and Hazardous Material

DANIEL B. FISHBEIN, M.D.

Medical Epidemiologist, Viral and Rickettsial Zoonoses Branch, Division of Viral Diseases, Center for Infectious Diseases, Centers for Disease Control, Atlanta, Georgia
Rabies

FAITH T. FITZGERALD, M.D.

Professor of Medicine, Division of General Medicine, University of California, Davis, School of Medicine, Sacramento, California
Magnesium Disorders
Phosphate Disorders

STEPHEN E. FOLLANSBEE, M.D.

Assistant Clinical Professor of Medicine, University of California School of Medicine; Attending Physician, Ralph K. Davies Medical Center and St. Luke's Hospital, San Francisco, California
Fever in the Adult

GARRETT FOULKE, M.D.

Assistant Clinical Professor, Division of Emergency Medicine and Clinical Toxicology, University of California, Davis, School of Medicine; Assistant Director, Department of Emergency Medicine, University of California, Davis, Medical Center, Sacramento, California
High-Altitude Illness

NOBLE O. FOWLER, M.D.

Professor Emeritus of Medicine and Pharmacology and Cell Biophysics, University of Cincinnati College of Medicine; Director, Division of Cardiology, University of Cincinnati College of Medicine and Chief Clinician, Cardiac Clinic, University Hospital, Cincinnati, Ohio
Nontraumatic Cardiac Tamponade

JACEK BRONISLAW FRANASZEK, M.D., F.A.C.E.P.

Associate Professor of Surgery, Emergency Medicine, Brown University Program in Medicine; Director, Department of Emergency Medicine, Rhode Island Hospital, Providence, Rhode Island
Response to Disaster

ILONA J. FRIEDEN, M.D.

Assistant Clinical Professor of Dermatology and Pediatrics, University of California School of Medicine, San Francisco; Chief of Dermatology, Kaiser-Permanente Medical Center, Oakland, California
Common Pediatric Rashes Without Systemic Illness

WESLEY FURSTE, M.D., F.A.C.S.

Clinical Professor Emeritus of Surgery, Ohio State University College of Medicine; Senior Attending Staff, Mount Carmel Medical Center and Riverside Methodist Hospital, Columbus, Ohio
Tetanus

MARY O. GABRIELSON, M.D., M.P.H.

Assistant Professor, Obstetrics and Gynecology, Medical College of Pennsylvania, Philadelphia, Pennsylvania
Contraceptive Problems

LORRAINE GATES, M.D.

Fellow in Pulmonary Diseases, Cardiovascular Research Institute, University of California School of Medicine, San Francisco, California
Pulmonary Embolism

J. LOUISE GERBERDING, M.D.

Fellow, Clinical Pharmacology and Infectious Diseases, Department of Medicine, University of California School of Medicine, San Francisco, California
Infectious Endocarditis

EDMUND W. GIEGERICH, M.D.

Assistant Professor of Medicine, State University of New York Downstate Medical Center; Chief of Endocrinology, Long Island College Hospital, Brooklyn, New York
Diabetic Ketoacidosis

PAUL C. GILLETTE, M.D., F.A.C.C.

Professor of Pediatric Cardiology and Director, Division of Pediatric Cardiology, South Carolina Children's Heart Center, Charleston, South Carolina
Pediatric Dysrhythmia and Other Cardiac Emergencies

BRUCE C. GILLILAND, M.D.

Professor of Medicine and Laboratory Medicine, University of Washington School of Medicine; Chief of Medicine, Pacific Medical Center, Seattle, Washington
Vasculitis

RICHARD B. GLASER, M.D.

Assistant Clinical Professor of Medicine and Instructor of Anesthesiology, University of California School of Medicine, San Francisco, California
Sedation and Rapid-Induction Anesthesia for Emergency Intubation

JEFFREY P. GOLD, M.D.

Assistant Professor of Surgery and Pediatrics, Division of Cardiothoracic Surgery, Cornell University Medical College; Attending Surgeon and Pediatrician, Division of Cardiothoracic Surgery, The New York Hospital, New York, New York
Penetrating Cardiac Trauma

STANLEY M. GOLDBERG, M.D., F.A.C.S.

Clinical Professor of Surgery and Director, Division of Colon and Rectal Surgery, University of Minnesota Medical School, Minneapolis, Minnesota
Anal Fissure, Anal Fistula, and Hemorrhoids

JEFFREY A. GOLDEN, M.D.

Associate Professor of Medicine, University of California School of Medicine, San Francisco, California
Pulmonary Problems in Acquired Immunodeficiency Syndrome

LEWIS R. GOLDFRANK, M.D.

Associate Professor of Clinical Medicine, New York University School of Medicine; Director of Emergency Services, Bellevue Hospital Center and New York University Hospital, New York, New York
Metabolic Acidosis and Alkalosis

FLAIR D. GOLDMAN, D.P.M., M.S.

Assistant Clinical Professor, Department of Basic Medical Science, California College of Podiatric Medicine, San Francisco; Chief, Division of Podiatric Surgery, Department of Orthopaedic Surgery, Kaiser Hospital, Santa Clara, California
Common Foot Disorders

H. WARREN GOLDMAN, M.D., Ph.D.

Associate Professor of Neurosurgery, Medical College of Pennsylvania, Philadelphia, Pennsylvania
Subarachnoid Hemorrhage

PHILIP C. GOODMAN, M.D.

Associate Clinical Professor of Radiology and Medicine,
University of California School of Medicine,
San Francisco, California
Mediastinal and Parenchymal Lung Masses

LEONARD GORDON, M.D.

Assistant Clinical Professor, Department of Orthopaedic
Surgery, University of California School of Medicine,
San Francisco, California
Hand Infections

JAMES H. GRENDELL, M.D.

Assistant Professor of Medicine and Physiology, University of California School of Medicine; Attending Physician,
San Francisco General Hospital, San Francisco, California
Mesenteric Vascular Occlusion

MICHAEL A. GRODIN, M.D.

Associate Professor of Pediatrics, Boston University
School of Medicine; Director, Pediatric Emergency
Services, Boston City Hospital, Boston, Massachusetts
Epiglottitis

JACK M. GWALTNEY Jr., M.D.

Professor of Medicine, University of Virginia School of
Medicine; Attending Physician, University of Virginia
Hospital, Charlottesville, Virginia
The Common Cold

RALPH W. HALE, M.D., F.A.C.O.G.

Chairman and Professor, Department of Obstetrics and
Gynecology, University of Hawaii, Honolulu, Hawaii
Diagnosis and Course of Normal Pregnancy

ALAN H. HALL, M.D.

Clinical Toxicology Fellow, University of Colorado
School of Medicine; Attending Staff, Rocky Mountain
Poison and Drug Center and Denver General Hospital,
Denver, Colorado
Prevention of Absorption in Overdose

J. ALEX HALLER Jr., M.D.

Professor of Surgery, Pediatrics and Emergency
Medicine, The Johns Hopkins University School of
Medicine; Pediatric Surgeon-in-Charge, The Johns
Hopkins Hospital, Baltimore, Maryland
The Pediatric Trauma Patient

STEVEN D. HANDLER, M.D., F.A.C.S.

Assistant Professor, Department of Otorhinolaryngology
and Human Communication, University of Pennsylvania
School of Medicine; Associate Director, Department of
Otolaryngology and Human Communication, Children's
Hospital, Philadelphia, Pennsylvania
Laryngitis and Croup

ANN HARWOOD-NUSS, M.D.

Associate Professor, Division of Emergency Medicine,
Department of Surgery, University of Florida College of
Medicine, Gainesville; Attending Staff, University
Hospital of Jacksonville, Jacksonville, Florida
Epididymitis and Orchitis
Toxic Shock Syndrome

JAMES P. HAYES, M.S.

Vascular Research, St. Anthony Medical Center,
Columbus, Ohio
Ateriosclerotic Popliteal Artery Aneurysm

BRUCE E. HAYNES, M.D.

Assistant Professor of Medicine, UCLA School of
Medicine; Director, Pre-hospital Care, Department of
Emergency Medicine, Harbor-UCLA Medical Center,
Los Angeles, California
Testicular Torsion

JERRIS R. HEDGES, M.D., M.S., F.A.C.E.P.

Assistant Professor, Department of Emergency Medicine,
University of Cincinnati School of Medicine,
Cincinnati, Ohio
Pharyngitis

JOHN P. HEGGERS, Ph.D.

Professor of Surgery, Division of Plastic and
Reconstructive Surgery, Wayne State University School of
Medicine, Detroit, Michigan
Frostbite and Local Cold Injury

DAVID B. HELLMANN, M.D.

Assistant Professor of Medicine, The Johns Hopkins
Hospital, Baltimore, Maryland
Arthritis

BRADLEY E. HENDERSON, M.D.

Former Christine Kleinert Fellow in Hand Surgery,
University of Louisville School of Medicine; Orthopaedic
Surgeon, Private Practice, Louisville, Kentucky
Laceration of the Hand: Fingertip Injury and Infection

BARRY H. HENDLER, D.D.S., M.D.

Clinical Professor of Medicine and Surgery, Medical
College of Pennsylvania and Clinical Professor of Oral
and Maxillofacial Surgery, University of Pennsylvania
School of Dental Medicine; Director of Oral and
Maxillofacial Surgery, The Medical College of
Pennsylvania, Philadelphia, Pennsylvania
Infection of the Head and Neck

GREGORY L. HENRY, M.D., F.A.C.E.P.

Clinical Assistant Professor, Section of Emergency Medicine, Department of Surgery, University of Michigan Medical School, Ann Arbor; Chief, Department of Emergency Medicine, Beyer Memorial Hospital, Ypsilanti, Michigan
Acute Cranial Nerve Lesions
Focal Neurologic Deficit

ALFRED D. HERNANDEZ, M.D.

Assistant Professor of Medicine, University of Tennessee College of Medicine; Chief of Dermatology, Veterans Administration Medical Center, Memphis, Tennessee
Fungal Infection of the Skin

CHARLES E. HESS, M.D.

Professor of Internal Medicine and Associate Head, Hematology-Oncology Division, University of Virginia School of Medicine, Charlottesville, Virginia
Lymphadenopathy and Malaise

MEYER R. HEYMAN, M.D.

Assistant Professor of Medicine, University of Maryland School of Medicine, Baltimore, Maryland
Blood Component Therapy

DAVID W. HILL Jr., M.D.

Clinical Instructor of Emergency Medicine, University of Illinois Affiliated Hospitals; Attending Physician, Emergency Medicine, Alexian Brothers Medical Center, Elk Grove Village, Illinois Masonic Medical Center, Mercy Hospital Medical Center, Chicago, Illinois
Chest Pain

SHALOM Z. HIRSCHMAN, M.D.

Professor of Medicine and Director, Division of Infectious Diseases, The Mount Sinai School of Medicine of the City University of New York; Attending Physician, The Mount Sinai Hospital and Director, Division of Infectious Diseases, The Mount Sinai Medical Center, New York, New York
Hepatitis

FRANKLIN T. HOAGLUND, M.D.

Professor, Department of Orthopaedic Surgery, University of California School of Medicine, San Francisco, California
Low Back Pain and Degenerative Disc Disease

ROBERT S. HOCKBERGER, M.D.

Assistant Professor of Medicine, UCLA School of Medicine; Director, Emergency Medicine Residency, Harbor-UCLA Medical Center, Los Angeles, California
Spinal Cord Injury

JEROME R. HOFFMAN, M.D.

Assistant Professor of Medicine, UCLA School of Medicine; Director, Emergency Medicine Residency Program, UCLA Center for the Health Sciences, Los Angeles, California
Wide Complex Tachycardia
Narrow Complex Tachycardia

ROBERT S. HOFFMAN, M.D.

Assistant Clinical Professor of Psychiatry, University of California School of Medicine, San Francisco; Attending Neurologist, Seton Medical Center, Daly City and Peninsula Hospital, Burlingame, California
Behavioral Emergencies

WILLIAM B. HOFMANN, B.A., M.D.

Assistant Clinical Professor, Department of Otolaryngology and Maxillofacial Surgery, University of Cincinnati Medical Center, Cincinnati; Director, Department of Otolaryngology, Administrative and Teaching Staff, Bethesda Hospital, Cincinnati, Attending Staff, Christ Hospital and Children's Hospital, Cincinnati, and Courtesy Staff, Clinton Memorial Hospital, Wilmington, Ohio
Mandibular Fracture and Dislocation

BENJAMIN HONIGMAN, M.D., F.A.C.E.P.

Assistant Professor of Emergency Medicine, Department of Surgery, University of Colorado Medical School; Director, Emergency Department, University Hospital and University of Colorado Health Sciences Center, Denver, Colorado
Ataxia

LEONARD D. HUDSON, M.D., F.A.C.P., F.C.C.P.

Professor of Medicine and Head, Division of Pulmonary and Critical Care Medicine, University of Washington, Seattle, Washington
Acute Respiratory Failure

J. STEPHEN HUFF, M.D.

Clinical Assistant Professor, Department of Emergency Medicine, University of Cincinnati College of Medicine, Cincinnati, Ohio
Syncope

JAMES C. HUNTER, M.D.

Chief Resident, Department of Emergency Medicine, University of Cincinnati College of Medicine; Staff Physician, University of Cincinnati Hospital, Cincinnati, Ohio
Anaphylaxis and Serum Sickness

KENNETH V. ISERSON, M.D., F.A.C.E.P.

Associate Professor and Residency Director, Section of Emergency Medicine, University of Arizona College of Medicine, Tucson, Arizona
Strangulation and Hanging

O. WAYNE ISOM, M.D.

Cardiothoracic Surgeon-in-Chief and Professor of
Surgery, Cornell University Medical College; Attending
Surgeon, Chief of Division of Cardiothoracic Surgery,
The New York Hospital, New York, New York
Penetrating Cardiac Trauma

RAO R. IVATURY, M.D., F.A.C.S., F.R.C.S.(C)

Assistant Professor of Surgery, New York Medical
College, Valhalla; Director of Surgical Intensive Care
Unit, and Associate Director of Trauma, Lincoln Medical
and Mental Health Center, Bronx, New York
Rib and Sternum Fracture
Flank and Buttock Trauma

RICHARD A. JACOBS, M.D., Ph.D.

Assistant Clinical Professor of Medicine, Co-Director,
Division of Clinical Infectious Diseases, University of
California School of Medicine, San Francisco, California
Sepsis in Adults

HAROLD A. JAYNE, M.D., F.A.C.E.P. (Deceased)

Former Assistant Professor of Clinical Emergency
Medicine, University of Illinois College of Medicine,
Chicago; Former Attending Physician, Illinois Masonic
Medical Center, Mercy Hospital and Medical Center,
Chicago, and Lutheran General Hospital,
Park Ridge, Illinois
Chest Pain

CAROL J. JESSOP, M.D.

Assistant Professor of Medicine, University of California
School of Medicine, San Francisco, California
Premenstrual Syndrome and Cramps

MARIE-LOUISE JOHNSON, M.D., Ph.D.

Clinical Professor of Dermatology, Yale University
School of Medicine; Attending Staff, Yale-New Haven
Medical Center, New Haven, Connecticut and Director of
Medical Education, Vice-President for Medical Affairs,
Benedictine Hospital, Kingston, New York
Inpatient Therapy in Skin Disease

ELAINE C. JONG, M.D.

Associate Professor, Department of Medicine, University
of Washington School of Medicine; Director, University
of Washington Travel and Tropical Medicine Clinic,
University Hospital, and Attending Physician, Division of
Emergency Medicine, University Hospital,
Seattle, Washington
Infectious Disease in Immigrants and Travelers

TIMOTHY T. K. JUNG, M.D., Ph.D.

Associate Professor, Division of Otolaryngology,
Loma Linda University School of Medicine,
Loma Linda, California
Dizziness

LEONARD B. KABAN, D.M.D., M.D., F.A.C.S.

Professor and Chairman, Division of Oral and
Maxillofacial Surgery, University of California School of
Medicine; Attending Surgeon, Oral and Maxillofacial
Surgery, Moffitt Hospital, San Francisco, California
Maxillofacial Skeletal Fracture

SHELDON L. KAPLAN, M.D.

Associate Professor, Department of Pediatrics, Baylor
College of Medicine; Chief, Infectious Disease Service,
Texas Children's Hospital, Houston, Texas
Sepsis in Children

RAYMOND H. KAUFMAN, M.D.

Ernst W. Bertner Chairman and Professor, Department of
Obstetrics and Gynecology and Professor, Department of
Pathology, Baylor College of Medicine, Houston, Texas
Vulvar Disease

JAMES S. KEENE, M.D.

Associate Professor of Orthopaedic Surgery, University of
Wisconsin Medical School and Clinical Sciences Center;
Co-Director, University of Wisconsin Spinal Injury
Center, Team Orthopaedic Surgeon, University of
Wisconsin Athletic Teams, Madison, Wisconsin
Acute Back Pain in Physically Active Individuals

EUGENE S. KILGORE, M.D.

Clinical Professor of Surgery, University of California
School of Medicine; Chief, Hand Clinics, University of
California School of Medicine, San Francisco, and the
Fort Miley Veterans Administration Hospital,
San Francisco, California
Dislocation of the Digits, Wrist, and Hand

EDWARD E. KIMBROUGH, M.D.

Professor and Chairman, Department of Orthopaedics,
University of South Carolina School of Medicine;
Attending Staff, Richland Memorial Hospital,
Columbia, South Carolina
Knee Dislocation

JEFFREY C. KING, M.D.

Assistant Professor of Obstetrics and Gynecology,
Georgetown University School of Medicine,
Washington, D.C.
Trauma in Pregnancy

THEO N. KIRKLAND, M.D.

Assistant Professor of Pathology and Medicine, University
of California School of Medicine; Staff Physician,
Veterans Administration Medical Center,
San Diego, California
Fungal Respiratory Disease

ROBERT KIWI, M.D., M.R.C.O.G., F.A.C.O.G.

Assistant Professor, Case Western Reserve University
School of Medicine; Head of Obstetrics, Mount Sinai
Medical Center, Cleveland, Ohio
Puerperal and Postabortal Infection

KENNETH W. KIZER, M.D., M.P.H., F.A.C.E.P.,
F.A.C.P.M.

Assistant Clinical Professor of Medicine, University of
California School of Medicine, Davis; Director,
California Department of Health Services,
Sacramento, California
Scuba Diving Accidents

MICHAEL KLEEREKOPER, M.B., B.S., F.A.C.P.

Clinical Associate Professor of Medicine, University of
Michigan Medical School, Ann Arbor; Head, Division of
Bone and Mineral Metabolism, Department of Internal
Medicine, Henry Ford Hospital, Detroit, Michigan
Hypercalcemia and Hypocalcemia

MARK W. KLINE, M.D.

Postdoctoral Fellow, Pediatric Infectious Diseases, Baylor
College of Medicine, Houston, Texas
Sepsis in Children

JAMES P. KNOCHEL, M.D.

Professor and Vice-Chairman, Department of Internal
Medicine, Southwestern Medical School; Chief, Medical
Service, Veterans Administration Medical Center,
Dallas, Texas
Heat Illness

ROBERT K. KNOPP, M.D.

Associate Clinical Professor of Medicine, University of
California School of Medicine, San Francisco; Chief of
Emergency Medicine, Valley Medical Center,
Fresno, California
Cervical Spine Trauma

BEVERLY L. KOOPS, M.D.

Professor of Pediatrics and Chairman, Department of
Pediatrics, Texas A & M University College of Medicine,
College Station; Neonatologist, Scott and White Hospital,
Temple, Texas
Resuscitation of the Newborn

ALAN D. KORNBLUT, A.B., M.S., M.D., F.A.C.S.

Associate Clinical Professor, Department of Surgery
(Otolaryngology), Georgetown University School of
Medicine, Washington, D.C. and Clinical Professor of
Surgery (Otolaryngology), Uniformed Services University
of the Health Sciences, Bethesda, Maryland
Tonsillitis and Peritonsillar Abscess

DAVID R. KRAUSS, M.D.

Associate Professor of Pediatrics, Texas A & M
University College of Medicine, College Station; Staff
Neonatologist and Director of Nursery Services, Scott and
White Hospital, Temple, Texas
Resuscitation of the Newborn

KARL H. KRIEGER, M.D.

Assistant Professor of Surgery, Division of
Cardiothoracic Surgery, Cornell University Medical
College; Attending Surgeon in Cardiothoracic Surgery,
The New York Hospital, New York, New York
Penetrating Cardiac Trauma

RONALD L. KROME, M.D., F.A.C.S.

Chief, Department of Emergency Medicine, William
Beaumont Hospital, Royal Oak, Michigan
Gastritis and Ulcer Disease

F. MARC LaFORCE, M.D.

Professor of Medicine, University of Colorado School of
Medicine; Associate Chief of Staff for Education,
Veterans Administration Medical Center,
Denver, Colorado
Syphilis

CHRISTOPHER M. LAHR, M.D.

Chief of Colon and Rectal Surgery, U.S. Air Force
Medical Center, Scott Air Force Base, Illinois
Anal Fissure, Anal Fistula, and Hemorrhoids

ROBERT LAMBERT, M.D., F.A.C.C.P.

Clinical Professor of Medicine, University Hospital,
Milton S. Hershey Medical Center, Pennsylvania State
University College of Medicine, Hershey, Pennsylvania
Avoidance of Malpractice

RICHARD L. LAMMERS, M.D., F.A.C.E.P.

Clinical Professor of Family and Community Medicine,
University of California School of Medicine, San
Francisco; Assistant Chief of Emergency Medicine,
Valley Medical Center, Fresno, California
Local Wound Infection

RUSSELL K. LAROS Jr., M.D.

Professor and Vice-Chairman, Department of Obstetrics,
Gynecology and Reproductive Sciences, University of
California School of Medicine, San Francisco, California
Normal Delivery

RICHARD C. LEHMAN, M.D.

Fellow in Sports Medicine, University of Pennsylvania
Sports Medicine Center, Philadelphia, Pennsylvania
Injuries in Runners

ROBERT E. LEVINE, M.D.

Associate Clinical Professor of Ophthalmology, University of Southern California; Chief of Ophthalmology Section, St. Vincent Medical Center, Los Angeles, California
Sudden Loss of Vision

RICHARD LEVY, M.D., M.P.H., F.A.C.E.P.

Professor, Department of Emergency Medicine, University of Cincinnati College of Medicine, Cincinnati, Ohio
Syncope

FRANK R. LEWIS Jr., M.D.

Professor of Surgery, University of California School of Medicine; Acting Chief, Department of Surgery, San Francisco General Hospital, San Francisco, California
Pulmonary Contusion

CHARLES S. LIEBER, M.D.

Professor of Medicine and Pathology, Mount Sinai School of Medicine of the City University of New York; Director, Gastrointestinal-Liver Training Program and Alcohol Research and Treatment Center, Veterans Administration Medical Center, Bronx, New York
Alcoholic Liver Disease

G. PATRICK LILJA, M.D., F.A.C.E.P.

Clinical Assistant Professor, Department of Family Practice and Community Health, University of Minnesota Medical School; Director, Emergency Medical Service, North Memorial Medical Center and Senior Associate in Emergency Medicine, Hennepin County Medical Center, Minneapolis, Minnesota
Esophageal Foreign Bodies, Trauma, and Perforation

CHRISTOPHER H. LINDEN, M.D.

Assistant Professor of Medicine, Department of Emergency Medicine, University of Massachusetts Medical School; Director, Regional Poisoning Treatment Center, University of Massachusetts Medical Center, Worcester, Massachusetts
Antidotes in Poisoning

TOBY LITOVITZ, M.D.

Associate Professor of Emergency Medicine, Georgetown University School of Medicine; Director, National Capital Poison Center, Georgetown University Hospital, Washington, D.C.
Sedatives and Opiates

ALAN B. LITTLE, M.D., F.R.C.S. (C)

Professor and Chairman, Department of Obstetrics and Gynecology, McGill University Faculty of Medicine; Chief of Obstetrics and Gynecology, Royal Victoria Hospital, Montreal, Quebec, Canada
Abnormal Uterine Bleeding

BERNARD LO, M.D.

Assistant Professor of Medicine and Clinical Director, General Medicine Practice II, University of California School of Medicine, San Francisco, California
Criteria for Withholding Emergency Resuscitation

ROBERT A. LOWE, M.D.

Assistant Clinical Professor, Department of Family and Community Medicine, University of California School of Medicine, San Francisco; Assistant Chief, Department of Emergency Medicine, Valley Medical Center, Fresno, California
Pharyngitis

STEPHEN LUDWIG, M.D.

Associate Professor of Pediatrics, University of Pennsylvania School of Medicine; Director, Emergency Department, Children's Hospital of Philadelphia; Educational Coordinator, Supportive Child-Adult Network, Philadelphia, Pennsylvania
The Abused Patient

SCOTT MANNING, M.D.

Assistant Professor, University of Texas Health Science Center, Southwestern Medical School, Dallas, Texas
Ear Trauma

ALAN J. MARGOLIS, M.D.

Professor of Obstetrics, Gynecology and Reproductive Sciences, University of California School of Medicine, San Francisco, California
Problem Deliveries

FRANK I. MARLOWE, M.D.

Professor and Chief, Division of Otolaryngology—Head and Neck Surgery, Medical College of Pennsylvania; Chief, Division of Otolaryngology—Head and Neck Surgery, Presbyterian-University of Pennsylvania Medical Center, Philadelphia, Pennsylvania
Epistaxis

GERARD R. MARTIN, M.D.

Fellow in Pediatric Cardiology, Department of Pediatrics and Cardiovascular Research Institute, University of California School of Medicine, San Francisco, California
Congestive Heart Failure in Infants and Children

BARRY M. MASSIE, M.D., F.A.C.C.

Associate Professor of Medicine, University of California School of Medicine; Director, Cardiac Care Unit, Hypertension Clinic, San Francisco, California
Pulmonary Edema

HANI S. MATLOUB, M.D.

Assistant Professor, Department of Plastic and Reconstructive Surgery, Medical College of Wisconsin; Attending Staff Physician, Froedtert Memorial Lutheran Hospital, Milwaukee, Wisconsin
Scalp, Facial, and Oral Laceration

RICHARD A. MATTHAY, M.D.

Professor of Medicine and Associate Director, Pulmonary Section, Yale University School of Medicine, New Haven, Connecticut
Cor Pulmonale

KENNETH L. MATTOX, M.D., F.A.C.S.

Professor of Surgery, Baylor College of Medicine; Chief of Surgery, Ben Taub General Hospital, Houston, Texas
Hemoptysis

KENNETH H. MAYER, M.D.

Assistant Professor of Medicine, Brown University Program in Medicine, Providence; Chief of Infectious Diseases Division, Memorial Hospital, Pawtucket, Rhode Island
A Scheme for Selecting an Antibiotic

JACK W. McANINCH, M.D.

Professor of Urology and Vice-Chairman, Department of Urology, University of California School of Medicine; Chief of Urology, San Francisco General Hospital, San Francisco, California
Kidney, Ureter, and Bladder Trauma
Urethra, Penis, and Testis Trauma

JOHN B. McCABE, M.D., F.A.C.E.P.

Associate Professor, Department of Emergency Medicine, Wright State University School of Medicine, Dayton, Ohio
Cystitis and Pyelonephritis

W. KENDALL McNABNEY, M.D.

Professor and Chairman, Department of Emergency Health Services, Truman Medical Center, University of Missouri–Kansas City School of Medicine, Kansas City, Missouri
Penetrating Cranial Trauma

ROBERT M. McNAMARA, M.D.

Instructor, Department of Emergency Medicine, Medical College of Pennsylvania, Philadelphia, Pennsylvania
General Approach to the Adult Trauma Patient

STEPHEN J. McPHEE, M.D.

Assistant Professor of Medicine, University of California School of Medicine; Attending Physician, Moffitt-Long Hospital, San Francisco, California
Anemia

NORMAN E. McSWAIN Jr., M.D., F.A.C.S.

Clinical Professor of Surgery, Uniformed Services University of the Health Sciences, Bethesda, Maryland, Professor of Surgery, Tulane University School of Medicine; Attending Staff, Surgery and Emergency Medicine, Charity Hospital, New Orleans, Louisiana
Blunt and Penetrating Great Vessel Trauma

HOUCK M. MEDFORD, D.D.S.

Assistant Professor, Department of Dentistry, Bowman Gray School of Medicine of Wake Forest University, Winston-Salem, North Carolina
Dental Trauma and Infection

HARVEY W. MEISLIN, M.D.

Professor and Chief, Section of Emergency Medicine, Department of Surgery, University of Arizona College of Medicine, Tucson, Arizona
Cutaneous Abscesses

DAVID R. MELZER, D.O.

Chief Resident, Division of Emergency Medicine, Department of Surgery, University of Florida, University Hospital, Jacksonville, Florida
Epididymitis and Orchitis

WILLIAM C. MENTZER, M.D.

Professor of Pediatrics and Director, Division of Pediatric Hematology-Oncology, University of California School of Medicine, San Francisco, California
Sickle Cell Anemia

WILLIAM L. MEYERHOFF, M.D., Ph.D.

Chairman and Professor, University of Texas Health Science Center, Southwestern Medical School, Dallas, Texas
Ear Trauma

MARVIN H. MEYERS, M.D.

Clinical Professor, Orthopaedic Surgery and Rehabilitation, University of California School of Medicine; Staff Physician, Division of Orthopaedics, Veterans Administration Medical Center, San Diego, California
The Multiply Injured Orthopaedic Patient

ROBERT B. MILLMAN, M.D.

Professor of Clinical Public Health and Associate Professor of Clinical Psychiatry, Cornell University Medical College; Director, Drug and Alcohol Treatment and Research Program, Payne Whitney Psychiatric Clinic–New York Hospital, New York, New York
Pain in the Emergency Department

JEROME H. MODELL, M.D.

Professor and Chairman, Department of Anesthesiology, University of Florida College of Medicine, Gainsville, Florida
Near-Drowning

GILLES R. G. MONIF, M.D.

Professor of Obstetrics and Gynecology, Creighton University School of Medicine, Omaha, Nebraska
Acute Salpingitis

HUGO D. MONTENEGRO, M.D., F.C.C.P.

Associate Professor of Medicine, Case Western Reserve University School of Medicine; Director, Medical Intensive Care Unit, University Hospitals and Co-Director, Medical Intensive Care Unit, Veterans Administration Medical Center, Cleveland, Ohio
Chronic Obstructive Pulmonary Disease

ERNEST E. MOORE, M.D.

Associate Professor of Surgery, University of Colorado Health Sciences Center; Chief, Department of Surgery, Denver General Hospital, Denver, Colorado
Penetrating Abdominal Wounds

FRED MORADY, M.D.

Associate Professor of Medicine, University of Michigan Medical School; Director, Clinical Electrophysiology Laboratory, University of Michigan Medical Center, Ann Arbor, Michigan
Ventricular Tachycardia

JOHN H. MORTON, M.D.

Professor of Surgery, University of Rochester School of Medicine and Dentistry; Senior Attending Surgeon, Strong Memorial Hospital, Rochester, New York
Hernia

PATRICK J. MULROW, M.D.

Professor and Chairman, Department of Medicine, Medical College of Ohio, Toledo, Ohio
Acute Adrenocortical Insufficiency

CHARLES MURPHY, M.D.

Clinical Assistant Professor of Medicine, University of California School of Medicine, San Francisco, California
Acute Dyspnea

JANE G. MURPHY, Ph.D.

Research Assistant Professor, Section of General Medicine, Department of Medicine, University of Pennsylvania School of Medicine; Research Director, Emergency Department, Hospital of the University of Pennsylvania and Senior Fellow, Leonard Davis Institute of Health Economics, University of Pennsylvania, Philadelphia, Pennsylvania
Quality Assessment of Emergency Care

DON K. NAKAYAMA, M.D.

Assistant Professor of Surgery, University of Pittsburgh School of Medicine; Pediatric Surgeon, Children's Hospital of Pittsburgh, Pittsburgh, Pennsylvania
Pediatric Gastrointestinal Problems

MANOHAR NALLATHAMBI, M.D., F.A.C.S.

Assistant Professor of Surgery, New York Medical College, Valhalla; Co-Director, Trauma Service, Lincoln Medical and Mental Health Center, Bronx, New York
Rib and Sternum Fracture

GARY A. NEWMAN, M.D.

Associate in Gastroenterology, Lankenau Hospital, Philadelphia, Pennsylvania
Lower Gastrointestinal Bleeding

WILLIAM L. NEWMEYER, M.D.

Associate Clinical Professor of Surgery, University of California School of Medicine, San Francisco; Faculty, San Francisco Orthopaedic Residency Training Program and Active Staff, St. Francis Memorial Hospital, San Francisco, California
Tendon Injury of the Hand and Wrist

CHRISTOPHER J.L. NEWTH, M.B., F.R.C.P.(C)

Associate Professor of Pediatrics, University of Southern California; Director, Pediatric Intensive Care Unit, Children's Hospital, Los Angeles, California
Pediatric Bronchiolitis and Asthma

LAUST H. NIELSEN, M.D.

Nephrology Fellow, University of Missouri School of Medicine; Nephrology Fellow, University of Missouri Health Sciences Center, Columbia, Missouri
Dialysis Emergencies

JAMES T. NIEMANN, M.D.

Assistant Professor of Medicine, UCLA School of Medicine, Los Angeles; Associate Chairman and Director of Research, Department of Emergency Medicine, Harbor-UCLA Medical Center, Torrance, California
Improving Systemic Perfusion During Cardiopulmonary Resuscitation

HIROSHI NISHIYAMA, M.D.

Volunteer Professor of Radiology, University of Cincinnati Medical Center; Chief, Nuclear Medicine Service, Veterans Administration Medical Center, Cincinnati, Ohio
Radiation Exposure

SANTHAT NIVATVONGS, M.D., F.A.C.S.

Associate Professor of Surgery, University of Minnesota Medical School; Attending Surgeon, University of Minnesota Hospitals, Minneapolis, Minnesota
Rectal Trauma and Foreign Bodies
Colonic Trauma

KARL D. NOLPH, M.D.

Professor of Medicine, University of Missouri School of Medicine; Director, Division of Nephrology, University of Missouri Health Sciences Center, Veterans Administration Hospital, Dalton Research Center, Columbia, Missouri
Dialysis Emergencies

FAROUCK N. OBEID, M.D., F.A.C.S.

Clinical Assistant Professor, Department of Surgery, University of Michigan Medical School, Ann Arbor; Director, Trauma and Emergency Surgery Section, Henry Ford Hospital, Detroit, Michigan
Penetrating Neck Trauma

THOMAS F. O'BRIEN, M.D.

Associate Professor of Medicine, Harvard Medical School; Director, Microbiology Laboratory, Brigham and Women's Hospital, Boston, Massachusetts
A Scheme for Selecting an Antibiotic

KENT R. OLSON, M.D.

Assistant Clinical Professor of Medicine, Adjunct Lecturer, Pharmacy University of California School of Medicine, San Francisco; Director, San Francisco Bay Area Regional Poison Center, Attending Physician, Emergency Department, Highland General Hospital, Oakland, California
Toxicology Screens and Asymptomatic Poisoning

FRANCIS J. OWENS Sr., M.D.

Staff, Department of Gastroenterology, Cleveland Clinic Foundation; Assistant Clinical Professor of Medicine, Case Western Reserve University School of Medicine, Cleveland, Ohio
Constipation and Impaction

GEORGE A. PANKEY, M.D.

Clinical Professor of Medicine, Department of Medicine, Division of Infectious Diseases, Tulane University of Medicine and Louisiana State University School of Medicine; Head, Section of Infectious Diseases, Department of Internal Medicine, Ochsner Clinic and Alton Ochsner Medical Foundation, New Orleans, Louisiana
Adult Infectious Diarrhea

ROBERT PAPADOPOULOS, M.D.

Chief Surgical Resident and Clinical Instructor, University of Colorado Health Sciences Center, Denver, Colorado
Penetrating Abdominal Wounds

MICHAEL M. PAPARELLA, M.D.

Clinical Professor and Chairman Emeritus, Department of Otolaryngology, University of Minnesota Medical School, Minnesota Ear, Head and Neck Clinic, Minneapolis, Minnesota
Dizziness

PAUL M. PARIS, M.D., F.A.C.E.P.

Assistant Professor of Medicine, University of Pittsburgh School of Medicine; Program Director, University of Pittsburgh Affiliated Residency in Emergency Medicine and Associate Medical Director, City of Pittsburgh Department of Public Safety, Bureau of Emergency Medical Services, Pittsburgh, Pennsylvania
Airway Obstruction
Drugs in Pregnancy

DAVID F. PAULSON, M.D.

Professor of Urology, Duke University School of Medicine; Chief, Division of Urology, Department of Surgery, Duke University Medical Center, Durham, North Carolina
Prostatitis

PAUL E. PEPE, M.D., F.A.C.P., F.C.C.P.

Assistant Professor of Medicine and Director of Emergency Medical Services, Baylor College of Medicine, Houston, Texas
Acute Respiratory Failure

SAMUEL W. PERRY, M.D.

Associate Professor of Clinical Psychiatry, Cornell University Medical College; Associate Director, Consultation–Liaison Division, The New York Hospital, New York, New York
Pain in the Emergency Department

ROBERT S. PETERS, M.D., F.A.C.P.

Director, Division of Gastroenterology, Central San Joaquin Valley Medical Education Program, University of California School of Medicine, San Francisco; Clinical Professor of Medicine, University of California School of Medicine, San Francisco and Los Angeles, California
Caustic and Corrosive Ingestion

NORMAN E. PETERSON, M.D.

Associate Professor of Surgery, University of Colorado Health Sciences Center; Associate Director, Department of Surgery and Division Chief, Urology, Denver General Hospital, Denver, Colorado
Urinary Obstruction and Retention

MICHELLE PETRI, M.D.

Assistant Professor of Medicine, The Johns Hopkins Hospital, Baltimore, Maryland
Arthritis

LINDA G. PHILLIPS, M.D.

Assistant Professor, Wayne State University School of Medicine, Detroit, Michigan
Frostbite and Local Cold Injury

LAURENS R. PICKARD, M.D., F.A.C.S.

Assistant Professor, Cora and Webb Mading Department of Surgery, Baylor College of Medicine; Associate, Surgery Service, The Methodist Hospital and Consulting Staff, Texas Children's Hospital, Houston, Texas
Hempotysis

LARRY K. PICKERING, M.D.

Professor of Pediatrics, Director of Pediatric Infectious Diseases, Program in Infectious Diseases and Clinical Microbiology, University of Texas Medical School, Houston, Texas
Pediatric Diarrhea

LAWRENCE H. PITTS, M.D.

Associate Professor and Vice-Chairman, Department of Neurosurgery, University of California School of Medicine; Chief of Neurosurgery, San Francisco General Hospital, San Francisco, California
Epidural, Subdural, and Intracranial Bleeding

M. ANTHONY POGREL, M.B., Ch.B, B.D.S.,
F.D.S., F.R.C.S.(Edin)

Assistant Professor, University of California School of
Medicine, San Francisco, California
Oral and Salivary Gland Infection

JAMES E. POINTER, M.D.

Assistant Clinical Professor, Department of Medicine,
University of California School of Medicine, San
Francisco; Associate Chief, Department of Emergency
Medicine, Highland General Hospital, Oakland and
Medical Director, Alameda County California Emergency
Medical Service District, California
Pancreatitis

MICHAEL S. POLICAR, M.D., M.P.H.

Assistant Professor of Obstetrics, Gynecology, and
Reproductive Sciences, University of California School of
Medicine; Medical Director, Women's Health Center, San
Francisco General Hospital, San Francisco, California
Vaginitis and Cervicitis

PETER T. PONS, M.D.

Assistant Professor of Surgery, University of Colorado
Health Sciences Center; Assistant Professor of Surgery
and Associate Director, Emergency Department, Section
of Trauma and Emergency Medicine, Department of
Surgery, University of Colorado Health Sciences Center,
Denver, Colorado
Concussion and Skull Fractures in Blunt Head Trauma

THOMAS C. QUINN, M.S., M.D.

Associate Professor of Medicine, The Johns Hopkins
University School of Medicine, Baltimore; Senior
Investigator, National Institute of Allergy and
Infectious Diseases, Bethesda, Maryland
Sexually Transmitted Enteric Infections

D. SUDHAKHER RAO, M.B., B.S., F.A.C.P.

Assistant Professor of Medicine, University of Michigan
Medical School, Ann Arbor; Staff Physician and Research
Associate, Division of Bone and Mineral Metabolism,
Henry Ford Hospital, Detroit, Michigan
Hypercalcemia and Hypocalcemia

JOSEPH H. RAPP, M.D.

Assistant Professor of Surgery, University of California
School of Medicine; Assistant Chief, Vascular Surgery,
San Francisco Veterans Administration Medical Center,
San Francisco, California
Abdominal Aortic Aneurysm

JAMES E. RASMUSSEN, M.D.

Professor of Dermatology and Pediatrics; Chief,
Dermatology Clinic and Inpatient Pediatric and Outpatient
Dermatology, University of Michigan Medical Center,
Ann Arbor, Michigan
Ectoparasites

ELLIOT J. RAYFIELD, M.D.

Professor of Medicine and Chief, Diabetes Section,
Mount Sinai School of Medicine; Attending Physician,
Mount Sinai Hospital, New York, New York
Diabetic Ketoacidosis

P. SUDHAKER REDDY, M.D.

Professor of Medicine, University of Pittsburgh School of
Medicine; Director, Cardiac Catheterization Laboratories,
Presbyterian University Hospital,
Philadelphia, Pennsylvania
Pericarditis

HERBERT Y. REYNOLDS, M.D., F.A.C.P.,
A.C.C.P.

Professor of Internal Medicine and Head, Pulmonary
Section, Yale University School of Medicine,
New Haven, Connecticut
Pneumonia Caused by Aerobic Gram-Negative Rods

MATTHEW C. RIDDLE, M.D.

Associate Professor of Medicine, Division of
Endocrinology, Metabolism, and Clinical Nutrition,
Oregon Health Sciences University, Portland, Oregon
Hypoglycemia

JAMES R. ROBERTS, M.D.

Assistant Professor of Emergency Medicine, University of
Cincinnati Medical Center, Department of Emergency
Medicine, Cincinnati, Ohio
Emergency Pacemaker Insertion and Malfunction

NORBERT J. ROBERTS Jr., M.D.

Associate Professor of Medicine, University of Rochester
School of Medicine; Senior Physician, Strong Memorial
Hospital, Rochester, New York

Bacterial Meningitis

MARTIN C. ROBSON, M.D.

Professor of Surgery and Chief, Division of Plastic and
Reconstructive Surgery, Wayne State University School of
Medicine, Detroit, Michigan
Frostbite and Local Cold Injury

MICHAEL ROHMAN, M.D., F.A.C.S.

Professor of Surgery, New York Medical College,
Valhalla; Chief, Cardiothoracic and Trauma Surgery,
Lincoln Medical and Mental Health Center,
Bronx, New York
Rib and Sternum Fracture

PETER ROLAND, M.D.

Assistant Professor, University of Texas Health Science
Center, Southwestern Medical School, Dallas, Texas
Ear Trauma

PETER ROSEN, M.D.

Professor of Emergency Medicine, Department of
Surgery, University of Colorado Health Sciences Center;
Director, Emergency Medical Services, Denver
Department of Health and Hospitals, Denver, Colorado
Blunt and Penetrating Chest Trauma

ROBERT J. ROTHSTEIN, M.D.

Adjunct Associate Professor of Medicine, UCLA School
of Medicine; Chairman, Department of Emergency
Medicine, Harbor-UCLA Medical Center,
Los Angeles, California
Adult Asthma

ERNEST RUIZ, M.D.

Assistant Professor of Surgery, University of Minnesota
Medical School; Chief of Service, Department of
Emergency Medicine, Hennepin County Medical Center,
Minneapolis, Minnesota
Percutaneous Transtracheal Ventilation and Cricothyrotomy

BARRY H. RUMACK, M.D.

Professor of Pediatrics, University of Colorado School of
Medicine; Director, Rocky Mountain Poison and Drug
Center, Denver General Hospital, Denver, Colorado
Prevention of Absorption in Overdose

DOUGLAS A. RUND, M.D., F.A.C.E.P.

Associate Professor and Director, Division of Emergency
Medicine, Department of Preventive Medicine, The Ohio
State University, Columbus, Ohio
Suicide Attempt

THOMAS R. RUSSELL, M.D., F.A.C.S.

Clinical Professor, Department of Surgery, University of
California School of Medicine; Chairman, Department of
Surgery, Pacific Presbyterian Medical Center,
San Francisco, California
Perirectal Infection and Abscess

THOMAS D. SABIN, M.D.

Professor of Neurology and Psychiatry, Boston University
School of Medicine; Director, Neurological Unit, Boston
City Hospital, Boston, Massachusetts
Acute Nontraumatic Spinal Cord Dysfunction

MARVIN L. SACHS, M.D.

Assistant Professor of Medicine, University of
Pennsylvania School of Medicine; Chief, Medical
Vascular Service, Hospital of the University of
Pennsylvania, Philadelphia, Pennsylvania
Thrombophlebitis

EUGENE L. SAENGER, M.D.

Professor of Radiology, University of Cincinnati College
of Medicine; Director, Eugene L. Saenger Radioisotope
Laboratory, University of Cincinnati Medical Center,
Cincinnati, Ohio
Radiation Exposure

MERLE A. SANDE, M.D.

Professor and Vice-Chairman, Department of Medicine,
University of California School of Medicine; Chief,
Medical Service, San Francisco General Hospital,
San Francisco, California
Infectious Endocarditis

ARTHUR B. SANDERS, M.D., F.A.C.E.P., F.A.C.P.

Associate Professor, Emergency Medicine, Department of
Surgery, University of Arizona School of Medicine;
Attending Physician, University Medical Center and Kino
Community Hospital, Tucson, Arizona
Eclampsia and Preeclampsia

JAMES R. SANGER, M.D.

Assistant Professor, Department of Plastic and
Reconstructive Surgery, Medical College of Wisconsin,
Attending Staff Physician, Froedtert Memorial Lutheran
Hospital, Milwaukee, Wisconsin
Scalp, Facial, and Oral Laceration

MELVIN M. SCHEINMAN, M.D.

Professor of Medicine and Chief, Electrocardiology and
Clinical Electrophysiology Section, University of
California Medical Center, San Francisco, California
*The Patient with S-T and T Wave Changes on
Electrocardiography*

DAVID S. SCHILLINGER, M.D.

Chief Resident, Division of Emergency Medicine,
Department of Surgery, University Hospital,
Jacksonville, Florida
Toxic Shock Syndrome

JEREMY D. SCHMAHMANN, M.B., Ch.B.

Instructor in Neurology and Research Associate in
Neuroanatomy, Boston University School of Medicine;
Staff Neurologist, Neurological Unit, Boston City
Hospital and Associate Neurologist, New England
Deaconess Hospital, Boston, Massachusetts
Acute Nontraumatic Spinal Cord Dysfunction

JAN SCHNEIDER, M.D., M.P.H., F.R.C.S.(C)

Professor and Chairman, Obstetrics and Gynecology,
Medical College of Pennsylvania,
Philadelphia, Pennsylvania
Contraceptive Problems

DAVID J. SCHNEIDERMAN, M.D.

Assistant Professor of Medicine, University of Arizona
School of Medicine; Director, Gastrointestinal Endoscopy
Unit, University of Arizona Health Sciences Center,
Tucson, Arizona
Upper Gastrointestinal Bleeding

STEPHEN C. SCHOENBAUM, M.D., M.P.H.

Associate Professor of Medicine, Harvard Medical
School; Deputy Medical Director, Health Practices,
Harvard Community Health Plan, Boston, Massachusetts
Infection in Pregnancy

MARK S. SCHREINER, M.D.

Assistant Professor of Anesthesiology, The University of Pennsylvania School of Medicine; Assistant Anesthesiologist, The Children's Hospital of Philadelphia, Philadelphia, Pennsylvania
Reye's Syndrome

MARSHALL B. SEGAL, M.D., J.D.

Clinical Associate Professor of Emergency Medicine, University of Chicago Medical Center and Pritzker School of Medicine, Chicago; President, Chicago Academy of Law and Medicine and Chairman, Department of Emergency Medicine, Little Company of Mary Hospital, Evergreen Park, Illinois
Consent and Restraint

WILLIAM C. SHOEMAKER, M.D.

Professor of Surgery, UCLA School of Medicine; Vice-Chairman, Department of Surgery, King-Drew Medical Center, Los Angeles, California
Evaluation and Resuscitation of Accidental and Surgical Trauma

ALAN R. SHONS, M.D., Ph.D.

Professor of Surgery, Case Western Reserve University School of Medicine; Director, Division of Plastic and Reconstructive Surgery, University Hospitals, Cleveland, Ohio
Replantation of Extremities

MARC A. SHUMAN, M.D.

Professor of Medicine, University of California School of Medicine; Attending Physician, University of California Medical Center, Head, Hematology Section, Cancer Research Institute, and Director, Adult Hemophilia Service, San Francisco, California
Hemophilia and von Willebrand's Disease

DONALD A. SHUMRICK, M.D.

Professor and Chairman, Department of Otolaryngology and Maxillofacial Surgery, University of Cincinnati Medical Center, Cincinnati, Ohio
Laryngeal and Tracheal Foreign Bodies and Blunt Trauma

KEVIN A. SHUMRICK, M.D.

Assistant Professor, Department of Otolaryngology and Maxillofacial Surgery, University of Cincinnati Medical Center, Cincinnati, Ohio
Laryngeal and Tracheal Foreign Bodies and Blunt Trauma

ERIC Z. SILFEN, M.D., F.A.C.P., F.A.C.E.P.

Clinical Assistant Professor, Emergency Medicine and Internal Medicine, Georgetown University Hospital, Washington, D.C.; Director, Emergency Services, Reston Hospital Center, Reston, Virginia
Non-infectious Colitis

ROBERT R. SIMON, M.D.

Associate Professor of Medicine, UCLA Emergency Medicine Center; Assistant Director, Residency Training, Los Angeles, California
Ligamentous Ankle Injury
Ligamentous Knee Injury

ROBERT SINE, M.D.

Assistant Professor, Department of Rehabilitation Medicine, Stanford University School of Medicine; Director, Department of Rehabilitation Medicine, St. Mary's Hospital, Stanford, California
Complications of Disuse and Immobilization

COREY M. SLOVIS, M.D.

Associate Professor of Medicine and Director, Emergency Medicine, Emory University School of Medicine; Director, Emergency Medical Services, Grady Memorial Hospital, Atlanta, Georgia
Foreign Body Ingestion

SCOTT J. SOIFER, M.D.

Assistant Professor, Department of Pediatrics and The Cardiovascular Research Institute and Acting Director, Division of Pediatric Critical Care Medicine, University of California School of Medicine, San Francisco, California
Congestive Heart Failure in Infants and Children

ALFRED M. SOLISH, M.D.

Assistant Clinical Professor of Ophthalmology, Jules Stein Eye Institute, UCLA School of Medicine; Director of Glaucoma Service, Wadsworth Veterans Administration Hospital, Los Angeles, California
Sudden Loss of Vision

GEORGE F. SOLOMON, M.D.

Professor of Psychiatry in Residence, University of California School of Medicine, Los Angeles, Adjunct Professor of Psychiatry, University of California School of Medicine, San Francisco; Chief, Drug Dependency Treatment Center, Veterans Administration Medical Center, Sepulveda, California
Assaultive Behavior

DANIEL SOOY, M.D.

Assistant Professor, Department of Otolaryngology, University of California Medical Center; Director of Clinics, San Francisco General Hospital, San Francisco, California
Otitis and Mastoiditis

HOWARD M. SPIRO, M.D.

Professor of Medicine, Yale University School of Medicine, New Haven, Connecticut
Lower Gastrointestinal Bleeding

WILLIAM M. STAHL, M.D., F.A.C.S.

Professor of Surgery, New York Medical College, Valhalla; Director of Surgery, Lincoln Hospital, Bronx, New York
Flank and Buttock Trauma

J. STEPHAN STAPCZYNSKI, M.D.

Assistant Professor of Medicine, University of Pittsburgh School of Medicine; Staff Physician, Emergency Department, University-Presbyterian Hospital, Pittsburgh, Pennsylvania
Cellulitis and Lymphadenitis

MARK G. STEIN, M.B., B.Ch., B.Sc.

Assistant Clinical Professor of Radiology, University of California School of Medicine; Chief of Thoracic Imaging, Fort Miley Veterans Administration Medical Center, San Francisco, California
Diagnostic Imaging in the Emergency Center

GEORGE L. STERNBACH, M.D., F.A.C.E.P.

Clinical Associate Professor of Surgery, Stanford University Medical School; Associate Director, Emergency Department, Stanford University Medical Center, Stanford, California
Bowel Obstruction
Herpesvirus

RONALD D. STEWART, B.A., B.Sc., M.D., F.A.C.E.P.

Associate Professor of Surgery, Assistant Professor of Anesthesiology and Critical Care Medicine, University of Pittsburgh School of Medicine; Medical Director, Department of Public Safety, City of Pittsburgh, Pittsburgh, Pennsylvania
Airway Obstruction
Endotracheal Intubation

ERIC STIRLING, M.D.

Assistant Professor of Medicine–Emergency Medicine, University of California School of Medicine, San Francisco, California
Chronic Venous Insufficiency and Ulcer

H. HARLAN STONE, M.D.

Professor of Surgery, University of Maryland School of Medicine, Baltimore, Maryland
Necrotizing Wound Infection

RONALD J. STONEY, M.D.

Professor of Surgery, University of California School of Medicine; Co-Chief, Vascular Surgery, University of California Medical Center, San Francisco, California
Abdominal Aortic Aneurysm

HARLAN A. STUEVEN, M.D.

Assistant Professor of Surgery, Medical College of Wisconsin, Milwaukee County Regional Complex; Chief, Emergency Medicine Department, Mount Sinai Medical Center, Milwaukee, Wisconsin
Electromechanical Dissociation and Asystole

MICHAEL STULBARG, M.D.

Adjunct Associate Professor of Medicine and Director, Chest Clinic, University of California School of Medicine, San Francisco, California
Pulmonary Embolism

RANDALL S. SUAREZ, M.D.

Chief Orthopaedic Resident, Richland Memorial Hospital–University of South Carolina School of Medicine, Columbia, South Carolina
Knee Dislocation

JOHN B. SULLIVAN Jr., M.D.

Associate Professor, University of Arizona Health Sciences Center; Staff, Department of Emergency Medicine, Clinical Pharmacology, and Toxicology, Arizona Poison Center, Tucson, Arizona
Snakebite

DAVID B. SWEDLOW, M.D.

Assistant Professor of Anesthesia and Pediatrics, University of Pennsylvania School of Medicine; Senior Anesthesiologist, Children's Hospital of Philadelphia, Philadelphia, Pennsylvania
Reye's Syndrome

SCOTT A. SYVERUD, M.D.

Assistant Professor of Emergency Medicine, University of Cincinnati Medical Center, Cincinnati, Ohio
Implications and Pharmacologic Treatment of Cardiac Conduction Block
Emergency Pacemaker Insertion and Malfunction

BERNARD TABATZNIK, M.D., F.R.C.P.

Assistant Professor of Medicine, The Johns Hopkins University School of Medicine; Chief, Department of Cardiology, North Charles Hospital, Baltimore, Maryland
Premature Ventricular Beats

RONALD B. TAYLOR, M.D.

Research Fellow, Ohio State University School of Medicine, Columbus, Ohio
Alcohol Intoxication and Withdrawal

HOWARD H. TESSLER, M.D.

Associate Professor of Clinical Ophthalmology, University of Illinois Medical School, Chicago, Illinois
Uveitis

CATHERINE S. THOMPSON, M.D.

Assistant Professor, Department of Internal Medicine, University of Texas Medical School; Attending Physician, Hermann Hospital, Houston, Texas
Hyponatremia and Hypernatremia

JUDITH E. TINTINALLI, M.D., F.A.C.E.P.

Clinical Assistant Professor of Surgery in Emergency Medicine, University of Michigan Medical School, Ann Arbor; Associate Director, Emergency Department, William Beaumont Hospital, Royal Oak, Michigan
Nontraumatic Pneumothorax

GILBERT J. TOFFOL, D.O.

Cerebrovascular Fellow, Division of Cerebrovascular Diseases, Department of Neurology, University of Iowa College of Medicine, Iowa City, Iowa
Cerebral Infarction and Transient Ischemic Attack

JOSEPH S. TORG, M.D.

Professor of Orthopaedic Surgery, University of Pennsylvania School of Medicine; Director, University of Pennsylvania Sports Medicine Center, Philadelphia, Pennsylvania
Injuries in Runners

JONATHAN B. TOWNE, M.D.

Professor of Surgery and Chairman, Department of Vascular Surgery, Medical College of Wisconsin, Milwaukee, Wisconsin
Arterial Insufficiency and Occlusion

JOSEPH J. TRAUTLEIN, M.D., F.A.C.P., F.A.A.I., F.A.C.A., F.C.P., F.A.C.U.R.P.

Associate Professor of Medicine, University Hospital, Milton S. Hershey Medical Center, Pennsylvania State University, Hershey, Pennsylvania
Avoidance of Malpractice

DONALD D. TRUNKEY, M.D.

Professor of Surgery and Chairman, Department of Surgery, Oregon Health Sciences University, Portland, Oregon
Hemorrhagic Shock
Air Embolism

TSU-MIN TSAI, M.D.

Assistant Clinical Professor of Orthopaedic Surgery, University of Louisville School of Medicine, Louisville, Kentucky
Laceration of the Hand: Fingertip Injury and Infection

MICHAEL V. VANCE, M.D., F.A.C.E.P.

Associate in Surgery, Section of Emergency Medicine, Arizona Health Sciences Center, University of Arizona College of Medicine and Associate in Pharmacology and Toxicology, College of Pharmacy, Arizona Health Sciences Center, Tucson; Associate Director, Central Arizona Regional Poison Management Center, Department of Medical Toxicology, St. Luke's Medical Center, Phoenix, Arizona
Toxic Inhalation and Burns

CHARLES W. VAN WAY, M.D.

Associate Professor of Surgery, University of Colorado School of Medicine, Denver, Colorado
Injury to the Diaphragm

DAVID W. VASTINE, M.D.

Assistant Clinical Professor, Department of Ophthalmology, Pacific Medical Center, San Francisco; Chairman, Department of Ophthalmology, Highland General Hospital, Oakland, California
Corneal Abrasion and Burn
Acute Eye Inflammation

PAUL A. VOLBERDING, M.D.

Assistant Professor of Medicine, Cancer Research Institute, University of California School of Medicine; Chief, Medical Oncology and Director, AIDS Activities, San Francisco General Hospital, San Francisco, California
Acquired Immunodeficiency Syndrome

JOEL D. WACKER, M.D.

Assistant Professor of Medicine, University of Wisconsin School of Medicine; Associate Director of Emergency Services, University of Wisconsin Hospital and Clinics, Madison, Wisconsin
Neurologic Assessment in the Emergency Setting

JOSEPH F. WAECKERLE, M.D.

Clinical Associate Professor, University of Missouri School of Medicine; Chairman, Department of Emergency Medicine, Baptist Medical Center, Kansas City, Missouri
Shoulder and Upper Extremity Injury
Disorders of the Hip

DAVID K. WAGNER, M.D., F.A.C.S., F.A.A.P.

Professor of Emergency Medicine and Chairman, Department of Emergency Medicine, Medical College of Pennsylvania, Philadelphia, Pennsylvania
General Approach to the Adult Trauma Patient
Approach to Acute Abdominal Pain

H. KENNETH WALKER, M.D.

Professor of Medicine and Associate Professor of Neurology, Emory University School of Medicine; Deputy Chief of Medicine, Grady Memorial Hospital, Atlanta, Georgia
Acute Weakness

ROBERT L. WALTON, M.D., F.A.C.S.

Professor of Surgery, University of Massachusetts School of Medicine, Worcester, Massachusetts
Wound Management

RICHARD E. WARD, M.D.

Associate Professor, Department of Surgery, University of California School of Medicine, Davis, California
Pelvic Fracture

DAVID G. WARNOCK, M.D.

Associate Professor of Medicine and Pharmacology, University of California School of Medicine; Chief, Nephrology Section, Department of Medicine, San Francisco Veterans Administration Medical Center, San Francisco, California
Potassium Disorders

CHATRCHAI WATANAKUNAKORN, M.D., F.A.C.P., F.C.C.P.

Professor of Internal Medicine, Northeastern Ohio Universities College of Medicine, Rootstown; Director of Infectious Disease Section, Department of Internal Medicine, St. Elizabeth Hospital Medical Center, Youngstown, Ohio
Community-Acquired Pneumonia

FRANK L. WEAKLEY, M.D., F.A.C.S.

Staff Surgeon, Department of Colorectal Surgery and Head, Section of Enterostomal Therapy, Cleveland Clinic Foundation, Cleveland, Ohio
Abdominal Mass

W. DOUGLAS WEAVER, M.D.

Associate Professor of Medicine, University of Washington School of Medicine; Director, Coronary Care Unit, Harborview Medical Center, Seattle, Washington
Ventricular Fibrillation and Torsades de Pointes

HOWARD A. WERMAN, M.D.

Instructor, Division of Emergency Medicine, Ohio State University College of Medicine, Columbus, Ohio
Uncommon Causes of Abdominal Pain

GERALD P. WHELAN, M.D., F.A.C.E.P.

Assistant Professor of Emergency Medicine, University of Southern California School of Medicine; Associate Director, Department of Emergency Medicine, Los Angeles County–USC Medical Center, Los Angeles, California
Atrial Dysrhythmia

ROBERT R. WHIPKEY, M.D.

Staff Physician, Department of Emergency Medicine, The Western Pennsylvania Hospital, Pittsburgh, Pennsylvania
Drugs in Pregnancy

BLAINE C. WHITE, M.D.

Associate Professor, Department of Surgery, Section of Emergency Medicine, Wayne State University, Detroit, Michigan
Ischemic Brain Injury

J. DOUGLAS WHITE, M.D.

Assistant Professor of Internal and Emergency Medicine, Georgetown University School of Medicine; Clinical Director, Department of Emergency Medicine, Georgetown University Medical Center, Washington, D.C.
Hypothermia

STEVEN J. WHITE, M.D.

Instructor, Department of Surgery, University of Pittsburgh School of Medicine and Faculty, Center for Emergency Medicine of Western Pennsylvania, Pittsburgh; Attending Physician, Emergency Department, Armstrong County Memorial Hospital, Kittanning, Pennsylvania
Airway Obstruction

HERBERT P. WIEDEMANN, M.D.

Staff Physician, Department of Pulmonary Disease and Head, Section of Respiratory Therapy, Cleveland Clinic Foundation, Cleveland, Ohio
Cor Pulmonale

JACOB T. WILENSKY, M.D.

Associate Professor of Ophthalmology, University of Illinois College of Medicine; Director, Glaucoma Service, University of Illinois Eye and Ear Infirmary, Chicago, Illinois
Acute Glaucoma

JAMES T. WILLERSON, M.D.

Professor of Medicine and Director, Cardiology Division, University of Texas Health Science Center, Dallas, Texas
Myocardial Infarction

TERRY M. WILLIAMS, M.D., F.A.C.E.P.

Physician, Emergency Services, Kaiser Hospital, Sacramento, California
Orthostatic Hypotension

WILLIAM H. WILSON, M.D., M.Sc., (Otorhinolaryngology)

Associate Clinical Professor of Otolaryngology, University of Colorado Health Sciences Center; Active Staff, Presbyterian-St. Lukes and The Children's Hospital, Denver, Colorado
Sinusitis and Rhinitis

TERENCE D. WINGERT, M.D.

Assistant Professor of Medicine, Division of Endocrinology and Metabolism, Medical College of Ohio, Toledo, Ohio
Acute Adrenocortical Insufficiency

THEODORE E. WOODWARD, M.D., D.Sc.(Hon)

Professor of Medicine Emeritus, University of Maryland School of Medicine; Physician, Veterans Administration Medical Center, Baltimore, Maryland
Rickettsial Infection

CHARLES F. WOOLEY, M.D.

Professor of Medicine, The Ohio State University College of Medicine; Professor of Medicine, Ohio State University Hospitals, Columbus, Ohio
Mitral Valve Prolapse

THERESA M. WORNER, M.D.

Assistant Professor of Medicine, Mount Sinai School of Medicine of the City University of New York, New York; Chief, Medical Section, Alcohol Dependence Treatment Program, Veterans Administration Medical Center, Bronx, New York
Alcoholic Liver Disease

CHARLES T. YARINGTON Jr., M.D., F.A.C.S.

Clinical Professor of Surgery, Uniformed Services University of the Health Sciences, Bethesda, Maryland and Clinical Professor of Otolaryngology, University of Washington School of Medicine; Chief, Otolaryngology –Head and Neck Surgery, Mason Clinic, Seattle, Washington
Nasal Fracture and Laceration

CONNIE WHITESIDE YIM, M.D.

Assistant Professor of Medicine, University of California, Davis, School of Medicine, Sacramento, California

Magnesium Disorders
Phosphate Disorders

N. JOHN YOUSIF, M.D.

Assistant Professor, Department of Plastic and Reconstructive Surgery, Medical College of Wisconsin; Attending Staff Physician, Froedtert Memorial Lutheran Hospital, Milwaukee, Wisconsin

Scalp, Facial, and Oral Laceration

PREFACE

Emergency medicine has come of age. It is not simply recognized as a specialty, but now has many mature and experienced full-time practitioners. It seemed to me there was now a need for a text for the experienced clinician (whether trained in emergency medicine or other specialties), as well as for the recent graduate. Such a text should reflect the new maturity of both the specialty and its practitioners by inviting contributors who possess an extraordinary degree of clinical, research, or publishing experience in their topic and not merely an interest in it. The increasing expertise of the emergency clinician and the reader would be addressed by in-depth discussion of management, often to a slightly further stage of therapy than is usually addressed in emergency medicine references.

In this text, the contributors have been selected on the basis of their expertise and reputation (which is usually national or international) and this is reflected in their chapter topics. Fulltime specialists in emergency medicine were preferentially chosen whenever they met these qualifications. However, owing to the youth of the specialty and the relative rarity of many of the conditions, there were many areas where only traditional specialists could provide the necessary expertise. Since clinical expertise was to be the hallmark of this text, that was always the final deciding factor, with my role being that of providing the orientation and perspective of emergency medicine.

Although the text is entitled Current Therapy, the fact is that in emergency medicine the most important "therapy" is proper recognition, diagnosis, and disposition of a clinical problem. Therefore diagnosis is discussed in all chapters and, in those where recognition and disposition are critical, is often the major topic.

The coverage of topics is comprehensive, and all major problems that might be seen by either an emergency physician or a traditional specialist in an emergency department, urgent care center, or office practice are covered in detail. There are two deliberate omissions. Toxicology is such a vast topic and changes so frequently that no text can do it full justice. Therefore, general principles of management are covered in depth, along with the three most common toxins (alcohol, opiates, and antidepressants) and emergency treatment and antidotes needed for any poison within the first hour. The reader is then referred to the local poison control center for further information. The other omission is the topic of extremity fractures needing reduction and casting, since this would add greatly to the size of the text, and the standard of care in most communities is that such fractures be treated by orthopaedic surgeons. Simple fractures not needing orthopaedic consultation are discussed, as are spine and pelvis fractures and all other orthopaedic injuries.

I want to thank once again all those authors who so kindly shared their many years of clinical and research expertise by contributing chapters, and the many clinicians, house staff, and patients over the years whose questions, arguments, rebuttals, and case management taught me what I know of the art of emergency medicine.

A final word. In the preface of the third edition of her *Russian-English Chemical and Polytechnical Dictionary*, my mother said that the only negative note in her career had been that having caused her children to observe her laboring at her desk all their lives, it had inspired them to go and do otherwise. The production of this text allows me the satisfaction of proving my mother wrong–a satisfaction seldom vouchsafed me, despite my valiant efforts.

Michael Callaham
San Francisco CA

CONTENTS

MANAGEMENT OF THE HEAD, NECK, AND UPPER AIRWAY

Management of the Pulmonary System

Management of the Cardiac System

Obstetric and Gynecologic Emergencies

Management of the Hemopoietic System

RESUSCITATION AND CRITICAL CARE

PRINCIPLES OF AIRWAY MANAGEMENT

DANIEL F. DANZL, M.D., F.A.C.E.P.

Adherence to airway management principles enables the emergency physician to ensure oxygenation and ventilation. Cornerstones of resuscitation also include protection of the airway, relief of obstruction, and suctioning capability.

Initially the airway is established by basic maneuvers including the head tilt, the jaw thrust, and the chin or neck lift. Relief of airway obstruction is the first priority. Ventilation is then initiated with mouth-to-mouth, mouth-to-mask, or other available mechanical devices. Finally the airway must be protected by use of oropharyngeal airway, intubation, or other devices (Table 1).

The techniques of oro- and nasotracheal intubation, rapid-induction anesthesia, percutaneous translaryngeal ventilation, cricothyrotomy, and relief of airway obstruction are reviewed in detail in other chapters.

RELIEVING OBSTRUCTION

The airway approach is initially dictated by the patient's level of consciousness and the possible presence of trauma (Fig.1). If obstruction is present (as it usually is to some degree in the obtunded patient), it must be relieved. The first step is the head tilt, the jaw thrust, or the chin lift. This elevates the tongue, which frequently falls back to obstruct the upper airway. However, these maneuvers cannot be used in the patient with suspected cervical spine injury. Secretions, blood, vomitus, and foreign bodies may also block the airway. The simplest method to clear the airway in patients without trauma who are comatose is direct laryngoscopic visualization with a McGill forceps or tonsil sucker in hand. The proper sniffing position for this laryngoscopic suction includes neck

TABLE 1 Summary of Airway Management Adjuncts

Technique	Indication	Contraindication	Advantages	Disadvantages
Head tilt	Relieve obstruction from tongue	Cervical spine trauma	Easy, effective	Does not clear material in airway
Jaw thrust or chin lift	Relieve obstruction from tongue	Cervical spine trauma (OK if *all* head movement is avoided)		Does not clear material in airway
Suctioning	Foreign matter in airway	None		Induces hypoxia Interrupts ventilation Raises intracranial pressure
Oropharyngeal airway	Obtunded patient without gag reflex	Active gag reflex	Protects upper airway from obstruction	
Nasopharyngeal airway	Obtunded patient with gag reflex	None	Tolerated by awake patients	Relatively small airway
S tube (pocket mask)	Obtunded patient without gag reflex	Active gag reflex	Allows mouth-to-tube ventilation without direct contact; oxygen supplementation possible	
Mouth-to-mouth ventilation	Hypoventilation	None	Good tidal volume, easy and effective	Room air only (FiO$_2$ = 20%) Very nonaesthetic Disease transmission risk
Bag-valve-mask ventilation	Hypoventilation	None	High FiO$_2$ possible ($\geq$80%)	Small tidal volume, difficult to maintain seal Gastric insufflation Aspiration risk
Manually triggered oxygen-powered devices	Hypoventilation	None	High FiO$_2$ (100%) Readily available	Problem with mask seal Gastric insufflation and aspiration Barotrauma

flexion with head hyperextension. This also alleviates obstruction by the tongue. If trauma is suspected, the upper airway is cleared while protecting the cervical spine. In-line cervical traction is constantly applied by an assistant, and then suctioning and oxygenation are carried out.

Suctioning

Adequate and repeated suctioning in the emergency department is often a neglected area of airway management. A rigid-tip plastic tonsil sucker should be kept handy in all resuscitation areas to rapidly remove large quantities of blood or vomitus. Use soft well-lubricated curved-tip catheters to suction the nasopharynx and tracheobronchial tree. Turning the head to the right while rotating the catheter facilitates passage into the left bronchus. Repeated right main stem bronchial intubation is more common with straight catheters.

Multiple suction catheter sizes should be available. To prevent pulmonic collapse from insufficient ventilation during suctioning, limit the suction catheter's size to half the diameter of the endotracheal tube (ET) tube. Always oxygenate before and after suctioning. Suctioning should be completed prior to administration of positive pressure ventilation so that breath sounds can be checked.

Tracheal stimulation may exacerbate intracranial hypertension. The cerebral perfusion pressure equals the mean arterial pressure minus the intracranial pressure, normally below 15 mm Hg. Lidocaine applied translaryngeally or transorally may be helpful. Results after intravenous administration, as reported in the literature, are mixed. Neither route of administration completely abolishes the cardiovascular response and reactive intracranial hypertension in nonparalyzed patients. Topical anesthesia in combination with intravenous lidocaine should be considered before the suctioning of patients with conditions

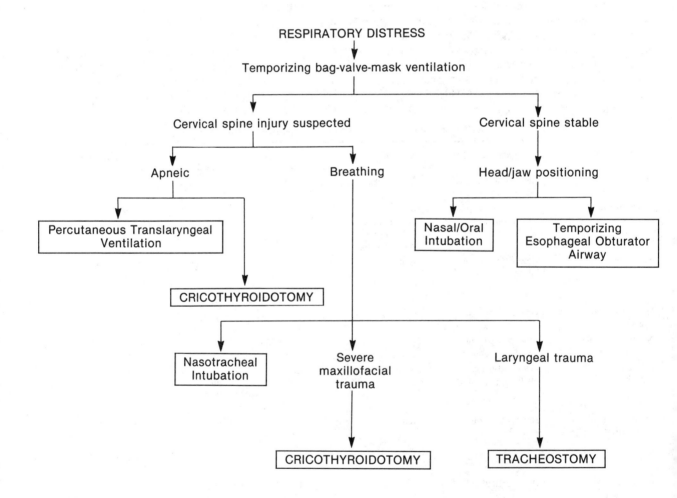

Figure 1 Approach to airway control. (From Textbook of Advanced Cardiac Life Support, American Heart Association, 1983.)

capable of elevating the intracranial pressure, such as stroke, head trauma, or intracerebral hemorrhage. Other common complications of suctioning include hypoxia, hypotension, arrhythmias, and direct mucosal damage.

Although the maneuvers differ, the principles of airway management are the same for infants and small children. Children under age 2 lack significant cartilaginous tracheal support. Thus hyperextension of the head may obstruct the airway. Avoid barotrauma from excessive tidal volume delivery, especially with manually triggered positive pressure devices.

PROTECTING THE AIRWAY

Oropharyngeal Airway

The oropharyngeal tube, or oral airway, elevates the base of the flaccid tongue off the hypopharynx. Several sizes should be kept available for temporary use in patients who have no protective airway reflexes. To insert the oral airway, either depress the tongue with a blade or rotate the airway after insertion from a convexity caudad position. If gagging occurs, remove the airway immediately. If the tongue is pushed backward, it blocks the airway (Fig. 2). Patients with oral airways should never be left unattended in the emergency department during preparations for intubation. A more functional use of this airway is as a bite block to prevent trismic occlusion of orotracheal tubes. A variation of the oropharyngeal tube is the S tube, which allows mouth-to-mouth ventilation without direct contact. Seal the flange against the lips and pinch the nose to ventilate.

Nasopharyngeal Airway

Patients with partially intact gag reflexes that prevent oropharyngeal airway use are good candidates for nasopharyngeal tubes, or nasal airways. After spraying the mucosa with a topical vasoconstrictor such as 0.25 to 1 percent neosynephrine, lubricate with lidocaine jelly. Insert the tube parallel to the palate. Insert the tip into the hypopharynx deep enough to free the base of the tongue from the posterior pharyngeal wall. Avoid inserting the tip too deeply, as it could enter the esophagus or stimulate laryngospasm (Fig. 3).

The insertion of a nasal airway is a temporizing maneuver. Patients with trismus, seizures, or cervical spine injuries are ideal candidates while they await nasotracheal intubation. Another indication is massive facial trauma with potential cribriform plate involvement, in which case orogastric intubation is often difficult and risky. Passage of the nasogastric tube through a nasopharyngeal airway can prevent the rare complication of intracranial tube placement. Slightly obtunded patients who may not require endotracheal intubation and are being closely monitored also tolerate nasopharyngeal tubes.

Esophageal Obturator Airway

An airway adjunct whose efficacy is controversial is the esophageal obturator airway (EOA). When endotracheal intubation is not a viable prehospital option, there is less gastric insufflation and regurgitation with the EOA than with the oral airway. Insertion does not require laryngeal visualization, and the cervical spine can be kept immobilized.

Oxygenation is easier than ventilation with this device. In a comparative study, the Pco_2 was significantly higher with the EOA than with the endotracheal tube. The results of several series evaluating this have been mixed, and vigilant reevaluation of oxygenation is indicated. The EOA appears more effective than an oral airway when endotracheal intubation is not possible, but requires constant attention and skill for effective ventilation.

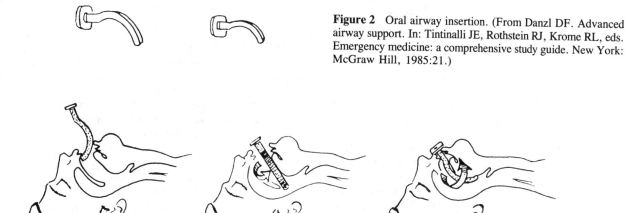

Figure 2 Oral airway insertion. (From Danzl DF. Advanced airway support. In: Tintinalli JE, Rothstein RJ, Krome RL, eds. Emergency medicine: a comprehensive study guide. New York: McGraw Hill, 1985:21.)

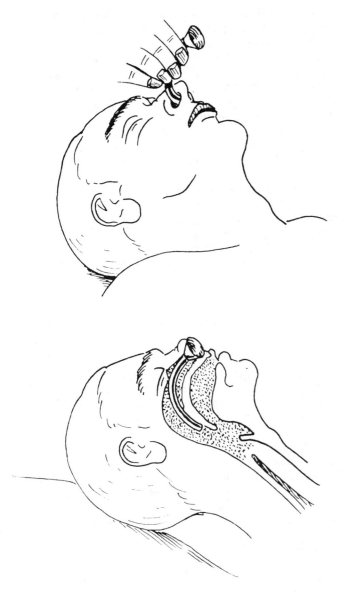

Figure 3 Nasopharyngeal tube insertion. (From Danzl DF. Advanced airway support. In: Tintinalli JE, Rothstein RJ, Krome RL, eds. Emergency medicine: a comprehensive study guide. New York: McGraw Hill, 1985:22.)

Contraindications include massive nasal or intraoral hemorrhage, caustic ingestion, esophageal disease, and upper airway obstruction.

Insertion of the lubricated EOA is done blindly. The mandible and tongue are pulled forward, with the head in a neutral position. Slight flexion of the stable neck decreases the incidence of inadvertent tracheal intubation. The cuff must be inflated below the carina, or partial tracheal compression may occur.

The original EOA has a rounded occluded distal tip. A transparent oronasal mask has a snap lock in the center that connects to the tube. Ventilation occurs through multiple ports in the proximal portion of the tube residing in the hypopharynx (Fig 4).

There are several variations of the original EOA. The esophageal gastric airway has an additional hole in the mask, which allows insertion of a nasogastric tube for gastric decompression. Another variation is the tracheoesophageal airway. A standard high-volume low-pressure cuffed ET tube is passed through the second hole in this device's mask. Insertion with the stable neck slightly extended while a Sellick maneuver (cricoid pressure) is performed facilitates the desired "inadvertent" tracheal placement of a functional ET tube. If the ET tube enters the esophagus, it allows gastric decompression during ventilation.

In patients with maxillofacial trauma, the EOA does not protect the lower airway from upper airway hemorrhage or secretions. In this setting, the experimental pharyngeo-tracheal lumen airway may prove useful (Fig. 5). A large low-pressure cuff, when inflated, seals the oropharynx at the proximal end of the airway.

With the standard EOA, inadvertent tracheal intubation occurs in 10 to 15 percent of insertions and must be instantly recognized to avert asphyxia. The incidence of esophageal rupture is not well established, but should be minimized if the esophageal gastric or tracheoesophageal airway is used. Complications increase if the patient does not remain deeply comatose. Vomiting, aspiration, laryngospasm, and Mallory-Weiss syndrome have been reported.

When the patient arrives in the emergency department, assemble assistants and necessary equipment including a tonsil sucker. Intubate the trachea prior to removal of the EOA. If the patient suddenly awakens with intact airway reflexes, roll the patient to the side and immediately deflate the cuff and remove the tube.

Observe conscious patients closely for symptoms or signs suggestive of esophageal injury. Symptoms of chest pain, dysphagia, or shortness of breath should not be ignored. Signs of Mallory-Weiss syndrome include hematemesis, Hamman's crunch, subcutaneous emphysema, or pneumomediastinum.

Tracheal Intubation

Skillful endotracheal intubation is the most reliable technique to prevent aspiration and provide adequate oxygenation and ventilation. In the emergency department setting, attempts to continously monitor patients who lack protective airway reflexes invite disaster. In nonfasting nonpremedicated patients, immediate intubation with an endotracheal tube may inadvertently cram foreign bodies and food into the glottis. Oxygen administration and suctioning should precede intubation. Orotracheal and nasotracheal intubation and extubation are discussed in the chapter on *Endotracheal Intubation*.

Immediate cricothyroidotomy may be lifesaving in patients with severe upper airway hemorrhage or when less invasive airway procedures fail. When surgical cricothyroidotomy is not feasible, a temporizing alternate approach to airway obstruction is translaryngeal positive pressure ventilation. See the chapters on *Airway Obstruction and Percutaneous Transtracheal Ventilations and Cricothyrotomy*.

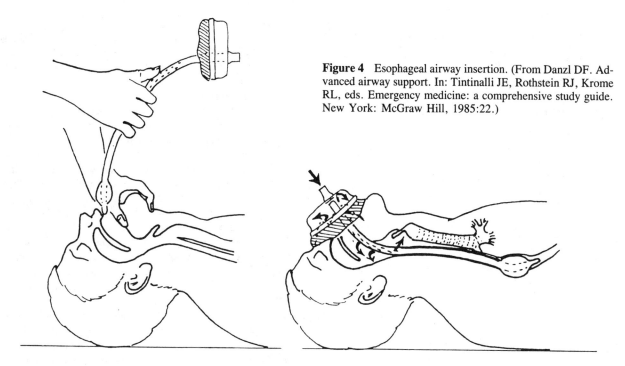

Figure 4 Esophageal airway insertion. (From Danzl DF. Advanced airway support. In: Tintinalli JE, Rothstein RJ, Krome RL, eds. Emergency medicine: a comprehensive study guide. New York: McGraw Hill, 1985:22.)

VENTILATION

The physician needs to evaluate respiratory function immediately in every case. The symptoms and signs of respiratory failure are often vague (Table 2). Any obtunded or comatose patient should have arterial blood gases drawn, as should those with unexplained dyspnea, restlessness, or confusion. Clinical estimations of adequacy of ventilation based on observation of chest movement and auscultation are notoriously unreliable and do not measure alveolar hypoventilation, shunting, or ventilation and perfusion defects. Thus, blood gases are mandatory. Ventilation should be initiated immediately whenever there is doubt, since blood oxygen saturation can fall 20 percent in 40 seconds in the apneic patient.

Bag-Valve-Mask Unit

The bag-valve-mask (BVM) apparatus consists of a self-inflating bag, a nonrebreathing valve, and a face mask. Avoid opaque masks, which can hide regurgitation. Adequate ventilation with this device requires con-

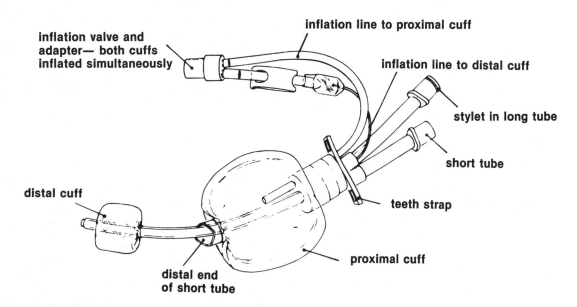

Figure 5 Pharyngeotracheal lumen airway. The distal cuff occludes the esophagus and the proximal cuff occludes the upper airway. (From Nieman JT, Rosborough JP, Myers R, et al. The pharyngeatracheal lumen airway: preliminary investigation of a new adjunct. Ann Emerg Med 1984; 13:591.

TABLE 2 Causes of Respiratory Impairment

Pulmonary—airways and lungs

Alpha-1 antitrypsin deficiency
ARDS/IRDS
Atelectasis
Bronchospasm
Bronchitis/bronchiectasis
COPD
Embolism/edema/effusions
Interstitial/cystic fibrosis
Pneumonia
Pneumoconioses
Tumor

Pulmonary—bellows action (bone, nerve, muscle, pleura)

Ascites
Botulism
Curariform agents
Demyelinating disease
Electrolyte abnormalities
Hypoventilation syndrome
Endocrinopathies
Myasthenia gravis
Metabolic derangements
Obesity
Poliomyelitis
Restrictive lung disease/kyphoscoliosis
Tetanus

Trauma

Asphyxia
Cervical trauma
Cranial trauma
Electrocution
Inhalation injury
Laryngotracheal trauma
Mandibular injury
Maxillofacial injury
Mediastinal emphysema
Poisoning
Pulmonary injury
Spinal injury
Thoracic injury

Obstruction

Anaphylaxis
Angioneurotic edema
Foreign body
Infection
Laryngospasm
Tumor

Neurologic causes

Cerebral edema
Cerebrovascular accidents
Encephalitis
Meningitis
Reye's syndrome
Seizure
Tumor

Cardiac causes

Insufficient cardiac output

siderable manual dexterity, and frequently a third hand. Mouth-to-mask ventilation is often more effective, particularly since the bag of the BVM unit is only 700 cc (thus delivering a much smaller tidal volume) and tidal volumes of 1000 cc are achievable with mouth-to-mask ventilation. However, high FIO_2 is not achievable with mouth ventilation methods.

Extend the stable neck and insert an oro- or nasopharyngeal tube. Clamp the proper size transparent mask snugly to the face, and estimate pulmonary compliance when ventilating. Air leaks around an improperly inflated mask seal are common, and are detected by hissing noises and unusually low resistance to ventilation. Adequate delivery of tidal volume is impossible when this happens. When ventilating, the tidal volume delivered should be 10 to 15 cc per kilogram, about twice the normal resting tidal volume. Greater tidal volumes produce gastric insufflation. Pay attention to the amount of resistance to airflow and bag compression. If resistance is high, reinspect for upper airway obstruction, or consider mechanical impediments to lung expansion such as hemothorax, pneumothorax, aspiration, or severe bronchospasm. Patients who are extremely difficult to bag become rapidly anoxic, and may require immediate cricothyroidotomy if obstructed, or decompression with a 16-gauge catheter over needle in the second or third intercostal space in the midclavicular line if absent breath sounds, hyperresonance, and tracheal shift suggest tension pneumothorax.

If prolonged ventilation with the BVM is required, attach a reservoir that is the same size as the bag volume. To deliver 100 percent oxygen, maintain an oxygen flow rate equal to the respiratory minute volume (at least 6 to 10 L per minute); attach a nonrebreathing valve to the unit. (Respiratory minute volume equals tidal volume times number of respirations per minute, and is about 6 L per minute at rest in an adult. However, a third of this is dead space, and so actual alveolar ventilation is only 4 L per minute).

Another option to reverse hypoxemia in spontaneously breathing patients is face-mask continuous positive airway pressure at 10 cm H_2O. This improves the intrapulmonary shunt fraction, although gastric dilatation may occur.

Masks are temporizing devices until more definitive management occurs. Direct complications include pulmonary aspiration and pressure injuries to the facial and trigeminal nerves.

Mechanical Ventilators

Manually triggered oxygen-powered breathing devices are commonly used in the prehospital arena, and are more flexible initially than pressure- or volume-cycled mechanical ventilators in emergency department resuscitations.

Coordinated positive pressure ventilation is obtained with valves (e.g., Flynn, Robertshaw, Elder) that go off at a set pressure. To avoid barotrauma, the usual settings are 50 cm water in adults and 25 cm water in children over 12. They should not be used on smaller children. The manual trigger button is released after the chest rises. An oxygen source with a flow rate of 100 liters per minute is required for adequate pressure and the proper FIO_2.

Before using this device, the physician should always "bag" the patient a few times; this gives a better feel for the actual pulmonary compliance. In the demand mode, patients with spontaneous respirations can trigger the valve with inhalation. Otherwise, a constant flow rate is delivered regardless of the patient's respiratory efforts. Unfortunately, the very high flow rate delivered in a short period of time does not optimally inflate the lungs, but preferentially inflates the stomach instead, causing distention and increased risk of aspiration.

SUGGESTED READING

Danzl DF. Advanced airway support. In: Tintinalli JE, Rothstein RJ, Krome RL, eds. Emergency medicine: a comprehensive study guide. New York: McGraw Hill, 1985:20.

DeGarmo B, Dronen S. Pharmacology and clinical use of neuromuscular blocking agents. Ann Emerg Med 1983; 12:48–55.

Kastendieck J. Airway Management. In: Rosen, et al, eds. Emergency medicine: concepts and clinical practice. St Louis: CV Mosby, 1983:26.

Natanson C, Shelhamer JH, Parrillo JE. Intubation of the trachea in the critical care setting. JAMA 1985; 253:1160–1165.

Nieman JT, Rosborough JP, Myers R, et al. The pharyngeotracheal lumen airway: preliminary investigation of a new adjunct. Ann Emerg Med 1984; 13:591–596.

AIRWAY OBSTRUCTION

STEVEN J. WHITE, M.D.
PAUL M. PARIS, M.D., F.A.C.E.P.
RONALD D. STEWART, B.A., B.Sc., M.D., F.A.C.E.P.

Airway obstruction is one of the few true emergencies in which a delay of mere seconds in recognition and treatment can have disastrous or fatal consequences. Many of its victims are healthy and many are young; the cost to society in productive years lost is immense. This unforgiving emergency requires the physician to be prepared with an array of airway control techniques; the ability to shout the phrase "Page Anesthesia!" is not enough.

TABLE 1 Causes of Upper Airway Obstruction

Intrinsic

    Posterior displacement of oropharyngeal soft tissues (decreased muscle tone, mandibular fracture)
    Laryngospasm/laryngeal edema
    Epiglottitis/croup/bacterial tracheitis
    Bilateral vocal cord paralysis
    Angioneurotic edema/anaphylaxis
    Laryngeal trauma
    Laryngeal tumors
    Arthritis of cricoarytenoid joint

Extrinsic

    Ludwig's angina/deep neck infections
    Hematoma (anticoagulation, trauma, surgery)
    Goiter/thyroid tumors
    Granulomatous diseases
    Esophageal foreign body/mass

Foreign body

    Food, especially meat in adults
    Any object in children or in mentally retarded or psychiatric patients
    Misplaced esophageal obturator airways
    Tracheostomy tube obstructions (mucous plug)
    Teeth/dental prostheses or appliances

ETIOLOGY; SIGNS AND SYMPTOMS

Causes of airway obstruction are listed in Table 1 in three distinct categories: intrinsic disorders of the larynx and supraglottic structures, extrinsic airway compression, and foreign bodies. Definitive therapy is directed to the reestablishment of air flow and to correction of the underlying cause.

The presentation of airway obstruction can be subtle or dramatic, depending on etiology and degree of obstruction. Generally, with partial obstruction, the patient is short of breath and demonstrates stridor. Isolated inspiratory stridor usually indicates supraglottic or glottic obstruction, whereas expiratory stridor is more characteristic of subglottic obstruction. Inspiratory stridor is often mistaken for the more common expiratory wheeze, especially by paramedics in the field, in which case the diagnosis may be missed and inappropriate therapy initiated.

Clinically, the patient may look apprehensive and may be diaphoretic and pale or cyanotic; he may lean forward, with head extended in the "sniffing" position in an attempt to decrease obstruction. There may be an alteration in voice, difficulty in phonation, difficulty in swallowing, pooling of secretions, and drooling. Retractions--suprasternal, substernal, and intercostal--may all be present and impressive. Coughing paroxysms are especially prominent in foreign body aspirations. Physicians must be especially wary of decreased mentation and combative behavior as indications of hypoxia and impending respiratory arrest.

Complete obstruction results in unconsciousness within seconds to minutes. Prior to that, the patient may exhibit signs and symptoms of partial obstruction or may suddenly become completely obstructed, unable to breathe, cough, or speak.

History and examination may be precluded by the need to establish an airway. Nevertheless, careful attention to activities surrounding the incident and time of onset provides important clues to the etiology of obstruction. Precipitating factors should be sought such as exposure to a bee sting or to a known food or drug allergen; eating food or holding an object in the mouth (foreign body); recent fever, cough, swollen glands, trismus, or sore throat (epiglottitis, croup, tracheitis, pharyngeal and oral infections); previous or recent neck surgery, neck trauma, or use of anticoagulants (hematoma, larynx fracture, vocal cord paralysis); or progressive hoarseness or weight loss (obstructing tumors, vocal cord paralysis).

The examination should focus initially on general appearance, since this best indicates whether immediate airway control is required. Posture, skin color, respiratory rate, degree of retractions, and any alteration in mental status should be noted. Beyond that, the examination should include the oral cavity, in search of glossal, mucosal, and uvular edema as well as swelling in the floor of the mouth or palate and tonsillar enlargement. The neck should be inspected for signs of trauma, hematoma, thyroid enlargement, adenopathy, and air crepitus, and for the presence of a tracheostomy. The chest should be auscultated to locate stridor and wheezes and to evaluate adequacy of air movement. The presence of urticaria is almost incontrovertible evidence of an allergic cause.

An exception to the foregoing should be noted in the pediatric patient with suspected epiglottitis: agitating the patient in any way, by examination or by show of needles, is likely to precipitate laryngospasm and respiratory arrest. Examination should consist of observation from a distance, and the child should never be out of sight of the physician. The remainder of the examination is conducted in the operating room under controlled conditions.

THERAPY

Airway management techniques exist at several levels of sophistication, from simple positioning maneuvers to involved surgical procedures. In dealing with airway obstruction, the physician progresses through these levels occasionally to procedures he has only read about. One can take comfort in the fact that the risk:benefit ratio is heavily weighted on the side of action. The potential complications of inaction are frequent, and often fatal; the usual complications of action are mostly temporary and bothersome. Having many options from which to choose makes success more likely, but the decision making more complex.

With the growth of emergency medical services systems, sophisticated airway control has expanded to include the field. Methods, techniques, and sequences described here for use in the hospital and emergency department are generally applicable to the pre-hospital environment as well. Some exceptions to this generalization will be noted.

In cases of partial obstruction (i.e., cases in which the patient is moving adequate air), supportive measures of reassurance and humidified oxygen should be applied. Monitoring by ECG should be instituted in all patients with airway problems, and intubation and suction equipment should be ready.

If obstruction is complete or if the patient is exhibiting signs and symptoms of hypoxia (e.g., cyanosis, air hunger, altered mental status), more definitive airway control is required. First maneuvers should include head tilt and jaw thrust to minimize possible soft tissue contributions to obstruction; jaw thrust alone should be used if cervical spine injury is suspected. The oropharynx and larynx should be inspected, and any vomitus, blood, or foreign material should be suctioned. Ventilation with 100 percent oxygen should be attempted with bag-valve-mask device (BVM); it is possible to overcome the obstruction at times, provided a good seal is obtained. The Seal-Easy mask is especially helpful in this circumstance. There is no role for the esophageal obturator airway (EOA) in the therapy of airway obstruction, since it does nothing to bypass the obstruction. In children with epiglottitis, sufficient airway pressure can usually be generated to ventilate despite the obstruction if one uses an adult-size bag with the correct-size pediatric mask; a definitive airway can then be established under circumstances less extreme than respiratory arrest.

Endotracheal intubation ensures a patent airway. Although not a simple procedure, it is even more difficult to perform in the setting of airway obstruction, in which edema and structural pathology create anatomic distortion, which in turn may prevent visualization of the glottis and passage of the tube. Orotracheal intubation under direct visualization is ordinarily first-line therapy, since it permits better visual assessment of the pathology, be it epiglottitis, laryngeal cancer, or foreign body. The issue of orotracheal intubation in the setting of possible cervical spine injury is complex at best; hyperextension should be avoided and in-line traction applied. The flexible fiberoptic laryngoscope is an excellent method of intubating the obstructed airway in the hands of someone skilled in this technique. If laryngoscopically guided intubation fails or if injury to the cervical spine is considered a possibility, several other alternatives are possible. The recently repopularized technique of tactile intubation can be employed and, like direct laryngoscopy may afford some insight into the anatomic pathology involved. The technique has limitations: it should not be used in patients with both teeth and an intact gag reflex, unless a bite block is also used. Orotracheal intubation with the lighted stylet (Tubestat) is a blind technique in which one transilluminates the soft tissues of the neck and observes a bright orange glow in the midline when the stylet (and endotracheal tube) enters the glottis. These and all other advanced airway techniques require practice. Fresh postarrest cadavers can be used to develop familiarity and facility with the techniques.

Endotracheal intubation under direct vision is the current standard for airway control in many EMS systems. Success rates seem acceptable, approaching 95 percent in some studies. A major complication is the problem of unrecognized esophageal intubation. However, strict attention to protocol for assessing tube placement minimizes the chance of this complication and makes endotracheal intubation the procedure of choice for securing the obstructed airway in the field. Paramedics can be trained to successfully perform the alternative methods of intubation as well, with success rates for tactile intubation approaching those of direct laryngoscopy. Preliminary data suggest similar rates for the lighted stylet.

In certain cases, such as fractured larynx or obstructing laryngeal tumor, intubation from above may not be possible, and access to the infraglottic airway is needed. Cricothyroid membrane puncture or percutaneous transtracheal ventilation (PTV) can be a lifesaving temporizing measure. This can be performed by introducing a 14-gauge over-the-needle catheter percutaneously through the cricothyroid membrane (see chapter on *Percutaneous Transtracheal Ventilation and Cricothyrotomy*).

An alternative measure for the field (or emergency department) is to use a 10-gauge catheter and attach the catheter hub to the 15-mm adaptor from a 3.0-mm internal diameter (ID) endotracheal tube (which happens to be the size that fits a standard catheter hub). Ventilation can be carried out by connecting the 15-mm adaptor to a BVM or to an oxygen-powered demand valve device. Critical diameter for ventilation with assistance in this manner is 2.5 mm ID; a 3.0-mm airway enables spontaneous respiration with maintenance of adequate blood gas parameters. A 10-gauge catheter has an ID of 2.25 mm, which suffices for temporary airway management.

In cases such as a crushed larynx or an infraglottic foreign body, one can place the catheter more inferiorly, through the tracheal rings, thus allowing a more ordered tracheostomy. Use in children is difficult, and complications, including bleeding and vascular, esophageal, and nerve injuries, must be weighted against possible benefit. Although most cases of complete airway obstruction allow sufficient exhalation to prevent barotrauma, the patient should be carefully observed for a rapidly accumulating tension pneumothorax.

Retrograde intubation, an under-utilized technique that can be used either alone or in conjunction with PTV requires introduction of a Seldinger wire through a catheter in the cricothyroid membrane, and placement of a clamp on the proximal end. The wire then is advanced cephalad into the oropharynx, and the distal end is removed from the mouth. It is then a fairly simple matter to thread a conventional endotracheal tube over the wire and into the trachea.

Cricothyrotomy is another technique that secures a definitive airway in cases in which less invasive methods fail. Requiring a surgical incision through the cricothyroid membrane, cricothyrotomy can be performed either with or without prior needle membrane puncture. The technique is described elsewhere in this book; it is perhaps the final option available currently to the emergency physician. Cricothyrotomy is difficult to perform in children, who, along with patients who have laryngotracheal disruption, may be the only patients who still require emergency tracheotomy. Otherwise the ''emergency tracheotomy'' is now obsolete.

The use of cardiopulmonary bypass (CPB) as a treatment for airway obstruction in the emergency department looms in the future. CPB units are becoming increasingly portable, and the skill required for emergency bypass is well within the abilities of emergency physicians. CPB has already been suggested for use in the treatment of cardiac arrest victims in the emergency department; its use in the operative therapy of tracheal tumors is documented. In those cases where an obstructing foreign body is at the level of the carina, where there is tracheal disruption, and in which the time to establish an airway is likely to be excessive, i.e., the time beyond which full neurologic recovery is not expected (10 to 20 minutes of asphyxia), CPB is a logical therapeutic measure that should be instituted early.

SPECIAL CASES OF AIRWAY OBSTRUCTION

Two topics deserve some elaboration: the obstructing foreign body, because of its frequency, and the obstructed tracheostomy tube, because of the difficulty it often presents to health care providers.

Foreign Body Obstruction. Obstructing foreign body, a common problem, is discussed in more detail in the chapter on *Laryngeal, Tracheal, and Oropharyngeal Foreign Bodies and Trauma.*

One should be alert to the possibility of foreign body in any case of collapse, but especially in certain circumstances: any small child found apneic, any person found apneic in a restaurant or found in a home during a meal, and any institutionalized person found not breathing. In one autopsy study, among 67 deaths occurring in restaurants, 66 were due to airway obstruction from food and only one was due to heart disease.

If the patient is coughing and actively moving air, no intervention should be attempted; the patient generates more expelling force from his own cough and there is always a danger of converting partial obstruction into complete obstruction. If the patient is moving air poorly, is unable to speak or make coughing efforts, quick action is in order, since he is likely to succumb to unconsciousness in seconds. A series of abdominal thrusts (Heimlich maneuvers) should be applied until the foreign body has been expelled or the patient has become unconscious.

If the patient becomes unresponsive, one should proceed immediately to direct laryngoscopy and removal of the foreign body with Magill forceps. This is usually successful, unless the foreign body is soft, impaled, or below the level of the cords. However, if the object can be seen below the cords, it is reasonable to make an attempt with forceps, since the alternative is death. Suction may be effective, especially in institutionalized patients, but in the field, one must appreciate the limitations of most mobile suction units. If the object is infraglottic, transcricoid membrane puncture may bypass the obstruction and allow ventilation. A more inferiorly placed cannula between the tracheal rings may be successful if the obstructing body is at the level of the cricoid ring; cricothyrotomy is an additional option in this case as it may permit retrieval of the object through the incision. Rigid bronchoscopy, in experienced hands, is an exceptional way of dealing with this problem; however, it is probably beyond the skills of most emergency physicians. Emergency tracheostomy also has a role here and can bypass a high infraglottic obstruction, but again it should be limited to experienced hands. Finally, as a measure of desperation, the physician can attempt to drive the foreign body beyond the carina with an endotracheal tube;

this would, of course, make subsequent retrieval efforts more difficult.

In those settings in which a laryngoscope is not available or in EMS systems in which paramedics do not intubate, and abdominal thrusts have failed, digital dislodging can be attempted. This differs from the finger sweeps that were a part of previous AHA guidelines, in which the posterior pharynx is swept from back to front. It requires pulling the tongue anteriorly with one hand and inserting the index and middle fingers into the mouth in an attempt to palpate the epiglottis and laryngeal structures.If a foreign body is encountered, one attempts to scissor it between the fingers. Care must be taken not to drive the object further into the airway. It is important to emphasize that prolonged rescue efforts should not be performed in the field and, if possible, should be performed while preparing for or during transport.

The initial treatment of choking and the sequence of maneuvers has been a subject of debate and controversy since the late seventies. Previous American Heart Association and American Red Cross guidelines (through 1985) called for the performance of four back blows followed by four abdominal thrusts followed by oral finger sweeps. Proponents of the Heimlich maneuver, most notably Dr. Henry Heimlich himself, have maintained that abdominal thrusts should be performed to the exclusion of other techniques, and that back blows are likely to drive the obstructing body deeper into the airway, or to convert a partial obstruction into a complete one. There is little experimental evidence (but some anecdotal evidence) to support back blows as an effective method and some literature that theoretically supports the possibility of retrograde movement, owing to Newton's Third Law of Motion. There are indications that this controversy, at least for the rescuer, will be coming to a close; it is expected that as this comes to print, AHA guidelines will no longer recommend back blows in the sequence for relief of obstructed airway.

Trachestomy Tube Obstruction. With advances in otolaryngology and oncology, more patients are in the community with tracheal stomas. With new tracheal appliances and advances in laryngeal prostheses for speech, it is often difficult to detect that a patient has a stoma. Emergency personnel must consider that a patient who cannot be ventilated by conventional means may be a neck breather.

A patient with a tracheostomy tube in place who presents with signs and symptoms of airway obstruction should be considered to have an obstructing mucous plug until proved otherwise. Sometimes the plug can be broken up by rapidly injecting 10 cc of normal saline down the tracheal tube. If this fails, however, the tracheal tube should be removed (or if a central cannula is present, that can be removed). If the patient is breathing spontaneously the problem may be solved, as most tracheostomy patients can breathe well through the stoma. However, the apneic patient must be reintubated and ventilated. This is accomplished most easily by inserting a conventional endotracheal tube through the stoma and into the trachea approximately 5 to 7 cm. Usually, a 5.0- to 6.0-mm ID tube works well; the minimum-size tube through which a normal-size adult patient can spontaneously breathe is 3.0 mm (2.5 mm with supplemental oxygen). This tube can then be replaced with a tracheal tube of the correct size at a later time.

Occasionally, emergency physicians are confronted by the problem of a dislodged tracheal tube from a recently (less than 1 week) created stoma. Replacement of the tube through the stoma runs a high risk of extratracheal placement, since the stomal tract is not mature. An attempt can be made to intubate orotracheally. Should this fail, one can ventilate over the stoma using a Seal-Easy mask to seal over the neck. The optimal method uses a flexible fiberoptic laryngoscope to verify intratracheal position; a tracheal tube can then be confidently inserted with the laryngoscope used as a stylet.

COMPLICATIONS OF AIRWAY OBSTRUCTION

As in any case in which hypoxemia has been present, patients should be expectantly observed for signs of cardiac and cerebral ischemia. In the at-risk population group, serial ECGs and cardiac isoenzymes should be obtained, and the patient should be monitored. Patients should also be watched for the development of tension pneumothoraces.

A well-described complication of airway obstruction is the development of pulmonary edema, occurring in as many as 7 percent of patients. It is believed to be secondary to the large negative intrathoracic forces that are generated as the patient attempts to inspire against the obstruction, and responds to conventional therapy, i.e., volume unloading, diuretics, and positive end expiratory pressure.

Finally, the therapy itself can have complications. Improperly performed abdominal thrusts can fracture ribs; there have also been cases of gastric rupture, liver laceration, and thrombosis of preexisting abdominal aortic aneurysm. Teeth can be loosened and aspirated in the process of airway management, and nasal, oral, and pharyngeal tissues can be damaged.

SUGGESTED READING

Marlowe FI, Aghamohamadi A. Acute upper airway obstruction. In: Tintinall J, et al, eds. Emergency medicine: a comprehensive study guide. New York: McGraw-Hill, 1985: 733.

Neff CC, et al. Percutaneous transtracheal ventilation: experimental and practical aspects. J Trauma 1983;23:84–90.

Safar P. Cardiopulmonary cerebral resuscitation: basic and advanced life support. In: Schwarz G, et al, eds. Principles and practice of emergency medicine. Philadelphia: WB Saunders, 1986:205.

Stewart RD. Tactile orotracheal intubation. Ann Emerg Med 1984; 13:175–178.

Stewart RD, et al. Influence of mask design on bag-mask ventilation. Ann Emerg Med 1985;14:403–406.

Vollmer TP, et al. Use of a lighted stylet for guided orotracheal intubation in the prehospital setting. Ann Emerg Med 1985; 14:324–328.

ENDOTRACHEAL INTUBATION

RONALD D. STEWART, B.A., B.SC., M.D.,
F.A.C.E.P.

Management of the airway should be a prime concern of emergency care providers, and this must take precedence over everything but safety. The practicing emergency physician or paramedic must be comfortable with and versed in the use of supplemental oxygen, mouth-to-mouth ventilation, positioning, clearing an obstructed airway, oro- and nasopharyngeal airways, and proper bag-mask ventilation. Without attention to these basic skills, the more advanced and sophisticated techniques of airway management are of little use and may do harm.

Although the emphasis of this chapter is on endotracheal intubation, it must be remembered that the skilled intubator is also a skilled basic airway manager. Endotracheal intubation is a psychomotor skill that can be relatively easily acquired, but one of the most difficult aspects of that skill is learning when *not* to use it. The decision to intubate the trachea is not to be taken lightly; although it can be life-saving, the procedure is not without complications.

The placement of an endotracheal tube bypasses the natural protective mechanisms of the upper airway and provides direct access to the vulnerable lung. The procedure can lead to trauma to the teeth and soft tissues; it can possibly aggravate a spinal cord injury; and the manipulation of the airway can set off reflexes that alter cardiovascular function and intracranial pressure. When improperly performed with prolonged attempts and inadequate monitoring, intubation can lead to hypoxia and even death.

WHEN TO INTUBATE

The indications for endotracheal intubation are usually readily apparent in the emergency setting. Few would argue that patients in respiratory or cardiopulmonary arrest require the controlled airway offered by intubation (Table 1).

Simply stated, patients who might require any of the benefits listed in Table 1 should be considered candidates for intubation. Patients with intact cough and gag reflexes and with adequate spontaneous ventilation may be "tided over" with careful monitoring and proper positioning.

TABLE 1 Benefits of Intubation

Control of ventilation (patency) and tidal volumes
Protection of the airway against aspiration
Easier ventilation compared to bag/mask, especially
  during transport
Direct access to the lungs for suction
A route for drug administration
An ability to apply positive end expiratory pressure

Patients in whom the cervical spine is not at risk from trauma should be placed in the left lateral position without pillow to allow drainage of upper airway secretions from the oropharynx and thereby reduce the likelihood of aspiration. In these patients, and in those immobilized with cervical collars in place and strapped to an extrication board or device, proper suction should be immediately available to remove vomitus or airway secretions.

NOTES ON BASIC ANATOMY

A knowledge of basic airway anatomy is essential for all clinicians who intubate the trachea. Not only should the landmarks be known by sight, but those who perform tactile (digital) intubation must be familiar with upper airway anatomy through palpation. The airway extends from the tip of the nose and lips to the alveolar-capillary membrane. The laryngeal prominence can be readily identified in most adult men, and in women it can usually be palpated if not readily seen. Pressure on this structure displaces the glottic opening and cords posteriorward to permit a better view during intubation.

Immediately inferior to this is the cricothyroid membrane, joining the inferior margin of the thyroid cartilage to the superior aspect of the cricoid cartilage. The thyroid cartilage has a muscular back wall; the cricoid is a complete cartilaginous ring. Puncture or incision of the cricothyroid membrane affords direct and ready access to the airway below the level of the cords. Pressure on the solid ring of the cricoid (Sellick maneuver) can occlude the esophagus, thus reducing the risk of regurgitation of stomach contents during the intubation procedure.

The tongue is the most common cause of airway obstruction in the unconscious patient and constitutes the major obstruction to proper visualization of the upper airway anatomy. The base of the tongue is attached to the mandible and connects to the epiglottis; a forward pulling or protrusion of the tongue can therefore lift the epiglottis upward and better expose the glottis.

The mucosa of the upper airway is vascular and delicate, and therefore it is particularly vulnerable to the trauma inherent in endotracheal intubation. The turbinates of the lateral nasal wall can obstruct the passage of a nasopharyngeal airway or nasotracheal tube, especially if the bevel of the device is directed laterally or superiorly. The tube should be well lubricated so that it can slide with the bevel placed against the nasal septum or floor of the nasal cavity. Avoidance of the turbinates reduces the risk of trauma and resultant bleeding.

The epiglottis is easily seen and palpated at the base of the tongue and is the most important landmark to identify during intubation. The trough between the base of the tongue and the epiglottis is known as the vallecula. On either side of the epiglottis are small recesses, the pyriform sinuses, and forming the posterior aspect of the laryngeal skeleton are the arytenoid cartilages, palpable in most patients as sharp projections.

A knowledge of the distances from the teeth to several important anatomic landmarks allows better judgement of the depth of placement of the endotracheal tube (Table 2). The numbers given in Table 2 represent averages and may be greater or less by a centimeter or two. For orotracheal intubation, therefore, a tube 25 cm in length is adequate for proper placement in the trachea, whereas a nasotracheal tube should be 30 to 33 cm in length.

The upper airway has three axes, all of which must be brought into alignment in order to view the glottis adequately (Fig. 1). These are the (1) axis of the mouth (a straight line passing through the mouth along the floor of the tongue), (2) axis of the pharynx (a line drawn along the posterior pharyngeal wall), and (3) axis of the trachea (passing along the trachea and intersecting with the others).

Flexion of the neck by elevating the occiput aligns the pharyngeal and tracheal axes. Extension of the head, by lifting up and back on the chin, brings the axis of the mouth in line with the other two axes. These maneuvers describe the "sniffing position," the position recommended for direct-vision orotracheal intubation with a laryngoscope.

The vagus and other nerves supply the upper airway, and manipulation can stimulate these nerves to produce cardiovascular changes such as bradycardia, hypertension, and in some, ventricular fibrillation. Manipulation of the airway by intubation or suctioning can cause a significant rise in intracranial pressure (ICP), particularly in those patients with head injury. These cardiovascular and ICP pressure changes persist beyond the time of the actual procedure. These changes can be blunted by topical local anesthesia applied to the mucous membranes or by the use of intravenous lidocaine.

EQUIPMENT

Endotracheal intubation equipment must be well maintained and ready to be used at a moment's notice. The proper functioning of each piece should be ensured daily. For field work, the airway control equipment should be provided in a portable kit, ideally in one lightweight, portable container (Table 3).

TABLE 2   Key Distances in Adults

15 cm:	Distance from incisors to the cords
20 cm:	Distance from incisors to sternal notch (thoracic inlet)
25 cm:	Distance from incisors to carina
30 cm:	Distance from nose to carina

TABLE 3   Contents of Endotracheal Intubation Kit

Laryngoscope handle: No. 3, No. 4 MAC blade,
  No. 4 MILLER blade
Endotracheal tubes: 33 cm in length; 7.0, 7.5 mm
  25 cm (precut); 7.5, 8.0, 8.5 mm
  1 Endotrol directional-tip tube
1 malleable stylet (SatinSlip preferred)
1 15-mm endotracheal tube adapter
1 10-cc syringe
Oropharyngeal airway (Guedel), nasopharyngeal airway
1 bite-block or mouth prod
2–3 tongue depressors
Adhesive tape: 1 1-inch roll
Tincture of benzoin ampule
Magill forceps
Packets of water-soluble lubricant
2 pairs rubber (nonsterile) examining gloves
1 Tubestat lighted stylet
4 × 4 gauze
2 needles: 18-gauge, 20-gauge
1 heparin lock
Lidocaine, 100 mg IV preload
Endotracheal tube holder

Note: Muscle relaxant, diazepam, etc. can be added before use. (See chapter on *Rapid-Induction Anesthesia.*)

Endotracheal Tubes

Recent improvements in the design and manufacture of endotracheal tubes have lessened the risk of intubation complications and provided a wider variety from which to choose. The modern endotracheal tube is constructed of clear or translucent plastic with a radiopaque line run-

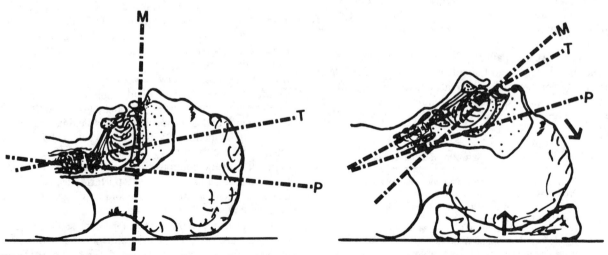

Figure 1   Axes of the upper airway; all must be brought into alignment for proper orotracheal intubation; M = Axis of the mouth; T = Axis of the trachea; P = Axis of the Pharynx.

ning lengthwise so that it can be clearly identified on the x-ray film. Clear plastic tubes have the advantage of permitting easy visualization of secretions and condensation of breath moisture, the latter an indication of correct intratracheal tube positioning. Tube cuffs to occlude the trachea are available in high-volume, low-pressure design and are said to protect the tracheal wall from damage by distributing less cuff pressure over a wider area of the tracheal mucosa.

Tube sizes are now given in millimeters, denoting the internal diameter of the tube. An average-size man should take an 8- to 8.5-mm tube, an average-size woman a 7.5-mm tube. Nasotracheal tube sizes are smaller and average 7.5 to 8 mm and 7 respectively. Choice of the correct size is important: too small a tube markedly increases airway resistance and makes for difficult suctioning, whereas too large a tube may lead to trauma to the cords. The standard length of endotracheal tubes is 33 cm and can be used for oro- or nasotracheal intubation. We advocate cutting the tubes used for orotracheal intubation to 25 cm prior to use, and in our Emergency Medical Services (EMS) system this has markedly decreased the incidence of right main stem bronchus intubations.

A specially designed endotracheal tube (Endotrol) incorporates into the tube a thin drawstring along the anterior aspect and a proximal loop that can be pulled to direct the tip of the tube anteriorly. This innovation was expected to provide a real advantage during nasotracheal intubation, but in clinical practice it has not been shown to be an overwhelming asset. The body temperature softens the plastic tube during use and its tip cannot be positioned accurately. In some hands it may still prove useful, especially in cases of abnormal or deformed anatomy.

Tubes should be well lubricated with a water-soluble jelly (K-Y, Lubifax, Surgilube). There is no advantage to using a local anesthetic cream or ointment. In fact, an ointment may become dry and sticky and actually irritate mucous membranes.

Laryngoscopes

The fact that so many laryngoscope blades are on the market would indicate that the ideal design has yet to be developed. The Macintosh or curved blade elevates the epiglottis to expose the cords with the tip placed in the vallecula; the straight or Miller blade is placed posterior to the epiglottis and "hooks" it up.

Most adults can be intubated with the No. 4 curved or "Mac" blade. A useful adaptation to the curved blade is the addition of a short extension at the tip. Because they have a relatively long and "floppy" epiglottis, infants and children are better intubated with the Miller (straight) blade.

Stylets

A malleable wire stylet to give firm shape to the tube for intubation may be useful when the upper airway is not clearly visualized. I prefer to use a plastic-coated stylet (Satin-slip) because of the reduced risk of tissue damage. These should not be reused too often, since in some reported cases the coating has broken, the result being a foreign body in the lung or airway obstruction.

Special Stylets

Stylets, specially designed to facilitate difficult or routine intubations, are commercially available. A controlled-tip stylet with a soft rubber covering (Flexiguide) protrudes beyond the distal tip of the tube and can be mechanically tilted anteriorly or posteriorly by means of a proximal handle. This is large and a bit unwieldy, however.

A lighted stylet, consisting of a 25-cm or 33-cm malleable wire connecting a distal bulb and proximal battery housing, can be used to perform orotracheal and nasotracheal intubation by means of the transillumination method (to be discussed). This stylet is useful in the following situations: (1) for guided transillumination orotracheal or nasotracheal intubation, (2) as a regular stylet to help with intratracheal placement during difficult laryngoscopic intubation, and (3) to check the position of an endotracheal tube. This stylet may be of particular value in trauma cases, in which the neck should be held immobile in the neutral position during intubation.

Other Equipment

Airways. Oropharyngeal and nasopharyngeal airways are useful in oxygenation of the patient prior to intubation. The oropharyngeal airway should be placed after intubation to act as a bite-block that prevents patients from biting down on the endotracheal tube and to help keep the airway open for suctioning of the oropharynx.

Magill Forceps. These are designed to direct the ends of endotracheal tubes as well as to remove foreign bodies from the airway.

Lubricant. A water-soluble jelly is recommended for lubrication of stylets, airways, and tubes. Surgilube, Lubifax, KY-Jelly, or equivalents are acceptable. However, overzealous use of lubricant may add more fluid that will have to be suctioned out of the airway. It has been well said that gentle insertion is the best lubricant.

Suction. A functioning suction unit within reach is mandatory for all intubations. In the field setting, a portable suction unit should be part of an airway kit or box that contains oxygen and other equipment. The frequency with which large amounts of blood and secretions are found in the upper airway of some patients dictates the need for a suction device with high displacement, wide-bore tubing, and large suction tips.

PREPARATION OF THE PATIENT

Ventilation

Providing supplemental oxygen to the patient prior to intubation should be considered absolutely basic to proper technique. Reducing the risk of hypoxia through adequate oxygenation decreases the likelihood of serious arrhythmias and other complications of intubation. If the patient is breathing spontaneously and has an acceptable minute volume, giving high-flow oxygen for 2 to 3 minutes through a tight-fitting face mask at 10 L per minute of hyperventilating with bag-valve-mask should ensure adequate oxygenation.

Patients who are apneic require positive pressure ventilation with supplemental oxygen. If a bag-valve-mask in order to provide 90 to 100 percent oxygen at the ventilating port. Recent improvements in the design of masks ating port. Recent improvements in the design of masks have reduced mask leak and ensured better ventilation. One of these designs consists of a partially filled balloon that fits over a specially designed oropharyngeal airway. The balloon mask is seated over the airway whose proximal end protrudes 1 to 2 cm outside the patient's lips. The balloon seals the nares and mouth, thus reducing dead space and allowing for a more efficient and easier mask seal. Laboratory and clinical studies have confirmed its effectiveness.

Premedication

Many intubations carried out in the emergency department or prehospital setting must be performed without much warning, and it is unusual to have time enough to medicate patients prior to the procedure. Patients can therefore be expected to have secretions, blood, or vomitus that may obscure anatomic landmarks in the upper airway. Most patients are unconscious and unable to control their airways; many are apneic. The need for adequate suction is therefore evident.

Drugs are often given to patients prior to elective intubation in the operating theater and can be of great help to (1) reduce upper airway secretions, (2) blunt the adverse physiologic effects of airway manipulation, (3) provide comfort to the patient, and produce an amnesic effect, and (4) facilitate intubation through chemical paralysis. Some of these goals may be appropriate to the emergency situation as well. These are discussed in detail in the chapter on *Sedation and Rapid Induction Anesthesia for Emergency Intubation.*

Airway Secretions

No intubation should be performed unless a reliable and adequate suction source is literally at the fingertips. Suctioning should be gentle, using a catheter or suction tip that is of a diameter sufficient to deal with the amount and type of material being removed from the airway. Since a dramatic fall in oxygen saturation may occur during suctioning and persist well beyond the procedure, the patient should be hyperoxygenated by increasing the rate and volume of ventilation for several minutes prior to the procedure.

Blunting Physiologic Reflexes

Although sometimes not possible in the emergency setting, premedication of the patient with lidocaine HCl, either topical or intravenous, can blunt the cardiovascular and intracranial pressure changes that may occur with instrumentation of the upper airway. Our preferred technique is to give intravenous lidocaine in a bolus dose of 1.5 mg per kilogram 4 to 5 minutes prior to intubation. As an alternative, lidocaine spray (4 to 10 percent) or other topical local anesthetic solutions (e.g., etidocaine) can be sprayed in the upper airway before and after insertion of the laryngoscope. The fact that the airway must be manipulated prior to applying the anesthesia represents the major disadvantage of this latter procedure.

Nasotracheal intubation is perhaps more stimulating to airway reflexes and can be painful to the patient. Local anesthesia of the nasal and posterior pharyngeal mucosa not only reduces the discomfort, but also can blunt the physiologic reaction to instrumentation of the upper airway. The best agent for topical application in nasotracheal intubation is cocaine (4 to 10 percent). Not only does it provide excellent anesthesia, but its vasoconstrictive properties, unique among the local anesthetics, shrink the nasal mucosa and reduce the risk of bleeding. A spray, or application of the 4 percent solution soaked in cotton applicators, is satisfactory. Toxic reactions have been reported with cocaine, and the dose should not exceed 200 mg. Cocaine is not so readily available as it once was, can be toxic, and may not be as effective as a mixture of 3 percent lidocaine HCl in 0.25 percent phenylephrine. For nasotracheal intubation, I recommend the latter solution sprayed or dripped into the nares.

Comfort and Amnesia

Some patients who are lightly unresponsive and at times combative may still require endotracheal intubation for a variety of reasons. An attempt to correct underlying hypoxia should be made before premedication is considered. Such patients can be provided comfort during the procedure by gentle technique and a combination of diazepam, 5 to 10 mg in adults, and local anesthesia applied to the mucous membranes of the nose and oropharynx (see chapter on *Sedation and Rapid-Induction Anesthesia for Emergency Intubation*).

Ketamine HCl has been used as an induction agent in elective anesthesia, and its possible applications to emergency medicine are being investigated. Low-dose intravenous or intramuscular ketamine (0.5 to 1.0 mg per kilogram) can produce in most patients a calm, dissociative state in which verbal contact is not lost, but the patient responds little to pain or the discomfort of airway manipulation. The incidence of reawakening hallucinosis, estimated for prolonged ketamine anesthesia to be 15 percent in adults, can be decreased with the use of midazolam or diazepam prior to or following the adminstration of the agent. Amnesia is almost complete with ketamine. The incidence of increased secretions, laryngospasm, or hypertension with low-dose ketamine deserves further investigation.

Muscle Relaxants

In about 5 percent of patients, the presence of straining, gag, or cough reflexes may make the smooth and atraumatic passage of an endotracheal tube difficult, if not impossible. In these situations, the use of a muscle relaxant may be justified. Currently, I recommend the use of intravenous diazepam, 5 to 10 mg given (if possible) 5 minutes prior to the use of intravenous succinylcholine, 1.5 mg per kilogram. It has been shown that diazepam can block the fasciculations, the heart rate changes, and the arterial pressure changes seen with succinylcholine.

Our protocol for the use of succinylcholine includes nitrogen desaturation of the lungs with 100 percent oxygen administration while diazepam (5 to 10 mg IV) is being administered. After 4 to 5 minutes of oxygenation, succinylcholine is administered over 5 to 10 seconds in a bolus dose of 1.5 mg per kilogram. During this time and until intubation is complete, cricoid pressure (Sellick maneuver) is applied by an assistant, and a transtracheal jet ventilator is immediately at hand for use in the event we are unable to promptly intubate the patient. Most patients can be safely managed if this protocol is rigidly followed.

Airway control in trauma patients, or in the patient who may require endotracheal intubation and yet may be somewhat responsive, presents a challenge to even the most experienced emergency care provider. Alternative intubation techniques, including tactile (digital), lighted stylet and transtracheal jet ventilation, may offer several advantages over use of the conventional laryngoscope, particularly in the trauma patient.

OROTRACHEAL INTUBATION

Emergency intubation in patients who are in cardiac arrest or deeply comatose usually means orotracheal intubation under direct vision using a laryngoscope; these are generally the easiest intubations. Recently several other methods have been evaluated (Table 4). The preparations for all intubations include (1) preoxygenation with 100 percent oxygen for 2 to 4 minutes, (2) an adequate suction at hand, (3) correct positioning of the patient, and (4) checking of the equipment.

Laryngoscopic Technique

This technique is the conventional and perhaps the first choice of intubation techniques. Other techniques are alternatives to this. There is really no substitute for seeing the tube pass through the cords and thus ensuring intratracheal placement. The essentials of the technique are as follows:

1. *Oxygenate.* Use a tight mask seal (the SealEasy mask is recommended) and assist ventilations with 100 percent oxygen or allow the patient to spontaneously breathe through a tight-fitting mask at 8 to 10 L per minute.

2. *Lidocaine.* Given intravenously in a bolus of 1.5 mg per kilogram, lidocaine has been shown to blunt both intracranial pressure and cardiovascular changes due to manipulation of the upper airway. To be effective, this should be administered 5 minutes prior to intubation.
   Note: If indicated, a sedative-analgesic can be given at this point.

3. *Check.* Laryngoscope, bulb, and the endotracheal tube should be checked for patency, cuff leak, and ease of deflation. Keep a 10-cc syringe attached to the one-way valve of the pilot tube; it should have the plunger drawn fully back to ensure that the cuff of the endotracheal tube is fully deflated, so as not to obstruct passage through the cords.

4. *Lubricate* the stylet, the end, and the cuff of the tube. Insert the stylet into the tube. (*Do not allow the end of the stylet to protrude beyond the distal tip.*) Bend the tube and stylet into the shape of a "hockey stick." Place the tube, with syringe attached, within reach on a clean surface.

5. *Position the patient.* If no trauma is suspected, place the patient supine with the occiput elevated 2 to 3 inches, resting on a towel or book, and extend the patient's head by pulling upward and back on the chin and gently pushing the forehead back (Fig. 2).
   Note: If a muscle relaxant is to be administered, it should be given at this point, and cricoid pressure should be applied.

6. *Continue to oxygenate.* Hyperventilate with an increased rate and tidal volume just prior to the intubation attempt.

7. *Count.* When the mask is removed from the patient, an assistant should continue cricoid pressure and should slowly count aloud.

8. *Insert laryngoscope.* Hold it in the left hand and avoid touching the teeth. The blade should be inserted on the right side of the oral cavity and used to push the tongue to the left. To save time, as the laryngoscope is advanced toward the epiglottis, the endotracheal tube in the right hand can now be inserted along the tongue on the right side. The tongue should be hooked forward in a "scooping" motion; *there is never a need to use the teeth as a fulcrum to "lever"*; the blade should not touch the upper teeth.
   Note: It is important to mention here that a common mistake is for the intubator to crouch down and get in as close as possible to the mouth in order to "see things better." This position distorts perspective, thus

TABLE 4 Intubation Techniques

Laryngoscopic orotracheal intubation under direct vision

Digital (tactile) intubation

Transillumination method (lighted stylet)

Blind nasotracheal intubation

Guided over fiberoptic laryngoscope

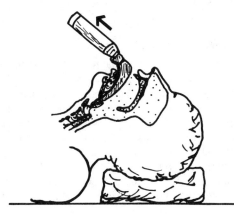

Figure 2 Correct position for orotracheal intubation ("sniffing position").

making visualization more difficult. In order to retain depth perspective and aid in intubation, the clinician should be a few feet or so from the oral cavity. As soon as the epiglottis is seen, the blade is placed in the vallecula (curved) or posterior to the epiglottis (straight) in an effort to lift that structure out of the way so that the glottis can be visualized.

9. *Visualize the cords.* When the cords are seen, the endotracheal tube, which has been advancing with the blade, can be slipped from the right side through the glottic opening. When the cuff is seen to pass, the laryngoscope can be removed and the tube inserted a centimeter or so more. *Note the centimeter marking on the tube at the incisors.* This helps one to predict how deep the tube may be and can aid in preventing right main stem bronchus intubations.

10. *Inflate the cuff.* Remove the syringe, all the while keeping hold of the tube.

11. *Begin ventilating the patient.* The total count by the assistant should not be greater than 30 to 45, measured *from ventilation to ventilation.*

12. *Check positioning.* This is a most important step in intubation, and should be carried out often, particularly in the field setting where patients tend to be moved more frequently. Signs of correct placement include persistent breath condensation on the tube, a firm compliance following cuff inflation, and absence of leak on ventilation. Intratracheal placement should be confirmed by auscultation of six sites: (a) right and left apical areas; (b) right and left mid-axillary lines; (c) the epigastrium—this is especially important; a silent epigastrium with breath sounds is a reliable sign of correct placement; and (d) the sternal notch, where "tracheal" sounds may be prominently heard. The chest wall should be watched and felt for movement.

A lighted stylet (to be discussed) can be used to check the position of the endotracheal tube. This is a reliable method which, when done carefully, does not disturb the tube. If in any doubt about placement, visualize the upper airway with a laryngoscope.

13. *Secure the tube.* Use tape or a commercially available endotracheal tube holder. There is no ideal version of the latter; avoid holders with Velcro fastening, since the small hooks can stick in the patient's lips and in the fingers of care providers.

14. *Continue to ventilate.* Recheck the position of the tube periodically.

Complications and Cautions

Intubation bypasses the natural defense mechanisms of the upper airway and can lead to dangers to the pulmonary tree that include dehydration of the mucosa, paralysis of ciliary action, and exposure to infection. Assuming the appropriate indications for intubation are present, the most common problems ascribed to the technique itself are hypoxia, trauma, and aspiration.

Hypoxia. This is one of the ever-present dangers of intubation and is usually due to prolonged attempts at placing the tube. There are few excuses that justify attempts beyond 30 seconds, and 45 seconds is the absolute maximum, measured from ventilation to ventilation. Ensuring adequate oxygenation and denitrogenation of the lungs by application of a tight-fitting oxygen mask at 8 to 10 L per minute or positive pressure ventilation with 100 percent oxygen can help to protect against this problem.

One of the most tragic complications of endotracheal intubation is an unrecognized esophageal placement of the tube. In the operating theater, this can be recognized more readily because of changes in the patient's color or vital signs. Many patients in the field or emergency department are perfusing poorly or in cardiac arrest, and any change for the worse is not so noticeable. We must therefore rely on other signs to prove intratracheal placement (to be discussed).

Laryngeal spasm, a serious complication of intubation, can result in serious hypoxia and even cardiac arrest. It usually responds to a relaxant, and transtracheal jet ventilation can be used as a life-saving measure in the face of this problem. Obstruction of the tube by blood, secretions, or kinking can lead to partial or complete respiratory obstruction. Constant vigilance is required to avoid these conditions. Inadequate ventilation can occur if the endotracheal tube is inserted too far into the endobronchial tree, and a right main stem intubation results. Hypoxia in patients undergoing intubation can predispose to serious cardiac arrhythmias culminating in arrest.

Trauma. The most common mistake of novice intubators is striking the upper teeth and "levering" in an attempt to visualize the cords. This may result in violation of the most basic tenet of intubation—that the patient should have the same number of teeth after the procedure as before. Trauma to the soft tissues, larynx, and other anatomic structures has been reported. Perforation of the mucosa is a particular danger with blind nasotracheal intubation. Gentleness and a knowledge of basic anatomy can protect against these serious complications.

Aspiration. Vomiting and aspiration of gastric contents can result from manipulation of the upper airway, with the attendant morbidity and mortality of aspiration pneumonitis. The Sellick maneuver, described as posteriorward pressure on the cricoid cartilage to occlude the esophagus, can be somewhat protective against this catastrophe.

Endotracheal Drug Administration

It has been our custom during cardiac arrest to administer the first doses of epinephrine and several other drugs through the endotracheal tube. Since this usually called for discontinuing ventilation while up to 10 cc of solution was squirted into the tube, and since some of the solution was lost during expiration, an alternative method had to be found. We now insert an 18-gauge needle capped with a heparin lock through the proximal endotracheal tube. Drugs can be administered by inserting the needle of any preload syringe through the rubber cap of the lock (Fig. 3). To pass a suction catheter, however, the needle needs to be withdrawn.

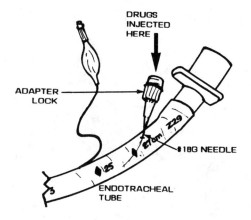

Figure 3 Set-up for endotracheal drug administration.

Transillumination With Lighted Stylet

During early bronchoscopic examinations with a fiberoptic bronchoscope, some physicians noted that the strong light at the end of the scope could be used to guide the tip through the glottis by observing the transilluminated light through the soft tissues of the neck. A surgical light, consisting of a 25-cm rigid copper wire connecting a proximal battery to a distal bulb (Flexilum, Concept Corporation, Clearwater, FL), was found to fit nicely into a 25-cm-long endotracheal tube.

The stylet and tube, when bent to about a right angle, could be used to lift up the epiglottis, and the position of the tip could be readily discerned by the transilluminated light. A circumscribed glow to the right or left of the midline laryngeal prominence indicates placement in the right or left pyriform fossa. The tube then needs only to be repositioned toward the midline, and a midline flow that shines through the laryngeal prominence signals correct placement at or below the level of the cords. This is the basis for guided endotracheal tube placement using a lighted stylet.

From clinical trials in patients undergoing elective surgery in the operating theater, the stylet has now been studied in the field and emergency departments and has performed well. It may be particularly valuable in patients with suspected neck injury, since it does not require special positioning of the head, or neck manipulation. In patients with small or deformed mouths, or in those with cervical spine abnormalities that restrict movement, it may prove invaluable.

The Stylet

The stylet has been improved and redesigned specifically for endotracheal intubation. The Tube-Stat intubating Stylet (Concept Corporation, Clearwater, FL) has the wire and bulb now encased in a plastic sheath, preventing the bulb from being dislodged and falling into the endobronchial tree. It has a brighter light as well.

Following lubrication, the stylet is slipped into a 25-cm-long endotracheal tube, and the two are then bent at about a right angle one or two fingerbreadths proximal to the tube cuff.

Technique

The patient is hyperventilated, and the neck and head can be placed in the "sniffing position" or held in neutral alignment. Gloves are suggested for the clinician, since there is a chance that the intubator's hands will come in contact with the patient's mouth and teeth.

1. *Check light.* Ensure that it is in working condition. If the stylet has been used previously, look directly at the light. If it is *not* uncomfortable to the eyes, it is probably not bright enough.
2. *Lubricate* stylet and tube. This makes for easier withdrawal of the stylet.
3. *Adjust stylet* by adjusting the proximal endotracheal tube adapter so that the end of the stylet is a few millimeters within the distal end of the tube.
4. *Bend stylet.* The patient's mandibular-hyoid measurement should be taken in fingerbreadths. While the tube-stylet combination is held with the dominant hand, the distal end is placed on the palmar surface of the fingers with the lightbulb-stylet junction at the index finger. To ensure this, grasp the wings of the endotracheal tube adapter to hold the proximal end of the tube firmly against the stylet's battery casing (proximal end). Bend the tube-stylet to the angles shown in Figure 4. *Note*: Attempt to create a gradual curve so that the stylet pulls out more easily following intubation.
5. *Approach the patient.* Face the head, with dominant hand nearest the patient. Turn on the stylet.
6. *Grasp the tongue* or, more easily, grasp the tongue and jaw as a unit and pull forward. Both techniques are designed to lift the epiglottis. *Note*: Darken the area as much as possible; shield the neck from direct light.
7. *Grasp the tube-stylet*, holding the battery casing flush against the proximal endotracheal tube adapter. Slide the tube along the tongue, "hooking up" the epiglottis and pulling the tongue forward with a "soup-ladle" action (Fig. 5).
8. *Identify location* of the tip of the tube by the transillumination of the soft tissues of the neck (Table 5).
9. *Release the tongue* when the midline glow is seen. *Hold stylet and tube firmly in place.* Do not force the stylet further into the trachea, since damage may be done due to the rigidity of the stylet.
10. *Support the tube* with the fingers placed along the tongue as the tube is slipped off the stylet and into the trachea. *Do not pull back on the stylet.* Advance the tube *off* the stylet.

Complete the intubation procedure, giving particular attention to confirming placement. Since this is a "guided" procedure and the cords are not directly visualized, the risk of unrecognized misplacement is greater.

The lighted stylet has proved to be a reliable alternative to the conventional laryngoscope for orotracheal intubation, particularly in trauma patients. It may well be the method of choice for orotracheal intubation in those at risk from cervical spine injury. The stylet can be help-

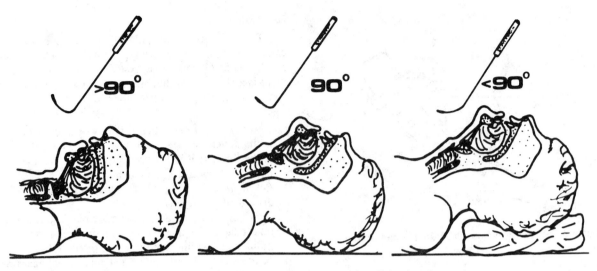

Figure 4 Patient positioning and appropriate lighted stylet angle.

ful as well in assisting placement during laryngoscopic technique and can be used to confirm correct intratracheal tube positioning. A special flexible nasotracheal stylet can be used for this.

Digital (Tactile) Intubation

Probably the first recorded method of intubation in humans in the eighteenth century required that the doctor feel for the epiglottis and guide the tube with the middle and index fingers. This technique, although seemingly primitive, is quick and reliable in selected patients, and should be considered an alternative to laryngoscopic intubation. It is particularly useful in deeply comatose patients at risk of a cervical spine injury, and in those with facial trauma in whom bleeding or anatomic distortion may prove difficult problems. As might be expected, only deeply unresponsive patients or those paralyzed with muscle relaxants are candidates for this method. The procedure is as follows:

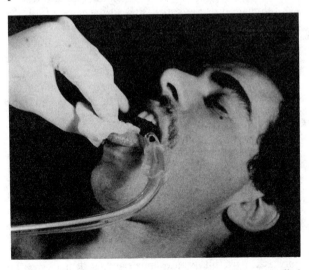

Figure 5 Insertion of the tube with stylet; jaw and tongue pulled forward to lift the epiglottis.

1. *Preoxygenate* as with direct-vision laryngoscopy, and administer other drugs that may be necessary.
2. *Glove.* Rubber examining gloves should be used for protection of the intubator.
3. *Prepare tube.* A standard endotracheal tube with lubricated stylet in place is bent in an "open-J" arrangement with the stylet recessed about 0.5 cm into the distal tip of the tube.
4. *Bite block.* Place a bite block or the distal end of an oropharyngeal airway between the molars to protect the fingers in case the patient awakens.
5. *Stand or kneel* at the side of the patient, facing the patient's head.
6. *Remove oxygen mask and insert fingers.* The left middle and index fingers are inserted into the mouth and "walk down" the tongue, pulling it forward and up. Open the patient's mouth wide. Slide the middle finger along the midline of the tongue, until the epiglottis is palpated. This is easily felt as the first firm structure past the base of the tongue.

Note: An assistant counts the seconds to 30, at which time the intubation should be completed or the patient reventilated.

TABLE 5 Interpretation of Lighted Stylet Location

Location of Light Seen*	Location of Tube
Bright, midline glow	Trachea, glottis
Glow under chin, well above larynx	Vallecula
Bright glow, right or left side of neck	Right/left pyriform fossa
Dull, midline glow	Esophagus

* If the light is seen in the lateral fossae, twist and lift the proximal shaft of the Tubestat to bring the tip toward the midline glottic opening. If a dull, esophageal glow is seen, bring the proximal shaft downward toward the chin and attempt to "hook" the epiglottis.

7. *Insert the tube.* Slide the tip along the side of the middle finger with the index finger supporting it behind. As the tip approaches the epiglottis, the side hole of the tube can serve as a landmark against the middle finger as the tip of the tube is slipped against the epiglottis in front, supported by the middle and index fingers behind.
8. *Advance the tube*, lifting the tube and epiglottis up and forward with the fingers. Maintain this forward pressure while the tube is advanced; otherwise it will slip posteriorward into the esophagus.
   Note: Resistance may be felt after the cords are passed. This is most likely due to the sharply curved tube abutting against the anterior larynx or tracheal wall. At this point the stylet should be pulled out and the tube advanced to a proper depth. Note the centimeter markings on the tube at the incisor line.
9. *Complete* the intubation, taking greater care to confirm correct tube placement, since this is a guided technique without direct visualization.

Other Methods

Several other techniques of orotracheal intubation are available to the emergency clinician, but can require relatively frequent use to maintain proficiency, or they may be somewhat more elaborate.

Fiberoptic Stylet or Laryngoscope

A fiberoptic stylet (or laryngoscope) can be inserted into an appropriately sized endotracheal tube and used to carry out oro- or nasotracheal intubation. Visualization of the cords is direct with these instruments, and the tube is simply slipped off the fiberoptic "snake" once the larynx is entered. The stylet is rigid, with a flexible (directional) tip. The laryngoscope can be used for both orotracheal and nasotracheal routes. A guide in the form of a modified Guedel airway (Berman, Williams) is useful if orotracheal intubation is done; this facilitates the procedure and protects the fiberoptic bundle from damage should the patient bite down.

The disadvantages of this method are several. A certain level of skill is required to successfully use the instrument. Second, the fiberoptic "window" at the distal tip of the tube is easily obscured with blood, secretions, or vomitus. Since at least one of these is usually present in patients in the emergency situation, the value of fiberoptic techniques for intubation in emergency medicine is limited.

Retrograde Techniques

The "retrograde" technique for oro- or nasotracheal intubation requires that a wire or long plastic catheter be passed first through the cricothyroid membrane upward past the cords and then drawn out through the mouth or nose. An endotracheal tube is then threaded over this guide. This technique, which requires some manipulation and can be considerably slower than more conventional approaches to intubation, has been superseded by the techniques already described.

Intubating Airways

Recent adaptations of the standard oropharyngeal airway have resulted in intubating airways that can guide an endotracheal tube through the glottic opening (Berman, Williams). The patient is placed in the "sniffing" position and the airway is inserted in the midline. After lubrication, the endotracheal tube is slipped down the large opening of the airway and guided gently into the larynx by visualizing the neck to detect lateral displacement. In the hands of experienced intubators, this method appears to work well, at least for elective surgical procedures.

NASOTRACHEAL INTUBATION

Nasotracheal intubation is a procedure whereby an endotracheal tube is passed through the nasopharynx into the trachea by blind, guided, or direct-vision technique. There are several advantages to this method, including the fact that it is perhaps better tolerated by patients who may not be deeply comatose. In addition, it does not require opening the mouth, and is therefore indicated in those who may have trismus or anatomic deformities of the oral cavity.

It has been said that this method should not be used in patients with head injury because of the possibility of intracranial placement of the tube through a basilar skull fracture. This complication is highly overrated; only one or two cases have ever been reported. In fact, nasotracheal intubation, if carefully and properly done, is considered by some to be the procedure of choice in head-injured patients, since the head and neck need not be manipulated.

Equipment

The equipment should be checked beforehand, as previously discussed.

Since the distance from the nares to the carina is approximately 27 cm in women and 32 cm in men, a 33-cm tube is used for these intubations. In addition, I prefer to prepare two endotracheal tubes of the same internal diameter (7.5 mm for a man and 7.0 mm for a woman) and 33 cm in length. Each tube is bent to form a circle by inserting its distal tip into its proximal adapter, and both are put aside while other equipment and the patient are prepared for the procedure. This ensures that the tubes retain an anterior curve, facilitating correct placement. Because the heat of the body tends to soften the curve of the tube, after two unsuccessful passes the first tube is removed, the patient is reoxygenated, and the second tube is used for the next intubation attempt. The Endotrol tube, the tip of which can be directed anteriorly by pulling on a string-and-loop arrangement, can be used as either a first-line or a backup tube if a conventional tube fails to pass after several attempts.

The distal end and the cuff of the tube are well lubricated with a water-soluble jelly (e.g., KY, Surgilube).

Preparation of the Patient

The patient is prepared for nasotracheal intubation as follows:

1. *Oxygenate* as previously described.
2. *The sniffing position* better ensures passage of the tube, although in patients with suspected C-spine injury, the neutral position with head and neck immobilization is preferred for first attempts.
3. *Inspect* the patient's nares for any obstruction and to determine which is larger.
4. *Drugs*(a) *Intravenous lidocaine* can be given as a bolus of 1.5 mg per kilogram, particularly in patients with a head injury to blunt ICP and cardiovascular reflex responses to the procedure.

   (b) *Local anesthesia* of the nasal mucosa and posterior pharynx should be carried out with a lidocaine-phenylephrine mixture (already discussed) placed by spray or drip. (Lidocaine, 4 to 10 percent spray, can be used as well.)

   (c) *Sedation-paralysis* can be carried out using diazepam (5 to 10 mg per kilogram), as previously described. Although it may be more difficult, nasotracheal intubation can be carried out in apneic patients.

Technique

Following ventilation and removal of the mask, nasotracheal intubation proceeds as follows:

1. *Insert the well-lubricated tube into the naris* with the bevel placed against the septum or the floor of the nasal cavity so that the tube does not catch on the laterally situated turbinates. The tube should be passed straight backward, not upward.

   Note: Again, an assistant should count aloud, and should perform the Sellick maneuver to occlude the esophagus. In addition, the assistant should pull the patient's tongue or jaw and tongue forward to aid in the passage of the tube.
2. *Pass the tube backward*, curving it gently around the posterior pharyngeal wall; the Endotrol tube is particularly helpful in this maneuver. This is a crucial point in the intubation procedure, since forcing the tube against resistance may result in laceration of the mucosa and submucosal passage of the tube.
3. *Watch the patient's neck.* The intubator places his ear and face close to the distal end of the tracheal tube as it is gently advanced toward the glottic opening. If the patient is spontaneously ventilating, the tube should be advanced until the breath sounds are heard and felt maximally, and the tube then thrust gently but quickly through the cords, preferably on inspiration. If the tube does not pass, the following observations may help to uncover the problem:

   (a) *Tenting of the skin in the midline above the laryngeal prominence.* The tube is most likely in the vallecula. Draw back on the tube, ensure that the tongue and jaw are pulled forward, and advance the tube again.

   (b) *Tenting of skin lateral to the laryngeal prominence.* The tip of the tube is most likely in the right or left pyriform fossa. Pull back on the tube, rotate the proximal end toward the midline, and advance the tube again.

A bulging of the laryngeal prominence usually indicates that the tube has passed through the glottic opening and into the trachea. The patient, unless deeply comatose, often bucks slightly or coughs. If the tube does not pass after two or three passes or within 30 seconds, remove it and ventilate the patient. Because the tube is now warmed by body heat, it usually does not retain a natural curve. For a second intubation attempt, use the second tube, which should have been kept at hand with the distal and proximal ends inserted into each other in order for it to retain its curve (already discussed).

4. *Inflate the cuff* of the tube, begin ventilation and check for correct placement. Secure the tube well with tape or with an endotracheal tube holder.

Problems and Complications

Since this is a "blind" technique, extra caution should be exercised in checking the position of the tube. All six sites should be auscultated and other maneuvers should be carried out to prove intratracheal positioning (already discussed).

Trauma to the nasal or oropharyngeal mucosa is one of the most common problems. Bleeding from the nose is usually not serious and stops on its own. Gentle technique reduces the risk of mucosal perforation and other major injuries to the upper airway structures.

Prolonged attempts present the most common problem with all intubations, particularly those carried out by the inexperienced or the careless. An assistant is helpful in preventing this, both by counting aloud and by insisting on ventilating the patient should the intubator be taking too much time.

Stimulation of the patient with this technique can lead to the complications of cardiac arrhythmias, blood pressure and heart rate changes, and increased intracranial pressure. The risk of these occurring can be reduced by the judicious use of topical anesthesia, intravenous lidocaine, or sedation if this is indicated.

Other Methods of Nasotracheal Intubation

The technique of blind nasotracheal intubation can be augmented by several maneuvers designed to facilitate the procedure.

Lighted Stylet. The rigid, 25-cm stylet now available for orotracheal intubation is not well suited to the nasotracheal technique, but a longer and more flexible device has been designed and shows promise. The transillumination method provides more accurate guidance of the tip of the tube toward the glottic opening.

Digital Guidance. The fingers can be used to guide the endotracheal tube toward the glottic opening as it passes down the posterior pharynx. The technique is the same as that described for tactile intubation via the orotracheal route.

Laryngoscope. The laryngoscope can be used to visualize the cords, and the tip of the tube can be advanced by an assistant while the intubator directs the tube anteriorly through the glottic opening using the Magill forceps or a hook.

Stylet. A regular semi-rigid stylet can be inserted into the tube once it passes the pharyngeal curve. The lubricated stylet should have been measured beforehand so that when inserted into the tube, the stylet comes within a few millimeters of the end of the tube, but not beyond. The stylet should assume a gentle curve in the mid-portion and a sharper anterior angle several centimeters from the distal end. The well-lubricated tube is inserted in the usual way, and the stylet can be advanced to the distal tip of the tube. When breath sounds are maximal, the tube can be slid off and its tip is usually directed anteriorly by the stylet. The stylet can then be withdrawn the rest of the way. Pulling forward on the tongue, or tongue and jaw, facilitates placement.

Retrograde Passage. The cricothyroid membrane can be punctured and a long catheter passed upward through the cords and attached to a second catheter that has been passed through the nose and into the mouth. The nasal catheter is then withdrawn, pulling the second catheter with it through the nose; the endotracheal tube is then advanced over the catheter and into the trachea. Although this method has been described, we have yet to use it in the emergency setting.

Fiberoptic Laryngoscope. Endotracheal tubes can be passed through the nose, using a fiberoptic laryngoscope inserted into the tube. The directional-tip distal end of the scope is particularly helpful in rounding the bend of the posterior pharynx. The cords can be seen directly through the fiberoptic bundle, and the tube can be slipped off the bundle into the trachea. In the nonmedicated patient with secretions, blood, or vomitus in the airway, the end of the laryngoscope can be easily blocked and the view of the airway obscured. The chance of this may be lessened by withdrawing the tip of the scope just slightly inside the distal tip of the tube in an attempt to protect it from fluid in the airway. A further disadvantage of this method is the fact that it requires a level of skill that might not always be present in only occasional users of the technique.

SEDATION AND RAPID-INDUCTION ANESTHESIA FOR EMERGENCY INTUBATION

RICHARD B. GLASER, M.D.

INDICATIONS FOR ADMINISTRATION OF ANESTHESIA IN THE EMERGENCY DEPARTMENT

The induction of anesthesia in the emergency department is often necessary in conjunction with laryngoscopic examination and endotracheal intubation and is achieved by the administration of muscle relaxants and/or anesthetic drugs. Patients who need airway management are frequently confused, combative, or unable to cooperate. Anesthesia overcomes these obstacles and blunts potentially damaging increases in blood pressures and heart rate induced by endotracheal intubation. Muscle relaxation facilitates laryngoscopic examination and prevents laryngospasm, coughing, bucking, and active resistance to positive pressure ventilation.

PREPARATION BEFORE ANESTHESIA AND INTUBATION

Each of the several approaches to managing the airway and accomplishing endotracheal intubation incorporates its own specific drugs and equipment. However, common to all approaches are the preparations prior to the administration of drugs or manipulation of the airway if death and other complications are to be avoided. Only when all of the equipment (Table 1), drugs (Table 2), and personnel are available should induction and intubation proceed.

Equipment

Irrespective of the route chosen for intubation, a laryngoscope, an assortment of laryngoscope blades, endotracheal tubes with fitted stylets, and oral and nasal airways should be available for establishing an airway in case problems arise during the intubation or the patient's condition acutely deteriorates. An Ambu bag or another means of delivering positive pressure ventilation and a well-fitting face mask should be in readiness along with an adequate source of oxygen. A functioning suction device may be life-saving in the event of emesis or profuse bleeding.

TABLE 1 Equipment for Induction of Anesthesia

Laryngoscope

Assorted laryngoscope blades

Stylets (fit into endotracheal tubes to increase stiffness)

Assorted endotracheal tubes, with syringes attached to cuff

Oral and nasal airways

Face mask fitted to patient

Suction device and tonsil tipped sucker

Ambu bag or soft rebreathing bag (preferable) attached to oxygen source

Functioning intravenous line

Syringes and needles

Necessary drugs, drawn and ready

TABLE 2 Drugs Use for Induction of Anesthesia

Drug	Dose	Comments	Onset	Duration
Sedative/hypnotics/analgesics				
Pentothal	0.5–4 mg/kg	Can cause hypotension in patients with hypovolemia (use lower dose range with hypovolemia or CHF)	IV:rapid	10–15 min
Ketamine	0.5–3 mg/kg	Sympathetic stimulant: maintains BP, causes tachycardia, salivation, bronchodilation, increased cerebral blood flow, hallucinations; useful in hypovolemia and for analgesia at lower dose ranges	IV:rapid IM:3–5 min	5–10 min 10–20 min
Etomidate	0.3 mg/kg	Useful in patients with severe myocardial dysfunction, hypovolemia; causes myoclonus; should be administered with a muscle relaxant	IV:rapid	2–3 min
Fentanyl	0.5–5 µg/kg	Short-acting narcotic with little effect on hemodynamics	IV:2 min IM:7–15 min	Variable
Muscle relaxants				
Curare	3 mg	Dose to block fasiculations in adults	IV:3–5 min	
Vecuronium	0.1 mg/kg	Intubating dose; smaller amounts, e.g., .02–.04 mg/kg, may be given to maintain relaxation; may "prime" using 10% of the intubating dose	IV: 3–4 min	30–40 min
Atracurium	0.5 mg/kg	Intubating dose; may cause hypotension attributable to histamine release	IV:4 min	30–40 min
Succinylcholine	IV:1.5 mg/kg IM:4 mg/kg	Beware hyperkalemia in patients with burns or neurologic disorders; also causes bradycardia and increased intraocular pressure	IV: 30–60 sec IM:2–3 min	7–12 min 10–20 min
Pressors				
Ephedrine	5–10 mg	Mild pressor with both alpha and beta adrenergic effects; may be given as bolus	IV:rapid	10–15 min
Neosynephrine	50–100 µg	Pure alpha-adrenergic agent; may be given as bolus (dilute 1 cc=10 mg with 9 cc of saline; discard all but 1 cc and dilute again to total of 10 cc; each cc then contains 100 µg)	IV:rapid	5–20 min
Dopamine	2–30 µg/kg/min	Primarily dopaminergic effects at 1–5 µg/kg/min; alpha and beta effects predominate at higher doses; titrate to effect	IV:rapid	
Other				
Atropine	.01–.02 mg/kg	Blocks bradycardia associated with succinylcholine; use routinely in children under 1 year; also useful to dry secretions	IV:rapid IM:2–5 min	15–20 min 30–60 min

DRUGS USED FOR THE INDUCTION OF ANESTHESIA

Muscle relaxants should always be available for the reasons already mentioned. A pressor agent, such as ephedrine or neosynephrine, should be accessible if not already drawn into a syringe. Atropine, which is routinely given to young children for prevention of bradycardia prior to administration of succinylcholine should be available for adults as well. Significant bradycardias are more likely to occur after multiple doses of succinylcholine, and atropine prophylaxis should be considered in such circumstances. Finally, in the event of cardiac arrest, a full complement of drugs for resuscitation (including epinephrine, sodium bicarbonate, and lidocaine) must be available along with a device for cardioversion. A functioning intravenous line, preferably large-bore, is mandatory.

Muscle Relaxants

Indications. Paralyzing agents relax the oropharyngeal muscles, facilitate laryngoscopy, and prevent laryngospasm caused by manipulation of the airway. They are also occasionally necessary to allow ventilation of a patient with chest-wall rigidity.

Choice of Muscle Relaxants. Muscle relaxants fall into one of two categories: depolarizing and nondepolarizing. Of the depolarizing variety, the only one in common use today is succinylcholine. Succinylcholine works by attaching to acetylcholine receptors at the muscle end-plate and depolarizing the muscle fibers. The drug must then be metabolized by plasma pseudocholinesterase before the muscle can repolarize. The effects of the drug are short-lived, with return of spontaneous ventilation in 5 to 10 minutes except in rare patients who have a pseudocholinesterase deficiency. The simultaneous depolarization of many muscle fibers results in fasciculations and the release of potassium. The fasciculations may raise intragastric and intraocular pressure, and in situations where this might be hazardous, a nondepolarizing relaxant is administered first to block fasciculations.

Nondepolarizing muscle relaxants work by competitively binding acetylcholine receptor sites so that acetylcholine cannot bind with the receptor and depolarize the muscle. Curare and pancuronium are the prototypical nondepolarizing relaxants. When given for intubation, their effects last for approximately 1 hour. They do not cause muscle depolarization and therefore are not associated with fasciculation or potassium release.

Two new nondepolarizing muscle relaxants have been recently released, atracurium and vecuronium. Both have a significantly shorter duration of action than the older agents and are generally associated with greater hemodynamic stability, although atracurium can cause hypotension, especially when administered rapidly. In situations in which succinylcholine is contraindicated or longer relaxation is desired, these are now the agents of choice for emergency intubation. The speed with which intubating conditions can be achieved following the full dose can be accelerated by using a "priming" dose, that is, giving approximately 10 percent of the intubating dose 3 to 4 minutes before administering the full dose. It should be cautioned that some people may complain of weakness and difficulty in breathing following the priming dose, and the intubator should be prepared to proceed with the induction and intubation.

Contraindications and Complications (Table 3). Muscle relaxants should not be used when there is reason to believe that intubation and/or mask ventilation might be unsuccessful. If such a situation prevails, relaxants should be used only if personnel and equipment are readily available to perform a tracheostomy or cricothyroidotomy.

Succinylcholine should not be administered to patients with significant neuromuscular disease. Denervated muscles release much more potassium when depolarized by succinylcholine, and hyperkalemic cardiac arrest following its administration has been noted in patients who have had strokes, spinal cord lesions, Guillain-Barré syndrome, and muscular dystrophy. The period of susceptibility following a neurologic injury starts at about 1 week, and lasts up to 6 months or longer for ongoing diseases.

The same problem exists for people with significant burns or soft tissue injury, and succinylcholine should be avoided from about day 7 following the burn or trauma until such wounds are completely healed (about 60 days after burn). Succinylcholine is relatively contraindicated in patients with an "open eye", such as might occur with a corneal laceration following eye trauma. In these patients, the increase in intraocular pressure that is seen following administration of succinylcholine may result in extrusion of intraocular contents. This increase in intraocular pressure can be ameliorated by blocking fasciculations with a subparalyzing dose of curare (3 mg for the average adult), given 3 minutes before the succinylcholine.

Malignant hyperthermia (MH) may be precipitated by succinylcholine, and the drug should be avoided in patients with the disease or a family history of MH. A corollary of MH, masseter spasm that results in a "locking" of the jaw, may follow administration of succinylcholine. Malignant hyperthermia frequently follows masseter

TABLE 3 Potential Complications of Muscle Relaxant Use

Complication	Comments
Succinylcholine	
Hyperkalemia	Occurs in patients with neurologic disorders (e.g., stroke paraplegia, Guillain Barré); susceptibility from about one week after event until 6 months or longer if disease is ongoing; also occurs following burns or soft tissue trauma (from about 1 week to 60 days following injury, or until the wound is completely healed)
Increased intraocular pressure (IOP)	May cause extrusion of intraocular contents in patients with a disrupted or lacerated globe; risk is diminished by giving "defasciculating" dose of a nondepolarizing relaxant (NB: IOP may also increase with coughing or bucking on tube)
Malignant hyperthermia (MH)	Rare complication; Familial occurrence; may be fatal unless treated with cooling, fluids, dantrolene; monitor temperature after succinylcholine, especially in children; consider MH in face of tachypnea, acidosis, hyperkalemia, increasing temperature
Masseter spasm	Corollary of malignant hyperthermia; usually resolves spontaneously; a proportion go on to develop MH
Nondepolarizing relaxants	
Loss of airway	These are long-acting drugs and should not be administered when there is concern about the ability to intubate or ventilate the patient; this is true for obstructing lesions of the upper airway, facial or laryngeal trauma, or unusual facial anatomy

spasm. If intubation and use of relaxants are still necessary, the patient should be ventilated until the masseter spasm resolves, and a nondepolarizing relaxant should be used in place of succinylcholine.

Anesthetics, Hypnotics, Sedatives

Hypnotic and/or anesthetic agents blunt unwanted reflex responses to intubation such as hypertension and tachycardia; in an awake patient, these agents prevent awareness of the noxious act of endotracheal intubation. It is critical to understand the pharmacology of these drugs and their potential interaction with the patient's disease before embarking on their use.

These drugs are most commonly used to render a patient unconscious or amnesic. All of the commonly used anesthetic agents have the potential to directly depress the myocardium and/or decrease sympathetic tone. These agents include pentothal, diazepam, narcotics, and ketamine. Patients with impaired myocardial function or who are hypovolemic should receive reduced doses or no anesthetic at all, depending on the severity of their condition. Such patients are usually maintaining perfusion and blood pressure by increased sympathetic tone, which diminishs when these agents are given. Patients who are hypovolemic should first undergo fluid resuscitation if possible. If fully rehydrated, they may be given a normal amount of drug. For mild degrees of volume deficit, reduced amounts of drug should be given. In this situation, ketamine is preferable because it causes reflex sympathetic stimulation. Etomidate, a drug recently introduced to the United States, is well tolerated in patients with hypovolemia or impaired myocardial function. It must be given with muscle relaxants such as succinylcholine because of its tendency to cause diffuse myoclonus. For severe degrees of volume deficit, an awake intubation is preferable, but if necessary, intubation can be performed with muscle relaxants only. The patient can then be given small amounts of sedative following rehydration if his or her blood pressure tolerates it. Narcotics can be useful for sedation, but morphine in particular releases histamine (causing hypotension), and although all of morphine's other actions are reversible by naloxone, histamine release is not.

Thiopental (Pentothal) has an advantage over most other hypnotics and/or anesthetics in its rapid onset and redistribution. The redistribution enables a patient to reawaken soon after intubation. The rapid redistribution also means that any deleterious effect on ventilation or hemodynamics quickly passes. Quickly is a relative term, however, and if the blood pressure plummets, even Pentothal may seem to last an eternity.

CONSIDERATION OF UNDERLYING DISEASE

Before anesthesia is induced, consideration must be given to any disease the patient may have that could be affected by the choice of drugs, airway manipulation, or body position. Some diseases warrant special precautions.

Head Trauma or Increased Intracranial Pressure (ICP). Hypoventilation results in hypercarbia and, secondarily, in increased cerebral blood flow. This vasodilation increases the volume of the intracranial contents. When intracranial pressure is elevated with trauma because of edema or bleeding, and the limits of intracranial compliance have been reached, this additional volume can have disastrous consequences, resulting in decreased perfusion and even herniation. In such a situation, a patient cannot be allowed to remain apneic for prolonged periods and ventilation may have to be supported (with cricoid pressure) while awaiting intubating conditions following administration of muscle relaxants. Prolonged head-down position or hypotension may also decrease cerebral perfusion pressure and should be avoided.

Cardiovascular Disease. Endotracheal intubation is a noxious stimulus and is frequently associated with hypertension and tachycardia. The drugs used to block this reaction (e.g., thiopental, benzodiazepines, narcotics) either cause direct myocardial depression or block sympathetic output and can lead to hypotension, especially in the hypovolemic patient who is dependent on maximal sympathetic tone to maintain blood pressure. These hemodynamic changes can be deleterious to patients with ischemic heart disease or vascular disease. Hypertension may contribute to myocardial ischemia and is also a threat to patients with an intracerebral, intrathoracic, or intraabdominal aneurysm. Hypotension likewise can result in myocardial or cerebral ischemia in patients with occlusive vascular disease. These hemodynamic consequences of drug administration should be anticipated with adjustment of dose and choice of the most appropriate drug for the situation. Ephedrine, 10 mg, or neosynephrine, 100 μg should be given by IV bolus to the acutely hypotensive patient who does not respond to volume administration or Trendelenburg position. More anesthetic should be given to the patient with a hypertensive response. It should be apparent from the foregoing that close monitoring of hemodynamic status is necessary immediately before and after intubation.

Reactive Airway Disease. Patients with asthma or bronchospastic lung disease are especially sensitive to airway manipulation. Bronchodilators should be available to treat the patient who develops severe bronchospasm following intubation. Bronchospasm is less likely to occur in the deeply anesthetized patient who is optimally treated with bronchodilators.

INDUCTION OF ANESTHESIA AND INTUBATION OF THE TRACHEA

Rapid-sequence Induction of Anesthesia

Indications. Rapid-sequence induction is undertaken when emergent orotracheal or nasotracheal intubation is indicated. This includes patients who are rapidly deteriorating and are at risk of dying if intubation is delayed. This form of controlled intubation is also indicated in confused or combative patients who have a

TABLE 4 Patients at High Risk for Post Intubation Complications

Condition	Complication	Reason	Therapy
Hypovolemia	Hypotension	Anesthetics decrease sympathetic tone and cardiac output	Avoid problem by using less drug, consider ketamine, etomidate Trendelenburg, volume infusion
		Positive pressure ventilation causes decreased venous return	Pressor (e.g., ephedrine, dopamine neosynephrine
Arteriosclerotic heart disease	Myocardial ischemia	Stress response to laryngoscopy (with hypertension, tachycardia)	More anesthetic, (e.g., Pentothal) Nitroglycerin: IV, sublingual, or paste
Asthma, COPD	Bronchospasm	Stimulation of airway reflexes with intubation	Bronchodilator, more anesthetic, especially ketamine

specific contraindication or intolerance to nasotracheal intubation. In the usual emergency situation in which most patients are assumed to have a "full stomach," rapid-sequence induction is the best way to minimize the risk of aspiration, since the application of topical anesthetics for nasotracheal intubation interferes with normal protective airway reflexes.

Contraindications. Rapid-sequence induction should not be undertaken in patients with major facial or laryngeal trauma. It is also contraindicated in any patient with upper airway obstruction, distorted facial or airway anatomy, or if a question exists about one's ability to visualize the larynx with direct laryngoscopy.

Technique and Preparation. The procedure is as follows:

1. In addition to the aforementioned general preparations, several special precautions are taken before a rapid sequence induction to minimize any loss of time between induction and intubation. An assortment of endotracheal tubes with *stylets in place* and a syringe attached to the cuff valve are kept at hand. Two functioning laryngoscopes and several blades of different length should also be available. Necessary drugs are drawn up in advance.
2. The patient is placed in the "sniffing position," i.e., with the head projecting forward and at an appropriate height for intubation.
3. An assistant is available to administer cricoid pressure and, if necessary, drugs.
4. A well-fitting face mask attached to 100 percent oxygen is positioned over the patient's nose and mouth so that there is no breathing of room air. If succinylcholine is to be used, a defasciculating dose of curare or another nondepolarizing muscle relaxant is given at this time. Oxygen is administered for at least 3 minutes.
5. Anesthetic, muscle relaxant, and cricoid pressure are administered simultaneously. Cricoid pressure should not be released until the trachea is successfully intubated and the position of the tube has been checked.
6. Approximately 60 seconds after the drugs have been administered, or about 30 seconds after the patient becomes completely apneic, laryngoscopy should be performed and the trachea intubated.

Preoxygenation. If attempts to intubate the patient fail, controlled mask ventilation is usually necessary until the patient resumes breathing. If mask ventilation is unsuccessful, the patient may then die from hypoxia. To help protect against this undesired eventuality, it is essential to "preoxygenate" a patient prior to induction of anesthesia. This replaces the air in the lungs with 100 percent oxygen, providing a reservoir sufficient to last up to 10 minutes in case the intubation fails. Preoxygenation is especially important in a patient with a "full stomach." It is preferable not to ventilate these patients when they are paralyzed, lest air forced into the stomach induce regurgitation of stomach contents.

Preoxygenation is accomplished by having the patient breathe 100 percent oxygen for 3 minutes prior to rendering them apneic with drugs. They must not be ventilated with ambient air until apnea occurs, lest they take a breath containing 79 percent nitrogen and defeat the purpose of preoxygenation. If the trachea cannot be intubated, the properly preoxygenated patient does not become hypoxemic for 5 to 10 minutes, which is usually adequate time for the patient to resume spontaneous ventilation. If there is concern that the patient is becoming hypoxic, ventilation with bag and mask should be attempted while cricoid pressure is maintained.

Cricoid Pressure. Muscle relaxants and anesthetics interfere with normal protective airway reflexes and increase the risk of aspiration of gastric contents, a potentially life-threatening complication. Partial protection against this eventuality is effected by means of cricoid pressure, the "Sellick maneuver." The cricoid cartilage, palpable just below the thyroid cartilage, is the only part of the airway where the cartilaginous skeleton is completely circumferential. By pressing on this cartilage, the esophagus is compressed between the cricoid and the spine, thus preventing passage of stomach contents. Cricoid pressure must not be released until it is certain that the tube is in the trachea and the cuff is inflated.

Nasotracheal Intubation

Indications. Patients who are hypoxemic, with tachypnea and air hunger, whose situation is urgent but not emergent, are usually the most appropriate candidates for an awake nasotracheal intubation. Patients with pulmonary edema, severe pneumonia, and asthma often fall into this category. The tachypnea keeps the glottis open a greater fraction of the time and greatly facilitates passage of the tube. This technique is also indicated for patients in whom prolonged intubation is anticipated. In a patient who is not critically ill, awake nasotracheal intubation is usually safer than intubation involving the use of anesthetics and muscle relaxants because the patient continues to spontaneously ventilate, and potential side effects of the drugs are avoided. This is especially true when the intubator is relatively inexperienced. It is important to continue the administration of oxygen to hypoxemic patients. This is accomplished by attaching a soft rebreathing bag (not an Ambu bag) and oxygen to the end of the endotracheal tube. When the glottis is entered, the bag moves with respiration, indicating proper placement of the tube. Alternatively, high-flow oxygen can be blown by the nose and mouth.

Contraindications. The most common contraindication to nasotracheal intubation is time. In a patient in critical need of ventilation and airway control, the added time for nasal preparation and blind attempts at entering the glottis may not be tolerated. Bleeding diathesis is the next most common contraindication. Patients who are taking anticoagulants or have renal failure, thrombocytopenia, or other problems of hemostasis should not be nasally intubated. Not only can the bleeding be profuse and a problem in and of itself, but it may further impair ventilation, obstruct the airway, and interfere with attempts to visualize the larynx and intubate the patient. A final contraindication to nasal intubation is facial trauma. With disruption of the nasopharyngeal mucosa or the facial bones, a blindly directed endotracheal tube can create a false mucosal passage and completely occlude the airway or even enter the cranium—with disastrous consequences.

Technique of Anesthesia. If nasotracheal intubation is performed in an awake, alert patient, it is best to topically anesthetize the oropharynx and glottis. Topical anesthesia of the nose can be accomplished with any local anesthetic such as cocaine, 4 percent, or lidocaine, 4 percent. The agent can be dripped into the nose or ap-

plied directly by means of cotton pledgets or cotton-tipped applicators. A saturated pledget can be introduced into the nose with bayonet forceps and allowed to stay there for 2 to 3 minutes. Alternatively, cotton applicators can be inserted into the nares and gradually advanced, dripping cocaine from a syringe onto the shaft of the applicator and allowing it to run into the nasopharynx. Cocaine can be administered in this way with little concern for a toxic central nervous system reaction because the peak serum level attained is blunted by mucosal absorption. The maximum dose administered should still be no more than 200 mg in an adult. Cocaine is ideal for nasal intubation because its vasoconstrictor properties enlarge the nasal passage and decrease the likelihood of epistaxis. Hypertension and tachycardia resulting from cocaine administration can be harmful to a patient with coronary artery disease. Topical lidocaine should be substituted for cocaine in this situation or in other cases in which the hemodynamic changes are unwanted. A transtracheal injection of 4 percent lidocaine (2 cc) can anesthetize the proximal trachea and the vocal cords. If a nasal intubation is to be done under direct visualization of the larynx in an awake patient, it is necessary to topically anesthetize the tongue and oropharynx by spraying a local anesthetic agent as the laryngoscope is advanced. It is important to realize that local anesthetics can interfere with protective airway reflexes. If properly administered, the local anesthetic will blunt the gag reflex. If the local anesthesia is incomplete, introduction of the endotracheal tube may stimulate the gag reflex and induce vomiting. Topical anesthesia is therefore best avoided in patients who are actively vomiting.

SUGGESTED READING

Goodman LS, Gilman AG. The pharmacological basis of therapeutics. New York: Macmillan Publishing Co, Inc, 1980.
Lebowitz PW, Newberg LA, Gillette MT, eds. Clinical anesthesia procedures of the Massachusetts General Hospital, 2nd ed. Boston: Little Brown and Co, 1982.
Miller RD. Anesthesia, 2nd ed. New York: Churchill Livingstone, 1986.

PERCUTANEOUS TRANSTRACHEAL VENTILATION AND CRICOTHYROTOMY

ERNEST RUIZ, M.D.

PERCUTANEOUS TRANSTRACHEAL NEEDLE VENTILATION

Many scenarios would call for the use of percutaneous transtracheal needle ventilation (PTNV), but the most common is as follows: a patient with a head injury and a possible cervical spine injury needs intubation and hyperventilation because of unconsciousness and presumed elevated intracranial pressure. The patient is not breathing well, and attempts at blind nasotracheal intubation fail. At this point the emergency physician could opt to perform an emergency cricothyrotomy or take his chances and orotracheally intubate the patient, thus risking a cervical cord injury. Fiberoptic laryngoscope techniques or the retrograde intubation technique is too time-consuming under these circumstances. This is a problem that can be solved with PTNV. The patient can be hyperventilated with this technique while a lateral C-spine roentgenogram is obtained. If no C-spine injury is seen, the patient can then be orotracheally intubated, avoiding a cricothyrotomy or tracheostomy.

Transtracheal needle ventilation is closely akin to the technique of needle aspiration of the trachea for purposes of obtaining a tracheal culture. Many years of clinical experience with this latter technique have taught us that tracheal puncture with a needle is relatively simple and safe. Bleeding from small arteries punctured by the needle is a rare but potentially fatal complication. There have been reports of asphyxia secondary to hematoma and/or bleeding as a result of needle aspiration. If the emergency physician always intubates the patient after temporarily using the PTNV technique, this complication can be avoided. The complication rate for transtracheal anesthesia was cited by Jacobs as less than 0.05 percent, and the incidence of serious bleeding would be considerably less than that. Nevertheless, PTNV is contraindicated in patients with a bleeding disorder unless no other method of airway control is at hand.

When the cricothyroid membrane is readily palpable, it is the puncture site of choice, since it is relatively superficial and free of an overlying thyroid gland. However, if it is not readily palpable, the proximal trachea can be used instead.

Equipment

The device used to ventilate the patient is simple, but must be assembled in advance (Fig.1). The device simply consists of:

1. High-pressure tubing with an adapter at one end to match the wall oxygen outlets. By convention, the pressure of wall oxygen (and oxygen cylinders supplied with pressure reducers) is 50 pounds per square inch.
2. The other end of this high-pressure tubing is connected to a hand-operated valve mechanism such as a two-way stopcock or, better, a push-button valve such as

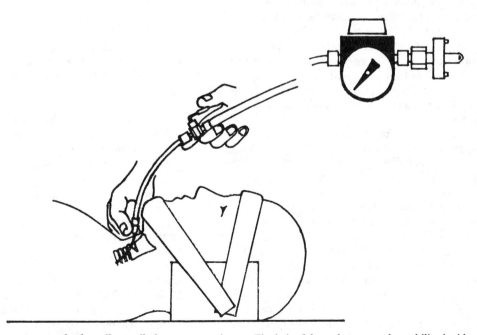

Figure 1 Percutaneous transtracheal needle ventilation apparatus in use. The hub of the catheter must be stabilized with one hand to prevent kinking and inadvertent withdrawal.

a Bird Rotary Valve No. 1813 (Bird Corporation, Mark 7, Palm Springs, CA 92263).

3. A short length of flexible plastic tubing with an inside diameter of about three-sixteenths of an inch is connected to the valve and the other end to a Luer-Lok male connector (Becton-Dickinson No. 3202, available from hospital supply houses).

Alternatively, a Sanders ventilation device (Pilling Company, 420 Delaware Drive, Fort Washington, PA 19034) for use with bronchoscopes is easily adaptable for this purpose. This device has the advantage of having an adjustable pressure valve that allows the operator to safely ventilate small children.

Technique

To identify the cricothyroid membrane, palpate the tracheal rings, the cricoid cartilage, and the larynx in that order. When there is still doubt about the landmarks, also palpate the hyoid bone, since the space between the hyoid bone and the larynx can be mistaken for the cricothyroid membrane. Attach a small syringe to a 14- or 16-gauge Teflon catheter-over-needle device, and while holding the trachea and/or larynx midline, advance the needle into the trachea via the cricothyroid membrane. If the cricothyroid membrane is easily palpable, the needle should be inserted through its more caudad portion, since there is sometimes a small artery that crosses it transversely through its cephalad portion. (In most cases it is not possible to make this distinction.) When it is judged that the needle is within the trachea, aspirate for air. The return of air confirms the needle's position. If the patient has aspirated blood, blood may return initially; when in doubt, therefore, empty the syringe and aspirate again. Advance the sheath over the metal needle until the hub of the sheath is at skin level. Remove the needle and reattach the syringe to the hub of the sheath. Aspirate for air once again. This is important, because the sheath may be kinked or the sheath may be misplaced. Remove or readjust the sheath if its position is in doubt before applying "wall oxygen" pressure. You will have to hold the hub of the sheath constantly while ventilating the patient to avoid kinking.

Once the tracheal catheter is connected to the high-pressure oxygen apparatus, the patient is ventilated by simply intermittently opening the valve until the chest wall rises suitably. This chest wall rise is the same rough estimation of the adequacy of ventilation used with the bag-valve-mask technique. I have monitored arterial blood gases in patients being ventilated with the PTNV technique and have found them to be ideal.

A further benefit of PTNV is that if there is aspiration or obstruction of the airway proximally, the foreign substance is blown out of the airway. Laryngospasm is not a contraindication because it may obstruct inhalation and not exhalation. If the obstruction is not cleared and the chest wall does not fall on closure of the valve, ventilation should be discontinued immediately to avert over-inflation of the lungs and its resultant air embolism, tension pneumothorax, or cardiovascular tamponade.

PTNV often results in a small amount of paratracheal emphysema in the neck and mediastinum that can be seen on x-ray examination. This emphysema is probably the result of oxygen leakage out of the trachea around the catheter and is of no consequence clinically. It does not necessarily mean that there has been bronchial disruption or esophageal perforation.

In small children, the trachea is so small and mobile as to preclude safe insertion of a needle. On the other hand, cricothyrotomy or tracheotomy may severely damage these small structures when performed under emergency conditions. However, the skin incision and blunt dissection used for cricothyrotomy and tracheotomy facilitate insertion of a needle into the trachea under direct vision. The correct combination of needle catheter size and oxygen pressure for use in children (less than about 40 kg) has not been systematically studied to my knowledge. Smith successfully used a 16-gauge catheter at 1,551 mm Hg (30 psi) pressure in a 6-year-old, 20-kg child and at 2,068 mm Hg (40 psi) in an 11-year-old, 46-kg child. Until more data are available, I would recommend a needle catheter proportionate to the size of the trachea and an adjustable pressure source to obtain satisfactory ventilation.

I would also caution against using catheters larger than the 16- and 14-gauge catheters already studied in adults. Problems that could arise are excessive intrapulmonary pressure and excessive leak of oxygen around the catheter.

CRICOTHYROTOMY

Cricothyrotomy has several advantages over tracheotomy in the emergency situation. The cricothyroid membrane lies relatively superficial in the neck as compared to the trachea. The technique requires few instruments and little technical assistance.

The most common clinical indication for cricothyrotomy in the emergency department is the patient with severe facial injuries who requires tracheal intubation (Table 1). Unfortunately, these patients are also at high risk for cervical spine injuries, and therefore the neck cannot be positioned for optimal palpation of the cricothyroid membrane. The patient is frequently making agonal or energetic efforts to breathe. It also seems as though all patients who require an emergency surgical airway have short, fat necks.

Technique

Given all the aforementioned difficulties, I recommend the following technique:

1. Briefly palpate the neck (as described for PTNV) and make a vertical incision about 2.5 to 5 cm in length (depending on the amount of subcutaneous fat present) midline over the cricothyroid membrane. Under emergency circumstances such as these, the vertically oriented veins in the subcutaneous tissue of the neck become dilated and capable of emitting gallons of blood

TABLE 1   Indications and Relative Contraindications for Percutaneous Transtracheal Needle Ventilation and Cricothyrotomy

	Indications	Relative Contraindications
PTNV	Difficult anatomy as in severe kyphosis; possible C-spine injury; laryngospasm blood and/or vomitus obscuring the airway; foreign body in the airway; acute epiglottitis	Bleeding diathesis; larynx fracture with obstructing hematoma; fixed airway obstruction as in laryngeal body in the airway; acute
Cricothyrotomy	Severe facial trauma; C-spine injury after temporizing with PTNV when fiberoptic technique not available or not practical because of blood or vomitus (blind nasotracheal intubation could also be used)	Bleeding diathesis; larynx fracture with obstructing hematoma

over the operating site, or so it seems. That is one reason for the vertical incision rather than a horizontal. Also, one can extend the vertical incision upward or downward for better exposure. A No. 10 scalpel blade is the blade of choice for this. Carry the incision through the platysma and subcutaneous fat down to the underlying strap muscles. Now palpate again for the trachea, cricoid cartilage, cricothyroid membrane, and larynx. If these structures are still difficult to palpate,

continue the dissection by spreading the strap muscles at the midline, using a clamp or dissecting scissors.

2. After the cricothyroid membrane becomes easily palpable, I prefer to use a tracheal hook to immobilize the larynx and trachea before continuing with the procedure (Fig. 2). Even if the patient is not making respiratory efforts, the puncturing of the membrane with a knife may stimulate coughing and cause the operator to lose the path of the knife into the trachea

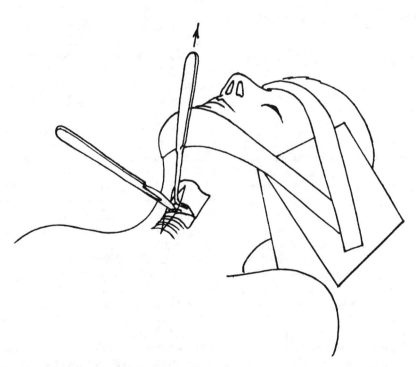

Figure 2   Cricothyrotomy using a tracheal hook. The straightened tracheal hook is used to immobilize the larynx while the cricothyroid membrane is opened transversely with a scalpel.

if countertraction and immobilization are not provided with a tracheal hook. Tracheal hooks have the wrong curve as they are supplied commercially. For use in cricothyrotomy they should be straightened with a clamp so that they form a right angle rather than a curve. This is necessary because the patient's jaw does not allow enough room to puncture the membrane with the point of the curved hook. The next step is to puncture the cricothyroid membrane with the tracheal hook and to apply firm traction cephalad on the hook so that the larynx is immobilized and under control.

3. The No. 10 scalpel is then used to stab into the airway through the cricothyroid membrane in a transverse fashion, just caudad to the tracheal hook. It can then be removed and the hole into the trachea enlarged with dissecting scissors. If a tracheal hook was not used, you have to leave the knife in the trachea and insert the dissecting scissors alongside it so that the path into the trachea is not inadvertently lost.

4. A Trousseau dilator can now be inserted into the trachea and spread transversally and longitudinally. A No. 4 (8.5 mm O.D.) Shiley tracheostomy tube (Shiley Inc., 17600 Gillette Avenue, Irvine, CA 92714) is used to intubate the trachea between the blades of the Trousseau dilator. Fracture of the cricoid cartilage should be avoided because it is the only complete ring of support for the trachea. Fracture of this cartilage may allow collapse of the trachea when the patient is extubated. Therefore, use only a size 4 tube in adults to avoid this complication. In larger children, sizes 00 (4.5 mm O.D.) to 3 (7 mm O.D.) can be used. In smaller children, temporize with PTNV until hands skilled in pediatric tracheostomy are available.

Any tube selected should have its balloon pretested for leaks. When the balloon is tested, it should be kneaded away from the tip of the tube as it is deflated; this greatly facilitates insertion of the tube into the trachea. When the tube is inserted, its obturator should be in place. If the tube is inserted from the side, there is less tendency for the tube to dissect anterior to the trachea. Place the tip of the tube and obturator in the trachea from the side, then twist the tube into its final position as it moves down the trachea. Replace the obturator with the inner sleeve of the tracheostomy tube, which connects to the ventilating equipment. This sleeve locks into the tracheostomy tube with a twist. Tying the tracheostomy tube in place and inflating the balloon cuff completes the procedure. If a tracheal hook was used in the procedure, do not remove it until you are sure the tube is in place and functioning. Do not pack the wound tightly or suture it closed because subcutaneous emphysema may result.

SUGGESTED READING

Dunlap LB. A modified, simple device for the emergency administration of percutaneous transtracheal ventilation. JACEP 1978; 7:42–46.

Jacobs HB. Emergency percutaneous transtracheal catheter and ventilator. J Trauma 1972; 12:50–55.

Schillaci RF, Iacovoni VE, Conte RS. Transtracheal aspiration complicated by fatal endotracheal hemorrhage. N Engl J Med 1976; 295:488–490.

Smith RB. Transtracheal ventilation during anesthesia. Anesth Analg 1974; 53:225–228.

Smith RB, Myers EN, Sherman H. Transtracheal ventilation in paediatric patients. Br J Anaesth 1974; 46:313–314.

Spoerel WE, Narayanan PS, Singh NP. Transtracheal ventilation. Br J Anaesth 1971; 43:932–938.

ACUTE RESPIRATORY FAILURE

PAUL E. PEPE, M.D., F.A.C.P., F.C.C.P.
LEONARD D. HUDSON, M.D., F.A.C.P., F.C.C.P.

This chapter discusses a generic approach to the early respiratory support of critically ill and injured patients. By having a sound understanding of the principles involved in early respiratory support, the emergency department practitioner is able to properly care for any patient with acute respiratory failure.

The term "respiration" refers not only to the act of breathing, but also to the process of cellular respiration (O_2 consumption and CO_2 production). Tissue function, particularly that of the brain and the heart, relies on the maintenance of cellular respiration, which in turn is largely dependent on adequate delivery of O_2 to the tissues.

$$O_2 \text{ transport (delivery) to the tissues} \pm$$
$$[1.34 \times \text{Hgb} \times \%O_2 \text{ saturation} + .003 \times PaO_2] \times \dot{Q}_T$$
$$\dots \text{ where Hgb} = \text{hemoglobin concentration}$$
(g per deciliter) and $\dot{Q}_T$ = cardiac output (L per minute).

This is immediately relevant to the basics of emergency care: (1) stop bleeding (preserve hemoglobin); (2) ensure an airway and ventilation with O_2 (facilitate adequate arterial oxygen tension); and (3) when appropriate give intravascular volume resuscitation, or pressor drugs, or perform external cardiac compressions (to maintain cardiac output).

In addition to ensuring adequate tissue O_2 delivery to support cellular respiration, one must also be concerned with the by-product of O_2 consumption, namely CO_2 production. If CO_2 is not removed as quickly as it is produced, the arterial CO_2 tension ($PaCO_2$) rises and contributes to acidity of the blood. Since CO_2 readily crosses the blood-brain barrier, this results in cerebral acidosis, a depressed level of consciousness, and cerebral vasodilatation that may significantly elevate intracranial pressure (ICP). Therefore, altered neurologic status in patients with overdose, stroke, or head injury may be in part due to hypoventilation and resultant CO_2 retention. Unlike impaired O_2 delivery, however, a high $PaCO_2$ in itself may not always constitute a major acute problem. For example, chronic CO_2 retainers usually have compensated for the acid contribution of CO_2 and often can tolerate high levels of $PaCO_2$, leaving them with a pounding headache at best during acute exacerbations.

Removal of CO_2 is a relatively simple process. As long as fresh air is continually reintroduced into alveoli, CO_2 is removed. The more O_2 is consumed, the more CO_2 is produced. With increased CO_2 production, more ventilation with fresh air needs to be delivered. Needless to say, patients can also be overventilated if CO_2 is removed faster than it is produced. For example, patients who are comatose from phenobarbital overdose or hypothermia often are initially overventilated as they require very little ventilation because of low metabolic rates. However, a shivering, awake patient with the stress of injury or acute illness may need a lot of fresh gas ventilation to adequately remove CO_2.

APPROACH TO THE PATIENT

The approach to assessing the need for early respiratory support is targeted at answering the following questions:

1. Will the patient need ventilatory support (manual or mechanical breaths to remove CO_2)?
2. Will the patient need oxygenation support (supplemental O_2, ventilator inflations, or positive end-expiratory pressure)?
3. What are the potential complications of these support interventions?

We make a specific point of distinguishing ventilatory support (VS) from oxygenation support (OS). Though the two are undeniably intertwined, some patients may require mechanical ventilator support for one but not the other. For example, an obtunded patient may be breathing comfortably without signs of distress and maintaining fairly normal blood pH and $PaCO_2$. However, the arterial O_2 tension (PaO_2) may be low because unoxygenated blood is being shunted past alveoli that are not being inflated owing to a progressive closing of airways in dependent regions of the lung. Inflated alveoli in less dependent areas still provide the route for clearance of CO_2. Therefore, a mild increase in respiratory rate (without change in tidal volume) can normalize the $PaCO_2$, but PaO_2 is not significantly affected because blood perfusing the open alveoli cannot be further saturated and blood perfusing the closed units remains unoxygenated (Fig. 1). The solution to this problem may involve delivering a certain volume of mechanical lung inflations. Although the size and rate of these inflations also affect pH and $PaCO_2$, the *need* for instituting such support would not depend on a need to ventilate (removal of CO_2). On the other hand, despite adequate oxygenation, some patients may need VS for acute respiratory acidosis due to CO_2 retention (chronic lung patient) or to lower $PaCO_2$ to decrease ICP (patients with severe head injury).

THE NEED FOR VENTILATORY SUPPORT

Minute ventilation ($\dot{V}E$) is the product of tidal volume (VT) and respiratory rate (RR). A patient's immediate "$\dot{V}E$ demand" can be considered the VT and RR required to maintain a normal blood pH. The need for VS generally arises when a patient is unable to ventilate adequately to maintain a normal blood pH. $\dot{V}E$ demand can be increased by (1) augmented CO_2 production by body tissues, (2) metabolic acidosis, and (3) an increased amount of wasted ventilation (increased dead space to tidal volume ratio or $VD:VT$). Most critically ill or injured patients have an increased $\dot{V}E$ demand, especially those with shock states who develop severe anaerobic acidosis. Shallow tidal volumes and increased CO_2 production because of stress and in-

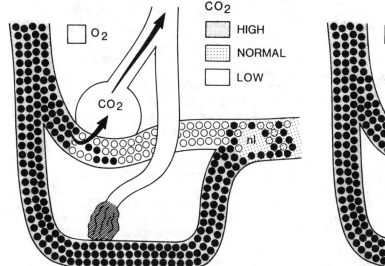
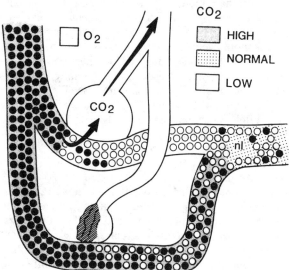

Figure 1 Pulmonary alveolar shunting. Left panel shows shunting (unoxygenated red cells) caused by collapsed or flooded alveoli even though ventilation (removal of CO_2) remains intact. Right panel shows how greater lung inflation allows better oxygenation. With 100 percent O_2 the remaining desaturated red cells may also be saturated. Therefore, one should initially provide 100 percent O_2 and ensure adequate lung inflation (15 ml per kilogram) in critically ill patients.

creased respiratory muscle use also increase ventilatory demand. Generally, most patients can briefly tolerate even large stresses in V̇E demand. But like prolonged exercise, prolonged increases in V̇E demand caused by injury may lead to respiratory muscle fatigue and eventual ventilatory failure, even in the healthiest of patients. Shock reduces the supply of metabolic nutrients to these muscles and exacerbates this problem. Respiratory failure with resulting hypoxemia and acidosis further depresses cardiac and cerebral function and the shock state is worsened, creating a vicious cycle. Therefore all severely ill or injured patients, particularly those with respiratory system impairment, are potential candidates for VS.

To meet ventilatory demand, a patient needs an intact bellows system. Such a system requires both the pump and the signal generator. The pump requires open airways, an intact, tightly sealed chest wall, and respiratory muscles capable of generating enough negative (outward-pulling) pleural pressure to expand the lungs to an inflated state. The chest wall is a particularly important component as it anchors respiratory muscles, including the diaphragm. The signal generator is the central nervous system (CNS), which determines the required V̇E and signals adjustments in the size and frequency of V̇T and RR via the brain stem and spinal cord. In severe injuries, all of these elements may be compromised or malfunctioning, but even when these elements are intact, VS may be necessitated by overwhelming demands. In cases of severe head injury, VS also may be indicated to lower $PaCO_2$ in order to decrease ICP.

THE NEED FOR OXYGENATION SUPPORT

The need for OS usually arises when a critical number of the patient's gas exchange units fail to remain inflated. (Inadequate ventilation can lead to hypoventilation and resulting hypoxemia by increasing the partial pressure of CO_2 in the alveoli, but this hypoxemia is not usually critical and reverses once VS or supplemental O_2 has been administered.) Hypoinflation (as opposed to hypoventilation) is more likely to result in serious hypoxemia (PaO_2 less than 60 torr). Shunting of blood past collapsed alveoli results in systemic arterial hypoxemia refractory to even a high inspired O_2 fraction (FiO_2) (see Fig. 1). Similarly, alveoli flooded with blood, vomitus, or pulmonary edema fluid block the pathway of O_2 from the airways to capillary beds. In the critically ill patient, all these factors are common occurrences.

Tidal volume (V̇T) size probably plays an important role in the maintenance of an adequate PaO_2 for victims of serious emergencies. Critically ill or injured patients, particularly those with severe head injury, often breathe with aberrant respiratory patterns and small tidal volumes. These patterns, by themselves, can result in significant hypoxemia refractory to administration of high inspired O_2 fraction. It is estimated that without intervention, 60 to 70 percent of patients with severe head injury have relative hypoxemia, and 30 to 40 percent have critical hypoxemia (PaO_2 less than 50 to 60 torr) despite apparently normal respiratory patterns and no sign of respiratory distress. The reasons may include aspiration of gastric con-

tents or accompanying lung contusion, but more often hypoxemia occurs because of clinically inapparent changes in the respiratory pattern. However, the hypoxemia often can be reversed with the initiation of effective positive pressure lung inflations alone with a V̇T of 10 to 15 ml per kilogram of lean body weight.

The lungs of patients in cardiac arrest rapidly deflate, and lung compliance diminishes fivefold or more. In many cases, endotracheal intubation and positive pressure ventilation are required to guarantee reinflation, particularly after a minute or two of apnea. The longer the deflation period, the longer it takes to reestablish an adequate state of static lung inflation. In patients who are conscious, such lung deflation is not a problem; in obtunded patients, stimulation or commands such as "take a deep breath", when successful, can often substitute for active ventilatory support (although airway protection still may be of concern).

Alveolar closure can also result from physical compromise of respiration by a collapsed or paralyzed chest wall, hemopneumothoraces, or by increased abdominal pressure. Aspiration of blood, vomitus, or foreign bodies can cause alveolar filling or atelectasis. Airway obstruction and distal collapse can occur from foreign bodies.

Certainly, without blood gas data, 100 percent inspired oxygen should be administered at high flows to critically ill and injured patients, particularly to those who are obtunded or comatose. Although after a day or so of 100 percent O_2 oxygen-induced lung injury can occur, emergency department practitioners should not be concerned with O_2 toxicity during the relatively brief period that they will spend with the emergency patient. As soon as it is feasible, inspired O_2 fractions should be lowered to "safe" levels (e.g., 0.5 to 0.6), when arterial blood gas measurements indicate that such levels (or lower) will maintain hemoglobin saturation (i.e., $PaO_2 > 60$ to 70 mm Hg). In the lung disease patient who chronically retains CO_2 and has lost the usual stimulus to breathe from rising CO_2 levels, the much weaker "hypoxic" stimulus to breathe helps to maintain the respiratory drive to some extent. Therefore, it is commonly taught that one should only give these patients low flow O_2 (1 to 2 L per minute). This consideration may be applicable if there is no acute exacerbation of lung disease such as when they are being evaluated for a foot injury. *However*, when dyspnea, increasing respiratory distress, or disorientation are involved, one should not withhold liberal O_2 flows while gauging the PaO_2. During acute exacerbations, in fact, these patients are very likely to be hypoxic, even while on low flow O_2.

Modes of FiO_2 administration include nasal cannula, face mask, and endotracheal (ET) tube. Because it helps to protect the airway and facilitates the provision of adequate lung inflation with a high FiO_2, endotracheal intubation should be emphasized in critically ill and injured patients. If intubation is precluded by a strong gag reflex, clenching of teeth or other such obstacles but delivery of a high FiO_2 is still desired, a face mask, with an O_2 reservoir attached, is a reasonable substitute. But even when endotracheal intubation or 100 percent inspired O_2 is not needed, low-flow O_2 (i.e., >2 L per minute) still should be administered, preferably by nasal prongs (see chapter on *Oxygen Therapy*).

To summarize the need for VS and the need for OS should be addressed independently: VS to acutely control pH (through $PaCO_2$) and OS to provide an adequate PaO_2 that saturates the available hemoglobin transported to the tissues. The means to accomplish these goals often overlap in terms of delivered tidal volume. Therefore a logical approach is to first choose an adequate delivered tidal volume (V_T) and then adjust respiratory rate (RR) accordingly to meet minute ventilation V_E) demands. The need for additional OS, that is, the appropriate level of supplemental FIO_2 and/or positive end-expiratory pressure (PEEP) then can be judged independently.

IDENTIFYING PATIENTS NEEDING RESPIRATORY SUPPORT

Experience and clinical judgment are the key to proper management of patients who may require VS and OS. In some situations, early intervention may be warranted despite normal arterial blood gas (ABG) analysis and clinical appearance. Elderly patients with rib fractures or head-injured patients with unstable neurologic signs may benefit from endotracheal intubation and mechanical ventilation with positive pressure breaths, particularly before they receive extensive evaluations such as radiologic examinations, peritoneal lavage, and computerized tomography (CT) scans. Often such patients become fatigued or deteriorate after initial evaluation, and this may not be recognized while multiple other diagnostic studies are carried out.

In identifying who needs VS and OS, four principles should be kept in mind:

1. Certain problems (e.g., airway obstruction, inadequate respirations or apnea, open or tension pneumothorax) require urgent attention prior to other assessments.
2. Some urgent problems, not obvious at first, can be detected by meticulous and repeated assessments (e.g., simple pneumothorax, flail chest).
3. The risk of late-appearing pulmonary complications (adult rerspiratory distress syndrome, pneumonia) often can be predicted by initial assessments.
4. Treatment of underlying conditions (asthma, COPD, CHF, overdose) must be addressed.

The initial assessment of the need for OS and VS should be directed at critical, life-threatening problems first. Later a more detailed evaluation can be done, but these critical areas must be constantly and frequently reassessed. Upper airway obstruction may not be obvious at first in a patient who has received blunt trauma to the head, neck, and chest. However, the trachea may become compromised by mechanical compression from an expanding deep hematoma in the throat. Such obstructions may not be discovered until stridor develops (a late sign) or, in some cases, until the unconscious patient turns cyanotic and apneic. Repeat assessments are the key. The most impor-

tant rule is to maintain a high index of suspicion for impending respiratory compromise. Normal chest examinations do not guarantee that active VS and OS are unnecessary.

Chest Films

Roentgenograms of the chest are a critical part of the evaluation of a severely injured patient. Even in an alert patient without dyspnea, the initial chest film may serve as a comparison film in case the patient develops late respiratory symptoms or signs. For example, traumatic pneumothorax may appear many hours after the initial injury. Even when not apparent on initial chest films, serial films usually reveal the source of any intrapulmonary shunt detected by arterial blood gas (ABG) analysis (e.g., pulmonary edema, pneumonia, atelectasis, right bronchus intubation, or pneumothorax). Aside from cardiac right-to-left shunts (congenital and traumatic), pulmonary emboli, and early hypoinflation, hypoxemia unresponsive to FIO_2 of up to 30 percent generally can be explained by an x-ray finding. Again, if not obvious on initial films, infiltrate progression is usually demonstrated on follow-up films, within a few hours in most cases. Even though infiltrates are noted on the chest film of the patient with severe hypoxemia, the severity of hypoxemia does not necessarily correspond to the amount of infiltrate seen. The chest film should also be repeated in any patient with sudden respiratory distress, development of asymmetric breath sounds, or abnormal or worsening ABG results.

Although proper ET placement can be gauged by markings on the tube (e.g., 21 to 22 cm H_2O at the teeth in the average adult), a chest film should quickly follow any ET tube (or attempted central venous catheter) placement. Studies have documented that as many as 15 percent of emergency room ET tube placements can result in right bronchus intubations despite the presence of bilateral breath sounds and regardless of the level of expertise of the intubator. Contralateral lung deflation can evolve in a short time (within 15 minutes) and can result in significant shunting. After chest tube placement, placement in the major fissure can be suspected by a frontal film alone, but if the tube is not functioning, a lateral chest film should be obtained to confirm the tube's position.

Arterial Blood Gases

Many patients at high risk of developing acute respiratory failure following trauma have good arterial oxygenation at first. For example, prediction of the development of the adult respiratory distress syndrome (ARDS) should not be based on initial blood gases. However, prediction can be aided by a careful accounting of the initial injuries and associated findings as well as *sequential* ABG analysis. Many cases of ARDS are not confirmed for several hours after injury,
but the physiologic (ABG) changes can evolve rapidly (usually within 3 to 4 hours). These ABG changes can occur without signs of respiratory distress or change in physical findings and are easily missed if the patient is

unable to communicate well or has other known injuries masking abnormal findings (e.g., diminished breath sounds from lung contusion masking the late onset of pneumothorax). In severely ill or injured patients, ABG measurements probably should be repeated every hour or two, at least in the early stages, particularly in those who are already receiving early VS and OS or are noncommunicative. In those with shock states, ABG measurements should be made frequently. In a sense, arterial blood gases are the end point of respiratory support. The immediate end point of OS is to maintain adequate saturation of hemoglobin (>97 percent) by maintaining adequate arterial O_2 tensions (e.g., PaO_2 >70 torr).

The immediate end point of VS is to deliver the $\dot{V}E$ that will maintain normal blood pH (7.35 to 7.45). Acutely, pH rather than $PaCO_2$ should be the focus of VS. An abnormal $PaCO_2$ itself is not harmful except for its effect on pH and ICP. However, pH variations of only ± 0.1 (>7.50 and <7.30) may result in life-threatening hypotension, seizures, and ventricular arrhythmias (alkalosis) or defective enzymatic function or drug responsiveness (acidosis). In a patient with shock whose $PaCO_2$ is 38 torr, the pH may be less than 7.10 owing to lactic acidosis. To correct the pH abnormality, the $PaCO_2$ should be temporarily lowered by deliberate hyperventilation. It is more advantageous in patients with severe injuries and acid-base abnormalities to manipulate acid-base status through changes in ventilation during the acute phases after injury because additional bicarbonate administration may result in an alkalosis after resuscitation. Among other things, this will shift the oxyhemoglobin dissociation curve to the left, thereby reducing oxygen delivery to the tissues. Alkali administration should be used only if VS is inadequate, and the acidosis is persistent or refractory to volume restoration, transfusion, and OS. In a patient who has received excess sodium bicarbonate or in a patient with chronic CO_2 retention, a high $PaCO_2$ should be left untreated if the pH is normal. Attempts to acutely lower $PaCO_2$ in this case elevates pH and increases the risk of life-threatening alkalotic complications. Occasionally, chronic CO_2 retainers who have become acutely hypoxic and who have developed a superimposed lactic acidosis, have a relatively normal pH when first ventilated to a normal $PaCO_2$. This is because the chronic bicarbonate retention is masked by the acute lactic acidosis in that the usually high serum bicarbonate level has been titrated back towards normal. As a result, when the hypoxia has been treated, the lactic acid is eventually cleared by the liver and the serum bicarbonate level rises again. This may cause an alkalosis if the patient is still being ventilated to a normal $PaCO_2$ level.

During the early hours following acute illness or injury, trends in PaO_2 (rather than a single result) should guide therapy. The variability of duplicate PaO_2 analysis alone can be as much as ± 10 percent. Artifacts in technique also can affect PaO_2 measurements, including lack of correction for body temperature, inadvertent venous sampling (or mixed sampling, when the needle tip is moved), laboratory error (technician error or miscalibration of the machine), misreporting (misunderstanding over the phone or poor handwriting), not placing the sample on ice, or the presence of air bubbles in the sample with

a long time elapsing before analysis. When in doubt, maintaining a high FIO_2 and repeating the sampling is the safest approach.

The success of supplemental O_2 therapy can be misinterpreted if the reported FIO_2 was inaccurate; for example, when sampling takes place during or soon after a transient increase to 100 percent inspired O_2 for transport or suctioning, or when the patient continually removes the O_2 face mask. Even 100 percent O_2 by a loosely fitting mask usually does not achieve much more than 50 to 70 percent inspired O_2. The patient who is receiving 100 percent O_2 with an endotracheal tube and resuscitation bag may not receive an FIO_2 of 1.0 if O_2 flows are not high enough.

Adequate PaO_2 does not guarantee O_2 transport to the tissues. A low hematocrit reflects a limited O_2 carrying capacity, which can be only partially overcome by very high PaO_2 (≥ 500 torr). Even with an acceptable hematocrit, adequate PaO_2, and good $\dot{Q}T$, adequate O_2 delivery to the tissues is not always ensured. When present, carbon monoxide preferentially occupies O_2 binding sites on the hemoglobin molecule and both carbon monoxide and cyanide interfere with the cytochrome oxidase enzyme system for O_2 metabolism. Therefore, PaO_2 should be viewed differently in smoke inhalation and fume victims because a PaO_2 that would normally saturate Hgb may no longer be adequate. PaO_2, however, should be elevated as high as possible: (1) to compete with CO binding, thereby decreasing the half-life of carboxyhemoglobin (CO-Hgb), and (2) to dissolve a certain (though limited) amount of O_2 in the blood for tissue oxygenation.

PATIENTS AT LATE RISK FOR OS AND VS

Patients who have aspirated gastric contents or who have been severely injured (two conditions which the emergency department practitioner often encounters), are at very high risk of developing ARDS. To date the exact pathophysiologic mechanisms have not been unraveled, however the risk of ARDS has now been correlated prospectively with several specifically defined clinical conditions including sepsis syndrome (serious infection and deleterious cardiovascular response), aspiration of gastric contents (documented by suctioning), pulmonary contusion, massive emergency transfusion (at a rate of >22 units every 12 hours) and several other diagnostic categories such as inhalation injuries and near-drowning. Risk increases with the number of risk factors simultaneously present. In addition, risk has been related to the injury severity score (ISS) and inversely related to the initial levels of oxygenation (initial PaO_2:FIO_2 ratios) in patients with one or more of the diagnostic risk factors. The criteria in Table 1 are usually used to diagnose ARDS. The period of risk for ARDS is highest during the initial 24 hours after the predisposing clinical event or trauma. Patients meeting criteria for pulmonary contusion, aspiration of gastric contents, massive emergency transfusions and multiple major long bone fractures should be monitored closely with ABG analyses, particularly during the initial 24-hour period. Other patients who are (and remain) alert, oriented, and spontaneously breathing without subjective

TABLE 1 Mandatory Criteria for Diagnosis of ARDS

Severe hypoxemia (e.g., $PaO_2 < 75$ torr on an FIO_2 of 0.5 or more)
New diffuse infiltrates involving all lung fields on chest film
Pulmonary artery wedge pressure (PAWP) less than 18 mm Hg
No other explanation for the above (such as pneumonia, atelectasis, heart failure)

dyspnea are unlikely to develop ARDS, however, and can be released within 3 to 4 hours if they remain asymptomatic and have no other indication for admission. This guideline is useful when applied to reliable patients who are being evaluated for possible toxic gas inhalation.

POSITIVE PRESSURE INFLATION

One of the decisions in early ventilatory management is whether to allow the patient to breathe spontaneously or to provide some form of ventilatory assistance.

When it is not clear that the patient is able to generate an adequate lung inflation, a self-inflatable bag-valve-mask system is usually employed. But even with a tight fit, ventilation may not be adequate, and is often complicated by gastric inflation. Whenever possible, this system should be replaced by endotracheal intubation and manual (or mechanical) inflations. The typical self-inflating, resuscitator-type bag commonly used for emergency ventilation generally has a volume of 1,200 to 1,600 ml, and using an endotracheal tube and average ventilatory technique, these bags usually provide a V_T of 800 to 1,200 ml, which meets the desired 10 to 15 ml per kilogram V_T for the average adult. With an endotracheal tube, the airway is theoretically sealed from the bag to the lungs, and the entire delivered V_T can be maintained in the system regardless of the inspiratory flow rate. On the other hand, using a bag-valve-mask (BVM) system, much of the V_T is usually lost (1) into the digestive tract (unless an esophageal obturator-type airway is used), (2) in leakage around the mask, or (3) in distending the oropharynx. If airway pressure rises above 15 to 20 cm H_2O, air preferentially goes into the digestive tract. The more the airway obstruction, the stiffer the lung, and the faster the breath is delivered, the higher the peak airway pressure and the less effective the V_T. Cardiac arrest or critical trauma patients usually develop noncompliant lungs as a result of closed airways, blood, or vomitus. They, in particular, will need provision of adequate inflation (and thus intubation). Therefore, when personnel resources are limited, and single-handed ventilation may be necessary, or when the patient has noncompliant lungs, a secured ET tube permits the most reliable and efficient means of delivering the best respiratory support. The use of continuous positive airway pressure (CPAP) by face mask has been suggested as a safe and effective method of treating hypoxemia in alert, spontaneously breathing patients. This technique has often been reputed as a method of early or prophylactic therapy to prevent progressive respiratory failure. However, although supportive of oxygenation, it is pro-

bably of no use in actually preventing the onset of acute respiratory failure or ARDS. Still, it may be useful in supporting oxygenation enough to obviate the necessity for endotracheal intubation. The major complication, facial sores, occurs only after prolonged use and can be prevented by cushioned edges around the mask. Aspiration, however, may be a problem if the patient is not alert and without an intact gag reflex.

Mechanically-assisted ventilation requires that an ET tube be in place. There are three basic types of mechanical ventilatory assistance currently used in the early phases of acute care:

1. Assisted mechanical ventilation (AMV), in which the patient initiates or "triggers" the positive pressure ventilator inflations.
2. Intermittent mandatory ventilation (IMV), in which the patient breathes spontaneously, but also receives mechanically delivered positive pressure ventilator inflations at pre-set (intermittent) intervals.
3. Controlled mechanical ventilation (CMV), in which all breaths are delivered by the ventilator at a set rate and no spontaneous or patient-initiated ventilator breaths are allowed.

A combination of (1) and (3), called "assist-control" (AC), is accomplished when a minimal number of pre-set mandatory ventilator inflations are given and the patient is still able to trigger additional ventilator breaths.

When mechanical ventilation is initiated, one must first choose a tidal volume. A volume-cycled respirator is preferable as it delivers a known inflation volume. Pressure-cycled ventilators do not always guarantee an adequate lung inflation, as the delivered volume is altered by any factors affecting airway pressure, such as changes in lung compliance or airway resistance.

The ideal V_T (10 to 15 ml per kilogram) refers to delivered V_T, not necessarily the V_T setting on the ventilator. A certain small amount of delivered gas volume is lost in the compliant ventilator tubing. This amount should be subtracted from the delivered V_T to calculate the effective V_T that the patient actually receives. For example, in a standard volume-cycled ventilator with a corrugated tubing system, 3 to 4 ml of volume is lost expanding the tubing for every centimeter of H_2O of peak airway pressure generated (as indicated by the ventilator manometer). This pressure is increased by several factors: (1) decreased lung and/or chest wall compliance, (2) increased airway resistance (e.g., a kinked ET tube or acute bronchospasm), and (3) rate of ventilator inflation (the faster the inspiratory flow, the higher the rise in airway pressure). All of these factors increase peak airway pressure and thus result in a somewhat smaller effective V_T. For example, a bronchospastic patient may develop a peak pressure of 50 cm H_2O with a V_T set at 1,000 ml. With 150 ml lost in the system due to tubing distention (3 ml per centimeter H_2O × 50 cm H_2O), the effective V_T is 850 ml. If the peak pressure had been only 15 cm H_2O pressure, 45 ml would have been lost and the effective V_T would be 955 ml.

Hypoinflation (less than 8 ml per kilogram lean body weight) predisposes to atelectasis, and overinflation (>20 ml per kilogram) predisposes to barotrauma (pneumothorax, pneumomediastinum, and subcutaneous emphysema). Therefore an effective V_T of 10 to 15 ml per kilogram is usually chosen. The larger the V_T, the greater the percentage of fresh gas reaching the alveolar spaces. Because V_D:V_T is decreased, these breaths are more efficient and $\dot{V}_E$ demand is decreased. Therefore it may be preferable to deliver the high end of this range (12 to 15 ml per kilogram), particularly if there is also hypoxemia unexplained by the chest film (i.e., possible underinflation of dependent zones). Patients with COPD, pneumonectomy, or chest injuries may be at a higher risk of barotrauma, and a lower V_T (8 to 12 ml per kilogram) might be selected. Obese patients have decreased chest wall compliance, and we suggest ventilation with 10 to 15 ml per kilogram of estimated lean body weight plus one-third of the extra weight. Another suggested formula is to deliver 20 percent of the patient's predicted vital capacity, which is based primarily on height alone and is therefore faster and easier to determine at the bedside. A patient with a pneumonectomy (whole lung) may require a smaller V_T (e.g., 8 ml per kilogram) but at a faster rate.

After an adequate V_T is chosen, respiratory rate should be adjusted to maintain the desired pH (and $PaCO_2$). Ventilator "breaths" are more efficient (decreased V_D:V_T) than spontaneous breaths, and the CO_2 production from the work of breathing is minimized, particularly in the patient with underlying respiratory impairment. Therefore a patient with pneumonia and a RR of 40 may need only 1,000 ml × 15 per minute. An unconscious patient who has taken an overdose of sedatives, who is otherwise healthy, has low $\dot{V}_E$ requirements and may need only 3 to 4 L per minute ventilation. On the other hand, an acidotic, stressed trauma patient may have increased ventilatory demand to maintain a reasonable blood pH. Therefore one must use clinical judgment when first choosing the proper rate. It may be better to initially err on the side of acidosis (which favors tissue oxygen delivery) and, in many cases, to initially choose a low rate (5 or 6 per minute) until the ABG analysis can be obtained, as long as the patient is also capable of "triggering" the ventilator.

Assisted mechanical ventilation or assist-control is often used initially because in most cases the patient can still trigger the ventilator enough to maintain a normal pH. This also makes sense because $\dot{V}_E$ demand varies from moment to moment in the early phases following acute illness or injury, owing to changes in body temperature, shivering, clearance of metabolic acid, and administration of drugs. In cases in which the patient is not triggering the ventilator (e.g., heavily sedated, paralyzed, or rate raised to therapeutically hyperventilate for head injury), the patient is effectively receiving controlled mechanical ventilation, and care should be taken so that one does not over- (or under-) ventilate. If the patient is receiving intermittent mandatory ventilation, the rate may be set too high and effectively becomes CMV. If the IMV rate is too low, the ill or injured patient may not be able to meet his or her own $\dot{V}_E$ demand since CO_2 production increases as the work of breathing increases. Intermittent mandatory ventilation can be used as an initial mode of ventilation, but care must be taken to monitor arterial blood gases. A trial of IMV is warranted in the patient with asynchronous breathing. The possible disadvantages of IMV compared with AMV, are that (1) it may not allow the patient to respond adequately to changes in clinical status and (2) it increases the work of breathing and oxygen consumption. IMV should be avoided in unstable patients whose ventilatory demands may suddenly change, in patients with impaired ventilatory drives, and in patients whose work of breathing should be minimized. Our rule of thumb for choosing an IMV rate is to find a rate that allows the patient to take 10 to 20 spontaneous breaths per minute since this would approximate a physiologic rate. Thus, the mode of ventilation should be adapted to the patient's individual needs, and the physiologic results evaluated whenever possible.

Hyperventilation is commonly suggested as a therapeutic modality for severe head injury. Lowering the $PaCO_2$ to 25 or 30 torr usually causes vasoconstriction in the cerebral vasculature. This decreases cerebral blood flow, which, in turn, shrinks brain size and lowers the ICP. However, this effect may be blunted by either hypoxemia or systemic arterial hypotension (Fig. 2). Therefore, the initial consideration is to ensure the best O_2 transport to the brain by providing (at least initially) 100 percent O_2 and adequate V_T and titrating arterial blood pressure to more than 100 mm Hg systolic. Hyperventilation to lower ICP can then be attempted, but care must be taken not to overventilate the patient. If alkalosis occurs (pH >7.50), the risk for seizures and ventricular arrhythmias increases. Neurosurgeons and neurophysiologists caution against hyperventilation below a $PaCO_2$ of 20 torr, since lower levels may produce local brain hypoxia in some patients, presumably by inducing too much vasoconstriction. Therefore, unless an ABG can be obtained immediately to confirm the $PaCO_2$, the initial respiratory rate probably should not exceed 20 when an adequate V_T (15 ml per kilogram) is provided. Taking into consideration the precautions for cervical spine injury, it *is* advisable to place an ET tube

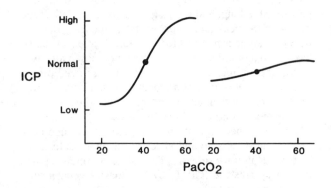

Figure 2 Effect of hypertension on intracranial pressure. *Left*: Normal intracranial pressure (ICP) response to alterations in arterial CO_2 tension ($PaCO_2$). *Right*: Blunting of this response occurs in the presence of hypoxemia and hypotension (decreased O_2 transport) or after diffuse cerebral anoxia.

and provide ventilation with 100 percent O_2, using a large V_T (15 ml per kilogram or 700 to 1,100 ml effectively delivered in the average 50 to 75 kg adult) and a RR of 16 to 18 per minute to ensure against hypoventilation until an ABG measurement can be taken. In the majority of patients, this regimen provides at least a mild degree of hyperventilation. Once ABG analysis is available, the $\dot{V}_E$ should be adjusted to maintain the $PaCO_2$ between 23 and 28 torr while increased ICP and metabolic acidosis are corrected. If the patient is deteriorating neurologically, the rate may be increased as needed.

There are several acute complications of intermittent positive pressure inflations. Positive pressure inflations (PPI) raise intrathoracic pressure, unlike spontaneous respirations, which decrease intrathoracid pressure during inspiration. Therefore PPI may impede venous return, especially in the intravascular volume-depleted patient, and this can result in diminished cardiac output. Positive pressure inflations increase the risk of pneumothorax, particularly in patients with penetrating or blunt chest trauma, rib fractures, COPD, or those who have had central venous catheterization attempts. Therefore certain patients at risk for pneumothorax who will be undergoing laparotomy or prolonged orthopaedic procedures often undergo "prophylactic" thoracostomy prior to surgery, since close intraoperative monitoring is often difficult.

Overinflation can occur when patients with high $\dot{V}_E$ requirements are not able to expel all of the delivered V_T before the next mechanical inflation is initiated. This is more common in patients with severe expiratory airflow obstruction (COPD, asthma), but also can happen in severely injured patients who are hyperventilated at rates higher than 20 or those with extremely high $\dot{V}_E$ demands such as the severely burned patient. When this occurs, air continues to be trapped in the lungs until elastic recoil becomes sufficient to allow complete expulsion of the selected V_T before the next breath. At this new state of equilibrium, the patient appears to be ventilating appropriately, but is now at a higher lung volume (increased functional residual capacity [FRC]). This results in an often unsuspected elevation of intrathoracic pressure throughout the ventilatory cycle known as occult PEEP or auto-PEEP. Not only does this auto-PEEP phenomenon diminish $\dot{Q}_T$, but transmission of this increased alveolar pressure raises vascular pressure readings (e.g., PAWP). If unrecognized, the auto-PEEP effects may lead to interpretation of high PAWP as reflecting a high intravascular volume status. The high PAWP and low blood pressure (or low $\dot{Q}_T$) might lead to a diagnosis of cardiogenic shock. However, the auto-PEEP phenomenon can be easily detected by finding an immediate rise in blood pressure (or $\dot{Q}_T$) several seconds after removing the patient from mechanical ventilation. IMV may alleviate auto-PEEP since occasional spontaneous breaths should lower mean intrathoracic pressure. More importantly, therapy should be directed at treatment for airway obstruction and decreasing $\dot{V}_E$. Occasionally, these patients are also volume depleted intravascularly due to infection or diuretic use, and fluid infusions may be helpful.

POSITIVE END-EXPIRATORY PRESSURE

Application of PEEP in appropriate patients increases functional residual capacity and usually results in improvement of arterial oxygenation. Areas of pure shunt are converted to areas in which there is some ventilation to the perfused lung units, even if small. This explains why PEEP can improve hypoxemia that is refractory to even 100 percent inspired O_2. Usually PEEP improves oxygenation only when the lung injury is relatively diffuse. PEEP applied to normal lungs or lungs with local disease (e.g., lobar pneumonia) also results in an increased FRC, but this occurs mainly in the areas of normal lung compliance, thereby resulting in three potential detrimental effects: (1) an increase in dead space and/or regions of high V/Q, (2) a regional increase in the pulmonary vascular resistance of the normal lung, resulting in a relative redistribution of blood flow to the diseased lung, thus creating an increased shunt, and (3) a reduction in $\dot{Q}_T$ (see below). Our experience has been that with unilateral disease, PEEP may initially increase the shunt at lower levels, but that at higher levels (>10 to 15 cm H_2O), an improvement in oxygenation often can be achieved. Therefore, PEEP trials should still be performed if critical hypoxemia ($PaO_2 < $ torr with $FiO_2 \geq 0.5$) is present, especially if the hypoxemia is progressing.

PEEP has important hemodynamic effects that can result in a significant reduction of cardiac output ($\dot{Q}_T$) owing to decreasing venous return. If hypovolemia exists or is induced, $\dot{Q}_T$ reduction is more likely to occur with the application of PEEP. If the $\dot{Q}_T$ does fall, fluid administration may result in its restoration. Routine application of up to 8 cm (H_2O) PEEP has no effect on blood pressure and heart rates in normovolemic patients. Diminished $\dot{Q}_T$ is rare below 10 cm H_2O in normovolemic patients, and demonstration of a decrease in blood pressure (or $\dot{Q}_T$) that reverses with low-level (<10 cm H_2O) PEEP removal is actually a good clinical test for hypovolemia!

Another potential problem with PEEP application is the effect on ICP. Because PEEP elevates intrathoracic pressure, the resulting impedance to venous return may impair cerebral blood drainage and cause a concomitant rise in ICP. Such increases are most pronounced in patients with severe head injury, but this effect is less apparent in patients with decreased lung compliance. Since these patients are the most likely to receive PEEP therapy, increases in ICP are not a major problem. PEEP should not be withheld when needed to maintain oxygenation in patients with head trauma and increased ICP. ICP monitoring can be used in these patients to help guide PEEP therapy. The risk of increased ICP from PEEP may be offset by lowering the mean airway pressure with IMV. In addition, elevation of the patient's head (when neck injuries have been ruled out) often alleviates any PEEP effects on ICP.

In a PEEP trial, the approach should always be systematic in order to allow an appropriate evaluation of the efficacy of each increment in PEEP. Since the goal of PEEP therapy is to maintain the maximum O_2 transport to the tissues at the safest FIO_2, it is necessary to evaluate all the components of O_2 transport (PaO_2, Hgb and $\dot{Q}T$) as PEEP is increased, and it is important to change only one variable at a time, namely the PEEP level. For example, since both PEEP and FIO_2 can affect the PaO_2, the FIO_2 should be held constant during the PEEP trial. Likewise, since VT can affect mean airway pressure (and therefore $\dot{Q}T$ and oxygenation), it also should be held constant. Time is an important variable since fluid requirements or metabolic requirements may change rapidly in a critically ill patient owing to bleeding, fever, or the syndrome of multiple organ failure (sepsis syndrome). These changes affect $\dot{Q}T$ and may confuse the issue of whether or not the PEEP itself has affected $\dot{Q}T$. Unless the emergency department is properly equipped, ICU admission is usually necessary for the trial. Generally, since ARDS does not occur for a few hours, patients should be admitted before PEEP trials are warranted. Patients with pulmonary edema from heart failure rarely have a PaO_2 less than 75 torr with a 50 percent FIO_2.

PEEP should be increased in small steps (for example, 5 cm H_2O), and the period of time at each step should be relatively short (15 to 30 minutes). Most evidence suggests that early in the course of ARDS, PEEP has a measurable beneficial effect within 10 minutes. With this concept in mind, our PEEP trial protocols are conducted in a manner that will facilitate their earliest completion. If significant BP or $\dot{Q}T$ falls occur, we lower the PEEP to the previous level and confirm that the fall in $\dot{Q}T$ or blood pressure is PEEP-related. However if there are no significant changes with PEEP, we draw blood samples at about 10 to 15 minutes and then immediately apply the next PEEP increment, repeating the same process. In order to facilitate the rapidity of the trial, we do not stop just to await ABG results. Instead we continue directly until the $\dot{Q}T$ falls by 20 percent or until we reach 15 to 20 cm H_2O PEEP, since most patients will have responded with these levels. As a result, our trials are usually complete within 1 hour. We raise our PEEP levels until a PaO_2 of 70 torr or more can be achieved with FIO_2 of 0.5 or until $\dot{Q}T$ falls by 20 percent from the $\dot{Q}T$ measured with no PEEP. If PaO_2 does not rise enough to saturate Hgb before $\dot{Q}T$ falls, we try other techniques such as IMV, red cell transfusion, fluid challenges, elevated FIO_2, and positioning.

SUGGESTED READING

Hudson LD. Ventilatory management of patients with adult respiratory distress syndrome. Semin Resp Med 1981; 2:128–139.

Jones PW. Hyperventilation in the management of cerebral oedema. Intensive Care Med 1981; 7:205–207.

Pepe PE. The clinical entity of adult respiratory distress syndrome: definition, prediction and prognosis. Crit Care Clin July 1986; 2(1):1–24.

Pepe PE, Copass MK, Joyce TH. Prehospital endotracheal intubation—rationale for training emergency medical personnel. Ann Emerg Med

Pepe PE, Hudson LD, Carrico CJ. Early application of positive end-expiratory pressure in patients at risk for the adult respiratory distress syndrome. N Engl J Med 1984; 311:282–286.

Pepe PE, Marini JJ. Occult positive end-expiratory pressure in mechanically ventilated patients with airflow obstruction: the auto-PEEP effect. Am Rev Resp Dis 1982; 26:166–170.

PRACTICAL ADVANCES IN CARDIOPULMONARY RESUSCITATION

CHARLES F. BABBS, M.D., Ph.D.

In recent years several experimental modifications of standard cardiopulmonary resuscitation (CPR) have been reported in the literature, including the use of simultaneous ventilation and compression, interposed abdominal compressions, and high-impulse compressions to improve systemic perfusion. Although each of these new methods has shown promising hemodynamic results in laboratory studies or in theoretical models, none has yet been shown to improve long-term survival in man compared to standard CPR. Hence, none of the experimental methods can be recommended for clinical use at this time. Indeed, there is recent evidence that *optimally performed* standard CPR is as effective as any of the newer experimental methods. Consequently, I believe that the quest for more successful resuscitation might well begin with optimization of standard CPR in four areas: electrical defibrillation, compression force, compression duration, and adrenergic drug therapy.

ELECTRICAL DEFIBRILLATION

Neglecting for the moment the legal and political issues of who is permitted to defibrillate, and focusing instead on the scientific evidence, it is clear that when the cardiac ventricles are fibrillating, all reasonable attempts should be made to defibrillate as soon as possible. In the animal laboratory, one can remove the electrical abnormality of ventricular fibrillation (VF) and restore spontaneous circulation virtually 100 percent of the time, if an adequately strong defibrillatory shock is given within 1 minute of the onset of VF. After 2 minutes of VF, a threshold shock continues to convert the electrocardiogram to a nonfibrillatory rhythm, but the likelihood of restoration of blood pressure diminishes sharply. After 3 or more minutes of VF, electrical defibrillation alone leaves the ventricles in a state of electromechanical dissociation; CPR and adrenergic drug therapy are necessary, but not always sufficient to restore spontaneous circulation.

Similar experience has been reported in animal models by Ewy, Yakaitis, and their co-workers. They found that for VF lasting less than 2 minutes in anesthetized dogs, defibrillation alone was always successful in restoring cardiac pumping and blood pressure. For VF lasting 3 to 4 minutes, both defibrillation and CPR were necessary. For VF lasting more than 4 minutes, defibrillation, CPR, and epinephrine were necessary, and the percent success diminished as the "down time" without therapy increased. In the laboratory, the best results are always obtained with prompt defibrillation.

The great effectiveness of prompt ventricular defibrillation is now established by clinical studies as well. The work of Eisenberg and co-workers in King County, Washington has clearly shown that the value of earlier defibrillation extrapolates from animals to man. They found that the probability of survival to discharge was more than twice as great (28 percent versus 13 percent) among patients defibrillated within 4 minutes of collapse as among those defibrillated after more than 4 minutes. When emergency medical technicians were trained to use defibrillators in the King County area, in order to shorten the time to defibrillation, long-term survival of patients with sudden cardiac death in ventricular fibrillation increased from 7 percent to 17 percent. Clearly, defibrillation by first responders is rational and effective therapy.

Moreover, from a public health standpoint, defibrillation by first responders is probably necessary to substantially improve outcome from sudden cardiac death, in view of the natural history of the condition. The Framingham study has taught us that fully 50 percent of deaths caused by coronary heart disease are sudden, that is, they occur within 1 hour of the onset of symptoms. In turn, the *majority of patients dying of coronary heart disease are not hospitalized at the time of death*. These epidemiologic facts mean that in a majority of cases the treatment for sudden cardiac death must be started in a pre-hospital setting and argue strongly for defibrillation by first responders.

Safety and Effectiveness of Countershock

A substantial body of literature exists to show that electrical ventricular defibrillation is both safe and effective, and the efficacy of relatively lower dose shocks (200 joules) in adult humans with spontaneous VF has now been established beyond doubt. Damage to the heart following defibrillator shock is minimal and unlikely at the lower energies that have now been shown to be effective.

The margin of safety for electrical defibrillation has been established by the author and Dr. Tacker, who determined the classic therapeutic index of single defibrillator shocks in dogs. The results, shown in Figure 1, indicate that compared to the defibrillation threshold, it takes about 30 times as much energy to produce any degree of microscopically detectable myocardial damage, and 500 times as much energy to produce death in a typical dog. Thus the classic therapeutic index (median lethal dose to median effective dose—LD_{50} to ED_{50})—is approximately 500 to 1. Indeed it is difficult or impossible to produce cardiac damage in dogs weighing more than 20 kg with a standard (400 joule max) commercial defibrillator. The study of the therapeutic index just described required a specially fabricated high-energy defibrillator capable of storing 5,000 joules. Considering the predicament of the patient, the benefits of prompt defibrillation far outweigh the risks.

The skill of administering a defibrillatory shock can be taught to qualified emergency medical technicians just as it has been taught to coronary care nurses and para-

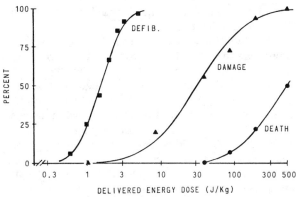

Figure 1 Margin of safety for single damped sine wave defibrillator shocks in anesthetized dogs. Percent of dogs responding is plotted as a function of delivered energy required to produce defibrillation, or microscopically detectable myocardial damage, or death.

medics. The requisite initial training is limited to about 10 hours initially, combined with close medical supervision. Moreover, for those who believe such training is too difficult or too expensive, "smart" *automatic defibrillators* are being developed by several companies. These machines are capable of automatically analyzing the electrocardiogram (ECG) signal sensed via the paddles and diagnosing the presence or absence of VF. If desired, they can be programmed to automatically deliver a defibrillatory shock. Thus, it is not only desirable but feasible to implement a program of early pre-hospital defibrillation. This is perhaps the single most important step that can be taken to improve long-term, neurologically intact survival of victims of sudden cardiac death, a step that can and should be implemented immediately.

Avoiding Errors in Technique

In addition to upgrading the performance of emergency medical systems for prompt defibrillation, it is important to maximize successful performance of individuals who operate defibrillators. The following is a list of eight correctable reasons for failure to defibrillate. Some of these represent simple lack of common sense; others represent concepts from recent research.

1. A line-operated defibrillator may not be plugged in to a power supply, or a battery operated defibrillator may not be charged.

2. There may be salt bridges of electrode paste between the paddle electrodes. These can form as electrode paste is smeared hastily over the chest and can shunt current between the electrodes via a low-resistance pathway that does not include the patient. The electrical dose delivered to the patient is therefore less.

3. A nonconducting gel such as those used in ultrasonic studies to couple the transducer to the chest wall may have been used by mistake for defibrillation. Such nonconducting gels or pastes have been shown by Ewy and co-workers to have substantially greater resistance to current flow than electrolytic gels and, in their opinion, have the potential to reduce defibrillation success.

4. Inadequate contact pressure may reduce the current entering the thorax and in turn increase chest resistance. Conversely, increased paddle pressure ensures

good contact and reduces the electrical resistance of the electrode-skin interface.

5. Defibrillation may have been attempted with improper paddle placement, as is common in everyday practice. If paddles are placed too close together on the precordium, shunting of current through electrode gel, skin, and subcutaneous tissue superficial to the heart may easily occur. Placement of paddles too low on the chest will "defibrillate the liver," not the heart. Sometimes defibrillation threshold is lower with the anteroposterior paddle position, as shown by Ewy, and this approach can be tried in an obese or emphasematous patient if the anterior-anterior approach fails.

6. If a shock is applied during inspiration rather than expiration, the defibrillation threshold is higher; the remedy is to deliberately shock during expiration.

7. Refibrillation may rapidly occur during the time of ECG blanking associated with electrode polarization and so mimic failure to defibrillate. This phenomenon is more common after epinephrine or calcium treatment.

8. Finally, there may be larger individuals who simply require more energy because of larger body size, previous antiarrhythmic drug treatment, or other factors. A mental checklist of these reversible causes for failure to defibrillate may help the individual practitioner achieve greater success.

COMPRESSION FORCE

One of the most neglected variables in CPR is the force of external chest compression; although it is common knowledge that the vigor of chest compression may vary widely among rescuers and may progressively diminish as a given rescuer tires. The first reference to compression force in the current (1980) Standards and Guidelines for CPR states "Efficient external chest compression requires sufficient pressure to depress an adult's sternum *a minimum* of 4 to 5 cm." Unfortunately, subsequent references to compression force in this document omit the word "minimum," leaving the impression that any degree of compression in the range of 4 to 5 cm is satisfactory. Such a recommendation would be rational if the true function relating blood flow and compression depth were of the form of the curved line in Figure 2. This hypothetical function rises to a plateau so that any degree of compression in the plateau region would be close to maximally effective. However, as shown recently in our laboratory (Ann Emerg Med 1983; 12:527–532) the function relating total flow during experimental CPR to compression depth in anesthetized dogs was much more like the straight line in Figure 2. Not only is artificial circulation a steep function of compression depth in the range of 4- to 5-cm sternal deflection, but there is also a range of compression below 2.5 cm in which no measurable flow occurred. That is, an "effective compression threshold" had to be exceeded to produce any flow at all. These two features of the true flow-compression curve mean that relatively small percentage change in compression can produce a relatively large percentage change in circulation. In dogs, flow is nearly doubled as chest compression is increased from 4 to 5 cm. Clinical practitioners

of CPR can profit from recognizing that chest compression force is a critical variable affecting artificial circulation.

Interestingly, when total blood flow (cardiac output) during CPR is plotted as a function of peak esophageal pressure, rather than compression depth, a curve similar to curve A in Figure 2 is generated. The esophageal pressure pulses may be recorded from a soft, fluid-filled tube in the midesophagus. When these pulses reach 50 mm Hg, near-maximal flow is obtained. Further increase in pressure above 50 mm Hg produces little added benefit, but does increase the risk of chest wall, cardiac, and hepatic trauma. I believe that clinical monitoring of esophageal pressure during CPR may prove to be a practical means of optimizing compression force in the future. The technique can help to prevent traumatic overcompression and can help to normalize the force of chest compression among patients of different size and chest resiliency.

COMPRESSION DURATION AND DUTY CYCLE

One of the issues in CPR for which there is abundant experimental and clinical evidence is the importance of compression duration or duty cycle. Compression duration may be thought of as the absolute compression time expressed in milliseconds, and duty cycle may be thought of as the ratio of compression time to cycle time expressed in percent. Several studies in animals and in humans have independently demonstrated that compression duration is an important determinant of blood flow during CPR. Fitzgerald and co-workers, in a comprehensive study of anesthetized dogs, investigated compression frequencies ranging from 20 to 140 per minute and duty cycles ranging from 10 to 90 percent. They found that there was little influence of compression frequency in the range of 40 to 140 per minute. However, there was a strong influence of duty cycle, with peak flow occurring in the range of 40 to 50 percent (Fig. 3). Studies in

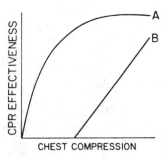

Figure 2 Alternative functions relating CPR effectiveness to the depth of chest compression. Curved line (A) indicates that CPR effectiveness is insensitive to small changes in compression over a large range, as seems to have been assumed by framers of CPR standards. Straight line (B) shows actual experimental results of an effective compression threshold, below which CPR is totally ineffective. In this case, CPR effectiveness is sensitive to small changes in compression. (From Babbs CF, et al. Relationship of artificial cardiac output to chest compression amplitude—evidence for an effective compression threshold. Ann Emerg Med 1983; 12:527–532.)

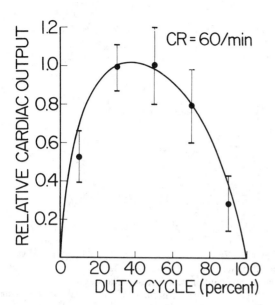

Figure 3 Dependence of total flow during CPR on the duty cycle of compression. Compression rate (CR) = 60 per minute. Maximal flow occurs with duty cycle in the range of 30 to 50 percent. The smooth curve represents the prediction of a mathematical model. (From Fitzgerald KR, et al. Cardiac output during cardiopulmonary resuscitation at various compression rates and durations. Am J Physiol 1981; 241:H442–H448).

humans demonstrated that the percutaneous ultrasonic Doppler flow velocity index was increased at longer compression durations for all compression frequencies investigated. The aforementioned studies were performed with a mechanical chest compressor and ventilator (Thumper R). Vaagenes' experience confirms that such experimental results can be reproduced in the clinical setting using manual technique as well.

The importance of duty cycle is worth stressing because use of a quick jabbing technique of chest compression is so common. One published account of this tendency was provided by Nagel, who recorded on video tape the technique of house staff performing CPR in 600 resuscitations in the emergency department of a Miami area hospital. The average duty cycle employed for CPR was 25 percent. Reference to Figure 3 reveals, that although flow at 25 percent duty cycle may be close to optimal, flow rapidly decreases if duty cycle falls below 25 percent. If the *average* duty cycle in Nagel's series was 25 percent, a substantial number of patients must have been resuscitated with duty cycles of chest compression less than 25 percent. Such quick jabbing technique is known to be ineffective.

The widespread tendency toward a quick jabbing type of chest compression is probably the result of emphasis in clinical training on obtaining a palpable pulse during external chest compression. Certain quick compressions can produce high peak pressures, but if these are not sustained, the net flow is small. Although high peak pressures or instantaneous flows are perceived as a palpable pulse, it is the area under the tracing of pressure or instantaneous flow as a function of time that is indicative of total flow. Presence of a palpable pulse is necessary,

but not sufficient, to guarantee good artificial circulation during CPR.

Finally, it is worth mentioning that a new experimental technique, "high impulse compression" CPR, developed by investigators at Duke university, does not violate the principle just discussed. This modification of standard CPR requires forceful compressions at high frequencies of 120 per minute delivered with short compression duration so that the duty cycle is about 30 percent. Fitzgerald's data for 120 per minute compression (Fig. 4) illustrate that this dependence of flow on duty cycle 120 per minute is similar to that at 60 per minute and that a duty cycle of 30 percent is not far from optimal. Thus, shorter compressions at a higher compression frequency may still be effective because cycle time is reduced enough so that duty cycle remains in a range compatible with good artificial circulation. If identical, short-duration compressions were performed at a lower frequency of 60 per minute, the duty cycle would be only 15 percent and flow would be seriously impaired. Thus, a thoughtful review of the literature suggests that jabbing compressions are effective only if combined with higher compression frequency.

AVOIDANCE OF PURE BETA-ADRENERGIC DRUGS

Pure beta-adrenergic drugs such as isoproterenol or dobutamine are not helpful when given during CPR and indeed may abolish all chance for return of spontaneous circulation. This principle derives from the work of the

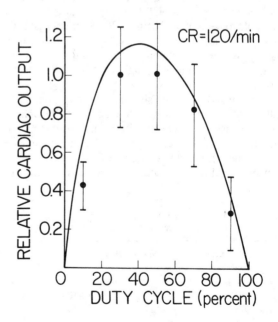

Figure 4 Dependence of total flow during CPR upon the duty cycle of compression. Compression rate (CR) = 120 per minute. Maximal flow occurs with duty cycle in the range of 30 to 50 percent. The smooth curve represents the prediction of a mathematical model. (From Fitzgerald KR, et al. Cardiac output during cardiopulmonary resuscitation at various compression rates and durations. Am J Physiol 1981; 241:H442–H448).

late Joseph S. Redding, his associate J.W. Pearson, their student Ron Yakaitis, and co-workers.* They have shown in repeated and consistent studies, that drugs with alpha-adrenergic activity promote return of circulation following experimental cardiac arrest and CPR, whereas pure beta drugs are of no benefit and appear to worsen the chances of survival. Typical results of their studies are summarized in Table 1. The results are the same for animal models in which cardiac arrest is induced either by ventricular fibrillation or by asphyxia.

Beta-agonists are not effective in CPR because the major site of action of adrenergic drugs during CPR is not the heart, but rather the peripheral vasculature. Constriction of peripheral systemic arterioles, an alpha-adrenergic response, raises diastolic arterial pressure during CPR and in turn coronary perfusion pressure. Constriction of peripheral systemic veins following drug administration improves cardiac filling as well, a phenomenon that can be demonstrated during open chest cardiac massage. The combined result is increased perfusion of the heart and brain. Isoproterenol, on the other hand, reduces coronary perfusion pressure and shunts flow from vital organs to skeletal muscle beds. The likely end results are reduced perfusion of the heart and brain and increased washout of metabolic acids from abundant skeletal muscle tissue.

The critical importance of achieving adequate systemic perfusion pressure and myocardial blood flow has been demonstrated recently, as illustrated in Figure 5. In class A animals, the circulation was restored with electrical defibrillation only. Class B animals required additional epinephrine and CPR. Class C animals were impossible to resuscitate. Figure 5 demonstrates that there was a strong correlation between myocardial perfusion during CPR and resuscitability; perfusion to organs other than the heart was not as strongly correlated with resuscitability.

Adrenergic drugs with significant alpha activity classically include epinephrine (alpha + beta), norepinephrine (alpha > beta), phenylephrine, methoxamine, and metaraminol (alpha). Very high-dose dopamine (alpha + beta + gamma), but not dobutamine (beta−1 > beta−), has been found to be similarly effective (see Table 1).

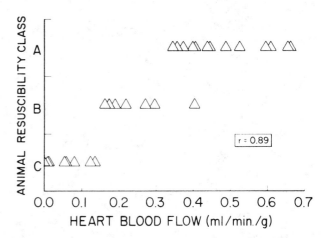

Figure 5 Results of resuscitation after 20 minutes of ventricular fibrillation and CPR in anesthetized dogs plotted as a function of myocardial blood flow. Class A animals recovered pulsatile blood pressure immediately after defibrillation; class B animals recovered with further adjunctive therapy; class C animals were impossible to resuscitate. (From Ralston SH, et al. Intrapulmonary epinephrine during cardiopulmonary resuscitation: improved regional blood flow and resuscitation in dogs. Ann Emerg Med 1984; 13:79–86.)

Epinephrine is still the drug of choice to promote restoration of the circulation during CPR, although currently recommended doses may be suboptimal. Its alpha activity induces peripheral vasoconstriction, whereas its beta activity tends to lower coronary vascular resistance. The result is a fivefold increase in coronary perfusion, as demonstrated in Holmes' study. However, use of pure beta-agonists in CPR is to be strongly discouraged. All available evidence suggests that they are lethal in this application, despite their appearance in some extant Advanced Cardiac Life Support (ACLS) protocols.

Opportunities for improvement of CPR techniques consistent within present guidelines emphasize practical measures for augmenting perfusion of the heart and brain and for restoring spontaneous circulation as quickly as possible. Prompt defibrillation, whenever and wherever possible, is a proven and effective means of enhancing long-term survival following sudden cardiac death and should be encouraged and practiced. Greater attention to optimization and consistency of chest compression is crucial for maximal benefit of external CPR. A 30 to 50 percent duty cycle of chest compression is essential for maximal artificial circulation, whereas any reasonable compression frequency above 40 per minute is satisfactory. Finally, choice of an adrenergic drug with adequate alpha agonist activity and avoidance of pure beta agents provides the most thoroughly tested adjunctive therapy, if CPR and defibrillation alone fail to restore the circulation.

TABLE 1   Outcome of CPR in Dogs After 6 to 8 Minutes of Asphyxia

Drug Therapy	Number Resuscitated/Number Studied
Saline (control)	1/10
Epinephrine	10/10
Phenylephrine	9/10
Dopamine (2 mg/kg bolus)	10/10
Isoproterenol	0/10
Dobutamine	2/10

* A recent review of Joseph S. Redding's contributions to resuscitation research may be found in the American Journal of Emergency Medicine 1985; 3:247–251.

SUGGESTED READING

Holmes HR, Babbs CF, Voorhees WD, deGaravilla B. Influence of adrenergic drugs upon vital organ perfusion during CPR. Crit Care Med 1980; 8:137–140.

Maier GW, Tyson GS, Kernstine KH, Olsen CO, Davis JW, Sabiston DC, Rankin JS. Coronary blood flow during high impulse external cardiac massage. Circulation 1982; 66:168.

Otto CW, Yakaitis RW, Redding JS, Blitt CD. Comparison of dopamine, dobutamine, and epinephrine in CPR. Crit Care Med 1981; 9:366.

Ralston SH, Babbs CF, Niebauer MJ. Cardiopulmonary resuscitation with interposed abdominal compression in dogs. Anesth Analg 1982; 61:645-651.

Ralston SH, Showen L, Carter A, Tacker WA. Comparison of en-dotracheal and intravenous epinephrine dosage during CPR in dogs. Ann Emerg Med 1985; 14:494-495.

Tacker WA, Neibauer MJ, Babbs CF, Combs WJ, Hahn BM, Barker MA, Seipel JF, Bourland JD, Geddes LA. The effect of newer antiarrhythmic drugs on defibrillation threshold. Crit Care Med 1980; 8:177-180.

Yakaitis RW, Ewy GA, Otto CW, Taren DL, Moon TE. Influence of time and therapy on ventricular defibrillation in dogs. Crit Care Med 1980; 8:157-163.

IMPROVING SYSTEMIC PERFUSION DURING CARDIOPULMONARY RESUSCITATION

JAMES T. NIEMANN, M.D.

Closed-chest CPR was introduced as an artificial circulatory and ventilatory support technique during cardiac arrest nearly a quarter of a century ago. Rhythmic closed-chest compression was rapidly accepted as a means of maintaining systemic perfusion during cardiac arrest until definitive therapy (electrical defibrillation) could be made available. Limited experimental and clinical investigation was carried out before the widespread acceptance and use of this technique. Mechanism(s) of action and efficacy were not well established and have been subjected to increasing scrutiny during the last half decade.

Traditionally, depression of the sternum of the supine patient in cardiac arrest was believed to selectively compress the cardiac ventricles between the sternum and the rigid posterior vertebral bodies. Selective ventricular compression during cardiac arrest should result in predictable hemodynamic changes and be reflected by cardiac valve motion and changes in cardiac chamber dimensions. Although time-honored and accepted, these concepts are not supported by past or recent experimental or clinical investigations. Contemporary studies also suggest that closed-chest CPR as currently practiced produces limited systemic perfusion. Cerebral and myocardial perfusion during CPR frequently fall below values necessary to meet metabolic demands. In addition, postreperfusion tissue injury may be a substantial cause for in-hospital postresuscitation morbidity and mortality.

BLOOD FLOW DURING CLOSED-CHEST RESUSCITATION

If sternal depression during cardiac arrest results in selective ventricular compression, left and right ventricular pressures should exceed those measured in the left and right atria during chest compression (CPR "systole"). Ventriculo-atrial pressure gradients should be evident and be accompanied by atrioventricular valve closure. Right and left ventricular pressures should also exceed those noted in the pulmonary arterial system and the proximal intrathoracic arterial circulation. The resulting intrathoracic arterial-venous pressure gradient would facilitate systemic perfusion during cardiac arrest.

This purported mechanism for blood flow during cardiac arrest and closed-chest CPR was questioned in the early 1960s. At that time, even limited hemodynamic observations failed to support the theory. The overwhelming majority of contemporary investigations in the experimental laboratory have also failed to support the selective ventricular compression theory. These latter studies have used state-of-the-art methods, e.g., extensive intravascular monitoring with solid-state catheters, pressure-synchronized cineangiography, and regional flow and perfusion assessed with radiolabeled microspheres and high-quality validation techniques. Corollary clinical studies during CPR in patients using two-dimensional echocardiography support findings in the experimental animal model.

At present, the majority of experimental studies and *all* clinical studies suggest that blood flow during closed-chest CPR is not the direct result of selective ventricular compression, but rather of changes in intrathoracic pressure. Sternal depression results in a generalized increase in intrathoracic pressure rather than direct ventricular compression. The rise in intrathoracic pressure is directly transmitted to all intrathoracic vascular compartments (cardiac chambers and great vessels) as evidenced by near-equivalent increases in pressures measured in these intravascular structures during CPR systole. Changes in intravascular pressures are directly dependent on changes in intrathoracic pressure. Systemic perfusion gradients are established between the arterial and venous circulation only in venous beds with functioning venous valves in close proximity to the intrathoracic venous circulation. It has been shown that closure of venous valves in the brachiocephalic circulation is responsible for cerebral perfusion. The absence of subdiaphragmatic venous valves in close proximity to the right heart limits subdiaphragmatic perfusion during closed-chest CPR. The abrupt rise in intrathoracic pressure results in venous valve closure and maintenance of an arterial-venous perfusion gradient in susceptible vascular beds.

Recent investigational studies have not only defined a new mechanism for blood flow during closed-chest CPR, but have also suggested that (1) cerebral perfusion during cardiac arrest can be improved by mechanical interventions, (2) cerebral and myocardial flow during cardiac arrest may be a substantial factor in resuscitation outcome, and (3) closed-chest CPR produces minimal perfusion during cardiac arrest.

DIFFERENCES IN CEREBRAL AND MYOCARDIAL PERFUSION DURING CLOSED-CHEST CPR

The perfusion gradient determinants of cerebral and myocardial blood flow during closed-chest CPR are graphically depicted in Figure 1. The cerebral perfusion gradient can be manipulated using several modified CPR techniques. To improve cerebral blood flow, the increase in aortic or carotid arterial pressure must exceed the effect on intracranial pressure or jugular venous pressure. Many modified closed-chest CPR techniques meet this requirement. However, few have been demonstrated to have a substantial effect on myocardial blood flow. Myocardial blood flow during cardiac arrest and CPR appears to be directly related to the coronary perfusion gradient, i.e., aortic minus right atrial pressure difference. This pressure difference has been shown to be a critical determinant of outcome after prolonged cardiac arrest and closed-chest CPR. No new CPR technique has been shown to consistently improve myocardial flow during cardiac arrest and none has been shown to substantially improve outcome in the clinical setting. With limited exceptions, closed-chest CPR mechanical manipulations do not improve CPR myocardial flow and therefore have a limited effect on resuscitation outcomes. However, the use of continuous pressor infusions during cardiac arrest and closed-chest CPR could substantially affect myocardial flow and outcome.

"NEW CPR" TECHNIQUES

Numerous modified or "new CPR" techniques have been described in the literature (Table 1). These new but unproven techniques have largely focused on cerebral per-

fusion during cardiac arrest and closed-chest artificial circulatory support. These new techniques have been shown to improve cerebral perfusion during cardiac arrest in experimental animal models. Few have been subjected to analysis using resuscitation outcome and long-term survival in humans as the critical and clinically relevant end point.

The contemporary theory of blood flow during closed-chest resuscitation suggests that changes in intrathoracic pressure are a critical determinant of systemic perfusion. Based on this model, greater fluctuation in intrathoracic pressure during closed-chest resuscitation should be accompanied by greater changes in arterial pressures, cardiac output, and vital organ perfusion. To increase intrathoracic pressure during closed-chest resuscitation, several techniques have been studied.

Simultaneous Chest Compression and Lung Ventilation (SCV-CPR)

Simultaneous compression of the sternum and positive pressure ventilation (producing peak airway pressures of 40 to 120 mm Hg) has been shown to improve cardiac output and cerebral perfusion during cardiac arrest and closed-chest resuscitation. Cerebral blood flow is dramatically improved, but myocardial blood flow is largely unaffected. A recently completed clinical trial has demonstrated that this technique offers no advantage over conventional CPR in the pre-hospital setting.

Abdominal Binding During Closed-Chest CPR

Tightly binding the abdomen with a pneumatic device (binder or military antishock garment) has been proposed as a means of improving cerebral perfusion during CPR. The efficacy of such an intervention has never been assessed using measurements of regional cerebral perfusion. Based on recent observations, abdominal binding should increase intrathoracic pressure during CPR chest compression by limiting the extent of diaphragmatic excursion. Observations made in the experimental laboratory should be considered preliminary at best. Several studies suggest that abdominal binding may impede effective ventilation, especially when endotracheal intubation and controlled volume ventilation are not available. In my opinion, abdominal binding using a specifically designed abdominal binder or a pneumatic antishock garment is contraindicated based on current available information.

Interposed Abdominal Compression CPR (IAC-CPR)

Manual compression of the abdominal cavity during CPR systole (CPR chest relaxation phase) has been proposed as a means of improving systemic perfusion during cardiac arrest. Direct and indirect measurements of cerebral blood flow and cardiac output in animal models support such a contention via poorly substantiated mechanisms. Although a CPR diastolic "counter pressure" effect has been suggested, it has not been well supported in the in vivo model. The technique does not substantially

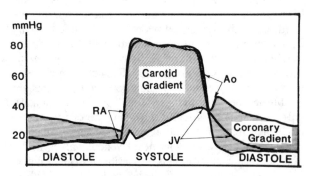

Figure 1 Pressures generated during CPR. RA = right atrium; JV = jugular vein; Ao = aorta. (From Cheng TO, ed. International practice of cardiology. New York: Pergamon Press, 1986.)

TABLE 1 Effects of Modified CPR Techniques in Animal Models

	Arterial Pressure	Cardiac Output	Cerebral Perfusion	Myocardial Perfusion
Simultaneous compression-ventilation CPR (SCV-CPR)	↑	↑	↑	NC
Abdominal binding during conventional CPR	↑	↑ or NC	↑	NS
Abdominal counterpulsation during conventional CPR (IAC-CPR)	↑	↑	↑	NC
Military antishock trousers during CPR (MAST-CPR)	↑	NS	NS	NS
Volume loading during conventional CPR	↑	↑	↓	↓
High-impulse CPR	↑	↑	↑	↑
Pneumatic CPR (vest and binder CPR)	↑	↑	↑	NC

↑ = increased; ↓ = decreased; NC = no change; NS = not studied.
From Cheng TO, ed. International practice of cardiology. New York: Pergamon Press, 1986.

improve artificial myocardial perfusion in a well-studied animal model. In a recently completed clinical trial in human victims of sudden prehospital cardiac death this new CPR technique did not significantly affect outcome when compared to closed-chest CPR as currently practiced.

Volume Loading During CPR

Intravenous volume loading during cardiac arrest and closed-chest CPR has theoretic advantage according to the traditional theory of blood flow during CPR. However, controlled observations in the experimental laboratory using state-of-the-art measurement techniques suggests that such an intervention may be detrimental. Intravenous volume loading improves left heart output, but decreases systemic arterial-venous perfusion gradients owing to a greater rise in venous pressure than in arterial pressure. The increased cardiac output is shunted to nonvital organs. Volume loading closed-chest CPR would appear to be contraindicated in the typical victim of pre- or inhospital nontraumatic cardiac arrest.

Sustained Pressor Infusion During Closed-Chest CPR

The use of alpha-adrenergic agonists has been shown to be beneficial in the management of cardiac arrest since the early 1960s. Several recent studies confirm that alpha-agonist agents are beneficial. No agent has been shown to be superior to epinephrine. Whether epinephrine is better given by infusion than as bolus, and in doses larger than currently used, is not known for certain, although preliminary studies suggest this is the case. The beneficial effect of alpha-agonists appears to be directly related to their increase of peripheral arterial tone and the myocardial perfusion gradient during CPR. Conversely, the use of beta-agonists (e.g., isoproterenol) is contraindicated based on available controlled experimental studies since such agents decrease peripheral vascular resistance, lower coronary perfusion pressure, and worsen outcome.

CARDIAC ARREST AND REPERFUSION TISSUE INJURY

A number of experimental studies suggest that ischemic damage may continue after restoration of circulation (reperfusion). Postreperfusion injury may substantially contribute to morbidity and mortality after seemingly successful cardiac resuscitation.

Postreperfusion injury largely results from the generation of hydroxyl and free-radicals after restoration of spontaneous circulation. Free-radical generation may produce lipid peroxidation, cell wall injury, altered cellular metabolism, and cell death. Appropriate interventions in the postreperfusion cellular cascade leading to cell death in the intact organism could substantially improve outcome of cardiac arrest without a modification in closed-chest CPR technique. Selected experimental models suggest that calcium-blocking agents, drugs that inhibit eicosanoid metabolism, and drugs that serve as free-radical scavengers may be of value in attentuating the postreperfusion syndrome. At present, the use of such therapeutic interventions must be considered experimental since there are insufficient data to support their use in the clinical population.

ROLE OF OPEN-CHEST CPR IN NONTRAUMATIC CARDIAC ARREST

Open-chest CPR and direct manual ventricular compression produce greater systemic perfusion during cardiac arrest than do conventional closed-chest techniques. The role and efficacy of more frequent use of the open chest technique in our contemporary frame of practice has yet to be determined.

In my opinion, the early use of electrical countershock for ventricular fibrillation will be effective regardless of the use of the open- or closed-chest artificial circulatory support technique. If early electrical defibrillation is not immediately available, there are no data to suggest that late use of open-chest CPR will improve outcome from pre-hospital or in-hospital cardiac arrest. Likewise, the efficacy of open-chest CPR in the management of cardiac arrest due to asystolic or pulseless idioventricular rhythms has not been established.

ISCHEMIC BRAIN INJURY

BLAINE C. WHITE, M.D.

In this chapter, ischemic brain injury is addressed primarily from the viewpoint of the complete ischemic-anoxic insult that occurs with cardiac arrest. Only about 5 percent of patients resuscitated from pre-hospital cardiac arrest ultimately go home neurologically intact; 50 to 60 percent of in-hospital deaths after resuscitation are related to neurologic injury, and thus this is a major clinical problem.

The insult of complete ischemic anoxia should be recognized as fundamentally different from that of primary anoxia (e.g. caused by airway obstruction) and severe incomplete ischemia (brain perfusion greater than 0 and less than 25 percent normal). In these latter two insults, the biochemical picture (to be described) is complicated both by somewhat longer persistence of significant ATP content and by the development of profound tissue acidosis due to a continuing supply of glucose in the face of inadequate oxygenation. Ischemic brain injury progresses through three phases: (1) ischemic phase, (2) early reperfusion phase, and (3) late reperfusion phase.

ISCHEMIC PHASE

Since the brain has limited stores of glucose or glycogen, initiation of complete ischemic anoxia is followed immediately by a precipitous decline in tissue ATP levels. These levels approach zero within 5 minutes. Degradation of the adenine to hypoxanthine accompanies this. About 80 percent of the brain's ATP is used to maintain ionic gradients (expressed in mM) across the cell membrane for K (130 in to 4 out), Na (5 in to 140 out), and Ca (10^{-5} in to 1 out). Therefore, it is not surprising that these also decay rapidly during complete ischemic anoxia. Equilibration of these ions between the interstitial and cytosolic fluid occurs within 5 to 10 minutes of the insult.

The accumulation of calcium during the insult appears to be the major trigger for the subsequent events leading to ultimate cell death. The greatly elevated cytosolic calcium levels result in the activation of membrane phospholipase and the accumulation of free fatty acids (FFA) during ischemia. The predominant FFA released is arachidonate. The high calcium loads also result in the conversion of normal xanthine dehydrogenase to xanthine oxidase in the endothelial cells by proteolytic cleavage during ischemia.

Thus the situation at the end of 10 to 15 minutes of complete ischemic anoxia in the brain includes ATP levels near zero, elevated hypoxanthine levels, moderate lactic acidosis, equilibrated transmembrane ionic gradients, activated phospholipase, elevated FFA and especially arachidonic acid, and the presence of the abnormal enzyme xanthine oxidase.

EARLY REPERFUSION

During the early phase of reperfusion at normal arterial pressures, brain blood flow is characterized by global hyperperfusion with scattered patches of poor reperfusion. Within 1 hour, global brain perfusion has dropped to levels of 20 to 40 percent of normal, where it remains for as long as 2 to 3 days. This is known as the progressive hypoperfusion phenomenon during reperfusion. This hypoperfusion phenomenon is inhibited by postresuscitation treatment with calcium antagonists such as flunarizine and nimodipine.

During early reperfusion, ATP recovers rapidly. If the duration of the ischemic insult is less than 20 minutes, the membrane ionic gradients also recover quickly. After much longer insults of 1 hour, total tissue calcium loads actually increase during reperfusion.

Arachidonic acid is rapidly metabolized via oxidation reactions by both cycloxygenase and lipoxygenase. The prostaglandins are the products of cycloxygenase, and the leukotrienes are the products of lipoxygenase. The production of the vasodilative prostaglandin, prostacyclin, is severely inhibited during early reperfusion. Thus, vasospastic compounds predominate in the leukotriene and prostaglandin products. Although the free arachidonic acid levels rapidly return to baseline during reperfusion, leukotrienes remain elevated for at least 24 hours. Since these products may be formed by nonenzymatic lipid peroxidation, it is currently believed that this process occurs during reperfusion.

There is a massive delocalization of iron from normal high-molecular-weight species to species weighing less than 30,000 daltons during the first 2 hours of reperfusion following a 15-minute cardiac arrest. Cellular levels of "free" iron are normally less than 10 to 18. This reflects tight biological control of this bivalent cation that readily catalyzes nonenzymatic oxidation-reduction reactions. Iron is rapidly delocalized by reduction out of ferritin by a number of different radical species, including O_2-, paraquat, and Adriamycin. There is reason to believe that O_2- is excessively present during early reperfusion. The classic substrate for xanthine oxidase is hypoxanthine, which has accumulated from adenine degradation during ischemia. O_2- is a side product of xanthine oxidase, lipoxygenase, and cycloxygenase, all of which are clearly active during early reperfusion. Moreover, brain mitochondrial superoxide dismutase is reduced to approximately 50 percent of normal during 15 minutes of complete ischemic anoxia.

Availability of a transitional metal, such as iron, is required for lipid peroxidation to occur, through formation of either the hydroxyl radical or perferryl species. Evidence of lipid peroxidation may be measured by assay of malondialdehyde, lipid conjugated dienes, or by demonstration of a loss of unsaturated fatty acids in the system. Malondialdehyde and conjugated dienes are elevated about 50 percent after 2 hours of reperfusion following a 15-minute cardiac arrest and resuscitation. However, at this time, brain tissue ionic content appears to be normal, and loss of unsaturated fatty acids is not yet evident. The iron chelator deferoxamine, when administered immediately postresuscitation, returns tissue concentrations of malondialdehyde and conjugated dienes to normal after 2 hours of reperfusion.

LATE EVENTS DURING REPERFUSION

After 4 hours of reperfusion following a 15-minute cardiac arrest, brain tissue ionic concentrations remain indistinguishable from normal. After 8 hours of reperfusion, the tissue iron is recovered into high-molecular-weight species. However, by this time, large shifts of the concentrations of CA, K, and Na have occurred. These shifts most likely reflect equilibration between the cytosol and the interstitial fluid for these ions. Malondialdehyde concentrations are about eight times normal, and there is a 35 percent loss of the total unsaturated fatty acids. Electron microscopic examination of brains fixed in vivo by bypass perfusion reveals an obvious general degradation of membrane structure and large holes in the nuclear and cytoplasmic membranes. This picture is consistent with ongoing membrane injury during reperfusion by mechanisms such as lipid peroxidation. This would produce degradation of membrane structure to the point that the membrane becomes freely permeable to ions.

Both deferoxamine and exogenously administered superoxide dismutase significantly inhibit malondialdehyde accumulation. However, only deferoxamine appears to retard the loss of unsaturated fatty acids and protect tissue Na/K ratios. We have found that the calcium antagonist flunarizine has no effect on products of lipid peroxidation, ultrastructural injury, or ionic gradient decay.

Considerable ultrastructural injury persists after 8 hours of reperfusion in animals treated with deferoxamine. This finding, the persistence of elevated leukotrienes, and the fact that deferoxamine treatment has not completely inhibited malondialdehyde accumulation after 8 hours reperfusion, have led to a reexamination of the possibility of continuing phospholipase activation during reperfusion. Lipid hydroperoxides, an intermediate product of lipid peroxidation, are powerful stimulators of phospholipase activity. Chloropromazine is a phospholipase inhibitor and has been found to have ultrastructural and biochemical protective effects in postischemic studies of the heart, kidney, liver, and isolated mitochondrial preparations. Examination of this agent alone and in combination with deferoxamine is currently under way.

CLINICAL IMPLICATIONS

The foregoing paragraphs indicate the complex nature of ischemic injury in the brain. However, the pattern of ATP and ionic recovery and the late decay of the ionic gradients during reperfusion suggest that there is probably a significant therapeutic time frame following reperfusion. Appropriate therapy during this time may minimize or prevent ultimate brain injury following resuscitation from even prolonged cardiac arrest. The biochemical sequence of brain injury from complete ischemic anoxia, as already described, represents a biomedical engineering problem of multiple dimensions. An effective therapeutic response to this problem can only be defined by urgent continuation of these studies. Such intervention will almost certainly involve a multiple-drug protocol. Clinical trials of single-drug regimens, in view of the pathochemistry and pathophysiology, are almost certainly doomed to negative outcomes, as has been the case, for example, with barbiturates. Such trials should perhaps be deferred until the pathologic picture is better defined and treatment protocols providing unequivocal benefit over a wide range of ischemic durations are identified.

In the meantime, the clinician can only rely on the known basics of brain protection—adequate but not excessive and maintenance of adequate vascular perfusion pressure. Despite a variety of studies in the literature on both new and old calcium-channel blockers, and on deferoxamine, none of these mechanisms or drugs is well enough understood to warrant therapeutic use. The clinician must stick to the basics and await the results of more exhaustive research and clinical trials.

SUGGESTED READING

Krause GS, et al. Ischemia, resuscitation, and reperfusion: mechanisms of tissue injury and prospects for protection. Am Heart J 1986; 111:768–780.

CRITERIA FOR WITHHOLDING EMERGENCY RESUSCITATION

BERNARD LO, M.D.

Cardiopulmonary resuscitation (CPR) and advanced cardiac life support may be effective treatment for unexpected sudden death. Between 20 and 40 percent of patients who suffer cardiac arrest outside the hospital are resuscitated successfully by bystanders and paramedics. However, in the emergency department questions often arise over whether it is appropriate to continue or start CPR. In some patients, CPR may seem medically futile. In addition, CPR is not appropriate for patients with terminal or chronic progressive illness whose death is expected. Guidelines have been established for "do not resuscitate" (DNR) or "no code" orders for inpatients in hospitals. In the emergency department decisions about withholding CPR are more difficult than in the acute care hospital, since information about the patient may be incomplete and there is little opportunity to gather further information. In case of uncertainty, CPR should be given.

PRIOR ARRANGEMENTS FOR WITHHOLDING CPR

Ethical and legal guidelines may guide decisions about withholding CPR. Any medical treatment may be withheld if an informed, competent patient refuses it. A competent, informed patient may indicate that he would not want CPR in case of cardiopulmonary arrest or would not want intubation and mechanical ventilation in case of respiratory failure. Usually, patients who refuse CPR or intubation have chronic or terminal illness. It is medically and ethically appropriate for care-givers to respect such refusal of CPR. For patients who have not expressed preferences while competent, the family may decide that treatment such as CPR is not in the patient's best interest.

Such general guidelines may be difficult to apply to particular patients in the emergency department. Emergency and paramedic personnel usually do not have information from the medical record, primary physician, and family members. Oral reports by family members or on-call physicians about "no code" orders may not be accurate. Emergency department staff who do not know the family or primary physician may not be sure that DNR orders were appropriately made. For example, the patient may not have been truly informed, or the family of an incompetent patient may have a conflict of interest with the patient. These practical problems with DNR orders may be addressed on a local level. Emergency departments, paramedic services, and organizations such as hospices and nursing homes in a referral area may wish to develop guidelines and standard forms for DNR orders. The durable power of attorney for health care may be a feasible method in some states for patients to ensure that their wishes against CPR are respected.

Futility Of Treatment

Another appropriate reason to withhold treatment is that the treatment is medically futile, with virtually no chance of success. Again, this general principle may be difficult to apply to decisions about resuscitation in the emergency department. Formerly, many patients were considered "dead on arrival." Resuscitation was not attempted because of the clinical judgment that CPR would not be successful. Although all would agree that CPR on a patient who has already undergone rigor mortis is futile, the American Heart Association suggests that in most cases the concept of "dead on arrival" may be an anachronism. Observers may not accurately report the time elapsed since the cardiac arrest or may not act in good faith. An apparently dead patient who has ingested drugs, who is hypothermic, or who has been struck by lightning can sometimes be successfully resuscitated even after prolonged efforts.

There are few sound clinical guidelines that identify patients for whom CPR would be futile. One prospective study found that no patient with metastatic cancer, pneumonia, acute stroke, or oliguria who suffered cardiac arrest in an acute care hospital was discharged alive after successful CPR. However, these findings have not been confirmed in other studies; in particular, they have not been validated in an emergency department. Moreover, their usefulness in the emergency department is limited because the patient's diagnosis may not be known at the time of the cardiac arrest.

Patients with asystole or electromechanical dissociation or traumatic cardiac arrest may have a low survival rate compared to those with ventricular fibrillation; nonetheless, some are successfully resuscitated. The likelihood of survival decreases as the time from arrest to initiation of CPR and advanced cardiac life support increases and as the duration of resuscitation increases. But there is no cut-off point that accurately separates patients who will die or have irreversible coma, even with maximal care, from those patients who have a chance of functional recovery. Other clinical variables, such as the age of the patient, serum chemistry tests, or nonreactive pupils during the arrest, do not accurately predict that further resuscitation would be futile. Even more sophisticated tests, such as an electroencephalogram (EEG) during the arrest, do not accurately identify patients who will not regain consciousness, since drug effects may confound the interpretation of EEGs. Even if tests like EEGs were completely accurate, halting resuscitation to run them would not be indicated.

POSSIBILITY OF BRAIN DAMAGE

A common reason to consider withholding CPR or advanced cardiac life support is the concern that severe irreversible brain damage has already occurred. Even if the heart is successfully resuscitated, the patient may remain in an irreversible coma or a persistent vegetative state. However, there are no reliable clinical guidelines for predicting neurologic outcome during resuscitation.

Taking a conservative position, the American Heart Association (AHA) syllabus about CPR recommends that only failure to restore circulation after basic and advanced cardiac life support is an appropriate criterion for stopping resuscitation efforts because of medical futility. The AHA, as cited by McIntyre, also points out the risk of legal liability:

> The argument that the patient could have collapsed ... and continued to have cardiac activity at a level sufficient to sustain the brain until the victim was rushed through the door of the emergency facility may be an insurmountable one. Armed with the experience that weak or slow pulses may be missed by inexperienced observers, a plaintiff's attorney may inquire as to the person upon whom the physician should reasonably rely as his witness to the onset and progression of the process of brain death.

It is not known whether these AHA recommendations are followed in practice. Anecdotal evidence suggests that resuscitative efforts may be terminated without applying all aspects of advanced cardiac life support. Moreover, it is not known whether these recommendations have adverse effects. If all patients in a poor-prognosis category receive maximal resuscitation but only a few patients obtain a good outcome, the resources of the emergency department may be inefficiently allocated, and other patients who may benefit more from the attention of the emergency department staff may be denied care.

LIMITED RESUSCITATION EFFORTS

The concern that resuscitation may lead to restoration of cardiac function in a patient who has suffered severe brain damage sometimes causes care-givers to consider intermediate steps between full resuscitation and a DNR order. Such efforts are variously called "limited," "slow," or "partial" codes. CPR is initiated, but drugs are not administered, intubation is not performed, and resuscitation is stopped after a predetermined period of time. However, the possibility of severe brain damage does not justify such "limited" codes, because the chance of successful resuscitation is compromised. The American Heart Association points out that even if basic CPR has failed, advanced cardiac life support, with administration of sodium bicarbonate, epinephrine, and other medications, may be successful. However, limited codes are appropriate if the patient had agreed to them. For example, a patient with severe chronic obstructive lung disease may not want intubation and mechanical ventilation in case of respiratory failure. Limited codes are sometimes intended to reassure the family that "everything was done." However, perfunctory CPR cannot be justified, since it offers no benefit to the patient and causes cynicism among the medical and nursing staff.

STOPPING RESUSCITATION

After resuscitation has been started or continued in the emergency department, care-givers may get additional information about the patient's wishes. They may learn, for instance, that a DNR decision had been appropriately made. With such additional information, it is appropriate to stop resuscitation. In some cases, the patient may have been successfully resuscitated but requires pressor agents or mechanical ventilation by the time care-givers learn about the DNR order. It is ethically, medically, and legally appropriate to respect the patient's wishes and discontinue life-sustaining treatment that has already been started. However, care-givers may be emotionally reluctant to discontinue life-sustaining treatment, even though they would have been willing not to start the treatment in the first place had they known the patient's preferences. Because of such reactions, it may be advisable in some cases for the patient's attending physician personally to turn off medications or disconnect the ventilator rather than require nurses or other physicians to do so.

After CPR is withheld or discontinued and the patient dies, the care-givers face the difficult task of talking with the family. Although this job is stressful for care-givers, spending time with relatives, providing emotional support, and helping with practical arrangements may help the survivors to deal with their grief.

SUGGESTED READING

American College of Emergency Physicians. Medical, moral, legal, and ethical aspects of resuscitation for the patient who will have minimal ability to function or ultimately survive. Ann Emerg Med 1985; 14:919–926.

Bedell SE, Delbanco TL, Cook EF, Epstein FH. Survival after cardiopulmonary resuscitation in the hospital. N Engl J Med 1983; 309:579–586.

Cummins RW, Eisenberg MS. Prehospital cardiopulmonary resuscitation: is it effective? JAMA 1985; 253:2408–2412.

Lo B, Steinbrook RS. Deciding whether to resuscitate. Arch Intern Med 1983; 143:1561–1563.

McIntyre KM. Medicolegal aspects of cardiopulmonary resuscitation (CPR) and emergency cardiac care (ECC). In: Mc Intyre KM, Lewis AJ. Textbook of advanced cardiac life support. American Heart Association, 1983.

Miles SH, Crimmins TJ. Orders to limit emergency treatment for an ambulance service in a large metropolitan area. JAMA 1985; 254:525–527.

MONITORING IN THE EMERGENCY DEPARTMENT

STEVEN C. DRONEN, M.D.

Critically ill patients, in many cases, experience the most acute phase of their illnesses while in the emergency department. Appropriate therapeutic interventions in these patients require assessment of variables such as the adequacy of oxygenation, ventilation, perfusion, and circulating blood volume. In some situations, monitoring of standard parameters such as the cardiac rhythm, arterial blood gases (ABGs), and blood pressure provides precise information on which reasonable clinical decisions can be based. Unfortunately, this is not always the case. Often the measurement of variables in the emergency department is relatively unsophisticated and results reflect imprecisely or indirectly the patient's true clinical state.

ARRHYTHMIAS

Continuous electrocardiographic monitoring of patients for the development of arrhythmias is commonplace in most emergency departments. It is simple, noninvasive, and relatively inexpensive and thus should be used liberally in patients at potential risk for the development of arrhythmias. This may include patients with chest pain, those with a potentially unstable cardiovascular status, and those with significant respiratory distress. Although it seems self-evident, it should be stressed that it does little good to provide continuous electrocardiographic monitoring if a system does not exist for the detection and prompt treatment of arrhythmias displayed on the oscilloscope.

BLOOD PRESSURE

Blood pressure (BP) is among the most common parameters monitored in critically ill patients, owing to the frequency with which it is abnormal and the ease with which it can be measured. A normal adult blood pressure is 120/80 mm Hg, but there is considerable variation. Young adults may have systolic pressures as low as 90 mm Hg. This increases with age to an upper limit of 160 mm Hg. Diastolic pressures are generally in the range of 60 to 100 mm Hg. The difference between systolic and diastolic pressures is the pulse pressure, and it may range from 30 to 50 mm Hg. Pulse pressure is a much better indicator of the adequacy of perfusion than either the systolic or the diastolic pressure. Significant changes in pulse pressure may accompany small and easily overlooked changes in blood pressure. This is particularly true of hypovolemic patients, in whom a falling pulse pressure is often the first sign of hypovolemia.

Blood pressure is maintained by the complex interaction of myocardial contractility, vascular tone, circulating blood volume, and various hormonal and neuroregulatory mechanisms. It is therefore subject to change in a host of pathophysiologic states including cir-

culatory failure, hypovolemia, central nervous system disorders, drug effect, and abnormal sympathetic discharge. There is little question that in many instances the BP provides useful information on which to base clinical decisions, but its value as a monitoring tool should not be overestimated. Blood pressure data are apt to be misleading, particularly when used in the evaluation of patients with suspected blood loss or those in shock. There are abundant data to show that blood pressure may be maintained in the normal range despite significant falls in cardiac output and tissue perfusion. In the hypovolemic patient, blood pressure is maintained through increases in heart rate and systemic vascular resistance, falls only after these compensatory mechanisms have been exhausted. Previously healthy patients may not experience a fall in systolic pressure until 20 to 25 percent of blood volume is lost. Paradoxically, diastolic pressure may rise owing to constriction of venous capacitance vessels. There is frequently a poor correlation between blood pressure and the more sophisticated indices of circulating blood volume and tissue perfusion. Thus, blood pressure should not be used as a primary index of the adequacy of resuscitation or restoration of circulating blood volume.

There are no set standards to determine the optimal frequency of blood pressure monitoring. In practice, the frequency varies considerably with the severity of the illness and the potential for sudden change. In the asymptomatic, acutely hypertensive patient, measurements every 30 to 60 minutes may suffice. However, in patients who are experiencing any degree of hemodynamic instability or are undergoing therapeutic intervention intended to rapidly change blood pressure, monitoring may need to be frequent or even continuous. The latter permits any changes to be documented as they occur. Continuous monitoring is of value in a number of clinical situations including hypertensive emergencies, shock of any cause, dissecting aneurysm, and head injury associated with hypertension.

The basic principles of blood pressure monitoring have not changed significantly since Korotkoff's original description. There have been technologic advances that permit measurement of arterial pressures continuously and without the use of a stethoscope. Automated pneumatic cuffs measure blood pressure noninvasively and at frequent intervals. They are of limited value in critically ill patients owing to their inaccuracy, particularly in the hypotensive range. Even when measured with a stethoscope, there is considerable potential for inaccurate blood pressure measurement in hypotensive patients. Moreover, frequent manual measurement is a laborious process.

These problems can be circumvented by direct intraarterial measurement with an indwelling catheter, generally placed in the radial artery. This site is generally chosen because of its accessibility, despite the fact that radial artery systolic pressure may be higher than aortic systolic pressure. However, mean radial artery pressure does correlate well with mean aortic pressure. Placement in the femoral artery is acceptable in an acute situation, but the issues of hygiene and access limit its usefulness as a long-term catheterization site.

Intra-arterial blood pressure monitoring requires a higher level of nursing care and technical skill than do simple noninvasive methods. Additionally, it is more expensive. However, it is the most reliable and accurate method of blood pressure determination in the critically ill patient, and therefore its use in the emergency department should be encouraged. Although the indications are not absolute, it should be considered (1) for hypotensive patients (in whom other methods are inaccurate), (2) when the potential for sudden change in pressures exists, and (3) during infusion of vasoactive drugs. Intra-arterial monitoring is particularly appropriate in those patients receiving either antihypertensive or vasopressor agents by the intravenous route.

CENTRAL VENOUS PRESSURE

In 1962 Wilson described central venous pressure (CVP) monitoring as a means of assessing the circulating blood volume. Subsequently the CVP was widely used as an index of the adequacy of resuscitation from severe hemorrhage and other hypovolemic states. Rapid acceptance of the CVP as a monitoring tool was based on the relative ease with which it is measured. Normal values are 4 to 10 cm H_2O when measured at end expiration, although there is some variation. Wilson was careful to point out in his initial description that there are not absolute CVP values that correlate with hypo- or hypervolemia. Trends in CVP values and responses to specific therapeutic interventions provide more information than absolute values.

The early use of CVP as a means of assessing blood volume led to a rather simplistic view of the process by which it is generated. Although certainly dependent on blood volume, CVP is also influenced by right and left ventricular function, vasomotor tone, intrathoracic pressure, pulmonary artery pressure, and drug administration. Because there are many factors that influence CVP, change in one factor is not always directly reflected by a proportional change in CVP. It does not necessarily correlate well with blood volume; nor do right-sided pressures consistently follow left-sided pressures. The latter statement is particularly true in patients with preexisting cardiopulmonary disease. In patients with cardiogenic or septic shock, CVP does not correlate with pulmonary artery wedge pressure (PAWP). The latter index is clearly more sensitive to changes in left ventricular function and blood volume.

The variation in normal and abnormal CVP values and the lack of correlation with more sophisticated measurements have led many clinicians to abandon the technique. This is unfortunate because more sophisticated monitoring tools such as right heart catheterization are not practical in most emergency departments. Furthermore, the CVP does provide useful information in specific clinical situations if one avoids the assumption that it is a substitute for the PAWP and is careful not to attach significance to any particular value. Rather, the pattern of change that occurs with therapeutic intervention should be used to guide further therapy.

Indications for CVP monitoring include the following: (1) massive volume replacement in hypovolemic shock, (2) volume replacement in hypovolemic patients with frail cardiovascular status, and (3) suspected cardiac tamponade. CVP monitoring is particularly useful during volume reinfusion early in the management of hypovolemic shock. Although it has been shown that absolute CVP values do not correlate with measured blood volume, a rise in the CVP from baseline values is generally seen in association with adequate volume reinfusion. Serial measurement of the CVP following administration of a fluid challenge is helpful in assessing the volume status, particularly in elderly and debilitated patients. A rise in the CVP of 5 cm H_2O 10 minutes after a fluid challenge is presumptive evidence that a patient is not hypovolemic; a rise in pulse pressure but not CVP suggests hypovolemia. The technique is not sufficiently sensitive to determine optimal fluid therapy. Measurements of cardiac output and blood volume are the preferred techniques, and these are best performed in the intensive care unit. Finally, CVP should be monitored in any patient suspected of having an acute pericardial tamponade. The rise in CVP above normal levels is one of the most sensitive indicators of the presence of an acute effusion.

Measurement of the CVP is not difficult. A thin flexible catheter is threaded into the superior vena cava (SVC) following percutaneous cannulation of the subclavian, or the internal jugular, or the antecubital vein. Right-sided internal jugular or supraclavicular subclavian vein cannulation is preferred because either route provides the most direct route to the SVC and minimizes the risk of catheter malposition.

URINE OUTPUT

Urine output is dependent on maintenance of renal blood flow and is therefore an indirect measure of the adequacy of perfusion. A drop in renal blood flow triggers release of aldosterone, which causes active tubular reabsorption of sodium and, secondarily, water. Release of antidiuretic hormone by the posterior pituitary is increased during low flow states, thereby causing increased water reabsorption. Thus, a decreased cardiac output is reflected in a urine output below the normal value of 0.5 to 1.0 ml per kilogram per hour.

Measurement of urine output is useful in patients with normal renal function who are not receiving diuretics. Placement of a urinary catheter and closed collection system permit accurate measurement over a fixed time interval, generally 30 to 60 minutes in the acute setting. Measurements at more frequent intervals are of questionable value because the kidney responds slowly to changes in perfusion. Failure to demonstrate any urine output is rare and suggests either an occluded or improperly positioned catheter.

ARTERIAL BLOOD GASES

Arterial blood gases contain a wealth of information about oxygenation, ventilation, and acid-base status and should be routinely monitored in most critically ill patients. This may be facilitated by the placement of an arterial line, particularly in patients admitted to an intensive care unit who would otherwise require repetitive arterial puncture. (See also chapters on *Metabolic Acidosis* and *Acute Respiratory Failure*.)

NONINVASIVE OXIMETRY

A recent advance in the monitoring of critically ill patients has been the ability to measure oxygen diffusing from capillary beds across the skin or conjunctiva. Transcutaneous and transconjunctival oxygen tensions ($PtcO_2$ and $PcjO_2$, respectively) are measured by the application of a modified Clark polarographic electrode to the skin or conjunctival surface. In healthy adult volunteers, $PtcO_2$ is about 80 percent and $PcjO_2$ is about 60 percent of simultaneous arterial oxygen tension (PaO_2). However, during periods of impaired tissue perfusion, these ratios fall in a predictable fashion. This limits the usefulness of these parameters as substitutes for PaO_2 in critically ill patients, but makes them accurate indicators of the adequacy of peripheral perfusion. Several studies have shown that the fall in $PtcO_2$ and $PcjO_2$ occurs early during hypoperfusion states and, most importantly, before changes in other commonly monitored parameters such as blood pressure.

Furthermore, these noninvasively measured oxygen tensions correlate well with other sensitive indicators of tissue perfusion, particularly cardiac output and oxygen delivery.

Noninvasive oximetry is ideally suited to the emergency department because it provides rapid, reliable, and continuous information. Its primary limitation as a monitoring tool is that it measures the end product of several different physiologic processes, including respiratory insufficiency, decreased cardiac output, hypovolemia, and increased vasoconstriction. Other parameters must be followed simultaneously in order to interpret the cause of an abnormal $PtcO_2$ or $PcjO_2$.

SUGGESTED READING

Dronen SC, Maningas PA, Foutch R. Transcutaneous oxygen tension during graded hemorrhage and reinfusion. Ann Emerg Med 1985; 14:534–539.

Morris AH, Chapman RH, Gardner RM. Frequency of technical problems encountered in the measurement of pulmonary artery wedge pressure. Crit Care Med 1984; 12:164–170.

Shippy CR, Appel PL, Shoemaker WC. Reliability of clinical monitoring to assess blood volume in critically ill patients. Crit Care Med 1984; 12:107–112.

Wilson JN, Grow JB, Demong CV, et al. Central venous pressure in optimal blood volume maintenance. Arch Surg 1962; 85:563–577.

APPROACH TO THE PATIENT IN SHOCK

EDWARD ABRAHAM, M.D.

Although hypotension has usually been included in the definition of shock, shock is best defined simply as a generalized decrease in perfusion and oxygen delivery to central organ systems and peripheral tissues. This limited definition of shock based on perfusion abnormalities correlates well with clinical situations in which a patient has a normal blood pressure, but clearly is physiologically unstable. For example, it is not unusual for a patient who has sustained multiple trauma to present with normal blood pressure even though the extremities are cold and mottled, the urine flow is decreased, and mentation is abnormal as a result of massive intra-abdominal or intrathoracic hemorrhage.

Decrease in tissue oxgenation can result from low cardiac output or from diminished oxygen content in the blood owing to hypoxemia or to decreased hemoglobin. Hemorrhage produces abnormalities in oxygen delivery to the tissues because both cardiac output and arterial blood oxygen content decrease; hypovolemia results in decreased ventricular filling volumes and decreased car-

diac output, whereas the anemia resulting from blood loss diminishes the oxygen-carrying capacity of the blood. Nontraumatic causes of diminished tissue oxygenation include decreased cardiac output during or after a myocardial infarction, chronic anemia, and hypoxemia from pulmonary diseases such as chronic obstructive lung disease or asthma.

Although cellular function can be maintained at minimal levels during hypoperfusion through utilization of anaerobic metabolic pathways, this is a physiologically unstable state that eventually results in cell death as energy stores are depleted and cell waste products accumulate. The therapy of shock states therefore is aimed at detecting and reversing these abnormalities in tissue perfusion and cellular metabolism at the earliest point possible.

DIAGNOSIS AND MONITORING

The sweaty, cold, clammy patient with anxious and confused mental state, peripheral cyanosis and mottling, decreased urine output, and hypotension is easy to recognize as being in shock. However, many cases are far more subtle, and it is critical to recognize them early.

The standard physiologic parameters followed in emergency medicine, namely the "vital signs," unfortunately are insensitive to abnormalities in clinical state.

For example, blood pressure does not start to fall until 30 percent of the total blood volume is lost. Similarly, heart rate is inaccurate in detecting hypovolemia, since many patients presenting to the emergency department have tachycardia as a result of pain or fear, making it difficult to detect the patient whose tachycardia is a result of blood loss. In the elderly, tachycardia may never occur because of sinoatrial node, autonomic, or conduction system dysfunction. In patients with diminished cardiac output as a result of myocardial infarction, it is not unusual to find a normal blood pressure even when cardiac output is only 60 percent of normal. Orthostatic vital signs are commonly used as a measure of hypovolemia (and by inference, shock), but are both insensitive and nonspecific (see chapter on *Orthostatic Hypotension*).

The invasive monitoring modalities used in intensive care units, such as pulmonary artery (Swan-Ganz) catheters, can measure cardiac output, left ventricular filling pressures, and mixed venous oxygen saturation, providing direct determination of the state of tissue perfusion and oxygenation. Unfortunately, placement of these invasive monitoring devices often is time-consuming and not generally performed in the emergency department. Measurement of central venous pressure (CVP) has been advocated as a diagnostic modality in the emergency department. Unfortunately, CVP values normally are low (i.e., less than 5 mm Hg), and so finding a value near zero in a trauma patient does not necessarily imply hypovolemia. Similarly, although an elevated CVP value (i.e., greater than 10 mm Hg) is present in hypervolemia, such values also are seen in situations in which the myocardial wall stiffness is increased, either from intrinsic causes such as myocardial infarction or from extrinsic causes such as pericardial tamponade. Therefore, although CVP measurement may provide important diagnostic information in selected critically ill patients, it probably is not of great utility when used indiscriminately. CVP measurement may be useful when this variable is measured frequently in a critically ill patient during a therapeutic intervention. For example, an increase in CVP from 1 mm Hg to 10 mm Hg during fluid resuscitation in a trauma patient may indicate that intravascular volume has been restored and that infusion of additional fluids risks producing pulmonary edema.

The recent development of noninvasive probes capable of providing a continuous measurement of tissue oxygenation permits assessment of tissue perfusion and early detection of physiologic instability in emergency department patients. Transcutaneous and conjunctival oxygen monitors place miniaturized oxygen electrodes on either the skin or conjunctival surface. These surface electrodes monitor oxygenation of the tissues beneath them; a decrease in tissue oxygen from previously normal values (approximately 60 to 80 percent of arterial oxygen tension [PaO_2]) indicates decreased perfusion to the monitored peripheral site. In a multiple-trauma patient, a sudden fall in tissue oxygenation may signal continuing hemorrhage. In a patient with chest pain and electrocardiographic changes, decreasing tissue oxygen is consistent with a fall in cardiac output as a result of an extending myocardial infarction. Clinical studies indicate that conjunctival and transcutaneous oxygen sensors can detect physiologic instability much earlier than vital signs. For example, loss of 15 percent of total blood volume results in abnormal conjunctival oxygen values; blood pressure usually is normal with this degree of hemorrhage.

CAUSES OF SHOCK

Shock, with associated abnormalities in tissue perfusion and oxygenation, can result from decreased cardiac output or from maldistribution of blood flow and oxygen to tissues even though the cardiac output is normal or even increased. In cardiogenic shock, the primary abnormality is a diminished cardiac output. The decreased cardiac output in cardiogenic shock usually results from myocardial ischemia, such as a myocardial infarction, but also may be caused by viral or idiopathic cardiomyopathy, pericardial tamponade, or myocardial contusion after blunt chest trauma. The patient is diaphoretic, pale, and tachypneic, and may complain of dyspnea. On examination, signs of biventricular heart failure, with rales, jugular distention, S_3 gallop, and hepatojugular reflux, are present. An electrocardiogram may show changes consistent with ischemia, or if pericardial tamponade is present, diffusely decreased voltage may be found. Placement of a central venous catheter or pulmonary artery catheter reveals elevated right atrial and left ventricular pressures.

The primary abnormality in hemorrhagic shock is decreased intravascular volume. This decrease in intravascular volume results in diminished ventricular filling and low cardiac output. Patients with hemorrhagic shock are pale, clammy, and tachycardic. Physical examination is relatively normal except for localized findings related to the sites of hemorrhage, such as abdominal tenderness after a traumatic splenic rupture. Central venous and pulmonary artery pressures are low and therefore may not be significantly different from normal values. Tissue oxygen tension values, measured at transcutaneous or conjunctival sites, are abnormally low (less than 50 percent of the PaO_2). An anion gap and metabolic acidosis secondary to lactate production from tissue hypoperfusion may be present on laboratory testing, but these abnormalities are not specific for hemorrhagic shock and are seen with other forms of shock as well.

In early septic shock, cardiac output usually is elevated, but a marked abnormality (shunting) in delivery of oxygen to peripheral tissues is present. The patient frequently presents with warm extremities despite hypotension. However, if intravascular volume also is diminished because of diarrhea, vomiting, or poor intake, the skin may be cold and pale. Physical findings may be unremarkable, but rales frequently are present on chest auscultation as a result of the development of noncardiogenic pulmonary edema (i.e., adult respiratory distress syndrome [ARDS]). A fever may or may not be present. Central venous pressures are usually normal. Laboratory testing may reveal either an abnormally high or low white blood count and often an increase in the number of immature or "band" forms of neutrophils. Tissue oxygenation is low as measured at the conjunctiva or skin.

Placement of a thermodilution pulmonary artery catheter usually reveals elevated cardiac output and decreased peripheral vascular resistance after intravascular volume has been normalized.

Anaphylactic shock results primarily from the release of vasodilative mediators associated with the allergic reaction. Intravascular volume is normal, but because the intravascular compartment has been suddenly increased, hypotension results. The skin may be either warm or cold and clammy. Wheezes often are present on chest auscultation. The history usually reveals the diagnosis because the patient suddenly became ill after taking a new medication or eating a new food.

TREATMENT

Therapy in shock is aimed at correcting the abnormalities in tissue perfusion so that cellular metabolism can be restored to appropriate physiologic levels. It is important to realize that tissue metabolic rates that are adequate in the normal, unstressed subject are inadequate in the hypermetabolic, critically ill patient. Critically ill patients have substantially higher resting energy expenditures, oxygen consumption, and carbon dioxide production than do normal subjects.

The underperfused state associated with shock produces a significant oxygen debt in tissues that are forced to utilize anaerobic metabolism for maintaining cellular integrity and metabolic processes. Correction of this oxygen "debt" and achievement of levels of tissue metabolism appropriate in the critically ill patient therefore require resuscitation to substantially greater cardiac output and oxygen delivery and consumption than are found in "normal" subjects.

Tissue oxygen delivery can be improved by increasing cardiac output or by improving arterial blood oxygen content. Blood transfusion in trauma serves two important functions, since cardiac output is increased through intravascular volume expansion and the oxygen-carrying capacity of blood is improved by the addition of extra hemoglobin. Crystalloid or colloid resuscitation in the patient with hemorrhage improves tissue oxygen delivery only by augmenting cardiac output without increasing the already diminished blood oxygen content. Colloid solutions, such as 5 percent albumin or 6 percent hetastarch, produce greater expansion of intravascular volume per milliliter administered than do crystalloid solutions such as normal saline or Ringer's lactate. However, colloids are significantly more expensive than crystalloids and generally are not available for the prehospital resuscitation of shock patients.

The recent development of resuscitation solutions (e.g., fluorocarbons) capable of carrying more oxygen than crystalloid or colloid solutions may permit more effective field resuscitation of trauma victims. Crystalline hemoglobin solutions that require no refrigeration and maintain long shelf lives have been developed; these solutions also may have an important future role in resuscitating trauma victims. Both fluorocarbons and hemoglobin solutions produce increases in oxygen delivery by augmenting cardiac output and increasing the oxygen-carrying capacity of the blood.

The pneumatic antishock trousers (MAST suit) have been advocated for the initial resuscitation of trauma victims. Experimental and clinical studies suggest that this device produces an increase in blood pressure primarily by raising peripheral vascular resistance. There appears to be little or no "autotransfusion" effect, and studies on critically ill patients show no improvement in tissue oxygenation after pneumatic trouser inflation. Recent clinical data support the minimal physiologic benefit of pneumatic trousers, since no improvement in outcome for trauma victims in large urban centers is seen with MAST use. Limited beneficial effect of the pneumatic trousers does seem to result from their ability to 'tamponade" bleeding sites beneath the inflated garment.

Medical patients generally have shock and decreased tissue perfusion as a result of diminished cardiac function. The oxygen content of the blood often is normal in these patients, but the abnormal cardiac output is unable to project this well-oxygenated blood to the tissues. Therapy in such patients, suffering from conditions as myocardial infarction or sepsis, is directed toward improving cardiac function. Unless rales are present, the initial therapy almost always is intravascular fluids in order to improve ventricular filling and cardiac output through advancement up a Starling curve. If fluid therapy appears unsuccessful in reversing shock, then pharmacologic agents (i.e., inotropes) that increase cardiac function are indicated. Dopamine generally is the first agent used in this situation, and has predominately inotropic (beta) effects in low doses (less than 10 μg per kilogram per minute), but produces vasoconstriction (alpha) effects as the dose is increased. Dopamine is usually mixed as 400 mg or 800 mg in 500 ml of 5 percent dextrose in water (D5W) or 500 ml of normal saline, and the dose is rapidly titrated to optimize mean arterial blood pressure. Doses below 5 μg per kilogram per minute generally have pure inotropic effects, preserve or even enhance renal blood flow, and produce minimal vasoconstriction. As the dose is increased, vasoconstriction becomes more prominent, and at doses greater than 20 μg per kilogram per minute, vasoconstriction is marked.

Norepinephrine (i.e., Levophed) has both alpha and beta effects at all dose ranges. This agent is usually mixed as 4 mg or 8 mg in 250 ml D5W. The infusion rate is titrated to maintain adequate blood pressure. Vasoconstriction can be intense with norepinephrine, and prolonged periods at high dosages can result in ischemic damage to the kidney and other organs.

Dobutamine acts as a pure inotropic agent throughout its dosage range (i.e., 1 to 30 μg per kilogram per minute.) Because this drug has strong beta effects, vasodilation occurs, resulting in little change in blood pressure despite improvement of cardiac output. Therefore, although dobutamine may be the drug of choice in the mildly hypotensive patient with a myocardial infarction because of its minimal effects on myocardial oxygen consumption, the markedly hypotensive patient requires therapy with either dopamine or Levophed. Dobutamine usually is mixed as 500 mg in 500 ml D5W and titrated to maintain an adequate cardiac output. Because blood pressure changes are minimal, invasive hemodynamic monitioring with a thermodilution pulmonary artery (Swan-Ganz) catheter usually is required to monitor the effects of dobutamine. The dosage range required to optimize cardiac output in myocardial ischemia is approximately 5 to 15 μg per kilogram per minute.

SUGGESTED READING

Chernow B, Raiwey TG, Lake CR. Endogenous and exogenous catecholamines in critical care medicine. Crit Care Med 1982; 10:409–416.
Shoemaker WC. Pathophysiology and therapy of shock syndromes. In: Shoemaker WC, Thompson WL, Holbrook PR, eds. Texbook of critical care. Philadelphia: WB Saunders; 1984; 52.

HEMORRHAGIC SHOCK

DONALD D. TRUNKEY, M.D.

Hemorrhagic shock is the result of decreased blood volume due to acute and severe loss of blood. Hemorrhagic shock accounts for nearly all of the shock seen within the first 24 hours of injury; however, tissue injury may also contribute to the pathophysiology.

The pathophysiology can be divided into four phases. The first phase is the compensation phase and represents the first response of the circulation to hypovolemia. This is a contraction of the precapillary arterial sphincters and causes the filtration pressure in the capillaries to fall. Since osmotic pressure remains the same, fluid moves into the vascular space with a corresponding increase in blood volume. If this compensatory mechanism is adequate to return blood volume to normal, the capillary sphincters relax and microcirculatory flow returns to normal. If shock is prolonged and profound, the next phase is entered.

The cell distress phase occurs when vascular volume has not been restored, the precapillary sphincters remain closed, and arterial venous shunts open up to divert arterial blood directly back into the venous system, thus maintaining circulation to more important organs such as the heart and brain. The cells in the bypassed segment of the microcirculation must rely on anaerobic metabolism for energy. The amount of glucose and oxygen available for the cell decreases, and metabolic waste products such as lactate accumulate. Histamine is released, resulting in closure of the postcapillary sphincters, and this mechanism serves to slow the remaining capillary flow and hold the red blood cells and nutrients in the capillaries longer. The empty capillary constricts almost completely; few capillaries remain open.

The third phase is the decompensation phase. Just before cell death, local reflexes (probably initiated by acidosis and accumulated metabolites) reopen the precapillary sphincters while the postcapillary sphincters stay closed. Prolonged vasoconstriction of the capillary bed damages endothelial cells and results in increased capillary permeability. When the capillaries finally reopen, fluid and protein are leaked into the interstitial space, the capillaries distend with red blood cells, and sludging occurs. Cells become swollen, they are unable to utilize oxygen, and they die.

The recovery phase is the final phase and follows initiation of resuscitation. If blood volume is restored at some point in the decompensation phase, the effects on the microcirculation may still be reversible. Badly damaged cells may recover, and capillary integrity may be regained. The "sludge" in the microcirculation is swept into the venous circulation and eventually into the lungs, where these platelet and white cell aggregates are filtered out and contribute to postshock pulmonary failure. Other capillaries may be so badly damaged and filled with sludge that they remain permanently closed; cells dependent on these capillaries die.

DIAGNOSIS

The patient may progress through a series of signs and symptoms if the hemorrhage is moderate, such as from a ruptured spleen. However, if the hemorrhage is exsanguinating by the time the patient is first seen, he is in profound shock. In general, the patient progresses through symptoms reflecting redistribution of blood flow as mother nature tries to protect the heart and brain.

The first signs and symptoms of shock are reflected in the skin and muscle as peripheral hypoperfusion. The hands and feet become cool and even mottled with weak or impalpable pulses. One of the first things that I do when I see the patient is feel an extremity (Fig. 1). If the patient is cool and pale or capillary filling is delayed, shock is assumed to be present until proved otherwise. Then, as I turn to assess and treat the airway, I look at the neck veins (see Fig. 1). If neck veins are flat, shock is assumed to be hypovolemic until proved otherwise. If, on the other hand, neck veins are distended, five conditions must be ruled out immediately: tension pneumothorax, pericardial tamponade, air embolism, myocardial contusion, and myocardial infarction. (These conditions are discussed in other chapters.)

The next reliable signs of hypovolemia represent decreased blood flow to the viscera. The easiest viscus to monitor is the kidney, and this can be done by inserting a Foley catheter and monitoring urine output. Urine output should always be greater than 0.5 cc per kilogram per hour.

At approximately 30 to 35 percent blood volume depletion, the patient manifests signs of hypotension.

Systolic blood pressure drops below 90 mm Hg. Obviously this occurs earlier in the older patient who cannot compensate than it does in the young, healthy adult. Orthostatic vital signs should be measured if equivocal blood pressure readings are found, with the caveat that patients with suspected back injury should not have this test performed.

The final signs and symptoms of profound shock occur when there is no longer enough blood volume to maintain perfusion to the heart and brain. Monitoring of the heart tends to be unreliable since electrocardiographic changes are essentially nondiagnostic. The primary manifestations of this late phase of shock is altered mental status. Initially the patient becomes restless, then agitated, confused, and lethargic, progressing into coma and ultimate death. Agitation and confusion are common findings in the injured patient and may represent hypoxemia, hypovolemia, brain injury, or drug or alcohol intoxication. It cannot be overemphasized that the primary priority in treating the trauma patient with an altered state of consciousness is to recognize and treat hypoxemia and shock if present. The second priority is to recognize and treat brain damage. The physician should never ascribe an altered state of consciousness to brain damage or inebriation until hypoxemia and shock have been either ruled out or treated.

Nontraumatic causes of hemorrhagic shock are common and include upper gastrointestinal hemorrhage, lower gastrointestinal hemorrhage, bleeding esophageal varices, ruptured abdominal aortic aneurysm, and spontaneous rupture of the spleen, to name a few. In the absence of a history of trauma, if the signs and symptoms of hemorrhage are present it is imperative to proceed aggressively as if the patient had been injured. In general, the patient or family can give some history of some antecedent cause for the massive hemorrhage.

TREATMENT

Approximately 10 percent of all trauma patients are at risk for losing their life or sustaining permanent disability. Of those patients who die in the pre-hospital set-

ting, approximately 30 percent die from massive hemorrhage. Since in most instances this hemorrhage occurs over a short period of time, it indicates that a large blood vessel has been injured. In a few cases, however, death from hemorrhage occurs over a longer period of time, which reflects delay in transport, delay in recognition, difficult extrication, or a simple factor of distance.

Pre-hospital Treatment

The pre-hospital treatment of life-threatening hemorrhage is controversial. If we define massive hemorrhage as more than 150 cc per minute and assume that it takes approximately 5 to 10 minutes to gain access to the circulation, simple arithmetic shows that the patient has lost between 750 and 1,500 cc of blood during the time that it takes to gain access to the circulation. Based on this analysis, many physicians have advocated that it is better to use this time in transporting the patient to definitive surgical care since surgical control of the hemorrhage is the only chance for survival. Obviously, such an analysis must be predicated on common sense and will depend on pre-hospital time, closeness of an appropriate facility, and the skill of the pre-hospital personnel in achieving venous access.

In the pre-hospital setting, I favor the use of balanced salt solution. Optimally, the patient should have the intravenous lines, preferably two, placed en route to the hospital. If extrication is prolonged, intravenous lines can be established during the extrication and balanced salt solution administered. In general, 2 L of balanced salt solution can be infused with impunity in the severely shocked patient. The older patient may not be quite so tolerant, and it is prudent to follow the neck veins when administering the fluid. As long as the neck veins do not distend above the clavicles, it is safe to give more fluid.

Even more controversial than intravenous fluid administration is the use of the pneumatic antishock garment in the pre-hospital setting. There is considerable anecdotal information to suggest that the device is effective, but no randomized study has done so. Studies in urban areas suggest that the device is not only ineffective, but may be harmful. Nevertheless, I feel that if the systolic blood pressure is below 70 mm Hg and transport time is longer than 10 minutes, the pneumatic antishock garment is indicated. If the hemorrhage appears to be arterial, as would be expected in a gunshot wound to the abdomen or a ruptured abdominal aortic aneurysm, the garment should be inflated to 90 to 100 torr. If, on the other hand, the injury is confined primarily to the pelvis and the hemorrhage is most likely to be venous, inflation to 40 torr may be more effective. More rational use of the pneumatic antishock garment will depend on future studies.

Pre-hospital professionals should stop obvious external hemorrhage by using direct manual compression. Blind clamping of vessels should be avoided, since it causes further injury. Tourniquets are rarely indicated except in traumatic amputation.

TABLE 1   Clinical Classification of Hypovolemic Shock

Mild shock (up to 20% blood volume loss)

   Definition: Decreased perfusion of nonvital organs and tissues (skin, fat, skeletal muscle, and bone)

   Manifestations: Pale, cool skin. Patient complains of feeling cold

Moderate shock (20–40% blood volume loss)

   Definition: Decreased perfusion of vital organs (liver, gut, kidneys)

   Manifestations: Oliguria to anuria and slight to significant drop in blood pressure, mottling in extremities (especially legs)

Severe shock (40% or more blood volume loss)

   Definition: Decreased perfusion of heart and brain

   Manifestations: Restlessness, agitation, coma, cardiac irregularities, ECG abnormalities, and cardiac arrest

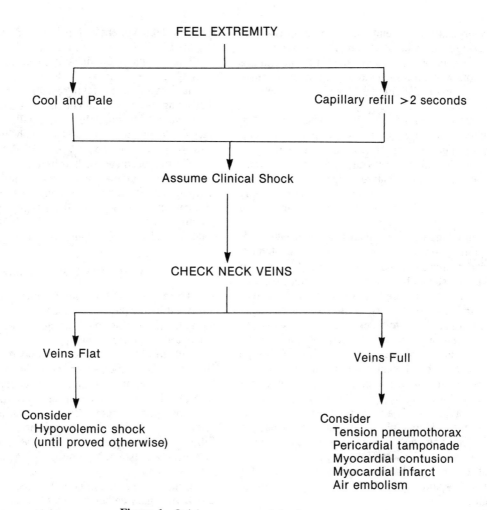

Figure 1 Quick assessment of shock.

In-hospital Treatment of Hemorrhagic Shock

General treatment measures include (1) placing the patient supine and level to maximize blood flow to the brain, and (2) preventing unnecessary heat loss by using blankets and warming all fluids when possible. Hypothermia is a common sequela of resuscitation and can be fatal. In the severely shocked patient an airway should be established, preferably by endotracheal intubation. Arterial blood gas measurements are obtained and serve as a guide both to the adequacy of oxygenation and to the severity of hypoperfusion, as indicated by the presence or absence of metabolic acidosis.

There are four priorities in treating hemorrhagic shock in the emergency department: (1) gain access to the circulation; (2) obtain some blood for typing and crossmatching for determination of the initial hematocrit, serial electrolytes, and chemistries (if indicated), and for toxicology; (3) determine the source of the blood loss; and (4) initiate fluid resuscitation.

In patients in mild shock a 16-gauge (or larger) catheter is placed percutaneously in an upper extremity vein. In patients in moderate-to-severe shock, access is gained by one or more cutdowns, the number depending on the clinical severity of the shock. The safest and quickest cutdown is on the long saphenous vein, over the medial malleolus. An additional cutdown on the basilic vein in the antecubital space, passing the catheter centrally, allows monitoring of the central venous pressure. Catheters inserted by cutdown should be as large as possible so as to maximize flow rates of the fluids administered; the size for the average adult is 14 gauge or larger. The catheters inserted in the saphenous vein at the ankle should be short, again to maximize flow, but a long catheter is used for the antecubital cutdown to produce the benefit of central venous pressure monitoring—I prefer a 5 F or 8 F pediatric feeding tube as the central venous monitoring line. Catheters should not be inserted in injured extremities. As fluid resuscitation proceeds, catheters may be placed percutaneously in upper extremity veins as they begin to distend. In some circumstances, as when a single physician is guiding the resuscitation or if a physician is uncomfortable with the surgical technique of a cutdown, percutaneous femoral vein punctures may allow rapid access to the circulation without major complications.

I discourage central percutaneous subclavian or internal jugular punctures in the hypovolemic patient. Although such punctures may be easy and safe in the quiet or hypervolemic patient, they can be difficult and dangerous in a restless or combative patient or in a hypovolemic patient. A severely hypovolemic patient has empty central veins, and such attempts at cannulation carry at least a 15 percent complication rate.

As soon as the first intravenous line is established, blood should be drawn for typing and crossmatching, hematocrit determination, and white blood cell count. Part of the specimen should be reserved to determine electrolytes, BUN, creatinine, amylase, blood sugar, and toxicology, if indicated by history or subsequent course.

The third priority is to determine the source of the blood loss. Hidden blood loss occurs in either of the hemithoraces, in the abdomen, or in the thigh. The thigh is easily ruled out by clinical examination. A fractured femur can sequester up to 8 units of blood. Treatment is straightforward: a traction splint. The one diagnostic test I require on all patients is a chest roentgenogram. If the chest film reveals hidden blood loss, tube thoracostomy should be done immediately and autotransfusion considered. However, if the chest film is negative, the physician must assume that the hidden blood loss is in the abdomen, and exploratory laparotomy is indicated as soon as possible.

The final priority is to begin immediately to restore blood volume. In mild or moderate shock, it makes little difference which fluid is used. In severe shock, the choice of fluid is important because endothelial permeability may be increased or microvascular forces altered, resulting in or augmenting "capillary leak," which compounds the problems if acellular colloid is given.

Crystalloids are preferred in the initial treatment of shock. They are readily available and effectively restore vascular volume for brief periods. Crystalloids also lower blood viscosity and enhance resuscitation of the microcirculation. Resuscitation and restoration of perfusion with balanced salt solution correct acidosis. Occasionally, some sodium bicarbonate may be required, and serial blood pH measurements are a guide. Overcorrection of acidosis is more harmful than the opposite. Recent animal experiments confirm that balanced salt solution, not normal saline, is the preferred crystalloid resuscitation.

Blood is available in emergencies as low-titer 0-negative or type-specific. 0-negative blood has the theoretic disadvantage of isoimmunization or later difficulty with typing and crossmatching; this is probably not a major consideration. Type-specific blood can be used until crossmatched blood becomes available (about 45 minutes). If shock persists after 2 liters of crystalloid have been infused, or if shock recurs after the patient initially responds, whole blood should be transfused immediately.

In the unstable patient with pelvic fractures, I also prefer to start blood as soon as possible.

Plasma and albumin solutions are detrimental in prolonged severe shock. These substances leak through capillary membranes, taking water with them, thus exacerbating the interstitial edema. Plasma and its components should be withheld until capillaries regain their integrity (about 24 hours) and should be used for specific indications such as factor V or VIII deficiency.

Plasma substitutes such as dextran interfere with function of the reticuloendothelial system and depress the already impaired immune mechanisms in shock patients. Clinical dextran coats red cells, making typing and crossmatching difficult; low-molecular-weight dextran coats platelets and may contribute to bleeding.

EVALUATION OF TREATMENT

The amount of fluid that a patient should receive is governed by the patient's response; there is *no* rigid formula. Constant close monitoring is essential. Urine output is a most useful sign.

Left atrial filling pressure is rarely measured directly. However, the pulmonary artery wedge pressure is a useful approximation and should be monitored in critical cases, but is probably impractical in the emergency department and operating room. Central venous pressure is sufficiently accurate in the great majority of patients. Atrial filling pressure, optimally, is kept at or near normal (3 to 8 torr) because higher pressures may aggravate interstitial edema.

Urine output should be monitored. If a patient is in shock, a urinary catheter should be placed during resuscitation if not contraindicated by urethral trauma. Urine output greater than 0.5 cc per kilogram per hour is a good index of visceral blood flow, specifically renal blood flow. Additional signs of successful resuscitation include an alert, oriented patient and adequate peripheral perfusion as judged by clinical criteria. Blood pressure, pulse rate, and respiratory rate should be recorded every 15 to 30 minutes. The hematocrit should be measured every few hours if continued bleeding is suspected. The hematocrit usually falls gradually over a period of 24 to 48 hours because of hemodilution even if bleeding has stopped. Blood gases should be determined repeatedly. Other measurements, obtained in certain circumstances, include cardiac output and oxygen consumption.

FAILURES OF RESUSCITATION

If both atrial filling pressure and urine output are increased, too much fluid is being given, and the infusion rate should be slowed immediately. If both atrial filling pressure and urine output are below normal, more volume is required. Additional intravenous access can be obtained. If perfusion cannot be improved, immediate control of bleeding is necessary.

High atrial filling pressure, low urine output, and high or normal cardiac output indicate deficient renal function. This may be further substantiated by urine plasma ratios of creatinine, sodium, and osmolarity. It is desirable to maintain the patient in a nonoliguric acute tubular necrosis (ATN) state, and I recommend giving mannitol (12.5 to 25 g IV) followed by an infusion of mannitol, 50 g in 500 to 1,000 ml of balanced salt solution. No more than 75 to 100 g of mannitol should be given in a 24-hour period. Lasix is contraindicated in the normovolemic or hypovolemic patient following hemorrhagic shock.

High atrial filling pressure, low urine output, and low cardiac output suggest that an inotropic agent is needed. Dopamine hydrochloride, 200 mg in 500 ml of sodium injection USP (400 μg per milligram), is given initially at a rate of 2.5 μg per kilogram per minute. These doses stimulate both the dopaminergic receptors, which increase the renal blood flow and urine output, and the beta-adrenergic cardiac receptors, which increase the cardiac output. High levels stimulate alpha-receptors to cause systemic vasoconstriction, and doses above 20 μg per kilo-gram per minute reverse the vasodilation of the renal vessels achieved at lower levels.

Finally, there is no convincing evidence that corticosteroids, naloxone, or ganglionic blocking drugs are of value in the treatment of hypovolemic shock.

SUGGESTED READING

Alexander RH, et al. The effect of advanced life support and sophisticated hospital systems on motor vehicle mortality. J Trauma 1984; 24:486.

Demling RH, Duy N, Monhar M, et al. Comparison between lung fluid filtration rate and measured Starling forces after hemorrhagic and endotoxic shock. J Trauma 1980; 20:856.

Demling RH, Manohar M, Will JA. Response of the pulmonary microcirculation to fluid loading after hemorrhagic shock and resuscitation. Surgery 1980; 87:552.

Smith BP, et al. Pre-hospital stabilization of critically injured patients. A failed concept. J Trauma 1985; 25:65.

EVALUATION AND RESUSCITATION OF ACCIDENTAL AND SURGICAL TRAUMA

WILLIAM C. SHOEMAKER, M.D.

Resuscitation in the emergency department is a complex process involving the management of unannounced, high-risk patients with a high-mortality rate and with a wide variety of emergency conditions who usually present themselves without previous background and history. Diagnosis, monitoring, and therapy must be coordinated during the rapid movement from the emergency department (ED), to the operating room (OR), and then to the intensive care unit (ICU). Until recently, decision-making rules for the management of these complex problems had not been formulated into decision trees or clinical algorithms.

A branched-chain decision tree for fluid therapy in the initial (first 30 to 60 minutes) resuscitation was developed and tested prospectively in the management of all 603 hypotensive (mean arterial pressure [MAP] less than 80 mm Hg) emergency patients entering our surgical ED over a 2½-year period (Fig. 1); 6 percent were admitted in arrest, 18 percent in severe shock (MAP <50 mm Hg), 52 percent in moderate shock (MAP <80 mm Hg), and 24 percent normotensive, the last-mentioned subsequently became hypotensive in the ED. Of the 28 percent with complications, 8 percent had shock-related complications including shock lung, acute renal failure, circulatory failure, sepsis in the uncontaminated patient, and fluid overload; half these patients died.

The fluid resuscitation algorithm, designed for these hypotensive emergency patients, provides a framework for fluid management that expedites resuscitation and reduces complications related to shock. In our prospective study of these patients, multiple deviations from the algorithm were associated with longer resuscitation times and a higher incidence of shock-related complications. Most of the delays in these patients and most of the shock-related complications could have been prevented. The resuscitation times were shorter and the shock-related complications were fewer in patients managed by the protocol. Delays in resuscitation were clearly related to an increased incidence of shock-related complications. When the algorithm was satisfactorily followed, there were faster resuscitations and less shock-related complications. In patients with severe associated illnesses, there were also shorter ICU stays, shorter hospitalizations, and a lower mortality rates when the algorithm was followed.

HEMODYNAMIC AND OXYGEN TRANSPORT VARIABLES

Monitored physiologic variables may now be readily and repeatedly obtained using systemic arterial and pulmonary arterial catheters (Table 1). From these directly measured variables, an array of hemodynamic values may be derived including cardiac index (CI), systemic and pulmonary vascular resistance (SVR and PVR), left and right ventricular stroke work, and cardiac work. More importantly, it is easy to determine the bulk movement of oxygen: O_2 delivery ($\dot{D}O_2$), O_2 consumption ($\dot{V}O_2$), O_2 extraction, the pulmonary venous admixture or shunting (Qsp/Qt), and the alveolar-arterial O_2 gradient (P[A-a]O_2). These variables are readily calculated by a computer or a hand-held programmable calculator.

RELEVANCE OF MONITORED PHYSIOLOGIC VARIABLES

The normal values of the commonly monitored variables including MAP, heart rate (HR), central venous pressure (CVP), wedge pressure (WP), and cardiac output provide rather poor criteria for monitoring, and normal values were restored equally in both survivors and nonsurvivors. Therefore, physiologic variables that are more closely related to outcome must be sought.

We evaluated the biologic importance of each cardiorespiratory variable based on its ability to predict outcome by a nonparametric predictive index; i.e., the capacity of each variable to predict outcome was considered to be a measure of its biologic relevance (see Fig. 1). Multivariate predictors provide a system for classification of outcome that is simple, objective, and physiologic. More importantly, they are able to define the goals of therapy. The predictive index was determined empirically from the frequency distributions of the survivors' and nonsurvivors' values. If a variable has little or no relation to outcome (e.g., HR, SVR, CVP, hematocrit [Hct], and PaO_2), then it is not important to therapeutic decisions. Variables reflecting oxygen transport in relation to red cell mass and red cell flow are, therefore, of the utmost importance to therapeutic management.

Blood volume restoration has been accepted as the most important goal in the treatment of shock and its sequelae, but reliable clinical criteria have not been well defined in the literature. In critically ill postoperative patients, the commonly used clinical criteria have been shown to be unreliable when compared with careful blood volume measurements.

GOALS OF FLUID THERAPY

Fluid therapy in acute catastrophes should first correct the specific underlying physiologic defects. Second, therapy should improve physiologic parameters, not to the full normal values, but to optimal values that are empirically defined by survivors of life-threatening critical illnesses. The most rigorous criterion for evaluation of the therapeutic effectiveness of various agents is their capacity to restore circulatory function and tissue perfusion. This is best evaluated by measured changes in flow, volume, $\dot{D}O_2$, and $\dot{V}O_2$; these variables were empirically found to be associated with outcome and were used to develop outcome predictors.

Criteria for fluid therapy were defined by the median values of survivors of life-threatening surgical conditions; they include (1) blood volume 500 ml in excess of the norm, i.e., 3.2 L per square meter for males, 2.8 L per square meter for females, (2) cardiac index (CI) 50 percent greater than the norm (4.5 L per minute per square meter), and (3) $\dot{V}O_2$ about 30 percent greater than normal (170 ml per minute per square meter). These supranormal valves are needed to supply the increased metabolism associated with the previous oxygen debt, fever, and the need for tissue repair of the critically ill post-trauma and postoperative patient.

TISSUE PERFUSION AND OXYGEN TRANSPORT AS CRITERIA FOR THERAPY

Tissue perfusion, which reflects overall circulatory function, may be evaluated in terms of oxygen transport, i.e., $\dot{D}O_2$ and $\dot{V}O_2$. Oxygen is the most flow-dependent blood constituent because oxygen has the greatest extraction ratio, and oxygen transport is strongly related to survival or death. The changes in oxygen transport after various therapeutic interventions provide more sensitive and specific criteria of circulatory performance than the gross overall mortality rates.

$\dot{V}O_2$, which represents the sum of all oxidative metabolic reactions, is therefore a measure of the body's total overall metabolism. It may be rate-limited by the circulatory alterations of trauma, surgical operations, anesthetic agents, postoperative states, and other forms of stress. Thus, $\dot{D}O_2$ and $\dot{V}O_2$ produce a useful means to assess both circulatory and metabolic functions.

PROSPECTIVE EVALUATION OF SURVIVOR VALUES AS PREDICTORS

Our study found that the median physiologic values of survivors of life-threatening postoperative conditions (rather than the norms of unstressed healthy volunteers) are the appropriate therapeutic goals for critically ill trauma patients.

SPECIFIC TREATMENT FOR THE CRITICALLY ILL TRAUMA PATIENT

In fluid therapy, the most important, as well as the most controversial, questions are the physiologic criteria for therapeutic goals. Unfortunately, however, the medical literature has few adequately designed, well-controlled studies in this important area. The efficacy of alternative fluid therapies is best evaluated by physiologic responses that are related to survival, rather than commonly monitored variables that are routinely used because of their convenience. If the effects of sodium (increased blood pressure and urine output) are selected as the criteria of efficacy, then sodium-rich solutions are likely to be judged efficacious. However, if cardiac output, blood volume, $\dot{D}O_2$ and $\dot{V}O_2$ are the appropriate outcome measures, then colloids and blood are clearly the most effective agents. In my view, the therapeutic goals are best defined by values of survivors of life-threatening shock and trauma conditions in their recovery stage. I believe that the high-risk critically ill patient requiring fluid resuscitation should have a pulmonary artery catheter to define physiologic problems and to titrate fluid therapy to the optimal goals defined by the pattern of the survivors of life-threatening accidental and surgical trauma. The therapeutic agent that is used is less important than is the achievement of these goals.

The branched-chain decision tree was developed for critically ill patients from outcome data of several previous series (Fig. 2). Criteria for assignment of priorities were based solely on survival statistics. My strategy is first a

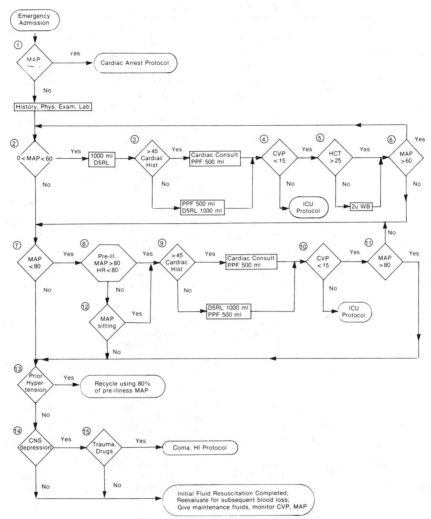

Figure 1 Clinical algorithm for initial (first hour) resuscitation of emergency admissions. This algorithm was designed for resuscitation of the acute emergency patient to restore circulatory integrity as rapidly as possible without producing fluid overload: (Step 1) If the MAP is zero or nearly zero, determine that there is a cardiac arrest and begin cardiopulmonary resuscitation immediately. If the patient has MAP less than 20 mm Hg, alert personnel for a possible cardiac arrest. (Step 2) If the MAP is less than 60 mm Hg, immediately start D5RL, 1,000 ml, and run as rapidly as possible, especially if the MAP is less than 50 mm Hg. (Step 3) If the patient is less than 45 years old and does not have a cardiac history, place a CVP line and start another D5RL, 1,000 ml, plus 500 ml of PPF or artificial colloid through a third intravenous line. (Step 4) Monitor the CVP at frequent intervals during the rapid infusion of these three solutions so as not to exceed values greater than 15 cm H_2O. If the CVP is greater than 15 cm H_2O, go directly to the ICU protocol. (Step 5) If the Hct is less than 25 percent, give 2 units of O-negative or type-specific blood. When cross-matched blood becomes available, transfusions of WB or PRBC should be given to maintain Hct higher than 33 percent. (Step 6) Rapid restoration of the MAP to 60 mm Hg is the titration end point for fluids in this section. If the MAP is less than 60 mm Hg recycle from steps 2 through 6. If an MAP greater than 60 mm Hg has been achieved, proceed to step 7. (Step 7) If the MAP is less than 80 mm Hg, go to step 8; if not, proceed to step 13. (Step 8) If the MAP is less than 80 mm Hg, consult the patient, the patient's family, or a previous hospital record to determine the patient's "normal" pre-illness control MAP. If the MAP is less than 80 mm Hg and the HR more than 80 beats per minute, measure orthostatic BP (see step 12). (Step 9) As in step 3, the cardiac patient requires less salt and water, but more colloid. If the age of the patient is greater than 45 years or there is a cardiac history, give 500 ml of colloid; if the age is less than 45 years and there is no cardiac history, give 1,000 ml of D5RL plus 500 ml of colloid. (Step 10) Fluids may be given safely if the CVP is less than 15 cm H_2O; if the latter is exceeded, go to the ICU protocol (Fig. 2) and continue to give fluids as needed to restore circulatory integrity, provided WP of 18 mm Hg are not exceeded. (Step 11) If the MAP is greater than 80 mm Hg and the CVP does not exceed 15 cm H_2O, the objective of this cycle has been achieved. If the MAP is less than 80 mm Hg, repeat steps 7 through 11. (Step 12) Orthostatic BP is measured. If there is a change in the MAP of less than 10 mm Hg on sitting or standing, this is presumptive evidence of at least 1,000 ml of BV deficit. (Step 13) After the MAP has been restored to the normal value (>80 mm Hg), it is still necessary to ascertain that the pre-illness BP was normal. If a prior hypertension was observed, steps 7 through 13 should be repeated using 80 percent of the pre-illness value as the criterion for the adequacy of resuscitation. (Step 14) Evaluate the patient for evidence of CNS depression, drug poisoning, or drug abuse. (Step 15) Evaluate the patient for evidence of head injury or other trauma. If positive, the patient should be treated in accordance with a coma-head injury protocol. (From Hopkins JA, et al. Results of a clinical trial on the use of an emergency resuscitation algorithm. Crit Care Med 1983; 11:621.)

TABLE 1 Cardiorespiratory Variables: Abbreviations, Units, Calculations, Normal Values, Preferred Values for Resuscitation, and Predictive Capacity

Variables	Abbreviations	Units	Measurements or Calculations	Normal Values	Preferred Values	Percent Correct
Volume-related						
Mean arterial pressure	MAP	mm Hg	Direct measurement	82–102	>84	76
Central vent pressure	CVP	cm H_2O	Direct measurement	1–9	<5	62
Central blood volume	CBV	ml/m²	$CBV = MTT \times CI \times 16.7$	660–1,000	>925	61
Stroke index	SI	ml/m²	$SI = CI/HR$	30–50	>48	67
Hemoglobin	Hgb	g/dl	Direct measurement	12–16	>12	66
Mean pulmonary artery pressure	MPAP	mm Hg	Direct measurement	11–15	<19	68
Wedge pressure	WP	mm Hg	Direct measurement	0–12	>9.5	70
Blood volume	BV	ml/m²	$BV = PV/(1-Hct)* \times$ surface area	Men 2.74 Women 2.37	>3.0 >2.7	76
Red cell mass	RCM	ml/m²	$RCM = BV - PV$	Men 1.1 Women 0.95	>1.1 >0.95	85
Flow-related						
Cardiac index	CI	liter/min/m²	Direct measurement	2.8–3.6	>4.5	70
Left vent stroke work	LVSW	g/M/m²	$LVSW = SI \times MAP \times 0.0144$	44–68	>55	74
Left cardiac work	LCW	kg/M/m²	$LCW = CI \times MAP \times 0.0144$	3–4.6	>5	76
Right vent stroke work	RVSW	g/M/m²	$RVSW = SI \times MPAP \times 0.0144$	4–8	>4.3	70
Right cardiac work	RCW	kg/M/m²	$RCW = CI \times MPAP \times 0.0144$	0.4–0.6	>1.1	69
Stress-related						
Systemic vasc resist	SVR	dynes/sec/cm⁵/m²	$SVR = 79.92(MAP-CVP)\dagger/CI$	1,760–2,600	<1.450	62
Pulmonary vasc resist	PVR	dynes/sec/cm⁵/m²	$PVR = 79.92(MPAP-WP)\dagger/CI$	45–225	<226	77
Heart rate	HR	beat/min	Direct measurement	72–88	<100	60
Rectal temperature	temp	°F	Direct measurement	97.8–98.6	>100.4	64
Oxygen-related						
Hemoglobin saturation	SaO_2	%	Direct measurement	95–99	>95	67
Arterial CO_2 tension	$PaCO_2$	torr	Direct measurement	36–44	>30	69
Arterial pH	pH	...	Direct measurement	7.36–7.44	>7.47	74
Mixed venous O_2 tension	$P\bar{v}O_2$	torr	Direct measurement	33–53	>36	68
Arterial-mixed venous O_2 content difference	$C(a-\bar{v})O_2$	ml/dl	$C(a-\bar{v})O_2 = CaO_2 - C\bar{v}O_2$	4–5.5	<3.5	68
O_2 delivery	$\dot{D}O_2$	ml/min/m²	$\dot{D}O_2 = CaO_2 \times CI \times 10$	520–720	>550	76
O_2 consumption	$\dot{V}O_2$	ml/min/m²	$\dot{V}O_2 = C(a-\bar{v})O_2 \times CI \times 10$	100–180	>167	69
O_2 extraction rate	O_2 ext	%	$O_2\ ext = (CaO_2 - C\bar{v}O_2)/CaO_2$	22–30	<31	69
Perfusion-related						
Red cell flow rate	RCFR	...	$RCFR = CI \times Hct$	0.6–1.8	>1.3	72
Blood flow/volume ratio	BFVR	...	$BFVR = CI/BV$	0.6–1.8	>1.7	75
O_2 transport/red cell mass	OTRM	...	$OTRM = \dot{V}O_2/RCM$	0.06–0.18	>0.25	79
Tissue O_2 extraction	TOE	...	$TOE = C(a-\bar{v})O_2/RCFR$	1.8–6.6	>5.7	75
Efficiency of tissue O_2 extraction	ETOE	...	$ETOE = C(a-\bar{v})O_2/RCM$	0.06–0.18	> .3	91
O_2 transport/red cell flow	OTRF	...	$OTRF = \dot{V}O_2/RCFR$	1–7	<3	71

* Hematocrit (Hct) value corrected for packing fraction and large vessel hematocrit to total body hematocrit ratio.
† Venous pressure expressed in mm Hg.
vasc resist = vascular resistance.

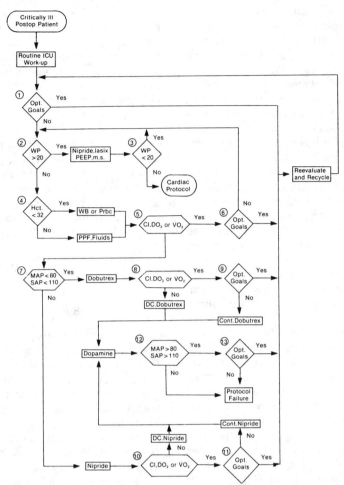

Figure 2 Preliminary evaluation of high-risk critically ill patients by routine ICU work-up that includes arterial blood gases, chest film, routine blood chemistries, ECG, and coagulation studies. These tests should be either performed or in process and the observed defects corrected, i.e., if PaO_2 is less than 70 torr, 7.3 > pH is greater than 7.5, $PaCO_2$ is greater than 55 torr, or respiration rate (RRO) is more than 30 breaths per minute, place on the respiratory protocol. If none of the above is present, proceed down the branched-chain decision tree: (Step 1) Determine whether the patient has reached the optimal goals. Measure CI, $\dot{D}O_2$, $\dot{V}O_2$, and blood volume (BV). If CI is less than 4.5 L per minute per square meter, $\dot{D}O_2$ is less than 600 ml per minute per square meter, $\dot{V}O_2$ is less than 160 ml per minute per square meter for men or 2.7 L per square meter for women, take Hct. If any of the preceding optimal values has not been reached, proceed to step 2. If the goals have been reached, the objective of the algorithm has been achieved. Reevaluate and recycle at intervals to maintain these goals. (Step 2) Take pulmonary WP. If greater than 20 mm Hg, proceed to step 3; if less than 20, proceed to step 4. (Step 3) If WP is greater than 20, give furosemide intravenously at increasing dose levels (20, 40, 80, 160 mg) if there is clinical or roentgenographic evidence of salt and water overload or clinical findings of pulmonary congestion. If not, consider vasodilators, nitroprusside, or nitroglycerin if MAP is greater than 80 and systolic pressure is greater than 100 mm Hg. Recycle up to 5 times to titrate the dose needed to reduce WP to less than 10 mm Hg, but maintain MAP above 80 mm Hg. If unsuccessful, place on cardiac protocol. (Step 4) If Hct is less than 32 percent, give 1 unit of WB or 2 units of PRBC. If Hct is greater then 32 percent give a fluid load (volume challenge) consisting of one of the following (depending on clinical indications of plasma volume deficit or hydration): 5 percent PPF, 500 ml; 5 percent albumin, 500 ml; 25 percent albumin (25 g), 100 ml; 6 percent hydroxyethyl starch, 500 ml; 6 percent dextran–60, 500 ml; D5RL, 1,000 ml. (Step 5) If the blood or fluid load improved any of the optimal therapeutic goals defined in step 1, proceed to step 6; if none is improved, proceed to step 7. (Step 6) If goals are not reached, recycle steps 2 through 6 until these goals are met or WP is greater than 20 mm Hg. (Step 7) If MAP is greater than 70 or SAP is less than 100 mm Hg, administer dobutamine in increasing doses. (Step 8) Titrate dobutamine, begin with 1 to 2 μ g per minute per kilogram and gradually increase doses up to 20 μ g per minute per kilogram, provided there is improvement in CI, $\dot{D}O_2$, or $\dot{V}O_2$ without further lowering of arterial pressure until goals are met. (Step 9) If goals are reached, reevaluate and recycle. If goals are not reached or it becomes evident that higher doses of the drug are not more effective or that they produce hypotension and tachycardia, continue dobutamine at its most effective dose range. (Step 10) If MAP is greater than 80 mm Hg and SAP is greater than 110 mm Hg, give sodium nitroprusside or nitroglycerin in gradually increasing doses. If MAP is less than 80 mm Hg and SAP is less than 110 mm Hg, give vasopressors. (Step 11) If there is no improvement in CI, $\dot{D}O_2$ or $\dot{V}O_2$ with the vasodilator, or if hypotension (MAP less than 80 mm Hg, SAP less than 110 mm Hg) ensues, discontinue the vasodilator. If there is improvement in CI, $\dot{D}O_2$, or $\dot{V}O_2$, titrate vasodilator to its maximum effect consistent with satisfactory pressures. (Step 12) If optimal goals are reached, reevaluate and recycle at intervals. If these goals are not reached and MAP is less than 80 mm Hg and SAP less than 110 mm Hg, give vasopressor. (Step 13) Titrate doses of vasopressor (dopamine) in the lowest doses possible to maintain arterial pressures (MAP > 80, SAP > 110). If pressures cannot be maintained, the patient is considered to be a protocol failure.

vigorous *volume load* without exceeding WP greater than 18 to 20 mm Hg. It is easier to achieve these goals with colloids, which expand the plasma volume without undue expansion of the interstitial water. After the maximum effect of fluids has been obtained, I then add an inotropic agent, such as dobutamine, beginning with 2 μg per minute per kilogram; the optimal dose is obtained by titration to achieve the optimal goals in terms of CI, DO_2, and VO_2. If the patient has high MAP and systemic vascular resistance index (SVRI), vasodilation with nitroglycerin or nitroprusside is considered; the optimal dose is obtained by titration to achieve improved CI without producing hypotension (i.e., MAP < 80, systolic arterial pressure < [SAP] 110 mm Hg). If fluids, inotropic agents, and vasodilators fail to achieve optimal goals, vasopressors such as dopamine are given in the smallest possible dose needed to maintain MAP at 80 and SAP at 110 mm Hg in patients who were normotensive before their illness. Vasopressors are given last because they increase venous pressure in addition to increasing MAP, and thereby may limit optimal fluid administration; no amount of dopamine can make up for blood volume (BV) deficits.

There is an average increase of 30 percent in VO_2 in the uncomplicated general surgical postoperative patient, but the increased VO_2 in both preoperative and postoperative patients with severe trauma, stress, sepsis and hypercatabolic states may be considerably greater and indicates further metabolic demands. However, the increased VO_2 does not mean that all the patient's metabolic needs have been met. Although the adequacy of therapy cannot be measured directly, tissue demand may be inferred indirectly by an empiric trial of therapy. If the therapy increases cardiac output and VO_2, it may be assumed that therapy opened up unperfused microcirculatory channels and that these hypoxic tissues then extracted more oxygen. Since tissues cannot take up more oxygen than they use, the increased VO_2 after fluid challenge means that an oxygen debt had been present and was at least partially relieved.

RESULTS OF PROSPECTIVE CLINICAL TRIALS

This therapeutic plan was prospectively tested in clinical trials against a control group; the traditional normal values were the goals of therapy. The only real difference between the groups was that the control patients had normal values of cardiorespiratory variables as their therapeutic goals, whereas the protocol group had as their therapeutic goals the median values of the survivors. The protocol group was at least as ill and probably more at risk than the control group. The results showed marked reduction in mortality from 35 percent in the control patients to 12.5 percent in the protocol patients as well as a significant reduction in morbidity.

Recently, our group has undertaken an additional preoperative prospective randomized trial of this concept. This trial was strictly randomized using one of three therapeutic systems (CVP catheter, pulmonary artery catheter with normal values as goals, and pulmonary artery catheter with optimal values as goals of therapy). The results showed no statistically significant difference between the ICU mortality of patients managed with a CVP catheter (23 percent) and that of patients with a pulmonary artery catheter (33 percent) with normal values as therapeutic goals; however, use of the pulmonary artery catheter with optimal goals led to significantly reduced (4 percent) mortality.

These prospective clinical trials suggest that as much as two-thirds of the postoperative and post-traumatic deaths may be attributable to physiologic problems that can be identified, described, predicted, and prevented. Therapy for critically ill patients should be defined by physiologic criteria, and therapy should be administered to obtain optimal physiologic goals rather than normal values; moreover, therapy should be given prophylactically rather than after deficiencies have occurred.

CHOICE OF FLUID IN CRITICAL ILLNESS

Albumin Metabolism in Stress

Critically ill trauma and septic patients cannibalize protein from body cells to maintain the metabolism and therefore may have rapid rates of disappearance of albumin from the plasma. It is not reasonable to interpret rapid equilibration and metabolism as a capillary leak, nor to withhold albumin therapy because increased catabolism has reduced serum albumin concentrations. "Leak" of albumin from the plasma must be distinguished from the normal "equilibration" of the body's albumin pool as well as from its normal or increased metabolism.

Albumin is normally secreted by the liver into the plasma, where it provides oncotic pressure; then it equilibrates in the interstitial water, where 55 to 60 percent of the body's albumin pool normally resides. Much of this extravascular albumin pool is tissue-bound and does not exert its full oncotic pressure. Subsequently, albumin enters body cells, where it is metabolized. The pathway of nitrogen from body cells back to the liver is by way of free amino acids. This nitrogen cycle may be accelerated during catabolic periods. Thus, the egress of albumin from the plasma volume may represent rapid equilibration as well as rapid turnover of the albumin pool associated with increased tissue demands rather than "leakage." The latter may occur in the late stage of shock, particularly with sepsis. When exogenous albumin is given, it promptly increases albumin concentrations and plasma oncotic pressure and drags interstitial water back into the plasma volume; this reduces excess interstitial water and restores BV. Subsequently, the albumin equilibrates in the body's miscible albumin pool and eventually is metabolized to replenish intracellular constituents as part of the nitrogen cycle.

Comparison of Physiologic Effects of Crystalloids and Colloids in Prospective Clinical Trials

Recent prospectively randomized studies comparing

crystalloids and colloids were conducted in critically ill postoperative patients, in burn patients, and in emergency hypotensive shock and trauma patients. These studies showed statistically significant advantages in colloid administration.

Our team has explored an approach that compares the relative effectiveness of alternative therapies using the patient as his own control. Figure 3 illustrates hemodynamic and oxygen transport values during resuscitation from burn shock in a series of burn patients who were given various colloids and lactated Ringer's solution alternately during the period of their critical illness. Increases in cardiac output, $\dot{D}O_2$, and $\dot{V}O_2$ were significantly greater after colloids than after twice or four times the volume of the crystalloids.

Hauser et al compared the changes after one liter of lactated Ringer's solution with changes following 25 g of 25 percent albumin (100 ml) given in random order to a prospective series of critically ill surgical patients with early shock lung. Albumin increased plasma volume by 465 ± 47 (SE) ml by shifting over 350 ml of water from the interstitial water to the intravascular water. Simultaneously, albumin increased CI, MAP, left ventricular stroke work, $\dot{D}O_2$, and $\dot{V}O_2$; lung function variables were not worsened, but in many instances actually improved. By contrast, one liter of lactated Ringer's solution expanded plasma volume only 194 ± 18 ml at its maximum, which was at the end of infusion, i.e., over 80 percent of the infused crystalloid almost immediately equilibrated or "leaked" into the interstitial water, and the small

proportion of fluid remaining in the plasma, then decreased exponentially. After administration of lactated Ringer's solution, $\dot{V}O_2$ decreased despite the slightly increased oxygen availability, and pulmonary oxygen transport deteriorated slightly. The hemodynamic responses to the administered fluid were directly proportional to volume expansion. Thus, colloids improve hemodynamics and oxygen transport by plasma expansion, whereas crystalloids principally expand interstitial volume; when tolerated, they may restore plasma volume if given in great excess.

Recently, this series was expanded to include 400 fluid therapy interventions in 211 patients with early adult respiratory distress syndrome (ARDS) occurring postoperatively and in sepsis. Figures 4 and 5 illustrate the flow and oxygen transport variables during respiratory failure, before or after the episode, and in a concurrent group of critically ill patients who did not develop ARDS. These data show significant increases in hemodynamic and oxygen transport values after colloid infusion, but no essential changes except increased arterial pressure and systemic (peripheral) vascular resistance after infusion of lactated Ringer's solution. There are no significant differences in cardiac output after infusion of colloids, whole blood, or crystalloids in patients in the preterminal stage of ARDS, defined as the last 24 to 48 hours of life. These data indicate that the capillary leak syndrome occurs after the clinical appearance of ARDS; it appears to be the result, not the pathogenic cause, of ARDS. Colloids

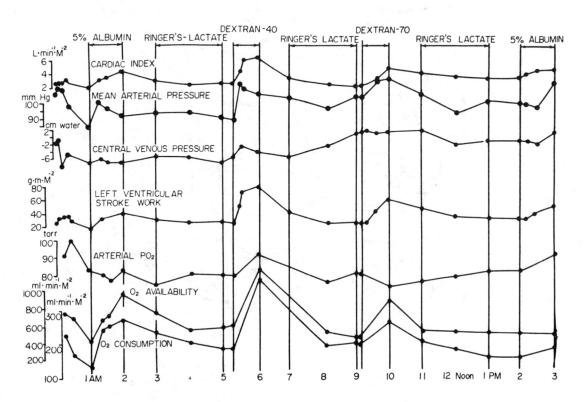

Figure 3 Cardiorespiratory values during resuscitation of a patient with severe burns. (From Shoemaker WC, Matsudo T, State D. Relative hemodynamic effectiveness of whole blood and plasma expanders in burned patients. Surg Gynecol Obstet 1977;144:909

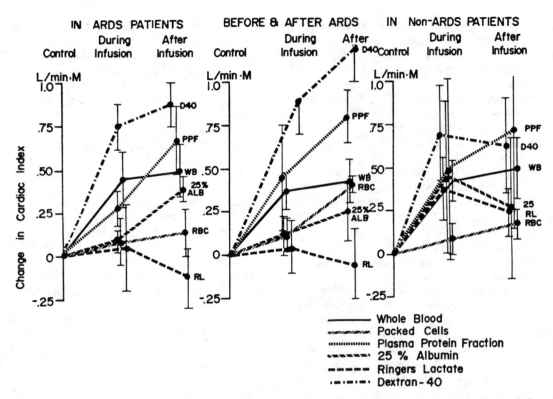

Figure 4 CI responses to various agents are shown in patients with ARDS during the episode of respiratory distress (left section), patients with ARDS who are not experiencing an episode of respiratory distress (center section), and patients without ARDS (right section). The data represent changes in CI ± SEM during and after the administration of each agent.

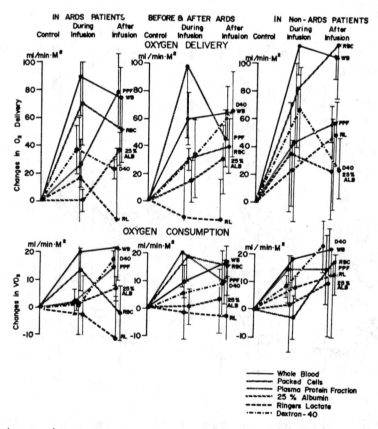

Figure 5 Changes in $\dot{D}O_2$ and $\dot{V}O_2$ during and after the administration of various agents.

may improve the physiologic variables that determine survival until they significantly increase $\dot{Q}sp/\dot{Q}t$ and $P(A-a)O_2$ or elevate WP inappropriately.

Summary of Fluid Therapy Recommendations

In general, red cell losses should be replaced with red cells, water loss from dehydration should be replaced with crystalloids, and plasma volume losses should be replaced with plasma or its colloidal equivalent (that is, plasma protein fraction [PPF] and 5 or 25 percent albumin, or artificial colloids such as dextran or hydroxyethyl starch, if cost is a problem).

Saline, glucose, and lactated Ringer's solution in various combinations are commonly used for initial resuscitation in mild degrees of shock and subsequent fluid replacement of daily losses. In general, 3 liters of fluid usually replace acute losses in mild or moderately ill patients who do not have extrarenal fluid losses and who are tolerating nothing by mouth. However, patients with enteric fistulas, diarrhea, vomiting, large volumes of nasogastric suction, and other extrarenal fluid losses may require several times this volume to replace the estimated fluid losses. After the estimated fluid losses are replaced, further fluid needs are determined by fluid balance studies, in which urinary, nasogastric suction, fecal, and enteric fistula losses are collected, measured, and recorded; estimated insensible losses are added to this.

In resuscitation from shock, at least one-third of the fluids given should be colloids in order to maintain the administered fluids in the blood volume compartment, since this is needed to maintain DO_2, $\dot{V}O_2$, and other perfusion variables at their optimal values. Whole blood or (WB) packed red blood cells should be given in sufficient quantities to maintain Hct over 34 percent.

SUGGESTED READING

Haupt MT, Rackow EC. Colloids osmotic pressure and fluid resuscitation with hetastarch, albumin, and saline solutions. Crit Care Med 1982; 10:159.

Hopkins JA, Shoemaker WC, Chang PC, et al. Results of a clinical trial on the use of an emergency resuscitation algorithm. Crit Care Med 1983; 11:621.

Jelenko C III, Williams JB, Wheeler ML, et al. Studies in shock and resuscitation. I: Use of a hypertonic, albumin-containing, fluid demand regimen (Halfd) in resuscitation: A physiologically appropriate method. Crit Care Med 1979; 7:157.

Modig J. Advantages of dextran–70 over Ringer's acetate solution in shock treatment and in prevention of adult respiratory distress syndrome: A randomized study in man after traumatic-hemorrhage shock. Resuscitation 1983; 10:219.

Shippy CR, Appel PL, Shoemaker WC. Reliablity of clinical monitoring to assess blood volume in critically ill patients. Crit Care Med 1984; 12:107.

Shoemaker WC, Appel P, Bland R. Use of physiologic monitoring to predict outcome and to assist in clinical decision in critically ill postoperative patients. Am J Surg 1983; 146:43.

Shoemaker WC, Hopkins JA. Clinical aspects of resuscitation with and without an algorithm: Relative importance of various decisions. Crit Care Med 1983; 11:630.

Shoemaker WC, Schluchter M, Hopkins JA, et al. Comparison of the relative effectiveness of colloids and crystalloids in emergency resuscitation. Am J Surg 1981; 142:73.

Shoemaker WC, Matsuda T, State D. Relative hemodynamic effectiveness of whole blood and plasma expanders in burned patients. Surg Gynecol Obstet 1977; 144:909

RESUSCITATION OF THE NEWBORN

BEVERLY L. KOOPS, M.D.
DAVID R. KRAUSS, M.D.

One of every 5 to 10 infants born on a typical delivery service requires the use of some resuscitative skills on the part of his or her attendant at the delivery. Since neonatal asphyxia is not an uncommon problem, delivery services should prepare in advance for the arrival of an asphyxiated infant by having appropriate equipment and a trained staff. In many situations, the birth of an asphyxiated infant can be anticipated. However, it can also follow an "uncomplicated" pregnancy and delivery. Therefore, a state of readiness is necessary if the asphyxiated infant is to receive optimal care.

PATHOPHYSIOLOGY OF ASPHYXIA

The asphyxiated infant is the result of conditions that interfere with the placenta's ability to function as the fetal organ of respiration or with the infant's ability to establish extrauterine respiration in spite of normal placental function. The end result, whatever the etiology, consists of hypoxemia, hypercapnia, and acidosis.

Many organ systems are affected by perinatal asphyxia. Necrotizing enterocolitis has resulted from the effects of asphyxia on the gastrointestinal tract. Renal failure, tubular necrosis, and cortical necrosis have all been reported as renal sequelae of perinatal asphyxia. Cardiac, pulmonary, and hematologic consequences of asphyxia have also been described in the literature.

Of greatest concern is the effect of asphyxia on the central nervous system (CNS). Although infants seem to tolerate asphyxia somewhat better than adults, absolute criteria are not available to define when irreversible brain damage has occurred.

A wide variety of conditions have been described following asphyxia, including intracranial hemorrhages, periventricular leukomalacia, and status marmoratus. Recent evidence suggests that CNS neurons can tolerate 20 to 60 minutes of anoxic ischemia without irreversible damage. Several mechanisms have been proposed to explain the damage that occurs following asphyxia of a duration less than that tolerated by CNS neurons. The failure of cerebral circulation to return to normal perfusion rates following an asphyxial event has lead to the concept of the "no reflow phenomenon." The loss of cerebral autoregulation, which occurs in severe asphyxia, makes the CNS particularly vulnerable to systemic blood pressure changes. Hypoxemia, hypercapnia, and acidosis all have direct effects on cerebral blood flow. There may be ongoing vasoconstriction and ischemia; in other areas of the brain, there may be vasodilatation, increased blood flow, and hemorrhage. Biochemical effects of asphyxia and ischemia include decreased brain glucose, accumulation of lactate and metabolites of high-energy phosphates, electrolyte derangements, and acidosis. The accumulation of arachidonic acid and production of oxygen free radicals may also contribute to injury. Calcium ion shifts may play a key role in these events. During an asphyxial event, the normal calcium gradient across the neuron membrane rapidly deteriorates. The calcium ion overload of the neuron may be responsible for post-ischemic hypoperfusion, arachidonic acid accumulation, and free-radical genesis. Calcium administration during resuscitation may not be as beneficial as previously thought.

ANTICIPATION OF THE DEPRESSED NEWBORN

In many cases, the arrival of a depressed newborn can be anticipated by a review of the maternal history. Table 1 lists high-risk factors known to be associated with the delivery of the depressed newborn. When there is an increased risk of having an asphyxiated infant, there should be a person in the delivery room, trained in neonatal resuscitation, who has no other responsibility aside from evaluating and caring for the newborn.

In preparation for neonatal resuscitation, resuscitative equipment should be available and its operating status determined. Table 2 lists essential equipment. All resuscitation equipment should be checked on a routine basis for both operational status and presence. Just prior to a high-risk delivery, the attendant responsible for resuscitation of the infant should again review and carefully check all the necessary equipment.

TABLE 1 Contributing Factors in Asphyxia

Antenatal factors

Maternal diabetes
Maternal hypertension
Maternal infection (chorioamnionitis)
Maternal hemorrhage
Maternal drug abuse
Maternal drug use (e.g., magnesium, reserpine, adrenergic blocking drugs)

Perinatal factors

Maternal eclampsia
Abnormal presentation
Multiple births
Maternal hypertension
Prolonged labor
Isoimmunization (Rh)
Excessive vaginal bleeding
Postmaturity or prematurity
Meconium-stained amniotic fluid
Cesarean section delivery
Abnormal fetal heart rate pattern

RESUSCITATION

There is one special situation that requires attention just prior to the delivery of the infant. If the amniotic fluid was noted to be meconium-stained just after delivery of the infant's head, but prior to the delivery of the thorax, the person assisting in the delivery should thoroughly suction the nasal and oropharynx of the infant using a DeLee suction catheter. This is the single most important step that can be taken to significantly reduce the risk of meconium aspiration syndrome in the infant. Following this procedure, the infant is delivered and transferred to a radiant warmer, already prepared for the impending resuscitation.

All infants should receive, as a minimum of attention following delivery, the following: they should be

TABLE 2 Resuscitation Equipment for the Newborn

Bag and mask with 100% oxygen source (should have multiple face mask sizes)
DeLee suction catheter with mucus trap or other suction apparatus
Laryngoscope with No. 0 and No. 1 Miller blade
Endotracheal tubes (2.5, 3.0, 3.5, and 4.0 mm ID) with adapters
Scissors, tape
Radiant warmer with good lighting
Intravenous fluid therapy equipment (including equipment for umbilical venous and/or arterial catheterization)
Stethoscope
Dextrose, 25 or 50%
Calcium gluconate, 10%
Atropine
Epinephrine (1:10,000)
Naloxone (neonatal vial)
$NaHCO_3$ (1 mEq/2cc)

placed in a warm environment, gently dried, and have their naso-oropharynx suctioned using a bulb syringe. During these procedures, the infant is being evaluated according to the Apgar score (Table 3). If the infant's total Apgar score is greater than 6, no further resuscitative efforts are necessary. When the infant has been dried, it is prepared for contact with the mother or transfer to the nursery.

If the total Apgar score is between 3 and 6, this represents mild neonatal asphyxia. If the infant was meconium-stained, at this time laryngoscopy should be performed and the trachea suctioned until it is free of meconium. When a face mask of proper size is used, most infants respond with regular respirations after receiving several manual ventilations by means of resuscitator or hand-bag. If the infant responds, finish drying the infant and prepare for evaluating the infant at 5 minutes.

Infants with Apgar scores less than 3 or infants that fail to respond to face-mask ventilation are usually moderately-to-severely asphyxiated. These infants deserve tracheal intubation for resuscitation (preceded by suctioning if meconium-stained).

Intubation is a skill learned only by experience. The infant should be placed in the ''flower sniffing'' position achieved by placing a small pad under the back of the infant's head, slightly elevating the head but not the shoulders. Although other positions can be used for intubation, we believe that this position makes the procedure the least complicated. After achieving this position, the laryngoscope blade is inserted in the infant's mouth. The No. 0 blade should be chosen for infants weighing less than 3 kilograms. For larger infants, the No. 1 blade usually is used. The proper endotracheal tube is selected as follows:

Infants 500 to 1,000 g, 2.5 mm
Infants 1,000 to 2,000 g, 3.0 mm
Infants 2,000 to 4,000 g, 3.5 mm
Infants 4,000 g + 4.0 mm

If secretions are obscuring the airway, suctioning should be done before intubation is attempted. Once the vocal cords are well visualized, the endotracheal tube is inserted. Care should be taken not to insert the tube too far into the trachea, thus occluding the left bronchus. Correct placement of the endotracheal tube should be ascertained by all of the following: (1) chest movement, (2) good breath sounds bilaterally, and (3) no sounds over the stomach.

If intubation and ventilation have been successful, in a vast majority of infants, the heart rate begins to increase and resuscitation is successful. The infant should remain intubated and ventilated until vigorous or until transferred to an intensive care facility.

If the infant has not responded to intubation and ventilation, the first consideration is to reevaluate the success of intubation. If it is certain that the infant has been successfully intubated and the heart rate remains less than 60 to 80 beats per minute, cardiac massage should be started. Both hands should encircle the chest with fingers over the back and thumbs over the midportion of the sternum. The midportion of the sternum is compressed one-half to three-fourths of an inch at approximately 100 beats per minute. With every third to fourth compression, the lungs should be inflated. If the infant continues to fail to respond, the use of drugs should be considered.

For drugs that are usually considered in the resuscitation of newborns, see Table 4. Access to the circulatory system can be achieved in an emergency by inserting a catheter into the umbilical vein. Epinephrine can be given intratracheally, via the endotracheal tube. It should be noted that the need for drugs during resuscitation is uncommon.

Hypovolemia may cause or accompany asphyxia. This problem should be considered if there is a history of excessive vaginal bleeding, persistent pallor, hypotension or weak pulses, tachycardia, or a poor response to resuscitation. Volume expansion should then be considered using one of the following solutions in incremental doses of 10 ml per kilogram:

0–negative blood (uncrossmatched if necessary to prevent delay)
Fresh frozen plasma
5 percent Albumisol
Lactated Ringer's solution

As soon as respiratory effort and heart rate have been stabilized, the infant should be transferred to an area where careful observation can be maintained. Infants that have required this degree of resuscitation are at high risk for numerous sequelae.

SEQUELAE OF NEONATAL ASPHYXIA

Asphyxiated infants are at high risk for sequelae following their asphyxial event. If the 5-minute Apgar score is less than 6 or 7, careful follow-up is essential. The more common sequelae after asphyxia are listed below:

TABLE 3 Apgar Score

	0	1	2
Heart rate	Absent	< 100	> 100
Respiratory effort	Absent	Slow, irregular	Good cry
Color	Blue, pale	Body pink, extremities blue	All pink
Tone	Limp	Some flexion	Well flexed
Reflex irritability	No response	Grimace	Cry

TABLE 4 Drugs Used in Resuscitation of the Newborn

Drug	Dose	Indications
Epinephrine 1:10,000	0.1 ml/kg	Bradycardia
Sodium bicarbonate	2 mEq/kg	Suspected acidosis
Naloxone	0.01 mg/kg	Respiratory depression secondary to narcotics
Dextrose, 25%	2 ml/kg	Hypoglycemia
Calcium gluconate, 10%	100 mg/kg	? low cardiac output ? (see text)

CNS insult
Myocardial dysfunction (especially papillary muscle
    dysfunction with tricuspid insufficiency)
Shock lung
Persistent fetal circulation
Hypoglycemia
Renal insufficiency, acute tubular necrosis, etc.
Necrotizing enterocolitis
Inappropriate antidiuretic hormone secretion
Thrombocytopenia

Nursery management should include no feedings, frequent monitoring of vital signs, intravenous fluids of 5 or 10 percent dextrose at 50 to 60 ml per kilogram per day, intermittent determination of blood sugar or blood glucose estimate, strict calculation of intake and output of fluids, and careful observation for abnormal neurologic signs, respiratory distress, or cardiac decompensation.

STABILIZATION AND TRANSPORT OF THE SEVERELY ASPHYXIATED INFANT

As soon as the infant is in the nursery, careful reevaluation must be done. She or he should be placed in an overhead warmer or incubator where normal body temperature can be maintained and good observation can continue. If the infant is allowed to remain or become hypothermic, there will be added metabolic stress.

The infant should be monitored frequently for all vital signs including temperature, pulse, respirations, and blood pressure. Arterial blood gases should be checked in any infant severely asphyxiated at birth. This can be done by arterial puncture or by inserting a catheter into one of the umbilical arteries.

If the infant remains hypoxic or hypercapnic, ventilation by bag or respirator should be done. For level I and II nurseries, this may require hand-bagging until the transport team arrives. Supplemental oxygen should be given until the infant's arterial oxygen is 60 to 80 torr. If arterial gases do not improve, or the infant's color remains poor, a chest roentgenogram should be obtained to evaluate the lungs and rule out air leaks.

If the arterial blood gases show a persistent metabolic acidosis or systolic blood pressure remains low, additional volume expansion should be considered. Normal blood sugar (40 to 120 mg per deciliter) should be maintained by means of appropriate glucose infusion.

Consultation with a neonatologist at a tertiary newborn center should be sought as quickly as possible. All efforts to stabilize the infant should continue until the transport team arrives. Neonatal transport is best achieved under controlled and stable conditions by a trained team. The family should be counseled by the primary physician regarding the infant's status and the need for transport.

SUGGESTED READING

Phibbs RH. Delivery room management of the newborn. In: Avery GB, ed. Neonatology: pathophysiology and management of the newborn. 3rd ed, Philadelphia: JB Lippincott, 1986.
Volpe JJ. Hypoxic–ischemic encephalopathy: basic aspects and fetal asphyxia. Hypoxic–ischemic encephalopathy: neuropathology and clinical aspects. In: Volpe JJ, ed. Neurology of the newborn. Philadelphia: WB Saunders, 1981; 141:180.

MANAGEMENT OF TRAUMA

GENERAL APPROACH TO THE ADULT TRAUMA PATIENT

ROBERT M. McNAMARA, M.D.
DAVID K. WAGNER, M.D.

Trauma is the leading cause of death among young Americans, and its economic impact in terms of medical costs and loss of productivity is staggering. Until recently, it was a neglected entity, and even today a large percentage of trauma deaths are considered preventable. The emergence of the specialist in emergency medicine has created the opportunity to provide these patients with the appropriate initial care so crucial to a successful outcome. This chapter presents in detail our approach to the unstable, multiply injured patient, focusing on the diagnostic and therapeutic steps necessary in the first hour of care.

BEFORE ARRIVAL OF THE PATIENT

Pre-hospital Phase

Through emergency medical systems (EMS), trauma patients are receiving advanced medical care earlier in the course of their injury. Ideally, rapid stabilization is brought about by attention to airway, oxygenation, and spine immobilization; initiation of large-bore intravenous lines; control of external hemorrhage; and, possibly, application of pneumatic trousers. Emergency physicians must exhort EMS personnel to avoid undue delay in the transport of these patients to definitive care. Prolonged attempts at vascular access and use of indadequate (small-bore) intravenous catheters must be forbidden.

Pertinent history should be provided including mechanism of injury, evidence of drug or alcohol use, presence of smoke and noxious gases, environmental factors, and, when applicable, the condition of the vehicle and other occupants. A brief presentation of the first responder's assessment, treatment, and subsequent changes in the patient's condition is also sought.

The Team Approach

These patients are most effectively treated by a well-organized team with preappointed responsibilities. The feasibility and make-up of this team are individual, depending on the institution. The leader should be the available person most experienced in resuscitating multiply injured patients and is responsible for assessing the patient, ordering therapeutic and diagnostic maneuvers, and monitoring fluid therapy and patient response. The team leader must control the resuscitation as well as the surroundings, ordering excess personnel aside. Ideally, he or she does not have to perform procedures or diagnostic maneuvers.

Other physicians, depending on their expertise, can be assigned to airway control, tube placement or venous access and need to follow orders closely, delaying discussion until the patient is stabilized. Nursing staff can monitor vital signs and intake and output, keep an orderly record of patient care, and provide medication, equipment, and venous access when appropriate. Orderlies and technicians can be used to provide cervical spine immobilization and retrieval of blood products and test results.

When possible, the trauma surgeon who will ultimately care for the should be present to observe the resuscitation and response to therapy. Early notification of consultants is beneficial, but extraneous consults can add to confusion in the trauma suite. In smaller settings, early activation of transport mechanisms, helicopter or otherwise, should be considered.

Preparing the Facility

Advance notification is becoming the rule in the effective management of multiply injured patients. The blood bank and operating room team should be put on alert and the trauma team and appropriate consultants notified. Intravenous fluids should be hung, catheters and surgical packs laid out, monitoring devices prepared, and airway equipment checked. We place pneumatic trousers on the trauma stretcher and prepare material for chest drainage and autotransfusion. Having portable radiologic equipment at hand can save valuable time. Infection and hepatitis transmission can be reduced if sterile gloves and antiseptic preparation materials are made available.

INITIAL HOSPITAL ASSESSMENT AND RESUSCITATION

This phase must be tailored to the individual patient, but the sequence should be establishing a patent airway, ensuring adequate respiratory exchange, and restoration of circulation. Patients must be completely undressed and all surfaces fully examined. Once identified, life-threatening problems must be immediately addressed and further assessment must then proceed rapidly. Treatment is often required before diagnosis is certain and should be aggressive, as the danger in waiting far outweighs the risk of invasive procedures.

Airway and Cervical Spine Control

An alert patient usually needs only supplemental oxygen and oropharyngeal toilet initially and should be periodically observed for deterioration. Less responsive patients require airway assessment by listening and feeling for air exchange. When inadequate, simple things are done first: finger swipe to clear debris, suction with a large tonsil sucker, perform a jaw thrust or chin lift, insert an airway, and then evaluate the result. If these methods fail, tracheal intubation is required. Patients who require urgent tracheal intubation are those with massive hemorrhage in proximity to the airway and patients with absent protective airway reflexes. Early intubation is considered when noxious inhalation or other injury has occurred that may later compromise the airway.

The cervical spine needs to be greatly respected in trauma patients. An alert, neurologically intact, nonintoxicated patient who has no cervical spine tenderness and can perform a full, painless active range of motion in our view is not at risk for significant cervical spine injury. All other trauma victims with a mechanism of injury that is unknown or one that could cause neck injury require constant cervical immobilization. This is usually accomplished with spine board and hard collar, bilateral sandbags, and taping of the forehead with one person assigned to control the head and neck. A good cross-table lateral roentgenogram showing the C7–T1 interface will rule out the vast majority of serious injuries. However, an inadequate film is a common problem. A single lateral roentgenogram may miss a certain percentage of pathology and neurologic damage. For example, the central cord syndrome commonly occurs without roentgenographic evidence. For this reason, undue manipulation is still avoided until a full roentgenographic series is accomplished or the neck is cleared of injury by other means.

How does one achieve tracheal intubation with a potential neck injury? First, be certain that the patient requires intubation, as all respiratory distress is not upper airway. Once it is determined that intubation is required, our preferred sequence of choices in preferential order is: (1) nasotracheal intubation, (2) cricothyrotomy, (3) tactile orotracheal intubation, and (4) orotracheal intubation with "in-line" traction. The nasotracheal route is omitted in apneic patients and in those with midfacial fractures. Remember, all these methods can move the neck unless axial orientation is maintained manually.

Depending on one's expertise, there are several additional "tricks" that can be employed including jet ventilation, lighted stylets, and fiberoptic intubation. A personal favorite involves passing a 70-cm catheter retrograde through the cricothyroid membrane to the pharynx, where it is retrieved and threaded through an endotracheal tube. Holding the catheter firmly at both ends, it serves as a guide wire over which the tube is slipped into the trachea. The catheter is then simply pulled out.

Ensuring Adequate Respiratory Exchange

Once an airway is established, the chest must be assessed to ensure adequate ventilation. This is easily done by feeling for air exchange, observing chest wall motion, and listening for breath sounds. Vigorous efforts with a patent airway and poor air exchange imply a mechanical defect, requiring immediate intervention. Lack of chest wall motion suggests neurologic deficit or profound shock and requires assisted ventilation.

In this initial phase, one must identify and address tension pneumothorax, open pneumothorax, and large flail chest segments.

Tension Pneumothorax. Patients present with shock from decreased preload and may show a combination of unilateral hyper-resonance to percussion, decreased breath sounds, tracheal deviation, and distended neck veins in the absence of hypovolemia. When the diagnosis of tension pneumothorax is entertained, immediate needle decompression is suggested. We prefer the fourth or fifth intercostal space in the anterior axillary line as the location for all aspirations and subsequent tube placements. This site avoids major vascular structures and functions well as a vent for both air and blood. In addition, by entering the thoracic cage posterior to the pectoralis muscles, difficulties in penetration of muscular individuals is avoided.

Open Pneumothorax. Also called a "sucking chest wound," this is easily detected and, if large enough, can seriously compromise ventilation. Covering with a flutter valve (such as Saran wrap taped on three sides) is effective immediate treatment, followed by a chest tube when available.

Flail Chest. When large enough, this injury can result in life-threatening hypoxemia from mechanical and underlying pulmonary contusion effects. Immediate intubation and assisted ventilation are required in some instances.

This initial assessment of the chest is rapidly done and when doubt exists, assisted ventilation should be undertaken until a more definitive evaluation is possible.

Restoration of Adequate Circulation

Shock is recognized by abnormal vital signs and observation of a cool, clammy patient with an altered sensorium. Its treatment is tailored to the cause and degree of shock.

Pump Failure

Shock of this category is due to cardiac tamponade, cardiac muscle dysfunction (usually from contusion), or tension pneumothorax. Elevated central venous pressure is key to the diagnosis, but may be absent with significant hypovolemia. Tamponade can often be diagnosed and temporarily treated by pericardiocentesis. A 3.5-inch 18-gauge spinal needle is inserted below the xiphoid at a 45-degree angle and directed toward the left shoulder. Aspiration of even a small amount of blood may yield dramatic improvement. Thoracotomy is the definitive treatment. This is best accomplished in the operating room, but must be done immediately in the critically unstable patient irrespective of location. An incision is made laterally from the sternum to the area below the left nipple, entering the thoracic cavity through the intercostal space. The adjacent costochondral cartilages are divided for better exposure as rib spreaders are inserted. The pericardium is incised longitudinally anterior to the phrenic nerve and the clot evacuated. Actively bleeding wounds are controlled with the fingers until definitive repair. Myocardial contusion is discussed elsewhere (see chapter *Myocardial Contusion*), and treatment parallels that of myocardial infarction.

Hypovolemic Shock

This is the most common form of traumatic shock, and therapy is directed to an estimate of blood loss. Blood volume (BV) is approximately 7 percent of body weight for adults (i.e., 70 cc per kilogram). Mild-to-moderate loss (<20 percent BV) may yield only slight tachycardia in the young, but in the elderly can cause more symptoms. Moderate-to-severe loss (20 to 40 percent BV) produces the classic signs of shock, including resting supine tachycardia, lowered blood pressure, and decreased mentation and urine flow. Severe loss (<40 percent BV) creates the pale, diaphoretic patient with thready pulse and life-threatening hypovolemia. The goal of treatment is the delivery of adequately oxygenated red cells to all tissues. Our initial therapy of hypovolemic shock is as follows:

Step 1: Stop Obvious Bleeding. Use direct pressure. Clamping is rarely done as it damages vital structures and is time-consuming. Pneumatic splints can help, and tourniquets are used only when needed in amputated limbs. Do not overlook the scalp!

Step 2: Establish Venous Access. Two large-bore lines, i.e., 16-gauge or larger, are a minimum. Uninterrupted flow to the heart must be ensured. Short and broad catheters yield the greatest flow. We initially attempt percutaneous catheterization of large arm veins, primarily in the antecubital fossa. Alternatively, 8 F catheters may be inserted in the femoral veins using the Seldinger (catheter over flexible guide wire) technique. Central vein catheterization accessed from the neck may be associated with significant complications in the emergency setting and is not recommended as an initial site of choice. We do cannulate these veins early to measure CVP when tamponade or cardiogenic shock is a possibility. The posterior approach to the internal jugular vein is preferred as it carries less risk of pneumothorax, and inadvertent arterial puncture can be directly compressed. Cutdowns are time-consuming and rarely needed except in pediatric cases. When used, flow-restricting long tubing (such as pediatric feeding tubes) should be avoided.

In the emergent situation, a reasonably sterile technique is usually possible. When initial stabilization is complete, other lines can be started, and cumbersome (antecubital) or problem (femoral, unprepped) sites can be discontinued. Remember, "any port in a storm," but be selective when possible.

Step 3: Deliver Fluid Volume. Initially, 2 to 3 liters of isotonic crystalloid is infused as rapidly as it can be administered and the response assessed. Partial responders or nonresponders usually have large losses and require blood and, often, urgent surgery. Those stabilized with this probably have minor losses, and further therapy depends on their evolution. Type-specific blood is safe and usually available within 10 minutes. In critically ill patients, blood is drawn for crossmatching as soon as venous lines are established, and the transport attendant is told to wait at the blood bank until two units of type-specific blood are available. These are immediately rushed back to the trauma suite. The team leader monitors volume resuscitation and assesses the patient's response.

Cardiac Arrest

This is usually secondary to hypovolemic shock, and external compression is ineffective with an empty heart. Immediate thoracotomy, with internal cardiac massage and compression of the descending aorta, is necessary. Vigorous volume replacement is also required.

Adjuncts to Circulation

Pneumatic trousers can augment blood pressure via an afterload effect. We find them most useful for hemorrhage control in patients with pelvic fractures. Their tamponade effect may be used prior to laparotomy for obvious intra-abdominal bleeding. Autotransfusion is highly effective in hemothorax, and simple devices are manufactured for emergency department use. Pressure infusion devices should be available.

FURTHER CARE

Complete Examination and Adequate History

A head-to-toe physical examination with complete neurologic examination is performed as early as possible. Explore all orifices. Problems uncovered are dealt with on the basis of priorities. Allergies, medications, pertinent medical history, last oral intake, and circumstances surrounding the event are elicited when possible.

Tubes

Chest tubes are inserted early in all cases of traumatic pneumothorax. A gastric tube detects blood, lessens the risk of vomiting, and treats gastric dilatation, which can compromise ventilation, especially in children. The oral route is preferred if cribriform plate integrity is questioned due to facial trauma. Bladder catheterization is indicated to monitor urinary output. If urethral rupture is suspected because of meatal blood, scrotal hematoma, or an abnormally positioned prostate, a urethrogram is performed first.

Diagnostics

These are indicated to identify injury, sites of blood loss, and direct therapy. The following is our initial approach.

Laboratory Studies. An initial low hematocrit is ominous; otherwise, the initial hematocrit determination serves only as a baseline. Chemistries, clotting studies, and urinalysis are routinely done. Toxicology studies are performed when indicated. Arterial blood gases are most useful to assess oxygenation in pulmonary contusion and possible aspirations.

Monitors. Electrocardiographic monitoring is initiated early on in all trauma patients. Subsequently, with chest injuries and older patients, a complete twelve-lead electrocardiogram is obtained. CVP and arterial pressure is serially evaluated as indicated.

Plain Roentgenograms. These are obtained as dictated by signs or symptoms. Chest and pelvic films are routinely obtained as they can reveal major sources of blood loss. Proper technique is essential to prevent confusing results. For chest films, a 6-foot view, with the principal ray centrally directed, is desirable.

Peritoneal Lavage. This is most useful in the abdominal evaluation of the patient with altered sensorium. Ideally, the surgeon responsible for the continuing care will participate in this procedure.

Other Studies. CT scan is invaluable for the head-injured patient and has shown increasing utility in blunt abdominal trauma. Arteriography may be required to identify certain vascular injuries, particularly when penetrating or sudden deceleration injuries have occurred. Any alteration in peripheral pulses requires definitive evaluation. A quick "one-shot" IVP prior to emergent laparotomy is frequently obtained to clarify renal function.

Immunoprophylaxis and Antibiotics

Tetanus antitoxin and antibiotics are addressed on an individual basis. The need for tetanus toxoid and tetanus immune globulin is dependent on the nature of the injury and patient immunization status. Early antibiotic therapy should be instituted for certain injuries, such as open fractures and penetrating abdominal trauma.

DISPOSITION

The decision to operate is made by the surgeon. The urgency of surgical intervention is dictated by the patient's response to initial therapy. Those who do not require initial surgical intervention must be closely observed for subsequent deterioration, preferably in an intensive care unit. The possible need for transfer should be recognized early. The referring physician is responsible for adequate resuscitation and stabilization for transport and must relay complete data to the receiving institution. The receiving physician must have the capabilities to handle the patient and be comfortable in the knowledge that appropriate stabilization has occurred prior to transfer. Direct communication is vital, and a complete written record with results of all diagnostic steps should accompany the patient. Adequately trained personnel must effect the transfer.

PATIENTS REFRACTORY TO TREATMENT

These patients demand close scrutiny. Their problems often lie with inadequate volume replacement due to unrecognized blood loss or a poor respiratory status. Cardiac causes, including myocardial infarction, contusion, and tamponade, should be considered. Acute gastric dilatation, especially in children, should be ruled out. Rare causes include adrenal insufficiency, anaphylaxis and severe acidosis from causes other than shock.

SUGGESTED READING

American College of Surgeons. Early care of the injured patient. Philadelphia: WB Saunders, 1982:1–44.
Committee on Trauma, Advanced trauma life support course manual. Chicago: American College of Surgeons, 1985:5–72.

MAXILLOFACIAL SKELETAL FRACTURE

LEONARD B. KABAN, D.M.D., M.D., F.A.C.S.
ROBERT CHUONG, D.M.D., M.D.

Fractures of the maxillofacial skeleton are common injuries since the face is relatively unprotected from trauma in automobile and industrial accidents, fisticuffs, and falls. Motor vehicle accidents are the most common cause of facial fractures in adults–accounting for 50 to 60 percent of such injuries. Approximately 70 percent of all patients injured in automobiles sustain some soft tissue or bony facial injury.

In children, the most common cause of facial fractures is a fall from a bicycle, steps, or jungle gym. Because the midface is less prominent than the skull in children, craniocerebral trauma is more common than isolated facial fractures in high-speed automobile crashes.

GENERAL EVALUATION

Facial injuries are often dramatic, and the inexperienced clinician may be distracted from more dangerous associated injuries. Assessment of the patient must proceed in an orderly fashion, dealing first with the most life-threatening problems. A careful history establishes the likely mechanism of injury and guides subsequent management.

Evaluation of the airway is the first priority in any injured patient. In the setting of maxillofacial trauma, airway obstruction may occur secondary to (1) posterior displacement of a fractured mandible or maxilla, (2) foreign body, such as food or other debris in the mouth, pharynx, or larynx, (3) severe hemorrhage from the nasomaxillary complex, and (4) laryngeal injury resulting in hematoma or fracture.

Airway control begins by clearing foreign bodies and blood clots from the mouth. If the airway is compromised, the anterior jaw thrust maneuver should be attempted, with minimal manipulation of the cervical spine. The mandible is moved anteriorly by applying digital pressure behind the angles of the jaw. This maneuver, when the anterior mandible is fractured, tends to restore the tongue, pharyngeal structures, and suprahyoid muscles to their proper location. If the tongue continues to fall back into the larynx, thereby causing obstruction, a suture or towel clip should be placed through the tongue and anterior traction applied. Unless contraindicated, the patient can be placed in the lateral or prone position to allow secretions and blood to drain and to assist in tongue positioning.

Intubation is indicated if there are labored respirations or when there is severe ongoing upper airway hemorrhage. Laryngoscopy may paradoxically be easier to perform when the mandible is fractured, since the anterior portion of the jaw can be displaced to allow visualization of the larynx. However, the possibility of anatomic distortion of the upper airway by hematoma and edema should always be considered.

Elective intubation, with the patient awake and/or sedated, is the most controlled aproach. In general, oral intubation is preferred in the emergency situation. However, nasal intubation, contrary to common misconception, is not absolutely contraindicated in the presence of nasal or midface fractures. The nasal airway is below the fractured nasal bones and oriented horizontally (Fig. 1). Indeed, nasal intubation is necessary at the time of definitive fracture repair. Oral or nasal intubation is preferrable to tracheostomy since long-term airway support is rarely necessary.

Hemorrhage from the maxillofacial complex is rarely the cause of significant hypotension. In the presence of hypovolemia, injuries to other organ systems must be assumed until ruled out by careful clinical evaluation. Active facial hemorrhage can be controlled in the emergency department by pressure dressings, e.g., nasal hemorrhage may require anterior and/or posterior packing. Blind clamping of bleeding points must never be done because

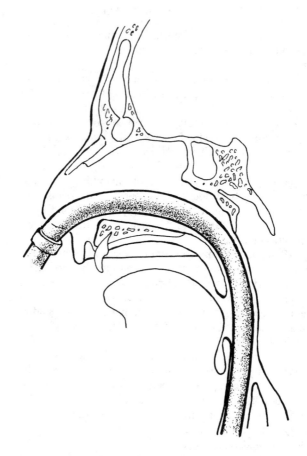

Figure 1 Relationship of nasal bones to nasal airway. The nasal airway is parallel to the palate, whereas the nasal bones are situated anteriorly and superiorly. A nasoendotracheal tube is shown in proper position. There is no impingement of the tube on the nasal bones or the region of the cribiform plate.

of potential injury to contiguous sensory or motor nerves, that is, branches of cranial nerve V or VII, or to the parotid or lacrimal ducts.

Once the airway is secure and hemorrhage controlled, injuries to other organ systems are systematically evaluated. Although facial injuries are often dramatic, they are rarely life-threatening and are usually of secondary importance in the acute setting. In addition, it is important to consider possible cranial, cervical, ophthalmologic, and laryngeal injuries in association with the maxillofacial trauma. Neurologic evaluation is mandatory to rule out focal sensory and motor deficits. Any periorbital injury requires careful ophthalmologic examination to rule out retinal detachment, hyphema, vitreous hemorrhage, or other global injury. Visual acuity must be documented at the initial evaluation. The cervical spine should not be manipulated until injury can be ruled out. Blunt injuries to the face may result in fractures of the cervical spine and one should not hesitate to obtain roentgenograms of this area. Laryngeal injury is uncommon, but should be suspected if there is ecchymosis, crepitus, or tenderness of the neck. Soft tissue films of the neck may reveal distortion of the airway and subcutaneous emphysema.

EVALUATION OF THE MAXILLOFACIAL COMPLEX

Diagnosis of facial injuries is established by history and physical examination, and confirmed by radiologic studies.

A careful history helps to establish the nature, direction, and point of contact of the injuring force. Particular patterns of injury may be suspected on the basis of such information. For example, blunt trauma to the chin point is often associated with fracture of the mandibular condyles and may be a clue to cervical spine injury. Paresthesia in one or more divisions of the trigeminal nerve suggests possible fractures of the mandible, maxilla, zygoma, or orbital floor. Discrepancies in the occlusion, no matter how minor, must be considered secondary to dentoalveolar, maxillary, or mandibular fracture until proved otherwise.

Systematic examination of the facial soft tissue, skeleton, and oral cavity must be carried out. In particular, it is important to assess and document injuries to (1) the seventh nerve when there are lacerations in the parotid region, (2) the parotid duct, which parallels and is adjacent to the buccal branch of the seventh nerve (Fig. 2), (3) the third, fourth, and sixth nerves and sensory branches of the fifth nerve, which may indicate fractures as these nerves traverse various bony canals and fissures of the maxillofacial complex, (4) adnexae of the eyes, including the canthal tendons, eyelids, and lacrimal system, (5) teeth and surrounding alveolar bone for fractures and mobility, and (6) oral mucosa and tongue for lacerations, bleeding, and ecchymosis.

Subcutaneous or submucosal hematoma may be a manifestation of an underlying fracture. The floor of the mouth and the periorbital area contain a loose, areolar tissue into which blood accumulates when the mandible or orbit has been injured.

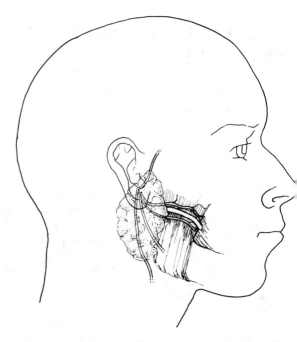

Figure 2 Relationship of facial nerve to parotid duct. The buccal branch of the facial nerve courses parallel and superior to the parotid duct. The duct is superficial to the masseter muscle and turns medially at its anterior border to enter the mouth. The duct can be located along a line from the tragus of the ear to a point approximately 1 cm above the oral commissure. (Adapted from Kaban LB, Goldwyn RM. Facial injuries. In: May HL, ed. Emergency medicine. New York: John Wiley and Sons, 1984:323-353.)

Epistaxis may indicate direct nasal injury, but the possibility of maxillary or zygomatic complex fractures must also be considered since these injuries cause bleeding into the maxillary sinus, which may then drain into the nose.

MANAGEMENT OF FACIAL FRACTURES

Maxillary (Midface) Fractures

Midface fractures occur most commonly as a result of high-speed automobile trauma or falls from a great distance, as from a window or scaffolding. Approximately 150 times the force of gravity is required to fracture the midface, significantly more than for any other facial bone.

Classification of maxillary fractures is based on cadaver experiments of RenQee LeFort, reported in 1901 (Fig. 3). He observed three general patterns of fracture in response to blunt midface trauma. *LeFort I* or transverse fracture is separation of the alveolar portion of the maxilla at the level of the nasal floor. *LeFort II* or pyramidal fracture is separation of the nasomaxillary complex from the zygomatic complexes. *LeFort III* fracture (craniofacial dysjunction) is separation of the entire midface, including zygomas, from the cranium. Both LeFort II and III injuries involve the orbits, and thus extraocular muscle entrapment and maxillary nerve injury are possible. Combinations of fractures at different levels are common; for example, a patient may have a

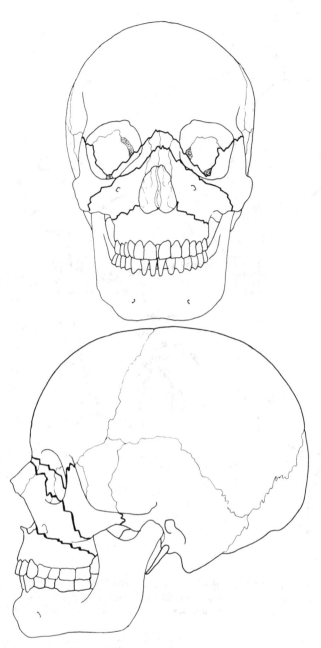

Figure 3 Midface fractures—LeFort classification. Frontal and lateral projections demonstrate the classic fracture lines of LeFort. Note that the LeFort II and III fractures involve the walls of the orbit. (Adapted from Kaban LB, Goldwyn RM. Facial injuries. In: May HL, ed. Emergency medicine. New York: John Wiley and Sons, 1984:323-353.)

transverse fracture (LeFort I) on one side and a pyramidal (LeFort II) fracture on the other.

Diagnosis is made by history to determine the mechanism of injury and by careful physical examination. With one hand, the examiner grasps the maxilla at the alveolar ridge and moves it up and down and side to side while palpating with the other hand for mobility at the piriform apertures, infraorbital rims, lateral orbits, and nasofrontal area (Fig. 4). Inspection classically reveals malocclusion, usually with an anterior open bite, elongation of the midface, epistaxis, periorbital edema and

ecchymosis, and subconjunctival hemorrhage. In LeFort II and III injuries, there may be infraorbital paresthesia as a result of injury of the maxillary nerve in the infraorbital canal.

Naso-ethmoidal-orbital fractures may be a component of severe midface injuries. Complex fractures of this type do not follow the simple patterns described by LeFort. Patients with naso-ethmoidal-orbital fractures exhibit traumatic telecanthus. Detachment of the canthal tendon from the frontal process of the maxilla results in rounding of the normally pointed medial canthal region. The nasolacrimal duct and lacrimal sac may be injured, and the nasal pyramid may be displaced into the interorbital region.

Roentgenograms are helpful to confirm the diagnosis of midface fracture and to determine the extent of comminution and degree and direction of displacement. A Waters' view shows the orbital rims, the lateral wall of the maxilla, the nasal pyramid, and the paranasal sinuses (Fig. 5). It is the most useful roentgenogram for midface and orbital injuries. The Caldwell (P-A) and lateral views are of limited value. Tomography may be helpful to assess injury at the cranial base and within the orbit.

Emergency department management of midface fractures consists primarily of airway management. Severe hemorrhage from the sphenopalatine or the internal maxillary arteries occurs rarely and may require packing. The airway may need to be secured by endotracheal intubation. Antibiotics (penicillin 500,000 to 1,000,000 units IV or a cephalosporin 500 mg to 1 g IV every 6 hours) should be administered routinely, beginning in the emergency department and continuing for at least 2 to 3 days.

Treatment consists of anatomic reduction of the midface in the transverse (horizontal), sagittal (lateral), and coronal (frontal) planes. Reduction and fixation of midface fractures may be performed as late as 10 days after injury, although earlier treatment minimizes the incidence of infection. The presence of cerebrospinal fluid (CSF) rhinorrhea is not a contraindication to treatment. In fact, early fracture reduction or at least immobilization may facilitate spontaneous sealing of the dural tear. CSF rhinorrhea precludes nasal packing because of the risk of ascending infection. The patient should be advised against blowing of the nose, which may force air intracranially or into the subcutaneous tissue.

ZYGOMATIC FRACTURES

Zygomatic fractures are best classified into zygomatic complex or zygomatic arch injuries. Fractures usually result from blunt forces (50 to 80 g) directed medially and superiorly. When the force is a punch, the left zygomatic complex is most often injured by a right-handed assailant. Zygomatic arch fractures result from a direct, localized, medially directed force producing a V-shaped, medially displaced, deformity of the arch.

Clinical signs and symptoms of zygomatic complex injury include infraorbital sensory disturbance, periorbital ecchymosis and edema, subconjunctival hemorrhage (typically lateral and inferior), chemosis, antimongoloid

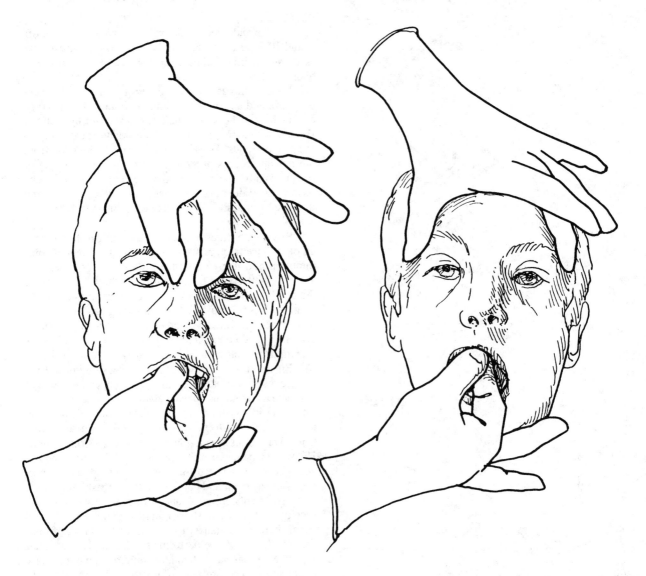

Figure 4 Bimanual palpation of the midface. The diagnosis of LeFort fractures can generally be established by bimanual palpation. The maxilla is grasped anteriorly and manipulated while the other hand palpates along the piriform aperture, nasofrontal area, and lateral orbital rims. (Adapted from Kaban LB, Goldwyn RM. Facial injuries. In: May HL, ed. Emergency medicine. New York: John Wiley and Sons, 1984:323-353.)

slant of the palpebral fissure, diplopia, trismus, and decreased lateral excursions of the mandible attributable to impingement of the zygomatic arch against the coronoid process of the mandible (Fig. 6). A palpable bony step-off may be found along the lateral or inferior orbital rim or lateral maxillary wall, intraorally, at the base of the zygoma. Ipsilateral epistaxis is common and is attributable to hemorrhage within the maxillary antrum. An isolated arch fracture presents as a depression over the lateral cheek and causes limitation of mandibular excursion. In contrast to the zygomatic complex fracture, there are no orbital signs.

Management in the emergency setting consists of diagnosis by clinical and radiologic examination,

ophthalmologic examination to rule out ocular injury, and referral for treatment.

Roentgenograms that are essential to determine the direction of displacement of the zygoma are the Waters', Caldwell, and submental-vertex ("jug handle") views. The latter allows assessment of arch displacement. To determine the extent of medial or lateral rotation, the Waters' view is most helpful. Finally, the Caldwell view assists in assessment of inferior-superior displacement of the zygomatic complex.

Edema and hematoma may hinder attempts to correct the deformity. Definitive treatment is therefore delayed for 3 to 5 days, until swelling subsides. Indications for reduction of zygomatic complex fractures are

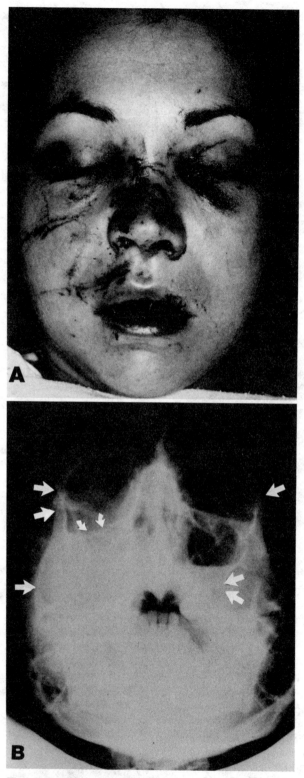

Figure 5 Midface (LeFort III) Fracture. *A*, Frontal appearance after blunt midfacial trauma. Note bilateral periorbital edema and ecchymosis and elongation of the middle third of the face. The midface was mobile to palpation. *B*, A Waters' view demonstrates fractures through the right inferior and lateral orbital rim, right zygomatic arch, left lateral maxilla, and left frontozygomatic suture. Note air-fluid level in left maxillary sinus and totally opaque right sinus. These findings are consistent with LeFort III fracture.

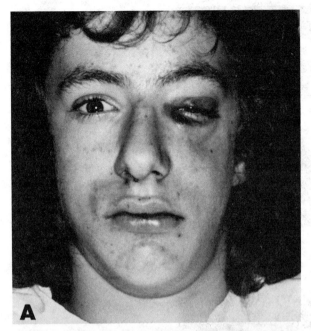

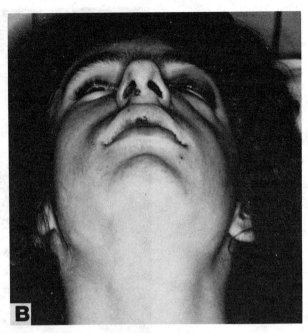

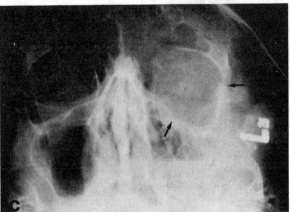

Figure 6 Zygomatic complex fracture. *A*, Frontal appearance shortly after blunt injury to the left zygomatic region. Note periorbital ecchymosis and edema, inferior displacement of the lateral canthus, flattening of the cheek, and dried blood in the left nares. *B*, Submental view more clearly demonstrates the marked flattening of the left cheek. *C*, Waters' view demonstrates a medially rotated left zygomatic complex fracture, that is, medial displacement at the frontozygomatic suture (lateral orbital rim) and inferior displacement at the zygomaticomaxillary suture (infraorbital rim). An air-fluid level in the maxillary sinus is noted.

facial asymmetry owing to flattening of the cheek, persistent diplopia secondary to entrapment, persistent paresthesia, and interference with mandibular excursions.

Blowout Fractures

"Blowout fracture," a term coined by Converse, is often inaccurately applied to fractures of the maxilla or zygomatic complex. The term is properly used to describe isolated fractures of the orbital floor or medial wall without violation of the orbital rim. Such injuries may occur by a hydraulic pressure mechanism. A blunt force applied to the globe drives it posteriorly in the orbital cone, thereby causing a sudden rise in intraorbital pressure. This results in a "blowout" of the thin orbital floor, typically posteromedially, or the medial wall in the thinnest portion, the lamina papyracea. It has been demonstrated that a "blowout" may occur without direct trauma to the globe, but by buckling of the orbital floor in response to a force at the orbital rim. The rim does not fracture, yet the orbital floor comminutes.

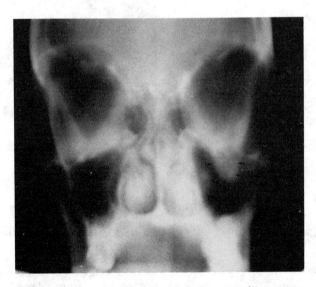

Figure 7 Blowout fracture. Coronal tomogram demonstrates herniation of orbital fat and muscle through the left orbital floor (arrows). Entrapment of this tissue results in restricted ocular motility.

The clinical signs are similar to those of zygomatic complex fractures, but without depression of the malar eminence or restriction of mandibular movement. The orbital rim is intact. There may be diplopia, enophthalmos, infraorbital paresthesia, ipsilateral epistaxis, periorbital ecchymosis and edema, and subconjunctival hemorrhage. Because of the marked periorbital swelling typically seen in zygomatic complex and blowout fractures, distinction between the two injuries may be difficult on clinical grounds alone in the acute setting.

The Waters' view, polytomography, and/or computed tomography may be necessary to define the injury. Tomograms demonstrate herniation of orbital soft tissues into the maxillary sinus (Fig. 7). Ophthalmologic consultation is essential to evaluate possible ocular injury and to measure the degree of enophthalmos.

Indications for treatment are controversial and cannot be comprehensively discussed here. We believe that reasonable indications for reduction of a blowout fracture are enophthalmos greater than 4 to 5 mm, radiologic evidence of a large orbital floor defect, and diplopia that does not resolve after 10 to 14 days. Persistent entrapment of the globe by forced duction test, which involves movement of the globe by forceps traction on the tendon of the inferior rectus, is another indication for operation.

SUGGESTED READING

Bertolami C, Kaban LB. Trauma to the chin and associated cervical spine injuries. Oral Surg 1981; 52:122.

Chuong R, Donoff RB, Guralnick WD. Retrospective analysis of 372 mandibular fractures. J Oral Maxillofac Surg 1983; 41:305.

Kaban LB, Mulliken JB, Murray JE. Facial fractures in children: an analysis of 122 fractures in 109 patients. Plast Reconstr Surg 1977; 59:15.

Wilkins RB, Havins WE. Current treatment of blowout fractures. Ophthalmology 1982; 89:464.

NASAL FRACTURE AND LACERATION

CHARLES T. YARINGTON Jr., M.D., F.A.C.S.

The occurrence of nasal trauma usually is not subtle, and from a historical standpoint as well as by physical examination does not present a diagnostic challenge. However, the assessment of the extent of nasal injury and associated trauma presents a significant problem. It demands sufficient physical examination skill, radiologic study, or other measures to rule out associated injuries to the facial structure, cranial cavity, cervical spine, and the eyes before injury to the nose itself can be evaluated and treated.

DIAGNOSIS

Diagnostic studies that should be considered are primarily limited to roentgenograms of the nose in the standard Waters view, lateral view, and occlusal view. In the pediatric patient, slight underexposure is necessary to delineate the nasal structures because of the lack of calcification in the younger age group. As it is sometimes difficult to distinguish between old and recent nasal fractures, correlation of the films with the physical findings on palpation and the history of injury is required. Frequently, physical findings are of more value than radiologic studies, but in significant injuries, the radiologic studies are required to rule out associated injuries to the maxillofacial skeleton. Baseline measurements of hemoglobin and hematocrit are helpful in consideration of possible blood loss or potential blood loss during surgery or manipulation. Other studies should be obtained as required in anticipation of hospitalization and surgery.

Lacerations and fractures of the nose may be classified simply as closed nasal fractures, open nasal fractures, and fractures involving other facial structures, either open or closed. In addition to the foregoing, lacerations involving the cartilaginous structure of the nose, with or without fracture, should be considered separately from simple lacerations involving neither cartilaginous nor bony structures. Finally, injuries involving the nasal septum should be considered as a separate entity. Any of the preceding injuries can occur in the adult or the pediatric patient, and differences in the care of these two groups will be outlined and the exceptions provided to the general recommendations that follow.

TREATMENT

Simple lacerations of the nose not involving the bony cartilaginous framework and closed fractures of the nose can usually be managed on an outpatient basis. A thorough evaluation of the nose, including external palpation and inspection, examination of the nasal vestibule and nostrils, and appropriate radiologic studies, is essential. Closure of simple uncomplicated nasal lacerations can be accomplished under local anesthesia by appropriately trained personnel utilizing fine suture material, with minimum debridement. Following initial closure, these lacerations can be cared for in the same manner as other facial lacerations, utilizing the principles of elevation and ice bag compress for the first 12 hours.

Simple closed fractures of the nose can be reduced immediately if appropriate personnel are available to accomplish this task, or reduction can await the resolution of initial swelling if necessary. In all cases, reduction should be accomplished within 5 days if possible, with elevation and ice packs used to minimize edema or hematoma. In most instances, hospitalization is not required, and the procedure can be carried out under local and topical anesthesia. The patient should be warned that with any fracture of the nasal pyramid, even the best reduction cannot guarantee restoration of the pretrauma profile, appearance and airway, and that secondary surgery to the pyramid or nasal septum may sometimes be required.

Exceptions to the above would include the pediatric patient with evidence of hematoma or significant fracture or malalignment of the nasal septum, or with significant comminution of the nasal pyramid, where adequate control and manipulation cannot be accomplished under local anesthesia, or where open reduction and exploration are deemed appropriate.

Lacerations involving the cartilaginous and/or bony structure of the nose, or open fractures of the nose in the pediatric patient usually require hospital admission and careful exploration, reduction, and closure by appropriate personnel under general anesthesia. Initial treatment should include careful cleansing of the wound, attention to tetanus immunization, and strict avoidance of any debridement or injury to remaining tissue. In the case of major avulsions of tissue, if this material is available it should be maintained in ice and saline for possible use as a free graft implantation. Application of a sterile saline-soaked compress as a dressing, a loose anterior nasal pack with saline-soaked cotton, and an external ice pack is recommended during the interim period before surgery. As noted previously, the presence of a septal hematoma or seroma or the presence of significant septal deformity even in the absence of external nasal trauma may require general anesthesia, exploration, and repair in the pediatric patient.

In the adult patient with an open nasal fracture or a laceration involving the cartilaginous structure of the nose, initial treatment should include cleansing the wound with sterile saline solution and the use of a sterile saline-soaked dressing with ice compresses. Bleeding is usually self-limiting, but can be controlled with saline-soaked cotton pledgets, a rolled Telfa tampon, or Vaseline gauze as required. The principles of repair require irrigation of the wound with normal saline, removal of foreign bodies, reapproximation of both the mucous membrane and cutaneous lacerations, and approximation of the cartilaginous and bony structures with appropriate stabilization. Further trauma or suturing through cartilaginous tissue in the external nose is avoided, although sutures are frequently used for stabilization of the septal cartilaginous and bony structures. The decision whether injuries to the adult nose require an operating room environment for an adequate reconstruction depends on the extent of the injury, the general health and cooperativeness of the patient, and the facilities available in the emergency room. Generally, however, these procedures can be carried out under local and topical anesthesia.

In summary, lacerations and fractures of the nose require immediate evaluation to determine whether hospitalization and surgery will be required. In the pediatric patient with significant fractures, open injuries, or septal derangement, open exploration and reconstruction are frequently carried out under general anesthesia within the first 24 hours. In the adult patient with similar injuries, therapy is usually carried out under local and topical anesthesia as soon after injury as possible. With simple closed fractures of the nasal pyramid, reduction can be carried out immediately, or at any convenient time when swelling has subsided during the first 5 days.

Finally, a word might be said concerning the selection of a consulting specialist to care for nasal lacerations and fractures. Although simple lacerations can frequently be cared for by emergency department personnel, a plastic surgeon or otolaryngologist should be selected for the care of most injuries. Both are well trained in the basics of nasal injuries and repair, but the otolaryngologist often is better prepared to deal with internal derangements of the nose. The emergency physician would do well to become familiar with the capabilities of available consultants and select individuals whose training and interests best fit the injury.

SUGGESTED READING

Larrabee WF. Nasal and nasalseptal fractures. In: Hold ED, Richard G, eds. Maxillofacial trauma. Boston: Little, Brown & Co, 1986.

EAR TRAUMA

SCOTT MANNING, M.D.
PETER ROLAND, M.D.
WILLIAM L. MEYERHOFF, M.D., Ph. D.

Otologic trauma covers a wide range of commonly seen injuries. The auricle, because of its exposed position, is frequently subject to blunt, thermal, chemical, and sharp trauma; the external canal is an inviting repository for foreign bodies; the tympanic membrane and middle ear are subject to penetrating and implosive injuries, and the inner ear is commonly involved in head injuries. While associated, potentially life threatening, injuries take precedence, careful attention to diagnosis and appropriate emergency therapy of ear injuries will go a long way toward prevention of potential long-term sequelae.

THE AURICLE

Soft Tissue Injury

Because of the excellent blood supply via the posterior auricular, superficial temporal, and deep auricular arteries, injuries to the auricle should be treated according to the principles of minimal debridement. Only unequivocally devitalized tissue should be removed. Simple lacerations with minimal wound gaping are best treated with 6-0 monofilament nonabsorbable nylon skin sutures after meticulous wound cleansing. Complex lacerations are best treated by proceeding from known to unknown areas with preservation of all but obviously devitalized tissue. An effort should be made to avoid placing sutures through cartilage. If the perichondrium remains intact, meticulous perichondrial closure usually suffices to approximate cartilaginous fragments. If absolutely necessary, catgut chromic sutures may be used to approximate cartilage where needed to reduce skin tension. Simple abrasions are best managed with vigorous cleansing followed by application of antibiotic ointment and sterile dressings. Full-thickness skin losses may be treated with primary skin grafting if the underlying perichondrium remains. In the absence of perichondrium and with exposed cartilage, therapeutic options include "wedging" out the area of injury with primary closure or removing the exposed cartilage with primary skin grafts applied to the underlying perichondrium. Leaving exposed cartilage to heal by secondary intention carries the risk of suppurative chondritis. Patients with heavily contaminated wounds or wounds in which there is exposure of cartilage should be given 5 days of oral antimicrobial therapy. Coverage should be directed against penicillinase-producing *Staphylococcus* and *Streptococcus*. Dicloxacillin, erythromycin, and second-generation oral cephalosporins are all reasonable choices.

Special consideration must be given to human bites, which comprise a large percentage of auricular injuries. These injuries are often best managed with vigorous wound cleansing followed by a course of systemic antibiotics and delayed definitive repair when danger of wound infection has passed. In these cases, antimicrobial therapy should be directed toward typical oral flora. A high percentage of anaerobic organisms are present in the oral cavity, and therefore clindamycin has been the drug of our choice for the treatment of human bites.

Tetanus toxoid and immune globulin should be administered to all patients with soft tissue injuries of the ear as with other soft tissue injuries. Consultation with a plastic surgeon or otolaryngologist is recommended.

Amputation

Complete auricular amputations are difficult problems whose definitive management is best left to the otolaryngologist. Every effort should be made to locate the detached part. It is best not to immerse the amputated part in iced saline as this promotes tissue maceration. The part should be wrapped in a sterile dressing and placed within an ice-filled container. Complete amputations have been managed with reattachment and reimplantation in a postauricular pocket following dermabrasion of the amputated part. Primary reattachment by microvascular anastomosis is occasionally undertaken.

Partial amputations, even if attached only by a small strip of auricular skin, are managed by primary wound closure. These have an excellent prognosis for full survival.

Thermal Injury

The external ear is particularly liable to thermal injury because of its exposed position and its paucity of subcutaneous tissue. Auricular burns are present in 90 percent of patients presenting with facial burns, and their treatment is aimed primarily at prevention of the complication of *Pseudomonas* chondritis. To this end the burned auricle should be cleansed and covered with antibiotic ointment and a sterile dressing. Pressure dressings should be avoided to prevent further compromise of cartilaginous blood supply. In patients who are hospitalized with severe burns or other injuries, care must be taken that inadvertent pressure is not applied to the auricles from pillows. Treatment of third-degree burns includes careful debridement and skin grafting as indicated.

The auricle is the most common area of the body to suffer frostbite. Treatment of frostbite is similar to that of burns. Acute frostbite injury should be treated by rapid warming with moist heat at about 40 °C. Surgical debridement should be delayed in any type of thermal injury for days to weeks as final demarcation may take this long. As with other facial injuries, debridement should be highly conservative.

Blunt Trauma

Auricular hematomas following blunt trauma generally occur on the anterior surface of the auricle in the plane between the cartilage and the perichondrium (Fig. 1). If untreated, the underlying cartilage, deprived of its perichondrial blood supply, undergoes degeneration and fibrosis, resulting in permanent deformity (cauliflower ear). Treatment consists of sterile aspiration followed by tight pressure dressings. It is essential that pressure be applied directly to the skin of the conchal bowl. Cotton, mechanic's waste, or dental rolls soaked in either sterile saline or sterile mineral oil should be pressed into the conchal bowl and a large mastoid-type pressure dressing placed over it. The wound should be checked on a daily basis for reaccumulation, which is common. When there has been no reaccumulation for a period of 4 days, the dressing may be removed, and the patient should be instructed to protect the ear. If hematoma has reaccumulated, it may be reaspirated. Reaccumulation after a second aspiration requires incision, drainage, and placement of a tie-over bolster dressing. The incision for drainage should be placed so as to closely parallel the greater helix.

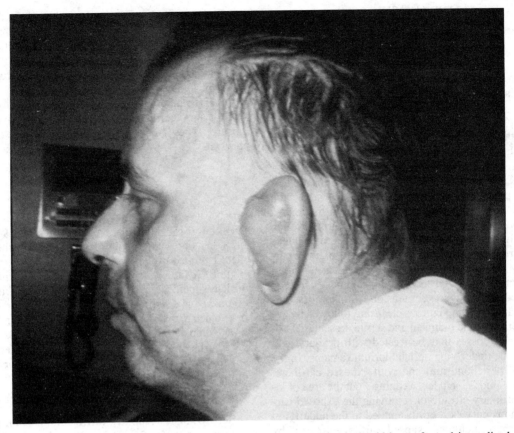

Figure 1 Auricular hematoma. Aspiration and/or incision and drainage should be performed immediately.

EXTERNAL AUDITORY CANAL

The external ear is subject to penetrating trauma from objects such as hairpins and pencil tips. The most important step in evaluating these injuries is careful inspection of the tympanic membrane for associated trauma. Most clean external canal lacerations can be treated expectantly with the patient admonished to avoid water in the ear. Contaminated wounds should be cleansed and treated with topical antibiotic drops. Severe injuries with tissue avulsion and profuse bleeding are best evaluated by an otolaryngologist with an operating microscope. Careful replacement of macerated skin with external canal packing may prevent development of canal stenosis in those cases in which there is severe disruption of the skin of the external auditory canal.

Foreign Bodies

External canal foreign bodies often present a difficult and frustrating problem for the emergency physician. The skin of the bony ear canal is exquisitely sensitive, and most foreign bodies are found in children who are frequently less than fully cooperative. Small foreign bodies can sometimes be removed with gentle irrigation, but this should be attempted only if the tympanic membrane can be visualized and seems to be intact. Insects one of the most common foreign bodies in adults, should be killed by instillation of mineral oil or topical 4 percent Xylocaine

prior to attempts at removal. Remember that attempts at foreign body removal with inadequate instrumentation and without anesthesia may lead to external canal bleeding, tympanic membrane perforation, and even ossicular injuries. Therefore, difficult foreign bodies are best removed with the aid of the operating microscope. It is prudent to abandon efforts in removing foreign bodies from awake children if initial attempts fail. It is almost impossible to hold the head of a distraught child completely still. Head movement leads to pain and bleeding, the result being a hysterical child with overwrought parents. It is far better to anesthetize the child for a few minutes and accomplish a traumatic removal. Patients who have had organic foreign bodies within the external auditory canal should be given otic drops for 48 hours to prevent external otitis caused by the irritant qualities of vegetable oils.

TYMPANIC MEMBRANE AND MIDDLE EAR

Tympanic membrane perforations may result from penetrating foreign bodies such as misguided cotton tipped applicators or from implosive forces as from a slap to the ear. Simple linear tears generally heal quickly. Antibiotic drops are not indicated for uncontaminated wounds and many otologists feel that steroid-containing drops may impair wound healing. All patients with tympanic membrane perforations need to be emphatically warned to keep water out of the affected ear. The presence of water within the middle ear space delays and sometimes prevents healing. Suppurative middle ear infection is common following contamination of the middle ear space with water. Cotton covered with Vaseline should be placed into the conchal bowl during bathing.

Two areas that warrant special attention because of their overall poorer outlook for healing are slag burns and water-skiing perforations. Both are highly likely to develop suppurative complications, the latter because of waterborn bacterial contamination and the former because of tissue necrosis from thermal injury. It is therefore recommended that these patients be placed on a regimen of antibiotic drops at the outset and followed closely by an otologist. Patients are seen who have had tympanic membrane disruption due to positive pressure applied over the external auditory meatus. The usual mechanism is a fall or a blow to the ear. Implosion from such an injury often causes inversion of the tympanic membrane, which may prevent healing. Many otologists believe that such injuries are best treated by operative eversion of the invaginated portion of the tympanic membrane, but such injuries should be evaluated on a case-by-case basis.

Any patient with tympanic membrane perforation from whatever cause must be evaluated for possible associated injuries of the ossicles, inner ear, or facial nerve. Gross evaluation of hearing can be performed in the emergency setting with Rinne and Weber tuning fork tests. If hearing loss is suspected, follow-up formal audiometric testing is mandatory. Ossicular disruption is suggested in patients who have a conductive hearing loss greater than 30 db, especially if it fails to resolve with tympanic membrane healing. Patients with injury to the inner ear, be it penetration or subluxation of the foot plate of the stapes, often present with true vertigo, nystagmus, and neurosensory hearing loss. Treatment consists of emergent surgical exploration and tissue seal to the oval window. Injury to the facial nerve, although uncommon with middle ear injuries, is another relative indication for immediate surgical exploration.

Barotrauma

In addition to penetrating and implosive injuries, the middle ear can be damaged via barotrauma. The usual mechanism is a failure of eustachian tube equalization of relative increase in ambient pressure similar to that which occurs with descent in an airplane or from a scuba dive. The resultant relative high negative middle ear pressure causes microvascular injury of middle ear mucosa with resultant edema, bleeding, and transudate causing middle ear effusion. The patient may present with hearing loss, aural fullness, and possibly unsteadiness. Physical examination reveals a retracted tympanic membrane with middle ear fluid. Frank bleeding into the middle ear space may result in hemotympanum. Initial therapy consists of use of systemic decongestants, decongestant nasal sprays, and oral antibiotics. Refractory cases may require placement of a tympanostomy tube.

TEMPORAL BONE FRACTURE

Fractures of the temporal bone make up the majority of basilar skull fractures. All patients will have sustained a forceful blow to the head, and most, but not all, will have lost consciousness. The majority have significant associated injuries of their central nervous system. The presence of blood behind an intact tympanic membrane following blunt trauma to the head is virtually pathognomonic of temporal bone (basilar skull) fracture. All patients should be hospitalized. Computed tomography should be performed as soon as the patient's condition warrants. Initial assessment and management should be directed toward ruling out and treating associated life-threatening central nervous system injuries.

Most fractures of the temporal bone are anatomically complex, but on a clinical basis, patients may be placed into one of two categories. Longitudinal temporal bone fractures account for 75 to 85 percent of patients and they extend from the squamous portion of the temporal bone across the posterior superior external canal, into the roof of the middle ear and along the long axis of the temporal bone through the cochlea and into the middle cranial fossa. Because of the location of the fracture line, physical examination reveals an external canal laceration and often a tympanic membrane perforation. The inner ear and facial nerves are generally spared. Transverse fractures account for only 15 to 25 percent of patients with temporal bone fractures. These fractures are characterized by fracture lines extending from the foramen magnum in the posterior fossa across the petrous pyramid into the middle cranial fossa. The fracture line extends either through the internal auditory canal or through the labyrinthine capsule itself. Patients with transverse temporal bone fractures are more likely to have severe sensorineural hearing losses and facial nerve injury. They are less likely to have frank hemotympanum, which occurs only when the lateral wall of the cochlea is fractured, resulting in bleeding into the middle ear space behind an intact tympanic membrane.

Many multiple trauma patients, when first seen, have blood filling their external auditory canal. If the patient's condition permits, blood should be removed from the external auditory canal so that the tympanic membrane can be examined. *Strict asepsis is essential.* Contamination introduced in the presence of a CSF leak could result in a preventable case of meningitis. In many cases, the blood filling the external auditory canal runs into the ear from a scalp or facial laceration and temporal bone fracture may be excluded. If there is a fracture of the roof of the external auditory canal with or without a torn tympanic membrane, basilar skull fracture is certain. In all cases of basilar skull fracture, CSF leakage into the middle ear space should be assumed.

All cases of head injury should be evaluated for facial nerve function. This is especially so in temporal bone fractures as the initial evaluation often determines definitive management. Patients with immediate onset of facial paralysis require complete facial nerve exploration as soon as they are medically stable. Patients with delayed onset of facial paralysis are managed nonoperatively with steroid therapy. Thus, the assessment of facial nerve function made by an emergency physician at the time of the patient's arrival in the emergency department often determines ultimate management.

It is frequently difficult to evaluate facial nerve function in the severely traumatized patient, especially if he is unconscious. Comparison of the two nasolabial folds can be helpful as the ipsilateral nasolabial fold is often lost with complete facial paralysis. Observation of nasal flaring during intubation procedures or as a result of other vigorous stimulation may show a loss of the nasal flare ipsilateral to paralysis. Evaluation of eye closure may demonstrate incomplete closure and a "Bell's phenomenon" if the periorbital soft tissues are intact. However, eye closure may be complete despite facial nerve paralysis with even minimal periorbital edema. All patients with facial nerve pareses should be followed carefully by means of electrophysiologic testing to detect degeneration at the earliest possible time.

Special mention should be made about facial paralysis secondary to gunshot wounds to the temporal bone. These injuries often involve extensive soft tissue destruction and therefore present a relative indication for early surgical repair so that the distal nerve stump can be located with a nerve stimulator before wallerian degeneration is complete at 72 hours. Also, gunshot wounds are associated with a high incidence of arterial injury, and these patients should be considered for arteriography.

PERILYMPH FISTULA

Leakage of perilymphatic fluid from the inner ear into the middle ear causes symptoms of labyrinthine dysfunction—neurosensory hearing loss, vertigo, and aural fullness. Total deafness may result. Diagnosis is difficult in cases in which leakage is episodic, and hearing loss and vertigo may come and go. The key to eventual diagnosis is the history. This condition should be suspected in any patient in whom the onset of symptoms occurred during a period of straining or marked change in ambient barometric pressure. Onset while lifting weights, straining at stool, or bending over are examples of the former. Accidental aircraft cabin depressurization and descent while scuba diving are examples of the latter. If the history suggests traumatic perilymph fistula, the patient should be hospitalized at complete bed rest. The patient's head should be elevated, and nose blowing, straining, and other activities causing elevation of CSF pressure should be avoided. If audiometric and electronystagmographic studies support the diagnosis, operative closure of the fistula should be undertaken.

SUGGESTED READING

Caruso VC, Meyerhoff WL. Trauma and infections of the external ear. In: Paparella MM, Shumrick DA, eds. Otolaryngology. Philadelphia: WB Saunders, 1980: 1345.

Gellucci RJ. Traumatic injuries to the middle ear. Otolaryngol Clin North Am 1983; 16/3:633–650.

Goodhill V, Harris I, Brockman S. Sudden deafness and labyrinthine window ruptures. Ann Otol Rhinol Laryngol 1973; 82:2–12.

Holland BA et al. High resolution CT of temporal bone trauma. AJR 1984; 143:391–395.

Hough JVD. Otologic trauma. In: Paparella MM, Shumrick DA, eds. Otolaryngology. Philadelphia: WB Saunders, 1980: 1656.

Makishima K, Snow JB. Pathogenesis of hearing loss in head injury. Arch Otolaryngol 1975; 101:426–432.

Marquet J et al. Computed tomograph in otoneurology. J. Otolaryngol 1984; 1364:241–246.

Schucnecht HF. Mechanism of inner ear injury from blows to the head. Ann Otol Rhinol Laryngol 1969; 78:253–262.

MANDIBULAR FRACTURE AND DISLOCATION

WILLIAM B. HOFMANN, B.A., M.D.

The auto accident is the most common cause of facial fractures including those of the mandible. Trauma to the mandible also occurs through the multiple expressions of man's inhumanity to man. Drivers under the influence of alcohol are responsible for at least 50 percent of motor vehicle fatalities, not to mention serious injuries. The chances that head trauma will result in death or injury after an auto accident are estimated at 70 percent. Injury is much more likely to occur if the automobile occupant involved in a traffic accident is not wearing a seat belt.

ASSESSMENT OF FRACTURE

There is always a history of trauma in mandibular fractures. If the patient is conscious, it is helpful to know as many details concerning the injury as possible. For instance, trauma to the point of the chin may lead to unilateral or bilateral condylar fractures. Force directed from the side may cause a contralateral condylar fracture with an ipsilateral body fracture. It is helpful to note sites of pain and whether or not the teeth feel normal when the jaw is closed.

Aside from other facial fractures, there are two diagnoses that should be kept in mind by anyone involved in the initial care of a mandibular fracture patient: fracture of the larynx and fracture of the cervical spine. A complete discussion of these injuries is beyond the scope of this chapter.

Physical Findings

The approximate incidence of mandibular fractures is as follows: 35 percent involve the condyle: 30 percent the angle, ramus, and coronoid; 25 percent the body, (usually near the mental foramen) and alveolar ridge, and 10 percent the symphysis area. Fractures may occur as single entities or in various combinations such as (1) both condyles, (2) body and contralateral condyle, (3) body and contralateral angle, (4) both sides of the body, or (5) both angles.

These injuries present with any or all of the following findings:

1. *Partial or complete airway obstruction.* With most mandibular fractures, this is usually not the case; however, rapid efficient airway management may save a life.
2. *Malocclusion of the teeth.* Any difficulty with dental occlusion suggests a fracture; however, certain injuries produce definite malocclusive problems such as the bilaterial condylar fracture, which results in an anterior open bite deformity, or a unilateral condylar fracture, which tends to give an open-bite on the side opposite the fracture and a crossbite on the involved side.
3. *Anesthesia or paresthesia* in the distribution of the inferior alveolar nerve.
4. *Gross fracture or mandibular asymmetry on inspection.* Asymmetry may be aggravated by displacement at the lines of fracture. The masseter, internal pterygoid, and temporalis muscles are mandibular elevators and are inserted behind the first molar; consequently, they tend to elevate posterior fragments unless the line of fracture prevents elevation. The digastric, geniohyoid, and mylohyoid muscles are inserted in front of the first molar. They are depressors of the mandible and will displace anterior fragments downward unless the line of fracture prevents displacement.
5. *Pain at the site of fracture.* Biting down on a firm surface such as a tongue blade may cause pain. The patient may be able to point to the fracture site.
6. *Tenderness and crepitation* over the site of the fracture, which may be best determined on bimanual examination.
7. *Difficulty in swallowing with drooling.*
8. *Fetor oris* a foul breath due to mixture of blood and saliva.
9. *Loose or missing teeth* and *separation of teeth* with intraoral laceration and compounding of the fracture. The possibility of aspiration of a tooth should always be kept in mind.
10. *Ecchymosis and swelling.* Severe swelling may ensue if the inferior alveolar artery is transected, causing increased hematoma at the fracture site.

X-Ray Examination

The best x-ray study for the diagnosis of mandibular fracture is a Panorex film, which gives a panoramic view of the mandible. Many hospitals are not equipped to take such films, and the patient's general condition may be a contraindication. In the absence of Panorex equipment, the following standard views should be obtained: (1) lateral oblique, (2) posteroanterior, (3) lateral view of the temporomandibular joint, and (4) modified Towne's view.

Photographs

Photographs are mentioned only to emphasize the importance of a pictorial record in case there is litigation subsequent to the injury. These may be obtained by emergency department personnel.

TREATMENT OF FRACTURE

Before Hospital Arrival

The person who is initially involved in the care of a patient with mandibular fracture—whether paramedic, physician, or other medical personnel—should evaluate the airway. Gentle suctioning of mucus and blood from the oral cavity and nose may be indicated. Bimanual lifting of the mandible in an anterior direction with the forefinger behind the ramus on either side may facilitate breathing. Use of an oral airway, esophageal breathing tube, or endotracheal tube may be necessary, depending on the needs of the patient and the training and experience of the treating individual. Gentle forward traction on the tongue may also improve the airway.

Dentures should be removed if they are present. Any and all dentures should be saved, even if they are broken, as they may be of great value to the surgeon responsible for the definitive treatment.

If there is no airway problem and the patient is uncomfortable, the paramedic may want to apply a Barton bandage to provide comfort and to partially immobilize the fracture until the patient arrives at the hospital.

This gauze-type bandage is wound under the mandible and over the top of the head to close the jaws together.

After Hospital Arrival

On arrival in the emergency department, the patient must undergo total evaluation. Facial fractures are often of secondary importance as a matter of life and death, and their management can reasonably wait until other more serious injuries are treated.

A reasonable plan of action for mandibular fractures would be as follows:

1. Secure the airway if this is a problem or has not already been done. Tracheotomy would rarely be necessary in this time frame.
2. Loose but reasonably stable teeth are left alone. Teeth hanging by a shred of tissue are removed. They can and should be saved as it may be possible in some instances to re-implant them at a later date.

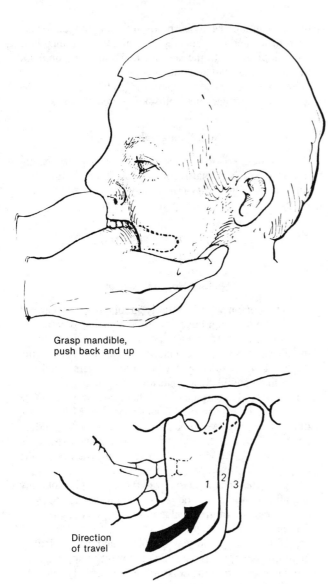

Grasp mandible,
push back and up

Direction
of travel

Figure 1 Mandibular reduction. (From May H, ed. Emergency medicine. New York: John Wiley and Son, 1984.)

3. A history should be taken if the patient is conscious and an accurate diagnosis established by signs, symptoms, and methods previously explained.
4. Tetanus prophylaxis should be given.
5. When swallowing is a problem, as in severe mandibular injury with intraoral compounding, an intravenous line should be inserted and intravenous antibiotics administered. My choice would be cefazolin (Kefzol) or cephalothin (Keflin). The dose of cefazolin would be 500 mg to 1 g IU piggyback every 8 hours, and a 1- to 2-g dose of cephalothin may be given in a similar fashion every 6 hours.
6. Elevate the head of the bed 30 to 40 degrees if possible.
7. The proper otolaryngologic or plastic surgical consultant should be called and a decision made as to whether or not the patient will be admitted. The patient who has simple fractures without much displacement and no question of airway problem may be discharged home on pain medication and antibiotics (if some com-

pounding of the fracture is suspected). Tylenol No. 2 or Tylenol No. 3 can be used for pain. The use of Ibuprofen (Motrin) in dosages of 400 to 600 mg every 4 to 6 hours may be helpful for pain, total dosage not to exceed 2,400 mg daily. The patient should be instructed in the use of mouthwash such as half and half saline solution and hydrogen peroxide. A liquid to very soft diet may be tolerated well and plans should be made for definitive treatment of the fracture, preferably within a few days of the injury.

Patients with severe mandibular fractures and other severe injuries may be admitted to a standard care floor or to an intensive care unit as is appropriate. Patients with compound fractures should be treated with antibiotics through the operative phase until healing starts to occur. Pain medication may be used as needed.

Mandibular fractures almost always require some type of open reduction and fixation. The teeth are placed in occlusion by means of arch bars and elastics for a period of 4 or 6 weeks. In the edentulous patient, intraoral splints may have to be fabricated, or the patient's own dentures may be used in the process of fixation.

Generally speaking, mandibular fractures in children are treated the same as they are in adults. Several points regarding fractures in children should be considered:

1. Early treatment is needed (in the first few days) as the healing process is well under way by 10 to 14 days.
2. A condyle fracture may affect the growth center of the mandible.
3. Many fractures are of the "greenstick" variety, and tooth buds may be in the fracture lines.

DISLOCATION OF THE MANDIBLE

Dislocation of the mandibular condyle in the absence of trauma can occur with any mandibular movement during eating, speaking, laughing, or yawning. The dislocation is anterior to the glenoid fossa and may be bilateral. This causes an "open anterior bite" deformity, which is unilateral or bilateral, depending on whether the dislocation is unilateral or bilateral. Dislocation is usually distressing to the patient as there may be significant pain with muscle spasm.

Treatment consists of mandibular manipulation to reduce the dislocation (Fig. 1). The patient is sedated and placed in the sitting position. The physician is in front of the patient and places his thumbs on the molar teeth—or alveolar ridge if no teeth are present. The hands grasp the mandible. The thumbs press down on the posterior portion while the hands are used to elevate the anterior part of the mandible and push it in a posterior direction. It may be helpful to place a sponge or towel between the thumbs and the posterior teeth or alveolar ridge to prevent the thumbs from slipping. Usually the condyle reduces itself over the articular eminence and resumes a normal postion. Occasionally, general anesthesia must be used to overcome muscle spasm.

SCALP, FACIAL, AND ORAL LACERATION

N. JOHN YOUSIF, M.D.
HANI S. MATLOUB, M.D.
JAMES R. SANGER, M.D.

To many patients, scars are the lasting signature of a past traumatic incident. Many of these patients judge the overall quality of their care by the final cosmetic appearance of their scars. Besides the obvious effort needed to achieve uncomplicated wound healing, lacerations around the head and neck require a concerted effort to achieve a final closure that produces the most inconspicuous scar possible.

PRIMARY CARE

The primary care of patients with head and neck injuries begins with appropriate triage. Patients with the most minimal injuries can obviously be treated with simple sutures. However, those with extensive soft tissue and/or osseous injuries or with multi-system injuries require further evaluation and treatment in the following priorities: airway control, C-spine control, treatment of hemorrhage and shock, and diagnosis of associated injuries. When this is done, treatment of the facial injuries can continue in a more controlled manner.

Hemorrhage

Obvious hemorrhage should be controlled as soon as possible. Digital pressure or pressure dressings are an effective temporizing measure. Final control is usually achieved by precise clamping followed by cautery or suture ligature with an absorbable suture such as 4–O Vicryl or 4–O chromic catgut for the smaller vessels and 3–O or 4–O nonabsorbable silk for the larger vessels. Blind clamping should be avoided to prevent permanent injury to important subcutaneous structures.

Wounds

Skin flaps that are distorted or twisted on themselves should be unraveled and placed back into their original position to prevent further vascular compromise. Other wounds should be covered with sterile dressings until definitive repair can be undertaken.

Diagnosis of Facial Injuries

A careful history should be obtained when possible from the patient, the observers, and the paramedical personnel. This historical review should include a detailed description of the mechanism of injury, time and place of injury, and pre-hospital treatment. A survey of the patient's past medical history should be included with specific emphasis on allergies, tetanus immunization, medications, as well as special problems that may increase the patient's risk of infection (e.g., diabetes, immunosuppression).

After the history is taken, and if the patient is stable and free of problems that necessitate more urgent attention, a comprehensive examination of the face should be performed. This begins with a thorough cleansing of the face and scalp of dried blood or dirt. Sterile gloves are worn and a systematic digital and visual examination is performed from the scalp to the neck. Notation is made of any abnormalities including hematomas, abrasions, particle tatoos, punctures, avulsions, and loss of tissue. It is important to remember that lacerations can be hidden in the scalp beneath the hair, behind the ears, within the oral cavity, or in the eyelids, and special attention should be given to these areas. Bony fractures are diagnosed by deep palpation (noting irregularities or asymmetries), by visualization through a wound, or by observation of instability or malocclusion. The thin calvarium of children is much more easily penetrated by sharp instruments or an animal's tooth and requires special attention.

The facial nerve becomes superficial beyond the limits of the parotid gland, and branches can be injured with even the most inconspicuous lacerations. The integrity of all five branches of the facial nerve (Fig. 1) should be ascertained by functional examination: (1) temporal branch—lifts eyebrows, wrinkles forehead; (2) zygomatic branch—closes eyelids; (3) buccal branch—wrinkles nose; (4) marginal mandibular branch—puckers lips, smiles, depresses lips; and (5) cervical branch—tenses platysma. Local anesthetics affect both sensory and motor branches, and evaluation of nerve functions should be done prior to achieving anesthesia. Nerve injuries need to be repaired as soon as possible, and a qualified microsurgeon should be consulted.

The parotid duct is another frequently injured structure in the face. Approximate location of the duct can be found by drawing a line from the tragus of the ear to the midpoint of the upper lip or its orifice within the mouth located opposite the second upper molar (see Fig. 1). Suspicion of injury is made when a deep laceration crosses this line, or when saliva is noted in the wound. Injuries to this important structure should be repaired as soon as possible and a qualified surgeon should be consulted.

Lacerations about the eye demand evaluation of the lacrimal duct, the eyelids, and the medial and lateral canthus (Fig. 2). These structures require immediate repair, and appropriate consultations should be initiated. Remember, any injury around the eye always merits, at the minimum, an examination of the cornea, globe, adnexa, and visual acuity.

TREATMENT

An initial decision must be made regarding complexity of the laceration. Can it be repaired in the emer-

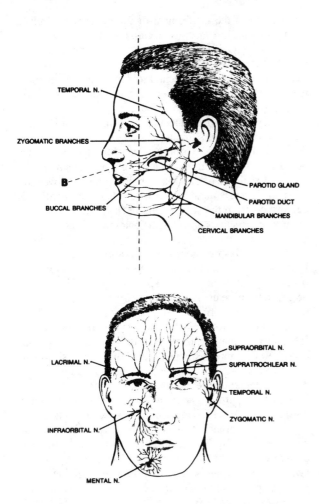

Figure 1 Nerves of the face. *Top*: Branches of the facial nerve and the parotid duct. *Bottom*: Sensory branches of the face amenable to regional blocks.

gency department or should the patient be transferred to the operating suite? Some patients may desire a plastic surgeon for even the most minimal lacerations. This in no way reflects on the primary care physician's competency, but rather the specific desires or biases of a particular patient. Those injuries most appropriately repaired in the operating room include extensive lacerations requiring a prolonged procedure for closure, lacerations in difficult anatomic areas, lacerations in uncooperative patients (children or adults), and particularly dirty wounds and lacerations, which require a more complicated procedure for repair. Other considerations include the availability of proper lighting and adequate instrumentation for closure as well as the need for assistance.

Anesthesia

The local anesthetic used universally in emergency departments today is lidocaine. It has a short time of onset, is effective up to 4 to 6 hours, and rarely elicits an allergic response. Available concentrations include 0.5 percent, 1 percent, and 2 percent with or without

epinephrine in concentrations of 1:100,000 or 1:200,000. Lidocaine, 1 percent with epinephrine 1:100,000, is most commonly used; however, if large areas are to be anesthetized, 0.5 percent is appropriate. There is no increase in hemostasis with increased concentrations of epinephrine and either or 1:200,000 or 1:100,000 achieve the same amount of vascular constriction. Both lidocaine and epinephrine can be toxic, and it is important to know and keep in mind the doses of these frequently used medications. The dosage of lidocaine is 5 to 6 mg per kilogram when used alone, and 7 to 8 mg per kilogram when used with epinephrine. Initial signs of lidocaine toxicity include tachycardia and lightheadedness. These effects may progress to seizures in severe cases. Epinephrine can cause tremors, hypertension, myocardial irritability and ischemia; it may also increase the incidence of local wound infection.

Anesthesia in the face can be achieved by either direct infiltration or local nerve blocks. In the case of nerve blocks, a small amount of anesthetic is instilled at the exit of the nerve from its bony foramen (see Fig. 1). Allow 10 to 15 minutes after injection, since nerve blocks take somewhat longer to achieve the desired effect. This anesthetizes a large area with a small amount of anesthetic; however, it does not provide assistance in hemostasis as would the direct instillation of an epinephrine-containing solution in the wound. When direct infiltration is the method used, injection should be done through the open wound to decrease the patient's discomfort.

Cocaine (4 percent) is the best topical anesthetic available for mucosal membranes (nose, mouth). Remember, it should never be injected into the tissues since subdermal injection can cause severe tissue necrosis. Cocaine can be applied with cotton pledges, cotton rolls, or cotton-tipped applicators. Only a small amount is required for maximal effect (toxic dose in adults is 200 mg), and anesthesia is achieved in 5 to 10 minutes.

When necessary and when there are no contraindications (i.e., head injuries, suspicion of abdominal trauma), administration of a systemic sedative can help the agitated

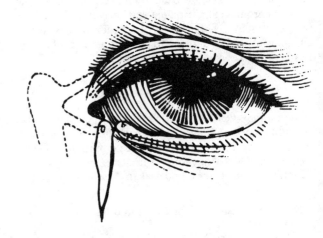

Figure 2 Structures around the eye. Lacerations of the lower lid may involve the lacrimal duct.

patient. Most hospitals have their own formula for pediatric sedation. If this is not available, slow, intravenous titration of diazepam, 0.5–0.1 mg per kilogram along with meperidine, 1 mg per kilogram per dose, can be used. This same concentration can be used in adults when necessary.

Draping

Valuable time and hours of frustration can be saved by washing the entire face and draping it free, even for the most minor lacerations (Fig. 3). This allows the patient added comfort and facilitates monitoring of the patient.

Conservative Debridement

For lacerations of the face, it is important that debridement be conservative. Tissues of questionable viability should be sutured back into place and re-examined in 1 to 2 days. Any tissue that is obviously necrotic should be removed. The wounds should be closed in two layers with a deep dermal suture of 4–O or 5–O chromic catgut or Dexon and a skin suture of 4–O or 5–O nylon. A running noninterlocking suture can be used for simple lacerations; however, with more complex lacerations, interrupted sutures are more likely to allow adjustment and positioning of the wound edges.

Where approximation of the wound edges produces some tension, a small amount of undermining beneath the wound edges may allow the wound to come together more easily (Fig. 4).

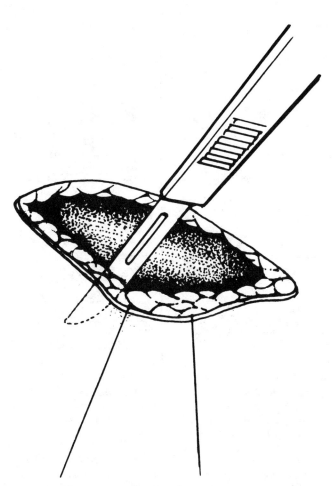

Figure 4 Undermining of the wound edges can be done with a scalpel or scissors. Hemostasis in the undermined area is important.

Suture Technique

The best results are obtained by remembering several key points. Gentle handling of the tissues prevents further injury. Meticulous alignment of both the skin and subdermal structures prevents irregularities of the final scar (Fig. 5). A layered closure is important to prevent tension and scar widening. This is accomplished by a deep layer of 4–O or 5–O chromic catgut and a final layer of nonabsorbable monofilament nylon for the skin. Chromic catgut dissolves quickly, and inflammation has not been a problem. Dexon or Vicryl used this way dissolves slowly, leaving palpable knots for some time. Sutures should be placed 2 mm apart and 2 mm from the wound edge on the face and 4 to 5 mm apart on the scalp. The size of suture ranges from 4–O to 6–O nylon, depending on the thickness of the skin being closed. Prevention of permanent suture marks depends more on the length of time the suture is in the wound rather than the size of the sutures. Sutures should be removed from areas around the face in 4 to 5 days and from the scalp in 10 to 14 days. Steri-Strips can be used in many wounds where the edges easily co-apt; however, their use on the face may be cum-

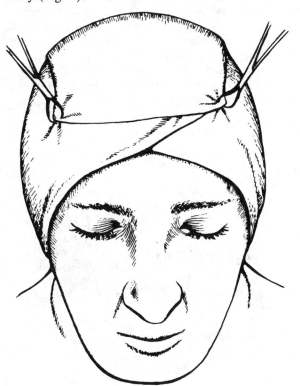

Figure 3 Sterile draping of the entire face allows added comfort for the patient.

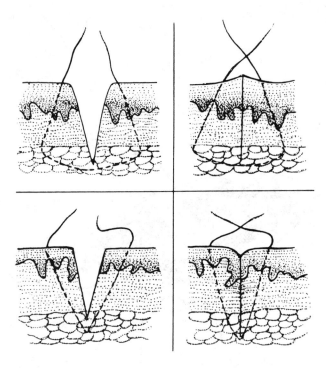

Figure 5 *Top*: The correct suture placement takes a greater amount of subcutaneous tissue, thus everting the wound. *Bottom*: Equal amounts of skin and subcutaneous tissue may lead to undesired wound inversion.

bersome because of poor adherence secondary to continuous motion, hair growth, and body secretions. In this setting, sutures are indicated. Principles to remember are (1) unhurried repair, (2) attention to detail, and (3) every stitch counts.

STELLATE LACERATIONS

These lacerations are difficult to suture and results are often unsatisfactory. If these lacerations are situated within mobile areas and sufficient debridement can be performed to eliminate the laceration without distortion, this should be done. However, if this is not possible, each element of the numerous flaps should be brought together to the best position possible.

AVULSION FLAPS

Avulsions of skin around the forehead or cheek may present different problems. The edges may be bevelled and it may be difficult to achieve an even wound closure. If the bevelled area is small, this can be excised on both sides of the wound, producing a right-angle laceration. When this is not possible, the flap should be returned to its position and small sutures used to reapproximate the edges as well as possible.

TISSUE LOSS

The best cosmetic results are obtained with immediate primary closure of wounds. However, when this is

not possible, and there is tissue loss in the face, these areas should not be unduly stretched in an attempt to bring them together. The area should be cleaned, covered with sterile dressings, and a plastic surgeon consulted for the possibility of either rotation flaps or application of a skin graft to these areas.

ORAL CAVITY LACERATIONS

Since lacerations of the oral cavity may be hidden, these areas should be examined thoroughly. Loose teeth should be sought. Intraoral injuries are exposed to numerous highly aggressive bacteria, and their care requires thorough debridement, irrigation, and antibiotic therapy.

LIP LACERATIONS

Cutaneous lacerations of the upper or lower lip may be through-and-through lacerations and therefore qualify as intraoral injuries. These injuries should be repaired in three layers including the mucosa, muscle, and skin. Mucosal repair is done either with silk suture or with an absorbable suture such as catgut or Dexon. Remember that these sutures tend to come untied, and at least 4 to 5 knots should be used. Repair of lacerations of the lip should always begin with one suture at the vermilion border since even minimal malalignment of this area is obvious (Fig. 6).

TONGUE

Lacerations of the tongue are difficult to repair, and in uncooperative children or adults this may necessitate general anesthesia. In the cooperative patient, the tongue can be grasped with a dry gauze and the area infiltrated with anesthetic (Fig. 7). The laceration should be cleaned of hematoma and bleeding points cauterized. Suture material can be either nonabsorbable 4–O silk or absorbable catgut or Dexon.

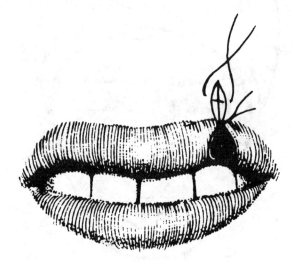

Figure 6 The first suture in the repair of a lip laceration should be at the vermilion border.

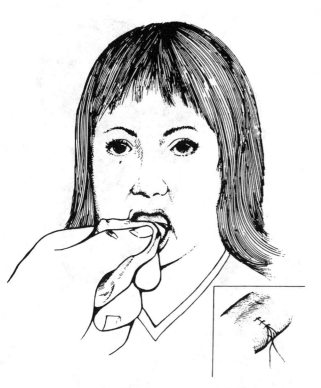

Figure 7 The tongue is grasped with a dry gauze and is cleaned, and sutured.

Patients with intraoral lacerations should be given antibiotics. The human intraoral flora is a large mix of aerobic and anaerobic bacteria. Cultures of wounds contaminated with human saliva most frequently culture strains of *Staphylococcus, Streptococcus, Eikenella*, and anaerobic bacteria. Most intraoral bacteria other than *Staphylococcus* are highly sensitive to penicillin, and therefore this antibiotic in an appropriate dosage for the patient's age and weight should be used. An addition of

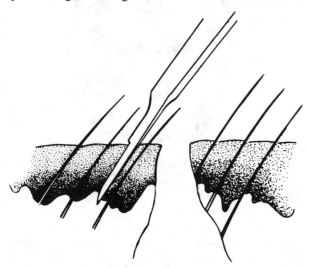

Figure 8 Incisions parallel to the hair follicles prevent deep injury to these structures.

TABLE 1   Summary of Management

History
    Time
    Place
    Mechanism
    Pre-hospital treatment
    Tetanus status

Diagnosis
    Thorough examination
    Facial nerve examination *prior to anesthetic*
    Parotid duct examination

Anesthesia
    Lidocaine, 5-6 mm/kg per dose along with 7-8 mg with
      epinephrine
    Cocaine, 4%, *topical* (2-3 mg/kg, not more than 200 mg)
    Meperidine, 1 mg/kg per dose
    Diazepam, slow IV titration 0.5–1.0 mg/kg
    Pediatric sedative. Combine 0.5 cc of each of the following;
      0.5 ml meperidine, (100 mg/ml), 0.5 ml Phenergan, (50 mg/ml).
      0.5 ml Sporine or chlorpromazine (50 mg/ml). Dosage is 0.1 to
      0.2 ml/10 lb body weight, PO or IM.

Treatment
  Scalp
    Look for hidden lacerations.
    Check for subperiosteal hematomas and skull fractures.
    Incisions should be parallel to hair follicles.

  Forehead
    Do not elevate eyebrow.
    Do not shave or cut eyebrows or eyelashes (very slow
      regrowth).
    Check for visual acuity.
    First stitch aligns hairline (Fig. 9).

  Eye
    Check the lacrimal system (see Fig. 2).
    Check visual acuity.
    Examine for through-and-through lacerations of eyelids which
      would necessitate consultation of a specialist.
    Excessive skin loss may require skin grafts.
    Check the medial and lateral canthus.
    Do not cut eyelashes.

  Face
    Perfect alignment of vermilion border of the lip.
    Excision of irregular edges.
    Every stitch counts.
    Suture removal at 4-5 days.

  Ear
    Lacerated ear parts can be viable even if they are retained on
      small pedicle, and these should be sutured back in place into
      good anatomic position.
    Hemostasis is of utmost importance.
    Perichondrial hematoma should be drained; once it is drained,
      suction drainage should be placed along with a pressure dressing
      (Fig. 10).

  Nose
    Through-and-through lacerations require a layered closure of
      the mucosa and then the skin.
    Amputated parts occasionally can be used as a composite graft
      if their size does not exceed 1.5 cm in greatest diameter.
    Meticulous realignment is important.

  Intraoral lacerations
    Diagnosis is important, requiring thorough examination (look
      for tooth and bony injury).
    Three-layer closure; mucosa, muscle, skin.
    Irrigation should be copious.
    Antibiotics should be given.

a penicillinase-resistant antibiotic such as dicloxacillin or a cephalosporin may be necessary to attack the staphylococcal strains; however, a cephalosporin alone is not effective against the frequently cultured *Eikenella* or anaerobic strains.

AMPUTATION OF FACIAL PARTS

Occasionally, amputated portions of the nose, ear, or scalp can be replanted. These parts should be placed in a dry plastic bag, which itself is placed on ice, and a microvascular surgeon should be called as soon as possible. At other times, small structures that are amputated and do not have a specific arterial or venous supply can be replaced as composite grafts, assuming their greatest diameter does not exceed 1.5 cm. This decision should rest with the plastic surgery consultant.

SCALP LACERATIONS

It is important to know some of the basic anatomy of the scalp in order to perform proper repair. The perio-

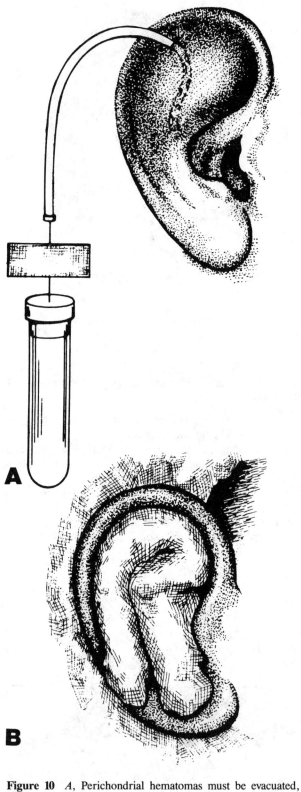

Figure 10 *A*, Perichondrial hematomas must be evacuated, followed by placement of a suction drain. This can be fashioned from a butterfly needle of which the hub is removed and small holes are cut in the plastic tubing. Suction is created by placing the needle in a vacuum tube. This tube should be changed regularly. *B*, Pressure dressing should include cotton anterior and posterior to the ear, tailored to the underlying structures to help maintain their definition.

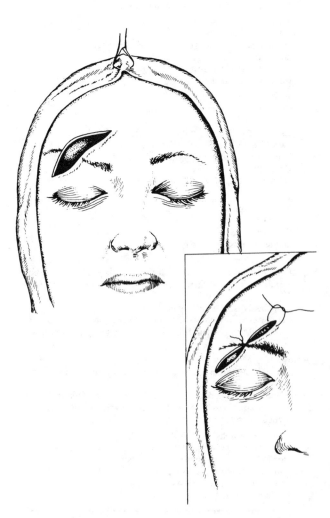

Figure 9 The first suture of an eyebrow laceration should align the hairline.

steum overlies the bony calvarium, above which there is a strong fascial layer called the galea, continuous with the temporoparietal fascia in the temporal region. Above the galea there is an areolar layer covered by a layer of dermal appendages where the deepest portion of the hair follicles is present. Within the dermis, there is a rich supply of vascular tissue which in itself can cause severe bleeding, at times difficult to control. Principles to remember are (1) examine the scalp, (2) palpate wound for subperiosteal hematomas, and (3) examine for skull fractures. For a complete summary of laceration management see Table 1.

Debridement

Most debridement of the scalp is achieved by a combination of vigorous irrigation and manual removal of obvious particles. This should be done after instillation of anesthetic in the wound edges. Irrigation can be performed using a 20 cc syringe and a 19-gauge needle held approximately 12 inches from the wound. Hair should be cut or clipped, never shaved. (Shaving creates microscopic nicks and increases risk of infection.)

Hemostasis

Bleeding from the scalp can be from either injured vessels within the depths of the wound or from a rich subdermal plexus present just beneath the skin. Large vessels within the wound should be clamped and cauterized, or ligated with absorbable sutures. Bleeding in the area of a subdermal plexus may be difficult to control. Exces-

sive cautery in this area may injure the base of the hair follicles. Specific bleeding points should be cauterized individually, and the remaining hemostasis obtained with pressure or the final closure of the skin.

Closure

Jagged edges are trimmed so that they are sharp and straight, allowing improved approximation of the edges. It is important to trim the scalp parallel to the hair follicles (Fig. 8), thereby preventing injury to the deep portions of these structures. A layered closure is performed by closing the galea with absorbable 3–O or 4–O chromic catgut, followed by closure of the skin with a nonabsorbable monofilament, usually 4–O nylon. The sutures are left in place for 10 to 14 days.

In dry wounds, drains usually are not necessary, but a compression gandage can provide additional hemostasis. If the wound continues to bleed slightly, a small Penrose drain can be placed through a separate stab wound. Large hematomas should not be permitted to accumulate, as they can easily become infected.

SUGGESTED READING

Converse J, ed. Reconstructive plastic surgery. 2nd ed. vol. 2, Philadelphia: WB Saunders, 1977.
Grabb WC, Smith JW, eds. Plastic surgery. 3rd ed. Boston: Little Brown, 1979.
Rowe NL, Williams JL, eds. Maxillofacial injuries. vol. 1. New York: Churchill Livingstone, 1985.

PENETRATING NECK TRAUMA

FAROUCK N. OBEID, M.D., F.A.C.S.
BRACK A. BIVINS, M.D., F.A.C.S.

Relative to its size, the neck has a greater concentration and contains a greater variety of organ systems than any other part of the body. These organ systems are not completely protected by the surrounding skeleton, although partial protection is provided by the investing musculature and by adjacent structures such as the spine, mandible, and shoulders. Penetrating wounds of the neck are commonly caused by knife, gunshot, or accidental impalement with any sharp object, and these wounds frequently result in injuries to the airway, esophagus, and vascular structures. These wounds have become a major interest to all involved in the care of trauma because of the increasing incidence of urban violence.

ASSESSMENT OF INJURY

After attending to the initial steps of resuscitation, one should proceed with a thorough history and physical examination and appropriate diagnostic studies for specific injuries. Injuries to structures in the neck can lead to considerable morbidity and possible mortality if not diagnosed and treated appropriately. These structures include the airway (trachea and larynx), the digestive system (pharynx and esophagus), the vascular structures of the neck including the carotid arteries and jugular veins, and last but not least, the spinal cord. Injury to any of the deeper structures of the neck usually leads to specific signs and symptoms, and these injuries can only exist if the superficial platysma muscle layer of the neck is violated; this can be determined by careful inspection of the wound. If the platysma is violated, serious injuries can be identified by a thorough and meticulous assessment performed by a team experienced in trauma. This evaluation becomes even more important if one follows a policy of selective rather than mandatory neck exploration.

Tracheal or laryngeal injury is usually manifested by hoarseness, hemoptysis, stridor, shortness of breath, obvious air leak from the injury site, or subcutaneous emphysema, which may be extensive and not explained by the presence of associated thoracic injury. In severe or obstructing injury to the airway, respiratory distress is usually obvious, necessitating immediate lifesaving intervention. In the more subtle cases of airway injury, laryngobronchoscopy may be of diagnostic value.

The common signs of pharyngeal or cervical esophageal injury include dysphagia, hematemesis, and crepitus. Neck infection and mediastinitis are late developments that usually require operative drainage. Soft tissue neck films, contrast esophagograms, and esophagoscopy may be obtained and usually demonstrate the presence and source of the infection.

Injuries to major cervical veins (even the internal jugular) rarely result in serious consequences. They usually present as a large or expanding hematoma. A significant pulmonary embolus from cervical venous thrombosis is rare. The most serious complication of cervical venous injuries is air embolism. The risk of air embolism is one of the reasons that the probing and exploring of neck wounds in the emergency department under less than ideal circumstances is prohibited.

Arterial injuries may result in exsanguinating hemorrhage with consequent hypotension or shock. Occasionally, hemorrhage in the neck may produce airway obstruction secondary to compression of the larynx or the trachea. Other signs of vascular injury in the neck include the absence or weakness of carotid or upper extremity pulses, the presence of vascular bruit, and hematoma formation. Once hemostasis and an adequate airway have been ensured, the main determinant of the outcome of cervical arterial injuries is the presence or absence of cerebral ischemia and, more specifically, the severity and duration of any preoperative neurologic deficit. In patients with neck injuries, a complete neurologic examination when the patient's condition allows is mandatory prior to the administration of muscle relaxants or general anesthesia. Documentation of the preoperative neurologic status is essential for diagnostic or therapeutic decision making, as well as for the medicolegal implications.

In general, injuries to the internal carotid artery are associated with a neurologic deficit. Injuries to the common carotid and innominate arteries less commonly produce a neurologic deficit, and injuries to the vertebral or subclavian arteries rarely cause neurologic sequelae.

Arteriography is desirable whenever an arterial injury is suspected in the upper and lower zones of the neck (zones 1 and 3) and if the patient's condition is stable. For lower neck injuries, arteriography is extremely helpful in dictating the type of surgical approach. The value of preoperative arteriography for upper neck wounds relates to the difficulty in obtaining exposure and hemostasis when high internal carotid injuries are present. Arteriography should also demonstrate thrombotic occlusion of the distal intracranial internal carotid and the adequacy of blood flow from one cerebral hemisphere to the other via the circle of Willis. The status of the collateral circulation determines the feasibility of ligation versus the necessity for a reconstructive procedure. For injuries located in the middle neck (zone 2), arteriography is not

generally needed since surgical exposure of vascular structures is easily obtained at this level.

Spinal cord injury causes various signs, depending on the extent of the injury; these include hemiplegia, paraplegia, or quadriplegia and even spinal shock syndrome. Neurologic findings related to spinal injuries should be differentiated from those resulting from cerebral arterial injuries.

Other neurologic injuries to be excluded include hypoglossal nerve injury, which is manifested by deviation of the tongue to the side of the lesion, and vagus nerve injury, which causes paralysis of the ipsilateral vocal cord and hoarseness. Cervical sympathetic nerve injury is manifested by the presence of Horner's syndrome, and phrenic nerve injury leads to paralysis of the hemidiaphragm. Less important injuries are those involving glandular structures, such as the thyroid and salivary glands, and are diagnosed on the basis of clinical suspicion and proximity of the injury to the anatomic location of the gland(s).

When the site of injury is the base of the neck, examination of the chest for the presence of pneumothorax or hemothorax is necessary because of the proximity of the pleura and the major vessels to this region. It is also important to examine the upper extremities for signs of vascular or neurologic injuries consequent to a wound at the base of the neck.

TREATMENT

All serious neck injuries should be treated as if the cervical spine were fractured. The head and neck should be immediately immobilized until films of the cervical spine have been obtained in the emergency department. Sand bags are preferable to a cervical collar; the latter interferes with physical examination and with a tracheostomy procedure, should it suddenly become necessary.

As with any traumatized patient, establishing an adequate airway is a primary concern. Direct trauma to the larynx, trachea, or pharynx may cause airway obstruction, and an expanding hematoma from vascular injury may compress the airway, necessitating urgent endotracheal intubation. Endotracheal intubation should be the primary method of establishing an airway. In rare instances, severe deviation of the trachea from massive hematoma, from concomitant maxillofacial trauma, or from laryngeal or tracheal fracture or separation may make orotracheal or nasotracheal intubation impossible. In that situation, emergency cricothyroidotomy or tracheostomy may be required. Injuries to the thorax may compromise respiratory exchange by production of hemothorax or tension pneumothorax, so that placement of a chest tube may be lifesaving.

After an adequate airway is secured, bleeding must be controlled, if present. External compression by finger or fist pressure is the method of choice and is usually effective. A rare exception is a vascular-enteric fistula, which may bleed massively into the trachea or esophagus when pressure is applied to control external bleeding. Intubation or tracheostomy followed by packing of the wound is required to control such bleeding and prevent fatal asphyxia from hemorrhage into the tracheobronchial tree. Probing of neck wounds and blind clamping to control bleeding may cause damage to various structures including major vessels. Probing and clamping usually result in more blood loss or may lead to a massive air embolism.

The introduction of a nasogastric tube is not an essential step in the initial management of the neck trauma patient and may be postponed until after the induction of anesthesia. Placement of a nasogastric tube may produce a severe reflex Valsalva maneuver, leading to increased venous or arterial pressure and release of a clot from an already tamponaded blood vessel, increasing the risk of hemorrhage.

Fluid resuscitation of the hemodynamically unstable patient with penetrating neck trauma requires special consideration in terms of site selection for intravenous lines. Normally, large-bore intravenous cannulas are placed in the upper extremities; however, if a vascular injury at the base of the neck or upper thorax is suspected, the intravenous lines should be placed away from the suspected injury site. Selection of an alternative site is necessary to prevent further damage to vessels, and also to prevent fluid or transfusion extravasation into the soft tissue or pleural cavity. Insertion of subclavian or internal jugular cannulas in a patient with a lower neck wound may lead to confusion in evaluation and difficulty in the surgical treatment of the neck injuries. In the presence of such injuries, the intravenous lines may be placed in the lower extremities.

After the initial evaluation and stabilization, a more thorough evaluation directed toward the identification of specific visceral injuries is appropriate. There is controversy as to whether mandatory or selective neck exploration should be performed. Advocates of mandatory exploration claim that some potentially lethal injuries cannot be diagnosed nonoperatively and that delayed treatment of occult injuries increases morbidity and mortality. Similarly, active observation needed for selective management is thought to require more professional time and greater utilization of special diagnostic procedures such as arteriography, contrast studies, and endoscopy than does mandatory exploration.

Proponents of selective management of neck wounds claim that most penetrating neck wounds do not cause significant visceral injuries. In their view, mandatory exploration is associated with a high rate of negative exploration. They claim that currect diagnostic techniques are highly accurate, and that some unsuspected injuries may be missed even on routine exploration. They also claim that morbidity and length of stay in the hospital are the same for patients who undergo negative exploration as for patients who are actively observed without undergoing exploration. Selective management should also encourage consultation in diagnosis and reduce the number of neck explorations performed by inexperienced surgeons. Selective management should encourage the transfer of patients who are likely to have occult injuries to hospitals with the required diagnostic facilities.

Our own experience at Henry Ford Hospital, after reviewing 180 patients with penetrating neck wounds, led us to change our mandatory exploration policy to a policy of selective exploration. We also found that special diagnostic studies such as angiography, gastrointestinal contrast studies, and endoscopy carry some potential for false results.

In our series, 10 percent of vascular injuries studied by arteriography were missed. Similarly, 20 percent of esophageal injuries were not seen on esophagography, and 50 percent of the esophageal injuries studied were not identified by esophagoscopy. None of our patients with a negative preoperative physical examination had any positive diagnostic study. These results raise some question about the need for these tests in patients with a negative clinical presentation. We believe that special studies should be reserved for patients who have a change in clinical status while under observation.

The need for prophylactic use of antibiotics also is an unresolved issue. Although most surgeons dealing with neck wounds, particularly wounds that require exploration, use antibiotics to cover different bacterial species including oropharyngeal anaerobes, we found no added advantage to the use of antibiotics in our series. Preoperative antibiotics were not effective in preventing postoperative infectious complications.

ADMISSION CRITERIA

Initial evaluation of any neck wound requires inspection to see if it penetrates the platysma muscle. The patient with a penetrating neck wound that has not penetrated the platysma may safely have that wound explored and closed in the emergency department and be discharged. If the wound penetrates the platysma and the clinical examination is otherwise completely negative, the wound may be closed, but the patient must be admitted for observation. The patient who has signs and symptoms of visceral neck injury needs operative exploration. Special diagnostic tests such as arteriography, esophagoscopy, and esophagography should be reserved for the patient who has an equivocal examination or a change in status under observation. These general recommendations assume that *all* patients with penetrating neck wounds, even if apparently trivial, will be seen and evaluated by an experienced surgeon prior to treatment and disposition.

SUGGESTED READING

Balkany TJ, Jafek BW, Rutherford RB. The management of neck injuries. In: Zuidema GD, Rutherford RB, Ballinger WF, eds. The management of trauma. Philadelphia: WB Saunders, 1979:342.

Bivins BA, Procter CD, Bell RM. Arguments against mandatory exploration of penetrating neck wounds. In: Daley RH, Callaham M, eds. Clinics in emergency medicine: controversies in trauma management. New York: Churchill Livingstone, 1985:163.

Obeid FN, Haddad GK, Horst HM, Bivins BA. A critical reappraisal of a mandatory exploration policy for penetrating wounds of the neck. Surg Gynecol Obstet 1985; 160:517–522.

CERVICAL SPINE TRAUMA

ROBERT K. KNOPP, M.D.

The term "cervical spine injury" describes several types of anatomic injuries occurring from direct or indirect trauma to the neck. Injury to the cervical portion of the spinal cord is the most serious injury; however, the vast majority of patients with cervical spine injury have no associated injury to the spinal cord. Two other anatomic structures can be injured from cervical trauma—the cervical vertebrae and ligaments that provide stability for the cervical spine (see Fig. 1) and protection for the cervical spinal cord. (Cervical vascular injuries can also occur, but are not discussed here.) The emergency physician must evaluate the patient with suspected cervical trauma to determine the integrity of both the bony and the ligamentous structures. This is imperative to prevent spinal cord injury from an unrecognized, unstable cervical spine injury.

Evaluation for spinal cord injury is accomplished by neurologic examination. If the patient has normal neuro logic function, the physician must attempt to determine whether a bony or ligamentous injury exists. It is not the role of the emergency physician to determine whether an injury is stable or unstable. This determination often requires further static (computed tomography [CT] scan, tomography) or dynamic (flexion and extension views) roentgenographic evaluation. Once a potentially serious injury is detected (e.g., neurologic deficit, cervical fracture, or subluxation), the patient requires neurosurgical evaluation.

DIAGNOSIS AND THERAPY

Patients with the following presentation require evaluation for possible cervical spine injury: (1) any patient with signs or symptoms of cervical trauma, or (2) patients with altered mental status and a history or suspicion of cervical trauma.

Pre-Hospital Measures

In the pre-hospital setting, paramedical personnel should immobilize the cervical spine of any patient in whom there is a suspicion of cervical trauma. This means that many, if not most, accident victims arrive in the emergency department with some form of cervical immobilization. Paramedics have neither the time nor the training to exclude a potentially serious cervical injury.

Table 1 lists the various types of immobilization techniques used alone or in combination in the pre-hospital setting for cervical immobilization. Although studies of cervical immobilization techniques differ in their findings, immobilization with a hard collar or the use of large sandbags and tape probably affords the best immobilization. The major problem involved in using these techniques is the danger of pulmonary aspiration after vomiting in patients with cervical immobilization. Patients with cervical immobilization require constant observation in order to avoid pulmonary aspiration should vomiting occur.

Emergency Department Measures

In the emergency department, the indications for cervical immobilization and method of immobilization vary depending on three factors: (1) signs or symptoms of cervical cord injury; (2) cooperation and level of consciousness; and (3) examination of the cervical spine.

Patients presenting with obvious paralysis involving the distribution of the cervical cord require immobilization with Gardner-Wells tongs. Although application of the tongs can be performed by an emergency physician

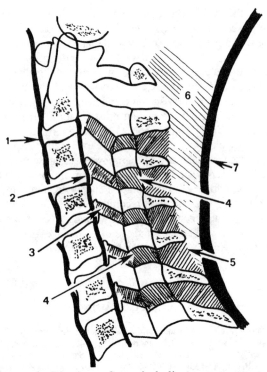

Figure 1 Diagram of cervical ligamentous structures (Squirre's): 1 = anterior longitudinal ligament; 2 = posterior longitudinal ligament; 3 = capsular ligaments; 4 = ligamenta flava; 5 = interspinous ligaments; 6 = ligamentum nuchae; 7 = supraspinous ligament. (From Gerlock et al. The cervical spine in trauma. Philadelphia: WB Saunders, 1978:22.)

TABLE 1   Prehospital Cervical Spine Immobilization Techniques

Short board
Sandbags
Tape and sandbags
Soft cervical collar
Extrication collar
Hard cervical collar
Philadelphia collar

experienced with this technique, insertion of the tongs and application of traction (when appropriate) is usually performed by the neurosurgeon.

Cooperation of the patient is essential for cervical immobilization. If a patient does not tolerate tape or a hard collar, but remains quiet with a "less effective" method of immobilization, common sense would indicate use of the method that allows maximum patient cooperation. Trauma patients with altered mental status should be considered to have a serious cervical injury until proved otherwise. A hard collar or tape with sandbags should be applied; constant nursing observation is essential

At this point, it would appear that virtually all patients involved in an accident require immobilization and complete cervical evaluation, including cervical roentgenograms. In patients with no signs or symptoms of cervical cord injury and no alteration in mental status, a neurologic examination and examination of the cervical spine are indicated. Normal mental status also means the absence of alcohol and mind-altering drugs, since these can mask the perception of pain. Evaluation of the neck (Fig. 2) consists of asking the patient if pain or discomfort is present. If not, the cervical spine should be palpated. If no tenderness is present, the patient should be asked to flex, extend, and then turn his head to each side. If none of these maneuvers elicits discomfort, the alert patient with no altered mental status requires no further evaluation. If any part of this testing elicits any positive response, the patient requires radiologic evaluation.

Radiologic Evaluation

The standard radiologic evaluation of patients with cervical trauma includes three views: (1) a cross-table lateral view (CTLV), (2) anteroposterior (AP) view, and (3) open-mouth (OM) view of the odontoid process (dens). Some institutions also include an oblique view in this series; however, the likelihood that this view will detect abnormalities not noted on standard views is extremely low (Knopp–unpublished data).

The CTLV is usually obtained as a portable examination in the resuscitation area. Several studies carried out during the past 5 years indicate that although the CTLV detects the vast majority of serious cervical injuries, it fails to detect 15 to 20 percent, including some unstable fractures. The fracture most often missed by the CTLV is the odontoid fracture.

The two most important technical factors in obtaining the CTLV are (1) visualization of all seven cervical vertebrae, and (2) a high-quality film (no patient movement) for accurate diagnosis. In some patients it is not possible to visualize all seven cervical vertebrae on the CTLV. In these cases, the physician has several options. More traction can be applied in pulling both arms toward the feet. If this maneuver is unsuccessful in improving visualization of all seven vertebrae, AP and open-mouth views should be obtained. The CTLV, AP, and open-mouth views can be obtained without requiring the patient to move. If these three views appear normal, but the physician cannot visualize all seven cervical vertebrae, then a "swimmer's" view is required. This view allows the

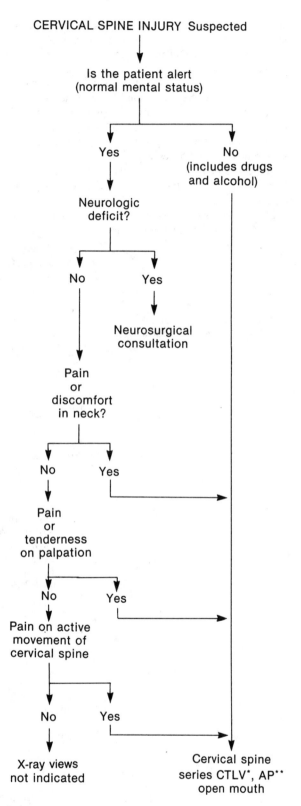

* CTLV = cross-table lateral view

** AP = arteroposterior view

Figure 2 Decision tree for determining need for radiologic evaluation of cervical spine.

lower cervical vertebrae to be visualized. Since the swimmer's view requires movement of the patient, the patient's condition may preclude its use. In such circumstances, the patient's cervical spine should remain immobilized in a hard collar until either tomography or CT scan can be obtained to visualize the lower cervical spine.

In uncooperative or unconscious patients, it may be difficult to obtain the open-mouth view. The best alternative for emergency department evaluation is the modified odontoid view, which usually allows visualization of the odontoid. If this view proves unsatisfactory, CT or tomography will be necessary.

When standard radiologic views have been completed, interpretation falls into one of three categories: normal, equivocal, or abnormal. One recent study evaluated the accuracy of the standard, three-view radiologic trauma series. In 7 percent of patients studied, the standard

radiologic views failed to detect a fracture that was subsequently noted on tomography. Most fractures that went undetected occurred at the C1 or C2 level.

Since the standard cervical trauma series do not always detect cervical fractures and ligamentous injuries, both(stable and unstable) injuries may go undetected, and unless subluxation is present, special studies may be required to accurately evaluate patients.It should be emphasized that this discussion is relevant for the emergency physician only in patients who have no neurologic abnormalities, obvious fractures, dislocations, or subluxations. Patients with the abnormalities described above require immediate neurosurgical consultation. Indications for the emergency physician to obtain special studies of the cervical spine are summarized in Figure 3.

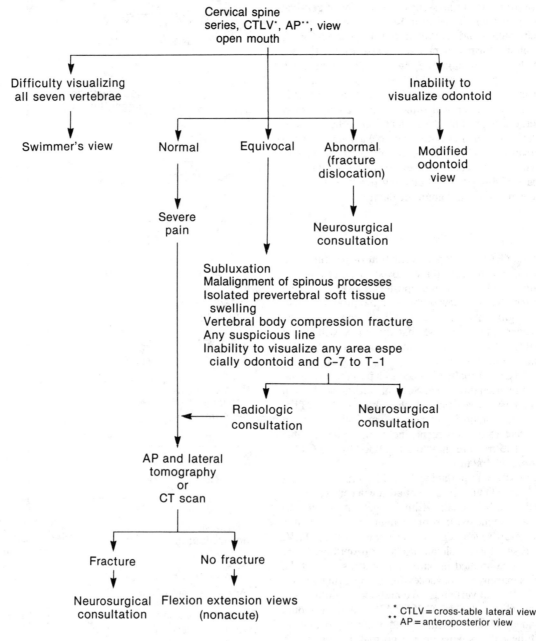

Figure 3 Radiologic evaluation of patient with no neurologic deficit.

Three special studies are used in evaluating patients with cervical trauma: (1) flexion and extension views, (2) tomography, and (3) CT. The emergency physician should not order flexion and extension views to evaluate the stability of the cervical spine in acute cervical trauma. These views may be inaccurate in the acute setting owing to cervical muscle spasm and lack of patient cooperation. Moreover, a potential danger exists for cervical cord injury during this procedure if sudden dislocation occurs during flexion or extension. Ideally, this examination should be performed several days after trauma; cervical spasm should subside during this interval. Fluoroscopy should be used for dynamic control of cervical stability. This is not possible in the emergency department.

Tomography and CT have been used to evaluate suspicious findings on standard views, inadequate visualization of certain structures of the cervical spine, patients with neurologic deficit and normal standard radiologic views, and patients with severe post-traumatic cervical pain despite a normal standard series. Studies by Binet and Maravella using tomography demonstrated that tomography can identify fractures not visualized on plain films, clarify suspicious findings on the plain films, and, most importantly, change patient management in 10 to 20 percent of patients studied.

Computed tomography allows more detailed visualization not only of bony structures, but of the spinal cord itself, thus affecting management decisions. The decision whether to use CT or tomography is made in consultation with the radiologist or neurosurgeon.

CERVICAL HYPEREXTENSION INJURY

Hyperextension injury of the cervical spine is sometimes associated with injury to the cervical cord, but most of these injuries produce no serious sequelae. The term "whiplash" has been used to describe an injury to the cervical spine or surrounding structures (e.g., muscles, ligaments) that occurs after trauma. However, it is not an appropriate diagnostic term. "Hyperextension injury" more accurately defines the mechanism of injury that actually occurs. The specific anatomic structures involved include the ligaments and muscles that provide support to the cervical spine.

Evaluation of the patient includes careful physical examination and neurologic evaluation of the cervical spine and cord. If the patient is entirely alert and cooperative, denies any pain, is not under the influence of alcohol or drugs that might mask pain, and was involved in a relatively minor accident, he should be put through a full range of motion of the neck. If this produces absolutely no pain or symptoms, roentgenograms generally are not needed. In all other situations, they should be obtained. It is only after serious injuries have been excluded that the diagnosis of hyperextension injury should be considered.

Treatment in the emergency department includes the application of ice packs to the area for a period of 24 to 48 hours. Analgesia and immobilization with a cervical collar is indicated if discomfort is severe.

The long-term prognosis for these patients is usually good. However, it may be days or weeks before the patient is asymptomatic. Occasionally, the clinical course is complicated by disability or legal claims related to the trauma. Orthopaedic or neurosurgical follow-up is indicated in patients with this injury.

SUGGESTED READING

Binet EF, Moro JJ, Marangola JP, et al. Cervical spine tomography in trauma. Spine 1977; 2:163–172.

Cline JR, Scheidel E, Bigsby EF. A comparison of methods of cervical immobilization used in patient extrication and transport. J Trauma 1985; 25:650–653.

Maravella KR, Cooper PR, Sklar FH. The influence of thin-skeletal tomography on the treatment of cervical spine injuries. Radiology 1978; 127:131–139.

Podolsky S, Baraff LJ, Simon RR, et al. Efficacy of cervical spine immobilization methods. J Trauma 1983; 23: 461–465.

Shaffer MA, Doris PE. Limitation of the cross-table lateral view in detecting cervical spine injuries: a retrospective analysis. Ann Emerg Med 1981; 10:508–513.

Streitwieser DR, Knopp RK, Wales LR, et al. Accuracy of standard radiographic views in detecting cervical spine fractures. Ann Emerg Med 1983; 12:538.

Wales LR, Knopp RK, Morishima MS. Recommendations for evaluation of the acutely injured cervical spine: a clinical radiologic algorithm. Ann Emerg Med 1980; 9:422.

DENTAL TRAUMA AND INFECTION

HOUCK M. MEDFORD, D.D.S.

LUXATIONS, EXTRUSIONS, INTRUSIONS: THE FIRST EIGHT HOURS

The two most common categories of patients who sustain dental injuries are victims of motor vehicle accidents and children who experience falls and playground accidents. Hemorrhage is usually present, and clots need to be removed with gauze sponges to allow the initial examiner to evaluate the extent of the injury. In cases of intraoral trauma, the teeth involved are usually lodged more deeply into the jaw (intrusions), partially extruded from the bone (extrusions), loosened from the alveolar bone (luxations), completely missing from the alveolar bone (avulsions), or a combination of the above. Treatment and prognosis vary with the type of injury and depend on whether the teeth involved are primary "baby" teeth or secondary "permanent" teeth. Cases involving intrusions, extrusions, and luxations should be treated by a specialty provider, and should be referred immediately to either a general dentist or an oral surgeon for definitive care.

AVULSIONS: PRE-HOSPITAL

Completely avulsed teeth require immediate and proper management by the primary care physician. For patients presenting with avulsed teeth, every effort should be made to replant the teeth in patients who are past the age of 6 or 7 years. This is the age when the teeth involved are more likely to be the permanent teeth. The first person to examine the patient is handicapped owing to the lack of proper radiologic diagnosis and comparison with the chart of the normal chronologic development of the permanent teeth; nonetheless, an attempt should be made to replant the involved teeth.

If contaminants such as blood and hemorrhage are present on the avulsed tooth it should be gently lavaged with any available saline or water to remove extraneous debris. The tooth should be immediately inserted into the alveolar bone and held in place until such time that the patient can be transported to the emergency department for more definitive stabilization.

In the event that the primary care provider is not comfortable with replantation procedures, the tooth (teeth) should be transported in a liquid medium; milk is the recommended transport medium. Saline, as a physiologic agent, is also acceptable, but does not have the advantage of physiologic osmolarity and protein enrichment.

The whole objective of immediate care for avulsed teeth is to maintain the vitality of the periodontal ligament i.e. the cells aligning the tooth root surface. The optimal time to accomplish this procedure for the best prognosis is within 30 minutes of the time of trauma.

AVULSIONS: THE FIRST EIGHT HOURS

In the emergency department the tooth may be stabilized with a periodontal dressing. Immediate referral to a general dentist or oral surgeon is indicated for more definitive stabilization and management.

Tetanus prophylaxis should also be provided. A moderate-to-strong analgesic should also be prescribed based on the patient's weight and tolerance.

INFECTIONS OF ODONTOGENIC ORIGIN

Infection at the Base of the Tooth: Periapical Abscess Secondary to a Necrotic Pulp

The patient indicates that the pain sensation is "throbbing." The tooth is sensitive to hot and cold and almost always sensitive to percussion. The percussion technique employs the handle of a small tuning fork which is used to tap the crown of the tooth in a vertical or horizontal direction. The patient complains of discomfort if there is periapical inflammation. Decay is generally obvious, and the apical area of the root is most always tender when palpated firmly with the fingertips on the buccal or lingual surfaces of the infected tooth. Swelling is more commonly generalized. Submaxillary and cervical lymph nodes may demonstrate tenderness and enlargement.

Treatment is palliative; an analgesic for moderate-to-severe pain is prescribed as well as an antibiotic. The antibiotic of choice is oral penicillin (Pen VK), the initial dose of 1 g being followed by 500 mg every 6 hours for at least one week.

The patient should be referred to the dentist for management and told that the medication will not cure the infected tooth.

Infection in the Gums: Periodontal Abscess

The patient describes a "gnawing" pain unlike the throbbing pain associated with a periapical abscess. Swelling is localized, usually at or near the gum line, rather than generalized, as with a tooth abscess. The tooth usually is discernibly mobile if the patient allows the examiner to touch it. Unlike a periapical abscess, hot and cold stimuli do not grossly increase or decrease the painful sensation.

The treatment is palliative; analgesics for moderate-to-severe pain and antibiotics are prescribed. The antibiotic of choice is oral penicillin (Pen VK), the initial does of 1 g being followed by 500 mg every 6 hours for approximately one week.

The patient should be referred to the dentist for management and told that the analgesics and antibiotic will not cure the abscess.

Infection With Erupting Third Molar (Wisdom Tooth): Pericoronitis

The patient, who complains of moderate-to-severe pain in the area of the most posterior mandibular molar, may present with trismus (difficulty in opening) and swelling. He or she is probably between the ages of 17 and 25, which is the eruption period of the affected molar. A tonsilar abscess should be considered in the differential diagnosis, which clinically shows the uvula deviated to one side.

Treatment consists of warm saline rinses in the infected area every 2 hours. On visual examination, a flap of soft tissue is usually noted overlying the most distal aspect of the posterior molar. Warm saline administered in a 10-cc syringe with a blunted needle is gently flushed into this area to remove food debris and other entrapped exotoxins of bacterial contamination. The antibiotic of choice is oral penicillin (Pen VK), which is administered as a 1-gram initial dose followed by 500 mg every 6 hours. Analgesics for moderate-to-severe pain should be prescribed.

The patient should be given the irrigation syringe and instructed in the self-administration of therapy every 3 to 4 waking hours. Referral to a dentist for prompt evaluation is indicated, and the patient should be told that this therapy will not relieve him of this chronic infection.

Infection After Extraction: Alveolar Osteitis

The patient complains of severe pain 2 to 3 days postoperatively after the extraction of a tooth, usually a lower posterior molar. During the healing process of the extraction site, the alveolar bone may incompletely heal because of possible bacterial contamination. The patient complains of severe pain in the area of the previous surgery.

Initial treatment consists of irrigating the extraction site with saline to flush out debris. Oral penicillin (Pen VK) is prescribed as the antibiotic of choice, the initial dose of 1 g being followed by 500 mg every 6 hours for one week. An analgesic for moderate-to-severe pain should be prescribed.

The patient should be immediately referred to a dentist for packing of the extraction site with a sedative and antibiotic dressing.

LIFE-THREATENING DENTAL INFECTIONS

Canine Swellings

When first seen, the patient has moderate-to-advanced swelling of the canine space (defined by the inferior orbital rim superiorly and nose medially) and symptoms of a periapical abscess at the base of the lateral incisor, cuspid (canine), or first premolar on the ipsilateral side. Even the periocular tissues may be swollen.

Swellings of the canine space are particularly dangerous because of a bacteremia communicating directly to the cavernous sinus via the angular vein and causing thrombosis.

Aggressive antibiotic therapy should be started immediately. The patient should be admitted to the hospital if any question of compliance is suspected or if the infection seems to be worsening. Two million units of aqueous penicillin G should be given, followed by one million units of aqueous penicillin administered every 6 hours until septic symptoms subside. A general dentist or oral surgeon is consulted regarding extraction of the infected tooth.

Submandibular Swellings

The patient has moderate-to-advanced swelling of the area under the lower jaw with symptoms of a periapical infection at the base of the lower tooth. On examination the tongue may appear elevated. The patient may have some difficulty in swallowing and even breathing.

The patient should be admitted to the hospital for intravenous antibiotic therapy and to maintain proper hydration. Penicillin G is the drug of choice, with 2 million units administered intravenously as the initial loading dose, followed by 1 million units every 6 hours. Consultation with a dentist should be obtained to localize the focus of infection and to arrange for extraction of the infected tooth. The patient should be monitored closely for potential airway obstruction.

SUGGESTED READING

Medford HM. Temporary stabilization of avulsed or luxated teeth. Ann Emerg Med 1982; 11:490–492.

EYE AND ORBIT TRAUMA

THOMAS A. DEUTSCH, M.D.

CLASSIFICATION OF OCULAR TRAUMA

When confronted with a case of eye trauma, the non-ophthalmologist's first tendency is to panic. However, the management of these patients is not difficult if the physician remembers basic principles of care.

The management of ocular trauma is based on the orderly classification of the type of injury and the careful evaluation of the eye. As seen in Table 1, injuries are classified according to location (periocular or ocular) and etiology (sharp, blunt, missile, or chemical).

Location of the injury is important because periocular trauma is rarely (though occasionally) a threat to visual acuity, whereas ocular trauma is associated with acute and often permanent visual morbidity. However, a casual examination to rule out ocular involvement is never suffi-

cient, and a thorough search for an ocular injury is always indicated. There is no excuse for overlooking an occult ocular injury, no matter how difficult the examination may be.

The specific cause of ocular trauma is an important prognostic indicator and should be sought in every case. Injuries caused by sharp objects have a uniformly better prognosis than those caused by blunt objects, and injuries caused by slow-velocity missiles (such as BBs) are well known to have the worst prognosis of all. Chemical injuries to the eye require instantaneous treatment to save vision.

TABLE 1 Classification of Ocular Injuries

Location	Etiology
Periocular	Sharp
Ocular	Blunt
	Missile
	Chemical

EXAMINATION

After obtaining the history of the injury, the physician immediately focuses on pertinent portions of the physical examination. Key points in evaluation are outlined in Table 2.

The presence of normal visual acuity does not rule out serious ocular injury, but the finding of reduced visual acuity is a condition that must be explained. The visual acuity should be evaluated at distance using an acuity chart or, at the very least, at near using a standard near acuity chart. If a near card is used, the patient's proper reading correction should be in place.

Broken facial or orbital bones portend complications of periocular or ocular trauma and should be evaluated with this in mind. There are three major clinical presentations of a blow-out fracture: (1) loss of upward gaze, which is caused by entrapment of the inferior rectus and inferior oblique muscles in the maxillary sinus, (2) enophthalmos (a sunken appearance of the eye), caused by expansion of the orbit with orbital contents prolapsed into the maxillary sinus, and (3) hypesthesia of the cheek under the involved eye, caused by damage to the infraorbital nerve. Any of these three signs should lead the physician to order orbital roentgenograms. The management of orbital fractures continues to be controversial, differing from specialty to specialty. Most ocular trauma surgeons currently treat expectantly in the early days after injury.

The finding that the globe is intact and uninjured is reassuring to both the patient and the evaluating physician. Likewise, abrasions of the exposed portions of the eye (the cornea and conjunctiva) are usually easily managed without referral and with minimal inconvenience to the patient. On the other hand, the suspicion of a perforation of the ocular coats is reason for concern. Signs that raise the index of suspicion include the presence of black tissue under the conjunctiva (suggestive of occult prolapse of the ciliary body), a pear-shaped pupil (suggesting occult prolapse of the iris), hyphema, a soft anterior chamber, and extensive hemorrhage under the conjunctiva. Indeed, any patient with a large subconjunctival hemorrhage should be suspected of having a ruptured globe. Any of these findings should prompt immediate referral to an ocular trauma specialist. A shield should be placed over the eye and no attempt made to remove "mucus" or "dead tissue," which may be part of the ocular contents.

All physicians should be able to screen for opacities in the ocular media. A direct ophthalmoscope, available in virtually every emergency department, is used in an attempt to visualize the posterior structures of the eye. A gross hemorrhage in the anterior chamber (hyphema) can readily be visualized with the light of the ophthalmoscope as a red layer. If a microscopic hyphema is suspected, high magnification examination with the slit lamp is necessary. A cataract may form within minutes or hours if the lens capsule is lacerated. More often, blunt trauma results in an anterior shield-like opacity of the lens, which appears days or weeks following the trauma. Dislocation of the lens causes opacity and trembling of the unsupported

TABLE 2 Key Points in Evaluation of Ocular Injuries

Visual acuity
    Normal or reduced

Facial and orbital bones
    Fractured or intact

Integrity of the globe
    Intact, abraded, or penetrated

Contents of the eye
    Ocular media clear, hemorrhage, or intraocular
        foreign body

iris on eye movement. Vitreous hemorrhage results in a diminished red reflex from the posterior segment and inability to see details of the fundus structures. Intraocular foreign bodies may sometimes be seen with the direct ophthalmoscope, but if suspected, referral to an ophthalmologist is suggested.

Blunt trauma occasionally causes damage to the iris and pupil. Most commonly, small ruptures in the iris sphincter result in an abnormally shaped pupil. Traumatic mydriasis may also occur, and the pupil may remain dilated for weeks or months.

STABILIZATION

Prior to the transfer of a patient to the emergency department, initial therapy should be given when necessary. In the case of eye trauma, only minimal care is necessary in most instances.

When penetration of the globe is diagnosed, placement of a metal or hard plastic "shield" is mandatory. The shield provides protection from further, inadvertent, trauma to the eye. There is no need to bilaterally patch any patient with a unilateral injury. Covering the uninjured eye only results in increased apprehension on the part of the patient and is of no medical benefit. In the case of a sharp perforation, if the offending weapon is available it should be retrieved and brought to the hospital. It can be cultured and, in some cases, tested for its magnetic properties if removal of a splintered piece from the eye is necessary.

In the case of a chemical injury, the eye should be copiously irrigated with any available noncaustic aqueous liquid. If possible, one liter per affected eye should be used immediately on making the diagnosis. When available, a sample of the chemical should be brought to the hospital for analysis.

INITIAL HOSPITAL CARE

If ocular penetration is suspected, cultures should be taken of the conjunctiva, the offending weapon (if available), and the wound edge if this can be accomplished without disrupting the wound. Broad-spectrum intravenous antibiotics should be started immediately and tetanus toxoid administered. If eyedrops are needed, they should be given from previously unopened bottles so as to avoid contaminating the wound. Appropriate roentgenographic studies should be ordered to rule out the presence of associated fractures or retained but unsuspected foreign bodies. Plain orbital films are usually adequate for screening, but there should be no hesitation in ordering a CT scan, utilizing thin cuts of 2 mm or less, if roentgenographic abnormalities are found. A shield should be in place over the injured eye at all times.

A patient with a hyphema (blood in the anterior chamber of the eye) should be evaluated by an ophthalmologist immediately. This injury is vision threatening, usually requiring hospitalization and careful follow-up. Patients with any hemoglobinopathy are at increased risk for complications of hyphema, and thus all black patients should have an immediate sickle cell screening test performed.

Surface corneal foreign bodies may be removed under magnification using a cotton applicator tip, a needle tip, or a specially designed drill that cannot perforate the eye. Irrigation in this instance is generally unrewarding as the foreign body has usually become embedded within the corneal epithelium.

When a corneal abrasion is suspected, fluorescein dye can be placed in the inferior conjunctival fornix. This dye then fills the tear film, spreading over the normal corneal epithelium, but staining the corneal stroma under any epithelial defect a brilliant green. The treating physician should then place a small amount of antibiotic ointment in the conjunctival fornix and apply two eyepads over the closed eye. Half-inch tape is then applied, with each piece running from the middle of the forehead to the maxilla in parallel fashion to create a firm (semipressure) dressing.

Lacerations of the eyelids can produce many complications when the lid margin, the canthal areas, or the medial portion of either lid (where the lacrimal ducts are located) is involved. If the palpebral ligament is injured, the canthus on that side of the eye sags and the lids are lax. These injuries require repair by an ophthalmologist or plastic surgeon. If referral will be delayed, ice packs should be placed over the injured area to minimize tissue swelling. Lacerations that do not involve the lid margin and from which no fat prolapses (thus indicating a lacerated tarsal plate of the lid) can be sutured with careful technique by the emergency physician.

The contralateral eye must be thoroughly examined in every case. It is worth the few extra minutes invested in this task to ascertain that the ''other eye'' is truly uninjured.

DISPOSITION

Uncomplicated corneal abrasions should heal within 48 hours. If fluorescein staining persists beyond this time, referral is indicated.

TABLE 3 Guidelines for Referral of Ocular Injuries

Injury	Guidelines
Chemical injury	
Severe	Stabilize and arrange for immediate admission.
Mild	Arrange for evaluation by an ophthalmologist prior to discharge from the emergency department.
Blow-out fracture	Arrange for early evaluation by an ophthalmologist. Admission and immediate surgery are rarely indicated.
Suspected ocular perforation	Arrange for immediate admission and prepare for surgery.
Hyphema	Arrange for evaluation by an ophthalmologist prior to discharge from the emergency department.
Corneal foreign body	The patient should be reexamined in 1–2 days and referred to an ophthalmologist if not healed.
Laceration of the eyelid	Arrange for evaluation by a specialist experienced in the care of lid lacerations.

Most patients suffering an ocular injury should be seen by an ophthalmologist. General guidelines for referral are given in Table 3. When a patient requires admission and no ocular trauma specialist is available, transfer to another hospital should be arranged. In most cases, a short delay will not result in significant visual morbidity. However, when undue delay in management occurs, the burden of proof in the explanation of any complications may fall on the referring physician. For this reason, it is wise to effect a transfer promptly.

Supported in part by grants from The Regenstein Foundation and The Louise C. Norton Trust.

SUGGESTED READING

Deutsch TA, Feller DB. Paton and Goldberg's management of ocular injuries. 2nd ed. Philadelphia: WB Saunders, 1985.

Deutsch TA, Feller DB. Injuries of the eyes, lids, and orbit. In: Zuidema G, et al, eds. The management of trauma. 4th ed. Philadelphia: WB Saunders, 1985:243.

CONCUSSION AND SKULL FRACTURE IN BLUNT HEAD TRAUMA

PETER T. PONS, M.D.

Blunt head trauma represents a wide spectrum of pathology for the emergency physician to evaluate, diagnose, and manage in the emergency department. As regards treatment, concussion or skull fracture requires little in the way of emergency intervention. However, it is critically important that the physician recognize life-threatening neurosurgical crises (e.g. subdural hematoma) that may be erroneously diagnosed as concussion or compatible with skull fracture. As with any patient who has a head injury, concern for associated cervical spine injury mandates protection of the spine until there is radiologic evidence to the contrary. A careful evaluation for other major life-threatening injuries should be performed and must take precedence over management of the head injury.

DEFINITION

Concussion

Although the classic definition of concussion is applied to any patient who has sustained blunt head trauma and a loss of consciousness with a gradual return to normal, the definition should really include any transient neurologic dysfunction with a subsequent return to a normal neurologic state. This then includes such symptoms as dizziness, nausea, vomiting, and headache, as well as loss of consciousness, as long as there is obvious improvement over time and resolution of the abnormality. No demonstrable pathologic lesions are noted on routine diagnostic studies.

Skull Fracture

Defined as disruption of the integrity of the calvarium, a skull fracture may be linear, depressed, or basilar. The serious nature of skull fracture relates not to the actual bone disruption, but to the potential for significant associated injury such as intracranial hemorrhage or direct injury to the brain.

ETIOLOGY

Both concussion and skull fracture may arise from similar mechanisms of trauma. Motor vehicle accidents, falls, and industrial mishaps account for a large number of these injuries, as a result of either deceleration (usually producing concussion) or direct trauma (causing either). A direct blow to the head, often during a fight or assault,

is another form of blunt head trauma. Of particular concern are those mechanisms capable of producing depressed fractures, such as blows with a fireplace poker, hammer, or high-heeled shoe, or large animal bites of the head in infants.

CLINICAL PRESENTATION

When a patient arrives in the emergency department with a history of having sustained some sort of head trauma, questions regarding neurologic abnormalities, such as loss of consciousness, should be asked of witnesses to the event and of the pre-hospital care personnel. In the case of suspected concussion, there should be a clear pattern of improvement over time. The patient with a skull fracture may have no specific historical findings. On occasion, a patient with a basilar skull fracture may present with the history of clear or serosanguineous drainage from his nose or ear.

On physical examination, the patient with concussion may have findings ranging from mild or no confusion to loss of consciousness without localizing signs. Repeat evaluations should reveal a gradual return to normal function over time. As an example, the patient who presents with confusion should demonstrate clearing over minutes to hours. Examination of the patient with skull fracture may reveal evidence of a hematoma over the fracture site, Battle's sign (hemorrhage over the stylomastoid area) or racoon eyes in some cases of basilar skull fracture, or cerebrospinal fluid otorrhea or rhinorrhea.

The differentiation between cerebrospinal fluid rhinorrhea and nasal rhinorrhea is often difficult; however, a number of tests may be applied. A drop of serosanguineous fluid applied to a piece of filter paper will reveal concentric rings of blood and clear cerebrospinal fluid after several minutes if, in fact, the fluid is cerebrospinal fluid. Testing the fluid discharge for glucose is also a valuable study. Cerebrospinal fluid rhinorrhea tests positive for glucose on Dextrostix. Another simple test consists of placing a drop of the discharge onto tissue paper. Nasal mucus dries and stiffens the paper, whereas cerebrospinal fluid does not cause it to stiffen.

The finding of blood behind the tympanic membrane or in the ear canal is presumptive evidence of basilar skull fracture. If the patient has an associated scalp laceration, careful visual and digital evaluation may demonstrate a fracture.

Neurologic examination in patients with concussion and skull fracture reveals no localizing findings.

DIAGNOSIS

By definition, the patient with concussion has no abnormal findings on diagnostic testing. Skull films and computed tomography, if performed, are normal.

The diagnosis of skull fracture is generally made on routine radiologic examination of the skull or by physical examination. Linear fractures are usually relatively easily recognized by their location, the "sharpness" of the margins, and the fact that they do not branch. Depressed skull fractures are frequently more subtle. The appearance is usually that of a small radiolucent area immediately adjacent to an area of increased density. If doubt exists as to the presence of a depressed fracture, a tangential view of the area in question should be obtained. The most difficult fracture to diagnose radiologically is the basilar skull fracture, and frequently there are no apparent abnormalities. Presumptive evidence is the finding of an air-fluid level in the sphenoid sinus.

The finding of multiple, complex, or depressed fractures on skull films of the pediatric patient should raise the issue of child abuse as a cause of the trauma.

The issue of when to obtain skull films has generated significant controversy. A number of authors have suggested various high yield criteria as indications for ordering these films in an effort to decrease the high incidence of negative studies. Recently, however, it has been shown that, of those patients who develop complications, patients with skull fractures are more likely to have a serious problem such as an intracranial hemorrhage. Therefore it is important to diagnose the skull fracture radiologically, and the indications for ordering the films should not be as stringent as previously suggested. Criteria for obtaining skull films include physical findings compatible with fracture (as discussed earlier), mechanism of trauma capable of producing a depressed skull fracture, and history of loss of consciousness or any significant head trauma.

Computed tomography generally is not necessary in these patients unless physical findings suggest an intracranial hemorrhage. In addition, a CT scan may be indicated when fractures that cross a vascular groove or location are noted on routine films.

THERAPY AND DISPOSITION

As a general rule, the patient with concussion may be discharged from the hospital if the concussion is thought to be mild, if the patient has no abnormalities in mental status, and if a responsible adult is available to watch the patient over the next 24 hours. If the patient has any continuing abnormality in mental status, he should be admitted for observation, and this should be explained to the person who will be observing him.

All patients with skull fracture should be admitted to the hospital for at least a 24-hour period. As mentioned earlier, skull fracture is associated with a higher incidence of intracranial hemorrhage, thus mandating observation in an appropriate environment with neurosurgical consultation.

Patients with depressed skull fracture require immediate neurosurgical consultation since elevation of the depressed fragment is usually necessary. The criterion used to determine operative intervention is depression greater than 5 mm or the width of the bony tables of the skull.

Patients with cerebrospinal fluid otorrhea or rhinorrhea are admitted and placed on bed rest. They are instructed not to blow their nose as this might introduce bacteria into the cerebrospinal fluid. Many of these leaks close spontaneously. The decision to initiate antibiotic therapy is a difficult one and remains controversial. It is thought that prophylactic antibiotics may predispose to infection with resistant organisms. The decision to start antibiotic therapy in the ED should be made only in consultation with the neurosurgeon.

COMPLICATIONS

The most common and most difficult complication of closed head injury is the post-concussion syndrome. Patients complain of persistent headache, dizziness, drowsiness, and inability to concentrate. These symptoms can last weeks or months. Although secondary gain from workmen's compensation or litigation may be a reason for persistence of this syndrome, most authorities now believe this to be a real pathologic entity. Patients may be warned that they will not return to full normal health immediately. Other diagnoses, such as chronic subdural hematoma, must be eliminated before making the diagnosis of post-concussion syndrome.

SUGGESTED READING

Henry RC, Taylor PH. Cerebrospinal fluid otorrhoea and otorhinorrhoea following closed head injury. J Laryngol Otol 1978; 92:743-756.

Hobbs C. Skull fracture and the diagnosis of abuse. Arch Dis Child 1984; 59:246-254.

Jennett B. Assessment of the severity of head injury. J Neurol Neurosurg Psychiat 1976; 39:647-655.

Ommaya AK. Nervous system injury and the whole body. J Trauma 1970; 10:981-990.

Ommaya AK, Gennarelli TA. Cerebral concussion and traumatic unconsciousness: correlation of experimental and clinical observations of blunt head injuries. Brain 1974; 97:633-654.

Parkinson D. Concussion. Mayo Clin Proc 1977; 52:492-496.

Rosner S. The diagnosis and treatment of cerebral concussion. Int Surg 1967; 47:371-376.

Ward AA Jr. The physiology of concussion. Clin Neurosurg 1964; 12:95-111.

PENETRATING CRANIAL TRAUMA

W. KENDALL McNABNEY, M.D.

The role of the emergency physician in cases of penetrating cranial trauma is one of early recognition, resuscitation or stabilization, and expediting transition to the care of a neurosurgeon, since all salvageable patients are managed operatively. Penetrating cranial injuries are associated with high mortality and disabling morbidity, self-infliction, and potential for organ donation if the patient is nonsalvageable. In most areas of the United States, gunshot wound is the most common etiology, impalement with various types of sharp objects contributing to the rest.

The disparity between physical damage and neurologic deficit is amazing. Large cranial defects can be compatible with recovery just as small missile wounds to a particular area can be fatal. The emergency physician must concentrate on rapid recognition and resuscitation. Application of the basic principles of trauma care should ensure minimal morbidity and mortality.

As in all cases, treatment begins with ensurance of an adequate airway. In the supine patient, the airway can be obstructed by the tongue, but the patient may also have penetration of the upper airway as well as the cranium. I therefore recommend that, if bleeding is occurring in the upper airway, the patient be transported lying on his side if awake and have endotracheal intubation with in-line cervical traction if unresponsive. A protected closed airway is also helpful if hyperventilation is judged to be desirable because of increased intracranial pressure.

If the patient is apneic or hypoventilating, mechanical ventilation through a closed airway system is preferred. Mask-valve bag may be used as a temporary expedient, but too often becomes associated with gastric dilatation. It should be remembered that penetrating cranial injuries frequently involve the upper airway.

Volume replacement can be critical, especially when there are associated injuries. Although shock is rarely associated with head injuries, penetrating injuries can lose a great deal of blood. A low perfusion state should alert you to two things: (1) to always look for associated injuries (multiple gunshot wounds) and (2) not to withhold volume, blood, or crystalloid because of the head injury. All patients with head injury fare better with adequate perfusion, and so shock should be corrected as quickly as possible. Although scalp bleeding is amenable to hemostasis, bleeding from within the brain is not in the emergency department setting. Impaled objects, if present, should be left in place.

When the patient is stabilized with adequate airway, ventilation, and perfusion, I request three portable x-ray views, assuming no other injuries are present: (1) AP skull, (2) lateral skull, and (3) cross-table lateral cervical spine. Most neurosurgeons request CT scans of the head if the patient's condition is stable. Patients in unstable condition should not be sent for a CT scan because of the physical movement necessary and the difficulty in monitoring the patient's status in the CT room. Unless there are associated injuries, no other diagnostic studies are needed.

Penetrating cranial trauma represents an open fracture as a minimum. Therefore, prophylactic antibiotics should be considered. The precise antibiotics vary with local preference, but oxacillin and tobramycin given intravenously are used at our institution. Efficacy of prophylactic antibiotics is always improved by early use. Therefore, early administration of antibiotics is an emergency department responsibility.

In patients who have evidence of increased intracranial pressure (coma, rostral-caudal progression of neurologic finding), several temporizing steps can be taken prior to definitive decompression. Frequently the penetrating injury is 'self-decompressing.' The nonsurgical maneuvers are hyperventilation and pharmacologic measures. Mild hyperventilation to the Pco_2 range of 25 to 30 mm Hg is quick and simple if the patient is intubated and on a ventilator. Intravenous mannitol, given as a 20 percent solution (1 mg per kilogram) over 20 to 30 minutes, is also rapid in action, but effect is short-lived. However, steroids have a slower onset and longer lasting effects. Decadron, 10 mg initially IV and followed by smaller doses, is recommended. Mannitol should be given in consultation with a neurosurgeon, preferably by protocol before the emergency, but also on a case-by-case basis. Because Decadron has a delayed effect, urgency of administration is not critical. Again, I believe use of Decadron, mannitol, and even prophylactic antibiotics represents a joint effort between the neurosurgeons and the emergency department physicians and should be discussed and agreed to by protocol prior to use.

The importance of associated injuries cannot be overstated, as regards both diagnosis and priority of treatments. Active bleeding elsewhere cannot be overlooked. It has been frequently stated that patients with isolated injuries to the head rarely present in shock. I also find this to be true of head injuries bleeding externally; therefore, I look for other causes. Penetrating cranial injuries are treated according to priority, the highest priority going to injuries that not only are the greatest threat to physiology, but also can be corrected. Many of these patients have irreversible brain damage.

What role does the emergency physician play after all remedies are unsuccessful? Patients with head injuries, especially young, otherwise healthy individuals, have historically made up the major pool of organ donors. Although the time frame in the emergency department is too short to fulfill criteria for brain death, relatives may have questions in this regard and these should be answered as candidly as possible. It is generally inappropriate to suggest this possibility in the emergency department, but the physician should be alert to inquiries by family members and direct them to the appropriate resources. Nearly all major metropolitan areas have a local agency that coordinates donor procurement and provides information for possible donors. The North American Transplant

Coordinators Organization (NATCO) provides a 24-hour service (telephone 1-800-24DONOR). This agency can provide the name of a local agency and provide information to potential donors.

A final consideration in regard to penetrating cranial injuries is the possibility that the wound is self-inflicted. Because a reliable history is not always immediately available, it is prudent to consider this possibility in dealing with the patient's family or law enforcement officers. From the forensic point of view, this means that clothing is carefully preserved and the washing or cleaning of the victim's hands is avoided as lead or nitrates can be reco- vered from a hand that has recently fired a weapon. Also, in patients who are awake, suicide precautions should be observed until deemed otherwise.

SUGGESTED READING

Giannotta SL, Weiss MH, Apuzzo ML, et al. High dose glucocorti- coids in the management of severe head injury. Neurosurgery 1984; 15:496–501.

Tsai FY, Teal JS, Hieshima GB. Neuroradiology of head trauma. Baltimore: University Park Press, 1984.

SPINAL CORD INJURY

ROBERT S. HOCKBERGER, M.D.

Spinal cord injuries from motor vehicle accidents, athletic endeavors, and falls result in permanent neuro- logic impairment for 8,000 to 10,000 young Americans yearly. Eighty percent of victims are between 18 and 25 years of age. The total cost of evaluating and caring for spinal injury victims exceeds two billion dollars annually in the United States, and the physical loss, psychological pain, and emotional distress suffered by the victims and their families is incalculable.

Spinal damage is often the least life-threatening in- jury sustained by trauma victims. Therefore, the general approach to the victim of multiple trauma should include (1) early spinal immobilization, (2) airway management and circulatory support, (3) assessment and treatment of potentially life-threatening non-neurologic injuries, (4) neurologic assessment, (5) radiologic evaluation of the spine, (6) initiation of therapy for spinal cord edema in patients with neurologic impairment, and (7) neurosur- gical consultation for consideration of cryotherapy, decompression, or stabilization procedures when indicated (Fig. 1). The assessment and treatment of non-neurologic injuries and the radiologic evaluation of the spine will not be addressed in this chapter.

SPINAL IMMOBILIZATION

Paramedical personnel should suspect spinal injury in all cases of trauma involving victims with complaints of neck or back pain, evidence of severe head or facial injury, or an altered sensorium. In addition, victims of high-speed deceleration accidents, falls from significant heights, near-drowning, and high-voltage electrical in- juries should be treated as though they had spinal inju- ries, regardless of complaints, until they reach the emer- gency department. Unguarded manipulation of an unstable spinal injury has been reported to have caused or wor- sened neurologic impairment in 3 to 25 percent of spinal injury victims. Spinal immobilization should be initiated by trained paramedical personnel in the field and should be maintained in the emergency department until the possibility of spinal injury has been eliminated or the vic- tim of spinal injury has been transferred to the care of a neurosurgeon.

Immobilization "in the field" should be initiated by placing the trauma victim on a spine board in the supine position with the head placed in a neutral position with respect to the longitudinal axis of the body. Once this is accomplished, the cervical spine can be kept immobile by placing sandbags on either side of the victim's head. Two-inch tape should then be used to anchor the victim's forehead to the sandbags and spine board. In addition, the victim's arms and torso should be anchored to the backboard with sheets or straps placed at the levels of the chest and pelvis to ensure normal alignment of the spinal axis during transportation and during evaluation in the emergency department. One study comparing "sandbags and tape" to other spinal immobilization modalities found the former to be equal to or better than all other recom- mended devices. Conscious and cooperative patients should be warned against spinal movement. Uncoopera- tive patients should have an individual assigned to hold head and neck in alignment with the remaining spinal axis. Such patients may have to be sedated once the possibility of other significant injuries has been eliminated.

Standard spinal immobilization recommendations must be altered in patients with ankylosing spondylitis in- volving the cervical spine. The brittle cervical spine of these patients becomes fused in a position of flexion. Attempts at 'straightening' the spine of such patients fol- lowing a cervical fracture may result in worsening pain and neurologic impairment. Therefore, patients with known ankylosing spondylitis of the cervical spine, as well as victims of spinal injury who voluntarily hold their heads in a position of flexion and complain of pain or neuro- logic impairment when a gentle attempt at normal align-

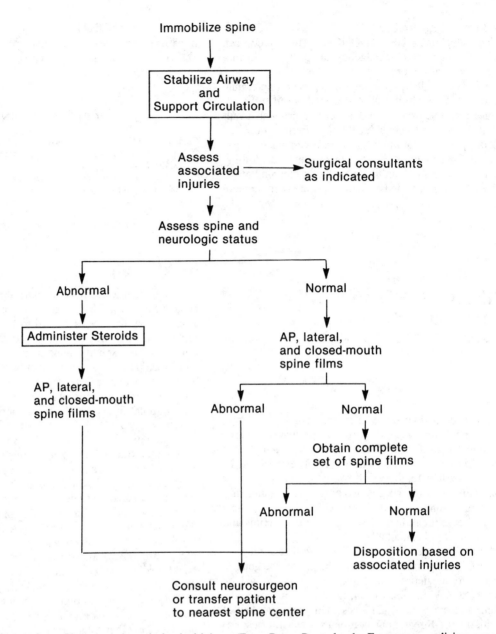

Figure 1 Approach to patient with suspected cervical spinal injury. (From Rosen P, et al, eds. Emergency medicine: concepts and clinical practice. St. Louis: CV Mosby, 1983.)

ment is made, should be maintained in a position of maximum comfort in both the pre-hospital and emergency department settings.

Definitive immobilization with Gardner-Wells or Trippe-Wells tongs and traction should not be attempted during initial emergency department resuscitative efforts. The placement and adjustment of such devices is time-consuming: the weight-and-pulley systems necessary for proper traction are not generally available in the emergency department, and most trauma gurneys are not adaptable for use with such devices.

AIRWAY MANAGEMENT AND CIRCULATORY SUPPORT

Maintenance of a patent airway in patients with neck injuries is crucial. Associated maxillofacial trauma,

retropharyngeal hemorrhage and edema from spinal injury, bleeding from facial injuries, and retained secretions often contribute to airway obstruction. In addition, low cervical injuries may result in ascending paralysis secondary to spinal cord edema and, occasionally, respiratory arrest secondary to delayed phrenic nerve paralysis.

According to the American College of Surgeons Advanced Trauma Life Support (ATLS) Guidelines, the preferred method of airway management for patients with traumatic cardiorespiratory arrest, even with evidence of spinal injury, is careful endotracheal intubation. Cricothyrotomy, in experienced hands, is a reasonable alternative. Nasotracheal intubation is the procedure of choice for patients with cervical trauma who do not have cardiac arrest but require respiratory support. When maxillofacial injuries preclude nasotracheal intubation, if a patient cannot cooperate for nasotracheal intubation, or when initial attempts at nasotracheal intubation are unsuccessful, cricothyrotomy should be performed. In patients without signs of respiratory embarrassment, repeated clinical assessment and monitoring of arterial blood gases, tidal volume, and vital capacity are essential for early detection of subtle signs of deterioration.

Patients with total transection of the spinal cord, as well as those in spinal shock (i.e., total absence of neurologic function distal to the level of a spinal injury secondary to spinal cord concussion and edema), lose peripheral autonomic tone and may present with neurogenic hypotension secondary to peripheral vasodilatation. In both instances, patients have flaccid paralysis below the level of their injury. Additional signs of spinal shock include (1) absence of peripheral signs of vasoconstriction usually seen in hypotensive states, (2) normal heart rate or bradycardia resulting from unopposed vagal tone, (3) normal or slightly decreased central venous pressure, and (4) rapid response to atropine (when heart rate is less than 60 per min), the Trendelenburg position, or the infusion of 500 to 1,000 ml of crystalloid fluid. In multiply traumatized patients, neurogenic hypotension can be diagnosed only after the exclusion of other causes of hypotension such as blood loss, pericardial tamponade, and tension pneumothorax. Neurogenic hypotension resulting from spinal shock is a self-limiting phenomenon lasting less than 24 hours. In patients with a spinal cord transection, autonomic tone usually returns within 3 to 7 days.

NEUROLOGIC ASSESSMENT

A rapid but complete neurologic assessment takes only minutes to perform and is mandatory to document the level and degree of damage (Table 1). The absence of neurologic impairment does not exclude significant and potentially unstable spinal column injury, and radiologic assessment of the potentially injured spine in neurologically intact patients must be completed before immobili-

zation attempts are discontinued. When neurologic impairment is identified, it can often be categorized as one of several commonly occurring spinal cord syndromes: complete cord syndrome, anterior cord syndrome, central cord syndrome, and Brown-Séquard cord syndrome(Fig.2).

A complete cord syndrome is defined as total loss of neurologic function distal to the site of a spinal cord injury and may occur as the result of total spinal cord disruption or the syndrome of spinal shock. The bulbocavernosus reflex can help differentiate these two conditions. The reflex is elicited by placing a gloved finger in the patient's rectum and then squeezing the glans penis or, alternatively, by tugging gently on an inserted Foley catheter. An intact reflex results in a sharp distinct rectal sphincter contraction. The absence of this reflex indicates the presence of spinal shock. No accurate estimate of a patient's prognosis for recovery can be made until this reflex has returned. In 99 percent of cases, spinal shock lasts less than 24 hours.

The central cord syndrome is seen most commonly in patients with degenerative arthritis of the cervical vertebrae whose necks are subjected to forced hyperextension. Compression of the spinal cord anteriorly by degenerative osteophytes and posteriorly by the hypertrophied ligamentum flavum results in a contusion of the central portion of the cord (see Fig.2). These patients have all motor and sensory tracts involved and exhibit greater neurologic deficit in the upper extremities than in the lower. A patient with a severe central cord syndrome may appear to have a complete cord syndrome, but on close examination exhibits evidence of sacral sparing. Signs of sacral sparing include persistent perianal sensation, good rectal sphincter tone, and slight toe flexor movement. Since this injury usually results from a spinal cord concussion or contusion, further investigative procedures (computed tomography or myelography) and surgery are rarely indicated. The prognosis for patients with this syndrome is directly related to how rapidly clinical recovery progresses and is, in general, good.

TABLE 1 **Neurologic Examination of the Spinal Trauma Patient**

Level of Lesion	Resulting Loss of Function	Resulting Loss of Reflex	Resulting Loss of Sensation
C2			Occiput
C3	Diaphragm		Thyroid cartilage
C4	Spontaneous breathing		Suprasternal notch
C5	Shrugging of shoulders		Below clavicle
C6	Flexion at elbow	Biceps	Thumb
C7	Extension at elbow	Triceps	Index finger
C8 to T1	Flexion of fingers		Small finger
T1 to T12	Intercostal and abdominal muscles*		
T4			Nipple line
T10			Umbilicus
L1 to L2	Flexion at hip		Femoral triangle
L3	Adduction at hip		Medial thigh
L4	Abduction at hip	Patellar	Knee
L5	Dorsiflexion of foot		Lateral calf
S1 to S2	Plantar flexion of foot	Achilles	Lateral foot
S2 to S1	Rectal sphincter tone		Perianal region

* Localization of lesions in this area is best accomplished with the sensory examination.
N.B. Most muscles are in fact innervated by several cord segments, so that the level determined is always approximate.

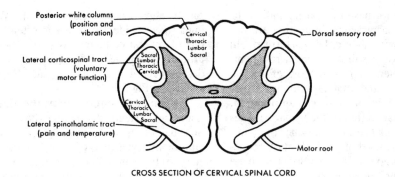

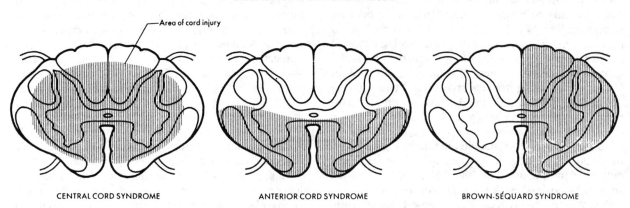

Figure 2 Incomplete spinal cord syndromes. (From Rosen P, et al, eds. Emergency medicine: concepts and clinical practice. St. Louis: CV Mosby, 1983:322.)

The anterior cord syndrome may occur as the result of cord contusion, from injury to the anterior spinal artery with resultant cord ischemia, or by protrusion of bony fragments or herniated intervertebral discs into the spinal canal causing spinal cord compression. This syndrome is characterized by paralysis and paresis and hypalgesia below the level of injury with preservation of posterior column functions including position, light touch, and vibratory sensations (see Fig. 2). Immediate myelography or computed tomography (CT) evaluation is indicated in such patients to identify surgical candidates who have evidence of cord compression. Following surgery, patients have variable degrees of recovery during the first few days, with little improvement thereafter.

The Brown-Séquard syndrome, or hemisection of the spinal cord, usually results from a penetrating lesion (bullet or knife), but may be seen following lateral mass fractures of the cervical spine. Such patients have ipsilateral motor paralysis and contralateral sensory hypesthesia distal to the level of injury (see Fig. 2). These patients are not candidates for surgery unless debridement of open wounds is necessary. Recovery is limited, but virtually all patients retain control of bowel and bladder function, and most eventually become ambulatory, occasionally requiring the use of a leg brace.

TREATMENT OF SPINAL CORD EDEMA

The maximal neurologic deficit following blunt spinal injury may not occur until several hours following the traumatic event. Research has identified the pathophysiology of this phenomenon. The initial traumatic event causes disruption of local intramedullary vessels with protein extravasation and edema. Increased endogenous catecholamine levels cause local vasoconstriction and ischemia, which worsens spinal cord edema and eventually extends the initial injury. There is no satisfactory treatment for acute spinal cord edema with proven efficacy in man. Nevertheless, recommended treatments include corticosteriods, naloxone, thyrotropin-releasing hormone, dimethylsulfoxide, hyperbaric oxygen therapy, surgical decompression, and hypothermia.

The use of corticosteroids in patients with spinal cord injuries remains controversial. Theoretically, steroids may act by preserving cellular and vascular membrane integrity, by exerting a strong anti-inflammatory effect to combat edema, and by reversing the sodium and potassium electrolyte imbalance resulting from tissue edema and necrosis. Although the efficacy of steroids in combating traumatic spinal cord edema in man has not yet been established, few contraindications to the use of steroids exist, and their routine use in spinal injuries associated with neurologic deficit is recommended by most neurosurgeons. Dexamethasone, 10 to 20 mg every 4 to 6 hours, can be administered by either the intramuscular or the intravenous route.

Large doses of both intravenous naloxone and thyrotropin-releasing hormone have been shown to improve neurologic recovery in experimentally traumatized cats. Treated animals do not exhibit the moderate drop in systemic arterial pressures seen after spinal injury in control animals, and the resulting improved spinal cord perfusion may aid neurologic recovery. There are, as yet, no reports addressing the efficacy of these drugs in humans, and the cost of employing them in the doses recommended (1 to 2 mg per kilogram) is prohibitive.

Dimethylsulfoxide (*DMSO*), with its anti-inflammatory, diuretic, vasodilatory, and cryoprotective properties, has been found to improve neurologic recovery in animals with experimentally induced spinal cord injury. As with naloxone, its efficacy in humans has not been established.

Hyperbaric oxygen therapy may improve tissue oxygenation and combat the cellular hypoxia seen after trauma to the spinal cord. Conflicting experimental and clinical data have precluded more widespread use of this potential treatment modality. Currently, otherwise stable patients with spinal injuries cared for in institutions employing hyperbaric oxygen chambers appear to benefit from treatment.

There does not appear to be clear evidence that surgical intervention in the form of decompressive laminectomy or durotomy is of any benefit in patients with acute spinal cord trauma in the absence of myelographic evidence of disc herniation or bony fracture-dislocation with acute cord compression. Laminectomy, followed by several hours of spinal cord bathing with cooled normal saline to prevent edema, has been advocated by some authors. Theoretically, hypothermia might lower metabolism and minimize the ongoing tissue destruction that occurs during the first few hours following spinal trauma. Thus far, experimental results in both animals and humans is conflicting. Several spinal centers are still in the process of studying the effects of controlled hypothermia in this setting.

Mannitol and other osmotic diuretics have been found to be effective in combatting post-traumatic cerebral edema, but have not been found to be effective in treating post-traumatic spinal cord edema. Alpha-methyl tyrosine, and other antiadrenergic compounds, which act by inhibiting norepinephrine synthesis or by depleting catecholamines, have been used experimentally with little success. Such drugs reduce central hemorrhagic necrosis significantly, but toxicity and the necessity of pretreatment in order to be effective are notable drawbacks. Epsilon aminocaproic acid (EACA), which functions in a synergistic manner with steroids to preserve the membrane integrity of cells, has been suggested, but not used clinically in humans for spinal cord injury because of the potential danger of inducing thromboembolic phenomena in bedridden victims of spinal injury.

NEUROSURGICAL CONSULTATION

All trauma patients with neurologic impairment and/or radiologic evidence of spinal injury should receive neurosurgical consultation. Acute operative intervention (within 6 to 12 hours) is indicated for the following reasons: (1) to relieve persistent spinal cord compression from bony fracture fragments, herniated intervertebral discs, or an epidural hematoma as demonstrated by myelography or computerized tomography, (2) to obtain an open reduction in patients with spinal column dislocations that do not relocate readily after attempts at closed reduction with traction, (3) to surgically augment the stability of markedly unstable cervical injuries, particularly above the level of C3.

MINOR SPINAL INJURY

Minor "whiplash" injuries of the cervical spine from motor vehicle accidents are a daily occurrence in our society and are frequently faced in the emergency department. Three types of symptoms may occur:

1. Hyperextension injury of the sternoceidomastoid, scalenus, and longus colli muscles and ligaments may result in pain and stiffness, starting immediately or up to several days following the inciting event. The mechanism of injury, degree of the patient's distress, and findings on physical examination are all factors that must be weighed in determining the need for radiologic assessment in such patients. Several days of immobilization with a soft cervical collar, local application of cold packs to injured ligaments and/or heat packs to injured muscles, and judicious use of muscle relaxants and anti-inflammatory medications are warranted. While many medications have been found to be superior to placebo in treating musculo-skeletal pain, no drug or combination of drugs has proved more effective or more cost-effective than aspirin (650 g every 4 hours) and diazepam (2 to 5 mg three times a day).
2. Severe hyperextension of the cervical spine may result in injury to the cervical sympathetic chain as it courses medially to the longus colli muscles, with resultant complaints of dizziness, nausea, blurred vision, and, occasionally, Horner's syndrome.
3. Flexion-extension injury of the cervical spine may occasionally cause radicular symptoms as the result of nerve root irritation. Such patients who are neurologically intact and have normal findings on cervical roentgenograms should have flexion and extension films performed. Such views should only be obtained on alert patients who can cooperate by actively flexing and extending their necks approximately 15 to 20 degrees. Patients should be warned to discontinue any movements if pain or radicular symptoms develop during the course of the examination. Roentgenographic instability is defined as greater than 3.5 mm of horizontal displacement of one vertebral body on another.

Symptoms may persist for 1 to 4 weeks. If symptoms last longer than 8 weeks, the following possibilities should be considered:

1. Occasionally minor unstable cervical ligamentous injuries may be masked initially by muscle spasm. Repeat flexion and extension cervical films should be considered to rule this out.

2. Continued pain and/or cervical radiculitis may be the result of cervical disc herniation; CT scan or myelography should be considered.
3. Only when all physical causes of continued symptoms have been eliminated, the possibilities of traumatic neurosis and secondary gain from litigation, workman's compensation, and attention of family and friends should be considered.

SUGGESTED READING

Cline JR, Scheidel E, Bigsby EF. A comparison of methods of cervical immobilization used in patient extrication and transport. J Trauma 25 (7):649:653.
De La Torre JC. Spinal cord injury: review of basic and applied research. Spine 1981; 6(4):315–335.
Podolsky S. Baraff LJ, Simon RR, et al. Efficacy of cervical spine immobilization methods. J Trauma 1983; 23(6):461–465.

STRANGULATION AND HANGING

KENNETH V. ISERSON, M.D., F.A.C.E.P.

ETIOLOGY AND TERMINOLOGY

There are approximately 3,500 deaths reported from suicidal strangulation and hangings in the United States each year. Strangulations account for 5 to 10 percent of criminally violent deaths in large urban areas. Hangings are responsible for approximately 5 percent of medicolegal autopsies. Most victims of suicidal hangings are males, usually white and elderly.

Strangulation is produced by pressure on the neck and takes four forms, depending on how the pressure is produced: hanging (the most common), ligature strangulation, manual strangulation, and postural strangulation. It can also be classified by the setting in which death occurs: suicide, accident, homicide, and judicial executions.

Injuries from pressure on the neck are described in relation to how the pressure was applied, how much force was used, and for how long the force was maintained. These are also the factors determining the time until death.

The body need not be suspended and hanging for death to occur. The term "complete hanging" is used when the feet do not touch the floor, and "incomplete" is used for all other positions. Hanging can occur from virtually any position, often from suspension points below the individual's standing height.

In ligature and manual strangulation, the constricting force is external; neither the weight of the body nor that of the head plays a part. Postural strangulation occurs when the victim's neck is placed over an object, with the weight of the body putting pressure on the neck. This is frequently seen in infants and toddlers.

In a classic judicial hanging, unless the drop was at least equal to the height of the victim, there was no injury to the cord, fracture of the spine, or fracture of the base of the skull. The most common spinal injury in judicial hangings was a significant disjointing of C2 from C3 with bilateral fractures of the C2 arch. Occasionally the disjointing occurred between C3 and C4.

Accidental hangings occur for two reasons. The first is either children "playing at hanging" or adults giving demonstrations of hanging. The second is the so-called "autoerotic" hanging whereby the victim dies while using hanging, self-strangulation, or both to enhance sexual self-gratification. The victims in this group are virtually all male.

Accidental ligature strangulation can occur from the umbilical cord during birth or by the tightening of clothing around the neck when caught on cribs or toys. Hair and clothing tangled in machinery have also caused this type of injury in adults. Accidental postural strangulation occurs most commonly in children when their neck is caught in crib rails or on a window ledge.

Suicide is the most common setting in which strangulation occurs. Hanging is by far the most common method. Suicide by ligature strangulation involves significant mechanical difficulties, making this method possible but uncommon. Suicidal and accidental manual strangulations are thought to be impossible.

PATHOPHYSIOLOGY

In nonjudicial near-hangings, the carotid arteries are compressed by direct pressure when they cross the transverse process of C6 (Fig. 1). A traction injury, reported in about 5 percent of these hangings, involves either slight bleeding into the walls of the carotid or a minimal tear in the intima at the level of the ligature, particularly if the victim is older and has severe atherosclerotic disease. Vertebral artery flow is rarely affected by the direct pressure, but this vessel is torn in as many as 40 percent of successful hangings.

The hyoid bone and the thyroid and cricoid cartilages compose the anterior semirigid neck structures. The U shape of the hyoid bone makes it vulnerable to fracture during hanging. In the thyroid cartilage, the superior cornua are most likely to be injured. Fracture of the thyroid cartilage is found in almost 50 percent of nonjudicial hanging deaths. The hyoid bone is fractured in about 20 percent of patients over 40 years of age. Virtually all are minimal fractures that would be clinically insignificant. The cricoid cartilage is rarely reported as having any injury in nonjudicial hanging or ligature strangulations.

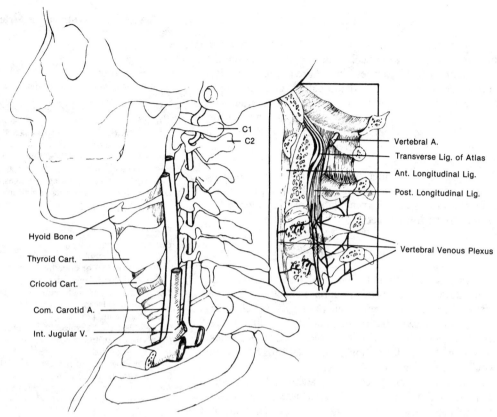

Figure 1 The vital anatomic structures in strangulations. From Iserson KV. Strangulation: a review of ligature, manual, and postural neck compression injuries. Ann Emerg Med 1984; 13:179–185.

However, in ligature strangulations, hyoid and laryngeal injury occur in nearly 50 percent of cases. Manual strangulation is most often associated with fracture of the larynx including the hyoid bone and thyroid cartilage.

Death from strangulation is caused in one of three ways: (1) by injury to the spinal cord and brain stem, (2) by mechanical constriction of the neck structure, or (3) by cardiac arrest, possibly caused by stimulation from carotid sinus and pericarotid sympathetic and parasympathetic networks. Spinal cord, medullary, and bony spine injuries are extremely unusual events. However, we do not know whether arterial occlusion, venous occlusion, or asphyxia plays the greatest part.

Venous compression, because of the low pressure required in any position, must be considered a factor in all nonjudicial hanging and ligature strangulation cases. The veins can be fully compressed while the arteries are not affected. Thus, the most likely pathophysiologic sequence in a nonjudicial hanging is that low pressure on the neck causes venous obstruction and loss of consciousness (Fig. 2). The body is then completely limp and muscle tone in the neck is decreased. This flaccid state results in an increased pressure on the neck, which may cause complete arterial occlusion, airway closure, or both, resulting in death.

Older people with atherosclerosis and carotid artery disease may die as a result of "reflex cardiac arrest" due to marked cardiac slowing from increased vagal tone following alterations in carotid sinus pressure. Similar deaths have occurred in persons subjected to "carotid sleeper" neck holds. However, these restraining maneuvers, used in law enforcement, also cause a direct decrease in carotid blood flow.

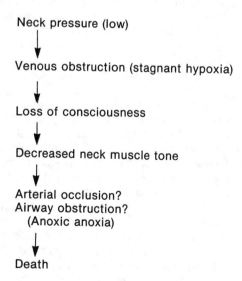

Figure 2 Pathophysiologic sequence in a nonjudicial hanging. From Iserson KV. Strangulation: a review of ligature, manual, and postural neck compression injuries. Ann Emerg Med 1984; 13:179–185.

INJURY RECOGNITION

After release of tension, there is often a brownish groove noted about the neck. These marks may remain visible for more than a week since there is often considerable small vessel trauma. If the patient is able to talk, severe hoarseness and stridor secondary to traumatic edema of the larynx in supraglottic tissue may be present. Aphonia may be present and there can be significant pain on swallowing. Subconjunctival petechial hemorrhages may also be apparent.

Abrasions from fingernails, bruising, or both may be present if the victim attempted to free himself prior to unconsciousness. Manual strangulation may also leave fingernail marks on the neck.

TREATMENT

Aggressive treatment of strangulation victims should be instituted regardless of the initial neurologic findings (Table 1). Even severe neurologic findings are often reversible in these cases. Victims of suicidal strangulation frequently have to be treated for other suicidal activities, including wrist lacerations, self-stabbing, gunshot wounds, and ingestion of toxins.

The neck should be externally stabilized. Appropriate radiologic evaluation should be performed, but in nearstrangulations, respiratory and neurologic support and assessment are usually critical to the patient's survival and must take priority. Soft tissue films may aid in assessing hemmorhage and edema of the neck, which may threaten the airway.

Aggressive respiratory management must be initiated immediately, including intubation and positive end expiratory pressure (PEEP) ventilation when appropriate. Most in-hospital deaths are due to pulmonary edema or bronchopneumonia. This may result from aspiration, a centrineurogenic cause, or both, and this responds well to PEEP. Neurologic support (e.g., hyperventilation, osmotic diuresis, and intracranial pressure monitoring) should be instituted as necessary to treat increasing intracranial pressure.

Absent or agonal respirations, absent heartbeat or the need for ventilatory assistance in the emergency department, a pH less than 7.2, or unsuccessful initial resuscitation in the field has an extremely poor prognosis. This may not be applicable in infants and children, some of whom have survived complete cardiopulmonary arrests following accidental strangulation. Initial electroencephalogram (EEG) assessment and neurologic findings have little prognostic significance.

Neurologic sequelae are the most significant aftermath of strangulation. Cerebral anoxia occurring during suspension may cause neurologic damage that is not immediately assessable. Conversely, patients often arrive with significant neurologic deficits that resolve over a period of days. Peripheral neurologic damage involving the spinal accessory nerve has been reported.

TABLE 1 Treatment of Strangulation Victims

Prehospital
  Cut off ligature
    Stabilize neck
    Do not cut knot (needed for possible medicolegal investigation)
  ABCs
    Ventilate if no/poor spontaneous ventilation
    If breathing spontaneously, position patient to prevent aspiration
    Use EOA (EGTA) if no spontaneous ventilation
    Cardiac monitor
  Start IV (D⁵ 0.45 NS) at TKO and draw baseline blood
  Begin treatment for increased intracranial pressure/herniation
    (hyperventilation, diuretic) if signs are present
  Get any history about patient's position, knot placement, drop, and type of ligature

Emergency Department
  Continue ventilation
    Replace EOA with NT tube (blind, fiberoptic, or retrograde intubations) or cricothyrotomy
    Use PEEP or CPAP
  Check for other self-induced injuries (gunshot wounds, poisoning, lacerations)
  Support systemic physiology
  Cross-table lateral C-spine film (probably negative)
  Do not cease efforts to make prognosis on the basis of initial neurologic findings
  Obtain photographs of any external neck injury
  Continue treatment of increased intracranial pressure
  Admit patient for observation, even with normal neurologic and pulmonary status

Hospital
  Continue ventilatory support
  Continue treatment for increased intracranial pressure (? intracranial pressure monitor)
  EEG at 48 hours or later
  Repeated neurologic assessment
  Psychiatric referral and suicide precautions when extubated

EOA = esophageal obturator airway;
EGTA = esophageal gastric tube airway;
TKO = to keep open; NT = nasotracheal tube

From Iserson KV. Strangulation: a review of ligature, manual, and postural neck compression injuries. Ann Emerg Med 1984; 13:179–185.

Delayed neurologic sequelae are rare. When they occur, they follow one of three patterns: (1) the comatose patient who, after minor neurologic improvement, dies; (2) the patient who appears to make an orderly neurologic recovery, including awakening and appearing close to his neurologic baseline, only to progress to an uncontrollable herniation syndrome with death or severe residua; and (3) the patient who appears completely normal neurologically, but develops a delayed encephalopathy and dies. This is consistent with the asymptomatic intervals that may follow any period of compromised oxygenation and circulation to the central nervous system with attendant increased intracranial pressure.

Even patients who appear neurologically normal in the emergency department should be admitted for observation of both respiratory and CNS dysfunctions. Arrangements must be made for a sequential neurologic follow-up.

BLUNT AND PENETRATING CHEST TRAUMA

PETER ROSEN, M.D.
MICHAEL W. BRUNKO, M.D.

Chest trauma is conveniently divided into blunt and penetrating mechanisms of injury. Since the pathologies are different, they will be discussed separately. Blunt forces impact upon the chest wall, but can be distributed to the contents of the thorax. Penetrating forces produce injuries varying with the degree of penetration, as well as the energy the penetrating missile imparts to the tissues it passes through.

PRE-HOSPITAL CARE

Care for the victim of chest trauma ideally begins at the scene of injury. Well-trained paramedics are an essential part of the trauma team. Early consideration must always focus on "the ABCs": the airway secured properly, obvious external bleeding controlled, and large-bore peripheral intravenous lines established to maintain adequate circulation. It is important to recognize that the patient with blunt chest trauma also has suffered innumerable combinations of blunt trauma to other parts of the body—the head, spine, abdomen, and pelvis being of primary concern. Initial field management must also concern itself with these other injuries.

The personnel at the scene must obtain details concerning the mechanism of injury. Information about the speed of the automobile and type of impact, the amount of interior and steering wheel damage to the car, the use and type of restraint devices (lap versus harness), whether the victim was found in the vehicle or out of the vehicle, the distance of a fall, and the condition of the patient at the scene are all useful in the evaluation and management of the patient in the emergency department. The patient with severe chest trauma receives no benefit from prolonged on-the-scene stabilization and management, but must be transported to the nearest "trauma center" where skilled trauma personnel are available.

INITIAL MANAGEMENT

On arrival in the emergency department, the patient with chest trauma should receive an initial total body assessment. Airway management is always the priority consideration in the patient with chest injury. The patient may require only passive supportive measures such as manipulation of the jaw or tongue to maintain an adequate airway, but in many cases, insertion of an endotracheal or nasotracheal tube is needed. If the patient has associated facial, laryngeal, or cervical soft tissue trauma, cricothyrotomy is advocated for airway management in the patient in respiratory distress. If a patient has a hematoma at the base of the neck (usually secondary to penetrat-

ing trauma, but also possibly caused by blunt trauma involving the large vessels), cricothyrotomy is less desirable and, if possible, should be avoided to avoid uncontrollable exsanguination.

Circulation management takes next priority. At least two peripheral intravenous lines should be inserted, preferably 16 gauge or larger. Central venous lines may be the only initial access in the hypovolemic patient, and large-bore 7 or 8 introducers can be inserted by means of the Seldinger technique. The central venous pressure (CVP) line in the chest trauma patient is also useful in the assessment of volume status. The CVP line should be placed on the side of the obvious chest trauma unless internal jugular or subclavian vessel trauma is suspected on that side. If the chest injury is below the clavicle, the central line should be placed on the side of the injury. If the injury includes penetration or signs of damage above the clavicle, or if there is large soft-tissue swelling around the clavicle, then the line should be placed on the opposite side of the chest. In this way, one can minimize complications for the patient. Saphenous, femoral, and brachial vein cutdown lines can also be placed for resuscitation, depending on the volume status of the patient and the extent of the injuries. The initial choice of fluid for resuscitation should be isotonic normal saline or lactated Ringer's solution. O-Negative blood should be used in the patient with massive blood loss if crystalloid solution, 50 ml per kilogram, has not stabilized the patient's condition.

If the patient continues to have respiratory difficulty after adequate airway management and volume resuscitation have been established, the cause of impaired ventilation may be pneumothorax, hemopneumothorax, or tension pneumothorax. Indications for immediate tube thoracostomy are penetrating gunshot wounds, as mentioned previously, decreased or absent breath sounds, hyperresonance to percussion of the chest, the palpable soft tissue crepitance of subcutaneous emphysema, the obvious appearance of a flail segment, and difficulty in the manual ventilation of an intubated patient.

If a sucking chest wound is discovered during the initial assessment of the patient, it should be closed immediately, in the field if possible, by means of sterile occlusive petrolatum gauze that is secured on three sides, allowing air escape when the patient exhales, but becoming "sucked" over the wound when the patient inhales, thus preventing more air from entering. Ultimately, a tube thoracostomy should be performed at another site—not through the wound, which may penetrate as far as the lung or diaphragm. Insertion of a thoracostomy tube through the existing wound increases the risk of contamination of the pleural space and subsequent empyema.

There is an understandable desire to obtain an early chest film, but this should be postponed until the patient is in stable condition. Even though the optimal study is done in an upright position, this position must be sacrificed if the patient is in unstable condition. Sitting the patient upright may induce an irreversible hypotension or cardiac arrest, should the patient be significantly volume-depleted. Often the only film possible to obtain is the portable supine anteroposterior view, and the trauma physicians must be able to interpret and act decisively on this view. In the case of penetrating missile wounds, it is wiser and safer to insert a thoracostomy tube and to delay x-ray studies until circulating volume is restored and ventilation is adequate.

Respiratory rate is a helpful clue to respiratory function, but since this is frequently altered by pain, alcohol intoxication, and procedures necessary for resuscitation, it is helpful to obtain early arterial blood gases. Even though diagnostic electrocardiographic changes are rarely seen after trauma, it is wise to have a baseline ECG for subsequent comparison.

SECONDARY ASSESSMENT

After initial assessment and stabilization of the patient with significant thoracic trauma, a more thorough survey of the patient should be performed with a view to possible multi-system trauma. Further evaluation of the chest may reveal injuries to the heart, lungs, mediastinal structures (vessels, esophagus, trachea, and bronchi), and associated bony structures. Proper evaluation and recognition of these injuries must be done without haste to maximize the patient's chances for survival. They include institution of treatment if necessary in the emergency department, diagnostic testing that usually requires personnel who are not immediately available, and obtaining consultants, especially from the trauma service.

BLUNT TRAUMA

Cardiac injuries from blunt trauma occur because of rapid acceleration-deceleration, direct compression, or an acute increase in intrathoracic or intra-abdominal pressure. The types of injuries to the heart that are the result of blunt trauma include myocardial concussion, myocardial contusion, valvular tears, and myocardial rupture, and these are discussed elsewhere in this text.

Myocardial Concussion

Myocardial concussion is the most acute form of blunt cardiac trauma and probably the most difficult to diagnose. A direct blow to the anterior chest wall and sternum causes a sudden transient dysrhythmia (ventricular fibrillation, ventricular tachycardia, or asystole) resulting in hypotension, loss of consciousness, and in many cases sudden death. This injury may be suspected if a patient is witnessed to sustain blunt trauma to the chest (e.g., from steering wheel, baseball, or helmet) and immediately afterward is found to be pulseless and without blood pressure, but may demonstrate spontaneous return of vital signs and consciousness. Autopsy usually shows no damage to the myocardium.

Myocardial Contusion

Myocardial contusion is estimated to occur in as many as 25 percent of patients with severe blunt chest trauma. The extent of the injury may vary from subendocardial cellular hemorrhage and edema to actual infarction.

Myocardial contusion is frequently missed in the patient with blunt chest injury because attention is directed toward the other obvious severe injuries. The diagnosis should be suspected in any patient with significant chest wall injury, as evidenced by history of steering wheel and automobile interior damage, multiple rib fractures, sternal fractures, or persistent tachycardia that is unexplained by the patient's other injuries or degree of blood loss. Other causes of persistent tachycardia may include drugs, alcohol, or a catecholamine release in response to the pain of the patient's injuries. These can be ruled out by appropriate diagnostic tests and analgesics for pain control. Although the best diagnostic tool in the emergency department is the electrocardiogram, this study still fails to diagnose myocardial contusion in about 50 to 65 percent of cases. The most frequent dysrythmias seen are persistent sinus tachycardia, atrial fibrillation, atrial and ventricular premature beats, and right bundle branch block. Any nonspecific S-T or T wave abnormalities that were not present on electrocardiograms prior to the injury (if available) or S-T or T wave changes that represent patterns of ischemia are diagnostic of myocardial contusion. Enzyme determinations (SGOT, LDH, CPK) are less helpful in the diagnosis because they are elevated in the patient with severe blunt chest trauma because of associated injuries. Creatinine phosphokinase-MB (CPK-MB) isoenzymes provide evidence of myocardial damage, peaking within 12 hours of the injury and absent or low by 72 hours after injury. However, isoenzymes are often unavailable or take a long turnaround time. Technetium pyrophosphate nuclear medicine scans, if immediately available, may demonstrate increased myocardial uptake if damage is present, but have been shown to be negative when there is other positive evidence of contusion.

Once the diagnosis is recognized in the emergency department, continuous cardiac monitoring is mandatory with institution of antidysrhythmic drugs, depending on the dysrhythmia present. Ventricular dysrhythmias, in particular, may be attributable to acidosis secondary to hypoxia and hypovolemia, and these conditions should be remedied first.

Overzealous fluid administration in the multiply injured patient with a myocardial contusion, especially the elderly patient with pre-existing heart disease, may precipitate congestive heart failure. In this situation, a central venous catheter should be inserted to help in the monitoring of volume status. Diuretics should be given to correct the fluid overload. If the patient continues to show signs of pump failure, an inotropic agent such as dopamine should be started at a dose of 2 to 5 μg per kilogram per minute and titrated upward until the desired response is seen. Patients who deteriorate nonetheless require cross-clamping of the descending aorta and open cardiac massage until an intraaortic balloon counterpulsation device can be inserted, usually in the operating room.

Valvular Tears

Patients with blunt chest trauma who suffer complete valve rupture usually die immediately. Small tears are seen most frequently involving the aortic valve, followed by the mitral. Any patient who presents after blunt chest trauma with a new heart murmur should be suspected of an aortic valve injury, which frequently causes a diastolic murmur described as "cooing dove" in character. Partial rupture of the mitral valve is less well tolerated because of the high pressures of the left ventricle. If it is not severe enough to cause death, a mitral insufficiency murmur is heard and there is rapid onset of pulmonary edema. While in the emergency department, the patient with partial aortic valve rupture may demonstrate worsening of aortic insufficiency: a decreasing diastolic blood pressure, visible capillary pulses, pistol-shot sounds over the brachial and femoral vessels, and a Corrigan's pulse.

Diagnostic aids in the emergency department are limited; physical examination is the most useful tool. A chest film may demonstrate pulmonary edema. An echocardiogram occasionally is diagnostic, but the definitive diagnostic test is cardiac catheterization.

Ultimately the patient needs cardiac catheterization followed by valve replacement. Immediate consultations with a cardiologist and cardiothoracic surgeon are necessary.

Myocardial Rupture

Blunt trauma to the heart may be severe enough to produce myocardial rupture; most patients succumb rapidly to exsanguination or tamponade. Less often, a low-pressure atrial chamber ruptures and is contained temporarily by the pericardium. A patient presenting with shock who is not responding to vigorous fluid resuscitation and has elevated central venous pressure and distended neck veins may have cardiac tamponade from a ruptured chamber. The classic signs of tamponade may not be present owing to blood loss from multiple-system injuries.

Pericardiocentesis is a temporizing procedure in resuscitation of the patient until thoracotomy and cardiac repair can be performed in the operating room. Emergency department thoracotomy and pericardiotomy are necessary if the patient loses vital signs. Once the pericardium is entered, direct finger pressure is applied to the area of rupture until definitive suturing can be performed in the operating room. If the injury is suspected early in a small community hospital where cardiopulmonary bypass and surgical staff are not immediately available, the patient should be transferred rapidly to another center where they are available. An indwelling pericardial catheter may be helpful in this situation to release pericardial blood as it re-accumulates during transport. There is no point in performing a thoracotomy in an emergency department that is not prepared to deal with the injuries.

Aortic and Great Vessel Injuries

Sudden horizontal deceleration accidents may result in traumatic rupture of the thoracic aorta. Laceration of the subclavian artery at the thoracic inlet is the next most common great vessel injury followed by avulsion or lacer-

ation of the innominate artery at the aortic takeoff. Occasionally, direct trauma in the region of the clavicles can cause sharp fracture fragments that can injure the subclavian veins and arteries and produce a large hematoma, venous thrombosis, or arteriovenous fistula. These injuries are discussed further in related chapters.

Clinical symptoms and signs are helpful if they are present. Damage to the car's steering wheel or steering wheel imprint on the chest, obvious chest bruising, sternal fracture or multiple rib fractures, upper extremity hypertension with loss of femoral pulses ("pseudocoarctation syndrome"), infrascapular murmur, a pulsatile mass at the base of the neck, carotid bruits or decreased carotid pulses, and paraplegia are observable signs. The patient may complain of ischemic-type extremity pain, dyspnea, stridor, and dysphagia. About one-third of these patients have little or no evidence of external chest trauma.

The most important clue to the presence of this injury is a knowledge of the mechanism of injury. The most useful study initially is the upright posteroanterior chest film. In many cases, the emergency physician has to be content with the portable supine anteroposterior view, which distorts the mediastinum. Unless the patient's condition becomes stable enough to permit the study to be repeated satisfactorily, the next diagnostic procedure is most likely to be the definitive aortogram. Any of the findings of Table 1 should increase the willingness to perform this study.

Tracheobronchial Injury

Injuries to the thoracic trachea and main stem bronchus are usually owing to rapid deceleration and shearing off the more mobile distal bronchi from the fixed proximal structures. They occur within one inch of the carina and may not be apparent for 3 to 5 days following injury. Forced expiration against a closed glottis or forced compression against the vertebral column may also cause tracheobronchial lacerations.

Tracheobronchial injuries should be suspected in the emergency department if massive subcutaneous emphysema is present. A chest roentgenogram may demonstrate mediastinal emphysema, pneumothorax, or other associated mediastinal injuries. If pneumothorax is present with a continued air leak that is not corrected by two large chest tubes connected to suction at 20 to 30 cm water, a

TABLE 1   Chest Film Findings Suggestive of Thoracic Aortic Injury

Widened mediastinum (>50%)
Deviation of trachea to right
Deviation of nasogastric tube to right
Loss of aortic knob contour
Left apical pleural "cap" (hematoma)
Loss of aortopulmonary window (lateral roentgenogram)
Depression of left main stem bronchus
Fractured first or second rib
Fractured sternum or scapula
Fracture-dislocation of the thoracic spine
Left pleural effusion or hemothorax
Anterior displacement of the trachea (lateral roentgenogram)

tracheobronchial tear should be suspected. Once the injury is detected, bronchoscopy is necessary to locate the origin of the tear.

The definitive treatment of a tracheobronchial tear is surgical repair. Lower tracheal and bronchial lacerations that involve more than a third of the circumference and are associated with continued air leak require thoracotomy and repair as soon as possible. Delay in bronchial repair may result in stricture formation, atelectasis, and pulmonary infection. A missed tracheal tear may result in a delayed and severe mediastinitis.

Esophageal Injury

Both blunt and penetrating injuries to the esophagus are rare; the majority of injuries are caused iatrogenically by endoscopy, biopsy procedures, or traumatic insertion of nasogastric tubes or esophagaeal obturator airways. Swallowed foreign bodies that perforate the wall or cause delayed ulceration and rupture can also be the cause of esophageal trauma. The recognition of these injuries usually depends on the history. The patient may complain of chest or neck pain, cough, dyspnea, or dysphagia. The presence of subcutaneous emphysema in the neck, fever, an auscultatory mediastinal "crunch" or mediastinal emphysema on chest films suggest esophageal injury. Esophageal injury, especially in cases of blunt trauma, may be overlooked because of associated injury to other structures, mainly the aorta and trachea. If these structures are injured, the esophagus should be assumed damaged also until proved otherwise.

Roentgenographic studies in the emergency department that may be helpful are the soft tissue lateral neck film and the chest film. The soft tissue neck film may show retropharyngeal soft tissue swelling or free air in the soft tissue if esophageal perforation has occurred. The chest film may show mediastinal emphysema, a foreign body, left-sided pleural effusion, pneumothorax, or a widened mediastinum. A spontaneous pneumomediastinum caused by extreme Valsalva maneuvers against a closed glottis is difficult to distinguish from a perforated esophagus. The patient usually has pain and dysphagia, but in general does not appear ill. Free mediastinal air is present on the chest roentgenogram. The patient with benign pneumomediastinum gives a history of an extreme valsalva performance, such as in the process of marijuana inhalation or following a minor unexpected trauma. If the patient appears well, no further diagnostic procedures are necessary. For the patient's comfort, the mediastinal air can be partially relieved by allowing him or her to breathe 100 percent oxygen. There is usually much symptomatic relief in 30 to 60 minutes.

Esophageal contrast studies are helpful in the diagnosis of more serious injuries. The water-soluble contrast Gastrografin is preferred by many because it causes less reaction to surrounding tissue if extravasation occurs. However, it is associated with false-negative results in approximately 25 percent of cases, a finding that is rare when insoluble barium contrast is used. The safest approach is to start with Gastrografin and, if the study is negative, to proceed with dilute barium for further delineation. Endoscopy occasionally may reveal the injury when radiologic procedures are inconclusive.

The pre-hospital and emergency department management should focus on recognition of the possibility of esophageal injury. The patient must not receive anything by mouth, should receive maintenance fluid support, have a nasogastric tube inserted carefully, and be started on broad-spectrum antibiotics in the emergency department. Surgical consultation is needed for repair of the lesion and drainage of the mediastinum.

PENETRATING TRAUMA

Stab Wounds

Stab wounds to the chest can range from serious cardiac and large vessel injuries to minor chest wall lacerations. Any wound of the chest, back, or upper abdomen is assumed to be serious, with possible cardiac, great vessel, or pulmonary damage, until proved otherwise. The trajectory of the knife and its length usually are not known at the initial encounter with the patient and must be assumed to have achieved full thoracic penetration.

Pre-hospital management of the patient with a stab wound to the chest should follow the protocol for any critically injured patient. In the emergency department, the patient should be fully undressed in a search for other wounds in less obvious places. Airway management, hemorrhage control, and volume resuscitation constitute the first priority, as discussed earlier. If the wound is precordial or epigastric in location, cardiac penetration is a possibility. Rapid deterioration of vital signs in the field or in the emergency department in the patient with a thoracic stab wound is indicative of large vessel or cardiac penetration, and in these patients pericardial tamponade should be considered and corrective measures must be undertaken promptly. The patient may initially be hypovolemic from blood loss and show signs of hypotension, tachycardia, and a normal or low central venous pressure. After adequate fluid and blood resuscitation, the patient then may demonstrate the classic signs of pericardial tamponade: decreased blood pressure, tachycardia, and increased central venous pressure ($>15cm$ H_2O). If this occurs, immediate pericardiocentesis should be performed. If blood is aspirated, causing improvement of vital signs, the diagnosis of pericardial tamponade is confirmed, and the patient should immediately be transferred to the operating room for thoracotomy and cardiac repair. If the patient loses vital signs, emergency department thoracotomy should be performed. If a rapid improvement in vital signs does not occur, the thoracic aorta should be cross-clamped and open cardiac massage begun. If a cardiac wound is apparent, digital pressure on the wound should be applied during rapid transport to the operating room. The myocardial injury may then be repaired with interrupted horizontal, mattress, pledge II nonabsorbable sutures. Once this is done, the back of the heart should be examined for further injury that should be repaired at this time.

Other indications for emergency department thoracotomy include other penetrating thoracic wounds with deterioration of vital signs, large vessel penetration with intrapleural exsanguination, and the presence of an air embolism. The patient with penetrating chest trauma whose vital signs are undetectable in the field is not likely to benefit from emergency thoracotomy.

The patient with a stab wound to the chest may also demonstrate respiratory difficulties. If active airway management and supplemental oxygen do not improve the patient's status, a hemopneumothorax or pneumothorax must be sought. If there are decreased breath sounds, subcutaneous emphysema, or hyper-resonance on the side of the wounds, an immediate tube thoracostomy should be performed.

In the unstable patient, a thoracostomy tube should be placed prior to diagnostic x-ray studies. Physical examination of the traumatized chest is often unreliable, especially early after injury. Breath sounds may seem normal, tracheal deviation is difficult to ascertain, and subcutaneous emphysema may take some time to develop. Vital signs are the best indicators of stability. If there is any question of the patient's stability, it is safer to insert a thoracostomy tube than to jeopardize that stability by the positional changes required for diagnostic studies.

Thoracostomy is performed using a 36 to 40 F chest tube inserted into the fifth intercostal space, midaxillary line. The procedure is made easier if the patient's arm is extended over his head. The use of 0.5 percent bupivicaine (Marcaine) for anesthesia makes the patient more comfortable and cooperative. Once the incision is made, a subcutaneous tunnel is made over the rib, directing the tract superiorly and posteriorly. Blunt dissection is used to enter the pleural space, and digital examination is used to document intrapleural penetration and to release any adhesions that may be present. Then, a blunt clamp is used to direct the chest tube through the incision posteriorly and superiorly into the desired position. It is sutured to the skin with a 1-0 suture wrapped several times around the tube. The tube should then be attached to a drainage system so that air leak and blood drainage can be assessed. A sterile petrolatum gauze dressing is wrapped around the wound and secured with elastic tape. Post-insertion intercostal nerve blocks two ribs above and two ribs below the insertion site, using 0.5 percent bupivicaine, provide prolonged anesthesia and assist in the prevention of pulmonary complications (e.g., atelectasis, infection).

Stab wounds to the chest that are below the nipples anteriorly and below the inferior border of the scapulae posteriorly require not only assessment of thoracic injury, but also evaluation of intra-abdominal and diaphragmatic penetration. Diagnostic peritoneal lavage should be performed in these patients with criteria for laparotomy lowered to 5,000 red blood cells per cubic millimeter in consideration of possible injury to the diaphragm.

The patient with a stab wound to the chest and stable vital signs should receive as thorough an evaluation as one with a more serious injury. After the initial examination, a chest roentgenogram should be obtained in search of hemopneumothorax or pneumothorax. It is a good rule of thumb to consider any pneumothorax caused by a penetrating injury serious enough to require a chest tube. It is difficult to assess from the initial chest roentgenogram the amount of blood, if present, in the pleural space. Any blood that may be present must be drained, and suspicion of a hemothorax warrants placement of a chest tube.

After thorough evaluation, including chest films, peritoneal lavage, if indicated, and placement of a central venous line for suspected cardiac injuries, the stable patient should be observed for 8 to 12 hours, either in the hospital or in an adequately staffed observation unit. Before discharge, repeat inspiratory and expiratory posteroanterior chest films should be obtained to rule out a delayed hemothorax or pneumothorax. A repeat hematocrit is also wise, and arterial blood gases may be useful, depending on the patient's clinical condition. The stab wound itself should be carefully cleansed and irrigated, but nothing should be inserted into the wound. It is impossible to determine the depth of a stab wound by probing with fingers or instruments, and in fact such probing may induce serious hemorrhage or an iatrogenic pneumothorax. It is safer and wiser to utilize the radiologic studies, and the passage of time, to eliminate injuries. The wound should then be left open and dressed with a sterile dressing with appropriate wound and infection precautions.

Gunshot Wounds

Gunshot wounds to the chest are managed in the same basic fashion as stab wounds. The indications for tube thoracostomy, pericardiocentesis, and emergency thoracotomy are the same as for stab wounds of the chest with one exception. If the chest is penetrated, one must assume that there is a hemopneumothorax; it is rare for the bullet to hit a rib and circle the chest without penetration. Since the vast majority of peripheral gunshot wounds of the chest can be managed by thoracostomy and by volume and blood replacement, it is wisest to immediately insert the thoracostomy tube without first proving its need with a chest film. In other words, assume that all patients with gunshot wounds of the chest are in unstable condition and need stabilization before diagnostic studies can be undertaken. Gunshot wounds, unlike stab wounds, are more likely to cause a through-and-through injury, tend to follow a straight path, and cause much more tissue and organ destruction because of the amount of energy associated with the impact of the missile.

Gunshot wounds are produced by two basic types of weapon: high-velocity and low-velocity. High-velocity weapons include most rifles, military weapons, and magnum-type pistols. Shotguns fired at close range may be considered high-velocity weapons because of the amount of mass imparted on the intended target and thus a large dissipation of kinetic energy. Low-velocity weapons include most hand guns, pellet guns, and small-caliber civilian rifles. When a bullet strikes human tissue, it does not follow a straight path because of cavitational effects, yawing, tumbling, and fragmentation, which all contribute to a dissipation of kinetic energy in the tissue and cause widespread tissue damage. High-velocity weapons, soft-nose or hollow-point bullets, and closely fired low-velocity weapons thus cause more tissue destruction than is apparent on external examination. A gunshot wound may well have caused extensive damage to other organs far away from the entrance site. Management should focus primarily on the clinical presentation of the patient and the assumption of serious injury rather than location of the missile and theorizing about the trajectory of the bullet. Surgical consultation should be sought immediately as thoracotomy and even possibly laparotomy may be necessary.

HEMOTHORAX

Hemothorax is usually caused by bleeding from lung parenchyma or intercostal vessel injury secondary to blunt or, more likely, penetrating trauma to the chest. The diagnosis should be suspected in the patient following trauma if breath sounds are diminished to auscultation, and dullness to percussion is present on the involved side, but often is present without these findings. If the patient is unstable and if a hemothorax is suspected, immediate tube thoracostomy should be performed. A chest roentgenogram is helpful in making the diagnosis, but 200 to 300 ml of blood must be present in the intrapleural space before a hemothorax can been seen on an upright chest film. If a subpulmonic hemothorax is suspected, a lateral decubitus film should be obtained to demonstrate fluid layering along the dependent lateral chest wall.

Treatment of a hemothorax requires early drainage, as the blood collection can cause both immediate and subsequent restriction of ventilation and venous return, and blood clots, if left in the pleural space, can release fibrinogenolytic and fibrinolytic substances that may cause continued bleeding from the original source of injury. A large chest tube should be placed to obtain drainage of blood and clots, and if this measure is not successful, a second tube can be placed to assist in removal of partially clotted or loculated blood.

The hemothorax of most peripheral injuries can be treated by tube thoracostomy alone, but occasionally patients with penetrating injuries continue to bleed and may require thoracotomy for control of the hemorrhage.

Thoracotomy is indicated if more than 1,500 ml of blood drains from the chest, if drainage of blood exceeds 200 ml per hour for 3 to 4 hours or longer, if the patient's vital signs remain unstable despite adequate resuscitation, or if the patient's clinical condition deteriorates after initial successful resuscitation. If rapid drainage of blood from a thoracostomy tube coincides with deterioration of the patient, fluid and blood transfusions must be aggressively administered and the patient made ready for surgery. If significant bleeding occurs and continues, autotransfusion may be used when available.

PNEUMOTHORAX

Pneumothorax, a collection of air in the pleural space, is a common complication of trauma to the chest. Traumatic pneumothorax is usually caused by a fractured rib that protrudes inward, causing a laceration of the pleura. Penetrating forces can also cause pneumothorax and may result in a communicating pneumothorax or "sucking chest wound." Blunt trauma to the chest can also cause pneumothorax by rupturing alveoli. If there is a one-way valve effect in the chest wound, not allowing air to escape with expiration, a tension pneumothorax is produced, leading to decreased cardiac output and eventually circulatory collapse.

Treatment of a traumatic pneumothorax usually requires a tube thoracostomy unless the pneumothorax is small and the patient asymptomatic. If only pneumothorax is present, tube thoracostomy should be performed with a small tube (24 to 28F). If an air leak persists after thoracostomy with one tube, a second tube should be inserted at a different site. If the patient continues to have an air leak after the insertion of two tubes and the lung is not seen to be fully expanded on a chest film, suction (20 to 30 cm H_2O) should be applied to the tubes to attempt to re-expand the lung.

SUGGESTED READING

Moore EE et al. Critical decisions in trauma. Chapters 31 to 38. St. Louis, Toronto, London: CV Mosby, 1984.

Rosen P et al. Emergency medicine—concepts and clinical practice. Chapters 16-23. St. Louis, Toronto, London: CV Mosby, 1983.

AIR EMBOLISM

DONALD D. TRUNKEY, M.D.

Systemic air embolism has not been commonly diagnosed and treated. Traditionally, air embolism was thought to be the presence of air on the right side of the systemic circulation that leads to ineffective right heart stroke volume and pulmonary hypertension. Systemic air embolism is most often associated with a bronchopulmonary venous fistula caused by blunt or penetrating trauma, primarily laceration of the lung from a fractured rib.

In my experience, systemic air embolism occurs in 14 percent of all major thoracic injuries. The incidence of air embolism following penetrating versus blunt upper torso trauma is 3:1. Patient survival is more likely following penetrating trauma (slightly >50 percent) than after blunt trauma, which has a survival rate of 20 percent.

DIAGNOSIS

The primary reason the syndrome is underappreciated and therefore undertreated is the subtlety of the presenting signs and symptoms. They fall into four categories, and the patient may present with any combination of these findings.

1. Lateralized focal neurologic findings in the absence of obvious head injury. This results from air in the cerebral circulation and can be confirmed by air seen in the retinal vessels during funduscopic examination.
2. Hemoptysis. Although hemoptysis is associated with many pulmonary injuries, when it is present, one must have a high index of suspicion for a bronchopulmonary venous fistula. With adequate blood volume and negative airway pressure, hemoptysis is not infrequent. With positive pressure ventilation, however, the pressure differential favors entry of air into pulmonary veins with resultant air embolism.
3. Sudden cardiovascular collapse shortly after endotracheal intubation. This represents air in the coronary circulation and is aggravated by the positive pressure ventilation that is usually applied immediately after intubation.
4. Froth that is obtained during aspiration of arterial blood for blood gas determinations. This is associated with 100 percent mortality.

Approximately two-thirds of patients have signs or symptoms of air embolism on, or shortly after, presentation to the emergency department. The remaining one-third usually manifest their symptoms within the first 24 hours of admission, although symptoms may occur as late as 5 days following injury.

SURGICAL MANAGEMENT

Treatment of patients who have definite signs and symptoms on admission is relatively straightforward; they require emergency thoracotomy. Ideally, the thoracotomy should be performed in the operating room, but if the patient is dead or dying on presentation, thoracotomy in the emergency department is indicated. In many instances, it is obvious which thorax is involved; I prefer to do the thoracotomy on the ipsilateral side. For example, if there is a penetrating wound of the left thorax or a flail chest involving the left hemithorax, a left anterior thoracotomy should be done. A left anterior thoracotomy is my preference for other resuscitative efforts. In some instances, the offending bronchopulmonary venous fistula is in the contralateral lung from the obvious injury, or it is difficult to determine which side is involved. If such is the case, a left anterior thoracotomy can be extended across the sternum into the right thorax so that bilateral anterolateral thoracotomies, which give excellent exposure, are used. The primary objective is to open the involved hemithorax as soon as possible so as to clamp the hilum of the lung and thus reduce the inoculum of air to the left atrium. After the hilum has been clamped, further resuscitation (which may include cardiac massage) should be carried out. Before cardiac massage is given, it should be noted whether or not there is air within the coronary circulation. This observation is not only to help confirm the diagnosis, but also to aid in treatment. If air is the suspected cause of circulatory collapse, it is prudent to administer epinephrine, either endotracheally or intravenously, to increase systemic pressure and empty the microcirculation of the microbubbles. If internal cardiac massage is being carried out, holding the ascending aorta with the thumb and index finger for two or three strokes helps to evacuate the coronary artery air. It is also important to vent the ventricle or the aortic arch, or both, with a needle to remove as much of the accumulated air as possible.

Once resuscitation has been achieved and the hilum of the lung is clamped, definitive surgery, in the majority of cases, consists of oversewing the pulmonary laceration. In instances of extensive trauma, lobectomy or even pneumonectomy may be necessary. The rest of the operative procedure is routine, as with any thoracotomy.

SUGGESTED READING

Graham JM, Mattox KL, Beall AC Jr. Penetrating trauma of the lung. J Trauma 1979; 1966:5.

Thomas AH, roe BB. Air embolism following penetrating lung injuries. J. Thorac Cardiovasc Surg 1973; 66:533.

Trunkey DD, Lewis FL. Current therapy of trauma-2, Toronto: BC Decker, 1986; 247–249.

PULMONARY CONTUSION

FRANK R. LEWIS Jr., M.D.

Pulmonary contusion is nearly always the result of blunt trauma, the only exceptions being penetrating trauma attributable to shotgun wounds, high velocity rifles (>2,000 feet per second muzzle velocity), or bullets that mushroom on impact (''dum-dum'' or hollow-point bullets). With blunt trauma, contusion is caused by high-speed impact, with high-energy dissipation. Mechanisms of injury that are typical are falls from heights, motorcycle injuries resulting from collision with a fixed object, or high-speed car accidents in which the passengers are unrestrained.

It is rare for the pulmonary contusion to exist in isolation; usually there are associated thoracic or upper abdominal injuries as well. Fractured ribs in the area of impact are almost universally present, and if the impact has been more severe, the spectrum of additional injuries may include myocardial contusion, lung laceration, ruptured diaphragm, aortic disruption, and liver or spleen laceration.

ETIOLOGY

The etiologic mechanisms are virtually always attributable to sudden rapid compression of the chest wall and underlying lung, thus producing direct traumatic damage to the lung parenchyma. Because the lung is mostly air-filled and is less dense than most solid organs, it can withstand major compressive forces more readily than other body tissues; this no doubt accounts for the infrequency of the lesion.

In addition to the direct tissue trauma, the rapid compression of the lung may produce severe but brief pulmonary vascular pressure elevation, which may be localized in the area of impact. This results in extreme capillary hypertension, causing fluid, protein, and red cell transudation into the pulmonary interstitium. It may also produce endothelial damage and a transient increase in capillary permeability.

Penetrating trauma that is of low velocity does not produce a significant contusion lesion; the damage being limited to the wound tract itself. However, as the velocity of the bullet increases, the energy increases exponentially, and tissue damage rises in parallel with energy transfer. As a result, tissue damage is produced at some distance from the primary tract. The higher the velocity, the greater is the radius of injury, and with military or high-velocity hunting rifles having muzzle velocities in excess of 3,000 feet per second (fps), the damage may extend several centimeters outside the primary tract. When the bullet "mushrooms," the tissue injury owing to direct damage as well as the energy transfer is also greater, and the contusion is correspondingly increased. The same is true when there are multiple projectiles, or when secondary missiles are created by a bullet striking a rib and fracturing it.

DIAGNOSIS

The diagnosis is generally made by the chest film in conjunction with a knowledge of the mechanism of injury. A lung contusion presents as a lung infiltrate of variable density with poorly defined borders in the area of maximal impact. With blunt trauma, it is peripherally based and tends to taper toward the hilum, thus presenting a roughly wedge-shaped appearance in many cases. Fractured ribs are usually present overlying the area of contusion, as it marks the area of maximal impact. Occasionally there is also a flail-chest segment overlying the contusion when fractures are particularly extensive. Because of the magnitude of force required to produce a contusion, other injuries should always be suspected and sought.

With penetrating trauma, the contusion corresponds to a cylinder of injured tissue surrounding the wound tract, or to the tissue injured directly when there are multiple fragments. The appearance may be somewhat altered by hemorrhage into the wound tract itself, and hemopneumothorax is universally present, in contrast to the cases of blunt trauma, where it is often absent.

In both blunt and penetrating trauma, the contusion does not conform to any anatomic boundaries in the lung.

If one sees a strictly lobar configuration, or if the infiltrative process is delimited by a major or minor fissure, it is likely to be something other than a contusion.

One characteristic of contusions is that they begin to develop within minutes and thus are present to some degree on the initial chest film taken in the emergency department. Classically, the infiltrates worsen for approximately 24 hours and then begin to resolve, disappearing in 3 to 4 days. Frequently pneumonia develops in the segment that was contused and supersedes the contusion on the chest film so that the infiltrate never fully clears. In such cases, one sees some initial clearing, then later worsening and evolution of the infiltrative process, the latter stages corresponding to the development of other signs of pneumonia.

There are no specific physical diagnosis signs of contusion, the most typical findings being tachypnea and splinting. If the contusion is severe, if there is a flail chest present, or if there are associated injuries such as pneumothorax, respiratory distress may be extreme. Cyanosis is rare, except in cases of crush injury to the entire chest, when a cyanotic discoloration of the head and neck, often in association with petechiae, is characteristic.

Blood gases should be obtained in any case of significant chest trauma, and when contusion is suspected, they are essential in the initial evaluation. Hypoxemia of moderate-to-severe degree is the usual finding, with normal carbon dioxide tension and pH. The magnitude of the hypoxemia parallels the severity of the contusion and, like it, generally worsens for the first 24 to 36 hours, before starting to improve.

There are no other laboratory tests necessary specifically for the contusion, although the frequency of associated injuries often requires more extensive work-up.

Differential Diagnosis

Pulmonary contusion is rarely confused with other diagnoses because it occurs only in immediate juxtaposition to major trauma. The other condition that may be suspected is aspiration pneumonia, which frequently occurs in traumatized patients who are comatose. It can usually be differentiated from contusion because the infiltrate is slower to develop, is more central, and usually corresponds to a segmental or lobar configuration.

Rupture of the left hemidiaphragm can give a confusing and ill-defined density in the left lower lobar area, and this can be confused with contusion, albeit infrequently.

TREATMENT

The majority of patients with pulmonary contusion require no specific treatment, only careful monitoring of the degree of respiratory compromise during the first few days until it resolves. When treatment is required, it is usually necessitated by either ventilatory failure or hypoxemia, each of which must be independently assessed.

Ventilatory Failure

Ventilatory failure by definition is compromise of the mechanical ability of the thoracic cage to move air in and out of the lung. When blunt thoracic trauma occurs, the pain from chest wall contusion or broken ribs causes marked splinting and impairs ventilation to a much greater degree than is generally appreciated, especially in older patients. The normal vital capacity (the amount of air that can be exhaled from full inspiration to full expiration) is in the range of 60 to 70 ml per kilogram body weight; hence for a 70-kg man, the normal vital capacity is about 4,600 ml. With moderate chest trauma, it is usual for this to be reduced to one-third or one-half of normal, i.e., 1,500 to 2,000 ml. It has been found empirically over many years that a minimal vital capacity of 12 to 15 ml per kilogram body weight is necessary to clear secretions and avoid progressive atelectasis. For a 70-kg man, this minimal vital capacity is 800 to 1,000 ml. It is clear if one compares these numbers that the margin between a dangerous level of vital capacity reduction and the level that is seen with moderate thoracic trauma is small. Patients who are operating near the failure level may be tipped over it relatively easily by a number of factors.

To evaluate ventilatory status, the simplest, quickest, and most definitive maneuver is to measure vital capacity. A number of inexpensive hand-held instruments are available for this measurement, and it can be done in less than 1 minute. All patients with moderate-to-severe blunt thoracic trauma should have this determination on admission, and if it is initially less than one-third of expected vital capacity it should be repeated at least daily until a rising trend is evident.

When their vital capacity is less than 20 ml per kilogram or when they demonstrate any evidence of respiratory distress, patients should be followed in an intensive care unit, where they can receive close monitoring and maximal nursing support to enhance ventilation and clearance of secretions.

When vital capacity falls below the range of 12 to 15 ml per kilogram, the patient usually requires tracheal intubation and ventilation because of inability to clear secretions, tachypnea, CO_2 retention, excessive work of breathing, or respiratory fatigue.

Hypoxemia

The second major reason for more aggressive treatment of pulmonary contusion is interference with oxygen exchange in the lung, thus resulting in arterial hypoxemia attributable to intrapulmonary shunting. Arterial oxygen tension is usually measured with the patient breathing either room air (oxygen concentration = 21 percent) or 100 percent oxygen. If room air is used, normal arterial Po_2 is 90 to 100 mm Hg, and significant compromise exists if Po_2 is below 75 mm Hg. If 100 percent oxygen is used, normal arterial Po_2 is over 500 mm Hg, and significant impairment is evidenced by a Po_2 below 300 mm Hg. Other standardized measures of hypoxemia can be used, with similar thresholds indicating the need for in-

tervention. The most common of these is the PaO_2 / FIO_2 ratio, with a value of less than 300 to 350 the cutoff, the $A-aDO_2$ gradient, with a value greater than 300 to 350 used as the threshold, and a shunt fraction (Q_s/Q_t) of more than 15 to 20 percent.

Patients with hypoxemia approaching any of the aforementioned thresholds should be placed in an intensive care unit so that conservative therapy can be maximized and monitoring intensified. The nursing measures employed are encouragement of deep breathing, suctioning if needed for removal of secretions, frequent postural changes, and administration of supplemental oxygen. If conservative measures fail, and patients develop clinical signs of respiratory distress, tachypnea in excess of 35 to 40, CO_2 retention, or hypoxemia significantly worse than specified by the aforementioned indicators, then intubation and ventilation are required.

Ventilatory Support

Endotracheal intubation with mechanical ventilation is the principal therapy available for the treatment of moderate-to-severe pulmonary contusion. The therapy is only supportive; it provides for adequacy of ventilation and oxygenation when the patient is unable to do it himself, and it prevents some of the complications of contusion, such as atelectasis and pneumonia.

A viewpoint has emerged in the last few years that intubation and ventilation of the patient with pulmonary contusion should be avoided at all costs, and that mortality is increased by such therapy. A full discussion of this question is beyond the scope of this chapter, but in my opinion this is a totally erroneous conclusion based on poorly documented and uncontrolled studies. Critical review of the literature fails to reveal a single paper in which detrimental effects of ventilation are shown where equivalent groups are being compared, and several papers are available in which beneficial effects are seen. No one advocates ventilation of all patients with the diagnosis of pulmonary contusion; as stated earlier, the majority of such patients do well with conservative treatment. However, when the contusion is more severe, or when there is associated chest wall damage producing compromise as defined by the indicators already listed, mechanical ventilation should be undertaken early instead of allowing the patient to develop progressive atelectasis or severe hypoxia, or to become exhausted in struggling to breathe.

Intubation may be undertaken by either the oral or nasal route, but the nasal route is preferable, as the tube, once placed, generally remains in place for several days before the patient can be successfully weaned. Tracheostomy is rarely necessary, and nasotracheal tubes may safely be used for periods of 8 to 12 weeks. The complications of tracheostomy—airway contamination, innominate artery erosion, tracheal stenosis, and tracheomalacia—greatly exceed the complications of nasal or oral endotracheal intubation, and tracheostomy should be avoided whenever possible.

Endotracheal tube selection is important. In adult

females, a No. 6 or No. 7 tube usually is the correct size, and in males, a No. 7 or No. 8 tube. In all cases, the tube should have a high-volume, low-compliance cuff and a device for controlling the cuff pressure at all times, so that it can be maintained in the range below 30 mm Hg. Tracheoesophageal fistulas result from excessive cuff pressure, but can be almost totally prevented by control of cuff pressure.

Ventilation of the patient can be done by any of a variety of excellent volume-cycled machines that are commercially available. The principles of mechanical ventilation that apply for all patients apply equally for those with pulmonary contusion, and will not be reiterated here. The duration of mechanical ventilation is governed by the natural progress of the patient.

Fluid Therapy

The second area in which the greatest misconceptions persist in regard to pulmonary contusion is the belief that crystalloid resuscitation is harmful, and that the patient benefits from fluid restriction or forced dehydration with diuretic agents. Based on the best evidence available, neither of these beliefs is correct.

The "crystalloid-colloid debate" has revolved around nearly every type of acute respiratory failure, and pulmonary contusion is not excepted. To critically review the voluminous literature would require several pages, but if I may summarize my own understanding of the current state of the literature, it is the following: As long as the patient is not overloaded with fluids (as gauged by measurements of left atrial or pulmonary wedge pressures), it makes no difference whether crystalloids or colloids are used for resuscitation, so far as the lung is concerned. Because of greater intravascular retention, less colloid solution is required to effect a given degree of volume replacement or intravascular filling. Quantitative studies have shown that isotonic salt solutions have to be given in approximately threefold greater volume than iso-oncotic colloid solutions to produce equivalent intravascular filling. However, if these equivalent quantities are given, as determined by dynamic monitoring of cardiac filling pressures, then there is no evidence of detrimental effects on lung function by either. Obviously, if either of the solutions is given in excess, and high pulmonary hydrostatic pressures are thereby produced, then either is capable of worsening lung function. In this regard, colloids are more hazardous because of their greater intravascular retention and, hence, smaller margin of error in administration.

The second belief, that pulmonary function is enhanced in pulmonary contusion by dehydration and fluid restriction, is also a complex subject, and the reader is referred to the most recent review of it (Am J Surg 1984; 148:145-151) for a full discussion. It can be fairly stated that unless the patient has fluid overload, as judged by high left atrial or pulmonary artery wedge pressures, there is no evidence whatsoever that he is helped by fluid restriction or forced dehydration. Indeed, recent evidence would indicate that it is in fact harmful if the diuresis or fluid restriction is carried so far as to produce hypovolemia, which is often the case with potent diuretics.

Patients with pulmonary contusion should be treated exactly the same as other traumatized patients: They should be given adequate fluids for the maintenance of normal cardiac filling pressures, peripheral perfusion, and urine output. They should not be overloaded, as cardiogenic edema can occur as easily as in any other group of patients, but neither should they have fluids restricted to the point of oliguria. Such therapy does no good and is probably harmful to organ perfusion, particularly in the kidney.

The Lesion

No specific therapies have ever been developed for pulmonary contusion, and no drugs have ever been shown to have benefit in preventing or reducing the lesion. Specifically, steroids have not been shown to be helpful, and are generally felt to be harmful by potentiating infection.

COMPLICATIONS

If it is uncomplicated, the pulmonary contusion resolves in a few days, and there is no residual anatomic or functional damage to the lung. It is interesting that pulmonary contusions resolve more quickly than cutaneous contusions and ecchymoses, at least based on the roentgenogram appearance. Some have speculated that this is attributable to the higher rate of blood flow per gram of tissue in the lung compared with the skin. Unfortunately, major complications may ensue, of which the most prominent are atelectasis and pneumonia.

Within the area of the contusion, interstitial edema and hemorrhage are seen, as is alveolar edema; combined with hypoventilation, atelectasis is the common result. If it is not extensive, it is well tolerated, but if it is progressive, it may require intubation and positive pressure ventilation to produce reexpansion.

There is also an apparent predisposition to pneumonia, usually at approximately the fifth or sixth day following injury, after the contusion itself has cleared. Prophylactic antibiotics should never be used for pulmonary contusion because they do not prevent infection, but only guarantee that the organisms that grow will be resistant ones.

SUGGESTED READING

Bongard FS, Leurs FR. Crystalloid resuscitation of patients with pulmonary contusion. Am J Surg 1984; 148: 145-151.

Tranbaugh RF, Elings VB, et al. Determinants of pulmonary interstitial fluid accumulation after trauma. J Trauma 1982; 22: 820-826.

Trunkey DD, Lewis FR. Chest trauma. Surg Clin North Am 1980; 60: 1541-1549.

RIB AND STERNUM FRACTURE

MICHAEL ROHMAN, M.D., F.A.C.S.
RAO R. IVATURY, M.D., F.A.C.S., F.R.C.S.(C)
MANOHAR NALLATHAMBI, M.D., F.A.C.S.

Fractures of the ribs and sternum usually are the consequence of blunt trauma from motor vehicle accidents, direct blows, and falls. In most instances the ensuing morbidity and mortality are directly related to the extent of the underlying injury to the lungs. However, trauma, even that limited to the rib cage, may produce major and even lethal consequences by interfering with ventilation and efficient coughing. Prompt diagnosis, effective relief or amelioration of chest pain and instability, and early specific treatment of parenchymal and pleural complications are the essentials of management of chest wall trauma.

SIMPLE RIB FRACTURE

DIAGNOSIS

The diagnosis is established by eliciting local tenderness on direct rib pressure in a patient who has sustained blunt thoracic trauma. Pain referred to the same area on bilateral chest wall compression and palpation of crepitation on ventilatory motion are additional diagnostic findings. Depending on the patient's pain tolerance, splinting of the chest wall, shallow ventilation, and tachypnea are observed to a varying degree. In the presence of pneumothorax or underlying parenchymal contusion, dyspnea and the use of accessory muscles of respiration are pronounced. In the setting of preexisting acute or chronic pulmonary disease, restriction of ventilatory effort due to pain may accelerate the onset of parenchymal complications. Derangements of acid-base balance may become increasingly severe with the potential for serious myocardial arrhythmias and other evidence of cellular derangements. X-ray examination usually confirms the site of fracture(s), but is not essential either for the diagnosis or to initiate treatment. In some cases x-ray identification may be difficult even though a variety of views are taken.

Management

Elderly patients, heavy cigarette smokers, and those with pulmonary disease must be observed closely and treated vigorously since they are more prone to pulmonary complications. They usually require hospitalization for treatment of pain, respiratory physiotherapy, repeat chest films for evidence of delayed complications (i.e., pneumothorax, hemothorax, atelectasis, pneumonia), serial arterial blood gas determinations, and sputum smears and cultures when indicated. Antibiotic administration rarely is necessary except to treat specific parenchymal infections. Younger patients may tolerate chest pain after the judicious use of analgesics and may be discharged from the emergency department, particularly if the home situation permits close observation. Medical follow-up in 24 to 72 hours is advisable.

A blow that fractures the *lower ribs* (i.e., eighth to twelfth) may be sufficiently severe to damage intra-abdominal organs. Careful evaluation of the abdomen is essential. The presence of upper quadrant tenderness and rigidity may be a reflection of the chest wall injury, but peritoneal irritation may also be responsible for these findings. Upright abdominal films for free air and changes in the splenic shadow are helpful. Peritoneal lavage may be essential, particularly in the hemodynamically unstable patient, to rule out splenic or hepatic lacerations and/or rupture of a hollow viscus.

Decreasing or eliminating pain is the cornerstone of care. In many cases this may be attained by doses of analgesic medication that reduce but do not actually eliminate all discomfort. The amount of narcotics required to relieve pain totally may affect the respiratory center adversely, blunt the cough reflex, and decrease mental alertness, further complicating management. Although splinting the thorax with adhesive tape may reduce pain on deep breathing and coughing, it also diminishes ventilation, burns and blisters the underlying skin, and is particularly uncomfortable for obese people and women; therefore, it is rarely used.

Intercostal Nerve Block. If pain does not respond to analgesic agents satisfactorily, an intercostal nerve block with 1 to 2 percent lidocaine or 0.25 percent Marcaine may be advisable. The technique is simple and should be mastered by all emergency physicians and surgeons. A skin wheal is made with the local anesthetic, using a 25-gauge needle, one inch posterior to the point of tenderness or at the posterior angle of the rib. A 20 to 22-gauge needle is inserted through the wheal and guided down to the inferior margin of the rib in question and is advanced an additional 0.5 cm under the rib. At this level, injection of 5 cc of the anesthetic agent will block the nerve effectively. To obtain complete anesthesia it is necessary to block one rib above and one below the fractured rib(s) as well. Care should be taken to avoid penetrating the pleural space and underlying lung. It is advisable to aspirate before injection to avoid intravascular administration of the medication. The block usually lasts 4 to 6 hours, during which time coughing and deep breathing must be encouraged to help in the expectoration of secretions and to maintain expansion of the lungs, particularly the lower lobes. It may be necessary to repeat the intercostal block once or twice before moderate analgesic therapy will suffice.

FIRST OR SECOND RIB FRACTURE

The shoulder girdle protects the upper ribs, particularly the first and second, from fracture in most blunt injuries. Therefore a fracture of one or both of these structures implies that the injury was unusually severe and raises the possibility that additional organ damage of major import may have occurred. Injuries of the subclavian artery, aorta, and tracheobronchial tree must be excluded.

Subclavian Artery Injury

Absence of pulses in the ipsilateral upper extremity with pallor, paresthesia of the hand, and slow capillary refill are suggestive of post-traumatic subclavian artery thrombosis. The presence of a pulsatile expanding hematoma above the clavicle is consistent with penetrating trauma of the artery by a rib fragment. Both conditions require prompt diagnosis by arteriography and/or operative intervention.

Aorta Injury

Sudden deceleration injuries, particularly those in which the victim's chest strikes the steering wheel or dashboard, may result in a shearing injury of the thoracic aortic intima and media. This may occur in any part of the aorta, but characteristically involves the descending portion at the junction of the intrathoracic arch and the retropleural continuation of the aorta (immediately distal to the left subclavian artery). It is estimated that 80 percent of these patients die immediately. The remainder arrive in the emergency department, frequently quite stable, only to experience completed aortic rupture unexpectedly with a fatal outcome. The x-ray findings in Table 1 should suggest the possibility of a contained aortic rupture and prompt immediate diagnostic aortography.

Since up to 5 percent of the patients who subsequently prove to have aortic rupture have no suggestive radiologic signs on admission, the severity of the accident as described by witnesses or the condition of the vehicle as reported by police or EMS personnel may provide sufficient information to warrant aortography. The documentation of a false aneurysm should prompt immediate surgical repair since the risk of exsanguination from complete rupture increases at the rate of 5 percent for every hour of delay.

Tracheobronchial Tree Injury

The presence of pneumothorax after severe blunt trauma is not unusual and may be managed by closed tube thoracostomy. The fifth interspace in the midaxillary line

TABLE 1 Roentgenographic Findings of Aortic Rupture

Widened mediastinum on upright film
Fracture of the 1st and/or 2nd rib
Obliteration of the aortic knob
Straightening of the left heart border
Deviation of the esophagus to the right
Apical capping
Infrapulmonary and intrapleural
  opacification (blood)
Downward displacement of the left main
  bronchus with deviation of the trachea
  to the right

is the preferred location because (1) it minimizes the potential risk of injury to the vertical portion of the diaphragm and subjacent organs, (2) the tube passes through a reasonable thickness of muscle mass which offers sufficient tissue to help seal the thoracotomy site after removal of the chest tube, and (3) it is a reasonably comfortable site from the patient's point of view.

Tension Pneumothorax

This usually presents with hypotension, severe dyspnea, cyanosis, deviation of the trachea to the contralateral side, and hyper-resonance to percussion. Decompression must be immediate because death may be imminent as a result of marked derangement in oxygenation of blood, carbon dioxide elimination, and reduced cardiac output. Tube thoracostomy usually provides definitive therapy; however, thoracentesis with a large-bore needle may be lifesaving, converting a tension into a simple pneumothorax and permitting some expansion and function of the lungs. Unusually large and/or persistent air leaks require surgical intervention for repair of the tracheobronchial tree or suture and/or resection of damaged pulmonary tissue.

MULTIPLE RIB FRACTURES

Flail chest is a consequence of multiple rib fractures in which the anterior and posterior bony continuity is disrupted or the costal attachments of the sternum are interrupted bilaterally. The resulting "floating" section of the chest wall is free to move paradoxically during the ventilatory cycle in response to changing pressure gradients between the atmosphere and the pleural space. During inspiration the flail portion is depressed, and during expiration the direction of motion is reversed. The efficiency of ventilation and coughing is compromised by severe pain. Hypoventilation leads to rapid retention of carbon dioxide and severe respiratory acidosis. Hypoxia, not necessarily apparent at first, may become a severe problem hours later. Retention of blood and secretions in the tracheobronchial tree may rapidly lead to focal atelectasis followed by segmental, lobar, or even total lung collapse from airway obstruction.

Perhaps the most important element in the pathophysiology of flail chest is the extent of the underlying pulmonary parenchymal damage. Actually it is this factor that may determine morbidity, mortality, or survival. The hemorrhage of severe contusion not only interferes with gaseous exchange, but also is an excellent pablum for infection. Death from sepsis is not infrequent, particularly in the elderly, and may reach as high as 50 percent in patients over 65 years of age.

Diagnosis

The diagnosis is made by the observation of paradoxical motion of the chest. Crepitation on palpation is a common finding. Respiratory distress and tachypnea usually are severe. Chest films and blood gas determinations should be obtained early in all patients to assess severity of pulmonary contusions and respiratory insufficiency.

Management

Stabilization of the chest by temporary measures may be lifesaving. At the scene of the accident and in transit to the hospital, the patient should be turned onto the side of injury to limit paradoxical respiration and pain and permit more efficient function of the contralateral lung. In the emergency department, closed thoracostomy to treat hemopneumothorax, if present, is essential. Relief of pain by intercostal block and mild analgesia may be all that is required for management of mild flails with minimal pulmonary contusion. However, serial arterial blood gas determinations are essential to detect significant hypoxemia and hypercarbia. Should the PaO_2 fall below 55 to 60 mm Hg on room air or the $PaCO_2$ rise above 42 to 45 mm Hg, endotracheal intubation and positive pressure ventilation with PEEP at 5 to 10 cm H_2O become necessary, using an FIO_2 as close to 35 to 40 percent as possible to maintain satisfactory oxygenation. Humidification of all inspired gases is essential. Not only does endotracheal intubation permit tracheal toilet, but positive pressure ventilation also provides internal splinting of the chest and expansion of the lungs, counteracting the effect of the flail. The use of antibiotics such as Cefadyl in this situation is probably wise, although the question of prophylactic antibiotics in the management of chest trauma generally is still controversial. It may be necessary to stabilize extensive flail segments of the chest surgically. Such procedures may shorten the period of intubation significantly and may reduce the frequency of tracheostomy which ordinarily is required if the patient remains intubated beyond 14 to 21 days.

FRACTURED STERNUM

This injury is occurring with increasing frequency as a consequence of motor vehicle accidents(MVAs). Direct blows and falls also may cause fractures of the sternum.

Diagnosis

Local tenderness, ecchymosis with crepitation, and/or overriding of the distal over the proximal portion of the sternum are the hallmarks of this injury. Portable and PA roentgenograms rarely confirm the diagnosis. If the injury is suspected, a lateral or oblique film is necessary.

The sternum in most people is a resilient structure and difficult to fracture. The presence of such an injury underscores the force involved in the accident and the possibility of underlying organ damage. It is mandatory that, among the other possible injuries, myocardial contusion be suspected. Ventricular arrhythmias and/or elevation of CPK-MB fractions require that the patient be hospitalized and treated in the same manner as a patient with suspected myocardial infarction. Careful ECG monitoring is essential. Intravenous lidocaine may be rerequired. Surgical repair of the fractured sternum is necessary if there is overriding, a serious flail, or severe pain.

SUGGESTED READING

Kirsch MM, Sloan H. Blunt chest trauma. Boston: Little, Brown and Co, 1977.
Trunkey DD, Lewis FR. Current therapy of trauma, 1984–1985. Philadelphia and Toronto: BC Decker, 1984.

INJURY TO THE DIAPHRAGM

CHARLES W. VAN WAY, M.D.

Injuries to the diaphragm are basically a diagnostic problem. They can present acutely, after trauma to the chest or abdomen, or chronically. The major intent of this chapter is to present a diagnostic strategy for detecting the acute injury. Diagnosis of the chronic diaphragmatic injury will also be reviewed.

About 80 percent of diaphragmatic injuries are from penetrating trauma to the lower chest or upper abdomen. Any injury between the nipples and the umbilicus must be suspected of involving the diaphragm. This means that one must either explore all such injuries routinely or use a strategy that will permit ruling out the diaphragmatic injury.

Diaphragmatic injuries produced by blunt trauma are usually associated with major injuries to the intra-abdominal and thoracic organs. Recognition is relatively easy, and most such injuries present other indications for abdominal exploration.

DIAGNOSIS AND THERAPY

Pre-hospital Phase

Diaphragmatic injuries can produce symptoms in only two ways. First, and most seriously, a large diaphragmatic injury may produce respiratory compromise because of loss of diaphragmatic function and because of the presence of intra-abdominal viscera in the chest. The initial therapy for this is positive pressure ventilation.

Although an endotracheal tube is best, mask ventilation is adequate.

Second, a smaller diaphragmatic injury may produce intestinal obstruction, like any other internal hernia. This is not common in the acute injury, although it is the usual mode of presentation of chronic diaphragmatic injury. This injury requires no particular pre-hospital treatment.

Emergency Department Treatment

The major problem is diagnosis. Large injuries are usually seen on the chest film. A major pitfall can be the tendency to read the chest film as "pleural fluid" or "atelectasis." These large injuries are usually produced by blunt trauma and are most often on the left side. The right side is protected by the liver, but if a right-sided injury is present, the film may show only a "high diaphragm." Thus it is possible to miss a large diaphragmatic injury.

A small diaphragmatic injury produced by penetrating trauma may be difficult to diagnose radiologically. Usually the only sign is fluid in the chest, and because the penetrating wound in these cases is usually in the lower chest, that fluid is usually diagnosed as ordinary hemothorax.

The diagnostic test of choice, assuming that the chest film fails to show the diagnosis, is peritoneal lavage, whereby the diagnosis is made in one of two ways.

First, the fluid may run up into the chest and be irretrievable. This may occur with either large or small injuries, but is more common and noticeable in large injuries. A post-lavage film confirms the presence of fluid in the chest.

Second, there may be small amounts of blood in the lavage return. My usual criteria mandate exploration for over 100,000 RBC per milliliter and strongly indicate exploration for 50,000 to 100,000. However, if a penetrating wound is near the costal margin, I would consider 5,000 RBC per milliliter to be ample indication for exploration. With an extremely liberal exploration policy, one can avoid missing diaphragmatic injuries.

The use of contrast studies is rarely indicated. Barium swallow or barium enema can be used to identify intrathoracic viscera. This is more strongly indicated if a chronic lesion is suspected. An "abdominogram," whereby contrast material is instilled into the abdomen in the hope of demonstrating passage into the thorax, is not very sensitive and is probably not worth doing.

More sophisticated studies, such as CT scanning, are not useful for the acute lesion. Identification of a puzzling intrathoracic mass as intrathoracic viscera may be done with the CT scanner. However, a barium enema is usually more effective.

Therapy is surgical in all cases. Because of the danger of late development of obstruction (to be discussed), surgical exploration is always indicated. There is rarely any reason to delay. Furthermore, if the diaphragm is injured, there may be other injuries requiring intervention. A chest tube is necessary because of the dangers of positive pressure anesthesia in the presence of possible lung injury. Whether the injury is transabdominal or transthoracic, the lung is likely to be injured.

Chronic Diaphragmatic Hernia

The patient may present with an asymptomatic mass above the diaphragm, which is thought to be viscera herniating through an old injury to the diaphragm. The diagnosis and management of asymptomatic masses is not usually an emergency medical problem.

The more dangerous presentation is intestinal obstruction. Because the hernia is typically small, strangulation obstruction is usual. The patient may be extremely ill, even in shock. The abdomen is distended, the patient vomits all he eats, and there may be dehydration, electrolyte disorders, and alkalosis. The chest film may show the herniated bowel or may show the same sort of nonspecific fluid or "high diaphragm" seen in the acute injury. A careful history may point to an old injury, perhaps years before. Any scars found near the costal margin, front or back, should be explained by the patient. If one of these is from an old knife wound that was treated without exploration, the presumptive diagnosis can be made, even without chest roentgenographic findings. If time permits, barium studies may be helpful. Barium enema is usually best, as the colon is involved in most cases.

Therapy for chronic diaphragmatic hernia from an old injury is always surgical. The situation is urgent if obstruction is present because of the danger of strangulation of the bowel.

SUGGESTED READING

Arendrup HC, Jensen BS. Traumatic rupture of the diaphragm. Surg Gynecol Obstet 1982; 154: 526–530.

Bajee A, Schepps D, Hurley EJ. Diaphragmatic injuries. Surg Gynecol Obstet 1981; 153: 31–32.

De la Rocha AG, Creel RJ, Mulligan GW, Burns CM. Diaphragmatic rupture due to blunt abdominal trauma. Surg Gynecol Obstet 1982; 154:175–180.

Waldschmidt ML, Laws HL. Injuries of the diaphragm. Trauma 1980; 20:587–592.

Williams RS. Traumatic rupture of the diaphragm. Med J Aust 1982; 1:208–211.

PENETRATING CARDIAC TRAUMA

JEFFREY P. GOLD, M.D.
LAWRENCE DURBAN, M.D.
KARL H. KRIEGER, M.D.
O. WAYNE ISOM, M.D.

DIAGNOSIS

The initial manifestations of penetrating cardiac trauma depend on the mode, site, and size of the injury as well as the state of the pericardial space at the time the patient is evaluated. Between 60 and 80 percent of all patients who sustain penetrating transmural cardiac injury, with or without associated injuries, die shortly after the injury from massive cardiac tamponade or from uncontrolled bleeding. Rapid recognition of patients in this group, exact diagnosis, and early effective intervention are essential to attempts to reduce this extremely high mortality.

In multiple reviews, stab wounds account for approximately 60 percent of all of the penetrating cardiac wounds; gunshot wounds account for the remainder. Approximately 75 percent of these wounds tend to be single. As with most other studies on trauma, the patient population tends to be overwhelmingly male with a mean age in the early thirties.

The relative frequency of the location of these wounds correlates directly with their respective area of exposure on the anterior chest wall. Therefore, the right ventricle is the site of penetration in 50 percent of most published series. Stab wounds tend to involve a single cardiac structure, whereas high-velocity missile wounds frequently involve more than one intracardiac structure at the time of injury. Well over 95 percent of penetrating cardiac wounds demonstrate a point of entry located between the midclavicular lines, below the clavicles, and above the xiphoid process of the sternum. As can be seen in Figure 1, the right ventricle is the chamber most commonly injured—followed in order of frequency by the left ventricle, the pulmonary arteries, and the right atrium—in these combined series of stab wound patients.

In a series of patients with gunshot wounds, the left ventricle was the most common chamber injured, four times more frequently than the next most common chamber involved, which was the right ventricle. This in part accounts for the much higher overall mortality from this group of injuries.

Early recognition of presenting signs and symptoms is important in this challenging group of patients. Eighty-five percent of such patients have a clearly demonstrable mediastinal entrance wound. Sixty to 70 percent also present with clear-cut signs of tamponade, which include a high central venous pressure, low arterial pressure, and distant heart sounds. Thirty-five percent of these patients present with profound hypotension as the sole feature; a significant percentage have no obtainable blood pressure on admission to the emergency department. There may or may not be significant chest tube drainage at the time of placement of an indwelling tube. Only 20 percent of such patients have chest tube drainage in excess of 500 ml, an important point. These diagnostic features are summarized in Figure 2.

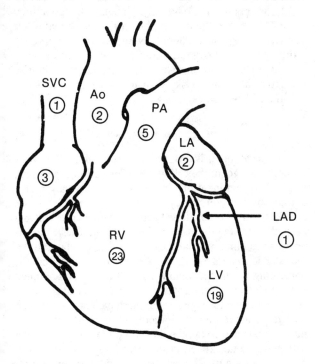

Figure 1 Regions of the heart most commonly injured in a series of 56 penetrating injuries. (SVC=superior vena cava; Ao=aorta; PA=pulmonary artery; LA=left atrium; LAD=left anterior descending; RV=right ventricle; LV=left ventricle.)

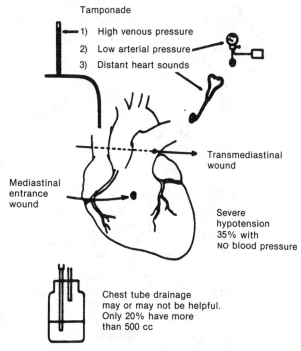

Figure 2 Clinical features of penetrating cardiac trauma at presentation.

PRINCIPLES OF INITIAL MANAGEMENT

As shown in Figure 3, the initial management consists of four basic steps once the appropriate diagnosis has been made. The volume losses are replaced with balanced salt solution and blood as necessary. The pericardial tamponade is relieved, the hemorrhage is controlled, and the injury repaired. Initially, intravenous access with large-bore lines should be established peripherally both above and below the diaphragm while assessment for multi-systemic injury is under way. Centrally placed subclavian vein or internal jugular vein lines should be avoided when possible as mediastinal anatomy may be greatly distorted, thereby increasing the risk of line-related complications. The placement of one or more tube thoracostomies may be indicated as well as a pericardiocentesis if there is any suspicion of pericardial tamponade. All patients should undergo immediate typing and crossmatching for large quantities (6 to 10 units) of blood. The cardiothoracic surgeon should be called immediately, even if the patient appears stable and cardiac injury has not yet been confirmed.

Pericardial tamponade—suggested by arterial hypotension, elevated central venous pressure, decreased heart sounds, agitation, air hunger, distended neck veins, paradoxical pulse, Kusmaul's sign, and others—increases the likelihood of a penetrating cardiac injury and should encourage the physician to perform an emergent pericardiocentesis. The aspiration of nonclotting blood is diagnostic; however, clotting blood does not rule out tamponade and may only indicate the rapidity of the bleeding. A negative pericardiocentesis does not rule out a significant cardiac wound. Aspiration of only small amounts of pericardial fluid can produce dramatic changes in cardiac function, only to later reaccumulate and cause a marked depression of cardiac output and all of the metabolic consequences attendant. Pericardiocentesis is itself truly diagnostic and only transiently therapeutic. However, the temporizing benefit should allow transfer of the patient to the operating theater for definitive therapy under more stable conditions.

The approach to pericardial decompression in the emergency department can consist of a subxiphoid pericardiocentesis, a subxiphoid pericardial window, a transdiaphragmatic pericardial window, or, more commonly, an emergent left anterolateral thoracotomy, which allows the physician to both decompress the pericardial tamponade and directly assess and address the cause of the hemorrhage.

Routine chest roentgenograms, chest fluoroscopy, electrocardiography, nuclear scans, and echocardiography may be of some value, but in the acutely ill unstable patient, these imaging tests are of little immediate utility. The time invested in these tests may actually adversely affect the outcome as it may prevent or delay immediate definitive therapy. The use of basic physical examination skills is much more rapid, and may be even more rewarding than any or all of the aforementioned studies.

Patients in whom a knife blade was the wounding agent, patients with single injuries particularly of the right ventricle or atrium, patients who are alert on admission with obtainable blood pressure, and patients who do not require thoracotomy in the emergency department comprise the group that is at lowest risk and in which the best results are obtained. Conversely, patients who are injured with a shotgun, patients with biventricular or major left ventricular injuries, patients who require emergency thoracotomy, and patients with severe hypotension or no obtainable blood pressure on admission clearly comprise the group at highest risk, with mortality rates between 65 and 100 percent.

SURGICAL MANAGEMENT

Surgical repair is ordinarily carried out by the cardiothoracic surgeon; the following information is pertinent only when imminent death forces an emergency thoracotomy by the emergency physician.

The patient is positioned and then widely prepped and draped, exposing the base of the neck, the chest, the anterior abdominal wall, and the upper thighs bilaterally in the sterile operative field. Access to the thighs for harvesting a venous conduit as well as to the abdomen for control of the intra-abdominal vena cava and aorta can be crucial in the management of these patients. A left submammary anterolateral thoracotomy is most commonly made, entering through the fourth intracostal space. If the patient has demonstrated sufficient stability, a median sternotomy incision may be preferable under certain circumstances (Fig. 4).

The interpericardial clot is immediately evacuated, allowing for subsequent control of the bleeding site by placement of a balloon-tipped catheter within the cardiac

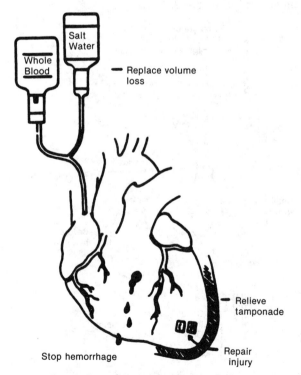

Figure 3 The principles and sequence of initial management of penetrating injuries of the myocardium.

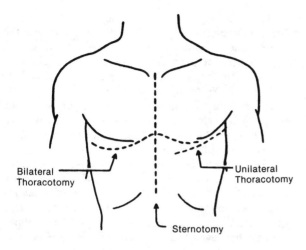

Figure 4 The most commonly employed surgical approaches to the mediastinal structures for management of penetrating injuries.

chamber or by placement of a finger or a partially occluding vascular clamp. At this time, the heart is allowed to regain normal action and the circulatory volume is repleted as necessary before any attempts are made to directly repair the cardiac wound. The anterior surfaces of the heart can be carefully inspected during this period. One should also look for associated injuries, in addition to posterior bleeding points, palpable thrills in any of the cardiac chambers, obvious congenital anomalies, or calcifications along the coronary arteries that can be appreciated and noted.

The majority of penetrating cardiac wounds can be closed by primary intention, with or without pledgeted sutures (Fig. 5). Multiple techniques such as sewing under one's finger, employing figure-of-eight stitches, or sewing underneath a partially occluding clamp with these permanent sutures have been utilized as well. Injuries of the myocardium in the immediate vicinity of the coronary arteries can be managed by placing relatively deep horizontal mattress sutures beneath the coronary vessel, thereby preventing occlusion of this vessel and simultaneously closing the wound.

Techniques such as cardiopulmonary bypass and inflow occlusion are rarely necessary to treat these patients. However, in the event the lesion cannot be primarily managed in the beating heart, or if an associated intracardiac lesion has been created, pump standby is sometimes useful. Should an intracardiac lesion be discovered at the time of emergent exploration for penetrating cardiac injury, this should be left, under most circumstances, for later evaluation and repair unless the magnitude of the deficit is such that the patient would most likely not survive.

Follow-up cardiac evaluation including catheterization and echocardiography can be performed in the immediate postinjury period in those patients with suspected intracardiac injuries with or without significant hemodynamic deficits. At a later time, reexploration with cardiopulmonary bypass under optimal conditions for valve replacement and/or reconstruction and closure of

septal defects can be done with much lower morbidity and mortality.

Direct injuries of the coronary arteries occur in 4 to 5 percent of all patients who experience penetrating cardiac trauma. The anterior descending is the coronary artery most frequently damaged, the right coronary artery ranking second in frequency. The circumflex artery is only rarely injured because of its deeply hidden posterior location and the high immediate mortality of patients sustaining injuries in this area. These vessels can be repaired, bypassed, grafted, or ligated, depending on the location and the nature of their injury.

RESULTS

The overall mortality of penetrating cardiac injuries varies directly with the mode of injury and the number of chambers that have been injured. Wounds of the right atrium alone carry only a 10 to 15 percent mortality in most series. Simple right ventricular wounds or left atrial wounds carry a mortality of 20 to 25 percent. Combined wounds of the ventricles or major wounds of the left ventricle are associated with mortality in excess of 50 to 70 percent.

The results in multiple series treated by immediate emergency department thoracotomy and cardiorrhaphy in patients sustaining penetrating cardiac injuries as their sole significant injury have varied over the last 10 years. The reported survival rates have varied from 0 to 100 percent. Most recent series are reporting overall survival in excess of 35 percent in this particular setting, with the best results in centers equipped for rapid intervention. This particular group of patients appear to have the strongest indications for this type of therapy. In almost all large studies, gunshot wounds carry a significantly higher mortality than do simple stab wounds, and close range shotgun wounds carry a near 100 percent mortality.

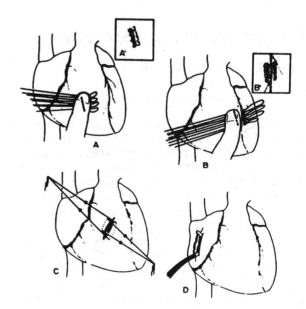

Figure 5 Four frequently used techniques for repair of penetrating myocardial injuries.

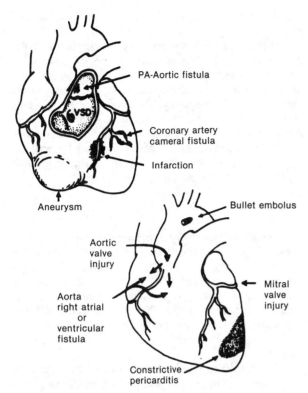

Figure 6 Some of the late sequelae of penetrating injuries of the heart and great vessels.

LATE SEQUELAE OF PENETRATING CARDIAC INJURIES

As is depicted in Figure 6, there are multiple potential late sequelae of penetrating cardiac injuries that may or may not be appreciated or anticipated at the time of initial exploration or hospital discharge. These include the development of a pulmonary-artery-to-aorta fistula, a coronary-artery-to-ventricle or -atrium fistula, a myocardial infarction, a ventricular or atrial septal defect, a true or pseudo-aneurysm of either ventricle or great vessel, an injury of the atrioventricular or semilunar valves, postpericardotomy syndrome, constrictive pericarditis, embolization of the projectile, and mural thrombosis with later embolization. Projectiles that are in the heart should therefore be removed if at all possible at the time of initial exploration. If they are subsequently found to protrude into the cardiac chambers, later re-exploration and removal employing cardiopulmonary bypass techniques are suggested to prevent late embolization and the development of bacterial endocarditis. This large group of unusual but relatively serious sequelae should form the basis for careful and long-term follow-up of these patients following their hospital discharge.

SUGGESTED READING

Evans J, Gray L, Rayner A, Fulton R. Principles for management of penetrating cardiac wounds. Ann Surg 1979; 189:777–784.

Ivatury R, Shah P, Ito K, et al. Emergency room thoracotomy for the rescuscitation of patients with "fatal" penetrating injuries of the heart. Ann of Thorac Surg 1981; 32:377–385.

Robbs J, Baker L. Cardiovascular trauma. Curr Probl Surg 1984; 21:1–87.

Symbas P. Traumatic heart disease. Curr Probl Cardiol 1982; 7:7–35.

Taveras S, Hankins J, Moulton A, et al. Management of penetrating cardiac injuries: the role of emergency room thoracotomy. Ann Thorac Surg 1984; 38:183–187.

MYOCARDIAL CONTUSION

MELVIN D. CHEITLIN, M.D., F.A.C.C.,

PROBLEMS OF DIAGNOSIS

Studies report an incidence of myocardial contusion after major thoracoabdominal trauma that varies from 9 to 76 percent. The variation in the frequency is attributable to the different criteria used in making the diagnosis. Pathologically, myocardial contusion occurs when there is injury to the myocardial muscle, usually by nonpenetrating trauma, resulting in bleeding, muscle injury, and myocardial cell death. The signs and symptoms of myocardial contusion are therefore related to myocardial dysfunction. Visceral-type chest discomfort similar to that of myocardial ischemia, orthopnea, shortness of breath at rest or with effort, and symptoms of low cardiac output, such as easy fatigability, should all suggest myocardial dysfunction. Signs such as tachycardia, an S_3 gallop, pulsus alternans, the murmur of mitral or tricuspid insufficiency, rales, elevated systemic venous pressure, hepatomegaly, and peripheral edema are all consistent with myocardial dysfunction.

Arrhythmias, both atrial and ventricular brady- and tachyarrhythmias, and AV block and intraventricular block or bundle branch block can occur as a result of myocardial contusion. Electrocardiographic evidence of myocardial damage can vary from simply nonspecific S-T and T wave changes to prolonged Q-T interval to evidence of myocardial injury with S-T segment elevation and/or Q wave development. Evidence of myocardial necrosis, especially the release of enzymes relatively specific for myocardial necrosis (such as the fast fraction of LDH or the MB fraction of creatine kinase), is considered to be specific for myocardial contusion.

Evidence of abnormal wall motion by 2-D echocardiography and radioisotope wall motion studies with measurement of ejection fraction have been used as more sensitive evidence of myocardial contusion. Finally, myocardial necrosis has been identified by radioisotope techniques using technetium-99 pyrophosphate scanning.

The problem with these myriad techniques for detecting myocardial damage and/or dysfunction is that they are all nonspecific for myocardial contusion. Pre-existing heart disease, such as coronary heart disease, can be aggravated by the excitement and effects of the trauma and result in acute myocardial infarction mimicking a myocardial contusion. Extensive skeletal muscle injury or small bowel injury can release significant amounts of MB-CK, and nonspecific S-T and T wave changes and arrhythmias can be the result of multiple factors other than myocardial contusion such as hypoxia, hyperventilation, sympathetic or vagal stimulation, hypotension with blood loss, acidosis with hypercarbia, central nervous system trauma, and electrolyte abnormalities.

When arrhythmias and ECG changes are considered diagnostic of myocardial contusion, the incidence is high. Using more specific markers, such as CK-MB release and pyrophosphate scanning, the incidence is much lower. Studies using the only "gold standard" we have, that of gross and microscopic examination of the heart, are difficult to carry out. The most significant report is that of Potkin et al, who comprehensively studied 100 consecutive patients after severe thoracoabdominal nonpenetrating trauma. CK-MB enzyme elevation occurred in 72 percent, ECG abnormalities in 70 percent, and 27 percent had grade III to V Lown arrhythmias. Clinically important cardiac damage did not occur in these patients. At autopsy on all 15 patients who died, it was found that none died of cardiac trauma; five had myocardial contusion, and ten did not.

The numbers were too small to permit firm conclusions to be drawn; however, there were no significant differences in the frequency of cardiac arrhythmias, ECG abnormalities, release of serum CK-MB, or pyrophosphate abnormalities between those with and those without myocardial contusion at autopsy.

DIAGNOSTIC APPROACH

Given the foregoing limitations, my present approach to the treatment of myocardial contusion rests on (1) the suspicion that myocardial contusion could have occurred and (2) evidence that myocardial injury or dysfunction is present. Thus, anyone involved in a thoracic compression injury or in a sudden deceleration accident, such as a fall, is suspect. Myocardial contusion is especially frequent in patients with multiple rib fractures and multisystem trauma.

Chest discomfort may be attributable to musculoskeletal and chest wall pain. If the discomfort is visceral and is not affected by breathing, by the position of the arms or body, or by compression of the chest wall, myocardial contusion should be suspected. In older patients who develop angina or myocardial infarction, the possibility of myocardial infarction or ischemia from preexisting coronary disease is greater.

Since the possible consequences of the myocardial contusion are serious, the possibility of myocardial contusion is an indication for hospitalization, if possible in an electrocardiographically monitored bed. This is especially important if the patient has ventricular arrhythmias or evidence of acute myocardial infarction. The presence of rales, especially if there is an S_3 gallop, suggests the possibility of extensive myocardial dysfunction. The presence of a murmur of mitral or tricuspid insufficiency, especially if the murmur is new, suggests the possibility of myocardial contusion. A pericardial friction rub or increased cervical venous pulse should suggest pericardial tamponade with myocardial laceration, and if the blood pressure is normal, an echocardiogram should be obtained immediately. If the patient is in shock without obvious blood loss and the cervical venous pressure is increased, especially with penetrating trauma, thoracotomy should be performed immediately. If the patient is stable, pericardiocentesis should be performed. If the patient is hemodynamically unstable, pericardiocentesis can be attempted first, but thoracotomy should be done as soon as possible, in the emergency department if the patient is in profound shock.

More commonly, the patient may be hemodynamically stable but have signs of congestive heart failure: rales, S_3 gallop, and pulsus alternans. The chest film may show pulmonary congestion, but this is not specific since many patients have pulmonary contusion. An elevated venous pressure with or without a right-sided S_3 gallop and clear lung fields can be seen with right ventricular contusion.

An electrocardiogram should be obtained, and although no finding is pathognomonic of myocardial contusion, in young patients elevation of S-T segments, inversion of T waves, or development of acute myocardial infarction with Q waves is nearly pathognomonic. In older patients, precipitation of an acute myocardial infarction in a patient with coronary disease is just as likely as myocardial contusion and is more likely than coronary thrombosis in an otherwise normal coronary artery.

TREATMENT OF SYMPTOMS

Any serious arrhythmias, such as ventricular tachycardia with hemodynamic instability or ventricular fibrillation, must be immediately treated with CPR and cardioversion. With conversion to sinus rhythm, lidocaine, 75 mg or 1 mg per kilogram stat IV and a repeat dose of 50 mg IV in 5 minutes, followed by a 1 to 4 mg per minute infusion should be given to pervent recurrent ventricular tachycardia. If lidocaine fails, procainamide, 20 mg per minute up to 1 g, or bretylium (5 mg per kilogram IV over 10 minutes followed by constant infusion of 1 to 2 mg per minute) should be given. With less serious arrhythmias such as atrial tachycardia, atrial flutter, and atrial fibrillation, an effort should be made to treat with a drug in order to convert to normal sinus rhythm or to slow the ventricular response. Such drugs as verapamil, 5 to 10 mg over a 1 minute period IV can convert atrial tachycardia to normal sinus rhythm. Beta-blocking drugs such as propranolol, 1 mg IV to a total of as much as 0.1 mg per kilogram IV, if heart failure is not present, or the calcium-channel blocker verapamil, 5 to 10 mg IV over a minute period, can slow the ventricular response. If the patient is unstable with these atrial arrhythmias, cardioversion should be done without delay. (See also other chapters on individual arrhythmias.)

For premature atrial contractions or premature ventricular contraction that are not causing hemodynamic problems, correctable causes such as hypoxia, hypo- or hyperkalemia, metabolic or respiratory acidosis or alkalosis, or other electrolyte imbalance should be addressed. If there is no obvious explanation for the ectopy, we do not treat PACs or occasional PVCs. Frequent PVCs and bigeminy or trigeminy, multiform PVCs, and PVCs that are early (R-on-T PVCs) are suppressed by lidocaine. If they persist, the patient is then converted to oral quinidine therapy, at least during his hospitalization and for the first week after possible myocardial contusion.

With first-degree AV block and second-degree AV block of the Wenckebach variety, observation is all that is needed unless there is a drop in blood pressure or multiple dropped ventricular beats. If atropine is not successful in increasing the ventricular response, a temporary pacemaker can be placed. If the patient has third-degree atrioventricular block, especially if the QRS is wide, placement of a temporary pacemaker on an emergent basis is required. Bundle branch block of any degree is observed closely for the possible development of Mobitz II AV block or complete heart block, which then requires a pacemaker.

In the presence of S-T and T wave changes, the patient is observed and CK-MB enzymes are drawn immediately, at 6 hours, at 12 hours, and at 24 hours after the injury. I find it valuable to obtain a 2-D echocardiogram to evaluate ventricular contraction for wall motion abnormalities, which must be interpreted in light of the patient's past history of cardiac disease, age, and the presence of other risk factors for coronary artery disease.

If the patient has signs of possible heart failure, I obtain, in addition to an echocardiogram, a radioisotope wall motion study with ejection fraction. At times an adequate echocardiogram cannot be obtained because of bandages, injury to the chest wall, pre-existing pulmonary emphysema, and inability to rotate the patient. Since the right ventricle is anterior, myocardial contusion of the right ventricular wall is more common than that of the left ventricular wall. In 77 patients with multi-system trauma studied by Sutherland et al by cardiac scintigraphy, 42 patients (53 percent) had focal abnormalities of wall motion; 27 involved the right ventricle, 17 the left ventricle, seven were biventricular, and one involved only the septum. With right ventricular contusion, the central venous pressure may be elevated and the pulmonary artery wedge pressure may be normal. In these cases, a radioisotope study is of great help since it will be obvious that the right ventricle is functioning poorly while the left ventricle is normal.

If there is any question of congestive heart failure, a Swan-Ganz catheterization with monitoring of the pulmonary artery diastolic pressure and wedge pressure and cardiac output is most valuable. This is especially important when large volumes of intravenous fluids or blood are to be given since a contused myocardium may handle excess volume load with marked increase in left ventricular filling pressure and pulmonary capillary pressure, thus causing pulmonary edema.

COMPLICATIONS

The complications of myocardial contusion are generally those of myocardial infarction: arrhythmias, rupture of necrotic myocardium, formation of either false or true ventricular aneurysm, development of intraventricular thrombus and embolism, and myocardial dysfunction and congestive heart failure. The management of these complications is similar to that of myocardial infarction caused by coronary artery disease, and the time course of recovery is also similar. The major difference is that the ultimate prognosis of the patient recovering from myocardial contusion is far more favorable than that of the patient who has had an acute myocardial infarction with coronary disease. For the most part, patients with myocardial contusion are younger, and have an entirely normal coronary tree before injury; therefore, the only problem is that part of the myocardium is not functioning. The remaining myocardium is normal and not in jeopardy from advancing coronary disease.

Myocardial necrosis can result in rupture of the myocardium from 3 days to the beginning of the second week after injury. If the rupture occurs into the pericardium, cardiac tamponade results and is usually fatal. In rare instances the rupture is limited by the epicardium or by the pericardium that is adherent to the epicardium, creating a false aneurysm. This may cause a bulge of the cardiac silhouette to be visible on the chest film. It can also be found by 2-D echocardiogram and radioisotope wall motion study. Once suspected, it should be studied angiographically and repaired since late rupture is common.

If the entire wall is infarcted and becomes aneurysmal, late rupture is rare, but ventricular arrhythmias and even congestive heart failure can be seen. Ventricular aneurysms may develop mural clots, and if embolization occurs or clot is seen by 2-D echocardiography, anticoagulation for a period of 3 months is recommended. If there are no complications with the true ventricular aneurysm, no specific treatment is necessary.

Thrombosis and thromboembolism can occur with or without the development of ventricular aneurysm and can affect the right and left atria and ventricles. Since injuries to the pelvis and legs are common, venous thrombosis and embolization can occur. If atrial fibrillation occurs, thrombosis can result in left or right atrial thrombus and embolization. If embolization occurs and the danger of bleeding from other injuries is minimal, anticoagulation should be instituted and continued for 3 weeks to 3 months after injury. The heparin can be started followed by coumadin for chronic anticoagulation.

If the patient ruptures the ventricular septum, a pansystolic murmur along the left sternal border or at the apex might result with evidence of left (with or without right) ventricular failure. If the papillary muscle is necrotic and ruptures, severe mitral insufficiency can result with a typical apical systolic murmur and severe pulmonary congestion with or without right heart failure. To differentiate these two complications, echocardiogram with contrast injection can show the abnormal left-to-right shunt and its location in the septum. Catheterization gives definitive evidence for the differential diagnosis by demonstrating left-to-right shunt in the presence of a ventricular septal defect, and the absence of shunt in the presence of a large pulmonary artery wedge "V" wave with acute mitral insufficiency.

If tricuspid insufficiency has resulted, there is evidence of right heart failure with increased cervical venous pressure, hepatomegaly, and eventually peripheral edema, ascites, and pleural effusion. Pathognomonic findings of right ventricular injury on catheterization, 2-D echocardiography and radioisotope studies include a small noninvolved left ventricle, small left atrium, a large hypocontractile right ventricle, large right atrium, a normal or decreased cardiac output, and a high right ventricular filling pressure. Doppler echocardiography is useful in finding and quantifying degrees of tricuspid or mitral insufficiency, although experience with the technique in cases of trauma is limited.

Finally, myocardial contusion in the patient who has congestive heart failure is treated with digoxin and diuretics. If there is no response to this treatment, afterload reduction with preload and afterload drugs is attempted; nitroprusside is given if the arterial pressure is normal or elevated. If chronic oral therapy is necessary, captopril, starting at 6.25 mg 3 times a day increasing to as much as 25 mg 3 times a day can be given. On rare occasions in the acute management of myocardial contusion with severe congestive heart failure, intra-aortic balloon counterpulsation has been lifesaving.

SUGGESTED READING

King RM, Mucha P Jr., Seward JB, Gersh BJ, Farnell MB. Cardiac contusion: a new diagnostic approach utilizing two-dimensional echocardiography. J Trauma 1983; 23:610–614.

Orlando R III, Drezues AD. Intra-aortic balloon counterpulsation in blunt cardiac injury. J Trauma 1983; 23:424–427.

Simon TR, Parkey RW, Lewis SE. Role of cardiovascular nuclear medicine in evaluating trauma and the postoperative patient. Semin Nucl Med 1983; 13:123–141.

Sutherland GR, Driedoer AA, Holliday RL, Cheung W, Sibbald WJ. Frequency of myocardical injury after blunt chest trauma as evaluated by radionuclide angiography. Am J Cardiol 1983; 52:1099–1103.

BLUNT AND PENETRATING GREAT VESSEL TRAUMA

NORMAN E. McSWAIN Jr., M.D., F.A.C.S.

Successful identification of vascular trauma is frequently done emergently by indirect methods of evaluation. Direct evidence, such as severe bleeding externally, absence of distal pulses, or pallor of an extremity, may not exist. However, its absence does not rule out these injuries. Indirect methods must include the detailed history of the injury process and an understanding of the mechanisms of injuries (kinematics) and of the potential structural damage that can occur. As in other illnesses, 90 percent of the diagnosis of trauma is history itself. The physician who neglects to take an adequate history or does not understand the significance of such a history may well miss injuries that, if picked up early, would significantly decrease the morbidity and mortality suffered by the patient.

KINEMATICS OF INJURY

Blunt Trauma

The mechanisms of injury in blunt trauma can be classified as either deceleration or compression.

Deceleration injuries occur as the body stops its motion and the vessel or the organ continues, until that motion is arrested by the vessel attached to the posterior abdominal wall. The shear forces across the point of a strong attachment adjacent to the point of weak attachments dictate both the location and the type of injury to be expected. In a head-on crash, the car stops its forward motion, the unrestrained occupant does not. The occupant continues forward (unless seat-belted) to crash into the frontal part of the passenger compartment. Inside the patient's body the same condition occurs. Although the body stops as it comes to an abrupt halt against the forward part of the passenger compartment, the organ continues in a forward motion, and at the same speed as the occupant (and the car) was traveling prior to the crash. This may produce an organ-body differential speed of 30 to 40 miles per hour. Since energy can be neither created nor destroyed, this forward motion must be absorbed in stretching or tearing of tissue.

The most frequently discussed such injury is deceleration of the thoracic aorta. The descending thoracic aorta, from approximately the point of the ligamentum arteriosum caudad, is firmly attached to the vertebral column. The arch of the aorta and the heart itself are fairly loosely suspended organs, and as the body and the attached descending thoracic aorta come to an abrupt halt, the arch and heart continue to move forward. The vessel shears just distal to the ligamentum arteriosum. Parmley's studies show that 80 percent of these patients exsanguinate in the first hour, another 6 percent in the first 6 hours, another 6 percent in 24 hours, and the remaining group survive up to 72 hours or longer. Only if the physician recognizes this potential, obtains appropriate studies, and treats the patient in a trauma center, can that 20 percent survive longer than the first hour.

Deceleration injuries to the *renal vessels* are further examples of the results of blunt trauma. The abdominal aorta, just like the descending thoracic aorta, is fairly tightly attached to the vertebral column; the kidney is not. As the body stops its forward motion, the kidney continues to move forward at the same speed as the automobile prior to impact, stopping only when constrained by the renal vascular pedicle. Stretch forces along this pedicle tear it free from the aorta, avulse it from the hilum, or stretch it along its length to the point of intimal damage, which will produce turbulence and clot formation.

Compression injuries can affect a vessel that is compressed between a hard external force, such as the steering column, and the continued moving vertebral column or a vessel that is stretched across a dislocated joint or fracture site where it is tightly adhered to the bone surrounding the point of injury. An example of the former is the typical ski-rope compression of the brachial artery against the shaft of the humerus. An example of the latter is popliteal artery damage that occurs with posterior dislocation of the knee produced as the tibia hits the dash in a frontal collision. The continued forward motion of the femur produces a posterior dislocation. The popliteal artery is tightly adhered to the femur above the knee and to the tibia below the knee by fascia as well as circumflex collateral arterial attachments. The forceful stretching of the artery across the proximal tibial surface produces an intimal disruption. This usually produces acute arterial obstruction; however, the onset of symptoms can be delayed 96 or more hours.

The astute examiner does not assume that the presence of pulses in such an injury indicates no vascular damage, but relies on a mechanism of injury to dictate the need for arteriography.

Penetrating Trauma

A missile fired from a weapon or a sharp object penetrating the skin is driven by force that was dictated by its originating source (Table 1). Once this energy has been imparted to the missile (since energy can be neither created nor destroyed), it remains a part of that missile until some other force slows it down (Newton's first law of motion).

As the missile penetrates the body, each tissue particle that it hits is imparted some of this energy. This energy exchange forces the tissue directly away from the pathway of the missile. The distance that it travels away is proportional to the amount of energy given up by the penetrating object. The number of particles impacted and, therefore, the amount of energy exchanged from the missile to the tissue are relative to the frontal surface of the missile itself as it passes through. The amount of frontal surface is dictated by three factors: profile, tumble, and fragmentation. This energy exchange produces a temporary cavitation as the tissue particles move away from

TABLE 1 Velocities and Energies of Common Bullets (≥1,000 ft/sec Causes Cavitation; ≥2,500 ft/sec Produces High-Velocity Shock Waves in Tissue)

Weapon	Bullet Weight (grains)	Muzzle Velocity (ft/sec)	Muzzle Energy (ft-lbs)
Handguns			
32	71	863	91
45	230	850	370
45 Colt	250	860	410
38 Special	158	1,090	425
357 Magnum	158	1,415	695
44 Magnum	240	1,470	1,150
Rifles			
22 Remington	40	1,180	124
M-16	55	3,200	1,248
22 Swift	45	4,140	1,825
30-30 Winchester	170	2,200	1,830
303 British	215	2,160	2,230
Russian 7.62	150	2,810	2,635
M-14	180	2,610	2,720
M-1	172	2,700	2,785
8-mm Mauser	170	2,530	2,415
Mauser Mod 98	198	2,650	3,031
357 H and H Magnum	270	2,720	4,440

From Ordog GJ, Wasserberger J, and Balasubramaniums. Wound ballistics. Ann Emerg Med 1984; 13:1113–1122.

the pathway of the missile. When they reach the limit of this imparted energy, the negative pressure within the cavity pulls them back toward the direction from which they came. The deformation of the tissue and the amount of the temporary cavity that becomes a permanent cavity depend on the compression and stretch of the tissue from the temporary cavity, the resiliency of the tissue, and its ability to return to its former position. These characteristics vary from tissue to tissue. On one end of the spectrum are vascular and muscle tissues, which contain a lot of elastic fibers and tend to return uniformly to the previous position: at the other end of the spectrum is bone, which contains little elastic tissue and does not return at all to its previous position. An intermediate tissue is the liver, which fractures as it spreads. Surrounding organ pressure returns it to its original position, although damaged. *Vascular tissues* are among the more elastic tissues in the body so that the compression wave of a temporary cavity may occur in the vicinity of the vessel, stretch the vessel, and produce micro or macro intimal damage without disruption of the vessel, but the vessel returns to its usual position. The pulse and perfusion may remain intact for several hours until the intimal disruption produces clot formation.

The physician examining the patient must base the need for arteriography on factors other than simple presence or absence of a pulse distal to the point of penetration. This section is certainly not an exhaustive discussion of the mechanisms of injury; it only covers the highlights. The reader is referred to other texts for more in-depth surveys of this important topic (see *Suggested Reading* at end of chapter).

THERAPY

Pre-hospital Management

As in all major trauma, time is of the essence in the treatment of vascular injury. Hemorrhage must be controlled immediately. Pre-hospital management consists of control of hemorrhage by pressure, appropriate airway management, volume replacement while en route to the hospital, and transportation of the patient to a facility capable of operative management within 1 hour after the onset of trauma. In general, this means transportation of the patient to a level-one trauma center, when such is available.

When exsanguinating hemorrhage or excessive blood loss originates in a vessel that communicates to the outside, direct pressure on the point of penetrating damage to the vessel and replacement of loss with intravenous Ringer's lactate should be instituted.

When blood is being lost into a closed space, such as the abdominal cavity, the pneumatic antishock garment (PASG) can decrease the rate of blood loss while the patient is transported to a major trauma center. The PASG should remain in place while resuscitation is continued and the patient is transported to the operating room.

Fluid replacement is accomplished en route by intravenous administration of Ringer's lactate solution. Transportation should not be delayed to start the intravenous infusion; rather, the infusion should be started while the patient is en route to the hospital.

Acute obstructive vascular trauma, such as that associated with direct penetration of the vessel with absence of distal flow or compression damage associated with fractures or dislocations, is managed by stabilization of a fractured bone, using standard stabilization techniques, and transportation to the appropriate trauma center. Simple manipulation of the fractured bone may restore blood flow and should be attempted on site or as soon as possible en route to the hospital.

Time limitations are related to the ischemia sensitivity of the particular tissue involved. The sensitivity to oxygen deprivation of the brain is certainly different from that of the extremity. Sensitivity also varies depending on collateral circulation. The collateral circulation around the brachial artery is far greater than that of the femoral. There may even be a distal pulse in the upper extremity with total disruption of the brachial artery because of such collateral circulation.

Emergency Department Management

Therapy of vascular trauma in the emergency department consists of a continuation of the direct compression initiated in the pre-hospital phase, resuscitation of the patient with Ringer's lactate and whole blood to restore lost vascular volume, and reestablished perfusion of all tissues of the body, particularly the heart, brain, and lung. Appropriate diagnostic steps should be taken to identify the injury, and the patient moved rapidly to the operating room. Patients who are alive on arrival in the emergency department should not remain there long enough to die of continued blood loss.

Reestablishment of adequate perfusion is determined by the usual parameters of return of pulse and blood pressure to within normal limits, urinary output exceeding 50 cc per hour, and signs of adequate tissue perfusion. One of the best methods of estimating the latter is good capillary refill and a pink, warm, dry great toe or thumb. There is little other definitive treatment that can be provided to an injured vessel in the emergency department; repair of vascular damage is an operating room procedure. However, when the emergency physician is not astute and does not have a high enough index of suspicion, such injuries are missed, and the morbidity and mortality rate can be excessive. Therefore, one of the major obligations of the emergency physician is identification for the need of adequate diagnostic procedures, such as arteriography. The final decision lies with the operating surgeon. The risk of delay in obtaining such studies as compared to the benefits of immediate operative intervention and arteriography on the operating table are individual to each case.

DIAGNOSIS

Thoracic Trauma

In the thoracic cavity, decelerating injuries to the aorta from blunt trauma and injuries to the heart, aorta, or pulmonary vessels from penetrating trauma must be excluded. The common signs associated with deceleration injuries to the thoracic aorta must be sought on the chest film (Table 2). Some of these abnormalities are extremely subtle and may be missed on casual review of a chest film. If at all possible, a 72-inch posteroanterior film should be obtained, as some of these findings may be difficult to evaluate properly on a supine AP film.

Major penetrating vascular trauma is suspected when the wounds of entrance are on opposite sides of the chest, when the penetrating missile appears to have crossed the midline, when there is more than 1,000 cc of blood in the chest on initial insertion of the chest tube, or when continued blood loss is in excess of 200 cc per hour.

The significance of penetrating thoracic trauma can be more definitively evaluated by use of the thoracoscope, either to identify the extent of hemorrhage when there is some question of when it may have stopped or to answer

TABLE 2 Roentgenographic Indications of Aortic Disruption

Fracture of 1st and 2nd ribs
Widening of the mediastinum
Obliteration of the pulmonary aortic window
Deviation of the left main-stem bronchus downward greater than 140 degrees
Deviation of the esophagus to the right
Deviation of the trachea to the right
Left pulmonary cap
Blurred aortic knob

the question of diaphragmatic penetration. Both pericardial tamponade and tension pneumothorax are critical potential thoracic injuries that require rapid diagnosis and management.

Intercostal artery hemorrhage, identified by continued blood loss from the chest tube, is managed by thoracotomy. Use of a thoracoscope to visualize and cauterize the bleeding vessel may render a formal thoracotomy unnecessary, but the thoracoscopy must be done in the operating room where the anesthesiologist can manage the airway and the pneumothorax, the latter being a necessary component of the procedure.

Extreme intrathoracic hemorrhage or penetration of the heart with rapid development of pericardial tamponade should be managed in the emergency department with resuscitative thoracotomy as the initial step. It must be emphasized, however, that the opening of the chest and clamping of bleeding vessels or the decompression of the pericardial tamponade is only the first step in a complicated thoracic procedure. This should not be attempted if the operating room is not in readiness to accept the patient immediately and the trauma surgeon is not present to continue management immediately when the initial steps have been accomplished. When the operating team is at home (including the trauma surgeon) and the physician in the emergency department has not had extensive training in thoracotomies, including a rotation through thoracic surgery, such a procedure carries a 100 percent mortality rate and should not be attempted. It is not a procedure for the beginner or the uninitiated; it is only a procedure for the physician who is experienced in the total management of thoracic trauma. Anyone can open a chest with a knife. Only with experience can a physician manage the problems that are identified once the chest is opened.

Abdominal Trauma

The diagnosis of abdominal vascular trauma is identified by a distended, tense abdomen, hypotension, tachycardia, and other signs of hypovolemia and intra-abdominal hemorrhage. Less rapid intra-abdominal hemorrhage is identified by peritoneal lavage.

Most major vascular injury in the abdomen affects retroperitoneal vessels. Penetrating trauma usually produces an access of these vessels to the free peritoneal cavity, which is diagnosable using the standard abdominal physical examination techniques plus peritoneal lavage. Retroperitoneal vascular injury, either from blunt trauma or from flank or back penetration, is much more difficult to diagnose. Because it does not create an aperture into the peritoneal cavity, peritoneal lavage is ineffective. Frequently, the hemorrhage is contained in the retroperitoneal space, and therefore the patient does not become hypotensive immediately. The IVP is frequently a helpful diagnostic tool, demonstrating nonfunction of a kidney (renal pedicle injury), deviation of the uterus or kidney from normal position (retroperitoneal hematoma), or deviation of the bladder, even into a light-bulb shape (pelvic hematoma). The contrast medium for this procedure can be infused as an intravenous bolus at the time of initial fluid resuscitation, so that initial films reveal abnormalities of kidney function or anatomy.

Pneumatic antishock garment application with inflation of the abdominal segment is highly effective in reducing intra-abdominal bleeding, either from the pelvic vessels or from those in the retroperitoneal space. Other management maneuvers, except fluid resuscitation, are not useful in the emergency department; hemorrhage control and vascular repair must be done in the operating room.

Extremity Trauma

Trauma to the extremities can injure the vessels either directly from the trauma itself or indirectly as compression damage from injured bone. The close proximity of the bone to the vessels in many portions of the extremities increases the likelihood of vessel injury. In blunt trauma, the fractured bone may lacerate the vessel entirely or compress it to cause clot formation or produce enough impingement to cause intima damage.

The popliteal artery at the knee and the brachial artery at the elbow are in such tight proximity that dislocations of these joints, especially in the adult, should all be evaluated with arteriography before definitive treatment is given to the joint injury. Supracondylar fractures of the elbow are sometimes associated with intimal tears that lead to ischemia. Many Volkmann's contractures are secondary to actual arterial damage and are not associated with cast applications. Almost all knee dislocations produce popliteal artery compression or intimal damage.

Fragments of bone broken loose by penetrating trauma become missiles themselves and can produce the same type of damage as if the vessel had been hit by the missile itself.

The importance of taking a good history of the event and relating this information, through an understanding of kinematics, to the possible types of injuries which may exist, must again be stressed.

Arteriography should be obtained when there is question of vascular injury or when the location of such an injury may influence the surgical procedure. It should not be attempted in the case of extensive hemorrhage or an absent pulse, when the diagnosis is apparent.

Indications for arteriography include penetrations in the vicinity of a large vessel, neurologic damage, decreased perfusion, decreased pulses, or penetrating trauma producing a fracture, even without other evidence of vascular damage. In the case of blunt trauma, patients with dislocations of the knee and elbow, fractures with decreased distal pulses, or other signs of decreased perfusion should undergo immediate arteriography.

Even in the most efficient radiology department, arteriography requires at least an hour to complete. On the weekend or at night, when major trauma most frequently occurs, much more time is generally required. If the radiologist and the vascular laboratory technician are at home when notified and must travel to the hospital, 2 or 3 hours are required from notification until the procedure is complete. This prolongs the ischemia and decreased perfusion of the extremity. In many instances, this delay can make the difference between a viable and a nonviable extremity, or the need for fasciotomy. Since fasciotomy is not without morbidity, if it can be avoided by moving the patient rapidly to the operating room when the diagnosis is well established, arteriography should not be attempted.

Neck Trauma

The controversy surrounding mandatory exploration of all penetrations of the platysma is discussed in the chapter *Penetrating Neck Trauma*. Because of the distinct possibility of stirring up bleeding after blood has clotted, the neck wounds should not be explored or probed in the emergency department. Indications for exploration include an expanding hematoma, a missile that crosses the midline, and a central neurologic deficit. An experienced surgeon is needed immediately and therefore all such injuries should be managed in a major trauma center if possible.

SUGGESTED READING

Fackler M. Penetrating trauma. In: McSwain NE, Kerstein M, eds. Evaluation and management of trauma. East Norwalk CT: Appleton Century Crofts, 1986.
McSwain NE. Kinematics of blunt trauma. In: McSwain NE, Kerstein M, eds. Evaluation and management of trauma. East Norwalk CT: Appleton Century Crofts, 1986.

KIDNEY, URETER, AND BLADDER TRAUMA

JACK W. McANINCH, M.D.

Traumatic injuries to the genitourinary system occur in approximately 10 percent of patients who experience abdominal trauma. These injuries create diagnostic dilemmas for the physician who initially evaluates the patient in the emergency setting. Only by correct diagnostic procedures can appropriate therapy be selected for management that will prevent the serious and complex complications that may develop.

KIDNEYS

Renal injuries may be divided into two broad categories: blunt trauma, accounting for approximately 80 percent of injuries; and penetrating trauma, accounting for approximately 20 percent. In rural areas, the incidence of blunt trauma is higher. Stab and gunshot wounds represent the majority of penetrating renal injuries, whereas motor vehicle or pedestrian accidents and falls account for the majority of the blunt injuries.

The essentials of diagnosis begin with examination of an adequate urine specimen in the emergency department. Any resuscitative measures, proper airway management, and stabilization of life-threatening injuries should be done before evaluating the urinary tract. A voided urine can be obtained if the patient is capable; however, in many circumstances urethral catheterization is required to ob-

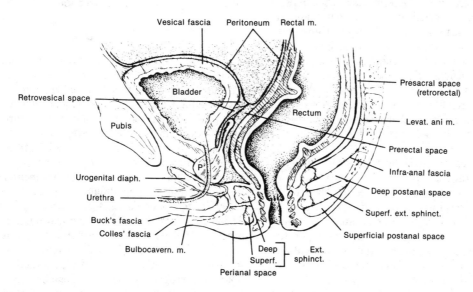

Figure 1 Anatomy of the pelvis. P = prostate gland. (From Pansky B, House EL. Review of gross anatomy. 3rd ed. New York: Macmillan 1975.

tain a specimen of diagnostic quality. The presence of gross or microscopic hematuria (>5 red blood cells per high-power field) is the best indicator of injury to the urinary system. In addition, one might suspect renal injury in the presence of lower rib fractures, flank contusions, upper abdominal tenderness, or evidence of entrance and exit wounds in the upper abdomen.

It should be emphasized that it is the presence of hematuria, not the degree, that is the most important consideration. Severity of injury does not always correlate reliably with degree of hematuria. For example, a finding of 10 to 20 red blood cells per high-power field in the urine of a patient who has sustained a rapid deceleration injury would be consistent with acute renal artery thrombosis. Gross hematuria, on the other hand, may be associated with a minor renal contusion.

The initial diagnostic study recommended in suspected renal injury with hematuria greater than 5 RBC per HPF is an excretory urogram (IVP). Although many patients with only microscopic hematuria have a normal IVP, significant injuries may be missed if all these patients are not so studied. When combined with nephrotomography, the IVP adequately stages 85 to 90 percent of renal injuries. The technique is important, since one of the common causes of diagnostic error is a study of poor quality. A high-dose contrast study should be done, with 2 ml per kilogram given as a rapid bolus injection. In patients with massive injuries, the contrast medium may be infused with the resuscitation fluids; the first plain roentgenogram of the abdomen then gives information regarding the presence of both kidneys, the location of the injury, and its extent.

In patients whose injuries are less acute, a more deliberate study should be done to gain maximal information. The IVP should show the presence of two kidneys with prompt, equal excretion; outline the parenchymal borders of the kidneys clearly; and demonstrate the renal collecting system of the pelvis and ureters well. When abnormal, indeterminate, or incomplete, and when poor renal visualization is present, additional studies are required to define the injury. At this point, urologic and surgical consultation should be obtained. Patients who are stable and in whom additional diagnostic studies are indicated should then undergo computed tomography (CT) to evaluate the extent of the renal injury. This study readily depicts renal lacerations, extravasation of opacified urine, and arterial injuries to the kidney. Arteriography also defines these injuries should CT not be available.

In the presence of persistent retroperitoneal bleeding, urinary extravasation, vascular injury, or large amounts of nonviable renal tissue, exploration and reconstruction of the kidney may be required. Surgery is necessary in less than 5 percent of cases of blunt renal injury and in approximately 75 to 80 percent of cases of penetrating injury. These decisions are based on defining the injury by good preoperative diagnostic studies and the clinical status of the patient.

Patients who have sustained mild blunt renal injury (contusion) and who have microscopic hematuria without associated injuries and a completely normal evaluation in the emergency department can be discharged and sent home. A follow-up visit should be arranged in about a week to ensure that hematuria has cleared and that secondary hypertension has not developed. Patients with gross hematuria after blunt trauma in whom diagnostic studies are normal should be hospitalized with bed rest until the gross hematuria clears. They may then be discharged with careful follow-up evaluation.

URETER

Stab and gunshot wounds are the most common causes of ureteral injuries seen in the emergency department. Blunt traumatic injuries are rare.

Any penetrating injury of the abdomen may be associated with complete or partial transection of the ureter. This is particularly true of stab wounds in the back and lower lumbar area and gunshot wounds that may demonstrate entrance or exit sites in these areas. Associated intra-abdominal injuries are present in 90 percent of these cases.

Suspicion of injury is the key to diagnosis. Hematuria is present in 90 percent of ureteral injuries, but in most cases it is microscopic. Even small degrees of hematuria (≥ 5 red blood cells per high-power field) warrant excretory urography for upper tract evaluation. A high-dose IVP (2 ml per kilogram contrast material) can demonstrate extravasation of opacified urine at the site of injury and establish a definite diagnosis. Small degrees of ureteral ectasia may be present proximal to the site of injury because of ureteral spasm. The ureter below the level of injury is seldom visualized.

These patients should be hemodynamically stabilized, and all associated injuries should be controlled and managed before the ureteral damage is corrected. Surgical consultation should be obtained once the IVP demonstrates the site of injury. All these patients should undergo surgical exploration and correction.

BLADDER

Trauma to the bladder occurs most commonly after blunt injury. However, bullet and knife wounds can penetrate the bladder, and this must be kept in mind when one is evaluating penetrating injuries. Approximately 10 percent of all patients who sustain pelvic fracture also have bladder or urethral rupture. Intraperitoneal bladder rupture is occasionally seen without pelvic fracture.

The clinical diagnosis of pelvic fracture can be established on the initial evaluation in the emergency department, and this finding should immediately remind the examiner that potential bladder or urethral injury exists. These patients have lower abdominal tenderness and at times generalized abdominal tenderness and rigidity. Most patients are unable to void; before catheterization, the urethral meatus should be carefully inspected. If blood is noted, urethrography should be done before catheterization. In the absence of blood, urethral catheterization can proceed, but if difficulty is encountered, the procedure must be stopped immediately and a urethrogram obtained. Gross hematuria is found in more than 95 percent of patients with bladder rupture after blunt trauma. At this point, urologic or surgical consultation is recommended before cystography is carried out.

Cystography is the best method of establishing the diagnosis of bladder rupture. The technique is important: incomplete bladder filling gives a false-negative result. Indeed, this is the most common diagnostic error. The bladder should be filled with 300 ml of contrast material; at the maximal point of filling, a plain, flat, abdominal roentgenogram should be obtained. After complete gravity drainage of the contrast material, a second plain, flat, abdominal roentgenogram should be obtained immediately. Oblique films and other views are unnecessary. The drainage film is important, since approximately 15 percent of such injuries can only be diagnosed on the drainage film. Approximately 60 percent of bladder ruptures are extraperitoneal, 30 percent intraperitoneal, and 10 percent combined. An IVP should be obtained in all patients to ascertain that concomitant renal injury has not occurred.

Bladder ruptures should be surgically corrected. In certain selected cases of extraperitoneal rupture, only catheter drainage may be necessary. However, this treatment mode must be chosen only after surgical consultation and careful assessment of the patient.

SUGGESTED READING

McAninch JW. Renal injuries. In: McAninch JW, ed. Trauma management. Vol. 2: Urogenital trauma. New York: Thieme-Stratton, 1985:27.

Carroll PR, McAninch JW. Major bladder trauma: mechanisms of injury and a unified method of diagnosis and repair. J Urol 1984; 132:254–257.

Krieger JN, Algood CB, Mason JT, Copass MK, Ansell JS. Urological trauma in the Pacific Northwest: etiology, distribution, management and outcome. J Urol 1984;132:70–73.

URETHRA, PENIS, AND TESTIS TRAUMA

JACK W. McANINCH, M.D.

URETHRA

The male urethra is divided into two major segments: the anterior urethra is that portion distal to the urogenital diaphragm; the posterior urethra is proximal to the urogenital diaphragm and includes the membranous and prostatic portions. Blunt trauma to the pelvis is the major cause of posterior urethral injuries. Pelvic fracture is present in more than 95 percent of cases, the impact of trauma exerting a shearing force on the urethra that causes rupture at the level of the urogenital diaphragm. Straddle injury, the most common cause of anterior urethral rupture, occurs during a fall or when blunt objects strike the perineum and scrotal area, crushing the urethra. The female urethra virtually never is significantly injured due to its short length.

The essential diagnostic sign of urethral injury is blood at the urethral meatus. Indeed, the most common error in diagnosis is failure to inspect the urethral meatus during the initial examination of any trauma patient. This finding is present in 80 to 90 percent of urethral injuries. In addition, scrotal and perineal hematomas may be noted, as well as evidence of injury to the lower abdomen. On careful inspection of the perineum, previously unrecognized hematomas may be detected, and a rectal examination in patients with suspected posterior urethral injury may help to determine whether the prostate is normally fixed or is disrupted and "floating."

If blood is noted at the urethral meatus or if a catheter does not pass easily, a urethrogram should be obtained. This is the key to diagnosis. Evidence of extravasation at the level of injury mandates urologic and surgical consultation.

A urethral catheter should not be passed in patients with known urethral injury because it may convert an incomplete laceration to a complete tear and introduce infection into the hematoma at the site of injury. The possible additional trauma from instrumentation may result in increased damage.

The initial treatment of urethral injuries is suprapubic cystostomy drainage, best accomplished in the operating room by surgical placement of a cystostomy catheter. In selected cases, percutaneous cystostomy drainage can be done, but only after urologic consultation. All these patients should be hospitalized for stabilization and observation. Most require cystostomy drainage until healing is complete and a delayed repair of the strictured area.

PENIS

The most common major traumatic injury to the penis is penile fracture. This occurs during the erect state and is most often associated with sexual intercourse, foreplay, or other sexual activity. Unusual stress on the penile shaft results in a transverse laceration of the tunica albuginea (the dense fascia surrounding the erectile bodies). Urethral rupture occurs in 20 percent of cases.

The patient reports hearing a loud cracking sound during sexual activity and experiencing immediate pain and detumescence. The initial examination reveals a large penile hematoma that usually involves the entire penile shaft. Patients with associated urethral injury usually have bloody urethral discharge. In many cases, palpation of the penile shaft reveals marked tenderness near the base of the penis–the common site of these ruptures.

Urethrography should be done in all patients to rule out possible urethral rupture. The diagnosis is based on history and physical examination; imaging studies are not helpful. Urologic consultation should be obtained as soon as the injury is suspected because surgical correction should be immediately performed. The patient can expect to regain normal sexual function.

TESTIS

Traumatic injuries to the testis occur primarily from blunt trauma. Assaults, contact sports, and motorcycle and bicycle injuries account for the majority.

These patients often have massive hematomas of the scrotum that prevent adequate palpation of the testis. On examination, the patient complains of marked tenderness on the involved side, which should raise immediate suspicion of testicular rupture, even in a patient with minimal hematoma. The most common diagnostic error is lack of suspicion on initial examination. Testicular rupture can lead to loss of the testicle.

Sonography of the testicle establishes the diagnosis. The characteristic sonographic pattern is altered echogenicity throughout the parenchyma of the involved testicle owing to hematoma accumulation and extruded parenchyma.

Once the diagnosis is established by sonography, testicular rupture should be corrected surgically. In cases in which massive hematoma exists without testicular rupture, surgical drainage of the hematoma decreases morbidity. Patients with small hematomas that are not associated with testicular rupture can be discharged and advised to remain at bed rest with scrotal elevation. When ambulating, these patients should maintain scrotal support and be seen frequently in follow-up to ensure that bleeding does not resume and that the hematoma is resolving.

AVULSION INJURIES

Skin and parts avulsion injuries of the genitalia most often occur when clothing becomes entangled in rotary machine equipment. They can also result from stab and gunshot wounds or self-inflicted injuries.

The extent of the injury is obvious at initial examination. Hemostasis should be obtained with compression bandages. Any skin or parts found at the scene of the incident should be preserved and brought with the patient to the hospital. In the emergency department, the skin and parts should be cleansed thoroughly and placed in saline solution and then in an ice-water bath. Preservation is important to provide the maximal opportunity for reconstruction and salvage.

Immediate consultation with a urologic surgeon is indicated because surgical correction is necessary. Properly preserved parts may be replaced by microsurgical techniques, and preserved skin may be debrided and grafted back into position. Small lacerations of the scrotum or penile skin may be cleansed and repaired in the emergency department.

SUGGESTED READING

McAninch JW. Injuries to the urinary system. In: Blaisdell WF, Trunkey DD, eds. Trauma management. Vol. 1: Abdominal trauma. New York: Thieme-Stratton, 1982: 199.
McAninch JW, Kahn RI, Jeffrey RB, Laing FC, Krieger MJ. Major traumatic and septic genital injuries. J Trauma 1984; 24:291–298.
Webster GD, Mathes GL, Selli C. Prostatomembranous urethral injuries: a review of the literature and a rational approach to their management. J Urol 1983; 130:898–902.

BLUNT ABDOMINAL TRAUMA

CHARLES APRAHAMIAN, M.D., F.A.C.S.

Trauma is a surgical disease. This is not to say that nonsurgeons cannot be involved, but rather that the decisions are surgical and need surgical involvement. The emergency management of blunt abdominal trauma should not be directed toward treating a specific abdominal organ injury (e.g., ruptured spleen or perforated viscus), but toward identifying (1) which patient will require operation (2) which patient will be admitted to the hospital for observation in the event of possible surgery, and (3) which patient may be discharged home.

MECHANISM OF INJURY

Traffic accidents, falls, and fights are only a few of the causes of blunt abdominal trauma, but represent the majority. Seat-belted front-seat riders would appear to do better then the unbelted since they avert head, torso, and pelvic injuries, but on occasion, improperly applied seat belts have caused injuries to the abdominal wall, small or large intestine, and pancreas. The potential for abdominal injury in rear-seat passengers may be less, although the unbelted are still exposed to abdominal injury when thrown against the car's interior. Principal injuries in pedestrian motor vehicle accidents are to the head, chest, and extremities, but abdominal trauma still occurs. Similar injuries, along with pelvic fractures, are prevalent in motorcycle accidents. Injuries from falls are associated with direct blows to the body on impact, but deceleration injuries to mobile viscera (e.g., renal pedicle) must be kept in mind. Injuries from assaults are the result of direct blows, principally to solid organs, although a blow to a distended urinary bladder may produce rupture.

EXTRA-ABDOMINAL INJURY

Extra-abdominal injuries, by their nature, may produce life-threatening problems that require major resuscitative efforts and preclude investigative efforts directed to the abdomen. These extra-abdominal conditions must be rapidly assessed and aggressively managed to stabilize the patient. When major resuscitative efforts are necessary, the delay in diagnosing intra-abdominal injuries is justified. However, when dramatic extra-abdominal injuries divert attention from assessment of intra-abdominal problems, increased and unnecessary morbidity and mortality result.

INTRA-ABDOMINAL INJURY

Intra-abdominal injury is manifested by blood loss or peritonitis. The degree of hemorrhage and physical evidence of hypovolemia is a reflection of the organ injured and the extent of that injury. Minor liver injuries may bleed, but eventually stop. Hollow viscera bleed, but not so severely as mesenteric vessels that supply that viscera. On the other hand, the injured hollow viscus can release the contents of the gastrointestinal or genitourinary tract into the peritoneal cavity, initiating peritonitis. The physical findings of peritonitis are more difficult to appreciate and evaluate in the patient who is unconscious or has a spinal cord injury.

SPECIAL CONCERNS AND DIAGNOSTIC PATTERNS

The hypotensive unconscious patient and the unconscious normotensive patient may need an airway and ventilatory support. A ruptured left diaphragm may present clinically as a left tension pneumothorax, and the rupture of the right diaphragm may have the radiologic appearance of a hemothorax. These conditions are associated with injuries to the spleen and liver. The inflation of the circumferential pneumatic compression suit (CPCS) on the hypotensive patient may cause the intra-abdominal contents to enter the chest through the ruptured diaphragm. On the chest film, fractures of the lower ribs may suggest injuries to the liver, spleen, and kidneys.

The number and site selection for venous access is dependent on the perceived severity of injury and the need for rapid fluid resuscitation. In many cases, patients treated by the EMT have CPCS applied, and peripheral line placement may be improved because of this garment. Saphenous venous access at the ankle in patients wearing the CPCS is still possible, and adequate volumes can be infused if a pressure pack is used to generate pressures greater than found in the garment. Newer models of the CPCS allow access to the groin should the need for such cutdowns exist. Central lines, whether subclavian or jugular, utilizing large-bore catheters are vital in selected patients.

The cardiac rate and rhythm must be monitored by ECG, and volume status is followed by monitoring urine output. Before the Foley catheter is inserted, a rectal examination should be performed to identify posterior urethral injury presenting as an elevated prostate. Hematuria is an indication of genitourinary tract injury and requires radiologic investigation. The more profuse the hematuria, the greater the likelihood that an injury will be identified. However, vascular disruption of the renal artery may occur with minimal or no hematuria.

EVALUATION OF ABDOMINAL TRAUMA

For purposes of evaluation, the blunt abdominal trauma patient falls into one of the following categories: (1) hypovolemic, whether conscious or unconscious, (2) normovolemic and unconscious, and (3) normovolemic, conscious, and with abdominal pain.

Abdominal pain includes the entire spectrum of peritoneal reaction to pain: tenderness, guarding, rigidity, abdominal distention, tympany, and decreased bowel sounds. Unconscious is defined as any decreased level of consciousness, whether due to trauma, alcohol, or drugs.

The Hypovolemic Patient

Occult intra-abdominal blood loss must be diagnosed early (Table 1). Visible blood loss from soft tissue injuries must be controlled. In the absence of hemothorax or a mediastinal abnormality, hypovolemia must be assumed to be due to continued blood loss from the abdomen or extremity. Application of CPCS to the lower extremities may control arterial and venous blood loss. Palpation of the pelvis may suggest a fracture and reinforce the physician's suspicion that there is an intra-abdominal injury with blood loss.

Peritoneal Lavage. While fluid resuscitation is aggressively pursued, the identification of intra-abdominal hemorrhage is also sought, the best means being peritoneal lavage. An incision is made just below the umbilicus at the midline. Local anesthetic supplemented with epinephrine is administered to minimize bleeding and provide comfort for the more alert patient. The incision is carried through the midline fascia and the peritoneum is entered so that the contents are clearly visible. The presence of gross blood calls for early exploration. If gross blood is not visible, the catheter is inserted into the peritoneal cavity, directed towards the pelvis, and aspirated. Easy aspiration of 10 cc of blood is an indication of intra-abdominal hemorrhage. If blood cannot be aspirated, the lavage fluid is instilled through the catheter while the wound is being closed. After the lavage fluid has been instilled, it is siphoned off, and a cell count is performed on an aliquot. A cell count of more than 100,000 RBC in the effluent is a positive sign of intra-

TABLE 1 Clinical Hypovolemia

Systolic BP <90 mm Hg

Systolic BP >90 mm Hg after fluid resuscitation or initial hypotension

Normal BP but with pulse ≥ 110, weak pulse, or pallor and peripheral vasoconstriction

abdominal hemorrhage, and exploration is indicated. Although the amylase determination in the lavage effluent has been recommended in the past, there is probably little need to do so since an injury sufficiently severe to cause release of amylase is associated with an abnormal RBC count.

The lavage only proves that there is an intra-abdominal hemorrhage and does not identify what organ or viscera has been injured, or to what extent. If the hypovolemic patient is unconscious, it is imperative to perform the peritoneal lavage early, while the ABC's are being performed. Early diagnosis of intra-abdominal hemorrhage expedites the ultimate operative management.

Patients who are found to have a pelvic fracture on clinical examination may have the peritoneal lavage performed above the umbilicus to prevent a false-positive examination. If the pelvic fracture, and not an intra-abdominal injury, is the cause of hypotension, early arteriographic evaluation and embolization may be necessary. If arteriography is negative, circumferential pneumatic compression may be applied at low pressures to minimize this venous bleeding.

The technique of peritoneal lavage is a skill that is easily learned and performed. Whether it is performed by the surgeon or the emergency physician is a matter of local and individual choice which should be determined in advance. In communities without surgical capabilities, the peritoneal lavage should not be performed since it would only delay the timely transport of the patient to a facility with the needed expertise.

Radiologic Examinations. If the peritoneal lavage dictates early surgery, the only radiologic examinations that are vital to the patient's care are the C-spine examination to identify fractures and a chest film to identify a hemopneumothorax that might necessitate thoracostomy. Skull, facial, abdominal, and extremity films can await control of the intra-abdominal hemorrhage. An IVP is not indicated, but an argument for a cystogram could be made in a patient with hypotension and associated hematuria. The hypotension would preclude an IVP.

The Unconscious and Normovolemic Patient

The intra-abdominal injury may be limited and may not be manifested early with hypovolemia, but later with delayed hemorrhage. Early diagnosis of occult intra-abdominal injury is critical and can be achieved with selective use of peritoneal lavage, flat plate of the abdomen, or abdominal CT.

If the patient's head injury is the most impressive and severe injury, peritoneal lavage should be done early to ensure a benign abdomen, especially if the general surgeon is not assuming final overall care. The lavage may be negative in patients with hepatic and splenic injuries who do not have disrupted capsules, or in those patients with injuries to the retroperitoneal structures (kidneys, ureters, pancreas, duodenum). A flat plate of the abdomen may suggest intra-abdominal injuries because of fractures to the lower ribs or retroperitoneal injury because of obliteration of the psoas shadow. On occasion, a splenic hematoma causes displacement of the stomach and splenic flexure of the colon.

A CT of the head often is needed in these patients. When it is done, an abdominal CT can be performed in lieu of the peritoneal lavage. Whereas the lavage suggests hemorrhage with no organ specificity, the abdominal CT has organ specificity but is limited in its assessment of ongoing intra-abdominal hemorrhage. Therefore, CT evidence of intra-abdominal injury, (e.g., liver, kidneys, spleen) must be clinically interpreted by the surgeon to determine the advisability of exploration.

Some communities have general surgeons but not neurosurgeons or CT capability. Under these circumstances, an unconscious trauma patient should be transferred to an institution with neurosurgical capability, but identifying occult abdominal injury by peritoneal lavage and correcting it prior to transfer may be lifesaving.

Abdominal Pain in the Conscious and Normovolemic Patient

The patient who presents only with abdominal pain but is conscious and normovolemic, with or without injuries requiring specialty surgical consultation, represents a true problem to primary physicians and general surgeons alike. The question is not what is the intra-abdominal injury, but rather, how far should you go to evaluate and treat the patient for intra-abdominal injury.

If the patient has major extra-abdominal problems that require surgery, a *peritoneal lavage* is in order. This can be performed in the operating room just prior to the performance of the other surgery and is intended to identify an occult intra-abdominal injury that could progress while the patient is under anesthesia.

If the patient has extra-abdominal problems or if there is sufficient concern about the abdomen to require admission to the hospital, the patient's abdominal findings and vital functions can be monitored closely to identify early changes. Peritoneal lavage is not indicated. Computerized tomography of the abdomen may be a consideration and can identify intrahepatic hematomas and subcapsular injuries to the liver and spleen.

Overnight hospital observation may be indicated for patients whose injuries do not appear to require admission, but who do not have ready access or ease of reentry into the EMS system in the event that symptoms progress.

SUGGESTED READING

Aprahamian C, Carrico CJ, Collicott PE, et al. Advanced trauma life support course, Instructor and Student Manual. American College of Surgeons Committee on Trauma, 1984.

Bouwman DL, Weaver DW, Walt AJ. Serum amylase and its isoenzymes: a clarification of their implications in trauma. J Trauma 1984; 24:573–578.

Davis JJ, Cohn I, Nance FC. Diagnosis and management of blunt abdominal trauma. Ann Surg 1976; 183:672–678.

Federle MP, Crass RA, Brooke J, Trunkey DD. Computed tomography in blunt abdominal trauma. Arch Surg 1982; 117:645–650.

Fortune JB, Brahme J, Mulligan M, et al. Emergency intravenous pyelography in the trauma patient: a reexamination of the indications. Arch Surg 1985; 120:1056–1059.

Marx JA, Moore EE, Jorden RC, et al. Limitations of computed tomography in the evaluation of acute abdominal trauma. J Trauma 1985; 25:933–937.

PENETRATING ABDOMINAL WOUNDS

ROBERT PAPADOPOULOS, M.D.
ERNEST E. MOORE, M.D.

Escalation of civilian violence in our country continues to make penetrating abdominal wounds a common problem in community emergency departments as well as in urban trauma centers. Salvage of these critically injured patients demands an efficient integrated team effort from the time of injury to definitive repair of intra-abdominal visceral and vascular injuries.

Although the pre-hospital management of the injured patient is basically generic and should be based on the clinical status of the patient, it is important to differentiate between the life-threatening potential of a stab injury and that of a gunshot wound. Approximately two-thirds of stab wounds to the anterior abdomen penetrate the peritoneal cavity, but less than half of these inflict significant visceral damage. Thus, approximately one-third of patients who sustain abdominal stab wounds require operative intervention.

Gunshot wounds, on the other hand, pose a much greater threat for serious visceral injury. Civilian low-energy missiles striking the anterior abdomen enter the peritoneal cavity 80 percent of the time, but 95 percent of the patients in whom the missile violates the peritoneum require emergent surgery. Accordingly, gunshot wounds to the abdomen warrant a more aggressive management plan, both in the field and in the emergency department.

PRE-HOSPITAL CARE

Resuscitation and evaluation of the acutely injured patient must begin at the scene. Prioritization of care is based on the physiologic ABC schedule (A for airway, B for breathing, and C for circulation) in the patient with a penetrating wound as well as the individual who sustains multisystem blunt trauma. The measures exercised to accomplish these management principles are governed by the training and expertise of the pre-hospital personnel as well as the geographic location of the closest trauma facility. At the scene, the first management consideration should be airway. The patient with adequate ventilatory effort should be given supplemental oxygen. The next consideration is volume restitution. Any external hemorrhage should be controlled with direct pressure. It is current practice in most pre-hospital systems to apply pneumatic antishock garment (PASG) if the patient has a systolic blood pressure less than 80 mm Hg. Although the ability of the PASG to "autotransfuse" the central blood volume from the periphery is probably limited to 250 to 500 cc, the major physiologic benefit of this device in the case of penetrating wound is tamponade of intra-abdominal major vascular bleeding. With experienced personnel, efforts should be made to initiate crystalloid fluid infusion by means of large-bore antecubital venous cannulas.

However, time committed to this advanced resuscitative technique must be based on the patient's clinical condition and the anticipated transport time to the receiving trauma facility. When a patient with a penetrating wound is in extremis, the secondary survey in the field should be brief and the patient transported expeditiously to the receiving hospital; only critical information should be conveyed, i.e., mechanism of injury, level of consciousness, ventilatory status, systolic blood pressure, heart rate, and arrival time. On the other hand, in the stable individual, a more thorough inspection should be completed in the field, particularly a search for additional penetrating wounds to the back, flanks, perineum, and axillae. Penetrating wounds to the lower chest, defined anteriorly as the nipple line to the costal margins and posteriorly as the tip of the scapula to the costal margins, are considered to be potential penetrating abdominal wounds. Conversely, penetrating wounds to the upper abdomen may enter the chest and cause life-threatening tension pneumothorax, major hemothorax, or pericardial tamponade.

A patient with a penetrating wound to the chest or abdomen should be triaged to a level I trauma center when this is geographically feasible. The mode of transportation depends on the patient's condition, distance to the regional trauma facility, and accessibility to the scene of injury. In urban regions, ground transportation with ambulances usually provides efficient transportation. However, in rural areas, rotary as well as fixed-wing transport should be considered.

EMERGENCY DEPARTMENT MANAGEMENT

A trauma team should be organized in the emergency department prior to the patient's arrival. The team varies considerably from hospital to hospital, but generally consists of emergency physicians, surgeons, nurses, and attendants. A predetermined team captain should be selected to optimally utilize individual talents.

Resuscitation and initial evaluation of the patient with a penetrating abdominal wound must occur simultaneously. As in the field, priorities in resuscitation are governed by physiologic rationale. The ultimate goal is to reestablish adequate oxygen supply to vital organs. If the patient is uncooperative owing to intoxication, hypoxemia, or profound shock, there should be no hesitation about using paralysis (succinylcholine, 1.5 mg per kilogram) to facilitate direct oral-tracheal intubation. Additionally, a tube thoracostomy (36 F) should be placed empirically on the side of a penetrating chest wound to vent a potential tension pneumothorax or to direct attention to an occult hemothorax.

The next physiologic priority is to restore circulating blood volume. Large-bore short intravenous cannulas in the antecubital veins are preferred. When the patient arrives with venous collapse due to protracted shock, we prefer saphenous vein cutdowns at the ankle with placement of 10-gauge intracaths. If additional venous access is required, 8 F introducer catheters are placed via central venous access routes. Ringer's lactate is the preferred initial resuscitation fluid. As the volume of crystalloid infusion approaches 50 cc per kilogram, blood should be transfused. Type-specific blood should be used when available; however, reconstituted O negative red cells may be required in extreme situations.

While resuscitation is in progress, a relevant history should be obtained from the pre-hospital personnel. Important features include confirmation of the data relayed during pre-hospital care, the type of weapon used, amount of blood loss at the scene, and a presumed time interval from injury to when they first arrived on the scene. Simultaneously, a rapid, but systematic, physical examination should be completed, literally proceeding from head to toe. Often neglected in this survey are inspection of the back, flanks, perineum, and axillae; neurologic assessment; rectal examination; and palpation of peripheral pulses. A nasogastric tube should be inserted to decompress the stomach and to look for occult blood, which suggests a penetrating gastroduodenal wound. A Foley catheter should be inserted to empty the bladder, monitor urinary output as an index of tissue perfusion, and search for hematuria.

Radiographic evaluation and laboratory testing should be individualized. Penetrating wounds to the lower chest and upper abdomen are indications for a chest roentgenogram to rule out associated intrathoracic injury, and to confirm positions of the endotracheal, thoracostomy, and nasogastric tubes as well as central venous lines. Following gunshot wounds, biplaner abdominal films are most useful to confirm missile trajectory and to demonstrate bullet fragments and foreign bodies. Intravenous urography should be done when any degree of hematuria is noted and when there are penetrating wounds in proximity to the urologic tract. As many as 25 percent of ureteral injuries do not manifest as microscopic hematuria. In addition, sigmoidoscopy should be performed when penetrating wounds are in proximity to the rectum. Initial laboratory screening usually includes a base-line hematocrit, white blood cell count, type and crossmatching, and a urinalysis.

Emergency department thoracotomy should be an integral part of the resuscitation of the patient who arrives in cardiac standstill or who continues to have a systolic blood pressure less than 60 mm Hg despite initial resuscitative efforts. The rationale for resuscitative thoracotomy in the patient with a penetrating abdominal wound is to permit (1) access to the descending thoracic aorta for temporary cross-clamping and (2) access to the heart for internal cardiac massage in the event of standstill. Additionally, a patient in extremis with a wound in proximity to the pericardium should undergo thoracotomy to release tamponade and control cardiac hemorrhage.

The need for emergent laparotomy is clear in approximately one-fourth of all patients with penetrating wounds. Hypovolemic shock, unexplained blood loss, absent bowel sounds, and abdominal rebound tenderness constitute indications for prompt abdominal exploration. In such patients, a broad-spectrum antibiotic in the form of a third-generation cephalosporin (cefoxitin, 2 g) or extended penicillin (mezlocillin, 4 g) should be administered in the emergency department. In the remaining three-fourths of

these patients, the need for laparotomy is not self-evident. The diagnostic approach to such individuals depends on the mechanism of injury and the location of the wound.

Stab Wounds to the Anterior Abdomen

Traditionally, laparotomy has been considered mandatory for all stab wounds to the abdomen. Although two-thirds of such wounds penetrate the peritoneum, less than half inflict significant visceral damage. An approach using mandatory exploration led to a negative celiotomy rate of 30 to 60 percent in civilian practice. Clearly, a selective policy for laparotomy is warranted for stab wounds entering the anterior abdomen.

One approach to ascertaining intraperitoneal injury has been serial physical examinations. Physical findings indicating visceral damage are lacking in roughly one-third of patients, and a needed laparotomy may thus be delayed. The other major disadvantage has been an inherent false-positive laparotomy rate in 15 percent of the patients.

In the absence of compelling indications for exploratory laparotomy, the first step is to determine whether the stab injury has violated the peritoneal cavity (Fig. 1). The gross appearance of the stab wound site is misleading unless evisceration has occurred. Sinography, the injection of contrast material via a catheter placed in the stab wound, once a popular technique to determine peritoneal violation, has subsequently been shown to be inaccurate. Direct wound exploration under local anesthesia in the emergency department is a rapid, safe, and reliable procedure to determine depth of stab wound penetration. The procedure is performed under standard asepsis with the providone-iodine preparation and sterile drapes. The area immediately surrounding the stab wound is generously infiltrated with 1 percent Xylocaine. The skin is usually incised an additional 4 to 6 cm to facilitate inspection, and the underlying subcutaneous tissue is dissected bluntly to ascertain fascial violation. Although there are two or three fascial layers to the abdominal wall, depending on location, the safest policy is to assume peritoneal violation when the anteriormost layer of fascia has been violated. If anterior fascia is intact, it is safe to assume that the knife has not entered the peritoneal cavity, in which case the extended portion of the skin may be closed by primary intention and the patient discharged from the emergency department. In our experience, this permits discharge of roughly one-third of patients with anterior abdominal stab wounds.

If peritoneal violation is proved or suspected, the next step is to determine whether visceral damage has resulted from the penetrating instrument. With few exceptions, most centers now rely on diagnostic peritoneal lavage to determine the need for laparotomy. We prefer the semi-open technique of peritoneal lavage performed at the infraumbilical ring level. Under sterile conditions, a standard peritoneal dialysis catheter is inserted into the pelvis. Initial aspiration of more than 10 cc of gross blood or fluid containing bile, feces, or particulate matter is an undisputed indication for laparotomy. If the aspirate is negative, an irrigation of 1,000 cc of normal saline (15 cc

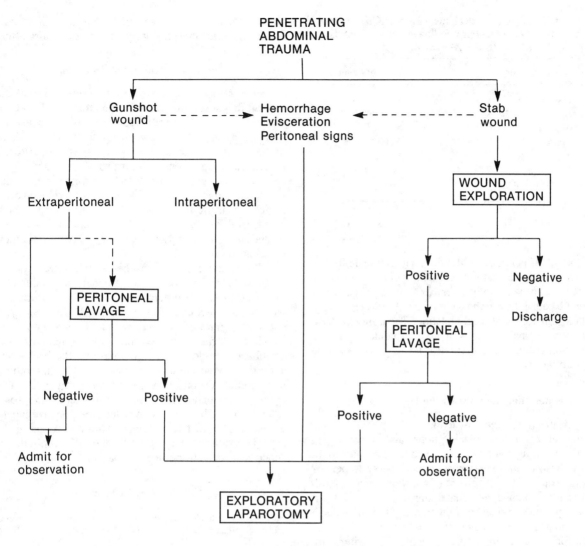

Figure 1 Decision making in penetrating abdominal trauma.

per kilogram in children) is instilled and returned by gravity. The red blood cell (RBC) count in the lavage effluent is the most useful index for predicting intraabdominal injury. Although the minimal RBC level indicating abdominal exploration remains controversial, most authorities use a minimum level of 100,000 per cubic millimeter. It must be stressed that although the aforementioned index avoids unnecessary laparotomy, it has an inherent 5 percent false-negative rate. Most such patients in whom the lavage red cell count is insensitive have isolated hollow visceral perforation, usually of the small bowel or stomach. Analysis of the peritoneal lavage fluid for white blood cells (WBC) and enzyme concentrations occasionally identifies these otherwise occult intestinal injuries. The commonly accepted criteria include a WBC count higher than 500 per cubic millimeter or elevation in the amylase or alkaline phosphatase above serum levels (Table 1). Because of the inherent 5 percent false-negative rate for diagnostic peritoneal lavage, all patients undergoing this procedure for an abdominal stab wound must be admitted to the hospital and followed with

serial abdominal examination over the ensuing 24 hours. Any deterioration in vital signs or physical findings suggesting evolving peritonitis warrant immediate abdominal exploration.

Gunshot Wounds to the Abdomen

Gunshot wounds to the abdomen are much more serious; a bullet entering the peritoneal cavity causes significant visceral damage 95 percent of the time. Thus, in the asymptomatic patient, the critical determinant for laparotomy is whether the bullet has traversed the peritoneum or has remained extraperitoneal. Missile trajectory is usually discernible by physical examination, corroborated by biplaner radiography. Local wound exploration is generally impractical for gunshot wounds because of the necessity for unroofing extensive bullet tracts. In the occasional patient in whom violation of the peritoneal cavity is in question, diagnostic peritoneal lavage is helpful. However in this situation, the RBC level considered to be an indication for exploration is reduced

TABLE 1 Diagnostic Peritoneal Lavage Criteria For Exploratory Laparotomy Following Stab Wounds to the Abdomen

Parameter	Positive Result
Red blood cells	$>100,000/mm^3$
White blood cells	$>500/mm^3$
Alkaline phosphatase	>6 IU/L
Amylase	>200 U/dl
Bile	Present
Gram stain	Bacteria
Vegetable stain	Fiber

to 5,000 RBC per cubic millimeter. The rationale for this change in policy is that such a quantity of blood (approximately 1 cc of whole blood per 1,000 cc of lavaged fluid) cannot be attributed to the technique of peritoneal lavage and thus implies peritoneal violation. The utility of WBC and enzyme analysis as well as a mandatory 24-hour admission for negative peritoneal lavage is the same as for stab wounds.

Penetrating Wounds of the Lower Thorax

The diaphragm may rise to the fourth intercostal space during full expiration, placing upper abdominal organs and the diaphragm at risk from penetrating wounds to the lower chest. In our experience, approximately 15 percent of stab wounds and 50 percent of gunshot wounds in this region are combined thoracoabdominal wounds. Not surprisingly, the physical examination in such patients is misleading. For this reason, diagnostic peritoneal lavage is performed in asymptomatic patients. The criteria for abdominal exploration is a count greater than 5,000 RBC per cubic millimeter. The reasoning for the relatively low count is similar to that applied to gunshot wounds, i.e., this number of red cells cannot be explained by the lavage procedure and thus implies at least a diaphragmatic defect. In a patient with tube thoracostomy, the accuracy of diagnostic peritoneal lavage can be enhanced by adding methylene blue or some other agent to the lavage fluid and observing for its exit from the chest tube. This phenomenon occurs because of the negative thoracoabdominal gradient created during normal respiratory effort.

Posterior Penetrating Wounds

Penetrating wounds entering the back and flank can present diagnostic difficulties. The injuries inflicted are often secluded anatomically in the retroperitoneal space. Clearly, patients with such wounds who manifest evidence of unexplained blood loss or signs suggesting peritonitis require early laparotomy. Unfortunately, telltale abdominal physical signs are often lacking when injuries are isolated in the retroperitoneal space. An overlooked colon perforation is life-threatening. On the other hand, the risk of visceral injury is only 10 percent for penetrating wounds to the back and approximately 25 percent for those entering via the flank.

Patient management must be individualized. For stab wounds, there is a role for occasional local wound exploration to ascertain depth of penetration. For gunshot wounds, this technique is impractical. Unfortunately, to date the accuracy of advanced radiologic techniques, such as triple-contrast computed tomography, remains to be established. Following a stab wound to the back, most authorities advocate a selective policy for laparotomy, using initial peritoneal lavage and serial physical examination as the major determinants. A selective approach to posterior stab wounds can reduce the negative laparotomy to approximately 10 percent. Gunshot wounds in this region merit a more aggressive policy if the missile has penetrated the retroperitoneal space.

SUGGESTED READING

Feliciano DV, Bitondo CG, Steed G, et al. Five hundred open taps or lavages in patients with abdominal stab wounds. Am J Surg 1984; 148:772–777.

Moore EE, Marx JA. Penetrating abdominal wounds: rationale for exploratory laparotomy. JAMA 1985; 253:2705–2708.

Peck JJ, Berne TV. Posterior abdominal stab wounds. J Trauma 1981; 21:298–306.

Shafton GW. Indications for operation in abdominal trauma. Am J Surg 1960; 99:657–664.

Thal ER. Evaluation of peritoneal lavage and local exploration in lower chest and abdominal stab wounds. J Trauma 1977; 17:642–648.

Thompson JS, Moore EE, Moore-Van Duzer S, Moore JB, Galloway AL. The evolution of abdominal stab wound management. J Trauma 1980; 20:478–484.

PELVIC FRACTURE

RICHARD E. WARD, M.D.
TIMOTHY J. BRAY, M.D.

The pelvis may be fractured in numerous places from myriad etiologies. It takes a tremendous amount of force to fracture the bony pelvis; thus, the incidence of associated injuries of both bone and soft tissue is high. Most pelvic fractures are the result of high-energy injury, although persons falling from heights or those involved in crushing industrial accidents are also at risk. Males between the ages of 20 and 40 are at highest risk. Small children are at low risk, although children who venture out on streets on bicycles can sustain this injury. It generally requires more force to break the pediatric pelvis because of its increased deformability.

DIAGNOSIS

A pelvic fracture should be relatively easy to detect, but often goes overlooked because of other more obvious or more dramatic but less important injuries. Pelvic fracture is frequently associated with closed head injury, long-bone fracture, and intraperitoneal visceral injury. All patients with the aforementioned injuries should be carefully evaluated for a pelvic fracture. Likewise, a large number of patients with pelvic fractures are hypotensive when admitted to the emergency department, and this finding should lead to careful evaluation of the patient's pelvis. All trauma patients should have AP radiologic views of the pelvis as part of the general approach to management, just as they routinely have lateral C-spine films.

Evaluation of the patient for pelvic fracture includes a number of straightforward physical examinations and anteroposterior roentgenograms of the pelvis. For examination, the multiply injured patient must be completely disrobed. Initial assessment should include examination of the pelvis for any signs of instability, hematoma, pain, or associated peripelvic injury. This is accomplished by first placing a hand on each anterior superior spine and, with firm pressure, attempting to force the spines outward and posterior. Second, one should apply pressure over the pubic tubercles bilaterally. If pain is elicited or if crepitus or movement is noted, the diagnosis of a fractured pelvis can be made with confidence. Further examination should include careful inspection of the urethral meatus in males for blood, inspection of the perineum and pelvic examination for any lacerations, and a rectal examination to test for the position of the prostate in males, to ascertain the presence or absence of sphincter tone and reflexes, and to test for the presence of blood in the rectum. The initial examining physician must look carefully for the smallest of puncture wounds about the pelvis, especially in the perineum. These are indicative of communications with the pelvic bones and are classified as open fractures until proved otherwise. Pelvic infections can increase the mortality rate for open pelvic fractures to 50 percent.

A number of common diagnostic errors such as missing hip dislocation, concomitant acetabulum fractures, and sacral nerve lesions are committed in these patients. Later rehabilitation will be helped if these problems are discovered early. The magnitude of blood loss may be severely underestimated. The pelvis contains not only the rectum and the bladder, but also the iliac arteries and veins. The rich plexus of veins that is adherent to the posterior pelvis is easily disrupted by posterior pelvic fractures and sacroiliac joint disruption. These veins are valveless and directly connected to the iliac veins and thus the vena cava. Disruption of these veins can account for massive amounts of blood loss limited to the extraperitoneal pelvis and not obvious on physical examination.

Another diagnostic error is that of overlooking a urethral or bladder injury. In the male, the membraneous urethra is firmly attached to the inferior margin of the pubic symphysis and is particularly vulnerable to injury in cases of anterior pubic rami fracture or symphyseal disruption. Blood seen at the urethral meatus is highly suggestive of urethral injury and is an indication for further evaluation with a retrograde urethrogram. If there is no evidence of meatal blood, a Foley catheter can be carefully inserted. If resistance is met, the catheter should be withdrawn and a urethrogram performed. If hematuria, either gross or microscopic, is noted on catheterization a cystogram should be performed to assess for bladder injury. Another error is that of failing to diagnose an open or compound pelvic fracture. This is defined as a fracture that communicates with the outside through the perineal skin, the rectum, or the vagina. To avert this error, one must be particularly attentive to visual inspection of the perineum, buttocks, natal cleft, and vagina. If there is evidence of rectal blood, anoscopy and/or sigmoidoscopy is necessary.

TREATMENT

Therapy in the field and in the emergency department should be aimed toward treating the major life-threatening aspect of pelvic fracture (hemorrhage) and preventing the consequent complications (coagulopathy, pulmonary and renal failure, sepsis). This can be accomplished by aggressive volume resuscitation and appropriate blood and blood component therapy. At least two large-bore (14- to 16-gauge) intravenous lines should be placed. The site of placement is not particularly critical. Lower extremity cutdowns in the saphenous vein at the ankle work as well as upper extremity lines despite the presence of the fracture and consequent venous injury in the pelvis. Lactated Ringer's solution is preferred for volume replacement and has theoretical advantages over normal saline or albumin products. Skin color and temperature, urine output, and central venous pressure are the common indicators of successful resuscitation. Hematocrit should be checked periodically, and after four liters of crystalloid have been administered, packed red blood cells should be infused. Every four units of cells should be followed by two units of fresh frozen plasma. Four platelet packs should be given after every eight units of cells.

Noninvasive methods that may be useful in decreasing the amount of bleeding are the pneumatic antishock garment (PASG) and the external fixation devices commonly applied by orthopaedists. Both modalities have been shown to decrease the amount of bleeding by either tamponade of the pelvis (PASG) or reducing the fractures into anatomic position (external fixators). The PASG should be applied and inflated in the field in the case of suspected pelvic fracture. This does not eliminate the need for intravenous volume and should be looked on as an adjunct to volume resuscitation. The external fixation devices can be easily applied in the emergency department, but are generally applied in the operating room or the intensive care unit.

If prompt resuscitation and maintenance of adequate hemodynamics are not possible in a patient with a pelvic fracture, hemorrhage in either the abdomen or the chest should be suspected. Chest roentgenograms can readily rule out major hemorrhage into the thoracic cavity. There is no good test in the face of a pelvic fracture that will do the same for the abdomen. Peritoneal lavage must be performed above the umbilicus to avoid any preperitoneal hematoma and may be useful. A negative lavage is indicative of no hemorrhage in the peritoneal cavity, but a positive lavage may not indicate intraperitoneal injury, since there is a high incidence of bleeding from the extraperitoneal hematoma into the peritoneum. Negative lavage does not rule out a large extraperitoneal hematoma and blood loss. Computerized tomography of the abdomen can rule out injury to the liver, spleen, or pancreas, but does not define the source of intraperitoneal fluid.

Because of the indecisive nature of noninvasive or minimally invasive evaluations in these patients, exploratory laparotomy may be the safest approach to the diagnosis of intraperitoneal hemorrhage. The final option is abdominal angiography with pelvic arteriography, which permits detection of bleeding in the solid abdominal viscera as well as the pelvis and may allow for transcatheter embolization of persistently bleeding pelvic vessels. This modality should probably be reserved for situations in which the preceding methods were not useful and the patient continues to bleed. Angiographic embolization is only possible in 5 to 7 percent of patients with pelvic fractures. The usefulness is higher in patients with persistent bleeding, especially when it does not abate after external fixation.

Operative intervention is necessary in patients with associated injuries elsewhere in the body as well as in patients with open fractures and genitourinary injury.

Patients with urethral disruption or with intraperitoneal bladder rupture require suprapubic urinary diversion. Those with extraperitoneal bladder disruption may be managed with urethral drainage alone. Urethral disruptions should not be repaired or manipulated in the acute phases after injury because of the high incidence of secondary complications late after repair. The patient with a pelvic fracture opening into either the perineum or the rectum should have a diverting colostomy, the distal segment of which should be copiously irrigated to minimize the incidence of sepsis and late osteomyelitis. External pelvic fixation has proved useful in this situation, allowing for ease in nursing care and wound management and for early mobilization of patients. Pelvic slings should never be used in the management of the open pelvic fracture.

SUGGESTED READING

Gilliland MD, Ward RE, Barton RM, Miller PW, Duke JH. Factors affecting mortality in pelvic fractures. J Trauma 1982; 22:691–693.

Gilliland MG, Ward RE, Flynn TC, Miller PW, Ben-Menachem Y, Duke JH Jr. Peritoneal lavage and angiography in the management of patients with pelvic fractures. Am J Surg 1982; 144:744–747.

Gylling SF, Ward RE, Holcroft JW, Bray TJ, Chapman MW. Immediate external fixation of unstable pelvic fractures. Am J Surg 1985; 150:721–724.

Ward RE, Clark DG. Management of pelvic fractures. Radiol Clin North Am 1981; 19:167–170.

ESOPHAGEAL FOREIGN BODIES, TRAUMA, AND PERFORATION

G. PATRICK LILJA, M.D., F.A.C.E.P.

Patients presenting to the emergency department with a history of a foreign body lodged in the esophagus and/or problems related to esophageal trauma are not unusual. It is necessary for physicians to understand the most common types of esophageal foreign bodies and causes of esophageal trauma. Esophageal foreign bodies should never be perceived as minor or trivial, since even the smallest and most asymptomatic can rapidly cause life-threatening complications.

Foreign bodies may completely or partially obstruct the esophagus, as well as lacerate it. Ninety percent of foreign bodies lodge high in the esophagus at the level of the cricopharyngeus muscle; the rest at the aortic arch and mainstem bronchus, the esophagogastric function, or at pathologic sites of narrowing caused by strictures or malignancy. The obstruction may also cause regurgitation of food, liquids, and saliva, resulting in aspiration and pneumonia. A common cause of esophageal obstruction is accidentally swallowing a chicken bone or a large piece of meat. Denture wearers are especially susceptible to only partially chewed boluses of food becoming lodged in the esophagus. Children may purposely swallow items such as buttons, rocks, coins, or small toy parts. The mentally handicapped may also ingest objects without realizing the consequences; prison inmates may do so deliberately to seek hospitalization. Finally, abnormal neuromuscular conditions or esophageal strictures may result in objects lodging in the esophagus.

Esophageal trauma may be the result of lodged foreign bodies, medical instrumentation, ingestion of caustics, and penetrating or blunt trauma to the neck. Sudden, violent, and usually repeated increase in abdominal pressure against a closed glottis, as in hiccuping, seizures, cardiopulmonary resuscitation, or vomiting (Boerhaave's syndrome), may also cause a perforation of the esophageal wall. Impacted foreign bodies that stay in place 24 hours or more may also cause perforation.

DIAGNOSIS OF ESOPHAGEAL FOREIGN BODIES

Most patients with esophageal obstruction present with the complaint of a swallowed object or food being stuck in the throat. This history, however, may be absent in a young child or the mentally retarded. The patient may point to where the object is stuck, although this is an inaccurate means of localization. Signs of obstruction include hypersalivation, drooling, dysphagia, and odynophagia. To confirm the diagnosis of esophageal foreign body, radiologic studies can be most helpful. Anteroposterior (AP) and lateral soft tissue roentgenograms of the neck may help localize radiopaque foreign bodies such as pins, bones, and small button batteries. Xerography can help locate more radiolucent substances. It is important that both the AP and lateral views be obtained, as small objects may only be seen in one plane. Radiolucent foreign bodies require a contrast esophagogram. Most clinicians initially use a soluble contrast medium such as Gastrografin since it carries less risk in case a perforation is present. However, care must be taken to avoid patient aspiration of this material, as it causes pneumonitis. Gastrografin may not be as successful as other contrast media in detecting small esophageal perforations. If a Gastrografin study is negative and perforation is suspected, follow-up films with barium may be needed. At times, with a very small object such as a fishbone, the initial work-up may be negative. It is important in these cases that patients be reexamined within 2 to 3 days to see if any symptom persists. If there is continued pain or other symptoms, endoscopy is probably indicated, as even small objects may go on to perforate and cause serious infection.

A very common complication of esophageal foreign body ingestion is a simple abrasion, which despite normal examination and esophagogram results causes a persistent foreign body sensation. This should gradually dissipate over the next few days. The physician must be very careful to have ruled out a laceration or missed foreign body, and persistent or worsening symptoms should be an indication for immediate endoscopy.

TREATMENT

Once an esophageal foreign body is located, one must decide on the appropriate method of removal. If there is complete obstruction, removal should be accomplished as soon as possible, since prolonged obstruction increases the risk of aspiration and perforation. If there is a partial obstruction, it should be removed within 12 to 24 hours. The method of removal depends on the type of object, availability of equipment, and the training of the physician. In general, objects may be mechanically removed or allowed to pass into the stomach by use of a spasmolytic or gas-forming agent. Each of these methods has certain advantages, but all also carry certain risks.

Mechanical Removal of Foreign Bodies

Endoscopy is the most commonly employed method of removing esophageal foreign body, since it allows for direct visualization. However, endoscopy requires the presence of a trained endoscopist, and even then, esophageal perforation can occur. Endoscopy is certainly the preferred method for removal of sharp or pointed foreign bodies such as bones, open safety pins, and razors. It also allows visual inspection of the esophagus for perforation.

An alternative to endoscopy is Foley catheter extraction. This works only if the foreign body is partially occluding the esophagus and has smooth or rounded edges, such as coins or buttons. In this method, a Foley catheter is advanced beyond the foreign body, the balloon inflated, and the catheter is then removed, forcing the foreign body ahead of the balloon. This maneuver does carry the hazard that the foreign body may fall into the larynx or trachea upon removal, causing upper airway obstruction. For this reason, the patient should be in a head-down position during this procedure. It is best performed under fluoroscopy. In addition, the esophagus must be inspected afterward, using radiologic contrast medium to rule out an unexpected perforation.

Spasmolytics

Spasmolytics relax the esophageal smooth muscle and the cardiac sphincter. This allows impacted food or other non-bony matter to pass from the distal esophagus into the stomach. Agents available include glucagon, anticholinergic agents, and nitroglycerin. Glucagon appears most efficacious, as it has a short duration of action and fewer side effects than anticholinergics. Glucagon should be administered intravenously as a 1-mg injection over 1 to 2 minutes. It must not be administered rapidly or it may cause nausea. Glucagon generally relaxes the esophageal smooth muscles in 45 seconds and its duration of action is approximately 25 minutes. If relief is not obtained within 20 minutes, a second administration of 2 mg intravenously may be given. If the object is still obstructing, other methods of removal must be utilized. Follow-up radiologic examination is important.

Gas-Forming Agents

One other method of dislodging lower esophageal foreign bodies has been described in the literature. It consists of giving the patient a tartaric acid solution followed immediately by a solution of sodium bicarbonate. This combination creates a gas that helps push the impacted food into the stomach. Radiologists stock a similar gas-forming solution for use in upper gastrointestinal contrast studies.

Enzymatic Digestion

Agents that dissolve meat have been used independently or in conjunction with spasmolytics. Papain, a potent digestive enzyme found in Adolph's Meat Tenderizer, has been used to partially digest impacted pieces of meat that do not contain bone. To prepare papain, mix 2 teaspoons of Adolph's Meat Tenderizer in 240 ml of water. Twenty-milliliter sips of this mixture should be given every 20 to 30 minutes for a maximum of six doses. A drawback to enzymatic digestion is that if left too long in an obstructed esophagus, papain may also dissolve the patient's esophagus, creating a perforation. Therefore, it is mandatory that a follow-up esophagogram be obtained to check for any abnormalities of structure or function. Patients who do not obtain relief of obstruction by this method in 6 hours or less should be admitted for further treatment.

ESOPHAGEAL TRAUMA AND PERFORATION

Perforation of the esophagus may follow obstruction with foreign bodies, manipulation in attempted foreign body removal, or other medical instrumentation. Small animal bones or other eaten objects that become lodged in the esophagus are the most common cause of perforation. There are even cases of corn chips causing esophageal laceration. In addition, severe vomiting, hiccups, seizures, and penetrating or blunt trauma may result in esophageal perforation. Perforation of the esophagus should be suspected whenever there is penetrating injury of the neck or upper chest. Special mention should be made of the small button batteries found in calculators and watches. If these become lodged in the esophagus, they will deteriorate and eventually cause esophageal perforation. Therefore, it is mandatory that these objects be removed as soon as possible.

The suspicion of esophageal perforation must be based on history and physical examination. When patients present late, pain is generally a symptom and often described as being worse when swallowing. Other symptoms, such as fever, hoarseness, dysphagia, and respiratory distress, are not uncommon. On physical examination the neck may be stiff and tender. In addition, subcutaneous emphysema may be felt. A mediastinal crunch may be heard on auscultation of the chest. X-ray examinations may show subcutaneous emphysema in the neck or chest as evidenced by mediastinal widening. Barium swallow should be performed if there is any suspicion.

Esophageal perforation is a true emergency, and the patient's chance of survival depends on early diagnosis and aggressive treatment. Intravenous antibiotics (cepoxitin and clindamycin) must be administered immediately, as it takes time to achieve adequate antibiotic tissue levels. Patients should receive nothing orally and have a nasogastric tube placed for gastrointestinal suction. Since shock is a common complication, a large-bore intravenous line must be established and volume replacement given as needed. Blood studies, including type and cross-match, should be obtained early in the course, just as one would do for any trauma patient. In addition, surgical consultation should be obtained immediately. To ensure survival, aggressive treatment for esophageal perforations must be started within 6 to 12 hours. Therefore, hospitalization and careful monitoring are essential whenever esophageal perforation is suspected.

SUGGESTED READING

Cutton PB, Williams CB. Practical gastrointestinal endoscopy, 2nd ed. Oxford: Blackwell Scientific Publications, 1982.

Glauser J, Lilja GP, Greenfield B, Ruiz E. Intravenous glucagon in the management of esophageal food obstruction. JACEP 1979; 8:228–231.

Merslin H, Kubernick M. Corn chip laceration of the esophagus and evaluation of suspected esophageal perforation. Ann Emerg Med 1983; 12:455–457.

Pope CE. The esophagus. In: Sleisinger MD, Fortran JS. Gastrointestinal disease: pathophysiology, diagnosis, management. 2nd ed. Philadelphia: WB Saunders, 1978: 196, 495.

Sawyers JL, Lance CE, Foster JH, et al. Esophageal perforation, an increasing challenge. Ann Thorac Surg 1985; 19:233–238.

RECTAL TRAUMA AND FOREIGN BODY

SANTHAT NIVATVONGS, M.D., F.A.C.S.

RECTAL TRAUMA

Rectal injuries are much less common than colonic injuries. The incidence is about 10 percent of all cases of large bowel trauma. As with colonic injuries, penetrating injuries from gunshot wounds are the most common, followed by stab wounds and blunt trauma.

Diagnosis

Good history taking helps to pinpoint the diagnosis and helps in the approach to management. If the patient is alert and conscious, specific questions should be asked about the type of injury, and how and when it occurred. In an unconscious patient, information from witnesses at the scene can be valuable.

A rectal injury is suspected in all casualties with wounds of the lower abdomen, buttocks, perineum, and upper thigh. Pelvic fractures frequently traverse the rectum. Rectal trauma from anal intercourse or intentionally inserted foreign bodies may be seen, particularly in homosexual men. Rarely, sources of relatively high pressure entering the rectum (such as compressed air or high-speed water skiing injuries) can produce rectal tears. Proctoscopy or flexible sigmoidoscopy must be done. A hematoma in the submucosa or blood in the rectum is indicative of rectal injuries. Its extent must be carefully evaluated. Gastrografin enema limited to the rectum is helpful to rule out or to locate the site of the perforation.

Management

The basic principles in the management of injuries to the intraperitoneal portion of the rectum are the same for injuries of the colon (see chapter on *Colonic Trauma*).

In the extraperitoneal portion of the rectum, if perforation occurs the contaminant enters the perirectal spaces and not the peritoneal cavity. The basic principles in the management of injuries to the extraperitoneal portion of the rectum are (1) antibiotics to cover both aerobes and anaerobes as soon as possible, (2) repair or resection, (3) diverting colostomy, (4) washout of stool in the rectum, and (5) presacral drainage.

Iatrogenic perforation of the extraperitoneal portion of the rectum, as from an enema tip, usually requires only adequate drainage transrectally through the perforation site. A colostomy to divert the fecal stream is indicated in selected cases.

Injuries of the Perineum and the Anal Canal

Direct trauma to the perineum occurs in victims of falls from high places who land on their buttocks, in those hit from behind by an automobile, or in those who experience a straddle–type fall onto an object. It is an uncommon injury, but is associated with a high morbidity and mortality. This type of injury can be deceptive in that the underlying skin may be intact or exhibit only ecchymosis or hematoma. Associated injuries to the bony pelvis, rectum, urethra, and prostate must be sought by means of careful physical examination (including rectal), urinalysis, and usually x-ray examination of the pelvis. Women are less likely to have significant urinary tract injury than men unless there is a fracture. This topic is further discussed in the chapters on *Kidney, Ureter, and Bladder Trauma* and *Pelvic Fracture*.

FOREIGN BODY OF THE RECTUM

Foreign bodies of the rectum can occur from many causes; they can be ingested or they can be the result of inadvertent breakage of instruments inserted into the rectum by medical personnel. Drug smugglers may carry cocaine wrapped in plastic in the rectum (body packing); this poses the additional hazard of fatal cocaine toxicity if the bag is ruptured spontaneously or by attempts at removal. This chapter, however, will describe only the foreign bodies resulting from autoeroticism, which has become increasingly common.

Type of Objects

Objects that are found or extracted from the rectum vary greatly. The shape of the objects is most commonly elongated, oval, or round. Among the common objects used by homosexuals are drinking glasses, bottles, light bulbs, broomsticks, rubber or wooden dildos, vibrators, and fruits and vegetables such as apples, carrots, cucumbers, and zucchinis. The fists and even feet of sexual partners may also be used.

Evaluation

The most common complaints of affected patients are rectal pain and bleeding. The patient may not reveal the truth about the foreign body in the rectum initially until tactfully asked. Patients should be placed in a private area to keep them at ease and then questioned regarding the type of the object inserted, the number, duration, and any attempts to remove it, as well as the occurrence of pain on insertion and the use of drugs that might mask pain. Since many homosexuals perform enemas before insertion, perforation of the rectum may occur without the usual prompt peritoneal warning signs, owing to the lesser degree of peritoneal soiling.

The next step is to perform a digital examination and, if the object is not palpable, proctoscopy or flexible sigmoidoscopy. Care must be taken not to push the object higher in the rectum. The purpose of this examination is to determine the level of the object. No attempt should be made to remove the foreign body at this time without anesthesia, unless it is small and can be grasped with forceps or a clamp.

Plain abdominal films are indicated to determine the type, level, and number of objects, and to observe any free air in the abdomen. Rubber, fruits, and vegetables are difficult to see. A Gastrografin enema should be done if perforation is suspected.

Management

Extraction of foreign objects from the rectum requires common sense in using appropriate instruments and maneuvers for their removal. Unless the object is small, the anal canal and the pelvic muscles must be completely relaxed. Local, spinal, or general anesthesia can be used.

Efforts should not be made to remove packets of cocaine or other smuggled drugs without prior consultation with the poison center to determine the safest method. If the object is low-lying and can be felt with a finger, extraction can be attempted in the emergency department, clinic, or office under local anesthesia. Bupivacaine, 0.25 percent (with 1:200,000 epinephrine), or lidocaine, 0.5 percent (with 1:200,000 epinephrine), is the anesthetic solution of choice. A 30-gauge needle with a 3-cc syringe is used to infiltrate the subcutaneous tissue of the anal verge all around and the submucosa of the anal canal just above the dentate line. The anal canal is gradually and gently dilated to admit the whole hand if necessary. Depending on the type and the shape of the object, fingers, hand, tenaculum, and forceps can be used to grasp the foreign body. For a short and round object, large spoons or delivery forceps may help. The main difficulty in extraction of an object transanally is the strong vacuum from above created by pulling the object down. This can usually be overcome by bimanual manipulation, with one hand or forceps on the object in the anorectum and the other hand pressing the upper part of the object at the pubis or rectosigmoid colon. Passage of a couple of Foley catheters along the sides of the object into the upper rectum as a vent has been reported to eliminate the vacuum effect. A low-lying object in the rectum rarely requires an exploratory celiotomy.

In the case of a high-lying object, if there is no clinical evidence of peritonitis or perforation, bed rest and sedation for 12 to 24 hours can be tried. Most objects descend into the lower rectum and thus can be removed transanally. When the patient is put under general or spinal anesthesia, the high-lying object frequently descends to the anorectum. If an exploratory celiotomy becomes necessary, the object in the colon should be milked down to the anorectum and removed transanally. A colotomy is rarely required.

Autoerotic insertion of foreign bodies into the rectum rarely causes perforation. Most perforations occur as the result of inappropriate and vigorous attempts to remove them by the patient, friend, or physician. After the foreign body has been removed, the rectum and sigmoid colon must be examined by means of a proctoscope, a flexible sigmoidoscope, or, if necessary, a Gastrografin enema to rule out injury or perforation. The patient should be admitted to the hospital for observation as indicated. Perforation is treated as described for trauma of the rectum.

SUGGESTED READING

Eftaiha M, Hambrick E, Abcarian H. Principles of management of colorectal foreign bodies. Arch Surg 1977; 112:691–695.
French GWG, Sherlock DJ, Holl-Allen RTJ. Problems with rectal foreign bodies. Br J Surg 1985; 72:243–244.
Haas PA, Fox TA Jr. Civilian injuries of the rectum and anus. Dis Colon Rectum 1979; 22:17–23.
Trunkey D, Hays RJ, Shires GT. Management of rectal trauma. J Trauma 1973; 13:411–415.

COLONIC TRAUMA

SANTHAT NIVATVONGS, M.D., F.A.C.S.

Management of colonic injuries is usually complex because of the multiple systems involved in most cases. A proper and logical approach to these patients requires an understanding of the type and location of injury, surgical options available, and morbidity and mortality that can occur.

Some of these patients are selected for primary repair; others are kept under close observation. Computed tomography of the abdomen in cases of abdominal trauma helps in the assessment of the extent of injury and permits more confident nonoperative treatment.

This chapter will discuss the injuries of the colon in civilians, but will exclude the iatrogenic injuries (Table 1).

The extent of injury and the incidence of associated organ involvement vary according to the types and the severity of the injuries. Knowing the mode of injury can help one to plan the evaluation and management of each case. Penetrating trauma of the large bowel is more common than blunt trauma. Gunshot wounds are the most common cause of injury, followed by stab wounds, blunt trauma, and shotgun wounds.

Typically, men are victims more often than women, the ratio being 5:1 to 10:1. Most injuries occur in the younger age group, between 20 and 35 years.

TABLE 1 Types of Colonic Injury

Penetrating trauma	Blunt trauma
Gunshot wounds	Crush injuries
Stab wounds	Seat belts
Shotgun wounds	

ASSOCIATED INJURIES

As important as, or even more important than, the injuries to the colon itself are the associated injuries to both intra-abdominal and extra-abdominal organs. These are the main determinants of outcome. The morbidity and mortality rates in patients with large bowel injuries rise steeply with the increase in number of organs injured. As a result, they have dictated the approach to management. The mortality of large bowel injuries is between 0 and 1 percent, compared with 3 to 14 percent when other organs are also involved. In 15 to 25 percent of cases, the colon is the only organ involved. In 95 percent, the colon is injured in single areas, and in 5 percent, multiple separated areas of the colon are involved. The incidence of multiple organ injuries depends on the type of injuries. With gunshot wounds of the large bowel, other organs are involved in 85 percent of cases; stab wounds, 46 percent; blunt injuries, 85 percent; and shotgun wounds, 100 percent.

The commonly associated intra-abdominal injuries are those of the small intestine, liver, stomach, major vessels, kidneys, spleen, pancreas, duodenum, mesentery, diaphragm, and urinary bladder.

The commonly associated extra-abdominal injuries are those of the chest, head and neck, soft tissues, and peripheral vascular system, and fractures.

INITIAL ASSESSMENT AND RESUSCITATION

The victim should be resuscitated in the usual fashion for trauma patients (see chapters dealing with resuscitation).

Broad-spectrum antibiotics (including an aminoglycoside) should be started as soon as the initial resuscitation has succeeded. Later, appropriate prophylaxis against tetanus is instituted.

DIAGNOSIS

A good history helps to pinpoint the diagnosis and helps in the approach to management. If the patient is alert and conscious, specific questions should be asked about the type of injury and how and when the injury occurred. If the patient is unconscious, information from witnesses at the scene can be valuable.

Examination of the entire body and systems will give clues to possible organ involvement and the severity of the injury. Seat-belt marks or even tire marks may be apparent. The sites of entrance and exit of the bullet and knowledge of the type of weapon used may give some indication of the organs that might be injured.

Roentgenograms may demonstrate intraperitoneal air under the diaphragm or air in the extraperitoneal tissues, an indication of a perforated viscus. Plain films of the abdomen may also reveal enlargement of organs such as subcapsular hematoma of the liver and spleen. Fractures of the spine and pelvis can usually be confirmed or ruled out. Bullets and certain kinds of foreign bodies also may be apparent. In many cases, x-ray examinations of other parts of the body are also indicated to rule out or confirm associated injuries. Gastrografin enema is rarely indicated in cases of colonic injury.

Peritoneal lavage is indicated when it is not obvious whether there is any intraperitoneal injury, particularly when patients have associated head injuries or when drugs preclude a dependable physical examination. The overall accuracy rate is about 97 percent. The false-positive and false-negative rates are less than 2 percent, and the complication rate is less than 1 percent. Most importantly, it is highly reliable when negative, providing strong evidence that there is no significant intraperitoneal injury. However, peritoneal lavage is not accurate in the diagnosis of retroperitoneal injuries, as in the retroperitoneal part of the colon, pancreas, duodenum, kidneys, and blood vessels. Therefore, injuries of the flank and back require a celiotomy (See chapter on *Trauma to the Flank and Buttocks*).

All gunshot wounds of the abdomen should be explored whether or not penetration is evident. Shock waves from nonpenetrating gunshot wounds of the abdominal wall can easily transect the bowel or lacerate the liver or spleen without entering the abdominal cavity.

CT scan of the abdomen has largely replaced radionuclide scintigraphy, angiography, and ultrasonography in the evaluation of blunt abdominal trauma. It should be done with intravenous infusion of contrast medium and orally administered diluted Gastrografin solution. The entire abdomen should be scanned. When properly performed, CT scan can define the source of injury and the extent of injury to both intra- and extraperitoneal organs.

MANAGEMENT

All stab wounds of the abdomen with obvious intraperitoneal insult, as noted on physical examination, require an immediate celiotomy. If the extent of injury is not certain, the wound should be explored under local anesthesia. If the depth of the wound shows no evidence of penetration of the abdominal wall fascia, the patient can be discharged. However, if the depth of the wound cannot be seen or if the anterior abdominal wall fascia is penetrated, peritoneal lavage is performed. If the lavage results show red blood cells less than 1,000 per milliliter, the patient can be observed for 24 hours. If there are more than 1,000 red blood cells per milliliter in the lavage solution, celiotomy should be performed. This approach has resulted in less than 10 percent negative celiotomies and no missed injuries.

Virtually all low-velocity gunshot wounds of the abdomen require a celiotomy, whether or not the penetration into the abdominal cavity is evident, because the shock waves and the blast effect of the bullets can injure the underlying organs. However, closed observations have been successfully reported in selected cases of low-velocity gunshot wounds of the abdomen in which careful examination showed no evidence of intraperitoneal insult.

Patients who have experienced blunt trauma to the abdomen and in whom there are no peritoneal signs and the peritoneal lavage is negative can be kept under observation.

Surgical management of colonic injuries must be tailored to the type and severity of injury.

The wartime policy of avoiding primary repair and anastomosis by doing resection and colostomy markedly improved the morbidity and mortality rates following colonic trauma. Recently, some experts have suggested primary repair of civilian colonic injuries in selected cases. Proper selection of patients for the primary repair must be largely confined to those with solitary injury and minimal intra-abdominal contamination.

The "gold standard" of resection, with the proximal end brought out as a colostomy and the distal end closed or brought out as a mucous fistula, must be observed in patients with severe injuries or with heavy contamination. The decision is made regardless of involvement of the left or the right colon. Circumstantial evidence suggests that the right colon injuries do not have a better healing capacity than the left colon, as was previously believed.

In cases in which the criteria are not well defined, the injured area is repaired and then brought out like a colostomy under a rod or a fascia bridge. The exteriorized segment of the colon must be brought out without tension. The transverse and sigmoid colon are more suitable to this technique. If there is no leak, the exteriorized segment of the bowel can be dropped back into the abdominal cavity within 1 to 2 weeks, and thus the morbidity and mortality associated with colostomy closure is avoided. If the exteriorized colon leaks, it can then be converted into a colostomy. The success rate in avoiding colostomy with this approach is 50 to 70 percent.

About 50 to 60 percent of colonic wounds lend themselves to primary closure; in about 30 percent of cases, an ileostomy or colostomy is indicated. The remaining 15 percent are suitable for exteriorization of the repaired segment.

Criteria for Obligatory Colostomy

There are certain conditions in which bowel anastomotic leaking is inevitable if primary repair is undertaken. A diverting colostomy must be done in the following circumstances: (1) shock; preoperative blood pressure lower than 80/60; (2) intraperitoneal blood loss more than 1,000 ml; (3) more than two intra-abdominal organ systems injured; (4) significant peritoneal soilage with feces; (5) time interval from injury to operation longer than 8 hours; (6) colon wound so destructive as to require resection; and (7) loss of sufficient abdominal wall to require mesh replacement.

SUGGESTED READING

Oreskovich MR, Carrico CJ. Stab wounds of the anterior abdomen. Ann Surg 1983;198:411—419.
Stone HH, Fabian TC. Management of perforating colon trauma. Randomization between primary closure and exteriorization. Ann Surg 1979; 190:430–436.
Walt AJ. Management of injuries of the colon and rectum. In:McClean LD, ed. Advances in surgery.Chicago:Year Book Med Publishers, 1983:277.

TRAUMA IN PREGNANCY

JEFFREY C. KING, M.D.

The reported increase in maternal trauma during pregnancy is a result of both heightened awareness by health care providers and increased exposure of the gravid woman to potential trauma-causing activities. The segment of the population most vulnerable to death from trauma includes those in the reproductive years, ages 15 to 40 years. Trauma is the leading cause of nonobstetric maternal death, and as therapy for other medical and obstetric conditions improves, it will account for a greater percentage of maternal and perinatal mortality. The exact incidence of trauma during pregnancy, ranging from minor to catastrophic, is unknown, but trauma is estimated to occur in 5 to 10 percent of pregnancies. Traumatic injury is most likely to occur during the third trimester (52 percent) compared with the second (40 percent) and first trimesters, (8 percent). The three major sources of injury are vehicular accidents, falls, and piercing instruments.

PHYSIOLOGIC CHANGES IN PREGNANCY

The emergency physician, trauma surgeon, and obstetrician obviously have to care for these patients with increasing frequency. The team approach is essential to optimize the outcome for both the mother and her unborn child. Although an extensive review of the anatomic and physiologic changes that occur during pregnancy is impractical, it is appropriate to point out those changes that may alter the types of injury pregnant women receive and the diagnosis and treatment of pregnant trauma victims compared with those of the nonpregnant victim.

Fetal loss resulting from trauma in the first trimester is rare because the developing fetus is protected by the bony pelvis, the uterus, and the amniotic fluid. During the second and third trimesters, the uterus expands beyond the pelvis, becoming an abdominal organ. The enlarging uterus is then vulnerable to abdominal trauma, which may injure either the uterus or the fetus, or both.

Pregnancy results in early and extensive alterations of the cardiovascular system, beginning with a 45 to 50 percent mean increase in blood volume and a corresponding decrease in peripheral vascular resistance. Cardiac output increases during the first trimester; it peaks at 40 percent above the nonpregnant level by the end of the second trimester and remains stable at that level until term. A 15 percent increase in pulse rate is expected with values of 80 to 95 beats per minute considered normal. Both systolic pressure and diastolic blood pressure decrease by 5 to 15 mm Hg during the second trimester, and then return to nonpregnant values near term.

These changes affect the evaluation of blood loss, the diagnosis of shock, and volume replacement in the pregnant victim. The classic sign of hypovolemia and hypoperfusion—cold and clammy skin—may not occur in pregnancy because of these physiologic changes. Up to 35 percent of the pregnant woman's blood volume may be lost before symptoms of hypotension develop. Similarly, the patient may maintain her own perfusion at the expense of uteroplacental perfusion, which leads to fetal asphyxia. The supine position should always be avoided because the growing uterus may obstruct inferior vena cava blood flow to the heart, thus resulting in the supine hypotension syndrome.

The most prominent changes in the respiratory system are an increase in tidal volume and a 50 percent increase in minute ventilation in excess of oxygen consumption and carbon dioxide production. Arterial blood gases reveal lower Pco_2 values (approximately 32 torr) and relative respiratory alkalosis, whereas Po_2 values are not substantially altered. Lung volumes and capacities are essentially unchanged by pregnancy, with the exception of functional residual capacity, which is decreased. The increased oxygen consumption and decreased functional residual capacity make the pregnant woman more susceptible to rapid induction of general anesthesia and to hypoxia resulting from oxygen deprivation.

Gastric motility is reduced, and emptying time is prolonged in the obstetric patient. These factors result in an increased risk of aspiration when the pregnant trauma victim is unconscious or when general anesthesia is induced. Insertion of a protective nasogastric tube is therefore necessary. The intestines are progressively pushed into the upper abdomen by the enlarging uterus. Although this tends to protect them from injury, when the upper abdomen is involved, the risk for damage to multiple bowel segments is higher. The sensitivity to peritoneal irritation from blood, feces, bile, urine, or bacteria may be diminished as a result of the stretching of the abdominal wall and loculation of abdominal areas by the enlarging uterus. This anatomic change may make paracentesis more dangerous and less diagnostic for the pregnant woman.

The uterus increases in weight from 70 g to 1,000 to 1,200 g during pregnancy, with blood flow approximately 500 to 700 ml per minute at term. Uterine blood flow has no autoregulating system and depends on maternal perfusion pressure. The growth of the uterus during the second and third trimesters predisposes it to a greater probability of injury resulting from either blunt or penetrating trauma. Additionally, such injury may result in extensive intraperitoneal or retroperitoneal hemorrhage or placental abruption.

ACUTE MANAGEMENT AND STABILIZATION

The basic principles of trauma management apply equally well to the pregnant and the nonpregnant patient. The most important action is to resuscitate the mother even before completing the diagnosis. The ABCs of resuscitation (airway, breathing, and circulation) are unchanged by coexistent pregnancy.

At the Scene of Injury

Avoiding the supine hypotension syndrome is essential. This is done by displacing the uterus off the inferior vena cava by positioning the patient on her left side or by placing a pillow or folded towel under her right hip. If a neck injury is suspected, the neck should be stabilized with a brace and the victim secured to a backboard. The entire backboard should then be tilted to prevent inferior vena cava compression by the uterus. Evaluation of ventilatory and cardiovascular status and initiation of appropriate cardiopulmonary resuscitation (CPR) are mandatory.

The airway should be cleared and oral endotracheal intubation should be performed if the patient is unconscious or has experienced a thoracic injury. Cricothyroidotomy may be necessary to establish an emergency airway. If no pulse is felt, external cardiac massage should be initiated using the standard technique. A large-bore peripheral venous catheter should be inserted, and in cases of overt hemorrhage, lactated Ringer's solution in a 3:1 replacement ratio for estimated maternal blood loss is essential to prevent fetal hypoxia or asphyxia. Vasopressors should generally not be used because they may further decrease uterine perfusion and worsen the fetal status. After adequate volume replacement, if a vasopressor becomes necessary, ephedrine, metaraminol bitartrate, or dopamine hydrochloride is the drug of choice. Obviously, all vascular injuries must be controlled by direct pressure with a gloved finger or by clamping. The use of pneumatic antishock garment (PASG) or military antishock trousers (MAST) is indicated to effect an autotransfusion of whole blood and increase peripheral vascular resistance. Only leg portions should be applied, since inflation of the abdominal section is likely to decrease uterine blood flow. At this point, transportation to the nearest trauma center by either helicopter or ambulance is indicated.

In the Emergency Department

As resuscitation proceeds, a careful history (often obtained from a family member or witness) and physical examination should be performed. Injuries to the head, chest, or abdomen, fractures, and entrance and exit wounds from gunshots or knives should be documented. Tension pneumothorax or cardiac tamponade should be sought and treated. Aspiration is avoided by placement of a nasogastric tube. However, if rhinorrhea from cerebrospinal fluid (CSF) leakage is suspected, the oral route should be used.

The adequacy of volume replacement can be assessed by insertion of either a central venous pressure catheter or Swan-Ganz catheter. A Foley catheter should be inserted not only to evaluate the adequacy of renal perfusion, but also to determine whether hematuria is present. Type-specific packed red blood cells should be transfused when blood loss in excess of 1,000 cc is estimated. Attention to Rh status is essential, since it relates not only to the current pregnancy, but also to possible future pregnancies. When time precludes the use of type-specific or cross-matched blood, type O Rh negative blood should be used.

The uterus should be carefully examined to evaluate fetal size and viability, to check for tenderness or rigidity, and to assess the presence of uterine contractions. Uterine rupture may occur in late pregnancy if a direct blow compresses the uterus against the spine, such as might occur if the victim is wearing a seat belt across the uterus. A narrow erythematous contusion matching the width of the belt often identifies the placement of the seat belt. Pelvic examination should be performed to determine cervical status and to assess for bleeding and/or rupture of membranes. Continuous electronic fetal monitoring should be instituted as soon as practical to provide a continuing evaluation of the fetal status.

After pregnancy has entered the second trimester, needle paracentesis is less accurate and more dangerous. The open peritoneal lavage technique is uniquely suited to the gravid patient and has a 98 percent accuracy in diagnosing occult intra-abdominal bleeding. A small infra- or supraumbilical incision, depending on uterine size, is made and the peritoneum is visualized. A peritoneal dialysis catheter is directed toward the pelvis and aspiration is attempted; if more than 10 cc of blood is obtained, the test is considered positive. If aspiration is unsuccessful, 1,000 cc of lactated Ringer's solution is infused into the abdomen and then drained through the dialysis catheter. Findings considered positive for intraperitoneal injury and hemorrhage include grossly bloody lavage fluid through either the Foley or chest tube, a red blood cell count greater than 100,000 per cubic millimeter, a white blood cell count greater than 500 per cubic millimeter, or an amylase level greater than 175 per deciliter. Negative findings are a red cell count less than 50,000 per cubic millimeter, a white cell count less than 100 per cubic millimeter, or an amylase less than 75 per deciliter.

The next special consideration for obstetric trauma patients is the appropriate use of diagnostic x-ray studies. Radiologic studies must not be withheld if their omission would compromise accurate diagnosis and optimal care. However, coordination of these studies is essential so that the least possible radiation exposure occurs. Attention must be paid to uterine shielding whenever possible. Utilization of various ultrasound techniques to evaluate the abdominal organs and major vessels can minimize ionizing irradiation.

Broad-spectrum antibiotics should be started in the case of obvious intestinal injury or an open fracture. Tetanus prophylaxis should be administered according to the guidelines proposed by the American College of Surgeons. Patients who had initial immunization but no booster within 7 to 10 years should receive 0.5 ml of toxoid. Previously immunized patients who have extensive tissue necrosis and nonimmunized patients should receive a complete toxoid schedule plus 250 mg of human tetanus immune globulin. If incomplete debridement or delay in therapy becomes evident, broad-spectrum antibiotics should be added to the treatment regimen.

Specific laboratory tests including complete blood count, platelet count, prothrombin time, partial thromboplastin time, fibrinogen, fibrin split products, electrolytes, liver function studies, blood urea nitrogen, creatinine, amylase, Kleihauer-Betke stain*, and type and crossmatch should be obtained, depending on the extent of trauma. Arterial blood gases are helpful to evaluate mental status and adequacy of cardiopulmonary function.

All personnel involved in the care of obstetric trauma victims should realize the high possibility for legal action. It is, therefore, essential that extensive, accurate records be kept regarding type of trauma, treatment at the scene, physical examination and laboratory findings,

---

* Kleihauer, Braun, and Betke developed an accurate, sensitive method to differentiate fetal red cells from adult red cells. This acid elution test is of great value in determining the incidence and size of fetal transplacental hemorrhage at various gestational ages, at delivery, and following various obstetric procedures and/or complications. The test is based on the fact that citric acid-phosphate buffer at pH 3.5 elutes hemoglobin from adult but not from fetal red blood cells. After smears of maternal blood have been processed by the Kleihauer test, 100 fields are scanned. Adult red cells are colorless; fetal red cells are bright purple-pink. The Kleihauer-Betke (K-B) test is particularly useful for identifying those Rh-negative mothers who have received a massive transfusion of Rh-positive blood from the fetus as a result of severe trauma or placental abruption.

therapeutic maneuvers, and the patient's response. Obviously, appropriate consultation should be made, depending on the extent of injury and organ system involvement.

DISPOSITION

After stabilization and treatment, patients requiring further evaluation and monitoring should be admitted to the intensive care unit. Once the mother has been stabilized, attention must be turned to monitoring the fetus for signs of premature labor or placental abruption. These complications are most likely to occur during the first 24 to 48 hours following the trauma episode. Continuous electronic fetal monitoring is recommended for the first 24 to 48 hours following significant trauma. Fetal distress diagnosed by means of electronic fetal monitoring may provide the earliest warning of maternal hypovolemia and shock. After even minor maternal trauma, fetal compromise and/or death may occur. Therefore, no pregnant trauma victim whose fetus is of potentially viable gestational age should be released before normal antepartum fetal heart rate testing is documented.

The incidence of fetomaternal hemorrhage following trauma is unknown, but fetal death may occur within 1 week, possibly owing to chronic fetomaternal transfusion. Serial Kleihauer-Betke tests should be obtained over the next 4 to 7 days to determine the extent of fetomaternal transfusion. If there is a fetomaternal bleed, and if the mother is Rh negative, an appropriate amount of Rh immune globulin should be administered.

A pregnant woman with minor trauma should be admitted when there is vaginal bleeding, uterine irritability, abdominal tenderness, abdominal pain, hypovolemia, leakage of amniotic fluid, or change in or absence of fetal heart tones. If admission is not deemed necessary, the mother should be instructed to record fetal movements over the next week. If the patient notes fewer than four movements per monitored hour, her obstetrician should be contacted immediately and a nonstress test should be performed. Fetal heart rate testing and a biophysical profile should be repeated approximtely 24 to 48 hours following the trauma episode.

Transfer of the patient should be considered if the original treating facility is not fully equipped to deal with the potential neurologic, cardiopulmonary, abdominal, orthopaedic, and obstetric complications that may develop. Additionally, plans must be made for the possible birth of a premature and/or traumatically injured neonate. Facilities and personnel to deal with this eventuality must be immediately available.

POSTMORTEM CESAREAN SECTION

Despite aggressive and exhaustive resuscitative efforts, a pregnant trauma victim may expire with her fetus alive and in utero. If the fetus has reached a potentially viable gestational age, rapid postmortem cesarean section may be life-saving for the unborn child. The chances for favorable neonatal outcome depend on fetal maturity, extent of fetal injury from the accident, and speed of delivery. If the interval between maternal death and delivery is less than 10 minutes, the chance for neonatal survival is good; however, with a delay of more than 20 minutes, a favorable outcome is rarely achieved. If maternal death has been confirmed, maternal CPR should be continued until delivery is performed. Open-chest CPR can provide much better cardiac output if the abdomen cannot be opened immediately.

The technique for the performance of a postmortem cesarean section should emphasize cautious speed, since the length of time between maternal death and delivery is prognostic of fetal outcome. Preparations for a postmortem cesarean section include consent of the family, gestational age of more than 28 weeks, immediate availability of personnel and equipment, continued postmortem ventilation and cardiac massage for the mother, and aggressive resuscitation of the infant. If possible, the consent of the next of kin should be obtained, but consent is implied in such a life-threatening situation when minutes count. A vertical midline incision is made from the umbilicus to the symphysis pubis. This is extended through the subcutaneous fat, rectus fascia, and rectus muscle, and the peritoneal cavity is entered. Delivery is rapidly ac-

complished by incising the uterine myometrium directly beneath the abdominal incision. This vertical incision into the thick upper uterine segment should be long enough to allow easy extraction of the fetus. Immediately following delivery, the fetus is suctioned and the umbilical cord is clamped and cut. The infant is then handed to the awaiting neonatologist or anesthesiologist for resuscitation. Infants delivered under these conditions invariably require extensive resuscitation, and appropriate neonatal consultation should be obtained as quickly as possible.

SUGGESTED READING

Buchsbaum HJ. Trauma in pregnancy. Philadelphia: WB Saunders, 1979.
Crosby W. Trauma during pregnancy: maternal and fetal injury. Obstet Gynecol Sur 1974; 29:683–699.
Haycock CE. Trauma and pregnancy. Littleton: PSG Publishing, 1985.
Katz M. Maternal trauma during pregnancy. In: Creasy RK, Resnick R, eds. Maternal-fetal medicine. Philadelphia: WB Saunders, 1984.
Levin JP Jr, Polsky SS. Abdominal trauma during pregnancy. Clin Perinatol 1983; 10:423–438.

THERMAL AND CHEMICAL BURNS

ALAN R. DIMICK, M.D.,F.A.C.S.

Most burns are minor and can be handled by most physicians. However, extensive burns usually require intensive long-term care in a specialized burn care facility. The initial treatment of these burns is often critical to their outcome, and that is the primary purpose of this discussion.

Roughly 90 percent of all burn injuries are due to thermal injuries such as flame and scald burns. Chemical burns account for 5 percent and electrical burns for 2 percent of all burns.

THE SKIN IN RELATION TO BURNS

Skin is composed of two layers, an outer epidermis and a deeper dermis. The epidermis is composed of flat cells that are impervious to water and therefore keep body fluids within the body and foreign materials such as bacteria outside the body. The dermis literally is the glue that holds the epidermis to the rest of the body. Within the dermis are blood vessels and nerves as well as collagen

and elastic fibers. At the deepest level of the epidermis is the germinal layer, which is constantly proliferating epidermal cells to replace those lost on the outer surface. It is estimated that approximately 40 percent of the surface epithelium is lost in the normal individual every 24 hours. Hair follicles and sweat glands are extremely important in the healing of second-degree burns, since they extend from the outer layer of the epidermis down into the depths of the dermis. They play a critical role in second-degree burns because they have epidermal cells lining them.

Depth of Burn

Classically burns are defined as first-, second-, and third-degree burns. An example of first-degree burn is a typical sunburn in which the skin is red, hot, swollen, and tender. The nerve endings are irritated, and therefore the area is hypersensitive to any stimulus. First-degree burns usually heal in 7 days with characteristic peeling of the dead skin.

Second-degree burns typically have blister formation and destruction of all layers of epidermis, including the germinal layer. However, the dermis is preserved; therefore this is also a partial-thickness burn. The epidermal lining of hair follicles and sweat glands provides foci for regeneration of the lost epithelium, a process that usually takes about 14 days. However, healing does not occur if infection occurs because infection destroys the hair follicles and sweat glands, converting the burn to a full-thickness third-degree burn. Second-degree burns are red, hot, swollen, and very tender with blister formation. The nerve endings are irritated and therefore the area is hypersensitive.

The third-degree burn involves all layers of the skin with coagulation and destruction; nerve endings are destroyed. Therefore, this burn, although it looks bad, is not painful initially. The patient has the sensation of touch, but does not have any pain in the area of the full-thickness third-degree burn. Since all skin layers have been destroyed (full-thickness burn), there is nothing from which to regenerate epithelium. After this dead tissue sloughs, the area must be covered by skin grafting.

Any patient may have all three depths of injury in the burn area, and the appearance may evolve over days. In actual experience, it is often difficult to distinguish between second- and third-degree burns. However, this usually makes little difference, since they are usually treated in the same way.

Estimation of Extent of Burn Injury

The usual estimation for surface area of burn in an adult is the Rule of Nines. The body surface is divided into areas of multiples of 9 percent: head and neck, 9 percent; each upper extremity from shoulder to fingertips, 9 percent; anterior surface of the trunk of the body, 18 percent; posterior surface of the trunk of the body, 18 percent; and each lower extremity from groin to toes, 18 percent. The perineum and genitalia make up the final 1 percent to total 100 percent.

In small children the head is larger in proportion to the lower extremities, and so in the newborn child, the head alone is 16 percent. As the child grows and develops into adulthood, the percentages are removed from the head and transferred to the lower extremities. The Lund and Browder chart for estimation of the extent of burn is more precise (Fig. 1).

FLUID RESUSCITATION

Burn shock is a form of hypovolemic shock. The natural reaction of the body to any kind of injury is edema formation. The edema fluid comes primarily from the circulating blood volume, specifically the plasma fraction. The larger the area of injury, the more fluid lost from the circulating blood volume. Early after the burn vasoconstriction occurs to compensate for this fluid loss, but as the loss continues, hypotension results. The larger the burn, the more severe the fluid loss. Burn shock starts immediately after the injury.

The fluid recommended for replacement of the lost plasma is Ringer's lactate. There have been numerous formulas for fluid replacement. The 1978 National Institute of General Medical Sciences (NIGMS) Burn Consensus Conference recommended a guideline for the first 24 hours after burn, which means it is calculated from the actual time of the injury, not from the time the patient arrives in the hospital emergency department. The formula recommends 2 to 4 ml of Ringer's lactate times the body weight of the patient in kilograms times the actual percent of body surface area burned. This gives the total amount of fluids that should be administered in the first 24 hours after burn. Half the calculated amount is given in the first 8 hours following the burn, one-quarter of this amount in the second 8 hours, and the final quarter in the final or third 8 hours following the burn.

The primary indicator of how well the fluid resuscitation is progressing is the hourly urine output, which ideally averages 50 ml per hour in adults and correspondingly less in children. The central venous pressure usually is negative or at least zero during the first 12 to 24 hours following burn, unless there is preexisting cardiac failure or another problem. Therefore, in general, the central venous pressure is not a good measure of the adequacy of early fluid resuscitation.

The urine should be evaluated carefully for its color. Deep burns may cause damage to red cells, releasing hemoglobin, or to muscle, releasing myoglobin. Should either of these pigments appear in the urine, it is important to flush them through the kidney as quickly as possible before they are precipitated in the renal tubules, causing acute renal failure. An osmotic diuretic is given, usually mannitol, 12.5 g by IV bolus and 12.5 g placed in each bottle of intravenous fluid until the urine has cleared. *Caution*: One must not be misled by an initial clear urine specimen since this may have already been in the bladder at the time the patient was burned. As the patient responds to treatment of shock, perfusion of damaged areas may pick up these pigments. It is important to observe the urine for the first several hours after initiating resuscitation to be sure that the urine remains clear.

CONSTRICTING BURNS OF EXTREMITIES OR CHEST

Eschar is the term used for coagulated skin in the third-degree burn. Constricting and circumferential burns of an extremity act as a tourniquet. The low-pressure venous system is occluded first by the constricting eschar; the higher-pressure arterial inflow continues until the tissue pressure from the edema equals the arterial pressure. This results in circulatory impairment with cyanosis and pain distally. If not corrected, this constriction results in ischemia, necrosis, and gangrene.

The simple procedure to prevent such a dreadful occurrence is basically the same as that used when an orthopaedic cast is too tight. The cast is usually split to remove this constriction. An opening in the eschar (escharotomy) is done with a scalpel in the area of the full-thickness third-degree burns. No anesthetic is necessary because all nerve endings have been destroyed. The incision is usually made on the medial and/or lateral aspect of the extremity. If one incision does not give adequate decompression of the constriction, a second incision is required. The incision is just through the eschar and not down into the subcutaneous tissue or fascia. Be sure there is full release of the constriction proximally.

Do not try to clamp or coagulate bleeding vessels immediately. The venous hypertension should be allowed to subside by elevating the extremity above heart level for 3 to 5 minutes. Then the extremity is lowered, and

Area	Age (Years)					% 2°	% 3°	% Total
	0-1	1-4	5-9	10-15	Adults			
Head	19	17	13	10	7			
Neck	2	2	2	2	2			
Ant. Trunk	13	17	13	13	13			
Post. Trunk	13	13	13	13	13			
R. Buttock	2½	2½	2½	2½	2½			
L. Buttock	2½	2½	2½	2½	2½			
Genitalia	1	1	1	1	1			
R. U. Arm	4	4	4	4	4			
L. U. Arm	4	4	4	4	4			
R. L. Arm	3	3	3	3	3			
L. L. Arm	3	3	3	3	3			
R. Hand	2½	2½	2½	2½	2½			
L. Hand	2½	2½	2½	2½	2½			
R. Thigh	5½	6½	8½	8½	9½			
L. Thigh	5½	6½	8½	8½	9½			
R. Leg	5	5	5½	6	7			
L. Leg	5	5	5½	6	7			
R. Foot	3½	3½	3½	3½	3½			
L. Foot	3½	3½	3½	3½	3½			
				Total				

Weight _____
Height _____

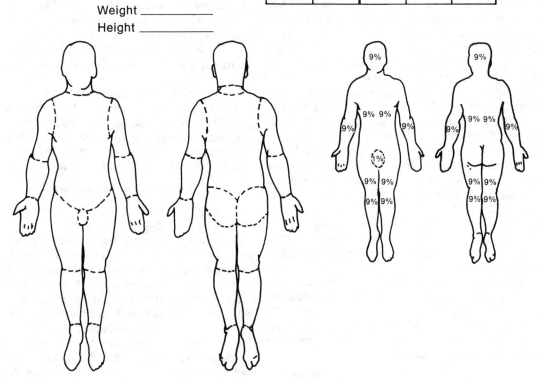

Figure 1 Lund and Browder chart. ''Rule of Nines'' divides the body surface into areas of approximately 9 percent or multiples of 9 percent; the head and neck and an upper extremity each represents 9 percent; a lower extremity and the front and back of the torso each represents 18 percent; the perineum one percent. This method of estimation is sufficiently accurate for emergency situations. It is modified in children from birth to 1 year of age to allow 19 percent for the head and neck and 13 percent for each lower extremity. One percent is subtracted from the head and neck and added to the lower extremities for each year from ages 1 to 10.

major bleeding points can be clamped or coagulated. Treatment of the escharotomy wound is the same as that for the adjacent burn wounds. No special treatment is required.

Constricting circumferential burns of the chest are extremely important because they limit chest expansion. The vital capacity may be almost zero, depending on the severity of the constriction. This is especially important in children who have soft, pliable rib cages and are therefore more susceptible. This should be suspected in children who are hypoxic and may be combative. Escharotomies on the chest are usually done in each midclavicular line and also transversely to allow expansion of the chest cage. Watch the chest expand during respiration to determine whether additional escharotomies are needed. The dressing for the escharotomies is the same as for the adjacent burn.

EMERGENCY MANAGEMENT

The airway must be patent, and oxygen should be administered for at least the first 24 to 36 hours after injury. Nasotracheal intubation may be necessary if upper airway edema is suspected or impending. It is better to intubate than to wish you had. Intubation is preferred to emergency tracheostomy.

Dry sterile dressings should be applied to the burn. Wet dressings, cold dressings, and ice should *not* be applied to burns because of the danger of frostbite. Wet areas also give bacteria easier access to the burn wound. After dry sterile dressings are applied, the patient should be wrapped in some type of insulation (e.g., blanket) to conserve the patient's body heat. If ice or cool compresses are applied, the patient's core body temperature may drop precipitously and hypothermia may occur.

The patient should be given nothing by mouth, and a nasogastric tube should be placed to decompress the stomach. Patients with extensive burns have a paralytic ileus for the first 24 to 48 hours following the burn. Anything he or she is given to drink is quickly vomited. Because the burn patient is apprehensive, anxious, and fearful, he or she swallows a considerable amount of air, causing gastric distention. The patient who is in shock is thirsty and begs for water, but if given anything to drink, vomits and loses more body fluid. Too often, well-intentioned helpers have given patients fluids to drink during their transfer, and this has resulted in vomiting, aspiration, and death.

Tetanus prophylaxis should be given to patients with burn injury, predicated on the previous immunization history of the patient.

It should be remembered that obvious injuries may not be the only injuries. Patients with burns should be checked carefully for other injuries.

Pain

Despite the terrible appearance of third-degree burns, no pain is felt in these areas because the nerve endings have been destroyed. However, first- and second-degree burns are painful. The ideal drug to alleviate fear, apprehension, and anxiety as well as pain in the initial stages is morphine, given intravenously only. Since the patient is in shock, he should not receive any medications intramuscularly. I usually give 2 to 4 mg morphine every 2 to 3 hours as needed for pain.

Management of Blisters

Many physicians believe that covering the blister accelerates wound healing. Others have seen infection of the blister fluid, and therefore advocate removal of all blisters and the application of dressings. Recently, it has been found that blister fluid has a high concentration of prostaglandins, which cause local vasospasm, possibly converting the burns to deeper burns. For this reason, many now advocate complete removal of the blister and application of a dry dressing combined with the use of systemic aspirin because of its antiprostaglandin activity.

Topical Therapy of Burn Wounds

There are bacteria on human skin at all times. Therefore all burn wounds are contaminated, but not necessarily infected. Systemic antibiotics are not needed in the early stages of burn care. What is attempted is to control the concentration of bacteria in the burn wound by applying topical antibacterial agents to the burn wound. Currently the topical antibacterial agent most frequently used in burn units is silver sulfadiazine (Table 1), a sulfa compound in a white cream which is placed on the burn wound and the dressing is changed either once or twice a day. It is a typical sulfa drug with broad bacteriostatic activity.

It is best *not* to apply creams to burns of a patient who is going to be transferred to a burn care facility within the first 12 to 24 hours because when he arrives at that facility all dressings, including the cream, must be removed for the purpose of assessment. Only sterile sheets should be applied before transfer.

Tar and Asphalt Removal

These two materials are considered as one, since the management is the same for each. First, the immediate need is not to remove it, but to cool it, because diminishing the amount of heat diminishes the amount of tissue damage. This cooling usually permits removal of large chunks of the solidified material. The many solvents that can be used to remove the smaller pieces include, but are not limited to, lard, polysporin or neosporin ointments, mineral oil, silver sulfadiazine, and cold cream. There are also many commercial solvents available. The patient usually has been working with tar and has a favorite way of removing it. Therefore, ask the patient! A recent survey by the union of roofing workers revealed no national consensus regarding the best method of tar removal. If necessary, removal can be accomplished over several days.

TABLE 1 Topical Antimicrobial Agents

Agent	Composition	Application	Bacterial Spectrum	Resistance	Advantages	Disadvantages
Silver nitrate	0.5% solution of the inorganic silver salt AgNO₃, in distilled water	Moist compresses changed b.i.d. and saturated q4h Painless	Bacteriostatic to entire spectrum	None	No sensitivities Not inactivated by specific antagonists	Does not penetrate eschar well Dilutional hyponatremia and hypokalemia due to leaching of electrolytes into wound Discolors wound, unburned skin, and environment Hypochloremia due to AgCl precipitation
Mafenide acetate	Methylated sulfonamide, 11.1% suspension in a water dispersible cream base	Applied topically b.i.d. as a cream; medication washed off daily Painful for 20–30 minutes following application to 2nd degree burn	Bacteriostatic to entire spectrum, but minimally effective against staphylococci and fungi	Occasionally to staphylococci	Penetrates eschar well	Potent carbonic anhydrase inhibitor Tends to produce acidosis Sensitivity in 5% manifested by a maculopopular rash
Silver sulfadiazine	1% suspension in a hydrophilic cream base	Applied topically b.i.d. as a cream; medication washed off daily	Bacteriostatic to entire spectrum	Occasionally to *Pseudomonas* and Enterobacter	No significant effect on fluids or electrolytes	Penetrates eschar poorly Can cause granulocytosis

From Bunkis J, Walton RL. Burns. In: Trunkey DD, Lewis FR, eds. Current therapy of trauma. Toronto and Philadelphia: BC Decker, 1986.

TABLE 2 Protocol for Transfer to Burn Care Facility

Establish and maintain airway. Give oxygen.

Treat shock

Protect the burn wound by applying sterile dressings. Apply blankets to conserve body heat. No creams or ointments are needed for transfer.

Relieve pain—morphine is best, but IV only in small doses.

Decompress stomach with nasogastric tube.

Record all therapy and send copy with patient.

Discuss patient with receiving physician at the burn center on the telephone before transfer.

Chemical Burns

These burns are frequently the result of accidents in industry, which uses strong acids and alkalis to treat or clean materials. Minor burns are sometimes caused by wet cement, which is highly alkaline. The most important treatment is to remove the chemical from the body surface as quickly as possible, usually by diluting the chemical with water. Remove all clothing saturated by the chemical, since the longer it stays in contact with the body surface the more severe the tissue destruction. Do not waste time looking for an antidote to mix with the chemical, because the resulting third chemical may be more damaging than the first. Certain exceptions to the use of water to dilute the chemical are (1) dry chemicals, which should be brushed off the body surface, and (2) hydrofloric acid, which requires the injection of calcium salts into the area involved. Once the chemicals have been removed, the treatment is the same as for any other burn.

Gasoline is a chemical that causes irritation of the skin. Prolonged contact may cause second-degree burns with blister formation. If significant gasoline is absorbed through the skin, it is then excreted through the lungs, possibly causing pneumonia. Cement and concrete, in their liquid forms, can also cause burns when skin contact is prolonged. They contain a strong alkali and may cause second- and even third-degree burn injury, depending on the duration of contact.

OUTPATIENT BURN MANAGEMENT

In general, burns of less than 15 percent of the body surface in adults and less than 10 percent of the body sur-

face in children can be treated on an outpatient basis. However, there are certain conditions that preclude outpatient treatment of burns: burns of the hands, face, feet, perineum, and genitalia; inhalation injury; electrical burns; and concurrent severe medical problems. Also to be considered is whether the patient can care for himself or has someone to provide the necessary care. The home environment must be adequate, with running water and other essentials required for wound care. If these requirements are not in place, the burn wounds cannot be cleansed properly and infection of the burn is likely. In children, the possibility of child abuse should always be considered, and if likely, immediate notification of authorities is imperative before the patient leaves the department.

The application of dressings to treat minor burns in the outpatient setting is essential. The initial dressing usually is applied with a topical antibacterial agent and includes an absorbent material. The type of topical antibacterial agent depends on the preference of the attending physician; Silvadene is a frequent choice. The dressing is changed in 2 to 3 days, depending on the amount of drainage. Dressing changes every other day are usually required initially, and then, as healing occurs, they can be done less frequently. The patient or the patient's family may be instructed in this procedure, and the patient advised to return at weekly intervals for follow-up care in the physician's office, in the outpatient clinic, or, if necessary, back in the emergency department.

TRANSFER TO BURN CENTER

In general, the more complicated and extensive burns are best treated in a special burn care unit. If the patient is transfered, the protocal in Table 2 should be followed.

SUGGESTED READING

Proceedings of the NIH consensus development conference in supportive therapy in burn care. J Trauma 1979; 19:855–936.
Proceedings of the NIH conference. Frontiers in understanding burn injury. J Trauma 1984; 24:S1-S204.
Second conference on supportive therapy in burn care. J Trauma 1981; 21:665-752.
Specific optimal criteria for hospital resources for care of patients with burn injury. American Burn Association, April, 1984.

FLANK AND BUTTOCK TRAUMA

WILLIAM M. STAHL, M.D., F.A.C.S.
RAO R. IVATURY, M.D., F.A.C.S., F.R.C.S.(C)

The flank is the area located between the anterior and posterior axillary lines extending from the sixth intercostal space to the iliac crest. The buttock is the anatomic area bounded by the iliac crest, inferior gluteal fold, greater trochanter, and intergluteal fold.

Injuries to these regions owing to blunt trauma (fall, motor vehicle accident [MVA], or assault) or penetration from stab or missile wounds, may result in injury to intraperitoneal, retroperitoneal, or pelvic organs (Fig. 1). Retroperitoneal and pelvic organ trauma pose difficult problems in diagnosis.

CLINICAL EVALUATION

After initial resuscitation and control of life-threatening emergencies (e.g., associated chest trauma, hypovolemia), the patients are rapidly assessed (Fig. 2). The mechanism of injury should be brought to light during the history, if possible, since it may provide a clue to the organs injured. Other important aspects of the history include tetanus immunization status, allergies, and significant medical illnesses.

Examination of the patient should follow the pattern of rapid initial evaluation and complete secondary survey. It is important to disrobe the patient completely since the back and the perineal and gluteal regions are often overlooked and may hide important clues such as wounds of entry, ecchymosis and/or hematomas. Palpation of the abdomen is carried out to elicit signs of peritoneal irritation: tenderness, rigidity, mass. The back is palpated for costovertebral tenderess and deformities of the spine. The pelvis is compressed to elicit tenderness from a pelvic fracture.

The secondary survey is a thorough examination of the total patient from head to toe. At this stage, a nasogastric tube is inserted and the nature of gastric contents noted. Rectal examination may provide important evidence of injury: blood at the anal orifice (rectal injury) and a high-riding prostate (urethral injury). Careful inspection for penile hematoma, blood at the urethral meatus, or scrotal hematoma should be routine. In the absence of these findings, Foley catheterization of the bladder is performed, and urine is examined for gross or microscopic hematuria.

DIAGNOSTIC INVESTIGATIONS

Sigmoidoscopy is indicated for all patients whose injury is associated with significant risk of rectal injury (e.g., bullet trajectory across the pelvis) and in patients with blood at the anal orifice or in the stool. It is the only definitive investigation for an extraperitoneal rectal perforation.

Other diagnostic tests that should be performed in all patients are summarized in Table 1.

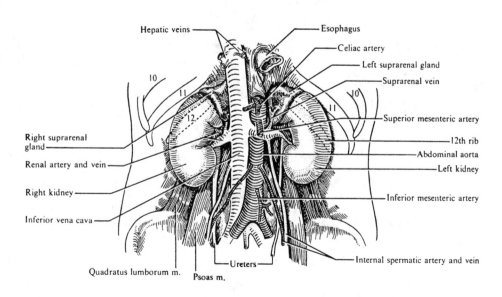

Figure 1 Retroperitoneal structures vulnerable to flank injury. (From Pansky, House. Review of gross anatomy. New York: MacMillan, 1975.)

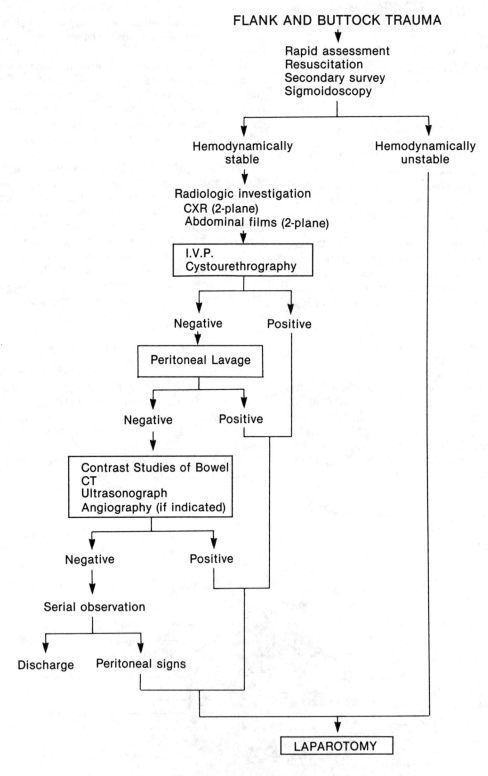

Figure 2 Management algorithm for flank and buttock trauma.

TABLE 1 Ancillary Diagnostic Tests

Biplanar chest roentgenograms

  Rib fractures: hemopneumothorax
  Indistinct diaphragmatic contour: rupture of diaphragm
  Free air under the diaphragm: viscus perforation

Biplanar abdominal film including pelvis

  Skeletal fractures: spine or the pelvic ring
  Abnormal gas pattern: duodenal rupture, free air from
    viscus perforation
  Soft tissue shadow: hematoma, obscuration of the psoas shadows
  Foreign bodies: bullet anterior to sacrum

TABLE 2 Radiologic Studies for Suspected Urologic Trauma

Study	Indications
Cystourethrogram (retrograde)	In all patients with blood at the meatus, penile or scrotal hematoma, or gross or microscopic hematuria
Intravenous pyelography	In all patients with gross or microscopic hematuria

The radiologic investigations in patients with gross or microscopic hematuria or clinical suspicion of genitourinary trauma are described in Table 2.

Patients with blunt trauma or stab wounds of the abdomen with no urgent indication for laparotomy should undergo peritoneal lavage (Table 3) after preliminary radiologic examination of the abdomen. All the patients with gunshot wounds with trajectory of the missile across the peritoneal cavity or pelvis require laparotomy.

Diagnostic laparotomy is indicated in patients with borderline hemodynamic stability, even in the face of negative diagnostic tests, and when a strong likelihood of significant retroperitoneal injury exists, as suggested by the trajectory of the bullet.

Other tests. Gastrografin series of the duodenum, contrast studies of the colon, and angiography should be carried out if there is a clinical suspicion of retroperitoneal injury to the duodenum, colon, and vascular structures. Computed tomography of the abdomen and ultrasonography are indicated in stable patients in whom retroperitoneal injury is suspected.

MANAGEMENT

In the pre-hospital phase, it is important that patients be transported to the hospital as expeditiously as is possible. Military Anti-Shock Trousers (MAST) is beneficial in splinting pelvic or extremity fractures.

TABLE 3 Peritoneal Lavage

Indications

  All patients with blunt trauma with disoriented mentation (e.g., alcohol or drug intoxication, severe head injury)
  All patients in whom physical signs cannot be relied on (e.g., spinal injury, extremely old or cachectic individuals)
  All patients with blunt injury or stab wound with clinical suspicion of intra-abdominal injury

Interpretation

  Positive if RBC count (spun) is more than 100,000 cells per mm³; WBC count, 500 cells per mm³; or effluent positive for bile, bacteria, or increased amylase

Caution

  In patients with pelvic fractures, a supraumbilical tap should be performed to reduce the incidence of false-positive results
  A negative lavage does not rule out retroperitoneal injury

TABLE 4 Indications for Laparotomy

History of hypotension or continuing hemodynamic instability

Peritoneal signs: tenderness and voluntary or involuntary guarding remote from the penetrating wound

All missile wounds of the abdomen traversing the peritoneal or pelvic cavity

Positive peritoneal lavage

Positive radiologic investigations for visceral injury

Sigmoidoscopic findings of rectal injury

High index of suspicion for retroperitoneal injury with or without positive ancillary diagnostic tests

As soon as the patient reaches the emergency center, he should be rapidly assessed. Initial resuscitation should follow the A,B,C, pattern with control of airway and ventilation. Circulation should be optimized by insertion of large-bore intravenous lines and volume resuscitation, initially with crystalloid solution, followed by type-specific blood, if necessary. Simultaneously, the patient's tetanus immunization status is ascertained and tetanus toxoid is administered, if indicated. Initial antibiotic therapy should be aimed at gram-negative and anaerobic organisms.

Once stabilization of the hemodynamic status is achieved, a complete secondary survey and diagnostic investigation should be performed. The objective of these procedures is only to determine whether the patient needs exploratory laparotomy (Table 4).

All patients with significant history of trauma to the flank and buttocks should be admitted to the hosptial. Repeated serial examination for development of signs of peritoneal irritation is mandatory.

THORACIC AND LUMBOSACRAL SPINE INJURY

DANIEL R. BENSON, M.D.

Thoracolumbar injuries occur when the vertebral column is subjected to either direct or indirect trauma. *Direct trauma* causes injury at the point of contact and is due to flying missiles, knives, or direct blows. This type of trauma usually does not produce unstable fractures, but neurologic damage is relatively common. The injuries are frequently open and complicated by laceration of nerve roots, dura, and the spinal cord. *Indirect trauma* causes the majority of thoracic and lumbar injuries. The result is a fracture or a dislocation at a distance from the point where the traumatic force was applied. Injuries due to indirect trauma are caused by an excessive load or motion being applied to the vertebral column. High-velocity vehicular accidents, motorcycle accidents, and falls from a height are some of the more common ways these fractures occur in our society. The abnormal forces associated with injury to the vertebral column include excessive flexion, extension, rotation, shear, and axial load. Each single or in combination, can produce specific types of fractures or dislocations. While in the individual patient, indirect trauma is less likely to produce neurologic damage than direct trauma, by sheer volume it produces most of the neurologic deficits. Many of the fractures and dislocations that result from indirect trauma are acutely unstable and could cause progressive neurologic damage if the spinal motion is not protected.

DIFFERENTIAL DIAGNOSIS

While fractures and dislocations are the most spectacular of the injuries to the spinal column, lesser degrees of violence might produce ligamentous, muscular, or soft tissue damage. The history, examination, and diagnostic tests will differentiate these injuries from true bone injury. If the degree of vertebral fracture is more severe than one would normally expect from the amount of trauma sustained, pathologic bone weakened by osteoporosis, infection, or tumor should be suspected. When neurologic changes occur and no bone pathologic changes are evident, an acute rupture of the anulus fibrosis of the intervertebral disc with herniation of the nucleus pulposus, causing cord or root compression, might be considered.

DIAGNOSIS

Patients with injury to the thoracic and lumbar spine will usually provide a clear history of a sudden violent episode of trauma followed by severe, persistent, and usually localized back pain. They may also be able to describe any loss of motor function or sensation which,

even if it is transient and now normal, gives clues as to degree of injury and stability of the spine. Because vertebral fractures are often associated with other injuries, including head trauma, sometimes a history is not available. In these cases, a description of the accident by the friends, family, or ambulance attendants, plus physical examination and roentgenographic tests may be the only basis for diagnosis. The patient will usually arrive at the emergency department lying on his back. If a thoracolumbar injury is suspected, the examiner should resist the temptation to move the patient into a prone or sitting position for a more convenient examination. A very accurate screening examination can be performed with the patient in a lateral or supine position. Clothing should be removed so observation and palpation are unhampered. The entire trunk should be inspected for any evidence of trauma. Any abrasions, ecchymosis, swelling, loss of normal spinal curvatures, or obvious distortion of the vertebral column is significant. Abrasions of the posterior thorax, particularly if they are unilateral, suggest an acute flexion-rotation injury of the thoracic or thoracolumbar spine. Abrasions or contusions traversing the lower abdomen indicate an acute flexion of the thoracolumbar or lumbar spine over a seat belt. Careful palpation of the entire thoracic and lumbar spine can be done starting superiorly and working progressively down to the sacrum. The spinous processes should be in a relatively straight line, evenly spaced, and not painful. If a gap or offset is felt, rupture of posterior ligamentous structures or fracture of the vertebral column is likely. If the damage is to the vertebral body, posterior palpation will usually produce some tenderness and may show paravertebral muscle spasm with loss of the normal spinal contours and motion. In a thin patient without accompanying abdominal trauma, deep abdominal palpation can help to make the diagnosis of the vertebral fracture. Spines with severe displacement will have acute angulation (gibbus) at the level of injury and should be considered highly unstable.

In all cases of suspected injury to the vertebral column, an accurate and complete neurologic examination should be performed and recorded. A good initial neurologic examination is invaluable later in determining any changes and the ultimate neurologic prognosis. This is, without doubt, the single most important diagnostic procedure that the emergency physician can perform in the patient with spinal injury. Take time to do it well. A form, if not already available, should be developed to record your findings. The voluntary movement and grade of strength of the trunk and lower extremity muscles are determined. Their strength is graded from 0 to 5. Zero strength indicates no contraction; grade 1 (trace) indicates slight contraction without joint motion; grade 2 (poor), complete range of motion with gravity eliminated; grade 3 (fair), complete range of motion against gravity only; grade 4 (good), complete range of motion with some resistance; and grade 5 (normal), complete range of motion with full resistance. Elevation or separation of the costal margins with deep inspiration indicates intact intercostal muscles. Abdominal bulging or cephalad migration of the umbilicus when coughing suggests abdominal muscle paralysis. Any voluntary control of toe flexors or extensors is important to record, as this may be the only clinical sign that the neurologic lesion is incomplete. A digital rectal examination will reveal whether voluntary and sphincter tone is intact or if it occurs when testing the bulbocavernous reflex. This reflex can be tested by pulling on the urethral catheter (if one is present), squeezing the glans penis, or applying pressure on the clitoris. The deep tendon reflexes, abdominal cutaneous reflexes, and the cremasteric reflex should also be tested.

Paralyzed muscles with intact deep tendon reflexes indicate a spinal cord or upper motor neuron injury, while paralyzed muscles with absent deep tendon reflexes suggest cauda equina or nerve root injury. The latter has a much more favorable prognosis. Initially, the examination of deep tendon reflexes may not be reliable. This is because post-traumatic spinal shock may create a temporary loss of all spinal reflexes. The absence of spinal reflexes due to spinal shock seldom lasts longer than 24 hours, and during this period the prognosis of neurologic recovery cannot be determined. If the bulbocavernous reflex returns, this is a reliable sign that spinal shock has passed. If this reflex returns with no documentation of motor or sensory function in the lower extremities, the patient can be predicted to have a complete neurologic lesion. Any motor or sensory sparing indicates an incomplete neurologic lesion with some hope for recovery. Sensory testing is less reliable because of its subjectivity and inconsistency. It should be done with particular attention paid to the perianal area, where many spinal cord levels are represented. Presence of a cutanous sensation in this area might be the only evidence that a suspected complete lesion is, in fact, incomplete. The minimal sensory examination should include sharp-dull discrimination with a needle, light touch, deep pain, and proprioception of the toes. Any discrepancy between the two extremities is important to note.

DIAGNOSTIC EXAMINATION

The minimal roentgenographic views in a suspected thoracic or lumbar fracture are anteroposterior and lateral views. By careful manipulation of the x-ray equipment or log rolling the patient as a unit, these views can almost always be safely obtained. The upper levels of the thoracic spine are particularly difficult to visualize and may require tomography for clarification. Oblique or spot views may help to evaluate a suspicious area completely. The roentgenograms are examined for any evidence of bony comminution, anteroposterior or lateral displacement, fracture of the neural arch or transverse processes, and loss of normal vertebral contours (i.e., thoracic kyphosis or lumbar lordosis). The posterior portion of the vertebral body, if fractured, is scrutinized for displacement into the spinal canal. Computerized tomography can assist in the evaluation of the suspected displacement of fragments into the vertebral canal. At times, the instillation of (metrizamide into the epidural space can help in discerning the relationship of the neural elements to the bony

and soft tissue compromise of the spinal canal. A myelogram alone is rarely indicated unless there is a post-traumatic neurologic deficit and no apparent skeletal damage. An unsuspected acute herniated disc may be detected by this study.

The lateral roentgeogram is studied for soft tissue injury. The spinous processes can be visualized using a bright light. Any abnormal widening between spinous processes indicates tearing of the intraspinous and supraspinous ligaments and potential instability of the spine.

Once a fracture or soft tissue lesion is detected, it can be further evaluated by more specific roentgenographic studies. In 10 percent of vertebral fractures, more than one vertebra is involved. Therefore, examine the roentgenograms an additional time to rule out injury at more than one level.

DIFFERENTIAL ROENTGENOGRAPHIC DIAGNOSIS

An old compression fracture, congenital scoliosis or kyphosis, and Scheuermann's disease (juvenile epiphysitis) can all be confused with acute trauma to the thoracic and lumbar spine. Patients with congenital scoliosis (hemivertebra) usually will have an extra pedicle and/or rib. Congenital kyphosis, which is caused by a congenitally absent vertebral body, may be very hard to differentiate from an acute fracture. Tomography may help to define the deformity. Scheuermann's disease typically involves more than one and usually several vertebral bodies causing anterior wedging, irregular end plates, and kyphosis. An old compression fracture is perhaps the most difficult differential diagnosis to make. The area of involvement should be nontender unless superimposed trauma has occurred. A technetium 99 bone scan will be positive if the fracture is new and negative if the fracture is old.

THERAPY

Suspected injury to the vertebral column should be treated as a potential unstable fracture from the scene of the accident until the final roentgenographic analysis is complete. An assessment of the circumstances and mechanism of injury may be helpful later in evaluating the spine. The patient may be able to relate transient neurologic symptoms directly after the accident which are later forgotten and are important for the examining physicians to know. The patient should be lifted as a unit by several persons or log rolled onto a hard stretcher or spine board. The body, including the head and neck, should be stabilized with straps or tape. When the patient reaches the emergency department, similar methods are used for transfer to the hospital emergency cart or x-ray table. Being in a hurry to retrieve ambulance equipment or obtain roentgenograms may place the spinal cord in jeopardy. The history and physical examination have already been described. Other organ systems are frequently injured when the vertebral column is fractured. The head, chest and ribs, abdomen, and genitourinary system should all be evaluated. Fractures of the thoracolumbar and lumbar spine will create a transient ileus with cessation of bowel sounds. Therefore, the patient should not be given anything by mouth until the gastrointestinal tract is operating once again. Medications are basically used to control the pain and anxiety of the patient. I do not feel that systemic steroids are helpful, and in fact they may be harmful in patients with spinal cord injuries. If the fracture is open, after cultures have been taken, antibiotics are started. These usually consist of a cephalosporin (Keflin) and an aminoglycoside (gentamicin), which are given intravenously. Tetanus toxoid is given if there is no history of the patient having received it in the past six years.

CONSULTATION AND BED CARE

The patient with an injury to the thoracic or lumbar spine is best treated by an orthopaedic surgeon and/or neurosurgeon, who is most familiar and interested in vertebral column trauma. Most can be nursed on a regular hospital bed, although some doctors prefer a turning frame (Stryker). Turning should be done every 2 hours to avoid pressure areas. This is especially true in the elderly or neurologically impaired patient. Neurologic examination is repeated frequently during the first 24 hours to assess any changes (progression for better or worse). The vital signs must be monitored, as the blood pressure can be affected by spinal cord injury. If transfer to another facility is required, it can be done after the patient is stable. Surgical treatment of vertebral fractures is usually not an emergency. The only absolute indications for immediate decompression and/or stabilization are progressive neurologic deterioration or an open vertebral fracture. Total paraplegia that is unchanged from the first examination or a myelographic block is not an indication to do immediate surgery.

STABLE FRACTURES OF THE THORACOLUMBAR SPINE

There are several fracture types which, although painful, are not likely to cause any neurologic damage. These include mild compression fractures and fractures of spinous or transverse processes. The compression fracture usually is the result of axial loading of the spine in flexion. The front of the vertebral body will be flattened or decreased in height. The compression, if less then 50 percent of the expected height, is considered to be stable. Avulsions of the spinous processes and particularly the transverse processes (lumbar spine) can be the result of violent muscle contractions or trauma. They may be combined with other vertebral or rib fractures. Avulsions of spinous and transverse processes have occurred in weight lifters, football lineman, and rugby players. These lesions, if isolated, can be treated symptomatically. Pain medication and abdominal splinting (lumbosacral corset) may be enough to make the patient comfortble. If bowel sounds are present (an ileus could complicate recovery) and the patient is reliable, he could be sent home. However, this should be done only if there is a friend or relative who can bring them back if any problems occur. This protocol is applicable only if one is absolutely sure of the fracture's stability. Any suspicion of instability would preclude sending the patient home.

SUGGESTED READING

Holdsworth F. Fractures, dislocations, and fracture-dislocations of the spine. J Bone Joint Surg 1970; 52-A:1524-1551.
Kaufer H, Kling TF, Stauffer ES. Fractures and dislocations of the spine. In: Rockwood CA Jr, Green DP, eds. Fractures in adults. Philadelphia: JB Lippincott, 1984:987.

REPLANTATION OF EXTREMITIES

ALAN R. SHONS, M.D., Ph.D.

The first experimental replantation was reported in 1903 by Hopfner who used a canine hind limb model. In 1960 Jacobson and Suarez reported a 100 percent patency rate in anastomoses of arteries 1.4 mm in diameter, using the operating microscope in the experimental laboratory. Decades of laboratory work thus set the stage for the world's first successful clinical replantation of an arm by Malt and McKhann in 1962. Komatsu and Tamai, in 1968, reported the first clinical digit replantation, bringing to the clinical setting the laboratory technical achievements in small vessel repair.

Many clinical replantation teams have been assembled in the last 10 years. With widespread technical expertise and the availability of sophisticated surface and air transport, the replantation of a part is a technique that is now available to virtually any patient in the United States. Primary physicians who receive emergency patients must understand current concepts regarding replantation.

Although small series of lower extremity replants have been reported, 97 percent of all reported amputations involve the hands and fingers. One-third of all lost-time industrial injuries involve the upper extremity, and 5 percent of such injuries are amputations. Guillotine injuries caused by a sharp blade occur in one-third of cases. Localized crush amputations caused by saws or presses occur in two-thirds of cases. A small minority of amputations are the result of avulsion, degloving, or diffuse injuries.

PATIENT EVALUATION AND SELECTION

Most patients know that parts can be replanted. Surgical teams are available to perform the operation. The legal profession has taken an interest in this area. For these reasons, in most cases I believe that the final decision regarding replantation should be made by a surgeon who does replants. If examination by a replantation team would involve long and expensive travel, and if the injury is definitely unfavorable for replantation, the primary physician in discussion with the patient and family may advise against replantation. A decision can be made without transfer if the patient and family are in agreement. There should be complete documentation in the patient's record of the discussion, and both physician and patient with family should sign the note. In the presence of uncertainty by either the patient or family, the decision should be deferred to a replant surgeon.

INDICATIONS

Patients with severe associated injuries requiring immediate and extensive treatment should not be considered for replantation. Chronically ill patients who could not tolerate prolonged operation are not candidates. Severe diffuse injury to the part is also a contraindication. The elimination of patients in the aforementioned categories leaves the vast majority of amputation cases. The remaining patients range from good to poor candidates for replantation.

Success rates of 95 percent can be achieved in survival of the part in ideal patients; 40 percent success can be expected in salvage cases. The proper goal of replantation surgery, however, is not simply survival of the part, but functional utilization. Critical analyses of success in functional utilization of replants has suggested relative contraindications for replantation. Patients over 55 years of age in whom joint stiffness and vascular degeneration are problems are not good candidates for replantation. Nerve regeneration potential decreases with age, as does the patient's ability to adapt to new sensory patterns, further compromising recovery potential in the elderly. In many cases, single digits should not be replanted. The index finger must function perfectly to be integrated into hand function. A less than perfect index finger will be bypassed, with opposition obtained between thumb and long finger. Poor function of long, ring, or little fingers will impair the function of the adjacent finger. Finally, avulsion injuries or other injuries involving multiple levels are relative contraindications to replantation.

Proximal replantations of the upper extremity at proximal arm or shoulder level are technically possible and always dramatic, but the long-term functional results are dismal owing to a lack of satisfactory reinnervation in most cases.

The thumb should be replanted in virtually all cases because of its importance in overall hand function. An attempt should be made to replant as many fingers as possible in a case of multiple finger amputations. Since it is impossible to predict which fingers will have good motor and sensory recovery, no finger that can technically be salvaged should be discarded. A more aggressive approach to replantation, including single-digit replants, is indicated in the child. The potential for excellent motor and sensory return is dramatically better in the young patient.

The best functional results are obtained with distal level replants in the upper extremity. Good results are seen in replants at the distal forearm and wrist level. Digital replants distal to the insertion of the flexor digitorum sublimis tendon at the proximal middle phalanx level exhibit the best range of motion and sensory recovery. Digital replantation at the distal interphalangeal joint level is technically possible. A very distal replant should be considered for cosmesis only since highly satisfactory finger function can be maintained with an amputation at the distal interphalangeal joint.

The indications for replantation of the lower extremity are limited. Leg length and adequate sensibility are critical to lower extremity functions of walking and weight bearing. A leg length discrepancy of only 2 to 3 cm can be compensated by pelvic obliquity and elevated shoes. The bone shortening necessary in many replants exceeds this short distance. Nerve regeneration and return of sensibility are poor in replants proximal to the ankle. A below-knee amputation with a prosthesis may be more satisfactory than a replanted insensate foot. In certain cases, reattachment of a segment of the amputated lower extremity may allow a below-knee amputation level rather than an above-knee level to provide a more functional extremity.

A final consideration in all replants is that, a technically successful replant is only the first step in a long period of rehabilitation. The initial hospitalization may be long. Secondary reconstructive procedures are necessary in about half the patients. The average disability time of patients with successful replants is 6 months, and 5 to 10 percent of patients never return to work. For some patients it is better to accept amputation with attendant short hospitalization and recovery and quick return to work if the former job can be performed after loss of the part.

PRE-HOSPITAL CARE

Medical personnel at the accident scene should be alert to the possibility of a replantation. All injured parts should be preserved as if for replantation in spite of what may seem overwhelming injury. In some cases, components of the injured part can be utilized in a salvage procedure even though the part itself cannot be saved. The part should be wrapped in a moist gauze or washcloth and placed inside a dry plastic bag. The plastic bag should be placed in an ice chest filled with regular ice. Recovery personnel should have ice available at the scene since prompt cooling of the part lengthens the time available for revascularization. Muscle, the most sensitive of the several tissues in a composite part, undergoes irreversible changes after 6 hours of warm ischemia. Digits have been successfully replanted after as much as 28 hours of cold ischemia. The more proximal the amputation, the shorter the available time for replantation owing to the greater muscle mass in proximal replants.

Life-threatening injuries must be appropriately managed at the accident scene. Hemorrhage from the amputation stump should be controlled with pressure and clean dressings. No manipulation or clamping of structures should be done because this may cause additional injury. A tourniqet should not be used. Intravenous fluids are given if necessary to maintain normovolemia.

HOSPITAL CARE

Emergency department preparation of the patient for replantation consists of the routine preparation of a patient for a long operation. Work-up must be adequate to rule out other significant injuries. Proximal extremity amputations are usually associated with other injuries, and a high index of suspicion is essential.

Laboratory work-up should include chest roentgenogram as well as roentgenograms of the amputated part and amputation stump. An electrocardiogram is obtained, and blood is drawn for complete blood count, electrolytes, blood urea nitrogen (BUN), glucose, and type and crossmatch. Monitoring lines are placed to include central venous catheter and urinary catheter. Temperature is monitored by rectal thermometer. Intravenous cephalosporin antibiotics are begun.

Very little should be done with the amputated part in the emergency department. Gross contamination may be irrigated off, but extensive washing should not be done because this will make identification of structures more difficult in the operating room. Nothing additional need be done to the amputation site as long as bleeding is controlled by the original dressing.

Transfer arrangements must be made if the replantation cannot be performed at the receiving hospital. It is imperative that the primary physician speak personally with the replant surgeon to inform him of the patient's status as well as any discussion or recommendations made regarding the advisability of replantation in this particular case. Complete records of treatment given must accompany the patient. Although time is critical in replantation surgery, even more critical is the overall care of the patient and the experience of the replantation team. The injured patient must be adequately stabilized for travel. A physician may have to accompany the patient. The patient must be directed to a capable team since the level of experience correlates with technical results. A few minutes extra travel time by jet air transport may be worthwhile to reach an experienced center since the difference between a poor and a good result may make a dramatic difference in initial medical care costs as well as lifetime productivity of the patient.

SUGGESTED READING

Chen ZW, Zeng BF. Replantation of the lower extremity. In: Shaw WW, ed. Symposium on clinical microvascular surgery. S Clin N Amer 1983; 10:103–113.

Cunningham BL, Shons AR. Current concepts in replantation surgery. In: Najarian JS, Delaney JP, eds. Emergency Surgery. Chicago: Year Book Medical Publishers Inc., 1982; 249.

Lister GD, Kleinert HE. Replantation. In: Grabb W, Smith J, eds. Plastic surgery-a concise guide to clinical practice. 3rd ed, Boston: Little, Brown, and Company, 1979; 697.

Wilson CS, Alpert BS, Buncke HJ, Gordon L. Replantation of the upper extremity. In: Shaw WW, ed. Symposium on clinical microvascular surgery. Clin Plast Surg 1983; 10:85.

LACERATION OF THE HAND: FINGERTIP INJURY AND INFECTION

TSU-MIN TSAI, M.D.
BRADLEY E. HENDERSON, M.D.

Sixteen million hand injuries per year occur in the United States, and 30 percent of these are seen in the emergency department. The result achieved after any hand injury depends, for the most part, on the efficiency of primary treatment. Secondary repair can never compensate for the time or the opportunity lost by neglect or improper primary procedure.

HISTORY

How Did the Accident Occur? The tidy wound is one in which a sharp item such as a knife, glass, or a razor has opened the skin. Often these tidy wounds may include laceration of many important deep structures including tendons, nerves, and vessels.

The untidy wound is one in which the hand has been crushed, torn, burned, or ripped by explosion. These injuries are often caused by compressing machines, high-pressure injection devices, or war missiles. The extent of venous thrombosis, edema, deep soft-tissue injury, necrosis, and contamination may be impossible to judge or predict on initial examination.

When Did the Injury Occur? If the injury is a tidy one and is seen within 6 hours, bones, tendons, nerves, and vessels may be repaired at the time of initial injury. If there has been a delay of 12 to 24 hours before treatment, an untidy wound will be grossly contaminated, despite thorough lavage and irrigation. In such a case, it is best to leave the wound open for delayed closure.

Where Did the Accident Take Place? When treating injuries contaminated by barnyard soil or street dirt, or those that have occurred in an environment such as a meat packing plant, the emergency physician should be aware of the danger of development of a severe infection despite early, thorough wound care. In such a severely contaminated case, closure of the wound must be delayed until the danger of infection has passed.

What Treatment Was Rendered at the Time of the Accident? Immediate treatment may include tetanus shot, intravenous antibiotics, dressings, cast, or splint.

EXAMINATION OF THE HAND

Open Wound Examination

A ring or bracelet may act as a tourniquet if the limb becomes swollen. Jewelry should be removed. Severe crush wounds or explosion injuries need not be exposed in the emergency department. The less severe wound may be examined if conditions are proper.

The purpose of the initial wound examination is to assess both the nature and the severity of the injury and to judge whether definitive care should be rendered in the emergency department. The skin, blood vessels, nerves, tendons, and bones must be examined. Roentgenographic examination (except in the case of trivial injuries) should be used to rule out fracture and foreign bodies (except wood or glass, which are seen often but not always).

Vascular Examination

The vascularity of the digits is partially determined by inspection of color and capillary refill. One may also perform a digital Allen test by exsanguinating the digit with graduated finger pressure starting at the tip and proceeding to the web. Both radial and ulnar digital vessels are then compressed and sequentially released. Vascular refill should be brisk from each side. More fundamental is the fact that a viable hand or digit actively bleeds distal to the laceration.

Most fingers have a dominant digital artery, as evidenced by the caliber of the vessel. When only one has been divided and the finger is well vascularized, repair is not required, but it should be done if a physician is available with experience in microsurgical repair. When the finger is nonviable, vascular repair is essential. Partial lacerations of arteries can produce considerable blood loss.

Nerve Examination

The sensation in each digit should be checked with both light touch and static two-point determination (S2PD). With S2PD, the ends of a paper clip are separated to 5 mm and then light pressure (just to blanch the skin) is applied to the distal pulp. The ends are oriented in the same longitudinal axis as the fingers and pressed on both the radial and ulnar sides. With nerve injury, the S2PD is usually greater than 10 mm.

Intrinsic motor function is examined when the patient actively flexes the metacarpophalangeal (MP) joint and extends the proximal interphalangeal (PIP) and distal interphalangeal (DIP) joints. This action is controlled by both the interossei and lumbrical muscles. The lumbricals are innervated by both the median and ulnar nerves,

so the patient will be able to perform these motions in at least the index and middle fingers despite injury to one of the nerves. To be more specific, the median motor branch should be tested by having the patient palmarly abduct the thumb against resistance to test the abductor pollicis brevis. The ulnar motor branch should be tested by resisted ulnar abduction of the little finger for the abductor digiti minimi and resisted radial abduction of the index finger for the first dorsal interosseous. The respective muscle belly should be palpated during this testing to feel for the normal contracted muscle.

Tendon Examination

With the wrist supinated, dorsiflexed, and relaxed, the digits are flexed at each joint increasingly from the index finger to the small finger. This is called the cascade, and if this natural flow of flexion is interrupted, there is cause for suspicion of discontinuity of the flexor tendons.

The patient's ability to move each joint actively and independently is then tested. Flexion and extension of the DIP joint is performed with the PIP and MP joints held by the examiner in extension. The PIP joint is flexed by the patient with the examiner holding the other digit's DIP joints in extension in order to block any contribution of the flexor digitorum profundus to this motion. MP flexion and extension are then determined.Resistance to each direction should be made. Weakness or pain with this maneuver may indicate a partial tendon laceration.

Bone Examination

Fracture is observed through fingernail position and hand position as well as roentgenographic examination (Table 1).

Skin Examination

The skin should be examined for simple lacerations, contusion, hematoma, viability of flap, skin loss, and other exposed tissue.

TREATMENT

General Principles

When evaluating hand wounds, one should always presume that all deeper structures in the region are severed until their anatomic continuity is confirmed by clinical examination or operative exploration.

TABLE 1   Indications for X-ray Examination

Significant trauma
Bone injury
Ligamentous injury
Suspicion of fracture
Foreign body or penetrating wound
Infection
Pain or swelling, cause unknown

One can rarely justify performing open reduction of fractures, flexor tendon repair, complex extensor tendon repair, nerve or artery repair, extensive exploration, or debridement of skin flaps in the emergency department. A split-thickness skin graft to small dermal wounds can usually be performed in a clean and efficient emergency department. As a general rule, the contaminated wound, the wound with necrotic tissue, or the wound that has occurred more than 6 hours previously should be allowed to remain open for secondary closure.

Most bleeding vessels can be controlled with gentle pressure. With brisk arterial bleeding some vessels may be clamped and tied, but care should be taken not to damage the nerve or jeopardize the repair to follow.

The choice of whether to use general, regional, or local anesthesia must be influenced by the nature of the surgery to be performed (never use epinephrine). Local digital block with 2 cc of local bupivacaine (Marcaine 0.5 percent) is useful.

If bones, tendons, nerves, or vessels are divided, the patient should be referred to a hand surgeon for definitive treatment (Table 2). A clean dressing can be applied, along with a splint if necessary, and the patient referred as soon as possible.

Prophylactic antibiotics are not effective in preventing infection in severe mutilating hand injuries such as those caused by farm-implements, but they are effective in home or industry-related injuries. In the recent literature, there are reports of tobramycin, penicillin, and cephalosporin combinations being used for this type of injury.

The patient should be given nothing orally. After the patient is stabilized, he can go to the operating room or be transferred to a hand surgery unit or a hosptial where he will receive more sophisticated care.

The Tidy Wound

The simple uncomplicated skin laceration caused by a sharp edge can be treated by local anesthesia and closure, and the patient can be discharged. No antibiotic is recommended except in the case of the wound that is over 6 hours old. A soft dressing is applied, immediate range of motion exercises are begun, and the patient wears a protective brace when he returns to work. Follow-up is usually in 2 weeks unless there is a problem.

Special Types of Injuries

Saw Injury. Saw injuries may be superficial to deep, depending on the type of saw; damage can be produced some distance from the skin wound. Mangled fingers result from power-driven saws, and the skin edge may not survive. Debridement is needed to provide a good viable edge (Table 3).

TABLE 2 Indications for Consultation with Hand Surgeon

Lacerations involving nerve, artery, tendon
Severe fracture or injury
Infection involving joint, tendon sheath, or deep space

TABLE 3 Principles of Debridement

Preserve neurovascular bundles
Preserve flexor tendons
Preserve bone and joint if possible
Preserve sufficient skin to allow closure without excess tension

Wringer Injury. Wringer injury consists of contusion, superficial abrasion or friction burns, and simple laceration. Simple lacerations may be debrided and closed under local anesthesia. Tendons, nerves, and vessels may be injured and the patient may have to be admitted. Another criterion for admission is the viability of the extremity (Table 4).

Power Mower Injury. Injuries caused by a lawn mower or snow blower usually consist of a partial or complete amputation of a toe or digit. Thorough cleaning and debridement with the wound left open for delayed closure is the safest procedure.

Flap Avulsions and Degloving Injury. Flap avulsions and degloving injuries are usually severe, and the patient should be admitted for wound debridement and delayed closure. A flap may be needed to close the defect.

Gunshot Wounds. A muzzle velocity of 2,000 feet per second or more is considered high velocity. This produces a high-energy injury with extensive soft-tissue injury and comminuted fracture. A low-energy wound often presents as little more than a foreign body in the hand. The bullet passing through the soft tissues alone leaves but a small entrance and exit wound and often leaves remarkably little damage through its track. More commonly there is a small entrance wound in the palm but a large destructive exit wound in the dorsal aspect, with comminuted fracture of the metacarpal.

Mangle Injury. Mangle injuries leave a deep thermal burn, usually on the dorsal surface of the hand. They are likely to be caused by a mechanically driven roller and a metal shoe, which supplies heat. Roller injuries commonly produce an avulsion flap, usually distally based and of questionable viability. There may be associated friction burn and fracture. Vessels are likely to be disrupted or thrombosed. Tendons and nerves may be contused or avulsed.

Punch Press Injuries. Punch press injuries can be moderate to severe. Comminuted fractures and carpal disruption, as well as soft tissue crushing, are the rule in these injuries.

Cornpicker Injury. A cornpicker injury usually involves crushing of the fingers but spares the thumb. The

TABLE 4 Indications for Admission

Viability of extremity is uncertain (vascular compromise, crush injuries, severe swelling)
High risk of infection (needs close observation, parenteral antibiotics)
Severe injury, pain, swelling
General condition of patient (especially multiple other injuries, diseases producing immune compromise)

hand or extremity may be trapped in the machine for a considerable period of time before its release. Soft tissue damage is extensive and characterized by crushing, avulsion, and burning of the tissue associated with fracture-dislocation and amputation.

Grease Gun Injuries. The finger is injected with grease under high pressure. Other fluids injected may include paint, turpentine, dry-cleaning fluid (trichlorethylene), and molten plastic (500°F, 4,000 psi). Through a small puncture wound, grease is injected through the soft tissues of the finger and often into the tendon sheath. These injuries may or may not be immediately painful. However, blanching and numbness of the digit usually occur. Grease or paint may exude from the minute wound. This injury causes an acute severe inflammatory reaction; immediate incision and evacuation of as much material as possible is the best method of treatment. Delayed treatment causes gangrene and infection, which leads to partial or complete amputation.

Penetrating Injury. Penetrating wounds may occur from wooden splinters, tacks or pins, needles, staples, and so forth. An unimpressive skin wound may hide a remarkable amount of damage to deep structures. Exploration in such situations is the absolute rule if there is a possibility of a foreign body being retained or if there is possible tendon, nerve, or vessel damage. The thinnest sliver of glass may divide the deep structure.

Diagnosis of a foreign body in the hand is made by history, physical examination and x-ray examination. Operative removal is indicated if the foreign body is palpable, if the foreign body has been localized by x-ray examination, or if infection is present.

Human Bite. Human bite wounds usually present as a nondescript laceration over the metacarpophalangeal joints and are commonly associated with serious morbidity.

Compressed Air Injection Injury. This injury causes skin trauma and emphysema of tissue, which usually subsides within 24 hours. The treatment is heat therapy and observation.

Welder's Injuries (Electrical). These injuries usually exhibit a small puncture wound at the site of entrance, beneath which there is an area of coagulated tissue and a minute foreign body. Symptoms are pain, abscess, and sinus formation.

Fingertip Injury

Injuries to the pulp should be carefully treated because adequate healing is needed for sensation, padding, and freedom from discomfort. A soft dressing is applied; later begin soaks and change the dressing within 1 week. If the bone is not exposed and the deficit is smaller than 1 cm², dressing changes are all that is required. If the deficit is larger than 1 cm², a free skin graft might be considered. Split-thickness skin grafts are used for small defects, particularly on the ulnar side of the digit, because contraction draws in normally sensitive skin. Full-thickness skin grafts are used in well-vascularized areas, especially the radial contact side of the finger. If bone is exposed, a flap is required. If the soft tissue loss is more from the palmar than the dorsal aspect, the local flap will be doomed to failure because of undue tension. Cross-finger flap, thenar flap, Moberg advancement flap, or dorsal neurovascular island flap may be considered; all should be carried out by a plastic or hand surgeon.

Nail Bed Injury

Subungual hematomas present as a ecchymosis under the nail and often are due to laceration of the nail bed. The intense pain can be relieved by heating the end of a paper clip and burning a hole through the cleansed nail to release the pressure of the hematoma underneath. If there is a significant nailbed laceration or the hematoma involves more than 25 percent of the visible nail, the nail bed should be removed. The nail bed should then be carefully repaired, primarily with a 6-0 or 7-0 absorbable suture, and the nail, Silastic sheet, or gauze dressing should be placed in the nail fold in order to prevent adhesions from forming between the cuticle and the nail germinal bed.

If the nail bed is missing, a split-thickness skin graft, nail bed graft, or reverse de-epithelialized cross-finger flap may be used. The dorsal half of the terminal phalanx should be present and if fractured, stably reduced, usually with a Kirschner wire. The more phalanx is missing, the greater the likelihood of a curved nail, and ablation should be considered.

SUGGESTED READING

Boyes J. Bunnell's surgery of the hand. 5th ed. Philadelphia: JB Lippincott, 1970: 635.

Flatt AE. The care of minor hand injuries. 3rd ed. St Louis: CV Mosby, 1983:93.

Flynn JE. Hand surgery. 3rd ed. Baltimore: Williams & Wilkins, 1982:85.

Lister GD. The hand: Diagnosis and indications. 2nd ed. Edinburgh: Churchill Livingstone, 1984:1.

Mittelbach HR. The injured hand (a clinical handbook for general surgeons). New York: Springer-Verlag, 1977:187.

TENDON INJURY OF THE HAND AND WRIST

WILLIAM L. NEWMEYER, M.D.

Extensor tendon injuries may be caused by either closed or open, usually incising, trauma. Almost all flexor tendon injuries are caused by lacerating trauma. The essential diagnostic tool is knowledge of specific tendon function (functional anatomy) and the ability to test for these functions (Figs. 1, 2, 3, and Table 1). The *most common diagnostic pitfall* in diagnosis of flexor tendon injury is failure to recognize either (1) a partial tendon laceration or (2) a complete tendon laceration in a location where the two flexor tendons, the superficialis and the profundus, lie in close proximity to one another. There may be apparent normal finger flexion on a cursory examination, but a detailed examination reveals loss of active flexion at the joint of primary action of the lacerated tendon.

On the extensor surface, one must keep in mind the function of the intrinsic and the extrinsic extensors to avoid the common error of missing a tendon injury. The intrinsics (i.e., the lumbricals and the interossei) can independently extend the interphalangeal joints with considerable force independent of the extrinsic extensors (Figs. 1 and 4). Therefore good interphalangeal joint extension in the presence of a laceration on the dorsum of the hand does not mean an intact extrinsic extensor ten-

don. Only by visualizing the tendon and noting active metacarpophalangeal extension can one conclude that there is no extrinsic extensor injury. The juncturae tendinum, bands interconnecting the extrinsic extensors on the dorsum of the hand, can also lead to a false sense of security because they allow weak active metacarpophalangeal extension in the presence of a lacerated extrinsic extensor tendon.

CLOSED INJURIES

The first two injuries to be discussed here, mallet deformity and boutonnière deformity, are usually closed injuries, but may be open injuries. For purposes of clarity, both the closed and open varieties of these injuries are discussed in this section.

The most common of these is the mallet or baseball finger, which is caused by a separation of the terminal extensor mechanism (TEM) from the distal phalanx. The cause is often fairly trivial trauma and the patient presents with an inability to extend the distal interphalangeal (DIP) joint. A roentgenogram should be obtained to rule out a fracture. If there is no fracture or if it is a small one (under 30 percent of the joint surface involved, with no palmar subluxation of the distal phalanx), treatment consists of application of a dorsal splint, which is kept in place for 8 weeks (Table 2). This can be fashioned from a tongue blade and a piece of adherent foam (Reston) or from a commercially available splint. The patient may remove the splint periodically to "air the digit," but the joint should be kept extended 100 percent of the time for 8 weeks. The proximal interphalangeal (PIP) joint is intentionally left

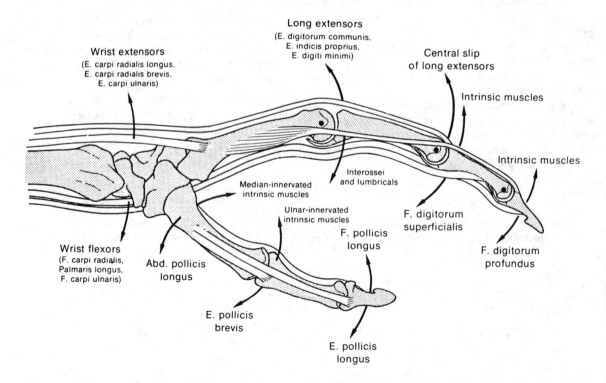

Figure 1 Tendons and muscles acting on the hand. (From Beasley RW. Hand injuries. Philadelphia: WB Saunders, 1981.)

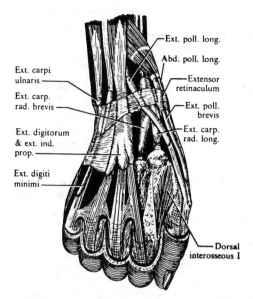

Figure 2 Extensor tendons and synovial sheaths. (From Pansky B, House EL. Review of gross anatomy. 3rd ed. New York: Macmillan, 1975.)

free, and the patient is encouraged to flex it to keep the finger limber.

If there is a fracture with over 30 percent of the joint surface involved or with subluxation of the distal phalanx, the injury is likely to require surgical repair. The digit should be splinted and the patient referred for early operative repair. If the injury is caused by laceration of the TEM, the tendon should be sutured, and it is generally advisable to support the DIP joint with a Kirschner (K) wire for 8 weeks.

The boutonnière deformity is an injury to the central extensor mechanism (CEM) at the PIP joint (see Fig. 4). With injury to the CEM, the lateral bands sublux volar to the axis of motion of the joint and become paradoxical flexors of the PIP and hyperextenders of the DIP joint.

This may result from end-on trauma to the finger (the so-called jammed finger), from a direct blow over the dorsum of the joint, or from a laceration. With closed trauma and a suspected boutonnière deformity, the joint should be supported by a dorsal splint taped in place, leaving the DIP and metacarpal phalangeal (MCP) joints free to flex. It should be kept in place for 6 weeks with the same admonitions as apply to the mallet deformity splint. If the injury is caused by a tendon laceration, the tendon should be repaired and the joint fixed with a K wire for 6 weeks.

An unusual closed injury, but one seen with enough regularity to merit mention, is the rupture of the flexor digitorum profundus (FDP) tendon. This injury occurs when the patient attempts to grasp something that is pulled from the grasp with great force. There is pain and swelling of the finger and an inability to flex the DIP joint. On the lateral x-ray film, a fleck of bone may be seen somewhere along the palmar surface, usually at the level of the PIP joint. This injury requires referral for early surgery (within a week).

Other closed tendon injuries are uncommon and may occur as a result of rheumatoid synovitis (usually extensors) or due to erosion of carpal bones into the carpal tunnel with fraying and rupture of one or more flexor tendons. An injury which may be seen several months following a Colles fracture is rupture of the extensor pollicis longus (EPL) tendon. It probably ruptures as a consequence of interference with its blood supply at Lister's tubercle, but rupture may be caused by a spicule of bone from the fracture. The patient presents with a rather sudden inability to extend with force the interphalangeal (IP) joint of the thumb.

OPEN INJURIES

In the examination of any open hand injury, certain basic principles must be observed. Mandatory are the positioning of the patient supine with the hand on a firm sup-

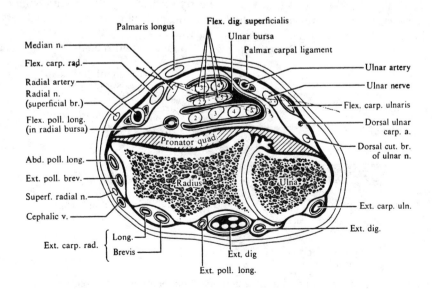

Figure 3 Cross section of the wrist showing tendons, arteries, and nerves. (From Pansky B, House EL. Review of gross anatomy. 3rd ed. New York: Macmillan, 1975.)

TABLE 1 Extrinsic Extensor Tendons of the Hand and Wrist

Tendon	Acronym	Number	Site of Action*
Flexor tendons			
Flexor digitorum profundus	FDP	4	Digits 2–5, DIP
Flexor digitorum superficialis	FDS	4	Digits 2–5, PIP
Flexor pollicis longus	FPL	1	Thumb, IP
Flexor carpi ulnaris	FCU	1	Wrist
Flexor carpi radialis	FCR	1	Wrist
Palmaris longus (present 85%)	PL	1	Wrist
Extensor tendons			
Abductor pollicis longus	APL	1	Wrist
Extensor pollicis brevis	EPB	1	Thumb, MCP
Extensor carpi radialis longus	ECRL	1	Wrist
Extensor carpi radialis brevis	ECRB	1	Wrist
Extensor pollicis longus	EPL	1	Thumb, IP
Extensor digitorum communis	EDC	4	Digits 2–5, MCP
Extensor indicis proprius	EIP	1	Index, MCP
Extensor digiti quinti minimus	EDQM	1	Little, MCP
Extensor carpi ulnaris	ECU	1	Wrist

* The site of primary but not necessarily exclusive action is shown.

port, the use of an arm tourniquet to render the wound bloodless, satisfactory limited regional anesthesia, the use of proper instruments and suture material, and correct dressing and splinting after treatment.

Flexor Tendons

Few, if any, flexor tendon injuries can be satisfactorily repaired in the emergency department setting; therefore, the emphasis must be on correct diagnosis, proper wound management, and arrangements for definitive treatment.

With any laceration on the palmar surface of a digit that penetrates through the flexor tendon sheath, one should assume that there is probably an injury to all or part of the flexor tendon or tendons. If, by functional testing, it can be determined that the flexor tendon or tendons are lacerated, the wound should be irrigated, loosely approximated with 4–0 or 5–0 nylon sutures on a plastic needle (Ethicon, P–3 or Davis & Geck PRE 2), antibiot-

ics started (erythromycin or an oral cephalosporin), a bulky dressing applied, and definite arrangements made for a consultant to take over responsibility for further treatment. It is usually not necessary for the patient to have definitive surgical care immediately, but it is best if tendon repair is accomplished within several days of injury. Probably the outside time limit for surgical repair is 3 weeks, but even that can be extended in certain instances.

If, by functional examination, the flexor tendons are found to be intact, recommended emergency treatment consists of the same steps as those just outlined. This is a difficult situation for the consultant surgeon because the tendon may not be injured, may be minimally injured, or may be nearly severed. Unless the tendon can be visualized, there is no way to determine which condition exists. The patient must be warned that the tendon may be nearly severed and may rupture with use. Therefore, a dressing and splint are advised and careful follow-up is mandatory.

With lacerations on the palmar surface of the digits,

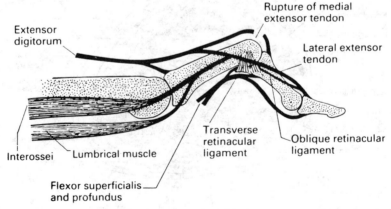

Figure 4 The finger extensor mechanism in boutonnière deformity. With the extensor tendon ruptured, the flexor superficialis and subluxed lateral bands of extensor tendon flex the PIP joint. (From Conolly WB, Kilgore ES. Hand injuries and infections. Chicago: Year Book Medical Publishers, 1979.)

TABLE 2 Summary of Treatment of Tendon Injuries in the Hand and Wrist

Type of Injury	Definitive Treatment	Timing of Treatment
Closed mallet injury	Splint	8 weeks
Closed boutonnière injury	Splint	6 weeks
Closed FDP rupture	Surgery	ASAP*
Closed, other flexor	Surgery	ASAP
Open flexor, total division	Surgery	ASAP or urgent (see text)
Open flexor, partial division	Surgery, observation	Judgment call (see text)
Extensors (zones I, II, III, distal IV)	Surgery	Often in OPD setting
Extensors (zone V)	Surgery	ASAP

* As soon as practical, usually within 3 or 4 days. Unless otherwise noted, surgery means in a major operating room under high regional or general anesthesia.

injury to digital nerves is common, and a careful examination of sensation is important.

Flexor tendon injuries are usually described as being in one of five zones. Zone I is that area from the level of the midportion of the middle phalanx to the terminal insertion of the FDP on the distal phalanx. In this area there is one tendon (the FDP) in a tendon sheath, and when it is lacerated it usually retracts into the palm unless held in position by its restraining mesentery-like structure called the vinculum.

Zone II lies between the midpalm and the proximal edge of zone I. Both the flexor digitorum superficials (FDS) and the FDP tendons lie in a fibro-osseous sheath. This is the so-called *no man's land* of tendon injuries, and the restoration of good active digital function after injury is difficult even in the best of circumstances. This is the area of the devastating infection, suppurative flexor tenosynovitis.

Zone III lies between the distal edge of the carpal tunnel and the midpalm. In the proximal portion of this zone, the superficial transverse vascular arterial arch and the median nerve at its terminal arborization lie superficial to the tendons, so that if there is tendon injury, there is also usually significant nerve and possibly vascular injury. In this zone, because of nerve and vascular injury, the need for surgical treatment is often urgent.

Zone IV is the carpal tunnel. Acute injuries in this area are rare because the thick volar carpal ligament affords good protection to the underlying structures. However, if penetrating or laceration injury does occur, the median nerve is often injured along with the tendons. With injury in this zone, as in zone III, the need for treatment may well be urgent rather than early elective.

The last zone, zone V, consists of the volar wrist and low forearm. The underlying structures, especially the median nerve and flexor tendons, but also the radial and ulnar arteries and the ulnar nerve, are vulnerable to penetrating or incising injuries. Self-inflicted injuries are common in this zone and may also occur following accidental falls into windows or onto glass or sharp metal. The need for surgical treatment of these wounds is usually urgent.

In any case of a hand wound for which the need for surgical treatment is urgent, the emphasis should be on preparation of the patient for surgery. Once the decision for immediate surgery has been made, the wound should be covered with sterile dressings and the extremity elevated and supported. The patient should be given nothing by mouth (NPO), an intravenous infusion started (with antibiotics administered via that route if there is any suggestion of contamination), and suitable preoperative blood and other tests initiated.

Extensor Tendons

Because most mallet and boutonnière deformities are from closed injuries, both the open and closed variations of these have been discussed under closed injuries (q.v.). These may be referred to as extensor zone I injuries (at DIP level) and extensor zone II injuries (at PIP level).

Injuries to the extensor mechanism between MCP and PIP joints and PIP and DIP joints may be called extensor zone III injuries. The extensor mechanism in these areas is a broad flat aponeurotic sheet. Injuries to it are almost always incising, and the entire mechanism is seldom lacerated. Lacerations to it may be readily repaired in an outpatient setting according to the principles previously outlined. Suture material of size 4–0 or 5–0 is used. A braided synthetic material is ideal, but monofilament nylon or even a polyglycollic acid suture may be used. Plain or chromic catgut or silk should not be used. A running suture should be used, and the digit is splinted for 3 weeks following repair.

On the dorsum of the hand (extensor zone IV), the tendons are discrete rather than aponeurotic bands. They are interconnected by bands called juncturae tendinum. The more distal the injury, the more readily is the repair carried out in the outpatient setting. With more proximal injuries, the proximal tendon stump may retract, and retrieval may be difficult for the uninitiated surgeon. If one elects to attempt an outpatient repair, all the general principles previously outlined should be followed. In addition, the traumatic wound should always be extended proximally for stump retrieval. The distal stump is readily found by passively extending the involved digit. Repair is done with a horizontal mattress suture of one of the materials already outlined, using size 4–0. The injured digit, the adjacent digits (except with a thumb injury), and the wrist should be immobilized for 3 weeks in an extended position.

Extensor tendon injuries at the wrist (zone V) are complicated problems because of the large excursion of the tendons and the presence of a restraining retinacular system. Injuries at this level are not amenable to outpatient repair except in rare instances. Wound toilet, dressing, and consultation should be carried out as for flexor tendon injury.

SUGGESTED READING

American Society for Surgery of the Hand: The hand: examination and diagnosis. 2nd Ed. New York: Churchill Livingstone, 1983.
American Society for Surgery of the Hand: The hand: primary care of common problems. Aurora, CO: Am Soc Surg Hand, 1985. Available at Am Soc Surg Hand, 3025 South Parker Road, Suite 65, Aurora, CO 80232, 1986.
Lampe EW: Surgical anatomy of the hand. CIBA symposium, vol 21, no 3, 1969. Available from CIBA Pharmaceutical Company, Summit, NJ 07901. Illustrations are by Frank Netter, M.D.

SHOULDER AND UPPER EXTREMITY INJURY

JOSEPH F. WAECKERLE, M.D.

SHOULDER INJURIES

The anatomy of the shoulder is extremely complex. The shoulder has more movement and range of motion than any other joint in the body. There are, in fact, four separate joints about the shoulder involved in upper-extremity movement: glenohumeral, acromioclavicular, sternoclavicular, and quasi-scapulothoracic. Full range of motion requires all these joints to function properly.

The following discussion will center on the more common shoulder joint injuries, that is, injuries to the glenohumeral, acromioclavicular, and sternoclavicular joints. For further information, the reader is referred to various orthopaedic texts, such as Rockwood and Green's *Fractures* or Simon and Koenigsknecht's *Orthopaedics in Emergency Medicine*.

Glenohumeral Dislocations

The glenohumeral joint is the most commonly dislocated major joint of the body in adults and the most commoly dislocated shoulder joint. Although its dislocation is rare in children, the treatment is the same.

The glenohumeral joint is almost always dislocated anteriorly. Although it is rare, dislocation may be posterior. A third, very rare dislocation is luxatio-erecta. As with all joints, the joint may be sprained, subluxed, or dislocated.

Roentgenograms. The standard views of the shoulder—anteroposterior (AP) and lateral—are helpful, as are the axillary views. It is essential for the AP roentgenogram to be the true anterior-posterior view of the joint, which requires that the x-ray tube be rotated 35 to 45 degrees towards the midline to properly detail the glenohumeral joint. A true lateral view of the glenohumeral joint requires the x-ray beam to be parallel to the scapula, shooting through its body. This trans-scapular view of the shoulder is the single most important view and in

all instances demonstrates whether the humeral head is anterior or posterior to the glenoid fossa.

Anterior Glenohumeral Dislocations

Classification. The subcoracoid is the most common of the four types of anterior dislocation. It is usually the result of indirect forces of abduction, extension, and external rotation. The subglenoid is the second most common type of anterior dislocation. The forces required to cause this are strong abduction associated with some extension and external rotation. The subclavicular, a rare anterior dislocation, is attributable to abduction and external rotation associated with a direct lateral force that displaces the humeral head medially. Intrathoracic dislocation is rare. It is also the result of abduction, external rotation, and lateral to medial forces.

Symptoms and Signs. The patient presents in severe pain. The extremity is guarded, slightly abducted, and externally rotated. The acromion process is prominent, the coracoid process is no longer distinct, and the shoulder takes on a "squared-off" appearance. The patient leans away from the injured side and will not abduct or externally rotate the shoulder. The neurovascular status must be checked immediately for impingement upon the brachial plexus or artery.

Roentgenograms. A true AP view is diagnostic of dislocation, but does not define if it is anterior or posterior. Trans-scapular and lateral axillary views will do so. The physician must look carefully for any bony defects in the humeral head, glenoid lip, or scapula.

Treatment. The prehospital treatment of a glenohumeral dislocation is immobilization in the position of least pain. (There is no "position of comfort" in orthopaedic injuries or there would not be an injury!) Ice may provide some analgesia. Neurovascular assessment should be recorded in the field and upon arrival in the emergency department.

Reduction of a dislocated shoulder joint should be done as soon as possible after a thorough history is taken and careful examination and appropriate roentgenograms are carried out. The patient should experience minimal trauma, which usually requires intravenous medication and possibly general anesthesia, although very early dislocations can be reduced quite easily in most instances.

There are a number of ways to reduce the glenohumeral joint by traction. The most commonly employed methods are traction-countertraction, Hippocratic traction-countertraction, and lateral traction. The simplest technique, which often does not even require analgesia, is to keep the humerus adducted against the chest wall and *slowly* externally rotate the forearm. Patient trust and muscle relaxation are critical, and thus smoothness and slowness are needed. By the time the arm is fully externally rotated, 80 percent of dislocations will be reduced—although often the probable sudden movement characteristic of other techniques is absent. The forearm is then returned to an internally rotated position against the chest wall. If this fails, I use the traction-countertraction technique. Unless there are contraindications, the patient receives parenteral narcotics prior to x-ray evaluation. When the patient returns, the narcotic effects should have begun. An intravenous line is established by heparin lock or intravenous fluid drip. This allows the administration of further muscular relaxants and narcotics if needed. I prefer diazepam because of its amnestic and relaxant effects.

One of the emergency department personnel grasps the two ends of a folded bedsheet which has been placed around the axilla of the injured joint and extended over and under the chest and opposite extremity. The assistant gradually applies countertraction in line with the traction being applied by the physician on the involved arm. With gradual, continuous force and good muscle relaxation, the humeral head will usually slip over the glenoid lip and into place. Occasionally, gently lateral traction on the upper humerus or external rotation of the extremity is helpful to direct the humeral head over the glenoid lip.

If these maneuvers are unsuccessful, I recommend orthopaedic consultation rather than use of any leverage techniques. Once the shoulder is reduced, neurovascular status should again be checked and documented on the chart and the patient sent for postreduction films. If the reduced joint is anatomically aligned, the patient should be placed in a swathe and sling or shoulder immobilizer and instructed to see his primary physician or orthopaedic surgeon in 2 to 3 days, or sooner if any problems arise. The emergency physician can inform the patient that he will be immobilized for a period of 1 to 8 weeks, and symptomatic treatment, such as ice and pain medication, may be required.

Complications. Recurrent dislocation is the most common complication of anterior glenohumeral dislocations and is age-related. The younger the patient, the greater the recurrence rate. Axillary nerve damage and axillary artery injury occur in about 10 to 30 percent of the patients, especially in the elderly population with anterior dislocations. Rotator cuff tears may occur with the subcoracoid or subglenoid injuries in 10 to 15 percent of the patients and always occur with subclavicular or intrathoracic dislocations. Fractures of the humeral head, glenoid, acromion, and coracoid processes may be seen on roentgenograms in approximately 20 percent of patients. The long-term complication is traumatic arthritis.

Posterior Dislocations

Incidence. A posterior dislocation is the rarest of all shoulder dislocations with an incidence of approximately 2 percent.

Classification. Anatomically, posterior dislocations are divided into subacromial (which accounts for 98 percent of all posterior dislocations), subglenoid, and subspinous; the latter two dislocations are rare.

Methods of Injury. A direct blow from anterior to posterior may force the humeral head out posteriorly. More commonly, the indirect forces of internal rotation, abduction, and flexion acting upon the humeral head force the head posteriorly. Bilateral posterior dislocations are often seen in patients with grand mal seizures or patients undergoing electric shock treatment.

Symptoms and Signs. Posterior dislocations are rare, and the diagnosis is frequently missed, especially the subacromial type, which is not an obvious injury. If the clinician is aware of the entity and performs a careful physical examination, a posterior dislocation will not be missed, as it is, in fact, a clinical diagnosis. The patient presents with adduction and internal rotation of the affected arm, but will not allow any external rotation or abduction because of severe pain. The posterior aspect of the shoulder is full, and the anterior aspect is flat. The coracoid process is prominent in these individuals.

Roentgenograms. Although the AP view is suggestive, a trans-scapular or true lateral view of the shoulder is required to make the proper diagnosis. This view shows the humeral head to be sitting posteriorly.

Treatment. Orthopaedic consultation is recommended upon arrival in the emergency department and prior to attempted reduction, as this is such a rare entity. The reduction technique is gentle, in-line traction with direct posterior pressure on the humeral head. This maneuver requires total muscular relaxation.

If there continues to be difficulty with traction and posterior to anterior pressure, the elbow may be flexed, gently internally rotated with continual traction, and then externally rotated slowly to allow the humeral head to slip back into the glenoid fossa. If this attempt requires any force, it is advisable to let the orthopaedic surgeon relocate the shoulder under general anesthesia. If the reduction is successful, the patient needs immobilization for approximately 4 weeks. The patient should visit the orthopaedic surgeon as soon as possible because of the different philosophies of postreduction care. Rest, ice, and analgesia are still essential. Rarely, open reduction is required to reduce posterior dislocations.

Complications. The incidence of associated fractures of the posterior glenoid rim, proximal humerus, and humeral head is high—approximately 50 percent. The prereduction x-ray films must be carefully scrutinized to document any fractures. Associated neurovascular and soft tissue injuries similar to anterior dislocations can occur as well and should be sought on initial physical examination. The postreduction physical examination and x-ray films should document new findings, if any, as the reduction itself may cause further injuries if not done gently.

Luxatio-Erecta Dislocations

Incidence. Luxatio-erecta is a rare type of glenohumeral dislocation in which the superior aspect of the humeral head is forced below the inferior rim of the glenoid. It is a severe injury.

Methods of Injury. The patient experiences an extreme hyperabduction maneuver of the affected arm. This causes the humeral head to be forced inferiorly under the glenoid, rupturing the capsule and all the attached muscles of the upper shoulder.

Symptoms and Signs. The patient presents in severe pain with the humerus overhead and locked. The patient is unable to move the affected arm, and the elbow is usually flexed with the forearm resting on the head. Neurovascular compression is almost always present.

Treatment. The prehospital treatment is support of the extremity and application of ice, if available. Orthopaedic consultation is recommended after evaluation in the emergency department. Reduction requires a traction-countertraction technique that uses upward traction on the affected arm. Then the arm is gradually brought into a less abducted position and finally placed at the patient's side.

Complications. There is always an associated rotator cuff tear or detachment of the greater tuberosity. There may be an inferior glenoid rim fracture, and neurovascular damage usually occurs. It is difficult to reduce luxatio-erecta glenohumeral dislocations, since the humeral head cannot be brought back into the joint space, as it has "buttonholed" through the capsule. In these instances, open reduction is required.

Acromioclavicular Injuries

Incidence. Acromioclavicular injuries are common (about 12 percent of all shoulder injuries) and are most often sustained during athletic events.

Anatomy. The acromioclavicular joint is a diarthrodial joint with an interarticular disc. It is supported by two sets of ligaments, the acromioclavicular and coracoclavicular, as well as the joint capsule (see Fig. 2, in the chapter *Shoulder Pain*). The coracoclavicular ligaments consist of the conoid and trapezoid ligaments, which are strong and essential to joint integrity.

Methods of Injury. Direct forces exerted on the acromioclavicular joint by the individual falling directly on the point of the shoulder with the arm adducted are the most common causes of injuries to this joint. Indirect forces, such as falling on an outstretched extremity and transmitting the force to the acromioclavicular joint, are less common.

Classification. Classification of acromioclavicular joint injuries is based primarily upon the degree of injury to the acromioclavicular and coracoclavicular ligaments, as well as the position and displacement of the clavicle.

Traditionally, the classification consists of type I, type II, and type III injuries, with types IV and V more recently described. The presentation and treatment of the various types will be discussed subsequently.

Symptoms and Signs. Type I injuries, or mild sprains, are associated with joint tenderness and swelling and minimal pain with movement. There is no displacement of the clavicle on the acromion. Type II injuries (moderate sprains or subluxations) are associated with moderate to severe pain, especially with movement. The distal clavicle may ride slightly higher on the acromion when compared with the opposite joint. Type III injuries (complete disruption of the acromioclavicular joint) are usually obvious. The normal appearance of the shoulder is distorted. The patient is in severe pain and guards against any movement of the affected extremity. There is movement and separation of the acromioclavicular joint on palpation. More severe type IV and type V injuries, which consist of complete disruption of the joint and displacement or fracture of the clavicle, cause severe pain with any movement and marked swelling. A complete neurovascular assessment must always be documented, especially in more severe injuries.

Roentgenograms. Acromioclavicular films require one-third to two-thirds less intensity than routine shoulder films; therefore, they should be ordered specifically. Stress films should also be ordered to assess the coracoclavicular ligament properly.

A type I injury appears on roentgenograms as a normal acromioclavicular joint. In a type II injury, the lateral aspect of the clavicle may be elevated by up to one-half of its width higher than the acromion. In a type III injury, the clavicle is elevated above the acromion by its entire width, and the joint space is widened. If there is associated coracoclavicular ligamentous disruption, the distance between the clavicle and the coracoid process is also widened, especially with the stress views. In the more severe type IV and V injuries, displacement or fracture of the clavicle in conjunction with the above findings is characteristic.

Treatment. Before admission to the hospital, the patient's injured extremity should be put at rest and supported by the use of a sling or shoulder immobilizer. Ice should be applied to the area as quickly as possible to provide analgesia and reduce swelling. After the appropriate physical examination, emergency department personnel should again immobilize the joint and apply ice to the injury while the patient undergoes further evaluation and roentgenograms.

Once the severity of the injury is determined, the treatment and discharge regimen will vary with the type of injury. The management of type I and II injuries is the noncontroversial conservative approach. Patients with type I injuries benefit from the local application of ice packs along with appropriate analgesia for the duration of acute pain, usually 2 to 3 days. More importantly, the patient should put the injured extremity at rest by using a sling until the acute pain subsides. The emergency physician should advise the patient to schedule follow-up evaluation with his primary care or orthopaedic physician in 2 to 3 days to ensure that no further injury will take place. It commonly takes 2 to 4 weeks to achieve normal, pain-free range of motion with full strength.

The discharge treatment of type II injuries is similar to the previously described treatment, except some clinicians recommend that the immobilization device provide continuous downward pressure on the superior distal clavicle to ensure that the stretched ligaments heal tightly. No matter what type of immobilization is used, follow-up in 2 to 3 days is important. The emergency physician may advise the patient to rest the joint for at least 1 to 2 weeks, depending upon age, symptoms, and circumstances. After this, rehabilitation should begin until full range of motion and strength are achieved.

In contrast to the above, there are two diverse approaches to patients with type III and more severe injuries; i.e., surgical repair versus conservative management. Orthopaedic consultation in the emergency department is needed. The orthopaedic surgeon may admit the patient for surgical repair, recommend immobilization for 6 to 8 weeks, or recommend immobilization for a few days and begin early functional use of the shoulder; the choice is based on the age, activity, and future plans of the individual.

Complications. Complications seen in the emergency department include neurovascular injuries and associated injuries to the clavicle, scapula, and humerus as well as the other shoulder joints themselves. If the patient is not allowed to heal for an appropriate length of time and proper rehabilitation is not undertaken, recurrence is common. Traumatic arthritis may also develop, especially in physically active patients. Such complications require orthopaedic evaluation and treatment.

Acromioclavicular Injuries in Children

Injuries to this joint in children are rare and usually confused with a fracture of the distal clavicle. The classification used to describe adult injury is not applicable for children because, in most instances, the coracoclavicular ligaments are not disrupted, since the stresses of the injury are placed on the periosteal tube of the distal clavicle and not on the ligaments. The symptoms and signs and roentgenogram techniques are essentially the same in the child as in the adult. Treatment is usually conservative and nonoperative. The prognosis in children is quite good if appropriate evaluation and treatment are done. It is recommended that the orthopaedic surgeon be consulted early.

Sternoclavicular Injuries

Incidence. This is a rare injury that usually results in one of two types of dislocation: the more common anterior dislocation and the posterior dislocation.

Anatomy. Joint integrity is attributable to various ligamentous structures: the interarticular disc ligament, the costoclavicular ligaments (which have an anterior and posterior component), and the anterior and posterior sternoclavicular ligaments. These ligaments are fairly strong and allow only a limited range of motion.

Methods of Injury. The sternoclavicular joint comes under a great deal of stress because it is subjected to motion with every movement of the upper extremity. Owing to its strong ligamentous support, however, the joint requires a tremendous amount of force to disrupt it.

Direct force will obviously cause a posterior dislocation as it drives the clavicle back on the sternum. Indirect force, which is the more common cause of injury, may cause an anterior or posterior dislocation. This occurs as follows: The individual is lying on the ground laterally with one shoulder in contact with the ground. The opposite, or upward, shoulder is then compressed into the ground. If a rotational effect occurs with the compression, i.e., if the upward shoulder is rolled forward, the ipsilateral sternoclavicular joint is forced backward so that a posterior dislocation occurs. If, however, the upward shoulder is rolled backward, then the ipsilateral joint is forced anteriorly.

Symptoms and Signs. A mild sprain is associated with minimal to moderate pain with movement of the ipsilateral extremity. There may be some local swelling and tenderness. A moderate sprain or subluxation is associated with marked swelling and decreased range of motion of the upper extremity. A dislocation is associated with severe pain and minimal range of motion. In anterior dislocations the medial aspect of the clavicle is visibly prominent and easily felt. Moreover, the medial clavicle may ride high and is usually mobile. In contrast, a posterior dislocation is usually associated with more pain, and the medial clavicle is less prominent and less palpable. The patient may complain of shortness of breath, choking, or dysphagia. Also, venous congestion and decreased circulation to the ipsilateral upper extremity may be evident upon examination, owing to impingement problems.

Roentgenograms. Interestingly enough, x-ray films are usually not helpful in diagnosing such injuries. Tomograms, and especially the computed tomographic scan for posterior dislocations, are more helpful. It is important to evaluate these injuries properly because there is a high incidence of medial clavicular epiphyseal fractures in individuals under 25 years of age.

Treatment. The treatment for sprains of the sternoclavicular joint is application of ice for the first 48 to 72 hours and immobilization for 3 to 4 days. The treatment for moderate sprains or subluxations is also ice and a clavicular strap or swathe and sling for 4 to 6 weeks. The treatment for dislocations is usually closed reduction under general anesthesia.

After the patient has been evaluated to rule out any vascular or airway compromise, the orthopaedic surgeon should be consulted to perform the appropriate reduction techniques under general anesthesia. Should the emergency physician be required to carry out such techniques, they should be done as follows: Sandbags are placed between the shoulders, and if the dislocation is anterior, the upper extremities are put in 90 degrees of abduction and extension. In-line traction is applied to the upper extremity, and posterior pressure is exerted over the distal clavicle. If the dislocation is posterior, lateral traction is applied to the abducted upper extremity, and the extremity is then extended. This should bring the clavicle out from behind the sternum; if it does not, a towel clip may be used to grasp the medial part of the clavicle and the physician may then pull it anteriorly.

Complications. There is a 25 percent incidence of vascular, esophageal, or airway complications with posterior dislocations. In contrast, anterior dislocations are associated with minimal problems, such as a cosmetic bump or movable medial tip.

Sternoclavicular Injuries in Children

The incidence, anatomy, mechanism of injury, classification, symptoms and signs, and treatment of sternoclavicular injuries in children are similar to those discribed for adults. Injuries of the sternoclavicular joint in children are treated nonoperatively. They are probably epiphyseal separations which heal and remodel without the need for surgical intervention.

ELBOW INJURIES

Incidence. Elbow injuries are the third most common dislocation in the human body after shoulder and finger injuries.

Anatomy. The elbow is a bicondylar joint with its strength in the humeral-ulnar joint. The radius provides stability and dexterity of the hand. The elbow joint is surrounded by a capsule and collateral ligaments—medial, lateral, anterior, and posterior. Between the synovial tissue and the fibrous capsule of the elbow are haversian glands, or fat pads, which lie in the coracoid and olecranon fossa. Normally, the anterior fat pad is barely visible, and the posterior fat pad is not visible on the roentgenogram of the elbow. Dislocations are classified by radial ulnar displacement in relationship to the distal humerus.

Posterior Dislocations Of The Elbow

Incidence. Eighty to 90 percent of all elbow dislocations are posterior or posterolateral, which is the more common of the two.

Methods of Injury. Falling on an outstretched hand with the arm extended and abducted causes this injury. This mechanism of injury forces the distal humerus through the anterior capsule, which tears the brachialis muscle and ligaments in the joint capsule and strips the triceps insertion off the ulna.

Symptoms and Signs. The patient presents with severe pain and swelling and limited range of motion. The arm is in mild flexion with the forearm appearing shortened. The olecranon is prominent and easily palpated posteriorly. Further palpation also reveals disturbance of the triangular relationship of the olecranon and epicondyles posteriorly. Neurovascular status must be checked immediately.

Roentgenograms. AP and lateral views prior to and after reduction are essential for proper evaluation and treatment.

Treatment. The prehospital treatment of elbow dislocations is the standard immobilization and ice after a neurovascular examination. Unless severe vascular compromise has occurred and no physician is available for a prolonged period, attempted reduction should be done in the emergency department and not in the field.

Once the patient has arrived in the emergency department, a physical examination with a detailed neurologic and vascular evaluation is carried out and documented. Roentgenographic assessment is then performed. Posterolateral and posterior dislocations are almost always reduced by closed means, but require complete muscular relaxation. No anesthesia may be needed if gentle reduction is attempted immediately after the injury. More commonly, spasm and swelling have occurred and the patient is apprehensive. Therefore, regional or general anesthesia becomes mandatory. However, treatment is not accomplished by simply reversing the mechanism of injury, so prior experience and knowledge are essential. Because of this, it may be in the patient's best interest to consult the orthopaedic surgeon immediately.

If vascular compromise is present, the physician must attempt to reduce the joint and relieve the vascular compromise. Traction-countertraction is the usual maneuver to reduce the dislocation, but the medial or lateral displacement must be corrected prior to correcting the anterior or posterior displacement. The easiest method is traction on the wrist and proximal forearm while countertraction is applied to the humerus. The medial-lateral displacement is corrected first. Then, with continued traction, posterior pressure on the forearm should disengage the coronoid from the olecranon fossa as the elbow is flexed. Hyperextension is always avoided. The physician should put the joint through full range of motion to ensure anatomic reduction, stability, and no mechanical block owing to an entrapped medial epicondyle.

The emergency department physician should not attempt reduction of a dislocated elbow more than twice, because in a majority of instances, if the elbow cannot be properly reduced with good analgesia after one or two attempts, general anesthesia is required. After clinical reduction, the neurovascular status is again evaluated and postreduction films are reviewed to ensure normal anatomy and no missed fractures. A long-arm splint is applied with the elbow flexed 90 degrees or more if possible. Orthopaedic follow-up in 24 hours is recommended to ensure neurovascular integrity.

The patient or family should also be instructed to observe the hand for circulatory changes. Ice and elevation are helpful. The emergency physician may instruct the patient that immobilization for approximately 1 to 2 weeks is the usual treatment. Active range of motion is then begun. Patients, especially older individuals, should not be immobilized longer than 3 to 4 weeks, as contractures will occur in the joint.

Complications. Myositis ossificans may occur as a result of the significant soft tissue injury. Also, these dislocations may rarely be unable to be reduced owing to interposition of soft tissue or bone. Nerve injuries, especially those of the median and ulnar nerve, may occur, as well as injuries to the brachial artery. These may be indications for surgical exploration. There can be associated fractures, with an incidence of 12 to 62 percent, usually involving the medial condyle or coronoid. Medial epicondylar fractures are more common in children and are rare in adults, but should be sought in both the prereduction and postreduction x-ray films. Prognosis for posterior dislocations is excellent in 75 to 80 percent of individuals, with the remainder having some loss of full extension.

Medial And Lateral Dislocations

Incidence. Medial-lateral dislocations do not occur often, the medial dislocation usually is a subluxation rather than a true dislocation.

Symptoms and Signs. The patient presents with pain and swelling, the elbow appears widened, and the forearm length appears normal. There may be some flexion and extension of the joint when the dislocation is lateral.

Roentgenograms. AP and lateral views are always required.

Treatment. The principles of treatment are similar to those for posterior dislocations described previously. Reduction is done by the traction-countertraction technique in mild extension with medial or lateral pressure to reduce the deformity. The physician should be careful to avoid converting this dislocation into a posterior dislocation.

Complications. Complications are similar to those of posterior dislocations, but since the medial injury is usually only a subluxation rather than a dislocation, soft tissue injuries are not as severe as with lateral dislocations.

Anterior Dislocations Of The Elbow

Incidence. This is a rare injury.

Methods of Injury. A blow to the flexed elbow will drive the olecranon forward, causing an anterior dislocation.

Symptoms and Signs. The patient presents with the elbow in extension, pain, swelling, and unwillingness to move the elbow. The forearm is lengthened and supinated.

Roentgenograms. AP and lateral views are again required.

Treatment. This is a severe injury associated with extensive soft tissue damage and vascular injuries. Some cases may present as open injuries. Orthopaedic consultation is recommended. Usually reduction is achieved easily by traction-countertraction in partial extension combined with posterior pressure on the forearm, however, knowledge and expertise are required.

Complications. Anterior dislocations have a high incidence of vascular compromise and may in fact present as open injuries.

SUBLUXATION OF THE RADIAL HEAD

Incidence. Subluxation of the radial head is an injury frequently seen in the emergency department.

Although it is difficult to obtain exact figures, one study documented an approximate 27 percent incidence of radial head subluxation when compared with elbow injuries. The average age at presentation is between 2 and 3 years, and the injury is rarely seen past the age of 7. The left upper extremity usually is involved in the majority of cases, and interestingly enough, the majority of patients are female.

Methods of Injury. The most widely accepted mechanism of injury is distal traction applied to the patient's wrist or hand when the forearm is pronated and the elbow is extended. The orbicular ligament partially slips proximally over the radial head.

Symptoms and Signs. If the emergency department physician is not familiar with this entity, diagnosis may be difficult because there is a lack of specific clinical findings and certainly a lack of roentgenogram findings. History is helpful in that there is usually an episode of longitudinal pull that is placed on the elbow of the child or infant. The child is reluctant to use the involved extremity, which hangs at the side with the forearm pronated. Any attempt to supinate the forearm or flex the elbow causes pain and distress. There may be some local tenderness over the radial head as well.

Roentgenograms. There are no roentgenogram findings which demonstrate subluxation or displacement of the radial head. However, it is still recommended that roentgenograms be taken to rule out other injuries.

Treatment. When the physician has diagnosed subluxation of the radial head, manipulation is performed to reduce it. The physician holds the patient's forearm with the elbow in the semiflexed position. The forearm is then supinated. If this fails to produce the characteristic popping associated with reduction, the elbow is then maximally flexed with the forearm supinated until the popping sensation occurs. The patient's arm does not usually need to be immobilized if this is a first or second injury. If it is a recurrent problem, the extremity should be immobilized in a sling and possibly a cast, and the patient referred to the orthopaedic surgeon for further consultation and rehabilitation. It is important to educate the family as to how the injury occurred so it does not happen again.

Complications. There are usually no long-term sequelae after subluxations. They are easily reduced in the emergency department or the physician's office. Recurrence has been reported to be 5 to 30 percent and is usually attributable to the same type of mechanism because the family has not been educated to avoid such pulling maneuvers.

SUGGESTED READING

Rockwood CA Jr, Green DP. Fractures in adults. 2nd ed. Philadelphia: Lippincott, 1984.

Rockwood CA Jr, Wilkins KE, King RE. Fractures in children. Philadelphia: Lippincott, 1984.

Simon RR, Koenigsknecht SJ. Orthopaedics in emergency medicine. Welsh RP, Shephard RJ. Current therapy in sports medicine. 1985–86. Toronto: BC Decker, 1985.

KNEE DISLOCATION

EDWARD E. KIMBROUGH, M.D.
RANDALL S. SUAREZ, M.D.

Dislocation of the knee, although it is an uncommon injury, is associated with a high incidence of vascular and neurologic complications. Because the results of these complications can be disastrous, the emergency medicine physician should be aware of the problems associated with knee dislocation and should be prepared to deal with it quickly.

CLASSIFICATION

Dislocation of the knee is classified by the position of the tibia in relation to the femur. There are five classifications: anterior, posterior, medial, lateral, and rotatory. Description of this injury may also include whether it is open or closed. If a fracture is associated with the dislocation, it may be described as a fracture-dislocation.

MECHANISM OF INJURY

Anterior dislocation is considered to be the most common form of knee dislocation, and most authors feel that anterior dislocation is a result of violent hyperextension of the knee. This results in tearing of the posterior capsule and anterior cruciate ligament and anterior displacement of the tibia on the femur. Posterior dislocation of the knee is often associated with motor vehicle accidents. This type of injury results from a blow to the anterior aspect of a flexed knee as in the "dashboard-knee" injury. Medial or lateral dislocations quite often occur in conjunction with a tibial plateau or femoral condyle fracture and may be associated with rotary stress, as is the case with rotatory dislocation.

ANATOMY

The ligamentous structures within the knee are complex, and the reader should refer to an anatomy text for a detailed review of these structures. However, one can easily see how the anterior and posterior cruciate ligaments could often be ruptured with any type of dislocation of the knee, especially in the anterior-to-posterior direction. It is also easy to understand that the collateral ligaments and the capsular structures are often torn because of the instability created by dislocation of the knee.

The popliteal artery is fixed proximally and distally as it passes posterior to the knee joint. Proximally, the popliteal artery is fixed as it passes through the adductor hiatus where the tendinous portion of the adductor magnus attaches to the femur. Distally, the popliteal artery is fixed to the posterior aspect of the tibia as it passes through the fibrous arch of the soleus muscle. The artery can frequently be injured as it is tethered on both ends, and when the knee is dislocated the artery can be easily stretched.

The popliteal artery gives off five arterial branches within the popliteal space. These branches include the superior and inferior medial and lateral genicular arteries and the middle genicular artery. These arteries anastomose with the anterior tibial recurrent artery; however, this is a tenuous anastomosis and usually does not provide an adequate blood supply to maintain the viability of the leg and foot in the event of popliteal artery disruption. In addition to this, the large amount of trauma that is necessary to disrupt the popliteal artery is also likely to disrupt these fine anastomotic vessels.

The nerves of the popliteal space; namely the tibial and the common peroneal nerves, are not as rigidly fixed as the posterior tibial artery to the posterior femur and posterior tibia. The nerve injury in this area is generally a traction-type injury as the popliteal nerves are stretched around the posterior aspect of the femoral condyles.

COMPLICATIONS

The most potentially devastating complication of dislocation of the knee is vascular disruption. The artery is tethered superiorly and inferiorly around the knee and is therefore prone to an injury with dislocation of the tibia on the femur; the frequency of injury is between 32 percent and 40 percent. In a study by Green and Allen, those people who had arterial disruption and did not have reestablished blood flow within a period of 6 to 8 hours had a below-knee amputation rate of 86 percent. Of the remaining 14 percent, two-thirds also had ischemic changes.

Incidence of neurologic injuries is between 30 percent and 35 percent. These injuries tend to be traction-type injuries and usually show at least partial return of function in 3 to 6 months without surgical intervention.

Almost by necessity, dislocation of the knee involves damage to the ligamentous structures. Therefore, ligamentous instability of the knee is a very common complication following this injury. The definitive management of this ligamentous injury is quite controversial and will be addressed later in this chapter. In general, if the knee appears to be stable following reduction, surgical intervention is not indicated. However, if the knee is grossly unstable after reduction, surgical intervention is generally indicated. It must be noted here that above all, vascular patency takes precedence. In the face of gross instability, if operative repair would jeopardize reestablishment and maintenance of blood flow, then operative repair should be postponed until the vascular status is stable.

DIFFERENTIAL DIAGNOSIS

When patients describe their knees as dislocated, this usually represents not a true knee dislocation but a patellar subluxation or patellar dislocation.

Several authors think that one reason that true knee dislocation is considered a rare injury is that quite often the knee dislocation is reduced spontaneously by the patient or by the emergency medical technician on the scene of the accident. Therefore, the emergency physician should always be suspicious of a vascular injury when confronted with a severely injured knee, particularly one with ligamentous disruption, because this may represent a reduced knee dislocation.

INITIAL MANAGEMENT

When confronted with a knee dislocation in the emergency department, it is imperative to perform a *neurologic and vascular assessment* immediately. If pulses are absent in the injured extremity, a reduction should be performed immediately and followed by a repeat vascular assessment. The presence of a warm foot with pulses and adequate capillary refill is not sufficient to assure popliteal-artery patency, and a damaged artery may be patent initially and later thrombose. A high index of suspicion is needed.

Reduction of a posterior dislocation is accomplished by traction on the lower leg and anterior movement of the tibia (Fig. 1) and should be accomplished as soon as possible. The patient should be examined initially and periodically for signs of impending compartment syndrome; if there is any suspicion of this syndrome, then compartment-pressure studies are recommended.

After initial assessment and reduction, the extremity should be splinted in a posterior splint in approximately 15 degrees of flexion. In order to leave the limb free to swell and to enable frequent vascular and neurologic

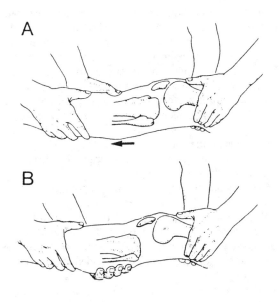

Figure 1 The reduction of a dislocation of the knee. *A*, The femur is stabilized proximally and the leg is pulled inferiorly. *B*, After traction the knee, which is posteriorly dislocated, is then lifted back in its anatomic position. (From Simon R, Brenner B. Procedures and techniques in emergency medicine. Baltimore: Williams & Wilkins, 1982.)

assessment, it is important not to apply a circumferential cast or restrictive dressing. Neurologic assessment must be done both prior to and after reduction, and both results should be documented. A changing neurologic picture can be evidence of a vascular injury or of a compartment syndrome.

After reduction, if an absent or diminished dorsalis pedis or posterior tibial pulse is evident, then further investigation is needed. This investigation can take one of two forms: immediate arteriography done either in the radiology department or in the operating room by the vascular surgeon, or immediate exploration by the vascular surgeon without the benefit of an arteriogram. One must always keep the 6-hour rule in mind; that is, blood flow should be reinstated in a maximum of 6 to 8 hours after the injury to afford the maximal chance of avoiding permanent ischemic injury. If obtaining an arteriogram would take too much of this 6-hour period of time, it is recommended that the arteriography be done on the operating table or the artery be explored directly without the benefit of the arteriogram. It should be noted that arteriography has been reported to increase vascular spasm. In light of this, arteriography should not be attempted unless the services of a vascular surgeon are readily available. If a vascular surgeon is not readily available, the patient should be quickly transferred to an institution that has one.

DISPOSITON

All patients with dislocation of the knee need admission and the evaluation described above for vascular sequelae. Patients with severe knee trauma or unstable knees in whom the possibility of dislocation with spontaneous reduction is suspected should be admitted and observed in the same fashion.

After prompt reestablishment and maintenance of adequate blood flow has been addressed, the issue of long-term management should be considered. There are a wide variety of opinions in the orthopaedic literature about the best form of treatment for ligamentous injuries of the knee. Some authors advocate early operative repair of all ligamentous injuries; other authors believe that in the majority of these cases immobilization is sufficient to ensure a stable knee. As stated previously, in general, an unstable knee following reduction should undergo operative ligamentous repair as soon as the vascular status permits. However, if the knee is stable following reduction, most authors consider cast immobilization for 8 to 10 weeks sufficient to provide a stable knee.

SUGGESTED READING

Allen S, Edmonson A, Crenshaw H, eds. Campbell's operative orthopaedics. New York: CV Mosby, 1980.
Connolly JF, ed. The management of fracutres and dislocations. Philadelphia: WB Saunders, 1981.
Evarts C, McCallister, ed. Surgery of the musculoskeletal system. New York: Churchill Livingston, 1983.
Larson RI, Jones DC. Dislocations and ligamentous injuries of the knee. In: Rockwood CA, Green DP, eds. Fractures in adults. Philadelphia: JB Lippincott, 1984:1502.

DISLOCATION OF THE DIGITS, WRIST, AND HAND

EUGENE S. KILGORE, M.D.

GENERAL PRINCIPLES

Acute dislocations are common hand injuries. They are easily diagnosed when a detailed history of the mechanism of injury is combined with the observation and palpation of a fresh deformity and roentgenographic abnormality. When treatment is delayed, swelling may obscure a deformity, which can then only be proved by a roentgenogram, although it may be suspected on the basis of an appropriate history and limitation of motion. Insidious and chronic dislocations caused by spastic, arthritic, and congenital states are not discussed here.

Most dislocations affect digital joints and are caused by direct or indirect force. Any dislocation, if recognized promptly, usually can be reduced fairly easily by appropriate distraction, combined with the simultaneous recreation and accentuation of the angle of the joint that favored the dislocation (the exception is subluxation of the metacarpophalangeal joint of the finger), and then careful manipulation of the dislocated bone back into normal alignment. This is often accomplished by a popping sound. Relaxation of the patient's muscles is imperative, and the reduction must not be a significantly painful experience, or else appropriate anesthesia should be administered. Force should never be used to accomplish a closed reduction. Instead, a gentle open reduction should be undertaken. The key to a successful reduction is the restoration of alignment and full, unrestrained passive and/or active range of motion without any axial rotatory abnormality. The presence of anesthesia and/or ischemia due to a dislocation means stretch, compression, or kinking of the neurovascular structures; this must be relieved by urgent closed or open means.

All open dislocations require local irrigation of the joint with antibiotics (e.g., 1 or 2 cc of Bacitracin at 1,000 U per cc), systemic antibiotics for 2 to 3 days targeted against *Staphylococcus* and *Streptococcus*, and up-to-date tetanus prophylaxis.

Concurrent fractures should be appropriately managed, and divided soft tissues accompanying open dislocations should be repaired whenever possible, particularly tendons and collateral ligaments. Whatever else needs repair is a matter of surgical judgment, as is the nature and duration of immobilization.

A roentgenographic confirmation of a reduction is advised immediately and 5 to 7 days later in follow-up. The prevention and reversal of edema are essential after all reductions. To this end, all jewelry and snug clothing should be removed and the hand comfortably elevated above the heart. Joint stiffness and pain are sequelae to most dislocations, and their magnitude and duration are unpredictable.

Any dislocation that does not reduce easily in the emergency department should result in prompt consultation with the hand surgeon. So should those that are open and those that are associated with significant fractures (e.g., more than a chip), ligamentous ruptures, and nerve, tendon, or circulatory impairment.

FINGER DISLOCATIONS

The distal bone invariably moves dorsal to the head of the more proximal bone. The reverse of this is rare. Interphalangeal joint dislocations are far more common and more easily reduced than those of the metacarpophalangeal joints. Most dislocations are closed, and most involve the proximal interphalangeal joint. The usual mechanism is abrupt hyperextension of the joint with simultaneous impaction as a result of a fall, carrying one's weight on the digit, or a sudden blow inflicted by someone's body during sports activity or by a fast-moving object, such as a basketball. There may or may not be considerable joint pain and/or distortion. If hyperextension is sudden and extreme, the palmar skin may be torn open in the flexion crease, and the phalangeal head may protrude in the wound.

Any dislocation involves a tear of periarticular tissues that normally restrain abnormal movement, dislocation, and angulation. Such tissues include the check-rein ligaments of the volar plate, the volar plate itself, the collateral ligaments, the dorsal joint capsule, and even the extensor hood. The tell-tale mark of significant rupture of a collateral ligament is laxity when the ligament is stress-tested after reduction of the dislocation. If pain prevents this test, the digit should be anesthetized to allow an adequate test.

Once the dislocation is reduced, there should be complete and unrestricted normal range of extension and flexion of the joint, without (1) a tendency of the finger joint to spring back into extension, (2) resistance to flexion, or (3) an abnormal plane of the surface of the nail plate when compared to adjacent digits and the opposite hand. Any of these three factors signals inadequate reduction, and the third one signals interposition of soft tissues (e.g., collateral ligament, volar plate, or portions of the extensor hood) inside the joint, causing a "trapped" dislocation. Such problems usually require surgery to accomplish the desired reduction.

Except when the injury is already open, the surgical approach is through a dorsal incision over the joint, and the soft tissues blocking reduction are then identified and gently retracted with a hand probe as the reduction is accomplished. Occasionally, one or both collateral ligaments must be partly or completely divided to accomplish the reduction. If the reduction remains unstable, particularly if there is an avulsion fracture of the volar lip of the base of the phalanx, the fracture fragments may have to be removed and the volar plate reattached to the bare surface of the bone. The adequacy of any reduction should be confirmed roentgenographically.

Postreduction immobilization must keep the digital joint in 20 to 30 degrees of flexion and guard against full

190

extension for 1 to 3 weeks, depending on how unstable the reduction was and whether volar plate advancement or fracture reduction was necessary. In many instances, a splint that blocks full extension, but allows active flexion, is desirable early on, so as to preclude the development of excessive joint stiffness. Whenever a collateral ligament has been divided, buddy-taping the finger to its neighbor for 3 weeks splints the ligament while it heals.

Any dislocated digital joint that is well reduced may leave in its wake an enlarged and stiff joint a month or more after the reduction. This merits a local injecton of a mixture of 1 ml lidocaine (1 percent) and 0.25 ml triamcinolone (40 mg per milliliter) about the collateral ligaments and the volar plate. This can be done at least twice in a period of 2 to 4 weeks and frequently results in reduction of soft tissue volume about the joint, increased range of motion, and decreased pain.

Dislocation of the metacarpophalangeal joint of a finger is uncommon and usually requires a surgical reduction. It usually involves the index finger. A partial dislocation (subluxation and locking of the proximal phalanx in 60 to 90 degrees of extension) may be easily reduced by simple distraction and joint flexion, avoiding any hyperextension that may convert an easily reducible into an irreducible dislocation. When the roentgenogram reveals the base of the phalanx to be dorsal to and overriding the head of the metacarpal, the dislocation is irreducible except by open reduction. The head of the metacarpal is trapped in a noose formed by the volar plate dorsally, the transverse fibers of the palmar fascia volarly, the lumbrical radially, and the long flexor tendons ulnarly. By exposing the volar plate dorsally and slitting it down the middle, as in unbuttoning the top buttons of a shirt, one can extract and easily reduce the head.

THUMB DISLOCATIONS

Dislocations of the thumb are diagnosed and treated according to the principles cited for the fingers: a careful history of the mechanism of injury, detection of deformity clinically and roentgenographically, and concomitant limitation of motion. At the interphalangeal joint, the principles of reduction are the same as for the finger. However, at the metacarpophalangeal joint, trapping of the acute dislocation does not occur, and in most cases, closed reduction is possible by traction and hyperextension followed by flexion. The collateral ligament (ulnar more often than radial) may be partially or completely ruptured, and this is ascertained by stress-testing and roentgenography after infiltrating the ligament with a small amount of lidocaine and then comparing the injured thumb with the uninjured one. A ruptured ligament should be repaired surgically, and when there is an associated avulsion fracture off the base of the phalanx, it should either be resected or reduced and pinned, depending on its size. The relocated thumb should be immobilized as described for the fingers.

CARPOMETACARPAL DISLOCATIONS

Dislocations of the carpometacarpal joints are seen most commonly at the base of the thumb, but may occur as single or multiple dislocations at any of the five digits, usually as a result of a violent impaction force. They may or may not be associated with a fracture. In the case of the thumb, a Bennett fracture of the thumb metacarpal is a common concurrent injury. The reduction may be easily accomplished by traction on the digit and downward pressure on the base of the metacarpal. However, these dislocations tend to be highly unstable and often require percutaneous pinning or open reduction and internal fixation to prevent recurrence. Consultation with a hand surgeon is advised.

WRIST DISLOCATIONS

Wrist dislocations are much less common than those of the digital and carpometacarpal joints. There is invariably a history of major trauma followed by pain, swelling, and some abnormality of motion. The injury may be open or closed. The dislocation or subluxation may only be proved by careful comparison of motion, stability, and roentgenograms of both the injured and uninjured wrists. Standard AP and lateral views, views in multiple planes and with forearm and wrist in extremes of motion, and particularly "reverse-oblique" views may be necessary to rule out the skeletal abnormality. Carpal dislocations may not be obvious on the x-ray films and are commonly missed in the emergency department; if the patient has marked swelling or pain, consultation with the radiologist or hand surgeon should be obtained before the patient is discharged.

Concomitant fractures must also be ruled out and may not show up until a follow-up roentgenogram is taken 7 to 10 days later. When there is no detectable roentgenographic abnormality of the wrist after the acute onset of pain from trauma, a diagnosis of "wrist sprain" must never be made until the wrist has been adequately splinted to eliminate pain with a short or long-arm cast for a week, and a follow-up roentgenogram confirms that there is no abnormality.

Any of the eight carpal bones as well as the radius and ulna can subluxate and dislocate. These dislocations may be with ligamentous disruption alone or combined with fracture such as (1) dislocation of the lunate, in which the lunate flips volarward out of its position between the capitate and the radius, (2) perilunar dislocation of the carpus, in which the lunate keeps its relationship to the radius, but the rest of the carpal bones pass to the dorsum of the lunate, and (3) several modifications of these two conditions with or without fractures, namely, dislocation of lunate and the proximal half of the scaphoid volarly, dislocation of the carpal bones dorsally while the lunate and proximal half of the fractured scaphoid remain in place (the so-called transscapho-perilunar dislocation, which usually has an associated fracture of the styloids of the radius and ulna), volar dislocation of the intact lunate and scaphoid, and periscapho-lunar dislocation, in which the scaphoid and lunate remain intact and the rest of the carpus moves dorsally, together with a fracture of the ulnar styloid. The most common of these dislocations are the anterior dislocation of the lunate and the transscapho-perilunar dislocation of the carpus dorsal to the lunate and proximal half of the scaphoid.

Closed reduction of these dislocations is generally fairly easy if it is not delayed, pain is relieved, muscles are relaxed, the wrist is distracted with traction and countertraction, and the displaced elements are manipulated back into place. The reduction must always be confirmed roentgenographically and the wrist immobilized in a well-padded cast that allows finger motion. If there is a fracture of the scaphoid, the thumb must be immobilized and a long-arm cast applied for at least 1 month, followed by a short-arm cast until there is roentgenographic evidence of union. Fractures that are not well approximated and reduced often need open reduction and internal fixation. Dislocations without fracture or with chip fractures require immobilization of the wrist for only 3 to 4 weeks. From the beginning, there should be daily active range of motion of all digital joints as well as the shoulder (and elbow if it is free) to prevent stiffness. Furthermore, the existence or development of sensory or motor nerve loss must be carefully assessed from the day of injury on, and a compression state dealt with by urgent or elective surgical decompression as the case warrants. Throbbing pain is a signal of venous congestion and possible compartment syndrome and requires unrelenting attention in the form of elevation, bivalving the cast and cast padding, or fasciotomy.

The distal radial-ulnar joint may subluxate and dislocate when a fall or sudden stress to the ulnar side of the wrist or torque force to the forearm tears the ligamentous structures. There are three such structures: (1) from the ulnar styloid to the triquetrum, (2) the capsular cuff-like ligament between the articular margins of the radius and ulna with a dorsal half that tightens with pronation and a volar half that tightens with supination, and (3) the triangular fibrocartilage originating from the dorsum of the radius to insert on the ulna between its head and its styloid.

Pain, tenderness, and a clinical and roentgenographic displacement of the head of the ulna in contrast to the normal wrist is diagnostic. There may be a significant "jog" (uneven movement) of the head of the ulna, interrupting the normal smooth rhythm when the patient alternates pronation and supination. This may be accentuated by compressing the radius and ulna during active rotation. The extent of subluxation may initially be obscured by swelling, pain, or failure of torn parts to be sufficiently attenuated. Therefore, immediate immobilization in a long-arm cast with the wrist and forearm in the neutral position for 3 to 4 weeks is essential. If dislocation is chronic, a surgical correction is needed to overcome existing symptoms, e.g., reconstruction of ligaments or resection of the ulnar styloid.

SUGGESTED READING

Eaton RG. Joint injuries of the hand. Springfield Ill: Charles C Thomas, 1971.

Green DP. Operative hand surgery. New York: Churchill Livingstone, 1982.

Kilgore ES, Graham WP. The hand: surgical and nonsurgical management. Philadelphia: Lea & Febiger, 1977.

Sandzen SD Jr. Atlas of acute hand injuries. New York: McGraw-Hill, 1980.

THE MULTIPLY INJURED ORTHOPAEDIC PATIENT

MARVIN H. MEYERS, M.D.

In most cases, the multiply injured orthopaedic patient has sustained injuries to several major body systems in a violent accident. The injuries may be life-threatening as a consequence of trauma to the respiratory, vascular, and central nervous systems. The management and successful treatment of multiply injured patients require the combined efforts of several specialists such as neurosurgeons, general surgeons, neurologists, and orthopaedic surgeons. For any patient with other than isolated limb trauma, consultation with a general surgeon is in order.

The primary consideration is the resuscitation of the vital functions of the patient. Therefore, it is essential to carefully evaluate the *airway, breathing, and circulation*. Appropriate ventilation must be maintained or reestab-lished by opening the airway. In many cases endotracheal intubation is required. This must be done carefully since it is a dangerous procedure in a patient with a fractured cervical spine. The head must be immobilized until instability of the cervical spine can be ruled out. Shock treatment should be pursued aggressively.

The examining physician then turns his attention to the brain, the abdomen, and the urinary system. Only after life-threatening problems are brought under control can attention be directed to the orthopaedic injuries.

The diagnosis and the philosophy of treatment of fractures in the multiply injured orthopaedic patient is not the same as in the patient with an uncomplicated extremity fracture. In the latter, closed treatment is frequently preferred; open reduction and internal fixation are the choice in multiply injured patients.

Immobilization and prolonged bed rest are detrimental to pulmonary physiology, often resulting in the death of a multiply injured patient. Early mobilization, which is possible after open reduction and internal fixation, aids in preventing pulmonary complications and thus is a necessary preventive measure for the trauma patient. Concomitant, ipsilateral extremity fractures are usually best treated by open reduction and internal fixation to mobilize major joints; thus the common complications of stiffness and contracture after prolonged immobilization are prevented.

Management of the orthopaedic patient with multiple injuries can be divided into three stages after the patient's medical condition has been stabilized. In the first stage, diagnosis is of paramount importance. All musculoskeletal problems must be identified. When this has been accomplished, the surgeon must determine the priorities in management of the injuries. Finally, definitive treatment is administered.

DIAGNOSIS

In most of these cases, the patient is unconscious because of an associated head injury and cannot participate in the evaluation of his musculoskeletal problems by indicating areas of pain and loss of function of the musculoskeletal structures. The examining physician must take careful note of any deformity, contusion, or abrasion in the extremities. He is obligated to conduct a careful physical examination and evaluation of all four extremities. Joint instability must be carefully evaluated. All areas of possible injury should be subjected to appropriate roentgenogram examination, but the patient must *not* be sent to the x-ray department for examination until his condition has stabilized and unless accompanied by a nurse or physician at all times.

It is absolutely essential that every patient with a head injury undergo roentgenogram examination of the cervical, thoracic, and lumbar spines. Evaluation of patients with abdominal or urinary tract injuries also should include x-ray film studies of the spine. Since it has been estimated that as many as 30 percent of spine injuries in multiply injured patients are missed, all multiply injured patients should probably undergo roentgenagram examinations of the spine and pelvis.

Joints above and below obvious fractures of the shaft of any long bone should be included in the radiologic evaluation. It is reasonable to expect that fractures may be missed in the multiply injured patient even after careful physical examination and x-ray film evaluation. Missed fractures are prevalent in any reported series of multiply injured patients.

A thorough physical examination must be repeated after the patient regains consciousness or within the first 24 to 48 hours after injury and initial treatment. New or unrecognized areas of swelling, ecchymosis, crepitation, deformity, false motion, and instability of joints raise the level of suspicion. X-ray film evaluation of suspicious areas at the second evaluation is required to detect previously unrecognized fractures.

There are many reports in the literature, especially regarding the multiply injured patient with a head injury, of long delays in diagnosis and permanent functional impairment due to untreated musculoskeletal injuries. Musculoskeletal injuries that are frequently overlooked include dislocations of the shoulder (especially posterior), carpus, and hip with concomitant fracture in the ipsilateral lower extremity.

PRIORITIES AND MANAGEMENT

There are few absolute musculoskeletal emergencies, but peripheral vascular injuries associated with extremity injuries require immediate attention. Major arteries in close proximity to fractured bones or dislocated joints are frequently blocked by pressure of the fracture surfaces or are torn. Ischemia, diminution of arterial pulses, or lack of arterial pulses distal to a fracture or dislocation requires the immediate attention of the physician in the emergency department. Severe hemorrhaging from open wounds must be stemmed by direct pressure until an adequate evaluation can be made. Reduction of the fracture or dislocation should be attempted to relieve arterial entrapment. The return of the pulses following these maneuvers signals the return of normal circulation. It should be kept in mind that return of the distal pulses does not rule out the possibility of arterial damage. Further evaluation must be carried out aggressively. The adoption of an expectant period of observation can have disastrous results. The golden period for the repair of major artery lacerations and blockage is 8 hours from the time of insult. The incidence of amputation for the severe arterial injuries that continue for more than 8 hours is unacceptably high.

Major arterial injury is characterized by (1) pulsatile bleeding in open wounds, (2) diminished or absent arterial pulses, and (3) the five Ps (pain, pulselessness, pallor, paralysis, and parasthesia). If there is any doubt concerning major arterial damage in the extremities, arteriography is mandatory for evaluation in most instances. In the evaluation of patients with ischemic episodes or questionable circulation, angiography may be time-consuming and occasionally accompanied by complications. However, this test can accurately demonstrate vascular disruptions and blockage. In many cases it can prevent unnecessary exploration of vessels.

Dislocated joints should be reduced as soon as possible and frequently can be relocated in the emergency department, where simple analgesia is given before the manipulation. Severe pain owing to the dislocation can be immediately alleviated by reduction of the joint.

All open fractures are contaminated. Delay in getting the patient to the operating room may convert a contaminated wound into an infected wound. Therefore, open fractures must be given a high priority, second only to life-threatening injuries. An open fracture involves skin, fascia, muscle, periosteum, and bone. Devitalization of the soft tissue in the region of the fracture may be massive, depending on the type of fracture and the force of the injury. The greater the amount of devitalized tissue, the better the milieu for bacteria to increase and gain a foothold.

At the scene of the accident, the fracture should not be disturbed. If bone is protruding from the wound, it should be covered with a sterile dressing and the limb splinted. The patient is then transferred to the emergency department where a complete inspection of the wound can be made. Cultures of the wound are obtained for correlation if later infection occurs. In almost all instances, bacteria cultured initially from open fractures correlates with the causative organism if infection ensues. Reduction of the fracture to relieve pressure on the tissues and decompress marginally vascularized areas is necessary; this is followed by adequate splinting. Appropriate tetanus prophylaxis should be instituted. Parenteral antibiotics are advised and should be started while the patient is being evaluated in the emergency area, even before he is taken to the x-ray department. A broad-spectrum antibiotic (a cephalosporin) is the drug of choice. This is continued for several days until the danger of infection has passed. If infection occurs, the organism must be identified, and following sensitivity testing, the appropriate antibiotic can be substituted.

The initial management of open fractures is the same regardless of the grade of the wound. Open fractures are classified into three grades. With grade 1 open fractures, usually caused by low-energy forces, the skin laceration is 1 cm long or smaller and is considered to be relatively clean. With grade 2 open fractures, caused by moderate-energy forces, there is usually more comminution of the fracture, and skin lacerations are over 1 cm long with some skin contusion and muscle damage. Grade 3 injuries are caused by high-energy forces and are characterized by marked fracture displacement with or without extensive skin loss and muscle damage. Examples of grade 3 open fractures are fractures with extensive lacerations, flaps, and severe crushing injury; segmental fractures; and open fractures with soil contamination, vascular injuries, or gunshot injuries.

Generally, it is inadvisable to provide definitive wound care and debridement of open fractures in the emergency department. Optimal sterile conditions and surgery require that open fractures be treated in a surgical operating room where strict asepsis, experienced personnel, and proper instruments are available.

Most surgeons allow open wounds to remain open after thorough debridement and perform secondary wound closure 5 to 7 days later when the wound is clean and granulating. Statistically, wound infection and osteomyelitis have a significantly lower incidence with this protocol; gas gangrene is almost nonexistent.

Stabilization of a pelvic ring injury has a high priority. An external fixator may not adequately fix some pelvic fractures, but this method effectively permits mobilization of the patient and may be lifesaving. Some believe that immobilization of pelvic fractures by external or internal fixation minimizes bleeding from pelvic blood vessels. In some cases, angiography for embolization of persistent bleeding pelvic vessels is required.

Injuries to the spine are common in the multiply injured patient. The examining physician must minimize inadvertent injury to the spinal cord. Traction, careful positioning of the patient, "log rolling" to change position, and avoiding flexion of the spine are all mandatory until the spine can be thoroughly evaluated by physical and roentgenogram examination. If there is an unstable fracture of the spine, traction can be helpful in reducing any deformity that may be present. The unstable spine must be stabilized by traction, a halovest, or internal fixation.

In conclusion, the multiply injured orthopaedic patient is best served by a skilled team of surgeons who are well versed in the care of trauma patients. After resuscitation of the patient, the orthopaedic surgeon can evaluate the musculoskeletal injuries, assign priorities, and carry out appropriate, definitive fracture care designed for early mobilization of the patient.

MANAGEMENT OF THE HEAD, NECK, AND UPPER AIRWAY

HEADACHE AND FACIAL PAIN

JOHN R. CUTLER, M.D.

Headache is one of the most frequent complaints for which patients seek medical advice; it is also a common feature of many primary medical, surgical, psychiatric, dental, and traumatic conditions. Each patient presenting for evaluation of acute or chronic headaches therefore, needs to be questioned and examined carefully for accompanying symptoms and signs that may suggest the presence of an underlying pathologic process (Table 1).

Chronic headaches with established patterns of frequency, severity, site and quality of pain, and associated symptoms rarely are symptomatic of other conditions; however, they may be associated with such disorders as temporomandibular joint (TMJ) syndrome, cervical spine disease, chronic sinusitis, chronic dental disease, and a myriad of chronic systemic illnesses. Recurrent headaches of more recent onset, varying from innocuous to severe, may be an early sign of an intracranial mass lesion, pseudotumor, infection, abscess, or another process. The presence of an intracranial mass lesion is often accompanied by signs such as change in personality or consciousness, focal neurologic abnormalities, stiff neck, fever, and papilledema. Tumors are most commonly seen in those over the age of 50; intracranial infection is more common in intravenous drug users, the immune compromised (e.g., AIDS patients), and those with known bacterial infection such as pulmonary infection, otitis, mastoiditis, or sinusitis. Such patients need a very complete neurologic examination in the emergency department and then prompt referral for computed tomography (CT) or magnetic resonance (MR) scan and further work-up.

Headaches of acute onset with a duration of hours or days are again most likely to be benign in all age groups, but it is imperative that each patient be evaluated carefully for symptoms and signs of conditions affecting other organ systems (such as malignant hypertension or pheochromocytoma) and for evidence of focal neurologic impairment (as caused by an intracranial mass). Acute, severe headaches can be symptoms of infectious diseases affecting the brain, meninges, or both, or infections of a more disseminated nature. Such headaches can also occur with intracranial hemorrhage, both subarachnoid and intracerebral. The former is commonly associated with the eventual development of meningismus (stiff neck and nerve root stretch signs), and the latter is commonly associated with focal findings on neurologic examination.

Certain patients presenting with headache need an emergency specialty consultation by a neurologist or neurosurgeon. Such patients are those in whom the

TABLE 1 Causes of Headache (In Approximate Order of Treatment Urgency)

Intracranial hemorrhage: subarachnoid, subdural, intracerebral
Intracranial infection: meningitis, encephalitis
Intracranial mass: brain tumor, abscess
Severe hypertension: hypertensive encephalopathy, pre-eclampsia, pheochromocytoma, hyptertensive crisis from monoamine oxidase inhibitors
Temporal arteritis
Glaucoma, iritis, uveitis
Stroke
Chemical: carbon monoxide, hypercarbia, many toxic inhalations and fumes
Increased intracranial pressure: pseudotumor cerebri
Post-lumbar puncture
Post-traumatic
Postictal
Extracranial causes: temporomandibular joint syndrome, sinusitis, otitis, mastoiditis dental infections
Herpes: premonitory to acute infection, or post-herpetic neuralgia
Tic douloureux
Glossopharyngeal neuralgia
Cluster headache
Tension headache
Migraine
Altitude sickness
Dietary: monosodium glutamate, chocolate, high-tyramine foods, caffeine, nitrite preservatives, alcohol
Nitrate medications

headache is accompanied by an alteration of consciousness, papilledema, or signs of focal neurologic dysfunction; rapid deterioration and death may be imminent. Patients with new severe headaches and patients with evolving or changing headache symptoms are best evaluated promptly by a specialist. If meningitis is suspected, a diagnostic lumbar puncture should be performed and the appropriate therapy initiated without delay. It is not necessary (and the delay may be deleterious) to perform a brain imaging study (CT or MR) prior to a lumbar puncture if meningitis is suspected in the absence of localizing neurological signs; i.e., if there is a headache and a depressed level of consciousness or papilledema.

EVALUATION

The patient's history should be carefully obtained, and should include background information such as family history and prior personal history of headache. The history includes details concerning the severity of the pain, its location, its quality, and the presence of any associated symptoms. The intensity and pattern of the headache should be noted and compared with prior ones. The frequency of attacks should be determined and careful inquiry should be made into any known provocative factors such as food, drink, environmental factors, time of day, and any other observed associations. A determination of any known relieving factors should be made and a list of current and previously employed methods of treatment obtained. The physical examination must include both a general examination with the determination of vital signs and an examination of the neurologic system. The neurologic examination should be thorough and should certainly include examinations for meningeal irritation, a careful funduscopic examination, and palpation of the carotid and superficial temporal arteries. Patients who have a long history of similar headaches generally need no further evaluation.

SPECIFIC HEADACHE DISORDERS

Migraine–Tension Headaches

There probably exists a spectrum between migraine and tension headaches with most headaches falling somewhere between the two extremes. Migraine–tension headaches are often familial and are not definitely associated with other pathology. It is now believed that their underlying cause is neurochemical and may, at least in part, be due to alterations in brain serotonin (5-hydroxytryptamine). The throbbing pain that characterizes migraine and has led to the appellation "vascular headache" may be nothing more than a secondary effect of some underlying neuronal alteration. This is also probably true of the muscle contraction that characterizes tension headaches.

Migraine is typically a unilateral, throbbing headache associated with photophobia, nausea, and vomiting and may be preceded or accompanied by visual changes (flashing lights, transient blind spots) or other neurologic signs. Commonly, the headache symptoms evolve over a period of minutes to hours and may last for several hours to a day. Migraine generally begins during the first 3 decades of life, and the headaches affect women more than men. They may be provoked by stress or other psychic phenomena, certain foods or drinks, menstruation, oral contraceptives, hunger, and particular environmental factors. Transient neurologic abnormalities such as hemiparesis, external ophthalmoplegia, brainstem dysfunction, and alterations of consciousness may be associated with migraine; however, such symptoms and signs should not be ascribed to migraine without a thorough investigation into other possible causes.

The treatment of migraine can be divided into three types: abortive drug therapy, prophylactic drug therapy, and nondrug therapy such as biofeedback, dietary alteration, relaxation training, and so forth. In the emergency department the major concern is for abortive therapy, and one of the most effective specific treatments of a severe, ongoing migraine headache is intravenous dihydroergotamine (DHE). This drug causes a considerable amount of nausea, so pretreatment with a parenterally administered antiemetic such as metoclopramide (Reglan) (10 mg intramuscularly or intravenously) or prochlorperazine (Compazine) (10 mg intramuscularly) is recommended. DHE is administered 0.5 mg by slow intravenous push and is repeated, if necessary, in 20 to 30 minutes. The use of this specific medication often obviates the need for parenteral narcotic administration for pain relief. DHE is contraindicated in patients with peripheral or cardiovascular disease, liver or kidney failure, hypertension, sepsis, or pregnancy.

Less severe migraine headaches can be treated with any of the many oral, sublingual, inhalant, and rectal preparations of ergotamine tartrate. Among these, the 2-mg sublingual and the 2-mg suppository forms have been used with the greatest success in my experience. With the sublingual tablets, begin with 2 mg and repeat every 20 minutes until relief is obtained, or a total of three tablets (6 mg) have been administered. The patient should be instructed to immediately take the entire amount of medication required to stop a headache at the onset of any subsequent headaches. The contraindications are the same as those for DHE. The accompanying nausea is best treated with a rectal or parenteral antiemetic, such as metoclopramide or prochlorperazine, rather than with an oral agent. Aspirin, acetaminophen, and narcotic medications (codeine and others) are useful for the symptomatic treatment of headache pain. If narcotics must be given, they should be given in adequate doses and parenterally, preferably intravenously (because this is by far the fastest route). Patients who present repeatedly to the emergency department for this problem need a formal pain management protocal as described in the chapter *Pain in the Emergency Department*.

Patients respond best to therapeutic intervention when they are kept in a quiet, dark room. Certain patients respond favorably to the application of ice packs or a damp cloth to the head or face region when they are suffering from acute migraine.

Useful prophylactic medications include ergonovine maleate, propranolol, amitriptyline, and cyproheptadine. The initiation and monitoring of these chronically administered medications are better left to a primary care physician or a specialist practitioner than to the emergency department staff.

Tension headache is also called depression, muscle contraction, or psychogenic headache. This is a chronic disorder that affects women more than men and is often associated with cyclic depression. The headaches tend to be more continual and chronic than migraine. The pain of tension headaches is likened by sufferers to a pressure or constriction of the head. The discomfort is generalized over the scalp, but predominates in the temporal, frontal and occipital regions, hence the association with muscle contraction. The headaches often occur daily and begin in the afternoon, gradually increasing over the balance of the day. There are no consistent external triggering or relieving factors. Depression and anxiety, which are often conspicuous, are frequently encountered symptoms and signs.

Therapeutic measures useful in the management of tension headache include behavioral techniques, psychotherapy, and pharmacologic treatment with anxiolytic and antidepressant agents. Rather than initiate therapy in the emergency department with these chronically administered medications, it is important to examine a patient carefully and to reassure him or her that there is no physical disturbance of consequence and to make an appropriate referral to a primary care or specialist physician. Treatment with analgesics or anxiolytics or both in the emergency department may be expedient, but the initiation of long-term therapy should be avoided and left to a physician who is in a position to monitor the patient and to deal with the psychological and behavioral aspects of this disorder and its treatment.

Cluster Headaches

Cluster headaches take their name from the characteristic grouping of the headache attacks that occur on a daily basis over several weeks, recurring in these groups (clusters) once or twice yearly. Cluster headaches begin to affect patients (men more than women) in the fourth or fifth decade of life and there is usually no family history of a similar disorder. The pain is described as a boring, severe, localized pain often centered on or around one eye or the temple. The pain is nearly always unilateral and occurs quite abruptly with a rapid rise to maximum intensity. The paroxysms of pain last from one-half to two hours and most often occur once or twice daily during a cluster. Another characteristic feature of cluster headaches is their periodicity; the pains typically come on at nearly the same time each day and often occur at night. This is the typical pattern; chronic and atypical varieties of cluster headache are frequently encountered.

Cluster headaches are commonly associated with ipsilateral Horner's syndrome (especially ptosis and miosis). Often conjunctival injection, lacrimation, and nasal stuffiness occur on the side of the pain. Apart from the presence of these signs and of tender superficial temporal arteries, physical and neurologic examinations are normal during a cluster headache. In the midst of a cluster, headaches can be triggered by the ingestion of alcohol and may be provoked by stress, glaring light, or other factors. These provocative factors are usually quite innocuous when they are encountered during a noncluster period.

The prophylactic treatment of cluster headache is generally more beneficial than abortive therapies. The treatment of an acute cluster headache in the emergency department principally involves the use of oxygen and ergotamine tartrate. Inhalation of 100 percent oxygen (through a nonrebreather mask at a flow rate of 7 L per minute for 10 to 15 minutes) is frequently effective in aborting an acute cluster headache. Ergotamine tartrate is administered by the inhalation (one to two puffs after thorough shaking) of the aerosolized preparation or by insertion of a suppository (1 to 2 mg rectally). The drugs that are most useful for prophylaxis are a combination of prednisone (given at a starting dose of 60 to 80 mg with a 10- to 14-day tapering course) and lithium carbonate (300 mg three to four times daily) to be continued over the expected duration of the cluster. Other drugs useful in the prophylactic management of cluster headache are chronically administered ergotamine tartrate, amitriptyline, cyproheptadine, and methysergide. Again, as in the long-term management of migraine, it is better to refer the patient to a specialist than to institute chronic prophylactic therapy in the emergency department.

Temporal Arteritis (Giant Cell Arteritis)

Temporal arteritis is an illness that affects older persons (sixth decade and beyond), particularly women, and is characterized by such symptoms as headache, visual loss, malaise, myalgia, low-grade fever, anorexia, and weight loss. The pathology of temporal arteritis is that of a sterile inflammation of the medium to large arteries, sometimes leading to vascular occlusion. Giant cells are often present on histopathologic examination, but are not required to make the diagnosis. Any vessels can be involved, but there is a predilection for the superficial temporal, vertebral, ophthalmic, and posterior ciliary arteries. Temporal arteritis is a medical emergency because it may rapidly result in visual loss. For this reason, the diagnosis of temporal arteritis should be established promptly and therapeutic intervention with corticosteroids should be initiated without delay.

The headache associated with temporal arteritis may develop early or late in the course of the illness, may be unilateral or bilateral, and is often located temporally on the scalp. The pain is usually not of great severity, it is localized to the scalp superficially, and is aggravated by touching the scalp, combing the hair, or putting any pressure on the scalp or temples. After headache, the next most common symptom elicited in patients with temporal arteritis is jaw claudication. This is a deep aching in or around the muscles of mastication. This pain occurs after chewing for a few minutes and is promptly relieved after the cessation of the chewing movements. The association of temporal arteritis and polymyalgia rheumatica is well known, and many of the systemic symptoms listed previously are shared by both conditions, especially myalgia and mild fever. The acute onset of visual loss or visual obscuration is an emergency and occurs in 10 to 40 percent of the cases. The visual changes are usually monocular and may be complete or incomplete at the time of presentation. As emphasized previously, no time should be lost in establishing the cause of this visual loss and in instituting appropriate therapy.

The most striking finding on physical examination may be diffuse corporal or cranial muscle tenderness. Tenderness and induration of the superficial temporal arteries may also be present. Elevation of the erythrocyte sedimentation rate (ESR) is the most reliable laboratory finding in temoral arteritis; however, there are many pathologically proven cases with normal or nearly normal ESR. Elevated liver function tests and mild anemia are commonly encountered in patients with temporal arteritis. Pathologic examination of superficial temporal artery biopsy specimens, if abnormal, can establish the presence of temporal arteritis unequivocally, a normal biopsy does not eliminate the diagnosis owing to the patchy nature of the pathologic involvement in this disease.

The treatment of temporal arteritis is with corticosteroids to prevent blindness, caused by ophthalmic artery occlusion, and for symptomatic relief. In suspected cases, even before pathologic confirmation of disease, therapy should be initiated with 60 to 80 mg of prednisone per day. For patients presenting with partial visual loss, this regimen may reverse the deficit. Once the diagnosis has been suspected and therapy undertaken, the patient should be referred to a neurologist or rheumatologist for evaluation, biopsy, and continued management. Temporal arteritis is usually self-limited, and therapy can be discontinued within 6 months to 2 years depending on the clinical response and the ESR.

Trigeminal Neuralgia (Tic Douloureux)

Trigeminal neuralgia in its primary or idiopathic form most commonly affects older persons (women more than men), but can begin at any age. When this illness has its onset in a younger person (below the age of 40), the possibility of secondary or symptomatic trigeminal neuralgia must be considered and a thorough investigation for a structural lesion of the posterior fossa or multiple sclerosis must be undertaken.

Trigeminal neurolgia is characterized by brief, intense, lancinating pains on one side of the face, most often confined to the territory of one of the divisions of the trigeminal nerve. These paroxysms of pain may occur without provocation or may be initiated by tactile stimulation of particular area on the face or scalp (trigger points). The pain has a brief intense phase that is succeeded by a longer period of less intense deep aching before final resolution. The physical examination in primary trigeminal neuralgia is typically normal; however, slight alteration in facial sensation is sometimes claimed by sufferers. Any definite abnormalities on examination require further investigation because the condition may be secondary rather than primary in nature.

The anticonvulsant medications carbamazepine and phenytoin comprise the mainstays of therapy. Carbamazepine is generally the more useful medication, but its usefulness may be limited by gastrointestinal side effects encountered at the onset of therapy. Treatment usually begins with one-half of a 200-mg tablet twice daily, increasing as tolerated by one-half-tablet increments until relief is achieved or side effects or toxic effects arise. This drug should be administered on a twice-daily or thrice-daily basis and serum levels measured to assure that a toxic dose is avoided. Carbamazepine is contraindicated in pregnant patients, patients with bone marrow suppression, patients taking monoamine oxidase (MAO) inhibitors, and in those with sensitivity to tricyclic compounds. Pretreatment and periodic blood counts are recommended while therapy with this drug continues. Phenytoin is also useful. This medication is better tolerated than carbamazepine and can be started at a maintenance dose of 300 mg daily (usually given at bedtime). Again, serum drug levels should be monitored to assure that toxic levels are avoided. Phenytoin is contraindicated in pregnant patients and in patients with known hypersensitivity to the drug or other hydantoins.

Patients with trigeminal neuralgia and those with other facial pain conditions should be referred to a neurologist for further evaluation and treatment.

Miscellaneous Headache Disorders

Post-traumatic headaches are frequently complained of by persons who have suffered from head trauma. (See chapter on *Blunt Head Trauma; Concussion and Skull Fractures*). These headaches may follow inconsequential or trivial blows to the head as well as more significant head trauma resulting in concussion and brain contusion. The pain may begin immediately after the injury or may be delayed for hours to days. The severity of the trauma often bears little relationship to the severity of the post-traumatic headache disorder. The characteristic feature of the headache is a nonlocalized, often throbbing pain with associated nausea, vomiting, and occasionally visual changes such as those reported with migraine. Post-traumatic headaches may also be dull and nonthrobbing and are often associated with other symptoms such as dysequilibrium, concentration difficulties, malaise, fatigue, irritability, and emotional disturbance.

Investigative procedures are generally unrevealing if the neurologic and general physical examinations are normal. Symptoms usually continue for several weeks to months before a gradual return to normal function occurs, but prolonged post-traumatic syndromes do occur. Treatment is best confined to symptomatic relief with analgesic, antiemetic, and anxiolytic agents in the acute setting. Sometimes antimigraine medications can be used effectively to treat post-traumatic headaches. For more prolonged syndromes, the use of tricyclic antidepressant agents has been found to be valuable. In any case, the patient should be reassured and supported emotionally.

Oral and Salivary Gland Infection / 199

Contrary to a commonly held belief, this is a real disorder, not an artifact of ongoing litigation. Care of such patients should be referred to a primary care provider or a neurologist. More severely injured patients should be evaluated by a neurosurgeon on an urgent basis.

Low intracranial pressure headaches most commonly follow lumbar puncture, but may occur following any rent of the dural investments of the nervous system. Such headaches occur within a few mintues after assuming an upright posture and are relieved by reclining. The pain is usually throbbing or dull, and a pulling sensation localized to the vertex of the skull or to the frontal or occipital regions may be reported. Frequently, globe tenderness, nausea, and vomiting are associated with these headaches.

If there is a history of a recent lumbar puncture or myelogram that accounts for the dural rent, the best treatment is to have the patient follow strict bedrest with oral fluids pushed for several days. If this is unsatisfactory and symptoms continue, the patient should be evaluated by an anesthesiologist, neurosurgeon, or neurologist. Definitive treatment involves performing a ''blood patch'' by the infusion of autologous whole blood into the spinal epidural space. In the case of orthostatic headaches with which no known recent dural puncture is associated, the patient should be evaluated by a neurologically sophisticated practitioner for diagnosis and management.

Cough headache (exertional headache) is a paroxysmal symptom of moderate to great severity brought on by coughing, sneezing, straining, bending, and so forth. Most often, this is a benign, self-limited problem for which no specific evaluation or therapy is required. However, in approximately 10 percent of cases, an abnormality of the central nervous system is associated with exertional headache. These are most often located in the posterior fossa and can be structural developmental abnormalities such as the Arnold-Chiari malformation, neoplasms, subdural hematomas, or other space occupying lesions.

Treatment of the benign form of exertional headache is best initiated with indomethacin at a dosage of 25 mg three times daily.

SUGGESTED READING

Caviness VS, O'Brien P. Headache. N Engl J Med 1980; 302:446–449.
Diamond S, Dalessio DJ. The practicing physician's approach to headache, 3rd ed. New York: Williams & Wilkins, 1982.
Raskin NH, Appenzeller O. Headache. Major problems in internal medicine. Vol. 19. Philedelphia: WB Saunders, 1980.
Saper Jr. Migraine (2 parts). JAMA 1978; 239:2380, 2480.

ORAL AND SALIVARY GLAND INFECTION

M. ANTHONY POGREL, M.B., Ch.B.
B.D.S., F.D.S., F.R.C.S. (Edin.)

ORAL INFECTION

Infections of the oral cavity are extremely common since the oral cavity has many natural flora which include many potential pathogens. Most oral infections are related to the teeth and the tooth-bearing structures. Infections arise because of dental caries (the world's most common disease) when it involves the pulp chamber of the tooth, which gives rise to acute pulpitis, usually leading to periapical abscess formation. The other site of infiltration of pathological organisms is down the periodontal ligament between the tooth, the gum, and the bone, thereby causing periodontal or paradontal infection. It has been estimated that 80 percent of all infections of the head and neck are dental in origin, and most are treated by dentists on an outpatient basis so that physicians and hospitals are rarely involved in their treatment. However, spread into the bone can occur and cause osteomyelitis; subsequent spread into the soft tissues can result in infections of the fascial spaces of the head and neck with potentially serious consequences. Even simple dental infections can have potentially serious side effects in persons who are in various susceptible categories, such as immunocompromised patients or those with cardiac valvular problems.

Teeth and Gingiva

Treatment of localized dental infections consists of simple local measures, including rehydration if necessary, rest, oral hygiene, and surgical drainage if pus is present. Drainage often involves pulpectomy or removal of an offending tooth. Antibiotics are not normally indicated in fit, healthy individuals with localized dental infections. Palatal abscesses from upper teeth can be very painful, but these rarely spread and respond well to drainage. However, the palatal artery is close by and bleeding can be troublesome.

The organisms commonly incriminated in dental and oral infections are streptococci and staphylococci (often penicillinase-producing). Gram-negative organisms such as *Proteus, Pseudomonas,* and *Enterobacteriaceae* can also cause infections. With more sophisticated culture techniques, anaerobic organisms such as *Bacteroides, fusobacterium* and *Peptostreptococcus* are being incriminated more frequently.

Pericoronitis is an inflammation of the gum around an erupting tooth. Pericoronitis around a partially erupted lower wisdom tooth can be severe and can cause trismus by irritation of the nearby muscles of mastication.

The infection can spread eaasily into the fascial spaces of the neck. Penicillin (500 mg orally 4 times daily in adults) is often used in addition to local measures such as warm saline mouth rinses. Double blind trials, however, have shown that metronidazole (250 mg 3 times a day) is equally effective since anaerobic organisms are frequently responsible. If trismus and swelling and systemic symptoms are severe, hospitalization and intravenous antibiotics may be necessary, as well as surgical drainage.

Acute necrotizing ulcerative gingivitis (Vincent's disease) is a unique form of gingivitis that causes characteristic craters of the interdental papillae between the teeth. A very unpleasant odor is characteristic. Vincent's disease normally occurs only in patients with very poor oral hygiene or in patients who are generally unwell; its presence may be a sign of an underlying disease process. In addition to local measures, including hydrogen peroxide (3 percent diluted to half strength) or sodium perborate (4 percent) mouthwashes and gentle brushing, antibiotics are frequently necessary. Penicillin (500 mg orally 4 times daily for adults) is recommended, but metronidazole has been shown to be equally effective.

Osteomyelitis

Emergency visits are usually the result of acute suppurative osteomyelitis or acute exacerbation of a preexisting chronic osteomyelitis. The mandible is more frequently involved in acute suppurative osteomyelitis than is the maxilla. The classic organisms are *Staphylococcus aureus* and *S. epidermidis*. Anaerobic organisms cause a foul-smelling exudate and are often associated with necrotic tissue and sequestrum formation.

The symptoms of acute suppurative osteomyelitis are intense pain and swelling in the affected area, pyrexia, and leukocytosis. If the mandible is involved, there may be anesthesia or paresthesia of the mental nerve. In the very eary stages, radiographs may be normal, though a technetium phosphate nuclear bone scan will show increased activity. Initially, there may be no swelling, loosening of teeth, or fistula formation.

At this point, the prompt and aggressive use of antibiotics may effect a cure. Narcotic analgesics may need to be given for the pain, and hospitalization may be necessary for general management and also for giving antibiotics intravenously. Antibiotics of choice include penicillin and penicillinase-resistant penicillins such as nafcillin if staphylococci are suspected. The adult doses are penicillin, 2 million units IV every 6 hours, or nafcillin, 1 g every 6 hours. The cephalosporins, such as cefazolin, and also erythromycin are useful. Clindamycin gives high bone levels and is extremely useful in the treatment of osteomyelitis despite its possible side effects, which include pseudomembranous colitis. The normal adult dosage for osteomyelitis is 150 to 300 mg IV 4 times daily.

In longer standing acute osteomyelitis, radiographs may show some rarefaction and even sequestrum formation. A sequestrum is an area of dead bone; it appears more dense on a radiograph than the surrounding bone.

Scintiscan is positive, and there may well be swelling, loosening of teeth, and discharging sinus, in addition to the early symptoms. If there is a discharging sinus, a specimen can be taken for culture and antibiotic sensitivity. Longstanding cases of osteomyelitis will almost certainly require surgical drainage and possible decorticaton of the bone and sequestrectomy if sequestra are present. If this surgical treatment is not carried out, the disease can become chronic and antibiotics will not effect a cure. Hospitalization is normally required for these patients.

Infections of the Fascial Spaces Around the Oral Cavity

The potential spaces between the layers of the cervical fascia provide an easy path for infections to track to vital structures. Most infections of these fascial spaces are of dental origin, in particular, from infected wisdom teeth. Treatment depends on their symptoms and site, but there are some factors common to all such infections. If the airway is compromised, its protection is the first priority, thereby necessitating passage of an endotracheal tube, a cricothyroidotomy, or a tracheostomy. If there is any fluctuation, it must be drained and a culture taken for Gram stain and antibiotic sensitivity.

If there are systemic symptoms, a blood culture should be taken (preferably at the height of pyrexia) and hospitalization may be necessary. A pyrexia greater than 38.4 °C (101 °F) coupled with cellulitis and lassitude may necessitate hospitalization, particularly if there are any signs of early airway compromise, e.g., dysphagia or painful swallowing. Systemic symptoms also make antibiotics mandatory. They can be given orally or intravenously depending on the severity of the infection. The antibiotic of choice is penicillin (250 to 500 mg orally 4 times daily in adults; the intravenous dose for more serious infections is 1 to 4 million units every 6 hours). Alternatives are the cephalosporins or erythromycin. If gram-negative organisms are seen on the Gram stain, an aminoglycoside can be added. Gentamicin is normally used in an adult dosage of 3 to 5 mg per kilogram of body weight 3 times per day. Serum levels are monitored to keep concentrations between 4 and 10 μg per milliliter. Clindamycin can also be substituted for a gram-negative infection in an intravenous dose of 150 to 600 mg every 6 hours.

Drainage can be by wide-bore needle aspiration (14 or 16 gauge), but is normally better done by Hilton's method, which involves a skin or mucosal incision at the site of maximal fluctuation and insertion of closed tissue forceps, which are opened in the tissues to open the fascial spaces. A corrugated or tube rubber drain is normally left in the incision for irrigation and until drainage ceases (usually in 2 to 3 days). Though it is tempting to carry out drainage under local anesthesia, more thorough drainage of fascial space infections is obtained under general anesthesia.

Infections around the oral cavity occur in a number of well-defined spaces related to the fascial planes, and these locations must be recognized since infections in some of them have potentially serious consequences. Following securing of the airway and drainage, the cause of the infection should be determined. Figure 1 shows how infected lower wisdom teeth can involve many of these spaces.

Buccal space infections occur between the mandible medially and the buccinator muscle laterally. These infections nearly always occur from lower teeth and virtually always remain localized to the oral cavity. Treatment is by penicillin and drainage if necessary.

Canine space infections occur between the maxilla medially and the buccinator and labial muscles laterally. They are the maxillary counterpart of the buccal space infection and treatment is similar. They normally remain localized and drainage and possibly antibiotics will cure most cases on an outpatient basis. Infections from upper teeth can also spread to the nasal cavity and maxillary sinuses. If the infection spreads to the infraorbital region, it can then spread via the angular vein to the cavernous sinus with serious consequences. In this case, more aggressive treatment with intravenous antibiotics and drainage is necessary.

Buccinator space infections occur between the buccinator muscle medially and the subcutaneous tissues laterally. They can arise from the teeth or from skin appendages and produce infection beneath the skin of the cheek. Infections usually remain localized and antibiotics on an outpatient basis, coupled with drainage if necessary, are the proper treatment.

The sublingual space lies in the floor of the mouth, deep to the mylohyoid muscle, between the muscle and the oral mucosa. Infections in this area cause elevation of the floor of the mouth with subsequent elevation of the tongue and possible difficulties with swallowing. These infections can be serious and may necessitate hospitalization for airway management plus intensive intravenous antibiotic administration and surgical drainage.

The submasseteric space is a potential space between the masseter muscle laterally and the ascending ramus of the mandible medially. Infection here usually arises from an infected lower wisdom tooth, and the major symptom is intense trismus with swelling and pyrexia. Treatment

is with antibiotics and intraoral drainage if necessary, coupled with subsequent removal of the tooth.

Pterygoid space infections arise between the ascending ramus of the mandible laterally and the medial pterygoid muscle medially. They result from an infected lower wisdom tooth or an infected inferior alveolar nerve block, which is one of the most common dental local anesthetic injections. Symptoms are trismus and swelling. Infection can spread to the adjacent parapharyngeal space with potential airway problems, so these infections must be treated aggressively. Treatment consists of antibiotics and surgical drainage if indicated via an intraoral approach with a drain left in situ for continued drainage and irrigation.

The submandibular space is the space formed by the splitting of the investing fascia to enclose the submandibular gland. Infections in this area can arise from the submandibular salivary gland itself or from the lower posterior teeth. They cause both intra- and extraoral swelling and can also cause elevation of the floor of the mouth and tongue and potential airway problems. Infection easily spreads to the other side or into the neck. These infections must be taken seriously; hospitalization for intense intravenous antibiotic therapy and surgical drainage is normally required. Even if there is no actual fluctuation, drainage is often carried out to relieve pressure in cases of cellulitis. If necessary, the airway is protected with an endotracheal tube or tracheostomy.

Parapharyngeal space infections can arise from pre-existing pharyngeal infections or can have spread from the submandibular or internal pterygoid space. Potentially they are extremely serious, since they can spread down the neck with ease and cause pressure symptoms in the pharynx and severe airway problems. Symptoms can include stridor, malaise, and pyrexia, and there is leukocytosis. Examination of the oropharynx may show medial bulging of the tonsillar fossa on the affected side and plain radiographs may show restriction of the airway, but this is more often seen on a coronal computed tomography scan. Hospitalization in a maxillofacial service is mandatory in these cases, and a tracheostomy is frequently required. If stridor is present the patient should not lie down, as the tongue may completely occlude the airway. Intensive intravenous antibiotics and surgical drainage via an intra- and extraoral approach may be necesary. Drainage is normally carried out under general anesthesia after the airway has been secured with a tracheostomy. A tracheostomy often has to be done under local anesthesia, so that the airway is entered and protected from any possible rupture of the parapharyngeal abscess with contamination of the airway.

Ludwig's angina is a term used to denote a spreading multiple space infection of the neck. It is normally bilateral, includes the submandibular and parapharyngeal spaces, and is a medical emergency since the airway is frequently severely compromised. Patients with Ludwig's angina may be cyanotic with stridor and elevation of the floor of the mouth and tongue. Hospitalization is mandatory with aggressive use of intravenous antibiotics, which are generally given in combination, such as penicillin G,

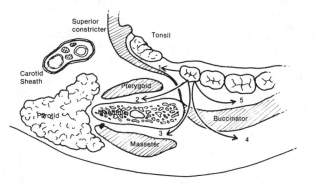

Figure 1 Coronal slight cut through the ascending ramus of the mandible just cephalic to the mandibular teeth. (1)=parapharyngeal space, (2)=internal pterygoid space, (3)=submasseteric space, (4)=buccinator space, (5)=buccal space.

2 to 4 million units every 4 hours, plus a penicillinase-resistant pencillin or aminoglycoside. Surgical drainage is necessary from both intra- and extraoral approaches. Even though frank pus is frequently not found, decompression occurs and multiple drainage sites are normally used. A tracheostomy to protect the airway is frequently required in these patients, and it often has to be very low to avoid making the incision through the infected area with potential contamination of the airway. Any attempt at endotracheal intubation may rupture an abscess with contamination of the airway. Following tracheostomy, the patient can be anesthetized for drainage.

Oral Viral Infections

The most common intraoral viral infection is herpes simplex virus type 1. The herpes simplex virus is a DNA virus, of which type 1 and type 2 infect man. Type 1 infection normally affects the oral cavity, whereas the type 2 infection affects the genital areas, though in some areas 20 percent of intraoral infections are caused by the type 2 virus. (See also the chapters on *Herpes Virus* and *Mucous Membrane Disease*.)

The primary herpes simplex type 1 infection normally occurs in childhood and produces a severe gingivostomatitis which causes shallow roofed vesicles on the gingiva and mucosa, particularly on that of the palate. There are systemic manifestations, including pyrexia and excessive salivation. As with most viral infections, there is no specific treatment; therapy is normally symptomatic, i.e., analgesics for the pain, antipyretics to lower the temperature, viscous lidocaine orally for the discomfort, and antibiotics in cases of secondary infection. The primary attack is normally self-limiting, ending after 1 to 2 weeks in healthy children, and leaves life-long circulating antibodies. These antibodies are not totally protective, however, in that the virus normally migrates to the trigeminal ganglion and from there can descend to cause recurrent attacks of herpes labialis or cold sores, against which the circulating antibodies are not protective.

In immunocompromised patients (and particularly patients with AIDS), the herpes simplex virus can become a life-threatening problem. These patients can get recurrent primary type herpes infections with recurrent intraoral vesicles which coalesce to cause shallow erosions, particularly on the tongue. Viremia also occurs, which can give rise to herpes encephalitis and other serious consequences. At the present time, the antiviral drug of choice for treatment of herpes simplex infection in the immunocompromised patient is acyclovir. This is administered intravenously in life-threatening infections, and the usual dosage is 5 mg per kilogram body weight 3 times daily for 7 days. Dosages for children up to 12 years are 250 mg per square meter of body surface every 8 hours for 7 days. Acyclovir ointment is also available, as are capsules, though gastrointestinal absorption of the drug is fairly poor (approximately 15 to 30 percent). The ointment is really indicated only for oral herpes in the immunocompromised patient; although the ointment has been used in normal herpes labialis, the results have been equivocal. It is generally felt that although viral shedding may be reduced, there is no real improvement in the symptoms or healing time unless the cream is applied during the prodromal phase. In this respect, it closely resembles idoxuridine, which proved equally disappointing for herpes labialis and has now been superseded by Acyclovir.

Another intraoral viral infection is infectious mononucleosis, or glandular fever, which is caused by the Eptsein-Barr virus. In addition to the enlarged cervical lymph nodes, there is frequently an exudative pharyngotonisillitis and petechiae of the palate, and a macular intraoral rash may occur, particularly on the palate. Systemic symptoms include headache, fatigue, malaise, and pyrexia. The incubation period varies between 30 and 60 days, and the disease is normally self-limiting, though serious complications can occasionally occur. There is no specific therapy; treatment is supportive and includes analgesics, antipyretics, viscous lidocaine mouth wash for the oral condition, and possibly an antibiotic if secondary infection is present. Ampicillin should not be used, since it virtually always causes a maculopapular eruption in patients with infectious mononucleosis.

Other viral infections that can affect the oral cavity include cytomegalovirus, measles (which causes the typical Koplik's spots on the buccal mucosa), herpangina, and hand-foot-and-mouth disease. Some of these infections can pose an intraoral diagnostic problem in that most of them cause shallow ulcers, but in general they do not constitute emergency problems. Treatment in all cases is symptomatic.

INTRAORAL FUNGAL INFECTIONS

The principal intraoral infection is candidiasis. The normal organism is *Candida albicans* though other *Candida* species are occasionaly incriminated. *Candida* is a component of the normal oral flora, so that suprainfections normally occur only in otherwise ill or immunocompromised patients, such as patients with AIDS. Candidiasis appears as a white curd-like plaque that forms on the oral mucosa, loosely adherent to an erythematous, inflamed mucosa. In newborn infants the disease is called thrush and it occurs in the throat. With the mucosa, particularly the tongue, an atrophic form also occurs which appears as a fiery red color. The disease can be painful and annoying but is rarely life-threatening on its own, though it can spread to form lesions in other organs and can denote an underlying illness or immunodeficiency. Local therapy normally consists of a nystatin vaginal tablet sucked as a lozenge 4 times daily. Miconazole and ketoconazole (Nizoral) are second choice drugs. Ketoconazole has been associated with hepatic damage, and liver function tests should be monitored in these patients. In severe infections, intravenous therapy with amphotericin B is the most usual treatment, though miconazole can also be given intravenously.

Actinomycosis

Actinomycosis in man is normally caused by *Actinomyces israelii*, though other subspecies are occasionally incriminated. *Actinomyces israelii* is a component of the normal oral flora, and the reason for its occasional pathogenicity is not entirely clear. The *actinomyces* species lie between the bacteria and the fungii, and have some properties of both. They are gram-positive and microaerophilic with branching hyphae that form a mycelium. The organisms can cause periapical infections, pericoronitis, osteomyelitis, and soft tissue infections. The soft tissue infections tend to produce chronic indurated swellings, which discharge from multiple sinuses. The pathognomonic finding is the so-called sulfur granule in the pus or exudate, which is a yellow granule 1 or 2 mm in diameter consisting of a matted mass of *Actinomyces* hyphae. Though it can produce a serious infection, actinomycosis rarely constitutes an emergency, since it tends to be chronic. The *Actinomyces* organism is quite sensitive to penicillin, but treatment must be prolonged because the antibiotic has difficulty penetrating to the center of the sulfur granule. Treatment should normally be given intravenously to start with, though oral medication can be substituted when there has been an initial response. Intravenous therapy would normally be 1 to 2 million units of penicillin every 6 hours; oral therapy, which can be substituted after 1 or 2 weeks, would be 500 mg 4 times daily. Most authorities state that treatment should be continued for at least 6 to 8 weeks, though others have claimed cures with shorter periods of therapy. If for any reason penicillin cannot be used, alternative drugs include: tetracycline, erythromycin, cephalosporins, streptomycin, and clindamycin. Necrotic tissue is frequently present, which may need to be removed surgically.

Other fungal infections that can affect the oral cavity include histoplasmosis, coccidioidomycosis, and blastomycosis. These do not normally present as emergency problems.

SALIVARY GLAND INFECTION

Acute Sialadentitis

Although originally seen as a staphylococcal infection in debilitated patients, sialadenitis is today caused by a wide spectrum of organisms. Presenting symptoms are pain (often severe), swelling, and tenderness of the affected gland with associated lymphadenopathy and mucopurulent discharge from the duct. Pyrexia and leukocytosis are frequently present. Immediate treatment is required.

The organisms most commonly incriminated today are *Staphylococcus aureus, Streptococcus viridans*, and pneumococci. The staphylococci are frequently penicillin resistant. Recently, various opportunistic and gram-negative organisms have been incriminated, including *Hemophilus influenzae, Escherichia coli, Proteus*, and *Klebsiella*.

The anatomical sites of the major salivary glands are so distinctive that there is really little doubt about the diagnosis when they are tense and swollen. The parotid gland lies in the pre-auricular region overlying the mandible, but the tail of the parotid gland continues caudally as far as the angle of the mandible, and the swelling is restricted in extent by the adherent parotid fascia. Similarly, sialadenitis of the submandibular salivary gland is contained within the submandibular fascial compartment, which lies beneath the mandible, extending from the angle region, forward to the region of the bicuspid teeth, and down into the neck as far as the hyoid bone.

The management of acute sialadenitis includes rest, antibiotic therapy, and possibly surgical drainage. If the systemic symptoms, i.e., pyrexia, malaise, and pain, predominate, hospitalization is necessary for rehydration, medical management, and possible surgical drainage. Because of the possibility of surgery, admission on an ENT or maxillofacial service may be necessary.

The sequence of management of the hospitalized patient should be as follows:

1. A specimen of the duct fluid should be obtained for staining, culture, and antibiotic sensitivity. It is not easy to obtain a pure specimen from the ducts of the parotid or submandibular gland, and it should be taken by someone with knowledge of this area. Otherwise, only normal oral flora is collected. The specimen can sometimes be milked from the duct, and on other occasions, the duct must be cannulated to obtain a good specimen.
2. If there are systemic symptoms, a blood culture should be taken, preferably at the peak of pyrexia. A complete blood count should also be performed.
3. Antibiotic therapy should be instituted as soon as the specimen has been taken. For hospitalized and seriously ill patients, a semisynthetic penicillin, such as Nafcillin, should be given, 1 g every 6 hours IV or by deep intramuscular injection. When the patient's condition improves, 500 mg of Nafcillin or dicloxacillin can be given orally every 6 hours. The aminoglycosides, such as gentamicin and tobramycin, can be used in addition to penicillin if gram-negative organisms are suspected. Gentamicin dosage is 80 mg 3 times daily for an adult, with monitoring to keep peak concentrations below 12 μg per milliliter. If a penicillin cannot be used, cefazolin (Kefzol or Ancef) can be given in a dosage of 1 g every 6 hours IV. When the patient has improved enough for oral medication, cephalexin, cephradine, or cefaclor can be given in a dosage of 500 mg 4 times per day. Clindamycin is present in high levels in saliva, unlike many other antibiotics, and is also effective, particularly when gram-negative organisms are suspected; it is given in a dosage of 150 to 300 mg 4 times daily IV. Patient's receiving clindamycin must be monitored carefully for the development of diarrhea and possible pseudomembranous colitis. If the Gram stain shows gram-positive organisms, then penicillin or a cephalosporin is probably appropriate, but if gram-negative organisms are seen,

an aminoglycoside should be added or clindamycin should be substituted while one awaits the definitive sensitivity report.

4. Surgical drainage may be necessary if there is obvious fluctuation or pus formation. If *S. aureus* is the causative organism, surgical drainage should be carried out sooner rather than later, since extensive destruction of the gland can occur due to suppuration. General anesthesia is usually needed.

Predisposing factors to acute ascending sialadenitis include almost anything that causes xerostomia or decreased salivary flow, including emotional conditions, e.g., fear, psychiatric conditions, depression; factors affecting autonomic nerve supply to the salivary glands, e.g., tumors, trauma, neurosurgical operations; salivary gland aplasia and hypoplasia; Sjögren's syndrome, an autoimmune condition; obstruction to salivary flow, most commonly due to calculus formation or fibrosis in the duct; post-irradiaton salivary atrophy; changes in fluid and electrolyte balance, e.g., dehydration and uncontrolled diabetes; and drugs, particularly the tricyclic antidepressants, monoamine oxidase inhibitors, and phenothiazines. Most appetite suppressants, antispasmodics, decongestants, and sedatives and tranquilizers also cause xerostomia. The most common are obstruction from calculus formation, Sjögren's syndrome, and drug-induced xerostomia.

There is an unusual condition called acute sialadenitis of childhood, in which there is recurrent painful swelling of the parotid glands and sialograms show sialectatic changes. The cause is unknown, but an autoimmune phenomenon has been suggested with superadded infection. Attacks usually cease during the midteens and there appear to be no permanent sequelae in most cases. Treatment consists of reassurance and orally administered antibiotics, with rest and rehydration. Hospitalization is not usually necessary.

Chronic Sialadenitis

The symptoms of chronic sialadenitis are recurrent low-grade pain and swelling in the associated salivary gland, normally without systemic involvement. The causes are similar to those of acute sialadenitis, though the most common cause is probably calculus formation. Treatment consists of antibiotics and removal of the offending cause if possible. The major complication is the development of acute ascending sialadenitis. Antibiotics can usually be given orally and hospitalization is unnecessary. The antibiotic of choice is a penicillinase-resistant penicillin such as dicloxacillin, 500 mg 4 times daily. Provided there is no caclulus or other obstruction in the duct, salivary flow should be encouraged by the use of a sialagogue such as citrus fruits and juices.

Viral Sialadenitis

The classic cause of viral sialadenitis is mumps. This acute infectious viral disease, which primarily affects the parotid glands, can also affect other salivary glands and other organs. It is normally a disease of children and young adults and affects the sexes equally. The disease has an incubation period of 2 to 3 weeks and sufferers develop malaise, headache, and preauricular pain followed, after 1 or 2 days, by acute swelling of the parotid glands. Both parotid glands are usually affected, though often one swells before the other. The swellings subside after about a week. There are normally no long-term complications, though in adults, orchitis and oophoritis as well as involvement of the pancreas, liver, kidney and nervous system can occur. Following the disease, a long-lasting immunity develops. As with most viral infections, there is no specific therapy and treatment is symptomatic only, though now there is an effective preventive vaccine. Hospitalization is normally unnecessary. Viral parotitis can also be caused by other viruses, including the coxsackie virus, echovirus, and choriomeningitis and parainfluenza viruses, and can cause symptoms very similar to mumps.

THE IMMUNOCOMPROMISED PATIENT

There is an ever-increasing number of people who are medically compromised, and in particular, who have incompetent immune systems. In some cases the immune system is incompetent due to a disease process, such as AIDS, whereas in other cases, it is incompetent because of a congenital immunodeficient status, which in an earlier era would have caused death. In most cases, however, incompetent immune systems occur for iatrogenic reasons in patients taking steroids or other immunosuppressive drugs as part of therapy. Infections in immunocompromised patients frequently cause symptoms all out of proportion to the degree of infection, and the causative organism is often gram-negative or anaerobic and not normally known to be pathogenic in healthy people. This applies as much, if not more, to oral infections as to those in other sites. A compromised host should be suspected if any of the following responses are noted: (1) a severe or life-threatening infection with no obvious cause; (2) recurrent or frequent infections that cannot be explained; (3) infections that do not respond to normally appropriate therapy; or (4) inappropriate responses to infections, e.g., a leukopenia instead of a leukocytosis, or lack of pyrexia. In immunocompromised patients exhibiting any of these signs, opportunistic infections should always be suspected, in particular, gram-negative and anaerobic agents including *E. coli, Pseudomonas, Klebsiella, Clostridia*, and anaerobic cocci. Appropriate antibiotics may need to be given in high doses intravenously together with surgical drainage. It is essential to obtain a culture and antibiotic sensitivity if possible, and only bactericidal antibiotics should be employed. Suitable antibiotics may include semisynthetic penicillins such as Nafcillin, carbenicillin, and ticarcillin, second- or third-generation cephalosporins, including cefoxitin, and aminoglycosides may need to be added against many opportunistic infections.

SUGGESTED READING

Mason DK, Chisholm WG. Salivary glands in health and disease. Philadelphia: WB Saunders, 1975.

Tapazian RG, Goldberg MH. Management of infections of the oral and maxillofacial region. Philadelphia: WB Saunders, 1981.

PHARYNGITIS

ROBERT A. LOWE, M.D.
JERRIS R. HEDGES, M.D., M.S., F.A.C.E.P.

Sore throat is the third most common symptom among patients who consult physicians in the United States, where the annual health care costs for pharyngitis exceed $300 million. Yet the literature on pharyngitis contains much debate on this superficially "simple" topic.

The frequency with which various pathogens cause pharyngitis varies according to the age of the patient, the season, and the local prevalence of specific agents. In half the patients with acute sore throat, no etiologic agent can be identified. The most commonly recognized causative agents and their incidence are shown in Table 1.

DIFFERENTIAL DIAGNOSIS

A rapidly fatal disease that may be confused with pharyngitis is epiglottitis, an entity that occurs most commonly in children aged 3 to 7, but that can also occur in adults. Many adults with epiglottitis are mistakenly discharged from the emergency department on their first visit, only to be diagnosed correctly on their return. They may present with a sore throat, difficulty in swallowing, drooling, or vague problems with breathing that rapidly progress to complete airway obstruction. Any stable patient with a sore throat that is out of proportion to findings on examination of the oropharynx or with drooling or midline anterior cervical tenderness should undergo soft tissue x-ray examination of the neck (see chapter on *Epiglottitis*).

Other diseases in the differential diagnosis of pharyngitis include infections of the facial spaces, such as peritonsillar or retropharyngeal abscess, and Ludwig's angina. Asymmetric swelling of the peritonsillar area, marked pharyngeal swelling, or other localized areas of facial swelling and tenderness should trigger the search for these potentially serious infections. Tertiary syphilis can cause gummas of the mouth and oropharynx, and these usually resemble ulcers or nodules. Tuberculosis can cause a solitary, irregular ulcer covered by persistent exudate on the tongue, tonsils, or soft palate. Erythema multiforme, bullous pemphigoid, systemic lupus erythematosus, Behçet's disease, Kawasaki syndrome, aphthous stomatitis, and Stevens-Johnson syndrome can all involve the oropharyngeal mucosa. Finally, the patient

TABLE 1 Microbial Causes of Acute Pharyngitis

Etiology	Syndrome/Disease	Estimated Importance*
Viral		
Rhinovirus	Common cold	20
Coronavirus	Common cold	≥5
Adenovirus	Pharyngoconjunctival fever, ARD	5
Herpes simplex 1 and 2	Gingivitis, stomatitis, pharyngitis	4
Parainfluenza virus	Common cold, croup	2
Influenza virus A and B	Influenza	2
EB virus	Infectious mononucleosis	<1
Cytomegalovirus	Infectious mononucleosis	<1
Bacterial		
Streptococcus pyogenes	Pharyngitis/tonsillitis	15–35
Chlamydia trachomatis	Pharyngitis, pneumonia	0–20
Mycoplasma pneumoniae	Pneumonia, bronchitis, pharyngitis	5
Mixed anaerobic infections	Gingivitis, pharyngitis (Vincent's angina)	<1
	Peritonsillitis/peritonsillar abscess (quinsy)	<1
Neisseria gonorrhoeae	Pharyngitis	<1
Corynebacterium diphtheriae	Diphtheria	<1
Corynebacterium hemolyticum and *C. ulcerans*	Pharyngitis	<1
Mycoplasma hominis	Pharyngitis (in volunteers)	Unknown

* Estimated percentage of cases of pharyngitis due to indicated organism in civilians of all ages

Modified from Gwalney JM. Pharyngitis. In: Mandell GL, Douglas RG, Bennett JE. Principles and practice of infectious disease. 2nd ed. New York: John Wiley and Sons, 1985.

with chronic sore throat that is unresponsive to the usual therapy deserves a careful evaluation by an otorhinolaryngologist for possible malignant tumor.

STREPTOCOCCAL PHARYNGITIS

The most common problem in the management of pharyngitis is distinguishing viral from streptococcal infection. Treatment of the latter is essential to minimize the risk of subsequent rheumatic fever.

Although the presentation of streptococcal pharyngitis is variable, streptococcal pharyngitis classically presents with the sudden onset of fever, chills (without rigors), and headache. These symptoms are followed by severe sore throat associated with exudate and tender anterior cervical lymph nodes. Children often have nausea, vomiting, and abdominal pain early in the illness. Streptococcal upper respiratory infections are less common in children under 2 years of age; cultures are positive in about 14 percent of children of this age with tonsilitis. Streptococcal infection can be subtle in this age group, sometimes with only a nasal discharge, anorexia, or other nonspecific symptoms developing over several weeks, and a physical examination showing only rhinitis and cervical lymphadenopathy without obvious oropharyngeal involvement. In nonepidemic settings, the peak incidence of streptococcal pharyngitis is at ages 6 to 14. Thirty-five to 40 percent of children with acute pharyngitis demonstrate group A beta-hemolytic streptococcus on culture, whereas about 15 percent of symptomatic adults have positive cultures.

Traditionally, clinicians have obtained throat cultures on all patients with pharyngitis and delayed treatment until the culture results were available. However, several reasons exist for initiating antibiotic therapy as soon as the diagnosis of streptococcal pharyngitis can be established with reasonable accuracy. Multiple studies have demonstrated that early antibiotic treatment of streptococcal pharyngitis shortens the duration of fever and other symptoms by at least 12 hours and possibly by as much as 3 days. Antibiotics appear to decrease the risk of suppurative complications such as parapharyngeal abscesses, suppurative cervical adenitis, and otitis media. Although antibiotic therapy is effective in preventing rheumatic fever even if initiation of therapy is delayed for 9 days after the onset of symptoms, maximal prophylaxis is achieved by early use of antibiotics.

Furthermore, the throat culture is not adequately reliable: 15 to 20 percent of children with pharyngitis and 5 to 10 percent of adults are "streptococcal carriers"; they have positive cultures, but no rise in antistreptococcal antibodies. These patients are at minimal risk for rheumatic fever and probably have viral pharyngitis with coincident streptococcal colonization. Conversely, dual-culture studies have demonstrated that single cultures miss streptococci in about 10 percent of cases. One study comparing cultures to serologies in children with sore throats found that cultures had a sensitivity of 88 percent and a specificity of 53 percent.

No clinical criteria can predict streptococcal pharyngitis with complete accuracy. However, the tools of decision analysis have demonstrated that diagnostic approaches other than the throat culture may be accurate enough to serve as the basis for therapy. Given the inaccuracies of the culture and the relatively low risk of penicillin therapy, oral penicillin therapy is justified if the probability of streptococcal infection is over 20 percent; parenteral therapy is justified when the probability is over 30 percent. Treatment thresholds are even lower if a large proportion of patients are not expected to follow-up on their culture reports.

Several approaches can predict the likelihood of positive throat culture accurately enough to justify immediate therapy. Walsh et al showed that adults with sore throats, if enlarged or tender cervical nodes are present and there is either a pharyngeal exudate or a history of recent exposure to streptococcal pharyngitis, have a high probability of a positive throat culture (predictive value of positive criteria for a positive culture approximately 28 percent for adults). Using these criteria, the physician can treat 55 percent of patients with streptococcal pharyngitis on initial presentation to the emergency department without obtaining throat cultures.

The pharyngeal Gram stain can also be used to identify patients who have a high probability of a positive streptococcal throat culture. A Gram stain of a direct smear from the area of pharyngeal inflammation is scanned at $100 \times$ magnification for areas having the most polymorphonuclear leukocytes. These areas are examined at $1,000 \times$ magnification for gram-positive ovoid cocci occurring singly or in longitudinal pairs. Although accuracy depends on the experience of the microscopist, approximately 67 percent of adult pharyngitis patients with a positive Gram stain have a positive culture, whereas about 10 percent of patients with a negative Gram stain have a positive culture.

In children a "nine-item streptococcal scorecard" has been recommended by Breese (Table 2). Breese found that 83 percent of his patients with a positive throat culture had scores of 30 or greater. Funamara, in a different geographic location and using the scorecard largely without the benefit of a leukocyte count, found that 40 percent of patients with a positive throat culture had scores of 28 or greater. The predictive value of a positive screen for a positive throat culture was over 40 percent for both studies.

A promising alternative to the foregoing screening tools is the latex agglutination test of a direct pharyngeal smear. Initial studies comparing latex agglutination techniques to throat cultures show these tests, which can be performed in 10 to 60 minutes, to have sensitivities of 77 to 95 percent and specificities of 86 to 100 percent. These studies need to be replicated, and the test results would have to be reported while the patient is in the emergency department for the latex agglutination test to replace clinical criteria or throat cultures.

During a true epidemic of streptococcal illness, all patients with pharyngitis should receive antibiotics; furthermore, patients with a history of rheumatic fever who

TABLE 2 Nine-Item Streptococcal Scoring System

Item	Score		
Month of illness:			
February, March or April	4		
January, May or December	3		
June, October or November	2		
July, August or September	1		
Age:			
5 through 10 years	4		
4, 11, 12, 13, 14	3		
3, 15 or more	2		
2 or under	1		
WBC:			
0–8.4	1		
8.5–10.4	2		
10.5–13.4	3		
13.5–20.4	5		
20.5 or more	6		
Not done	3		
	Yes	No	Unknown
Fever 38 °C or more	4	2	2
Sore throat	4	2	2
Cough	2	4	4
Headache	4	2	2
Abnormal pharynx	4	1	3
Abnormal cervical glands	4	2	3

From Breese BB. A simple scorecard for the tentative diagnosis of streptococcal pharyngitis. Am J Dis Child 1977; 131:514–517.

are not currently on penicillin prophylaxis and present with pharyngitis should receive antibiotics because of the great risk of recurrent rheumatic fever in the presence of a streptococcal infection. Walsh's criteria in adults or Breese's criteria in children are sufficiently specific to justify antibiotics without a throat culture. The Gram stain is even more accurate, when physician time or technician skill level allows. If antibiotics are prescribed at the first emergency department visit, there is no need to obtain a throat culture. If the "screening tests" are negative, however, a throat culture should be obtained and therapy should be guided by the results.

Therapy of streptococcal pharyngitis consists of penicillin or erythromycin. Intramuscular benzathine penicillin G (e.g., Bicillin L-A) is recommended by the American Heart Association. Patients weighing over 60 pounds receive 1.2 million units: smaller children receive 600,000 units. In patients with little muscle mass, local reactions to the injection can be decreased by using a combination of benzathine and procaine penicillin (e.g., Bicillin C-R 900/300); however, the proper dose is the above-stated amount of benzathine penicillin, ignoring the procaine penicillin in the preparation.

Oral penicillin is slightly less effective than parenteral therapy for eradicating streptococci, but may be associated with fewer allergic reactions. The dose is 400,000 units of penicillin G or 250 mg of penicillin V 3 or 4 times daily for adults, or half this dose for children. Therapy must be continued for a full 10 days, and

compliance is often a problem, since the patient usually becomes asymptomatic much sooner. In patients allergic to penicillin, erythromycin, 250 mg 4 times daily or 500 mg twice daily (10 mg per kilogram per day in divided doses for children), is prescribed for 10 days. Children with streptococcal pharyngitis should be considered infectious and kept out of school until they have received antibiotics for at least 24 hours.

Patients with pharyngitis, regardless of etiology, generally benefit from symptomatic therapy, such as warm saline gargles, commercially available lozenges or gargles, rest, analgesia, and liquids.

INFECTIOUS MONONUCLEOSIS

Mononucleosis, usually caused by the Epstein-Barr virus, but occasionally by the cytomegalovirus, is the cause of a much smaller percentage of sore throats. The illness usually occurs in patients between 15 and 25 years of age. After an incubation period of 30 to 50 days, patients develop a prodrome of mild symptoms, including headache, malaise, and fatigue. Three to 5 days later, more classic symptoms begin to manifest themselves. These symptoms are variable in presence and severity, but usually include fever, sore throat, and cervical lymphadenopathy.

Sore throat is the most common feature of infectious mononucleosis and usually begins in the first week. Most patients have hyperplasia of pharyngeal lymphoid tissue along with inflammation and edema. About half the patients develop a grayish-white exudative tonsillitis along with a gelatinous appearance of the uvula and palatal arch. Tonsillar enlargement and pharyngeal swelling may occasionally compromise the airway. Palatine petechiae are common, although they are also seen in streptococcal pharyngitis. Fever is typical, usually peaking in the afternoon, and may reach 103 °F (39.4 °C) daily for 1 or 2 weeks. Over 90 percent of patients with infectious mononucleosis have posterior cervical adenopathy, and generalized enlargement of lymph nodes frequently occurs, the nodes being firm and moderately tender. Splenomegaly occurs in about half the patients, being greatest during the second and third weeks of illness. Although only 10 percent of patients have clinical signs of hepatic involvement, most have abnormal liver function tests. Rashes of various types occur in about 10 percent of patients. Transient bilateral supraorbital edema may also occur early in the illness.

The most rapidly lethal complication of infectious mononucleosis is splenic rupture. The presence of abdominal pain in a patient with infectious mononucleosis should raise a strong suspicion of impending splenic rupture. Other complications of infectious mononucleosis include hemolytic anemia, thrombocytopenia, myocarditis, pericarditis, and a variety of neurologic abnormalities, including aseptic meningitis, encephalitis, coma, cerebellar symptoms, and Guillain-Barré syndrome.

Children may have a milder form of infectious mononucleosis. The incubation period may be as short as 10 to 14 days, and the fever may be mild or absent. About half the children with the clinical syndrome of infectious mononucleosis never develop heterophil antibodies.

Laboratory studies helpful in the diagnosis of suspected infectious mononucleosis include the complete blood count with differential and the heterophil antibody test. Early in the illness, the total WBC count is normal, or depressed owing to neutropenia. About 70 percent of patients have a relative and absolute lymphocytosis at presentation. During the second and third weeks of illness, the total leukocyte count usually rises to 10,000 to 20,000, with approximately 60 percent lymphocytes and monocytes. The percentage of atypical lymphocytes ranges from 0 to 90 percent. Sixty percent of patients have a positive heterophil antibody test within the first 2 weeks of illness, whereas 80 to 90 percent have positive tests by the end of the first month. In equivocal cases, liver function tests may be useful, since 90 percent of patients have some abnormalities. Antibodies to Epstein-Barr virus are elevated in almost all patients, but this test is not often readily available.

Since heterophil antibodies are often negative early in the illness and since there is no specific therapy for infectious mononucleosis, it seems reasonable to withhold these studies in the patient with recent onset of pharyngitis unless the suspicion of mononucleosis is high. The physician should evaluate as previously discussed for streptococcus and may then instruct the patient to return for further evaluation (i.e., CBC with differential and heterophil antibodies) only if symptoms persist longer than 1 week.

Treatment includes bed rest during the febrile period and symptomatic therapy as outlined for streptococcal pharyngitis. Patients with splenomegaly should avoid heavy lifting or contact sports. Most patients recover within 2 to 4 weeks. Strict isolation is not necessary, but the virus can be transmitted through saliva or blood.

On rare occasions a patient with exudative pharyngotonsillitis and *severe* pharyngeal edema may benefit from a course of steroids. When used, prednisone 40 to 80 mg should be given on the first day and tapered over a 7- to 14-day period. Patients with airway obstruction, neurologic complications, hemolytic anemia, severe thrombocytopenia, or cardiac involvement should be admitted and given steroids.

Some patients with infectious mononucleosis have throat cultures positive for group A beta-hemolytic streptococcus. Although it is unclear whether these are carriers or victims of two simultaneous infections, it is safest to treat them with penicillin or erythromycin. Ampicillin should not be used, since it frequently induces a rash in patients with mononucleosis.

MYCOPLASMAL AND CHLAMYDIAL PHARYNGITIS

Recent data indicate that *Mycoplasma pneumoniae* causes pharyngitis in 5 to 8 percent of cases. *Mycoplasma* commonly produces extrapharyngeal symptoms including cough, pulmonary findings, and bullous myringitis. When mycoplasmal infection presents as pharyngitis alone, it cannot be distinguished clinically from streptococcal or viral infection. The symptom complex for chlamydial pharyngitis has not been defined, and investigators attempting to determine the frequency of *Chlamydia trachomatis* infections in patients with pharyngitis have reported conflicting data, with frequencies ranging from 0 to 20 percent.

Although tetracycline or erythromycin has been advocated for extrapharyngeal mycoplasmal and chlamydial infections, pharyngeal infections by these organisms are probably self-limited. Furthermore, when erythromycin was used extensively in Japan for empiric treatment of pharyngitis, the incidence of streptococcal resistance to this antibiotic increased dramatically. The uncertainties about the significance of these organisms do not justify widespread empiric use of broad-spectrum antibiotics.

GONOCOCCAL PHARYNGITIS

Gonococcal pharyngitis is usually asymptomatic, but can present with subtle complaints such as itching, burning, dry mouth, or as an exudative pharyngitis. This diagnosis should be considered in patients with a history of recent fellatio (especially homosexual men and other patients with multiple sexual partners), and in patients with symptoms of genital gonorrhea. Diagnosis is made by culture. The physician should not use a cotton-tipped swab, as cotton inhibits the growth of the gonococci. The specimen must be promptly plated out on Thayer-Martin or "chocolate" agar and placed in a high-CO_2 atmosphere by the physician. Since some *Neisseria* species are normal oral flora, the specific species must be identified prior to initiation of therapy. Alternatively, signs consistent with genital gonorrhea may make the presence or absence of an additional focus of infection a moot point. However, not all antibiotic regimens that are effective against genital gonorrhea are adequate for pharyngeal infection. Satisfactory treatment consists of ceftriaxone 250 mg intramuscularly. Alternative regimens include procaine penicillin 4.8 million units intramuscularly (half the dose in each hip), along with 1 g of oral probenecid, or trimethoprim-sulfamethoxazole (80 mg and 400 mg per tablet respectively), nine tablets once a day for 5 days.

DIPHTHERIA

Early in its course, pharyngeal diphtheria is indistinguishable from streptococcal pharyngitis, with low-grade fever and pharyngeal erythema or a small amount of nonspecific exudate. Later, the pharyngeal exudate coalesces into a thick membrane—bluish white, gray, or black, depending on the degree of hemorrhage. The membrane becomes so firmly attached to underlying tissues that attempts to remove it result in bleeding. Although membranes can occur with streptococcal pharyngitis, *Corynebacterium hemolyticum*, viral pharyngitis, or mononucleosis, a membrane extending beyond the tonsils should raise a strong suspicion of diphtheria. The membrane may extend to involve the larynx and trachea, producing severe airway problems. Edema can spread to the submandibular glands and anterior neck, resembling Ludwig's angina. Later, a systemic toxin can produce myocarditis or peripheral neuritis with diffuse weakness, progressing to paralysis and death in severe cases. This disease has become rare owing to immunization, but it can be seen in immigrants and other inadequately immunized groups.

Diagnosis can be confirmed by demonstration of the organism on methylene blue-stained smears in about 80 percent of cases or by a fluorescein-labeled diphtheria antitoxin technique. If the patient has not been receiving antibiotics previously, the organism can be reliably cultured on Loeffler's medium within 8 to 12 hours. Patients with suspected diphtheria must be admitted and kept at bed rest and in strict isolation. Specific treatment includes antitoxin, penicillin or erythromycin, and a search for contacts in need of prophylactic therapy.

OTHER BACTERIAL INFECTIONS

Other bacterial infections presenting as pharyngitis include *Yersinia enterocolitica*, *Corynebacterium hemolyticum*, non-group A streptococcus, *Staphylococcus*, and anaerobes. Antibiotic susceptibility varies with these different pathogens. These are probably rare diseases. Therefore, complete throat cultures (as opposed to screening cultures for group A beta-hemolytic streptococcus and occasionally gonococcus) are rarely indicated. However, when pharyngitis remains symptomatic for more than 1 week and a diagnosis has not been established after "strep screen," culture for gonococcus on Thayer-Martin medium, evaluation for infectious mononucleosis, and complete laryngoscopy, either a complete aerobic and anaerobic culture or empiric antibiotic therapy may be appropriate.

OTHER CAUSES

Vincent's angina can involve the throat and/or the gum margins. The patient may complain of a mild unilateral sore throat and a bad taste. Examination reveals a foul odor to the breath and a purulent pharyngeal exudate overlying a tonsillar ulcer. It is caused by a combination of anaerobic bacteria and spirochetes. Treatment consists of penicillin in the same doses as for streptococcal illness.

Hand, foot, and mouth disease causes painful vesicles on the oropharynx, mouth, palms, and soles, along with fever, malaise, and headache. It is caused by a coxsackievirus and resolves within 2 to 4 weeks with symptomatic therapy.

Other viral infections are listed in Table 1. These infections are frequently associated with other upper respiratory symptoms, tracheobronchitis, conjunctivitis, and constitutional complaints.

SUGGESTED READING

Brancato FP. Microbiological procedures: direct preparations of clinical materials, stained and unstained, in emergency medical care. In: Roberts JR, Hedges JR, eds. Clinical procedures in emergency medicine. Philadelphia: WB Saunders, 1985.

Breese BB. A simple scorecard for the tentative diagnosis of streptococcal pharyngitis. Am J Dis Child 1977; 131:514–517.

Funamara JL, Berkowitz CD. Applicability of a scoring system in the diagnosis of streptococcal pharyngitis. Clin Ped 1983; 22:622–626.

Gwaltney JM. Pharyngitis. In: Mandell GL, Douglas RG, Bennet JE, eds. Principles and practice of infectious diseases. 2nd ed. New York: John Wiley and Sons, 1985.

Lowe R, Hedges JR. Early treatment of streptococcal pharyngitis. Ann Emerg Med 1984; 13:440–448.

Rapid office diagnostic tests for streptococcal pharyngitis. Medical Letter on Drugs and Therapeutics 1985; 27:49–51.

Walsh BT, Bookheim WW, Johnson RC, et al. Recognition of streptococcal pharyngitis in adults. Arch Intern Med 1975; 135:1493–1497.

TONSILLITIS AND PERITONSILLAR ABSCESS

ALAN D. KORNBLUT, A.B., M.S., M.D., F.A.C.S.
MARY E. BOTTONE, M.D.

Each palatine tonsil is an accumulation of lymphoid tissue located in a fossa that is bounded by three muscles—the palatoglossus (the anterior pillar), the palatopharyngeus (the posterior pillar), and the superior pharyngeal constrictor (the posterior wall of the fossa). The tonsil is separated from these muscles by a capsule through which pass small vessels, nerves, and efferent lymphatics.

The surface area of each tonsil is increased by numerous invaginations or crypts that contain lymphocytes and various immune substances. However, these crypts also serve to entrap foreign organisms or particles from ingested foods as well as surface epithelia. As a result, the crypts are a significant source of tonsillar inflammations and infections.

ACUTE TONSILLITIS

Acute tonsillitis is an acute febrile illness and is frequently self-limiting. Examination of the throat invariably reveals enlarged inflamed tonsils that are sometimes covered with multiple pustules or a whitish-gray exudate. This exudate is usually limited to the tonsillar fossae and tends to be soft and friable. Although parenchymal ulcerations can also occur, this exudate is usually nonadherent to underlying tissues.

Etiology. Tonsillitis varies in severity depending on the virulence of the infecting organisms and the resistance of the patient. The most common bacterial organisms cultured from patients with acute tonsillitis are the beta-hemolytic streptococci, although staphylococci, pneumococci, and *Haemophilus* species also can be found. In addition, such viral pathogens as influenza, parainfluenza, herpes simplex, coxsackie, ECHO, rhinovirus, and respiratory syncitial viruses are common. More recently, anaerobic organisms have become recognized as other significant causes of acute tonsillitis. Tonsillitis attributable to other causes tends to be chronic, although certain persons may experience acute tonsillitis as a consequence of mucoid drainage from the nose or nasopharynx. These latter inflammations are frequently sterile or contain anaerobic organisms.

Clinical Manifestations. Acute tonsillitis usually occurs in adolescents and in young adults, and is relatively less common in older age groups (but still occurs). Certain conditions can predispose patients to tonsil infections, such as fatigue, inadequate diet, pre-existing upper respiratory infections, or exposures to persons with such infections.

The clinical onset of tonsillitis can be sudden and associated with fever and chills. Sore throat soon follows, as does difficulty in swallowing (as a result of inflammation of the pharyngeal constrictor muscles). There may be concomitant pharyngitis along with coating of the tongue and thick tenacious mucus in the oral cavity. Tender cervical adenopathy is also relatively common. Systemic complaints such as headache, joint pain, and malaise are common in these patients.

Symptoms may persist for 4 to 6 days and gradually resolve unless complications occur. Viral tonsillitis as well as certain bacterial infections are usually self-limited. However, by definition, infections lasting longer than 48 to 72 hours should be considered "chronic" rather than "acute." Persistent infections may also be complicated by peritonsillar abscesses as well as by infections of the deep neck. Septicemia from tonsillitis may also seed infections to the heart, lungs, brain, and other distant sites.

Diagnostic Work-up. When possible, initial laboratory studies should include a complete blood count with differential and a throat swab of the affected tonsils. When indicated, a Gram stain preparation can be useful in diagnosing bacterial causes of tonsillitis. If viral tonsillitis is suspected, specific viral agglutination studies may be ordered, although such testing tends to be impractical under most clinical circumstances. Similarly, cultures for bacteria are *most* useful for the diagnosis (and treatment) of infections that are refractory to initial therapies. These latter cultures are best taken when patients are *initially* seen (if clinically warranted) so that medications can be promptly adjusted as necessary without incurring further delays in therapy.

Treatment. The usual treatment of acute tonsillitis is directed toward eliminating bacterial infection and providing immediate supportive care. Adequate fluid intake, rest, warmth, and proper hygiene are important. Oral lavages with diluted hydrogen peroxide or warm saline solutions are helpful in keeping the oral cavity clean. Analgesics should be given as required, and aspirin or the acetaminophen preparations are useful as both analgesics and antipyretic agents. Topical analgesic medications have some value, but certain products contain cetylpyridium and sodium phenolate. Examples are Cepacol and Chloraseptic, which either contain or can act as astringents and may further irritate the pharyngeal mucosa.

Systemic antibiotics are necessary for the treatment of acute symptomatic bacterial tonsillitis, and penicillin, the sulfonamides, erythromycin, and tetracycline are still useful clinically. Dosage is dependent on the age and weight of the patient. However, tetracycline should *not* be used in children (especially children with non-erupted teeth) because of the dental staining produced. Assessment of the individual patient's history of drug allergies is also important. Antibiotic therapy is generally given for 7 to 10 days to prevent production of antibiotic-resistant bacteria. As indicated previously, specific bacterial cultures should be obtained for antibiotic sensitivities when patients remain refractory to treatment, and this should be done *before* any adjustments of medications are made.

Hospital treatment for patients with acute tonsillitis is not usually required, but should be considered for those patients with dehydration and when proper home care is unavailable.

Differential Diagnosis. A number of diseases can be included in the differential diagnosis of acute tonsillitis. Prior to the prevalent use of routine vaccinations and availability of antibiotics, diphtheria was a major clinical problem. However, such infection has a more gradual onset with less pronounced initial systemic symptoms. Hoarseness, stridor, and croupy cough develop later, with the tonsils exhibiting a firm, leathery gray, adherent membrane that is pathognomonic.

Vincent's angina, or trench mouth, is characterized by ulcerative gingivitis and stomatitis with pharyngitis. It is caused by concomitant infection with a spirochete and *Bacteroides* species in patients with poor oral and dental hygiene, but may also mask an underlying malignant disease.

Patients with infectious mononucleosis can exhibit mild inflammations or frank ulcerations of the oral cavity and tonsils. Posterior cervical adenopathy and palatal petechiae may be present as well.

Other disease states that may produce membranous or pseudomembranous tonsillitis include leukemia, agranulocytosis, pemphigus, and epithelial neoplasms.

CHRONIC TONSILLITIS

Chronic tonsillitis is the result of chronic inflammation of the tonsils following recurrent acute or subclinical infections. Tonsillar enlargement may occur as a result of parenchymal hyperplasia, or scarring may result with obstruction of the tonsillar crypts.

Etiology. Organisms cultured from chronically infected tonsils are similar to those involved in acute tonsillar infections, but are generally gram-positive. Viral pathogens and fungi are also frequently found in infected tissues.

Clinical Manifestations. Although chronic tonsillitis can occur in any age group, it is most frequently found in an adult population. Its occurrence is invariably the result of recurrent episodes of acute tonsillar inflammation and infection.

Affected patients commonly experience chronic recurrent sore throat, which may be partially relieved by supportive measures. Halitosis is a frequent complaint, and many patients also note chronic postnasal drainages. Patients also note recurrent febrile episodes as well as such systemic complaints as malaise and joint pain. Enlarged cervical nodes are relatively common and are sometimes more prominent during active periods of infection.

On examination, tonsillar size may vary: some tonsils are large, while others are small as a result of chronic scarification. Caseous debris or concretions are frequently seen in the tonsillar crypts, and the presence or absence of infection or inflammation depends on whether or not empiric treatments have been used prior to examination. Most importantly, unilateral enlargement of either tonsil should be suspect for possible malignant change.

Diagnostic Work-up. Any of the causes of acute tonsillitis should be considered in the diagnosis of chronic tonsillitis. The most cost-efficient diagnostic evaluation in patients with chronic tonsillitis consists of a careful history and physical examination. When warranted, complete hemograms should be done, as well as urinalyses, cultures (inclusive of bacteria, mycoses, and acid-fast organisms), blood sugars, and serologic studies. Chest films also should be obtained as needed, and biopsies of tissues obtained when clinically indicated.

Treatment. The treatment of patients with chronic tonsillitis is essentially symptomatic and includes those measures used in the management of patients with acute tonsillitis—adequate rest, appropriate hygiene, sufficient fluids, analgesics,and antibiotics as warranted. Underlying causes for the tonsillitis must also be treated. However, recurrent episodes of inflammatory or infectious tonsillitis are best treated by surgical removal of the tonsils. In addition, any tissues removed, especially in the adult patient, must be examined microscopically for possible neoplasia.

Differential Diagnosis. The possible causes of chronic tonsillitis include disease processes that can produce a pseudomembrane over the tonsils (e.g., Vincent's angina, infectious mononucleosis). Granulomatous diseases also may occur and include tuberculosis, syphilis, leprosy, mycoses, and certain of the collagen diseases. In addition, lymphomas and squamous carcinomas in the tonsils may present as chronic tonsillar enlargements and inflammations.

PERITONSILLAR ABSCESS

The peritonsillar abscess, or "quinsy," is a localized accumulation of pus within the peritonsillar tissues and is invariably the result of suppurative infection within the adjacent tonsil. Infection penetrates the tonsillar capsule, commonly at the superior pole, and extends into the connective tissue space between the capsule and the posterior wall of the tonsillar fossa.

Etiology. Any of the organisms causing acute or chronic tonsillitis may be the cause of a peritonsillar abscess. More recently, anaerobic organisms have come to be recognized as frequent causes of these abscesses. Since many patients who are seen in the emergency department have already received initial therapy with penicillin, coagulase-positive or beta-lactamase producing organisms must also be considered.

Clinical Manifestations. Patients with peritonsillar abscesses commonly give a past medical history of persistent sore throat that progressively worsens in spite of treatment. Pain usually becomes localized to one side of the throat, although bilateral abscesses (infrequently) occur. Fever is present, with temperatures ranging from 102 to 105 °F, unless patients are taking antipyretic medications or are immunosuppressed. Other complaints are chills, malaise, nausea, and difficulty in swallowing. Patients commonly have trismus and are unable to swallow any diet or even their secretions so that dehydration results. In these patients, drooling is commonly seen, and the breath becomes rancid. Speech also becomes difficult, and the voice tends to have a nasal or thickened "hot potato" quality. Tender cervical adenopathy is also common.

Examination of the throat in affected patients can be difficult if trismus is present, and an oral analgesic lavage may be required (such as 2 to 4 percent lidocaine or benzocaine solutions) before an adequate examination can be done. When the oral cavity is examined, there is almost always marked edema and infection of the involved peritonsillar tissues, with bulging of the tonsillar pillar and soft palate. The tonsil itself may not be visible because of adjacent tissue edema or the mucopus present. Swelling of the uvula results in its displacement to the unaffected side. If pus extends inferiorly behind the tonsil, retro- or parapharyngeal infections occur and may also produce supraglottic edema and airway obstruction.

Diagnostic Work-up. Initial laboratory studies should include a complete blood count with differential, a urinalysis, and determinations of blood urea nitrogen, blood sugar, and serum electrolytes. Throat cultures should be obtained for aerobic and anaerobic organisms. Useful radiologic studies include AP and lateral soft tissue views of the neck and a chest film to evaluate the airway and possible further involvement of the deep tissues of the neck. However, the diagnosis of an actual abscess is established by needle aspiration of pus from behind or adjacent to the affected tonsil, and is preferably done by a clinician who is experienced in treating such infections. This avoids unnecessary complications, such as the inadvertent spread of infection to uninvolved tissues or the puncture of an aberrant major vessel. The actual technique of aspiration is not difficult, and can usually be accomplished by having patients gargle with an anesthetic solution and then carefully inserting an 18–gauge needle that is *firmly* fixed to a 5 or 10 cc Luer-Loc type syringe. The return of pus in the aspirate is diagnostic, but a Gram stain and culture may also be indicated. In some cases, the aspirate may also be therapeutic (to be discussed).

Treatment. Medical measures alone may abort an early peritonsillar abscess or cellulitis, and occasional spontaneous rupture of the abscess may also occur through the tonsil or tonsillar pillars. However, effective drainage of loculated pus requires surgical drainage. This incision and drainage procedure has traditionally been done on an outpatient basis under topical or local anesthesia. Certain patients—especially very young or uncooperative patients—require admission and general anesthesia for the drainage procedure to be safely done.

General treatment after drainage of an abscess includes saline or peroxide lavages for oral hygiene, enforced hydration, and sufficient analgesics to relieve discomfort. Elevation of the head protects the airway from edema and secretions. Preferably, bedside suction should be made available to remove pooled secretions and to help maintain oral hygiene. Parenteral antibiotics are mandatory and should be selected with a view to avoiding drug allergies and adjusting prior antibiotics used (as based on smears and cultures). When antibiotics are begun empirically, broad-spectrum antibiotics may be preferable, especially when penicillin has been used previously. It should also be realized that (as previously discussed) some organisms produce penicillinase or beta-lactamase, inactivating penicillin and many of its derivative antibiotics. The cephalosporins or clindamycin might be the best choice in these patients. However, whatever antibiotic is given should be based on the age and the weight of the patient, should be adjusted according to cultures and sensitivities, and should be used for 7 to 10 days to avoid the production of antibiotic-resistant organisms.

A sizable literature is now accumulating about the value of tonsillectomy *a chaud*, i.e., abscess tonsillectomy. This is useful in managing patients with recurrent episodes of tonsillitis or recurrent peritonsillar abscesses, although patients must be carefully selected. Patients can be toxic when seen initially and may fare poorly if a general anesthetic is required and no attempt is made to begin parenteral fluids and antibiotics before surgery.

More recently, several reports have indicated that peritonsillar abscesses may be adequately treated by needle aspiration alone and appropriate antibiotics. Again, we would stress that patients so treated be carefully selected and closely followed since failures of such therapies do occur.

Differential Diagnosis. The usual problem in diagnosing a peritonsillar abscess is differentiating the abscess from acute suppurative tonsillitis and peritonsillar cellulitis. Management may require a specialist's assistance. Other lesions presenting as peritonsillar swellings include congenital cysts, aberrant vessels, and benign and malignant neoplasms.

SUGGESTED READING

Herzon FS. Permucosal needle drainage of peritonsillar abscesses. A five-year experience. Arch Otolaryngol 1984; 110:104–105.

Kornblut AD. Non-neoplastic diseases of the tonsils and adenoids. In: Paparella MM, Shumrick DA, eds. Otolaryngology. Vol. 3. Head and neck. 2nd ed. Philadelphia: WB Saunders, 1980:2263.

Lee KJ, Traxler JH, Smith HW, Kelly JH. Tonsillectomy: treatment of peritonsillar abscess. Trans Am Acad Ophthalmol Otolaryngol 1973; 77:417–421.

Maisel RH. Peritonsillar abscess: tonsil antibiotic levels in patients treated by acute abscess surgery. Laryngoscope 1982; 92:80–87.

FOREIGN BODIES OF THE EAR, NOSE, AND OROPHARYNX

SABINO T. BALUYOT, M.D., F.A.C.S.

FOREIGN BODY IN THE EAR

Commonly found in children, foreign bodies in the ear range from a piece of toilet paper, napkin, eraser, crayon, cotton ball, seed, silly putty, sponge, plastic, styrofoam, stone, or anything small enough to be pushed into the ear canal by either the child or someone else. Such foreign bodies frequently do not attract immediate attention unless inserted with such force as to lacerate the ear canal or rupture the eardrum. When bleeding occurs, the patient or family is alarmed and the problem is brought to immediate attention.

Live insects on the other hand, when they get into the ear, cause such tremendous discomfort and pain that urgent attention is needed. Each time the insect moves, extreme discomfort is experienced. It has to be killed. The ear canal should be filled, preferably with alcohol, lidocaine, or ether, and the solution is allowed to remain in the canal for 1 to 3 minutes until the insect dies. If these solutions are not available, scotch, bourbon, or any alcoholic drink will suffice. Once killed, removal is accomplished by the same means as are used for removal of inanimate foreign bodies.

Foreign bodies in the ear are often discovered by an examining physician during a routine check-up. By the time it is discovered, the foreign body may already be encrusted in cerumen and mistaken for impacted wax.

In adults, with the exception of the mentally retarded, foreign bodies in the ear are less frequent. Insects and flying objects, e.g., metal particles from welding or grinding, are more frequent offending agents and require immediate attention. Slugs, for example, are painful and frequently cause perforation of the eardrum that may require surgical closure if it does not heal spontaneously. In an unconscious or debilitated person, a roach or any other crawling insect can enter the ear.

What does one need to do as soon as the foreign body is recognized? If there is bleeding, instilling a few drops of hydrogen peroxide into the ear canal generally stops the bleeding until the removal process is instituted. A live foreign body must be killed by filling the ear canal with alcohol, lidocaine, or ether; if neither is available, scotch or any alcoholic beverage can be used.

For removal, good lighting is essential; it should allow freedom of both hands and be easily directed and focused into the ear. A flashlight held by a nurse is definitely not adequate. A reflecting head mirror or a battery or electrically operated headlight is the ideal choice. An ear speculum is necessary to open the ear canal and bring the object into view. One must use the largest size that fits the canal. The foreign body can be flushed out with an irrigating syringe and lukewarm water, a special pressure irrigation set, or a Water Pik, with the water current directed along the ear canal, not on the foreign body. The idea is to direct the current to hit the eardrum so that as the water exits, it pushes out the object as well. If there is any question whether the eardrum is perforated, flushing with water must not be done. Perforation should be suspected if there is loss of hearing, history of previous perforation, or an ear discharge of long duration.

Suctioning with a finger-controlled Frazier or brain suction tip can also be employed. The foreign body can also be grasped with a pair of alligator forceps or pulled out with an ear curet.

The patient must keep still. In an uncooperative patient, whether child or adult, active restraint with the help of a nurse or a papoose board is essential. General anesthesia may be necessary if neither of the aforementioned is feasible. One must avoid trauma to the ear canal, the eardrum, or the ossicles. During the attempt at removal, if bleeding occurs, it is a good idea to stop the attempt and complete the removal under anesthesia to avoid further trauma.

In the case of a small insect in the ear canal, once it is killed and the eardrum is deemed intact, removal can be effected by irrigation or by grasping with micro alligator forceps as previously described. If the insect is large and is totally impacted in the ear canal, removal under general anesthetic with microinstruments and microscope is the rule.

Following removal of the foreign object, antibiotic steroid ear drops in suspension form are instilled into the ear to prevent infection. If the eardrum has been perforated, the patient is advised to keep the ear dry and consult an otolaryngologist. Most traumatic eardrum perforations, if they involve less than 30 percent of the surface of the tympanic membrane, heal spontaneously.

FOREIGN BODY IN THE NOSE

If one finds a foreign body in the ear of a child, it pays to check the nose and perhaps even the other orifices for foreign body.

Children, out of curiosity, put things in their noses. If they cannot remove them, they become frightened and do not tell their parents. If someone observes the child in the act, immediate removal can be instituted. In most cases, however, the child presents with a unilateral foul-smelling nasal drainage. The alert examiner cleans the drainage and finds the offending object, which could be a variety of things, such as an eraser, piece of paper, plastic, wheels from a small toy, cotton, piece of rubber sponge, styrofoam, bean, seed, bead. If you can name it, it has been in the nose somehow, sometime.

There is no rush in removing a foreign body from the nose. Immediate care is most often necessary for the person or parent who discovers the foreign body, not the patient.

As with foreign bodies of the ear, removal is best accomplished with adequate lighting, as previously described. It is necessary to anesthetize and shrink the nasal lining, and for this I prefer 5 percent cocaine and equal parts of 0.25 percent Neo-Synephrine. Five drops of this combination instilled into the nostril is enough in most cases. It is instilled into the nostril with the patient recumbent and the nostril pointing upward. I have yet to subject a child to general anesthesia to remove a foreign body in the nose. With a little talk and play these children cooperate enough to remove the foreign body without inflicting trauma on the nasal lining.

A nasal speculum is indispensable for good visualization. The foreign body is grasped and pulled out with an alligator forceps or a thumb forceps. If a circular object, like a bead, is stuck in the nose, it can be sucked out with a finger-controlled No. 10 Frazier or brain suction with a piece of rubber tubing attached to its end.

FOREIGN BODY IN THE OROPHARYNX

The oropharynx is bounded above by the soft palate and below by the tip of the epiglottis.

The most common foreign body found in the oropharynx is a fish bone. Any other foreign object with the shape and pliancy of a fish bone, such as a piece of metal, plastic, or glass, can also be lodged there. The history is typical and simple. Someone eating fish feels something caught in his throat, and the sensation persists even after he gulps water and swallows hard bread. The examiner should ask the patient to point to the area where he feels the foreign body and concentrate there during the examination. The tongue is depressed with a curved metal tongue blade. If the foreign body is stuck to the faucial tonsil, one can easily see it and remove it with grasping forceps (e.g., bayonet or alligator type). In a patient who gags readily, it is necessary to anesthetize the throat with either Cetacaine spray or 5 percent cocaine solution in an atomizer or with a Xylocaine topical solution. Occasionally, 5 mg of Valium given by intravenous push may sedate the gag reflex.

A common mistake in examining the oropharynx is to ask the patient to put out his tongue. This obstructs the examiner's vision. The tongue should be in its relaxed anatomic position. Another important point is to use a curved metal tongue depressor to keep the depressing hand out of the line of vision.

If the fish bone is in the lingual tonsil, visualization is accomplished indirectly with a laryngeal mirror. Topical anesthetic with the previously mentioned agents is essential. The patient is asked to hold his tongue out, and it is wrapped with a gauze sponge. The examiner introduces the laryngeal mirror with one hand and grasps and removes the foreign body with curved Kelly forceps with the other hand.

Once in a while, the foreign body is not localized with the above maneuver. Occasionally, oropharyngeal abrasions may cause a persistent foreign body sensation, but this should not last long. If the patient continues to complain of a sensation of foreign body after 12 to 24 hours, the physician is absolutely obligated to perform an examination and remove the object under general anesthesia. This can be done on an outpatient basis. Failure to do this may result in life-threatening mediastinal infection. X-ray film studies generally are not useful if the foreign body cannot be seen on direct examination.

INFECTION OF THE HEAD AND NECK

BARRY H. HENDLER, D.D.S., M.D.
JAMES T. AMSTERDAM, D.M.D., M.D.

The complexities of the maxillofacial area and its proximity to the central nervous system, airway, and thorax mandate a clear understanding of infections occurring in this region. Spread of infection from this region throughout the head and neck may have devastating local and/or systemic effects.

The most common focus of infection is odontogenic. An overwhelming percentage of head and neck infections are bacterial in origin.

DIFFERENTIAL DIAGNOSIS

A number of other conditions can cause facial swelling. Tumors may initially present as routine head and neck infections because they can become secondarily infected and drain pus. Viral infections rarely cause facial swelling, but occasionally infections such as actinomycosis or tuberculous lymphadenitis (scrofula) occur. These may cause secondary infections that may initially appear to be bacterial; therefore, appropriate cultures must be obtained.

A patient with head and neck swelling may also have submaxillary or parotid gland disease. Such patients often have a history of increasing pain and swelling when they eat. Submandibular gland infections are usually caused by streptococci and blockage by stones; most parotid gland infections are caused by Staphylococcus. Diabetics, too, can have parotid swelling, but it is usually bilateral and unaccompanied by leukocytosis or fever. Additionally, there are autoimmune phenomena, such as Sjögren's syndrome and Mikulicz's disease, that can cause facial swelling associated with the salivary glands.

Mucormycosis is among the most frequently fatal fungal infections, particularly in severe diabetics. Forty percent of reported cases demonstrated ophthalmologic or rhinologic findings. Phycomycetous fungi are the cause. There are four forms of the disease: rhinocerebral, pulmonary, alimentary, and disseminated. The organism is believed to enter the nose and paranasal sinuses by inhalation. It sporulates in tissues that have lost their natural resistance to fungi, particularly when bacterial ecology has been changed by antibiotic therapy. The diagnosis is best made by an appropriate biopsy or tissue scraping and a high index of suspicion. The only treatment is wide surgical resection of all devitalized tissues and the intravenous administration of amphotericin B.

Actinomycosis is a fungal infection caused by *Actinomyces israelii*, usually after injury; it is characterized by formation of multiple fistulas. The most frequently involved region is the cervical area. Primary actinomycosis has been reported in the lacrimal gland, orbit, tongue, hypopharynx, larynx, and parotid gland. Clinically, patients have an indurated swelling located near the mandible. The infection burrows extensively, forming deep abscesses, and drainage develops through multiple sinuses. The discharge contains diagnostic "sulfur granules." Treatment should include high doses of penicillin administered for as long as 6 months.

FASCIAL PLANES OF THE HEAD AND NECK

Cellulitis of odontogenic origin, including maxillary teeth, involves the mid and lower half of the face and neck owing to lymphatic and dependent drainage patterns. In the nondebilitated host, most untreated infections tend to localize and drain spontaneously. If a particularly virulent strain of microorganism is involved or host defenses are compromised, infections rapidly spread with potentially lethal morbidity.

Treatment is based on an attempt by the emergency physician or the oral and maxillofacial surgeon to compartmentalize the spread of infection. The head and neck are divided into fascial spaces, which are potential spaces normally filled with loose areolar tissue that readily breaks down when invaded by infection.

In therapy, knowing the compartment involved helps to determine whether incision and drainage procedures should be done inside the mouth or externally on the neck or facial area. Compartmentalization can also be invaluable in determining an infections's potential morbidity, such as the likelihood of upper airway obstruction and mediastinitis.

The deep cervical fascia lies beneath the platysma muscle and runs from the clavicle and sternum to the inferior border of the mandible and zygomatic arch, mastoid process, and superior nuchal line of the occipital bone. Anteriorly, it is attached to the symphysis menti and the hyoid bone and posteriorly to the ligamentum nuchae and the spine of the seventh cervical vertebra. It thickens in three areas: the pretracheal fascia in front of the trachea; the prevertebral fascia in front of the vertebrae; and the carotid sheath, which surrounds the carotid artery, vagus nerve, and jugular vein. The masticator space—so called because it invests the muscles of mastication—is formed where the deep cervical fascia attaches to the inferior border of the mandible, splitting laterally and medially around both ascending rami, enclosing the parotid gland, the masseter muscle, and the internal pterygoid muscle. Above the zygomatic arch, some authors further divide the masticator space into superficial and deep temporal pouches.

The deeply situated parapharyngeal space lies medial to the masticator space and lateral to the pharynx. It extends from the base of the skull to the level of the hyoid bone and is bounded medially by the superior constrictor of the pharynx, laterally by the mandible and internal pterygoid muscle, superiorly by the petrous portion of the temporal bone, and inferiorly by the submandibular gland and the posterior belly of the digastric muscle.

Any infection that resides in the masticator space has the potential for moving superiorly into the superficial and deep temporal pouches and medially into the parapharyngeal space (Fig. 1). Once infection involves the parapharyngeal space, it poses an immediate danger of upper airway obstruction and mediastinal descent.

DIAGNOSIS AND THERAPY

Pre-hospital Phase

Pre-hospital management consists of airway management, establishment of an intravenous line, and supportive therapy. Patients generally prefer to sit upright in a semi-Fowler position or with the head forward. Visualization of the oropharynx should be attempted to exclude the possibility of gross airway obstruction from the tongue or secretions. No tongue blades should be used in this setting as laryngospasm may be precipitated.

A soft nasopharyngeal airway may be helpful. Intubation may be required if the patient develops significant airway compromise; a nasotracheal technique is preferred.

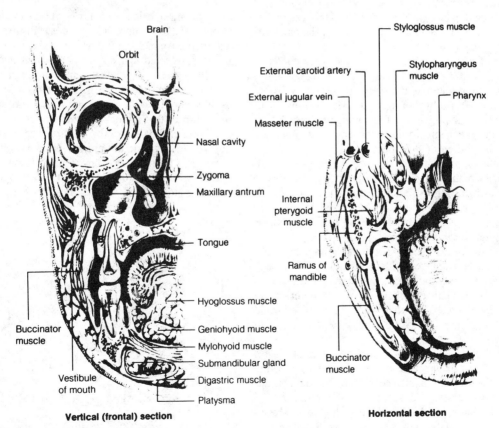

Vertical (frontal) section

Horizontal section

Figure 1 Pathways of infection. The pathways by which such infections travel are the postzygomatic (from the canine fossa in the cuspid and bicuspid region); vestibular; facial; submandibular; sublingual; palatal; antral; pterygomandibular; parapharyngeal; and masticator. (From Rose LF, Hendler BH, Amsterdam JT. Temporomandibular disorders and odontic infections. Consultant 1982; 22:125.)

Aside from the usual complications of intubation, an additional complication of rupture of an abscess with aspiration is possible. Therefore, if possible, intubation should be performed in a more controlled environment. If intubation cannot be performed successfully, a needle or complete cricothyrotomy is necessary in the emergency setting.

The First 8 Hours

Depending on the compartment in which the infection resides and the extent of its progress, a patient with head and neck infection may require only primary antibiotic therapy, or antibiotic therapy and adjunctive incision and drainage procedures on an outpatient basis. Treatment varies because there is a progression of swelling attributable to bacterial contamination that can best be thought of as the stages of early-to-late cellulitis, and the effectiveness of antibiotic therapy changes throughout these stages.

An oral examination is imperative to check for swelling of the oropharynx and elevation of the tongue, both of which can cause upper airway obstruction. If the oropharynx cannot be visualized, hospitalization is mandatory. The next step is to determine whether an infection is fluctuant.

In the early stages of cellulitis, most patients run fevers of about 101° F with a leukocytosis of 10,000 to 15,000 cells. The swelling is usually soft, warm, and red. Antibiotics tend to be extremely effective at this stage because of increased vascular permeability in the early inflammatory reaction.

Antibiotic therapy is much less effective in the later stages of cellulitis. As the infection progresses, the tissue becomes indurated as the body attempts to wall off the infection from further spread. This, along with decreased blood supply to the area owing to compression of the tissue, mechanically impedes antibiotics from arriving at the source of the infection.

Eventually, liquefaction necrosis takes place leading to the formation of pus. Since the body attempts to eliminate pus as soon as possible, it moves along a path of least resistance through either bone or tissue until eventually the pus makes its exit internally in the mouth or externally on the face or neck.

One of the first clinical signs that this stage has been reached is the appearance of fluctuance. In head and neck infections, especially those attributable to an intraoral focus, intraoral fluctuance is characterized by reverse curvature of the mucolabial or mucobuccal gutters. External or facial fluctuance shows a skin surface that is stretched and shiny.

In later stages of cellulitis, there is often at least a temporary drop in the patient's temperature and white count. By the time the fluctuance appears, antibiotics cannot usually penetrate the dense tissue or eliminate all the thick pus that has formed unless there are high tissue blood levels that are usually achieved parenterally. There is quicker and more complete resolution of infection if antibiotic therapy is combined with surgical evacuation of pus.

Culture of the pus is important before therapy is initiated; the best way is by fine-needle aspiration. In an external incision and drainage procedure, the pus can be cultured directly with a swab. Intraorally, contamination often occurs. For a diagnostic culture, prepare the skin and directly insert the needle into the infected space. If the cavity that is entered is large and filled with pus, the best culture is obtained and need for incision and drainage is confirmed.

Although antibiotic therapy and incision and drainage procedures may resolve the patient's immediate problem of facial swelling, long-term treatment requires establishment of the etiology of the infection. Usually, facial films, especially a panoramic view, are adequate to evaluate any intraoral or perioral focus of infection. A lateral view of the neck may also be helpful on occasion.

It is axiomatic that one should *not* focus on facial infection and distortion and forget about other systemic infectious foci. Before starting antibiotics, one should obtain blood cultures (aerobic and anaerobic), a CBC and differential, urinalysis, electrolytes, and a rectal temperature. Chest roentgenograms are imperative along with computed tomography (CT) scan of the head, neck, and mediastinum whenever there is a potential for mediastinal descent of infection or for upper airway obstruction.

Incision and Drainage

The anesthesia for an intraoral incision and drainage is provided by a superficial mucosal infiltration of local anesthetic. An incision is then directed through the mucosa into the infected space (Fig. 2). When needed, drains should be placed dependently and consist of a 2-inch strip of quarter-inch iodoform gauze or a half-inch Penrose drain secured with a single suture. Drains should be removed in 24 to 48 hours and the area copiously irrigated at least once a day until the incision site closes spontaneously. Although the initial incision and drainage may be performed in the emergency unit, follow-up by the oral and maxillofacial surgeon should be arranged. Most infections show initial resolution in 48 hours.

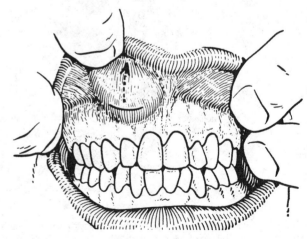

Figure 2 Intraoral incision for labial space infection showing dependency for drainage and pathway of blunt dissection.

When incision and drainage procedures are performed externally, aesthetics are an additional concern. Since the skin that shows fluctuance is devoid of subcutaneous fat, placing a blade in the center of the fluctuant area causes the skin to collapse and results in invagination of the skin and a poor scar on healing. If the incision is made about 1 or 2 cm below the area of fluctuance and blunt dissection is carried upward with a small hemostat, an aesthetically acceptable scar is created.

Antibiotic Therapy

Patients with severe stages of cellulitis normally require aqueous penicillin in doses of 15 to 20 million units a day IV. Penicillin is bactericidal and effective against most of the common causative organisms: *streptococcus* A,B, and *viridans*; anaerobic streptococci, particularly microaerophilic *Streptococcus*; and oropharyngeal strains of *Bacteroides*. Although a relative increase in resistance to penicillin among certain oral *Bacteroides* species has been reported, it has not yet proved to be much of a problem. Anaerobic organisms such as Vincent's organisms are also adequately treated by penicillin. Staphylococcus is not usually a strong contaminant in head and neck infections, although it is occasionally present.

Other antibiotics provide reasonable alternatives. The cephalosporins are excellent alternatives for the penicillin-allergic patient in doses of 1 or 2 g IM or IV every 6 hours. Moreover, cephalosporins have antistaphylococcal activity.

If a patient has an anaerobic infection owing primarily to *Bacteroides*, clindamycin, 600 to 900 mg IM or IV every 8 hours, is the treatment of choice. Patients should be monitored for drug-related side effects. Chloramphenicol, although highly effective against obligate anaerobes, is potentially toxic and should be reserved for situations in which the pathogenic role of *B. fragilis* is of prime importance or for patients who are allergic to penicillin, cephalosporins, or clindamycin.

Erythromycin is generally active against most indigenous oral bacteria, but is comparatively less active than penicillin. Its limited parenteral use makes it unsuitable for patients with severe infections. Ampicillin is another alternative, but it does not have the same clinical effectiveness as penicillin. Carbenicillin and ticarcillin appear to be promising agents for mixed orofacial infections, although clinical experience with them is still limited.

Major Infections: Inpatient Therapy

Infection, particularly in the lower molar teeth, commonly invades the area between the internal pterygoid and the masseter muscles and most often presents as swelling at the angle of the mandible, usually accompanied by external fluctuance.

Patients with these masticator space infections often run low-grade fevers in the range of 100 to 102° F and white cell counts of 12,000 to 20,000. The characteristic feature is trismus (Fig. 3) because the muscles that open and close the jaw are essentially frozen by infection. Trismus, pain, and swelling usually develop within a few hours of the abrupt onset of infection and reach a peak in 3 to 5 days.

It is essential to look into the mouth to see whether the parapharyngeal wall is swollen toward the midline, indicating spread to the parapharyngeal space. Trismus often makes this difficult, and so most patients should be admitted to the hospital. Most masticator space infections need to be drained externally in the region of the angle of the mandible to achieve complete drainage.

A parapharyngeal space infection usually obliterates not only the angle of the mandible, but any indentation normally present below the ear to the midpoint of the neck (Fig. 4). Once the infection descends into the neck, it cannot be drained intraorally; a submandibular incision anterior to the sternocleidomastoid muscle is needed.

Because of the danger of upper airway obstruction and mediastinitis, all patients with suspected parapharyngeal space infections should be admitted for a complete diagnostic work-up and treatment. Airway precautions such as aspirators, endotracheal tubes, and tracheostomy sets at bedside should be maintained in an environment in which the patient can be observed closely. The patient should be kept in a semi-Fowler position so that

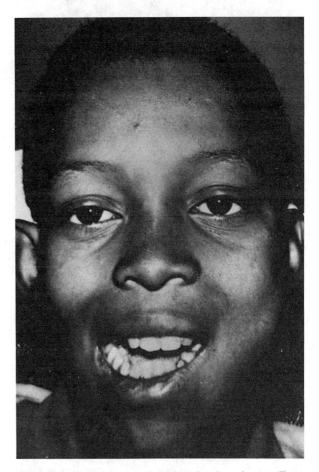

Figure 3 Masticator space infection showing trismus. (From Hendler BH, Amsterdam JT. Infection of dental origin. Curr Top Emerg Med 1981; 2:1. By permission.)

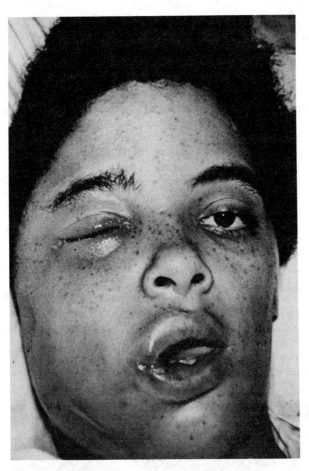

Figure 4 Combined fascial space infection involving the masticator, parapharyngeal, and temporal spaces.

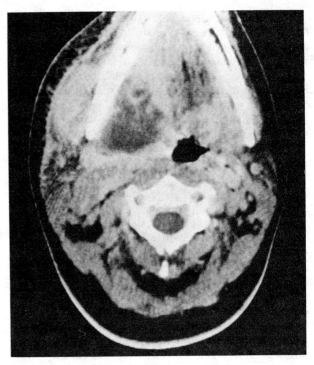

Figure 5 CT scan showing abscess cavity medial to the angle of the mandible. Note constriction of airway and massive swelling of the masseter muscle.

oropharyngeal secretions can be evacuated. Obtaining arterial blood gases ensures that no compromise of the airway goes unnoticed. Once appropriate cultures have been obtained, monitoring of the patient and antibiotic therapy are started, as already described.

In a significant percentage of patients with parapharyngeal space infection, the infection descends into the mediastinum. The best diagnostic test is a CT scan of the neck and mediastinum (Fig.5). Lateral neck films are sometimes helpful, but often equivocal. Mortality and morbidity are high.

An entity that is often confused with parapharyngeal space infection is *Ludwig's angina*. Ludwig's angina is a bilateral boardlike swelling involving the submandibular, submental, and sublingual spaces accompanied by elevation of the tongue. The upper airway obstruction that often accompanies Ludwig's angina is largely attributable to this elevation, which pushes the tongue against the posterior pharyngeal wall.

Ludwig's angina is usually secondary to infection of the lower second and third molars, the predominant organisms being hemolytic streptococci, staphylococci, or combined aerobes and anaerobes. Ludwig's angina is much less rapid in progression than paraphyaryngeal space infection. It commonly begins as a unilateral swelling and progresses across the midline over a period of 5 to 7 days. The swelling is not associated with intense pain, and so the patient delays seeking care. Fever of about 101° F, chills, difficulty in swallowing, stiffness of tongue movements, and trismus are commonly present. As the tongue becomes increasingly elevated, respiration becomes difficult since the oropharynx becomes occluded. The larynx may also become edematous. Airway obstruction and mediastinitis may ensue.

Recently, some physicians have recommended combined antibiotic therapy or high-dose intravenous, penicillin rather than surgical treatment. Although many patients with Ludwig's angina respond to antibiotic therapy alone, a certain percentage still require incision and drainage procedures. If a patient does not respond to antibiotic therapy within a short time, it is best to go ahead with incision and drainage procedures even if there is incomplete clinical evidence that pus is present. Such procedures are performed in the operating room under general anesthesia.

SUGGESTED READING

Amsterdam JT, Hendler BH, Rose LF. Emergency dental procedures. In: Roberts J, Hedges J, eds. Clinical procedures in emergency medicine. Philadelphia: W.B. Saunders, 1985:946.

Hendler BH, Amsterdam JT. Infection of dental origin. Curr Top Emerg Med 1981; 2:1.

Osbon DB. Facial trauma. In: Irby WB ed. Current advances in oral surgery. St. Louis: C.V. Mosby, 1965: 214–241.

Rose LF, Hendler BH, Amsterdam JT. Temporomandibular disorders and odontic infections. Consultant 1982; 22:110-117.

EPISTAXIS

FRANK I. MARLOWE, M.D.

With the exception of menstrual bleeding, epistaxis or nosebleed is the most common type of spontaneous hemorrhage. The most common cause is spontaneous erosion of one of the superficial mucosal blood vessels near the anterior end of the nasal septum (Fig. 1). There seems to be a "nosebleed season," especially in the elderly; it occurs in winter when poor hydration and poor humidification of living spaces (especially with forced air heat) produce mucosal drying and spontaneous bleeding. It is usually an isolated incident, but can be a presenting symptom of systemic disease. A brief but appropriate history may establish the underlying etiology or pathology (Table 1).

HISTORY

The patient should be questioned with regard to trauma, whether major trauma sufficient to cause a fracture of the nasal bones (usually obvious) or minor trauma such as nose picking or excessive blowing. It is also use-

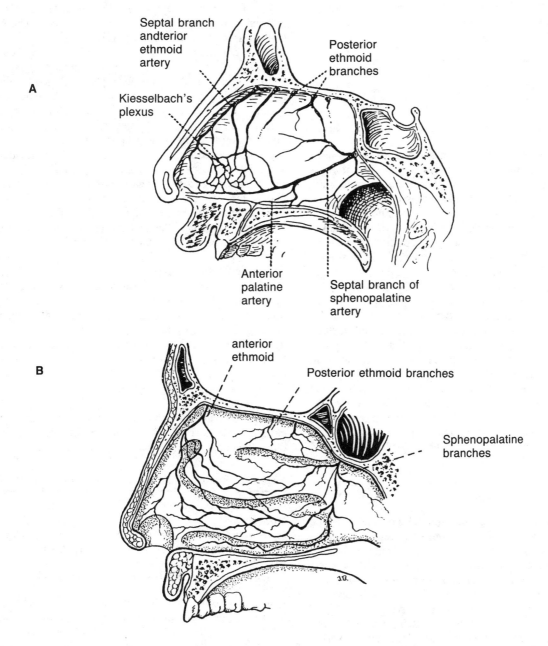

Figure 1 A, Blood supply of septal and B, lateral wall and turbinates of the nose. (From DeWeese DD, Saunders WH. Textbook of otolaryngology. 6th ed. St. Louis: CV Mosby, 1982.)

TABLE 1 Evaluation of the Patient with Epistaxis

History

Easy bleeding or bruisability
Family history
History of trauma or surgery
History of anemia (possibly due to blood loss)
Medications (anticoagulants, aspirin)

Physical examination

Location of site using proper light, suction, and anesthesia;
may not be possible in case of deviated nasal septum.

Laboratory tests

Screen
Prothrombin time (PT)
Partial thromboplastin time (PTT)
Hematocrit
Platelet count
Detail
Specific factor assay

Other measures

Angiography
Hematologic consultation

---

ful to inquire about previous nasal surgery or previous nosebleeds that required cauterization. The line of questioning should pertain to a possible bleeding disorder, that is, whether the patient recalls excessive bleeding from minor cuts or excessive bruising from minor bumps. A history of drug ingestion such as excessive aspirin intake, anticoagulant therapy, or chemotherapy must be sought, especially in older individuals, and possible substance abuse, such as cocaine use, in younger individuals. Despite arguments to the contrary in the literature, clinical evidence points to a higher incidence of epistaxis in the hypertensive population than in the normal population. In the elderly, hypertensive, and possibly arteriosclerotic patient, epistaxis, more particularly posterior epistaxis, is common. Nosebleed also may be noted in bleeding disorders such as hereditary hemorrhagic telangiectasis (Osler-Weber-Rendu syndrome), idiopathic thrombocytopenia, or some of the leukemias. Finally, nosebleed can occur as a result of a neoplasm of the nasal cavity, nasopharynx, or paranasal sinuses, usually preceded by purulent nasal drainage or localized pain and swelling.

EXAMINATION

Emergency treatment of "simple" nosebleed may be carried out by the patient and consists of remaining in the upright position with nose "pinched" shut for 5 to 10 minutes by the clock, with the soft side walls of the nasal alae exerting firm pressure on the nasal septum. Many nosebleeds can be terminated at home in this fashion. Other home treatments are not effective.

Patients whose epistaxis persists and brings them to emergency care are often anxious. They require verbal reassurance and sometimes judicious use of sedatives such as diazepam, although care must be taken to avoid induc-

ing respiratory depression. Once it has been determined that the patient's vital signs are stable and there is no imminent danger of shock, and an intravenous route of access has been established, examination may be undertaken with the patient in a comfortable, upright position with the head bent forward so as to allow blood to drain from the nose and not down the pharynx.

Satisfactory examination requires the use of special equipment including an adequate source of coaxial light to leave the examiner's hands free for manipulation. A set of "helping hands" is often indispensable (Table 2).

Spontaneous nasal hemorrhage arises from three major areas:

1. The anterior septal area, known as Little's area, is the site in approximately 90 percent of cases and contains a vascular network known as Kiesselbach's plexus. Bleeding commonly arises from a prominent vessel at the mucocutaneous junction or in the mid-anterior septum, and this area should always be inspected first. Bleeding in the septal area may also occur from the sharp edge or "spur" of a deviated nasal septum or from a nasal septal perforation, one of the few causes of true bilateral bleeding. Arising from the thin, friable mucosa covering the edges of the perforation, the source usually is obvious, and treatment consists of cautery or packing.

2. Bleeding from the anterior ethmoidal artery area may be intermittent and profuse, and the patient may actually volunteer that he can feel the onset of the bleeding and point externally to the medial canthus area. The bleeding point can rarely be visualized, and combined anterior-posterior packing is usually required with arterial ligation reserved for refractory cases.

3. Posterior epistaxis occasionally presents as bleeding into the pharynx only; however, it most commonly presents as combined anterior bleeding and pharyngeal bleeding. The precise site of bleeding is extremely difficult to visualize, and once the general site of bleeding is determined, packing and/or arterial ligation is almost always required.

TREATMENT

The general approach to anterior epistaxis begins with cleansing the nose of all accumulated blood, including clots. The patient may blow his nose to expel the clots,

TABLE 2 Equipment Needed for Examination in Epistaxis

Light source (head mirror or head light)

Nasal speculum

Suction with Frazier nasal tip (not a nasal suction catheter with tip and cover hole separated by 12 inches of limp tubing)

Bayonet forceps

Topical and local anesthesia (4% lidocaine with epinephrine; 2–4% cocaine)

Cautery source (silver nitrate, chromic acid, or electrocautery)

Nasal packing (petrolatum gauze, ½ inch × 72 inches, adaptic gauze, ½ inch × 4 yards, or ribbon gauze, ½ inch, impregnated with antibiotic ointment)

Assistant

and the remainder may be removed by suction. On occasion this reactivates bleeding, and the source can be more easily identified and controlled directly. The nasal mucosa may then be anesthetized and decongested using a maximum of 2 cc of 10 percent cocaine or 5 cc of 4 percent cocaine solution in a spray nebulizer or on cotton pledgets or gauze strips. Cocaine is both an excellent topical anesthetic and a powerful vasoconstrictor, and therefore use of the one agent accomplishes both goals. Since record-keeping and storage is a problem with this material, combinations of 4 percent topical lidocaine with epinephrine solution may provide a satisfactory alternative. The interior of the nasal cavity is then carefully examined using appropriate light, speculum, and suction, and if the bleeding site is identified and easily accessible, it may be cauterized with chemical agents (silver nitrate or chromic acid beads) or electrocoagulation using a suitable electrosurgical unit. When bleeding is controlled, inspect the remainder of the nasal cavity to rule out the possibility of another lesion such as a neoplasm. Light nasal packing or a topical lubricant ointment such as Cortisporin may be used to protect the cauterized area from airflow desiccation and promote healing. It is also acceptable to use a small pledget of hemostatic material (Gelfoam, Surgicel) to protect the bleeding site, but is is not advisable to fill the nasal cavity with these materials as they are difficult to remove should rebleeding occur.

Although methods such as injection of the greater palatine foramen with Xylocaine or other substances have been suggested as a way to stop bleeding, the benefit is temporary, the complications are significant, and the technique is difficult. This procedure is best left to the specialist.

When an anterior source of bleeding cannot be identified or is noted to be in an inaccessible position, or when the bleeding is determined to be posterior, a *posterior pack* has to be placed, and additional items are required, including rubber or polyethylene catheters (10 or 12 F), grasping forceps such as hemostats, preferably a metal tongue depressor, and a posterior pack of appropriate configuration. The most easily employed posterior packs are the commercially available pneumatic or hydrostatic balloon devices available from numerous manufacturers. These are specially designed devices for insertion into the nasal vault with balloons that are then inflated with air or fluid to maintain pressure against the nasal mucosal areas and to retain the balloon in place. A commonly employed alternative to this is use of a Foley catheter, which is placed into the nasopharynx through the nasal cavity, inflated so as to impact in the posterior aperture of the nose (the choana), and used as a buttress against which to place an anterior gauze pack. Securing of the Foley catheter is critical and requires careful cushioning of the Hoffman or "C" clamp used, so that no metal comes in contact with the nostril margins, as alar necrosis can occur in as little as a few hours, and a permanent deformity is a distinct possibility. The patient with an anterior pack needs follow-up and pack removal in 2 to 3 days. Since in most cases the pack prevents adequate sinus drainage, prophylactic antibiotics such as a cephalosporin are often given.

Placement of a posterior gauze pack requires fashioning an appropriate pack from a rolled 4 × 4 gauze sponge. Three strings of heavy suture material such as No. 2 black silk or umbilical tape are secured to the sponge, and it is inserted as follows: a rubber or flexible polyvinyl catheter, 10 to 12 F, is passed through the nostril on the bleeding side until it becomes visible in the oropharynx. It is grasped through the mouth with a clamp and brought out through the mouth so that now the tip of the catheter lies outside the mouth and the end of the catheter lies just outside the nostril. Two of the strings of the pack are tied to the tip of the catheter, and the catheter is withdrawn through the nose, bringing the strings of the pack retrograde into the mouth, behind the palate, and out through the nasal passage to be grasped outside the nostril. It is important that the strings be long enough to be easily retrieved without dragging the packing into the mouth at this point. The patient is instructed to open his mouth wide and breathe through the mouth while the operator simultaneously pulls on the nasal strings and guides the pack into the mouth and up behind the palate. Tension is maintained on the strings, and the pack lodges firmly in the posterior choana. The uvula should be hanging free in the posterior pharynx, and an appropriate nasal packing of lubricated ribbon gauze is inserted through the nostril. The strings are finally tied over a gauze roll or a dental cotton roll at the nostril opening. The third string that exits from the mouth, is taped to the cheek and is used to facilitate later removal of the packing from the nasopharynx and mouth. This type of pack is easily modified to provide bilateral posterior packing by withdrawing one string from each nostril using two catheters rather than both strings through the same nostril. Following this procedure, bilateral anterior nasal packing is placed.

With the bleeding controlled, attention must be directed to *further supportive care*, which, in the case of a minor bleed that was easily controlled without resort to packing, might consist of only screening tests to rule out serious coagulation defects. Most commonly, this would consist of complete blood chemistry, prothrombin time (PT), partial thromboplastin time (PTT), bleeding time, and platelet count. If vigorous bleeding was noted and/or control of the bleeding was difficult, hospital admission for further supportive care, especially in the elderly individual, is probably advisable, and admission studies would include electrocardiogram (ECG) and appropriate blood chemistries for hepatic or renal disease. Appropriate consultation for hypertension or diabetes would be obtained, and possibly x-ray films of the paranasal sinuses to rule out a possible neoplastic lesion or to serve as a prelude to trans-sinus arterial ligations, which might become necessary. Hematologic consultation and specific factor assay are indicted if screening tests are abnormal. Local measures such as cautery and packing, although occasionally employed in epistaxis owing to coagulation defects as a last resort, may well aggravate the situation, and primary treatment must be directed toward correction of the clotting defect with specific blood factors or fresh plasma.

Otolaryngologic consultation should be obtained in all patients who require a posterior pack. In general, hospital admission, intravenous fluids, bed rest, sedation, and appropriate narcotic analgesics are required because posterior nasal packing is uncomfortable and makes eating, sleeping, and breathing difficult. Particularly in older individuals, reflex pulmonary changes result in hypoxemia of dangerous degrees, and the packs may have to be removed and arterial ligation performed. Humidified oxygen should be administered, and if any question with regard to oxygenation occurs, arterial blood gas studies should be obtained. Since sinusitis and otitis media are almost universal complications of this treatment, antibiotic therapy is usually instituted at the time of pack placement, and although penicilln and erythromycin were once widely used, it is more common to employ the cephalosporin antibiotics at this time owing to their broader coverage and fewer problems with resistant organisms. If brisk bleeding was noted initially, or if the patient has sustained significant blood loss as evidenced by a drop in hematocrit, or if further bleeding is anticipated, the patient's blood should be typed and crossmatched for several units of blood. Packing is usually left in place for 2 to 3 days to allow formation of a stable clot that is unlikely to be lost owing to the effect of thrombolytic enzyme activity.

An extensive discussion of the operative treatment of epistaxis is beyond the scope of this paper. Suffice it to say that the procedure involves ligating the closest feeding vessels. The closer the ligation to the bleeding site, the better its chance of establishing definitive control, as there is less chance of continued bleeding from retrograde flow and anastomotic flow, which is not uncommon in the nasal area owing to its diffuse and extensive blood supply. This ligation most commonly involves the anterior ethmoidal artery, which is approached through a small incision in the area of the medial canthus, and the internal maxillary artery and its branches, which are approached through an incision in the gingiva, traversing the maxillary sinus to obtain access to the pterygopalatine fossa. Although ligation of the external carotid artery in the neck is technically easier and more direct, its distance from the nasal bleeding site makes it much more prone to failure. Following satisfactory ligation, which is usually done under general anesthesia, utilizing the operating microscope and hemostatic clips, the nasal packs are removed immediately, and in most cases the patient may be discharged from the hospital the following day or the day thereafter.

Patients who require nasal packing to control epistaxis should be re-evaluated in 3 to 4 weeks to ensure proper healing of areas of mucosa subjected to cautery or damaged by pressure from the packing. This also allows a further chance to rule out the possibility of any nasal tumor or ongoing nasal or sinus infection.

SUGGESTED READING

DeWeese DD, Saunders WH, eds. Nosebleed. In: Textbook of otolaryngology. St Louis: CV Mosby, 1982.

Rosnagle R. Epistaxis. In: English GM, ed. Otolaryngology. Philadelphia: Harper and Row, 1978.

Saunders WH. Epistaxis. In: Paparella MM, Shumrick DA, eds. Otolaryngology. Philadelphia: WB Saunders, 1980.

OTITIS AND MASTOIDITIS

DANIEL SOOY, M.D.

ACUTE OTITIS MEDIA

Acute otitis media (AOM) is the most common localized infection in children, accounting for most acute visits to the pediatrician. Seventy to eighty percent of all children have one episode before school age, and in the pre-antibiotic era AOM was responsible for most cases of meningitis.

AOM is defined as an infectious process of the middle ear cavity and is usually secondary to an upper respiratory infection. The cause is believed to be an obstruction of the eustachian tube. Normally the eustachian tube opens and closes with swallowing or yawning, admitting a small amount of air into the middle ear cleft. The air is then reabsorbed by the blood vessels in the lamina propria of the mucosa. Unless there is periodic opening and closing of the eustachian tube, the resorbtive process creates a negative pressure. Viral infections or allergies cause swelling of the mucosa and a relative obstruction when the reabsorption of air occurs. This is followed by retraction of the tympanic membrane with reduced mobility. As the negative pressure increases, a transudate from the blood fills the middle ear (serous otitis media), and secondary infection by direct extension of bacteria from the nasopharynx results in purulent otitis media.

Diagnosis

Most AOM occurs between birth and the age of 6 years, though infection in adults is not uncommon. In children as well as adults, fever, pain, and hearing loss are the major symptoms. Small children frequently pull at their ears; however, this is not always a reliable sign of infection. Any history of previously treated bouts of otitis media as well as allergy, immunologic abnormalities, and structural abnormalities predisposing to ear infections, such as cleft palate, should be elicited.

Initially otoscopic examination usually shows hyperemic vessels along the handle of the malleus with a retracted drum, decreased mobility, and a slight conductive hearing loss. As infection progresses, the entire drum becomes hyperemic and bulging. There is loss of normal landmarks, a marked conductive hearing loss, and pain. If this process goes unchecked, there is often a spontaneous rupture of the drum with blood-tinged pus flowing from the ear and relief of pain.

In the differential diagnosis of acute ear pain, one needs to consider other causes. Pain on motion of the auricle or tragus suggests external otitis (Figure 1 and Table 1). Bullous myringitis consists of blisters containing clear or hemorrhagic fluid on the tympanic membrane. When the pain is more gradual in onset or associated with pharyngeal pain or there is a normal otoscopic examination, a complete head and neck examination is indicated to rule out referred pain secondary to tumors or infections of the pharynx or larynx.

Treatment

Pure viral otitis does occur, but a secondary bacterial otitis is the more common clinical problem. The typical causative organisms of acute otitis are beta-hemolytic *Streptococcus*, *Streptococcus pneumoniae*, and *Haemophilus influenzae*. The role of *Staphylococcus aureus* in AOM is debated; *Branhamella catarrhalis* is becoming more common, reaching perhaps one in ten infections. Some strains of *H. influenzae*, *B. catarrhalis*, and *S. aureus* produce beta-lactamase. This is an important clinical consideration because these organisms can be resistant to penicillin and ampicillin. Gram-negative bacteria like *Escherichia coli* are more common in the neonate, the immunosuppressed, and patients with chronic otitis media. *H. influenzae* is more common in the under-5 age group but does also occur in older age groups. Antibiotic treatment (Table 2) should be aimed at the specific organisms and continued for a period of 10 to 14 days.

Ideally, antibiotics are selected by culture. This can be obtained from aural drainage or by tympanocentesis (see Table 2). This may not be possible in the busy emergency department and may be best left to the consultant. Initiating antibiotics on an empiric basis is frequently necessary. Amoxicillin or ampicillin covers most *H. influenzae*; however there might be resistant *H. influenzae*, *S. aureus*, or *B. catarrhalis*. With patients who have failed to respond to previous treatment or in whom one

suspects a resistant organism, a drug with broad coverage like erythromycin-sulfisoxazole (Pediazole), cefaclor, or amoxicillin with Clavulanate (Augmentin) should be selected. If there is not significant clinical improvement within 48 hours, tympanocentesis with culture should be considered.

Decongestants are traditional and can be used, but they are controversial because several recent large studies have found them ineffective.

Myringotomy provides prompt and complete relief of pain in otitis media with a bulging eardrum (Table 3). It is best performed under optimal conditions of magnification and anesthesia to minimize the risk to ossicles and middle ear structures. Anesthesia can be achieved through a four-quadrant subcutaneous injection of the canal with 1 percent lidocaine using a 27-gauge needle. An alternative and very effective technique for anesthesia is to use iontophoresis to introduce a topical solution of epinephrine and lidocaine through the intact skin by electric charge.

In performing myringotomy, careful attention should be paid to the location of the incision, which should be in the anterior inferior quadrant. This can be assured by visualizing the long process of the malleus and dropping an imaginary line from that down to the annulas. The incision should be made in front of this line and in the lower portion of the drum. Great care must be taken not to make the incision in the posterior superior portion, because disruption of the ossicles could occur with permanent conductive hearing loss.

The fluid should then be aspirated from the middle ear sterilely if a culture is being taken. Because of the possibility of contamination from the external auditory canal, a culture should be obtained from the canal prior to myringotomy so that contaminating organisms can be identified.

Complications of otitis media result from the direct or hematologic spread of the infection to the structures that surround the middle ear. The extracranial complications of otitis media include mastoiditis, labrynthitis, and facial paralysis, so facial symmetry should be checked and noted. These complications should be treated with myringotomy, culture, and intravenous antibiotics.

Meningitis is the most common intracranial complication of AOM, with 80 percent of cases in children being of otologic origin. Brain abscess, extradural abscess, sigmoid sinus thrombosis, and petrositis with sixth-nerve paralysis also occur.

CHRONIC OTITIS MEDIA

Chronic otitis media is a term used to indicate a persistent or recurrent infection usually associated with perforation of the tympanic membrane. These patients often present with aural drainage, which may be purulent, mucoid, or foul smelling. Pain is infrequent. The exacerbations of chronic otitis media usually occur secondary to upper respiratory infections or water contamination of the middle ear. *S. aureus* or gram-negative bacteria are frequently the predominant organisms. When drainage is the primary complaint, these infections often respond

TABLE 1 Distinguishing Features of Otitis Media and Externa

	Otitis Media	*External Otitis*
Symptoms (in order of appearance)	Decreased hearing; pain; discharge	Pain; discharge; decreased hearing
History	Upper respiratory infection	Swimming
Examination	Ear canal open	Ear canal swollen
Ear movement	No pain	Painful
Discharge	Mucoid	Watery
Treatment	Antibiotics; decongestants; avoid water	Antibiotics; ear drops; avoid water

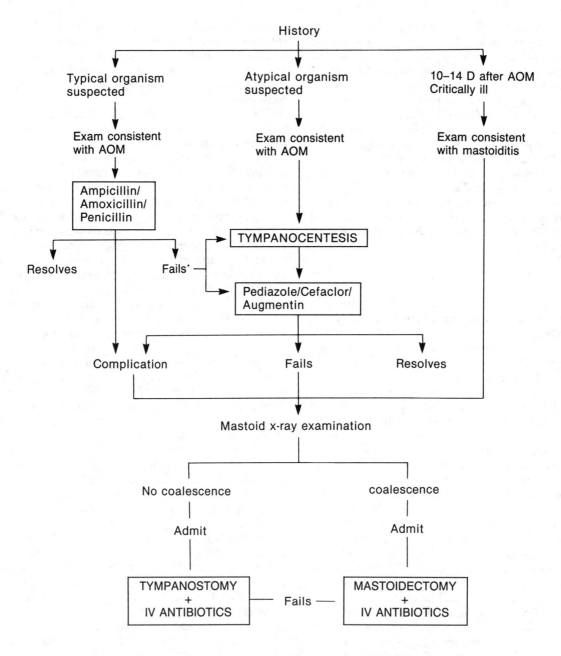

Figure 1 Treatment of acute otalgia.

* If toxic, consider both; if not, consider drug therapy.

to treatment with antibiotic drops alone. Follow-up with a specialist is important because there may be an underlying cholesteatoma.

OTITIS EXTERNA

Otitis externa (swimmer's ear) is the most common ear infection in adults. This infection starts initially as a dermatitis of the external auditory canal, which is typically infectious but may be allergic in nature. Allergic dermatitis may be due to a contact dermatitis from hair spray or due to seborrheic dermatitis; both respond nicely to 0.1 percent Triamcimlone (TAC) cream.

Infectious etiologies can be either fungal (most typically *Aspergillus*) or bacterial (typically staphylococci or *Pseudomonas aeruginosa*). Infectious otitis externa starts with entry of the pathogen through macerated skin secondary to prolonged water exposure or trauma to the external canal from cleaning. Clinically there is swelling, purulent discharge, and exquisite tenderness elicited by movement of the pinna. Hearing is normal, although with accumulation of debris, there may be a conductive hearing loss.

Treatment should consist of removing all bacterial, fungal, and squamous debris, followed by the application of topical medication. For fungal infection, clotrimazole

TABLE 2 Antimicrobial Therapy for Acute Otitis Media

Patient	Antimicrobial Agent	Dosage	Administration
Pediatric	Ampicillin	50 mg/kg/day	Divided doses q6h
	Amoxicillin	40 mg/kg/day	Divided doses q8h
	Erythromycin/	50 mg/kg/day‡	Divided doses q6h
	sulfisoxazole *†	150 mg/kg/day	
	Amoxicillin/potassium*		
	clavulanate	40 mg/kg/day	Divided doses q8h
	Cefaclor*†	40 mg/kg/day	Divided doses q8h
Adult	Penicillin	500 mg	Dose q6h
	Ampicillin	500 mg	Dose q6h
	Clavulanate potassium		
	(Augmentin)	500 mg	Dose q8h
	Cefaclor*†	500 mg	Dose q8h

* Atypical organisms expected
† Penicillin Allergic
§ Can be calculated on either erythromycin or sulfisoxazole dosage.

(Lotrimin) drops or Castellani's paint should be used. In bacterial infections, a combined steroid and antibiotic otic preparation like Cortisporin Otic or Pyocidin-Otic, is most effective. Should the drum not be visible because of swelling, it may be necessary to use a small cotton wick to conduct topical medication medially. Should there be any question as to whether there is concomitant otitis media, coverage with oral antibiotics should be added. The patient should be seen daily until the start of resolution.

Malignant external otitis is an invasive variant of otitis externa that occurs in diabetics and immunosuppressed patients. This is an aggressive and fulminant osteomyelitis of the base of the skull, secondary to infection with *P. aeruginosa*. Neuropathy of the seventh, ninth, tenth, and eleventh cranial nerves can occur and is the harbinger of a poor clinical course. On examination there is granulation tissue at the junction of the bony and cartilaginous canal or exposed bone. Immediate hospitalization and consultation with otolaryngology and infectious disease specialists is required.

MASTOIDITIS

Suppurative otitis media can extend to the mucosa of the mastoid air cell system owing to the close proximity of the middle ear to the mastoid. Usually when inflammation of the middle ear subsides under treatment, so does that in the mastoid.

Infection when untreated or insufficiently treated may smolder, leading to demineralization and necrosis of the bony septa (coalescence) of the mastoid bone. When un-

checked, the infectious process may escape into contiguous structures.

Diagnosis

The signs and symptoms of edema and pain over the mastoid may indicate spread of infection through the mastoid cortex. The tympanic membrane may be bulging with only moderate inflammation, or a draining perforation may be present. Additional findings might include sagging of the posterior superior portion of the external ear canal; lateral displacement of the ear, which is out and down (subperiostial abscess); and occasionally swelling over the mastoid tip (Bezold's abscess). The diagnosis is confirmed by x-ray films showing opacification of mastoid air cells and breakdown of their bony septae.

Treatment

Acute mastoiditis without radiographic evidence of coalescence can be treated by in-hospital tympanotomy and intravenous antibiotics. However, when radiologic evidence of coalescence is present, intravenous antibiotics and surgical drainage by mastoidectomy are indicated in order to prevent complications such as meningitis, brain abscess, extradural abscess, and labrynthitis.

The bacteriology in acute mastoiditis is similar to that in AOM. However, in subacute or chronic cases, *S. aureus* and gram-negative bacteria can be expected. In chronic otitis media and mastoiditis, *Pseudomonas* and *Proteus* are common pathogens. Therefore, broad intravenous coverage with multiple antibiotics or cefuroxime (Zinacef) 100 mg per kilogram per day, or 1.5 g IV, given every 6 to 8 hours, is necessary until smear and culture information is available from tympanocentesis or mastoidectomy to narrow therapy.

TABLE 3 Indications for Considering Myringotomy with Tympanocentesis

Persistent pain
Persistent fever
Patients that are under 6 months
Patients that are immunosuppressed
Failure of antibiotic therapy
Evidence of mastoiditis
Evidence of complications

SUGGESTED READING

Bluestone CD, Stoole SE, eds. Pediatric otolaryngology. Philadelphia: WB Saunders, 1984.
Paparella MM, Shumrick DA, eds. Otolaryngology. Philadelphia: WB Saunders, 1980.
Shambaugh GE, Glasscock ME III, eds. Surgery of the ear. Philadelphia: WB Saunders, 1980.

SINUSITIS AND RHINITIS

WILLIAM H. WILSON, M.D., M.Sc.
(Otorhinolaryngology)

The majority of patients seeking professional help for nasal complaints do so on the assumption that they suffer from "sinus trouble." Most have neither acute nor chronic sinus disease. Complaints of headache, facial pressure, coryza, and intermittent nasal obstruction generally rise from a seasonal or perennial nasal allergy.

Purulent drainage from one or both nasal airways suggests sinus infection, but may occur secondary to a wide range of potentially serious pathologic processes. A thorough examination of the sino-nasal tract is mandatory to rule out a foreign body or more rare and dangerous conditions such as benign or malignant neoplasia, fungal infections (e.g., mucormycosis, actinomycosis, moniliasis), or necrotizing midline granuloma and Wegener's granulomatosis.

EXAMINATION

Examination of the nasal cavity generally reveals the presence of pus or mucopus in the middle meatus or on the nasal floor. Purulent drainage demonstrable only on the posterior wall of the nasopharynx suggests an infection of the sphenoid sinuses if accompanied by other classic signs and symptoms. The absence of purulent drainage does not rule out acute involvement of the sinuses. Edema of the frontal duct or the natural ostia may prevent the flow of excretions. Shrinkage of the middle meatus with a vasoconstrictor followed by suction may produce a diagnostic show of pus, thereby indicating its source.

Patients with an acute infection may complain of pain localizing over the frontal or maxillary sinuses. Pain over the frontal bones need not indicate involvement of those sinuses, but may be referred from the maxillary area. A decrease in the degree of pain on rising is relatively common and gives the patient a false sense of improvement. An exacerbation of the pattern of pain typically occurs midmorning. Sphenoid sinusitis, a relatively rare condition, causes pain referred to the occipital portion of the skull.

Localized tenderness to percussion over one or both frontal sinuses is highly suggestive of an acute inflammatory process. Tenderness over the maxilla may suggest dental disease as well as localized sinus disease, since the roots of the maxillary teeth are located there.

Transillumination with a bright light in a dark room may reveal reduced light transmission in sinusitis if the sinus is filled with pus, but light transmission is also reduced by the changes of chronic sinusitis and other conditions.

The course of sinus disease is generally afebrile, but low-grade fevers may occur. Higher fever in the presence of an acute frontal empyema, particularly if accompanied by chills, strongly suggests local phlebitis.

Examination of the sino-nasal tract frequently requires supplemental roentgenography. However, x-ray examination of the paranasal sinuses should not become a routine procedure. A history suggestive of infection of short duration, which is localized to one or more areas and accompanied by percussion tenderness and demonstrable pus in the nasal cavity, should allow for a definitive diagnosis without the benefit of x-ray examination. Indications for roentgenography include (1) a difficult diagnostic problem, (2) infection persisting after a reasonable period of therapy, (3) a suspicion of chronicity, and (4) the presence of a demonstrable oral-antral fistula.

Episodes of acute paranasal sinusitis are a common complication of viral upper respiratory infections. Other causes include swimming and diving, dental apical abscesses and extractions, nasal packing for epistaxis or nasal surgery, and acute allergic rhinitis.

RHINITIS MEDICAMENTOSA

Seasonal and perennial allergic rhinitis account for most coryzas, followed in frequency by acute viral upper respiratory infections. Rhinitis medicamentosa may complicate either of these conditions. Vasoconstricting nasal inhalers, sprays, and drops, if used for more than a few days, generally create sufficient rebound vasodilatation to result in an addicting cycle of increased frequency of use. This cycle may persist weeks or months after the original cause of rhinitis has passed.

Exacerbation of symptoms commonly occurs when vasoconstrictors are withdrawn and the patient should be alerted to this in advance. Patients suffer greatest discomfort during the first 2 nights of withdrawal. Use of the vasoconstrictor in only one nostril for 48 hours generally allows a return to normal physiologic function on the untreated side. This can be supplemented by nocturnal sedation with antihistamines such as diphenhydramine hydrochloride (Benadryl) or promethazine hydrochloride (Phenergan).

ALLERGIC RHINITIS

Dust, chemicals, mold spores, and pollens account for most nasal manifestations of allergy. Nasal symptoms from the ingestion of a food to which the patient is hypersensitive present a particularly difficult diagnostic problem. For temporary relief, oral antihistamine-decongestants may be prescribed. Supplemental local nasal therapy includes the use of flunisolide (Nasalide), beclomethasone depropionate (Beconase or Vancenase), and cromolyn sodium nasal solution (Nasalcrom).

MAXILLARY SINUSITIS

The maxillary sinuses are most frequently infected. An early dental infection may offer a differential diagnostic problem (Table 1). Dental consultation obtained at the onset of discomfort occasionally rules out dental disease. A dental source of pain becomes more apparent if the physician rules out sinus disease and the discomfort localizes to a tooth.

ACUTE FRONTAL SINUSITIS

Acute empyema of one or both frontal sinuses can present a misleading roentgenographic picture. Paranasal sinus films occasionally show essentially normal frontal sinuses in the presence of acute empyema, whereas the sinuses appear opaque by transillumination through the floor of the sinus. This may occur when frontal sinuses are shallow in their anterior-posterior diameter. Inflammation and edema in the region of the frontal duct orifice, possibly accompanied by a thin line of mucopus, offer additional confirmation of the presence of infection. Chills and fever should heighten the concern of the physician.

Edema of the frontal duct may prevent a flow of mucopus, contributing to the prospect of a complicating infection. Moderate-to-severe pain associated with tenderness over the involved frontal sinus should confirm the diagnosis.

Possible *complications* of empyema of the frontal sinuses include retrograde bacterial phlebitis with the potential for osteomyelitis of the frontal bones and epidural, subdural, or frontal lobe abscess. Chills and spiking fever with pitting edema over the frontal bone warn of serious involvement, which requires immediate hospitalization and trephining of the sinus.

ETHMOID SINUSITIS

Extension of infection into the orbit affords great concern in acute ethmoiditis, a complication more commonly seen in children. Orbital extension may range from simple inflammatory edema to orbital cellulitis with the potential for subperiosteal or orbital abscess. Acute ethmoiditis in children frequently occurs without involvement of other sinuses. It is generally associated with a pansinusitis in adults. Pain centering between the medial ocular canthi, associated with demonstrable pus in the middle meatus, suggests involvement of the ethmoid labyrinth. Close monitoring of visual acuity is mandatory in children and affords a reliable indicator of clinical progress in infection of the orbit. Progressive loss of acuity while under adequate medical management demands surgical intervention.

THE ROLE OF CULTURES

An established diagnosis of acute infection of one or more of the paranasal sinuses requires definitive therapy. Cultures furnish data in planning a therapeutic regimen, but obtaining an accurate culture generally requires needle aspiration of a maxillary sinus. The discomfort and impracticality of this procedure preclude its routine use.

Cultures of purulent excretions from the nose and nasopharynx may fail to reveal the same pathogen as that responsible for the infection in the sinuses. This occurs through bacterial contamination of the nasal airway. Anaerobic pathogens produce negative cultures unless strict anaerobic sampling techniques are employed. The difficulty inherent in culturing this group, plus the slowness with which such cultures grow, makes dependency on the technique impractical. The Gram stain furnishes a more rapid determination of the pathogen.

The majority of successful cultures reveal *Streptococcus pneumoniae* or *Haemophilus influenzae*. Cultures obtained from the nasal middle meatus prove significant if they reveal one of these pathogens or, in children, *Branhamella catarrhalis*. Contamination may account for the presence of other organisms. Only the more severe acute episodes necessitate a culture. Instigation of antimicrobial therapy should not await the report.

Anaerobic growth suggests an acute exacerbation of chronic sinus infection or infection of dental origin. Maxillary sinus aspirate in a well-controlled study of acute sinusitis revealed the presence of *Streptococcus pneumoniae* in 43 percent, *Haemophilus influenzae* in 31 percent, anaerobes in 9 percent, and *Branhamella catarrhalis* in 5 percent.

TREATMENT

Amino-penicillin therapy offers a logical first choice in view of likely involvement by one of the first two pathogens. Both ampicillin and amoxicillin are specific, but the latter affords better gastrointestinal absorption and maintains efficacy in the presence of gastric acids. The 3-times-a-day dosage schedule for amoxicillin adds another practicality to this allowable scheduling irrespective of meals. Most infections respond with unit dosages of 250 to 500 mg.

Body weight determines the dosage regimen for children: ampicillin dosage is 50 to 100 mg per kilogram per

TABLE 1 Maxillary Sinusitis Versus Dental Disease

Signs and Symptoms	Acute Maxillary Sinusitis	Acute Dental Crisis
External swelling of maxillary area	Absent	Possible
Swelling over upper alveolar ridge	Absent	Frequent
Tenderness with digital pressure over maxilla	Present	Possible
Sensitivity to oral, hot liquids	Absent	Frequent
Sensitivity of a premolar or molar to tapping	Absent	Frequent
Lessening of pain first few hours after awakening	Frequent	Never
Clouding or opacity on transillumination of paranasal sinuses	Significant if unilateral or of suspected sinus	Significant if transilluminate clearly
X-ray studies of paranasal sinuses	Diagnostic with opacity or air-fluid level	Significant if negative
Dental x-ray studies	Negative	Frequently inconclusive

day; amoxicillin dosage is 30 to 40 mg per kilogram per day. Dosage requirements for both antibiotics depend on the severity and potential seriousness of the infection.

In communities where there is a relatively high incidence of beta-lactamase-producing *Haemophilus influenzae*, treatment with a potassium clavulanate amoxicillin combination as a beta-lactamase inhibitor (Augmentin) should be considered. The availability of this combination allows for specific therapy for many anaerobic as well as aerobic infections. *Branhamella catarrhalis* infections respond to trimethoprim-sulfamethoxazole (Bactrim or Septra) or erythromycin. The former has proved equally specific in treating ampicillin-resistant *Haemophilus influenzae*.

There exists a degree of cross-reactivity in all penicillins. A history of rash from previous administration should alert the physician to the potential of an adverse reaction to the amino-penicillins. A history of an anaphylactic response is an indication for therapy with a completely unrelated antimicrobial. Cefaclor (Ceclor) offers a safe alternative to the amino-penicillins unless a history of a serious reaction to previous penicillin therapy exists.

Should the severity of the sinus infection require parenteral therapy, intramuscular ceftriaxone sodium (Rocefin), among other third-generation cephalosporins, provides an excellent alternative for the amino-penicillins. Its advantage lies in its dosage schedule (every 12 to 24 hours). Outpatient therapy may be possible with this regimen. Dosage ranges from 1 to 2 g every 12 to 24 hours. Children require 50 to 75 mg per kilogram per day. Precautions apply regarding previous adverse reactions to penicillin.

An erythromycin-sulfonamide combination (Pediazole) offers an additional substitute for the amino-penicillins when resistance is found or suspected. Its efficacy against *S. pneumoniae* and *B. catarrhalis*, in addition to *H. influenzae* makes it a logical alternative, particularly for children.

Supplemental therapy includes shrinkage of the mucosa of the middle meatus with local vasoconstrictors followed by suction. The establishment of drainage by this means may appreciably hasten resolution of the infection. The frequent use of heat applied locally over the involved sinuses provides both therapeutic benefit and symptom relief.

Often, the oral administration of antihistamine-decongestants helps to establish drainage by lessening mucosal edema at the sinus ostia. Considering their propensity to produce rebound vasodilation, opinion varies as to the efficacy of local vasoconstrictors.

Failure to respond to these regimens after a reasonable period necessitates inclusion of a rhinologist in the therapeutic team. Acute maxillary sinusitis may require a needle or trochar perforation through the lateral wall of the inferior nasal meatus followed by an evacuating lavage. Aspiration before lavage provides an opportunity for culture. The procedure also affords the opportunity to instill an appropriate antimicrobial directly into the maxillary sinus.

Considering the potential of intracranial complications, acute empyema of one or both frontal sinuses may necessitate immediate consultation with a rhinologist. This concern occasionally results in a decision to directly perform a trephine of the frontal bone to establish drainage. The procedure also allows a sampling of the sinus content for culture.

Well-selected antimicrobial therapy should carry the majority of acute sinus infections to total resolution. Those that do not respond may represent chronic disease with acute exacerbation. A rhinologist can offer additional diagnostic and therapeutic assistance should chronicity appear to complicate the care of the patient.

SUGGESTED READING

Fairbanks DNF. Pocket guide to antimicrobial therapy in otolaryngology–head and neck surgery 3rd Ed. The American Academy of Otolaryngology—Head and Neck Surgery, Inc. 1985–1986:6–60.

Wald ER. Sinusitis and its complications in pediatrics. Pediat Clin North Am 1981; 28:777–796.

EPIGLOTTITIS

MICHAEL A. GRODIN, M.D.

Inflammatory processes of the upper respiratory tract may be classified into those affecting primarily the supraglottic structures (epiglottitis) and those affecting the infraglottic structures (laryngotracheitis). Upper airway obstruction may lead to respiratory compromise, hypoxemia, and subsequent cardiac arrest. Epiglottitis is more accurately described as supraglottitis in that the pathology reflects involvement of the aryepiglottic folds and arytenoid soft tissues as well as the epiglottis. It is this extensive involvement of the upper airway that places the pediatric patient in danger.

Supraglottitis is seen chiefly in children, but affects all age groups from the newborn to the elderly. Statistics reveal an attack rate of 0.5 to 0.9 cases per 1,000 pediatric hospital admissions. A higher proportion of cases are seen in the winter months.

Acute infectious epiglottitis is caused almost exclusively by the bacterial pathogen *Haemophilus influenzae*, Type B. Blood cultures are positive in approximately 60 percent of children, whereas only 35 percent of adults with the disease are found to be bacteremic. *Haemophilus influenzae*, Type B may also be obtained from the epiglottis, trachea, posterior pharynx, and nasopharynx, but the organism is not a common isolate from the nasopharynx of healthy children. Other organisms that have on rare occasions been suggested as causes of epiglottitis include *Streptococcus pneumoniae*, *Staphylococcus aureus*, and *Haemophilus parainfluenzae*. Viruses, which are the primary cause of infraglottic laryngotracheitis, have not yet been proved to cause supraglottitis.

CLINICAL FINDINGS

The clinical presentation of children with epiglottitis is usually characteristic. The signs and symptoms relate to acute obstruction of the upper airway. Airway resistance is a function of the fourth power of the radius of the trachea. Children with smaller upper airways are compromised with proportionately less supraglottic edema and swelling than might be seen in the adult airway with its larger radius. The most characteristic symptom complex found in young children is the toddler with a history of a mild antecedent cold proceeding to an acute toxic illness within a few hours. Prominent features include fever to 102° F or higher and respiratory distress with inspiratory stridor. The duration of the illness is usually measured in hours and is almost always less than 24 hours. The older child or adult with the larger supraglottic airway may complain of a severe sore throat and difficulty in eating and in swallowing his secretions. The older child may assume the "sniffer's" position, hyperextending the neck and protruding the chin in an attempt to open and maintain the upper airway. Hypoxemia may lead to agitation and anxiety.

On physical examination the patient is found to be stridorous and to have decreased ventilation. The child should be observed for signs of airway obstruction by looking, listening, and feeling for air movement at the mouth. Direct visualization of the epiglottis, aryepiglottic folds, and false vocal cords would reveal a large swollen edematous "cherry-red" epiglottis, but such examination is contraindicated as there are reports of acute obstruction of the airway following manipulation of the posterior pharynx. If the examiner believes that the patient may have epiglottitis, visualization of the supraglottic structures should be postponed and accomplished either noninvasively radiologically or only under controlled circumstances in the operating room at the time of intubation.

LABORATORY FINDINGS

If the patient is having respiratory compromise but is unobstructed, the child should not be separated from his or her parent, and laboratory evaluation should be delayed until an airway has been secured. As establishing an adequate airway is imperative, diagnosis as well as therapeutic intervention should be carried out in the operating room under controlled conditions at the time of intubation.

Following intubation, blood cultures and supraglottic cultures can be obtained. A complete blood count usually reveals a white blood cell count greater than 10,000 per cubic millimeter, and one often sees counts exceeding 20,000 per cubic millimeter. The white blood cell differential generally reveals a shift to the left, often with 80 percent or more polymorphonuclear cells. The only clinical tests that should be obtained prior to securing of a fixed airway, and then only in patients who have mild-to-moderate distress, are x-ray studies of the upper airway. These films are helpful in differentiating supraglottic epiglottitis from subglottic laryngotracheitis or croup. Because attempts at visualization of the posterior pharynx may lead to obstruction, as noted previously, a noninvasive roentgenographic assessment of the airway may be helpful. If the child is in severe or progressive distress, however, this diagnostic test must be bypassed and the child urgently transferred to the operating room for direct visualization.

Roentgenographic studies, when obtained, are done with the child in the upright position to avoid obstruction. One film is taken in the posteroanterior position, preferably on expiration and with phonation; this view allows for opposition of the vocal cords and adequate visualization of any subglottic narrowing. A second lateral neck film is taken, preferably on inspiration; this allows air to fill the supraglottic structures above any obstruction and easily outlines the soft tissues. Patients with epiglottitis have evidence of inspiratory obstruction, narrow valleculae, and a thick mass of tissue (smudge or thumb sign) extending from valleculae to arytenoids. This tissue mass consists of the swollen epiglottis, aryepiglottic folds, and arytenoid soft tissues. (See chapter on *Laryngitis and Croup*.)

DIFFERENTIAL DIAGNOSIS

The major differential diagnostic consideration in the patient with the acute onset of upper respiratory distress is infraglottitis or croup. Croup usually occurs in children less than 3 years of age who have a viral illness of gradual onset characterized by fever, barking cough, hoarse voice, and inspiratory stridor. Spasmodic croup is recurrent and usually self-limited. Finally, in any patient with stridor, aspiration of foreign bodies, toxic ingestions, or inhalations should be considered. There is a great deal of overlap between these syndromes, and it is difficult to make a diagnosis based purely on symptoms and signs.

TREATMENT

The most important aspect of treatment of the child with epiglottitis is a well-constructed and well-understood hospital-based protocol. This protocol should be established by the team of physicians who will take care of these children, that team representing emergency medicine, pediatrics, radiology, anesthesia, otolaryngology, and surgery (Table 1). Although therapy may vary depending on available personnel, hospital locale, and experience of the examining physician, the pediatric patient with acute infectious epiglottitis is optimally managed by a team of clinicians. *The patient should never*

TABLE 1   Initial Management Protocol

The protocol must reflect the level of respiratory distress and obstruction and the facilities and expertise immediately available. *Never leave the patient unattended. Equipment for surgical airway intervention should always be available.*

Remain calm and keep patient calm and with parent.

Administer humidified oxygen by hand-held nebulizer.

Call the following departments: ENT, anesthesia, surgery, nursing supervisor, radiology, and transport; and alert operating room.

If patient is in *severe distress*, arrange transport kit (laryngoscope, ET tubes, 14-gauge angiocath, No. 11 blade, tracheostomy tray, portable monitor and O_2, Mapelson bag and masks) and transport with team to operating room for intubation.

If patient is in *moderate distress*, transport kit to accompany patient and team to the radiology department for posteroanterior and lateral neck films.

  If *epiglottitis*, transfer to OR for intubation.

  If *croup* and *stable*, transfer to ICU.

  If *croup* and increasing *respiratory distress*, transfer to OR for intubation.

---

be left unattended from the moment of entry into the emergency medical system. Oxygen and personnel capable of establishing an adequate airway should accompany the patient wherever he or she is transported.

The goals of therapy are two: (1) secure an airway (in all patients), (2) begin antibiotic therapy.

If the patient is in respiratory arrest when first seen in the field or in the emergency department, positive pressure ventilation by means of a bag-mask apparatus may be successful as a temporizing maneuver for oxygenating the patient. Only rarely is cricothyrotomy required as an emergency procedure in respiratory arrest.

The need for establishment of a secure airway in all patients has been well studied. The incidence of total airway obstruction associated with "watchful waiting" is 50 percent and the attendant sequelae of hypoxic encephalopathy and death is unacceptable. The only question is whether a tracheostomy or intubation should be performed. Whether to perform a tracheostomy or intubation is based somewhat on hospital locale and the staff's experience and capability for maintaining a nasotracheal tube in place. Though nasotracheal intubation has been shown to be safe, effective, and associated with fewer complications than tracheostomy, this assumes an anesthesiologist and pediatric and nursing staff who are prepared to assure that this "life-line" remains intact. A tracheostomy tube is less likely to be dislodged, but is associated with a greater complication rate, is usually left in for a more prolonged period, and leaves a scar.

Intubation is best carried out in the operating suite. Maintaining parental contact with the agitated child is often beneficial, and if possible, the mother or father may carry the child to the area outside the operating room and help by holding the anesthetic mask to the child's face. Once the child is sedated, a stable intravenous line is placed, and blood chemistries and cultures of blood can be obtained. In the operating room, the epiglottis may be visualized and oral intubation completed. A small tube is utilized in an attempt to reduce added trauma and edema to the airway. Oral intubation is followed by a controlled nasotracheal intubation. The nasotracheal tube is secured and stabilized. This tube is less likely to be dislodged or to move up and down and thus further irritate inflamed tissues. Short-term intubation of this kind, usually lasting less than 72 hours, has not been associated with long-term sequelae. Once the tube is in place, the patient is restrained, particularly at the elbows, and sedated as necessary with chloral hydrate. Humidified oxygen is administered via a T-piece. The patient is transferred to an isolation room in the intensive care unit for the first 24 hours (Table 2). In many cases, extubation is possible within 24 to 48 hours, depending on clinical course and response to antibiotics.

Antibiotics directed at *Haemophilus influenzae*, Type B should be started in the operating room. These should be administered as soon as the airway has been established, cultures of blood have been drawn, and venous access established. The increasing prevalence of ampicillin resistance in this organism (5 to 20 percent) has necessitated the use of chloramphenicol or other suitable agents. Chloramphenicol should be given intravenously at a dose of 50 to 75 mg per kilogram per 24 hours in four divided doses given every 6 hours. Blood chloramphenicol levels and complete blood counts should be obtained at regular intervals. Several third-generation cephalosporins have activity against ampicillin-sensitive and ampicillin-resistant *Haemophilus influenzae*, Type B and have also been licensed for treatment of infections in childhood, includ-

TABLE 2   Intensive Care Protocol

Cardiorespiratory monitor

At least 1:1 nursing

Ventilator or T-piece to deliver humidified O_2 (30-35% FIO_2)

Frequent suctioning with available help

Arterial blood gas when stable

Chest film to ascertain tube placement

Intravenous fluids at 1½ times maintenance

Sedate and restrain patient to avoid extubation; use chloral hydrate or morphine sulfate

Tracheostomy kit at bedside

With air leak at 48 hours, consider return to OR for controlled extubation

Post-extubation mist tent and observation for 24 hours in ICU

Continue antibiotics (chloramphenicol, 50 to 75 mg per kilogram per day in divided doses every 6 hours) for 7 days (see Table 3)

ing meningitis (Table 3), and are acceptable alternatives to chloramphenicol. Older cephalosporins, including cephalothin and cefamandole, are likely to be less effective and should not be given.

COMPLICATIONS

Complications of epiglottitis result from extraepiglottic foci of infection and from therapeutic mishaps. Though rare, secondary foci of *Haemophilus* infection have been seen in the form of pneumonia, meningitis, septic arthritis, and pericarditis. Therapeutic complications include aspiration, tube dislodgement, irritation or erosion, and extubation. It is probably best to keep the patient NPO for the 2 to 3 days of intubation and to observe closely for glottic competence following extubation.

CASE CONTACTS

Contacts of children with invasive *Haemophilus influenzae*, Type B disease are at increased risk of subsequent or concomitant *Haemophilus* infections. The Committee on Infectious Diseases of the American Academy of Pediatrics has recommended prophylaxis for all household (adult and child) contacts in households where there are children (other than the index case) less than 4 years old. Nursery or day school contacts who are in close daily proximity to the index case are considered by some authorities as household contacts, and the same protocol should be followed. Rifampin, 20 mg per kilogram, is

TABLE 3 Antimicrobial agents against Haemophilus Influenzae, Type b (ampicillin-sensitive and resistant strains)

Agent	Dose (patients without meningitis)	Interval
Chloramphenicol	50–75 mg/kg/day	q6h
Cefuroxime	75–150 mg/kg/day	q8h
Cefotaxime	100–200 mg/kg/day	q6h
Ceftriaxone	50–75 mg/kg/day	q12h

given orally (except in pregnancy) once daily for 4 days (maximum dose 600 mg per day). Nasopharyngeal cultures of contact are not helpful in assessing susceptibility or need for prophylaxis. Children who are contacts and who develop a febrile illness should be evaluated by medical personnel, and if indicated, appropriate antimicrobic therapy against invasive *Haemophilus influenzae*, Type B should be started.

SUGGESTED READING

The present review is a modified version of an article which appeared in *The Journal of Emergency Medicine* 1:13, Grodin MA: Epiglottitis, 1983. Pergamon Press Ltd. and is reprinted with permission.
Bates JR. Epiglottitis: diagnosis and treatment. Pediatr in Review 1979; 1:173.
Daum RS, Bates JR, Smith AL. Epiglottitis (supraglottitis). In: Feigan RD, Cherry JO, eds. Textbook of pediatric infectious diseases. Philadelphia: W.B. Saunders, 1981:138.

LARYNGITIS AND CROUP

STEVEN D. HANDLER, M.D., F.A.C.S.

LARYNGITIS

Laryngitis is usually a benign, self-limited condition of the larynx that seldom results in emergency department visits. Strictly speaking, laryngitis is an inflammatory lesion of the larynx; however, many health professionals and patients equate laryngitis with hoarseness, which is really only one of its components. The patient with laryngeal inflammation usually presents with sore throat, cough, hoarseness, fever (occasionally), and respiratory distress (rarely).

Viral Laryngitis

The most common cause of laryngitis is a viral agent, usually the same one that is responsible for a concomitant upper respiratory infection (URI). Since the laryngeal component of the process is more of an annoyance than anything else, medical attention is seldom directed to the laryngitis. However, if the cough persists and/or is particularly violent, the patient may come to the emer-

gency department. The examining physician must extract a complete history of this illness together with any other information that might shed some light on the cause of the laryngeal problem. Recent exposure to infectious agents, concomitant URIs, and so on, all help to pinpoint a viral cause for the laryngitis. Physical examination should include a careful evaluation of the head and neck, with special attention to the nose, oral cavity, pharynx, neck, and chest. Indirect examination of the larynx would be helpful in this evaluation, but is really necessary only in the atypical case of laryngitis.

The patient whose laryngitis has lasted for 3 weeks, or who has associated serious symptoms (such as weight loss, malaise, hemoptysis) or respiratory distress must have an indirect examination of the larynx. If the emergency physician is unable to perform this examination, an otolaryngologist must be consulted to examine the larynx. Neoplasms, foreign bodies, and unusual infections can all present initially with what seems to be a simple, uncomplicated case of laryngitis. However, any symptom, such as one of those mentioned, should trigger further investigation and evaluation of the patient.

Emergency department treatment of simple, uncomplicated laryngitis is supportive. The patient is reassured, and recommendations are made for oral hydration, humidification (vaporizer, humidifier, nebulizer), rest, and antipyretics: aspirin (650 mg orally every 3 to 4 hours) for adults, or acetaminophen (10 to 15 mg per kilogram of body weight every 3 to 4 hours) for children. Voice rest, while helpful in resolving an inflammatory process of the larynx, is almost impossible to accomplish. The laryngitis should subside within 5 to 7 days and resolve without any sequelae. If it does not resolve within that amount of time, however, the patient should return to the emergency department for another evaluation. This time, otolaryngologic consultation must be obtained for indirect and possibly direct examination of the larynx.

Radiographic evaluation of the larynx and chest is not part of the routine evaluation of the patient with laryngitis. However, if either the history or physical examination suggests something more than the routine URI as the cause of the laryngitis, anteroposterior and lateral neck, and posteroanterior and lateral chest radiographs should be ordered. Once again, what at first glance may have seemed to be uncomplicated laryngitis may ultimately turn out to be a neoplasm (of larynx or lung), a foreign body, or an unusual (fungal, mycoplasmal) infection.

Bacterial Laryngitis. Bacterial causes of laryngitis are uncommon, especially in adults, but are usually part of a more generalized URI. The presenting symptoms and physical examination are almost identical to those of a patient with viral laryngitis. Some of the things that might help to identify a bacterial cause for laryngitis in the emergency department include an elevated white blood cell count with a shift to the left, productive purulent cough, enlarged tender cervical lymph nodes, the presence of an associated acute follicular tonsillitis, and of course a positive throat culture. Organisms responsible for bacterial laryngitis include *Hemophilus, Pneumococcus, Streptococcus, Staphylococcus,* and *Mycoplasma.*

Treatment of bacterial laryngitis is the same as for viral laryngitis with the exception of antimicrobial therapy. Penicillin (250 to 500 mg orally 4 times daily) and amoxicillin (25 to 50 mg per kilogram of body weight orally every 24 hours in 3 divided doses) are the drugs of choice for adults and children, respectively, to cover the bacterial pathogens usually responsible for bacterial laryngitis. Erythromycin (200 to 400 mg orally every 6 hours for adults; 30 to 50 mg per kilogram of body weight per day orally in 4 doses for children) is an alternative drug in patients allergic to penicillin or in whom staphylococcal or mycoplasmal infection is suspected. If the patient does not respond to this regimen or if the symptoms worsen, he must be seen again in the emergency department and otolaryngologic consultation obtained.

One type of bacterial laryngitis that has a high incidence of respiratory obstruction is supraglottitis or epiglottitis. While this is usually a disease seen in children age 2 to 6, cases in adults are not uncommon. The diagnosis and management of this entity are discussed in the chapter *Epiglottitis.*

Fungal and Mycoplasmal Laryngitis. Fungal and mycoplasmal laryngitis are very uncommon. They are most often part of a more generalized process involving the upper and lower airway. Patients with laryngitis who are from or have traveled to places where *Mycoplasma (M. tuberculosis)* or fungal infections (histoplasmosis, coccidioidomycosis) are endemic should be checked carefully for any signs of extralaryngeal (pulmonary, neck, etc) involvement. Indirect laryngoscopic examination of the larynx is very important in evaluating a patient with possible fungal or mycoplasmal laryngitis. The laryngeal mucosa is often red, granular, and polypoid in nature.

Varying degrees of respiratory distress may be present in patients with fungal or mycoplasmal laryngitis. Humidified oxygen (30 to 40 percent) administered by mask may help to relieve some of the distress while the patient is in the emergency department or during transport. If the obstruction is moderate to severe, intravenous corticosteroids (dexamethasone, 0.5 to 1.0 mg per kilogram of body weight) may be used to decrease laryngeal edema. In the rare case of severe airway obstruction secondary to the laryngeal involvement, intubation may have to be performed in the emergency department.

If a fungal or mycoplasmal laryngitis is suspected, the patient should be admitted for further evaluation and treatment. During the first several hours of hospitalization, attention should be directed to confirming the diagnosis and maintaining an unobstructed airway. The patient should be placed in respiratory isolation in a setting where he can be watched for signs of respiratory compromise. Humidified oxygen and intravenous steroids (as discussed previously) may be helpful in decreasing the amount of laryngeal obstruction. Direct laryngoscopy under general anesthesia is usually required to make the diagnosis of fungal or mycoplasmal laryngitis. Biopsy specimens of the affected mucosa are sent for bacteriologic and histologic studies to confirm the diagnosis. In the case of severe laryngeal involvement, the otolaryngologist may be required to perform a tracheostomy to bypass the obstruction until the inflammatory process resolves. Antimicrobial treatment depends, of course, upon the results of the bacteriologic and histologic studies.

Diphtheria. Diphtheria is a rare cause of bacterial laryngitis. With an increase in the number of unimmunized children and immigrants into the United States, diphtheria is being seen with increasing frequency. The characteristic membrane of diphtheria may be present anywhere in the pharynx or larynx and leaves a raw, bleeding surface when separated from underlying structures. This membrane may cause significant respiratory distress in the patient with laryngeal involvement. A high index of suspicion must be maintained when treating a patient at risk for diphtheria when he presents with laryngitis with or without airway compromise. While the diagnosis is suspected based on observation of the diphtheria membrane, confirmation rests on bacteriologic and pathologic studies of the membrane.

Erythromycin (1 g IV every 6 hours for adults, 20 to 50 mg per day IV in 4 divided doses for children) is the drug of choice for *Corynebacterium diphtheriae.* Diphtheria antitoxin (20,000 to 100,000 units) should be given intramuscularly or intravenously. In the patient with diphtheria laryngitis who has significant respiratory distress, emergency laryngoscopy with removal of the obstructing membrane, intubation, or tracheostomy may be required.

Traumatic Laryngitis. Another common cause of laryngitis is trauma, specifically vocal abuse or misuse. Patients (usually children) who yell, scream, or generally strain their voices may develop inflammatory changes on their vocal cords. The pathologic characteristics can range from mild edema of the vocal cords to the formation of distinct vocal nodules. Small areas of hemorrhage occasionally occur as a result of a single episode of severe vocal abuse, such as singing or cheering at a sports event.

The patient with traumatic laryngitis presents with tory distress, and other constitutional symptoms are usually absent. While traumatic laryngitis is usually suspected on the basis of a careful history, indirect laryngoscopy may be required to confirm the diagnosis. Treatment is on an outpatient basis and involves voice rest and humidification. In acute episodes in patients for whom resolution of the process is very important (singers, teachers), a short course of steroids (Medrol dose pack) may be given to reduce the vocal cord edema. Chronic cases may require intensive vocal therapy to help train the patient not to strain his voice. Rarely, nodules that do not respond to the aforementioned conservative maneuvers require surgical excision.

Arthritic Laryngitis. Cricoarytenoid arthritis is an inflammatory condition of the larynx associated most often with generalized rheumatoid arthritis. Presenting symptoms are hoarseness and a sore throat. Stridor or airway obstruction are rare but exceedingly serious complications mandating admission. Indirect laryngoscopy is needed to make the diagnosis of this entity based on the detection of bright red, swollen arytenoids with reduced mobility upon phonation. Anti-inflammatory drugs may help to decrease symptoms, but surgical treatment with arytenoidectomy is usually required for a more complete and permanent cure.

CROUP

Viral Croup. Croup, or laryngotracheobronchitis, is an inflammatory condition of the airway that causes a hoarse, barky cough, fever, and variable degrees of respiratory distress. The condition most often occurs in children between the ages of 1 to 5 years and is caused by viral agents, usually parainfluenza, influenza A, and respiratory syncytial virus. Differential diagnosis includes laryngitis, subglottic stenosis, foreign body, and vocal cord paralysis. While the viral agent affects the entire respiratory tract, the involvement of the larynx and subglottic space causes the morbidity and mortality associated with croup. Subglottic edema is responsible for the characteristic inspiratory stridor and brassy or barky cough seen in croup.

The diagnosis of croup is most often made on the basis of the history and physical examination. The child usually presents with a history of a URI, low-grade fever, slowly progressive difficulty in breathing, stridor, and the characteristic brassy or barky cough. Anteroposterior and lateral neck films will demonstrate subglottic narrowing (Figs. 1–4). Indirect or direct laryngoscopy is seldom required to make the diagnosis of croup.

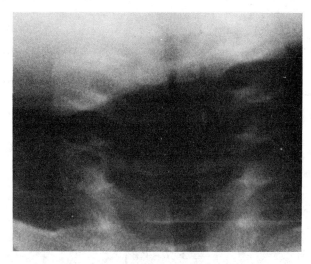

Figure 1 Posteroanterior chest roentgenogram showing symmetric narrowing (pencil or steeple sign) of the subglottic airway (arrows). (Figures 1 and 2 reproduced by permission from Potsic WP, Hander SD. Primary care: pediatric otolaryngology. New York: Macmillan, 1986:143.)

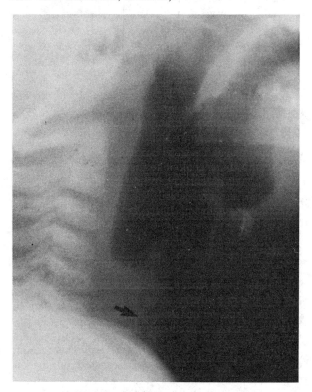

Figure 2 Lateral neck roentgenogram demonstrating narrowing of subglottic airway (arrow).

At the time of presentation in the emergency department, the child with croup must be assessed with respect to the degree of respiratory compromise. The vast majority of cases of croup are mild and self-limited and these children usually do not require emergency department treatment. If the child is having no difficulty breathing, treatment can be given at home with humidification, hydration, and antipyretics. Those children who have significant trouble breathing and demonstrate chest retractions, cyanosis, or hypoxia must be hospitalized for further

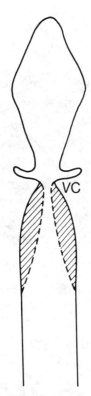

Figure 3 Drawing of posteroanterior view of airway showing normal subglottic airway (solid line) and steeple sign (dotted line) caused by edema (lined area) of the subglottic space. VC=vocal cord.

observation and treatment. Once again, hydration and humidification (usually via a mist or "croup" tent) are the mainstays of treatment.

Racemic epinephrine (0.5 ml in 4 ml of saline) nebulized and administered by mask is extremely helpful in reducing the subglottic edema of croup and its associated respiratory distress. The first treatment can be given in the emergency department or during transport. Improvement is usually quite rapid and dramatic. However, one should not be lulled into complacency by a good response to racemic epinephrine and send the child home after the treatment. The beneficial effect may be short-lived, and the child can suffer a rebound and recurrence of symptoms at home. My rule is: Any child who requires a racemic epinephrine treatment for croup is admitted for inpatient observation and care.

The use of corticosteroids in the management of croup is controversial. While some studies have shown significant improvement in symptoms of patients treated with corticosteroids, others have found no effect at all. I feel that a short course of corticosteroids (dexamethasone, 1.0 mg per kilogram of body weight every 24 hours IV in 2 to 4 doses) is indicated in the child who does not respond to conservative measures before resorting to airway intervention with intubation or tracheostomy. Antimicrobials do not play any role in this viral disease.

If the child shows signs of increasing respiratory distress and/or worsening fatigue, an artificial airway is re-

quired. Oral intubation is the emergency method of choice. The emergency department physician or transport personnel must be ready and able to intubate the child with croup should the need arise. Because of the subglottic edema, the endotracheal tube should be one-half to one size smaller than what would be appropriate for the same child under normal circumstances. It is necessary to ensure a tube small enough for a slight leak to prevent subsequent subglottic stenosis. The tube should be well secured to prevent inadvertent extubation. The child may require arm restraints and/or sedation. Sedation, however, should only be given once the airway is secure. Often the oral endotracheal tube is electively replaced by a nasal tube because this is better tolerated by the child.

If the child cannot be intubated with an endotracheal tube of sufficent caliber to allow ventilation and/or suctioning, or if there is no leak around the tube, a tracheostomy is required to secure the airway until the subglottic edema subsides.

Bacterial croup is being recognized with increasing frequency. This process has also been called membranous croup or bacterial tracheitis. The agent responsible for bacterial croup is usually *Staphylococcus aureus*. In addition to subglottic edema, there is thick, inspissated mucus or "membrane" formation within the tracheal lumen. It is this mucus that causes the significant respiratory distress usually seen in this disease. The patient with bacterial croup is usually more toxic and febrile and in more respiratory distress than the child with viral croup. The response to racemic epinephrine is also less pronounced because of the presence of the "membrane." Lateral neck roentgenograms show subglottic narrowing and often

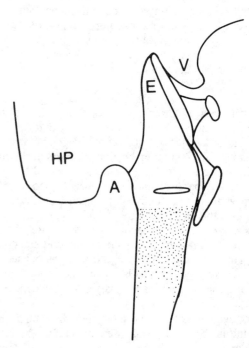

Figure 4 Lateral representation of upper airway. Stippled area is the subglottic space that becomes hazy on the roentgenogram of a patient with croup. A=arytenoid, HP=hypopharynx, V=vallecula, E=epiglottis.

demonstrate soft tissue densities within the tracheal lumen that represent the inspissated mucous casts.

Treatment in the emergency department is identical to that for viral croup with the addition of intravenous antistaphylococcal antimicrobial agents. Humidification of the airway is particularly important to help the patient loosen and clear the inspissated mucus.

The child with bacterial croup, once admitted to the hospital, needs the same intensive care and respiratory therapy as the child with viral croup. However, many of the children with bacterial croup need some type of airway intervention: intubation, bronchoscopy and removal of obstructing mucous casts, or tracheostomy.

Spasmodic Croup. The condition of spasmodic croup is thought to be allergic in origin. In cases of spasmodic croup, the child is well when he goes to bed, but wakes up in the middle of the night with a barky cough and inspiratory stridor. The condition responds to humidification and subemetic doses (15 ml) of ipecac; the mechanism by which ipecac works is not known. The child

is then usually able to resume sleeping without stridor. The next day he is well again, but the same process repeats itself on two or three successive nights. The repetitive nature of this problem along with the absence of any signs of an upper respiratory infection separate this entity from acute infectious croup. The child with spasmodic croup is seldom ill enough to require evaluation or treatment in the emergency department. However, emergency department management of spasmodic croup is identical to that for viral croup.

SUGGESTED READING

Denneny JC, Handler SD. Membranous laryngotracheobronchitis. Pediatr 1982; 70:705–707.

Denny FW, Murphy TF, Clyde WA, et al. Croup: an 11-year study in a pediatric practice. Pediatr 1983; 71:871–876.

Vrabec DP, Davison FW. Inflammatory diseases of the larynx. In: English G, ed. Otolaryngology. Vol 3. Philadelphia: Harper and Row, 1984.

LARYNGEAL AND TRACHEAL FOREIGN BODIES AND BLUNT TRAUMA

KEVIN A. SHUMRICK, M.D.
DONALD A. SHUMRICK, M.D.

LARYNGEAL AND TRACHEAL FOREIGN BODIES

The larynx arose not as an organ of phonation, but rather as a primitive sphincter to separate the two passages for food and air. Despite this teleologic effort to keep foreign bodies out of the airway, over 1,000 deaths per year are attributed to foreign body aspiration. These are the "café coronaries" in which a person who has been eating rapidly, with excessive alcohol intake, suddenly clutches his throat and dies on the spot without uttering a sound. This is almost always attributable to a piece of meat lodged firmly in the glottis causing complete airway obstruction.

Etiology

There are several situations in which the protective reflexes guarding the airway may be overcome. The most common is in infants under the age of 3, whose reflexes are not fully developed and who lack the dentition for effective mastication. Among this group, a prime offender is the peanut, so much so, that it is recommended that a household with small infants avoid peanuts completely. Any child under 2½ years of age who is found with peanuts on his person, whether choking or not, should be suspected of possible foreign body aspiration and be observed closely. This is because peanuts, with their

smooth surface and oblong shape easily travel to the distal portion of a main stem bronchus and become impacted at the primary bronchus. After an initial coughing spell (which may be unobserved), the child is asymptomatic until pneumonia or pneumonitis sets in. Less common than peanuts are any number of objects that infants may ingest and aspirate, but they too tend to have a smooth surface and oblong shape. Typical offenders are doll's plastic bottle caps, doll's imitation lipstick, buttons, kernels of corn, and slices of carrots.

A major cause of foreign body aspiration in adults is an impaired sensorium or reflex. This can take many forms: drug or alcohol ingestion, stroke, decreased tactile stimulation from dentures, senility and organic brain disease, epilepsy, and trauma. Special note should be made of the trauma patient, who is especially susceptible to foreign body aspiration either at the initial traumatic event or from a clouded sensorium afterward. The foreign body usually consists of teeth, bridgewear; or dentures. Every trauma patient should have these accounted for and, if not, should be highly suspect for foreign body aspiration.

The last group of patients have normal mentation and reflexes, but have a foreign body in the mouth or lips when startled or surprised and inhale the object. The classic case is that of the carpenter with finishing nails or tacks in his mouth.

History and Symptoms

The history depends on the age and sensorium of the patient. As mentioned, this is often insufficient and frequently is supplied by an observer or concerned parent. The clinician's index of suspicion should always be high when dealing with any of the previously mentioned patients at risk for foreign body ingestion. A child's statement that he swallowed or choked on something should never be ignored.

With the first contact of the foreign body with the respiratory mucosa, a cascade of reflexes designed to protect the airway are initiated. These consist of choking, gagging, coughing, and wheezing, all of which can be violent to the point of paroxysms. Eventually, however, the mucosal sensation adapts, the reflexes fatigue, and symptoms abate. This quiescent period, when both patient and clinician may dismiss the possibility of a foreign body, lasts until complications with their attendant symptoms arise, in the form of obstruction with pneumonia and atelectasis, chemical pneumonitis, or erosion with hemorrhage or tracheoesophageal fistula.

Physical Examination

The physical status of the patient with a foreign body in the airway may range from "in extremis" to asymptomatic, depending on where the foreign body has lodged (i.e., larynx, trachea, or bronchus) and the degree of airway obstruction it is causing.

The larynx represents the narrowest point in the airway, and it is here that the foreign body presents the greatest threat to life. Complete obstruction, as in the "café coronary," leaves the patient aphonic with no movement of air. Thus, it is a fallacy that all patients choke or cough after foreign body aspiration. However, in cases of complete obstruction, examination of the chest wall shows inspiratory efforts with suprasternal and intercostal retractions. Unconsciousness, cyanosis, and death follow rapidly. Partial obstruction, which is compatible with life, causes symptoms related to the vocal cords. If above the cords, it causes muffling of the voice; at the cords, hoarseness; and below the cords, a normal, but weaker voice. There may also be a croupy cough, wheezing, dyspnea, and possibly hemoptysis.

Tracheal foreign bodies tend to move with respiration, since this is the widest portion of the airway. This movement may produce an audible "slap" or palpable "thud" with respiration. In addition, there may be an asthmatic wheeze.

Bronchial foreign bodies are the most common of the three, but produce the fewest physical findings. If air can pass the foreign body, a wheeze is audible and there may be signs of air-trapping (hyperresonance). If the obstruction is complete, the only signs are decreased breath sounds and possibly consolidation with pneumonia. These findings may vary with time owing to the migration of the object or local tissue reaction. The signs of a bronchial foreign body are identical, at least initially, to those of an asthmatic attack or pneumonia and may improve somewhat if treated with bronchial dilators, steroids, or antibiotics.

Radiologic Evaluation

Although x-ray studies are often helpful, and sometimes diagnostic, they cannot replace a careful history and examination in the evaluation of airway foreign bodies. This is especially true in cases of vegetable foreign bodies, which are not seen on roentgenogram and only become apparent after a complication has arisen.

The basic radiologic approach is to outline the airway and demonstrate the nature and location of the suspected foreign body. The screening examination consists of slightly overpenetrated anteroposterior and lateral films of the neck and chest. These should be done in both full inspiration and full expiration; the inspiratory film being important to demonstrate obstructive atelectasis and the expiratory film to show possible check-valve emphysema. If a question remains, a more sensitive test of disparate chest wall motion can be obtained by fluoroscopic monitoring of the entire respiratory cycle.

Treatment

Airway foreign bodies tend to present in one of two ways: either as complete obstruction, which is rapidly fatal, or as partial obstruction, which is stable. It is rare, in our experience, to lose an airway once a foreign body has stabilized without some iatrogenic interference. The point is not to convert the second situation into the first by an imprudent attempt at therapeutic intervention.

Without a doubt, the single most important advance in the treatment of complete airway obstruction is the development of, and the public education in the use of, the Heimlich maneuver. If this fails, the situation is then so desperate as to warrant a "slash" tracheostomy. The physician's only intent should be to establish an airway, and since this is being performed in the field with improvised materials, a high tracheostomy aiming for the cricothyroid membrane should be performed. However, one should recognize that entry through the cricothyroid membrane is not always as easy as described, and the physician should be willing to incise the cricoid cartilage if necessary. He or she does this with the knowledge that it can be repaired if the patient survives. One should also remember that the cricothyroid membrane is directly inferior to the glottis, and foreign bodies may extend to that point. Once the airway is entered a variety of tubular objects may serve as temporary tracheotomy tubes. The most commonly reported is the shaft of a ballpoint pen.

The treatment of choice of partial airway obstruction is an orderly work-up and evaluation of the foreign body's location with removal under general anesthesia by rigid endoscopy. We mention only to condemn several methods currently advocated as these may convert a stable situation to an unstable one. One should avoid trying to "fish" foreign bodies out of the hypopharynx because of the possibility of impacting them at the glottis. Similarly, one should avoid turning the patient upside down and pounding him on the back. This may dislodge the foreign body only to have it migrate to the glottis and cause complete obstruction. Finally, we mention two dangerous methods of managing esophageal foreign bodies. First, the administration of papain to dissolve impacted meat; this has resulted in esophageal necrosis and at least two deaths. Second is the use of a distended Foley catheter to remove foreign bodies in the cervical esophagus. This goes against every principle of foreign body management, namely, there is not adequate visualization (there may be nonradiopaque foreign bodies in addition to those seen on film, with possible sharp points), and the airway is not controlled. We know of at least two deaths caused by extraction of foreign bodies from the esophagus only to have them aspirated from the hypopharynx to completely obstruct the glottis.

BLUNT LARYNGEAL AND TRACHEAL TRAUMA

After intracranial injuries, obstructive damage to the airway is the second most common cause of death associated with trauma of the head and neck. There are two main types of laryngotracheal injury: open and closed. Open injuries are serious and life-threatening, and should be handled in the operating room as soon as the patient is stabilized. Blunt trauma, on the other hand, although usually not life-threatening initially, if misdiagnosed or mistreated may also prove fatal and is the cause of considerable long-term adverse sequelae. This takes the form of laryngeal or subglottic stenosis, frequently requiring extensive surgical correction. Early diagnosis and treatment of laryngeal and tracheal injuries are crucial to their successful management and prevention of these late complications, but delay still occurs in a distressingly large number of cases.

Etiology

Blunt trauma to the larynx is usually caused by motor vehicle accidents, but may be sustained in a variety of contact and semi-contact sports such as karate, basketball, and football. In the common situation of sudden deceleration, a person who is not wearing a seatbelt would be thrown forward with the hyperextended neck striking the dashboard, steering wheel, or windshield, the result being injury to the vulnerable laryngotracheal complex. We have also noted an increasing incidence of laryngotracheal trauma among riders of two- and three-wheel off-road vehicles and snowmobiles. These patients strike branches or ropes strung across their trail and sustain a severe "clothesline" type of injury.

History and Symptoms

These injuries are almost exclusively the result of a high-speed deceleration type of injury, with the laryngotracheal complex bearing the brunt of the force. The history may be significant to explain a change in voice or actual aphonia and in ascertaining the development or progression of dyspnea. Hoarseness and dysphonia indicate at least a moderate amount of laryngeal trauma and warrant further investigation. Dyspnea, shortness of breath, and stridor are serious symptoms that may not be present initially, but develop as swelling and edema progress. If present, these indicate moderately severe trauma and represent a compromise of the airway of 60

to 70 percent. Patients with these symptoms should never be left unattended, and plans should be made for securing the airway. A history or finding of hemoptysis usually means a mucosal tear of either the larynx or hypopharynx. It is present only in moderately severe or severe injuries and should prompt a thorough investigation of the patient's airway and hypopharynx. Dysphagia and odynophagia usually indicate a fracture of the hyoid or concomitant esophageal bruising, but can represent an actual laceration of the mucosa of the hypopharynx or esophagus.

Physical Examination

In closed laryngeal injuries, the appearance of the neck may be misleading, and a potentially fatal laryngotracheal injury may exist beneath the apparently normal overlying tissue. However, several findings are distinctive. Deformity of the anterior neck with loss of part or all of the laryngeal prominence (Adam's apple) indicates severe trauma. Palpation over the larynx may reveal the crepitance of cartilage fractures or subcutaneous emphysema. Palpation over the hyoid may reveal tenderness and/or fracture. Indirect or fiberoptic-assisted direct examination of the larynx should be attempted in subacute cases. This often shows signs of internal derangement such as mucosal lacerations, avulsion of a true vocal cord, displaced arytenoids, displaced epiglottis, and hematomas. Under no circumstances should a patient in whom trauma is suspected be placed in the prone position and the larynx examined directly. Patients who were partially obstructed may now become completely obstructed with the tongue, mandible, larynx, and hyoid falling posteriorly. Fiberoptic evaluation with the patient in the upright position is of immense help.

Radiologic Assessment

Radiologic studies may be invaluable in assessing these cases, but are not warranted in an unstable patient. A member of the trauma team should accompany these patients to the radiology suite. The standard radiologic study consists of anteroposterior and lateral neck films. These should be reviewed for endolaryngeal swelling, shift in the position of the epiglottis, fracture of an ossified cartilage or hyoid, and presence of subcutaneous emphysema. In addition, there is a significant association of blunt laryngeal trauma with cervical spine injuries due to hyperextension and direct compression, and separate cervical spine films should be obtained, with all seven cervical vertebrae being visualized. In complete tracheal transsection, the tracheal air column is disrupted and the hyoid is sitting higher in the neck than usual. Occasionally, a barium swallow is performed if a laceration of the hypopharynx or esophagus is suspected. However, we believe that a water-soluble contrast medium such as Gastrografin is a preferable alternative.

Although CT scan evaluation is probably the definitive study in evaluating these injuries, it is not indicated on an emergent basis and, owing to the manipulation required, may even be dangerous.

Management

Management of these patients depends on the severity of the laryngotracheal injury. A trauma victim who has minimal symptoms, but signs of mild bruising or edema, should be admitted to the hospital and observed because of the well-known propensity for delayed swelling and edema to cause late airway compromise. Absolute bed and voice rest should also be instituted along with a cool mist tent. Steroids (IM or IV decadron, 10 mg every 6 hours for 24 to 36 hours) and antibiotics are often added, the latter especially in cases of mucosal lacerations. Any sign of deterioration of the airway, no matter how slight, is an indication for tracheostomy, since the complication rate is much lower with an orderly tracheostomy than with an emergency tracheostomy.

In severe cases, the *maintainence of an adequate airway* takes precedence. The airway must be established without flexion or extension of the neck to avoid aggravating a possible cervical fracture. Laryngeal intubation is of limited value in severe blunt laryngeal trauma because of the difficult anatomy, the possibility of further damage to the larynx, and inability to extend the neck. We also believe that a cricothyrotomy is best avoided because the cricoid is often involved in the traumatic event, landmarks are often obscured, and there may be an obstructed airway below the tracheostomy site. Percutaneous transtracheal ventilation with a large-bore (14-gauge) needle has been described, and advocated, to gain time while stabilizing the patient. We believe that this is contraindicated in patients with blunt laryngeal trauma because (1) if done superiorly, one might encounter the problems already mentioned, and (2) if done inferiorly, several large veins and the thyroid must be traversed, giving rise to bleeding with no exposure to control it. A low tracheostomy without extension of the neck is the best approach. Again, this is easier said than done and should be performed, in this critical situation, by the most experienced person available, often with the patient sitting upright. Once the tracheostomy is performed, direct laryngoscopy, bronchoscopy, cervical esophagoscopy, and, if indicated, surgical exploration of the larynx should be undertaken.

SUGGESTED READING

Shumrick DA, Gluckman JL. Trauma of the larynx and lower airway. In: Paparella M, Shumrick DA, eds. Otolaryngology. Philadelphia: WB Saunders, 1980:2438.

Snow JB. Diagnosis and therapy for acute laryngeal and tracheal trauma. Otolaryngol Clin North Am 1984; 17:101–106.

Tucker GF. Foreign bodies in the esophagus and respiratory tract. In: Paparella M, Shumrick DA, eds. Otolaryngology. Philadelphia: WB Saunders, 1980:2628.

Turtz MG, Stool SE. Foreign bodies in the pharynx and esophagus. In: Bluestone CD, Stool SE, eds. Pediatric otolaryngology. Philadelphia: WB Saunders, 1983:1095.

MANAGEMENT OF THE EYE AND ORBIT

APPROACH TO OCULAR EMERGENCIES

MICHAEL V. DRAKE, M.D.

The first step in managing an ocular emergency is to conduct a careful history and physical examination. Many emergency departments are not equipped with sophisticated ophthalmic instrumentation, so the amount of information the physician gathers can be limited. By taking a pertinent history and by conducting an examination with a penlight or flashlight, the emergency physician can generally arrive at a tentative diagnosis and initiate treatment, consultation, or referral as the situation warrants.

HISTORY

A decrease in vision and pain are the two most important ocular symptoms to evaluate in the emergency setting. In evaluating loss of vision, one should determine whether the loss was sudden, over minutes or hours, or gradual, over days or months. How did the patient first notice his visual loss? Was it associated with a catastrophic event, or did he discover it while testing the vision in each eye separately by covering the other eye?

Sudden Visual Loss

If the patient reports sudden visual loss, it is important to determine whether the visual loss actually occurred suddenly or whether the patient simply noticed it suddenly. A patient with unilateral macular degeneration may experience a gradual loss of central vision in the affected eye. The peripheral vision is not affected, and the loss of central vision in the affected eye is not noticed because the central visual fields of both eyes overlap. The unaffected eye essentially compensates for the affected eye. Only when an unusual event causes the patient to use his eyes separately does he notice that the vision in the affected eye is poor.

Progressive Visual Loss

With visual loss that has taken place over days to weeks, one should determine whether the loss is progressive. Is the rate of progression constant, or has the vision waxed and waned during the period in question? Patients with temporal arteritis or other causes of optic nerve disease may report that the quality of their vision changes throughout the day. A patient with diabetes may experience changes in refractive error associated with changes in blood sugar level. Is the vision the same at all times during the day under all lighting conditions? A posterior subcapsular cataract, for example, tends to affect the vision more when the patient is exposed to bright oncoming light, such as the setting sun or headlights, than when he is in dim light such as one might find in a movie theater or an ophthalmologist's office. Does the loss affect the whole visual field, or are specific areas spared? Did the visual loss begin in one area and spread like a curtain or veil to involve other areas, as might be the case with retinal detachment or vitreous hemorrhage? Was the visual loss preceded by a scintillating scotoma, consistent with ocular migraine? If the visual loss is regional, are the same or similar areas involved in both eyes? A patient may report poor vision in the right eye but, in fact, be experiencing poor vision to the right side because of a defect involving the right hemifield of both eyes. Does the patient have diplopia or double vision? Does the diplopia go away when either eye is covered? Is it better or worse in certain gaze directions or at particular times during the day? Was the diplopia sudden in onset or gradual? Was it associated with pain in or about the eye? Has the patient experienced headache, dizziness, nausea, or vomiting? Is there a history of trauma?

Systemic Illness

The patient's history should include inquiry into systemic illnesses the patient may have, such as diabetes or hypertension. A list of all medications that the patient is taking may reveal drugs that are associated with loss of vision.

Finally, the character of the visual loss should be explored. Is the vision blurry or fuzzy? Are objects bright but distorted, or is the vision dim or gone entirely?

Pain

The nature and character of pain associated with ophthalmic emergencies should be evaluated in much the same way as pain elsewhere in the body. One should determine whether anything relieves or exacerbates it and whether it is worse at certain times of the day or under certain circumstances. If possible, one should determine whether the pain is originating from the eye itself or from the ocular adnexa. Commonly, asthenopia is caused by referred pain from the musculature of the neck or face and is associated with tension rather than specific ocular pathology. Is there a scratchy, foreign-body sensation, or is the pain dull and throbbing? Although many patients will complain of light sensitivity, few have true *photophobia* or pain on exposure to light. Patients should be questioned carefully about this, and a distinction should be made between those patients who find light uncomfortable and those patients who fine light intolerable.

Trauma Involvement

If trauma has been involved, one should inquire specifically into the activities that led to the injury. Was explosive force involved, as might be the case with fireworks injuries or exploding car batteries? Were power tools involved? Was the patient hammering metal on metal? If a chemical injury is suspected, was a strong acid or alkaline solution involved? Was the patient wearing glasses at the time of the injury? If so, what was the fate of the glasses? Were they shattered or knocked free? Did the patient lose consciousness?

PHYSICAL EXAMINATION

Although a thorough ophthalmic examination requires expensive and complicated equipment generally not found in an emergency department, one can often assess adequately the condition of the eye by physical inspection, penlight examination, vision assessment, and funduscopic examination.

Physical Inspection

Physical inspection begins with the ocular adnexa and lids. In cases in which severe chemosis or swelling is present, one must determine whether the globe itself is involved. If the patient cannot open his eye, or if the lids are so swollen that they cannot be gently pried open with the fingers, then a Desmarres retractor or similar instrument can be used to separate the lids. A reasonable facsimile of a Desmarres retractor can be fashioned from a large paper clip if a manufactured lid retractor is not available. The paper clip is unfolded at its center, and then the larger end is folded perpendicular to the long axis to make an angle of 100 to 150 degrees. The smooth base of this folded *U* makes an effective retractor. *Extreme* caution should be exercised not to put pressure on the globe while separating the lids. If a perforating injury is present, intraocular contents may be expelled by slight pressure and the eye may be damaged irreparably. In some cases, when the patient cannot cooperate with an attempt to examine the eye and continues to squeeze the lids shut at any attempt to pry them apart, a short-acting facial nerve block may facilitate the examination. Among the many techniques for facial nerve block, the O'Brien block is convenient and easy to use in the emergency setting. The technique is as follows: 8 or 10 cc of 1 percent lidocaine is drawn into a 12-cc syringe. The area just anterior to the temporomandibular joint is cleansed with an alcohol swab. A small skin wheal is raised with the lidocaine using a 25-gauge disposable needle. Once this is accomplished, approximately 6 cc of anesthetic is injected slowly, superficially over the anterior temporomandibular joint. This raises a palpable wheal approximately 2 cm in diameter. Next, the needle is withdrawn and gentle pressure is applied to diffuse the anesthetic and to stop any bleeding from the injection site. The O'Brien block takes effect within a few minutes and lasts approximately 1 hour.

If lacerations are present, one should determine whether they go through and through the lid or the lid margin. Lacerations that go through and through the lid have the potential of continuing through to the globe and thus must be handled with extreme caution. Lacerations of the lid margin are difficult to repair cosmetically. Lacerations in the medial one-third of the lower lid can be especially troublesome if they involve the lacrimal-drainage apparatus. If the laceration is not repaired adequately, the patient may be left with an eye that tears chronically or a lacrimal system that is prone to repeated infection.

Conjunctiva and Sclera Examination

With the lids parted adequately, one can examine the conjunctiva and sclera. If the eye appears red, is it because of injected or dilated vessels as in conjunctivitis or iritis, or is there a subconjunctival hemorrhage? Is the conjunctiva boggy and edematous (chemotic)? Chemosis is important because it can be an indicator of severe injury or perforation of the globe. The severity of the injury may not be apparent at first inspection because the edematous conjunctiva tends to obscure deeper pathology. If purulent material is present, it should be collected for culture and microscopic examination.

Penlight Examination

A penlight or flashlight is helpful in examining the cornea and anterior chamber. The cornea should be completely transparent and have a glassy, smooth surface. If a corneal foreign body is suspected, a drop of fluorescein solution can be instilled and the eye examined immediately. The fluorescein will stain the tear film uniformly green. If a superficial corneal foreign body is present, the fluorescein does not stain it, and it stands out as a dark island in a light-green sea of fluorescein. If no foreign body is seen, the fluorescein can be washed out with a balanced saline irrigating solution. The fluorescein stains areas of corneal abrasion; therefore, such areas remain green when the fluorescein has been washed from the eye. If normal corneal clarity is present, it is easy to see iris detail in the anterior chamber. If the cornea is hazy, the iris detail is difficult to discern; in severe cases, the iris may not be visible at all.

If the iris can be seen, one should assess the position and function of the pupil. The pupils should be equal, round, and reactive to light and accommodation. Anisocoria, or unequal pupils, can be physiologic or pathologic. In most cases of physiologic anisocoria, the pupillary diameters are within 1 mm or, at maximum, 2 mm of one another. They are round and react normally. Important pathologic causes of anisocoria include iritis, Horner's syndrome, traumatic mydriasis (pupillary-sphincter rupture), and serious intracranial events, such as uncal herniation. A teardrop-shaped pupil can indicate a corneoscleral perforation with peripheral iris herniated into the wound. The swinging flashlight test for an afferent pupillary defect (the Marcus Gunn pupil sign) is useful in separating pathology to the retina or optic nerve from other causes of visual loss (such as cataract). In this test, a penlight is shone into one eye, and then it is moved rapidly to the other eye and back. Normally, the direct and consensual pupillary reactions are equal, and both pupils constrict in response to the light. If an afferent defect is present (of the optic nerve or rarely the retina) then the pupil in that eye can have a greater consensual reaction than a direct one. This can be seen as a paradoxical dilation in response to direct illumination as the pupil reacts more strongly to the dilatory influence of the consensual response than to the constrictive stimulus of direct light.

The anterior chamber is usually clear, but in cases of trauma or severe infection it may be partially filled with blood (hyphema) or purulent material (hypopyon). If the patient has been seated before he is examined, the hyphema or hypopyon will layer out and can be described as 10 percent, 50 percent, total, and so on.

Vision Assessment

In all ocular emergencies, it is imperative to make every effort to assess the vision. This is best done as early as possible in the examination. A patient who did not realize the extent of his visual loss prior to the examination may incorrectly believe that the examination in some way made his vision worse, and this may lead to an uncomfortable or unproductive confrontation. There are a few essential points to remember when assessing vision. The first is that the vision should be measured with the patient's glasses on. Although refractive errors are important, they are not emergencies. If the patient is middle-aged or elderly, the near-correction or bifocal portion of the glasses must be used as he is attempting to read a near target. If the patient has a refractive error but his glasses are not available, he should be asked to look through a pinhole during his vision measurement. The vision should be measured in each eye separately. If a standard eye chart is not available, any reading material is acceptable, as long as the size of the target and the dis-

tance from the patient are specified. For instance, one may record the patient's vision as "reads standard newsprint at 20 inches," "reads headlines at 12 feet," or "reads physician's name tag at 6 feet." Alternatively, one can create an eye chart by printing block letters of different sizes on a piece of paper. The patient is then asked to read the block letters at various distances. The patient's vision can then be noted as "reads ¼-inch block letters at 15 feet," and so on; alternatively, the temporary eye chart can be placed in the patient's medical record with the distance at which the patient was able to see a given size of printing noted directly on the eye chart. If a patient cannot read English, then an *E* can be printed on a piece of paper and turned with the arms pointed up (like a *W*), down (like an *M*), and so on. The patient is then asked to reproduce the direction of the arms on the *E* with the fingers on his hand. If the *E* is held with the arms up, the patient points his fingers toward the ceiling, and so on. If the acuity is so poor that the patient cannot read any size print or headlines, then the examiner should hold his fingers in front of the patient to see whether the patient can count his fingers. If the patient can do this, then the vision is recorded as "counts fingers at 3 feet," "counts fingers at 6 feet," and so on. If the patient's vision does not enable finger counting, he is asked whether he can see a hand moving in front of him. If he cannot see this, he is asked whether he can perceive light and dark. If he cannot perceive light and dark, the vision is recorded as "no light perception."

Extraocular Movement

Extraocular movements are recorded by asking the patient to look right, left, up, and down and then asking the patient to follow a target throughout these gaze positions. Each eye should be examined separately, and then both eyes should be examined together.

Visual Field Examination

A cursory visual-field examination is done by sitting approximately five feet in front of the patient and asking him to cover one eye. The patient is asked to fixate on the examiner's eye or nose. While the patient maintains steady fixation, the examiner slowly moves (about two to three inches per second) his hand or other target in from the periphery toward the central field. This is done for four to eight meridians per eye. For example, using clock hours as a reference, one could begin testing at the 12-o'clock position, or superior vertical meridian, and test the field at 1½ clock-hour intervals, for a total of eight meridians. If the patient's vision is normal, he sees the hand as soon as it starts to move. In the case of a large visual-field defect, the examiner's hand is not visible to the patient throughout a significant portion of the visual field.

Visual-field defects may be isolated to one eye, indicating disease anterior to the optic chiasm. Defects involving corresponding areas of both fields (e.g., right, temporal, superior) indicate disease at or posterior to the chiasm. Subtle defects such as those present in early glaucoma are missed by the type of examination described here, but these defects are unimportant in the emergency setting.

Funduscopic Examination

Diseases of the retina, vitreous, and optic nerve are covered in other chapters. However, there is one particular ocular fundus disease that deserves mention here.

Papilledema

Papilledema is one of the most important ophthalmoscopic findings. Unfortunately, even the ophthalmologist finds it difficult to diagnose papilledema at times. Probably the best way to ensure that one does not miss the diagnosis of papilledema is to examine normal optic nerves routinely. If one has a clear appreciation of the normal-appearing optic disk, one stands a good chance of being able to detect the sometimes subtle abnormalities of early papilledema.

We use the term papilledema to describe disc edema associated with increased intracranial pressure. Papillitis is inflammation of the optic nerve. Disc edema is a swelling of the optic nerve head not associated with papillitis or increased intracranial pressure.

A pertinent history of a patient with papilledema focuses on the symptoms of increased intracranial pressure. Headache is a common symptom of increased intracranial pressure, but it is also thoroughly nonspecific. The patient may or may not have an altered state of consciousness. Some patients may experience so-called transient obscurations, which are brief (about 15-seconds) episodes of blurring or graying out of vision. Because of the transient nature of this symptom, it does not always make a strong impression on the patient. When detected, however, it can be a useful diagnostic finding. An isolated sixth-cranial-nerve palsy is sometimes seen with increased intracranial pressure. In chronic cases the eye may become increasingly esotropic with time. Finally, pupillary abnormalities may be seen, ranging from a mildly sluggish pupil to a fixed dilated one.

There are several ophthalmoscopic findings in papilledema. The first is that the optic disc is swollen. One may not be able to see the central optic cup. Spontaneous venous pulsations are lacking. (Spontaneous venous pulsations do not always occur in normal individuals. However, spontaneous venous pulsations almost never occur in the presence of significant elevation of intracranial pressure.) The disc margin is often blurred. In papilledema, the disc-margin blurring almost always begins nasally. If one observes a disc in which only the temporal margin is blurred, one should suspect a local problem. The disc is often hyperemic because normal venous drainage is impaired by increased intracranial pressure. One may see flame-shaped hemorrhages around the disc or scattered throughout the retinal periphery. A large

preretinal or intravitreous hemorrhage extending from the disc may be a sign of subarachnoid hemorrhage. If significant papilledema is present, the optic disc may be pushed forward into the eye such that a series of concentric reflexes is seen along the temporal margin of the disc progressing out into the retina.

Finally, visual acuity is usually spared in papilledema. Careful mapping of the visual field may reveal an enlarged blind spot, but central vision will be approximately normal unless a macular hemorrhage or some other abnormality is present.

Any or all of the aforementioned signs and symptoms may be present in varying degrees. It is important to evaluate the entire constellation of findings before rushing to the conclusion that papilledema is present.

Pseudopapilledema

There are many conditions that may be confused with papilledema or cause pseudopapilledema. Two of the more common of these are papillitis, or optic neuritis, and optic nerve head drusen. In acute papillitis the optic nerve head may appear swollen and hyperemic. Signs of inflammation may include localized hemorrhage and exudate. There may be inflammatory cells in the vitreous, especially just over the optic nerve. The most important hallmarks of papillitis, however, are that the visual acuity is usually impaired and that the Marcus Gunn sign is present. In some cases the acuity may approach normal, but there is a dense unilateral visual-field defect.

Optic nerve head drusen appear as yellow-white refractile bodies located within the substance of the disc. The disc may appear slightly swollen, and its margins can be indistinct. Although central acuity is unaffected, optic nerve head drusen can cause localized visual-field abnormalities. However, the disc does not appear hyperemic, there are no inflammatory signs or evidence of localized retinal edema, and there may be spontaneous venous pulsations.

Because it may be difficult to diagnose papilledema in subtle cases, it is wise to consult opthalmologists or neurologists when in doubt. From the patient's standpoint, there are significant drawbacks both to missing the diagnosis of papilledema and to making the diagnosis inappropriately.

Using the foregoing guidelines and performing an examination without using specialized ophthalmic equipment, the emergency physician can usually obtain information sufficient to allow appropriate triage referral and treatment of most common ocular emergencies.

SUGGESTED READING

Freeman HM, ed. Ocular trauma. New York: Appleton-Century-Crofts, 1979:1.

Gambos CM. Handbook of ophthalmic emergencies. Flushing. New York: Medical Examination Publishing Co, 1973.

Paton D, Goldberg MF. Management of ocular injuries. Philadelphia: WB Saunders, 1976.

CORNEAL ABRASION AND BURN

DAVID R. DEMARTINI, M.D.
DAVID W. VASTINE, M.D.

CORNEAL ABRASION

The cornea is one of the most sensitive tissues in the body. When altered by loss or injury to the surface epithelium and exposure of the underlying nerve endings there is immediate pain, foreign body sensation, photophobia, and reflex tearing. Within a few minutes the conjunctiva will turn red. Later the lids will swell. This common symptom and sign complex is the same for any type of corneal surface injury. The conjunctiva is much less sensitive and can be almost asymptomatic, even with severe injuries.

Most corneal injuries involve high velocity or surprise, which defeats the rapid protective blink reflex. The most common causes of such injuries include tree branches, infant fingernails, contact lenses, foreign bodies projected by power equipment, wind, or explosions. Whenever a high-speed missile injury is suspected, the patient should be investigated for occult ocular perforation by dilated fundus examination, roentgenogram, computed tomography, and/or ultrasonography. Occasionally, when the history does not correlate with the abrasion seen on examination, the *recurrent erosion syndrome* may be the explanation. It occurs in patients who have had a previous corneal injury or disease, even many years prior to the most recent episode. It is caused by faulty epithelial basement membrane that allows a precipitous slough of the same area of corneal epithelium and acute recurrence of the painful symptom complex. It is treated in a manner similar to an acute corneal abrasion.

Most patients with a corneal abrasion will be rapidly relieved of symptoms if given one drop of topical anesthetic, thus making examination easier. If they are not relieved rapidly, another, more complex problem may exist and an ophthalmology consultation should be requested. Once pain is relieved, vision in both eyes should always be tested and recorded for all patients with eye complaints.

The diagnosis of corneal abrasion is easily made using sterile fluorescein dye and a cobalt blue light source (Wood's lamp or slit lamp). The dye is adsorbed to the corneal or conjunctival areas denuded of epithelium. With the cobalt blue light the excited orange fluorescein dye turns bright yellow-green. These areas are usually linear, if caused by abrasive forces, or round, if surrounding a foreign body (Fig. 1). The area of dye uptake should be stationary on the eye and not move with blinking (e.g., mucus) or change with tear pooling. A herpes simplex virus infection can be differentiated from a corneal abrasion by its characteristic dendritic ("Chinese letter") configuration.

Treatment

The treatment of corneal abrasion is best initiated by one or more drops of topical anesthetic to renew patient comfort. (Topical anesthetics are extremely toxic to the corneal epithelium when used chronically and should never be given to patients for home use.) The maximum duration of the common topical ocular anesthetics (proparacaine, tetracaine) is only 20 to 30 minutes and the patient should be warned that the pain and foreign-body sensation will return after this medication wears off and will persist until the epithelial defect fully heals (approximately 24 hours).

To improve the chronic aching periorbital discomfort of secondary ciliary body spasm, one drop of a short-acting cycloplegic (cyclopentolate 1 percent, homatropine 5 percent) should be applied. The patient should be alerted that this medication will also dilate the pupil and paralyze accommodation (near focusing ability) for approximately 24 hours.

Prior to patching, all eyes should be instilled with an antibiotic ointment to prevent bacterial contamination. Aminoglycoside, erythromycin, or chloramphenicol is adequate for common conjunctival flora. Steroids or combination antibiotic and/or steroid preparations should be avoided to prevent the risk of provoking or exacerbating a herpes simplex virus infection. Steroids should never be administered if herpes is present or even remotely suspected.

A pressure patch is the most important form of therapy for a corneal abrasion. When appropriately applied it improves comfort and promotes healing. A stiff, tight application works best. This is best accomplished by first tearing six to eight strips of 1-inch tape and folding over one end to allow a small nonsticky tab for easier removal later. One or more sterile eye patches are placed over the gently closed lid and the strips of tape are applied diagonally beginning on the forehead, across the patch(es), and onto the cheek. Elevation of the cheek prior to application of the tape can cause continued tightness of the patch as the cheek is pulled down by gravity. The remaining pieces of tape are applied adjacent to and on top of the original layers to add stiffness to the dressing. The patch should feel tight to the patient. There is usually no need for elastic dressings. Too much pressure might infarct the ocular vasculature.

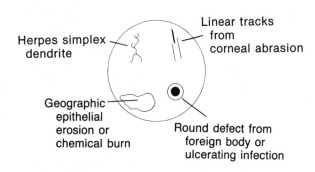

Figure 1 Identifying corneal epithelial staining defects.

All patients should be seen every 24 hours until the epithelial defect(s) has disappeared. If a white inflammatory infiltrate appears in the cornea or poor healing of the epithelium is observed the patient should be sent for ophthalmology consultation.

CORNEAL BURN

Burns of the cornea and conjunctiva are usually caused by acute changes in pH, temperature or absorption of ultraviolet light. The degree of damage depends on the intensity, duration, and type of burn. Most burns are minor and elicit the same acute painful symptom complex described for abrasions. When the intensity or penetration of the burn kills the nervous tissue no pain is experienced because the ocular surface is rendered anesthetic. The severity of the burn and the prognosis are worse when ocular ischemia (blanching), anesthesia, and/or immobility are present. These signal necrosis and eventual replacement by scar tissue responsible for visual loss.

The most common burns are probably pH burns. Of these, *alkali burns* are the most damaging. The fat-soluble nature of these chemicals gives them the ability to penetrate rapidly into the eye. Once inside they are difficult to remove and cause rapid necrosis of the intraocular structures. *Acid burns* are generally less damaging owing to their poor fat solubility and tendency to coagulate protein, creating their own barrier. However, any strong chemical can cause extensive ocular damage regardless of its chemical nature, and such burns should be considered ocular emergencies and the agent removed immediately.

Heat or *ultraviolet damage* to ocular surfaces can be as serious as chemical damage. Fortunately, conscious patients cannot tolerate long exposures to intense heat, making these injuries less common. When intense exposures to heat (e.g., fireball explosions) do occur, however, they can lead to ocular necrosis equal to that from any pH exposure.

Short bursts of intense *radiant energy* can be asymptomatic when initiated (e.g., welders' flash burns or "snow blindness"), but cumulative burns can later become very symptomatic. This form of superficial ocular surface burn is best treated as a corneal abrasion.

Extreme *cold injuries* are uncommon, but probably best tolerated of all. Gentle warming of the ocular tissues is all that is required.

Treatment

Time is of the utmost importance in treating chemical burn injuries. Immediate irrigation with any clean neutral pH fluid is essential and should be continued for at least 30 minutes, using as much irrigant as possible. The irrigation is essential for either alkali or acid burns. With the arrival of emergency response personnel, irrigation fluid should be switched to isosmolar fluids and continued until tear pH can be tested (with litmus paper) and confirmed normal. If available, at least 1 L of normal saline should be irrigated constantly through each burned eye before the pH is tested. Conjunctival fornix pH should be frequently retested after cessation of irrigation to be sure that neutral pH is maintained, especially for alkali burns. A drop of topical anesthetic (tetracaine, proparacaine) improves comfort in the minimally burned patient during the irrigation and subsequent examinations. The severely burned ocular surface is usually anesthetic. Thermally burned ocular surfaces require irrigation immediately also, but only until the normal body temperature is reestablished. In general, further irrigation after normal pH and temperature are established and constant is probably only irritating to the epithelium.

Only after adequate irrigation is accomplished should the eye(s) be examined for extent of injury. The conjunctival fornices should be explored first to remove any residual solid particles of caustic material. Then a full ocular examination is always advisable, including visual acuity, pupillary reactions, extraocular movements, and slit lamp and fundus examinations. Fluorescein dye will show areas of epithelial loss and extent of surface injury. Poor acuity and pupillary paralysis may indicate intraocular penetration of injurious chemicals. All patients with ocular burns should receive ophthalmology consultation immediately.

Acutely burned ocular surfaces should be observed frequently, as the natural barriers to infection are absent. Collagenases are liberated, causing melting of the tissue collagen and subsequent perforation. The tear composition is markedly altered and will probably be significantly reduced as conjunctival healing and scarring progress.

SUGGESTED READING

Deutsch TA, Feller DB. In: Paton, Goldberg, eds. Management of ocular injuries. 2nd ed. Philadelphia: WB Saunders, 1985.
Duane TD, Jaeger EA. Clinical ophthalmology. Vol 4. Philadelphia: Harper and Row, 1984.
Newell FW, Ernest JT. Ophthalmology principles and concepts. 5th ed. St Louis: CV Mosby, 1982.
Scheie HG, Albert DM. Textbook of ophthalmology. 9th ed. Philadelphia: WB Saunders, 1974.

ACUTE EYE INFLAMMATION

DAVID R. DEMARTINI, M.D.
DAVID W. VASTINE, M.D.

The normally white conjunctiva responds to ocular disease by vasodilation (redness), fluid exudation (swelling), and cellular migration (discharge). The intraocular tissues respond by similar pathologic mechanisms which manifest as blurred vision (corneal edema, aqueous flare, or retinal disease), or photophobia (aqueous cells or ciliary spasm). Diagnosing and treating the acutely inflamed red eye involves understanding and interpreting these symptoms and signs as they relate to conjunctivitis, iritis, acute glaucoma, and acute keratitis (Table 1).

Most patients seek acute medical care for symptomatic red eyes; the causes of asymptomatic nonacute red eyes are too numerous for this discussion.

Prior to examining any patient with eye problems, visual acuity should be routinely tested and documented in both eyes. Medicolegally, this is imperative. The only exceptions should be those cases in which withholding treatment will significantly alter clinical outcome (e.g., chemical burns); these patients should be tested after sufficient treatment has been rendered to allow safe testing of visual acuity.

Viral conjunctivitis ("pink eye") is the most common cause of redness with ocular inflammation. Either one or both eyes may be involved. There is often an associated history of other systemic viral complaints (e.g., upper respiratory infection (URI), gastrointestinal upset) or recent viral exposure. Adenovirus is the most common pathogen and promotes intense redness with conjunctival hemorrhage and edema. The lids will also swell with edema and produce a "bumpy," inflammatory infiltrate or pseudomembrane on the palpebral conjunctival surface. Preauricular or submandibular adenopathy is commonly present. The discharge is usually watery ("tears") without purulence. Three to 7 days later a keratitis (corneal inflammation) may develop, causing symptoms of foreign body sensation, photophobia, and decreased vision. The decrease in vision concerns patients and may bring them in for acute care. This keratitis is best seen with fluorescein dye applied to the tear film, causing the multiple superficial punctate corneal lesions to stand out (fluoresce). In most patients, this self-limited disease will resolve without specific therapy. Symptomatic relief can be promoted with artificial tear drops or ointment. Topical antibiotic drops may help prevent secondary bacterial infection. The disease is extremely contagious, and patients (and medical staff) should be made aware of this danger. Occasionally significant corneal scarring can result from adenoviral disease and all patients should be warned and later followed by an ophthalmologist.

Bacterial conjunctivitis is much less common than viral conjunctivitis. The discharge is usually more purulent and tenacious, with a tendency to obscure vision or stick the lids together. The conjunctival redness is less intense and there is less lid edema. Preauricular adenopathy is less prominent or absent. Monocular disease is more common, but not pathognomonic. Contagion is minimal (except in gonococcal infection). Gram stain of conjunctival discharge will yield a rapid bacteriologic diagnosis. Giemsa stain will uncover more difficult diagnoses, such as *Chlamydia*, allergy, or fungi. Conjunctival culture and appropriate antibiotics bring quick resolution. A chloramphenicol, sulfacetamide, aminoglycoside, or neomycin antibiotic drop every 2 to 4 hours while the patient is awake is usually adequate. Infants are probably better treated with erythromycin ophthalmic ointment 4 times daily, as it is more adherent than drops and has a longer contact time.

Neisseria gonorrhoeae conjunctival infections are aggressive and can quickly result in corneal perforation. They should be treated systemically (procaine penicillin, 4.8 million IU intramuscularly) and topically (hourly tetracycline 1 percent ointment; or chloramphenicol, 0.5

TABLE 1 Major Causes of the Acute Red Eye

	Conjuctivitis	Iritis	Acute Keratitis	Closed-Angle Glaucoma
History	URI, infectious exposure	Trauma (or unprovoked)	Trauma, previous infection, contact lens use	Unprovoked or pupil dilation
Onset	Gradual	Gradual	Sudden	Sudden
Major symptoms	Discharge	Photophobia, aching pain	Foreign body, pain, photophobia, tearing	Severe ache, nausea, vomiting
Vision	Normal	Slight blur	Usually normal	Very blurred
Cornea	Clear	Clear	Abrasion, suppuration	Hazy
Anterior chamber	Normal	Aqueous cells and flare (normal depth)	Normal	Narrow, flashlight sign positive
Pupil	Normal	Sluggish, irregularly shaped	Normal	Unreactive, mid-dilation
Intraocular pressure	Normal	Normal	Normal	Very high
Treatment	Antibiotics	Cycloplegics	Patching or antibiotics	Hyperosmotics, miotics, carbonic anhydrase inhibitors

percent drops; or penicillin drops 100,000 IU per milliliter). Irrigation every 15 minutes to remove discharge will help prevent corneal perforation. All gonorrheal conjunctivitis should be immediately referred for ophthalmologic consultation and probably admitted to hospital. Patients with more routine bacterial conjunctivitis should be referred for ophthalmologic evaluation within five days to check on treatment progress.

Ocular allergy is characterized by acute swelling and itching with only minimal redness (without hemorrhage) and a mild watery discharge. There may be other systemic or local signs of allergy (e.g., rhinitis, dermatitis, asthma). One or both eyes may be involved. There is usually a history of allergies and a recent suspected exposure. Resolution depends on the intensity of exposure and host response. Avoidance is the best therapy. Topical antihistamine drops relieve most acute symptoms. Protection from, or treatment of, systemic manifestations during the acute attack by systemic antihistamines (diphenhydramine hydrochloride 25 to 50 mg 3 times a day or 5 mg per kilogram every 24 hours) or steroids should be considered.

Iritis (acute inflammation of the iris or ciliary body) usually manifests with the triad of pain, redness, and severe photophobia (see also the chapter *Uveitis*.) Usually only one eye is involved. Vision is often slightly blurred. Onset may be spontaneous or after blunt trauma. There is no foreign body sensation and topical anesthetics do not bring relief. The conjunctival redness may be in a ring pattern surrounding the cornea overlying the ciliary body ("ciliary flush"). The intraocular pressure is low (< 12 mm Hg), normal, or only minimally elevated (< 30 mm Hg). The diagnosis is made by the typical history and slit lamp observation of cells (white blood cells) and flare (protein) suspended in the aqueous humor.

Acute closed-angle glaucoma is rare, but is one of the most significant eye emergencies (see also the chapter *Acute Glaucoma*). Tonometry should always be tested in the painful acute red eye, as elevated pressure is diagnostic. Immediate ophthalmologic referral and treatment are mandatory to preserve vision.

Acute keratitis (corneal inflammation) is a common cause of acute symptomatic red eye(s) because of the remarkable pain response from an injured cornea. An intense foreign body sensation is characteristic and differentiates a keratitis from the pain, redness, and tearing of the other red eye conditions. Trauma is the most common cause, but corneal infection and foreign body also need to be considered. Any patient with corneal infection should be referred for immediate ophthalmologic evaluation, while corneal abrasions can be treated primarily (see the chapter *Corneal Abrasion and Burn*.)

Herpes simplex virus infection of the cornea is not uncommon and is a special problem for ophthalmologists. Most herpetic disease is recurrent virus, but new contaminations are also common. The characteristic "dendrite" (see Fig. 1 in the chapter *Corneal Abrasion and Burn*) is the sign of active live virus and also considered diagnostic. Contagion is present only when live virus (dendrite) is present. Decreased corneal sensation, preauricular adenopathy, and unilateral infection are almost always present. Antiviral medications (idoxuridine 0.5 percent or trifluridine 1 percent drops every 2 hours while awake, or idoxuridine 1 percent or vidarabine 3 percent ointment 5 times daily) are available, but the complexity and potential for significant visual loss require ophthalmologic supervision. Topical steroid medications can cause the virus to penetrate, scar, and/or perforate corneal stroma and should never be used acutely when *herpes simplex* is suspected.

Eyelid infections and inflammations are common and also cause the eye to turn red secondary to local inflammation, irritation, or spread of infection. The common stye, termed "chalazion" when internal or "hordeolum" when external, is a small acute bacterial abscess in the sebaceous glands of the lid. Most will mature through increased swelling, redness, and tenderness, and will eventually open and drain, causing quick resolution. This process can be accelerated by applying a hot compress (for 15 minutes 4 times a day) to the local area. Heat will also act as a preventive treatment for patients with chronic or recurrent disease. Except for pointing external lid abscesses, incision and drainage is not recommended, as lid notch or scarring could develop or the infection could spread. Systemic tetracycline (250 mg orally daily) will also help resolve chronic or recurrent disease. Most cultures from the lids reveal Gram-positive cocci or *Propionibacterium* species.

Herpes simplex skin disease can also be found on the eyelids and the eye should be protected by the application of topical anti-herpetic ointment to the suspected lesions. Skin herpes cultures or immunofluorescent antibody testing should be obtained whenever possible to confirm the diagnosis.

Orbital cellulitis is uncommon, but is potentially a vision- or life-threatening disease. Two separate syndromes are possible in orbital cellulitis, depending on the location of the nidus of inflammation or infection: anterior (preorbital septum) or posterior (posterior to the orbital septum). Infectious orbital cellulitis is more common than sterile orbital inflammations. Only infectious orbital cellulitis will be considered in this discussion.

Anterior orbital cellulitis is located primarily in the skin and muscle layers of the lid skin and will usually not involve or inflame the contiguous eye or posterior orbital tissues. There is no proptosis, motion restriction, pupillary signs, or decreased vision. Opening the involved lid(s) will usually reveal a normal quiet eye underneath. Treatment consists of systemic antibiotics (ampicillin, erythromycin, or a cephalosporin) in appropriate dosages. The abscess will usually drain anteriorly. Local hot compresses may speed the process. Daily monitoring is mandatory to ensure steady improvement.

Posterior orbital cellulitis is a true medical emergency, as the infection can spread to the cavernous sinus of the brain. Signs usually include red and swollen lids, orbit, and conjunctiva; proptosis; decreased vision; afferent pupillary defect; ocular movement restrictions; and systemic signs of illness (fever, elevated white blood cell count, malaise, etc). Often there is a current or past history of contiguous (sinus, dental) or blood-borne infection. Blood cultures, orbit and skull computed tomographs, and white blood cell count should be obtained. Ear, nose, and throat (ENT) consultation with local orbit and/or sinus drainage and culture is helpful. Immediate high-dose intravenous antibiotics are mandatory. Locally derived infections are caused by nasopharyngeal microbiologic flora and are usually covered by intravenous ampicillin and cephalosporins. More distant or traumatic sources of infection make the choice of antibiotics more difficult, and they should cover a broader spectrum. Fungi also should be considered. Hospital admission and close monitoring are imperative.

All red eyes are significant, since they reveal ocular inflammation and pathology. Many can be acutely treated adequately by the emergency physician, but all should eventually be seen by an ophthalmologist. In most cases (except where noted otherwise previously), ophthalmologic evaluation a few days later is ideal.

SUGGESTED READING

Deutsch TA, Feller DB. In: Paton, Goldberg, eds. Management of ocular injuries 2nd ed. Philadelphia: WB Saunders, 1985.

Duane TD, Jaeger EA. Clinical ophthalmology. Philadelphia: Harper and Row, 1984.

Kolker AE, Hetherington J. Becker-Schaffer's diagnosis and therapy of glaucomas. 4th ed. St. Louis: CV Mosby, 1985.

Newell FW, Ernest JT. Ophthalmology principle and concepts. 5th ed. St. Louis: CV Mosby, 1982.

Scheie HG, Albert DM. Textbook of ophthalmology. 9th ed. Philadelphia: WB Saunders, 1977.

UVEITIS

HOWARD H. TESSLER, M.D.

Strictly defined, uveitis refers to an inflammation of the middle vascular coat (uvea) of the eye. In practical usage, uveitis refers to any endogenous inflammation of the eye that is not attributable to external perforation or trauma.

CLASSIFICATION

Uveitis is actually a group of diseases. The type of uveitis is defined in several ways. The time course is one way. Acute disease begins abruptly with symptoms of pain, redness, and photophobia (light sensitivity). On the other hand, chronic uveitis, has an insidious onset, often with minimal symptoms of blurring or a sensation of vague discomfort or floaters.

The location of the inflammation is also a way to define uveitis. Uveitis involving the anterior part of the eye is often referred to as iritis. When uveitis involves the posterior portion of the eye, it is referred to as choroiditis or retinitis. If the uveitis is secondary to corneal or scleral disease, it is called keratouveitis or sclerouveitis.

The etiology of the ocular inflammation can often be determined by the presentation of the uveitis. Acute iritis is often related to ankylosing spondylitis and to the presence of HLA-B27. Posterior uveitis is frequently infectious and can be associated with toxoplasmosis, tuberculosis, syphilis, or the ocular histoplasmosis syndrome.

Nonophthalmologists should not be expected to diagnose and treat the various types of uveitis. However, it is worthwhile for them to suspect ocular inflammatory disease and to institute the proper ophthalmic referral.

RISK OF CORTICOSTEROIDS

Because many cases of uveitis are treated nonspecifically with corticosteroids, nonophthalmologists should be aware of the risks of these drugs. One should be absolutely certain of the diagnosis before initiating treatment of a patient with ocular inflammation by means of topical or systemic corticosteroids. Topical corticosteroids are associated with side effects such as cataracts, the induction of glaucoma, and the risk of precipitating bacterial, fungal, or viral overgrowth. Unless it is impossible to obtain ophthalmologic consultation, it is probably unnecessary for nonophthalmologists to use topical or systemic corticosteroids for ocular inflammatory disease. For example, if the patient has a herpes simplex keratoiritis, the use of topical corticosteroids may worsen that patient's condition. Also, certain types of keratomalacia associated with rheumatoid arthritis may become much worse with the use of topical corticosteroids. In these cases, topical corticosteroids may literally melt away corneas.

ACUTE IRITIS

Patients with acute iritis usually develop pain, redness, and photophobia in one eye. They do not have the purulent or mucopurulent discharge that is common with conjunctivitis (Table 1). The inflammation of iritis is deeper than that of conjunctivitis. Thus, if 2.5 percent or 10 percent phenylephrine drops are placed in an eye with iritis, there is not much blanching of the erythema. This is especially true around the limbus of the eye. Conversely, in conjunctivitis, there should be almost total blanching of the conjunctival blood vessels.

With acute iritis, the eye is sore to the touch, and there is a deep ache (analogous to a toothache). This is the opposite of conjunctivitis, in which there may be discomfort about the eye, but not usually a tremendous amount of pain in the eye itself.

In acute iritis, the pupil is usually small (miotic) and poorly reactive to light. Conversely, the pupil is commonly normal in conjunctivitis and may be fixed and slightly dilated in acute glaucoma.

The intraocular pressure in acute iritis is frequently low. On occasion, the pressure may be elevated, but usually does not reach the high levels seen in acute glau-

TABLE 1 Differential Diagnosis of Red Eye

Diagnosis	Conjunctiva	Discharge	Iris	Intraocular Pressure
Conjunctivitis	Blanches with phenylephrine	Purulent, mucopurulent	Normal	Normal
Uveitis	Only partial blanching occurs	Watery	Constricted, poorly reactive	Usually low
Acute glaucoma	Only partial blanching occurs*	Watery	Mid-dilation, fixed	Elevated

* Phenylephrine may further dilate the pupil in acute glaucoma and make the disease worse. If acute glaucoma is suspected, do not place phenylephrine or other dilating agents in the eye.

coma. In conjunctivitis, the intraocular pressure is normal.

With the slit lamp, the cornea is seen to have cellular precipitates on the endothelium. The anterior chamber shows cells and protein exudation (flare).

The *therapy* for acute iritis (acute anterior uveitis) is directed at dilating the pupil in order to promote comfort by paralyzing the ciliary body and stopping ciliary spasm. Dilation of the pupil also tends to break and prevent synechiae (adhesions between the iris and the lens). Dilation may worsen acute glaucoma. Thus, if the diagnosis is uncertain, it may be risky to dilate the patient's pupil. Topical corticosteroids control acute iritis in most cases. As mentioned, unless one is certain of the diagnosis and has no ophthalmologic consult, it is probably wrong for the nonophthalmologist to initiate corticosteroids for this type of eye disease.

CHRONIC IRIDOCYCLITIS (IRITIS)

This type of inflammation usually begins insidiously. Patients have vague discomfort, mild redness, and blurring of vision. Usually, this is bilateral, unlike acute iritis, which is frequently unilateral. The eyes may show various amounts of redness. Some patients have almost white eyes, whereas others have highly injected conjunctivae. The pupils in these patients, when untreated, tend to be small. Often, the pupils are irregular from synechiae (adhesions) that have formed. Slit lamp examination reveals a clinical picture similar to that of acute iritis. The intraocular pressure is often low in cases of chronic iritis, but may be elevated.

Sarcoidosis is a common cause of chronic iritis and iridocyclitis. Patients with juvenile rheumatoid arthritis are also at risk. Often, no etiology can be determined for chronic iritis.

Since these patients do not experience a great deal of pain, it is not an emergency situation, and treatment can be deferred until they are seen by an ophthalmologist. Treatment is similar to that for acute iritis.

INTERMEDIATE UVEITIS

Intermediate uveitis is a type of inflammation that tends to occur in young adults. It is usually bilateral and begins insidiously. The patients often complain of floaters and blurred vision. There is almost never any redness. The pupils appear normal. The slit lamp examination demonstrates the anterior chamber and cornea to be relatively free of inflammation. The vitreous behind the lens is usually loaded with cells. These patients commonly develop cystoid macular edema, which results in decreased visual acuity. Cystoid macular edema may be suspected when the patient reports that objects viewed directly cannot be seen, but when they are viewed off-center, objects become more clear. When patients with cystoid macular edema read a line of print, they have trouble keeping an entire word or line in focus. They are forced to scan back and forth across a word or line to see it entirely.

Intermediate uveitis (one form of which is called pars planitis) generally is not an emergency situation, and treatment may be delayed until the patient is seen by an ophthalmologist. Occasionally, these patients present with a vitreous hemorrhage and a sudden loss of vision. They may have been unaware of any ocular problem until this occurs. On examination, the fundus is difficult to see, and the vitreous is loaded with blood and reddish in appearance.

The management of intermediate uveitis is difficult and controversial. Corticosteroids, either injected periocularly or taken systemically, are often required. Patients with a vitreous hemorrhage should be instructed to keep their head elevated, to refrain from bending over, and to avoid lifting heavy items. They should sleep propped up on two pillows. Ultrasonography may disclose the presence of a retinal detachment as well.

RETINITIS

Inflammation of the retina usually occurs without much pain or discomfort. Patients commonly complain of blurred vision. Occasionally, there may be so much inflammation in the retina that anterior uveitis is present as well. Thus, symptoms of pain, redness, and photophobia may also be associated with a retinitis. It is important, therefore, to examine the fundus in every patient with iritis to detect any underlying retinitis.

The pupil is often normal with retinitis, and the eye is not usually very red. Examination with a direct ophthalmoscope may disclose a white area in the retina, which usually represents necrosis and inflammation of retinal tissue. Frequently, the vitreous is hazy owing to the influx of white blood cells. Examination of the fundus with an indirect ophthalmoscope often shows the clinical picture more easily than a direct ophthalmoscope. Slit lamp examination demonstrates few cells in the anterior chamber, but many cells in the vitreous.

Toxoplasmosis

The therapy for retinitis depends on its etiology. *Toxoplasma gondii*, a common cause of retinitis, is usually treated with appropriate antibiotics and often systemic steroids to prevent inflammatory damage to important portions of the retina. Current therapy includes triple sulfa (trisulfapyrimidine), 2 to 6 g per day, daraprim (pyrimethamine), 25 to 50 mg per day, and sometimes clindamycin, 300 mg 4 times a day. Systemic corticosteroids are often added as well. This therapy is usually required for at least 3 weeks.

Syphilis

Another cause of retinitis may be syphilis. A fluorescent treponemal antibody absorption test should be done on any patient with uveitis. Syphilis may cause inflammation in almost any part of the eye and can produce retinitis. There have been cases reported in which the Veneral Disease Research Laboratory (VDRL) test and rapid plasma reagin test were nonreactive and the fluorescent treponemat antibody absorption (FTA-ABS) was reactive in patients with ocular syphilis. In patients with luetic retinitis, 20 million units of intravenous penicillin daily for 10 days may be considered. Many cases of ocular syphilis do not respond to the usual dose of oral or intramuscular penicillin.

Viral Retinitis

Patients who are immunocompromised, such as those receiving chemotherapy or those who have acquired immune deficiency syndrome, may develop viral retinitis. Retinal inflammation with herpes simplex and cytomegalovirus is becoming more common than previously. In these cases, there are usually large areas of whitening of the retina with hemorrhage. Unfortunately, unless the immunosuppression can be reversed, most of these patients do poorly. The new systemic antiviral agents have not proved particularly useful in the treatment of viral retinitis.

CHOROIDITIS

Inflammation of the choroid occurs more posteriorly in the eye than inflammation in the retina. Thus, patients often have fewer cells in the vitreous. However, their complaints are usually similar to those of patients with retinitis, but there are fewer signs of inflammation such as redness or discomfort about the eye.

Histoplasmosis

The ocular histoplasmosis syndrome, which is believed to be related to previous infection by *Histoplasma capsulatum*, usually presents as inactive choroidal inflammation. Affected patients frequently have small atrophic scars scattered throughout the fundus, in which abnormal blood vessels develop. Hemorrhage in these scars at the macula causes a sudden decrease in vision. Patients with this syndrome complain of blurred vision or a spot in front of one eye. It is believed that the ocular histoplasmosis syndrome is either an allergic reaction or a degenerative change in an old scar. It has nothing to do with active fungal replication. Thus, antibiotic therapy has no use in this disease. If the abnormal vessels are in a location where they can be eliminated without damaging visually important retina, therapy can be given with an argon or krypton laser. In a few patients, systemic corticosteroids may have some use. In histoplasmic choroiditis, there are usually no cells in the anterior chamber or vitreous, and the eye is painless and shows no redness.

Tuberculosis

Tuberculosis choroiditis is rare, but may occur in the absence of active pulmonary disease. The clinical features of tuberculous choroiditis may be similar to those of histoplasmosis. With ocular tuberculosis, however, there are usually cells in the vitreous. The eye may be irritated and red. When tuberculous choroiditis is suspected, a therapeutic trial with antituberculous medication often produces dramatic clearing of inflammation and improvement in vision within 1 or 2 weeks. Tuberculous choroiditis should always be considered in the differential diagnosis because it is one of the few types of uveitis that can be "cured."

Most cases of posterior uveitis, including intermediate uveitis, retinitis, and choroiditis do not require therapy in the emergency department.

DISPOSITION

Most patients with uveitis do not need to be admitted to the hospital. Unless visual acuity has decreased to bare light perception or no light perception, the ophthalmologist can usually see the patient within 6 to 12 hours rather than immediately. Unless the patient has severe pain or a very high intraocular pressure (symptoms of acute glaucoma), he or she can also wait for 6 to 12 hours to be seen by an ophthalmologist. Because irreversible synechiae (adhesions) can occur with acute iritis and chronic iritis, it is important to note the state of the pupil. If the pupil is normal, the chance of synechiae forming may be less than with a small 1-mm pupil. Patients with small 1-mm pupils should be seen sooner by the ophthalmologist than those with normal pupils.

SUGGESTED READING

Smith RE, Nozik RA. Uveitis: a clinical approach to diagnosis and management. Baltimore: Williams & Wilkins, 1983.

Tessler HH. Diseases of the uvea. In: Duane TD, ed. Clinical ophthalmology. Philadelphia: JB Lippincott, 1978–1984.

ACUTE GLAUCOMA

JACOB T. WILENSKY, M.D.

Glaucoma is the term used to describe a group of ocular diseases that are caused by an elevation of pressure inside the eyeball and that lead to the death of retinal nerve cells and, consequently, blindness. The causes of glaucoma can be primary or secondary. Most of the time glaucoma develops gradually, (open-angle glaucoma), frequently with few or no signs or symptoms. Occasionally, however, the presentation is acute (angle-closure glaucoma). When this occurs, the patient may have signs and symptoms such as tearing, hazy vision, corneal edema, injection of the globe, a mid-dilated nonreactive pupil, headache, and even nausea and vomiting. Three particular types of glaucoma account for the majority of the acute glaucomas: angle-closure glaucoma, uveitic glaucoma, and neovascular glaucoma.

TYPES OF ACUTE GLAUCOMA

Angle-closure glaucoma occurs most commonly in patients who are genetically predisposed. These patients have eyeballs that are shorter than average and a somewhat anteriorly placed and fatter than usual lens, thereby resulting in a shallow anterior chamber. Almost all of these patients are farsighted. Events such as the dilation of the pupil or certain pharmacologic agents can produce a relative pupillary block that increases the pressure in the posterior chamber behind the iris. This in turn causes the iris to push forward against the peripheral cornea, thereby occluding access to the normal drainage mechanism for the aqueous humor. When this occurs, the intraocular pressure rises rapidly, causing signs and symptoms of acute glaucoma (Table 1). Other causes of angle-closure glaucoma include an intumescent cataractous lens that pushes the iris forward, a dislocated lens (particularly if it occludes the pupil), tumors in the posterior segment of the eye, and central retinal vein occlusion.

In *uveitic glaucoma*, several different mechanisms can cause the acute rise in intraocular pressure. Among these are acute inflammation of the trabecular meshwork with localized edema, obstruction of the trabecular meshwork by inflammatory cells or macrophages, and increase in the viscosity of the aqueous humor attributable to a breakdown of the blood-aqueous barrier or leakage of the lens protein. Secondary forms of angle-closure glaucoma also can result from uveitis caused by adhesions, either between the lens and iris (posterior synechiae) or between the peripheral iris root and cornea (peripheral anterior synechiae).

During the course of a number of systemic or ocular disease processes, new vessels may begin to grow on the iris surface (*rubeosis iridis*). This *neovascularization* of the iris is seen most commonly in patients with diabetes mellitus or following an ischemic central retinal vein occlusion. As these new vessels grow across the iris surface, they form a fibrovascular membrane that bridges the angle between the iris root and the peripheral cornea. As this membrane grows and contracts, it pulls the peripheral iris up against the trabecular meshwork, thereby occluding the outflow channels.

DIFFERENTIAL DIAGNOSIS

When a patient presents with a red or painful eye and some decrease in visual acuity, several conditions in addition to glaucoma must be considered in the differential diagnosis (Table 2). These include herpes simplex keratitis, some form of iritis or uveitis, and retrobulbar neuritis. In herpes simplex keratitis, the predominating feature is usually pain. There is profuse tearing, but often only mild-to-moderate conjunctival injection. Fluorescein staining of the cornea commonly reveals a dendritic figure, and the corneal changes are localized to one area of the cornea rather than being diffuse. Often the pupil is miotic.

In uveitis the amount of conjunctival injection can vary from minimal to severe. Small clumps of white cells (keratic precipitates) may be present on the corneal endothelium, and inflammatory cells may be seen in the anterior chamber on slit lamp examination. Depending on the type of uveitis, there may be adhesions of the iris to the lens, which may cause distortions of the pupil. If there are no adhesions, usually the pupil is miotic. The amount of visual disturbance in uveitis is commonly minimal unless there is an extremely heavy inflammatory reaction in the anterior chamber or secondary lens changes (cataract) have already occurred. In retrobulbar neuritis the eye is almost always quiet and the cornea is clear. The pupil may be mildly dilated, particularly in comparison with the other eye. There may be pain on motion of the globe. The visual loss is frequently profound, from 20/200 to the finger-counting range.

TABLE 1   Signs and Symptoms of Acute Glaucoma

Blurred, foggy vision with halos around lights
A mid-dilated, nonreactive, and oval pupil
Conjunctival injection
Loss of corneal luster
Tearing
Eye ache, brow ache, or headache
Nausea and vomiting

TABLE 2   Differential Diagnosis of a Red or Painful Eye

Herpes simplex keratitis: pain usually predominates
Uveitis: more photophobia; pupil may be irregular
Retrobulbar neuritis: usually no injection
Glaucoma: more corneal edema
  Angle closure: mid-dilated, nonreactive pupil
  Uveitic: same as other uveitis, but with corneal edema
  Neovascular: abnormal vessel on iris, may have blood in the anterior chamber

One of the major *problems in making the diagnosis* of acute glaucoma is that many patients do not exhibit the classic symptoms. Visual symptoms may be minimal or not noticed because of good vision in the other eye. Headache, runny nose, or nausea may be the predominant symptoms. Unless the eyes are examined for signs of glaucoma, an incorrect diagnosis of "flu," sinus infection, or even common cold may be made.

The key to the diagnosis of acute glaucoma is the measurement of the *intraocular pressure*. Currently, the preferred method of measuring the intraocular pressure is with the Goldmann applanation tonometer on a slit lamp biomicroscope. In the absence of a slit lamp, a Schiotz tonometer can be used, although caution must be taken to adequately clean and sterilize the instrument after use to avoid the spread of infection from patient to patient. A value of 4.0 or above with a 5.5 g weight or 6.0 or above with a 7.5 g weight indicates an intraocular pressure of 22 mm Hg or less. In acute glaucoma, pressures are usually 40 mm Hg or more, which would produce a zero reading by Schiotz with either weight. If no tonometer is available, the fingers can be used to palpate the globe. It may be possible to detect an elevated intraocular pressure even by this gross method, particularly if there is a marked difference between the two eyes.

Once an elevation of intraocular pressure has been detected, it is necessary to differentiate among the different types of acute glaucoma since the treatment varies considerably with type. A slit lamp biomicroscopic examination is often necessary to make this differentiation. Usually this means that the emergency physician must immediately consult with an ophthalmologist.

TREATMENT

Prompt treatment of acute glaucoma is essential to prevent significant visual loss or even blindness. The highly elevated intraocular pressures that can occur during an acute attack (70 to 80 mm Hg) may rapidly decrease vision within hours or days. This probably occurs through one of two mechanisms: infarction of the immediate postlaminar optic nerve head or a central retinal artery occlusion. Moreover, if an acute-angle closure attack is appropriately treated promptly, the intraocular pressure can be normalized with little or no sequelae, whereas if the attack is allowed to persist for a day or two, permanent scarring of the outflow channel can lead to a chronic form of glaucoma even though the acute attack is resolved.

In *angle-closure glaucoma*, the goals of therapy are to pull the iris away from its contact with the trabecular meshwork and to reopen the drainage channel. The simplest way to do this is to place the iris on stretch by constricting the pupil with a miotic agent such as 1 percent pilocarpine. Unfortunately, the sphincter muscle of the iris is sensitive to ischemia. If the intraocular pressure has been elevated for even a relatively short period of time, this muscle becomes unresponsive to stimulation. Therefore, medication must be given to lower the intraocular pressure and to restore circulation to the sphincter muscle before the miotic agent can work. This is accomplished by giving a hyperosmotic agent such as glycerol, 1.0 to 2.0 ml per kilogram of body weight orally,

or mannitol, 1 to 2 g per kilogram of body weight in a 20 percent supersaturated solution given intravenously. These hyperosmotic agents increase the osmolarity of the intravascular compartment, thereby leading to a bulk flow of water from the extravascular compartment (including the eye), thus reducing the volume of fluid inside the eye and, thereby, the intraocular pressure. Optionally acetazolamide (Diamox), 500 mg, may be given by slow IV push to lower the pressure.

Once the iris sphincter becomes responsive, it responds to the miotic agent, places the peripheral iris on stretch, and pulls it away from the chamber angle. In some cases, particularly when the attack has been in progress for a day or more, the eye does not respond to this therapy, and the attack cannot be broken medically. Surgical treatment then becomes necessary, and an iridectomy or some other form of glaucoma surgery is performed.

Usually, however, the medication successfully breaks the attack. As the intraocular pressure decreases to the normal range, any corneal edema noted during the acute attack partially or totally resolves in an hour or two. At this point, a laser iridectomy can be performed, which is curative for most cases of this type of glaucoma. However, some patients may subsequently require chronic antiglaucoma eye drops.

In *uveitic glaucoma*, the precise treatment varies depending on the type of uveitis. In general, the main goal of therapy is to control the inflammatory disease through the use of topical, periocular, or systemic corticosteroids. Atropine or one of its shorter-acting synthetic analogs may also be used. Timolol (0.25 percent, one drop every 12 hours) and a systemic carbonic anhydrase inhibitor, such as Neptazane (50 mg every 8 hours) or Diamox sequels (500 mg every 12 hours), are used to try to lower the intraocular pressure until the uveitis can be brought under control.

The management of *neovascular glaucoma* is generally the most difficult of these three groups of diseases. In many cases, the patient already has extensive permanent closure of the chamber angle at the time of presentation. Often timolol and the carbonic anhydrase inhibitors may help lower the intraocular pressure, but usually not to a normal level. Panretinal photocoagulation therapy may cause the rubeosis iridis to regress, but cannot reopen a scarred outflow channel. If the pressure remains significantly elevated, either glaucoma filtering surgery or cyclocryotherapy (depending on the visual status of the eye) may be required.

When a patient presents with acute glaucoma, the most important thing is to recognize the disease and obtain prompt consultation with an ophthalmologist. If an opthalmologist is not available, the physician should institute treatment. It is critical that definitive treatment be instituted as quickly as possible, because just a few hours delay can change the prognosis from good to poor.

SUGGESTED READING

Chandler PA, Grant WM. Glaucoma. Philadelphia: Lea and Febiger, 1979.

Kolker AE, Hetherington J. Becker-Shaffer's diagnosis and therapy of the glaucomas. St. Louis: CV Mosby, 1983.

SUDDEN LOSS OF VISION

ROBERT E. LEVINE, M.D.
ALFRED M. SOLISH, M.D.

Patients who believe they have suddenly lost vision are frequently frightened and often near panic by the time they reach the emergency department or physician's office. Even if one eye is normal, a patient may have fears of living out his or her life as a blind person and will often ask "Am I going to become blind?" Indeed, in certain situations, sight may be lost needlessly in the involved eye if appropriate treatment is delayed. A systematic approach to the problem of sudden blindness is therefore imperative for the physician who initially sees the patient.

It would seem most logical to take a careful history and to examine the eye, structure by structure from front to back, to look for the etiology of the visual loss. From a practical viewpoint, however, the approach must be somewhat modified. In the case of a vascular occlusion, even minutes count. The patient with acute glaucoma may be acutely ill, and the patient with severe corneal injury is really hurting. The possibility of one of these conditions can be ruled in or out in about two minutes; we therefore recommend a brief triage-type examination as soon as the patient arrives. The triage examination also clarifies what points in the history need to be emphasized.

HISTORY

Onset of Visual Loss

Frequently, what the patient presents as a sudden loss of vision is really a sudden discovery of visual loss. Typically, something happens that causes the patient to suspect the eye has been affected or injured—e.g., blunt trauma or a foreign body. The patient then covers one eye at a time and becomes aware of a difference in vision between the two eyes. That difference may have existed for a long time, but the patient had no occasion to discover it.

Specific inquiry should be made as to when the patient was last sure the vision in the eye was good. Aside from prior medical testing, the patient may have had an eye test connected with a driver's license examination or a school or work physical.

Etiology of Visual Loss

Under what circumstances did the patient note the visual loss? Was there any antecedent old or recent cranial or ocular trauma (especially if blood is present in the anterior chamber)? Does the patient wear contact lenses? Was there any exposure to ultraviolet radiation such as a sun lamp or staring at the sun? Was the onset truly sud-

den, or did it progress over a period of time? Is there any associated pain or redness of the eye? Did the entire visual image disappear at once, or was there a progressive loss of field, like a shade coming down or up as might be seen in a slowly detaching retina? Are there any paraocular or systemic problems such as diabetes, hypertension, collagen disease, or drug use or abuse? Is all vision lost, or is some still retained? Is there a significant difference between distance and near vision?

PHYSICAL EXAMINATION

Visual Acuity

Acuity should be measured for each eye, separately, at distance and near, using any of the standard charts, as well as whatever glasses the patient has available. If the patient is unable to see even the largest letter, acuity should be noted as the distance at which the patient can count fingers and if that, too, is not possible, the distance at which he or she can see hand movements. If the acuity is still worse, it should be noted whether or not the patient can see light with each eye. It is important to use a bright light for this test and to make sure the contralateral eye is securely covered.

External Examination

Look for evidence of trauma, inflammation (perilimbal injection, miosis of the pupil, tenderness of the globe, pain on ocular movement) and corneal involvement (photophobia, lacrimation, corneal haziness, irregularity, or fluorescein staining).

Pupillary Responses

Examine the pupillary responses especially looking for an afferent pupillary defect* in the involved eye.

Red Saturation and Light Brightness Tests

Ask the patient to cover each eye separately for the red saturation and light brightness tests. In cases of optic nerve involvement, the brightness of all images decreases and red vision becomes desaturated. When a red test object (e.g., label or bottle top) is shown to the affected eye,

---

*An afferent pupillary defect is a useful sign of optic nerve disease or decreased function of a large area of the retina. Testing for this defect is based on the fact that the direct pupillary reflex (utilizing afferent pathways from the tested eye) is stronger than the consensual reflex. Normally, shining a flashlight into an eye constricts the pupil in that eye and elicits a consensual reflex in the other eye. When the light is switched to the second eye, its pupil, which is now experiencing a direct reflex, should become even more miotic. Similarly, when the light is switched back to the first eye, that pupil should be in a mildly miotic state due to the consensual reflex and should become even more miotic with the direct reflex. If the direct reflex is impaired, however, the pupil in the impaired eye, instead of constricting further when the light is moved from the contralateral eye to the impaired eye, will dilate.

the patient describes the red as "not as bright" or "darker," compared to the normal eye. Next, show a penlight to the patient and say, "If the brightness of the light you see in my hand is worth a dollar with the good eye, what is it worth with the bad eye?" In optic neuritis they might answer, "Fifty cents."

Ophthalmoscopy

Do not assume that if you cannot see the fundus through the undilated pupil that you are dealing either with cataract or vitreous hemorrhage as a cause of visual loss. A moderately dense nuclear cataract that precludes fundus visualization through a small undilated pupil may still be consistent with reasonably good vision. Comparison with the view through the contralateral pupil is often helpful. Dilation may be required to see the fundus or to localize the opacification in the media.

PROBLEMS THAT CAN CAUSE SUDDEN VISUAL LOSS

Eyelid Including the Visual Axis

In general, patients with swollen lids due to trauma, allergic reactions, infections, insect bites, etc. are aware of their lid problem and realize they can see from the eye if they open the lid manually; therefore, they do not present complaining specifically about their vision. However, an elderly patient with preexisting senile ptosis, which already lowers the lid margin to the upper aspect of the pupil, may not be aware of a sudden increase in that ptosis (e.g., partial third-nerve palsy) that makes vision impossible. Once it is established that the eye is, indeed, functional with the lid raised, further work-up would be directed to separate out the causes of the ptosis, e.g., partial third-nerve palsy, Horner's syndrome, myasthenia gravis, progressive thinning of the levator aponeurosis, etc.

Anterior Segment Problems

Loss of Corneal Clarity

This condition most often occurs acutely, as a result of trauma to the corneal epithelium. Common causes are corneal abrasion and overwearing of contact lenses (which may cause epithelial haze without actual loss of the corneal epithelium). Damage from sun lamps may not manifest for a number of hours after the treatment was carried out with inadequate eye protection. Similarly, corneal infection by such agents as herpes simplex or zoster may be severe enough to reduce vision significantly. The actual degree of visual loss in the cases of corneal epithelial involvement may vary from loss of a line or two on an eye chart in mild cases to visual reduction to 20/400 or even finger counting in severe cases. Corneal epithelial damage causes pain, photophobia, lacrimation, acute redness, fluorescein staining of the cornea (which may be subtle enough to require a slit lamp for visibility in mild cases or gross enough to be seen without the aid of blue light in severe cases), and, in the case of herpes simplex keratitis, decreased corneal sensitivity. As a result of the axon reflex response to corneal injury, the pupil may be miotic compared with the other eye.

The clarity of the corneal stroma depends on its ability to maintain a state of relative dehydration by virtue of active transport mechanisms in the corneal endothelium. Acute rises in intraocular tension, prior corneal disease, or ocular surgery, as well as the effects of blood or inflammatory cells in the anterior chamber can impair the function of the corneal endothelium, resulting in corneal edema and resultant decreased vision.

Treatment possibilities include patching the eye with an antibiotic for epithelial damage, antivirals for herpes keratitis, and treatment of the underlying problem for corneal edema.

Glaucoma

Glaucoma, a disease of the optic nerve related to elevated intraocular pressure, occurs in two forms—acute and chronic. Either form can cause sudden loss of vision. Immediate ophthalmologic examination and treatment is mandatory in acute glaucoma and advisable in the early minutes or hours of visual loss in chronic glaucoma. (See chapter on *Acute Glaucoma*.)

Blood in the Anterior Chamber

Blood in the anterior chamber (hyphema) is most commonly seen with trauma to the eye. It can also occur in conditions in which neovascularization of the iris (rubeosis iridis) occurs. These include diabetes mellitus, chronic ocular inflammation, carotid insufficiency, and prior ocular injury or surgery. There may be loss of corneal clarity due to the effect of blood and/or associated ocular inflammation on the corneal endothelium. If enough blood is present, a definite blood level can be seen. Smaller amounts of blood may require a slit lamp for visualization. Sometimes a small blood level will develop if the patient is kept seated or with the head upright in bed for a period of 60 minutes. Otherwise, the presence of a small amount of blood may be appreciated by virtue of the loss of clarity of iris detail or by slit lamp visualization.

The treatment for hyphema depends on its etiology. In those cases arising from rubeosis iridis, pan-retinal photocoagulation may be of value in reducing the production of vasoproliferative factor. This can be accomplished only after substantial clearing of the hyphema. For the short term, control of intraocular tension by medical and/or surgical means may be required. In the case of traumatic hyphema, the major concerns are the possibility of prolonged elevation of intraocular pressure with subsequent optic nerve damage, blood staining of the cornea, and re-bleeding (which usually occurs within the first 5 days after injury). The treatment consists of management of the intraocular pressure by medical and/or surgical means, bed rest, cycloplegics, topical steroids, and possibly epsilon-amino caproic acid to reduce the incidence of re-bleeding.

Any eye that has even minimal hyphema secondary to trauma should be assumed to have had a substantial injury. Ophthalmologic consultation and subsequent evaluation of the filtration angle with a gonioscope lens are mandatory. Many of these eyes have an angle recession that can lead to glaucoma many years later. Angle recession, when present, must be diagnosed so that patients can be adequately advised about the necessity for careful ophthalmologic follow-up throughout their lifetime.

Cataract

Cataract never develops acutely (except in traumatic rupture of the lens capsule, as can occur with a perforating injury). Rather, a patient may suddenly discover poor vision in the eye due to a preexisting cataract.

Treatment consists of lens extraction with possible intraocular lens implantation.

Inflammation or Infection

Decreased vision due to inflammation or infection results from haziness of the aqueous or vitreous, or both, caused by the presence of inflammatory cells. Ocular infections do not have to be endogenous to the eye (e.g., secondary to perforating traumas, ocular surgery, or corneal ulceration), but can result from metastatic dissemination from a primary source elsewhere (e.g., an infected kidney causing blood-borne pyrogenic emboli).

Anterior or posterior uveitis is associated with a wide range of systemic illnesses, principally arthritis, collagen disease, sarcoid, toxoplasmosis, lues, tuberculosis, nematode infestation, or sensitization to various microorganisms (e.g., lues).

Inflammatory signs include lid edema, conjunctival injection, chemosis, and tenderness of the globe.

Antimicrobial therapy is directed at the infection, when present, and cycloplegics and steroids (topical, subconjunctival, or systemic, as required) are used to treat the uveitis.

Vitreous Hemorrhage

When attempting to view the fundus with the ophthalmoscope, vitreous hemorrhage may be appreciated as a reddish haze in mild cases or as a black reflex in severe cases. It is usually associated with bleeding from the retinal neovascularization (proliferative diabetic retinopathy, prior vascular occlusion, sickle cell disease), retinal tear or detachment, or an ill-defined bleeding point in the retina associated with hypertensive retinopathy. When the hemorrhage is severe enough to prevent fundus examination even with the indirect ophthalmoscope, review of the history and the contralateral fundus may give a clue as to the etiology. Ultrasonography can be used to determine whether or not the retina is detached.

Treatment consists initially of bed rest and possibly bilateral patching to speed resorption of the hemorrhage. If the retina is attached, a decision to do vitrectomy is not usually made for 6 months, to allow for possible spontaneous resorption to occur. If the retina is detached, combined vitrectomy and retinal surgery is usually undertaken promptly. If the cause of the hemorrhage was neovascularization, photocoagulation may be done after the hemorrhage clears or at the time of the vitrectomy.

Retinal Detachment

Retinal detachment can occur secondary to blunt ocular trauma or spontaneously. Traction detachments can occur in patients with proliferative diabetic retinopathy. Additional rare causes of detachments include choroidal melanomas or extensive choroidal effusion associated with severe posterior uveitis (Harada's disease). Detachments are more common in patients with aphakia and high myopia and in those with family histories of retinal detachment. Typically, the patient will experience light flashes (which represent traction on the retina from the vitreous) and floaters or a cobweb (representing vitreous hemorrhage) caused by a retinal tear. As the retina detaches, the patient will become aware of a loss of the field of vision, which he or she may describe as a shade coming up or down or from the side. When the detachment extends to the macula, central vision is also lost.

The diagnosis is often suspected on the basis of history and confrontation visual fields and is readily confirmed by direct ophthalmoscopy (except when vitreous hemorrhage or other opacities are present in the ocular media, in which cases indirect ophthalmoscopy or ultrasonography may be required). If there is extensive retinal detachment, an afferent pupillary defect may be present.

Treatment consists of a gas bubble injection or scleral buckling procedure, combined with cryotherapy or diathermy, to reattach the retina. Traction detachments require vitrectomy as well. The diagnosis requires immediate ophthalmologic consultation and often admission to the hospital.

Maculopathies

Central vision may be compromised as a result of transudation of fluid or bleeding into the macular area. The patient may report distortion of images (metamorphopsia). On ophthalmoscopy, loss of the sharp foveolar reflex due to transudation of fluid may be seen. There may be a diffuse reflex and possibly even a clearly delineated fluid blister. Hemorrhage in the macula may appear red if it is anterior to the pigment epithelium and black, or green, or gray if it is subepithelial. The cause may be an idiopathic maculopathy (senile macular degeneration, serous retinopathy, subretinal neovascularization) or related to another problem in the eye (macular hemorrhage secondary to myopic degeneration, macular edema secondary to an old toxoplasmosis, blunt trauma to the eye, or ocular histoplasmosis syndrome). The condition may clear spontaneously in some patients (serous retinopathy, macular hemorrhage secondary to myopic degeneration) whereas others may require fluorescein angiography to identify a specific leaking vessel or neovascular tuft, which may be amenable to laser photocoagulation.

Vascular Occlusion

Central Retinal Artery Occlusion

This is the ocular equivalent of myocardial infarction or cerebral vascular stroke and requires urgent and intensive treatment by the first physician to see the patient. Treatment may be rewarded by restoration of vision. The condition is generally associated with atherosclerotic disease elsewhere and may, in fact, result from an atheromatous plaque coming into the central retinal artery from the carotid circulation. It can also be a manifestation of cranial (temporal) arteritis, which must be considered in every case, as it requires immediate specific treatment (intensive steroids). Inquiry should be made concerning other symptoms of cranial arteritis (scalp tenderness, pain on chewing, transient ischemic attacks). Temporal artery pulses should be palpated. Measurement of temporal artery circulation times, thermography, or ocular plethysmography may be helpful if cranial arteritis is suspected. Erythrocyte sedimentation rate measurement (which is markedly elevated in cranial arteritis) should be performed by the Westergren method. Histologic confirmation by temporal artery biopsy may be required.

Occlusion of the central retinal artery causes vision to be markedly reduced or extinguished. On viewing the fundus, the arteriolar tree may appear empty, narrow, or show very slow flow (''boxcaring''). The posterior pole appears white as a result of cloudy swelling of the ischemic retina. Because the inner layers of the retina (which are supplied by the central retinal artery) are not present at the fovea, the normal choroidal tint shows through, resulting in the so-called cherry-red spot. Because there is no way to distinguish between cloudy swelling, which is potentially reversible, and ischemic necrosis of retinal cells, which is not reversible, treatment is indicated even if hours or days have passed from the onset of visual loss.

The principles of therapy are to dislodge or dissolve the clot if possible, to dilate the artery to allow flow around the obstruction, to facilitate whatever flow may be present, and to reduce the intraocular pressure, thereby increasing the perfusion gradient. Treatment should be begun immediately by the emergency physician (Table 1). Intermittent manual massage of the globe may occasionally dislodge a clot or a plaque. Although experience with them is limited, streptokinase or other new agents capable of dissolving clots should be considered if one is still within the time frame of effectiveness of such therapy. Heparin and low-molecular-weight dextran have been used to improve the flow of the affected vessel.

The central retinal artery is thought to be affected by agents that dilate the cerebral vascular circulation, and therefore carbon dioxide has been used (either by rebreathing in a paper bag or as carbogen). The use of papaverine and similar agents is not well established, but such drugs may reasonably be considered.

The intraocular tension can be lowered by paracentesis of the anterior chamber, osmoglyn, timolol eye drops, or acetazolamide administered parenterally (500 mg IV

TABLE 1   Immediate Emergency Department Treatment of Central Retinal Artery Occlusion

If there are no contraindications to any of these procedures, perform the following:

1. Give Osmoglyn, 4 to 6 oz (depending on body weight).
2. Instill Timoptic 0.5%. I drop in the affected eye (or Betoptic or Betagan).
3. Give acetazolamide 500 mg IV over 5 minutes, then orally 250 mg q6h.
4. Check blood pressure, then start Carbogen (95% oxygen, 5% carbon dioxide) inhalation. Recheck blood pressure in 20 minutes. If no unacceptable pressure rise has occurred, continue Carbogen 20 minutes every hour, and run oxygen inhalation between Carbogen doses. If Carbogen is not immediately available, have the patient rebreathe into a paper bag for 20 minutes each hour until Carbogen can be started.
5. Massage the globe intermittently.
6. Call an ophthalmology consultant.
7. Call a cardiology consultant for advice on possible use of streptokinase or similar agent.
8. Plan to heparinize the patient as soon as the medical work-up and laboratory work are complete.
9. Arrange to admit the patient.

given over five minutes) and/or orally (500 mg initial dose, then 250 mg 4 times a day)(Table 1).

Central Retinal Vein Occlusion

Central retinal vein occlusion occurs with increased frequency in patients with hypertension, diabetes mellitus, and glaucoma. In incomplete occlusions, vision at the level of 20/100 or 20/200 may be obtained. In complete occlusions, more severe visual loss is possible.

Through the ophthalmoscope, the picture is one of venous engorgement and increased venous tortuosity with deep hemorrhages (dot and blot) in all four quadrants.

Whether any treatment is truly of value is questionable in cases of complete occlusion. In incomplete occlusion, measures to improve flow may be of help (e.g., aspirin, Persantine, heparin).

Branch Arteriolar or Venous Occlusion

Occlusion of an arteriole or branch vein in the retina may go unnoticed by the patient if it involves only the peripheral retina, but it can markedly reduce central vision if the macular area is involved. The ophthalmoscopic appearance is essentially similar to that described under central retinal artery and central retinal vein occlusion, except, or course, that the pathology is much more limited. The principles of treatment are essentially the same, except that therapies designed to increase vascular flow by vessel dilation have no role because retinal arterioles have no ability to dilate.

Inflammatory Diseases of the Retina or Choroid

Inflammatory diseases of the retina and choroid (toxoplasmosis, tuberculosis, nematode infestations, cytomegalic inclusion virus, etc.) can decrease vision by effusion into the macula, opacification of the vitreous, or direct destruction of retinal elements.

Diagnosis is made on the basis on inflammatory signs and, when possible, laboratory confirmation of the presence of an offending agent (e.g., rising serial antibody titers).

Treatment consists of therapy directed against the specific infectious agents, when known, in addition to intensive steroid therapy. In selected cases, infectious agents (e.g., toxoplasmosis or nematodes) may be destroyed by photocoagulation or cryotherapy.

Optic Neuropathies

Ischemic Optic Neuropathy

This condition is characterized by sudden loss of field of vision or central vision, or both, as the result of microvascular occlusions in the optic nerve. An afferent pupillary defect (Marcus-Gunn pupil) may be present, and red vision may be decreased. In some cases, there is blurring of the optic nerve margins. Hemorrhage at the nerve head may be present. It is doubtful that any treatment is helpful.

Retrobulbar Neuritis and Optic Neuritis

These entities, which are often described as if they were one condition, probably represent the end result of multiple etiologic pathways. In about one-third of the cases other signs of multiple sclerosis are eventually manifested. In some cases these entities may be a manifestation of cranial arteritis (check the sedimentation rate), whereas in others they may have a collagen vascular disease etiology or idiopathic cause not related to any of the foregoing.

Typically, there is sudden loss of vision, an afferent pupillary defect, and decreased ability to see red. Depending on the level at which the problem occurs, papillitis with cells in the vitreous and blurring of the optic nerve margins may or may not occur. Papillitis may be confused ophthalmoscopically with papilledema, but the latter is not associated with suddenly decreased acuity. If the process occurs further back (retrobulbar neuritis), there is pain on movement of the eye because of involve-

ment of the muscle cone. Immediate ophthalmologic consultation is needed.

Recommendations for treatment range from no treatment to intensive oral steroids. The latter therapy has been employed with dramatic apparent success in certain cases, but it has not been proved effective in any large series. There may very well be specific cases that are steroid sensitive (e.g., those secondary to a collagen disease), and it is not always possible to sort these out clinically. In our personal experience, if there are no overriding contraindications, we prefer a short trial of high-dose steroids (100 mg of prednisone a day for several days). If there is no therapeutic response, steroid therapy is abandoned. Where it is helpful, the dosage is gradually tapered.

NON-OCULAR CAUSES OF SUDDEN VISUAL LOSS

Cortical Blindness

Cortical blindness may be caused by trauma, stroke, or meningitis involving the occipital lobe. It is bilateral. Diagnosis is made on the basis of associated neurologic findings, visual field testing, computerized tomography (CT) scan, and possibly spinal fluid findings.

Treatment depends on the etiology.

Conversion Reactions, Hysteria, and Malingering

These are diagnoses of exclusion and should not be made, even when suspected, without ruling out organic disease. Malingering may be identified by specialized testing that makes it impossible for the patient to know what the correct responses should be (e.g., separation of prism images in such a way that the patient cannot tell which image is coming from which eye). Psychiatric consultation may be needed in those cases that are not self-limited.

SUGGESTED READING

Newell FW, Ernest JT. Ophthalmology principles and concepts. 3rd ed. St Louis: CV Mosby, 1974.

Vaughn D, Asbury T. General ophthalmology. 8th ed. Los Altos, CA: Lange Publishers, 1977.

MANAGEMENT OF THE CENTRAL NERVOUS SYSTEM

NEUROLOGIC ASSESSMENT IN THE EMERGENCY SETTING

JOEL D. WACKER, M.D.
MICHAEL BOWMAN, M.D., M.S.

In the emergency department the physician is called on to evaluate a wide spectrum of neurologic complaints. These conditions can range from acute to chronic, from relatively minor to life-threatening. The emergency physician must be able to evaluate the patient rapidly yet completely, to localize and diagnose the condition in order to begin therapy promptly.

In the bustle of the emergency department the examiner must develop an organized, systematic approach to the patient with neurologic complaints. The purpose of this chapter is to provide such a structural framework to enable the physician to obtain relevant information in a short period of time.

ESSENTIAL OF THE NEUROLOGIC EXAMINATION

Table 1 outlines the areas to be evaluated in any patient with neurologic complaints. Each area will be discussed in more detail subsequently.

History

A history of the patient's neurologic status prior to arrival in the emergency department and the time course of events is necessary in attempting to determine the cause of the patient's problem. History obtained from family and friends should also be sought, as the patient may be unable to give correct answers because of a depressed level of consciousness or dementia.

Events that occur over a period of *seconds to minutes* are almost always vascular in nature. Neurologic signs associated with transient ischemic attacks may have resolved by the time the patient has arrived at the emergency department. The diagnosis, though historical, must be made promptly and the patient treated aggressively to prevent a permanent, possibly disastrous cerebrovascular event.

Neurologic deterioration over a *period of days* should alert the physician to the possibility of central nervous system infection, metabolic derangement (e.g., dehydration, uremia, overmedication), or subdural hematoma. Toxic-metabolic insult should especially be considered if the patient has nonfocal, variable findings on examination.

Patients with a history of slowly progressive or chronic neurologic changes over a *period of months* cannot usually have a definitive diagnosis made in the emergency department and can be referred for a more comprehensive neurologic evaluation.

Mental Status

The screening neurologic examination is used to localize the level of nervous system involvement to

TABLE 1 Screening Neurologic Examination

Area	Assessement
History	Time course of events, previous neurologic status
Mental status	Orientation, level of consciousness
Cranial nerves	Pupillary response, funduscopic examination, extraocular movements, corneal reflex, facial movements, gag reflex
Motor response	Strength, tone, mass
Sensory examination	Pain, vibratory, position sense
Reflexes	Deep tendon, pathologic (Babinski, grasp, snout)
Coordination and gait	Gait, finger-to-nose

cerebral cortex, brain stem, cerebellum, spinal cord, or peripheral nerves.

Mental status is best assessed by engaging the patient in normal conversation to assess speech, orientation, memory, or cognitive skills (see also chapter on *Behavioral Emergencies*). While more objective assessments of cortical function can be made, these add little information to the initial mental status screening. In patients with a more severe depression in level of consciousness, the use of an objective, reproducible assessment such as the Glasgow Coma Scale is helpful in describing the patient's mental status and in identifying further deterioration on repeat examinations.

Cranial Nerves

While the olfactory nerve is not formally tested, the nose should be examined for the presence of cerebrospinal fluid (CSF) rhinorrhea. CSF may be differentiated from nasal secretions by the finding of a positive glucose dipstick response if the fluid is CSF.

Examination of the eyes and ocular movements allows the physician to assess the second, third, fourth, and sixth cranial nerves. Pupillary size and symmetry should be assessed along with direct and consensual response to light. Pupillary asymmetry of greater than 1 mm is seen in 5 percent of the normal population; however, if the asymmetry is associated with a depressed level of consciousness, the likelihood of increased intracerebral pressure with herniation is high. The fundi should be examined for papilledema and changes in the retinal vessels from diabetes or hypertension. Visual fields should be checked, as some cerebral tumors can cause field loss before any other neurologic signs. Visual fields can be assessed by having the patient and examiner look directly into each other's eyes while the examiner brings his or her fingers from the periphery to the center between them. The patient is asked to say when the fingers are first seen and this is compared with the examiner's field. The test should be performed in all four visual quadrants.

Conjugate ocular movements are controlled by the mid-brain and brain stem, and the eyes should be put through the full range of motion into the six cardinal positions of gaze. Nystagmus should also be sought. The nystagmus may be horizontal, vertical, or rotatory and, except for horizontal nystagmus on extreme lateral gaze, is abnormal.

The fifth cranial nerve is assessed by the corneal reflex. The cornea is lightly touched with a wisp of cotton and blinking of the eye is a positive response. The examiner should have the patient look away from the side the stimulus approaches and must take care to touch only the cornea; response to touching the sclera or eyelashes does not count.

The seventh cranial nerve controls the muscles of facial expression and is assessed by having the patient shut his eyes tightly, smile, or show his teeth. Peripheral lesions of the seventh nerve cause complete paralysis of the entire ipsilateral side of the face, while upper motor neuron lesions paralyze only the lower ipsilateral portion of the face.

The eighth nerve is assessed by normal auditory acuity and, if necessary, Weber and Rinne tests to differentiate conductive from neural hearing loss. In Weber's test, the handle of the vibrating tuning fork is placed upon the midline of the skull. The patient is then asked to compare the sound in the two ears. Lateralization of the sound to one ear indicates a conductive loss in that ear or a perceptive loss in the opposite ear. In the Rinne test, the handle of the vibrating tuning fork is placed over the mastoid process while the patient covers his opposite ear with his hand; the patient signals when the sound ceases, at which time the vibrating tuning fork is placed near the uncovered ear; then the patient signals when the sound ceases. Rinne-positive occurs when air conduction is greater than bone conduction. Rinne-negative occurs when bone conduction persists as long or longer than air conduction.

The external auditory canal should be examined for CSF or hemotympanum seen with basilar skull fractures in the temporal area.

The presence of a gag response is used to assess the ninth, tenth, and eleventh cranial nerves. Abnormality of the twelfth cranial nerve can be demonstrated by having the patient protrude his tongue. The tongue will deviate toward the affected side.

Motor

Muscle strength can be assessed by letting the patient actively move the muscle. If range of motion is intact, then test contraction by asking the patient to move against your resistance. The pattern of muscle weakness will help localize the lesion (Tables 2 and 3). Standing from the kneeling position or rising from a sitting position can also grossly test muscle groups for strength. Pronator drift is a sensitive screen for weakness of the upper extremity. The patient holds both arms fully extended in front of him with the palms up and maintains this with eyes closed. A drift of one palm toward pronation indicates weakness.

In addition to assessment of muscle strength, the examiner should also assess muscle mass and tone. Spasticity is indicative of an upper motor neuron lesion, while flaccid paralysis is seen with lower motor neuron lesions. The presence of fasciculations also indicates a lower neuron injury. Of far more importance than generalized weakness is the finding of asymmetry between sides of the body or between upper and lower extremities.

Sensory

The pattern of sensory changes can help delineate the location of the neurologic abnormality. Changes involving the entire half of the body are associated with lesions above the brain stem. Brain stem abnormalities are associated with facial findings on one side with involvement of the body on the other side. Complete loss of sensation below a vertebral level is seen with spinal cord injuries which are outlined in Table 4. It is important to assess perianal sensation and rectal tone in patients with suspected cord lesions. Loss of sensation or function across the upper chest and arms to a greater degree than the legs

TABLE 2 Summary of Muscle-Nerve Relationships in Upper Extremity

Segment	Muscle	Named Nerve
C5–C6	Biceps brachii	Musculocutaneous
C5–C6	Brachialis	Musculocutaneous and radial
C5–C6	Brachioradialis	Radial
C5–C6	Coracobrachialis	Musculocutaneous
C5–C6	Deltoid	Axillary
C5–C6	Infraspinatus	Suprascapular
C5–C6	Subscapularis	Upper and lower subscapular
C5–C6	Supraspinatus	Suprascapular
C5–C6	Teres major	Lower subscapular
C5–C6	Teres minor	Axillary
C6–C7	Abductor pollicis longus	Deep radial
C6–C7	Extensor carpi radialis brevis	Deep radial
C6–C7	Extensor carpi radialis longus	Radial
C6–C7	Extensor pollicis brevis	Deep radial
C6–C7	Flexor carpi radialis	Median
C6–C7	Palmaris longus	Median
C6–C7	Pronator teres	Median
C6–C7	Supinator	Deep radial
C6–C7	Extensor carpi ulnaris	Deep radial
C6–C7	Extensor digitorum	Deep radial
C6–C7	Extensor indicis	Deep radial
C6–C7	Extensor pollicis longus	Deep radial
C6–C7	Triceps brachii	Radial
C7–C8	Anconeus	Radial
C7–C8	Extensor digiti minimi	Deep radial
C7–C8	Flexor digitorum profundus	median and ulnar
C7–C8	Flexor digitorum superficialis	Median
C8–T1	Abductor digiti minimi	Deep ulnar
C8–T1	Abductor pollicis brevis	Median
C8–T1	Abductor pollicis	Deep ulnar
C8–T1	Flexor carpi ulnaris	Ulnar
C8–T1	Flexor digiti minimi	Deep ulnar
C8–T1	Flexor pollicis brevis	Median
C8–T1	Flexor pollicis longus	Median
C8–T1	Interossei	Deep ulnar
C8–T1	Lumbricales	Deep ulnar and median
C8–T1	Opponens digiti minimi	Deep ulnar
C8–T1	Opponens pollicis	Median
C8–T1	Palmaris brevis	Superficial ulnar
C8–T1	Pronator quadratus	Median

Reprinted with permission from Pansky, B, House EL. Review of gross anatomy. 3rd ed. New York: Macmillan, 1975.

is seen in traumatic central cord syndrome. Loss of sensation in the "stocking-glove" distribution is seen with peripheral neuropathies of many causes.

Reflexes

Both deep tendon and pathologic reflexes should be assessed. Again, the important finding is asymmetry of reflexes and this is associated with lesions in the reflex arc or central nervous system. Hyperreflexia and clonus are seen with upper motor neuron lesions, while absent or depressed reflexes indicate peripheral nerve or spinal cord abnormality.

Coordination and Gait

While frequently assumed to assess cerebellar function, assessment of gait involves motor and sensory con-

trol as well. Similarly, the Romberg test assesses not only cerebellar function, but also proprioception. If the patient can stand with the eyes open, but not closed, a proprioceptive abnormality is present; however, if the patient has difficulty standing with the eyes open, it points toward cerebellar dysfunction. Another useful test of cerebellar dysfunction is finger to nose testing. The examiner should tell the patient to rapidly alternate touching his nose and the examiner's finger. Provocation of tremor at the end of the movement is associated with cerebellar lesions.

Asymmetric Weakness

All too often the emergency physician is called on to evaluate the patient with complaints of paresthesias or weakness of one or more extremities. While evaluation of the peripheral nervous system seems simple, precise diagnoses of peripheral neuropathies can be time-

TABLE 3   Summary of Muscle-Nerve Relationships in Lower Extremity

Segment	Muscle	Named Nerve
L2–L3	Adductor brevis	Obturator
L2–L3	Adductor longus	Obturator
L2–L3	Gracilis	Obturator
L2–L3	Sartorius	Femoral
L2–L4	Illiacus	Femoral
L2–L4	Psoas	Nn. to psoas
L3–L4	Obturator externus	Obturator
L3–L4	Pectineus	Femoral
L3–L4	Quadriceps femoris	Femoral
L3–S1	Adductor magnus	Obturator and sciatic
L4–L5	Tibialis anterior	Deep peroneal
L4–S1	Gluteus medius	Superior gluteal
L4–S1	Gluteus minimus	Superior gluteal
L4–S1	Inferior gemellus	N. to guadratus femoris
L4–S1	Lumbricales	Medial and lateral plantar
L4–S1	Plantaris	Tibial
L4–S1	Popliteus	Tibial
L4–S1	Quadratus femoris	N. to quadratus femoris
L4–S1	Tensor fascia latae	Superior gluteal
L4–S2	Semimembranosus	Sciatic
L4–S2	Semitendinosus	Sciatic
L5–S1	Extensor digitorum longus	Deep peroneal
L5–S1	Extensor hallucis longus	Deep peroneal
L5–S1	Peroneus brevis	Superficial peroneal
L5–S1	Peroneus longus	Peroneal
L5–S1	Tibialis posterior	Tibial
L5–S2	Gluteus maximus	Inferior gluteal
L5–S2	Obturator internus	N. to obturator internus
L5–S2	Soleus	Tibial
L5–S2	Superior gemellus	N. to obturator internus
L5–S2	Biceps femoris	Sciatic
S1–S2	Abductor digiti minimi	Lateral plantar
S1–S2	Abductor hallucis	Medial plantar
S1–S2	Adductor hallucis	Lateral plantar
S1–S2	Extensor digitorum brevis	Deep peroneal
S1–S2	Extensor hallucis brevis	Deep peroneal
S1–S2	Flexor digiti minimi	Lateral peroneal
S1–S2	Flexor digitorum brevis	Medial plantar
S1–S2	Flexor digitorum longus	Tibial
S1–S2	Flexor hallucis brevis	Medial plantar
S1–S2	Flexor hallucis longus	Tibial
S1–S2	Gastrocnemius	Tibial
S1–S2	Interossei	Lateral plantar
S1–S2	Piriformis	N. to piriformis
S1–S2	Quadratus plantae	Lateral plantar

Reprinted with permission from Pansky B, House EL. Review of gross anatomy. 3rd ed. New York: Macmillan, 1975.

TABLE 4   Patterns of Spinal Injury

Cord Level	Motor Response	Sensory Area	Reflex
C3–5	Diaphragm	—	—
C6	Arm flexion	Thumb	Biceps
C7	Arm extension	Middle finger	Triceps
C8	Hand grasp	Little finger	—
T4	—	Nipple line	—
T10	—	Umbilicus	—
L2–4	Knee flexion	Anterior thigh	Quadriceps
L5	Foot dorsiflexion	Great toe	—
S1	Foot plantarflexion	Lateral foot	Gastrocnemius
S2–4	Rectal tone	Perianal area	Anal wink

consuming and elusive. The emergency physician must employ a systematic and logical approach when dealing with complaints referrable to the peripheral nervous system.

First, the physician must rule out central nervous system lesions as the cause of the patient's complaints. Careful history and neurologic examination with attention paid to cranial nerve findings is essential to exclude central lesions.

Second, the physician should attempt to localize the peripheral lesion to the nerve root, nerve itself, or nerve endings and determine whether one or more of these structures is involved. Lesions of the nerve roots will have physical findings in a dermatomal pattern. Nerve root injury is most commonly attributable to compression by a herniated disc, osteophytes, or neoplasm. Close attention must be paid to the autonomic nervous system (poor rectal tone, bowel or bladder changes) to rule out spinal cord compression, which requires prompt therapy.

Lesions of specific peripheral nerves will cause motor and sensory changes localized to well-defined areas. The motor and sensory areas of enervation of peripheral nerves are available in many sources and will not be outlined here. The causes of these mononeuropathies include traumatic disruption, compression (''Saturday night'' paralysis of the radial nerve with wrist drop, carpal tunnel syndrome), infection (herpes zoster), vasculitis, or tumor invasion.

More often the emergency physician must deal with diffuse polyneuropathies. In these cases the neurologic findings are less well defined, with sensory changes usually in a ''stocking-glove'' distribution and diffuse muscle weakness. The differential diagnosis of this disorder is quite broad, and up to as many as one-third of patients defy specific diagnosis after extensive work-up. Principal causes include toxins (heavy metals, botulism, tetanus, drugs), metabolic disorders (diabetes, uremia, amyloidosis, porphyria), alcoholism, infection (Guillain-Barre, diphtheria, leprosy) vascular disease and sarcoidosis. The physician must also differentiate between neuropathies and myopathies. Myopathies will usually involve proximal musculature to a greater degree, sensory changes are usually absent, and deep tendon reflexes are preserved. In addition, laboratory changes are more common in patients with myopathies, with elevated sedimentation rate and muscle enzymes often seen.

Finally, the emergency department physician must remember that examination of the peripheral nervous system is imprecise with subjective input on the part of both the patient and examiner. A brief neurologic assessment in the emergency department is not sufficient to make a diagnosis of a functional disorder. In doubtful cases the patient should be instructed to return if symptoms worsen or should be referred for a more detailed neurologic evaluation.

ACUTE CRANIAL NERVE LESIONS

GREGORY L. HENRY, M.D., F.A.C.E.P.

The cranial nerves constitute a diffuse group of structures that originate from the various portions of the brain itself and extend out to provide the body with specialized sensory information, motor control in the head and neck region, and certain types of autonomic innervation. When considering emergency situations involving the cranial nerves, it is important that they be viewed individually. The cranial nerves may all be affected by intrinsic central nervous system problems or may be involved by both anatomic and metabolic problems along their course after leaving the brain proper.

BASIC RULES OF ACUTE CRANIAL NERVE LESIONS

Although each cranial nerve is a distinct entity, some general principles can be stated for evaluating cranial nerve problems that have a sudden onset.

1. The sudden onset of multiple cranial nerve abnormalities is generally an acute vascular event, either hemorrhage or infarct.

2. Acute cranial nerve findings on one side of the head and neck with motor or sensory findings on the opposite side of the body constitute an alternating pattern that is virtually always a vascular lesion at the level of the brain stem.

3. The sudden onset of cranial nerve lesions with accompanying motor or sensory findings on the same or ipsilateral side of the body generally constitutes a cerebrovascular accident, either infarct or hemorrhage located above the midbrain level, usually in the region of the internal capsule or cortex.

4. Acute sixth-nerve palsies, either unilateral or bilateral, may be the result of increasing intracranial pressure, giving the false impression of a localized lesion. Whenever a sixth-nerve palsy is found, particularly with alterations of mental status, an immediate search for the presence of increased intracranial pressure is essential.

5. The slow onset of multiple cranial nerve lesions may be from various causes but should be considered neoplastic until proven otherwise.

SPECIFIC VASCULAR LESIONS OF THE BRAIN STEM

Because of the extremely complex neuroanatomy of the brain stem, relatively minute vascular lesions may cause a complex assortment of clinical signs and symptoms. A detailed knowledge of brain stem neuroanatomy and reference to a standard text may be required to delineate the precise localization of all lesions, but the most common clinical presentations are outlined in Table 1. The sudden onset of any of these syndromes is most generally the result of vascular occlusion or microhemorrhage.

Emergency Department Evaluation and Treatment

Acute brain stem dysfunction leading to suspicion of a vascular lesion requires a computed tomography (CT) scan for proper etiologic diagnosis. Because each vascular lesion in the brain stem is different, minor variations in presenting signs and symptoms may exist. By reference to standard texts, precise localization of the brain stem vascular lesions can be made. Control of hypertension or hypotension benefits the patient, as does control of any bleeding diathesis should CT scan reveal an acute hemorrhage. Consultation with a neurologist or neurosurgeon is desirable before starting any further treatment. Most cases warrant admission.

Table 1   Clinical Presentations of Vascular Lesions by Location

Clinical Findings	Anatomic Location
Paralysis of upward gaze without affecting other eye movements (Parinaud's syndrome)	Lesions of the superior colliculi (pineal tumor most frequent cause)
Ipsilateral external strabismus and ptosis with contralateral loss of vibration, pain, and temperature and contralateral ataxia and tremors (Benedikt syndrome)	Tegmentum of the midbrain affecting the oculomotor nerve, the medial lemniscus, the red nucleus, and fibers of the superior cerebellar peduncle
Paralysis of the contralateral arm and leg combined with ipsilateral external strabismus and ptosis along with ipsilateral pupillary dilatation (syndrome of Weber)	Lesion of the basal portion of the midbrain
Paralysis of the contralateral arm and leg with paralysis of the ipsilateral jaw musculature and ipsilateral anesthesia of the face (alternating trigeminal hemiplegia)	Basal portion of the pons affecting the paramedian tract and fibers of the trigeminal nerve
Contralateral paralysis of the arm, leg, tongue, soft palate, and lower portion of the face with ipsilateral jaw muscle paralysis and facial anesthesia	Basal pons extending to destroy the medial lemniscus and uncrossed fibers of the cortico-bulbar and cortico-mesencephalic tracts
Distorted or loss of hearing and cerebellar ataxia ipsilateral with progression to include ipsilateral decreased facial sensation and paralysis of all ipsilateral facial musculature	Pontocerebellar angle expanding lesion, usually tumor
Contralateral paralysis of the arm and leg, ipsilateral internal strabismus of the eye, and ipsilateral facial muscle paralysis (Millard-Gubler syndrome)	Lesion in the basal portion of the caudal pons
Contralateral paralysis of the arm and leg, ipsilateral internal strabismus of the eye, ipsilateral facial muscle paralysis, and contralateral loss of position and vibratory sense (Foville's syndrome)	Lesion in the basal portion of the caudal pons with involvement of the right medial lemniscus and right medial longitudinal fasciculus
Ipsilateral cerebellar ataxia and hypotonia, ipsilateral facial anesthesia, and contralateral body anesthesia for pain and temperature; alternating analgesia with ipsilateral loss of gag reflex and conjugate deviation of the eyes (Wallenberg's syndrome; syndrome of the posterior/inferior cerebellar artery)	Dorsal lateral portion of medulla and inferior cerebellar peduncle
Contralateral loss of pain and temperature of the body, not involving the face, with ipsilateral paralysis of the gag reflex and abnormal palate movement	Lesion in the lateral portion of the reticular formation of the upper medulla including the nucleus ambiguous and lateral spinothalamic tract
Paralysis of the ipsilateral tongue and contralateral arm and leg; alternating hemiplegia	Lesion of the basal medulla

SPECIFIC CRANIAL NERVE LESIONS

I—Olfactory

Function and Anatomy. The olfactory nerve provides the sense of smell and proceeds from the posterior portion of the nose through the ethmoid bone and back along the olfactory groove to enter the base of the brain.

Common Presenting Problems. Complaints of anosmia or decreased sense of smell are unusual in the emergency department. The olfactory nerve is an extremely difficult nerve to test in the ambulatory care setting. The most common cause of decreased olfaction is upper respiratory infection involving the nose; the other major cause is severe trauma.

Evaluation and Treatment. Traumatic loss of smell smell should be viewed in relationship to the patient's entire level of trauma. If there has been severe trauma and there is any question of cerebrospinal fluid leak, CT scanning may be required to delineate fractures in the region of the basilar skull involving the ethmoid bone. Nontraumatic alterations in the sense of smell are rarely medical emergencies.

Disposition. Patients with severe trauma resulting in anosmia require neurosurgical consultation as part of the management of potentially serious intracranial injuries. Patients with nontraumatic olfactory problems can generally be managed on an outpatient basis through consultation with an otolaryngologist or neurologist.

II—Optic Nerve

Function and Anatomy. The optic nerves are derived from the diencephalon of the brain, and pass out of the superior orbital fissures to enter the posterior portion of the orbits. They initially convey light impulses into the brain and are therefore intimately involved with vision and control the afferent limb of the pupillary light reflex.

Common Presenting Problems. Disturbances of the visual system must initially be divided into unilateral loss of vision, bilateral loss of vision, and visual field defects (see also chapter on *Sudden Loss of Vision*). A list of drugs commonly causing altered vision appears in Table 2.

Acute Visual Field Defects. Field defects, either

Table 2　Common Drugs Causing Altered Vision

Ethyl alcohol
Methyl alcohol
Quinine and quinidine
Digitalis
Iodoform
Methyl chloride
Methyl bromide
Chloramphenicol
Sulfanilamide
Ergot medications
Salicylates
Ethambutol
Isoniazid

bitemporal hemianopsia or homonymous hemianopsia and quadrantanopsia, indicate disease of the visual system at the level of the optic chiasm or posterior to it (Fig. 1). This indicates intrinsic brain disease and requires prompt neurologic evaluation to determine the cause of the visual defect. Such patients invariably require neurologic or neurosurgical consultation and rapid evaluation.

III—Oculomotor

Function and Anatomy. The oculomotor nerve exits the brain stem and proceeds through the superior orbital fissure to supply four of the six extraocular muscles of the eye, the inferior rectus, inferior oblique, medial rectus, and superior rectus and give parasympathetic innervation to the pupil (causing constriction).

Common Presenting Problems. Isolated involvement of the third cranial nerve is uncommon, but not rare. The important differentiation in looking at any third-nerve lesion is to determine whether it is complete or incomplete. A complete third-nerve palsy is one that involves extraocular muscular control, resulting in an eye that is deviated laterally and downward, accompanied by dilatation of the pupil. Incomplete third-nerve palsies are also referred to as "pupil-sparing" third-nerve palsies. In these cases the patient has the extraocular muscle involvement but the pupil remains reactive to light both directly and consensually.

Evaluation and Treatment. Patients with complete third-nerve palsies are generally suffering from lesions that are directly compressing the third-nerve along its course. This can be seen in severe head injury, in which the uncus of the temporal lobe pushes on the third-nerve, but such cases are rarely missed owing to the severe nature of the trauma received. Sudden complete third-nerve palsy without signs of major trauma should be considered an immediate neurosurgical emergency. The most likely cause is from compression of the third nerve by an aneurysm. Such patients require immediate neurosurgical referral and arteriography.

Incomplete third-nerve palsies, i.e., those that spare the pupil, are generally the results of small infarcts of the nerve. This is almost always due to diabetes mellitus. In known diabetics who present with painless incomplete third-nerve palsies, the diagnosis is essentially assured, but in any patients a blood glucose should be obtained to diagnose occult diabetes mellitus.

Disposition. Disposition depends on the diagnosis. A diabetic with incomplete third-nerve palsy may require admission for control of diabetes mellitus; a complete third-nerve palsy invariably requires further radiologic study, including CT or arteriography looking for surgically treatable lesions. No specific medication therapy is required.

IV—Trochlear Nerve

Function and Anatomy. The fourth cranial nerve (trochlear nerve) supplies motor function to the superior oblique muscle of the eye, which produces medial and

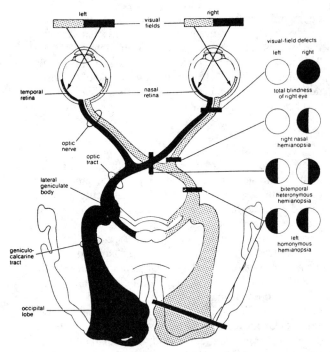

Figure 1 Lesions in the optic pathways. (Reproduced by permission from Henry GL. Seeing nothing or double. Emerg Med 1984; 160):154.

downward gaze (as in crossed eyes). It passes out of the brain stem through the superior orbital fissure and into the orbit.

Common Presenting Problems. Isolated fourth cranial nerve palsies are rare. They are generally seen in severe trauma, when the nerve itself or the trochlea of the muscle are involved. Very occasionally the vasculature of the nerve is infarcted with diabetes mellitus. In rare cases, severe hypertension, multiple sclerosis, and sickle cell anemia have been reported to cause isolated fourth-nerve palsies.

Evaluation and Treatment. Emergency evaluation should be aimed at the patient's underlying disease. Fourth-nerve palsies as a result of trauma are rarely missed owing to the extensive degree of injury required to produce such a lesion. In nontraumatic cases, not showing any signs of hypertensive encephalopathy, the vast majority of fourth-nerve palsies are the result of diabetes mellitus. Blood glucose tests should be performed on all such patients. In patients with normal blood glucose and no history of trauma who have the genetic potential for sickle cell anemia, a peripheral blood smear should be examined.

Disposition. Admission depends on etiology. Patients with diabetes that is not under control or with severe hypertension may require admission. In patients in whom a microvascular occlusion or multiple sclerosis is considered likely, further evaluation can generally be performed on an outpatient basis.

VI—Abducens Nerve

Function and Anatomy. Cranial nerve VI is considered at this time because it, along with cranial nerves III and IV, is responsible for the extraocular movements of the eyes. The sixth cranial nerve has the longest intracranial course of any of the cranial nerves and is subject to compression with diffuse increases in intracranial pressure. A sixth cranial nerve finding should be considered a sign of diffuse increased intracranial pressure until proven otherwise. Because the sixth cranial nerve innervates the lateral rectus muscle, its dysfunction produces a medially deviated eye and paralysis of lateral gaze.

Evaluation and Treatment. Sixth-nerve palsy has many potential causes (Table 3). While the various causes are being worked up, it is prudent that the patient receive thiamine 100 mg intravenously to prevent the possible onset of Wernicke's syndrome. Evaluation to determine the possibility of increased intracranial pressure, diabetes mellitus, or severe hypertension should proceed rapidly. In cases of suspected myasthenia gravis, Tensilon testing may be performed. In adults, 2 mg may be infused rapidly intravenously and, if no side effects are noted, the remaining 8 mg may be given. A positive Tensilon test produces resolution of any cranial nerve weakness for a variable period of time (from 2 to 10 minutes). Most patients with true myasthenia gravis return to their cranial nerve abnormalities within the 10-minute time frame. An isolated sixth-nerve palsy should be viewed as a lateralizing finding, therefore, lumbar puncture should be avoided until a mass lesion and increased intracranial pressure are ruled out.

Disposition. Acute sixth-nerve palsies require definitive diagnosis, which usually requires hospitalization.

V—Trigeminal Nerve

Function and Anatomy. The fifth cranial nerve divides intracranially into three principal branches: opthalmic, maxillary, and mandibular. It exits the skull to supply sensation to the face and innervation to the muscles of mastication.

Common Presenting Problems. Isolated lesions of the fifth cranial nerve resulting in complete dysfunction are rare. The fifth cranial nerve may be involved in tumors that involve the brain stem, but multiple cranial nerves are usually affected. When three divisions are involved, it is generally a massive injury. Irritative lesions of the fifth cranial nerve may include constant hemifacial pain

Table 3 Causes of Unilateral Sixth Nerve Palsy

Increased intracranial pressure: tumor, trauma, infection (meningitis)

Arteriosclerosis: hypertension

Diabetes mellitus

Multiple sclerosis

Myasthenia gravis (early)

Syphilis

Wernicke's syndrome due to thiamine deficiency

Post-lumbar puncture

Arteriovenous malformations

with decreased sensory loss on the involved side and partial Horner's syndrome; this syndrome is called Raeder's paratrigeminal syndrome. Various other irritative conditions of the fifth cranial nerve can cause intermittent severe pain (tic douloureux).

Evaluation and Treatment. In patients with Raeder's paratrigeminal syndrome, evaluation revolves around isolating the cause for irritation of the nerve, which generally requires sophisticated x-ray evaluation. Pain control in Raeder's syndrome may be obtained with the use of phenytoin 200 to 400 mg daily or carbamazepine 400 to 1,200 mg daily. Surgical correction of the underlying process is often required.

Tic doulourex patients often undergo devastating amounts of pain. Narcotic agents such as meperidine (Demerol) or codeine may be required during an attack. Long-term improvement in trigeminal neuralgia can often be provided by (1) phenytoin 200 to 400 mg daily; (2) carbamazepine 400 to 1,200 mg daily; or (3) baclofen 5 to 10 mg 3 times a day. Perhaps 20 percent of trigeminal neuralgia patients do not receive adequate relief of pain with medications. Such patients may respond well to surgical intervention with electrocoagulation of the gasserian ganglion or microsurgical decompression of the trigeminal nerve.

Disposition. Management of trigeminal neuralgia patients may be handled on an outpatient basis once pain is controlled. Raeder's syndrome patients may require inpatient evaluation depending on the availability of sophisticated studies and the degree of pain the patient is experiencing.

VII—Facial Nerve

Function and Anatomy. The seventh cranial nerve provides innervation to the facial musculature. It also provides taste to the anterior two-thirds of the tongue, sound-dampening control through the innervation of the stapedius muscle, and parasympathetic fibers to various salivary glands.

Common Presenting Problems. Upper motor neuron seventh-nerve problems involve only the musculature to the lower half of the face and are almost always seen in conjuction with cerebrovascular accidents that affect motor fibers involving other portions of the body. Lower motor neuron seventh-nerve lesions (complete seventh-nerve lesions) represent involvement of the nerve after it exits the brain stem. Depending on the localization of the compression, all of the nerve functions can be impaired.

Evaluation and Treatment. Upper motor neuron seventh-nerve lesions require prompt evaluation for intracranial lesions. No specific therapy should be initiated until a proper diagnosis is made.

Lower motor neuron seventh-nerve lesions require careful evaluation for the involvement of other cranial nerves. Compressive lesions, such as tumors almost always involve the fifth, sixth, or eighth cranial nerves as well. Once isolated involvement of the postnuclear seventh nerve has been established, treatment may be given. Idiopathic facial palsy (*Bell's palsy*) has a greater than 90 percent incidence of spontaneous improvement. Therapy with corticosteroids recommended, and may be started with prednisone 60 mg for 5 days and gradually tapered over 10 to 14 days. Facial spasms can occur as a late complication of idiopathic facial palsy. Sedation with diazepam 5 to 10 mg 4 times a day or phenobarbital 30 to 60 mg 3 times a day has been advocated. In patients with Bell's palsy, artificial tear solutions as well as taping of the eyelid during sleep should be used to prevent drying of the cornea and subsequent ulceration.

Disposition. Patients with isolated seventh-nerve lesions and no evidence of other cranial nerves involved, can usually be started on their steroid therapy, and with proper follow-up, assured can be followed in an outpatient setting.

VIII—Auditory Nerve

Function and Anatomy. The eighth cranial nerve carries sensation from the inner ear structures to the brain stem. The auditory nerve has two distinct components: a vestibular nerve and a cochlear nerve. The vestibular branch of the auditory nerve is involved in carrying information about body position from the semicircular canals into the vestibular nuclei. The cochlear division of the eighth nerve carries information about sound from the cochlea to its respective brain stem nuclei.

Common Presenting Problems. Acute involvement of the cochlear division may present with abnormally loud sounds with a recruitment phenomenon and gradually progressive decrease in hearing. Acute loss of hearing may be the only finding in certain lesions of the cochlear branch of the nerve.

Acute *vestibular symptoms* are somewhat dependent on their location along the end-organ semicircular canals and the nerve, but usually include vertigo and nausea.

Nystagmus. All forms of nystagmus require some brain stem deviation mechanism with a cortical correction component. Acute nystagmus problems are usually related to chemical ingestants, such as alcohol or drugs, or may be related to stimulation of the vestibular nuclei through the eighth cranial nerve. This may be due to irritation of the semicircular canal or lesions along the nerve itself. In certain patients, even middle ear infections, or pressure against the tympanic membrane from cerumen impactions can cause nystagmus.

An important point in diagnosing new-onset nystagmus is that chemically induced nystagmus from ingested drugs is generally horizontal in nature, and can be reproduced by lateral gaze. Nystagmus secondary to irritation of the eighth nerve, and semicircular canals, is generally reproduced only by movement of the head, and such patients often feel considerably better when the head is at rest. Nystagmus secondary to structural lesions in the brain stem itself is rarely associated with feelings of vertigo, usually is nonfatiguable, may be multidirectional, and is not dependent on the movement of the head.

Evaluation and Treatment. Sudden hearing loss may be divided into bilateral and unilateral causes (Table

4). The emergency department evaluation essentially involves ruling out treatable causes of hearing loss. Meniere's disease should include treatment with an anti-motion sickness drug. Meclizine 12.5 to 25 mg twice a day, dimenhydrinate 25 to 50 mg 4 times a day, or scopolamine as a transdermal preparation 0.5 mg may all be effective. Patients with incapacitating symptoms often respond to diazepam 2 to 5 mg given slowly intravenously, which inhibits the brainstem centers. Patients should concomitantly be treated with a low-salt diet and evaluation by an otolaryngologist should be obtained. Severe cases of Meriere's disease may require surgical ablation of the nerve. Other causes of peripheral vertigo such as acute viral labyrinthitis may also be treated with the same drug regimens.

Disposition. Patients with acute Meniere's disease or vestibular-type vertigo from other causes may require hospitalization for control of their nausea and vomiting. Further work-up, however, for underlying etiologies can usually be performed on an outpatient basis.

IX—Glossopharyngeal Nerve

Function and Anatomy. The glossopharyngeal nerve leaves the skull through the jugular foramen and along the musculature of the pharynx and larynx to supply the sensory nerve from the mucosa of the tonsil, soft palate, and posterior one-third of the tongue. Cranial nerve IX also supplies motor innervation to the stylopharyngeus muscle, and to the striated muscles of the pharynx.

Common Presenting Problems. The ninth cranial nerve is rarely involved as an isolated entity. Compressive lesions of the lower brain stem may involve multiple cranial nerves, causing problems with swallowing. Problems with swallowing require, however, that causes of esophageal dysfunction and obstruction, and life-threatening causes of weakness, such as myasthenia gravis, be ruled out first. An unusual entity, similar to tic douloureux of the fifth nerve, is called glossopharyngeal neuralgia. This syndrome gives intense short bursts of pain to the sensory distribution areas in palate and throat.

Evaluation and Treatment. When cranial nerve IX dysfunction is suspected, evaluation of the lower brain stem is necessary, looking for concomitant cranial nerve and cerebellar lesions. Without other findings, an isolated glossopharyngeal tic may be treated with phenytoin 200 to 400 mg daily or carbamazepine 400 to 1200 mg daily.

Disposition. Patients with acute isolated cranial nerve glossopharyngeal tic may be treated as outpatients following control of their initial pain. Patients with lower brain stem findings in conjunction with their glossopharyngeal involvement require evaluation to determine the exact cause of the brain stem lesion.

X—Vagus Nerve

Function and Anatomy. Isolated lesions of the vagus nerve are extremely rare. Lesions of the nerve are usually seen in conjuction with other brain stem symptoms, but may present early on with dysarthria and dysphonia. With bilateral involvement of the lower brain stem swallowing and breathing may constitute such a problem that tracheostomy is required.

Evaluation and Treatment. Evaluation of the exact nature of the brain stem lesion is required before any specific therapy can be instituted.

Disposition. Patients with tenth cranial nerve lesions are generally admitted for sophisticated posterior fossa studies. It should be noted that in severe syringobulbia, and in the last stages of amyotrophic lateral sclerosis, the vagus nerve can be severely involved.

XI—Accessory Nerve

Function and Anatomy. The accessory nerve exits through the jugular foramen and supplies innervation to the sternocleidomastoid and trapezius muscles. Along with its bulbar component, the eleventh cranial nerve has a large spinal component derived from the upper cervical segments. Isolated involvement of the accessory nerve is extremely rare. The accessory nerve is generally injured by vascular syndromes involving the lower four cranial nerves, or compressive lesions affecting the brain stem or the jugular foramen.

Evaluation and Treatment. Evaluation in the emergency department basically involves looking for other lower cranial nerve lesions.

Disposition. Patients with accessory nerve lesion require extensive studies of the posterior fossa.

Table 4 Sudden Loss of Hearing

Sudden Bilateral Central Neurologic Hearing Loss	Sudden Unilateral Hearing Loss
Meningitis	Direct head trauma and acoustic trauma
System infections	Meniere's disease
Ototoxic drugs	Viral illness
Multiple sclerosis	Spontaneous rupture of the round-window membrane or inner ear membrane
Congenital syphilis	Vascular disorders
Idiopathic	Postsurgical
Hysterical	Postanesthesia

XII—Hypoglossal Nerve

Function and Anatomy. The hypoglossal nerve leaves the brain stem, exits the skull through the hypoglossal canal, and then passes to the muscles of the tongue.

Common Presenting Problems. The hypoglossal nerve can occasionally be injured in severe basilar skull fractures or dislocations of the upper cervical vertebrae as well as through the usual peripheral neuropathic mechanisms. Nuclear and supernuclear lesions are the result of brain stem pathology and generally involve the lower four cranial nerves.

Evaluation and Treatment. Evaluation revolves around examination of the lower brain stem for neoplastic or vascular disease injuries.

Disposition. Patients with acute hypoglossal nerve injuries either isolated or in combination with injuries, to the other lower cranial nerves, need immediate evaluation for the possibility of brain stem or cortical damage.

SUGGESTED READING

Daly DD. Cerebral localization. In: Baker AB, Baker LH, eds. Clinical neurology. New York Harper Row, 1985.

DeJong RN. The neurological examination. 4th ed. New York: Harper Row, 1979.

Henry G, Little N. Neurological emergencies: a symptom oriented approach. New York: McGraw-Hill, 1985.

Toole JF, Cole M. Ischemic cerebrovascular disease. In: Baker,Baker. eds. Clinical neurology. New York: Harper Row, 1985.

Youmans JR, Albrand OW. Cerebral blood flow in clinical problems. In: Youmans JR, ed. Neurological surgery. Philadelphia: WB Saunders, 1973.

FOCAL NEUROLOGIC DEFICIT

GREGORY L. HENRY, M.D., F.A.C.E.P.

Whenever a focal deficit is found during an ambulatory or emergency department evaluation, the physician should be immediately suspicious of a structural neurologic lesion. There are occasional focal deficits caused by metabolic illness, but these are the exception and not the rule. The first obligation of the emergency physician is to rule out a rapidly progressing anatomic lesion that might be arrested or reversed by immediate surgical or medical therapy. This chapter will describe the rapid evaluation of focal deficits, with the exception of the special sense organs, i.e., vision, hearing, and smell, which are covered in other chapters.

Once a reasonable history has been taken and a general physical and neurologic examination performed, the physician must proceed along a structured, algorithmic approach. The first question to ask is whether the patient's neurologic deficit can be defined by one anatomic site, or whether it must be the result of multiple unrelated anatomic sites. For example, numbness in one arm with a lack of strength in the opposite leg cannot easily be explained by one lesion in the central nervous system. Similarly, diplopia and weakness in one leg cannot be explained by one lesion. When such diverse findings are encountered, the possibility of multiple anatomic sites must be entertained. *Mononeuritis multiplex* is the term given to the involvement of multiple nerves appearing simultaneously. This is generally caused by exacerbations of systemic diseases that cause vascular compromise to the peripheral nerves. Such injury to the blood vessels may cause unusual patterns of widely diffuse focal deficits. The causes of mononeuritis multiplex include diabetes mellitus, rheumatoid arthritis, polyarteritis nodosa, sarcoidosis, tuberculosis, and Waldenström's disease.

Another possibility whenever multiple anatomic sites are noted is *multiple sclerosis*. The diagnosis of multiple sclerosis generally cannot be made on a first visit to an emergency department, but it can certainly be suspected when diffuse neurologic complaints are noted which generally involve sites both above and below the foramen magnum. Multiple sclerosis can usually be differentiated from mononeuritis multiplex in that it involves deep central nervous functioning, such as vision and coordination of eye movements, and is generally not associated with specific peripheral nerve lesions.

The third diagnostic possibility, and one that may vary from patient population to population, is the functional or *psychiatric patient*. Extremely sophisticated patients may mimic multiple neurologic deficits and pose a difficult diagnostic dilemma in the emergency department.

SINGLE ANATOMIC SITES

Patients may have multiple areas of neurologic loss which can be explained by one anatomic lesion. An entire side of the body may be left without sensation or motor function based on a single intracerebral vascular event. The function of the emergency physician is to rapidly localize the site of anatomic loss and proceed to identify the most appropriate differential diagnosis, searching for those causes that are most amenable to therapy. Table 1 lists the various areas of focal deficit and their most probable anatomic location.

Cerebral lesions that lie on the *cortex* or in the *internal capsule* generally produce loss of motor function, sensation, or both on the contralateral side of the body, including the face, neck, and trunk. Such obvious findings rarely represent diagnostic dilemmas to the emer-

TABLE 1 Focal Weakness

Area of Weakness	Location
Unilateral face, arm, leg (hemiplegia)	Cortex, internal capsule, rarely brain stem
Unilateral face, contralateral arm and leg	Brainstem
Bilateral arm and leg without neck and head (quadriplegia)	Cervical spinal cord, rarely medulla or pons
Weakness in arms bilaterally without involvement of the head, neck, or legs (diplegia)	Central cord syndrome or syringomyelia of the cervical spinal cord
Legs bilaterally without involvement of upper body or head (paraplegia)	Thoracic or lumbar spinal cord
Contralateral weakness one leg, with decreased pin and temperature sensation in ipsilateral leg	Hemisection of spinal cord (Brown-Séquard syndrome)
Unilateral or bilateral single dermatome weakness with associated sensory changes	Spinal-nerve-root lesion
Specific peripheral nerve, with associated sensory findings	Isolated peripheral nerve
Isolated arm or leg (monoplegia)	Pons, occasionally central cortex, spinal cord; small lesion, extremely rare

Reprinted by permission from Henry G, Little N. Neurologic emergencies: a symptom oriented approach. New York: McGraw-Hill, 1985:111.

gency physician when the completed syndrome is present. Of greater importance in the well-being and prognosis of the patient, however, is the transient ischemic attack. If a patient presents with a history of short-term loss of functioning, whether it be motor or sensory, which rapidly clears and sounds as if it may involve a cerebral or cortical pattern, the possibility of a transient ischemic attack must be considered. Such patients are at risk of progressing to a full cortical infarct and deserve rapid evaluation for the possibility of a surgically correctable lesion and/or anticoagulation therapy. Because of the highly regional nature of the brain, small structural lesions may cause extremely specific neurologic loss. Table 2 illustrates some common neurologic deficits associated with specific anatomic sites on the cerebral cortex.

Structural lesions in the brain stem may lead to extremely diverse and sometimes confusing symptoms. Because of the nature of crossed and uncrossed fibers at the various levels of the brain stem, tracts may be involved in both a crossed and an uncrossed fashion. Thus, patients may have sensory or motor findings on one side of the face and on the opposite side of the body. This crossed pattern, whether it be motor or sensory, should always be thought of as a brain stem type lesion until proven otherwise. Many of these patterns have been well recognized and described. Table 3 lists the most common brain

TABLE 2 Selected Functional Losses with Localized Cortical Lesions

Area of Involvement	Functional Loss with Destructive Lesion
Frontal lobes:	Contralateral:
Motor area	Loss of voluntary motor control
Premotor area	Paresis, mostly distal and mostly in fine, skilled movements
Frontal eye fields	Inability to turn eyes to contralateral side
Motor speech area (Broca) (dominant hemisphere)	Expressive dysphasia-aphasia
Parietal lobe:	
Sensory receptive area (postcentral gyrus)	Raised threshold, or poor discrimination, but not loss of sensation to pin, hot, cold
	Impairment of two-point discrimination
	Inability to recognize letters or numbers written on skin (agraphesthesia)
	Inability to localize tactile sensation (topagnosis)
	Sensory extinction to simultaneously applied stimuli
	Inability to recognize form and nature of objects by touch (astereognosis)
	Inability to identify or orient body parts (somatotopagnosia)
	Inability to recognize disease or dysfunction of body part (anosognosia)
Optic radiations	Inferior quadrant visual field defect
Angular gyrus	Loss of visual guidance for such functions as writing or drawing (constructional apraxia)
Angular gyrus (dominant hemisphere)	Loss of meaning for printed words (alexia)
Temporal lobe:	
Auditory receptive area (transverse temporal gyrus)	Poor sound localization (never deafness)
Wernicke's area (superior temporal gyrus of dominant hemisphere)	Loss of ability to understand spoken words (auditory receptive aphasia)
Optic radiations	Contralateral superior quadrant visual field loss
Occipital lobe:	
Visual receptive area (calcarine fissure)	Contralateral visual field loss

Reprinted by permission from. Henry G, Little N. Neurologic emergencies: a symptom oriented approach. New York: McGraw-Hill, 1985:75

TABLE 3 Named Focal Brain Stem Syndromes

Common Name	Area Involved	Symptoms	Eponym	Common Causes
Lateral medullary syndrome	Lateral medulla	Whirling dizziness Dysarthria Dysphagia (Ipsilateral palate weakness) Ipsilateral facial numbness and loss of coronal reflex Contralateral body numbness Rarely diplopia Ipsilateral facial paresis	Wallenberg's syndrome	Vertebral artery occlusion; posterior-inferior cerebellar artery occlusion
Medial medullary syndrome	Medial medulla	Contralateral hemiparesis Contralateral loss of position and vibration Retention of pain and temperature Ipsilateral tongue paralysis		Vertebral artery occlusion
	Lateral mid pons	Ipsilateral facial paralysis Ipsilateral paralysis of gaze Contralateral hemiplegia ±Contralateral proprioceptive loss	Foville's syndrome	Anterior-inferior cerebellar artery occlusion; multiple sclerosis
Ventral pontine syndrome	Lateral inferior pons	Ipsilateral lateral rectus palsy Ipsilateral facial paralysis Contralateral hemiplegia ±Contralateral proprioceptive loss	Millard-Gubler syndrome	Anterior-inferior cerebellar artery occlusion; pontine glioma
	Lateral inferior pons	Ipsilateral lateral rectus palsy Contralateral hemiplegia ±Contralateral proprioceptive loss	Raymond's syndrome	Anterior-inferior cerebellar artery occlusion
	Oculomotor nucleus and corticospinal tract, midbrain	Ipsilateral third-nerve palsy Contralateral hemiplegia	Weber's syndrome	
	Tegmentum and base of midbrain	Ipsilateral third-nerve palsy Ipsilateral hyperkinesis (tremor, chorea, athetosis) Contralateral hemiplegia	Benedikt's syndrome	Small-vessel vascular occlusion
Syndrome of superior colliculus	Midbrain–superior colliculus	Paralysis of conjugate Upward gaze ±Eyelid retraction	Parinaud's syndrome	Posterior third-ventricular tumors; pinealomas; multiple sclerosis
Syndrome of medial longitudinal fasciculus	Medial longitudinal fasciculus from medulla to midbrain	Paralysis of adduction of contralateral eye on attempted ipsilateral gaze Normal convergence of same eye Nystagmus–mild paresis of abducting ipsilateral eye	Internuclear ophthalmoplegia	Isolated bilaterally; multiple sclerosis isolated unilaterally; small-vessel vascular occlusion
	Sympathetic fiber pathways in lateral brain stem; spinal cord; cervical sympathetic chain; postganglionic fibers	Ipsilateral miosis Ipsilateral ptosis Ipsilateral anhydrosis Apparent enophthalmos	Horner's syndrome	Many causes depending on location of involvement

Reprinted by permission from Henry G, Little N. Neurologic emergencies: a symptom oriented approach. New York: McGraw-Hill, 1985:79, 80 stem syndromes and their anatomic locations. The important thing to remember is that whenever crossed findings are located, a vascular problem of the brain stem should be assumed.

Lesions of the *spinal cord* may be complete or incomplete, but generally present with either a specific level or involvement of specific tracts. An example of tract involvement is weakness of the arms bilaterally but sparing of the legs, which can be seen in traumtic central cord syndrome or syringomyelia. Compressive lesions on the cervical cord generally involve arm function bilaterally, as well as motor and sensory function in the trunk and legs. Lesions of the thoracic and lumbar spine generally spare the arms but will involve the trunk and leg depending on their anatomic location. Lesions of the spinal cord can usually be isolated within two disc segments at examination when a definitive sensory level can be found. Rarely, lateral hemisection or compression of the cord may occur, causing a classic Brown-Séquard syndrome, which is delineated by an ipsilateral weakness and decrease in vibratory and position sense with a contralateral loss of pin and temperature sensation. Specific anatomic levels of spinal cord involvement require immediate diagnosis to prevent further injury to the cord. The principal rule overlying an emergency physician's response to spinal cord lesions should be rapid evaluation to rule out the possibility of reversible disease. Although traumatic compression, compression from tumors, and infection are the most common causes of spinal cord injuries, many other etiologic agents may be involved less frequently. The possible causes of acute myelitis or myelopathy include primary infections (viral, bacterial, rickettsial, fungal, parasitic); postinfectious; toxic; radiation; electrical injury; trauma; cancer; compression or spondylosis; nutritional deficit; or congenital defect.

Nervous tissue can also be involved at the root, plexus, or specific *peripheral nerve* level. Whenever a nerve root is involved, the findings generally follow the segmental sensory dermatomes. Isolated peripheral nerves are generally injured by direct trauma, compression, or through vascular compromise. Careful physical examination is often required to separate what is a true peripheral nerve from a more proximal root or plexus lesion (Fig. 1). The common nerve entrapments are listed in Table 4.

CAUSES OF ACUTE FOCAL NEUROLOGIC DEFICITS

Once the anatomic site has been localized, the exact cause needs to be determined (Table 5). Here, the *rapidity of onset* is very helpful. The overriding rule should be that anything that occurs over seconds to minutes in the nervous system is vascular in origin. Such patients often have evidence of vascular disease throughout the body, and may have had previous episodes. The *anatomic site* also helps determine the cause. Sudden central nervous system disease of a cortical or subcortical or brain stem nature is almost always vascular. Such knowledge does not differentiate acute infarction from hemorrhage, but does determine the necessity for a rapid study that can evaluate the brain for acute vascular damage.

Tumors, in and of themselves, are rarely the cause of acute deficits in the central nervous system. Sudden hemorrhage into a tumor, however, may cause expansion or exacerbation of a mass lesion. Tumors may also reach a critical size at which they begin to compromise the vascular supply of other surrounding areas. Acute hydrocephalus, caused by an expanding tumor, may also present as a focal deficit.

Abscess may present a confusing picture. They may or may not cause signs and symptoms of an acute infection suggesting meningoencephalitis, and will most always have features suggesting a mass lesion. A brain abscess is one of the most rapidly expanding lesions inside the intracranial cavity and may cause abnormally increased pressure. Patients suspected of brain abscess should have a computed tomography scan or brain scan to rule out its presence before a spinal tap is attempted.

Seizure patients will frequently present to the emergency department in a postictal state. As the brain recovers, those areas most involved with the seizure focus may retain dysfunction even after the patient has regained full consciousness. Such transient paralyses, known as Todd's paralysis, may give clues as to the location of the patient's seizure focus. Such a paralysis may be very short-lived, but in certain patients the Todd's paralysis may last for days. A postictal paralysis implies

TABLE 4 Nerve Entrapment Syndromes

Syndrome	Signs and Symptoms
Carpal tunnel syndrome (median nerve)	Tingling in the hand–first, second, third, and one-half of fourth digit; late muscular wasting, thenar area
Pronator syndrome (median nerve at the muscle	Pain from the elbow to the wrist; weakness in thenar muscles
Ulnar nerve–wrist	Paresthesias, fourth and fifth fingers; atrophy, intrinsic muscles of the hand
Ulnar nerve–elbow	Same as ulnar nerve–wrist, plus decreased strength in ulnar deviation of the hand at the wrist
Radial nerve	Weakness of the finger extension and wrist extension
Lateral cutaneous nerve of the thigh	Numbness in the lateral part of the thigh
Posterior tibial (tarsal tunnel)	Numbness of the soles of the feet; decreased sensation
Bell's facial-nerve palsy	Weakness of facial musculature all divisions of the seventh cranial nerve ipsilateral to the lesion

Reprinted by permission from. Henry G, Little N. Neurologic emergencies: a symptom oriented approach. New York: McGraw-Hill, 1985:112

a focal or structural source of the seizure and should be followed aggressively. The patient who seizes for the first time and is left with any focal deficit residual requires evaluation for the possibility of an intracranial mass or vascular lesion.

Metabolic disorders only rarely result in focal neurologic lesions. This usually occurs in the setting of previous neurologic damage where there are marginal areas of recovery that are sensitive to substrates that control immediate brain metabolism, i.e., glucose and oxygen. Likewise, areas that are highly susceptible to osmolar changes and swelling may be affected by changes in blood glucose and sodium concentrations.

Multiple sclerosis is essentially a diagnosis of exclusion. Multiple sclerosis may cause dysfunction at one anatomic site which clears rapidly. Without a previous history of multiple such events in many areas of the body a diagnosis of multiple sclerosis in the patient with a focal neurologic lesion is essentially impossible in the emergency department.

Finally, the *psychiatric patient* who is both medically wise and convinced of his own illness may present a difficult diagnostic dilemma in the emergency department. Again, a psychiatric cause for a focal neurologic lesion should always be a diagnosis of exlusion and thought of only after treatable conditions have been considered and ruled out.

TREATMENT

The causes of specific focal neurologic deficits are as varied as the deficits themselves. Some general rules of therapy can be listed, however. Definitive therapy can be based only on an accurate diagnosis. Sudden intracerebral deficits require immediate evaluation for the possibility of neurosurgical repair.

TABLE 5 Causes of Acute Focal Neurologic Deficit

Vascular (arterial thrombosis, intra- and extracranial vasculitis compression)
   Venous thrombosis
   Arterial embolism
   Intracerebral hemorrhage; aneurysm, (AVM), hypertension, coagulopathy
   Subdural hematoma
   Epidural hematoma
Tumors
   Primary (gliomas, meningiomas, pituitary)
   Metastatic (lung, breast, melanoma, choriocarcinoma, renal)
Abscesses (subdural intracerebral and spinal epidural)
   Bacterial
   Parasitic
   Fungal
Postseizure
Migraine
Bell's palsy
Cardiovascular (to marginal flow areas)
   Hypovolemia
   Arrhythmia
Metabolic (locally susceptible areas)
   Hypoxia
   Hypoglycemia
   Hyponatremia
   Hyperosmolar-nonketotic hyperglycemia
Psychogenic
Multiple sclerosis

Reprinted by permission from. Henry G, Little N. Neurologic emergencies: a symptom oriented approach. New York: McGraw-Hill, 1985: 81

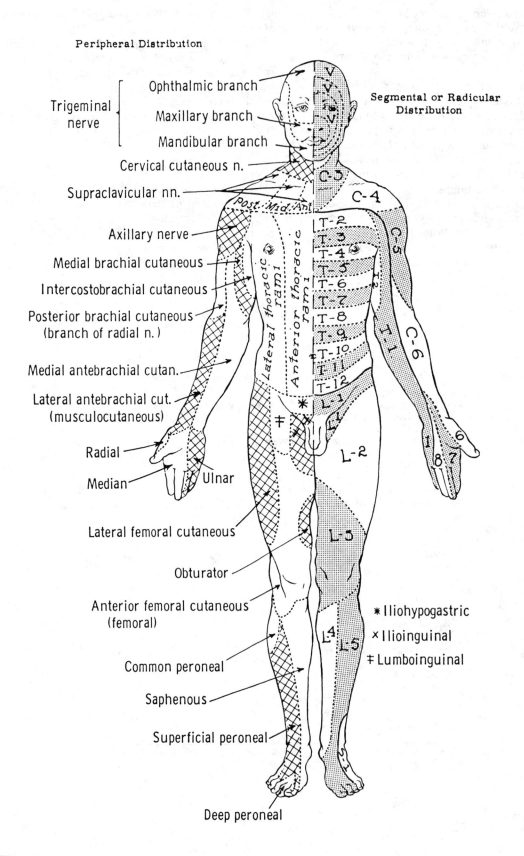

Peripheral Distribution

Segmental or Radicular Distribution

Trigeminal nerve
- Ophthalmic branch
- Maxillary branch
- Mandibular branch

Cervical cutaneous n.

Supraclavicular nn.

Axillary nerve

Medial brachial cutaneous

Intercostobrachial cutaneous

Posterior brachial cutaneous (branch of radial n.)

Medial antebrachial cutan.

Lateral antebrachial cut. (musculocutaneous)

Radial

Median — Ulnar

Lateral femoral cutaneous

Obturator

Anterior femoral cutaneous (femoral)

Common peroneal

Saphenous

Superficial peroneal

Deep peroneal

Post. Mid. Ant.

Lateral thoracic rami

Anterior thoracic rami

C-3
C-4
T-2
T-3
T-4
T-5
T-6
T-7
T-8
T-9
T-10
T-11
T-12
L-1
L-1
C-5
C-6
L-2
L-3
L-4
L-5

* Iliohypogastric
× Ilioinguinal
‡ Lumboinguinal

Figure 1 *A,* and *B,* Cutaneous innervation. From Chusid JG: Correlative neuroanatomy and functional neurology. 17th ed. Los Altos, California: Lange Medical Publishing, 1979:210,211.

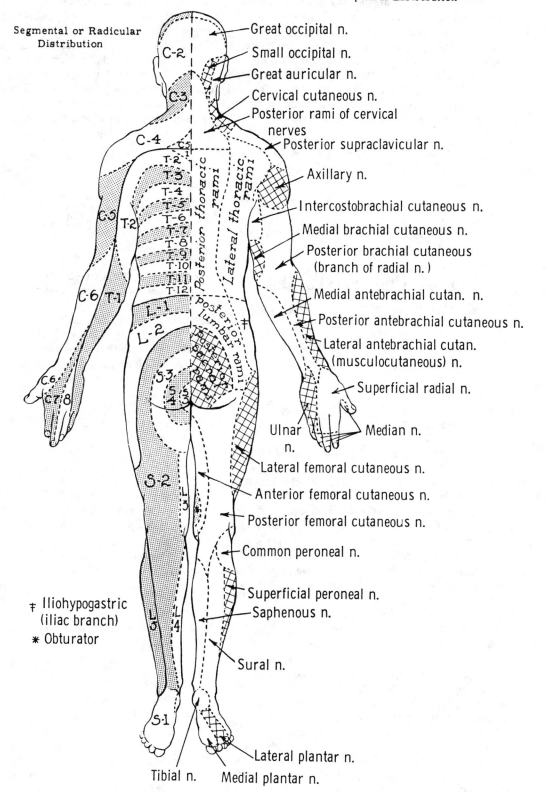

Peripheral Distribution

Segmental or Radicular
Distribution

Great occipital n.

Small occipital n.

Great auricular n.

Cervical cutaneous n.

Posterior rami of cervical
nerves

Posterior supraclavicular n.

Axillary n.

Intercostobrachial cutaneous n.

Medial brachial cutaneous n.

Posterior brachial cutaneous
(branch of radial n.)

Medial antebrachial cutan. n.

Posterior antebrachial cutaneous n.

Lateral antebrachial cutan.
(musculocutaneous) n.

Superficial radial n.

Median n.

Ulnar n.

Lateral femoral cutaneous n.

Anterior femoral cutaneous n.

Posterior femoral cutaneous n.

Common peroneal n.

Superficial peroneal n.

Saphenous n.

Sural n.

Lateral plantar n.

Medial plantar n.

Tibial n.

† Iliohypogastric
(iliac branch)
* Obturator

It is always worthwhile to make certain that general oxygenation of the patient is good and that blood pressure control is neither too low nor dangerously high. In the normotensive patient without obvious signs of hypovolemia, overhydration should be avoided.

The use of anticoagulation therapy in presumed vascular occlusive disease should await definitive diagnosis so that an acute hemorrhagic disease has been ruled out. A definitive study to exclude bleeding is appropriate prior to beginning any medications. There is little or no reason to perform a spinal tap for a focal neurologic lesion in the awake patient in the emergency department, and to do so for a focal lesion in an obtunded patient can cause brain stem herniation and death.

Lastly, the true nature of a patient's focal deficit may be lost without frequent re-examinations. The waxing and waning character of focal deficits, such as seen in Bell's palsy, migraine headache, seizures, and metabolic disease, will help to define the location and cause of the patient's problem more clearly and will help the emergency physician determine the speed with which medical therapy or neurosurgical evaluation is required.

THE COMATOSE PATIENT

JOHN J. CARONNA, M.D.

Coma is a symptom of a broad spectrum of life-threatening conditions that depress or injure the central nerous system (CNS). The locus of CNS dysfunction may be in the cerebral hemispheres, the brain stem, or a combination of both. Appropriate therapy of coma is dependent on accurate analysis of the underlying cause of the unconscious state.

Diagnosis in the unconscious patient presents a major challenge. Often there is little information available concerning either the circumstances of coma or the previous medical history of the patient. The physical examination and the response of the patient to simple diagnostic and therapeutic maneuvers, in most cases, will enable the clinician to limit the differential diagnosis to one of several major categories and to institute appropriate management.

DEFINITION OF COMA

When a toxic-metabolic process or structural lesion interrupts impulses from the ascending reticular formation to the hemispheres, making arousal impossible, stupor or coma results. The comatose patient maintains a sleep-like unresponsiveness from which he cannot be aroused; eye opening does not occur; no comprehensible speech is detected; and the extremities move neither to commands nor appropriately to localize or ward of noxious stimuli. Nonpurposive reflex movements such as flexor or extensor posturing may be present. Stupor resembles coma except that the patient remains rousable if strong external stimulation is applied. In stupor or coma, the defect in arousal predominates, and the potential of the unaroused hemispheres for cognition cannot be determined.

Some patients with severe brain damage recover from the sleep-like state of coma, but never interact meaningfully with their environment. It seems improper to describe these awake unconscious patients as being comatose or in coma. The terms akinetic mutism, vigilant coma, and, recently, vegetative state have been applied to this condition. Coma should not be described by arbitrary levels, but by specific descriptions (e.g., reacts purposefully to noxious stimuli only) or by the Glasgow Coma Scale.

DIFFERENTIAL DIAGNOSIS

Coma is the most serious complication of acute brain failure and always requires immediate therapeutic intervention. The clinician first must determine whether the lesion causing coma is diffuse or discrete, and whether it is of metabolic or structural origin. This distinction can be made more easily if all types of coma are divided into three pathophysiologic categories: toxic-metabolic encephalopathy, supratentorial lesions, and subtentorial lesions. Each of these causes of coma has a characteristic clinical presentation and evolution (Table 1).

Toxic-Metabolic Coma

Noncerebral disease may affect consciousness by diffusely impairing the metabolism of the cerebral cortex and brain stem. Brain metabolism may be depressed by exogenous toxins, as in sedative drug poisoning, or by endogenous toxins, as occurs in uremia and hepatic failure. In hypoxia and hypoglycemia, the supply of extrinsic energy sources is insufficient for brain requirements, and coma occurs. Neuronal excitability may also be altered by electrolyte and acid-base imbalances and changes in serum osmolality.

In metabolic encephalopathy, symmetrical neurologic abnormalities are usually difficult to attribute to a regionally restricted lesion. No physical sign is pathognomonic of metabolic coma; however, pupillary light reflexes are generally preserved (except in patients who have ingested glutethimide, atropine-like agents, or barbiturates in high doses) even when signs of lower brain stem depression, such as apnea, ophthalmoplegia, and motor flaccidity with areflexia, are present. In severe sedative drug poisoning, nearly all brain and spinal cord functions may be absent, including electrocerebral activity.

Alcohol and drugs are frequently present in patients presenting in coma; they may or may not be the cause of it. The work-up for a cause should be thorough, lest an underlying electrolyte disorder or subdural hematoma be the real culprit. Alcohol levels may be useful only after a complete work-up has ruled out other causes of coma; elevated levels provide a plausible cause for coma. The patient must then be regularly assessed (preferably with the Glasgow Coma Scale) at 30-minute intervals. If the patient does not begin to awaken over the next several hours, the diagnosis should be re-assessed and other causes of coma sought. Missed intracranial bleeding after occult trauma is common in intoxicated patients, and a common cause of malpractice liability.

Supratentorial Lesions

Mass lesions of the cerebral hemispheres produce coma by herniating beyond the confines of the supratentorial compartment and compressing the brain stem reticular formation. Two syndromes of herniation associated with supratentorial lesions are recognized clinically: central downward herniation and temporal lobe herniation.

Central Downward Transtentorial Herniation. Deep or midline masses may compress and displace the supratentorial contents caudally through the tentorial opening into the subtentorial compartment. Unless herniation is checked by treatment, there is a progressive failure of the rostral brain stem and then the pons and medulla. The initial stages of cerebral herniation are marked by symmetrical signs which may be mistaken for metabolic encephalopathy. Clinically, the first signs reflect failure of the hemispheres and subcortical structures: reduced consciousness, small pupils with preserved reaction to light, bilateral signs of corticospinal and extrapyramidal tract dysfunction, grasp reflexes, decorticate, flexor posturing, and periodic (Cheyne-Stokes) respirations. At this stage, downward herniation is potentially reversible by osmotic agents and surgery if a tumor or hematoma is present, but when signs of midbrain failure appear (fixed, dilated or midposition pupils, and decerebrate rigidity), it is likely that distortion and compression have led to hemorrhagic infarction (Duret hemorrhages) of the subtentorial brain stem. The Cushing reflex, a late sign of herniation, consists of hypertension and bradycardia.

Herniation of the Temporal Lobe. This easily recognized syndrome occurs when an expanding mass in one hemisphere or in the lateral middle fossa displaces the uncus of the temporal lobe medially over the edge of the tentorial opening and compresses the third cranial nerve, the adjacent midbrain, and the posterior cerebral artery. The earliest sign of uncal herniation is unilateral pupillary dilatation with a sluggish or absent reaction to light attributable to compression of pupilloconstrictor fibers of the third cranial nerve. As the medial temporal lobe progressively compresses the midbrain, the patient becomes deeply comatose and manifests a complete ipsilateral third cranial nerve palsy and contralateral decerebrate, extensor posturing. If treatment cannot halt brain displacement at this point, brain stem dysfunction progresses caudally in a manner clinically indistinguishable from that caused by central herniation.

Subtentorial Lesions

Two types of posterior fossa lesions produce coma: lesions intrinsic to the brain stem that destroy the reticular activating system (e.g., pontine hemorrhage and paramedian infarction of the midbrain or pons) and lesions

---

TABLE 1 Causes of Coma

Toxic-metabolic causes

    Postictal
    Hypoglycemia
    Hypoxemia
    Electrolyte disorders (hyponatremia, hypercalcemia)
    Hyper- or hypo-osmolality
    Hypothermia
    Heat stroke
    Uremia
    Hepatic encephalopathy (hepatic failure, Reye's syndrome)
    Myxedema
    Postanoxia (cardiopulmonary arrest)
    Hypertensive encephalopathy
    Wernicke's encephalopathy
    Air, fat, or amniotic fluid embolism
    Decompression illness
    Cerebral vasculitis
    Meningitis
    Encephalitis or cerebritis (viral, toxoplasmosis, rickettsial, malaria)
    Meningeal carcinomatosis
    Toxins: carbon monoxide, cyanide, alcohol, narcotics, sedative-hypnotic drugs, antidepressants

Supratentorial lesions

    Subdural or epidural hematoma
    Intracerebral hemorrhage (hypertension, [CVA]) cerebral vascular accident
    Brain abscess
    Brain tumor
    Cerebral infarction (CVA)
    Cerebral edema and increased intracranial pressure
    Subarachnoid hemorrhage

Subtentorial lesion

    Brain stem hemorrhage
    Brain stem infarction and thrombosis (includes thrombotic thrombocytopenia purpura [TTP])
    Brain stem concussion
    Ruptured cerebral aneurysm
    Basilar artery occlusion (thrombus, embolus)
    Posterior fossa (cerebellar) bleeding or tumor

extrinsic to the brain stem that compress and distort it (e.g., cerebellar tumor and hematoma). In addition, unconsciousness follows acute distortion or direct blows to the brain stem tegmentum as occurs in cerebral concussion and rupture of a cerebral aneurysm. In cases of intrinsic brain stem dysfunction, it is important to distinguish between brain stem infarction due to basilar artery thrombosis and pontine hemorrhage. In the former, heparin anticoagulation may be indicated; in the latter, anticoagulation would be catastrophic. Computed tomographic (CT) scan is the best means of making this distinction.

Compressive lesions of the brain stem are often difficult to distinguish from intrinsic lesions, and cerebellar hemorrhage may mimic brain stem stroke clinically. In other cases, the caudal-to-rostral evolution of neurologic signs may resemble the patchy brain stem depression of metabolic coma. Asymmetrical motor signs, active deep tendon reflexes, and hypertension owing to the Cushing reflex usually serve to distinguish acute brain stem compression from brain stem depression caused by sedative drug intoxication. Surgical evacuation of a cerebellar hematoma may be life-saving and may restore consciousness if instituted promptly.

TREATMENT

The intial management of the comatose patient is directed toward stabilization. The first step is to ensure an adequate airway by intubation if necessary (Table 2). Intubation raises intracranial pressure; if this is already a problem, measures must be taken before intubation to blunt this response (see chapter on *Sedation and Rapid-Induction Anesthesia*).

The respiratory rate and its pattern should be noted before they are obscured by therapeutic measures such as intubation and mechanical ventilation. Disordered respiration is one of the best indicators of brain dysfunction. Depressed respiration is a usual concomitant of excessive dosage of opiates, sedative-hypnotics, or tranquilizers. In addition, hypoventilation may follow excessive dosage with tricyclic antidepressants, anticonvulsants (including phenytoin), and aspirin, the latter producing hyperventilation followed by respiratory depression. Severe hyperventilation occurs when brain damage, subarachnoid hemorrhage, or ingestion of acidic substances produces a lactic acidosis in cerebral spinal fluid (CSF) that stimulates the medullary receptors controlling respiration. Hyperventilation also may be of extracerebral origin, as is the case when neurogenic pulmonary edema complicates an intracranial catastrophe. Periodic respiration implies bilateral hemisphere dysfunction; ataxic breathing heralds impending medullary failure and apnea.

When adequate ventilation has been established, the following procedures are mandatory. Blood should be drawn for a determination of blood glucose, routine chemistries, and toxicology. At this point, arterial blood

TABLE 2 Management of the Comatose Patient

Immediate Steps

1. Ensure and protect airway patency.
2. In case of trauma, stabilize neck.
3. Institute resuscitative measures.
4. Draw blood for stat determinations of glucose, electrolytes, urea nitrogen, creatinine, complete blood count, prothrombin time, partial thromboplastin time, liver function, and osmolality; administer dextrose, 25–50 g IV.
5. Monitor respiratory rate and pattern, blood pressure, pulse, rectal temperature, and cardiac function.
6. Obtain ECG; measure arterial blood gases.
7. Administer naloxone 0.4 to 0.8 mg IV and thiamine 100 mg IV.
8. In case of recurrent seizures or status epilepticus, stop seizures with diazepam 5–10 mg IV, then administer phenytoin in IV loading dose of 15–20 mg/kg (1,000–1500 mg).
9. Briefly examine patient for signs of trauma and meningitis. Complete motor and neurophthalmologic examinations; treat any metabolic derangements.
10. In suspected cases of bacterial meningitis, perform lumbar puncture (LP) promptly; do not delay until after CT scan.
11. If a mass lesion is suspected or signs of herniation are present a CT scan should be obtained *before* LP is preformed.
12. If herniation present: hyperventilate, administer mannitol, obtain CT scan, and consult neurosurgeon.
13. Regular re-evaluation for change in status.

Subsequent Measures

1. Insert nasogastric tube and Foley catheter. Perform gastric lavage with large orogastric tube if overdose is suspected.
2. Send blood and urine specimens for toxicologic screening.
3. If seizures continue, administer phenobarbital in IV loading dose of 10 to 15 mg/kg (750 to 1,000 mg).
4. Obtain films of chest, cervical spine, abdomen, as indicated.
5. Perform CT scan to rule out space-occupying lesion in stabilized patient.
6. If no evidence of space-occupying lesion and diagnosis uncertain, perform lumbar puncture (cells, protein, glucose, culture cytology) to rule out subarachnoid hemorrhage, hepatic encephalopathy, herpes simplex, encephalitis.
7. Obtain an electroencephalogram (EEG) if you suspect metabolic encephalopathy or seizures.

gases should be analyzed to confirm that oxygenation is adequate. Immediately afterwards, 25 to 50 grams of dextrose should be administered intravenously. Even in cases of hyperosmolar coma, the administration of one ampule of dextrose will not be harmful. Naloxone hydrochloride (0.4 to 0.8 mg) and thiamine (100 mg) should be administered intravenously to all patients regardless of whether opiate or alcohol abuse is suspected.

In the usual clinical dosage, naloxone reliably reverses opiate-induced respiratory depression and also can reverse ethanol-induced coma in some patients. Much higher doses (1 to 5 mg per kilogram) in animals have reversed the depressant effects of barbiturates, benzodiazepines, and some inhalation anesthetics. The duration of action of naloxone is 2 to 3 hours; therefore, patients who have taken an overdose of a long-acting narcotic such as methadone may relapse after an initial period of improvement. Administration of thiamine will reverse coma in those patients with Wernicke's encephalopathy.

During this initial stabilization and assessment of the vital signs, the patient should be checked quickly for signs of head trauma (scalp laceration, bleeding from the ears, CSF rhinorrhea) and spontaneous movements (seizures or posturing).

Concurrent with these therapeutic procedures and other diagnostic efforts, a history should be obtained. In every case, it is important to determine the circumstances in which coma occurred and, if possible, the details of the medical history. These facts must be obtained from relatives, friends, police, ambulance attendants, or anyone who may have observed the patient prior to admission. A history of psychiatric illness, depression, alcoholism, drug abuse, previous head injury, seizures, or underlying chronic illness may indicate the cause of coma.

Placement of a nasogastric (NG) tube may be indicated to examine the stomach contents. This procedure always places the patient at risk for aspiration because the NG tube dilates the gastroesophageal sphincter and permits regurgitation of gastric contents around the tube. Regurgitation is especially likely in cases of drug overdose coma when a dilated and atonic stomach filled with pills is encountered; therefore, any patient in coma or with a depressed gag reflex should have a cuffed endotracheal tube in place prior to passage of an NG tube for gastric lavage. The patient should be placed on the left side with the head down and rotated to the side. This position places the pylorus uppermost and diminishes propulsion of poisons from the stomach to the small bowel (most drugs are not absorbed from the stomach but from the small bowel). After the stomach has been emptied as completely as possible, tap water should be instilled slowly with constant suction to prevent stomach distention. In most adults, one or two liters of water, followed by saline if necessary, can be used. Lavage should be continued as long as ingested material is recovered, and then 100 g activated charcoal should be administered.

Use of the Vital Signs to Guide Treatment

The blood pressure will often provide the *first* clue to the etiologic diagnosis of coma. Hypertension can be a reflex response to increased intracranial pressure (ICP) (Cushing reflex) or brain stem ischemia and commonly accompanies an intracranial hemorrhage. Rarely, hypertension *per se* may cause coma, as in hypertensive encephalopathy. Hypotension may indicate myocardial infarction, hemorrhagic shock, sepsis, or sedative-hypnotic drug overdosage.

The immediate reduction of ICP may be required while awaiting definitive surgical therapy (e.g., the removal of an intracranial hematoma or abscess). Hyperventilation by Ambubag or mechanical ventilator should be used first to reduce PCO_2 to 32 mm Hg or lower. An osmotic agent (Mannitol 1 g per kilogram as a 20 percent solution initially, followed by 0.25 to 0.5 g per kilogram every 2 to 3 hours) will further reduce ICP. If these fail to reduce ICP, a single bolus of a short-acting barbiturate (pentobarbital 1.5 to 3 mg per kilogram) may be administered to a mechanically ventilated patient, but hypotension is an undesirable side effect.

The pulse rate and rhythm may give additional clues to the cause of coma and should be recorded and monitored. Bradycardia associated with an elevated blood pressure is an ominous sign of brain stem compression, and reversible causes of transtentorial herniation (e.g., subdural hematoma) should be immediately considered before cardiovascular collapse ensues.

The morphology of the electrocardiogram (ECG) may indicate the presence of acute myocardial infarction (MI) which in up to 10 percent of patients is accompanied by a neurologic event (cerebral embolism or anoxic ischemic coma due to cardiac arrest). The presence of the peaked, tall, so-called "cerebral T waves" and a concave type of elevated ST segment, distinct from the ST segment pattern associated with MI, may indicate the presence of a subarachnoid hemorrhage or increased intracranial pressure due to a cerebral mass lesion. Prolongation of the QRS complex can occur in the presence of an overdosage with tricyclic antidepressants; a shortened or prolonged QT segment may indicate the presence of hyper- or hypocalcemia, respectively.

The patient's rectal temperature should not be neglected in the initial evaluation. Hypothermia can be secondary to Wernicke's disease, exposure, overdosage with sedative drugs, near-drowning, and hypothyroidism. This important sign often is not detected because either the rectal temperature measurement is omitted or an ordinary thermometer is used that cannot detect temperatures below 35 °C. Hypothermia below 26 °C will produce coma by itself; therefore, warming and resuscitative measures are indicated in all hypothermic patients even if all vital signs are absent.

The presence of fever in a comatose patient demands an investigation for possible meningitis. If there is no history of trauma, the neck should be flexed to assess the presence of *meningismus* (positive Kernig and Brudzinski signs). When head trauma is a possible cause of coma, the presence of cervical spine injury should be assumed until the cervical spine can be examined radiologically. The neck should be stabilized immediately by sandbags or headboard to prevent movement during the physical and radiologic examinations.

Meningismus may indicate bacterial meningitis or subarachnoid hemorrhage; but, in the latter case, there is often a delay of up to 12 hours before blood in the subarachnoid CSF pathways has produced enough chemical irritation of the meninges to be detected by neck flexion. In deep coma, meningismus may be absent despite the presence of bacterial or chemical meningitis.

DISPOSITION

Virtually all patients who present in coma need hospital admission and neurologic or neurosurgical consultation. Patients who are still in coma need respiratory support and intensive care unit (ICU) admission.

A few patients may present in coma and fully recover in the emergency department (e.g., alcohol or heroin intoxication, hypoglycemic reaction). It is safe to discharge such patients only if they have a complete recovery to normal mental status within a few hours and if there is no chance of either delayed drug absorption or prolonged half-life that could cause relapse (for example, methadone overdose treated with naloxone, or accidental overdose of long-acting insulin). Otherwise, they should be admitted for observation.

SYNCOPE

J. STEPHEN HUFF, M.D.
RICHARD LEVY, M.D., M.P.H., F.A.C.E.P.

In the largest sense, syncope can encompass all transient losses of consciousness. The term syncope may be employed when the interruption of consciousness occurs within seconds, when the return to alertness is rapid, and when the restoration of consciousness is complete. It may occur as a result of several well-defined disease states or it may represent a physiologic event without a specific cause. The differential diagnosis of brief loss of consciousness includes several diagnoses other than syncope (Table 1).

The fleeting brain failure implied by syncope reflects loss of substrate availability necessary for neuronal function. Glucose, oxygen, and other essential nutrients must be supplied continually to the brain, and interruption of these substrates for as little as 2 to 3 seconds may impair consciousness. Most frequently the temporary interruption is attributable to a disruption of supply, i.e., the cerebral blood flow rather than depletion of nutrients (Table 2).

In the clinical studies that examine large groups of patients with transient loss of consciousness, fully 30 to 50 percent of the patients have no known etiology for their syncope at the end of evaluation. The next largest category is that of vasovagal or reflex syncope (25 to 40 percent). Cardiac causes vary widely and occur in 8 to 25 percent of cases in different studies. A final diagnosis of seizure disorder also varies greatly in frequency (5 to 30 percent).

PRE-HOSPITAL MANAGEMENT

The emergency physician's approach to the patient mandates rapid identification and intervention to stem possible threats to life. This begins in the field. For the patient who has "passed out," the ABCs of emergency care must be initiated. If the patient does not rapidly regain consciousness, the diagnosis of syncope is excluded and other conditions such as cerebral trauma, shock, intoxication, or seizures should be considered. Airway and breathing status must be addressed initially. Pulse and blood pressure should be obtained, and if abnormal, rapid venous access should be secured. If the pulse is irregular or tachycardia or bradycardia is present, cardiac monitoring should be initiated. If the patient's condition permits, historical information may be obtained at the scene. Appropriate communication with medical control is necessary since the constellation of disease entities encompassed by syncope is too complex to be managed by protocol.

EMERGENCY DEPARTMENT MANAGEMENT

Reassessment

The initial field assessment should be repeated when the patient arrives at the emergency department. Airway, breathing, and circulation should be reevaluated and appropriate intervention initiated. If triage detects symptoms of chest pain, dyspnea, abdominal pain, or a history of cardiac disease, the patient should be moved to an area where careful observation and cardiac monitoring are possible. Otherwise the patient may be placed in an area of the emergency department where reasonable observation is possible until seen by a physician (Fig. 1).

History

When evaluating a stable patient with an episodic loss of consciousness, the exact historical information sur-

TABLE 1 Differential Diagnosis of Transient Loss of Consciousness

Seizure
Head trauma
Intoxications
Transient hypoxia
Transient hypoglycemia
Hyperventilation
Psychogenic factors
Factitious causes
Syncope

TABLE 2   Causes of Syncope*

Cardiac causes

  Decreased heart rate
    Bradyrhythms
    Complete heart block
    Sick sinus syndrome
    Pacemaker dysfunction

  Increased heart rate
    Supraventricular tachycardia
    Ventricular tachycardia

  Obstruction
    Aortic stenosis
    Idiopathic hypertrophic subaortic stenosis
    Atrial myxoma
    Pulmonary embolism

Systemic vascular causes

  Decreased filling or decreased vascular resistance
    Blood loss
    Postural hypotension
    Volume depletion
    Reflex syncope
      Vasodepressor or vasovagal syncope (simple faint)
      Carotid sinus hypersensitivity
      Tussive syncope
      Micturition syncope
      Valsalva maneuver syncope/hyperventilation
      Glossopharyngeal neuralgia
      Breath-holding
    Drug effect
    Orthostatic hypotension

Cerebrovascular obstructive causes

    Arteriosclerosis, usually with diffuse and severe disease
    Subclavian steal

---

* Please note that the exact mechanism of syncope is incompletely understood in many of the above etiologies and that multifactorial processes are often involved. The grouping above is for instructional purposes and, by necessity, arbitrary in places.

---

rounding the event must be elicited from the patient and, if necessary, from any observers. Has the patient experienced any similar events in the past? Often patients volunteer that they "faint" easily. What was the patient doing just before loss of consciousness occurred? A precedent coughing episode or history of urination provides suggestive evidence of tussive syncope or micturition syncope. Witnessing venipuncture or some other psychologically noxious event may trigger a vasovagal faint. Upper extremity exertion classically precedes loss of consciousness in the subclavian steal syndrome. A history of sometimes subtle manipulation of the neck before the syncopal episode may point to carotid sinus hypersensitivity. Facial pain immediately prior to loss of consciousness may lead to the suspicion of glossopharyngeal neuralgia. Again, historical information should focus on the activity immediately before and after the event. Was there a change in position? Loss of consciousness when assuming the upright position is common and often innocent; however, it may reflect orthostatic hypotension from volume depletion or autonomic neuropathy. Was there any prodrome? Syncope patients typically remember a few seconds of light-headedness or visual disturbances. In contrast, the seizure patient may report an aura, but this may involve specific sensory or motor abnormalities. The color of the face prior to the event is valued by some as another way to distinguish seizure from syncope; a pale face is thought to reflect poor facial perfusion paralleling the impaired cerebral perfusion immediately prior to a syncopal attack. Other clues to the diagnosis of seizures include incontinence, a postictal state of confusion, or the witnessing of motor movements. Unfortunately, not even motor movements can reliably distinguish seizure from syncope; "convulsive syncope," in which the patient is observed to have a few irregular movements of the extremities, is common and is sometimes seen as part of a venipuncture-induced vasovagal episode.

Medication history is also important. Several antihypertensive drugs have orthostatic hypotension as a side effect. Alcohol or other intoxicants may be consistent with a transient loss of consciousness.

History of other medical illnesses may lead to a diagnosis. Hypoglycemia should be suspect in the diabetic, although the loss of consciousness is most often sustained. Autonomic neuropathy with orthostatic hypotension is also common in diabetics. A history of other endocrine diseases or steroid use may be present and suggests adrenal insufficiency.

Physical Examination

Physical examination should include measurement of blood pressure and pulse with the patient supine then upright. Auscultation for carotid bruits and heart murmurs should be done. Provocative maneuvers, such as hyperventilation or carotid massage, should be performed in patients who have a suggestive history. A neurologic examination emphasizing new focal findings or neuropathy should be performed. A persistent, new neurologic finding is indicative of a disease process other than syncope.

Laboratory Evaluation, Monitoring, and Disposition

Patients with blood loss, volume depletion unrelated to bleeding, clear cardiac problems, or intoxication are usually readily identified. If the loss of consciousness is thought to be from a seizure, further action is required. There still remains a group in whom no underlying medical problem is evident. The clinician faces a dilemma with this group of patients. Inpatient evaluation of syncope is notably cost-ineffective, yet some patients do have life-threatening causes for their syncope. For the young patient who seems to have suffered a simple faint or other reflex syncope, no further evaluation is necessary. Follow-up with his or her family physician is recommended. The patient with no prior history of brief loss of consciousness and no clear precipitating factor poses an even more difficult problem. For persons at risk for cardiac disease or over age 35, an electrocardiogram (ECG) is obtained, though the yield is low in patients who have no historical clues of cardiac disease. Serum glucose and electrolyte evaluations are commonly obtained, again with low yield. Any abnormalities may dictate admission or other follow-up.

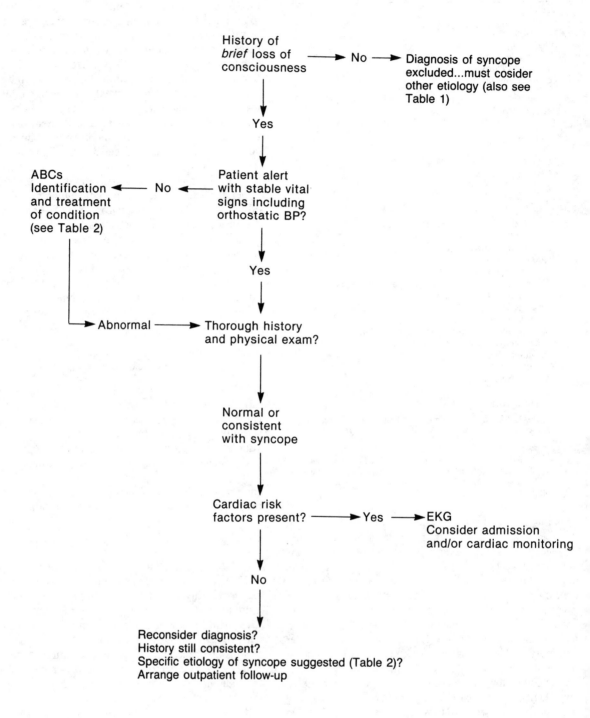

Figure 1 Emergency department approach to patient with transient loss of consciousness.

The main function of the emergency physician after identifying specific causes of loss of consciousness is to identify those patients who seem to have a cardiac etiology of their syncope. Heart murmurs may suggest the rare cardiac obstructive lesion. The primary problem is arrhythmia identification, and cardiac monitoring may be indicated. Prior cardiac history, palpitations, and suspicion of new myocardial ischemia or pulmonary embolus should prompt admission and monitoring of this group at high risk for sudden death. Patients with a cardiovascular cause of syncope have a high mortality rate. Outpatient evaluation can be undertaken with Holter monitoring if the suspicion of arrhythmia is more remote.

SUGGESTED READING

Day SC, Cook EF, Funkenstein H, Goldman L. Evaluation and outcome of emergency room patients with transient loss of consciousness. Am J Med 1982; 73:15–23.

Kapoor WN, Karpf M, Wieand S, Peterson JR, Levey GS. A prospective evaluation and follow-up of patients with syncope. N Engl J Med 1983; 309:197–204.

Kapoor WN, Karpf M, Maher Y, Miller RA, Levey GS. Syncope of unknown origin: the need for a more cost-effective approach to its diagnostic evaluation. JAMA 1982; 247:2687–2691.

Martin GJ, Adams SL, Martin HG, Mathews J, Zull D, Scanlon PJ. Prospective evaluation of syncope. Ann Emerg Med 1984; 13:499–504.

Noble RJ. The patient with syncope. JAMA 1977; 237:1372–1376.

Riley TL. Syncope and hyperventilation. In: Riley TL, Roy A, eds. Pseudoseizures. Baltimore: Williams and Wilkins, 1982:34.

DIZZINESS

TIMOTHY T.K. JUNG, M.D., Ph.D.
MICHAEL M. PAPARELLA, M.D.

When a patient complains of dizziness, it is essential to differentiate true vertigo from a feeling of faintness, weakness, light-headedness, unsteadiness, or disequilibrium. Vertigo is defined as a hallucination of motion in which the patient feels he is spinning or his surroundings spin. An imbalance between the two vestibular systems is believed to be the cause of vertigo. For example, any disorder such as tumor, infection, or trauma that causes unilateral reduction of vestibular function may cause vertigo. Most vertigo originates from peripheral disorders in the vestibular system (85 percent), and the rest from central disorders (15 percent).

Once it is determined that the patient has vertigo, the next step is to localize the source of the disorder by separating peripheral or ear problems from central nervous system (CNS) disorders. Usually, vertigo caused by peripheral disorder has a sudden onset, a paroxysmal pattern, and severe symptoms of short duration (Table 1). In addition, horizontal or rotatory nystagmus is present along with fatigable positional effects with 1 to 2 seconds of latency. Nausea and vomiting are commonly present as well as symptoms of ear problems such as hearing loss and tinnitus. On the other hand, vertigo caused by CNS disorder is characterized by slow and seldom paroxysmal onset and by less severe symptoms of longer duration. Nystagmus may or may not be present. It is seldom associated with nausea, vomiting, tinnitus, or hearing loss. Disturbance of consciousness and other neurologic signs are frequently present.

DIAGNOSIS

It is essential to make an accurate diagnosis before appropriate treatment can be initiated (Table 2). The history is the most important single diagnostic tool. A careful history differentiates vertigo from other "dizziness," separates peripheral vertigo from central vertigo, and leads to at least a working diagnosis.

The next step in evaluating a dizzy patient is a careful general medical, otologic, and neurologic examination. Special attention should be given to the presence or absence of postural hypotension, nystagmus, ataxia, otoscopic or tuning-fork abnormalities, or any abnormal-

TABLE 1 Differentiation of Peripheral from Central Vertigo

Symptoms	Peripheral	Central
Onset	Sudden	Less frequently sudden
Pattern	Paroxysmal	Seldom paroxysmal
Intensity	Usually severe	Seldom severe
Duration	Usually short	Longer
Nystagmus	Present	Present or absent
Positional effects	May be present, latency, fatigue	May or may not be present, no latency, no fatigue
Nausea and vomiting	Usually associated	Unusual
Tinnitus	Frequently present	Seldom present
Hearing loss	Frequently present	Seldom present
Disturbance of consciousness	Seldom present	More frequently present
Other CNS signs	Usually absent	Frequently present

ities in the cranial nerves. In otoscopic examination of the tympanic membrane, a careful search for perforations, cholesteatomas, granulomas, or tumors should be made. Tympanic membrane mobility should be examined by pneumatic otoscopy and by observation of mobility following Valsalva inflation. Pneumatic compression may induce a positive fistula response, thereby producing nystagmus with or without a sensation of dizziness.

A simple vestibular function can be tested in any emergency department by the caloric test, which determines whether one ear is less active than the other. If both ears are equally active, balance is intact and unilateral vestibular hypofunction is ruled out. This procedure requires only a syringe with a metal tip covered with a rubber tubing at the end and hot (120 °F) or ice water. The patient's head is tilted backward, about 60 degrees and 2 to 5 cc of hot or ice water is used to irrigate the tympanic membrane. It is important to use exactly the same method of

stimulation in each ear and to wait at least 5 minutes before the opposite ear is stimulated. When the ear is stimulated with cold water, a horizontal rotatory nystagmus occurs with the fast component of the nystagmus toward the opposite ear. Characteristics of nystagmus such as duration, frequency, amplitude, and direction should be noted.

Basic laboratory studies including urinalysis, blood count, serology, blood sugar, and other chemistry; chest films; electrocardiogram; and other indicated tests are helpful in the detection of potentially treatable metabolic or medical causes of dizziness. Special tests such as standard and impedance audiometry, auditory brain-stem response audiometry, electronystagmography (ENG), and tomography of the internal auditory canal may be necessary before a final diagnosis can be made.

TREATMENT

When the cause of dizziness becomes evident during the initial work-up, the specific medical problem should be treated. The diagnosis and the natural history of the disease should be completely explained to the patient in order to help allay fears and anxieties and establish rapport with the patient. Only the patient with a severe and persistent form of vertigo needs admission to the hospital. The majority of patients can be started on treatment for symptomatic relief of vertigo in the emergency department, and depending on their symptoms, referred to an otolaryngologist or a neurologist on an outpatient basis.

Nonspecific Symptomatic Treatment

Several categories of pharmacologic agents such as antihistamines, anticholinergic drugs, sedatives, antiemetics, and vasodilators are in use for nonspecific symptomatic relief of vertigo. When the oral route (PO) is not feasible, suppositories (SP) or intramuscular (IM) or intravenous (IV) injection may be used.

Antihistamines. The sedative effect of antihistamines is utilized in the treatment of vertigo. Commonly used antihistamines and their dosages are as follows: (1) diphenhydramine (Benadryl), 25 to 50 mg PO, IM, or IV 3 to 4 times a day; (2) dimenhydrinate (Dramamine), 50 to 100 mg PO, IM, or IV 4 times a day; (3) meclizine (Antivert, Bonine), 12.5 to 25 mg PO 3 times a day; (4) cyclizine (Marezine), 50 mg IM 4 times a day; and (5) promethazine (Phenergan), 25 mg PO, SP, IM, or IV 3 times a day.

Anticholinergic drugs. The anticholinergic drugs, especially scopolamine, are the best agents for the prevention of motion sickness. The dosage regimen for scopolamine is 0.6 mg PO or subcutaneously (SQ) every 4 to 6 hours. The side effects of scopolamine include dry mouth, drowsiness, headache, blurred vision, and ataxia. These side effects, except for dry mouth, can be eliminated by the combination of d-amphetamine (10mg). Scopolamine can also be given transdermally (Transderm-scop).

TABLE 2 Differential Diagnosis of Vertigo

Central nervous system causes

   Circulatory: basilar-vertebral insufficiency, postural hypotension, anemia
   Demyelinating disease: multiple sclerosis
   Trauma: concussion syndrome
   Tumors: cerebellar or brain stem, primary or secondary
   Infection
   Epilepsy
   Migraine
   Drugs

Otologic causes

   Associated with acute otitis media: serous or suppurative labyrinthitis
   Associated with chronic otitis media: labyrinthine fistula, cholesteatoma
   Trauma: fracture of temporal bone, labyrinthine concussion, perilymph fistula
   Endolymphatic hydrops: Menière's disease, allergic, luetic
   Benign positional vertigo
   Vestibular neuronitis
   Acoustic neuroma
   Ototoxic drugs

Proprioceptive causes—peripheral neuropathy

   Vitamin deficiency
   Chronic alcoholism
   Diabetes mellitus
   Tabes dorsalis
   Cervical vertigo

Metabolic causes

   Hypoglycemia
   Hypothyroidism
   Hyperventilation

Ocular causes

   Refraction errors
   Simple glaucoma

Psychogenic causes

Nonspecific causes

Sedatives. Diazepam (Valium), 2.5 to 5 mg PO, IM, or IV 3 times a day, has been found to have direct vestibular suppressant activity in addition to its sedative effects.

Phenothiazines (Antiemetics). The phenothiazines have minimal effects on the vestibular system, but are used to control nausea and vomiting. Some preparations and their dosage regimens are (1) prochlorperazine (Compazine), 10 mg PO or IM 3 times a day; (2) trimethobenzamide (Tigan), 200 mg PO, SP, or IM 3 times a day; and (3) chlorpromazine (Thorazine), 10 to 25 mg PO or IM every 3 to 4 hours.

Droperidol (Inapsine). Droperidol is a tranquilizer and is effective in the treatment of acute vertigo. It should be given in the hospital setting with an intravenous line in place. Dosage should be individualized. The usual adult dosage is 2.5 to 5 mg (1 to 2 ml) IV or IM every 4 to 8 hours. Vital signs should be monitored routinely to watch for hypovolemic hypotention.

Vasodilators. Vasodilators have sometimes been used empirically in the treatment of patients who complain of dizziness. They probably have no effect on the cerebral blood flow and have minimal effects on the vestibular system. The following drugs are marketed as vasodilators: (1)nylidrin hydrochloride (Arlidin), 3 to 12 mg PO 3 times a day; (2) cyclandelate (Cyclospasmol), 200 mg PO 4 times a day; (3) nicotinic acid (Niacin), 100 mg PO 4 times a day; and (4) papaverine hydrochloride, 150 mg PO 4 times a day.

Treatment of Specific Vertigo Syndromes

Diagnostic points and therapeutic regimens for specific vertigo syndromes are to be discussed.

Meniere's Disease. About three-quarters of patients with vertigo attributable to an ear disorder have Meniere's disease or idiopathic endolymphatic hydrops. Meniere's disease is unilateral most of the time, but bilateral 30 to 50 percent of the time. In Meniere's disease, endolymphatic spaces are distended either because of an overproduction of endolymph or because of interference with absorption or drainage. Patients with Meniere's disease present with episodic vertigo, fluctuating hearing loss, tinnitus, and a sense of fullness or pressure in the ear. The vertigo is usually violent, of abrupt onset, and associated with nausea and vomiting. Symptoms of hearing loss, tinnitus, and pressure are more pronounced during the attack of vertigo. Hearing deteriorates progressively, affecting lower frequency first with a peak at 2 kHz as documented by audiogram, then affecting all frequencies as time passes.

In many cases, the diagnosis of Meniere's disease can be made on the basis of history alone. Otoneurologic examination, audiometric and vestibular tests, and laboratory tests are helpful to confirm the diagnosis. Electronystagmography is helpful in quantifying and documenting vestibular function. Acoustic neuroma should be ruled out with a computed tomography (CT) scan if clinically indicated.

The patient should be treated conservatively and reassured that he or she does not have a more serious disease. The more the patient understands the self-limiting, waxing and waning characteristics of Meniere's disease, the better he can cope with it. Medical therapy includes diuretics, low salt diet, and trial of one of the antivertiginous drugs such as diazepam (Valium), dimenhydrinate (Dramamine), or meclizine (Antivert). During the acute episode of vertigo, droperidol (Inapsine) can be used in the hospital setting or one of the antihistamines on an outpatient basis. Vasodilators and histamines are used with variable results.

If the patient continues to have incapacitating vertigo in spite of extended medical management, several surgical procedures may be considered. Surgical procedures may be either conservative (endolymphatic mastoid shunt) or destructive (labyrinthectomy), depending on the patient's symptoms and hearing level.

If the patient's hearing is acceptable (50 decibels and 80 percent discrimination) and an adequate trial of medical treatment has failed, an endolymphatic mastoid shunt would be the procedure of choice. If the patient's hearing is poor and tinnitus is not a problem, transmastoid labyrinthectomy is advised. If the patient has severe tinnitus in addition, a translabyrinthine cochleovestibular neurectomy is recommended. When incapacitating vertigo persists after conservative therapy in patients with bilateral Meniere's disease, ablation of both vestibular labyrinths through parenteral administration of streptomycin can be considered.

Benign Positional Vertigo. This disorder occurs when the patient's head is placed in a certain position, and diagnosis can be made by placing the patient in different positions until symptoms occur. Vestibular and hearing tests are usually normal.

Since this disorder is commonly self-limited, reassurance is an important part of the treatment. Sedatives, antihistamines, or antiemetic drugs may be helpful. If an extended medical therapy fails, section of the singular nerve can be considered.

Labyrinthitis. Labyrinthitis can be a bacterial or viral infection and can develop from infection of the middle ear or mastoid (otogenic labyrinthitis) or meningitis (meningogenic labyrinthitis). The most violent type of vertigo develops when vestibular function of one ear is suddenly lost, as in otogenic labyrinthitis.

It is important to identify the cause of labyrinthitis before treatment can be planned. If the cause is an ear infection, the infection must be eliminated by means of appropriate antibiotics and emergency surgery. Acute symptoms of vertigo accompanying labyrinthitis should be treated by the same method as an attack of Meniere's disease.

Vestibular Neuronitis. Vestibular neuronitis usually follows a viral upper respiratory infection and may occur in epidemic form. The patient presents with intermittent vertigo, normal hearing, and reduced caloric response. The symptoms usually subside within 6 months. It is important to assure the patient that he does not have a serious disease such as a brain tumor. Nonspecific medications for symptomatic relief of vertigo—either antihistamines or sedatives—are usually all that is necessary.

Trauma. Vertigo can be caused by trauma such as a blow to the ear, a basal skull fracture, or a fracture of the temporal bone. In longitudinal temporal bone fracture, the fracture line usually spares the labyrinth, but extends through the middle ear and the external auditory canal, thus causing blood in the middle ear and conductive hearing loss. A transverse fracture of the temporal bone may extend across the bony capsule of the inner ear and result in complete loss of hearing with or without facial nerve paralysis. Treatment is directed toward symptomatic relief of vertigo. After the patient is stabilized, conductive hearing loss can be corrected by an ossiculoplasty.

Perilymphatic fistulas can occur in the round window and in the oval window area as a result of traumatic events such as flying and diving barotrauma, tubotympanic compression, acoustic or blast trauma, penetrating ear trauma, head or blunt ear trauma, and poststapedectomy or other otologic procedures. The patient with perilymph fistula presents with sudden hearing loss and vertigo. The fistula test may be positive. Initial treatment consists of bed rest and antivertiginous medications. Surgical repair of fistulas should not be delayed when spontaneous healing does not occur with rest. Hearing may return only partially even after a successful repair of fistulas.

Drugs. Many drugs (e.g., streptomycin, ethacrynic acid, gentamicin, kanamycin, nitrogen mustard, and aspirin) are capable of inducing vertigo. Drug induced vertigo usually is not the violent type seen in labyrinthitis or Meniere's disease. Treatment consists of withdrawal of the offending drug.

Tumors. Tumors can invade the inner ear and cause vertigo with or without hearing loss and facial nerve palsy. Tumors of the temporal bone may be primary or secondary. Primary tumors include glomus jugulare tumors, acoustic neuromas, and carcinomas of ear canal and middle ear. Treatment is surgical removal. Radiotherapy is combined with surgery, especially in squamous cell carcinoma.

Secondary tumors are metastatic tumors from distant sites, such as the lungs, breasts, kidneys, or prostate, or from adjacent tumors. Treatment for secondary tumors is symptomatic and palliative at best.

Vertigo Attributable to Central Disorders. Central (neurogenic) vertigo may be caused by epilepsy, multiple sclerosis, vascular accidents, posterior fossa tumors, and vertebrobasilar artery insufficiency.

In vertiginous epilepsy, vertigo can be severe, episodic, or mild. It is usually associated with hallucinations of music or sound. The patient may exhibit daydreaming and purposeful or purposeless repetitive movements.

Vertigo may be the inital symptom of multiple sclerosis in 5 to 10 percent of the cases. As many as 50 percent of these patients complain of vertigo at some time during the course of the disease. Diagnosis of multiple sclerosis is based on a detailed analysis of clinical pictures and cerebrospinal fluid abnormalities. Electronystagmography is also helpful in the diagnosis.

One of the most common brain stem vascular accidents, which causes vertigo, is Wallenberg's syndrome. This syndrome is caused by an infarction in the posterior lateral area of the medulla, which is supplied by the posterior inferior cerebellar artery. The dominant symptom of Wallenberg's syndrome is vertigo, which is associated with nausea, vomiting, hiccups, dysphagia, dysphonia, and blurring of vision. Characteristic neurologic signs include nystagmus, Horner's syndrome, loss of pain and temperature sensation on the same side of the face and on the opposite side of the body, homolateral ataxia, and paralysis of the pharynx and larynx. Usually there is no hearing loss or tinnitus.

Vertebrobasilar artery insufficiency is one of the most common disorders of elderly patients, and vertigo is the most common symptom. Other symptoms include hemiparesis, visual disturbances, dysarthria, headaches, and vomiting. Tinnitus and deafness are unusual symptoms. Drop attacks, without losing consciousness, are one of the characteristics of this disorder.

When symptoms of vertigo are suspected owing to central disorders, a neurologic consultation should be obtained. Treatment may depend on the particular disorder. Nonspecific medications for symptomatic relief of vertigo may be used as well as a specific treatment.

SUGGESTED READING

Finestone AJ, ed. Evaluation and clinical management of dizziness and vertigo. Boston: John Wright PSG Inc., 1982:45.

Goodhill V. Ear diseases, deafness, and dizziness. New York: Harper and Row, 1979:218.

McCabe BF, Ryu JM. Vestibular physiology in understanding the dizzy patient. Rochester (Minnesota): American Academy of Otolaryngology, 979:1.

Paparella MM, Shumrick DA, eds. Otolaryngology. Volume 2. Philadelphia: WB Saunders, 1980:241, 1878.

ATAXIA

BENJAMIN HONIGMAN, M.D., F.A.C.E.P.

Ataxia is a failure of coordination of voluntary movements. The term is most often used to describe unsteady walking, but it also applies to disturbances affecting other coordinated motor functions. Important causes of ataxia that require consideration in the emergency setting include mass lesions (e.g., subdural or epidural hematomas, cerebral neoplasms, cerebellar hemorrhages, or infarcts), drugs (e.g., alcohol, phenobarbital, benzodiazepines), and metabolic or infectious causes (e.g., cerebral abscess, infectious mononucleosis, Guillain-Barré syndrome, or hypothyroidism). Less common causes are noted in Table 1.

Other difficulties in walking that should be distinguished from an ataxic gait are the shuffling gait of the patient with Parkinson's disease; the waddling gait of the patient with muscular dystrophy; the theatrical, bizarre gait of the hysteric; and the gait of advanced age; as well as simple diffuse weakness of all muscles (see the chapter *Acute Weakness*).

Many causes can be determined from the history and physical examination, but analysis of the patient's gait may reveal important clues to the diagnosis. Grossly, the patient should be assessed in the sitting position. If truncal ataxia is present, consider an emergent cause, such as cerebellar hemorrhage. More refined gait examination should be done with the patient barefoot and walking toward and away from the examiner. Conclusions about gait should not be made from the side. During the examination the patient may need to be protected from falling. The arm swing, which should be the same on both sides, the width of the gait, and any limp or other abnormality should be noted during ordinary walking.

PHYSICAL EXAMINATION

The three major forms of ataxia are cerebellar, sensory, and toxicologic. Each can be characterized by different findings on physical examination and can help point to a general category of illness. The clinical findings that suggest cerebellar or vestibular causes partly depend on the anatomic location of the abnormality and whether adjacent neurologic structures are involved. For example, a hemisphere lesion produces ataxia in the ipsilateral limbs with less effect on truncal muscles; a midline lesion of the cerebellum tends to affect the trunk more than the limbs. An unsteady, wide-based, stiff-legged gait with jerky progression is common with cerebellar disorders; the arms may be lifted away from the body for balance. The unsteadiness may be more prominent upon arising quickly from a sitting position, stopping suddenly while walking, or turning quickly. With bilateral disease, reeling from side to side occurs. With unilateral lesions, the individual reels or lurches to the ipsilateral side; this may be accentuated by asking the patient to walk around a chair. When the patient is turning toward the affected side, he tends to fall into the chair, when to the normal side, the patient moves away from the chair in a spiral.

The patient with cerebellar ataxia is also often conspicuously tremulous. Some degree of tremor may be observed at rest or when the patient is walking, but it is most noticeable during voluntary movement. In cerebellar ataxia it is not only the gait and posture which are uncoordinated, but the eyes (nystagmus) or speech may also be affected.

TABLE 1 Causes of Ataxia

Sensory	Cerebellar

Lesions of:
  Peripheral nerves
  Dorsal roots
  Dorsal columns of spinal cord
  Medial lemnisci
  Both parietal lobes
	Lesions in the cerebellum or vestibulosensory system
	Neoplastic lesions e.g., medulloblastoma, glioma, hemangioblastoma, cerebellopontine angle tumor, metastatic disease—commonly lung, ovary, lymphoma
	Vascular lesions e.g., cerebellar hemorrhage, cerebellar infarct

Examples:
  Spinocerebellar degeneration—lack of Vitamin E
  Syphilitic tabes dorsalis
  Syphilitic meningomyelitis
  Vitamin B_{12} myelopathy
  Multiple sclerosis
  Friedreich's ataxia
  Chronic sensory neuropathy, e.g., diabetic neuropathy
	Traumatic disorders e.g., subdural hematoma, cerebellar contusion, posthyperthermia
	Metabolic disorders e.g., Hartnup disease, maple syrup disease, hypothyroidism, pyruvate dehydrogenase deficiency, ornithine transcarbamylase deficiency, lipoproteinemia
	Infectious disorders e.g., cerebellar abscess, acute cerebellar ataxia of children, infectious mononucleosis, Fisher variant of Guillain-Barré

Therapeutic and Toxic Substances 100 percent O_2 at 2 atm pressure, vinblastine, 5-fluorouracil, thallium, diphenylhydantoin, carbamazepine, benzodiazepines, glutethimide, lithium, alcohol, piperazine, barbiturates	Degenerative diseases e.g., chronic alcoholism, multiple sclerosis, olivopontocerebellar atrophy, parenchymatous cerebellar degeneration Hereditary or congenital anomalies e.g., ataxia-telangiectasia, hereditary spastic ataxia, Friedreich's ataxia, hereditary ataxia with muscular atrophy

The gait of a patient with *sensory* ataxia may have many features in common with that of cerebellar ataxia, but it has some distinguishing characteristics. Again, the gait is wide-based with swaying from one side to another. Slapping of the feet and clumsiness may be more common with a sensory deficit. Patients have no joint-position sense so they usually watch their legs so that they will know where they are. A smooth surface is negotiated better than a rough one and removing the shoes may aggravate the ataxia. The strength of movement may not be diminished. With the eyes closed (Romberg's sign) or in the dark the ataxia is much worse. Patients with sensory ataxia are subjectively aware of their deficit.

Ataxia secondary to *toxic or therapeutic substances* is characterized by swaying and reeling in many directions and possibly falling; no effort is made to correct the staggering. Steps tend to be irregular and uncertain; vertigo and dizziness may accompany the ataxia.

Several additional features of the gait examination may point to the cause, e.g., toe-walking. This tests the strength of the plantar flexors and, to a lesser degree, the patient's cerebellar function, since this exaggerates a broad-based gait. Tandem gait walking, on the other hand, greatly accentuates a cerebellar disorder. Heel-walking tests should also be performed; this may elicit cerebellar ataxia. Also, patients with any degree of weakness of the dorsiflexors are unable to do heel-walking.

Romberg's test (the patient standing with his feet together and eyes closed) can also be helpful. Patients who display a wide-based gait or who are unable to walk tandem may have trouble assuming this position, and may be allowed to stand with feet slightly apart. If Romberg's sign is present, the patient begins to weave and then falls with the body fairly straight, which suggests loss of proprioception in the legs. This may be the best assessment of a sensory ataxia. A great deal of body shaking suggests either cerebellar dysfunction or a psychogenic problem.

In addition, with the patient seated, cranial nerves and strength of the upper arms should be tested. Leg strength and coordination should be assessed and a sensory examination performed with the patient lying down. With a sensory deficit, the incoordination of the lower limbs may be observed.

WORK-UP AND DISPOSITION

The emergency department work-up of the patient with ataxia should focus on the gross neurologic examination and some minimal refined tests to help identify acute disease that requires immediate treatment, such as cerebellar hemorrhage or subdural hematoma. Truncal ataxia in the presence of hypertension and headache should arouse suspicion of a cerebellar hemorrhage; they are the most common early signs. The truncal ataxia may be elicited by having the patient sit unassisted. Cerebellar

TABLE 2 Work-up of Ataxia in Children and Young Adults

Age of Onset Under 5 Years	Useful Investigations
Acute or Subacute Presentation:	
Postinfectious, usually viral, Fisher variant of Guillain-Barré	Viral titers, drug screens, heavy metal screen, blood ammonia urinary VMA excretion, EEG, CT scan CSF examination
Posterior fossa tumors Drug intoxication Hyperthermia	
Episodic Course:	
Metabolic disorder, e.g., ornithine transcarbamylase deficiency, Hartnup disease Drug ingestion	Blood ammonia, pyruvate, lactate, amino acids, drug levels, urinary amino acids
Chronic Nonprogressive Course:	
Congenital cerebellar ataxias	

Age of Onset Between 5 and 25 Years	
Acute or Subacute Presentation:	
Multiple sclerosis	CT scan, EMG, nerve conduction studies, EEG, neuro-otologic and neuro-ophthalmo-logic assessments, muscle and nerve biopsy
Chronic Progressive Course: Friedreich's ataxia Ataxia telangiectasia Posterior fossa tumors Hydrocephalus Multiple sclerosis Spinocerebellar degeneration	assessments, muscle and nerve biopsy

hemorrhage requires urgent computed tomography (CT) scanning, neurosurgical consultation, and surgery for hematoma evacuation.

Subdural hematoma should be suspected in any comatose patient with evidence of trauma or in any alcoholic with an altered mental status. Common presenting features include headache, confusion, personality change, or altered consciousness, in addition to ataxia. CT scanning followed by surgical evacuation should be performed on an emergent basis. Temporizing measures such as intubation with hyperventilation or diuretics may reduce intracranial pressure in severe cases.

Other helpful tests that will rule out rapidly progressive causes of ataxia include drug screens for toxic causes, CT scans for cerebral mass lesions, and lumbar punctures for potential infectious causes. Table 2 analyzes several causes of ataxia in children and young adults and includes investigational tools that will be helpful in reaching the diagnosis. Less urgent causes may be difficult to elucidate in the emergency department, and referral is essential for more elaborate testing. The primary function of the emergency department physician is to rule out acute and life-threatening causes, begin expeditious management, and refer less urgent cases to a neurologist for management.

SUGGESTED READING

Erzurum S, Kalavsky SM, Watanakunakorn C. Acute cerebellar ataxia and hearing loss as initial symptoms of infectious mononucleosis. Arch Neurol 1983; 40:760.

Garcin R. The ataxias. In: Vinken PJ, Bruyn GW, eds. Handbook of clinical neurology. Vol 1. Amsterdam: North-Holland, 1969:309.

Jenkyn LR, Reeves A, et al. Neurologic signs in senescence. Arch Neurol 1985; 42:1154.

McLachlin RS, Bolton CF, et al. Gait disturbance in chronic subdural hematoma. CMA 1981; 125:865.

Walton JN, ed. Brain's diseases of the nervous system. Toronto: Oxford University Press, 1977.

Wyngaarden JB, Smith LH Jr, eds. Cecil's textbook of medicine. Philadelphia: WB Saunders, 1985.

ACUTE WEAKNESS

H. KENNETH WALKER, M.D.

True acute weakness is an urgent problem. It is the final common manifestation of many disorders of diverse etiology that threaten either life or the quality of life. Proper diagnostic and therapeutic measures need to be begun in a short time interval. The diagnosis is often suggested by the history, so it is fortunate that many of the patients remain conscious. The examiner can take the essential history as initial therapeutic measures are begun. A number of disorders are suggested by the pattern of weakness, although a few disorders can be diagnosed only by laboratory results. Because of the number of heterogeneous disorders that may be involved, the examiner must attack on several fronts at once. Prioritization of actions is important, since most patients with the complaint of weakness do not have true, acute, life-threatening weakness.

The initial set of actions is aimed at urgent supportive measures and rapid diagnosis of conditions whose presence or absence will determine what follows. Table 1 summarizes these actions. Airway adequacy must be determined first, with vital signs a close second. Many of the causes of weakness affect the pulse, the blood pressure, and the diaphragm. Ascertaining the status of the cervical cord is important because movement without its immobilization is absolutely contraindicated. A history of a fall, the presence of bruises anywhere, or a history of rheumatoid arthritis (causing spinal ligamentous laxity) is highly suggestive. The electrocardiogram (ECG) is important because hyperkalemia, hypokalemia, and hypocalcemia can be revealed and therapeutic measures undertaken at once. Blood gases may be deranged owing to diaphragmatic dysfunction in a number of disorders producing acute weakness; an even earlier finding of respiratory failure is decreased pulmonary function tests on bedside spirometry (FEV_1 or PEFR).

As the examiner continues working with the patient and concomitantly taking the history, he or she must be exquisitely alert for clinical manifestations that are highly suggestive of what might be termed *etiologic clusters*. For example, several etiologies produce diaphragmatic dysfunction. This is a good time to start thinking in terms of these clusters, since airway and ventilatory adequacy are being determined at this point. Table 2 lists various helpful clues that may suggest specific diagnostic possibilities. The anatomic pattern of involvement can be particularly helpful.

Table 3 organizes the causes of acute weakness according to *neuroanatomic localization*. This is a logical way to organize one's thoughts about the problem of acute weakness. Diagnosis and immediate therapy are included. The majority of these conditions require immediate admission to an intensive care unit and the attention of an appropriate specialist. Transfer to another hospital can be

---

TABLE 1 Actions for Initial Assessment of the Acutely Weak Patient

Vital signs (including accurate respiratory rate)
Airway adequacy (gag reflex, secretions, drooling. In less obvious cases, bedside spirometry can document clinically inapparent respiratory embarrassment).
Ascertain if cervical cord injured
ECG for potassium, calcium
Draw blood for
    Electrolytes
    BUN/creatinine
    Blood gases
    CBC
Intravenous access establishment

TABLE 2 Clues to Diagnosis of Acute Weakness

Observation
  Fasciculation
    Organophosphates
    Electrolyte imbalance
  Tetany
  Alkalosis (usually respiratory)
  Tetanus
  Hypocalcemia
  Hypomagnesemia

Anatomic Pattern of Dysfunction
  Ocular dysfunction (ptosis, ophthalmoparesis)
    Myasthenia
    Botulism
    Organophosphates
    Guillain-Barré syndrome (Miller-Fisher variant)
  Bilateral facial paralysis
    Myasthenia
    Botulism
    Organophosphates
    Guillain-Barré syndrome
    Tick paralysis
  Bulbar involvement (dysphonia, dysarthria, impaired gag
    reflex, difficulty swallowing, drooling, decreased respira-
    tory function)
    Botulism
    Myasthenia
    Guillain-Barré syndrome
    Organophosphates
    Necrotic myopathies
    Tick paralysis
    Diphtheria
    Polio

Prominent proximal weakness
  Necrotic myopathies
  Alcoholic rhabdomyolysis
  Endocrine myopathies
  Guillain-Barré syndrome
  Myasthenia (rare)
  Porphyria
Ascending paralysis
  Guillain-Barré syndrome
  Hyperkalemia or hypokalemia
  Diphtheria
  Porphyria
  Triorthocresylphosphate (TOCP)
  Thallium poisoning
  Tick paralysis
Painful weak muscles
  Rhabdomyolysis
  Necrotic myopathies
  Toxoplasmosis
  Trichinosis
  Toxic shock syndrome
  Hypokalemia
  Hypophosphatemia
  Certain drugs (clofibrate, emetine)
Rhabdomyolysis and myoglobinuria
  Heavy exertion
  Muscle ischemia or infarction
  Alcoholic rhabdomyolysis
  Toxic infections
  Hyperthermia
  Hypokalemia
  Hypophosphatemia
  Heroin use
  Amphetamine abuse
  Phencyclidine use
  Neuroleptic side effects
  Snake bite
  Spider bite (brown recluse)
Electrolyte disturbances
  Hyperkalemia or hypokalemia
  Hypocalcemia
  Hypermagnesemia or hypomagnesemia
  Hypophosphatemia

accomplished after stabilization of vital signs and electrolyte management when appropriate. When indicated, ventilatory support and cardiac monitoring are necessary during transfer.

Since the emergency physician sees many patients with the complaint of weakness, and a very few will have potentially life-threatening weakness, *triage of patients* who complain of weakness is best done by thinking of these categories of patients:

1. Neurologic disorders in which weakness is a prominent manifestation. Weakness here is usually a motor or muscle problem, and it may increase unpredictably and cause respiratory failure (e.g., myasthenia gravis).
2. Systemic disorders that may present as weakness. Gastrointestinal bleeding is a good example. Many patients who have lost blood chronically through the gut, e.g., to a hematocrit of 18, will have a chief complaint of "I feel very weak."

3. Depression and other emotional disorders with weakness mentioned prominently.

Any patient presenting to an emergency department with the complaint of weakness must have a careful and thorough history, physical examination, and screening laboratory tests (complete blood count, SMA 18). Many of the serious causes of weakness will be revealed by the time these data have been collected, and appropriate measures can be taken based on the diagnosis. Certain situations must be taken seriously even when no obvious diagnosis is discovered.

1. Any previously healthy patient who has developed the inability to walk over a period of time up to several months.
2. Patients with recent onset of difficulty swallowing or talking, as evidenced by gagging on food, drooling, or whispering.
3. The complaint of weakness with areflexia in a young person, even without objectively decreased strength (Guillain-Barré syndrome).

TABLE 3 Disorders Causing Acute Weakness

Disorder	Clinical Features	Aids in Diagnosis	Immediate Therapy
Muscle			
Electrolyte disturbances			
Hypokalemia	Symmetric often ascending weakness. Deep tendon reflexes (DTRs)↓ or zero. Bulbar involvement in severe cases.	ECG Serum K+ Admit ICU	Respiratory support if indicated. Close observation. Repletion.
Hyperkalemia	Symmetric often ascending weakness. DTRs ↓ or zero. Often owing to renal or adrenal insufficiency.	ECG Serum K+	ECG monitoring. Respiratory support if indicated. 1) Calcium gluconate 10% IV with ECG monitor; 2 cc/min up to 20-30 cc. 2) Sodium bicarbonate 44-88 mEq IV. 3) Glucose 10% 200-500 cc mixed with 15 units regular insulin. 4) Kayexalate. 5) Dialysis if needed. 6) Treat associated conditions. 7) Admit ICU.
Necrotic myopathies	Proximal then generalized weakness. Painful, tender muscles. Occasionally myoglobinuria. Immune, infectious, and drug causes. Acute alcoholic rhabdomyolysis owing to hypophosphatemia fits here.	CPK Biopsy EMG	Respiratory support if indicated. Monitor vital signs and watch for arrhythmias. Search for specific cause. Admit ICU.
Neuromuscular junction			
Myasthenia gravis	History of fluctuating weakness. Involves extraocular muscles (sparing pupils), masseters, and face, bulbar, and proximal muscles.	Tensilon test EMG	Respiratory support. Admit ICU. Call neurologist.
Botulism	Eating spoiled food followed in 6-72 hours by GI symptoms (50% patients) then dysphagia, dysphonia, diphonia, ptosis, face and jaw weakness, blurred vision, dry mouth, unreactive pupils (50%), and trunk, respiratory, and limb weakness.	Suspicion EMG Call CDC or State Health Department	Respiratory support. Trivalent (ABE) antiserum (Health Department or CDC). Admit ICU. Call neurologist.
Drugs	Apnea, paralysis, ptosis, ophthalmoplegia, and bulbar weakness, following certain antibiotics, adrenergic blockers, membrane stabilizers, psychotropic and anti-inflammatory drugs.	Drug history	Respiratory support as drug is metabolized.
Organophosphate and carbamate insecticides	GI symptoms, sweating, agitation, twitching, small pupils, paralysis.	Exposure history	Respiratory support. Washing and gastric lavage if indicated. Atropine 2 mg IV every 3-5 minutes until bradycardia reversed. Pralidoxime (PAM) 1 g IV over 2 minutes; may repeat once in 20 minutes if no improvement.
Hypercalcemia	Literature scanty. Genuine muscle weakness may not occur. Some reports stress weakness, others spasticity and hyperactive reflexes.	Serum calcium	Hydrate generously, rapidly with normal saline. Lasix 80 mg IV. ICU admission.
Paralytic shellfish poisoning	Thirty minutes after eating toxic shellfish species, paresthesias of mouth, lips, face, then neck, arms, and legs, numbness, then paralysis, including diaphragm. GI signs, salivation, abdominal pain may occur. Mental status normal. Mortality about 10%. Epidemics occur.	History	Respiratory support if necessary. ICU admission. Effects diminish and vanish over 1-2 days.
Tick paralysis	Flaccid ascending paralysis, areflexia, nausea and vomiting, bulbar involvement.	Find tick (often at hairline) and remove it	Respiratory support.

TABLE 3 Disorders Causing Acute Weakness

Porphyrias	Abdominal pain, vomiting, fever, mental disturbances followed by weakness of variable pattern is common presentation. Cramps and muscle tenderness may be present. May mimic Guillain-Barré syndrome	History of previous attacks Heredity Precipitating drug Delta aminolevulinic acid and urine porphobilinogen	ICU admission. IV glucose. IV hematin. Other supportive measures.
Paint thinner or glue sniffing	Predominantly motor neuropathy with rapid onset, respiratory paralysis, muscle atrophy owing to long exposure, persistent sensory complaints.	History	Respiratory support. Admission
Diphtheria	Polyneuropathy appearing 6–12 weeks after onset of disease, seen especially in patients with palatal paralysis occurring during second week. Weakness of limbs (often ascending as in Guillain-Barré syndrome), trunk and neck paresthesias, and areflexia.	History of diphtheria, onset 6–12 weeks earlier	Respiratory support. ICU admission.
Motor neuron Polio and other enteroviruses	Aseptic meningitis picture (fever, headache, stiff neck), aching, then twitching "tight" muscles followed by weakness and then flaccid paralysis and areflexia. Pattern variable: any trunk or limb muscles, bulbar muscles	History Lumbar puncture Electrodiagnosis Virologic studies	Respiratory support. ICU admission.
Paralytic (dumb) rabies	Syndrome mimicking Guillain-Barré syndrome 7–90 days after animal bite (but no bite history in 20%). Pain and paresthesias at bite site, then weakness of same limb with rapid spread to other extremities. Flaccid paralysis with areflexia. Mentation normal until late.	History of animal bite. Lumbar puncture Electrodiagnosis	Respiratory support. ICU admission.
Spinal Cord Cervical cord	Trauma or compression or subluxation. Signs variable depending on location and extent of lesion. Complete lesion gives quadriparesis, sensory level, sphincters out, diaphragm paralysis. CT–C6: biceps and brachioradialis reflexes decreased or absent, triceps and finger-jerks increased, diaphragm affected, spastic paraparesis, sphincters out, sensory level.	History Evidence of trauma Presence of diseases such as cancer or rheumatoid arthritis Cervical spine films	Immobilization of neck. Respiratory support if necessary. Call neurosurgeon.
Transverse myelitis	Thoracic (67%), cervical (22%) or lumbar (11%) level. Back or radicular pain, sensory and motor level, sphincters out, paraparesis developing over hours or days.	Lumbarpuncture with myelogram to rule out compressive lesion	Support. Call neurologist for diagnostic tests.
Epidural abscess	History of skin furuncle, back pain, radicular pain, paraparesis and signs as listed above, fever, headache.	Suspicion and examination	Call neurosurgeon. Do not do lumbar puncture.
Metastases	Cancer history, especially prostate, lung, lymphoma, sarcoma. Local or radicular pain (90%) present for days to weeks followed by evidence of compression that proceeds with striking rapidity: symmetrical weakness, feet paresthesias, sphincter dysfunction, Babinski's, sensory level.	History ofcancer and clinical findings	Call neurosurgeon.

TABLE 3 Disorders Causing Acute Weakness

Acute disk	Pain extending into shoulder or arm or down leg. Examine as under "Cervical cord." Lumbar disc: loss of ankle jerk (or knee jerk): positive straight leg raising	CT scan Myelogram	Call neurologist or neurosurgeon.
Anterior spinal artery occlusion	Due to embolus (e.g., cardiac), aortic dissection, vascular malformation, vasculitis or atherosclerosis. Thoracic cord usually. Sensory and motor level; sphincters out.	Clinical manifestations Search for cause	Admit to ICU.
Ateriovenous malformation or hemorrhage	Vascular malformation or hemorrhage with anticoagulant therapy. Acute pain, motor and sensory level.	History and physical	Admit to ICU. Call neurosurgeon.
Tetanus	Infection of wound or skin ulcer (but none can be found in 25%) followed in 4–20 days by difficulty opening jaws, dysphagia, neck muscle stiffness, then generalized muscle rigidity and spasms, laryngospasm common, even with mild symptoms.	Wound. Suspicion Clinical picture	Be ready to intubate at once (succinylcholine or similar drug needed). Admit to ICU. Diazepam (10 mg IV (q4–6h) and chlorpromazine (25–50 mg IV q4–6h) or similar drugs.
Hypermagnesemia	Level of 3 mEq/L: smooth muscle paralysis, nausea and vomiting, hypotension. 5–10 mEq/L: heart block and cardiac arrest	Serum Mg	Respiratory support. ECG monitor. Calcium gluconate 10%, 10 cc IV followed immediately by dialysis depending on level.
Neurotoxic snake bite	Paralysis 1–10 hours after bite. Eye muscle weakness, facial and jaw weakness, bulbar paralysis, limb paralysis, seizures.	History and signs of bite	Specific antivenin, respiratory support.
Peripheral nerve Guillain-Barré syndrome	Presenting symptom paresthesias (50%), paresthesias and weakness (25%), or weakness (25%). Weakness often begins in legs and ascends but may be diffuse or spotty. Decreased to absent reflexes. Respiratory involvement and autonomic hyperreflexia with cardiac arrhythmias are life-threatening. Many patients come to emergency room at least once before diagnosis is made. Complaint of mild weakness with areflexia in previously healthy individual highly suspicious.	Electrodiagnostic studies Elevated CSF protein	ICU admission. ECG monitoring. Respiratory support.
Hypophosphatemia	Paresthesias (lips, feet) followed by generalized weakness including cranial nerves and respiration. Seen most often in patients on hyperalimentation and alcoholics. Symptoms can be fulminating.	Serum phosphorous below 1.0 mg/dl: usually 0.6 mg/dl or lower	Respiratory support if necessary. Admit to ICU. ECG monitoring. Replace 20–40 mm phosphate IV q8h adding other electrolytes if they are low (calcium, potassium, magnesium). Monitor serum values of all these electrolytes closely.
Hypocalcemia	Tetany without actual paralysis. Laryngeal spasm can cause death. Seen post-thyroidectomy, post-hypoparathyroidectomy, in alcoholics with pancreatitis, renal failure	Hyperventilation Trousseau's test (blood pressure cuff) Chvostek's sign Serum calcium	Observe carefully for laryngeal spasm (emergency intubation if possible or cricothyrotomy may be necessary). ECG monitoring. IV repletion of calcium.

4. Weakness in a patient with cancer.
5. Trauma followed by weakness.
6. Weakness in a patient with a disease known to produce spinal cord compression, e.g., rheumatoid arthritis.

There will remain a number of patients, many of whom fit into the third category (those with emotional disorders). These patients should be given explicit instructions about immediately returning to emergency should there be any change in or addition to their symptomatology, and they should be referred to their primary physician. In addition, the physician should be sure that patients discharged have a home situation that provides reasonable support and the ability to return to emergency if deterioration occurs.

SUGGESTED READING

Layzer RB. Neuromuscular manifestations of systemic disease. Philadelphia: FA Davis, 1985.
Ringel SP. Clinical presentations in neuromuscular disease. In: Vinken PJ, Bruyn GW, eds. Handbook of clinical neurology. Vol. 40, Diseases of muscle. Amsterdam, North-Holland: Elsevier, 1979; 295.
Walker HK. Neurological disorders. In: Hurst JW ed. Medicine for the practicing physician. Boston: Butterworth 1983; 1539.

GRAND MAL (MAJOR MOTOR) SEIZURES

ROBERT H. DAILEY, M.D.

DIAGNOSIS AND ETIOLOGY

Most seizure patients who are brought to the emergency department are not actively seizing, and it may not be immediately apparent that a seizure has occurred. To clarify this situation, an understanding of the natural history of a seizure is helpful. A major motor seizure has several phases. The first is sudden loss of consciousness; the second, generalized rigidity of all muscle groups (tonic phase), lasting less than a minute; and the third, rhythmic generalized jerking movements (clonic phase) of variable duration. During the first phase, a fall may result in trauma to the elbows, shoulders, or head, especially the occiput or supraorbital ridges. During the last two phases, the patient hypoventilates (secondary to ineffective intercostal and diaphragmatic motion) and may chew the tongue. Immediately following the seizure, all muscle groups relax (including sphincters) with consequent common urinary incontinence and uncommon fecal incontinence. After the seizure (postictal phase) there is coma, gradually lightening to stupor and confusion. Postictally, hyperventilation compensates for respiratory and lactic acidosis. Muscular hyperactivity and increased sympathetic tone cause fever, leukocytosis, and hyperglycemia. The postictal phase lasts minutes to hours, depending on the severity and duration of the seizure. Some rare patients consistently manifest hemiparesis postictally (Todd's paralysis); this hemiparesis often takes many hours to clear. However, unless the patient is known to regularly have postictal paralysis, it must immediately be evaluated by computed tomography (CT) scan. When no history is available, the most pathognomonic indicator of a prior major motor seizure is a chewed tongue; the tongue is rarely bitten (occurring only when the patient falls with the tongue accidentally protruding), but rather the lateral margins and tip are chewed. However, a significant minority do not chew their tongue.

The foregoing description is classic; many patients with legitimate seizure disorders present with complex, atypical, or confusing pictures that make the diagnosis less apparent. Petit mal, temporal lobe seizures, and behavioral abnormalities should be considered. Some hysterical patients learn to effectively imitate grand mal seizures in order to draw attention to themselves and their problems. Characteristically, such *"pseudo-seizures"* predicted by the patient, occur in settings with secondary gain, have no tonic phase, are associated with emotion, tears, screaming, or anger, and are goal-directed, especially assaultive. However, even the most sophisticated clinician sometimes has difficulty in differentiating between true seizures and pseudo-seizures, and indeed these entities are not mutually exclusive.

Once it has been determined that a grand mal seizure has occurred, the physician should formulate a differential diagnosis. Table 1 lists some of the more common etiologies. It is important to note that poor control of seizures is usually attributable to noncompliance with treatment regimens. The history is of overwhelming importance in evaluating seizures; a determined attempt must be made to question relatives or observers of the patient.

On *physical examination*, special attention must be made to rule out head trauma (unfortunately acute head trauma may be a cause *or* a result of the seizure). Atten-

TABLE 1 Causes of Grand Mal Seizures

Discontinued anticonvulsant medication

Alcohol withdrawal

Head trauma and neurosurgery (immediate and delayed)

Metabolic: hypoxia, hyponatremia, uremia, hypoglycemia, hypomagnesemia

"Toxic": eclampsia, heat stroke

Drugs: ASA, INH, lidocaine, cocaine, amphetamines, tricyclic antidepressants (TCAs), phenothiazines, aminophylline, camphor, zephirin, propoxyphene (Darvon), codeine, ergot, boric acid, many others

Infections: meningitis, encephalitis, brain abscess

CVA: especially with infarction and hemorrhage

Brain tumors: both primary and metastatic

Idiopathic

tion should be paid to the pupils, fundi, tympanic membranes, tongue, and neck. A formal neurologic examination is usually neither possible nor helpful, but careful observation for differences in limb movement in the immediate postictal period is important. Most patients are flaccid and have positive Babinski signs.

Certain *laboratory and other studies* are indicated. All patients should have a bedside glucose analysis strip performed to rule out hypoglycemia. Although the return is low, measurements of electrolytes and blood urea nitrogen are indicated when hyponatremia and uremia are possible causes. Magnesium or calcium levels should be only selectively ordered. Toxicology screens should be considered if epileptogenic drugs may have been ingested. Skull films are seldom indicated; CT scans have largely supplanted them. Cervical spine films should be obtained if significant head trauma may have occurred.

The decision whether a *lumbar puncture* (LP) should be performed is often difficult; seizures alone may cause fever, headache, confusion, and lethargy. Therefore, an LP to rule out meningitis is indicated only if there is no rapid postictal improvement in mental status. The LP is no longer used as the primary means to rule out subarachnoid hemorrhage, since a noncontrast CT scan is positive in over 75 percent of cases. Criteria for emergency CT scans following a seizure are difficult to establish. Some are as follows: focal seizure or central nervous system (CNS) findings, status epilepticus without toxic or metabolic explanation, prolonged postictal state, signs of increased intracranial pressure, associated head trauma, or unexplained coma. What is considered a "prolonged" postictal state? Most patients with a single grand mal seizure awaken to confused lethargy within minutes; a longer period—even hours—can be expected following multiple severe seizures or status. The most important consideration is that the patient's mental status should continues to improve.

TREATMENT

Why should a seizure be treated? The answer is because brain damage occurs, both from the seizure itself (primary factors) and from the metabolic or traumatic consequences (secondary factors). Among the primary factors are impaired autoregulation of cerebral blood flow; excessive brain glucose utilization, which exceeds glucose transport across the blood brain barrier; and the nonspecific deleterious effect on the brain of tetanic electrical discharge. Secondary factors include direct brain trauma occurring with falls; lactic acidosis generated by excessive skeletal muscular contraction; and hypoxia and hypercarbia from ineffective ventilation and partial upper airway obstruction. Thus, seizures must be controlled.

General Measures

During seizure activity the patient's *airway* must be ensured and any *further injury avoided*. Specifically, the gurney side rails must be up and padded, the patient turned on his side, leather waist restraints applied (no limb restraints, since fractures and dislocations can occur), oxygen given by nasal cannula, and pillows placed appropriately. Tongue blade insertion should be avoided since it is unnecessary and difficult, and may cause gagging, vomiting, and aspiration. If the tongue obstructs the upper airway, even though the patient is on his side, a soft nasopharyngeal airway may be placed. While these general measures are being performed, seizure activity generally subsides spontaneously, and then further specific treatment can proceed in an organized and orderly fashion.

An intravenous catheter should be placed and blood specimens drawn; the catheter must be well secured in the event of another seizure. Then intravenous antidotes should be considered: glucose for hypoglycemia, naloxone for propoxyphine (Darvon) overdose, pyridoxine for isoniazid intoxication, thiamine for any alcoholic (consider Wernicke's syndrome), and physostigmine for anticholinergic poisonings. A word of caution: some antidotes (e.g. physostigmine) have their own toxicity and therefore should be given only for proven specific intoxications.

Anticonvulsant Drug Therapy

Once basic supportive therapy has been instituted, anticonvulsive therapy should be considered. The specific drug, route of administration, and urgency of administration must be determined by the specific clinical circumstances. First, oral or intramuscular drug delivery is usually inappropriate in the emergency department. Delayed or inconsistent drug absorption by such routes makes rapid and predictable blood levels unachievable; rather, drugs should be given intravenously. More than 95 percent of motor seizures can be controlled by diazepam (Valium), phenytoin (Dilantin), or phenobarbital. The pharmacology of these drugs is summarized in Table 2. All three drugs are poorly water-soluble and so are suspended in propylene glycol. This vehicle may, of itself, cause respiratory depression, hypotension, and electrocardiographic changes, but only with phenytoin loading is the amount of propylene glycol sufficient for such potential side effects. Despite the insolubility of these three drugs in routine intravenous solutions, there has been uniformly adequate delivery when they are injected into rapidly flowing solutions of normal saline.

Diazepam is packaged in a disposable syringe, 10 mg in 2 cc. It should be injected into the intravenous line no faster than 5 mg per minute. Its anticonvulsant activity is immediate; however, because it rapidly distributes into tissues, its effective duration is only about 20 minutes. Elderly patients, especially those with toxic or metabolic problems, are sensitive to its respiratory depressant effect, and so should be given smaller initial doses. Should hypoventilation occur, however, bag/mask ventilation for 10 or 15 minutes is usually adequate ventilatory support. Lorazepam is another useful benzodiazepine; it is probably at least as effective as diazepam and has a longer duration of action. More experience is needed before its place in therapy can be determined.

TABLE 2 Principal Emergency Department Drugs for Grand Mal Seizures

		Half-Life	Diluent	Loading Dose	Rate of Administration	Time to Peak Brain Level	Therapeutic Blood Level	Maintenance Dose	Complications		
									Resp	CV	Other
Diazepam (Valium) (10 mg/2 cc)	IV	20 min*	40%	5–20 mg	<5 mg/min	1 min	300 µg/ml	5 mg q30–45min post-loading	4+	2+	
	PO	30 hours		N/A	N/A	N/A					
Phenytoin (Dilantin) (100 mg/2 ml) (250 mg/5 ml)	IV	Approx. 25 hours	40%	15–18 mg/kg Same (approx. 1 g)	<50 mg/min Best in divided doses	6 min 6–14 hours less in low doses	10–20 µg/dl (mg/L)	100 mg IVP q6h 200–400 mg daily ? divided	3+	4+	CNS 2+ GI and CNS
	PO										
Phenobarbital (130 mg/ml) tubex	IV	±100 hours	75% propylene glycol	? 10–15 mg/kg	<50 mg/min in 250 mg increments?	3 min	10–30 µg/dl (mg/L)	Virtually un-necessary in ED	3+	2+	CNS 4+
	PO			Same	Divided doses	12–18 hours		120 mg/day			2+ CNS

* Distribution (not elimination) half-life.

Phenytoin is packaged variously, but always in a concentration of 50 mg per milliliter. The loading dose is considered 15 to 18 mg per kilogram. However, most alcoholic patients require and tolerate less. Because of low serum albumins in alcoholics, a given dose of phenytoin is less protein-bound and results in higher levels of the free drug than in nonalcoholics. Also, alcohol markedly potentiates the cerebellar toxic signs of phenytoin. Phenytoin can be given intravenously in one of three ways: first, as with diazepam, by injection into the intravenous line; second, by utilizing a Harvard infusion pump to inject into the intravenous line; and third, by diluting the phenytoin with small amounts (50 to 100 ml) of normal saline in an on-line chamber (Volutrol, Buritrol) and delivering by an infusion-regulating device (e.g., Ivac). All three methods are practical and effective, and every physician should become comfortable with one of them and its use according to a standardized protocol. The rate of administration should not exceed 50 mg per minute. Problems of crystal precipitation have been greatly exaggerated: what precipitation does occur is harmless, does not influence dosing, and is minimized by the on-line 0.45-micron filter of standard intravenous tubing.

Diazepam and phenytoin are a logical combination to provide rapid, smooth control of seizure activity. Diazepam provides control for the 20 minutes necessary for phenytoin loading.

Phenobarbital is an excellent anticonvulsant and, if given intravenously, is safe and rapidly effective. However, the relationship between intravenous doses and serum blood levels in adults has been unclear. This has recently been studied, and a mean loading dose of 550 mg reliably results in a mean blood level of 15 mg per deciliter (therapeutic). Although most patients would be heavily sedated by such a loading dose, sedative-resistant patients in alcohol withdrawal remain alert. Furthermore, with the advent of CT scans, wakefulness is no longer important as a parameter of CNS function in scanned patients. When the drug is given at rates less than 50 mg per minute, cardiovascular or respiratory depression are rare.

SPECIAL CIRCUMSTANCES

Alcoholic Withdrawal Seizures

Major motor seizures often occur as an early sign of alcohol withdrawal. Whether they should be treated and, if so, with what drug remain two active controversies. However, some rational judgments may be made when one considers the natural history of alcohol withdrawal seizures: patients have only a few seizures, 90 percent of them within a 6-hour period; most patients with prior alcohol withdrawal seizures seize again in the same setting; and conversely, patients who have not seized before in a setting of alcohol withdrawal are unlikely to do so during a subsequent episode. Thus, if the patient is seen soon after convulsing in a setting of alcohol withdrawal, and seizures have occurred during previous alcohol withdrawal, seizure control is probably warranted. As regards

the effectiveness of the three aforementioned drugs: diazepam is effective, but requires multiple dosing over the 6-hour "risk" period; although some data have suggested the effectiveness of phenytoin, two more recent studies have not supported this conclusion. Phenobarbital is probably effective, but this remains to be proved.

Seizures due to Noncompliance With Anticonvulsant Therapy

This situation is commonly encountered in many emergency departments, where in one must decide whether to await blood levels before instituting therapy or to treat "blindly." If clinical noncompliance and other circumstances indicate high risk for more seizures in the immediate future, it is prudent to administer a submaximal loading dose of phenytoin intravenously (350 to 500 mg); if the risk of seizures appears small, and turn-around time on anticonvulsant blood levels is short, await the blood levels.

Status Epilepticus

Seizure activity that is continuous or near-continuous constitutes a true medical emergency that must be promptly and aggressively treated. The same supportive care and specific drug therapy discussed previously is pertinent here. While directing primary attention to ruling out serious underlying disorders in need of immediate correction (such as meningitis, traumatic hematomas, and metabolic and drug conditions), one must pay careful attention to adequate ventilation and oxygenation.

If status epilepticus cannot be promptly controlled, the patient should be intubated and ventilated. Often blind nasotracheal intubation is successful, but if not, the patient should be paralyzed and intubated orotracheally. Following intubation, diazepam, phenytoin, or phenobarbital should be given aggressively, and the patient checked frequently for hypoventilation and hypotension. It is rare for full loading doses of all these three drugs to fail to control status epilepticus. However, should this be the case, and toxic/metabolic causes ruled out, other agents, such as paraldehyde (10 to 20 cc PO, diluted, by nasogastric (NG) tube), valproic acid (1 to 1.5 g as the syrup, by NG or rectal tube), lidocaine (1 mg per kilogram load, then 2 to 3 mg/min infusion), general anesthesia, or long-term paralysis, must be considered. Since uncontrollable status is unusual, no single author has a large experience with any of these secondary modalities.

SUGGESTED READING

Bauer LA, Edwards WAD, Dellinger EP, et al. Importance of unbound phenytoin serum levels in head trauma patients. J Trauma 1983; 23:1058–1060.

Cloyd JC, Gumnit RJ, McLain LW. Status epilepticus. JAMA 1980; 244:1479–1481.

Ernest MP, Marx JA, Drury LR. Complications of intravenous phenytoin for acute treatment of seizures. JAMA 1983; 249:762–765.

Leppik IE, Derivan AT, Homan RW, et al. Double-bind study of lorazepam and diazepam in status epilepticus JAMA 1983; 249:1452–1454.

Wilbur R, Kuiik FA. Anticonvulsant drugs in alcohol withdrawal. Am J Hosp Pharm 1981; 38:1138–143.

EPIDURAL, SUBDURAL, AND INTRACRANIAL BLEEDING

LAWRENCE H. PITTS, M.D.

Trauma is by far the leading cause of intracranial hemorrhage. Traumatic hemorrhage occurs much more frequently than does bleeding from vascular anomalies or intracranial tumors. There are more than 100,000 coma-producing head injuries in the country each year, nearly 50 percent of which are fatal and significantly more which are accompanied by severe head injuries, virtually all of which have some degree of intracranial hemorrhage. Bleeding can occur into any of the intracranial spaces and not uncommonly into more than one space in one patient. Whereas small amounts of blood in the subarachnoid, epidural, subdural, or intracerebral compartments may not require specific therapy, progressive hemorrhage and brain compression after head injury is a life-threatening emergency that must be diagnosed and treated as quickly as possible to reduce the morbidity and mortality of head injury.

ETIOLOGY

Traumatic subarachnoid hemorrhage (SAH) occurs commonly after injury, even with relatively minor impacts, probably from tearing of small pial arteries or veins. This type of SAH can be seen in some patients on computed tomography (CT) scan, is almost always self-limited, and in the acute situation, is of no importance.

Epidural hematomas (EDHs) are exceedingly rare without a skull fracture. At the time of fracture, the dura is stripped from the inner table of the skull, thereby allowing bleeding into the space between skull and dura from either the fracture itself or from torn meningeal arteries or veins. A torn artery can bleed with sufficient pressure to continue to strip the dura from the skull, thereby giving rise to an expanding EDH, sometimes of large size with subsequent brain compression. Fractures through thin parts of the skull, especially in the temporal region, can occur with little concomitant instrinsic brain injury. As many as one-third of patients who develop EDHs are not rendered unconscious at the time of impact and may have remarkably good brain function until the EDH expands sufficiently to cause brain compression. Although these patients may be able to open their eyes and possibly follow commands, they generally complain of significant headache that may be accompanied by nausea or vomiting; they begin to deteriorate neurologically as the EDH expands. Since EDHs often occur in the absence of instrinsic brain damage, these are important traumatic lesions to recognize promptly since their treatment can result in a normal outcome.

Subdural hematomas (SDHs) are the most common post-traumatic intracranial mass lesions that require sur-

gery. They occur more frequently in older patients suffering low velocity injuries such as falls and may be present in as many as 50 percent of patients with coma-producing head injury. SDHs are somewhat less common in younger patients and those suffering injuries as motor vehicle occupants. SDHs typically occur with laceration of veins, that travel from the cortical surface through the subarachnoid space to join the superior saggital sinus. Antero-posterior movement of the skull in the saggital plane carries a significant risk of tearing these bridging veins with venous hemorrhage collecting in the subdural space. SDHs are somewhat more frequent in the frontal and temporal regions, but can extend from front to back over the cortex and can achieve remarkably large sizes of 100 to 200 cc or more. The energy necessary to cause a SDH often also cause diffuse brain injury at impact so that many patients with acute SDH are rendered unconscious at impact and remain so as the SDH enlarges. Because of the intrinsic brain damage, the outcome after SDH formation is significantly worse than with other kinds of brain hemorrhage.

Traumatic intracerebral hematomas (ICHs) also are more common in older than younger patients, although they can occur at any age. About one-third have accompanying SDHs or EDHs and can occur any time after injury although only 25 percent are present within 6 hours of injury. Early CT scans typically show areas of contusion that later coalesce into formed hematomas, but occasionally the initial CT scan shows no brain abnormality where an ICH eventually develops. Since ICHs are somewhat slower to form than SDHs or EDHs, they usually do not require treatment in the early hours after injury.

Brain hemorrhage can occur with compound depressed fractures directly from brain laceration and tearing of superficial arteries and veins. The compartments into which bleeding occurs include all of those already listed.

PRE-HOSPITAL THERAPY

Since the brain injury that occurs at the time of impact (primary injury) cannot be treated specifically, therapy necessarily is limited to the recognition and the prevention or reversal of those insults that can further damage the injured brain (secondary injury). Therefore, pre-hospital treatment is directed to systemic abnormalities with control of hemorrhage, reversal of shock by leg elevation, or intravenous fluid administration, and treatment of hypoxia or hypercarbia by mask ventilation with 100 percent O_2. In a few circumstances, when highly skilled personnel are available, endotracheal intubation allows optimal control of arterial gases. However, it should be noted that intubation can cause increased intracranial pressure with additional brain ischemia, if intracranial hypertension already exists after injury.

EMERGENCY DEPARTMENT MANAGEMENT

Vigorous fluid resuscitation and airway management should be continued as soon as the patient arrives in the emergency department. The injured brain is particularly vulnerable to hypoxia and shock so that securing an airway, controlling ventilation and hemorrhage, and restoring normal blood pressure are of vital importance in the head injured patient. If a lethargic patient appears to be breathing comfortably, arterial blood gases should be determined to ensure adequate spontaneous ventilation. Comatose patients should be intubated to prevent vomiting or aspiration and to reverse hypoventilation. In comatose patients there is always the possibility of an intracranial hematoma with sufficient size to cause a mass effect and intracranial hypertension. Hyperventilation to Pco_2 of 25 to 30 mm Hg causes cerebral vasoconstriction with a reduction in intracranial blood volume and intracranial pressure (ICP). (Also see chapters *The Comatose Patient* and *Rapid Sedation and Rapid-Induction Anesthesia for Emergency Intubation*).

After external hemorrhage is controlled, shock must be vigorously treated with crystalloid fluid replacement in sufficient volumes to establish normal blood pressures. If arterial pressures cannot be returned to, and maintained at, normal levels, intrathoracic or intra-abdominal bleeding should be suspected and evaluated by chest x-ray film and appropriate abdominal examinations or diagnostic tests, possibly including peritoneal dialysis or abdominal CT scanning. Few lesions are as damaging to the injured brain as hemo- or pneumothorax, which both raise venous and intracranial pressures, promote hypoxia, and cause hypercapnia with cerebral vasodilitation and increased ICP. It is imperative these secondary injuries are treated promptly.

Only after initial resuscitation is deemed satisfactory is a baseline *neurological evaluation* conducted. The examination must provide sufficient data to allow later comparison examinations to determine whether the patient is improving, deteriorating, or remaining stable. Determination of level of consciousness using the Glasgow Coma Score (Table 1) can be done quickly and reliably and offers a much more exact description of consciousness than such ill-defined descriptions as lethargic, stuporous, or poorly responsive. Other initial observations must include evaluation of brainstem responses. Pupillary size, quality, and responsiveness to light should be documented. Assessment of eye movements can provide important information about the integrity of the brainstem—including the majority of the pons and midbrain. Conjugate horizontal eye movement indicates that the III (medial rectus) and the VI (lateral rectus) nerves are intact and their nuclei are joined by a functioning medial longitudinal fasciculus. If spontaneous eye movement is not present, cold water caloric testing should be done with up to 100 cc of ice water instilled in the external auditory canal, provided the tympanic membrane is intact. This should cause conjugate gaze toward the irrigated ear. After lateral x-ray films exclude cervical spine fractures, smooth, but fairly brisk, lateral rotation of the head should provoke eye movement opposite to the direction of head movement (doll's eyes maneuver) again indicating intact brainstem reflexes. The gag reflex should be ascertained as well as a cough reflex in intubated patients. The Glasgow Coma Score determi-

TABLE 1 Glasgow Coma Scale

Eyes open	Never	1
	To pain	2
	To verbal stimuli	3
	Spontaneously	4
Best verbal response	None	1
	Incomprehensible sounds	2
	Inappropriate words	3
	Disoriented and converses	4
	Oriented and converses	5
Best motor response	None	1
	Extensor posturing (decerebrate rigidity)	2
	Flexor posturing (decorticate rigidity)	3
	Complex flexion	4
	Localizes pain	5
	Obeys	6
Total (Eye + verbal + motor scores)		3–15

nation of level of consciousness, and the entire brainstem examination can be done in 3 to 4 minutes.

At times with head injury, a patient's level of consciousness is depressed owing to alcohol, other intoxication, or perhaps owing to a recent seizure. Since an inebriated patient should improve over 3 to 4 hours and the postictal patient in an hour or less, serial neurologic examinations can be used to document a patient's improvement or lack thereof. If a patient fails to improve or if a patient deteriorates below the initial baseline examination, an *emergency CT scan* without contrast should be obtained. A CT scan should be promptly obtainable on an around the clock basis in facilities where significant head injuries are treated. A CT scan is the easiest, most available, and most reliable intracranial study in patients with traumatic cerebral lesions. Hemorrhage of any significant volume in any of the brain compartments is readily seen. In addition, mass effect is demonstrated by deformation or collapse of the ventricles, shifts of the pineal, and compromise of the basal cisterns. In the event of patient deterioration, immediate *neurosurgical consultation* should be obtained so that the most rapid definitive treatment of mass lesions can be started.

An intracranial hematoma should be suspected and a CT scan obtained in all patients in traumatic coma (Glasgow Coma Score 8 or less) or in those with focal neurologic abnormalities such as hemiparesis or dysphasia. When such patients are enroute to the CT scanner or the operating room for bur-hole exploration for an extracerebral mass lesion, *mannitol* (1.5 g per kilogram of an intravenous 20 percent solution) should be given rapidly. Mannitol should not be used in patients undergoing serial observation without CT scanning since mannitol can cause brain dehydration and temporarily allow a mass lesion to enlarge without neurologic progression. However, when the mass becomes sufficiently large enough to cause symptomatic brain compression, further medical management with mannitol or hyperventilation is less effective than if used earlier in the patient's course. Thus, *mannitol should only be used when the patient is "going somewhere", specifically for a CT scan or surgery.*

The risk of *post-traumatic seizures* is increased by the presence of a subdural or epidural hematoma so that *phenytoin* loading should be done early in the patient's course, either in the emergency department or in the operating room. An appropriate initial dose is 15 mg per kilogram given intravenously with continuous monitoring of the electrocardiogram (EKG) and arterial pressure, the latter preferably by an indwelling arterial catheter connected to a pressure transducer and a bedside monitor. At least five prospective randomized clinical trials of *corticosteroids* in head injury have failed to demonstrate any improvement in outcome after coma-producing head injury, and they are being used progressively less by neurosurgeons for craniocerebral trauma. Prophylactic antibiotics generally are not used except in penetrating head injury.

Treatment of *infants and children* is not substantially different from that of adults. Subdural hematomas are less common than in older patients, but intracranial hemorrhage of all types can occur even in infants. Nausea, vomiting, and early seizures are more common in young patients, but their presence or absence correlates poorly with intracranial hematomas. Because orientation is difficult to document in young children, CT scanning should be used fairly liberally in their evaluation. Whereas a negative early CT scan does not preclude later hematoma formation, it gives a substantial safety margin to a course of expectant observation; this is true in infants and children as well as in adults.

HOSPITAL ADMISSION

Patients with normal neurologic function after head injury are extremely unlikely to develop intracranial com-plications and can be discharged from the emergency department after adequate instructions are given to a responsible family or friend regarding the danger signs of neurologic deterioration. Patients with severe nausea, vomiting, or headaches often cannot be managed satisfactorily at home and are admitted for observation and sometimes intravenous hydration. As mentioned above, patients in coma with focal findings require CT scanning, which also may be warranted in lethargic patients who do not improve within 6 hours of their injury. Intoxicated patients can be observed initially in the emergency setting, but CT scanning should be considered in these patients if they do not improve within 3 to 4 hours after injury. The risk of intracranial hematoma formation is markedly higher in patients with skull fractures so that consideration should be given to admitting for observation those patients with recognized new fractures of the skull base or vault. In many cases, overnight observation allows a patient to clear sufficiently to be discharged, although hospitalization for a few days is common in patients who have been rendered unconscious at the time of injury and who are initially lethargic in the emergency department. Patients admitted to the hospital should be under the care of a neurologist or neurosurgeon, or a primary care physician or trauma surgeon with a close working relationship with a neurosurgeon so that changes in neurologic status can be assessed and treated expeditiously.

SUGGESTED READING

Bowers SA, Marshall LF. Outcome in 200 consecutive cases of severe head injury treated in San Diego County: a prospective analysis. Neurosurgery 1980; 6:237–242.
Jennett B, Teasdale G, Galbraith S, et al. Severe head injuries in three countries. J Neurol Neurosurg Psychiat 1977; 40:291–298.
Miller JD, Butterworth JF, Gudeman SK, et al. Further experience in the management of severe head injury. J Neurosurg 1981; 54:289–299.

BACTERIAL MENINGITIS

NORBERT J. ROBERTS Jr., M.D.

Bacterial meningitis is a relatively common infection which, if unrecognized and untreated, is almost uniformly fatal. If recognition and treatment are delayed, the patient is often left with severe neurologic sequelae. Although history and physical examination are useful, the diagnosis of meningitis ultimately depends on findings in the cerebrospinal fluid (CSF), and whenever the diagnosis is seriously considered, a lumbar puncture is indicated.

The majority of cases of bacterial meningitis in both children and adults are due to *Streptococcus pneumoniae*, *Haemophilus influenzae*, and *Neisseria meningitidis*. A variety of factors, including age and presence of underlying diseases, determines whether these or other organisms are involved. For example, *H. influenzae* is responsible for over 40 percent of cases in children under 5 years of age, but less than one percent of cases in adults. Neonates are frequently infected with streptococci or gram-negative bacilli, which are unusual in adults. The patient with a CSF shunt is more likely to be infected with *Staphylococcus epidermidis*, *Staphylococcus aureus*, or (to a lesser extent) streptococci, diptheroids, gram-negative enteric bacilli, or other organisms. The immunosuppressed host is susceptible to a wide variety of organisms, including *Listeria monocytogenes*, enteric gram-negative organisms, staphylococci, strepotococci, and others. In this setting, any organism is a potential pathogen and should not be dismissed as a contaminant. A postoperative neurosurgical patient is more likely to have meningitis due to staphylococci or gram-negative enteric bacilli. It should be noted that patients routinely may have nuchal rigidity, headache, and neurologic findings after neurosurgery. Thus, these signs are not as useful in determining the presence of bacterial meningitis. Fever in a postoperative neurosurgical patient, even with an obvious alternate source, warrants additional evaluation of CSF.

Bacterial meningitis must be distinguished from nonbacterial meningitis although, in an individual patient, this is not always possible in the initial evaluation. In viral meningitis the prodrome is usually prolonged and the patients are less toxic. Fungal and mycobacterial meningitides commonly have an even longer pre-diagnosis history. Nonbacterial meningitis may even exhibit marked signs similar to those of bacterial meningitis. Hence, a small proportion of patients with aseptic meningitis present with coma and localizing neurologic signs. Patients with fungal and tuberculous meningitis tend to have more chronic progressive signs; such patients are often immunocompromised. All patients require examination of CSF to make the diagnosis.

DIAGNOSIS

A typical history suggesting meningitis consists of headache, fever, lethargy, confusion, and stiff neck. The presentation may be variable, so that meningitis should be considered in any patient with fever and even minimal neurologic signs and symptoms. The onset of symptoms may be rapid, without prior known respiratory illness, or slower (1 to 7 days), often with preceding upper respiratory infection and symptoms. Occasionally, the symptoms of meningitis may appear as late as 3 weeks after respiratory illness. In addition to recent upper and lower respiratory tract infections, otitis media and/or sinusitis, underlying debilitating diseases, or recent neurosurgical procedures may predispose to development of bacterial meningitis. If a family member or close contact (enclosed environment) has had meningitis recently, the risk for development of meningitis may be greater than for the population at large.

The diagnosis of bacterial meningitis cannot be reliably established or excluded by physical findings, although they are helpful. Neurologic findings include nuchal rigidity and associated signs (Kernig's or Brudzinski's), altered level of consciousness, and neurologic deficits. However, nuchal rigidity may be absent. Physical findings may suggest associated diseases such as otitis media. Petechiae or other types of rashes (such as purpura or vasculitic lesions) are common signs in meningococcal infection, but are not pathognomonic of meningococci, being observed occasionally in other bacterial meningitides as well as in viral infections.

General laboratory tests are helpful in supporting, but not in excluding, the diagnosis of meningitis. Blood cultures are often positive in bacterial meningitis. If a space-occupying lesion is suspected clinically rather than meningitis, computerized tomography (CT) should be performed to detect such a lesion before a *lumbar puncture* is done. However, such a procedure should not substantially delay the performance of a careful lumbar puncture (with a small-bore needle) if meningitis is suspected. Clearly, CSF examination is the most important investigation and should be performed promptly so that therapy can be started. There are few contraindications to a carefully performed lumbar puncture and even these are relative. If the patient is critically ill and bacterial meningitis is a good possibility, careful lumbar puncture may have to be performed without delay. Precautions to avoid herniation include the use of a small-bore needle and the availability and use of mannitol and/or steroids to prevent herniation if elevated pressures are found. Herniation is a risk chiefly in seriously ill patients with obtundation and localizing neurologic signs; it is much less likely to occur in the awake patient without such signs.

Four to 5 ml of CSF are required from adults for routine initial studies. However, having more CSF available for culture enhances the probability of establishing a microbial etiology. If the opening CSF pressure is normal, that is, less than 20 cm H_2O, 10 to 15 ml of CSF can usually be obtained safely. The results of CSF examination may vary widely, depending on the clinical circumstances. Thus, rigid application of common value ranges to the data from an individual patient is inappropriate and can lead to error. Bacterial meningitis is usually associated with (1) a CSF white blood cell count that is elevated (commonly > 1,000), consisting predominantly (> 60 percent) of polymorphonuclear leukocytes; (2) a depressed glucose (< 45, or < 60 percent of blood glucose); (3) elevated protein (> 80); (4) a positive Gram stain (80 percent of cases); and (5) a positive bacterial culture (> 90 percent of cases). Typical CSF findings in other intracranial infections are listed in Table 1. Blood glucose levels are important especially in detecting the confounding feature of an elevated blood glucose level (e.g., in diabetics or with intravenous glucose administration), which could produce a "false normal" absolute CSF glucose value. Early in bacterial meningitis, the CSF values can be entirely normal, or mononuclear leukocytes or lymphocytes may be predominant. Careful observation with repeat lumbar puncture may be indicated in a minimally ill individual if bacterial meningitis remains a possibility.

The CSF values may be altered by partial treatment of bacterial meningitis, and a history of prior antibiotic use should be sought in all patients. In such cases, although the white blood cell count and percent polymorphonuclear leukocytes may remain elevated, there may be less prominent depression of glucose values, elevation of protein values, and even a relatively increased percent of mononuclear leukocytes. With partial treatment of meningitis, a decreased percent of cases have positive Gram stains and cultures. Partially treated bacterial meningitis is a particular concern in pediatric cases, in which oral antibiotic therapy may have been initiated prior to consideration of meningitis. Such oral doses of antibiotics

TABLE 1 CSF Parameters in Meningitis

Laboratory parameter	Bacterial meningitis (untreated)	Bacterial meningitis* (partially treated)	Viral meningitis	Fungal meningitis	Tuberculous meningitis	Carcinomatous meningitis	Brain abscess	Endocarditis
White cell count	↑(>1000)††	↑(>1000)	↑(<1000)‡	↑(<500)	↑(<1000)	0—500	↑(10—500)	↑(<500)
Polys	↑(>60% PMN)	↑(>60% PMN)	↑(10% of Pts.)*		↑*	0—95%		↑(28% of patients)
Lymphs			↑	↑				↑(25% of patients)
Red blood cells	0	0	Variable	0	0	Variable	Variable	Occasionally↑
Glucose	↓(<45)†	↓(<45) Variable	Normal§	Normal; slight↓	↓(<45)	↓; Normal	Normal; ↓ (25%)	Normal; ↓
Protein	↑(>80)	↑(Variable)	Normal; slight↑§	↑(>60)	↑↑(>100)	Usually ↑	↑(75%)	Normal; ↑
Gram stain	+(80%)	+(60%)	Negative	Negative	+ AFB Stain (80%)**	Negative	+(<10%)	Unknown
Bacterial culture	+(>90%)	+(65%)	Negative	Negative	+ AFB (85%)	Negative	+(16%)	+(16%)

From Reese RE, Douglas RG Jr. A practical approach to infectious diseases. 2nd ed. Boston: Little Brown, 1986.
* See text for discussion; if polymorphonuclear leukocytes (PMN) >90% on serial exams, viral etiology is not likely, especially with low (<500) white cell count (WBC); an average of 13% of patients with TB meningitis will have PMN predominance.
† Or< 50—66% of blood glucose. As many as 40—50% of patients with bacterial meningitis may have normal CSF glucose.
‡ 85%<1000; rare >2800.
§ See text for discussion of major exceptions.
** High percentage is smear positive if 10 cc of CSF is centrifuged and examined for 30—90 min.
†† If>50,000, brain abscess with rupture should be considered.
Sources: Carpenter RR, Petersdorf RG. The clinical spectrum of bacterial meningitis. Am J Med 1962; 33:262.
Karandanis D, Shulman JA. Recent survey of laboratory findings in bacterial, tuberculous, and aseptic meningitis. South Med J 1976; 69:449.
Lepow ML et al. A clinical and laboratory investigation of aseptic meningitis during the four-year period, 1955-1958. I. Observations concerning etiology and epidemiology, N Engl J Med 1962; 266:1181. II. The clinical disease and its sequelae. N Engl J Med 1962; 266:1188.
Swartz MN, Dodge PR. Bacterial meningitis—a review of selected aspects. N Engl J Med 1965; 272:725, 779, 842, 898, 954, 1003.

are not likely to affect all CSF findings, however, and one or more of the values is likely to remain abnormal. In such a setting, special CSF studies such as counter-immunoelectrophoresis (CIE)—for the common organisms—may be especially helpful.

If initial studies of CSF in a patient suspected of having bacterial meningitis are not diagnostic, other special studies may be indicated. If the Gram stain is negative, CIE may provide an early diagnosis in *S. pneumoniae*, *H. influenzae* type B, and *N. meningitidis* infections, and is especially useful in evaluating patients who have received oral antibiotics. Negative CIE tests do not rule out bacterial meningitis, since not all strains are reactive with the commercially available test preparations. However, these tests often remain positive for the common infecting organisms even when the Gram stains have been rendered negative by partial treatment. Follow-up studies on CSF, especially if initial studies are less suggestive of bacterial meningitis, would include serial leukocyte counts and differentials, India ink preparations and cryptococcal antigen testing, acid-fast smears and mycobacterial cultures, or potentially fungal cultures, depending on the clinical situation. It should also be remembered that foci of infection that are close to the meninges may result in clinical findings suggestive of meningitis. Thus, a meningeal syndrome may be associated with paraspinal abscesses, subdural empyema, soft tissue ab-

scesses, and sinus space infections. Appropriate roentgenographic and other studies for such processes or etiologies should be done if indicated.

TREATMENT

Rapid institution of antibiotic therapy is vital. The choice of antibiotics for treatment of bacterial meningitis is determined by organisms that (1) are seen on the Gram stain, (2) are identified by CIE, (3) are subsequently isolated, or (4) are probably present as suggested by the clinical findings (Table 2). Antibiotics should be administered intravenously in high doses. If the Gram stain of CSF suggests one or another of the aforementioned common pathogens, therapy can be more specifically directed toward that organism. In the absence of that information, therapy in adults is directed against *S. pneumoniae* and *N. meningitidis*, e.g., penicillin (chloramphenicol in the allergic patient, or perhaps a third-generation cephalosporin if the allergy has been of a delayed type). With an immunosuppressed host, other organisms must be considered, such as *Listeria* (for which ampicillin, perhaps with an aminoglycoside, would be the drug of choice) or other organisms (see Table 2). In children 6 weeks of age or older, therapy should also be directed against *H. influenzae*, e.g., chloramphenicol and ampicillin. For neonates, therapy is directed in particular against *E. coli*, group B

TABLE 2   Initial Antibiotic Therapy and Suspected Bacterial Etiologies When the CSF Gram Stain Is Negative*

Setting/Patient	Antibiotic(s)	Suspected Etiology
Neonate (<3 weeks of age)	Cefotaxime or similar agent, plus ampicillin	Group B streptococci, *E. coli*, and *Listeria*
Child (community-acquired)	Ampicillin, plus chloramphenicol	*N. meningitidis, S. pneumoniae*, and *H. influenzae*
Adult (community-acquired)	Penicillin or ampicillin	*N. meningitidis*, and *S. pneumoniae*
High-risk patient		
Postoperative neuro-surgical patient, penetrating head trauma, hospital-acquired	Cefotaxime or similar agent, plus nafcillin†	*S. aureus*, gram-negative bacilli
Immunosuppressed host	Cefotaxime or similar agent, plus nafcillin, plus ampicillin†	*S. aureus*, gram-negative bacilli, and *Listeria*, as well as the common pathogens

* See Table 3 for appropriate intravenous doses of the antimicrobial agents listed. See text for discussion of alternate agents.
† An aminoglycoside should be added if the possibility of *P. aeruginosa* infection is increased.

streptococci, and *Listeria*. Therapy can be modified and made more specific as information from the laboratory evaluation of CSF becomes available. In children in whom *H. influenzae* is a consideration, ampicillin and chloramphenicol are generally used until results of beta-lactamase studies are available. An alternative that has become available recently is use of one of the third-generation cephalosporins, such as cefotaxime or ceftriaxone. Such agents have the advantage of being active against the common pathogens as well as *E. coli* and group B streptococci, and therefore could be used in neonates as well as in older children. The appropriate intravenous doses for the antibiotics are provided in Table 3.

Several conditions may alter the anticipated organisms noted above and suggest alternate therapeutic regimens. For example, in the individual who has recently undergone neurosurgery, *S. aureus* and gram-negative bacilli are common pathogens. (Such an individual is unlikely to be seen in the emergency department, but may be seen on the floor in the postoperative setting.) The third-generation cephalosporins are the agents of choice in enteric gram-negative meningitis, but many would include an aminoglycoside (gentamicin or amikacin, depending on local susceptibility patterns) because of the possibility of *Pseudomonas aeruginosa*, which is often resistant to an agent such as cefotaxime. In such a setting, it is also wise to cover staphylococci effectively by addition of nafcillin.

When antibiotics have been used prior to patient presentation, the decision whether to use or withhold antibiotics in the emergency department setting can be difficult, especially if the CSF values are not diagnostic.

TABLE 3   Doses (Intravenous) for Initial Antibiotic Treatment of Bacterial Meningitis*

Agent	Adults	Children
Aqueous penicillin G	18–24 million units/day q4h	200,000–300,000 units/kg/day q4h
Ampicillin	12 g/day q4h	200–400 mg/kg/day q4–6h
Chloramphenicol	75–100 mg/kg/day q6h	75–100 mg/kg/day q6h
Nafcillin	9–12 g/day q4h	200 mg/kg/day q4–6h
Cefotaxime	8–12 g/day q4–6h	200 mg/kg/day q6h
Ceftriaxone	1–2 g/day q12h	100 mg/kg/day (not to exceed 4 g) q12h
Gentamicin†	4.5–6.0 mg/kg/day q8h	7.5 mg/kg/day q8h
Amikacin†	15 mg/kg/day q12h	15–30 mg/kg/day q8h

* See text and Table 2.
† Antibiotic levels should be obtained to determine appropriate dosing for efficacy and avoidance of toxicity.

If the CSF reveals only a few mononuclear cells, the glucose is normal, the Gram stains and CIE studies are negative, and the patient looks good and had received oral antibiotics in relatively low doses, it may be reasonable to observe the patient carefully with a repeat lumbar puncture in 6 to 24 hours (depending on the clinical course). If the CSF glucose is low, or if there is a predominance of polymorphonuclear leukocytes, the patient is likely to need a full course of antibiotics.

The duration of antibiotic therapy generally ranges from 7 to 14 days and depends on the organism and the clinical response. Staphylococcal or gram-negative bacillary meningitis may require therapy of longer duration. Response is usually evaluated by monitoring the patient's clinical signs and symptoms, particularly mental status changes, neurologic signs, and temperature response. In the adult who is responding well to antibiotic therapy for a specific bacterial pathogen, routine follow-up lumbar puncture is not indicated. However, repeat studies are indicated if the initial diagnosis was unclear, if there is new fever and clinical progression, if there is an inadequate or atypical clinical response, or if there has been isolation of an unusual bacterial organism for which assurance of CSF sterilization is warranted. The need for routine follow-up lumbar puncture in pediatric patients is controversial, but similar principles would apply in general.

DISPOSITION

The patient strongly suspected or shown to have bacterial meningitis needs to be admitted to the hospital. (The unit, regular or intensive care, depends on the patient's condition on admission.) Performance of the lumbar puncture and initiation of therapy should not be delayed by transfers to the appropriate floor. If the patient is seen in an emergency department or "satellite facility" without facilities for admission, cultures should be obtained and appropriate therapy initiated prior to transfer to another medical facility. It is crucial not to delay therapy in the acutely ill patient with clear community-acquired meningitis; that is, the patient with fever, meningismus, and a rapidly deteriorating course over the preceding 24 hours. It is reasonable to start therapy after the CSF sample has been obtained, but not fully examined, in such seriously ill patients.

PROPHYLAXIS

Patients with bacterial meningitis in whom the causative organism is unknown should be placed in respiratory isolation (a private room, masks for individuals entering, and good handwashing) until a firm diagnosis is established. Meningococcal meningitis is the only diagnosed bacterial meningitis for which patients routinely should be placed in isolation until adequately treated for 24 hours. In addition, with identified meningococcal meningitis, prophylaxis is indicated for several groups once the index case has been diagnosed: household contacts (residing with the index patient); nursery school or day school contacts (i.e., young children); other close day-to-day contacts of the index case (e.g, boyfriend, girlfriend); and those in unusual hospital situations with close contact (for example, mouth-to-mouth resuscitation in the emergency department). Nasopharyngeal cultures of these contacts is not needed. Prophylaxis is not indicated for routine contacts of the hospitalized patient, casual school contacts, or casual contacts at work or in the home. Rifampin, the preferred agent when susceptibility studies and/or serotypes are not known, should be administered for 2 days (600 mg orally twice a day for adults; 10 mg per kilogram twice a day for children). The role for prophylaxis of contacts of individuals with *H. influenzae* type B meningitis is controversial, although rifampin has been shown to eradicate the carrier state effectively. It has been recommended that if there is a sibling less than approximately 4 years old in the household of an index case, all household contacts should receive rifampin.

SUGGESTED READING

Garvey G. Current concepts of bacterial infections of the central nervous system: bacterial meningitis and bacterial brain abscess. J Neurosurg 1983; 59:735–744.
Van Voris LP, Roberts NJ, Jr. Central nervous system infections. In: Reese RE, Douglas RG Jr, eds. A practical approach to infectious diseases. 2nd ed. Boston: Little Brown and Company, 1986; 123.

SUBARACHNOID HEMORRHAGE

WILLIAM F. BOUZARTH, M.D., F.A.C.S.
H. WARREN GOLDMAN, M.D., Ph.D.

Spontaneous subarachnoid hemorrhage (SAH) is most often due to intracranial aneurysmal (ICA) rupture. This pathologic entity accounts for 8 percent of patients with "stroke" or 16 per 100,000 persons in the United States per year, with approximately half under the age of 50. There is little dispute that neurosurgical operations are the only definitive treatment. In contrast to most other strokes, early recognition and successful surgery can return the patient to his previous style of life; otherwise, early death is nearly certain. Unfortunately, approximately 40 percent of patients are not referred for neurosurgical evaluation after the first symptom, which is usually headache (Table 1). Part of the reason is that the presenting symptom may not be severe enough for the patient to seek medical help. Of those who do report to an emergency department on an ambulatory basis, nearly half are

TABLE 1 Common Symptoms of Spontaneous Subarachnoid Hemorrhage

Headache, usually sudden and generalized
Nausea and vomiting
Brief loss of consciousness (includes seizures)
Neck pain and/or stiffness
Oculomotor palsy
Transitory weakness and/or speech disturbance
Progressive coma

TABLE 2 Uncommon Symptoms and Incorrect Diagnoses

Hearing loss	Otitis
Malaise and diffuse aches	"Flu"
Neck and/or arm pain	Cervical strain or disc
Low back and/or leg pains	Lumbar disc
Confusion/ataxia	Acute alcoholism
Photophobia/visual disturbance	Glaucoma
Diarrhea (especially with vomiting)	Gastroenteritis
Agitation	Anxiety reaction
Head injury (secondary to SAH)	Head injury

not properly diagnosed (Tables 2, 3). This chapter will stress the pitfalls in diagnosis and management of such patients with mild "warning" leaks.

The second most common cause of SAH is trauma. Since the apoplectic nature of ICA rupture may cause the patient to fall and strike the head, the differential diagnosis may be difficult. Indeed, previous cranial trauma can produce ICA. Other causes of spontaneous SAH are hypertension, nonaneurysmal vascular malformations, coagulopathy, and angiitis, often associated with drug abuse. Tumors that bleed usually do not produce SAH. No cause is found in 10 to 20 percent of patients despite four vessel angiography. Depending upon the cause, the cerebral location, and the magnitude of the SAH, brain disruption with major neurologic deficits can occur. Intracerebral hemorrhage associated with SAH will not be discussed here.

There is a strong correlation between physical stress and SAH. Nearly 10 percent of ICA ruptures occur during sleep, but at least one-third of patients are awake in a resting state at the time of the rupture. Because emotional crisis can elevate blood pressure, the associated headache of SAH is often erroneously considered psychological.

SYMPTOMS IN AMBULATORY PATIENTS

The cardinal complaint is *headache*, which occurs in more than 90 percent of patients in whom a history of onset can be obtained. In cases of trauma there is no clinical characteristic(s) to differentiate between the local effect of injury and SAH. The pain is described as "the worst headache of my life" or "it struck like lightning." The head pain rarely starts off as a mild headache and builds up in intensity over hours. It usually is generalized, but a frontal location or pain concentrating posteriorly involving the neck is common. Indeed, these locations often suggest a tension headache. Although hemicranial pain similar to migraine is rare in SAH, when it does occur, the patient will be mistakenly treated for migraine, especially if the first such headache was 14 days earlier or less (the "warning" leak). Bitemporal or vertex headaches are less likely to be due to SAH. The pain may be throbbing in nature, but it is more commonly steady and intense. The patient frequently tries to sleep, but the pain may prevent this. On the other hand, SAH can cause lethargy. When the severity of the headache, in the physician's judgment, requires a narcotic to bring relief, SAH is a likely possibility. When there is a history of chronic

and/or intermittent headache, we cannot stress enough that the acute onset of a different type of head pain may be due to SAH.

Associated symptoms often suggest that the headache is due to SAH. Nausea and vomiting are believed to be the result of increased intracranial pressure, especially if there is a tendency to be sleepy or lethargic. When the patient is retching, the emergency physician may tend to minimize the headache and concentrate on "the virus that is going around." Surprisingly, diarrhea may also occur, and distracts from the proper diagnosis. Since SAH is associated with a temperature elevation, the combination of frontal headaches and fever sidetracks the diagnosis toward a "sinus problem." An enlarging ICA may produce face and/or eye pain prior to rupture. The complaint of photophobia with headache rarely suggests, as it should, an SAH; 'flu'' does the same and this becomes the mistaken diagnosis of choice.

Diplopia may precede a SAH. This is usually due to a posterior communicating artery aneurysm compressing the ipsilateral and uncrossed third cranial nerve (oculomotor). It can produce extraocular muscle weakness, ptosis, and/or pupillary dilatation. Similar third nerve palsy is seen in viral encephalitis and diabetes, but impending aneurysmal rupture or actual SAH must be considered in the differential diagnosis. A sixth nerve (abducens) palsy may produce weakness of lateral deviation of one or both eyes, presumably owing to increased intracranial pressure. This usually occurs a week or more after onset and the subsided headache receives little attention from the physician, who directs the patient to an ophthalmologist instead of a neurosurgeon.

Preexisting hypertension adds to the likelihood of ICA formation and SAH; indeed, it is the most important factor in explaining multiple ICA. Hypertensive crisis is associated with headache and retinal vascular changes (preretinal hemorrhages also can be the result of sudden increase in intracranial pressure). What is not appreciated is that SAH can cause or worsen preexisting hypertension. In

TABLE 3 Common Errors in Physician Diagnosis

Migraine	13%
Meningitis	10%
Cerebral ischemia	8%
Myocardial infarction	8%
Tension headache	7%

Modified from Table 4 in Kassell NF, Kongable GL, Tosner JC, et al. Delay in referral of patients with ruptured aneurysms to neurological attention. Stroke 1985; 16:587.

such patients the next step is electrocardiography, especially if bradycardia due to the bleed is present. It must be stressed that electrocardiographic changes, such as large and often inverted T waves, prolonged Q-T interval, and large ("cerebral") U waves, may be totally due to the SAH in an otherwise healthy heart. Usually any electrical abnormality leads the physician toward a cardiovascular problem. Too often such patients are admitted with a cardiac diagnosis such as acute myocardial infarction.

The ambulatory patient may also complain of confusion, irritability, dizziness, and/or rotational vertigo. A syncopal attack may have been the first symptom and the headache that follows often is considered as an unimportant head bump and easily explained in the context of the mistaken diagnosis. A transitory mild hemiparesis and/or speech disturbance may suggest a transitory ischemic attack, but when associated with headache SAH is more likely.

MORIBUND PATIENTS

Acute SAH can be immediately devastating. It is estimated that nearly half such patients will either die within 30 days of the ictus or remain in coma for months to years. Autopsy and/or computed tomography (CT) may demonstrate only SAH and not brain disruption. What accounts for such severe neurologic loss? The magnitude of the bleed can acutely increase intracranial pressure to such a degree that large subhyaloid hemorrhages occur. This high intracranial pressure diminishes cerebral blood flow and cerebral function. Cellular anoxia results and the brain can be irreversibly damaged.

Another mechanism is cerebral vasospasm. The exact mechanism of vasospasm is controversial. It is thought that vasospasm that occurs immediately following SAH is a result of an intrinsic muscular contraction of the arterial wall as a response to the injury itself (conceivably a protective mechanism). Spasm occurring after 24 hours is considered the result of biochemical changes due to breakdown products of cellular elements or changes in serum characteristics on a molecular or protein level.

Regardless of the cause of vasospasm, it can be devastating depending on in which vessels and to what degree spasm occurs. For example, middle cerebral spasm can produce a typical hemiplegia, and in the dominant hemisphere, an aphasia. The anterior cerebral artery spasm mainly affects the leg, less so the arm. Posterior cerebral circulation spasm can cause homonymous hemianopsia. When spasm is generalized to both hemispheres the patient goes into coma, since the reticular activating system cannot arouse the ischemic cerebrum.

NEUROLOGIC SIGNS

The neurologic abnormalities associated with SAH include changes in the level of consciousness ranging from lethargy and confusion to a total areflexic coma with dilated fixed pupils. These are nonspecific neurologic signs that are totally compatible with an SAH. On the other hand, third nerve palsy, especially without a major decrease in the level of consciousness, is highly suggestive of an ICA of the posterior communicating artery. As the ICA enlarges or ruptures, the adjacent third nerve is injured. The eye can only move laterally and downward owing to paralysis of the four other extraocular muscles, and the dilated pupil, hidden by the complete ptosis, is highly suggestive whether headache is present or not. Nuchal rigidity is a very common abnormality and indeed may be the only neurologic abnormality. If a temperature elevation is also present, as can occur with SAH, meningitis is often the mistaken diagnosis.

CONFIRMATORY TESTS

When there is a reasonable index of suspicion the diagnosis can be confirmed only by two tests i.e., CT demonstrating blood within the subarachnoid space and analysis of the cerebrospinal fluid for red blood cells and/or xanthochromia (after 2 weeks an elevated protein level strongly indicates previous SAH). We believe that CT should be done first as quickly as possible. If CT is not immediately available or transportation of the patient to such a unit is not logistically feasible, telephone consultation with the neurosurgeon is recommended so that this specialist will be involved in the decision about a lumbar puncture (the same recommendations apply when meningitis is suspected).

Cranial CT can also be falsely negative, depending on the number, the thickness, and the projection of the slices. Missing a view of the chiasmal cistern, for example, may mean missing the SAH. Sagittal midline reconstruction may be required to see blood in the interhemispheric fissure. Movement artifacts can obscure a small localized SAH. In an anemic patient, the diagnosis may be missed even with an adequate CT scan, since hemoglobin concentration is as important as the amount of blood. With the passage of time, hemoglobin concentration diminishes, giving a false sense of security that SAH did not occur.

If the CT demonstrates SAH, *lumbar puncture* (LP) need not be done. LP should not precede CT because a clot may be present in a nondominant temporal lobe or sylvian fissure without neurologic signs. Removing cerebrospinal fluid for analysis (and the seepage into the epidural space which may follow) can hasten the impending herniation, resulting in rapid deterioration and death. (If the patient has meningitis, an accompanying cerebritis or abscess can usher in the same complication.) Herniation is less likely to occur when a small gauge needle (22 to 24) is used, but even this is not a total safeguard. Too often the physician performing LP has little experience; after multiple attempts, one cannot be sure if the blood was due to "a traumatic tap," SAH, or infection. On the other hand, LP soon after a SAH may not demonstrate red blood cells, for it can take some hours for the cells to reach the lumbar region. A finding of "normal" cerebrospinal fluid usually results in prescription of an antibiotic and a referral to the patient's personal physician. However, when there is high suspicion of SAH and the CT is normal, LP is warranted.

Leukocytosis tends to parallel the severity of the SAH, so do not be led toward the diagnosis of an infectious process. Hyperglycemia may follow SAH.

MANAGEMENT OF SAH

After a baseline neurologic examination, frequent mini-neurologic examinations should be done once the diagnosis is confirmed. This aids the neurosurgeons in their selection of medications. Neurosurgical consultation, if not already requested, should be obtained regarding admission to the hospital best staffed and equipped for aneurysmal surgery. The timing of arteriography (and surgery) varies from immediate to a delay of days to weeks, depending on the philosophy of the neurosurgeon. Prior to admission or transfer, management can begin in the emergency department.

If the onset was ushered in by a seizure(s), phenytoin (Dilantin) is the first drug of choice. A 70 kg person usually requires 1 g IV (never intramuscularly) at a rate no faster than 50 mg per minute. Persons over age 50, or with known cardiac disease or acute electrocardiographic changes, should be closely monitored, with the rate of infusion reduced by 50 percent or more should ECG changes occur. If seizures occur in the emergency department, diazepam (Valium) is the drug of choice (10 mg IV over a 2-minute period). In patients who have not had seizures, phenobarbital, 100 mg IM is suggested. Its sedative effect also is beneficial.

The patient should be placed in a quiet area, reassured, and family visitors kept to a minimum. History is best taken from the family. When head or neck pain is so intense that the patient appears agitated, narcotics may be required. Intramuscular meperidine (Demerol), 50 to 100 mg, can be considered by itself or to supplement phenobarbital sedation.

Vomiting should be vigorously treated. Trimethobenzamide (Tigan), 200 mg deep in the gluteal muscles, in the average adult is suggested. Although one of the side effects is convulsions, we believe this to be a minimal problem as compared with rebleeding from retching. This is not true for prochlorperazine (Compazine), which is contraindicated because it can cause seizures. It should be obvious that rectal manipulations such as a digital examination, suppositories, or enemas are contraindicated, as they may cause increased intracranial pressure.

Hypertension may be the cause or the effect of SAH. Regardless, every effort should be made to reduce blood pressure to normal. The following protocol has served us well for initial therapy in the emergency department—for blood pressure over 150 mm Hg, parenteral hydralazine, 10 mg every 3 to 4 hours as needed, and for blood pressure over 200 mm Hg, intravenous sodium nitroprusside titrated to maintain a pressure below 160 mm Hg.

Dexamethasone and/or hyperosmolar agents, such as 20 percent mannitol, have been widely used to combat cerebral edema. Deliberate intravascular volume expansion and/or antifibrinolytic agents also have their advocates in the treatment of aneurysmal problems. It is our opinion that these treatments are best left to the neurosurgeon.

Obtunded patients can hypoventilate, retaining CO_2 and increasing intracranial pressure. Such patients should have blood gases assessed; a PCO_2 of 40 mm Hg or more is an indication for intubation and ventilation. When *endotracheal intubation* is required, rapid, smooth insertion is required. Intubation causes increased intracranial pressure, and topical pharyngeal lidocaine, intravenous lidocaine, and/or paralyzing agents should be used (see the chapter *Sedation and Rapid-Induction Anesthesia for Emergency Intubation.*)

Routine blood tests should include coagulation screening if there is any question as to the cause of the SAH. We also suggest that an intravenous fluid line be connected to the needle or catheter used for blood sampling rather than as a separate procedure, since needle sticks may agitate the patient. Regardless, the infused volume of 2.5 percent glucose in 0.5 N saline should be no faster than 50 ml per hour.

An English pathologist (Gull) 125 years ago reported on the close relationship between ICA and SAH. Yet even today, the correct diagnosis of "warning" leaks represents a major challenge to emergency physicians. To prevent the second and usually devastating rebleed by rapid referral for neurosurgery is today's goal.

SUGGESTED READING

Bouzarth WF, Dhopesh VP. The subtle subarachnoid hemorrhage. Emerg Med 1982; 13:203–217.

Gascin P, Ley TJ, Toltzis RJ, et al. Spontaneous subarachnoid hemorrhage simulating acute transmural myocardial infarction. Am Heart J 1983; 105:511–513.

Kassell NF, Kongable GL, Tosner JC, et al. Delay in referral of patients with ruptured aneurysms to neurosurgical attention. Stroke 1985; 16:587–590.

Leblanc R, Winfield JA. The warning leak in subarachnoid hemorrhage and the importance of its early diagnosis. Can Med Assoc J 1984; 131:1235–1236.

CEREBRAL INFARCTION AND TRANSIENT ISCHEMIC ATTACK

HAROLD P. ADAMS Jr., M.D.
GILBERT J. TOFFOL, D.O.

Cerebral infarction is the most common form of stroke, affecting approximately 250,000 Americans annually. Cerebral infarction results primarily from large artery atherosclerosis, small artery disease (lacunar stroke), or cardiac embolism. In addition, stroke can complicate a number of other diseases such as sickle cell anemia, thrombocytosis, fibromuscular dysplasia, or vasculitis (Table 1). During the last 25 years, there has been a remarkable decline in the incidence and mortality of cerebral infarction. This decline is largely attributable to improved treatment of risk factors such as heart disease and hypertension. However, early recognition and treatment of patients with transient ischemic attacks (TIA) and advances in treatment of cerebral infarction are also having an impact on mortality.

TRANSIENT ISCHEMIC ATTACK

A TIA is a transient episode of focal neurologic dysfunction of vascular origin that lasts fewer than 24 hours. The usual duration of a TIA is 5 to 20 minutes. A TIA results from a microembolic event or a hemodynamic disturbance. A TIA is important because there is a 20 to 35 percent risk of cerebral infarction if no treatment is instituted. The first few hours and days are the period of highest risk. A recent TIA is a medical emergency. Therefore, a patient with a recent TIA deserves hospitalization, frequent observation, prompt evaluation, and early treatment.

Recognition of a TIA is not easy. Misdiagnosis is frequent. The differential diagnosis of TIA includes seizures, syncope, migraine, and masses such as a brain tumor or a subdural hematoma, which can produce waxing and waning symptoms. It is important to determine whether the symptoms reflect ischemia in the distribution of the internal carotid or the vertebrobasilar circulations. Symptoms of carotid TIA include ipsilateral, painless, transient monocular visual impairment (amaurosis fugax) or contralateral clumsiness, and numbness or weakness of the hand, arm, or face. Other symptoms may include brief episodes of aphasia, dysarthria, or hemiparesis. Symptoms of vertebrobasilar TIA include vertigo, dysarthria, ataxia, diplopia, or binocular visual disturbances. Motor or sensory impairment may be unilateral, bilateral, crossed, or alternating. Isolated vertigo without other symptoms is not specific for TIA, and one should be cautious about attributing vertigo to vascular disease. Transient loss of consciousness, syncope, giddiness, light-headedness, confusion, dizziness, and wooziness are not symptoms of TIA. Patients with TIA should not have neurologic residuals. Asymmetries of neck or cranial pulses, presence of cranial or neck bruits, and differences in blood pressures should be sought. The fundi should be visualized for the presence of emboli. These examinations can be easily performed in an emergency department. However, the diagnosis of TIA should not be entertained in a patient who has atypical symptoms just because a carotid artery bruit is heard.

Much of the *evaluation* of a patient with a recent TIA can be expeditiously performed in an emergency department. Because conditions other than cerebral ischemia can cause transient neurologic dysfunction, neurologic consultation should be obtained. Most patients also need a computed tomographic (CT) examination. Other investigations should include a search for the cause of the TIA (Table 2). Noninvasive studies of the carotid artery, cerebral arteriography, electroencephalography, and sophisticated hematologic studies can be done after admission. Arteriography is the most important diagnostic procedure; it demonstrates the sites and extent of extracranial and intracranial arterial lesions. In most large hospitals the risk of complications of the procedure is 1 percent or less. Digital intravenous subtraction angiography is not yet a useful alternative to conventional arteriography.

Patients who have experienced a TIA in the preceding 48 to 72 hours need emergency, preventive therapy.

TABLE 1   Nonatherosclerotic Causes of Cerebral Infarction or TIA

Hematologic causes: polycythemia, thrombocytosis sickle cell disease, lupus anticoagulant

Arteriopathies: vasculitis, drugs, fibromuscular dysplasia, moyamoya, dissections, trauma, saccular aneurysms

Acute alcohol intoxication

Peripartum conditions

Postoperative complications

Oral contraceptives

Cardiac causes: atrial fibrillation (valvular and nonvalvular), recent myocardial infarction (mural thrombosis), ventricular aneurysm, cardiomyopathy, mitral valve prolapse, prosthetic valve, atrial myxoma, infective endocarditis, paradoxical embolism

TABLE 2   Laboratory Evaluation Studies for Patients with TIA or Cerebral Infarction

Emergency studies: complete blood count, platelet count, erythrocyte sedimentation rate, coagulation studies, blood sugar, serum chemistries, electrocardiogram, chest roentgenogram, CT (without contrast enhancement)

Later studies: electroencephalogram, echocardiogram, noninvasive carotid studies, luetic screening, vasculitis screening, coagulation studies, arteriogram

Patients who have had several TIAs or events that were increasingly severe are at greatest risk. Definitive medical or surgical treatment should be initiated as soon as possible. Coincident heart disease, hypertension, diabetes mellitus, and chronic obstructive lung disease need treatment. Antihypertensives should be initiated slowly and cautiously because a patient with TIA may have a high-grade stenosis. Cerebral infarction can be precipitated by sudden lowering of blood pressure in such a patient.

Interim treatment with intravenous *heparin* may be useful for high-risk patients. It acts quickly, and its effects can be easily reversed. The efficacy of heparin for patients with recent TIA has not been established, but it appears to be a reasonable choice. Heparin is given as a constant infusion following a loading bolus. Most patients require 800 to 1,200 units per hour. The therapeutic goal is an activated partial thromboplastin time twice control values. Heparin should not be administered until after the CT has been reviewed. Heparin treatment should be limited to a brief duration.

Early treatment may also be instituted with *aspirin*. Aspirin is the best medical therapy for long-term prevention of cerebral infarction, and it may be useful in patients with recent events. However, some surgeons are reluctant to operate on a patient who has received aspirin, and if a patient has a lesion demonstrated by arteriography, which would benefit from surgery, it should be performed as soon as possible. Carotid endarterectomy is indicated for a patient with a carotid TIA and a stenosis of the internal carotid artery that exceeds 50 percent of the luminal diameter. A patient should not be referred for carotid endarterectomy if the surgeon's combined rates of morbidity and mortality exceed 3 percent. Anastomosis of the superficial temporal artery with the middle cerebral artery has not proved to be superior to medical treatment.

The optimal long-term medical therapy is *aspirin*, 1,300 mg per day. A lower dose may be better, but this has not been proved. Warfarin may be an alternative, but is associated with several management problems. New antiplatelet aggregation drugs, such as ticlopidine, may prove to be superior. Dipyridamole is not useful in the prevention of stroke among patients with TIA. Even though aspirin is the standard treatment, physicians are in error if they prescribe aspirin without doing a thorough evaluation.

CEREBRAL INFARCTION

Most patients with cerebral infarction do not have a warning TIA. These patients present with major, evolving neurologic deficits, usually of a few hours duration. The symptoms and evaluation of the acute event provide clues if it is of embolic or thrombotic origin. Convulsions, headache, or disturbances in consciousness may accompany the focal neurologic signs. Thrombotic infarctions often have a course punctuated by fluctuations, steps, and temporary improvements. When cerebral flow is sluggish, collateral circulation may be inadequate to permit perfusion of a focal area that was originally supplied by an occluded artery. This phenomenon may explain why thrombotic events are more likely to occur during the night or while the patient is taking a nap. Embolic infarctions produce neurologic deficits that are sudden and maximum at onset. However, owing to migration of the embolus, a stepwise course can result. Headache before the appearance of neurologic signs can develop with a thrombotic stroke. Headache accompanying the onset of symptoms favors intracerebral or subarachnoid hemorrhage, or embolic infarction. Convulsions are more common with embolic infarction or intracranial hemorrhage. Vomiting suggests a hemorrhagic event. Depressed consciousness usually means massive brain injury or increased intracranial pressure; it follows hemorrhage or large infarctions. Coma may occur with basilar artery thrombosis. The differential diagnosis of acute cerebral infarction includes intracranial bleeding, brain tumor, brain abscess, complicated migraine, or a postictal state.

Pre-hospital Care

Patients with acute cerebral infarction deserve emergent evaluation and treatment, which can begin when ambulance personnel arrive on the scene. A brief assessment, including measurement of vital signs and blood pressure, checking the integrity of the airway, and observation of the neurologic state, can be performed quickly. The level of consciousness, pupillary reactions, extraocular movements, motor function, and speech function can be measured. The Glasgow Coma Scale (see chapter on *Epidural, Subdural, and Intracranial Bleeding*, which is useful for patients with head trauma, can be applied to patients with acute infarction. Early assessments by an emergency medical technician are critical for documentation of progression of neurologic deficits, a scenario that occurs in 25 to 40 percent of patients. Cardiac monitoring is important because many of these patients have had a silent myocardial infarction or have cardiac arrhythmias. An intravenous access for a slow infusion of normal saline is started mainly as a route to administer any necessary drugs. In addition, many stroke victims have an element of dehydration. If there is a fear of cardiac decompensation, small volumes of saline can be given. The airway should be secured in any obtunded patient. Hypoventilation, atelectasis, and aspiration are potential complications. Ventilatory assistance may be required. Unless the patient has chronic lung disease, supplemental oxygen is warranted. It probably is not safe to routinely give glucose to every patient with a stroke. A large bolus of glucose may induce further damage to brain tissue that lacks adequate perfusion and oxygenation. If there is specific reason to believe that hypoglycemia is the cause of symptoms, 50 g of 50 percent dextrose combined with 100 mg of thiamine can be administered. Intravenous diazepam may be used to stop frequent convulsions, but one must guard against respiratory compromise. The administration of naloxone, volume expanding agents, antihypertensives, or anticoagulants should be reserved until after the patient is in the hospital.

Hospital Treatment

The emergency physician's approach to a person with an acute cerebral infarction should be the same as to any other critically ill patient. Further deterioration secondary to propagation of the clot, recurrent embolization, failure of collaterals, or development of cerebral edema occurs during the first few hours after the ictus. The first steps are stabilization of the airway and support of cardiac and respiratory functions. Continuous cardiac monitoring and frequent assessments of the vital signs are necessary. In exceptional cases, apnea monitors or continuous blood pressure measurements are indicated.

Unless the patient has severe pulmonary disease, oxygen should be given. If an intravenous line is not in place, it should be started with infusion of normal saline. Patients with acute or evolving cerebral infarction often have moderate-to-severe arterial hypertension. These elevations may be compensatory to the acute neurologic process. The response to quickly lower blood pressure should be avoided. Unless the blood pressure measurements are extremely high (systolic 200 torr or mean 140 torr), the blood pressure should be cautiously lowered or not at all. Overzealous treatment of hypertension in patients with acute cerebral infarction can extend the size of the ischemic lesion.

Evaluation should be expeditious. However, documentation of the patient's history and course by the physician should precede any rush toward obtaining an emergency CT examination. Queries about any antecedent events, the onset of illness, and any progression are critical. The prognosis and early treatment of an embolic infarction differs markedly from those of thrombotic arterial occlusions. Specific therapy should be withheld until the diagnosis is solidified.

Diagnostic studies that can be obtained in the emergency department include electrocardiogram, chest roentgenogram, complete blood count, platelet count, prothrombin time, partial thromboplastin time, erythrocyte sedimentation rate, and blood glucose and serum electrolyte levels. If the patient is febrile or has leukocytosis, blood cultures should be obtained because of the possibility of infective endocarditis. Computed tomography without contrast enhancement should be performed as soon as possible. Although CT is usually negative during the first few hours after cerebral infarction, it does help to eliminate the possibility of intracerebral hemorrhage or other focal mass lesions. If the question of a mass, such as a tumor, persists after CT without contrast, a contrast study should be performed. Unless there is a strong suspicion of either meningitis or subarachnoid hemorrhage, lumbar puncture does not need to be performed.

All patients with acute cerebral infarction merit *hospitalization*, preferably in a monitored bed or in a skilled care unit. Early neurologic consultation is warranted. Diagnostic studies that can be obtained in the first few hours after admission include coagulation studies, platelet function studies, blood serology, and tests for systemic vasculitis. Other examinations that are often indicated are cerebral arteriography, echocardiography, electroencephalography, and noninvasive carotid imaging.

The chief *causes of death* during the first few hours following cerebral infarction are cerebral edema or direct consequences of massive brain injury. Deaths from cerebral infarction during the first 24 hours are exceptional. The patients at highest risk are those with major neurologic deficits and depressed levels of consciousness. Endotracheal intubation secures the airway and allows for ventilatory support. If intracranial pressure is markedly elevated, hyperventilation to a PCO_2 of 25 to 30 torr is useful. Hyperventilation is supplemented with 20 percent mannitol (0.25 to 0.5 g per kilogram body weight) every 4 to 6 hours. Intracranial pressure monitoring expedites the use of these therapies. The diuresis resulting from the mannitol is replaced by a comparable volume of parenteral fluid. Dexamethasone or methylprednisolone are not useful in patients with intracranial hypertension secondary to cerebral infarction.

Less critically ill patients are kept at bed rest during the first few hours after admission. The head of the bed is kept flat. Vital signs and blood pressure are measured frequently. The nurses should also closely watch the patient for changes in neurologic status. Cardiac monitoring is continued. Food and fluids are not given orally during the first 24 hours. Intravenous normal saline is administered in a volume sufficient to maintain urinary output. Some patients need a condom or Foley catheter.

Diabetic patients are a special therapeutic problem. If marked hyperglycemia is found, insulin is given. Hypoglycemic levels should be avoided; normalization of the blood sugar is the goal. Glucose-containing fluids are avoided.

Anticonvulsants are not routinely prescribed. If the patient has had convulsions with the ictus, either phenytoin or phenobarbital can be given. There is no evidence that barbiturate-induced coma ameliorates the effects of acute cerebral infarction.

Antihypertensive drugs are cautiously administered to patients with sustained marked hypertension. Sodium nitroprusside is a reasonable choice because the dose can be titrated and it has a short duration of action. If a patient deteriorates commensurate with lowering of the blood pressure, the antihypertensive is discontinued.

Heparin is the most commonly prescribed drug for patients with acute or progressing cerebral infarction. Its efficacy is the subject of lively debate, but it remains the customary treatment. It is given as a constant intravenous infusion following a loading bolus dose (usually 5,000 to 7,000 units). Most patients require 800 to 1,200 units of heparin per hour to maintain an activated partial thromboplastin time twice control values. Heparin is not given until after the CT examination has been reviewed; neither is it given within 2 hours of lumbar puncture. Patients who are medically unstable and those who have uncontrolled hypertension or severe infarctions should not be given heparin. Patients with embolic cerebral infarction are a special concern because they are at high risk of recurrent embolism. Early use of heparin is particularly justified in these patients. Heparin is discontinued when long-term treatment has commenced, after 24 to 36 hours without improvement, or if there is neurologic deterioration. Oral anticoagulants are not useful for the acute setting. The potential value of aspirin in the treatment of cerebral infarction is not known.

An alternative therapy is *hypervolemic hemodilution*. Recent reports are promising. The goals are to increase cerebral blood flow and perfusion by augmenting cardiac output and improving the rheologic characteristics of the blood. Fluids such as plasmanate or albumin can be given. Low-molecular-weight dextran, 500 ml in 6 hours followed by another 500 ml over 12 hours, is most commonly prescribed. Complications of this therapy include anaphylaxis or congestive heart failure. Volume expansion combined with removal of a unit of blood reduces the blood hematocrit to approximately 40 percent. Lowering the hematocrit optimizes cerebral circulation. Venesection also helps to reduce the risk of cardiac decompensation. If hypervolemic hemodilution is selected, careful cardiac monitoring and measurements of central venous pressure are necessary. Treatment is usually continued for 2 to 5 days.

Naloxone in conventional doses (0.4 to 1.2 mg) is not useful in reversing the effects of cerebral infarction. Calcium-channel blockers, large doses of naloxone, heparin fragments, fibrinolytic agents, aminophylline, or hypertensive drugs may become valuable. These treatments are being evaluated.

Some investigators have reported successful reversal of cerebral infarction by emergency carotid endarterectomy for acute carotid artery occlusion. However, most surgeons are reluctant to undertake this operation.

SUGGESTED READING

Adams HP Jr, Kassel NF, Mazuz H. The patient with transient ischemic attacks. Is this the time for a new therapeutic approach? Stroke 1984; 15:371–375.

Berguer R, Bauer RB. Vertebrobasilar arterial occlusive disease. New York: Raven Press, 1984.

Kistler JP, Ropper AH, Heros RC. Therapy of ischemic cerebral vascular disease due to athero thrombosis. N Engl J Med 1984; 311:27–34 (Part 1); 311:100–105 (Part 2).

Strand T, Asplund K, Eriksson S, et al. A randomized controlled trial of hemodilution therapy in acute ischemic stroke. Stroke 1984; 15:980–989.

Warlow C, Morris PJ. Transient ischemic attacks. New York: Marcel Dekker, 1982.

ACUTE NONTRAUMATIC SPINAL CORD DYSFUNCTION

JEREMY D. SCHMAHMANN, M.B., Ch.B.
THOMAS D. SABIN, M.D.

The outcome of potentially reversible nontraumatic spinal cord disease is most closely correlated with the patient's clinical condition at the initiation of treatment. Therefore, early recognition may be the single most critical factor in determining the prognosis.

IS IT SPINAL CORD?

When it malfunctions, the spinal cord has a limited repertoire of symptoms and signs. Completed acute transecting lesions cause spinal shock with flaccid paralysis, areflexia, sensory loss, and autonomic dysfunction at and below the level. Chronic transecting or extrinsic lesions below the T1 segment cause leg weakness of upper motor neuron type (spasticity, hyperreflexia, and upgoing toes), whereas those at the C5 to T1 region cause lower motor neuron weakness (hypotonia, areflexia, atrophy, and fasciculations) at that level, and upper motor neuron weakness below. The signs may ascend more proximally over time with a single thoracic or cervical lesion by virtue of the lamination of the cord (Fig. 1). A transverse sensory level on the trunk is essentially diagnostic of spinal cord disease. Dissociated sensory deficit with loss of pin and temperature sensation, but preservation of vibration and proprioception in the same area, indicates an intrinsic cord lesion. Loss of bladder sensation and motility in acute lesions results in a distended painless bladder with overflow incontinence. Bowel involvement manifests with constipation early on, overflow fecal incontinence becoming a problem later. Cauda equina lesions present with multiple lumbosacral nerve root signs of weakness, sensory loss, areflexia, and absent plantar responses, in addition to bowel and bladder incontinence when severe and bilateral. The classic Brown-Sequard syndrome caused by hemisection or asymmetric extrinsic compression of the cord produces ipsilateral upper motor neuron signs and loss of vibration and proprioception, with contralateral loss of pin and temperature appreciation. Early lesions of the cord present only with subjective complaints of paresthesias, difficulty with gait, and change in urinary habits, rather than the obvious findings of paraparesis and a sensory level. One especially perplexing group are those patients who have a rather bizarre, seemingly functional, ataxia with no elementary neurologic signs and who go on to develop unequivocal cord compression.

Symmetrical weakness of the lower extremities suggests spinal cord disease, but may also result from bilateral anterior cerebral artery occlusion, ruptured anterior communicating artery aneurysm, proximal myopathy, and the Guillain-Barré sydrome. The patient's history, sensory level, state of tendon and plantar reflexes, and autonomic disturbances should narrow the differential diagnosis. Some who present with acute spinal cord disease may appear less than appropriately concerned, and there is a danger of misdiagnosis as hysteria.

PRINCIPLES OF MANAGEMENT

The general management is similar to that of patients with traumatic injury. Destabilization of possible fractures is prevented by immobilizing the patient during transit and initial evaluation. Skin ulceration—which can occur within hours after the loss of protective sensory, motor, and autonomic mechanisms—is prevented by frequent turning and protective padding. Marked fluctuations in pulse rate and blood pressure require careful monitoring and fluid homeostasis. The insensitive, paralyzed, and distending bladder provides an excellent medium for local infection and septicemia. An indwelling catheter is usually necessary before massive distention occurs, although prophylactic antibiotics are not routinely recommended. Dexamethasone in high doses of 20 mg to 100 mg as a bolus, followed by 6 mg every 6 hours intravenously or by mouth, is indicated in many instances. The concomitant use of cimetidine, 300 mg intravenously or by mouth every 6 hours, prevents gastrointestinal ulceration. Paralytic ileus occurs in many acute situations affecting the cord and necessitates early nasogastric drainage with intravenous fluid support. The newly immobilized lower extremities provide an opportunity for deep venous thrombosis, and prophylactic subcutaneous low-dose heparin, 5,000 units twice daily, lessens this risk. These patients are usually aware of the surrounding medical commotion, and talking frankly with them is often reassuring.

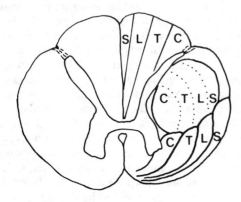

Figure 1 Diagrammatic representation of the cervical-to-sacral lamination of the major clinically pertinent spinal cord tracts. Represented here are the dorsal columns, the corticospinal and spinothalamic tracts. C-cervical; T-thoracic; L-lumbar; S-sacral. (Adapted from Walker EA. Arch Neurol Psychiat 1940; 43:294.

COMPRESSIVE EMERGENCIES

The Clinical Problem

Two fundamental principles in this setting affect management directly. First, the intradural space is small, and volume added suddenly produces a precipitous rise in pressure with acute neurologic decompensation. Compressive lesions that have been present for several months may unpredictably reach a point on the volume-pressure curve where compensatory mechanisms fail, and dramatic deterioration ensues. Second, when occlusion of the subarachnoid space by a mass is suspected, a spinal tap should be obtained only at myelography, and then only after neurologic and/or neurosurgical consultation. There is a danger of exaggerating the clinical state by spinal cord herniation, and also of making it impossible to define the subarachnoid space with contrast material subsequent to removal of the cerebrospinal fluid below the level of the block.

Tumor

Neoplasms most frequently complicated by metastatic compressive myelopathy are carcinoma of the lung, breast, prostate, and colon-rectum, as well as lymphoma and leukemia. Once there are findings of myelopathy in this setting, the likelihood of significant recovery of function is diminished. Therefore early diagnosis and treatment make the difference between an ambulatory and a bedridden state.

If there are clear signs of a myelopathy, one should proceed directly to myelography. Spinal fluid obtained at myelography is tested for cell count, cytology, glucose, protein, VDRL, and bacterial, fungal, and tuberculous pathogens.

If there are no signs of a myelopathy, but a history of recent onset of localized, persistent back or radicular pain, particularly in a patient with cancer, this should be viewed as a precursor of compressive myelopathy and managed accordingly. The first investigation is a plain film of the affected region. If this shows metastatic disease, the next and immediate step is myelography. If the roentgenographic findings are negative, the next step, which should be performed as soon as feasible, is a bone scan. If vertebral metastases are detected, the next and immediate step is myelography. If both the plain films and bone scan are negative, epidural metastasis is unlikely, and one can observe these patients and reevaluate their status at a later date if indicated.

The emergency treatment of documented epidural metastases includes dexamethasone. The definitive therapy is decompressive laminectomy or radiation, singly or in combination. This decision is made on an individual basis, depending on residual cord function, the patient's general condition, the type of tumor, and individual preference. Completed cord lesions are usually treated with palliative radiation for pain.

Tumors arising around the cord (meningioma,

schwannoma, neurofibroma) usually present a more protracted course, but may decompensate rapidly, and the immediate management is essentially as has been described.

Epidural Abscess

Localized back pain and tenderness in an ill, febrile patient with leukocytosis suggests the diagnosis of epidural abscess. The manifestations of cord compression may be subtle or overt from the start. Predisposing factors vary from furuncles to pneumonia, endocarditis, and septicemia. *Staphylococcus aureus, Streptococcus,* and gram-negative organisms are the most common pathogens. Fungal, tuberculous, and other granulomatous diseases have a more protracted course, but may decompensate rapidly.

Plain roentgenograms may or may not show vertebral osteomyelitis, although bone scan is usually positive. Emergency myelography is the test of choice and demonstrates partial or complete block, and the spinal fluid shows pleocytosis, elevated protein, and sometimes xanthochromia and decreased glucose. Dexamethasone is helpful, but surgical decompression is required in most cases combined with high doses of antibiotics appropriate for the isolated organism.

Herniated Intervertebral Disc

Herniation of the nucleus pulposus of the intervertebral disc is most frequently directed laterally, but may be directed posteriorly in the midline. Back and often radicular pain, exacerbated by the Valsalva maneuver, occurs together with findings referable to the affected segment. Multiple nerve root entrapment in the cauda equina may resemble cord compression, but the loss of reflexes and asymmetry are distinguishing features.

The patient's spine should be immobilized by the emergency team both prior to reaching the hospital and during the clinical and radiologic examinations. Evaluation of the acute presentation includes plain roentgenograms and emergency myelography. The spinal fluid should be evaluated for other causes (epidural abscess, metastatic tumor) of acute back pain and compressive myelopathy. Narcotic analgesics are used to relieve severe pain, and dexamethasone minimizes edema from the acute compression. The decision to treat conservatively or by early decompression is usually made by the neurosurgeon and attending physicians once the patient has been admitted to the hospital.

Rheumatoid Arthritis

Laxity of the transverse ligament of the atlas in rheumatoid arthritis permits subluxation of the odontoid process and the development of cervico-medullary compression. This may be subacute, but has the explosive potential for sudden death or major neurologic impairment. Patients with signs referable to a high cervical lesion require neck immobilization in the emergency department, plain films, and neurologic and neurosurgical consultation to guide further clinical and radiologic (CT and/or myelogram) management.

Hemorrhage

Hemorrhage in and around the spinal cord typically occurs in the setting of a bleeding diathesis, trauma, or local vascular malformation, or it may be spontaneous with no precipitating cause isolated. A screen for coagulopathies includes a personal and family history of bleeding disorders and a full list of drugs currently being taken. A complete blood count, platelet count, prothrombin, and partial thromboplastin time and bleeding time are standard. If all these parameters are normal in the absence of a history of trauma, a vascular malformation is possible. There may be clinical clues such as cutaneous nevi in the dermatomal distribution of the affected segment.

With an epidural hematoma, the development and worsening of prominent local back pain and the signs of compression are rapid. Dexamethasone is given as a bolus. Correction of the coagulopathy should be promptly instituted with the appropriate agent (platelets, vitamin K, fresh frozen plasma, factor VIII), as indicated by the etiology in each case. Computerized tomography may demonstrate the hemorrhage, but emergency myelography is still the procedure of choice. Treatment is operative decompression. Subdural hematoma is uncommon, and although the presentation is less rapid than the epidural, management is essentially the same.

Intraparenchymal hemorrhage is frequently devastating and only minimally reversible. Severe back pain, dramatic loss of cord function, autonomic instability, and hemorrhagic or xanthochromic cerebospinal fluid suggest the diagnosis. Computerized tomography may be diagnostic. Therapeutic options are limited and rarely include surgery.

NONCOMPRESSIVE EMERGENCIES

Subacute Combined Degeneration of the Cord (Vitamin B₁₂ Deficiency Syndrome)

Progression of the myelopathy in vitamin B_{12} deficiency may be unpredictably rapid. Intense paresthesias in the hands and feet are followed by a disturbance of equilibrium and gait, loss of vibration and position sense, and weakness, spasticity, and upgoing toes. Deep tendon reflexes are variable. Autonomic dysfunction is distinctly unusual.

Diagnosis is straightforward when associated with macrocytic anemia, multilobed polymorphonuclear leukocytes, and a megaloblastic marrow. However, the neurologic syndrome may be an early manifestation, and the hematologic signs may also have been masked by prior folic acid administration. If doubt exists as to the diagnosis, a myelogram should be obtained.

After drawing blood for vitamin B_{12} assay, one should administer 1,000 μg of vitamin B_{12} immediately. This does not adversely affect the later definitive diagnosis of pernicious anemia, as the Schilling test requires prior B_{12} administration. The other causes of B_{12} deficiency should be apparent from the history and investigations.

Acute Transverse Myelitis

This immune-mediated demyelinating disease of the white matter of the spinal cord affects predominantly the mid to upper thoracic segments. In 40 to 60 percent of cases it follows 10 to 14 days after viral infections (particularly measles), mycoplasmal and occasionally bacterial infections, vaccinations against smallpox, and earlier rabies vaccines that are no longer used in the United States. It occurs as a complication of systemic lupus erythematosus, as a nonmetastatic paraneoplastic phenomenon, and after the first reuse of heroin following prolonged abstinence. It is a frequent manifestation of multiple sclerosis, but an isolated attack is only occasionally a precursor of future disseminated white matter disease. Clinical manifestations may progress over hours to days. Patients are frequently ill at the time of presentation with back and radicular pain, fever, malaise, nuchal rigidity, and leukocytosis. Sphincter disturbance is almost invariable, but respiratory embarrassment rarely occurs. A negative myelogram helps to confirm the diagnosis. Spinal fluid varies from normal to a sterile pleocytosis with elevated protein. High-dose adrenocorticoid therapy is of value in reducing the duration of an attack and perhaps improving final recovery. Intramuscular ACTH gel is our choice, although intravenous ACTH and prednisone by mouth are possibly as effective. We start with 80 units daily for 3 days, then rapidly taper by using consecutively 60 units, 40 units, 20 units, and 10 units, each given daily for 3 days. Antacids are essential. We use cimetidine in the dose already described.

Acute Infectious Myelopathy

Bacterial infection of the cord with intramedullary abscess formation develops over hours to days in a systemically ill patient in whom a primary source can usually be found. Local back pain occurs with dissociated sensory loss, weakness, and autonomic dysfunction. Spinal fluid obtained at myelography reveals pleocytosis and elevated protein. Myelography may demonstrate partial or complete block. Treatment includes surgical drainage and maximal doses of antibiotics appropriate for the suspected or identified organism.

Poliomyelitis (poliovirus and, less frequently, coxsackie and echovirus) characteristically presents with acute asymmetric lower motor neuron dysfunction and preserved sensation in a systemically ill patient. The spinal fluid shows a pleocytosis and elevated protein, and the stool culture reveals the poliovirus in 90 percent of cases within days of the onset of symptoms.

Treatment is supportive. Secretion and excretion precautions should be followed. Intramuscular injections and muscular exertion should be avoided because of an apparent lowering of resistance to viral attack of the anterior horn cells innervating sites of trauma. Public health authorities should be notified of the case once the clinical diagnosis is made.

Fungal infections, parasites, and tuberculous and sarcoid granulomas are usually chronic, but may decompensate rapidly. Subsequent to the myelogram and spinal fluid examinations, the diagnosis may be confirmed by the surgical specimen.

Meningovascular syphilis causes an infective vasculitic infarction of the cord.

Schistosomiasis (Bilharziasis)

This disease is rampant throughout Africa, Asia, and South America. The diagnosis is suggested by the history of recent immigration to the United States or of travellers who were exposed to slow running water in appropriate geographic areas, followed by an acute systemic illness, eosinophilia, and a progressive spinal cord, cauda equina, or anterior spinal artery syndrome. In S. mansoni infection, there is an interposed second stage of fever, diarrhea, urticaria, lymphadenopathy, and splenomegaly (Katayama fever). The presence of ova in the stool confirms infection, but not necessarily causality. Myelography with spinal fluid evaluation is usually indicated.

Treatment needs to be instituted immediately, as evolution, particularly of the necrotizing transverse myelitic form, can be aggressive. The drug of choice is praziquantel, a relatively nontoxic agent with activity against the adult form of all schistosomal strains. The dose is 20 mg per kilogram given orally 3 times for one day. A short course of dexamethasone combined with antacids may help to diminish the acute manifestations of ova-induced granulomas, but the immunosuppression of protracted steroid use may adversely affect the host response to toxins released by dead and dying ova.

Infarction

Ischemic infarction of the spinal cord results from aortic aneurysmal dissection with occlusion of spinal arteries; surgical clamping of the aorta; aortic, renal, and spinal cord arteriography; diffuse hypoperfusion; emboli from infective endocarditis, left atrial myxoma, and small thrombi at the origin of spinal arteries; vasculitic infarction in systemic lupus erythematosus, polyarteritis nodosa, and meningovascular syphilis; and vascular encasement in meningeal carcinomatosis. Clinically significant atherosclerotic thrombosis of the spinal arteries probably does not occur.

The single anterior spinal artery is most often affected, resulting in back pain, symmetric flaccid weakness, a sensory level to pin and temperature with preservation of proprioceptive and vibratory sense, and autonomic involvement. Posterior cord infarction is rare, with a sensory level to vibration and transient mild weakness. Transverse infarction of the cord produces spinal shock. Blood should be drawn for erythrocyte sedimentation rate, antinuclear antibody determination, blood cultures, coagulation parameters, and VDRL (or equivalent), unless the cause is obvious. Spinal fluid obtained at myelography is tested for pleocytosis, protein content, malignant cells, and syphilis. Contrast-enhanced computerized tomography of the aorta and selective spinal artery angiography are occasionally indicated.

There is no specific treatment for completed infarction. Use of heparin to maintain the partial thromboplastin time at 1½ times normal is confined to cases with a clear embolic source.

It is worth stressing that meningovascular syphilis has become harder to diagnose because frequent antibiotic use has attenuated the presentation and there is a generally lowered level of awareness of this condition. Treatment consists of 2 to 4 million units of aqueous crystalline penicillin G intravenously every 4 hours for 10 days. An acceptable alternative is a 10 day course of aqueous procaine penicillin G 2.4 million units intramuscularly daily, administered concomitantly with probenecid 500 mg by mouth 4 times daily. In either case, the initial treatment should be followed by weekly intramuscular injections of 2.4 million units of benzathine penicillin G for 3 doses. Tetracycline 500 mg orally every 6 hours for 30 days, is used in penicillin-allergic patients.

Decompression Sickness

Severe cases of acute atmospheric decompression present with diffuse joint and back pain, headache, confusion progressing to coma, and spinal cord signs of sensory loss, para- or tetra-paresis, areflexia, and sphincter paralysis. Less fulminant cases begin with warm prickly paresthesias in the hands or feet, followed in minutes to hours by proximally progressive loss of sensation with weakness and occasionally paralysis of the affected limbs. Involvement is commonly unilateral. Dizziness, nausea, mild headache, and ataxia are associated nonspecific features.

Treatment is by recompression as soon as possible, with gradual restoration of normal atmospheric pressure. Management and transportation to a recompression chamber should be coordinated with the local Coast Guard units and paramedical teams. Breathing 100 percent oxygen as a temporary measure has achieved relief in some reported cases and should be used, although clinical trials documenting its efficacy are awaited.

Electrical Injury

Electrical injury to the spinal cord most commonly affects the cervical segments when current passes from one hand to the other. The resultant myelopathy may be physiologic, transient, and acute or demyelinating, severe, and delayed for hours to days. Paresthesias, local or radicular pain, weakness, and disturbances of micturition herald the onset.

It is prudent to observe patients with significant electrical injury for the development of this syndrome. The need for hospital admission depends on such factors as associated injuries and the possibility of observation at home.

Toxins

Acute segmental spinal cord syndromes occur sporadically after intrathecal cytotoxic agents, exposure to arteriographic and myelographic contrast media, spinal anesthetics, the first reuse of heroin after prolonged abstinence, and oral ingestion of clioquinol and the industrial lubricant orthocresylphosphate.

In cases attributable to arteriography and direct injection of agents into the thecal sac, it has been recommended that the offending agent be removed by repeated draining of the cerebrospinal fluid and replacement with sterile saline. Steroids have been used in these toxic myelopathies, but have not been proved effective. In most instances, the management is supportive.

SUGGESTED READING

Adams RD, Victor M. Diseases of the spinal cord. In: Adams RD, Victor M, eds. Principles of neurology. 3rd ed. New York: McGraw Hill, 1985:665.

DeMyer W. Anatomy and clinical neurology of the spinal cord. In: Baker AB, Joynt R, eds. Clinical neurology. Vol. 3. Philadelphia: Harper and Row, 1984: Ch. 43.

Kincaid JC, Dyken ML. Myelitis and myelopathy. In: Baker AB, Joynt R, eds. Clinical neurology. Vol. 3. Philadelphia: Harper and Row, 1984: Ch. 48.

Moosey J. Vascular diseases of the spinal cord. In: Baker AB, Joynt R, eds. Clinical neurology. Vol. 3. Philadelphia: Harper and Row, 1984: Ch. 19.

Mulder DW, Dale AJD. Spinal cord tumors and discs. In: Baker AB, Joynt R, eds. Clinical neurology. Vol. 3. Philadelphia: Harper and Row, 1984: Ch. 44.

GENERAL APPROACH TO BEHAVIORAL EMERGENCIES

BEHAVIORAL EMERGENCIES

MICHAEL J. BRESLER, M.D., F.A.C.E.P.
ROBERT S. HOFFMAN, M.D.

People with behavioral disorders are seen in the emergency department (ED) for three principal reasons: aggressive behavior; acute depression, perhaps with suicidal ideation; and the acute onset or exacerbation of obviously

After ensuring the physical protection of the medical staff, the task of the emergency physician is to rule out the possibility of serious medical illness; evaluate the potential for suicide, homicide, or grave mental disability; institute initial treatment if indicated; and provide for appropriate disposition.

Although management may be initiated in the emergency department, treatment of psychiatric disorders is often a long-term process. However, diagnosis is crucial. It is particularly important to recognize underlying medical illness presenting with primarily psychiatric symptoms, which has accounted for more than a third of patients hospitalized on psychiatric wards in some studies. Delayed diagnosis of subdural hematoma, toxic encephalopathy, or metabolic disturbance may result in permanent disability or death.

Because emergency department treatment modalities for behavioral disorders are limited, and because evaluation is the critical task of the emergency physician, methods for evaluation of behavioral disorders will be discussed in some detail in this chapter.

PHYSICAL PROTECTION

Injured physicians and nurses are of little value to anyone. The most common cause of injury to health professionals is the premature removal of restraints applied in the field by law enforcement officers. Restraints should be removed from potentially violent patients only after thorough evaluation *and* observation, and only in the presence of sufficient personnel to subdue unexpected violent behavior.

If violence is demonstrated, adequate force must be employed to subdue the patient. Ideally, five staff members should be used to restrain the violent patient: one for each extremity and one for the head. Sometimes the mere display of several muscular staff members is sufficient to convince the potentially violent patient that resistance would be futile. If physical restraint is necessary, however, this should be accomplished definitively, but humanely. Remember that the patient is frequently suffering from acute brain dysfunction; a judgmental or punitive attitude on the part of the medical staff is inappropriate.

Because psychoactive medications may confuse evolving neurologic signs, these drugs should be avoided if possible until a diagnosis is achieved. When necessary, diazepam may be administered to nonpsychotic patients, 10 mg by mouth (PO), intramuscularly (IM), or, if necessary, intravenously (IV). Psychotic patients may respond to haloperidol, 5 mg PO or IM every hour until calm. In unusual circumstances, haloperidol can be given intravenously 3 to 5 mg over 1 minute every 20 minutes. Monitoring for hypotension is essential. Chlorpromazine may also be used, 50 mg PO or IM every hour as needed. Chlorpromazine should *not* be administered intravenously.

EVALUATION

Although a history should be obtained from any conscious emergency patient, additional information from family and friends is crucial in cases of behavioral disturbance. Important factors are the time course, prior episodes, associated physical symptoms, and medications. Physical, and particularly neurologic, examination should be performed on all psychiatric patients evaluated in the emergency department, with the possible exception of those suffering mild symptoms from obvious situational anxiety (e.g., domestic argument).

The mental status examination (MSE) is a mandatory part of ED evaluation. The MSE includes assessment of behavior, mood, thought, and cognitive function. The first three are usually evaluated automatically during conversation; cognition must be tested specifically.

Abnormal behavior may include agitation, psychomotor retardation, inattentiveness, or unusual posturing. The mood may be anxious, depressed, euphoric, hostile, or "speeding." Thought disorders may involve abnormal thought process such as looseness of association or faulty logic. Abnormal thought content may involve delusions, ideas of reference (the TV broadcaster is sending secret messages), feelings of influence (thoughts controlled by outside forces), or suicidal or homicidal ideation. Abnormal perception may include illusions (false interpretation of actual perceptions, e.g., a cloud is radioactive) or hallucinations (false perception in the absence of external stimuli).

Cognitive function testing is the most critical part of the emergency evaluation of behavioral disorders. This is the principal means of separating ''purely psychiatric'' disorders from the organic disorders—those due to toxic, metabolic, pharmacologic, neurologic, or surgical pathology. *Impaired cognitive function is the hallmark of organic mental disorders.*

Cognitive function testing includes evaluation of the level of consciousness, orientation, attention, memory, and fund of information. Level of consciousness may range from fully alert through various degrees of obtundation to frank coma. Orientation is grossly abnormal if the patient is not oriented to person, time, place, and situation. ''Orientation times four'' does not preclude organicity, however. Attention may be obviously abnormal, but subtle dysfunction may be present if the patient cannot remember six digits in order, or four in reverse order. Two-digit arithmetic can also be used. Memory can be evaluated by taking a medical history, inquiring as to the events of the past few hours, or asking the patient to remember three words or objects at 1 and 5 minutes. Fund of information may include current events, public figures, and the like. Remember that you are testing knowledge appropriate to the patient's education and social situation—not your own.

DIFFERENTIAL DIAGNOSIS

Figure 1 is an algorithm for the evaluation of behavioral emergencies. Psychiatrists may utilize the entire American Psychiatric Association's *Diagnostic and Statistical Manual of Mental Disorders* (DSM-111). Figure 1 contains only the general diagnostic categories necessary for emergency department evaluation.

People with behavioral disorders may be divided into two broad categories; those who are neither confused nor psychotic, and those who are either confused or frankly psychotic. The nonconfused, nonpsychotic conditions frequently seen in the emergency department include acute anxiety states such as the hyperventilation syndrome, situational reactions to stress or loss, and chronic drug or alcohol dependence.

Confused or psychotic conditions result in an abnormal mental status examination. They may broadly be divided between organic and nonorganic disorders. Organic mental disorders also cause specific impairment of the cognitive function portion of the MSE. They include senile and presenile dementias, acute substance-induced intoxication or withdrawal, and medical or surgical illness presenting psychiatrically, such as endocrine disorders, infection, infarction, tumor, or trauma. Organic dysfunction may be attributable to acute encephalopathy

(sometimes referred to as delirium) or may reflect longstanding dementia. Nonorganic disorders include the schizophrenias and the major affective illnesses: bipolar disorder and major depression. People with affective disorders may not be overtly psychotic or confused between acute episodes.

TREATMENT OF SPECIFIC DISORDERS

Nonconfused, Nonpsychotic Disorders

If the patient presents with somatic complaints, these must be evaluated. Particularly common are headache, nausea, muscle cramps, dizziness, fainting, and chest or abdominal discomfort. The hyperventilation syndrome consists of dyspnea, paresthesias, dizziness, agitation, occasionally chest tightness, and, if severe, carpopedal spasm or even syncope. The hyperventilation syndrome may be confirmed by blood gas studies revealing respiratory alkalosis with excellent oxygenation, a pattern reflecting either tachypnea or hyperpnea or both. Care must be taken not to assign this diagnosis to all hyperventilation without considering the differential; the patient who is hypoxic owing to a pulmonary embolus, for example, can look like this, and bag rebreathing can be highly dangerous in such patients. Treatment consists of reassurance and bag rebreathing, which allows the recycling of carbon dioxide and reduction of pH toward normal levels. Although treatment of any acute emotional disturbance requires reassurance and empathy, pharmacologic intervention is sometimes necessary: chlordiazepoxide, 25 mg PO, or diazepam 10 mg PO, may be used. The benzodiazepines are unique in that oral absorption is generally faster than intramuscular. Single-dose treatment in the ED, or occasionally 1 or 2 days of treatment, may be helpful. But long-term pharmacologic therapy should be instituted only by a psychiatrist with the opportunity for continuing evaluation and treatment of the underlying causes of agitation or depression. It is crucial that people with acute emotional disturbances be given adequate referral for continuing care.

Organic Mental Disorders

Although all confused or psychotic patients demonstrate abnormalities on mental status examination, those with organic mental disorders have specific impairment of the cognitive function section of the examination. Organic dysfunction may reflect chronic dementia or acute encephalopathy. Among the causes of chronic organic brain syndromes are senile or presenile dementia of the Alzheimer type, multi-infarct dementia, and posthypoxic encephalopathy. Rapid deterioration in such a patient, or the acute onset of new symptoms, may reflect a separate—often reversible—acute encephalopathy attributable to toxic, metabolic, or structural abnormality. Common causes of acute encephalopathy, which may occur in a previously healthy person or may be superim-

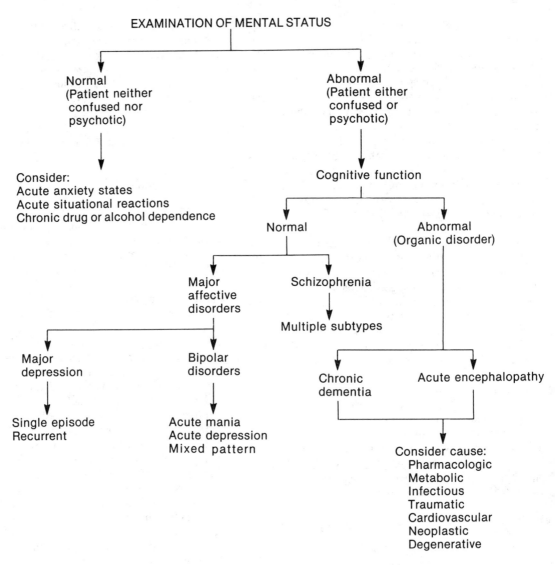

Figure 1 Diagnosis of behavioral emergencies.

posed on chronic dementia, include electrolyte disturbance, infection, subdural hematoma, infarction, drug intoxication or withdrawal, and medication effect owing to overdose or the interaction between multiple medications. It is thus crucial that the emergency physician not dismiss new symptoms, particularly in the elderly, as a reflection of underlying chronic dementia. Emergency department evaluation of acute encephalopathy may allow reversal of many disorders. Specific treatment in the ED depends on diagnosis.

Table 1 is a partial list of "medical illnesses" which may present "psychiatrically" as organic brain dysfunction. Some of the diagnostic tests that might be considered in evaluating organic mental disorders are complete blood count (CBC), glucose, electrolytes, calcium, magnesium, renal function, liver function, thyroid function, blood gases, urinalysis, electrocardiogram (ECG), serum levels of prescribed medication, serum and urine toxicology screen for abused drugs, computed tomography (CT) or

magnetic resonance imaging (MRI) scan, lumbar puncture, sedimentation rate, syphilis screen, B_{12} and folate levels, skin tests for tuberculosis, coccidioidomycosis, chest roentgenogram, and electroencephalogram (EEG).

Perhaps the most frequent cause of organic mental disorders seen in the ED is acute alcohol or drug intoxication or withdrawal. We will discuss briefly some of the more common substances.

Alcohol is the most frequently abused drug and is further discussed in the chapter on *Alcohol Intoxication and Withdrawal*. Acute intoxication may result in violent behavior, the management of which has been described previously. Severe intoxication may cause respiratory suppression, but rarely requires intubation. Respiratory problems are more often owing to aspiration of gastric contents into the lungs of the comatose patient. No pharmacologic agent can reverse alcoholic intoxication; close observation and support are necessary. If the serum ethanol level is too low to account for the degree of seda-

TABLE 1   Common Medical Illnesses Presenting as "Psychiatric" Disorders

Metabolic disorders: glucose, sodium, calcium, or magnesium imbalance, acid/base imbalance; acute hypoxia or posthypoxic encephalopathy, renal failure, hepatic failure, anemia, copper disorders (Wilson's disease)

Endocrine disorders: thyroid disease, parathyroid disease, adrenal hormone imbalance (corticosteroids, mineralocorticoids, catecholamines [pheochromocytoma]), other catecholamine disorder (carcinoid), insulinoma

Infectious diseases: encephalitis, meningitis, brain abscess, tertiary syphilis, generalized sepsis or any severe systemic infection

Trauma: concussion or postconcussive syndrome, intracranial hematoma (especially occult subdural hematoma)

Cardiovascular disorders: cardiac dysrhythmia, hypotension, TIA, CVA, migraine, vasculitis (temporal arteritis, lupus, periarteritis nodosa), hypertensive encephalopathy, multiinfarct dementia

Neoplastic diseases: CNS tumors or metastases, remote tumors with hormonal secretion (insulin, ADH, ACTH)

Degenerative diseases: senile or presenile dementia of the Alzheimer type

Drug abuse: alcohol, barbiturates, sedative hypnotics, amphetamines and other stimulants, hallucinogens

Drug reactions: L-Dopa, steroids, beta-adrenergic blockers, antihypertensives (reserpine, αmethyldopa, hydralazine), cardiac drugs (digoxin, quinidine, procainamide, lidocaine), bronchodilators (methylxanthines [aminophylline], beta-adrenergic agonists [ephedrine, terbutaline]), anticonvulsants, thyroid preparations, cimetidine, isoniazid, rifampin

tion, or if the obtundation does not resolve as expected, other conditions such as subdural hematoma must be considered.

Alcoholic withdrawal causes increasing tremulousness, agitation, confusion, and often visual or tactile hallucinations and seizures. Full-blown untreated delirium tremens may have a mortality rate as high as 15 percent. Benzodiazepines are used prophylactically to prevent progression of alcohol withdrawal to delirium tremens and convulsions: either chlordiazepoxide, 50 to 100 mg PO, or diazepam, 10 to 20 mg PO, every 2 to 4 hours as needed. The intravenous route can be utilized, but dosage must be decreased. Diazepam can be administered intravenously in 5-mg increments, repeated until effective, with careful monitoring of blood pressure and respiratory status.

The Wernicke-Korsakoff syndrome may be seen in chronic alcoholics. Signs are confusion, memory deficiency, ataxia, and particularly nystagmus and ocular palsies. The onset of acute Wernicke's encephalopathy may follow a drinking binge, but prompt treatment with thiamine, 100 mg IV, may prevent the acute, reversible Wernicke's encephalopathy from progressing to the chronic, irreversible Korsakoff anamnestic syndrome. A blood specimen for serum thiamine level determination should be drawn first. Thiamine, 100 mg IM or IV, is frequently given prophylactically to chronic alcoholics in order to prevent the syndrome. Prophylactic thiamine may be particularly important when alcoholic hypoglycemia

is reversed with intravenous dextrose, an intervention that is occasionally associated with the precipitation of acute Wernicke's encephalopathy.

Opiate intoxication causes respiratory suppression and pinpoint pupils. Reversal may be achieved with naloxone, 0.8 mg IV, repeated as needed to maintain adequate ventilation. Large doses may be required to reverse synthetic opiates such as fentanyl and propoxyphene, or the non-narcotic agent pentazocine. Unlike withdrawal from alcohol or barbiturates, opiate withdrawal is not medically dangerous, although it is exceedingly uncomfortable. Medically managed withdrawal may be assisted with methadone or morphine.

Barbiturate intoxication may require ventilatory support, and some of the long-acting preparations can be dialyzed. Withdrawal from barbiturates resembles alcohol withdrawal. Signs may include agitation, toxic psychosis, tremulousness, vomiting, fever, hypotension, and potentially fatal seizures. Treatment consists of reintoxication with barbiturates and staged withdrawal in the hospital.

Central nervous system (CNS) stimulant (amphetamines, cocaine) intoxication may cause agitation, euphoria, belligerence, panic, paranoia, hallucinations (particularly visual and tactile), hypertension, dysrhythmias, fever, seizures, or coma. Immediate treatment is frequently required in the ED and may include the oral or intramuscular administration of diazepam, 10 mg; chlorpromazine, 50 to 75 mg; or haloperidol, 5 to 10 mg. Fever may signal impending medical deterioration. If fever or other significant physical (as opposed to purely behavioral) signs occur, reversal may be achieved with antipsychotic agents that have dopaminergic-blocking properties, such as haloperidol or chlorpromazine. Withdrawal may be associated with weakness and severe depression, which may respond to tricyclic antidepressant medication. Such agents generally should not be prescribed in the emergency department. In-hospital withdrawal, or at least intensive outpatient psychiatric care, is required.

Hallucinogen (PCP, LSD, marijuana) intoxication rarely causes serious medical complications, but behavioral sequelae may be extremely severe. Although marijuana intoxication is usually relatively benign, LSD (lysergic acid diethylamide) and PCP (phencyclidine) can result in lethal behavior. People on LSD are not typically violent, but they may suffer fatal accidents (e.g., trying to fly out a window). PCP intoxication can cause extremely violent behavior, resulting in homicide.

Mild intoxication may be treated in the ED by "talking down" and reassurance. Severe reactions require hospitalization and often sedation. Antipsychotic medication should ideally be withheld for 24 hours to ensure accurate diagnosis, but benzodiazepines (diazepam, 10 mg PO or IM) may be used. Haloperidol, 5 mg IM, may be useful for severe PCP intoxication, particularly if the patient is violent.

Patients who are confused or psychotic and have abnormalities of mental status on examination—but who have normal cognitive function—may fall into several broad nonorganic categories. Although transient, non-recurring psychotic episodes can happen, the presence of chronic or recurrent psychotic episodes generally indicates either schizophrenia or an affective disorder.

Schizophrenia

The schizophrenias are a group of disorders characterized by recurrent episodes of psychotic behavior that may include abnormalities of thought process (e.g., loose association), thought content (e.g., delusions), perception (e.g., hallucinations), and judgment. Auditory hallucinations are particularly common in schizophrenics, whereas tactile or visual hallucinations are more typical of organic disorders. Schizophrenics often function poorly between frank psychotic episodes and frequently have a prior history of eccentricity or of difficulty interacting with other people. There is often a family history of schizophrenia. The disorder usually becomes apparent during adolescence or early adulthood. Middle-aged patients with new-onset psychosis do not have schizophrenia; an organic cause must be excluded.

Severely impaired schizophrenics should be hospitalized, but mild excerbations of abnormal behavior may be treated in an outpatient setting so long as close psychiatric follow-up is available. In the past, schizophrenic patients have frequently been maintained on long-term antipsychotic medication. Because of the risk of tardive dyskinesia with prolonged usage, however, there is now a tendency to use these drugs, if possible, only during acute episodes. The severely impaired schizophrenic may be treated in the emergency department with chlorpromazine, 50 mg PO or IM, or haloperidol, 5 mg PO or IM. This dose may be repeated every hour if necessary, but blood pressure must be monitored because of the risk of postural hypotension. If dystonic reactions occur, these may be reversed with diphenhydramine, 50 mg PO, IM, or IV, or benztropine, 2 mg PO or IM. Postural hypotension is more common following chlorpromazine; dystonic reactions are more frequent after haloperidol.

Affective Disorders

These are grouped primarily into two general types: bipolar disorders and major depression. People with chronic bipolar affective disorders may have acute episodes of mania or depression, or a combination of the two. Patients with major depression only do not develop manic episodes, but may have either single or recurrent episodes of depression. Between acute episodes, people with affective disorders are typically normal as opposed to schizophrenics, who often display some degree of abnormal behavior between acute exacerbations.

During a manic episode, the patient may be euphoric or irritable. Typical signs are pressured speech, flight of ideas, grandiose delusions, reckless behavior with loss of judgment, and even hallucinations or incoherence.

Major depressive episodes are characterized by obviously depressed affect, often with psychomotor retardation, but sometimes with agitation. Suicidal ideation is not uncommon (see the chapter on *Depression and Suicide*).

Acute episodes of either mania or major depression often require hospitalization. Assessment for suicide potential is crucial. Although definitive therapy may include lithium for mania, or antidepressant medication or electroconvulsive therapy for major depression, the initial use of antipsychotic agents in the emergency department may be helpful; chlorpromazine or haloperidol may be used in the same dosages given for schizophrenia.

DISPOSITION

Patients with behavioral disorders who demonstrate abnormal cognition on mental status examination have organic disorders attributable to neurologic, metabolic, toxic, endocrine, or structural disease. The condition may represent a chronic dementia or an acute encephalopathy. Acute deterioration in a patient with underlying chronic dementia may reflect a potentially reversible disorder unrelated to the underlying disorder. Medical or surgical (as opposed to psychiatric) work-up is essential, and acute nonpsychiatric hospitalization is often required.

Patients with normal cognitive function, but other abnormalities on mental status examination, are frequently suffering from schizophrenia or the affective disorders. The initial use of antipsychotic medication may be required in the emergency department, but acute psychiatric hospitalization is often indicated.

Patients with acute anxiety or minor situational depression, who have no significant abnormalities on the MSE, may respond to verbal reassurance and referral for a brief course of outpatient counseling. Short-term medication with a benzodiazapine preparation may be helpful.

Regardless of the diagnosis, however, there are three specific indications for urgent psychiatric hospitalization: suicidal risk, homicidal risk, and grave mental disability.

Suicidal risk is greatest when there is a specific plan, prior serious attempt, advanced age, chronic physical illness, major depressive illness, schizophrenia, or a feeling of intense hopelessness. It is appropriate to ask the depressed patient about thoughts of suicide. Such discussion does not increase the risk, but may allow the patient's life to be saved by appropriate intervention.

Homicidal risk is often associated with formulation of a specific plan, a past history of violent behavior, delusions of persecution, acute alcohol or drug intoxication (particularly amphetamines and phencyclidine), or a provocative, taunting victim.

Grave mental disability may prevent the patient from finding shelter and food or otherwise attending to the daily functions of life. Specific questioning about plans may reveal the patient's inability to care for himself.

These three conditions may require involuntary hospitalization.

SUGGESTED READING

American Psychiatric Association. Diagnostic and statistical manual of mental disorders. 3rd ed. Washington, D.C.: American Psychiatric Association, 1980.
Hoffman RS. Psychiatric emergencies. In: Eliastam M, Sternbach GL, Bresler MJ, eds. Manual of emergency medicine. Chicago: Yearbook Medical Publishers, 1983:131.
Kaplan HI, Sadock BJ. Comprehensive textbook of psychiatry. 4th ed. Baltimore: Williams and Wilkins, 1985.

THE ABUSED PATIENT

STEPHEN LUDWIG, M.D.

The abused patient is a manifestation of what Dr. C. Everett Koop, the United States Surgeon General, has called the nation's number one public health problem: violence. Child abuse and spouse abuse are two common forms of violent behavior. They are seen daily in many emergency departments and present medical, legal, and interpersonal challenges to the emergency physician. It may be difficult even to establish the diagnosis of child abuse or spouse abuse. An abused child may be preverbal, or even if able to communicate, may be reluctant to betray the abusive parent for fear of the consequences. The abusive parent is likely to be in crisis, and thus torn between being detected and being controlled. In spouse abuse there often are unrealistic expectations that the abuser will reform and fear of social stigma which impede making an accurate diagnosis. It is clear in both conditions, however, that failure to intervene places the victim at greater risk for more serious or fatal injury. Thus, what is difficult for the emergency physician is essential for the victims. In addition to this ethical and moral responsibility, the physician can be (and has been) held legally liable for failure to diagnose and report abuse.

CHILD ABUSE

The cause of child abuse is a complex interaction among individual, family, community, and societal factors. Theorists have proposed a list of four essentials for child abuse to occur: (1) a parent who is stressed and poised to respond to stress with a loss of control; (2) a child who is provocative and perceived by the parent as different or special; (3) a crisis that throws the family unit into a state of dysfunction; and (4) a society that permits or condones a certain level of violent behavior. There are other factors that impinge on each of these essentials. For example, parental use of drugs or alcohol may add to parental stress while lessening parental control. There are times in the child's life when developmental factors make the child more provocative to the parents, such as during the period of colic or toilet training. The societal belief in the use of corporal punishment as a preferred discipline technique increases the potential for destructive discipline.

Just as the causes of abuse are multiple, so are the definitions. We use the term ''child abuse'' to describe many different parental behaviors. The emergency physician must realize this and not expect abuse to fit one stereotype. Abuse is used to describe a parent who repeatedly beats, starves, and confines the victim. It also describes a parent who leaves a child unattended for a short time and a parent who loses control on one occasion while attempting to instill the child with admirable values. Any behavior that results in injury to the child may be considered as abusive. Each state has a child abuse law that defines the parameters of acceptable parental behavior within that state. Most of the state laws recognize four conditions as subsets of child abuse: (1) physical abuse, (2) physical neglect, (3) emotional or psychological abuse, and (4) sexual abuse. The emergency physician must also be aware of his or her own personal definition of abuse; some situations require the physician to make a value judgment based on personal factors and experiences.

The manifestations of child abuse are varied. Virtually any traumatic injury seen in a child may have been caused by abuse. This is yet another factor that makes identification difficult. Abuse may be manifested as cardiac arrest, a bruise, a toxic ingestion, an electrolyte imbalance, a psychological disturbance, or a nutritional deficiency. In sexual abuse the only manifestation may be a detailed history of sexual contact given by the child.

Of the *physical manifestations* of abuse the most common injuries are to the skin and soft tissue. Integument injuries include not only bruises, hematomas, and lacerations, but also burns from hot objects and immersion. The next most common form of abuse is skeletal injury. Central nervous system trauma, both direct trauma and shake injuries, account for the high mortality and morbidity associated with abuse. Other forms of life-threatening abuse are abdominal trauma, thoracic trauma, and intentional drowning. The child who is brought to the emergency department requiring resuscitation may be the victim of homicide if no other cause is apparent. Homicide is now the fourth leading cause of death in the 1- to 14-year age group in the United States.

The *manifestations of neglect* span a wide range. Physical abandonment of a child is the most extreme form. Other signs of neglect are found in the examination of the child's state of nutrition, hygiene, or health care. The distinction between noncompliance with medical care and actual medical neglect is made when there is injury to the child. If a parent fails to comply and that noncompliance results in injury, then the criteria for neglect are met.

Psychological or emotional abuse is difficult to identify in the emergency department. The findings of extreme psychological maladjustment may be apparent, for example, in the suicidal child; however, it is difficult to establish that this is the result of parental behavior. With regard to *sexual abuse*, again the manifestations are varied. Physical injury following sexual abuse is present in approximately 15 percent of cases. Included in this small group with physical manifestations are those with sexually transmitted disease. Most sexually abused children will have only a detailed history of the encounter and some nonspecific behavioral manifestations, such as fears, changes in adaptation, and sleep or eating disturbances.

Management

The management of child abuse includes the following: (1) maintain a high index of suspicion, (2) establish a reporting threshold, (3) consider a differential diagnosis, (4) consider the need for crisis hospitalization, (5) notify the parents of your report, and (6) file the report and arrange follow-up.

The first step in the management plan is to maintain a high *index of suspicion*. Any practicing physician who has not identified at least one case of abuse has not entertained the possibility. Abuse is so prevalent within our society that it is virtually inescapable unless the physician has a closed mind about it. Some estimate the incidence of abuse to be 1 to 3 percent of the population. More than 4,000 deaths per year are caused by abuse in the United States.

To reach a *reporting threshold* the emergency physician must gather all the important data about the child and the family. The data sources are the physical examination, the history, laboratory information, and impressions gained from observing and experiencing the family's interaction. These pieces of data are used like building blocks to build a level of suspicion that will satisfy a reporting threshold. In some cases the abuse will be obvious and only an examination of a child with multiple whip marks is necessary to suspect the diagnosis. In other situations one may be puzzled by an unusual pattern of injury. Then the minimal suspicion will be strengthened by an inadequate or inconsistent history. Laboratory information may rule out the presence of an organic disease (Table 1).

The fourth building block, *family interaction*, attempts to identify some of the causes that lead to abuse, such as stress, crisis, or perception of the child as special.

TABLE 1 Laboratory Studies Useful in Cases of Child Abuse

Study	Target Problem
Complete blood count	Blood loss
	Nutritional anemia
Platelet count	Coagulation status
Prothrombin/partial	
thromboplastin time	
Blood urea nitrogen	
Urine specific gravity	Dehydration
Toxic screen: serum, urine,	
gastric contents	Poisoning
Urine hematest	Urinary tract trauma
	Myoglobinuria
	Muscle trauma
Creatinine phosphokinase	Pyoderma
Bullae culture	Pancreatic trauma
Serum amylase	Bone disease
Serum calcium	
Phosphorus	
Alkaline phosphatase	
Sexually transmitted	Sexual abuse
disease cultures	
Urinalysis	
Urine pregnancy test	
Pap smear	
Seminal fluid analysis	
RPR test for syphilis	
Foreign pubic hairs, fingernail	
scrapings	
Clothing analysis	

When the four building blocks are added in varying combinations, a level of suspicion may be met such that the physician feels that reporting is justified. Because the evidence of abuse is difficult to obtain, it is often helpful to obtain consultation from a social worker or a specially trained nurse. These consultants may have special skills in observing family interactions and assisting with some of the difficult value judgments that may need to be made. Indeed, the multidisciplinary approach is helpful throughout the management of child abuse cases.

Before making a final determination about the need to report a case of suspected abuse, it is wise to consider a *differential diagnosis* (Table 2). Most state laws require the reporting of "suspected" abuse rather than confirmed abuse. This distinction is drawn in order that the reports are made often and easily enough to include all cases. Thus, the laws tend to encourage over-reporting. Nonetheless, because of the social stigma that parents may face, and the potential future involvement that the physician may face, it is wise to consider a differential diagnosis carefully. In most cases the differentiation between accidental trauma and nonaccidental trauma must be made. Other more sophisticated distinctions may usually be made with the aid of laboratory tests. At times the actual diagnosis may be established only by the passage of time and repeated physical observations of the child.

Prior to notification of the parents, it is important to try to determine whether or not *crisis hospitalization* is indicated. This issue should be resolved in the minds of the treatment team prior to approaching the parents with a plan. Crisis hospitalization must be instituted if there is a feeling that the child will be in danger if returned to home. In order to determine if the home is safe one needs to know: (1) the whereabouts of the suspected perpetrator, (2) the stability of the extended family available to protect the child, (3) the response time of the child protective services agency and/or police, (4) the age and vulnerability of the child, (5) the intensity of the crisis leading to the abuse, and (6) evidence of repetitive abuse in the past. If it is determined that the child is unlikely to be safe, then crisis hospitalization must occur regardless of the child's medical condition, the parent's health insurance status, or the hospital's utilization practices. Protection of a vulnerable child comes first. In some states physicians are given virtual police power to do this; in others the physician may need to make a plea for protection from a local judge or child protective services worker.

The next step in the management process is perhaps the most difficult for the physician. At this point the *parents must be told* of the physician's suspected diagnosis and about the ensuing report to the designated reporting agent. The best approach to the parents is one that stresses the physician's concern for the welfare of the child. An approach that accuses or admonishes the parents is to be avoided. By using the former approach the physician and the parents start from a point of agreement, namely, that we are all concerned about the health and safety of the child. With the latter approach, one is more likely to encounter defensiveness, denial, and at times hostility directed toward the staff. Failing to notify the

TABLE 2 Differential Diagnosis of Abuse

Diagnosis	Confirming Study
Accidental trauma	History, physical examination, laboratory results, observed interaction
Scurvy	Long-bone radiograph
Rickets	Wrist radiography, calcium phosphorus, alkaline phosphatase levels
Secondary hyperparathyroidism	BUN, creatinine levels, long-bone radiograph
Kinky hair syndrome	Long-bone, rib radiograph, hair analysis
Mucolipidosis II (T-cell diseases)	Long-bone, rib radiograph, analysis of facial features, fibroblast studies
Congenital syphilis	Serum test for syphilis
Osteomyelitis	Bone culture, blood culture, sedimentation rate
Osteogenesis imperfecta	Skeletal radiographs, bone biopsy
Infantile cortical hyperostosis	Long-bone mandible radiograph
Skeletal sclerosis	Long-bone radiograph
Hypophosphatasia	Long-bone radiograph, serum alkaline phosphatase

parents at all sets up an impossible situation for those who must follow in the care of the child. Most parents who have abused their children and bring them to the emergency department are looking for help. Most are sorry about their loss of control. We should seek a posture that allows them to accept help and restraint. Direct accusation and confrontation will build higher walls of isolation and mistrust around the abusive parent. If crisis hospitalization has been decided upon, then parents must be told that the child's current condition warrants it.

The final step in the process is actually *filing the report* with the proper agency in your local area. In some places reports go to the child protective service agency, which is a branch of the child welfare agency. In other areas police accept such reports. In a few jurisdictions there is joint reporting. In addition, it is important to arrange for some form of *follow-up*. This may occur at the hospital or at the child's primary care provider. Never should a case of suspected child abuse leave the emergency department without a comprehensive and specific follow-up plan.

Common Pitfalls

There are several pitfalls in the management of child abuse that one should be sure to avoid.

First, the seriousness of abuse does not correlate with the degree of injury. What appears to be minor injury may be a sign of severe family dysfunction. Through your own inquiry or with the consultation of a social worker try to determine how the family is functioning.

Second, beware of people "like us." If the parents are like us as far as their appearance, socioeconomic status, or intellectual level, we tend to feel that they could not be abusive to their child. This is a self-protective mechanism for the physician. The reality is that anyone has the potential to abuse if placed in the right situation.

Third, remember that suspicion equals reporting. One does not need to document an "airtight" case of abuse before reporting. If the physician uses such a strict definition, many cases will go unreported.

Fourth, remember that reporting equals help. There is a natural tendency to feel that reporting on someone is destructive. It means getting someone in trouble. In cases of child abuse this is reversed. Reporting leads to help for the child, and hopefully for the parents if they have been prepared to accept help.

Finally, if you did not document it, it did not happen. Child abuse cases may result in legal actions either in criminal or civil court. These actions may not evolve for weeks or months. Therefore, it is very important to document carefully everything that is done. Sketches or photographs of the physical injuries, results of laboratory tests, reports of x-ray readings, and consultations with other physicians or social workers must all become a permanent part of the medical record. It is wise for the physician to copy these records for his or her own file. Extra time taken to document the findings in the emergency department will be of great benefit in the future.

Child abuse is an unfortunate fact of life in our society. The emergency physician may have little impact on the incidence of the disorder. However, the early detection and reporting of abuse is of great consequence in the ultimate morbidity and mortality associated with this unfortunate human behavior.

SPOUSE ABUSE

Violence against women, like violence against children, is a problem of massive proportion. Estimates of this form of abuse indicate that as many as six million wives may be abused annually. Some 2,000 to 4,000 women are beaten to death annually in the United States.

There are also a growing number of men who have been abused by their wives, either as a primary response or in retaliation for their own abusive behavior. Other estimates indicate that family violence may occur in one-third of American families. Domestic violence accounts for more police emergency telephone calls and investigations than any other form of criminal complaint.

Spouse abuse occurs in all age groups. In a study by Goldberg and Tomlanovich the victims ranged from age 16 to 79; the mean age in several studies is 30 to 33 years. All socioeconomic groups and individuals with all levels of education are affected. Abuse happens not only to those legally married but also to many couples in nonmarital relationships. An abusive episode often occurs when one or both partners have been using alcohol or drugs. Spouse abuse is often difficult for the emergency physician to diagnose. However, failure to diagnose may lead to more severe injury or death.

The barriers to diagnosis are many. The average victim of spouse abuse has had many episodes of injury prior to identification. In one study there were between 2 and 60 previous attacks, with a mean of 11 (Table 3). In another study 50 percent of domestic violence victims were abused at a frequency of once a month or more. Often the victim's chief complaint will disguise the abuse. Common complaints include other forms of trauma, such as motor vehicle accidents or falls, or nonspecific psychiatric complaints.

There are other barriers as well. The victims may have such low self-esteem that they may feel unworthy of help and unable to accept a helping relationship. Often there are unrealistically optimistic views that the perpetrator will reform. The victim is often in a dependent position in relation to the abuser both in emotional and financial terms. The abuser may be excused because "this only happens when he drinks" or because the abuser may be contrite and loving in between episodes of violence. As in child abuse, there are strong societal beliefs that set up the potential for spouse abuse, such as that women like to be dominated by a strong male figure, and that the victim gets what she deserves. In addition, there is a strong societal belief that we should not interfere with any domestic situations and that the home is a sanctuary. The sum of these forces makes it difficult for the emergency physician to recognize abuse and for the victim to accept help once the abuse is recognized.

It should be noted that there is a strong interaction between spouse abuse and child abuse. This is the result of two mechanisms. The most common is that the abusive spouse has injured both his spouse and their children and that the violence is losing any focus. Through the second mechanism the wife may be abused by her spouse and then pass on her frustration and anger to the children. Long-term studies of children living in homes of violence show high rates of educational and emotional deficits. Thus, in managing one form of family violence always look for and ask about other forms.

When the victim does seek help it is imperative that the opportunity not be lost. Some of the factors that have been correlated with motivation for seeking help are sustaining of serious physical injury, endurance of chronic pain, realization of an overall negative relationship, concurrent child abuse, and the use of weapons. When these factors play a role, the victim is in crisis, and during crisis appropriate management can result in significant improvement in handling both this episode and future crises.

Management

The management of spouse abuse requires a *multidisciplinary approach*. This starts with the registration clerk being sensitive to the issue of domestic violence. It continues with the emergency department nurse, physician, and social worker all having an established protocol for case management. If there is no established plan of action and clear definition of roles, the victim's crisis spreads to the staff rather than being alleviated by the staff. The first step is to obtain *detailed documentation* of the abuse as it occurred during this episode and in the past. Careful documentation is very important for both medical and legal reasons. The physician must carefully describe and document the injuries, both old and new. Laboratory tests, radiographs, and photographs are often indicated. The social worker or nurse must document the social history in depth and gauge the victim's motivation for change. The victim and the health care workers will need to explore a number of important questions in order to guide further management (Table 4).

The next step in management is to determine what *support system* is needed to carry the management past the identification stage. Identify any natural support systems in the form of friends, neighbors, or relatives. Frequently the victim's passivity and low self-esteem will have resulted in isolation and relatively few natural supports. The next level of intervention may be a shelter run either by the community or by a private agency. If no outside shelter exists, the hospital may have to serve this function. *Psychiatric consultation* may also be needed prior

TABLE 3 Characteristics of Acutely Battered Women

Age	Mean, 31.2 yr
Previous abuse	Mean, 11.2 times
Sought help in past	53%
Children abused	47%
Partner use of alcohol	86%
Partner use of drugs	13%
Father abused mother	53%
Complaint on admission	
Altercation	63%
Fell	20%
Motor vehicle accident	6.6%
Psychiatric crisis	6.6%
Physical examination	
Contusion face left	23%
Contusion face right	6.6%
Contusion face both sides	53%
Sprained ankle	20%
Pregnant	6.6%

Adapted from Appleton W. The battered woman syndrome. Ann Emerg Med 1980; 9:2, 84–91.

TABLE 4   Questions to Explore with Victim of Spouse Abuse

Where does he or she live? With whom?
Are there children living in the home?
Who is aware of the violence there?
Has this sort of thing happened before?
Has it happened with this spouse before or with other persons?
Is it safe to return home?
Is the assailant in the home? Will he or she cause further harm?
Are the children safe? Where are they now?
Are family members in the area? What kind of relationships exist?
Are they aware of the violence?
Are there friends or neighbors who could offer safety?

Adapted from McGrath PE, Schultz PS, Culhane PL. Monograph 5. Rockville. MD: National clearinghouse on domestic violence. 1980

to the patient leaving the emergency department. The victim may be suffering from severe anxiety or depression and may require ongoing psychotherapy.

The emergency department must also be aware of the existing *legal ramifications* of spouse abuse. There may be specific legal "treatments" that will need to be applied. Also, there may be specific reporting requirements that the emergency department physician will not want to overlook. It is important for the emergency department staff to develop a working relationship with the police and the district attorney's office, as there are many legal issues surrounding these cases. Some jurisdictions have developed specific protection from abuse. In other situations an existing criminal code will have to be applied.

Other legal issues have to do with filing of divorce or separation actions, the obtaining of support, the protection of children, and the issues of custody and visitation.

Before the domestic abuse victim leaves the emergency department, there should be a clear plan of *follow-up*. Many hospitals have established follow-up teams to make sure that the many forces bearing on this problem do not act to persuade the victim to let the episode drop and re-expose him - or herself and possibly the children to further abuse.

SUGGESTED READING

Child Abuse

Burgess AW, Groth NA, Homstrom LL, et al. Sexual assault of children and adolescents. Lexington, MA: Lexington Books, 1978.
Ellerstein NS. Child abuse and neglect: a medical reference. New York: John Wiley and Sons, 1981.
Jason J. Child homicide spectrum. Am J Dis Child 1983; 137:578–581.
Ludwig S. Child abuse. In: Fleisher G, Ludwig S, eds. The textbook of pediatric emergency medicine. Baltimore: Williams & Wilkins, 1983.

Spouse Abuse

Appleton W. The battered woman syndrome. Ann Emerg Med 1980; 9:12, 84–91.
Goldberg W, Tomlanovich M. Domestic violence victims in the emergency department: new findings. JAMA 1984; 251:24, 3259–3264.
Goodstein RK. Situational emergencies. 1984; 169–207
McGrath PE, Schultz PS, Culhane PO. The development and implementation of a hospital protocol for the identification and treatment of battered women. Monograph 5. Rockville: National Clearinghouse on Domestic Violence, 1980.

SUICIDE ATTEMPT

DOUGLAS A. RUND, M.D., F.A.C.E.P.

SUICIDE

Although suicide undoubtedly caused human death long before recorded history, it currently represents one of our most serious epidemics. Cause of death statistics consistently rank suicide among the ten leading causes of death for our population. The problem is even more serious for our young. Self-destruction is the *second* leading cause of death for teenagers and young adults.

The emergency physician encounters the problem of suicide in two types of patients. The patient who threatens but has not attempted suicide, and the patient who arrives in the emergency department for medical and psychiatric management following a suicide attempt.

Skillful management of both situations by the emergency physician requires mastery of the following: maintaining a nonjudgmental attitude toward the attempter;

accurately assessing suicide risk to determine need for hospitalization; establishing suicide precautions; and arranging proper consultation, hospitalization, or outpatient referral.

Attitude

The negative attitudes of emergency physicians, emergency nurses, and emergency medical technicians toward the person who requires treatment for attempted suicide are well documented. Attempted suicide represents a self-inflicted injury or illness that seems to load the emergency team with more work. An attitude often expressed is that painful, punitive treatment will "teach the patient a lesson" not to repeat self-destructive behavior. Such an attitude, of course, is clearly incorrect. The suicide attempter actually feels a greatly diminished self-worth yet maintains an ambivalence about dying. Harsh treatment rendered by an authority figure, the physician, further diminishes the patient's self-esteem and thus intensifies his suicidal tendencies. Initial negative attitudes conveyed by the emergency team also complicate the mission of the social worker, psychologist, or psychiatrist who must establish a trusting, communicating relationship. If the attitudes of the emergency staff cannot be supportive they should at least be nonjudgmental.

Assessment of Suicide Risk

The conscientious assessment of suicide risk constitutes one of the most important suicide management skills for emergency physicians. The full assessment of suicide risk includes several variables that have been found to help the physician accurately predict who is most likely to commit suicide, and distinguish high-risk patients from those who actually represent a low risk of committing suicide.

Psychosis

One of the most clearly identifiable features of a suicide attempter that virtually mandates hospitalization is psychosis. The psychotic patient has a substantial impairment of thinking processes. The elements of his conversation are frequently rambling and thoughts and speech are loosely associated. The typical psychotic patient experiences hallucinations. When the psychosis is functional (psychiatric) in origin, these hallucinations are more likely to be auditory. In the case of a patient attempting suicide, such auditory hallucinations may be threatening or may ''command'' suicide. Psychotic patients also experience delusions; they may feel things about themselves or others that have no basis in fact. Since the psychotic patient is unable to distinguish true reality from the reality that exists within the mind, the risk of suicide by the psychotic is almost completely unpredictable. Whenever the physician encounters a psychotic patient who has either made a suicide attempt or seems to have a clear plan for suicide, psychiatric consultation must be obtained and the patient must be hospitalized. Whether the psychosis is due to schizophrenia, affective disorder (depression or mania), or a disorder of shorter duration, such as brief reactive psychosis, the patient can usually be treated successfully with antipsychotic agents and psychiatric care.

Risk-Rescue Ratio

One method that helps assess suicide risk involves the concepts of risk and likelihood of rescue. In general, the higher the risk of dying from an attempt, the more likely the patient is to be a serious suicide risk. Risk factors include the agent used, degree of impaired consciousness, nature of the lesions, toxicity of the overdose, reversibility of the process, and treatment required. When the likelihood of rescue is low the risk is even higher. The ratio of risk to likelihood of rescue increases with more lethal attempts. Rescue factors include location of the attempt, the person initiating rescue, the probability of discovery by any rescuer, the accessibility to rescue, and the delay until discovery. The patient who jumps from a high bridge or building is considered to be at risk of dying. The person who takes a small overdose of over-the-counter medication, by contrast, is considered to be at low risk of dying. With regard to the likelihood of rescue, the patient who takes an overdose and immediately telephones a close friend or family member can expect a high probability of rescue. Someone who makes an attempt in an isolated area or abandoned building would expect a low probability of rescue. In most cases, merely documenting both of these features is an important part of record-keeping for the emergency physician.

Thoughts and Feelings at the Time of the Attempt

One of the most important features of the assessment of the suicide attempter is to determine the patient's *feelings* and *thoughts* at the time of the attempt. Some patients equate a suicide attempt with other forms of emotional discharge like crying, talking to a friend, or getting drunk. They don't really perceive it as an attempt to end their life. Those patients who report feeling angry or feeling that they wanted to get back at someone in a revengeful frame of mind have a much better prognosis than patients who say that they feel hopeless or helpless. When such a person feels that there is no way out of his situation except suicide, the relative overall risk is higher.

Hopelessness

Feelings of hopelessness or helplessness are proven predictors of high suicide risk. When the patient tells the physician that there is simply no other way for him to go because life holds nothing for him and he can see no solution of his major problems, this represents a serious suicide risk.

Future Plans

The future plans of the suicide attempter are quite important for risk assessment. No physician should be reluctant to ask whether the patient still feels that he would like to end his life. For most people the suicide attempt is an act of catharsis. They typically discharge quite a bit of self-destructive energy. Most patients report that they no longer feel the impulse to kill themselves. The patient who continues to state a wish to die, however, should be asked about the details of ending his life. If the plan is well organized, the patient should be considered a serious risk. For instance, if the patient plans to take a known lethal quantity of medication or has a weapon such as a gun and plans to use it, the risk if high. The physician may want to check on the feasibility of the patient's plans, but in general if the physician hears about a plan that seems feasible, then the patient should receive prompt psychiatric counseling and hospitalization.

Age and Sex

Certain demographic features, particularly age and sex, have traditionally been used as predictors of likelihood of suicide. In general, the likelihood of being able to complete a suicide attempt successfully increases with age. For men, risk keeps increasing with age, and the rule of thumb is that a man over 45 who makes a suicide attempt should probably be hospitalized. For women, the likelihood increases to approximately age 60 and then seems to plateau as the years advance. Any woman over 45 who makes a suicide attempt should probably be hospitalized unless she has had extensive psychiatric evaluation that shows a history of frequent minor manipulative suicide attempts and other aspects of the evaluation do not reveal significant risk. In the past women attempted suicide more often than men and men successfully completed suicide more often than women. While these patterns still hold true, the number of successful suicides by women is increasing. Teenagers and young adults are also at risk. The number of suicides by adolescents has risen significantly in the past several decades.

Physical Illness

The physician should consider whether the patient has a serious physical illness. Suicidal patients with a serious medical illness, especially a painful, incurable illness, must be taken seriously. The helplessness, despair, and unrelenting pain understandably drive these patients to seek a way out. Although this often represents a difficult ethical problem for the physician and family, the immediate management by the emergency physician is straightforward. The emergency physician must complete a medical and psychiatric assessment to detect any reversible or palliative features that may make life more bearable for these patients and act to interfere with any suicide plans.

Social Support System

Persons who are single, divorced, separated, or widowed seem to have a higher likelihood of attempting suicide. If a suicide attempter has a truly supportive spouse or other family members, they constitute an important element of the social support system. When such support is available the physician may feel more reassured about sending the patient home after an attempt.

The patient who seems to be successfully employed and who has a reasonably good relationship with co-workers has an effectively functioning social support system. Unemployed persons, by contrast, have a higher risk of suicide. Some suicide attempters seem to have no apparent support system. In such patients the sense of loneliness or despair may be the overwhelming motive to commit suicide. Community mental health centers, churches, or other charitable organizations might represent the best social support option for such persons. Sometimes it is difficult to determine the degree of support a family will give to a suicide attempter. In general, the physician's judgment is probably the best guideline to use. If the family truly does want to help the patient, and other aspects of the risk assessment indicate a low suicide risk, the physician can probably safely discharge the patient to the care of the family.

Secondary Gain

The suicide attempt may have been made to achieve some secondary gain, such as increased attention from parents, friends, or others. This seems particularly true when the issue involves a boyfriend or girlfriend. When the goal of getting attention or revenge has been achieved, the need for an additional attempt is considerably diminished. In some cases the secondary gain is obvious. The rejected girlfriend who slashes her wrists in her boyfriend's home or the daughter who takes a handful of sleeping pills in her bathroom and then informs her mother represent fairly common examples of suicide attempts where the gains are obvious. The patient wants attention, revenge, or affection. The physician can usually easily judge whether the gain has been accomplished. In some cases, determining the secondary gain is more difficult, but the physician should use common sense in ascertaining whether there was a need for secondary gain and whether that gain has been achieved. In cases where the only gain is death and apparent relief from a seemingly hopeless situation, the risk of suicide is much greater than when the attempt involves anger or revenge.

Prior Attempts

A history of prior suicide attempts is sometimes an indicator that there is risk of a subsequent attempt. In general, a recent attempt or series of attempts within a short period of time is a serious omen. If these attempts have involved serious physical risk of harm for the patient, there is greater likelihood that the patient once again will make a serious attempt. A particularly ominous pattern is one in which the intensity and apparent lethality escalate with each subsequent attempt.

If, for instance, the initial attempt involved a drug overdose and a more recent attempt involved attempted hanging, the pattern of attempts shows escalating risk and thus greater lethality.

Psychiatric Diagnosis

There is both agreement and disagreement about the importance of psychiatric diagnosis in determining suicide intent.

Alcoholism

Alcoholism is a well-recognized risk factor for suicide. The alcoholic may be attempting to treat his own depression by drinking ethanol, but may eventually become aware that this is no permanent solution to his problems. Perhaps of greater importance is the fact that the intoxicated patient has diminished emotional control and diminished self-protective reflexes. Such a patient may commit suicide on impulse. In fact, some patients become suicidal only when intoxicated. Their inhibitions are lessened while drinking and they can proceed with a suicidal act. At least 25 percent of all suicides are associated with alcohol.

Drug Abuse

When the diagnosis is drug abuse, it is sometimes difficult to tell whether the drug overdose was intentional or accidental. A person used to taking drugs may regard them with diminished fear and see the overdose by ingestion of drugs as a rather painless solution to his problems. Drug users accustomed to recreational drug use may also have a steady supply or source of drugs that can be used for suicidal purposes.

Schizophrenia

When the psychiatric diagnosis is schizophrenia, suicide risk is increased. Some estimates indicate that as many as 10 percent of schizophrenics end their lives by suicide.

Depression

Depression has always been regarded as a serious risk factor. Depressed persons make more serious attempts than those with other psychiatric diagnoses. The mnemonic *in sad cages* shown in Figure 1 may be helpful in making a preliminary diagnosis of major depression.

Attitude and Affect

The patient's attitude and affect following the attempt are helpful in assessing lethality and the likelihood of a subsequent attempt. If the patient, for instance, sits quietly with eyes cast to the floor and answers questions slowly and expresses overall feelings of fatigue, failure, and exhaustion he may claim that he just can't go on. Such a person may be at high risk. In general, the patient who seems to be able to vent hostility and anger; who expresses hostility toward parents, spouse, or a friend, for instance, seems to have a better prognosis than the tight-lipped, apparently depressed patient. In general, the risk is lower if the patient is embarrassed, angry, or remorseful.

Suicide Precautions

Once the decision that the patient requires hospitalization has been made, the physician can proceed with voluntary hospitalization or involuntary holding and mandatory hospitalization. The emergency physician's further obligation is to take suicide precautions while the patient is in the emergency department. In general, this means that the patient is observed continuously by a staff member and that all potentially harmful objects such as glass, bottles, or needles are out of the patient's reach.

The Emergency Physician's Duties Regarding Involuntary Hospitalization

Emergency physicians have an ethical, moral, and legal responsibility to interfere with a suicidal patient's self-destruction. When psychiatric consultation is immediately available, the psychiatrist nearly always formulates and implements the specific strategy that should prevent a suicide. When such consultation is not readily available, the emergency physician should institute suicide

In	Interest
S	Sleep
A	Appetite
D	Depressed mood
C	Concentration
A	Activity
G	Guilt
E	Energy
S	Suicidal intent

Figure 1 *In Sad Cages.* When five of these nine items (must include depressed mood or sadness) are abnormal, a diagnosis of major depression is likely. (From Rund DA, Hutzler JC. Emergency psychiatry. St. Louis: CV Mosby, 1983:144.

precautions and arrange for hospitalization pending psychiatric consultation. The emergency physician must thoroughly document his or her findings justifying the impression that the patient is in imminent danger, try to obtain cooperation from the patient's family, and detain or restrain the suicidal patient as needed. It is hard to conceive that the physician acting in good faith on behalf of the patient's survival would face civil or criminal charges. On the other hand, a physician who releases a clearly suicidal patient could certainly be held liable for the consequences.

Consultation and Disposition

Once the physician has determined the degree of suicide risk using the variables described, it is clearly in the best interests of everyone that such variables be carefully documented in the chart. The ultimate decision is then to obtain psychiatric consultation, hospitalize, or discharge the patient. Most authorities recommend that the physician not be afraid to hospitalize a person believed to represent a suicide risk even when the likelihood of risk seems equivocal. The risk-benefit ratio of hospitalizing the patient who may attempt suicide is great. A subsequent suicide attempt could take that patient's life; the risk of hospitalization involves only the financial cost, time missed from work, and perhaps loss of some self-esteem. In cases like this, the legal considerations and the ethical considerations are the same. The physician clearly does not wish the patient to end his life, and therefore a careful, perhaps overcautious, attitude about hospitalizing these patients is appropriate. Many emergency departments have psychiatric emergency areas and similar caution should be used by the psychiatrists or psychiatric social workers who see suicidal patients in such settings. A supportive attitude, careful risk assessment, suicide precautions, and an overcautious consultation-hospitalization policy form an approach that will benefit both the suicidal patient and the emergency physician.

PAIN IN THE EMERGENCY DEPARTMENT

SAMUEL W. PERRY, M.D.
ROBERT B. MILLMAN, M.D.

Pain is the most common reason for seeking emergency care. The first step in its management is to assess the pain's severity and duration. Patients generally fall into four groups: (1) those whose pain is *severe* and *acute* (as in myocardial infarction, bone fracture, renal stone); (2) those whose pain is *moderate* and *acute* (as in ankle sprain, headache, cellulitis); (3) those whose pain is *moderate* and *chronic* (as in backache, arthritis, causalgia); and (4) those whose pain is *suspect* (e.g., malingerers, substance abusers, and those who are psychiatrically disturbed). The pain management for each of these four groups is somewhat different.

ACUTE SEVERE PAIN

Acute severe pain can be managed successfully with narcotic analgesics without producing excessive central nervous system depression. For most patients, intramuscular morphine (10 mg per 70 kilograms) is the drug of choice. If adequate relief has not been achieved 20 to 30 minutes after administration, 5 to 10 mg of intramuscular morphine can be given and repeated every 2 to 4 hours as necessary to provide sustained relief.

Five common misconceptions must be overcome in managing acute severe pain.

1. Physicians may be understandably so preoccupied with treating the underlying emergency problem that they neglect the pain management. This neglect increases the patient's anxiety and psychophysiologic responses to pain and decreases the patient's cooperativeness and ability to provide a history.

2. Physicians are unduly concerned that diminishing the pain will *interfere with the diagnostic assessment*. With the exception of acute abdominal pain, this "masking" is rarely a problem; more often patients are able to describe their symptoms more accurately and in greater detail when they are not in acute distress.

3. Physicians are not well informed about the pharmacologic action of narcotic analgesics and consequently tend to *undertreat for pain*. They are unaware that patients vary enormously in their response to a given dosage of a narcotic, and as with anticonvulsants, antihypertensives, and antiarrhythmics, the dosage of analgesics must be adjusted according to clinical response.

4. Physicians are unduly concerned about *respiratory depression*, fearing that this side effect will occur before adequate pain relief is provided. Actually, if the patient's analgesic response is monitored, the severity of the pain is likely to be greatly reduced before respiratory depression occurs; as a result, patients stop splinting and take deeper breaths. Even if this rare complication of narcotic administration should develop, 0.5 to 3 mg intravenous naloxone (Narcan), a narcotic antagonist, can reverse the respiratory depression and increase the respiratory rate within 30 to 50 seconds. Naloxone's effects persist for 2 to 3 hours.

5. The greatest concern about using narcotic analgesics generally stems from unwarranted *fears of iatrogenic addiction*. No studies have ever documented that providing adequate pain relief with narcotic analgesics in the emergency situation has lead to drug dependency, whereas many studies have documented that this concern has lead to the undermedication for pain that is often associated with a disruption of the doctor-patient alliance.

Meperidine (Demerol), though more widely prescribed, has few advantages over morphine. It can prevent the smooth muscle spasm that occasionally is seen with morphine, but its duration of action is shorter (2½ to 3 hours), it has no advantage with respect to toxicity or dependence, and its metabolite (normeperidine) can accumulate (especially in those with renal disease) and cause myoclonic jerks, multifocal seizures, and confusion. Other narcotics, such as pentazocine (Talwin) and the newer agonist-antagonists produce a withdrawal syndrome in patients being maintained on agonists (e.g, terminal cancer patients on morphine or methadone). These drugs also may be contraindicated in patients with cardiac disease because of the negative ionotropic effect on cardiac muscle. If narcotics other than morphine must be prescribed because of an individual patient's susceptibility to its side effects, care must be taken to prescribe an equianalgesic dosage (Table 1).

When prescribed in therapeutic doses in the emergency situation, narcotic analgesics rarely produce severe side effects. They have little effect on blood pressure or heart rate or rhythm in the supine patient. Acute urinary retention may occur in individuals with prostatic hypertrophy, and some patients, especially the elderly, may experience confusion, dysphoria, nausea, and abdominal cramps. Adjunctive medication (e.g., psychotropics, amphetamine, or hydroxazine) usually are not necessary acutely and may only complicate the clinical situation.

ACUTE MODERATE PAIN

Aspirin and acetaminophen are the drugs of choice for acute moderate pain (600 mg PO). For additional analgesia, these drugs can be combined with 30 mg oxycodone (Percodan, Percocet) or 30 mg codeine; however, these additional drugs will increase the incidence of nausea and abdominal cramps. Although patients frequently request medications stronger than aspirin, controlled studies have repeatedly demonstrated that the analgesia produced by aspirin is equal to the usual doses of commonly used weak narcotic drugs, such as 30 mg codeine, 50 mg meperidine, or 65 mg propoxyphene (Darvon). A problem is that patients do not take the aspirin or acetaminophen wisely: they do not increase the dosage (up to 600 mg)

TABLE 1 Narcotic Analgesics for Acute Severe Pain

Drug	Equianalgesic Dose	Usual Frequency	Comments
Morphine	10 mg IM 60 mg PO	q3–4h	Subcutaneous route inconsistent; poor oral efficacy
Meperidine (Demerol)	75 mg IM 300 mg PO	q3h	Slightly shorter effective duration than morphine; underdosage common by oral route
Hydromorphone (Dilaudid)	1.5 mg IM 7.5 mg PO	q4h	Fast acting; good oral efficacy; rectal route available
Levorphanol (Levo-Dromoran)	2 mg SC 4 mg PO	q4–5h	Potent oral analgesic; long plasma half-life; accumulation with repetitive dosing
Methadone (Dolophine)	10 mg IM 20 mg PO	q5–6h	Similar to levorphanol with even longer plasma half-life (17–24 hours)
Pentazocine (Talwin)	60 mg IM 180 mg PO	q3–4h	Psychotic-like side effects; may produce withdrawal syndrome in patients maintained on other narcotics
Oxymorphone (Numorphan)	1.5 mg IM	q4h	Like morphine
Butorphanol (Stadol)	2 mg IM	q4h	Like pentazocine, except fewer psychotomimetic reactions
Nalbuphine (Nubain)	12 mg IM	q4h	Like pentazocine, except fewer psychotomimetic reactions

when necessary. They often wait until the pain has increased in severity before taking the medication rather than anticipating the pain by taking the medication before the pain increases. Moreover, in a situation of persistent pain, patients "forget" to take the medication regularly every 4 hours to insure that adequate blood levels are maintained; this may sometimes even include awakening from sleep to take the analgesic. Since many patients with acute moderate pain are sent home and not hospitalized, the emergency physician must inform these patients regarding the optimal dosage and the schedule for nonnarcotic medication.

For patients who are unable to take aspirin (usually because of adverse gastrointestinal effects or idiosyncratic hypersensitivity reactions), *nonsteroidial anti-inflammatory agents* (NSAID) are indicated. These agents (e.g., phenylbutazone, indomethacin, diflunisal) are really no more effective than aspirin, are considerably more expensive, and have severe potential toxicities of their own, particularly gastric ulcerations, aplastic anemia, neutropenia, thrombocytopenia, azotemia, and various dysphoric reactions. One advantage of these agents over aspirin is their long duration of action, which requires that fewer pills be taken daily and improves compliance.

CHRONIC MODERATE PAIN

Although many patients come to the emergency department with a chief complaint of chronic pain, this problem cannot be treated in such a setting. The pharmacologic and behavioral management of chronic pain, even when its etiology is clear, requires an ongoing relationship with a physician who can dissect the organic and functional components, monitor the use of and response to medications, and prescribe nonpharmacologic interventions.

Attempts to manage chronic pain in the emergency room situation can be frustrating for both the physician and the patient and may cause considerable harm, including "the three Ds"—drug dependency, depression, and doctor-shopping. The unsystematic "hit and run" treatment of chronic pain may be associated with the abuse of or dependence on a variety of oral analgesic preparations including oxycodone, codeine, and propoxyphene. Because the emergency physician cannot provide the sustained supportive behavioral methods of teaching their patients how to cope with their pain syndrome, the depressogenic effects of the chronic pain worsen as the patients become increasingly discouraged and resentful. Even if the physician carefully explains that the emergency prescriptions are only a temporary measure, chronic pain patients may misconstrue this maneuver, take whatever is prescribed until the pills run out, then return to one or another emergency room without even following through with the referral to the appropriate physician or a pain clinic.

For many chronic pain patients in the emergency room, the toughest pill to swallow is the idea that *no* pain pill will be presribed. To appease such patients, the physician is tempted to prescribe an antianxiety or an antidepressant drug in place of an analgesic. The physician justifies such a prescription by noting that the patient is anxious and/or depressed—most chronic pain patients are. There are at least four reasons why giving psychotropic drugs to these patients in the emergency room setting is unwise:

1. The *psychotropic probably will not be effective.* Except for relatively high doses of hydroxyzine (Vistaril), psychotropics do not have analgesic properties of their own. Tricyclic antidepressants, such as amitriptyline, have proven helpful for certain chronic pain patients who are

closely monitored over a period of several months, but in an emergency situation this kind of sustained treatment and dosage titration cannot be provided.

2. Whereas physicians are unduly wary of using high dosages of narcotic analgesics for acute severe pain, they are at times rather casual about prescribing certain *anti-anxiety drugs*, such as diazepam (Valium), even though the abuse of and dependency on these psychotropic drugs is a major problem in the United States. The emergency physician has little assurance that the chronic pain patient will not use up such a prescription and then obtain a renewal from some other source.

3. Prescribing a *psychotropic medicine tends to label the problem* in both the physician's and patient's minds as "psychiatric," rather than viewing the problem as chronic pain with psychological consequences. The perception by the patient and by others is that he or she is now "a crock," which only fuels the patient's anguish and resentment.

4. The prescription of a psychotropic may deflect attention from the emergency physician's primary task, namely, to inform the patient tactfully, yet directly, that chronic pain can be successfully managed, even if not totally cured, only if the patient is offered comprehensive, coordinated care by a physician or in a clinic setting. A multidisciplinary, multifaceted approach may be necessary (e.g., biofeedback, self-relaxation, hypnosis, behavioral modification, acupuncture, nerve block, physical therapy) in the quest for the best method or methods to improve a particular chronic pain problem and to help the patient cope with the pain that still remains.

PAIN THAT IS SUSPECT

Since pain is by definition a *subjective* unpleasant experience, all pain is "real." Even when no organic basis for the pain is found and even when psychological factors are playing a major role, the patient in pain hurts. To say that the pain is "all in the head" defines the location of the pain but not its severity. Furthermore, many physicians mistakenly believe that they know how much a given injury or disease "should hurt" even though studies have shown repeatedly that the severity of pain varies enormously between individuals. Nor can physicians determine the severity of pain by observing the patient; some patients in severe pain remain stoically silent whereas others wince and thrash wildly with pain they themselves rate as only mild or moderate. Studies have also shown that the psychophysiologic response to pain (diaphoresis, elevated blood pressure and skin temperature, increased heart and respiratory rate) do not reliably correlate with the severity of pain. Therefore, for the majority of patients—well over 90 percent—the best way to determine pain severity is simply to ask the patient such a question as, "If "1" is very mild pain and "10" is the worst pain you can ever imagine experiencing, what number would you give your pain now?" This number can be recorded, and after an analgesic has been given and has taken effect, the patient can then be asked to again rate the pain's severity. The drug's dosage and frequency can then be adjusted accordingly.

In the emergency situation, however, there are three groups of patients whose subjective rating of pain is not reliable: (1) malingerers, (2) the psychiatrically disturbed, and (3) drug abusers.

Malingerers. There is no clinical test for malingering. It is a diagnosis based on careful clinical judgment. Although obvious secondary gain must be present (e.g., workman's compensation, disability insurance, welfare), the presence of secondary gain is not in itself sufficient to make the diagnosis. Nor can the diagnosis be made simply because no organic disease has been found. If the physician strongly suspects that the patient's pain complaints are attributable to malingering, no pain medicines should be given, and the patient should be told that the reasons for the pain are not at all clear and will therefore require an evaluation over time in a nonemergent setting. An explicit referral should be made. The physician should then note in the chart that malingering was suspected, but could not be confirmed without a more extensive, ongoing knowledge of the patient. This chart notation is important because the diagnosis of malingering is best supported by a past history of this behavior. Future physicians, at least in that same emergency department, will be forewarned.

Psychiatrically Disturbed. As already stated, most patients in pain are anxious or depressed. Most often these emotional disturbances are the result and not the cause of pain; physicians should not presume that the pain problem is psychological merely because the patient appears upset. Nor should the diagnosis of psychogenic pain be primarily based on the absence of discernable organic disease. The diagnosis of psychogenic pain should be one of inclusion rather than only exclusion, that is, it should be based on (1) a documented history of psychiatric problems, (2) bizzare thoughts or appearance, (3) fixed irrational ideas, or (4) signs and symptoms of affective illness (e.g., sleep disturbance, weight loss, profound hopelessness or helplessness, suicidal ideation). When a psychiatric problem is strongly suspected as the cause of the pain complaints, analgesics should not be prescribed. The physician can state that because the patient is emotionally upset, bodily sensations are being distorted and misperceived, *but* the physician should then reassuringly add that he understands that the patient is experiencing pain and will vigorously pursue a solution to the underlying problem.

Drug Abusers. Patients with either a history or physical evidence of drug abuse (particularly narcotic addicts) pose difficult problems with respect to pain management. Some drug abusers lie about the existence of pain in order to receive an injection or a prescription for narcotic drugs. In fact, however, drug abusers use the emergency department relatively rarely for this purpose since physicians usually deny the drug-dependent patient narcotic analgesics or they prescribe a route and dosage of the narcotics that offer little relief to a heavily-dependent patient (e.g, 50 mg intramuscular meperidine or aspirin with codeine). In those instances in which a drug-dependent person does present at the emergency department complaining of pain with no discernable basis for the symptoms, the physician should not enter into an adversarial relationship with the patient, nor should he prescribe an inappropriate medication simply to get rid of the undesirable. Rather, a stance of supportive and concerned curiosity should prevail, and the patient should be referred to a drug treatment program. Profound pessimism about such a referral is unwarranted. The patient may actually be seeking rehabilitation, but has chosen a roundabout, face-saving way of asking for help.

A more common problem concerns the *drug abusing patient who has a clear-cut reason for the acute pain* (e.g., a bone fracture, stab wound, renal stone, or sickle cell crisis). Because it is often difficult to assess the degree of tolerance that exists as a result of the drug dependency, it is difficult to determine the dosage of narcotics that will provide sufficient relief. The patient may claim that he has a habit of "$100 a day," which cannot be translated into tolerance terms. For these reasons, it is practical to institute analgesia with a moderately high dose of narcotic (e.g., 15 mg intramuscular morphine) and continue to administer 10 mg intramuscular morphine every 20 to 30 minutes thereafter until adequate pain relief is obtained or until the patient has become heavily sedated and the respiratory rate has decreased below 13 respirations per minute. In rare cases, the physician might overshoot the mark substantially, and naloxone, intravenously or intramuscularly, is required, or in the worst case, ventilation has to be briefly supported mechanically. Providing adequate analgesia to drug abusers in the emergency situation in no way adversely affects the severity of their drug dependence, and it may possibly be a first step toward forming a therapeutic alliance that might help motivate the patient to enter a drug rehabilitation program. The minor risks of moderate-to-high narcotic dosages is far less than the major risks of inadequate analgesia, which may eventuate in an agitated patient who is likely to have poor impulse control, and poor tolerance for pain, and to be uncooperative and even combative.

Narcotic-dependent patients pose an additional problem. They may have conditioned the experience of drug craving to the experience of pain. As a result, even though they may have an organic basis for the pain, they perceive the pain as a signal that they are "sick" and need a "fix." For them the pain is experienced as inordinately severe and even life-threatening. This kind of perceptual confusion in drug abusers rarely responds to admonition ("You don't hurt that much!"). The drug-abusing patient with a documented emergency illness is better served with moderate-to-high dosages of narcotics and an explanation that the confusion between drug craving and physical pain would improve in a comprehensive drug-rehabilitation program that corrects this kind of response to any physical discomfort.

EDUCATING THE STAFF

The emergency physician, in many cases, must institute life-saving procedures immediately. In those situations pain management understandably cannot be a primary concern of the physician. Educating other staff members, especially nurses, about the basic principles of pain management and about the dosages and effects of the various analgesics can be extraordinarily helpful for the physician who simply does not have the time to closely monitor the patient's response to a given analgesic and adjust the medication accordingly. As we have emphasized throughout, effective pain management requires this kind of comprehensive, individualized approach to each patient.

Supported in part by NIH grant #P50GM26145 (Perry) and the New York State Division of Substance Abuse Services (Millman).

SUGGESTED READING

Jaffe JH, Martin WR. Opioid analgesics and antagonists. In: Gilman AG, Goodman LS, Rall TW, Murad F, eds. Pharmacologic basis of therapeutics. 7th ed. New York: Macmillan Publishing Co, 1985:491.
Stimmel B. Pain, analgesia and addiction: the pharmacologic treatment of pain. New York: Raven Press, 1983.

CONSENT AND RESTRAINT

MARSHALL B. SEGAL, M.D., J.D.

A MINOR PRESENTING TO THE EMERGENCY DEPARTMENT WITHOUT PARENTS

A minor is chronologically incompetent to give consent for nonemergency treatment. The right to consent belongs to the parents or legal guardian. However, when a licensed physician renders emergency treatment to a minor, consent of the minor's parent or legal guardian need not be obtained if, in the sole opinion of the physician, the obtaining of consent is not reasonably feasible under the circumstances without adversely affecting the condition of the minor's health. This rule is applicable throughout the United States and Canada although it may be phrased differently in various state laws. The important thing to note is that the threshold that establishes the physician's right and duty to proceed with treatment in the absence of parental consent is not that the child's "life or limb" is at stake, but that the failure to treat could "adversely affect the minor's health."

A minor presenting to an emergency department without parents should immediately be sent to triage so that an initial determination of the minor's condition can be made. Then, in the temporal order established by triage, the minor should be seen by a physician.[1] The physician should obtain a medical history and perform a physical examination in order to assess whether the minor's health may be adversely affected if not treated. Of course, to determine this, the physician must determine what is wrong with the minor patient. Blood tests, x-ray studies, CT scans, invasive procedures, even exploratory surgery may be necessary to make this assessment. Should a determination be made that the minor's health may be adversely affected without prompt treatment, the physician should proceed to provide the minor with all appropriate treatment.

During assessment and treatment, attempts should be made to contact the minor's parents. However, these efforts to contact the minor's parents should not interfere with the minor being processed through the emergency department's triage, diagnosis, and treatment routine in a regular and timely fashion.

The emergency department staff should document on the emergency record that the minor is in the emergency department without parents and should serially document all the steps that are taken to contact the minor's parents. The physician should also document the minor's condition on the chart so that it is clearly established that the minor's health might be adversely affected by delay of treatment.

Most minors presenting to an emergency department have a medical condition that might adversely affect their health if not promptly assessed and treated. There is no way to determine whether a minor has such a condition without triage, a medical history, and physical examination, and the indicated diagnostic tests. Failure to carry out at least this much puts the minor's health at risk and exposes the emergency department's staff to allegations of negligence in their care of that minor should the child subsequently and consequently suffer harm from not being promptly diagnosed and treated.

There is no known recorded appellate law case where any physician or nurse has been held liable for treating a minor in an emergency situation in the absence of parental consent.[2]

What If the Minor Refuses Treatment

A minor does not have the legal capacity to explicitly consent to treatment, but his medical condition gives the emergency department staff his constructive consent for treatment. Constructive consent is not actually the consent of the minor, but is a legal replacement for consent that is founded on common law, statute, and social necessity.

If the minor cannot give consent, then the minor cannot hold back consent. The emergency department staff, in the absence of the minor's parents, stand *in loco parentis*, charged with the rights, duties, and responsibilities of the parents. Since a minor is incompetent to say yes to treatment, he is also incompetent to say no.

What If Both Parents Are Present and One Parent Gives Consent While the Other Parent Refuses Consent for Their Child To Be Treated?

Any parent, including a parent who is a minor, may consent to having a medical or surgical procedure performed on his or her child by a licensed physician. Only one parent's consent is necessary, not both. The law encourages the preservation of life and health, especially of minors. Given two parents, one giving consent, the other denying it, the physician has the requisite consent of a parent and may proceed with treatment. Besides, should there be a subsequent legal action, the emergency physician is in the better position, having gone forward to protect the minor child by treating that minor rather than allowing the minor to suffer some disastrous consequence by following the wishes of the refusing parent. Conceivably the refusing parent, in the face of a subsequent medical disaster severely affecting the minor child, may claim that he or she did not really understand the consequences of refusing consent, had not received an informed explanation from the emergency physician, or was in such a state of agitation or grief that he or she did not even intend to refuse consent. The better legal and medical course of action, faced with two conflicting parents, one requesting treatment, the other refusing consent, is for the physician to opt for treatment.

What If Both Parents Are Present and Both Refuse Consent for Their Child To Be Treated?

Here the legal test to judge the physician's right and duty to treat changes. No longer will the possibility that the minor's health may be adversely affected by lack of treatment be a sufficient reason to proceed with treatment, as it is when both parents are absent. When both parents are present (or one parent is present and the other is not available) and both parents wish to remove the child from the emergency department without treatment, the physician may physically take the child away from the parents and proceed with treatment only if, in the physician's sole judgment, the child is in "imminent danger." This criterion is established in the abused and neglected child reporting acts (i.e., the child abuse laws). These laws establish the right of the physician to treat a child whose health is in imminent danger, and they also create a duty for the physician to go forward to protect that child. Should the physician fail to treat a child who is in imminent danger, the physician could later be held liable to compensate the child for any harm the child may subsequently suffer at the hands of his abusive parents or even an abusive third party in the child's home or school environment.

The medical chart must document the child's condition and clearly state why the child was in imminent danger. Also, the proper state administrative agencies must be notified initially by phone and subsequently in writing.

Financial Responsibility for Unaccompanied Minors

The parents of a minor are responsible for the necessities of life supplied that minor by others. Emergency medical care, like food and lodging, is a necessity of life for which the parents have a legal obligation to the provider to pay the reasonable value of the medical products supplied and professional services rendered. The fact that the parents are not present when the minor patient is treated in the emergency department does not shield the parents from financial responsibility for such treatment.

UNCONSCIOUS ADULTS

Unconscious adults are incompetent to care for themselves and are unable to make decisions affecting their care. When an unconscious adult is brought to the emergency department, the emergency department staff have that patient's constructive consent for treatment. Constructive consent is not like explicit consent, which a patient gives verbally. Nor is it like implied consent, which is implied by the patient's action. Rather, constructive consent is the child of necessity, created to care for those who cannot care for themselves. The emergency department staff have the same obligation to treat an unconscious patient as they do to treat an unaccompanied minor—even more so, as no finding need be made that an unconscious patient's health may be affected if treatment is withheld. The patient's unconscious condition defines the necessity for the emergency department staff to go forward and treat.[3]

What If the Spouse or Relative of the Unconscious Patient Refuses Consent?

The unconscious patient's spouse or relative has no legal right to endanger the patient's life. The physician's obligation to the unconscious patient is a duty the physician directly owes that patient. The consent of a spouse, relative, or friend is not necessary or relevant to the emergency staff's obligation to protect and treat the unconscious patient. The emergency staff must treat an unconscious patient regardless of the express directions of third parties.[4]

However, the patient's prior competent refusal is effective refusal; just because the patient is now unconscious does not mean that a physician can treat the patient against the patient's clearly and competently expressed prior refusal.

PATIENTS WITH DIMINISHED CAPACITY

The most difficult consent and disposition problems arise with regard to patients with diminished capacity. The physician should treat patients with diminished capacity in emergent situations when consent is not possible owing to the patient's condition. The emergency staff can easily conceptualize the necessity of restraining a patient in shock or with a head injury against his will so that he

can be treated. The intoxicated alcoholic also has diminished capacity when he presents to the emergency department. However, it is difficult to determine the precise point at which the intoxicated patient becomes competent. The law establishes the alcohol blood level at which one driving a motor vehicle is under the influence of alcohol, but does not define a reciprocal level of competency to guide the emergency physician in determining when it is safe to discharge the patient. The legislature has left the problem to the judgment of the physician. The physician should document in the chart that the patient appears to be competent, oriented, and in a satisfactory mental and physical condition to leave the emergency department. Giving the patient to a responsible friend or relative who will care for the patient at home is desirable, but not always practical or even possible.

The physician must always keep in mind that should an intoxicated patient elope from the emergency department and subsequently, while still intoxicated, be involved as a driver in an automobile accident, the people injured in that accident might have a cause of action against the emergency department staff for negligently allowing that patient to leave the emergency department while a danger to others.[5]

The emergency physician must also consider the problem that is posed by the patient who wakes up from an apparent heroin overdose after receiving Narcan. Often such a patient declares an immediate inclination to leave the emergency department to "go downtown to do some business." The patient is awake, but is probably not competent to understand his condition and what may soon happen to him. There is the danger that in less than 30 minutes the patient could again become unconscious. A physician cannot explain the pharmacology and pathophysiology of narcotic antagonists to this patient in a reasonable amount of time so that the patient fully understands the dangers facing him should he now leave the emergency department; in such a situation it is virtually impossible to obtain the patient's informed consent. He or she may have to be refused discharge and even restrained until the danger passes.

THERAPEUTIC RESTRAINT

The emergency department staff may use reasonable methods to restrain a patient who has diminished capacity in order to protect the patient from harming himself or others. Therapeutic restraint should not be confused with false imprisonment. False imprisonment requires that one have the intent to deprive a person of his liberty without legal justification. Should the emergency staff prevent a patient from leaving the emergency department because the patient has not paid his bill (for instance by not returning his clothes) that could be false imprisonment. In contrast, restraining a shocky, intoxicated, toxic, hypoxemic, metabolically deranged, or cerebrally injured patient is simply good medical care, not false imprisonment. The duty of the emergency department staff to protect the patient creates the legal justification that prevents their actions from being considered false imprisonment. In fact, to restrain a patient with diminished capacity could expose the emergency department staff to liability for negligence.[6]

CITATIONS

1. See *Distad v. Cubin*, 433 P.2d 167 (Wyo. 1981) and United States Federal Code of Regulations, 42 CFR 405.1032(4): "[All] Patients, on their initial visit to the department, [shall] receive a general medical evaluation...."; 405.1033(c)(3): "A physician shall see all patients who arrive for treatment in the emergency service."

2. See *Luka v. Lowrie*, 171 Mich. 122, 136 N.W. 1106 (1912), (amputation of child's foot); *Jackovach v. Yocum*, 212 Iowa 914, 237 N.W. 444 (1931), (amputation of child's arm); *Sullivan v. Montgomery*, 155 Misc. 448, 229 N.Y.S. 575 (1935), (administration of ether while setting a young man's broken ankle resulting in death); *Wells v. McGehee*, 39 So. 2d 196 (La. 1949), (administration of chloroform while setting child's arm resulted in death).

3. See *Cotnam v. Wisdom*, 83 Ark 601 (1907) (physician finds injured patient on the street); *Bennan v. Parsonnet*, 83 N.J.L. 20, 83 A. 948 (1912), (hernia operation).

4. See *Collins v. Davis*, 51 Misc.2d 616, 273 N.Y.S. 624 (1966), (spouse attempts to prevent emergency surgery by refusing consent); *J.F.K. Memorial Hospital v. Heston*, 58 N.J. 576, 279 A.2d 670 (1971), (parents of hemorrhaging 22-year-old woman attempt to prevent transfusion at emergency surgery by refusing consent).

5. See *Tarasoff v. Regents of the University of California*, 17 Cal.3d 425, 551 P.2d 334, 131 Cal.Rptr. 14 (1976), (psychiatrist fails to warn third party about his dangerous patient); *Clark v. State of New York*, 99 A.D.2d 616, 472 N.Y.S.2d 170 (A.D.3 Dept. 1984), (the state may be liable for the release of a psychiatric patient who shoots an emergency physician).

6. See *Cook v. City of New York*, 441 N.Y.S.2d 104 (1981), (an example of the consequences of the emergency department staff's failure to restrain a patient).

ASSAULTIVE BEHAVIOR

GEORGE SOLOMON, M.D.

Adequate treatment of the actively assaultive individual requires prompt assessment of the variety of reactive, psychopathologic, characterologic, neurologic, and pharmacologic factors that can lead to loss of control over hostile-aggressive impulses. Obviously, initial measures to ensure safety to staff, patient, and/or others may need to take precedence over even the most preliminary of assessments.

ETIOLOGY

Theories of aggression, hostility, and violence fall into three major categories, none mutually exclusive: instinctual, frustration-aggression, and learning. Causation can never be determined accurately in the emergency setting.

Adult conditions, as defined by the Diagnostic and Statistical Manual of Mental Disorders, Third Edition (DSM III), associated with assaultive behavior include (but are not limited to):

1. *Adjustment disorder with disturbance of conduct.* This is a maladaptive "acute situational reaction" to an identifiable stress such as is attributable to separation or to provocation. If the situational stress is of sufficient intensity, even the otherwise stable person may show symptoms or "blow up" (a "classic" example being the "trusting" husband who comes home early to find his wife in bed with his best friend!)

2. *Intermittent explosive disorder.* This disorder is characterized by episodic loss of control over aggressive impulses out of proportion to any precipitating stress, with little or no provocation, and in the absence of generalized impulsiveness or aggressivity. The aggressor is remorseful following the episode. The pattern is repetitive and may result in serious injury or destruction, but can be infrequent and irregular in occurrence. The episode may be a surprise even to the perpetrator and may be attributed to a force beyond one's control such as a "spell" (but not to "voices" or other persons). Symptoms appear and remit quickly.

3. *Isolated explosive disorder.* This disorder is a discrete episode of breakthrough of rage, which had been conscious or unconscious to varying degrees, leading to a single, violent catastrophic act. Violence toward an idealized love object may ensue in an episode of dyscontrol following failure of frantic attempts to repair the relationship. (Homicides commited while suffering from this disorder are usually not considered first-degree murder, which requires premeditation and deliberation, and may even be found nonculpable in those jurisdictions with a volitional ("irresistable impulse") standard for insanity). The act seems "out of character."

4. *Antisocial personality disorder* (sociopathy, psychopathy). This disorder is characterized by, among other features, a lack of internalized principles and values (superego, conscience), lack of acceptance of social norms, varying degrees of impulsivity and aggressiveness, and frequently is accompanied by substance abuse. The individual lies, cheats, manipulates, "cons," and coerces. The victimizer lacks a capacity for empathy. "I wouldn't have beat him up if he'd only handed over his wallet."

5. *Schizophrenic disorder, paranoid type.* Although assaultive and violent behavior is rare in psychotic individuals, when it does occur it is generally perpetrated by distrubed individuals with this diagnosis, who are subject to persecutory delusions, even terror, and may perceive themselves to be acting in "self-defense." Hallucinatory "voices" may "command" aggressive behaviors, and these may or may not be resisted. By its nature, the schizophrenic process disrupts ego functions and reality testing.

6. *Paranoid personality disorder.* This disorder is characterized by suspiciousness and mistrust and often by

readiness to take offense and to counterattack any perceived threat. Pathologic jealousy is common. Such individuals are predisposed to assaultiveness.

7. *Major (psychotic) depressive disorder.* Suicidal impulses may be in part murderous as well as self-destructive. (Examples: A depressed mother may wish her children not to have to endure a world perceived as hellish. A man threatening (and intending) to kill himself in front of his rejecting lover shot her instead when she refused to promise to take care of his dog).

8. *Delirium* or acute brain syndrome. In this clouded state of consciousness, perceptual disturbances can include misinterpretation and can occasionally result in assault, which is also made possible by the irritability and hostility that can be part of the syndrome. (Delusional disorders predisposing to assaultiveness can also be based on dementia or chronic organic brain syndromes). The individual is not oriented to time, place, and/or person and has defects in recent memory as, for example, difficulty in doing "serial sevens" (subtracting 7 from 100, 7 from 93, etc.)(see chapter on *Behavioral Emergencies*).

9. *Temporal lobe epilepsy.* This uncommon condition can, in rare instances, involve aggressive behavior during seizure episodes, but also may be accompanied by an interictal behavioral syndrome including aggressiveness and emotionality. Generally a history of prior seizure episodes can be elicited from patient or family. There may be an "aura," altered perceptions or feelings, immediately preceding the episode. (Without clear history, this diagnosis is difficult to establish in an emergency setting, particularly in differentiation from dyscontrol syndromes such as episodic explosive disorder).

10. *Post-traumatic stress disorder (PTSD), chronic or delayed*—particularly that following violence-related stress such as the Vietnam conflict—can result not only in re-experiencing the trauma (as in recurrent dreams or intrusive thoughts) and emotional numbing, but in dyscontrol of aggression, particularly when exposed to events that symbolize or resemble the traumatic event. A Vietnam veteran with concurrent marital conflict assaulted a Chinese laundryman who had lost his clothing, as if he were a member of the Viet Cong.

11. *Substance abuse disorders.* Alcohol intoxication, like that with other central nervous system depressants such as barbiturates, is disinhibitory and may "release" otherwise controlled aggressive impulses (the "mean drunk"). Such drugs do not "cause" violence; they "permit" it. Amphetamine or cocaine abuse can result in a paranoid-like delusional disorder with ideas of reference, aggressiveness, and hostility as well as panic, emotional lability, and lowered impulse control. Psychotomimetic or hallucinogenic compounds such as phencyclidine (PCP) and lysergic acid diethylamide (LSD) can result in delusions, agitation, anxiety, confusion, misinterpretation of perceptions, grandiosity ("can do no wrong"), belligerence, impulsivity, lability, impaired judgment, delusions, hallucinations, and frank delirium, all conducive to assaultiveness. Effects of such drugs are variable in length and can be long-lasting, at times waxing and waning. The opiates generally are not associated with violence or as-

saultive behavior during intoxication, but may lead to such behavior in states of withdrawal.

A high incidence of prior self-destructive behavior, early deprivation and neurologic impairment is found in habitually violent and assaultive individuals. In view of close psychodynamic links between hostile and self-destructive motivations, it must be kept in mind that "aggression-out" can readily be "retroflexed"; thus, the assaultive patient often represents a real suicidal threat.

Childhood and adolescent assaultive behaviors are generally associated with one of two conduct disorders:

1. *Conduct disorder, undersocialized, aggressive* is the pattern of the delinquent, who may go on to become the antisocial "psychopath." Such youngsters may commit vandalism, set fires, and/or steal as well as assault without guilt or remorse and in the absence of meaningful, affectional interpersonal bonds. These children themselves generally are the victims of rejection, neglect, and often abuse, but occasionally represent "spoiled" youngsters who lack limit-setting parental figures.

2. *Conduct disorder, socialized, aggressive* is characterized by violence and/or thefts in the presence of evidence of meaningful social attachment to others, some capacity for concern, and appropriate guilt or remorse (although perhaps not in relation to "outsiders"). Such "acting out" is generally symptomatic of problems at home and emotional conflict.

EMERGENCY MANAGEMENT AND TREATMENT

Treatment of the patient who is or has been engaged in assaultive behavior can be divided into behavioral, psychological, and pharmacologic categories. Short-term tactics are best based on quick diagnostic assessment.

Behavior Management. Since much violent behavior is perceived as self-defense by frightened, panicked, or deluded individuals, the examining physician and ancillary personnel should attempt to be non-threatening and generally need to maintain some distance between the patient and themselves. It is an error to assume that appearing unfrightened by a threatening individual will lessen aggression. On the other hand, panic by treatment personnel can lead to an escalating feedback. Gentle firmness and acknowledgement of the fear and rage of the patient, as well as acknowledgement of one's own concerns for safety of self and others, is called for. Try to withdraw any objects or persons from the immediate environment that appear to frighten the patient. Verbally provide reassurances and calmly express an attitude of helpfulness. If it can be established, verbal communication based on empathic understanding is helpful and can abort nonverbal acting-out.

In the presence of *physical assault*, a sufficient number of personnel to ensure an obvious ability to subdue and restrain must be promptly assembled. Five are optional, one person for each limb and one free to obtain help, medication, and the like. Medical "uniforms" such as white coats are helpful to convey perceptually a benevolent intent. If subjugation becomes necessary, as is rarely the case, it should be done as firmly and gently as possible by several individuals. Restraining ties should be avoided if possible, but should be adequate and not painfully constricting if applied. The clear inability to be destructive is generally reassuring to the patient as long as it is not accompanied by terror of being harmed. (Only verbal and physical, not pharmacologic, methods of control should be used prior to arrival at a medical facility). Precautions against suicide (including elopement), especially continuous observation, are generally indicated in addition to providing protection of others, particularly in the depressed patient or the individual who is feeling guilty over immediate prior assaultiveness.

Rapid Assessment. It is helpful to understand assaultive behavior by dividing it into three phases: pre-assault, assault and post-assault. What was the provocation? Was there ingestion of drugs and/or alcohol? How much? When? Is there a history of prior assaultiveness, criminal behavior, bizarre behavior, mental illness, head injury, neurologic disease, or recent physical illness? Was assaultive behavior goal-directed toward a particular victim(s)? What was the response of the patient immediately subsequent to attack? Does he or she remain belligerent? Is there remorse? Does withdrawal or passivity follow? Quick ascertainment of basic mental status should determine orientation, memory of behavior and events leading up to assaultiveness, confusion, and especially, any delusional ideation. Is there agitation, slurring of speech, incoordination? If available, Breathalyzer determination of the presence and level of alcohol intoxication is always useful. Has the patient calmed down spontaneously? Does verbal reassurance and support and, if necessary, physical control produce a calming effect? Patients whose aggression was reactive and situational or explosive in nature generally are not imminently in danger of further assaultiveness (but may be in danger of suicide). Does the behavior seem a manifestation of an antisocial pattern requiring prompt law enforcement intervention? Should psychiatric or neurologic consultation be obtained as quickly as possible? (Generally, the answer is "yes.") If the patient is no longer behaviorally belligerent, are there verbal threats or abusiveness? If not spontaneously expressed, does questioning elicit threats to others or self?

Pharmacologic Management When Alcohol Has Been Ingested. Administration of medication is best after physical control has been established and before moving the patient to a seclusion area (with *frequent* observation) or for definitive disposition. Ascertaining the presence or likelihood of existing intoxication with alcohol or other substance is essential prior to administration of any medication, in which case *extreme* caution must be exercised if any drug is utilized to control, calm, or sedate. In view of danger of respiratory depression, no drug should be used if blood alcohol is above 0.4 percent in an alcoholic or 0.2 percent in an occasional drinker who appears otherwise in good physical condition. Paraldehyde is excreted by the respiratory route, is malodorous, and nowadays often is not available, but it remains a relatively safe drug in the presence of alcohol

(or for withdrawal seizures). As much as 5 cc can be administered intramuscularly or 20 cc can be given orally. The other relatively safe drug, moderately effective as a sedative in the presence of modest amounts of alcohol, is magnesium sulfate, 1 g of which can be injected intramuscularly in each buttock, with a repeat of 1 g in 4 hours. Although benzodiazepines should be avoided in the actively intoxicated patient, in the post-assaultive, agitated patient in an acute alcohol withdrawal syndrome, clorazepate dipotassium (Tranxene), 30 mg PO, can be given.

Pharmacologic Management When Alcohol Has Not Been Ingested. No drug is specific for violent behavior. The most effective, and those with least lowering of seizure threshold, are the high-potency, low-dose neuroleptics, which can also be expected to ameliorate paranoid thought disorder. Chlorpromazine (Thorazine), thioridazine (Mellaril), and especially promazine (Sparine), which has the lowest effectiveness/toxicity ratio, should *not* be used. In the absence of CNS depressant drugs such as alcohol, haloperidol (Haldol) is generally the drug of choice; an intramuscular dose of 5 mg can be repeated every 30 to 60 minutes up to a dose of 30 to 50 mg in 24 hours. Fluphenazine hydrochloride (Prolixin) (HC1, *not* decanoate or enanthate, which are designed for weekly or semi-weekly "depot" use), 5 mg IM, or thiothixene (Navane), a thioxanthene rather than an aliphatic phenothiazine, 4 to 5 mg IM, is also satisfactory. Because of the strong possibility of akathisia or dystonia following parenteral high-potency neuroleptics and because of documented instances of akathisia-associated violence, an anti-parkinsonian medication, such as benztropine mesylate (Cogentin), 2 mg, should be concurrently administered parenterally. (*Any* psychotic patient, especially one with a history of violence, should remain under observation after the administration of a neuroleptic). Benzodiazepines have little use in the treatment of assaultive behavior, but may be helpful in stimulant-induced aggressiveness, e.g., diazepam (Valium), 10 to 20 mg IM or IV. A benzodiazepine or anticonvulsant is indicated parenterally in the rare case of seizure-induced aggressiveness.

Occasionally, the reaction to a neuroleptic is paradoxical. For example, it can occur, in the *extremely* rare case of catatonic excitement, which is accompanied by mute terror and sometimes by nondirected assaultiveness (and can even be life-threatening to self, probably as a result of endogenous catecholamine-induced cardiac arrhythmias).

If a parenteral neuroleptic drug, even if repeated once following at least a half-hour of observation, is ineffective in halting (especially if the initial dose exacerbates) severely assaultive, violent, dangerous behavior, a radical intervention such as anesthesia may be necessary. Anesthesia or deep sedation by intravenous barbiturate such as sodium amobarbital (Amytal), 150 to 400 mg, must be carried out while the necessary equipment for intubation and support of respiration and circulation is readily available. Antidepressant drugs and lithium, which are slow to act and have dangerous complications, have no place in emergency treatment. Pharmacotherapy should be utilized more conservatively in children and adolescents, and dosage must be adjusted for body size.

DISPOSITION

Most assaultive patients who are not released to the custody of law enforcement authorities require continued *observation and treatment* within an acute, locked psychiatric facility. Generally, short involuntary "holds" are desirable to prevent prompt attempts at discharge against medical advice. Such petitions for brief involuntary hospitalization, usually 72 hours, are available in most jurisdictions for use by authorized persons, such as physicians or police officers, without court hearing (subject to petition of habeas corpus). The emergency physician, preferably following psychiatric consultation, can sometimes safely release the no-longer intoxicated individual or the person with an isolated explosive disorder or adjustment disorder, who is not subject to criminal charges, provided there is assurance of outpatient follow-up. The rare assaultive epileptic should be admitted to a neurologic or medical service once the assaultive behavior is under control. Verbal assurances of nonviolence on the part of a patient are, per se, insufficient reason for release, which must be based on medical, behavioral, and psychological assessment. It is better to err on the side of caution.

Generally, continued observation, once adequate diagnostic assessment has been made, is best within a facility that is better designed to cope with disturbed individuals than an emergency department. The patient should be transported to a facility with capacity for restraint. If transportation by ambulance is necessary following stabilization, the number of persons in attendance should be adequate. The patient who is not mentally or physically ill, but is character-disordered (antisocial), must be turned over to appropriate authorities, preferably after behavioral stabilization, and always after adequate diagnostic assessment to rule out serious intoxication.

A somewhat problematic issue is the "duty to protect" (often misinterpreted as a "duty to warn") as exemplified by the California Supreme Court Tarasoff decision. Threats to specific individuls must be seriously considered, and if the patient is being released or leaves, the intended victim should be notified (informing the police can be deemed insufficient). Release of a mentally ill person, dangerous to others or to self, can be the basis of medical liability action for consequences of the *patient's subsequent* behavior. If an assaultive patient elopes from an emergency medical setting, notification of law enforcement authorities to return the patient for completion of evaluation and appropriate disposition is generally necessary.

Disposition of *children or adolescents* can present special problems. The undersocialized youth often requires transfer to juvenile authorities. Child protective services may have to be called in for other out-of-control youths. Extreme caution should be exercised in returning a child to his or her parents before a careful psychosocial assessment can be made of the parents and the home situation, to which the assaultive behavior itself may be a reaction. The aggressive child may become a victim. Again, consultation is indicated, preferably by a child psychiatrist.

COUNTERTRANSFERENCE ISSUES

The abusive, assaultive individual, particularly one who has already done harm, can often elicit therapeutically inappropriate attitudes and behaviors in the treating medical personnel. Counterhostility and counteraggression are the most obvious. Fear, while possibly appropriate and adaptive, can have antitherapeutic consequences. Calm, assertive, unequivocal behavior that is as gentle and understanding as possible is the rule.

PSYCHIATRIC INPUT

Prompt neuropsychiatric consultation is imperative. Moreover, it is strongly advised that all emergency personnel undergo some psychiatric training in dealing with such difficult patients, including, when feasible, some psychodrama, role-playing, and practice. Written policies and guidelines regarding the handling of such patients, particularly in terms of use of restraint and seclusion within an emergency facility, are desirable.

SUGGESTED READING

Diagnostic and Statistical Manual of Mental Disorders 3rd ed. Washington: American Psychiatric Association, 1980.

Hanke N. Handbook of emergency psychiatry. Tunbridge Wells (U.K.): Castle House Publications, 1984.

Hays JR, Roberts TK, Solway KS, eds. Violence and the violent individual. New York: SP Medical & Scientific Books, 1981.

Sandler M, ed. Psychopharmacology of aggression. New York: Raven Press, 1979.

MANAGEMENT OF THE PULMONARY SYSTEM

ACUTE DYSPNEA

CHARLES MURPHY, M.D.

Dyspnea is defined here as an "inappropriate awareness of breathing" by the patient. An athlete completing a marathon does not seek out a physician because of labored breathing, yet a 45 year old person may present complaining of feeling "tired" and "out of breath" after his usual five mile jog, or a 22 year old person may complain of "shortness of breath" at rest, relieved with exertion.

The pathophysiology that produces the symptom of dyspnea is imperfectly understood, and a detailed discussion is beyond the scope of this article. However, the following observations can be made. Control and awareness of respiration depend upon the complex integration of the peripheral and central nervous systems involving J receptors, irritant receptors, baro- and chemoreceptors, muscle spindle-tension appropriateness, work of breathing, tissue oxygenation, and more. Generally respiration is an unconscious activity, but it may impose itself on awareness in both physiologic and pathophysiologic conditions. Though the work of breathing and the amount of tissue hypoxia may at times be greater in the former, they are not perceived as abnormal. Furthermore, as with Kussmaul respirations, the patient may not experience dyspnea and yet the work of breathing is great, tissue hypoxia exists, and an active disease process is present.

Still more vexing to the clinician is the observation that the complaint of dyspnea may be unassociated with any disorder beyond anxiety or may be associated with disease primarily outside the cardiopulmonary axis, e.g., anemia, thyrotoxic states, sepsis, and poisonings. It is hardly surprising that Kenneth T. Bird observed, "A medical chest specialist is long-winded about the short-winded."

GENERAL CONSIDERATIONS AND PRINCIPLES

What Is Acute?

Any definition is going to be arbitrary, if not dangerous. Three minutes is acute. Three hours is acute. Is 3 days acute? Or 3 weeks? Can the physician confronted by a patient with a 3 week or 3 month history feel confident that the problem is not serious simply on the basis of the duration of symptoms? No, though the need for urgent intervention is less likely in situations of longer duration.

Urgency of Management and Initial Therapy

Within the first few minutes the clinician must judge the gravity of the dyspneic patient's condition and decide whether to initiate therapy (with an imperfect understanding of the patient's problem) or to initiate the serial approach in which the history, physical examination, and laboratory data are collected in the traditional order and a rational therapeutic plan is instituted.

In either event oxygen should be promptly administered. In patients with carbon dioxide retention, lower FIO_2 concentrations should be used initially, but higher concentrations should never be withheld if required to correct hypoxemia, and the patient's respirations should be assisted as needed. The distinction between "prompt" and "crash" intubation-cricothyrotomy-tracheostomy must be understood (see Figure 1). A "crash" intubation simply means that there is no other way to manage the airway, even for several minutes, without subjecting the patient to severe morbidity or death. "Prompt" indicates that the patient's airway can be managed safely within the constraints of the situation for several minutes or more and that, consequently, the procedure or intubation can be performed in a more orderly and more controlled manner. The majority of intubations should be prompt and not crash. The emergency medicine specialist must be facile with a bag and mask; otherwise many intubations that would otherwise be prompt are converted to a crash situation with a significant increase in morbidity. Also, all bags should have an oxygen reservoir such that they deliver an FIO_2 of 0.9 or more; bags without reservoirs seldom deliver an FIO_2 of more than 0.5 and frequently deliver less.

History

Beware of the patient presenting with an established diagnosis consistent with the complaint of dyspnea; such patients cause physicians to jump to easy (and often wrong) conclusions. Consider, for example, a patient with chronic obstructive pulmonary disease who presents with

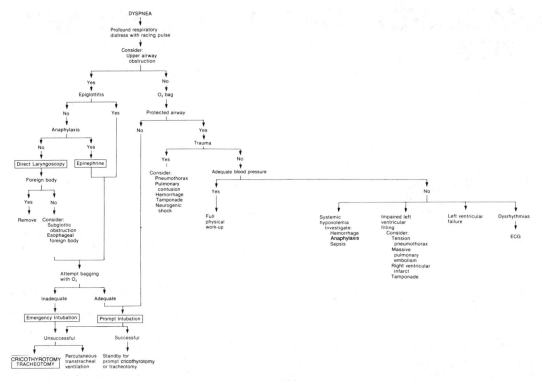

Figure 1 Management and initial therapy in dyspnea.

an increase in shortness of breath over the preceding 24 hours. His deterioration may be attributable to nothing more than a recent viral syndrome or poor compliance with prescribed therapy. However, the same patient may be at risk for a spontaneous pneumothorax or a silent myocardial infarction. An established diagnosis sometimes serves a physician as blinders serve a horse.

The development or worsening of dyspnea over minutes to hours should lead the physician to seek the following causes (see Tables 1 and 2): acute myocardial ischemia or infarction, acute dysrhythmias, acute valvular insufficiency, pulmonary edema, cardiac tamponade, pulmonary embolism, pneumothorax with or without tension, massive aspiration-inhalation, upper airway obstruction, or psychogenic hyperventilation.

Psychogenic hyperventilation can be a particularly misleading ''established'' diagnosis, which ends all serious medical evaluation. Patients with pulmonary embolism may look exactly the same. The technique of having the patient rebreathe into a paper bag can be dangerous unless oxygen supplementation is given, as it can worsen hypoxia and precipitate cardiac arrest.

Physical Examination

Examination of the lungs may reveal normal or misleading findings in the presence of severe and even life threatening pulmonary or cardiac disease. A large pneumothorax may not be detectable by physical examination. Extensive interstitial lung disease whether owing to infection or other causes can present with minimal or no lung findings. In patients suffering chronic cardiopulmo-nary diseases (e.g., chronic obstructive pulmonary disease, congestive cardiomyopathies), little or no change may be found in the lung examination during an acute exacerbation compared to when they are compensated.

Rales, though often associated with congestive heart failure, are seen in a variety of other diseases, and though much is made of wet and dry rales, the distinction may be more oral than aural to the clinician. Wheezing suggests bronchospasm but should suggest more than asthma, especially in patients with known heart disease, in those without known heart disease who are dyspneic and have a markedly elevated blood pressure (cardiac asthma in both cases), and in patients with a history consistent with foreign body aspiration, toxic inhalation-ingestion (e.g., chlorine gas, scombroid food poisoning), or anaphylaxis. Rubs can be heard in pleurisy, pneumonia, pulmonary infarction, and pericarditis.

Tachypnea, defined as a respiratory rate greater than 15 per minute in an adult, is a totally nonspecific sign, more important by its absence than its presence. Judging severity of illness by the degree of tachypnea may be extremely misleading. Respiratory rate gives no indication of tidal volume, minute volume, ventilation, or oxygenation, and little regarding the work of breathing.

Chest pain has been well described in patients with acute myocardial infarction and in those with acute pulmonary embolism. The clinician should be chary of dismissing these diagnoses because of the presence of chest wall tenderness. Patients are often baffled in trying to describe their pain and by the distinctions that the physician is trying to elicit. The presence of chest wall pain offers minimal comfort to the physician unless palpation

TABLE 1 Causes of Severe Dyspnea of Sudden Onset (Within One Hour of Seeking Medical Help)

Upper airway
  Angioedema (separately, or part of anaphylaxis)
  Caustic burn
  Epiglottitis (onset of symptoms >1 hr, but usually <1 day)
  Foreign body

Cardiac
  Acute ischemia
  Acute valvular insufficiency (including prosthetic valves)
  Dysrhythmia
  Pulmonary edema (often secondary to one of the above)
  Cardiac tamponade (decompensation can be sudden and dramatic)

Pulmonary
  Aspiration
  Asthma
  Pneumothorax
  Noncardiac pulmonary edema, (drugs, neurogenic)
  Toxic inhalations: smoke, chlorine gas
  Pleurisy (dyspnea is seldom severe; restriction of deep
    inspiration due to pain is characteristic)

Trauma
  Flail chest
  Hemo- and pneumothorax
  Pulmonary contusion
  Ruptured bronchus, trachea, and air embolism
  Cardiac tamponade)

Poisonings
  Carbon monoxide
  Cyanide
  Salicylates
  Scombroid food poisoning
  Sedatives, hypnotics, narcotics (can cause profound respiratory
    depression, but patients do not present with dyspnea)

Allergic-immunologic
  Anaphylaxis

Miscellaneous

  Psychogenic hyperventilation (a diagnosis of exclusion)

TABLE 2 Causes of Dyspnea as a Secondary Complaint

Anemia
Neurologic disease
  (Guillain-Barré syndrome, myasthenia gravis)
Hyperthyroidism
Metabolic acidosis (diabetic ketoacidosis,
  ETOH ketoacidosis, lactic acidosis)
Pregnancy
Sepsis
Infections-toxins: botulism diphtheria, tetanus

of the affected area of the chest precisely reproduces the symptom complex (see *Chest Pain*).

Laboratory Tests

The ability of the physician to estimate hypoxemia is poor. Therefore, arterial blood gas levels are often essential in evaluation of the dyspneic patient. In patients with chronic cardiopulmonary disease or the elderly, arterial blood gas levels should always be obtained. They also provide useful information about pH, ventilation, Pco_2, and alveolar-arterial gradients (see Table 3). However, not every patient complaining of dyspnea requires blood gas level determinations; the age, underlying diseases, primary diagnosis, and condition of the patient after initial therapy may all affect the decision to obtain such information.

Chest X-ray Examination

The chest x-ray film findings can be totally unremarkable in the presence of severe illness manifesting as dyspnea. The obvious examples of pulmonary embolus, myocardial infarction, and anemia come to mind, but patients may sustain massive aspiration, toxic inhalation, or pulmonary contusion with normal x-ray film findings during the first 24 hours after insult. In the presence of significant dehydration a patient may have extensive pneumonia with normal chest x-ray film findings. Also, patients with longstanding chronic obstructive pulmonary disease or heart disease, e.g., congestive cardiomyopathy and mitral stenosis, may suddenly decompensate without demonstrating any x-ray film changes, including the typical roentgenographic findings of congestive heart failure.

SPECIFIC CAUSES OF DYSPNEA

Myocardial Ischemia

The literature clearly documents that dyspnea may be an anginal or infarct equivalent. In one series of 102 myocardial infarctions, 14 presented with dyspnea without chest pain. If the patient gives a history of previous bouts of dyspnea that in other respects (e.g., relation to exertion, or duration) resemble angina, the diagnosis may be obvious. However, the absence of such a history does not exclude the diagnosis. Ischemic dyspnea seldom lasts un-

TABLE 3 Calculation of A-a Gradient

Definitions:

A = alveolar partial pressure of oxygen (150 torr at sea level)

a = arterial Po_2 (measured by blood gases)

BP = barometric pressure (approximately 760 torr at sea level)

FIo_2 = fraction of inspired gases that is oxygen; on ambient air it is 0.21; on 100% oxygen it would be 1.0

Formula for A-a gradient:

$$A = [FLo_2 \times (BP - 47^*)] - [1.2 \times Pco_2]$$
$$A = [0.21 \times (760 - 47)] - [1.2 \times Pco_2]$$
$$A\text{-}a = [150 - (1.2 \times Pco_2)] - \text{arterial } Po_2$$

Normal values: A-a at age 20 = 3 ± 11 torr
  at age 60 = 17 ± 11 torr

Formula for estimating normal arterial Po_2 on ambient air:

$$Po_2 = 100.1 - 0.323 (age) \pm 5 \text{ torr}$$

---

* 47 = the partial pressure of H_2O in the lungs at sea level.

remittingly for days, and it seldom lasts for only several seconds. An S3 gallop may be present on physical examination in both acute and chronic heart disease, but the presence of an S3 during a bout of dyspnea when it is absent without dyspnea is highly suggestive of an ischemic origin. An absolutely normal electrocardiogram while the patient is suffering an attack of dyspnea favors rejecting ischemia if pseudonormalization can be excluded. In most situations in which myocardial ischemia is being considered, the electrocardiogram is never absolutely normal. A normal electrocardiogram when the patient is not experiencing dyspnea is of no help; and an abnormal electrocardiogram taken while symptoms are present that shows no change from previous tracings is of limited value. In one study 17.2 percent of the patients with angiographically proven unstable angina had electrocardiograms that showed no change during their attacks when compared to those taken when the patient was asymptomatic.

During the first 4 to 6 hours after myocardial infarction the MB band of creatine phosphokinase may not be elevated above normal, and the total creatine phosphokinase level may never be abnormal. What if the patient has been suffering symptoms for more than 6 hours? Unfortunately for the clinician, though the patient may have been symptomatic for more than 6 hours, actual infarction may have been in progress for a far shorter length of time. Consequently, with rare exceptions, if a physician feels compelled to order cardiac enzyme levels, the patient should be admitted.

Though appropriate for control of pain, the use of nitroglycerin as a diagnostic tool in the emergency setting should generally be condemned. If the patient fails to respond, it proves little; and if the patient does respond, the effect may be attributable to the relief of esophageal spasm, which can perfectly mimic myocardial ischemia, or to a placebo effect, or to coincidence. After evaluating the history, physical examination, laboratory data, and x-ray views the physician may seriously question the diagnosis of ischemic dyspnea, and the decision to pursue it further depends on how convincingly the data support an alternative diagnosis. It is safest to err on the side of caution and admit the confusing patient.

Dysrhythmias

Both bradycardia and tachycardia may present as acute or subacute dyspnea. Provided the patient is symptomatic at the time of presentation, the electrocardiogram confirms the presence of the dysrhythmia, but the following caveats should be heeded:

1. Supraventricular dysrhythmias with ventricular heart rates between 50 and 160 generally do not produce dyspnea at rest unless there is also an advanced cardiomyopathy, mitral stenosis, or advanced aortic valvular disease, or unless the cardiac status is so impaired that the patient cannot tolerate a moderate increase in rate.

A supraventricular heart rate of 160 may be totally appropriate for a patient in congestive heart failure complaining of dyspnea. The physician may be unsure whether the rhythm is sinus or paroxysmal supraventricular tachycardia. The solution to this quandary is not the intravenous administration of verapamil or cardioversion. Rather, vagal maneuvers, Lewis leads or esophageal or intra-atrial leads should be utilized to help establish the correct diagnosis.

A heart rate of 160 may be totally appropriate for a patient with acute pulmonary embolism, pneumothorax, pneumonia, or thyrotoxicosis. Supraventricular dysrhythmias with ventricular rates between 50 and 160 should, with the foregoing exceptions noted, prompt the physician to seek other reasons for dyspnea that is present at rest.

2. Accelerated idioventricular rhythms (50 to 100 per minute) certainly can cause dyspnea, but if the patient's blood pressure is adequate, consideration should be given to withholding pharmacologic or electrical cardioversion until temporary pacing is available. In this situation cardioversion may reveal a heart without any other spontaneous rhythm.

3. Bradycardia is frequently the harbinger of respiratory arrest and not the cause. Attention should be directed to the bag valve mask, not the electrocardiogram.

Even when the dyspnea is clearly related to the dysrhythmia, the physician must inquire as to the cause of the rhythm disturbance. Consider the association of new atrial fibrillation with myocardial infarction as well as its association with pulmonary embolism or hyperthyroidism.

Pulmonary Embolism

Pulmonary embolism is the nemesis of every physician who has ever struggled to diagnose the dyspneic patient, and few subjects generate more controversy. In the acute stage it presents in one of three ways (see also *Pulmonary Embolism*).

It can manifest as massive occlusion resulting in systemic hypotension and symptoms of shock, and when associated with chest pain, it may be confused with massive myocardial infarction. However, the findings on physical examination of acute cor pulmonale, absence of pulmonary findings consistent with congestive heart failure, a chest x-ray view demonstrating no failure, and an electrocardiogram consistent with acute cor pulmonale or failing to support a diagnosis of massive myocardial infarction suggest the correct diagnosis. Unfortunately right ventricular infarction may present with similar physical and roentgenographic findings, and on occasion the electrocardiographic findings may be similar. Fortunately the therapy available to the emergency physician for both these conditions is essentially the same: oxygen and support of blood pressure with fluids until one can make a definitive diagnosis and therapy can be instituted.

Embolism may present as infarction with acute pleuritic pain, shortness of breath, a friction rub, sometimes hemoptysis, and an effusion. Only 10 percent of emboli manifest this way. The pleuritic nature of the pain and the electrocardiogram aid in distinguishing it from myocardial ischemia. Fever (generally less than 102°), leucocytosis, and elevated sedimentation rate also can occur.

The majority of pulmonary emboli occur as multiple peripheral occlusions without large areas of infarction. The most common symptom is dyspnea, and the most common sign is tachypnea, defined as a respiratory rate greater than 16 to 20, depending on the study cited. The manifestations of this entity are protean and it is easily misdiagnosed.

The predominant risk factors are those conditions known to predispose the patient to venous stasis and to a lesser degree hypercoagulable states, but pulmonary embolism also occurs in patients without evident risk factors. Physical examination may be misleading: chest wall or rib tenderness is well described.

Elevated white cell counts are common with pulmonary embolism. Arterial blood gas levels with arterial Po_2 levels greater than 90 mg Hg while the patient is breathing ambient air have been described in the presence of acute pulmonary embolism. However, the presence of a normal alveolar-arterial oxygen gradient is uncommon (see Table 3).

The chest x-ray view is useful when it shows pneumothorax or consolidated pneumonia; otherwise it is of limited value. Most commonly the chest x-ray view in acute pulmonary embolism is either normal or unchanged from previous films. A normal ventilation-perfusion scan excludes the diagnosis of pulmonary embolism with extremely few exceptions.

Ultimately the vigor with which the clinician pursues the diagnosis of pulmonary embolism depends on the index of suspician, which should always be high when he or she is confronted with a patient without a convincing explanation for the dyspnea. It should be relatively high in patients with previously stable cardiopulmonary disease who become decompensated without an identifiable cause.

Pneumothorax

The complaint of dyspnea coupled with decreased breath sounds and increased tympany over the affected area should suggest pneumothorax. The soft tissues should also be checked for crepitus. If hypotension or mediastinal shift is present, tension pneumothorax should be considered. However, what deserves re-emphasis is that in the case of an uncomplicated pneumothorax, the physical examination, with surprising frequency, fails to suggest the diagnosis. Moreover, in patients with tension pneumothorax the only physical clue may be hypotension. Therefore, when a patient presents with poorly or unexplained hypotension, prompt consideration should be given to this diagnosis, particularly in patients receiving positive pressure ventilation. The clinician should also keep in mind that pneumothorax occurs spontaneously in patients without evidence of pulmonary disease. Finally, do not mistake a bulla for pneumothorax.

Psychogenic Dyspnea

The main pitfall in making the diagnosis of psychogenic dyspnea is that it is too readily made, thus missing the real disorder. On the other hand it is time consuming, expensive, and frustrating to belabor this diagnosis in the pursuit of organic disease that does not exist. The following observations are offered as help in avoiding a pitfall.

1. A history of relief of dyspnea with exertion strongly favors a psychogenic etiology. This history should not be confused with "walk through" angina or its ischemic equivalent, "walk through" dypspnea. Here the patient complains of shortness of breath with the initiation of exertion, but notes that it abates 5 to 10 minutes after beginning the activity when his body has had time to make the compensatory changes associated with exercise and consequently myocardial oxygen consumption has fallen and symptoms have resolved. The history of circumoral and digital paresthesias helps support the diagnosis of psychogenic dyspnea and hyperventilation.

2. The presence of arterial respiratory alkalosis does not establish the diagnosis of psychogenic dyspnea even in the presence of a "normal" Po_2 level. Pulmonary embolism, myocardial infarction, metabolic acidosis, occasionally pneumonia, moderate to severe anemia, hepatic cirrhosis, salicylism, carbon monoxide poisoning, and pregnancy can all present with respiratory alkalosis and a "normal" Po_2 level. The combination of the history, physical examination, and an analysis of the entire arterial blood gas spectrum often eliminates many, but not all, of these diagnoses. Furthermore, it should be recalled that some patients with psychogenic dyspnea have been hyperventilating for more than 24 hours and consequently have a mild compensatory metabolic acidosis. It is particularly interesting that in one study half the patients diagnosed as having psychogenic hyperventilation in fact had high normal to elevated salicylate levels.

AIDS

Though the number of cases has increased dramatically during the past 5 years, many physicians with a vast amount of clinical experience have had little or no experience with the acquired immunodeficiency syndrome. This diagnosis (and specifically, *Pneumocytis* pneumonia) should be entertained in any patient at risk for AIDS who presents complaining of dyspnea. A careful history and physical examination are critical. In particular the physician should not be misled by the frequent youth or apparent fitness of the patient. All such patients should undergo chest x-ray examination. If the findings are normal, an arterial blood gas level determination is mandatory, since the initial symptom of *Pneumocystis carinii pneumonia* may be dyspnea without any physical signs, and the only routine test abnormality is an increased alveolar-arterial oxygen gradient (elevated sedimentation rate values are extremely common with *Pneumocystis* pneumonia but nonspecific). An increased gradient or an abnormality in the chest roentgenogram, or the presence of fever, necessitates consultation with someone familiar with diagnosing AIDS.

It is important that physicians inexperienced with this disease not make the diagnosis of AIDS, despite their suspicions. Remember that the patient at risk for AIDS may have any of the "usual" causes of dyspnea and that the inaccurate or premature diagnosis of AIDS produces a tremendous amount of unnecessary suffering for the patient and his family and friends.

Upper Airway Obstruction

The topic of airway obstruction is considered in another section of this book. Nevertheless a few observations will be made here. Physicians are familiar with the presentation of complete or nearly complete upper airway obstruction: a patient in obvious distress, who is possibly grasping at his throat, displaying suprasternal, supraclavicular, and intercostal retractions. Impaired or absent speech, drooling, and cyanosis may be present. The presence of inspiratory or expiratory stridor is always ominous. However, its absence does not exclude imminent collapse. Air flow varies directly with the fourth power of the internal airway diameter, and consequently a small change (e.g., a slight increase in edema, slight laryngospasm) in an already impeded airway can produce profound reductions in air flow.

What is less frequently appreciated is that significant upper airway disease may exist without any of the foregoing signs. For example, in adults epiglottitis may present with minimal to mild dyspnea, fever, and a sore throat. The physical examination offers no clues unless the clinician palpates the anterior neck and elicits midline tenderness; unexplained dyspnea in a patient with fever and with either a complaint of sore throat or the finding of anterior midline neck tenderness on examination should prompt the physician to consider epiglottitis.

Patients with epiglottitis can often be effectively ventilated with a bag valve mask, and consequently this modality should always be attempted prior to crash intubation, cricothyrotomy, or tracheostomy.

SUGGESTED READING

Clausen JL. Finding the cause of shortness of breath. J Resp Dis 1982; 3:11.

Diaz JH, Lockhart CH. Early diagnosis and airway management of acute epiglottitis in children. South Med J 1982; 4:399 (104 of 106 cases managed with nasotracheal intubation).

Glicklich M, et al. Steroids and bag and mask ventilation in the treatment of acute epiglottitis. J Pediatr Surg 1979; 14:247.

Hull D, et al. Pulmonary angiography, ventilation lung scanning, and venography for clinically suspected pulmonary embolism with abnormal perfusion lung scan. Ann Intern Med 1983; 98:891.

Lucke WC, Thomas H Jr. Anaphylaxis: pathophysiology, clinical presentations and treatment. J Emerg Med 1983; 1:83.

CHEST PAIN

HAROLD A. JAYNE, M.D., F.A.C.E.P.
DAVID W. HILL Jr., M.D.

This chapter provides an overview of chest pain; specific treatment of various diseases is discussed in the relevant chapters.

All patients seen in an emergency department complaining of chest pain should be approached as having a potential life threat. Most people are concerned that their chest pain connotes serious heart disease. Thus it is important that physicians not only be expedient in the diagnosis and treatment of serious causes of chest pain, but also alleviate the anxiety of patients with less serious causes of chest pain.

ETIOLOGY

The causes of chest pain are multi-system and range from simple muscle strain requiring rest to cardiovascular and pulmonary catastrophes. Possible causes of chest pain are listed in Table 1. Even with the extensive diagnostic armamentarium available today, evaluation of acute chest pain remains a challenge to the most astute physician.

DIFFERENTIAL DIAGNOSIS

Chest pain of cardiac origin, i.e., myocardial ischemia or *infarction* (MI), should be suspected on the basis of the presenting history. The pain of infarction is usually described as a dull, aching, or pressure sensation located in the substernal or parasternal area or epigastrium, often radiating to the jaw, left shoulder, or neck and down the left arm. These symptoms occur when the oxygen requirements of heart muscle exceed the supply of oxygen arriving at the muscle, usually because of narrowed coronary arteries. Other associated symptoms include nausea, vomiting, lightheadedness, diaphoresis, or dizziness. Any patient presenting as above should be treated with urgency, regardless of the presence or lack of supporting diagnostic data such as electrocardiogram (ECG). It is important to remember that patients with diabetes often have "silent MIs" or present with unusual symptoms; many patients have normal ECGs when first seen. The same symptoms can be produced by esophageal or gastric disease.

Anginal or *ischemic chest pain* is different from infarction chest pain in that the duration is usually shorter and often associated with activity. It is divided into stable

TABLE 1 Causes of Chest Pain

Cardiac causes: angina pectoris, unstable angina, myocardial infarction, valvular disease (especially mitral valve prolapse, aortic stenosis, aortic insufficiency), pericarditis

Vascular causes: dissecting thoracic aneurysm, leaking upper abdominal aortic aneurysm, pulmonary hypertension

Pulmonary causes: pulmonary embolism, pleurisy, pneumothorax, pneumomediastinum, pneumonia

Musculoskeletal causes: muscle strain, costochondritis, rib fractures (bone or cartilage), early herpes zoster (before rash)

Gastrointestinal causes: peptic ulcer, pancreatitis, biliary colic, esophageal reflux and spasm, esophagitis, mediastinitis, ruptured esophagus, cholecystitis and unstable angina, the major point of difference being the increase or change in the patient's symptomatology. Stable angina is the patient's usual type of chest pain and is readily relieved with rest or medication. Unstable angina is defined as a change in the character of the pain including an increase in severity, duration, or frequency.

The pain of acute *pericarditis* is often identified as that of angina pectoris or myocardial infarction, but it has some distinguishing features. The pain in pericarditis is usually sharp, nonradiating, and increased in the supine position. It may be accentuated with deep inspiration as well as coughing or yawning. The pain may be relieved when the patient sits up or leans forward. The most characteristic finding is the pericardial friction rub, which can be intensified by having the patient hold his breath.

Signs of an associated cardiac tamponade should be sought. These are jugular venous distention, systemic hypotension, and pulsus paradoxus. The ECG may show diffuse ST segment elevations, which can be differentiated from ischemic changes in the cardiogram by the upward concavity and P-R depression in both pericardial and limb leads. The chest film may show a globular heart with loss of hilar markings. If a pericardial effusion is suspected, an echocardiogram is indicated.

Patients with *aortic dissection* describe their pain variously as a crushing, ripping, or tearing, often felt in the back. Patients are elderly and have a history of hypertension; assessment and stabilization must occur immediately.

Pulmonary embolism should be suspected in patients who present with chest pain and shortness of breath. The chest pain is pleuritic in nature and exacerbated by inspiration. Other symptoms include apprehension, cough, and hemoptysis. Clinical findings include tachycardia, tachypnea, and increased intensity of the pulmonic component of the second heart sound. Historical information that places the patient in the high-risk group includes history of heart disease, thrombophlebitis, previous pulmonary embolism, recent pregnancy, use of oral contraceptives, malignant disease, or chronic lung disease.

When a young, healthy patient presents with sudden onset of sharp chest pain radiating to the shoulder or back with or without dyspnea, *spontaneous pneumothorax* should be strongly considered. The diagnosis can sometimes (but not always) be made clinically on the basis of decreased breath sounds and hyper-resonance over the affected lung; the chest roentgenogram is diagnostic.

Severe stabbing chest pain, increased with inspiration and coughing, is often indicative of *pleural inflammation.* A pleural friction rub is sometimes present. One of the major causes is pneumonia. The presentation may also include cough—productive or nonproductive—fever, chills, night sweats, myalgias, and dyspnea.

By far the most common cause of chest pain, and the least likely to be fatal, is pain of musculoskeletal origin. A pertinent history and meticulous physical examination are essential so that a more serious cause of chest pain is not overlooked. The hallmark of musculoskeletal pain is the ability to reproduce it with palpation. Common causes are rib fracture (detected by localized tenderness and crepitus) and costochondritis, with localized tenderness over a costochondral junction. Rarely there may be occult injuries or osteomyelitis of the sternum. Although radicular chest pain from spinal compression of an intercostal nerve is rare, occasionally herpes zoster is seen as unilateral chest pain before any rash appears.

PRE-HOSPITAL THERAPY

A brief but pertinent history should be obtained while basic maneuvers are initiated. The paramedics should immediately start oxygen, place the patient on a monitor, and establish an intravenous line. Historical points of diagnostic and treatment value include onset, character, location, radiation, duration, and relief of the pain as well as identification of risk factors. The initial vital signs dictate the direction of the physician in his initial treatment. Another factor to be considered is the estimated time of arrival. One should remember that the emergency department is the optimal site for treatment.

If the patient is suspected of having chest pain caused by ischemia, nitroglycerin is indicated as the first intervention. The side effect of hypotension must be anticipated and the physician be prepared to treat the patient with intravenous fluids and Trendelenburg positioning. The patient presenting with an initial blood pressure (BP) of 110 systolic or less is at risk of having hypotension secondary to nitroglycerin. In this situation, the use of morphine sulfate, 2 to 3 mg IV, would be preferable as it has less hypotensive effect. The most common arrhythmia associated with the chest pain is that of premature ventricular contractions or PVCs. Ischemic chest pain and five to six PVCs per minute are indications for intravenous lidocaine—an initial bolus of 1 mg per kilogram followed by a drip of 2 mg per minute.

In the case of aortic dissection, after the basic field treatment has been initiated, the patient must be rapidly transported because of his or her unstable condition and need for surgical intervention.

If the patient is suspected of having a pulmonary embolism, high-flow oxygen by mask rather than nasal cannula is indicated. The hypoxic insult resulting from a shunt requires high-flow oxygen to compensate.

The patient with pneumothorax should receive high-flow oxygen, and the field team should be prepared to intubate the patient if severe respiratory deterioration occurs. If intubation is needed, development of tension pneumothorax requiring needle decompression should be anticipated. Needle thoracostomy by means of a 14-guage angiocath in the anterior chest wall should be reserved for patients in severe respiratory distress. Once again, rapid transport to the hospital is mandatory for definitive treatment—tube thoracostomy.

INITIAL APPROACH IN THE EMERGENCY DEPARTMENT

All patients should be disrobed to allow for detailed examination of neck, heart, lungs, abdomen, and extremities. While initial vital signs are being obtained, the patient should be attached to a monitor. For all patients experiencing respiratory distress, diaphoresis, or chest pain, oxygen therapy should begin without delay. Usually 3 to 4 liters by nasal cannula are adequate, except in the case of patients with severe chronic pulmonary disease, for whom a Venti-mask is recommended to better regulate and monitor oxygen administration.

An intravenous infusion should be started. Many physicians advocate the use of D5W to avoid the possible sodium load that is a potential hazard when normal saline is given to patients who are prone to congestive heart failure. However, there is one advantage to the use of normal saline in patients with chest pain—it is the solution of choice in a hypotensive patient who requires fluid resuscitation. Given at a to keep open (TKO) rate, the sodium load should be minimal.

Whenever the suspicion of medical catastrophe is present, a stat ECG, arterial blood gases (ABG), and portable chest film should be ordered. Cardiac enzyme, electrolyte, glucose, blood urea nitrogen (BUN), and creatinine determinations should also be performed.

Nitroglycerin is the cornerstone of therapy for patients who present with chest pain of cardiac origin (i.e., myocardial infarction, stable and unstable angina). Nitroglycerin dilates coronary and systemic vessels; however, it also relaxes smooth muscle and can relieve pain from esophageal spasm. It is important to know the blood pressure and to have intravenous access prior to administration of nitroglycerin. Initial therapy should consist of nitroglycerine gr 1/150, every 10 to 15 minutes until resolution of the pain or until the patient becomes hypotensive. If hypotension occurs, the patient is placed in the Trendelenburg position and given a fluid challenge with normal saline. If the patient's blood pressure can be maintained at an adequate level with fluids, nitroglycerin may be continued. It is imperative that the physician realize that repeated hypotensive episodes may increase cardiac ischemia and possibly increase infarct size.

The other alternative is the use of intravenous *morphine sulfate* (MS). This may be administered in doses of 2 to 3 mg IV every 5 to 10 minutes. One must remember that MS is a respiratory depressant, and cessation of breathing is a potential complication. Another alternative is the use of beta-blockers, especially in patients with tachycardia. It is important to recall that both the heart and the upper gastrointestinal tract are served by the vagus nerve, and both areas can cause identical pain. Chest pain relieved by nitroglycerin may in fact be attributable to esophageal spasm, which is also relieved by this drug. Although pain relieved by antacids is probably gastric in origin, usually oxygen and reassurance are being given at the same time and may alleviate cardiac pain. Whenever one is in doubt, it is wisest to assume the existence of cardiac ischemic pain.

Failure of chest pain to respond to initial therapies requires the use of more aggressive intervention such as intravenous nitroglycerin or even placement of a balloon pump. Both require close monitoring of the patient clinically. When intravenous nitroglycerine is being used, the blood pressure should be rechecked at least every 5 minutes. Ideally, an arterial line should be placed with continuous pressure monitoring. If an aortic balloon pump

is needed, consultation should be obtained and the patient transported to the critical care unit as quickly as possible.

The use of lidocaine in patients presenting with cardiac pain continues to be controversial. Many studies have documented the increased incidence of arrhythmias associated with the "reperfusion" of ischemic cardiac muscle. We recommend that patients who are suspected of having an MI be placed on prophylactic lidocaine for the first 24 to 48 hours. The patient should receive an initial bolus of 1 mg per kilogram followed by one-half the initial dose approximately 10 minutes later to avoid the pharmocologic subtherapeutic period. Then the patient should be started on a lidocaine drip at 2 mg per minute to be titrated to cessation of ectopy or development of toxic symptoms.

When treating a patient with a possible aortic dissection, the most important contribution of the emergency physician is to suspect the diagnosis and initiate proper diagnostic maneuvers. The pulses and blood pressures of all four extremities should be checked and compared; evidence of cardiac tamponade should be sought. An ECG should be done to differentiate the pain from ischemic cardiac pain. A chest film should be studied for (1) left pleural effusion, (2) mediastinal widening, and (3) calcification of the aorta. Blood should be typed and crossmatched for 6 to 10 units. Special attention must be paid to stabilizing the blood pressure at the lowest possible level that will provide adequate perfusion of vital organs. Once this diagnosis is considered, an immediate cardiovascular or surgical consultation is mandatory.

In the patient with a suspected pulmonary embolism the initial studies include chest film, ECG, and arterial blood gas determinations. The initial management requires high-flow O_2 to overcome hypoxia. Intravenous access is essential for two reasons: (1) these patients are at risk for shock, and (2) the early treatment of choice is intravenous heparin. The diagnosis can be made by ventilation-perfusion (V-Q) scanning or angiography. An initial prothrombin time/partial thromboplastin time (PT/PTT) should be drawn prior to starting anticoagulation therapy.

Pleurisy and *costochondritis* are both treated with anti-inflammatory agents. Chest wall pain secondary to musculoskeletal problems is treated with analgesics and/or anti-inflammatory agents. In cases with severe but well-localized pain, local injection with lidocaine or bupivacaine, or an intercostal nerve block, may provide excellent relief. (See chapter on *Blunt and Penetrating Chest Trauma*, for the technique). Musculoskeletal causes can be treated on an outpatient basis with close follow-up.

SUGGESTED READING

Goldman L, Lee TH. Chest pain: infarction or not? Acute Care 1985; 2:10–18.

Lee TH, Cook F, et al. Acute chest pain in the emergency room. Arch Intern Med 1985; 145:65–69.

Parrish NL. Evaluation of acute chest pain. Nurs Clin North Am 1981; 16:25–35.

Schneider RR, Seckler SG. Evaluation of acute chest pain. Med Clin North Am 1981; 65:53–66.

Selker HP. Sorting out chest pain. Emergency Decisions 1985; 1:8–17.

OXYGEN THERAPY

HILLARY DON, M.D.

Reduction of the partial pressure of oxygen in arterial blood (hypoxemia, Table 1) is potentially immediately lethal; its correct and effective treatment is therefore essential. Hypoxemia causes two separate problems. First, arterial oxygen content is reduced, hindering the transport of oxygen from lung to capillary bed; this can be partially or completely compensated for by an equivalent increase in cardiac output. Second, hypoxemia lowers the oxygen pressure gradient for diffusion of oxygen from capillary to tissues; this effect is not improved by changes in cardiac output, and the only treatment is to increase arterial oxygen partial pressure (PaO_2). Although the fundamental treatment of hypoxemia is correction of the underlying cause, the immediate response must be management of the low PaO_2 itself.

INDICATIONS FOR OXYGEN THERAPY

The first objective of oxygen therapy is to increase an existing low PaO_2 to a normal or adequate level (Fig. 1). The levels of PaO_2 that should be treated are disputed, but PaO_2 less than 40 mm Hg must be increased, as cerebral function is usually impaired below that level. To create a margin of safety, it is advisable in most patients to maintain PaO_2 at 60 mm Hg or greater; the exceptions to this rule are patients with a tendency to develop hypercapnia when given added oxygen, and when the prolonged administration of oxygen may produce oxygen toxicity.

Hypoxemia is documented only by measurement of the oxygen tension in an arterial blood sample. However, there are clues to its presence: certain clinical settings (e.g., postoperatively, following myocardial infarction or pulmonary embolism, and in patients with severe hypotension); the presence of cyanosis; low mixed venous oxygen content (less than 75 percent saturated); decreased cerebral function; abnormal cardiac rhythms; oliguria; and metabolic acidosis.

The second objective of oxygen therapy is to produce a higher-than-normal PaO_2. This is indicated either to treat nonhypoxemic hypoxia (e.g., carbon monoxide poison-ing, methemoglobinemia, anemia, decreased oxygen transport attributable to reduced cardiac output and/or increased oxygen demand, and histotoxic problems such as sepsis) or to correct a pathologic state that is actually treated by an elevated PaO_2 (e.g., reduction of elevated pulmonary resistance, hastened elimination of carbon monoxide, reduced sickle forms in homozygous sickle cell disease, decreased size of a pneumothorax or pneumomediastinum, treatment of pneumatosis cystoides intestinalis, management of anaerobic infections, and possibly reduced infarct size during myocardial ischemia). Elevation of PaO_2 may also aid wound healing.

HAZARDS OF OXYGEN THERAPY

The first category of hazards consists of physical problems, such as fire, tank explosions, and trauma from dry gas or equipment (mask or cannula). Ironically equipment failure or errors in administration (e.g, the delivery of nitrous oxide instead of oxygen) can aggravate the very problem being treated.

The second category consists of functional hazards such as atelectasis or reduced alveolar ventilation. Atelectasis is thought to be produced by the absorption of oxygen beyond closed airways. Alveolar ventilation may be reduced if the administration of oxygen removes a hypoxemic drive to breathe. Depression of ventilation by the administration of oxygen is unusual unless baseline hypercapnia exists, and it does not always occur even then.

The third category consists of cytotoxic hazards, which are thought to be produced by an increased rate of generation of partially reduced oxygen products within the cell. Minor changes of pulmonary oxygen toxicity are seen as diminished vital capacity and substernal chest pain. More prolonged exposure may result in changes in the interstitium of the lung accompanied by reduced pulmonary compliance, severe hypoxemia, and a diffuse bilateral infiltrate on the chest roentgenogram—the so-called adult respiratory distress syndrome. In premature neonates, retrolental fibroplasia and permanent visual impairment may result from hyperoxia.

CONTRAINDICATIONS TO OXYGEN THERAPY

There is no contraindication to the administration of oxygen to patients who are hypoxemic, or who suffer nonhypoxemic hypoxia, which would potentially be aided by an increase in FIO_2. Carbon dioxide retention is not a contraindication when the patient is hypoxemic. Recognition of the hazards of oxygen therapy dictates that its administration must be undertaken with these potential complications in mind.

TECHNIQUE OF ADMINISTRATION OF OXYGEN THERAPY

As with any therapeutic modality, oxygen must be administered in a dose that is appropriate to the achieve-

---

TABLE 1 Predicted Normal Arterial Oxygen Partial Pressure (PaO_2) in Adult Patients with Normal Arterial Carbon Dioxide Partial Pressure, Breathing Air at Sea Level

Sitting: PaO_2 = 100 minus ⅓ age in years mm Hg
Supine: PaO_2 = 100 minus ½ age in years mm Hg

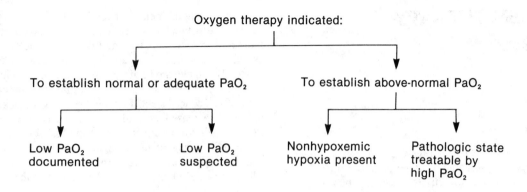

Figure 1 Categories of indications for oxygen therapy.

ment of the stated objective of treatment, with guidelines to document achievement of the objective, and with prompt discontinuation of therapy when treatment is no longer necessary. Precautions must be taken to prevent hazards (e.g., no smoking when oxygen is in use, periodic measurement of oxygen concentrations in the delivered gas, humidification of dry gas, and appropriate care of equipment). The patient must be monitored for the development of complications (e.g., measurement of arterial carbon dioxide partial pressure).

Figure 2 shows an algorithm for the choice of method of administering oxygen. In the following text, capitalized letters refer to the letter in the algorithm.

A. The *objective of the treatment* must be defined and methods of determining the achievement of the objective outlined. If the indication for oxygen is to treat hypoxemia, it is preferable to measure PaO_2 before beginning therapy. It is acceptable practice, however, to begin therapy without measurement of PaO_2 when delay in augmenting inspired oxygen may be an unacceptable hazard for the patient. Achievement of the objective is ideally documented by measuring or remeasuring PaO_2. If there is reason to suspect that hypercapnia may result from the administration of oxygen, it is essential that both arterial carbon dioxide tension ($PaCO_2$) and PaO_2 are measured following alterations in inspired oxygen. Hypercapnia may be suspected in patients with chronic lung disease (particularly chronic bronchitis), obesity, kyphoscoliosis, central nervous system diseases such as infection or trauma, metabolic alkalosis, and in the presence of drugs that depress ventilation centrally (e.g., narcotics). However, it is unusual for $PaCO_2$ to rise with the giving of oxygen if there is not baseline hypercapnia.

It is not always possible to measure arterial blood gas tensions in patients in the emergency department. Estimates of PaO_2 can be made from ear oximetry, which measures hemoglobin saturation, from transconjunctival electrodes, or from transcutaneous electrodes. The latter technique has not been documented to be a reliable indicator in adult patients. The clinical state of the patient can also be used as a guide to the success of therapy (reversal of cyanosis, improved mental state, disappearance of cardiac arrhythmias, reduction of metabolic acidosis, and increase in urine output).

B. A *nasal cannula* has the advantages of being more comfortable for most patients and is easier to keep in place. The Venturi mask operates as a high-flow device, maintaining an inspired oxygen (FIO_2) that is close to the fraction delivered by the apparatus (FDO_2). The high flow is created by the entrainment of air with the negative pressure created by oxygen passing through a narrow orifice (Table 2).

C. A *simple oxygen mask* delivers a flow of 5 to 10 liters per minute of dry gas to the patient. The FIO_2 is lower than the FDO_2 because of the low delivered flow compared to the patient's inspired flow rates. The FIO_2 necessary to achieve a defined PaO_2 is variable. In general, in the presence of acute lung disease (e.g., acute pneumonia), hypoxemia is resistant to changes in FIO_2 owing to the presence of intrapulmonary shunting. Hypoxemia associated with chronic lung disease such as chronic bronchitis or emphysema is easily correctable by small increases in FIO_2, but may bring with it worsened hypercapnia. The FIO_2 can be increased by the use of a partial rebreathing mask. With this apparatus, the first part of the exhaled gas is collected in a plastic reservoir; this gas,

TABLE 2 Entrainment Ratio for a Set Flow of Oxygen in a Venturi Mask Oxygen Device

FDO_2*	Entrainment Ratio	Usual Set Flow (liters/minute)	Total Flow (liters/minute)
0.24	25:1	4	104
0.28	10:1	4	44
0.35	5:1	8	48
0.40	3:1	8	32

* FDO_2 is the oxygen fraction delivered to the patient.

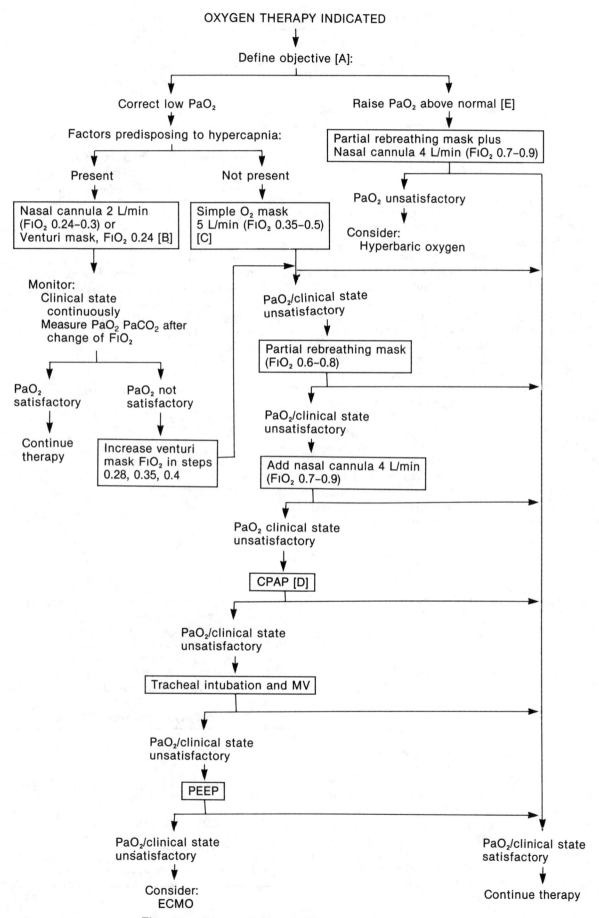

Figure 2 Algorithm for the administration of oxygen.

TABLE 3 Contents of Commonly Used Tanks of Compressed Oxygen

Size of Cylinder	Oxygen Content When Full		Pressure When Full lb/sq inch	Minutes Available When Full, With 5 Liter/Minute Flow
	Liters	Cubic Feet		
E	624	22	2,000	125
H	6,907	244	2,000	1,382

rich in oxygen but without carbon dioxide, is then rebreathed during the initial portion of the subsequent inhalation.

D. If hypoxemia persists in the presence of the maximum achievable FIO_2, continuous positive airway pressure breathing (CPAP) can be employed. This technique is difficult to maintain in a patient in whom there is no endotracheal tube present. A more reliable, but more hazardous, method for the administration of oxygen is to combine endotracheal intubation with controlled or assisted mechanical ventilation (MV). If hypoxemia persists, positive end-expiratory pressure (PEEP) should be added. Finally, if hypoxemia is resistant to these maneuvers, extracorporeal membrane oxygenation (ECMO) can be used. Although ECMO almost invariably increases PaO_2, overall survival does not seem to be increased, at least in a large study of adult patients with acute lung disease. The use of ECMO in the emergency department has been reported, but requires extensive equipment and personnel.

E. Indications for the achievement of a higher-than-usual PaO_2 are given in an earlier section. Treatment with hyperbaric oxygen within the first few hours of admission is not common, but it has been reported for the management of patients with carbon monoxide poisoning; the high oxygen achieved not only helps to correct the nonhypoxemic hypoxia, but also hastens the release of carbon monoxide from the blood. It has also been employed in the emergency treatment of air embolism.

It is important that oxygen therapy be *given continuously* and not intermittently. This is particularly important if a patient must be sent from the emergency department to the radiology department or other departments in the hospital. Before the patient is sent to another department, it must be ascertained that there is sufficient oxygen available for the duration of the test requested as well as for the return trip. Knowledge of the capacity of a tank of oxygen is essential in computing whether sufficient oxygen will be available (Table 3). When oxygen is compressed, the gas available is proportional to the pressure in the tank.

SUGGESTED READING

Bone RC, Pierce AK, Johnson RL Jr. Controlled oxygen administration in acute respiratory failure in chronic obstructive pulmonary disease. A reappraisal. Am J Med 1978; 65:896–902.

Don HF. Oxygen therapy. In: Don HF, ed. Decision making in critical care. Toronto: BC Decker, 1985:102.

Fulmer JD, Snider GL. ACCP-NHLBI national conference on oxygen therapy. Chest 1984; 86:236–247.

Gross R, Israel RH. A graphic approach for prediction of arterial oxygen tension at different concentrations of inspired oxygen. Chest 1981; 79:311–315.

TOXIC INHALATION AND BURNS

MICHAEL V. VANCE, M.D., F.A.C.E.P.

As aerobic organisms, we are forced to breathe constantly; as a result, we are at the mercy of toxic substances that may contaminate our atmosphere. When we are exposed to harmful substances in significant concentrations or for significant periods of time, illness and injury follow. These harmful substances may include specific gases, fumes, or vapors, or they may represent very complex mixtures in smoke inhalations (Table 1). Because of the large numbers of chemicals that may be involved and because the exact substances may not be known, a patient presenting with toxic inhalation poses a difficult problem for the emergency physician.

Whether damage occurs in toxic inhalation is a function of the concentration of the toxins involved and duration of exposure to the toxins. Obviously, any exposure in an enclosed space (building, room, vat, tank, pit, pipe, ditch) suggests a greater concentration, and any delay in

TABLE 1 Toxic Products of Combustion

Toxin	Source
Acrolein	Cellulose, polyolefins
Ammonia	Fabrics
Hydrogen chloride	Chlorinated acrylics, polyvinylchloride
Hydrogen cyanide	Polyacrylnitrite, polyurethane
Hydrogen fluoride	Polyfluorinated hydrocarbons
Hydrogen sulfide	Hair, hides, wools
Isocyanate	Polyurethane
Nitrogen oxides	Celluloid, fabrics
Phosgene	Chlorinated hydrocarbons, plastics
Sulfur oxides	Sulfur-containing materials

the patient's escape (including the requirement for rescue by another) indicates a prolonged exposure. In addition, patients with asthma or other chronic pulmonary disease are at greatly increased risk for the acute and delayed effects of toxic inhalations and require much closer and prolonged observation.

Despite the potential complexities, toxic inhalations produce illness and injury through only four primary mechanisms: *asphyxiation* (due to displacement or consumption of oxygen); *pulmonary injury* (due to direct thermal or chemical injury to the upper airways, lower airways, or alveoli); *hematologic toxins* (carboxyhemoglobin and methemoglobin); and *cellular toxins* (cyanide and hydrogen sulfide). These major pathophysiologic mechanisms result in abnormalities of aerobic metabolism, including impairment of oxygen supply (asphyxiation), oxygen absorption (pulmonary injury), oxygen delivery (hematologic toxins), and oxygen utilization by the cells (cellular toxins). All diagnostic and therapeutic efforts should be directed toward the evaluation and correction of abnormalities in oxygen supply and use.

PRE-HOSPITAL CARE

Pre-hospital care of any toxic inhalation is simple and straightforward. Removing the patient from exposure limits concentration and duration of exposure, although rescuer protection (including self-contained breathing apparatus) is a must. Airway and ventilatory status should be closely evaluated and artificial airway maintenance and ventilatory support should be initiated at the first sign of impairment. As the common pathophysiologic mechanisms involve oxygen deprivation, supplemental oxygen should be provided empirically in all cases of known or suspected toxic inhalations, preferably at moderate to high flow (6 to 8 L per minute or more). Because oxygen deprivation primarily affects the central nervous system and cardiovascular system, aggressive management of complications such as seizures and dysrhythmias should be initiated as soon as possible.

PATIENT ASSESSMENT

The clinical presentation of the patient in the emergency department may provide valuable information in the evaluation of victims of toxic inhalation. Because collision, explosion, or fire may be the precipitating event, burns and other associated injury may be present. Toxic inhalation should always be presumed to accompany significant burn injury, and it is in fact responsible for many more fire deaths than is actual burn injury. Particular concern is required in the patient with obvious facial burns, singed facial hair, or black carbonaceous secretions and sputum.

Early signs and symptoms suggestive of toxic inhalation include mucous membrane irritation (redness, edema, rhinorrhea, tearing) and occasionally actual skin irritation. Cough, hoarseness, and substernal chest pain (due to acute tracheitis or bronchitis) are also suggestive of pulmonary exposure. More serious problems are likely if the patient is complaining of subjective dyspnea or appears tachypneic or even cyanotic. The presence of abnormal auscultatory findings such as stridor, wheezes, or rales indicates severe pulmonary involvement.

Less obvious but perhaps more ominous signs of significant toxic inhalation may include effects on the primary target organs of oxygen deprivation: the brain and the cardiovascular system. Toxic inhalation should always be one consideration in the differential diagnosis of a patient presenting with an altered level of consciousness, seizure disorder, or hemodynamic instability. Other findings that suggest toxic inhalation are considered in the discussion of specific exposures.

EMERGENCY DEPARTMENT DIAGNOSIC TESTS

As the patient arrives in the emergency department, supportive care (oxygen, ventilatory assistance, and so on) are continued. At this point, *the single most important step* is to obtain arterial blood gases. Arterial blood gases provide virtually all the information the emergency physician needs to make a reasonable determination of the most likely pathophysiologic mechanism involved.

The Po_2 is the primary value of interest, because it indicates the current status of oxygen supply, absorption, and delivery into the blood from the lungs. If oxygen tension is lower than would be expected (depending on FIO_2), a primary pulmonary injury should be suspected, because this is the only pathophysiologic mechanism that produces persistent hypoxemia by the time the patient arrives in the emergency department. It should be particularly emphasized that oxygen tension is measured as the partial pressure of oxygen dissolved in the serum; it does not reflect the real oxygen content, which depends on the quantity and quality of hemoglobin-related oxygen transport. Thus a normal or elevated Po_2 indicates only that the supply and absorption systems are functioning well, but does not provide any information as to delivery or utilization by tissues.

The Pco_2 is the next most important value, because it indicates the status of alveolar ventilation. Naturally, if CO_2 retention is present, more aggressive means of ventilatory support should be initiated. If the Pco_2 is decreased, indicating alveolar hyperventilation, the Po_2 and pH values must be considered in relation to the level of ventilation.

The pH is the third value of concern and is particularly significant if metabolic acidosis is present. A simple asphyxiation results in metabolic acidosis, but this should be largely resolved by the time the patient arrives in the emergency department unless other complications are present (such as seizures or hypoperfusive states). Pulmonary injury should not result in metabolic acidosis unless very severe hypoxemia is present. Therefore, a persistent metabolic acidosis indicates a deficit in oxygen delivery or utilization.

At many institutions, arterial blood gases automatically include a *carboxyhemoglobin level.* If this is not the case, a carbon monoxide (CO) determination should be drawn simultaneously (carboxyhemoglobin results should be available within the same time frame as the blood gas results, because it is a simple determination that can be incorporated easily into most standard blood gas machines). A significantly elevated carboxyhemoglobin level may well be responsible for persistent neurologic and metabolic abnormalities, although careful correlation of the severity of the exposure and the clinical presentation is necessary (for example, a carboxyhemoglobin of 20 to 30 percent should not be assumed to be responsible for a persistent metabolic acidosis).

Some laboratories also automatically provide a methemoglobin level with arterial blood gases. However, this is not necessary as a screening procedure, because the typical chocolate-brown appearance of blood that has a significant methemoglobin concentration should provide adequate evidence of methemoglobinemia.

Thus the simple determination of a single diagnostic test allows for a rapid elimination process for most pathophysiologic mechanisms in toxic inhalations. An adequate Po_2 rules out the asphyxiation environment and pulmonary injury as reasons for persistent or progressive metabolic or neurologic abnormalities (assuming the patient has not suffered a severe hypoxic neurologic insult initially). The absence of a significant carboxyhemoglobin level or of chocolate-brown blood indicates (assuming a reasonable hemoglobin) a normal delivery system. Therefore, the patient with persistent metabolic acidosis or neurologic abnormalities not otherwise explained should be presumed to have a defect in oxygen utilization at the cellular level.

The only other standard diagnostic test that should be routinely performed in toxic inhalation is a chest x-ray examination. In many cases, abnormalities may be found on physical examination that warrant the study, but in many other instances it should be a baseline study, anticipating delayed pulmonary complications. Other studies (electrocardiogram, blood count, and so on) may be ordered on a case-by-case basis. However, these studies should not interfere with or delay the provision of continued supportive care and the initiation of definitive care, which will be dictated by the available history, physical examination, and arterial blood gases.

TREATMENT

The remainder of this chapter deals with specific therapies for each of the primary toxins related to the pathophysiologic mechanisms described above.

Asphyxiation Injury

Simple asphyxiation is the easiest of the "toxic inhalation" injuries to care for in the emergency department, because the severity of the injury is determined by the response of the patient to appropriate pre-hospital care. Therapy is directed toward supportive care and treatment of hypoxic encephalopathy. Generally, the ultimate outcome and need for specific therapy are determined by the condition of the patient on arrival in the emergency department. Patients arriving with intact cardiovascular activi-

ty and neurologic recovery at the treating facility have an excellent outcome with few complications. Patients who arrive with intact cardiovascular activity, but persistent neurologic impairment obviously have a much worse prognosis, and patients who arrive in persistent cardiopulmonary arrest have little chance for survival, assuming that they do not have a major component of hematologic or cellular toxin. If there is a strong suspicion that a substance such as CO or cyanide is present, empiric treatment has virtually no adverse effect on the eventual outcome but may be life-saving in some instances. (One other therapeutic consideration is the initiation of "brain resuscitation" techniques; although these techniques are controversial, the brain is the primary target organ in an asphyxiant environment and is really the only organ that is likely to suffer long-term damage in survivors.)

Pulmonary Injury

Pulmonary injury is divided into upper airway injury, lower airway injury, and alveolar injury, primarily depending on the water solubility of the chemical involved. However, very high concentrations or very long exposures to any of the typical gases or fumes may produce damage throughout the respiratory tract.

Upper airway injury results from exposure to highly water-soluble chemicals such as ammonia and chlorine. The local tissue response consists of airway edema and occasionally laryngospasm, resulting in mechanical airway impairment. Therapy is easily directed to airway maintenance by the standard techniques. Upper airway injury has a very rapid onset and rarely progresses for more than 20 to 30 minutes once the exposure is terminated. In addition, any patient who has not also experienced severe mucous membrane irritation (nose, eyes) is at virtually no risk for upper airway problems. In fact, these highly water-soluble substances are so irritating that the patient attempts to escape the environment by any means. A patient who has been trapped in such an environment and exposed for more than a few breaths is very likely to develop serious lower airway and alveolar injury as well, and should be watched very closely.

Lower airway injury results from exposure to less water-soluble substances such as sulfur oxides and nitrogen oxides. Because these gases are not as irritating, patients may tolerate much longer exposures unless very high concentrations are encountered. These patients present with chest tightness, cough, and dyspnea due to bronchial irritation; the symptoms may increase over several hours or even days as the chemical injury and tissue response progress. Most individuals develop symptoms due to increased mucous production, ciliary dysfunction, and edema of the respiratory epithelium, and sensitive individuals may experience significant bronchospasm. Therapy with aerosolized beta-agonists (terbutaline, isoetharine) is very effective at reducing the acute bronchial irritation, and severe coughing may be managed by adding 3 cc of 2 percent lidocaine to the small-volume nebulizer. Patients with true asthma may require additional bronchodilators, such as intravenous theophylline, and those with severe cases may require steroids (as any severe asthmatic). These patients require much longer periods of emergency department or in-hospital observation (6 to 12 hours) because of their increased risk of delayed-onset alveolar injury.

Alveolar injury results from exposure to substances with very low water solubility (or prolonged exposure to highly and moderately water-soluble substances, but with a much more rapid onset), usually with a delay in onset of symptoms of 24 hours or more. (Classic examples are phosgene and nitrogen dioxide.) Alveolar injury develops due to two primary mechanisms.

The first is a chemical injury to the type I alveolar (squamous) cells, which results in increased permeability of the alveolocapillary membrane. As serum, plasma, and even cellular components escape from the pulmonary vasculature into the alveoli, the clinical and x-ray pictures look exactly like pulmonary edema in congestive heart failure. However, this must be recognized as true *noncardiogenic pulmonary edema,* because the pathologic process is increased alveolocapillary permeability instead of increased pulmonary vascular pressures. The treatment of choice for noncardiogenic pulmonary edema is high-flow oxygen, positive pressure ventilation if necessary, and adjuncts such as positive end expiratory pressure (PEEP) in severe or refractory cases. The use of standard therapeutic modalities for *cardiogenic pulmonary edema* (such as morphine and furosemide) for preload reduction is effective and inappropriate.

The second mechanism of alveolar injury is chemical injury to type II alveolar (cuboidal) cells, which leads to gradual and progressive depletion of surfactant production and activity (as well as other local effects). This results in local alveolar and small airway collapse and the other classic changes associated with the development of the adult respiratory distress syndrome (ARDS). Although ARDS is a condition that requires long-term therapy and is beyond the scope of this chapter, it is important for the emergency physician to be aware of this potential in a toxic inhalation exposure, because it may be necessary either to admit patients for observation or to recognize ARDS if the patient presents 24 to 48 hours after an exposure.

To summarize the pulmonary injury mechanism, the emergency physician must be attuned to the common early presentations of highly water-soluble and irritating exposures such as chlorine, but must also anticipate the delayed presentations of the more insidious chemicals and provide for appropriate observation and follow-up.

HEMATOLOGIC TOXINS

Carbon monoxide is without a doubt the single most important substance encountered in the evaluation and treatment of toxic inhalations. It is always a component of any smoke inhalation incident and is a common culprit in many residential and industrial exposures. Carbon monoxide produces injury by two primary mechanisms: its strong affinity for hemoglobin reduces the oxygen-carrying capacity of the blood, and it interferes with normal aerobic metabolism at the cellular level. This latter effect is frequently not well appreciated but is actually the primary mechanism responsible for the neurologic and other tissue injury associated with both acute and chronic carbon monoxide poisoning.

The clinical presentation of CO poisoning is related to the effects of oxygen deprivation (both supply and utilization) on the organ systems most susceptible: the central nervous system and the cardiovascular system. Toxicity correlates reasonably well with carboxyhemoglobin levels in acute exposures, but poorly in chronic or recurrent, subacute poisoning (Table 2).

Carbon monoxide is a competitive inhibitor of oxygen at carrier and metabolic sites. Because it has a much higher affinity at these sites than does oxygen, the treatment is directed at saturating the system with an excess of oxygen molecules. The standard treatment of choice is to provide 100 percent oxygen with a tight-fitting non-rebreathing mask. This markedly enhances the elimination of carbon monoxide, reducing the half-life to 60 to 90 minutes from the usual 4 to 5 hours on room air. Serial carboxyhemoglobin levels should be monitored along with clinical condition to evaluate response to therapy. In no case should oxygen administration be delayed while waiting for carboxyhemoglobin levels to return from the laboratory.

Patients who have extremely high (above 50 to 60 percent) carboxyhemoglobin levels or who show severe or persistent neurologic effects benefit from treatment with *hyperbaric oxygen.* All emergency physicians should be aware of hyperbaric facilities available to them and have a transfer plan at hand. There is no doubt that hyperbaric oxygen may be life-saving in acute carbon monoxide poisoning, and there is some evidence that it may reduce the neurologic sequelae of chronic and subactue exposures as well.

Methemoglobin represents the other hematologic toxin produced by toxic inhalations. It is formed by substances that can oxidize normal ferrous (Fe^{2+}) iron in hemoglobin to ferric (Fe^{3+} (methemoglobin), which cannot carry oxygen. Thus methemoglobinemia is a true hematologic toxin, one whose only biologic effect is to decrease oxygen delivery to the cells.

In addition to the typical chocolate-brown color of methemoglobin, this condition may also be identified by the cyanotic appearance of the patient at even low levels (10 to 20 percent) of methemoglobin. Because the patient retains most of his oxygen-carrying capacity, these cyanotic patients are surprisingly free of typical hypoxic symptoms, and the cyanosis does not respond to oxygen administration as would be expected in true desaturated but normal ferrous hemoglobin. Because there is no tissue toxicity except that related to decreased oxygen delivery, it requires higher levels of methemoglobin to produce clinical symptoms: headache, nausea, and dizziness may occur with 20 to 30 percent methemoglobin; tachycardia, dyspnea, and syncope usually require 40 to 60 percent; severe effects (seizures, coma, death) typically require very high levels (up to 70 to 80 percent).

Treatment is initially supportive and, of course, in-

TABLE 2   Carbon Monoxide Levels and Symptoms

Severity of Poisoning	Level	Symptoms
Mild	15–25 %	Headache, nausea, dizziness
Moderate	30–40 %	Dyspnea, tachycardia, syncope
Severe	≥ 50 %	Seizure, coma, cardiovascular collapse, death

cludes high-flow oxygen because of the cyanotic appearance of the patient. The body has a normal enzymatic pathway, methemoglobin reductase, that converts the ferric iron of methemoglobin back to normal ferrous hemoglobin. However, this reaction proceeds very slowly unless a catalyst is provided in the form of methylene blue. In patients with significant symptoms related to cellular oxygen deprivation, methylene blue may be administered as a slow intravenous dose (1 mg per kilogram over 5 to 10 minutes), and doses may be repeated hourly until improvement is noted. It is *extremely* important to ensure proper administration, because if methylene blue is given too rapidly or in too high a dose, it may produce additional methemoglobin and may prove to be fatal, especially in children.

CELLULAR TOXINS

Cyanide represents the classic cellular toxin. It may be encountered as a cyanide salt, but in toxic inhalations cyanide poisoning results from the combustion of cyanogenic substances such as polyurethane (from insulating foams that are polymers of organic isocyanates). Hydrogen cyanide gas is, of course, easily absorbed by the respiratory tract and rapidly diffuses into all body tissues. At the cellular level, it combines with ferric iron in the cytochrome oxidase system, effectively inhibiting normal electron transport and adenosine triphosphate production. Thus it is known as a cellular asphyxiant, capable of bringing normal aerobic metabolism to a sudden halt.

Exposure to cyanide is usually assumed to be rapidly fatal, although the severity of symptoms depends on the concentration, duration of exposure, and extent of interference with normal cellular metabolism. Signs and symptoms are indistinguishable from the usual effects of hypoxia on the central nervous system and the cardiovascular system, but the level of metabolic acidosis is usually much greater than in the syndromes previously described. Many references emphasize the importance of the aroma of "bitter almonds" in the diagnosis of cyanide poisoning, but less than half of the general population has the genetically determined ability to sense that particular odor.

The treatment of cyanide poisoning is very simple once the diagnosis is known or suspected. However, it is important that the emergency physician maintain a high index of suspicion of a cellular toxin such as cyanide in patients who present with a persistent metabolic acidosis and neurologic or cardiovascular effects that cannot be explained by any of the previously described pathophysiologic mechanisms (asphyxiation, pulmonary injury, or hematologic toxins). Although a number of alternatives have been described, the treatment of cyanide poisoning is still most effectively accomplished by the use of the Lilly Cyanide Antidote Kit (see chapter on *Antidotes in Poisoning*).

Hydrogen sulfide is the other cellular toxin that is commonly encountered in toxic inhalations. It may be encountered in any situation in which sulfur products are involved, especially in any sewage tank or sewer pipe exposure. Hydrogen sulfide is especially dangerous because although virtually everybody can detect a low concentration of "sewer gas" or "rotten egg" odor, concentrations above 150 ppm result in olfactory fatigue, or loss of ability to sense the presence of dangerous levels.

Hydrogen sulfide is just like cyanide in that it combines with ferric iron in cytochrome oxidase and paralyzes cellular respiration. A single exposure to 1,000 ppm ("one-breath knockdown") may affect cortical function to the point at which escape is impossible, and subsequent prolonged contact is rapidly fatal. However, lesser concentrations produce the typical wide range of clinical symptoms, and its water solubility results in mucous membrane and even pulmonary injury as does any typical, water-soluble inhalation toxin.

Because hydrogen sulfide has a pathophysiologic mechanism similar to that of cyanide, it stands to reason that the treatment should follow the same approach: induction of methemoglobinemia to pull the active sulfide groups out of the cellular sites. However, most clinical experience suggests that nitrite therapy is effective only if used in the immediate postexposure phase, and treatment is questionable at best if there is any delay in transporting the patient to the emergency department. In addition, if sodium nitrite is given, subsequent use of the sodium thiosulfate in the Lilly Cyanide Antidote Kit is contraindicated, because the sulfmethemoglobin formed by nitrite therapy is rapidly metabolized naturally without chemical adjuncts.

DISPOSITION

One of the most difficult decisions for the emergency physician in the evaluation and management of toxic inhalations relates to the length of observation in the emergency department or the necessity of admission. Obviously, any patient with progressive pulmonary, neurologic, or cardiovascular dysfunction requires admission, usually to an intensive care unit. At the same time, patients who have no initial or progressive symptoms, but who present for evaluation of possible exposure can be managed as outpatients in almost every situation. The decision to observe or to admit is otherwise dependent on the pathophysiologic mechanisms involved, the severity of initial symptoms, and the response to treatment.

Victims of simple asphyxiation who regain consciousness at the scene usually do not require any prolonged care following initial supportive measures, assuming that no underlying organ damage (myocardial injury, for example) has occurred owing to preexistent risk factors. Patients exposed to highly water-soluble substances tend to develop their injury within a few hours and progressively improve. It is extremely unlikely that any late complications will develop except in those individuals with significant underlying chronic pulmonary disease. On the other hand, patients exposed to moderately or poorly water-soluble substances (Table 3) have a high risk of late complications such as noncardiogenic pulmonary edema and ARDS. Patients with a history of high concentration or prolonged duration of exposure to these substances, or who have significant mucous membrane irritation *shortly* after exposure, should usually be hospitalized for 24 to 48 hours for close observation of delayed complica-

TABLE 3 Delayed Symptoms

Chemical	Reaction
Hydrogen fluoride	Gradual fluoride ion effect
Nitrogen oxides	Conversion to nitric acid
Phosgene	Conversion to hydrochloric acid
Phosphorus oxides	Conversion to phosphoric acid
Sulfur dioxide	Conversion to sulfuric acid

tions. Patients with exposures to hematologic toxins or cellular toxins require observation or admission only if the complications of organ-system hypoxic insult require continued treatment. Assuming there is no reason to suspect further exposure, mild to moderate exposures can usually be treated entirely in the emergency setting, and severe poisoning almost always results in complications requiring prolonged hospitalization.

PLEURAL EFFUSION

STEPHEN L. ADAMS, M.D.

A pleural effusion is an abnormal accumulation of fluid in the pleural space. It may be indicative of intrathoracic, extrathoracic, or systemic disease. The fluid accumulation may be attributable to mechanical factors such as changes in hydrostatic or oncotic pressures (transudation), or to inflammatory factors causing changes in the permeability of the pleura (exudation).

The causes of pleural effusions are many. Some of the causes of transudative effusions include congestive heart failure, cirrhosis with ascites, and nephrotic syndrome; causes of exudative effusions include neoplasm and infection (Table 1). Massive pleural effusions are most commonly caused by malignancies, in particular lung and breast carcinomas.

The patient with a pleural effusion may present with pleuritic chest pain, shortness of breath, chest tightness, or other symptoms related to the pleura. He may also present with systemic or extrapleural disease and have no symptoms referable to the pleura. The signs of pleural effusion may include an increased respiratory rate, decreased breath sounds, dullness to percussion, decreased fremitus, and a pleural friction rub.

DIAGNOSIS

The diagnosis of a pleural effusion is made most often by *chest radiograph*. Chest roentgenogram, posteroanterior and lateral views, will reveal as little as 250 to 600 ml of fluid. Blunting of the costophrenic angle is the most common observation. A lateral decubitus film will reveal as little as 5 to 50 ml, and by use of ultrasound as little as 3 to 5 ml of fluid may be discerned.

An attempt to diagnose the cause of a pleural effusion may be assisted by the evaluation of the fluid removed from the pleural space by thoracentesis. Thoracentesis is

TABLE 1 Common Causes of Pleural Effusions

Transudates
  Congestive heart failure
  Cirrhosis with ascites
  Nephrotic syndrome
  Hypoproteinemia
  Myxedema

Exudates
  Neoplasm
  Infection (tuberculosis, bacterial, viral, fungal)
  Connective tissue disease
  Pulmonary embolus
  Pancreatitis
  Lymphatic disease
  Uremia

also used as a therapeutic procedure to remove fluid from the pleural space when its accumulation causes respiratory embarrassment.

A thoracentesis is usually performed in the area of the posterior thorax, mid-scapular line; the exact location is determined by radiographic evidence of fluid and evidence of dullness to percussion in the area. The lowest level that should be entered for thoracentesis is the eighth intercostal space. After preparing the area of thoracentesis, local anesthesia is applied. A needle is inserted over the rib (to avoid the intercostal vessels and nerves that run beneath the rib) into the pleura and fluid is removed. Unless respiratory embarrassment is present, about 50 to 100 ml should be removed for diagnostic evaluation. The fluid is then analyzed for causes of the pleural effusion.

Errors and complications that may occur during thoracentesis include the following:

1. "Dry tap." This is due to a lack of fluid in the area tapped, either because a lateral decubitus film to document fluid movement was not obtained, or because the wrong intercostal space was entered.
2. Bleeding. This may be attributable to an injury to the lung or intercostal vessels as a result of the procedure, or as a result of abnormal coagulation parameters.
3. Unilateral pulmonary edema. This has been reported as a result of removing too much fluid too rapidly from an area of massive pleural effusion. Some authors recommend that the quantity of any pleural fluid aspiration be limited to less than 1,500 ml on any one occasion, and to 1,000 ml if there is any indication that the effusion has been present for more than one week.
4. "Pleural shock." This has been attributed to a vasovagal response during the procedure.
5. Air embolism.
6. Pneumothorax.
7. Infection.
8. Hypoxemia. This appears predictably following thoracentesis, is usually self-limited, and rarely attains clinical significance. The degree of hypoxemia appears to be related to the volume of aspirate removed. In one study, the Po_2 was reported to decrease from 5 to 18 mm Hg. This may not be seen immediately, but is usually apparent from 20 minutes to 2 hours after the procedure and usually resolves within 24 hours. The cause is unclear, but has been postulated to be due to a worsened ventilation-perfusion mismatch in areas of the re-expanded lung with the resumption of perfusion and inadequate ventilation. Oxygen administration may be indicated in patients with limited pulmonary reserve.
9. Hemoperitoneum. This is a result of the puncture of the liver or the spleen through the diaphragm.

Relative contraindications to thoracentesis include mechanical or manual ventilation, as either may be associated with a tension pneumothorax following inadvertent lung puncture. Others are bleeding disorders, which should be corrected before attempting a thoracentesis, and a ruptured diaphragm.

After fluid has been removed, appropriate diagnostic tests may be obtained (Table 2). The diagnostic tests performed will depend on the clinical picture. In the initial evaluation it is important to distinguish between a transudate and an exudate, as this will help the clinician assess the cause of the effusion.

Analysis of the fluid to determine whether the cause of the effusion is a transudate or an exudate should include specific gravity, concurrent serum and pleural fluid LDH, and concurrent serum and pleural fluid protein tests. If the specific gravity of the pleural fluid is greater than 1.016, or the protein level exceeds 3.0 g per 100 ml, then the fluid has classically been described as an exudate. More recently it has been shown that if the following criteria are met, the fluid is considered to be exudative: (1) pleural fluid to serum protein ratio >0.5; (2) pleural fluid LDH >200 IU; (3) pleural fluid to serum LDH ratio >0.6. Most exudates have at least one of these three characteristics, and very few transudates meet any of these criteria. No single test is diagnostic.

Other pleural fluid diagnostic tests that may be helpful in determining the cause of an effusion include those listed below:

1. Glucose. A low value relative to the serum may be seen in rheumatoid arthritis, tuberculosis, empyema, and malignancy.
2. Complete cell count with differential. A white cell count of greater than 10,000 per cubic millimeter is most commonly seen in parapneumonic effusions, but may also be seen in other conditions. Grossly bloody pleural effusions will have red cell counts above 100,000 per cubic millimeter. This is suggestive of

TABLE 2 Laboratory Tests Useful in Evaluating Pleural Effusions

Specific gravity
Protein
LDH (lactate dehydrogenase)
Glucose
Complete cell count with differential
Culture and sensitivity
  Aerobes
  Anaerobes
  Acid-fast bacillus
  Fungus
Stains and smears
  Gram stain
  AFB smear
  Other
pH
Cytology
Others
  Complement
  Rheumatoid factor
  Antinuclear antibody

trauma, malignancy, or pulmonary embolus. A differential of greater than 50 percent lymphocytes may be seen with tuberculosis or lymphoma.

3. Culture and sensitivity. These may include aerobes, anaerobes, acid-fast bacilli (AFB), and fungal cultures.
4. Smears and stains. These may include Gram stain, AFB smear, India ink preparation and direct fluorescent antibody (DFA) for *Legionella*.
5. Cytology. Pathologic evaluation of the fluid may be diagnostic for various neoplasms.
6. Amylase. This may be elevated if pancreatitis is the cause of the effusion. It may also be elevated in a rupture of the esophagus.
7. pH. This may be useful in distinguishing between an empyema or parapneumonic effusion that requires tube thoracostomy drainage and a parapneumonic effusion that will resolve without drainage. A pH of less than 7.30 may indicate the need for drainage, whereas a pH of greater than 7.30 is generally seen in a benign parapneumonic effusion.
8. Complement levels, rheumatoid factor, antinuclear antibody. These may be helpful in evaluating connective tissue diseases.

The physician should not discard the excess pleural fluid but rather save it, as further diagnostic uses for it may emerge as results of laboratory studies are evaluated.

TREATMENT

Appropriate therapy is dictated by the patient's clinical condition. Oxygen therapy may be warranted. Therapeutic thoracentesis may be indicated if the amount of fluid causes respiratory embarrassment. Appropriate antibiotics are indicated if the effusion is thought to be due to an infection. A therapeutic tube thoracostomy may be indicated if the pleural fluid is due to an empyema. Pleural biopsy may be indicated in the further evaluation of the pleural effusion.

A patient who has undergone a diagnostic thoracentesis with no complications should be observed for a period of time (2 hours may be reasonable). A post-procedure chest radiograph should be obtained to exclude the presence of a pneumothorax.

SUGGESTED READING

Black LF. The pleural space and pleural fluid. Mayo Clin Proc 1972; 47:493–506.

Brandstetter RD, Cohen RP. Hypoxemia after thoracentesis. JAMA 1979; 242:1060–1061.

Light RW, Macgregor MI, Luchsinger PC, et al. Pleural effusions: the diagnostic separation of transudates and exudates. Ann Intern Med 1972; 77:507–513.

Ross DS: Thoracentesis. In: Roberts J, Hedges J, eds. Clinical procedures in emergency medicine. Philadelphia: WB Saunders, 1985: 84–98.

Sahebjami H, Loudon RG. Pleural effusion: pathophysiology and clinical features. Semin Roentgenol 1977; XII:269–275.

Storey DD, Dines DE, Coles DT. Pleural effusion: a diagnostic dilemma. JAMA 1976; 236:2183–2186.

Trapnell DH, Thurston JGB. Unilateral pulmonary oedema after pleural aspiration. Lancet 1970; 1:1367–1369.

HEMOPTYSIS

LAURENS R. PICKARD, M.D., F.A.C.S.
KENNETH L. MATTOX, M.D., F.A.C.S.

Hemoptysis presents three considerations to the clinician which require immediate attention. The first is the possibility of evolving or imminent cardiorespiratory embarrassment, which can occur with massive hemoptysis as a result of airway compromise from blood and/or blood clots. The second is establishing a diagnosis, which is necessary early in the event it is of an infectious nature. The third is localization of the bleeding site, so the surgeon will know what area to be prepared to resect if emergency pulmonary resection becomes necessary.

EVALUATION

In evaluating the patient with hemoptysis, answers should be sought to the following questions: (1) Does the patient truly have hemoptysis? (2) Is there frank, massive hemoptysis or merely blood-streaked sputum? (3) What is the volume per unit time of expectoration? (4) Is there any associated upper respiratory tract bleeding?

(5) Is there any coagulation abnormality? (6) Is there any history of acute upper respiratory tract infection, smoking, or other relevant medical history? (7) Can the patient locate the site of hemoptysis?

The causes of hemoptysis can be grouped into six categories (Table 1). The most common causes in patients under the age of 40 are cardiovascular disease, tuberculosis, foreign bodies, and bronchiectasis. Over the age of 40, neoplasms and lung abscesses become prominent causes in addition to the causes seen in the younger age group. The particular type of infection varies according to geographic location, ethnic concentration, and patient groups seen at a given institution. Tuberculosis has been reported to be the most common cause of massive hemoptysis. An increasingly common cause of hemoptysis is pulmonary hemorrhage associated with balloon flotation catheters. Only 5 percent of cases are idiopathic.

An underlying condition exists in 90 percent of patients with hemoptysis. One should pursue any history of thrombophlebitis, exposure to tuberculosis, chronic or recurrent bronchitis, past or present cigarette smoking, and personal and family history of bleeding disorders. It is essential to be aware of any medications that the patient is taking, especially anticoagulants or any platelet inactivating drugs, and these should be specifically asked about.

DIAGNOSIS

Physical Examination

One should note the characters, duration, and volume of the bleeding as thoroughly as possible. An oral or nasal source of bleeding should be ruled out by examination. At times it may be difficult to distinguish between true hemoptysis and the aspiration of vomited blood from upper gastrointestinal tract bleeding or swallowed blood from epistaxis. Blood in patients with true hemoptysis is usually bright red and frothy, whereas blood from the stomach is usually darker and may be mixed with food. The bloody material can be tested for pH; sputum is generally alkaline, and gastric contents acidic. Hemoptysis is almost invariably accompanied by vigorous coughing; gastrointestinal bleeding usually has an antecedent history of gastrointestinal symptoms. The patient with hemop-

TABLE 1 Categories of Causes of Hemoptysis

Trauma and Foreign Bodies
 Lung contusion, tracheobronchial trauma

Cardiovascular Lesions
 Arteriovenous malformations, congenital heart disease, pulmonary hypertension pulmonary edema, pulmonary infarction

Inflammations and Infections
 Bronchiectasis, bronchitis, lung abscess, mycetoma, pneumonia, tuberculosis, polyarteritis nodosa, parasites

Blood Dyscrasias

Mass Lesions
 Granulomas, carcinoma, others

Idiopathic

tysis will often prefer to lie "on the bleeding lung," that is, with the lung from which the bleeding is originating in a dependent position. Occasionally, patients will have an accurate impression of which side of the chest is bleeding and the general location of the bleeding site within the chest. Physical examination may reveal signs of consolidation of the abnormal lung from which the bleeding is originating and rales and rhonchi may also be present. There is often a "spillover" of blood into the opposite lung which may produce abnormal physical findings on the contralateral side; this may make localization on the basis of physical findings impossible. Clubbing may be present in patients with chronic lung disease and pulmonary neoplasms. If thrombophlebitis is present, one may suspect the development of a pulmonary embolism causing hemoptysis. Cardiac examination may reveal abnormalities that may establish a cardiovascular basis for the hemoptysis, such as the murmur of mitral stenosis.

Sputum Examination

Examination of the sputum is fundamental. Gross blood is often seen with infectious conditions. Acid-fast smears should be performed immediately, since tuberculosis may be the diagnosis; antituberculous treatment should be started as soon as possible, and the patient should be appropriately isolated. Many patients with tuberculosis will need no specific therapy for the hemoptysis per se. Specimens should also be submitted for cytopathologic studies.

Laboratory Examinations

Coagulation studies should be performed, including the basic screening tests of prothrombin time, partial thromboplastin time, and platelet count. Other relevant laboratory examinations include serum lactic dehydrogenase which, when elevated in the presence of a normal SGOT, is suggestive of pulmonary infarction. An elevated white blood cell count suggests infections, and the hemoglobin and/or hematocrit may indicate the extent of the bleeding and may reflect any chronic disease state. Routine cultures of the sputum and cultures for fungi and acid-fast organisms should be done at the time of the initial examination.

Roentgenogram

The chest roentgenogram may reveal evidence of cardiovascular disease, such as an abnormal cardiac silhouette and aneurysms; compression of the trachea or main stem bronchi; or primary pulmonary pathologic changes, such as neoplasms, infiltrates, cavities, and foreign bodies. The finding of a single lesion or abnormality, however, does not guarantee that the bleeding is from this site. An infiltrate may be due to aspirated blood from an occult cause that will not produce an abnormality on the plain chest x-ray film itself. Chest tomograms may pinpoint specific disease processes more accurately than the plain chest x-ray film. Pulmonary angiography and selective bronchial artery catheterization can pinpoint bleeding sites in the lung under special circumstances, and in certain patients, vessels supplying the bleeding sites can be occluded with autologous clot, or occluding or clot-producing devices or materials.

Bronchoscopy

It is important to consider the need for bronchoscopy early in the patient's evaluation for several reasons. Patients will often stop bleeding spontaneously after an initial episode of hemoptysis, and it is advantageous to carry out the bronchoscopy while the bleeding is still active so that the endoscopist can localize the site of bleeding. If the bleeding has stopped, the bronchoscopy will be helpful to remove any residual blood in the tracheobronchial tree and to identify any visible lesions. Definitive localization may not be possible. It has been noted on many occasions that bronchoscopy may be "therapeutic" in that bleeding will often stop during bronchoscopy. Various bronchoscopic techniques have been described for clearing the airway of blood and tamponading bleeding at the level of the main stem, lobar, and segmental bronchi.

MANAGEMENT AND TREATMENT

Management

The patient presenting to the emergency department with massive, life-threatening hemoptysis requires minimal work-up prior to therapeutic intervention. This includes an expeditious history and physical examination, arterial blood gases, complete blood count, blood urea nitrogen, urinalysis, prothrombin time, partial thromboplastin time, posteroanterior and lateral chest roentgenogram, type and cross-match for blood, and, if necessary, transfer to a facility where both flexible and rigid, "open tube" bronchoscopy can be performed. Bronchoscopy should be performed as soon as possible to control the airway and localize the origin of the bleeding.

Treatment

The optimal work-up for the patient with nonmassive or non-life-threatening hemoptysis includes sequential steps as illustrated in the algorithm (Fig. 1). The emergency department physician should approach these patients with an eye toward concomitant airway control, establishment of cause, localization, and specific therapy as soon as possible (Table 2). If the bleeding site is known, the patient should be placed with the bleeding site in a dependent position. This will help prevent "spillover" and protect the normal lung. Cough suppressant medications such as codeine should be prescribed. Sedation may result in decreased pulmonary artery and bronchial artery pressures and a decrease in the bleeding may result. However, one should be careful not to oversedate a patient and oversuppress a cough reflex. The patient with sputum positive for acid-fast bacilli on initial acid-fast smears should immediately begin to receive antituberculous chemotherapy. Antimicrobial therapy directed toward the treatment of bronchitis should be started at once in patients with clinical evidence of bacterial infections. Patients with penetrating injuries of the lungs resulting in pneumothorax and hemoptysis will often stop coughing up blood after a chest tube has been placed and the lung is reexpanded appropriately. Patients with pulmonary edema should be treated for this accordingly. Use of endotracheal intubation and assisted ventilation should be based on the usual criteria used for respiratory failure. Blood transfusions should be administered according to the usual guidelines. One should recall again, however, that the usual immediate threat to life is airway compromise from the sheer physical presence of the obstructing blood in the airway, rather than major blood loss.

Consultations. Immediate consultation with both pulmonary specialists and thoracic surgeons is appropriate for the patient with life-threatening hemoptysis. Indications for urgent operation include life-threatening hemoptysis and situations in which airway compromise is imminent. Contraindications to pulmonary resection include poor pulmonary function, evidence of an inoperable pulmonary tumor, poor general medical condition, grossly abnormal coagulation, and evidence of extensive metastatic disease from a malignant lesion. Patients with massive hemoptysis should undergo immediate resection upon localization of the bleeding site, provided of course that there are no contraindications.

Methods of Airway Control. Methods of airway control start with suction assisted ventilation and traditional endotracheal intubation and include the use of special double-lumen endotracheal tubes, selective intubation of the main stem bronchus on the side that is not bleeding, the use of tamponading balloon catheters, and bronchial packing. Balloon catheters used to tamponade a bronchus require placement during bronchoscopy with an open-tube, rigid bronchoscope. Rarely, in patients in whom an airway cannot be maintained due to severe hemorrhage, cardiopulmonary bypass may be considered as an adjunct to definitive therapy. Patients who develop hemoptysis from a pulmonary vascular injury caused by a pulmonary artery catheter may require a thoracotomy and pulmonary resection.

In patients in whom operation is contraindicated some other modalities may be helpful, including tamponade of the bleeding area with endoscopic packing of the bronchus, closure of the bronchus through a thoracotomy without a resection, and ligation or embolization of a pulmonary or bronchial artery and percutaneous drainage of pulmonary cavities such as those seen with *Aspergillus* infections. A new tool that is becoming an extremely effective mode of therapy for severe hemoptysis from tracheal and bronchial tumors is laser photoradiation. Referral to a surgeon or pulmonary internist who is involved with laser treatment of airway lesions should be sought for patients in whom operation is contraindicated.

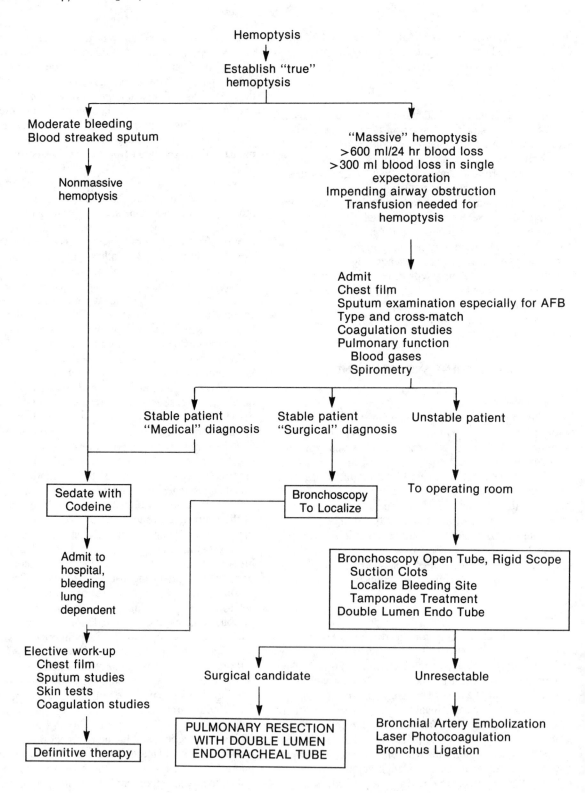

Figure 1 Algorithm for decision-making in treatment of hemoptysis.

TABLE 2 Some Causes of Hemoptysis with Supportive History, Physical Findings, Evaluation, and Treatment

Cause	History	Physical Examination	Diagnostic Studies	Treatment
Mitral stenosis	Dyspnea, fatigue	Dependent edema, heart murmur	Chest x-ray film, ECG, echocardiogram, cardiac catheterization	Salt restriction, diuretics, etc, mitral valve operation if indicated
Pulmonary infarction (pulmonary embolus)	Postoperative patient, phlebitis, pleuritic chest pain, shortness of breath	Phlebitis, cyanosis, hypotension	Hypoxemia, LDH, positive lung scan, or pulmonary arteriogram	Supportive, with O₂ supplement; no anti-coagulants; caval inter-ruption may be indicated
Infection	Fever, other constitutional symptoms	Rales, consolidation	Sputum examination, culture, chest x-ray film	Antimicrobial therapy, isolation
Carcinoma	Weight loss, smoking	Consolidation, lymphadeno-pathy, neurologic signs, clubbing	Chest x-ray film, tomograms sputum cytopathology bronchoscopy	Pulmonary resection, laser, bronchial artery embolization
Foreign bodies	Sudden dyspnea, wheezing, stridor, cough	Stridor, wheezing, may be localized	Chest x-ray film	Bronchoscopy, occasionally thoracotomy
Coagulopathy	History of coagulation disorder, chemotherapy, anticoagulant therapy	Petechia, purpura	Coagulation profile	Specific therapy for coagulation defect

SUGGESTED READING

Bobrowitz ID, Ramakrishna S, Shim YS. Comparison of medical vs surgical treatment of major hemoptysis. Arch Intern med 1983; 143:1343–1346.

Edmondstone WM, Nanson EM, Woodcock AA, Milland FJC, Hetzel MR. Life-threatening hemoptysis controlled by laser photocoagulation. Thorax 1983; 38: 788–789.

Feloney JP, Balchum OJ. Repeated massive hemoptysis—successful control using multiple balloon-tipped catheters for endobronchial tamponade. Chest 1978; 74: 683–685.

McElvein RB, Zorn G. Treatment of malignant disease in trachea and main stem bronchi by carbon dioxide laser. J Thorac Cardiovasc Surg. 1983; 86:858–863.

Sebhat S, Oreizie M, Moinedine K. Massive pulmonary hemorrhage: surgical approach as choice of treatment. Ann Thorac Surg 1978; 25: 12–15.

Wholey MH, Chamarro HA, Rao G, Ford WB, Miller WH. Bronchial artery embolization for massive hemoptysis. JAMA 1976; 263:2501.

MEDIASTINAL AND PARENCHYMAL LUNG MASSES

PHILIP C. GOODMAN, M.D.

A chest roentgenogram demonstrating a mediastinal or pulmonary mass always generates excitement because of its dramatic visual appearance. And yet in the emergency department, as elsewhere, there is in almost all instances no need to hurry the evaluation of the lesion.

In some patients, clinical signs or symptoms may direct a search for a particular mass, as in patients with myasthenia gravis and thymomas or patients with weight loss and bronchogenic carcinoma. In other patients, the finding of a mass is purely incidental and unexpected. In any case, the radiologic work-up of a mass is directed at determining the nature of the lesion and, in particular, whether the lesion is benign or malignant. In this regard, the radiologic evaluation of mediastinal or pulmonary masses should proceed along fairly well-established paths. For the sake of clarity in the following discussion, the routine for investigating masses in each of these areas is discussed separately.

MEDIASTINAL MASSES

A mediastinal mass should be suspected when there is distortion or enlargement of the normal contours of this compartment. The concept of a 'large mediastinum'' is one that is firmly implanted in the mind of anyone who attempts to interpret chest films, yet there are no universally accepted measurements to define what is large. Instead, one should become familiar with the normal left and right silhouettes of the mediastinum so that alterations in the contour of these interfaces with lung are appreciated. Thus, on the left in a craniad to caudad direction, the usual structures that create the roentgenographic mediastinum are spine, left subclavian artery, aortic arch, aortopulmonary window, main pulmonary artery, left atrium, and left ventricle. Each of these regions has a common convex or concave orientation with adjacent lung. A change in the usual shape warrants an explanation. If, for example, the normally concave aortopulmonic window becomes straight or convex, an underlying mediastinal mass, such as an enlarged lymph node, should be suspected regardless of whether there is an impression of a "large mediastinum." Conversely, the aortic arch may become ectatic and tortuous, appearing "large" on the chest film, yet if positioned normally with a usual rounded and well-defined edge, this atherosclerotic change should not be construed as evidence of a mediastinal mass. The sophisticated observer may take time to learn some of the other less commonly appreciated normal radiographic anatomy (e.g., anterior and posterior mediastinal lines, aortopulmonic line, azygoesophageal recess), and be prepared to diagnose more subtle mediastinal abnormalities.

Since the advent of computed tomography, the workup of suspected mediastinal lesions has been simplified. Unless otherwise dictated by compelling clinical findings, a CT scan is the first and often last radiographic procedure required to diagnose or direct the diagnosis of such abnormalities. Computed tomography has distinct advantages over other forms of investigation. It is relatively noninvasive (intravenous iodinated contrast material is generally administered prior to scanning), provides excellent anatomic information regarding location and extent of the mass, and permits a preliminary assessment as to the nature of the lesion by densitometric analysis. For instance, a teratoma may be strongly suspected if fat and bone are seen in a characteristically positioned anterior mediastinal lesion. In this regard, CT is far superior and much more sensitive than conventional chest roentgenograms. Vascular anomalies such as coarctation of the aorta or acquired vascular lesions such as aortic aneurysms or dissections may be diagnosed without the need for angiography. The enhanced contrast-resolving potential of CT permits easy demonstration of entities such as mediastinal lipomatosis and bronchogenic cysts. If a precise answer as to the nature of a mediastinal mass is not possible, CT provides a road map that can guide percutaneous or direct visual biopsy of the lesion. Along this line is the increasing use of CT to guide the appropriate mediastinoscopic approach for lymph node biopsy during the staging of bronchogenic carcinoma.

Angiography of the great vessels of the mediastinum may be performed conventionally or with digital subtraction technique and may be required in certain complex vascular anomalies. The diagnosis of traumatic rupture of the aorta should only be attempted by angiography. CT is not the appropriate modality for this situation!

Current investigation into the value of *magnetic resonance* for mediastinal imaging suggest that this new modality may in time supplant CT from its primary diagnostic role. MRI is totally noninvasive (no contrast material is necessary) and is extremely accurate in discerning mediastinal vascular and cardiac anatomy. At present it suffers from poorer spatial resolution than CT, from the lack of availability, and from certain other features such as the inability of MRI to detect calcium as a unique density.

PULMONARY MASSES

Pulmonary masses, benign or malignant, are often asymptomatic. Their discovery comes frequently as a surprise that provokes significant consternation in both clinician and patient. An orderly approach to diagnosis follows a few tested directions, the ultimate path being determined by various patient parameters (e.g., underlying COPD or heart disease, age, operability).

Perhaps the most important thing to do subsequent to finding a lung nodule or mass is to make a careful, exhaustive search for old films. It has often been my experience that primary physician and radiologist alike would prefer to perform a CT, biopsy, or operate on these lesions rather than telephone, write, or drive to the patient's other hospital or doctor's office in order to procure prior films. From both medical and economic standpoints, it makes sense to find the old studies even if this is not perceived as practicing medicine. If the nodule or mass can be shown to be unchanged in size over a 2-year period, it can safely be assumed that the lesion is benign, and no further work-up is necessary. If the mass is unchanged in a comparison examination less than 2 years old, further study is necessary. This may take the form of repeat examinations at 3-month intervals until two years have elapsed during which no enlargement of the nodule is observed, or it may involve more direct relatively noninvasive techniques.

Conventional tomography, low-KV radiography, or CT may reveal central, concentric, or popcorn-like calcification, which in itself indicates with an extremely high degree of confidence the benign, probably old, granulomatous nature of the mass. CT densitometry using a newly devised phantom is currently being evaluated in an effort to determine benignity of nodules based on calcium content when no visible calcification is evident. Conventional tomography, films exposed while the patient performs certain respiratory maneuvers, or contrast-enhanced CT may occasionally reveal the presence of an arteriovenous malformation.

If the preceding options fail to yield a diagnosis, the invasive modality of percutaneous transthoracic needle biopsy can be employed. This procedure has a 90 to 95 percent accuracy in the diagnosis of malignant processes. According to one report, benign lesions may be diagnosed with approximately 80 percent accuracy.

Nodules or masses that increase in size from one film to the next should generally be considered malignant. An exception to this is when growth is extremely rapid (e.g., doubling of the diameter within one month), a circumstance that suggests an acute infectious process. In the other cases, the most expeditious procedure would be excision of the mass following appropriate determination of resectability. Prior to resection of a suspected solitary metastasis, one might first obtain full-lung CT. While in many circumstances additional nodules will represent metastases, one should remember that in an older individual, these could be benign granulomatous lesions. Final disposition of the patient (follow-up films, percutaneous needle biopsy, surgery) should depend on the entire clinical picture and not solely on the radiographic findings.

In conclusion, the evaluation of a mediastinal or lung mass is not generally a hurried undertaking. Time spent searching for prior chest films and organizing subsequent radiographic procedures will be rewarded by less cost and disruption to the patient.

SUGGESTED READING

Heitzman ER. The mediastinum. Radiologic correlations with anatomy and pathology. St. Louis: CV Mosby, 1977.

Khouri NF, Statik FP, Erozan YS, et al. Transthoracic needle aspiration biopsy of benign and malignant lung lesions. AJR 1985; 144:281–288.

Zerhouni EA, Boukadoum M, Siddiky MA, et al. A standard phantom for quantitative CT analysis of pulmonary nodules. Radiology 1983; 149:767–773.

NONTRAUMATIC PNEUMOTHORAX

JUDITH E. TINTINALLI, M.D., F.A.C.E.P.

Pneumothorax is the development of a collection of air in the pleural space, owing to rupture of an alveolus or bronchus. In spontaneous pneumothorax, there is no pulmonary trauma or instrumentation responsible for the development of the disorder. Spontaneous pneumothorax is most likely to occur in those with preexisting lung disease. Chronic obstructive lung disease, emphysema, asthma, pneumoconiosis, and smoking, are the most common predisposing conditions. Systemic disorders such as Marfan's syndrome, cystic fibrosis, eosinophilic granuloma, tuberous sclerosis, endometriosis, pulmonary malignant tumor and scleroderma have also been associated with spontaneous pneumothorax. The most common underlying condition associated with neonatal pneumothorax is idiopathic respiratory distress syndrome and assisted ventilation. In healthy individuals, an extreme and acute elevation of intra-alveolar pressure, such as can occur with screaming or vomiting, or during labor and delivery, can result in spontaneous pneumothorax. It can be a complication of intubation or airway ventilation with excessive pressures. In some individuals, potential channels exist between the peritoneal and pleural cavities, so that pneumothorax has been described as a complication of laparoscopy.

ESSENTIALS OF DIAGNOSIS

Symptoms of spontaneous pneumothorax are the sudden development of sharp chest pain and shortness of breath. Chest pain is usually pleuritic and unilateral, but can be described as precordial and pressure-like. Pain can also be localized to the neck or shoulder. Hemoptysis can be present also.

On physical examination, tachypnea and tachycardia are invariably present if there is tension pneumothorax. If there is severe hypoxia, cyanosis may be evident. Jugular venous distention is present as a result of the increase in pleural pressure. Subcutaneous emphysema and crepitus may be demonstrated along the thorax, even extending into the neck. The diagnosis is clinically confirmed by the detection of decreased or absent breath sounds in a hemithorax, along with hyperresonance to percussion on the affected side. However, small degrees of pneumothorax can present with a virtually normal physical examination.

The development of tension pneumothorax is characterized by increasing respiratory distress, more pronounced tachycardia and tachypnea, and hypotension. The trachea is noted to be deviated away from the affected side, and hyperresonance to percussion is increased on the affected side, since the time of initial examination. Jugular venous distention is more pronounced.

The diagnosis is confirmed by *chest roentgenogram*, in which the visceral pleura can be seen detached from the parietal pleural surface. Posterior-anterior or anterior-posterior films are sufficient to detect all but the smallest pneumothoraces. An inspiratory-expiratory film demonstrates a small pneumothorax in the expiratory phase. For neonates, children, or uncooperative patients, a lateral decubitus film with the affected side upward is equally satisfactory for diagnosis.

Differential diagnosis includes (depending on presentation) severe emphysema with little air exchange; large emphysematous bullae; acute myocardial infarction; pulmonary embolus; and pulmonary infiltration or consolidation. Every patient with preexisting pulmonary disease and acute respiratory distress should be quickly evaluated for the presence of spontaneous pneumothorax. With severe emphysema, breath sounds can be so poor that decreased breath sounds on one side may not be detectable clinically. Furthermore, pneumothorax could be bilateral, in which case there is no variance in breath sounds on either side. An emphysematous bleb appears as a "loculated pneumothorax," and pulmonary marking is visible on the periphery of the lung. In the patient with acute myocardial infarction, a normal chest film, diagnostic electrocardiogram, and absence of pneumothorax on chest film point to the correct diagnosis. Chest roentgenogram, arterial blood gases, and possibly ventilation-perfusion scanning are necessary for the diagnosis of pulmonary embolus or infiltration.

Although the diagnosis of simple pneumothorax can usually wait for roentgenographic confirmation, the diagnosis of tension pneumothorax is always based solely on clinical findings. To postpone treatment until the chest film is obtained guarantees deterioration of the patient's condition and may hasten demise.

TREATMENT

Tension pneumothorax must be treated by tube thoracostomy. If equipment is not ready, needle aspiration must be accomplished without delay, to be followed by tube thoracostomy.

Treatment of simple spontaneous pneumothorax can follow several regimens: observation, inspiration of high concentrations of oxygen, needle aspiration, outpatient Heimlich valve, or tube thoracostomy with suction drainage. Treatment options depend on the amount of pneumothorax, amount of underlying pulmonary function, amount of lung collapse, and amount of respiratory reserve.

Small pneumothoraces in relatively asymptomatic patients with good pulmonary reserve can be treated by observation in the hospital, although this method is not widely practiced. The patient should be admitted to an area where close nursing observation is the rule, and some institutions utilize a step-down unit for this purpose. Chest auscultation and vital signs should be repeated every hour, and interval chest films every 4 hours or so. Equipment for management of tension pneumothorax should be at the patient's bedside.

Another inpatient treatment option is the inhalation of 100 percent *oxygen*. Inhalation of a high concentration of oxygen results in a decrease in tissue gas tension in comparison to that in the pleural space, enhancing the absorption of the pleural collection. Also, the high concentration of oxygen and very low, or no, nitrogen in the inspired air enhances the absorption of nitrogen from the pleural space. The major drawbacks to this technique are the development of absorption atelectasis and oxygen toxicity, need for prolonged treatment (days), and impracticality for the emergency physician.

Larger pneumothoraces can be treated by simple *needle aspiration*. A 16-gauge intravenous cannula connected to a stopcock with one port under water-seal drainage, is inserted into the pleural space. Any accepted location for entry is satisfactory, whether the second intercostal space anteriorly, the anterior axillary line at the fifth intercostal space, or just below the tip of the scapula posteriorly. The first location is the one most commonly employed. Air is gently aspirated from the pleural space, and this is documented by noting air bubbles under the water seal. If air is aspirated and inadvertently reintroduced into the pleural cavity, tension pneumothorax can be created. The major disadvantage to this technique is the fact that the lung can brush against the aspirating needle or catheter, resulting in pulmonary laceration or contusion. In addition, patients still require admission and observation for reaccumulation of the pneumothorax. This technique is less painful and, at least theoretically, offers less chance for infection.

A recent technique utilizing the insertion of a Heimlich flutter valve and management as an outpatient has been described, but has not been widely accepted. Tube thoracostomy is still the standard mode of therapy for pneumothoraces greater than 20 to 30 percent. A 22 to 28 F tube is inserted into the fifth or sixth space at the anterior axillary line. The tube is connected to 5 to 10 cm underwater suction, and repeat chest film confirms re-expansion and proper tube placement. Complications of tube thoracostomy include laceration of an intercostal artery, pulmonary contusion or laceration, laceration of liver, spleen, or diaphragm, insertion into the wrong hemithorax, re-expansion pulmonary edema, hypotension, and infection. The first three complications can be avoided by strict adherence to surface anatomy when placing the thoracostomy tube. It is safest to utilize the fifth intercostal space because, in the supine position, and in obese patients or those with ascites, the dome of the diaphragm can rise to the fifth interspace. Once the pleural cavity has been entered, careful digital exploration is necessary to ascertain that the tube is not directed into viscera. Re-expansion pulmonary edema is most likely to occur in the elderly patient with prolonged pneumothorax, with bronchial obstruction, and with application of high pressures for re-expansion. The cause is believed to be an increase in pulmonary capillary permeability.

DISPOSITION

Patients with pneumothorax should be admitted after appropriate therapy has been instituted. Generally, a regular medical or surgical bed is sufficient, unless complications from tube thoracostomy have developed. *Re-expansion chest films* should always be obtained before the patient is admitted. Precise localization of the chest tube cannot be determined unless both PA and lateral films have been obtained. Patients with pneumothorax generally should not be transferred to another facility for care until the pneumothorax has been treated, as it is impossible to predict which particular individual may develop tension pneumothorax en route. If helicopter or air ambulance is the mode of transfer, tube thoracostomy or insertion of a Heimlich flutter valve is necessary before transfer to prevent development of tension pneumothorax.

SUGGESTED READING

DeVries WC, Wolfe WG. Management of spontaneous pneumothorax and bullous emphysema. Surg Clin North Am 1980; 60:851–865.

Hoffer FA, Ablow RC. The cross-table lateral view in neonatal pneumothorax. Am J Roentgenol 1984; 142:1283–1286.

Pavlin DJ, Raghu G, Rogers TR, et al. Re-expansion hypotension. Chest 1986; 89:70–74.

Pavlin DJ. Lung re-expansion—for better or worse? Chest 1986; 89:2–3.

ADULT ASTHMA

ROBERT J. ROTHSTEIN, M.D.

According to the American Thoracic Society, asthma is a disorder of respiratory function characterized by dyspnea, paroxysms of cough, and wheezing caused by episodic, reversible impedance of the movement of air into and out of the lungs. Although this simplistic definition has served the literature well for years, it in no way reflects the complexity and variability of this disease process. An understanding of the pathophysiology, clinical presentation and management of this problem is essential for the practicing emergency physician.

PATHOPHYSIOLOGY

Many factors are responsible for the disease, including allergic and nonallergic stimuli, irritants, cold, exercise, cholinergic nervous stimulation, psychogenic factors, and the endogenous mediators formed and released by the sensitive individual. Over a period of time ranging from minutes to days, these factors produce the narrowing of small and large airways through smooth muscle spasm, bronchial edema, mucous hypersecretion and inspissation, and inflammatory changes, resulting in the clinical picture of obstructed airways and wheezing.

PHYSICAL EXAMINATION

As soon as the physician is convinced of the diagnosis and has decided on a line of therapy, treatment should begin, but the examination should eventually be completed in order to assess severity and rule out other causes of wheezing. Many other disorders cause wheezing (Table 1), and the physician should be careful to rule these out before accepting the diagnosis of asthma, particularly if it is the patient's first episode.

First, look at the patient and get a sense of the degree of respiratory distress. Cyanosis, diaphoresis, altered mental status, tachycardia (>130), and tachypnea (>30), especially with pursed lip breathing and accessory muscle use, may correlate with severity. A fever suggests infection, but breathing rapidly past an oral thermometer may falsely lower the temperature. Some hypertension is a natural response to the attack, but major blood pressure elevations may preclude parenteral sympathomimetic therapy. The pulsus paradoxus should be measured.

Listen to the chest for both inspiratory and expiratory wheezes, rales and rhonchi, and mediastinal "crunch" (indicating pneumothorax or pneumomediastinum). Jugular venous distention, rales, an S_3 gallop, and peripheral edema suggest "cardiac asthma" failure, which sometimes can present with virtually no findings except bronchospasm. Other common causes of wheezing such as pulmonary embolism, toxic inhalation, and occupational exposure can usually be excluded by careful history, physical examination, and response to therapy (see Table 1).

ASSESSMENT OF THE PATIENT

Historically, it is important to recognize what may have precipitated the attack: (1) Is the patient allergic to something (pollen, plants, molds, animal hair, insects, arthropods, mites)? (2)Was the patient exposed to an irritant (smog, aldehydes, gases)? (3) Is there an infection? (4) Is there an environmental influence (exercise, cold air)? (5) Any psychological stresses? (6) Any problem with medications (e.g., inhaler abuse, supply of medications ran out, decreased steroids) or sensitivity to aspirin or nonsteroidal anti-inflammatory drugs? (7) Is there a history of gastroesophageal reflux?

Ask about what medications the patient is currently taking. Is the dose adequate? When was the last dose? Is the patient abusing an inhaler? Ask what medications the patient has been on in the past, with specific reference to steroids.

When did this attack begin? Acute bronchospasm may be severe, but may be more easily reversible than an attack that has been slowly increasing in severity over several days. Ask the patient how he would rate this attack, i.e., mild, moderate, or severe. Has he been hospitalized in the past with attacks like this? Finally, don't be afraid to ask the patient, "What helps?"

SEVERITY ASSESSMENT

Signs such as cyanosis, altered mental status, severe diaphoresis, and inability to speak are probably indicative of a severe attack; however, subjective impressions of the clinician or patient fail to correlate with objective signs of severity. Severity should be determined, objectively, using initial values of pulmonary function tests and response to therapy.

TABLE 1 Causes of Wheezing (Bronchospasm)

Infections: pediatric bronchiolitis, bronchitis, pneumonia, parasites (*Ascaris, Strongyloides,* hookworm, *Brugia, Trichinella*)

Irritants: particles (cotton, red cedar and other aromatic lumbers, grains), chemicals (toluene, metal fumes, ammonia, sulfur dioxide, smoke inhalation, chloride, other toxic gases)

Allergic causes: allergic reactions, anaphylaxis, vasculitis (and polyarteritis nodosa), aspergillosis, allergic alveolitis (farmer's lung)

Upper airway obstruction: tumor, edema, foreign body, volitional (pseudo-asthma)

Cardiac causes: cardiac asthma (failure), pulmonary edema, occult mitral stenosis

Noncardiogenic pulmonary edema (CNS, ARDS)

Pulmonary causes: asthma, COPD, cystic fibrosis

Embolus: pulmonary embolus, fat embolus, amniotic fluid embolus, injected foreign body embolus

Other causes: Loeffler's syndrome (pulmonary infiltrates with eosinophilia), chronic eosinophilic pneumonia, carcinoid syndrome

Every patient who presents with an asthma attack should have the peak expiratory flow rate (PEFR) or 1-second forced expiratory ventilation (FEV_1) measured at the initial evaluation. Absolute numbers are not so helpful as the percent of predicted normal. Initial values less than 25 percent of normal represent a severe attack and correlate well with normalizing arterial PCO_2 initial values less than 15 percent of normal correlate with hypercarbia. Often, a normal PCO_2 in a dyspneic patient is an ominous sign, suggesting rising PCO_2 owing to respiratory failure. This strong correlation between PCO_2 and pulmonary functions obviates the need for routine arterial blood gases (ABGs). A PEFR of less than 60 to 100 L per minute or an FEV_1 less than 0.6 to 1 L is in the moderate-to-severe range. If the FEV_1 does not improve to more than 1.6 L, or if the PEFR is greater than 160 L after one dose of epinephrine (or the equivalent), or the FEV_1 does not improve more than .4 L or to more than 2.1 L, or if the PEFR is less than 300 L after 4 hours of therapy, there is a 67 to 92 percent chance that the patient will need admission or will relapse if sent home.

Fischl et al devised an index of severity based on multiple parameters observed in asthmatics. Patients received 1 point for each of the following on presentation: PEFR less than 120 L per minute, respiratory rate (RR) greater than 30 per minute, moderate-to-severe wheezing, dyspnea and use of accessory muscles, pulse greater than 120 per minute, and paradox greater than 18 mm Hg. They claimed that four or more points correlated with a 95 percent need for admission, or relapse if discharged. The obvious advantages of such an index are that the parameters are easy to recognize, and they are measured on admission to the emergency department. Unfortunately, this index did not perform successfully or reproduce the author's claims in two independent prospective trials that later attempted to validate the criteria.

Thus, although there are still no validated, absolute criteria, it is clear that the status of patients with poor initial function studies and minimal response to therapy is to be considered severe. None of these studies considered the variables of age, previous or current therapy or, perhaps most importantly, the duration of the attack. The patient with an acute onset who has an FEV_1 of 1 L is not the same as the patient of an equivalent age and FEV_1 who has had an attack for 3 days. Nevertheless, the clinician should be aware of the utility of objective parameters and use some consistent guidelines.

OTHER LABORATORY STUDIES

Routine laboratory studies are relatively unhelpful in the acute attack. The white blood count (WBC) has never been correlated with severity of asthma, and generally is raised substantially both by stress and steroids. The differential count may demonstrate eosinophilia, but absolute eosinophil counts are more accurate in determining an allergic component to the asthma. Arterial blood gases should be drawn only if pulmonary function tests indicate severe obstruction. Significant metabolic acidosis (not just respiratory acidosis from hypercarbia) is a poor prognostic sign and may warrant treatment with bicarbonate. Routine chest films are of low yield unless pneumonia, pneumothorax, or pneumomediastinum is clinically suspected. More than 10 eosinophils per high-power field on the sputum examination suggests allergy, whereas more than 10 neutrophils on a good specimen (i.e., one containing <3 epithelial cells) suggests infection. Theophylline levels should be obtained *stat* on all patients who have taken theophylline preparations. Routine electrocardiograms (ECGs) are not helpful unless cardiac ischemia is suspected. Changes such as tachycardia, ST segment alterations, cor pulmonale, and axis shifts usually revert to baseline with therapy.

TREATMENT

The treatment of an acute asthmatic attack depends on the severity of the attack, the duration of symptoms, previous medications, and an understanding of the pathophysiology, although there are some basic principles that apply to all cases.

Oxygen is indicated as the initial therapy in all asthmatics. Dehydration is another concern in asthmatics. Since they are usually breathing rapidly and the work of breathing is increased, their insensible water loss is greater than normal. In addition, they may be diaphoretic, febrile, and unable to replace fluid losses. For these reasons, rehydration is appropriate. Although bronchial edema and mucous inspissation do occur, dilating the bronchi, providing humidified O_2, and preventing further detrimental effects will correct these changes more rapidly than pushing intravenous fluids.

Currently available drug therapy for the acute attack can be divided into sympathomimetics, methylxanthines, steroids, anticholinergics, and others. Despite an incredible amount of research regarding all aspects of asthma therapy, there is still no cookbook approach and no ideal therapy available. To discuss medical therapy in a rational way requires an understanding of the pathophysiology and pharmacology.

The goal, simply stated, is to reverse the pathophysiologic process, dilate the airways, and prevent further release of mediators capable of producing narrowing of the airways. The first goal is accomplished by elevating levels of cAMP and/or reducing levels of cGMP.

Sympathomimetic Drugs

Sympathomimetic drugs have been the initial therapy for asthma for many years. Isoproterenol is the prototype nonspecific beta-adrenergic stimulant. Although it is the most potent drug available in its class, it also has prominent and undesirable beta$_1$ (cardiovascular) side effects. Newer drugs have supplanted this medication in adult asthmatics. Epinephrine (epi) has both beta$_1$ and beta$_2$ adrenergic stimulating properties. Because the beta$_2$ receptors predominate in the lung, epinephrine results in bronchodilatation, but peripheral alpha and beta$_1$ stimulation produce significant side effects. Epinephrine traditionally is given subcutaneously as a 1:1,000 solution, in a dose of 0.01 cc per kilogram to a maximum of 0.5 cc per dose, every 20 minutes, for a total of three doses. Although still used as initial therapy by many, there doesn't appear to be a good reason for using it in adults. Recent studies have shown that a single dose of Sus-Phrine, an oil-based sustained-release epinephrine preparation (at one half the dose of epinephrine), has equivalent bronchodilatory effects to those of epinephrine, except that (1) its onset is in 10 minutes as compared to 3 to 5 minutes for epinephrine; (2) it has fewer side effects, and (3) it is longer lasting (up to 6 hours). Epinephrine (or Sus-Phrine) is relatively contraindicated in patients who are elderly, are diabetic, have thyroid disease, are hypertensive, are on monoamine oxidase (MAO) inhibitory drugs, have coronary artery disease, or abuse sympathomimetic inhalers.

Terbutaline was one of the first drugs released in this country as a selective $beta_2$ stimulator. Clinical studies have failed to support the contention that this drug, at doses producing an equivalent therapeutic effect, has any fewer side effects than epinephrine. There are advantages to it, however. In doses of 0.25 mg, subcutaneously given twice at 30-minute intervals, terbutaline has a duration of 4 hours. In addition, it can be given orally or by metered-dose inhaler and thus can be used for outpatient management.

Isoetharine (Bronkosol) has $beta_2$ selectivity when nebulized in a dose of 0.5 cc in normal saline. Its onset of action is 5 minutes and duration is 30 to 90 minutes. It can be repeated every 60 minutes. Metaproterenol may be given orally or by inhalation. By nebulized inhalation, 0.3 cc of a 5 percent solution has an onset of 15 minutes and duration of 4 hours. Its longer duration and oral administration may be desirable. Albuterol, available now in this country as a metered-dose inhaler and tablet, is a popular drug in Europe because of its $beta_2$ selectivity and a potency nearly equal to that of isoproterenol. The onset is within 15 minutes and duration is 3 to 8 hours. It is not yet available in nebulized form in this country, which limits its emergency use. Fenoterol is another $beta_2$ selective drug that is widely used in Europe with excellent results.

Numerous studies suggest that sympathomimetic drugs given by inhalation have several advantages over parenterally administered drugs. The side effects are significantly less by inhalation because a far smaller dose is needed when delivered directly to the airways, resulting in minimal absorption. Furthermore, many drugs are $beta_2$ selective when inhaled. Finally, the studies fail to demonstrate any therapeutic advantage of the parenteral sympathomimetics.

Methylxanthines

Methylxanthines (theophylline) were first introduced for the treatment of asthma in 1900, although use did not become widespread until 1936. Now, aminophylline, the prototype preparation, contains 85 percent theophylline and is a mainstay in asthma therapy. The therapeutic range of 10 to 20 μg per milliliter of serum provides a narrow

therapeutic index, and toxicity occurs relatively frequently.

Clearance is reduced in infants, but increases rapidly until adolescence, and then begins to decline throughout adulthood. Since clearance is by the liver, it is reduced by anything that produces hepatic dysfunction, including primary liver disease, congestive heart failure, viral diseases, and certain medications. On the other hand, patients with cystic fibrosis and smokers have nearly double the clearance of age-matched controls.

Aminophylline should be administered as a loading dose of 5 to 6 mg per kilogram of total body weight (less in markedly obese patients). Maintenance is based on ideal body weight. The following are recommendations for maintenance: children and healthy smoking adults, 0.9 mg per kilogram per hour; healthy nonsmoking adults, 0.5 mg per kilogram per hour; patients who are over 60 years of age or have cor pulmonale, 0.3 mg per kilogram per hour; patients with congestive heart failure or liver disease, 0.2 mg per kilogram per hour. Any patient who has taken a theophylline preparation in the previous 24 hours should have a maintenance drip started and a *stat* theophylline level drawn. A loading dose may be given empirically based on clinical judgment, but levels cannot be accurately predicted. Serious cardiovascular toxicity and seizures can occur at levels over 20 μg per milliliter and are not always preceded by minor toxicity such as headache, nausea, vomiting, and tremulousness. Every 1 mg per kilogram load raises the serum level 2 μg per milliliter. Loading is usually done intravenously, but can also be done orally with theophylline elixir, which is rapidly absorbed and usually well tolerated. Oral tablets are too slowly absorbed for emergency loading.

Corticosteroids

Steroids are controversial only in their mechanism of action; clearly they are effective in the acute and chronic management of asthma. The effects will be delayed; thus, most of the activity of steroids will not be evident for at least 4 to 6 hours.

The optimal dose of steroids in an acute attack has not been established; nor is it altogether clear that the intravenous route is superior to the oral route. Most authorities recommend a dose of 3 to 4 mg hydrocortisone phosphate or succinate or the equivalent, to be given intravenously every 6 hours, although doses as high as 1,000 mg are recommended by some. Methylprednisolone, 4 mg per kilogram, has been proved to reduce relapse and return visits to the emergency department. Other commonly used steroids are prednisone (about 4 to 5 times the antiflammatory potency per milligram of hydrocortisone) and methylprednisolone (5 to 6 times the potency). Neither has any significant sodium-retaining effect, unlike hydrocortisone.

Anticholinergics

Parasympathetic-cholinergic stimulation of the lung produces smooth muscle contraction, bronchoconstriction, and mucus secretion. Bronchomotor tone is dependent on a balance between sympathetic and parasympathetic activity or between levels of cAMP and cGMP. Stimulation of nasopharyngeal, laryngeal, or tracheal receptors results in reflex vagal stimulation and bronchospasm in susceptible individuals and is thought to be the mechanism for cold-induced and exercise-induced asthma.

Although knowledge of this aspect of asthma has been available for a long time, anticholinergic therapy has not been used clinically in the past simply because the only drug available, atropine, has significant anticholinergic side effects when given in doses necessary for bronchodilation.

In terms of relative effectiveness, this class of drugs is fully effective in reversing cholinergically induced bronchospasm and partially effective in reversing histamine- and prostaglandin-induced bronchospasm. They may be effective in reversing beta blockade-induced bronchospasm, but have a variable effect in reversing bronchospasm from irritants, antigens, exercise, and cold air. Psychogenically induced asthma responds well to anticholinergics. These drugs are probably most effective in chronic bronchitis and emphysema with reversible components.

Inhaled, nebulized atropine can be given in a dose of 0.015 mg per kilogram in adults. Ipratropium bromide, an effective anticholinergic with minimal side effects, is not yet available in this country.

Other Drugs

Numerous drugs under investigation inhibit various steps in the mediator synthesis/release process, but are unlikely to be available for clinical use in the near future. However, calcium-channel blocking agents have been receiving attention lately because of their ability to inhibit calcium influx. It has been shown that nifedipine may significantly inhibit exercise-induced asthma. The role of calcium-channel blockers in the treatment of acute asthma remains to be determined.

Rational Drug Therapy

When approaching the asthmatic in the emergency department, the key considerations are severity and duration of the attack, age of the patient, previous medications, and response to initial therapy.

Oxygen is indicated for all these patients. Initial therapy should probably be a nebulized sympathomimetic-like isoetharine or metaproterenol. If the attack is severe, as judged by pulmonary functions, Sus-Phrine may be added and/or an intravenous infusion started for aminophylline

therapy. If the patient has severe initial indices and does not improve significantly after sympathomimetics, steroids should be given and admission arranged. If the patient has previously received steroids or is receiving tapering doses of steroids, early administration of corticosteroids is indicated.

Severely dyspneic, cyanotic, diaphoretic, or somnolent patients and patients who are in respiratory failure (i.e., hypercarbic) and do not respond to therapy rapidly should be intubated and attached to ventilator support. Morphine and succinylcholine should be avoided in the treatment of asthmatics.

Therapy of the pregnant asthmatic is directed at preventing or correcting maternal hypoxemia. All currently used antiasthmatic medications are "probably" safe; a great deal of experience is lacking with many of the newer drugs, but no teratogenic effects have been directly attributed to epinephrine or aminophylline.

Medications Prescribed at Discharge

Asthmatics who improve enough to be discharged must be referred for urgent follow-up. Adjusting previous medications is appropriate (e.g, increasing theophylline or steroids dose). For the patient who was not taking medication before the attack, an albuterol or metaproterenol inhaler, 2 puffs every 4 to 6 hours as necessary is probably adequate. Careful instruction in its proper use is important. Substitution or addition of a theophylline preparation is acceptable. Typical aminophylline dosage is 3 to 6 mg per kilogram orally every 6 hours. Long-acting theophylline preparations are best tolerated because of compliance; the daily dose is 24-hour maintenance, in divided doses. If the patient has been "loaded," blood should be drawn immediately to determine therapeutic levels; otherwise steady-state levels will not be reached for 5 to 7 days. The test should be repeated to monitor levels and dosage.

Terbutaline or metaproterenol tablets may be given, but are not much more effective than inhalers. Outpatient steroids should be prescribed in consultation with the patient's primary physician.

SUGGESTED READING

Corre K, Rothstein RJ. Assessing severity of adult asthma and need for hospitalization. Ann Emerg Med 1985; 14:45–52.

Goldstein RA, ed. Advances in the diagnosis and therapy of asthma. Chest 1985; 87(suppl): 1S–112S.

Hendeles L, Weinberger M. Theophylline; a "state of the art" review. Pharmacotherapy 1983; 3:2–44.

Metcalfe DD, Donlon M, Kaliner M. The mast cell. CRC Crit Rev Immunol 1981; 3:23–74.

CHRONIC OBSTRUCTIVE PULMONARY DISEASE

HUGO D. MONTENEGRO, M.D., F.C.C.P.
NEIL S. CHERNIACK, M.D.

The term chronic obstructive pulmonary disease (COPD) refers to a group of disorders characterized by airflow limitation. The two most common disorders associated with airflow limitation are chronic bronchitis and emphysema. Chronic bronchitis is characterized clinically by excessive bronchial mucus secretion; emphysema is a permanent abnormal enlargement and destruction of the air spaces distal to the terminal bronchioles. Because these disorders frequently overlap, they are commonly described by the term chronic obstructive pulmonary disease. Although the etiology and pathogenesis of COPD is still unclear, important risk factors are cigarette smoking, environmental pollution, occupational exposure, and pulmonary infectious processes during childhood.

DIAGNOSIS AND DIFFERENTIAL DIAGNOSIS

Common symptoms of COPD include a productive cough and dyspnea. In the absence of other obvious causes, cough and sputum production usually indicate the presence of chronic bronchitis. Dyspnea is also an important symptom and may be present in either emphysema or chronic bronchitis. The onset of dyspnea may be insidious, and in patients who are not active, dyspnea may not be a signficant symptom.

The physical findings in patients with COPD are those of airway obstruction and hyperinflation. Airway obstruction is manifested by wheezes or a prolonged expiratory phase. Hyperinflation is evidenced by a "barrel-shaped" chest, hyperresonance, and limited excursion of the diaphragm. Other physical findings include rhonchi, and crackles that occur mainly at the beginning of the inspiration. In patients who have cor pulmonale, distended neck veins, leg edema, hepatomegaly, a prominent pulmonic second sound and a right ventricular gallop may be noted. Additional clinical features are those of hypoxemia and hypercapnia. Hypoxemia is manifested by euphoria, irritability, and abnormalities in higher cognitive intellectual functions. Hypercapnia may be manifested by confusion, obtundation, and coma.

Because the clinical signs and symptoms of hypoxemia and hypercapnia are variable and nonspecific, measurement of *arterial blood gases* is the only way to determine whether they are abnormal and to what degree. Fatigue of the respiratory muscles may occur in patients with COPD and contribute to hypoxemia and hypercapnia. In patients with respiratory muscle fatigue, the use of accessory muscles and an inward movement of the abdomen during inspiration may also be present. *Bedside Spirometry* in the form of simple devices to measure peak expiratory flow rate or the forced expiratory volume in 1 second (FEV_1) not only document obstruction, but are useful for comparison to previous values. However, spirometry does not measure the amount of respiratory work needed to exchange air.

During acute exacerbations of COPD, cough and dyspnea worsen, and the main *differential diagnosis* is heart failure. Orthopnea is more suggestive, but not pathognomonic, of ventricular failure; distended veins may be seen in patients with COPD owing to an increase in intrathoracic pressure. The rales found in bronchitis may be confused with rales of cardiac failure. Because of hyperinflation, heart sounds may also be difficult to auscultate. In general, the diagnosis of left ventricular failure during acute exacerbations of COPD may be difficult, and in some instances it seems advisable to treat the patient as if he had both conditions.

THERAPY

Therapy in COPD patients is aimed at improvement of airflow limitation and *correction of hypoxemia*. It is important to remember that hypoxemia is the major threat to the patient's life. Patients with COPD who are hypoxemic require low (24 to 28 percent) concentrations of inspired oxygen. High concentrations of inspired oxygen are not only unnecessary, but in some patients may also worsen hypercapnia. One should aim at maintaining PaO_2 between 55 and 60 mm Hg or oxygen saturation of 85 to 90 percent. Although several methods of delivering oxygen at low concentrations are available, the safest and most effective method of delivery is the Venturi mask. One should start with inspired oxygen concentrations of 24 percent and then change the concentration appropriately after determination of arterial blood gases. The administration of oxygen in COPD patients should always be on a continuous basis. When the inadvertent administration of high inspired oxygen concentrations induces a significant degree of CO_2 retention (more than 15 mm Hg per hour), the concentration of oxygen should be diminished but not stopped.

The management of airflow limitation is accomplished with the use of bronchodilators, mainly *theophylline* derivatives and adrenergic agents. The most commonly used theophylline derivative is aminophylline, which must be given intravenously during acute exacerbations. A loading dose is not necessary if the patient has been on a maintenance dose of theophylline. However, in patients who have not received aminophylline previously, a loading dose of 6 mg per kilogram given over a 20-minute period by intravenous drip is indicated. The maintenance dose is 0.8 mg per kilogram per hour in smoking adults, but in critically ill patients, 0.5 mg per kilogram per hour is more appropriate. Because of the multiple factors that affect the pharmacokinetics of theophylline in critically ill patients, blood levels are essential in adjusting the dose of this agent. Measurement of drug levels should be performed at 8 to 12 hours and then at 18 to 24 hours. Caution should be used in patients who are already being treated with theophylline preparations, as levels are unpredictable and toxicity can easily be induced. Additional theophylline should await results of a drug serum level; 1 mg per kilogram IV increases serum levels by 2 mg per deciliter.

Bronchodilatation can be enhanced by the use of adrenergic agonists. The use of *beta₂*-adrenergic agents minimizes the undesirable cardiac effects commonly found when nonselective beta-adrenergic agents are used. Newer agents such as metaproterenol, terbutaline, and albuterol are most commonly used. These agents can be administered by aerosol, orally, or by a metered-dose inhaler. The safest and most efficacious route is by aerosol using an air-driven nebulizer. By this route, the medication is deposited in the obstructed bronchial tree and systemic side effects are minimized. Although aerosolized adrenergic agents can be delivered by IPPB or by metered-dose inhaler (MDI), there is no advantage in using IPPB machines, and the patient may be incapable of the degree of coordination required to effectively use the MDI inhaler. The recommended doses of aerosolized bronchodilators are isoetharine, 5 mg every 4 hours; metaproterenol, 15 mg every 6 hours; albuterol, 2.5 mg every 6 hours. Beta-agonists such as metaproterenol, terbutaline, and albuterol are also available as oral agents. Although they are effective orally and have a long duration of action, when given by mouth they also produce more side effects, mainly tremor, palpitations, and nervousness. The role of these oral agents in acute exacerbations of patients with chronic airway obstruction is unclear.

Corticosteroids are not indicated as part of the routine treatment of acute respiratory failure in COPD patients. However, they may be beneficial in patients with an allergic component, as evidenced by family or personal history of allergies or by the presence of eosinophils in the sputum or nasal smears. The recommended steroid dose is methylprednisolone, 0.5 mg per kilogram every 6 hours. The response to corticosteroids should be assessed with some measurement of pulmonary function before steroids are continued. If improvement is noticed during the first 3 days of steroid administration, one can switch to oral prednisone in the range of 30 to 40 mg and again repeat the pulmonary function tests to assess the need for long-term therapy.

Early recognition and treatment of *precipitating factors* are important in the management of acute exacerbations of COPD because they are usually not only reversible, but also preventable. Respiratory infection is one of the most common precipitating factors. *S. pneumoniae* and *H. influenzae* are commonly found during acute exacerbation. The administration of broad-spectrum antibiotics early in the course may prevent deterioration of clinical status. Ampicillin (500 mg every 6 hours), amoxicillin (250 mg every 6 hours), or trimethoprim-sulfamethoxazole (80 mg and 400 mg respectively every 12 hours) can be administered. If the patient is febrile, has signs consistent with pneumonia, or has been receiving long-term antimicrobial therapy, a sputum Gram stain (and culture with sensitivity) should be done to guide specific antibiotic therapy.

Another important precipitating factor is ventricular failure. *Right ventricular failure* may be already present in patients with long-standing COPD, particularly in those with persistent hypoxemia. The management of right ventricular failure in these patients consists of oxygen administration and an aggressive treatment of airway obstruction. Digitalis is not recommended in the management of right ventricular failure in the absence of overt left ventricular failure.

Left ventricular failure may pose a diagnostic problem in the patient with COPD. Signs and symptoms of left ventricular failure such as dyspnea and rales are common in patients with chronic airway disease, whereas gallop rhythms may be masked by hyperinflation or by respiratory sounds. Noninvasive techniques for evaluating left ventricular function in patients with COPD are under active investigation, but usually are not available as bedside techniques. If a definitive diagnosis of left ventricular failure must be established, measurement of pulmonary capillary wedge pressure may be obtained by use of a balloon-tipped catheter. On the other hand, when the presence of left ventricular failure is strongly suspected, digitalis should be started. Patients with failure of the left ventricle also have a history of coronary artery disease or hypertensive cardiovascular disease.

Other precipitating factors include the injudicious use of narcotics, sedatives, tranquilizers, and high concentrations of inspired oxygen, all of which may induce hypoventilation.

The *decision to hospitalize* a patient with an acute exacerbation of COPD requires judgment. Patients with severe hypoxemia (40 mm of mercury or less), tachypnea (respiratory rate 30 or above), hypotension, pneumonia, or signs of respiratory muscle fatigue (paradoxical inward movement of the abdominal wall with inspiration) should be considered for hospital admission. Although the use of bedside spirometry in the assessment and management of the asthmatic patient is well established, its value in the emergency room assessment of the patient with COPD has not yet been determined.

The decision to use *mechanical ventilation* in a patient with COPD relies on clinical assessment. Patients with signs of respiratory muscle fatigue may benefit from a trial of mechanical ventilation to rest the respiratory muscles. Patients with obvious signs of tachypnea and respiratory distress with severe hypoxemia are also candidates for mechanical ventilation. The development of metabolic acidosis is also considered an indication for mechanical support. Hypercarbia alone, even if severe, is not an indication for artificial ventilatory support as long as the patient remains alert and able to cough.

SUGGESTED READING

Bake M. Medical management of emphysema. Clin Chest Med 1983; 4:465–482.

Weinberger M, Hendeles L, Ahrens R. Pharmacologic management of reversible obstructive airways disease. Med Clin North Am 1981; 65:579–583.

PNEUMONIA CAUSED BY AEROBIC GRAM-NEGATIVE RODS

HERBERT Y. REYNOLDS, M.D., F.A.C.P., A.C.C.P.

Gram-negative pneumonia is chiefly a hospital-acquired (nosocomial) disease, but since the organisms are common colonizers of the pharynx, the patient with underlying disease may become infected as an outpatient as well. Particularly at risk are those with chronic obstructive pulmonary disease, congestive heart failure, diabetes, alcoholism, intravenous drug abuse, debility, recent surgery, prior antibiotic use, immunosuppression, and increased risk of aspiration. Nosocomial pneumonia occurs in 1 to 5 percent of all hospital admissions, but in 25 percent or more of patients in medical intensive care units. It causes considerable morbidity and has a high mortality (30 percent). The seriously ill patient is particularly susceptible to aspiration of naso-oropharyngeal secretions and to aerobic gram-negative rods. Certain clinical situations may suggest specific lung infections, e.g., *Pneumocystis carinii* or mycobacterial infection in those with the acquired immunodeficiency syndrome, fungal pneumonia in granulocytopenic leukemia patients, or an atypical viral pneumonitis that turns out to be caused by *Legionella* species. However, lung infection with a gram-negative rod is always part of the differential diagnosis in these high-risk patients.

The aerobic gram-negative bacilli that commonly cause pneumonia are in the families of Enterobacteriaceae (principal species are *Klebsiella pneumoniae, Escherichia coli, Serratia marcescens*) and Pseudomonadaceae (*Pseudomonas aeruginosa*). Normally these bacteria are part of the bowel flora or can reside on moist, intertriginous skin areas, but they are found infrequently on the pharyngeal and nasal mucosa (occurrence is about 15 percent in area swabs taken from the mouths of healthy people). Normal flora of the naso-oropharynx are dominated by anaerobic bacteria and common commensals such as *Neisseria* species, streptococcus *Branhamella catarrhalis*, and perhaps *Haemophilus* species and *Streptococcus pneumoniae* in people with chronic bronchitis. Almost any form of stress (hospitalization, intensive care stay, or a surgical procedure), metabolic derangement (uncontrolled diabetes mellitus, renal or hepatic failure), chronic illness, or immunosuppressive therapy with antineoplastic chemotherapy or anti-inflammatory agents is associated with a striking increase in colonization of bowel, skin, and upper respiratory tract mucosa with the gram-negative rods mentioned. This has been well documented in medical and surgical intensive care units where acquisition of these organisms in the oropharynx is rapid, occurring within 1 to 3 days of admission, and frequent, as more than half these patients can become colonized. Thus, the stage is set for a hospital-acquired or so-called nosocomial pneumonia to develop. Aspiration of secretions into the lung probably provides the inoculum. Inhalation of bacteria from contaminated aerosol or ventilatory equipment is not such a common means now that more care is being given to changing tubing on ventilators and better cleaning methods are generally used.

ANTICIPATING THE SUSCEPTIBLE PATIENT

Almost any unusual stress, serious illness, and hospitalization, especially in an intensive care facility, promotes rapid acquisition and oropharyngeal colonization with common but potentially pathogenic gram-negative rods. The origin of these bacteria is probably the patients themselves, who may autoinoculate their upper respiratory tracts with their hands or bodily secretions; health care personnel and such innocuous things as uncooked food, salad, or even flowers and plants in the room can also be vehicles. Colonization develops quickly and may not be preventable. What consequence it ultimately has depends somewhat on the integrity of host defenses and individual resistance of the patient. Therefore, it is important to know what the patient's baseline microbial flora is, to monitor its change so that when the potential culprits appear one knows where they are residing, and to obtain preliminary antibiotic sensitivities.

As part of the admission laboratory evaluation of the high-risk patient, nasal, oropharyngeal, perirectal, and axillary skin swabs should be obtained for routine bacterial cultures. Any potential pathogens isolated can be tested for antibiotic sensitivities, especially if the hospital is having any problems with resistant species. The cotton-tipped applicators should be dipped in transport medium first (Stuart's bacterial transport medium containing glycerophosphate and thioglycolate, Culturette, Marion Scientific, Kansas City, MO) to moisten them before they are rubbed over the skin sites or in the nares. A daily naso-oropharyngeal culture should be obtained for the first 3 days of hospitalization, for the majority of patients will acquire the potential pathogen and colonize the nose and throat quickly. If the potential pathogen is recovered in the initial nasopharyngeal or sputum culture, then subsequent daily cultures that have been planned can be cancelled.

When colonization with a potentially pathogenic gram-negative rod has developed in the oropharynx of a patient at risk enhanced surveillance is indicated. Usually, attempts to manipulate bacterial flora with aerosol antibiotics are not successful.

In summary, anticipating respiratory infection in high-risk patients may be the best approach to diagnosing it quickly and treating it promptly. Unfortunately, nothing can completely prevent colonization, but severe respiratory infection often follows the acquisition of certain bacteria in the oropharynx which are later aspirated into the lungs. An appropriate strategy for coping with nosocomial respiratory infection should include: (1) assessing which patients are likely to develop colonies of potentially pathogenic organisms in their oropharynx; (2) monitoring the patient when colonization occurs; (3) concentrating special care on the highly susceptible patient, giving special attention to control of secretions and increasing general surveillance; and (4) knowing which organisms are sensitive to which antibiotics.

RECOGNIZING THAT PNEUMONIA MAY EXIST AND FINDING AN ETIOLOGIC AGENT

In elderly, severely ill, or immunocompromised patients in whom nosocomial pneumonia is most likely to occur, early detection of respiratory infection may not be easy, nor is its onset always obvious. The usual clinical variables, including fever and leukocytosis, can be trivial and respiratory symptoms may be subtle. Patients may cough little, have scant expectoration if any, and often are intubated and on assisted ventilation so they cannot speak and communicate their chest complaints readily. Fever can be deceptively absent, especially if renal or liver failure exists, or bone marrow insufficiency precludes the anticipated whole blood cell count rise and blunts the inflammatory response so that an infiltrate on a chest radiograph may be slow to blossom. Agitation or altered mentation frequently ushers in the infection; an elevated pulse rate and more difficulty with fluid balance, especially diminished urine output, are clues. The point is that the presentation can be atypical and a high index of suspicion plus subtle clues often suggests the diagnosis. When respiratory signs are minimal, only after excluding infection systematically in other organ systems (urinary tract, wound or catheter sites, decubitus areas, occult meningitis) does the respiratory tract receive more consideration. One may be reluctant to make (or to accept) a diagnosis of nosocomial pneumonia without definite radiographic changes, for a new infiltrate is considered as prime evidence. Unfortunately, auscultation of the chest may not reveal an early pneumonitis if secretions are scant or the patient is attached to a ventilator. The question of occult aspiration causing the pneumonia inevitably arises, which can never be decided with certainty. As normal people during sleep can aspirate oropharyngeal secretions, patients with a disoriented sensorium from many causes, including prescribed sedation, can aspirate. Suctioning up hyperalimentation liquid or small food particles from the endotracheal tube may strengthen the diagnosis. Measuring pH of respiratory fluid or the glucose content to identify tube feeding material is touted as helpful in picking up small, recurrent aspiration. In my experience, this has rarely proved decisive.

When one realizes that a pneumonitis exists, the most expeditious means for making a microbial diagnosis must be decided on. This may precipitate the most controversial step in patient management which can turn into the weakest link in the health care process. The issue focuses on how invasive to be to obtain an adequate specimen for bacteriologic diagnosis, for it seems that these patients invariably never make much sputum or cannot cough well. Although the initial choice of antibiotics will be somewhat empiric to cover the spectrum of probable infectious agents responsible, the crucial step of narrowing the antibiotic coverage later, based on recovery of a specific infectious agent, will be difficult unless adequate specimens were cultured originally. Of course, several blood cultures are an indispensable part of the work-up, but their yield will not be known for a few days. Here we can rely on the baseline surveillance cultures to reveal some of the flora of the patient and to identify which of the potentially pathogenic gram-negative rods have already colonized the naso-oropharynx or are present in expectorated secretions. Such bacteria are likely to be the culprits, or certainly are involved in the infection, and initial antibiotic coverage should include such probable pathogens.

Still, the issue usually remains how to proceed to get actual lung secretions or tissue. For the intubated patient, deep tracheal suction with a firm curved catheter than can be advanced into a major bronchus may suffice. Attempts to aerosol nebulized water particles into the airways to stimulate secretions are usually worthless and at best provide a stimulus for coughing which might produce some sputum. In many cases this dilemma arises: Should transtracheal aspiration (if a skilled person is available) or a fiberoptic bronchoscopy be done or should one go straight to an open lung biopsy, if the diagnosis is not going to be obtained with one of the first procedures and if the patient can tolerate a mini-thoracotomy?

Transtracheal aspiration avoids most of the oropharyngeal flora that can confuse sputum culture results. The procedure seems to be good based on literature reports, yet its use varies from none to frequent in different medical centers. Fear of acute cricothyroid artery bleeding and the patient's reluctance to have a procedure done too close to his throat are inhibiting factors. However, transtracheal aspirates should be obtained more frequently for they provide reliable cultures. A small amount of subcutaneous air in the neck and some blood-tinged sputum with coughing may occur after the procedure, but are self-limited and considered minor complications.

Fiberoptic bronchoscopy can be done readily, even if the patient is on a ventilator, through a side port attachment to the endotracheal tube (minimal size of 8 mm needed). If the patient is thrombocytopenic, platelet transfusions given just before bronchoscopy will largely prevent endobronchial bleeding. The brush catheter seems to cause the most trouble with bleeding. Transbronchial biopsies can be done in this setting with care. Oxygen should be given through the bronchoscope. With a combination of cultures from a telescoping protected tip catheter, brushings and transbronchial biopsies, the yield of a probable pathogen is approximately 50 percent in the immunocompromised host. There will be upper airway flora included in the culture reports, too, for it is virtually impossible not to pick up some pharyngeal secretions during passage of the bronchoscope and the various specimen catheters. Often the bronchoscopy provides additional help by permitting a view of the bronchial orifices to rule out endobronchial obstruction. Serious complications from bronchoscopy are not frequent. With transbronchial biopsy, a pneumothorax will occur in about 5 percent of patients and may require placement of a chest tube.

Open lung biopsy is often necessary in the immunocompromised patient with an advancing, undiagnosed pulmonary infiltrate and pneumonia. However, two failings often are observed with the procedure. Medical personnel procrastinate and wait too long to get the biopsy, thus delaying appropriate antimicrobial therapy, or they do not coordinate the handling of the tissue with the microbiologist and pathologist to ensure optimal analysis. A brief presurgical consultation with all the principals is most helpful.

INITIAL TREATMENT

The initial therapy must be chosen on the basis of the skillful interpretation of essentially clinical phenomena. Appropriate ancillary support is necessary with parenteral fluids, antipyretic drugs, supplemental oxygen, airway suction or postural drainage for secretions, and bronchodilator therapy for some patients. Intubation is often required for ventilatory support and better oxygenation, and also to facilitate good pulmonary toilet measures. The minimal amount of inspired oxygen needed to keep blood gases acceptable is the goal, plus judicious use of positive end-expiratory pressure and parenteral fluids, guided by Swan-Ganz catheter data. Bronchospasm can complicate pneumonitis, so nebulized bronchodilators may be needed. Frequent but careful endotracheal suctioning, which does not abrade the mucosa, must be stressed.

For the bacteria under consideration—aerobic gram-negative bacilli—a broad selection of antibiotics exists: aminoglycosides (gentamicin, tobramycin, and amikacin); semisynthetic penicillins that are active against *Pseudomonas* principally (carboxypenicillins such as carbenicillin and ticarcillin) or have an extended spectrum (ureido penicillins including piperacillin and mezlocillin); and cephalosporins, which are divided into three generations based on general features of antimicrobial activity. Representative cephalosporins most active against the bacteria under discussion are first generation agents such as cephalothin, second-generation choices such as cefamandole or cefoxitin, and third generation agents represented by cefotaxime and moxalactam. Several third generation cephalosporins have especially good antipseudomonal activity (cefoperazone and cefsulodin). A newer group of beta-lactam antibiotics called thienamycins are not included; however, these agents do have activity against certain Enterobacteriaceae and *Pseudomonas* species that are resistant to cephalosporins, but laboratory susceptibility testing is required for their selection. Suitable antibiotics for anaerobic organisms in the lung include penicillin G, clindamycin, and perhaps metronidazole. Finally, an old standby antibiotic, ampicillin, is often used to treat unknown respiratory infection because of its gram-positive and gram-negative antibacterial activity and general efficacy as a respiratory tract antibiotic. If urosepsis is contributing to the infective process and *E. coli* is a possible lung pathogen, ampicillin may be used.

This list of antibiotics is not inclusive, only representative. New cephalosporins continue to proliferate, seemingly more potent and active against certain bacteria such as *Pseudomonas*, but still broad in overall coverage and more expensive to prescribe. Some of these agents need more clinical study. As the higher generations of cephalosporins have been developed with greater activity against gram-negative bacteria, some of their effectiveness against gram-positive ones has been lost, so these drugs may not offer suitable treatment for species of staphylococci, enterococci, and *Streptococcus pneumoniae*. On the other hand, much of the commercial literature about these newer cephalosporins suggests that a single agent will give broad coverage and alone may suffice for treatment of a serious infection. As a caution, a single antibiotic has not generally proved to be adequate in eradicating or curing pneumonia caused by a *Pseudomonas* or *Klebsiella* species, especially if the host is in any way immunocompromised and granulocytopenic. Dual or multiple antibiotics are still recommended for predictable coverage.

Let us consider the treatment for a patient with a pneumonia, possibly nosocomial in origin and very likely to be caused by a pathogenic gram-negative rod. The patient's oropharynx is colonized by a probable pathogen, so there is a reasonably certain bacterial etiologic agent for which a rational selection of initial antibiotic(s) is possible. However, it was necessary to obtain better samples of respiratory secretions, so fiberoptic bronchoscopy was done and specimens obtained have been cultured appropriately. Blood cultures are incubating as well. Keep in mind that we want to treat the most probable infectious agent, based on our surveillance cultures and current analysis of a carefully Gram stained smear of the respiratory secretions, but one must also cover the patient for the unsuspected bacterium that could be the most devastating in this clinical setting. I am always concerned about covering for *Pseudomonas* infection because it is the most frequent cause of nosocomial pneumonia. It becomes an extremely virulent infection in the elderly or immunocompromised host and can progress rapidly. If *Pseudomonas* is judged to be a reasonable infectious agent, then initial antibiotic coverage must be adequate for *Pseudomonas*, until culture results rule out this cause. Concomitant septicemia with pneumonia has to be considered. If gram-negative sepsis exists, a nonpulmonary nidus of infection is likely (urinary tract or bowel), and attention must be directed to treating the primary source also. Urosepsis and *E. coli* pneumonia often are coupled in this way.

For treatment of a newly diagnosed nosocomial pneumonia, the initial antibiotic combination should include an aminoglycoside and a semisynthetic broad-spectrum penicillin to cover the aerobic gram-negative rods. If aspiration is evident, then penicillin G or clindamycin should be given, too. The need for antistaphylococcal coverage must be weighed also. Gentamicin is preferable because of its broad activity and good general efficacy, plus the desire to save other aminoglycosides for later use, should resistance to gentamicin develop. A loading dose of 1 mg per kilogram of body weight IV is given, followed by doses of about 1.7 mg per kilogram every 8 hours. Intermittent (given over 30 minutes diluted in saline or 5 percent dextrose solution), not continuous, intravenous administration is preferred. The aim is a daily total of about 5 mg per kilogram a day, assuming that the patient has normal renal function. After 2 to 3 days at this high dose, it is scaled down to 3 mg per kilogram a day total dose for the duration of therapy, which is usually 7 to 10 days. However, if *Pseudomonas* is a likely possibility from the start, use of tobramycin is better because it is more potent on a molar weight basis against this bacterial species. After a loading dose of 1 mg per kilogram IV, subsequent doses of 1.7 mg per kilogram are given every 8 hours for a total daily dose of 5 mg per kilogram. This total dose should be reduced to 3 mg per kilogram daily in several days for the duration of treatment, which is also 7 to 10 days. As all aminoglycosides are excreted by the kidneys, nephrotoxicity can occur. With renal insufficiency the daily dose in terms of amount and frequency of administration must be adjusted according to the degree of renal impairment. Nomograms and formulas based on serum creatinine and/or urine creatinine clearance must be consulted to determine the appropriate dose. After gentamicin or tobramycin therapy is under way for about 48 hours, the peak level (serum sample obtained at completion of dose) and a trough level (before next dose) should be measured. It is desirable not to exceed 12 μg per milliliter at the peak. It is important to know the trough value, for it gives a clue to how well antibiotic levels are maintained between doses. The lower value should be at least 3 to 4 μg per milliliter, to ensure continuous bactericidal activity against the gram-negative rods. Generally, these organisms are sensitive to a mean inhibitory concentration of 2 to 4 μg per milliliter or less.

Amikacin should not be used in the initial antibiotic combination unless specific microbial resistance is known which dictates its use, because this is the back-up, last resort aminoglycoside. This antibiotic does not perform better than the others discussed, but it is likely to be active if resistance to gentamicin and tobramycin has occurred. Save it if possible, especially in the immunocompromised patient or one with cystic fibrosis who may have repeated respiratory infections with *Pseudomonas*. When used, amikacin is given in three divided doses for a total daily dose of 15 mg per kilogram of body weight. The same caution about renal toxicity and side effects applies for amikacin as for the other aminoglycosides.

As the choice of a broad-spectrum semisynthetic penicillin, mezlocillin is now preferred to the others listed in this category. It is a bactericidal antibiotic with a potent and impressive range of activity against important gram-positive and gram-negative bacteria. With an aminoglycoside it has a synergistic effect against *P. aeruginosa* and *K. pneumoniae* and perhaps against *Serratia* too. One of these broad-spectrum penicillins is a necessity in patients with granulocytopenia, if they are to have a reasonable chance of survival. Whereas the original antibiotic in this category, carbenicillin, and ticarcillin both provide good activity, mezlocillin has several desirable qualities that make it preferable. Mezlocillin is more active against streptococci and *Haemophilus influenzae*, it inhibits more *Klebsiella* isolates at lower concentrations than the others, it is the least likely of the broad-spectrum penicillins to alter bleeding times, and it is relatively low in sodium content. The intravenous dose is 200 to 300 mg per kilogram of body weight per day given in four divided doses (or about 4 g every 6 hours). In patients with renal failure the dose intervals should be lengthened to 8- to 12-hour intervals.

The question may arise about using a cephalosporin as a single drug or in combination with an aminoglycoside for one of the serious gram-negative pneumonias under consideration—*Pseudomonas, Klebsiella,* or *Serratia.* The combination of cephalothin and gentamicin has been an acceptable one for *K. pneumoniae* for some time. The first generation cephalosporins have some activity against gram-negative organisms which might be considered adequate (versus *E. coli, K. pneumoniae,* and *Proteus mirabilis*), and this activity gets more potent with the second and third generation drugs. Only a subset of third generation agents are active against *P. aeruginosa* and the clinical experience with them is still limited. One use of these cephalosporins is that they are a good antibiotic option for a patient with penicillin allergy in whom there is a reasonable possibility that cross-reactions will not occur acutely. In my judgment they should be used in combination with an aminoglycoside and not be relied upon as a single agent. This holds for a primary *K. pneumoniae* or *Pseudomonas* respiratory infection. For *Pseudomonas* pneumonia, sole use of cefoperazone, for example, would seem to be insufficient and it should be combined with an aminoglycoside. However, the substitution of cefoperazone for mezlocillin in the combination already discussed may be equally good, but will need further laboratory and clinical assessment.

Finally, once the patient's therapy is underway, the physician must remain alert for complications that may develop. A resurgence of fever after an initial period of defervescence is a frequent clue. One of a number of problems could be the cause. Poor coughing and an accumulation of secretions or a mucous plug can obstruct an airway, leading to partial collapse of a lung lobe or segment. Vigorous postural drainage and endotracheal suction may remove secretions and help reexpand the lung portion and if possible should be tried for 24 hours before resorting to bronchoscopy. The development of loculated pleural fluid could be the cause and usually requires thoracentesis and possible chest tube drainage. As microbial culture results return, the broad spectrum coverage must be tailored to fit the specific organisms, and doses of antibiotics may need adjustment. Secondary bacterial infection or superinfection occurring after broad-spectrum antimicrobial therapy may cause fever and worsening of the patient's condition; thus reculturing sputum and blood is necessary. Drug allergy causing mild blood eosinophilia and lingering fever is a frequent and often unsuspected complication that requires discontinuation or substitution of the antibiotic regimen. Complete resolution of the pneumonic process or closure of a lung abscess, for example, must be observed, for failure of this part of the healing phase may require additional attention. Sputum cytologies and bronchoscopy might be indicated to rule out a partially obstructing airway lesion or endobronchial tumor.

SUGGESTED READING

Reynolds HY. Pneumonia due to *Klebsiella*. In: Wyngaarden JB, Smith LH, eds. Cecil's textbook of medicine. 17th ed. Philadelphia: WB Saunders, 1985:1509.

Reynolds HY. Pneumonia caused by aerobic gram-negative bacilli (*Pseu-domonas, Escherichia coli, Serratia*). In: Wyngaarden JB, Smith LH, eds. Cecil's textbook of medicine. 17th ed. Philadelphia: WB Saunders, 1985:1510.

Reynolds HY. Respiratory infections may reflect deficiencies in host defense mechanisms. Disease-a-month 1985, 31:1–98.

COMMUNITY-ACQUIRED PNEUMONIA

CHATRCHAI WATANAKUNAKORN, M.D., F.A.C.P., F.C.C.P.

ETIOLOGY

Historically, pneumonia has been classified anatomically according to the appearance of roentgenograms: lobar pneumonia, bronchopneumonia, interstitial pneumonia, and others. With the advent of antimicrobial agents, it is more appropriate for clinicians to consider pneumonia in terms of the etiologic agent because effective therapy depends largely on the knowledge of the specific infecting organism. Table 1 lists the organisms that may cause community-acquired pneumonia in the United States. The list is not an exhaustive one and does not include bacteria, fungi, viruses, and parasites that are unlikely to cause pneumonia in adults and that are acquired outside the hospital in the United States. When pneumonia develops in patients in nursing homes or in patients who have had recent hospitalization, it should be considered hospital-acquired pneumonia.

The two most common types of pneumonia are caused by *Streptococcus pneumoniae* and *Mycoplasma pneumoniae*. The clinical features of these two types of pneumonia are distinctly different (Table 2). Since mycoplasmal pneumonia does not respond to penicillin therapy, it is imperative that *Mycoplasma* as the cause of pneumonia be excluded if penicillin is to be used to treat a patient with community-acquired pneumonia.

Pneumococcal pneumonia is usually associated with an acute onset of fever with or without a sudden chill. Pleuritic chest pain is also common. Often there is cough productive of purulent sputum, and the sputum may even be bloody or rusty. Physical signs of consolidation are common, but may be absent. Rales and pleural friction rub may be heard. In addition, there may be lobar, seg-mental, or patchy infiltrates. Pleural effusion is common, and empyema may occur. There is usually leukocytosis.

Mycoplasmal pneumonia, on the other hand, is usually associated with an insidious onset, with predominantly constitutional symptoms such as headache, sore throat, malaise, myalgia, and sometimes earache. There may be low-grade fever. The cough is usually nonproductive and may be "hacking." Occasionally, there may be some clear sputum. Physical examination may disclose rash and bullous myringitis, and there are usually rales unilaterally or bilaterally. Roentgenograms may show unilateral or bilateral pulmonary infiltrates and sometimes show more extensive involvement than physical findings indicate. There is usually no leukocytosis. Pleural effusion may be present, but it is not common.

Table 3 lists some useful clues in considering the etiology of community-acquired pneumonia. *Haemophilus influenzae* has increasingly been shown to cause pneumonia in adults, usually in patients with chronic obstructive lung disease who smoke. Onset is usually acute, as in pneumococcal pneumonia, and there may be unilateral or bilateral lung involvement.

Community-acquired pneumonia caused by *Klebseilla pneumoniae* is not common and usually develops in alcoholics. The patient with *klebsiella* pneumonia is usually toxic with high fever, and sputum is purulent.

Mixed aerobic-anaerobic (aspiration) pneumonia is more common in alcoholics, in patients with seizure disorders, and in patients with swallowing disorders. These patients usually have poor dental hygiene. The fever is generally high, and the patient looks toxic. Sputum production is usually copious, purulent, and foul-smelling. Roentgenograms of the chest may disclose abscess formation.

Staphylococcus aureus pneumonia is uncommon. It may present as a superinfection in patients who have influenzal pneumonia with sudden onset of high fever and purulent sputum. More commonly, it occurs in intravenous drug abusers as a result of septic pulmonary emboli from tricuspid valve endocarditis. It typically presents with high fever, chills, dyspnea, tachypnea, tachycardia, and pleuritic chest pain. There may be scanty sputum production that may also be bloody. Chest films usually show multiple patchy infiltrates with or without cavities. Blood cultures invariably yield *S. aureus*.

Pneumonia caused by *Legionella pneumophila* has increasingly been diagnosed in patients who acquire pneumonia in the community. Cases of this type of pneumonia occur in a sporadic manner, but a history of exposure to dust at a construction site may be a helpful clue to *Legionella* as the cause. The onset is usually abrupt with high temperature. Mental confusion, abdominal pain, and diarrhea are common symptoms. There is usually scanty mucoid sputum with many pus cells and no organism on Gram stain. Chest roentgenograms may show lobar dis-

TABLE 1 Organisms That May Cause Community-Acquired Pneumonia

Common bacteria	Other important organisms
Streptococcus pneumoniae	(list is not exhaustive)
Mycoplasma pneumoniae	Influenza virus
	Adenovirus
Less common bacteria	Varicella virus
Haemophilus influenzae	Measles virus
Legionella pneumophila	*Histoplasma capsulatum*
Mixed aerobic-anaerobic bacteria	*Blastomyces dermatitidis*
(aspiration pneumonia)	*Coccidioides immitis*
Staphylococcus aureus	*Cryptococcus neoformans*
Klebsiella pneumoniae	*Chlamydia psittaci*
Mycobacterium tuberculosis	*Coxiella burnetii*
Other mycobacteria	*Pneumocystis carinii*

TABLE 2 Clinical Features Differentiating Pneumococcal Pneumonia and Mycoplasmal Pneumonia

Features	Pneumococcal Pneumonia	Mycoplasmal Pneumonia
Onset of symptoms	Acute; fever, often with a sudden chill	Insidious, low-grade fever
Cough	Productive of purulent, sometimes rusty, sputum	Nonproductive, hacking cough, sometimes minimally productive of clear sputum
Other symptoms	Pleuritic chest pain	Headache, sore throat, malaise, myalgia, earache
Physical findings	Rales, signs of consolidation, pleural friction rub	Rash, bullous myringitis, rales, rhonchi often bilateral
Leukocytosis	Present	Absent
Chest roentgenogram	Often lobar or segmental, pleural effusion common	Patchy, may be bilateral, may have pleural effusion
Sputum Gram stain	Polymorphonuclear leukocytes and gram-positive diplococci	If available, few polymorphonuclear leukocytes and no bacteria
Diagnostic work-up	Blood culture, sputum Gram stain and culture	Cold agglutinins, complement-fixing antibodies (acute and convalescent)
Response to penicillin	Yes	No
Response to erythromycin	Yes	Yes

tribution early, progressing bilaterally. Analysis of arterial blood gas shows severe hypoxemia. There is mild leukocytosis. There may be hyperbilirubinemia with elevated levels of transaminases. Elevated levels of serum creatine phosphokinase, myoglobinuria, hematuria, and renal failure may be found. If the diagnosis is not made and the patient is given beta-lactam and/or aminoglycoside antibiotics, the clinical condition deteriorates, sometimes rapidly.

Pulmonary tuberculosis is uncommon in the United States. However, it should be suspected when patients, especially the elderly, are not responding to appropriate antibiotic therapy for bacterial pneumonia. Other species of *Mycobacterium* may also cause pulmonary infiltrates, usually of a subacute or chronic nature.

Influenza virus may cause hemorrhagic pneumonia in some patients during an influenza epidemic. Adenovirus pneumonia is uncommon, occurring mostly in people housed in closed quarters, such as armed forces recruits. Varicella pneumonia may occur as a serious complication in some adults with chicken pox. The measles virus may also cause pneumonia in adults with clinical measles.

Histoplasma capsulatum seldom causes acute pneumonia except when a large number of spores are inhaled, usually in a unique setting, e.g., cleaning chicken coops, demolishing old barns. Dyspnea, low-grade temperature, and nonproductive cough are usual symptoms. The areas endemic for histoplasmosis in the United States are along the Ohio and Mississippi rivers. *Blastomyces dermatiti-*

TABLE 3 Useful Clues in the Etiology of Community-Acquired Pneumonia

Clues	Etiology To Be Considered
Sudden onset of high fever with one chill	Pneumococcus
Sore throat, headache, malaise, earache, hacking cough	Mycoplasma
Chronic obstructive pulmonary disease	Pneumococcus, *Haemophilus influenzae*
Alcoholics	Pneumococcus, *Klebsiella*, mixed aerobic-anaerobic (aspiration)
Seizure disorder, bad dental hygiene	Mixed aerobic-anaerobic (aspiration)
Copious, foul-smelling sputum	Mixed aerobic-anaerobic (aspiration)
Purulent sputum, leukocytosis	Bacterial pneumonia
Intravenous drug abuser	*Staphylococcus aureus*
Mental confusion, high fever, diarrhea, abnormal hepatic function, unresponsive to beta-lactam drugs	*Legionella pneumophila*
Contact with parakeet, parrot, working in turkey processing plant	*Chlamydia psittaci*
Not responding to appropriate antibiotic therapy	*Mycobacterium tuberculosis*, fungi
Male homosexual	*Pneumocystis carinii*
Severe hypoxia	*L. pneumophila*, *P. carinii*

dis may cause pulmonary infections with or without cutaneous lesions. If cutaneous lesions are present, diagnosis can easily be made by a potassium hydroxide preparation and culture of pus from these lesions. However, the diagnosis may not be obvious if there are no cutaneous lesions. The areas endemic for blastomycosis are similar to those for histoplasmosis. Coccidioidomycosis should be considered if a patient has a history of travel to the southwestern United States. *Cryptococcus neoformans* may cause symptomatic pulmonary infection in patients who have a history of taking corticosteroids or have Hodgkin's disease or diabetes mellitus.

Psittacosis and Q fever should be considered in the differential diagnosis of atypical pneumonia. *Chlamydia psittaci* may be transmitted from parakeets, parrots, and turkeys to humans, causing pneumonia. *Coxiella burnetii* can be found in materials from contaminated cows in this country, especially in California. Inhalation of *C. burnetii* can cause pneumonitis.

Recently, acquired immunodeficiency syndrome (AIDS) has been reported in male homosexuals and, to a lesser extent, in intravenous drug abusers and hemophiliacs. *Pneumocystis carinii* pneumonia may be the initial presenting problem in AIDS patients. The pneumonia is usually bilateral and diffused. Lung biopsy is usually required for diagnosis.

DIAGNOSIS

A detailed history is imperative in the diagnosis of community-acquired pneumonia. Most patients have pneumonia that is attributable to pneumococcus or mycoplasma. Table 2 lists the important differential features of pneumococcal pneumonia and mycoplasmal pneumonia. There are also other clues listed in Table 3 that may be helpful in considering other causes of pneumonia. Table 4 lists the laboratory methods of diagnosis of major pathogens causing community-acquired pneumonia.

Beside chest roentgenography, the Gram stain and culture of sputum are the most important laboratory procedures in the diagnosis of bacterial pneumonia. A good sputum specimen from deep cough is essential. In general, a good sputum sample should contain at least 25 neutrophils and fewer than 20 epithelial cells per high-power field. For a diagnosis of bacterial pneumonia, bacteria of a predominant type should be seen on the Gram stain. If the Gram stain shows many leukocytes and mixtures of different types of bacteria, a mixed aerobic-anaerobic aspiration pneumonia should be suspected. Two to three blood cultures should be obtained, since some patients with bacterial pneumonia have bacteremia. If the blood cultures are positive, the etiology of the pneumonia is further confirmed.

The diagnosis of mycoplasmal pneumonia is based mainly on clinical features. Although *Mycoplasma pneumoniae* can be cultured from sputum specimens, many patients do not have productive sputum. Furthermore, most clinical microbiology laboratories are not capable of doing mycoplasmal cultures. The diagnosis of

TABLE 4 Diagnostic Methods for Community-Acquired Pneumonia

Etiologic Agents	Diagnostic Methods
Pyogenic bacteria	Blood cultures Sputum Gram stain Sputum culture
Mycoplasma pneumoniae	Serology
Legionella pneumophila	Sputum culture for *Legionella* Sputum immunofluorescence stain Serology
Mycobacteria	Sputum acid-fast stain Sputum culture for mycobacteria PPD skin test
Virus	Sputum culture for virus Serology
Fungus	Sputum culture for fungus Potassium hydroxide preparation of sputum Serology
Chlamydia psittaci	Serology
Coxiella burnetii	Serology
Pneumocystis carinii	Methenamine-silver stain of lung specimen

mycoplasmal pneumonia can be confirmed by serology, i.e., a fourfold rise in complement-fixing antibody to *Mycoplasma pneumoniae*. Cold-agglutinin antibody is a nonspecific test, but a high titer in a patient who has clinical features of mycoplasmal pneumonia supports the clinical diagnosis.

Legionella pneumonia should be diagnosed and therapy started on clinical grounds. Some laboratories are equipped to do *Legionella* immunofluorescent antibody stain of sputum and also sputum culture for *Legionella*. Otherwise, the diagnosis can be confirmed by a fourfold rise of indirect fluorescent antibody.

Acid-fast stain of sputum is a rapid method for the diagnosis of mycobacterial infection, which should be confirmed by sputum cultures for mycobacteria; a PPD skin test should be done. Potassium hydroxide preparation and fungal cultures should be done in the diagnosis of deep fungal infection; serial serology may be helpful. Viral pneumonia can be diagnosed by sputum culture for virus and serial serology. Psittacosis and Q fever should be diagnosed by serology. *Pneumocystis carinii* pneumonia is usually diagnosed by methenamine-silver stain of a lung biopsy specimen.

THERAPY

Specific antimicrobial therapy depends on the infecting agent or on the most likely infecting agent based on clinical features. Table 5 lists the antimicrobial drugs of choice and alternative drugs for infecting agents most likely to cause community-acquired pneumonia.

Parenteral penicillin G is the drug of choice, and oral penicillin V may be used in mild cases of pneumococcal pneumonia. If a patient is allergic to penicillin, erythromy-

TABLE 5 Antimicrobial Therapy for Community-Acquired Pneumonia

Etiologic Agent	Drugs of First Choice	Alternative Drugs
Streptococcus pneumoniae	Penicillin G 600,000 units IV q6h *or* Penicillin V 500 mg PO q6h (mild cases)	Erythromycin 500 mg IV, *or* PO q6h (penicillin allergy)
Mycoplasma pneumoniae	Erythromycin 500 mg PO q6h	Tetracycline 500 mg PO q6h
Haemophilus influenzae	Ampicillin 1–2 g IV q4h	Cefuroxime 750–1,500 mg IV q8h (resistant strain) *or* Tetracycline 250 mg IV q6h (penicillin allergy)
Mixed aerobic-anaerobic (aspiration)	Penicillin G 1 million units IV q4h	Clindamycin 300–600 mg IV q6h (penicillin allergy or no response to penicillin)
Staphylococcus aureus	Nafcillin 1–2 g IV q4h *or* Cefazolin 1–2 g IV q8h *or* Penicillin 5 million units IV q6h (if organism is sensitive)	Vancomycin 1 g IV q12h (first choice drug if organism is methicillin-resistant)
Klebsiella pneumoniae	Cefazolin 2 g IV q8h	Gentamicin 1.7 mg/kg IV q8h (penicillin allergy or resistant organism)
Legionella pneumophila	Erythromycin 0.5–1 g IV q6h	
Chlamydia psittaci	Tetracycline 500 mg PO q6h	
Coxiella burnetii	Tetracycline 500 mg PO q6h	
Pneumocystis carinii	TMP/SMZ 20 mg/kg of TMP plus 100 mg/kg of SMZ IV per day in 4 divided doses	Pentamidine (iethionate 4 mg/kg per day given in one dose IM)

cin is a good alternative drug. Mycoplasmal pneumonia may be treated with either erythromycin or tetracycline. In a patient whose clinical features are not definitive for either pneumococcal or mycoplasmal pneumonia, erythromycin is the preferred drug, since it is effective against both types of pneumonia.

The drug of choice for *Haemophilus influenzae* pneumonia is ampicillin. If the infecting strain is resistant to ampicillin, cefuroxime, a new second-generation cephalosporin, may be used. In patients with severe penicillin allergy, tetracycline may be used. Nafcillin or cefazolin are the drugs of choice for *Staphylococcus aureus* pneumonia. Penicillin G should be used if the infecting strain is sensitive to it. If the infecting strain is resistant to methicillin and therefore resistant to all beta-lactam antibiotics, or if a patient has a severe penicillin allergy, vancomycin should be used.

For pneumonia caused by *Klebsiella pneumoniae*, cefazolin is the drug of choice. If the organism is resistant to cefazolin, or if the patient has a severe penicillin allergy, gentamicin is a good alternative drug. Some authorities suggest the combination of cefazolin and gentamicin for the treatment of *Klebsiella* pneumonia, but there is no good clinical study showing better results than those obtained with a single drug. The new second- and third-generation cephalosporins (cefamandole, cefuroxime, cefonicid, ceforanide, cefoxitin, cefotaxime, moxalactam, cefoperazone, ceftizoxime, ceftriaxone, ceftazidime) may be used if the infecting strain is resistant to cefazolin.

For aspiration pneumonia that is caused by mixed aerobic-anaerobic bacteria, penicillin G is the drug of choice. Clindamycin is a good alternative drug in patients who are allergic to penicillin or who fail to respond to penicillin G.

The drug of choice for the treatment of pneumonia caused by *Legionella pneumophila* is erythromycin. Although some authorities empirically add rifampin to erythromycin for patients who are seriously ill, there has been no clinical study to show that this is beneficial. For psittacosis and Q fever, tetracycline is the drug of choice.

Trimethoprim-sulfamethoxazole (TMP/SMZ) is the drug of choice for the treatment of *Pneumocystis carinii* pneumonia. Unfortunately, many patients with AIDS cannot tolerate TMP/SMZ because of severe adverse drug reactions. Pentamidine is the alternative drug. Pentamidine administration is associated with multiple side-effects and toxicities, e.g., phlebitis, sterile abscess with intramuscular injection, hypoglycemia, leukopenia, renal toxicity, hepatic toxicity.

DISPOSITION

Patients need to be admitted to the hospital whenever there is a virulent infection in a normal host, manifested by consolidation of an entire lobe, high fever and toxicity, hypoxemia, multilobar pneumonia, abscess, or strong suspicion of bacteremia. In addition, relatively minor pneumonias in compromised hosts warrant admission—as in the severe asthmatic, the patient with emphysema, the alcoholic, the elderly, or any patient with immunosuppression.

Patients with mild-to-moderate pneumonia who are otherwise well can be followed closely on an outpatient basis; a first check-up within a day or two is ideal.

THE COMMON COLD

BARRY M. FARR, M.D., M.Sc.
JACK M. GWALTNEY Jr., M.D.

The common cold remains the most frequent cause of acute morbidity and of visits to physicians in the United States. Adults average two to four colds per year, and children have six to eight colds per year.

The disease is actually a syndrome of symptoms produced by respiratory infections with any one of more than 100 antigenically distinct viruses (Table 1). A viral etiology has been determined in two of three colds by use of currently available cultural and serologic techniques; the remaining one-third of colds is presumed to be caused by currently unidentified viruses. Colds caused by the various etiologic agents are usually indistinguishable from one another except by viral isolation or serology, but viral culture and serology are both unavailable and unnecessary for routine patient care.

DIAGNOSIS

The manifestations of the common cold are so characteristic that the patient's self-diagnosis is usually correct. The key symptoms are nasal discharge, nasal obstruction, sneezing, sore throat, and cough. Similar symptoms attributable to allergic conditions are usually easily distinguished by their chronic or recurrent pattern and also by relationship to allergen exposure. Fever is usually absent except in the colds of infants or young children. The median duration of symptoms is one week, but colds last as long as 2 weeks in 25 percent of patients. The severity and duration of cough are often increased in cigarette smokers with a cold.

Physical findings are usually unremarkable except for the occasional presence of visible rhinorrhea or nasal voice. The physicians's most important challenge is to differentiate the uncomplicated cold from the 2 percent of cases with otitis media (mostly children) and the 0.5 percent of cases developing secondary bacterial sinusitis (mostly adults) requiring antimicrobial therapy. A history of change in auditory acuity or earache should be evaluated with pneumatic otoscopy. Pain or tenderness in the maxillary or frontal bones suggests the need for sinus transillumination and/or roentgenograms. Severe sore throat or tonsillar pharyngeal exudate indicates the need for throat culture to exclude streptococcal pharyngitis.

TREATMENT

The uncomplicated cold is self-limited and best treated by reassuring the patient and prescribing only those medications needed to relieve the individual patient's symptoms. Combination products containing remedies for all possible symptoms are usually less effective and cause more adverse effects than does specific therapy.

Nasal congestion is best treated with topical vasoconstrictors, such as 0.25 to 0.5 percent phenylephrine or 1 percent ephedrine drops or sprays. These nasal drops or sprays must be used regularly every 4 hours for 3 to 4 days. Longer-acting compounds, such as oxymetazoline (Afrin) drops or spray, may be used twice a day. Oral administration of decongestants, such as pseudoephedrine (Sudafed), 60 mg by mouth four times a day, offers an

TABLE 1 Etiologies of the Common Cold

Agent	Number of Antigenic Types	Approximate Percentage of Cases
Rhinovirus	89 numbered (plus 20 more awaiting enumeration)	30
Coronavirus	≥ 3	≥ 10
Respiratory syncytial virus	1	
Influenza virus	3	
Adenovirus	33	10–15
Parainfluenza virus	3	
Other viruses (enterovirus, varicella, rubeola)		5
Presumed undiscovered viruses		30–40
*Streptococcus pyogenes**		5

* Streptococcal pharyngitis is not always clinically distinct from viral pharyngitis.

alternative that is less effective than topical therapy and may be complicated by increased blood pressure. This may be a significant hazard in patients with prior hypertensive or cardiac disease. Patients should also be warned about the danger of rhinitis medicamentosa following prolonged usage of decongestants. Antihistamines have not been shown to relieve the nasal congestion of colds, which correlates with recent research that did not find elevation of histamine in the nasal secretions of patients with experimentally induced rhinovirus colds. The drying effect of antihistamines on nasal secretions is attributable to an anticholinergic effect. This benefit must be weighed against antihistamines' other frequent side effect of drowsiness.

Malaise, aches, and low-grade fever are best treated with bed rest and analgesic/antipyretics such as aspirin or acetaminophen. Sore throat is relieved by warm saline gargles and mild analgesics. Cough usually does not require treatment, but moderate-to-severe coughing may be suppressed with codeine, 15 to 30 mg orally every 4 to 6 hours, after the possibility of pneumonia is excluded by history, physical examination, and, if necessary, chest roentgenogram. The patient should be warned that this dosage of codeine may result in constipation, which may be counteracted by increasing dietary bulk. Proprietary cough syrups containing dextromethorphan are also effective. The usual adult dose of dextromethorphan is 15 to 30 mg 3 to 4 times daily. Smokers should always be advised to stop smoking.

Antibiotics should never be prescribed prophylactically for a patient with an uncomplicated cold as they have no effect on the natural course of the viral infection, they alter the patient's flora to more resistant bacterial species, and they expose the patient to unnecessary risks ranging from mild side effects such as rash and diarrhea to more severe, life-threatening complications such as pseudomembranous colitis and anaphylaxis.

Large-dose therapy with vitamin C has not been shown effective as either prophylaxis or therapy for the common cold. No specific antiviral agent is yet available for prophylaxis or therapy, and vaccines have proved impractical because of the many different viruses involved. Since some cold viruses may be spread by direct hand contact and self-inoculation, handwashing and avoidance of finger-to-nose or finger-to-eye contact is recommended after exposure to a cold sufferer.

PULMONARY PROBLEMS IN ACQUIRED IMMUNODEFICIENCY SYNDROME

JEFFREY A. GOLDEN, M.D.

ETIOLOGY AND PATHOGENESIS

There is no laboratory test for the acquired immunodeficiency syndrome (AIDS). It is the manifestation of immune deficiency implied by the presence of opportunistic infections, tumors, and other processes that heralds the presence of this syndrome. AIDS is defined for surveillance purposes of the Center for Disease Control (CDC) as the presence of disease at least moderately predictive of an unexplained, underlying cellular immunodeficiency, such as Kaposi's sarcoma in a patient less than 60 years old or *Pneumocystis carinii* pneumonia (PCP).

It has been estimated that half a million to one million Americans test positive for serum human T-lymphotrophic virus, type III (HTLV-III), the reputed cause of AIDS. Although its significance is unclear, the presence of antibody to HTLV-III does not constitute a diagnosis of AIDS. Similarly, the presence of HTLV-III itself is not a diagnostic criterion for AIDS. Although the virus can be detected in blood, saliva, bronchial lavage secretions, and semen, it cannot be identified in half the patients with AIDS. This is consistent with the T-cell depletion characteristic of advanced disease. The virus is harbored in T cells and depletion of these cells could relate to the decreased ability to isolate the virus. Further, analyzing subsets of T cells and detecting a decreased helper to suppressor T cell ratio also does *not* constitute a diagnosis of AIDS. Transient viral infections among otherwise healthy people causes a temporary decrease in helper to suppressor T cell ratio similar to that found in patients with AIDS. At the present time it is the manifestation of immune suppression that constitutes the diagnosis of AIDS.

The syndrome may have other related manifestations, including unexplained diffuse lymphadenopathy, fever, diarrhea, idiopathic thrombocytopenia, lymphopenia, anemia, and a "wasting illness", which are generally referred to as AIDS-related complex, or ARC. Defining patients with ARC as being "pre-AIDS" is controversial. However, up to 20 percent of patients with lymphadenopathy syndrome developed AIDS by CDC criteria over a 3-year period. Furthermore, serologic evidence of prior infection by HTLV-III is present in more than 90 percent of patients with ARC. Between 1978 and 1984, among a cohort of 6,875 homosexual men, the prevalence of serum antibody to HTLV-III increased from 4.5 percent to 67 percent and almost one-third developed AIDS or ARC over this six-year period.

Patients at high risk for AIDS include homosexual or bisexual men, intravenous drug abusers, hemophiliacs or anyone who has had a transfusion of blood or blood products within the previous five and a half years, Haitians, and children whose mothers have AIDS. Although appropriately exposed heterosexuals are likely to have AIDS in some regions of the world, such as Central Africa, in the United States thus far only heterosexual women who are exposed to men with AIDS are at increased risk for this syndrome. However, it is likely that soon all appropriately exposed heterosexuals will be at risk for AIDS, as in Africa.

PULMONARY COMPLICATIONS OF AIDS

Pneumocystis Carinii Pneumonia

The lungs are the most common site of disease owing to immune suppression, and pulmonary problems are the most common cause of death among AIDS patients. PCP is the most common pulmonary problem afflicting patients with AIDS; 60 to 85 percent of AIDS patients develop PCP and half of these patients have recurrent PCP within 12 months. Although PCP is the most common treatable infection among AIDS patients, each episode of PCP is associated with a 30 to 50 percent mortality rate. In view of the epidemic nature of AIDS, physicians should be familiar with the presenting clinical and laboratory characteristics that suggest the presence of PCP. Patients who are diagnosed and treated early are more likely to survive a particular episode of PCP; in general, patients with less hypoxia and lower respiratory rate do better with therapy than patients who are diagnosed later in their course when PCP has resulted in more severe respiratory dysfunction.

Clinical Presentation Suggestive of PCP

The symptoms of PCP are dyspnea on exertion and nonproductive cough. Unlike PCP among patients without AIDS, PCP in the context of AIDS often presents insidiously, with a duration of illness prior to diagnosis of 2 to 10 weeks and a mean duration of illness of 1 month.

Shortness of breath and cough are nonspecific symptoms. When such symptoms are elicited from a patient in a risk group for AIDS, the possibility of PCP must be considered. Other symptoms that may more strongly suggest PCP and AIDS include sore throat or dysphagia caused by thrush or *candida* esophagitis, as well as prolonged unexplained fever, diarrhea, weight loss, lymphadenopathy, and the other manifestations of ARC.

The physical examination of patients who complain of shortness of breath and cough may help further define who is likely to have AIDS. Examination of the oropharynx may detect thrush. Thrush is uncommon in adults without immunodeficiency or recent use of steroids or antibiotics. In one study, 60 percent of patients with thrush in a high-risk group for AIDS subsequently developed this syndrome. The oropharynx may reveal lesions of Kaposi's sarcoma. Further, "hairy tongue" may be associated with AIDS. Skin findings other than Kaposi's sarcoma which may suggest AIDS include seborrheic dermatitis and herpetic anogenital lesions. Eye findings suggestive of AIDS includes herpes zoster ophthalmicus,

conjunctival Kaposi's sarcoma, and on fundoscopic examination, cotton wool exudates and findings consistent with cytomegalovirus chorioretinitis. Also, the presence of lymphadenopathy in more than two anatomic regions suggests the diagnosis of lymphadenopathy syndrome. Pulmonary auscultation may reveal interstitial type "Velcro" rales, but two-thirds of our patients with PCP had a normal pulmonary auscultation.

The chest roentgenogram may be helpful if the classic diffuse ground glass pattern of PCP is present. However, focal abnormalities and even a normal chest roentgenogram (which occurs in 8 to 25 percent of patients) are also consistent with PCP. Nodular parenchymal infiltrates and/or pleural effusions are more consistent with pulmonary Kaposi's sarcoma; Kaposi's sarcoma is virtually always evident on physical examination by the time this tumor is visible on the chest film. Finally, chest film evidence of hilar or mediastinal adenopathy does not imply PCP and cannot be ascribed to lymphadenopathy syndrome. In my experience such adenopathy has been attributable to other processes, including lymphoma, Hodgkin's disease, tuberculosis, and cryptococcosis.

The routine laboratory evaluation available in the acute or semi-acute setting may suggest the presence of PCP in patients who present with cough and shortness of breath. Based on my experience, at initial presentation patients with PCP have anemia (80 percent), lymphopenia (42 percent), thrombocytopenia (6 percent), increased lactate dehydrogenase (78 percent), increased erythrocyte sedimentation rate (100 percent), and increased immunoglobulin A (86 percent). Unfortunately, these findings are nonspecific and not universally present among patients with PCP. Finally, analysis of arterial blood gases on room air often reveal hypoxia and hyperventilation. These findings are also nonspecific, and 10 to 30 percent of patients with PCP have been reported to present with normal arterial blood gases at rest.

Additional Laboratory Evaluation

For patients whose acute clinical evaluation is equivocal for the presence of PCP, there are several additional tests that may be helpful, especially if there is a normal or near normal chest film. In the emergency department or office, spirometry can be easily performed. By virtue of increased lung elastic recoil, most diffuse peripheral pulmonary processes (including PCP) are associated with increased airflow as measured by spirometry and reflected by an increased forced expired volume in 1 second (FEV_1) expressed as a percentage of the forced vital capacity (FVC) (FEV_1 percent of $FVC = FEV_1 \div FVC \times 100$). This abnormality is not diagnostic of PCP, but is extremely suggestive in the appropriate clinical setting. We have performed spirometry on all homosexual men who presented with respiratory symptoms consistent with possible PCP. There was a statistically significant difference between the mean FEV_1 percent of FVC for the group of patients subsequently found to have PCP compared with those found not to have PCP; 86 ± 5.3 percent versus 78 ± 2 percent, respectively ($p < .001$). Comparing each individual PCP patient with his predicted FEV_1 percent of FVC, 16 of 17 patients had an increased FEV_1 percent of FVC, and the one patient without an increased flow rate had asthma. Further, although the diffusing capacity cannot be tested in the emergency department or office, it is noteworthy that the diffusing capacity was decreased in all but one of the first twenty patients with PCP studied with pulmonary physiology.

The gallium lung scan is another test helpful in determining the presence of diffuse parenchymal disease in patients with undiagnosed respiratory symptoms and normal chest roentgenograms. Although not available on an acute basis, and never specific for any disease, virtually all our patients with PCP have a diffuse grade III or IV gallium lung scan, even in the presence of a normal chest roentgenogram (a grade III scan implies lung uptake equal to that of liver; grade IV scan implies gallium uptake in the lung more intense than that in the liver).

Diagnosis of PCP

Once a patient is felt possibly to have PCP, a specific diagnosis must be made. Empiric therapy is acceptable for several days while specific diagnostic tests are undertaken. However, empiric therapy without a specific diagnosis should be discouraged for several reasons. The clinical presentation of PCP is nonspecific and a different agent may be identified. Also, specific diagnosis of PCP is a simultaneous diagnosis of AIDS by definition. Given the ultimate lethal nature of AIDS and possible future effective therapy for this condition, the diagnosis of PCP and AIDS should be as accurate and specific as possible. Finally, therapy for PCP is commonly associated with significant side effects and makes a specific diagnosis of this entity mandatory.

The diagnostic approach to PCP is undergoing constant revision at the present time. Bronchoscopy is currently the preferred approach in terms of high yield and low morbidity. Bronchoscopy, by combining both transbronchial biopsy and bronchoalveolar lavage (BAL), has a diagnostic accuracy for PCP that approaches 100 percent. However, transbronchial biopsy may result in serious complications: hemoptysis (5 to 10 percent) and pneumothorax (5 percent). In our recent prospective study, BAL alone using the bronchoscope detected PCP in 34 of 35 patients (97 percent). We are now performing BAL with a disposable catheter using a semidisposable fiberoptic stylet (Microvasive, Inc, Boston, MA). The diagnostic yield of PCP with this inexpensive, safe bedside technique is at least 90 percent.

Recently sputum induction has resulted in a diagnosis of PCP in 60 percent of cases. Whether induced sputum testing misses other pathogens and whether laboratory personnel in other hospitals are as adept at identifying PCP in sputum remains unknown. If sputum and/or lavage continue to be effective diagnostic modalities, patients suspected of PCP will probably be studied directly with these modalities, obviating the expense and delay of screening evaluation such as gallium scanning, pulmonary function test, and diffusing capacity.

Our present initial approach to patients with possible PCP is to perform a lavage or sputum induction on an outpatient basis if possible. After a negative lavage, a full fiberoptic bronchoscopy employing both transbronchial biopsy and repeat lavage is undertaken. If the bronchoscopy with biopsy and BAL is negative and the patient's clinical course is the same or worse, we repeat the bronchoscopy. Using this approach, we have never had to go on to an open lung biopsy in the context of AIDS.

Treatment of PCP

Hospitalization of patients with a diagnosis of PCP and AIDS should be kept to a minimum. With appropriate monitoring, they can be treated as outpatients for some or all of their 3-week treatment course. Prospective and retrospective studies have shown that pentamidine and trimethoprim-sulfamethoxazole (TMP/SMZ) are equally effective; with either compund, roughly 70 percent of patients survive a particular episode of PCP. Surprisingly, TMP/SMZ, when used in patients with AIDS, is associated with significant side effects in at least half of them. Nevertheless, initial treatment with TMP-SMX is recommended, especially as this therapy lends itself to outpatient management; pentamidine must be given parenterally.

The oral dose of TMP/SMZ is 20 mg per kilogram of body weight of trimethorprim and 200 mg per kilogram of sulfamethoxazole in four divided dialy doses, which usually equals 4 single strength tablets (or 2 double strength tablets) 4 times a day. Patients with severe PCP and/or diarrhea must be hospitalized for parenteral therapy. It has been recommended that patients receiving oral TMP/SMZ should have a blood level test $1 1/2$ hours after a dose; the blood level of trimethoprim should be at least 5 μg per milliliter and for sulfamethoxazole 100 μg per milliliter.

Patients receiving treatment for PCP should be monitored for both drug effectiveness and toxicity. Response to therapy is completely unpredictable, although patients with an initial room air Po_2 of 70 mm Hg and above tend to do much better than those who present with a Po_2 below 70 mm Hg. In general, there are three patterns of therapeutic response: recovery, rapid downhill course, and slow downhill course. A positive response is usually heralded by a decrease in the fever by day 5 or 6, a increase in the Po_2 compared with baseline of at least 10 mm Hg by day 8 to 10, and an improvement in chest roentgenogram by day 12 or 13. If the patient is not improved or is worse by day 5 or 6, therapy should be changed to pentamidine (4 mg per kilogram daily IM or IV in 250 ml of D5W slowly infused over 2 to 3 hours). Patients who are switched from TMP/SMZ still must be dine because of failure to improve have only a 10 to 12 percent chance of survival.

Patients who respond to TMP/SMZ still must be monitored twice a week for drug toxicity: fever, rash, decrease in white blood cell count or platelet count, increase in transaminase levels, and azotemia. Addition of folate has not minimized hematologic side effects. Also, in patients in whom TMP/SMZ is discontinued because of the development of rash or fever, the subsequent reinstitution of this compound can result in life-threatening anaphylaxis. In contrast to patients switched from TMP/SMZ to pentamidine secondary to drug failure; patients responding to TMP/SMZ who are changed to pentamidine because of drug toxicity are very likely to survive that particular episode of PCP. At least 50 percent of patients suffer side effects of pentamidine, including hypotension, fever, azotemia, neutropenia, rash, and sterile abscess formation at the intramuscular injection site.

Because of the side effects of conventional therapy, new therapeutic modalities are being studied. Dapsone (diaminodiaphenylsulfone), 100 mg orally once a day, has been combined with trimethoprim (20 mg per kilogram a day) with some effectiveness but is still associated with toxicity (pancytopenia, hemolytic anemia, and rash). Also, protective prophylactic therapy has been reported using a tablet of Fansidar (pyrimethamine and sulfadoxine) once a week.

Kaposi's Sarcoma

In addition to PCP, Kaposi's sarcoma is the other hallmark of AIDS as defined by the CDC. Roughly half the patients with Kaposi's sarcoma have pulmonary involvement with this tumor. In one autopsy series, 25 percent of patients with pulmonary Kaposi's sarcoma were felt to have died as a result of that tumor. Symptoms of pulmonary Kaposi's sarcoma include cough and shortness of breath, but unlike patients with PCP, those with Kaposi's sarcoma also complain of hemoptysis, pleural pain, wheezing, and stridor. Moderate-sized pleural effusions are attributable to pleural Kaposi's sarcoma or mediastinal tumor (often evident only at autopsy). In addition to pleural effusions, pulmonary edema may result from lumphatic obstruction owing to mediastinal involvement by Kaposi's sarcoma. Kaposi's sarcoma lesions line the airway mucosa and cause hemoptysis and pulmonary hemorrhage which can mimic the classic radiologic manifestations of PCP. Airway lesions can cause airway obstruction, giving rise to stridor and wheezing.

Cytomegalovirus

Cytomegalovirus (CMV) is frequently present in conjuction with PCP in patients immunosuppressed with or without AIDS. It is an untreatable infection. However, it is not clear what pathogenetic role its presence in the lung implies. Among AIDS patients with PCP, the presence or absence of pulmonary CMV has no effect on the clinical course following PCP therapy. Occasionally patients with large amounts of virus may have a shorter life span, possibly owing to pulmonary CMV.

CMV may cause adrenal necrosis. Patients with AIDS may present with hemodynamic instability because of a hypoadrenal state possibly secondary to CMV.

Atypical Mycobacterium Avium Intracellulare

Another common pulmonary manifestation of AIDS is atypical *Mycobacterium avium intracellulare*. Patients with AIDS develop poorly formed granulomas, so biopsy material from AIDS patients should be stained appropriately for mycobacterial organisms even in the absence of granulomas. It is difficult, if not impossible, to treat this infection. In nonimmunosuppressd patients with this infection, the therapeutic success is about 50 percent because of drug resistance. In AIDS patients, in addition to the problem of drug resistance, the organism is usually widely disseminated: lung, blood, stool, bone marrow, liver, etc. Two new antituberculosis therapies, ansamycin (a rifampin derivative) and clofazamine, may prove effective against this organism.

Fungi

Fungal infections account for only a few percent of pulmonary infections among AIDS patients. Most commonly, cryptococcosis presents with diffuse involvement of many organs including the lung and brain. Treatment is with amphotericin B. After a l-mg test dose, initial therapy is 0.25 mg per kilogram per day, which is increased to 0.5 mg per kilogram per day subsequently. Unfortunately, after therapy is discontinued, cryptococcal relapses are common. Other fungal infections not classically considered "opportunistic" include histoplasmosis and coccidioidomycosis; the latter has recently been reported with simultaneous PCP.

Miscellaneous Additional Pulmonary Problems Among Patients with AIDS

Other pulmonary problems related to AIDS include recently reported pulmonary cryptosporidiosis. Although acknowledged as a cause of severe diarrhea, cryptosporidiosis has only recently been associated with diffuse interstitial lung disease which mimics PCP. Patients who present with copious sputum production should be suspected of having this infection. An acid-fast smear of sputum or lung secretions can identify this organism.

Non-Hodgkin's lymphoma has been reported as a possible consequence of AIDS. Virtually all 90 cases recently reported had extranodal involvement, including brain, eye, rectum, and lung. Pulmonary involvement by lymphoma occurred in 15 percent of cases with radiologic expressions that included adenopathy, parenchymal nodules, masses, and interstitial infiltrates. Finally, diffuse lung involvement can be secondary to lymphocytic interstitial pneumonitis. Lung pathologic studies reveal fine nodular lymphoplasmacytic infiltrates around bronchioles extending into the alveoli. This process may be a pulmonary expression of a generalized phenomenon of reactive lymphoplasmacytosis involving lymph nodes, bone marrow, liver, kidney, salivary glands, etc. Lymphocytic interstitial pneumonitis may be associated with the development of lymphoma.

SUGGESTED READING

Broaddus C, et al. Bronchoalveolar lavage and transbronchial biopsy for the diagnosis of pulmonary infections in the acquired immunodeficiency syndrome. Ann Intern Med 1985; 102:747–752.

Fauci AS, et al. The acquired immunodeficiency syndrome: an update. Ann Intern Med 1935; 102:800–813.

Kovacs JA, et al. Pneumocystis carini pneumonia: a comparison between patients with the acquired immunodeficiency syndrome and patients with other immunodeficiencies. Ann Intern Med 1984; 100:663–671.

Murray JF, et al. Pulmonary complications of the acquired immunodeficiency syndrome. Report of a National Heart, Lung and Blood Institute Workshop. N Engl J Med 1984; 310:1682–1688.

FUNGAL RESPIRATORY DISEASE

THEO N. KIRKLAND, M.D.

All the common fungi capable of causing deep mycoses are respiratory pathogens. Since millions of people in the United States have immunologic evidence of prior infection with one of the pathogenic fungi, fungal respiratory infections must be fairly common. However, most of these infections are subclinical and either are not recognized by the patient at all or are thought to be a "cold." Occasionally, one of these infections causes more serious disease, which prompts the patient to seek medical attention. The spectrum of disease in this subset of patients is broad, ranging from bronchitis to severe pneumonia. Even in these patients, most infections resolve spontaneously, but a few disseminate to other organs or cause chronic pneumonia.

Only a few species of fungi are capable of causing respiratory infections in immunocompetent patients. These organisms can be divided into two groups: (1) dimorphic filamentous fungi and (2) yeast. The dimorphic filamentous fungi share the common property of growing as a mold in the soil and converting to a yeast-like form with the body. The common pathogenic filamentous fungi of North America listed in Table 1 are all found in the soil, and infections result from inhaling the spores from dust. Once inside the lung, these fungi differentiate into their parasitic forms. For *Histoplasma capsulatum* the parasitic form is a small (2 to 4 μ) oval yeast that buds from its narrow end. The parasitic form of *Coccidioides immitis* is the spherule, which is a round structure ranging in size from 20 to 80 μ. The spherule divides internally to generate hundreds of endospores, each of which has the capacity to develop into a new spherule. *Blastomyces dermatitidis* develops in a large, fairly round yeast that has a broad-based bud.

Table 1 lists the endemic areas for each of these fungi. Histoplasmosis and blastomycosis are endemic in the Mississippi and Ohio River valleys, whereas coccidioidomycosis is limited to the southwest. *H. capsulatum*

is also occasionally found outside the endemic area. All these organisms thrive within microenvironments within the endemic areas. *H. capsulatum* grows particularly well in soil contaminated by bird or bat droppings, and *C. immitis* seems to grow much better in some areas of the desert than in others.

Cryptococcus neoformans is not dimorphic; it grows as a yeast both in the soil and in infected tissues. It is the only yeast that commonly infects people by the respiratory route. Although cryptococcal infections do occur in normal hosts, about 50 percent of serious cryptococcal infections occur in the immunosuppressed, a much higher percentage than is found with the filamentous fungi. In addition, cryptococcal disease presents most frequently as meningitis, though symptomatic lung infections also occur. *C. neoformans* is not limited to any area of the United States and occurs throughout the world.

In severely immunocompromised individuals many fungi can cause pulmonary infections. The most common cause of invasive pulmonary disease in the immunocompromised host is *Aspergillus fumigatus*, but other species of *Aspergillus*, as well as a wide variety of other filamentous fungi, can cause disease in neutropenic patients. These less virulent organisms rarely cause invasive pulmonary disease in patients with normal numbers of neutrophils, and will not be considered further here.

DIAGNOSIS

The clinical presentations of pneumonias due to the primary pathogenic dimorphic fungi are similar and will be discussed together. As already mentioned, the spectrum of severity of the illness is wide. However, the patient usually presents with a flu-like illness character-

TABLE 1 Primary Pathogenic Fungi

Filamentous Fungi	Parasitic Form	Edemic Area
Histoplasma capsulatum	Small, oval, budding yeast	Mississippi and Ohio River Valleys
Coccidioides immitis	Spherule	Southwest
Blastomyces dermatitidis	Large, round, budding yeast	Mississippi and Ohio River Valleys

ized by nonproductive cough, pleuritic chest pain, headache, fever, myalgias, and arthralgias. The typical patient is not as toxic as most patients with bacterial pneumonia, and the onset of the illness is usually more insidious, frequently developing over 5 to 7 days. The cough is most often nonproductive, but some patients develop purulent sputum. Pleuritic chest pain and nonpleuritic chest discomfort are common symptoms, but pleural effusions are uncommon. The systemic symptoms of myalgias, fever, night sweats, and malaise are often prominent, even when the infection appears to be limited to the chest. In severe cases, these symptoms can take weeks to months to resolve.

In most cases the physical examination of the chest is either normal or remarkable only for rales. Signs of lobar consolidation are unusual. The general physical examination should include a careful examination for evidence of disseminated infection. Some of the most common sites of dissemination for each of the fungi are listed in Table 2. Erythema nodosum or erythema multiforme is a complication of acute histoplasmosis or coccidioidomycosis. These responses are most often seen in young women and can be associated with reactive arthritis. The most common roentgenographic feature of acute fungal pneumonia is a patchy, nonsegmental infiltrate, although lobar infiltrates or miliary patterns may be seen. Pleural effusions are relatively uncommon. In histoplasmosis and coccidioidomycosis, mediastinal and hilar lymphadenopathy are common and should be a diagnostic clue.

Respiratory infections due to *Cryptococcus neoformans* do not present a distinctive clinical picture. The infection is frequently asymptomatic, even when large lung masses are present. The patient who is symptomatic should undergo bronchoscopy and transbronchial biopsy to establish the diagnosis. A search for skin lesions should also be made because scrapings or biopsies of these lesions frequently reveal the diagnosis. Blood cultures generally are not useful, but can be positive for *C. neoformans* and *H. capsulatum* in some cases.

A number of immunologic tests are available to help establish the diagnosis. The most specific tests are available for *C. immitis*. Precipitating antibodies develop soon after symptoms develop in approximately 75 percent of patients. Only 25 percent of patients with self-limited pneumonia develop complement-fixing (CF) antibody, and these are usually of low titer (less than 1:16). A high titer of complement-fixing antibody suggests that dissemination has occurred. Most patients develop a positive skin test for *C. immitis* antigens within several weeks of infection. The serologic tests for histoplasmosis are less specific, and false-positive results are a problem. Nonetheless, a complement-fixing titer of 1:32 against the yeast phase is suggestive of acute disease, although a fourfold rise in titer is of more diagnostic value. In histoplasmosis, the level of CF antibody has no prognostic significance. The agar gel precipitation test is simpler and easier to perform, but is of less diagnostic value. The histoplasmin skin test should not be done until serologic testing is completed, since skin testing can cause rises in antibody titers. It is of limited usefulness in the highly endemic area (because almost everyone has a positive reaction), but it is useful outside the endemic area. Serologic tests for blastomycosis are of limited value. The finding of cryptococcal antigen in the serum or spinal fluid is diagnostic of cryptococcal disease, if false-positives due to rheumatoid factors are excluded.

TREATMENT

The decision to treat any individual patient is a complex one, and many factors must be considered. If there is evidence of disseminated disease, treatment should be started promptly because disseminated lesions rarely resolve spontaneously. If no evidence for disseminated disease can be found, one must consider the immunocompetence of the patient and the severity and duration of the lung disease. Patients who are immunocompromised are unlikely to resolve their infections. Infants with histoplasmosis are likely to require drug treatment, as are patients with coccidioidomycosis with high titers of complement-fixing antibody ($> 1:32$). Anyone with pneumonia that is severe enough to compromise oxygenation should also be treated promptly. The majority of cases do not fall into one of these categories, and individual decisions must be made based on the severity and duration of the illness. If patients are clinically ill for more than 3 weeks, initiation of treatment should be strongly considered, if only to ameliorate symptoms.

The drugs that are available to treat invasive fungal disease are listed in Table 3. Amphotericin B is the most toxic of the drugs listed, but it is also the drug that has the most proven value. Amphotericin B treatment is effective for all primary pathogenic filamentous fungi, as well as *C. neoformans*; it should always be the drug of first choice in acute life-threatening disease. Amphotericin B has both acute and chronic toxicities (to be discussed). It usually causes fevers and chills during the period of drug infusion, as well as thrombophlebitis at the site of infusion. Since patients usually become somewhat tolerant of the acute systemic toxicity, the drug is initiated slowly. All patients should be given a 1-mg test dose over 1 hour, and their vital signs closely monitored for several hours after the infusion because a small per-

TABLE 2 Common Manifestations of Disseminated Infection

Histoplasmosis: oropharyngeal ulcers, hepatosplenomegaly, Addison's disease, gastrointestinal ulceration, endocarditis

Coccidioidomycosis: verrucose skin lesions, arthritis, meningitis osteomyelitis

Blastomycosis: ulcerative skin lesions, osteomyelitis, genitourinary involvement

Cryptococcosis: meningitis

centage of patients develop shock when treated with the drug. If the test dose is well tolerated, a second dose of 0.3 mg per kilogram can be given over a period of 1 to 2 hours. If the test dose was poorly tolerated, a smaller second dose should be given. Pretreatment of the patient with aspirin and Benadryl, as well as incorporation of 10 to 25 mg of hydrocortisone and 1,000 units of heparin into the infusion, may also help to ameliorate the acute toxicity. In the rare case of fulminant pneumonia, the dose of amphotericin B should be escalated as quickly as possible. In less pressing circumstances, the dose is increased by 10 mg per day, until a dose of 0.7 mg per kilogram (maximum of 50 mg per day) is reached. I prefer to switch to an every-other-day regimen once maximum doses are achieved because the drug has a long half-life and the organisms multiply slowly. An every-other-day regimen also gives the patient a respite from the acute toxicities of amphotericin B.

The total amount of amphotericin B needed to treat the various mycoses has, by and large, been empirically determined. A total of 2 to 3 g are recommended for disseminated histoplasmosis and coccidioidomycosis; 1.5 to 2.5 g of amphotericin B is recommended for blastomycosis. A 2- to 3-week course of 40 to 50 mg per day has been shown to be effective in acute pulmonary histoplasmosis. The clinical course should influence the duration and total amount of drug. Meningitis and endocarditis require additional therapy, which will not be considered here.

The major limitation in the amount of amphotericin B that can be used to treat an infection is the renal toxicity of the drug. As higher cumulative doses are achieved, the glomerular filtration rate gradually falls to 20 to 50 percent of normal. In some cases, rapid deterioration of renal function occurs. When this happens, the drug should be stopped for a few days, if possible, and restarted at a lower dose. Frequently, this slows the deterioration of renal function. Some patients tolerate amphotericin B poorly; in these cases one either constantly adjusts dosages or

chooses an alternate drug. In most cases renal function slowly improves after the drug is stopped, but some patients have permanent severe kidney damage. Amphotericin B also causes renal tubular acidosis and potassium wasting, and so electrolytes should be monitored. Anemia, caused by impaired erythrocyte production, is also a frequent side effect of therapy.

Of the fungi we are considering, only *Cryptococcus neoformans* can be treated with 5-fluorocytosine (5-FC). However, 5-FC should not be used as a single drug to treat the *cryptococcus,* since resistance develops rapidly. The combination of 5-FC and amphotericin B is more effective than amphotericin B alone in the treatment of cryptococcal meningitis. I prefer to use this combination for the treatment of any cryptococcal disease that requires therapy. Amphotericin B is given at a lower dose (0.3 mg per kilogram per day) for 6 weeks when it is combined with 5-FC, 150 mg per kilogram per day divided into four equal doses. The 5-FC dose must be adjusted for renal function and may need to be changed during the course of therapy as renal function deteriorates. Hematopoietic and gastrointestinal toxicity may be caused by 5-FC, especially if high blood levels are achieved. One should monitor 5-FC blood levels, if possible, and keep the blood level below 75 μg per milliliter.

Ketoconazole is another drug that is active against some pathogenic fungi. This drug is given orally and is much less toxic than amphotericin B. Experience with ketoconazole is still limited, and its usefulness is still being defined. However, ketoconazole appears to be effective for the treatment of histoplasmosis if the infection is not immediately life-threatening; 400 mg per day of ketoconazole seems to be about as effective as amphotericin B, and much less toxic. Ketoconazole should not be used in conventional doses to treat fungal meningitis or endocarditis. For the majority of cases of indolent disseminated disease, or histoplasmosis pneumonia that is slow to clear, ketoconazole is a reasonable alternative to amphotericin B. Experience with blastomycosis is more limited, but the drug appears to be effective therapy for this infection as well. Coccidioidomycosis does not respond as well to ketoconazole as does disease caused by the other two primary pathogenic dimorphic fungi. Many patients have a temporary response, but the relapse rate is high. I think that amphotericin B is the drug of choice for disseminated coccidioidomycosis. However, ketoconazole treatment may suppress chronic skin, bone, and joint lesions that have not been eradicated by amphotericin B therapy. Whether primary pneumonia due to *C. immitis* is responsive to ketoconazole therapy is unknown.

Ketoconazole requires an acid stomach for absorption, and so it should be given before meals. The usual dose for an adult is 400 mg per day in a single dose. Higher doses cause more side effects, and it is unclear whether they are more effective. For histoplasmosis and blastomycosis, the drug is usually given for 6 months. If the disease is not responding to treatment, one should switch to amphotericin B treatment. The guidelines for treatment of coccidioidomycosis with ketoconazole are

TABLE 3 Antifungal Agents

Drug	Activity Against Respiratory Fungi	Toxicity
Amphotericin B	Dimorphic pathogenic fungi	Acute: fevers, chills, hypotension (rare), thrombophlebitis
	C. neoformans	Chronic: renal insufficiency, anemia, hepatitis
5-Fluorocytosine	C. neoformans	Gastrointestinal and hematologic
Ketoconazole	Dimorphic pathogenic fungi	Nausea, vomiting, endocrine abnormalities, hepatitis

less clear, but prolonged treatment is often necessary to suppress the disease. The most frequent side effects of ketoconazole are nausea, vomiting, and occasionally diarrhea. Frequently, these side effects clear over time, especially if the dose is temporarily reduced. Transient, asymptomatic elevations of liver function tests are common. Symptomatic hepatitis is rare, but can be fatal. The drug should be stopped promptly if clinical hepatitis develops.

SUGGESTED READING

Kirkland TN. Newer antifungal agents. Petersdorf RG, Adams RD, et al, eds. In: Harrison's principles of internal medicine. Update VI. New York: McGraw Hill Books, 1985:19.

Medoff G, Kobayashi GS. Strategies in the treatment of systemic fungal infections. N Engl J Med 1980; 302:145–155.

PULMONARY INFECTION CAUSED BY AEROBIC GRAM-POSITIVE COCCI

JOHN G. BARTLETT, M.D.

Gram-positive cocci that are important pulmonary pathogens include the pneumococcus, *Staphylococcus aureus*, and *Streptococcus pyogenes* (group A beta-hemolytic streptococci). Occasional reports suggest that the enterococcus, *Streptococcus viridans*, and *Staphylococcus epidermidis* may cause lower airway infections, but either these are very rare or the occasional anecdotal reports do not provide compelling evidence of their pathogenic role. Anaerobic and microaerophilic streptococci are relatively common organisms in aspiration pneumonia or lung abscess.

The *pneumococcus* is the most frequently recognized bacterial pathogen of the lower airways, accounting for 40 to 60 percent of infections in adults over the age of 35 years who acquire their disease in the community. *S. aureus* accounts for about 2 percent of community-acquired infections and 10 to 20 percent of nosocomial pneumonias. *S. pyogenes* is a relatively rare pulmonary pathogen, but it has been implicated in some epidemics of pneumonia, particularly in military recruits.

Management strategies include selection of an antibiotic. This is best when based on reliable microbiologic data such as cultures of an uncontaminated specimen source, including blood, pleural fluid, transtracheal aspirates, transthoracic aspirates, or a site of distant dissemination such as cerebrospinal fluid or joint fluid. The diagnosis is considered tentative when based on a Gram stain of expectorated sputum showing a dominance of an appropriate bacterial morphotype accompanied by a large number of neutrophils, or on the recovery of this type of organism in culture in large concentrations.

DIAGNOSIS

Nearly all patients with acute infections of the pulmonary parenchyma have fever, symptoms referable to the lower respiratory tract (e.g., cough, dyspnea, sputum), and an infiltrate exhibited on chest x-ray film. The major noninfectious conditions to consider with this type of presentation are pulmonary embolism, pulmonary edema, adult respiratory distress syndrome, chemical pneumonia (Mendelsohn's sydrome), and bronchial obstruction (e.g., foreign body, neoplasm). Factors that assist in the differential diagnosis are that nearly all patients with the noninfectious lesions have associated predisposing conditions that are readily recognized, that fever is almost invariably present with pneumonia and tends to be higher than that associated with alternative conditions, that purulent sputum favors infection, that rigors favor pneumonia, and that the patterns of changes seen on x-ray film are often helpful.

When the diagnosis of pneumonia appears confirmed, the next challenge is to identify a specific etiologic agent. This is a much harder task. A good-quality expectorated sputum culture for *Gram stain*, cytologic screen, and culture should be obtained (Table 1). Experience from our hospital indicates that the Gram stain of the expectorated specimen shows a dominant organism with the morphologic characteristics of a likely pulmonary pathogen in about one-half of patients with community-acquired pneumonia. Cytologic screening is done with low-power (10×) examination to determine the relative proportions of neutrophils and epithelial cells. In specimens that show a dominance of polymorphonuclear cells, the organism suggested by Gram stain is cultured in 90 to 95 percent of cases.

A likely etiologic agent can be identified in about half of the cases with expectorated sputum Gram stain. This information is immediately available and should form the basis for initial antibiotic selection. The other half of the patients have no good specimen or expectorations that show a "mixed flora," "normal oral flora," or "sparse bacteria." Diagnostic considerations here include all of the organisms listed in Table 1 (including *S. pneumoniae*), aspiration pneumonia (involving oral flora, especially anaerobic bacteria), atypical pneumonias (especially *Mycoplasma pneumoniae* or *Legionella pneumophila*), viral pneumonia, pulmonary infections involving pathogens that require nonroutine diagnostic techniques (mycobacteria, Q fever, chlamydia, *Bordetella pertussis*, *Nocardia*, *Francisella*, fungi, and *Pneumocystis carinii*), and the noninfectious conditions reviewed subsequently.

Patients who lack a diagnostic expectorated-sputum sample may be considered candidates for *specialized methods to obtain lower airway secretions*. These include nasopharyngeal, transtracheal, bronchoscopic, and transthoracic aspirates. All of these procedures have advocates and skeptics regarding indications, value, and morbidity. In my view, invasive tests should be reserved for cases that satisfy the following criteria: (1) the diagnosis cannot be established with noninvasive tests (sputum, nasopharyngeal aspirate, blood or pleural fluid cultures); (2) the severity of the disease must justify the risk involved; (3) for infections with suspected bacterial pathogens, the test should be done prior to antibiotic therapy; (4) technical expertise must be available; and (5) there must be no patient contraindications.

CLINICAL PATTERNS OF DISEASE

Microbiologic findings must obviously be correlated with clinical findings. The following patterns of illness are seen with the various gram-positive cocci:

1. *S. pneumoniae* is classically described as an acute pneumonia with a single rigor, rusty sputum, and a consolidated (lobar) infiltrate revealed on x-ray film. However, most cases are atypical and lack these classical features. Poor prognostic findings are multiple lobe involvement, bacteremia, debilitated host, and leukopenia. The mortality rate with bacteremia is 20 to 30 percent despite penicillin therapy. Antibiotics have not altered mortality rates during the first 5 days of treatment. Clinical deterioration does not necessarily indicate an erroneous diagnosis, and controlled trials show no advantage to high doses of penicillin (20 million units per day) compared to the modest doses commonly advocated (2 million units per day) for seriously ill patients with uncomplicated disease.

2. *S. aureus* is a rare cause of pneumonia except in the cases of infants, hospital-acquired pneumonia, pneumonia superimposed on influenza, and selected hosts (those with cystic fibrosis, chronic granulomatous disease, or neutropenia). Contrary to popular belief, most patients simply have x-ray films showing bronchopneumonia; cavitation is the exception rather than the rule, and lobar pneumonia is distinctly rare. Symptoms may be acute or chronic. Response to therapy is slow. Unlike patients whose disease is caused by the pneumococcus, nearly all patients have a positive sputum culture; thus, the failure to recover this agent from a good pretreatment specimen is strong evidence against the diagnosis.

3. The most characteristic feature of pneumonia attributable to *group A beta-hemolytic streptococci* is the early and often large associated pleural effusion that may be hemorrhagic fluid or pus. This disease is rare.

Supportive Care

Clearance of pulmonary secretions with adequate hydration, encouragement of coughing, and, if necessary, use of a steam vaporizer or water nebulizer are important. Expectorants are of questionable benefit. Available data do not show convincing evidence that recovery is promoted by pulmonary physiotherapy including intermit-

TABLE 1   Gram Stain Identification of Pathogens in Pneumonia

Gram Stain Finding	Suspected Pathogen	Comment
Gram-positive cocci in chains	*Streptococcus pneumoniae*	Should be lancet shaped and quellung positive. Most common mistake is to fail to distinguish *S. viridans* that is a dominant component of oral flora
Gram-positive cocci in clusters	*Staphylococcus aureus*	Anaerobic gram-positive cocci (peptococci) resemble staphylococci
Gram-negative coccobacilli (small)	*Haemophilus influenzae*	One of the most commonly overlooked pulmonary pathogens
Gram-negative diplococci (large)	*Branhamella catarrhalis*	Newly recognized pathogen
Gram-negative bacilli (large)	Enterobacteriaceae or *Pseudomonas*	All organisms in this group appear similar

tent positive pressure breathing. A possible exception is that of patients with large volumes of secretions, particularly those with large abscesses or severe bronchiectasis, in whom postural drainage may prove useful when supervised by a pulmonary physiotherapist. Additional methods to facilitate drainage in this setting include nasotracheal suction and bronchoscopy. Patients with a debilitating cough may have this suppressed with codeine in doses of 45 to 60 mg as necessary. This drug or similar agents may also be used to relieve severe pleuritic pain. The use of sedatives or large amounts of narcotics for pain relief may cause suppression of respiration and should be avoided.

Patients who have hypoxia may benefit from oxygen therapy, which may be delivered with a nasal cannula at a flow rate of 6 L per minute; however, this must be done with caution in patients with chronic lung disease. Patients with a history of respiratory insufficiency who require supplemental oxygen should receive this using 24 to 28 percent oxygen by Ventimask or a nasal cannula with a flow rate of 1 to 2 L per minute. Small-bowel ileus or gastric dilatation may cause elevation of the diaphragm and further compromise pulmonary function. Patients with this complication may benefit from nasogastric suction or a rectal tube.

The decision to use antipyretics is often difficult, particularly in patients under home care, because these drugs are widely available in virtually all nonprescription remedies for respiratory infections. There are disadvantages to eliminating fever. Elevated temperatures appear to enhance the immune response to a microbial infection. Fever is also a major parameter used to judge response to treatment, and the intermittent use of antipyretics may result in wide fluctuations in the temperature profile, which may contribute to patient misery. Antipyretics are best used for patients with high fever who do not tolerate temperature elevations well or who have medical contraindications to high fever, as with myocardial ischemia. In these settings, the usual regimen is acetaminophen or aspirin in doses of 0.6 g every 4 to 6 hours. Corticosteroids are not advocated for the patient with severe pneumonia, but patients who have previously received these agents chronically should have an increased dosage to prevent addisonian crisis, using doses as high as the equivalent of 300 mg of hydrocortisone during the period of acute illness. Other supportive measures for the seriously ill patient include intravenous fluids for dehydration, correction of electrolyte imbalance, intravenous sodium bicarbonate for lactic acidosis, and digitalis or diuretics for congestive failure and fluid retention.

Pleural Effusions

Pleural effusions should be aspirated for culture, cell count, and pH determination. With large effusions, the thoracentesis is done for both diagnosis and therapy. The decision for chest-tube drainage depends on multiple interrelated factors, but the usual criteria are positive pleural fluid cultures, a pH under 7.0, purulent collections that do not flow readily with needle aspiration, and large effusions that reaccumulate rapidly or in loculated collections.

Epidemiologic Considerations

The source of infection in patients with bacterial pneumonia is often difficult to etablish, although the possibility of transmission within the hospital setting is a subject of considerable concern. My policy is adherence to the guidelines of the Centers for Disease Control (CDC), which provide a medicolegal document with at least some rationale. No particular precautions are necessary in patients with pneumococcal pneumonia except for those with penicillin-resistant strains. Patients with penicillin-resistant *S. pneumoniae* are placed in a single room with secretion precautions until 24 hours after initiation of appropriate antibiotic therapy. Patients with staphylococcal pneumonia receive strict isolation for the duration of the illness.

ANTIBIOTIC SELECTION

Antibiotic treatment is summarized in Table 2.

S. Pneumoniae

Penicillin is the drug of choice for *S. pneumoniae* although major controversies exist over the route of administration, dosage, and duration of treatment. The only possible exception to penicillin treatment is the patient with an isolate that is resistant to penicillin. Such strains are unusual except in children who have received multiple or extensive courses of penicillin. Most of these strains are only "moderately" resistant (minimum inhibitory concentration ([MIC] values of 0.1 to 1.0 μg per milliliter) and presumably should respond to penicillin given parenterally at somewhat higher dosages. The alternative agent for strains that are highly resistant to penicillin and to other agents is vancomycin.

The dosage and route of administration for the usual patient with pneumococcal pneumonia depend on the severity of illness, the decision for inpatient versus outpatient management, and the presence or absence of extrapulmonary, suppurative complications. Most patients are treated with either procaine penicillin G, 600,000 units every 8 to 12 hours or aqueous penicillin G, about 2 million units per day. Treatment is continued until the patient has been afebrile for 2 to 5 days, although this course may be completed for an outpatient using oral penicillin V, 500 mg 4 times a day. High doses of penicillin (10 million to 20 million units of aqueous penicillin G per day) are reserved for patients who have cases complicated by pneumococcal meningitis, septic arthritis, or endocarditis.

The preferred alternative agents for parenteral use are cephalothin (1 g IV every 4 hours) or cefazolin (1 g IV every 8 hours). Patients with a contraindication to beta-lactam antibiotics may be treated with clindamycin (600 mg IV every 8 hours) or any of several other agents listed in Table 2.

TABLE 2 Initial Treatment of Staphylococcal and Streptococcal Pulmonary Infections

Agent	Preferred Regimen	Alternatives	Comments
S. pneumoniae Outpatient therapy	Penicillin V 250–500 mg PO q.i.d.	Erythromycin 250–500 mg PO q.i.d.	Acceptable alternatives: Ampicillin, penicillin G, tetracycline, clindamycin, sulfamethoxazole-trimethoprim
Hospitalized patients	Moderately ill: Procaine penicillin G 600,000 units q8–12h Severely ill: Aqueous penicillin G 500,000 units IV q4-6h Complicated: Aqueous penicillin G 3–5 million units q4–6h	Cephalothin 0.5–1 g IV q6h Cefazolin 0.5 g IM or IV q8h	Acceptable alternatives: Other cephalosporins, clindamycin, nafcillin, chloramphenicol, vancomycin "Complicated" refers to patients with meningitis, septic arthritis, or endocarditis
S. aureus Methicillin-sensitive	Nafcillin 1–3 g IV q 4–6h	Cephalothin 1–2 g q 4–6h Clindamycin (erythromycin and clindamycin-sensitive strains) 600 mg IV q8h Vancomycin 500 mg IV q6h	Strains sensitive to penicillin at 0.1 μg/ml may be treated with penicillin G 1–2 million units q4–6h Oxacillin and methicillin are considered equivalent to nafcillin Cefamandole and cefazolin are considered equivalent to cephalothin
Methicillin-resistant	Vancomycin 500 mg IV q6h	None	For overwhelming or refractory cases: nafcillin, cephalothin, or vancomycin plus rifampin (300 mg PO b.i.d.) *or* an aminoglycoside
S. pyogenes	Aqueous penicillin G 600,000 units IV q4–6h	Cephalothin 0.5–1 g IV q6h Clindamycin 600 mg IV q8h	Acceptable alternatives: Ampicillin, clindamycin, other cephalosporins (preferably cefazolin, cefotaxime or cefamandole), erythromycin, vancomycin, chloramphenicol

S. Aureus

Penicillinase-resistant penicillins are regarded as the drugs of choice for methicillin-sensitive strains. Nafcillin and oxacillin are considered therapeutically equivalent and are given intravenously in relatively high doses (2 g every 4 to 6 hours) for rather extended periods. As a general rule, patients with staphylococcal bronchopneumonia are treated parenterally until they have been afebrile for at least 7 days, and this may be followed by an oral agent, such as dicloxacillin (2 g per day), cephalexin (2 g per day), or clindamycin (1.2 g per day) following discharge. Parenteral antibiotics are usually given for 4 to 6 weeks for patients with lung abscess, empyema, or suspected or established endocarditis, which includes patients with staphylococcal right-sided endocarditis and septic emboli to the lung (commonly seen in association with intravenous drug abuse). Rifampin (600 mg per day) or an aminoglycoside (usually gentamicin) may be added to the penicillinase-resistant penicillin or cephalosporin for patients who do not respond or who are critically ill.

Cephalosporins are considered therapeutically equivalent to penicillins in the treatment of serious staphylococcal infections, particularly cephalothin (2 g every 4 to 6 hours), cefazolin (1 g every 8 hours), or cefamandole (2 g every 4 to 6 hours). Most third-generation cephalosporins have reduced activity against *S. aureus,* although cefotaxime and ceftizoxime are usually considered acceptable when used for mixed infections. The first-generation cephalosporins may be preferred for the patient with a possible hypersensitivity reaction to penicillins or poor tolerance to intravenous administration of penicillins, which is particularly common with nafcillin. Cefazolin is the preferred agent when intramuscular treatment is necessary. Patients who have a history of IgE-mediated allergic response as indicated by anaphylaxis or giant urticaria, or who have a positive skin test to penicillin major or minor determinants, should receive an agent other than beta-lactam agents. Clindamycin (600 mg IV every 8 hours) has established efficacy, but it should be reserved for strains that are sensitive to both erythromycin and clindamycin. The reason is the high probability of rapid emergence of clindamycin resistance in erythrombycin-resistant strains. Vancomycin is another alternative to the beta-lactam drugs that is active against virtually all strains.

In recent years there has been an alarming increase in the incidence of methicillin-resistant strains of *S. aureus.* These strains are also resistant to virtually all cephalosporins, although they may appear sensitive with the routine in vitro sensitivity tests. Some of the strains are susceptible to aminoglycosides, sulfa-trimethoprim, or tetracycline, although there is limited clinical experience with these drugs. The only agent that can be advocated is vancomycin (500 mg IV every 6 hours using slow infusion over 60 minutes for adults with normal renal function). This drug is advocated for all patients with pneumonia involving methicillin-resistant strains, and it is often the preferred drug for empiric treatment for nosocomial infections where *S. aureus* is an established or suspected pathogen in hosjpitals where these strains are highly prevalent. In such situations, the antibiotic choice may be changed when in vitro sensitivity data are available.

S. Pyogenes

The preferred regimen is aqueous penicillin G given intravenously in doses of 2 to 4 million units given daily for initial treatment. This is continued until the patient has been afebrile for 2 to 5 days, and it may be followed by oral penicillin G or penicillin V (2 g per day) following discharge. There are multiple agents that may be given as alternatives, including cephalosporins and clindamycin. Many patients have pleural effusions or an empyema that requires an appropriate drainage procedure.

ADMISSION CRITERIA

Most patients, perhaps 70 to 75 percent, with infections of the lower airway may be managed as outpatients. This decision is largely based on the severity of the infection according to the history and physical examination. Initial laboratory tests advocated for all patients include a chest x-ray examination and a complete blood count. Chest roentgenography is the definitive test to distinguish pneumonia with involvement of the pulmonary parenchyma from infections limited to the major airways (bronchitis) or infection to the upper airways (e.g., sinusitis, upper respiratory infection, allergic rhinitis). Occasionally there are patients with pulmonary infections who do not demonstrate an infiltrate during the first day of the infection, but this is uncommon. Most adult patients with a pulmonary infiltrate and systemic findings compatible with a lower respiratory tract infection have an infection involving a treatable agent, whereas those with a negative chest x-ray examination and otherwise typical findings usually have bronchitis, which is most commonly caused by viruses, or have their major pathology in the upper airways. The purpose of the complete blood count is to determine the presence of anemia, which would indicate a systemic disease necessitating investigation, a very high or very low peripheral leukocyte count, or a prevalence of eosinophils, which would introduce many additional considerations in the differential diagnosis of the patient with a pulmonary infiltrate. There are three general indications for hospitalization: a patient who is seriously ill and requires either supportive care or intravenous antibiotics; a patient who by history or by screening laboratory tests has evidence of an underlying disease that requires diagnostic evaluation; and a patient whose social circumstances merit hospitalization simply

because the resources for supervised care as an outpatient are limited. Critical factors in outpatients include observation for evidence of response, compliance with the treatment regimen, and adequate long-term follow-up.

FOLLOW-UP

One of the most important facets in the treatment of pneumonia is to know what to expect in terms of response. The published experience with pneumococcal pneumonia shows that penicillin therapy has not altered the natural mortality rate of this disease during the first 3 to 5 days following treatment, and about 20 percent of patients with pneumococcal bacteremia die despite appropriate use of antibiotics. For those who do respond, about one-third become afebrile in 24 hours, one-third become afebrile in 1 to 3 days, and one-third require a longer time. Patients appear clinically improved with decreased temperatures within 24 to 48 hours. There is less information about pneumonia attributable to *S. aureus* or *S. pyogenes*, except that these patients tend to respond more slowly. The best parameters to follow are the temperature profile, leukocyte count, and clinical appearance. Serial chest x-ray examinations are not very helpful because there may be progressive infiltrates or new cavities in patients who are otherwise doing well. I recommend follow-up roentgenography early in the treatment course only in patients who are doing poorly by clinical criteria or to evaluate pleural effusions. Nevertheless, long-term follow-up x-ray examinations are important to document clearance of changes and detect any underlying lesions. The following factors should be considered in evaluating patients who fail to respond to the initial antibiotic regimen:

1. *Inappropriate antimicrobial agent*: This depends largely on the security of the etiologic diagnosis as defined previously. The sensitivity of *S. aureus* to methicillin should be confirmed. Sensitivity of pneumococci to penicillin should also be confirmed in the appropriate setting.
2. *Inadequate dosage or route of administration*: This is seldom a problem when using the regimens enumerated in Table 2.
3. *Compliance*: This is a major concern in outpatients.
4. *Inadequate host*: Some patients simply do not respond despite optimal management. This is most common in patients with overwhelming infections, patients who are treated relatively late in the course of disease, and patients with inadequate host defenses such as those with chronic granulomatous disease, neutropenia, or severe chronic lung disease.
5. *Associated lesions or complications*: Major concerns are empyema requiring drainage, an underlying obstructing lesion, and a distant metastatic site of suppuration. Pleural effusions should be aspirated and bronchoscopy should be performed whenever bronchial obstruction is suspected.
6. *Superinfection*: Patients with this complication usually respond and then deteriorate. Cultures of sequentially collected sputum are of limited value except to pro-

vide guidelines for treatment when clinical observations clearly support the impression of superinfection.

7. *Infection at another anatomic site*: This may include urinary tract infections, phlebitis at intravenous infusion sites, and tracheitis in patients with tracheostomies or endotracheal intubation.

8. *Alternative diagnoses*: Included are infections due to alternative agents (e.g, mycobacteria, chlamydia, fungi, rickettsiae, viruses, mycoplasma, *L. pneumophila*, aerobic gram-negative bacilli, anaerobes) and noninfectious diseases (e.g., hypersensitivity pneumonitis, tumor infiltrates).

9. *Adverse drug reaction*, especially drug fever: Affected patients often appear deceptively well compared with their temperature profile. The most likely antibiotics are sulfonamides and beta-lactam antibiotics, although almost any drug may be responsible. Eosinophilia may or may not be present.

SUGGESTED READING

Bartlett JG, O'Keefe P, Tally FP, et al. The bacteriology of hospital-acquired pneumonia. Arch Intern Med 1986; 146:868–871.

Dans PE, Charache P, Fahey M. Management of pneumonia in the prospective payment era. Arch Intern Med 1984; 144:1392–1397.

Donowitz GR, Mandell GL. Empiric therapy for pneumonia. Rev Infect Dis 1983; 5:540–554.

PULMONARY EMBOLISM

LORRAINE GATES, M.D.
MICHAEL STULBARG, M.D.

Among the most challenging tasks encountered by the emergency physician are the diagnosis and initial management of acute pulmonary embolism (PE). This chapter emphasizes the following: (1) pulmonary embolism is a common, potentially lethal entity that should be considered in the initial assessment of any patient with unexplained acute dyspnea, chest pain, hemoptysis, or syncope; (2) the diagnosis is frequently difficult to establish without the invasive "gold standard" procedure, pulmonary angiography; and (3) making a correct diagnosis is crucial, since, although it is likely that treatment with anticoagulation improves outcome in patients with acute pulmonary embolism, such treatment carries a small but definite morbidity and mortality.

There are approximately 650,000 cases of acute pulmonary embolism per year in the United States. An estimated 10 to 30 percent of patients with acute PE die within an hour of the event, many never reaching medical care. Although the efficacy of immediate and long-term treatment of those who survive beyond that first hour has not been established with certainty, most authorities believe that anticoagulation therapy reduces morbidity and mortality significantly.

PATHOGENESIS AND PATHOPHYSIOLOGY

More than 95 percent of clinically significant pulmonary emboli arise from the deep veins of the lower extremities and pelvis. The major risk factors for deep venous thrombosis and PE are conditions associated with venous stasis, endothelial injury, and hypercoagulability, namely, immobilization (including travel), congestive heart failure, varicose veins, vascular injury (including leg trauma), oral contraceptives, pregnancy, the postpartum period, major surgery (especially pelvic and orthopaedic), malignancy, and antithrombin III deficiency. Less common sources of pulmonary emboli include tricuspid valvular vegetations in infective endocarditis, septic thrombophlebitis (which may, of course, occur in the upper as well as the lower extremities), infected arteriovenous fistulas (in chronic hemodialysis patients), and tumors.

When a thrombus dislodges from its deep venous source and migrates to the lung, one of three acute syndromes may occur. If the embolus is large, it may lodge in a proximal pulmonary artery and produce the syndrome of massive PE. Because of sudden major mechanical obstruction to blood flow through the lungs, cardiac output diminishes significantly; hypotension, often accompanied by syncope or by a sensation of impending doom, may ensue. Immediate survivors of massive PE may present with acute cor pulmonale and shock.

Smaller emboli, whether originating directly from the deep venous system or from the fragmentation of a large, proximal embolus, produce the syndrome of pulmonary infarction in a minority of patients. This syndrome is characterized by pleuritic chest or back pain, and sometimes a peripheral infiltrate on the chest roentgenogram. Hemoptysis and/or a pleural effusion (which may or may not be hemorrhagic) may also be present. When small or medium-sized emboli do not cause pulmonary infarction, the patient may present with only acute dyspnea, nonspecific chest pain, and/or apprehension; the chest roentgenogram may be normal or unchanged from baseline.

An increase in the alveolar-arterial oxygen difference almost invariably accompanies clinically apparent acute PE, and is caused by intrapulmonary shunting, nonshunt ventilation-perfusion mismatch, or a combination of the two. Both processes are mediated at least in part by vaso- and bronchoactive substances released by thrombus-associated platelets. The symptom of dyspnea and the laboratory finding of a low $PaCO_2$ may occur in response to hypoxemia, but may also be present in the setting of a normal or only mildly widened alveolar-arterial oxygen difference, owing to a primary increase in ventilatory drive.

DIAGNOSIS

Unfortunately, there are no symptoms, signs, or simple laboratory tests that are specific for pulmonary embolism. The key to making the diagnosis is to consider it in patients who present with any of the common (albeit nonspecific) symptoms of PE. On the basis of history, physical examination, chest roentgenogram, and electrocardiogram findings, the physician must decide if it is likely that the patient has had a PE. If the likelihood is reasonably high, the diagnosis should be pursued with one or both of the special diagnostic procedures that will be discussed later in this chapter.

Symptoms

Dyspnea is the most common symptom of acute PE, occurring in 80 to 85 percent of patients. Pleuritic chest pain occurs in about half the patients (and is not necessarily accompainied by a pleural effusion); hemoptysis (usually scant) is present only 15 to 30 percent of the time. Syncope occurs in 10 to 15 percent of patients and is usually the result of massive embolism. Nonpleuritic chest discomfort and cough are common, but too nonspecific to be helpful in the diagnosis of PE.

Physical Examination

Physical findings are similarly nonspecific. Tachypnea occurs in more than 90 percent of patients. Tachycardia (heart rate greater than 100) is a surprisingly insensitive finding, occurring on initial presentation in only one-half to two-thirds of patients. Fever occurs at presentation one-half to two-thirds of the time. A pleural friction rub is present in no more than 20 percent of patients. An accentuated pulmonic component of the second heart sound suggests massive embolism.

Laboratory Tests, Electrocardiogram, and Chest Roentgenogram

Routine laboratory tests may or may not be helpful in the initial assessment of the patient with suspected PE. While the majority of patients with acute pulmonary embolism are hypoxemic, 10 to 15 percent have a PaO_2 on room air above 80 mm Hg, and in about 5 percent the PaO_2 is 90 mm Hg or more. In the vast majority of these patients, however, the $PaCO_2$ is reduced, so that, as previously discussed, the alveolar-arterial oxygen difference is abnormal (see the chapter *Acute Dyspnea*). Hypercapneic respiratory failure is not a feature of pulmonary embolism (in the absence of severe underlying cardiac or pulmonary disease), and suggests another diagnosis.

The electrocardiogram is usually abnormal in acute PE. Findings tend, again, to be nonspecific, and usually consist of minor S-T segment and T wave abnormalities. Findings of acute right heart strain (tall, peaked p-pulmonale, right bundle branch block, right axis deviation, and/or an $S_1 Q_3 T_3$ pattern) correlate strongly with the presence of acute PE.

The chest roentgenogram is abnormal in the majority of patients with acute PE. Findings that support the diagnosis of acute PE include elevation of the dome of one hemidiaphragm (seen in 20 to 45 percent of patients with acute PE), a localized infiltrate (in up to 50 percent of patients), and pleural effusion (in 15 to 50 percent of patients and almost always unilateral). Hampton's hump is a pleural-based, wedge-shaped density with a rounded convexity toward the hilum, attributed to pulmonary infarction; while uncommon, its presence in the proper clinical context strongly suggests pulmonary embolism. Westermark's sign, a region of hyperlucency caused by hypoperfusion distal to an embolus, is a common finding, although often appreciated only in retrospect.

The Ventilation-Perfusion Lung Scan

If the clinical picture suggests pulmonary embolism, a ventilation and perfusion (V-Q) lung scan should usually be the next diagnostic step. Even when significant underlying pulmonary disease makes it unlikely that the results of a V-Q scan will be diagnostic (see later), most angiographers prefer that it be performed prior to angiography, in the hope that it will guide selective dye injection.

If the patient's clinical status is such that he would not be admitted to the hospital if PE were ruled out, it is appropriate to perform a V-Q scan in the emergency department. A normal perfusion scan rules out acute PE.

Abnormal perfusion scans are considered in conjunction with the ventilation scan and the chest roentgenogram. Although various combinations of V-Q scan and chest roentgenogram findings are most correctly considered as representing a probability spectrum that acute PE is present, for convenience these findings are usually classified as having high, intermediate (or indeterminate), or low probability for PE. The interpretation of V-Q scans is summarized in Table 1. A ''high probability'' scan may occur in the absence of PE up to 10 percent of the time; conversely, a ''low probability'' scan does not exclude acute PE with certainty.

Pulmonary Angiography

Pulmonary angiography remains the gold standard for the diagnosis of acute PE. The findings of an intravascular filling defect or an arterial cutoff are diagnostic. Because this procedure is expensive and not without some

TABLE 1 Interpretation of Ventilation-Perfusion Lung Scans

Probability of Pulmonary Embolism	Findings
Very low	Normal perfusion scan
Low	Matched perfusion and ventilation defects
	Perfusion defect smaller than a corresponding chest roentgenogram abnormality
	Single subsegmental ventilation-perfusion mismatch
Intermediate/ indeterminate	Single segmental ventilation-perfusion mismatch without a corresponding chest roentgenogram abnormality
	More than one subsegmental ventilation-perfusion mismatch
	Perfusion defect similar in size to a corresponding chest roentgenogram abnormality
	Diffuse ventilation abnormalities
High	One or more lobar or more than one segmental ventilation-perfusion mismatch

risk, however, it is not performed routinely in all patients with suspected PE. The decision to perform pulmonary angiography must take several factors into account: the level of clinical suspicion of pulmonary embolism; the results of the V-Q scan; the presence of risk factors for complications of pulmonary angiography; and the presence of risk factors for complications of anticoagulation therapy. For example, in a patient in whom the clinical suspicion of pulmonary embolism is high and who is not at increased risk for complications of pulmonary angiography, angiography might justifiably be performed in the setting of a "low probability" V-Q scan. As another example, in a patient with a "high probability" V-Q scan who has had recent active gastrointestinal bleeding (a relative, but not absolute, contraindication to systemic anticoagulation), a pulmonary angiogram should probably also be performed. In general, angiography is not necessary in the setting of a high probability V-Q scan in a patient without relative contraindications to anticoagulation. However, if either thrombolytic therapy (see discussion later in chapter) or vena caval interruption is planned, angiography must be performed to be as certain as possible of the diagnosis.

Relative contraindications to pulmonary angiography include chronic pulmonary hypertension (the major risk factor for death from the procedure) and renal insufficiency (serum creatinine concentration greater than 2 mg per deciliter). Overall mortality from pulmonary angiography is approximately 0.01 percent.

If a patient is felt to be at high risk for complications of pulmonary angiography, computed tomography scanning or magnetic resonance imaging may be used to visualize proximal emboli. Unfortunately, the latter procedure is currently available only in specialized centers; furthermore, the sensitivity and specificity of these techniques for the diagnosis of acute PE have not been established.

THERAPY

The immediate treatment for suspected pulmonary embolism is supportive. Supplemental oxygen should be administered; fluids and pressors are given as necessary to support blood pressure. To treat shock in the setting of suspected massive PE, isoproterenol may be administered as a continuous intravenous infusion, beginning at a dose of 0.5 μg per kilogram per minute, and increasing cautiously to a maximum dose of 5 μg per kilogram per minute as needed to achieve hemodynamic stability. Alternatively, dopamine may be administered at an initial rate of 2 μg per kilogram per minute; the usual maximum dose is 20 μg per kilogram per minute.

Heparin

The cornerstone of therapy for acute PE is immediate systemic anticoagulation with intravenous heparin. If there is a strong clinical suspicion of PE, and there is no contraindication to anticoagulation, intravenous heparin may be administered in the emergency department, pending results of definitive diagnostic procedures. Absolute contraindications to systemic anticoagulation therapy include a history of craniotomy, cerebral hemorrhage, or large stroke within the past month; active gastrointestinal bleeding; and severe uncontrolled hypertension. Relative contraindications include recent major surgery, recent active gastrointestinal or genitourinary bleeding, and the presence of a hemorrhagic pericardial effusion or uremic pericarditis. Continuous infusion of heparin is associated with a lower risk of major bleeding complications than is intermittent intravenous bolus heparin therapy. A loading dose of 5,000 to 10,000 units, depending on body weight, is followed by an initial maintenance dose of 800 to 1,200 units per hour. The maintenance dose should then be adjusted to keep the activated partial thromboplastin time (PTT) one and one half to two and one half times normal.

Thrombolytic Therapy

Most pulmonary emboli lyse spontaneously over a period of days to weeks, so that in the vast majority of cases, supportive care and anticoagulation alone are adequate therapy for acute PE. (Heparin works, in part, by preventing formation of new clot, but does not directly aid in the lysis of existing clot.) Because of the potential for severe bleeding complications, thrombolytic therapy with streptokinase or urokinase is indicated only in the treatment of life-threatening massive PE (i.e., if immediate lysis of clot is believed to be necessary to restore hemodynamic stability). Streptokinase and urokinase cause lysis of clot by combining with plasminogen; this complex then converts other plasminogen molecules to plasmin, leading to fibrinolysis. The advantage of urokinase over streptokinase is that it is less antigenic; however, streptokinase is much less expensive, and is the more commonly used agent in the United States. Absolute contraindications to thrombolytic therapy are a history of craniotomy, intracerebral hemorrhage, or stroke within the previous two months; and active bleeding. Relative contraindications include a history during the previous two weeks of surgery, trauma, childbirth, a biopsy in an inaccessible site (including pleural or peritoneal biopsies), or external cardiac massage. A standard loading dose of 250,000 units of streptokinase is given intravenously over 30 minutes, followed by a maintenance intravenous infusion of 100,000 units per hour, for 24 hours only. One hundred milligrams of intravenous hydrocortisone should be administered prior to streptokinase infusion, and then every 12 hours, to prevent allergic reactions. The latter occur in 5 to 10 percent of patients. Heparin and streptokinase (or urokinase) should not be administered simultaneously; heparin therapy should, however, be initiated after infusion of the thrombolytic agent has been stopped.

If thrombolytic therapy is anticipated, and while it is being administered, arterial puncture should be performed only in the radial artery; pressure must be applied to the site afterward for at least 20 to 30 minutes, and the site must be observed carefully during the time that the streptokinase is being administered. When deep venous access is necessary, it should be gained prior to administration of the thrombolytic agent, and preferably via an antecubital or external jugular vein rather than a subclavian, internal jugular, or femoral vein.

In the rare situation in which massive pulmonary embolism has been proven by angiography, but anticoagulation is absolutely contraindicated, emergency embolectomy combined with vena caval interruption should be considered.

DISPOSITION

Patients with suspected or proven submassive pulmonary embolism who are hemodynamically stable can usually be admitted to a general medical ward, unless there is severe underlying cardiac or pulmonary disease. In the latter situations, an intensive care setting may be more appropriate. A patient with suspected or proven massive pulmonary embolism must be admitted to an intensive care unit for careful monitoring and adjustment of hemodynamic support and anticoagulation therapy.

SUGGESTED READING

Hyers TM, Hull RD, Weg JG. Antithrombotic therapy for venous thromboembolic disease. Chest (Suppl) 1986; 2:26S–35S.

Matthay RA, Matthay MA. Pulmonary thromboembolism and other pulmonary vascular diseases. In: George RB, Light RW, Matthay RA, eds. Chest medicine. New York: Churchill Livingstone, 1983; 323.

Moser KM. Pulmonary embolism: state of the art. Am Rev Respir Dis 1977; 115:829–852.

MANAGEMENT OF THE CARDIAC SYSTEM

MYOCARDIAL INFARCTION

JAMES T. WILLERSON, M.D.

Myocardial infarction is the term used to describe irreversible cellular injury that occurs as a consequence of prolonged ischemia. Infarction may occur with coronary arterial thrombosis or spasm or because of an insufficient increase in coronary blood flow relative to regional oxygen demand.

RISK FACTORS

Several epidemiologic studies have indicated that hyperlipidemia, especially hypercholesterolemia, represents a major risk factor predisposing to the development of premature atherosclerosis. Approximately one-third of survivors of acute myocardial infarction who are under 60 years of age have some form of hyperlipidemia, defined as serum cholesterol and/or triglyceride level above the ninety-fifth percentile for the control population. Systemic arterial hypertension, smoking, lack of regular physical activity, and emotional stress represent additional risk factors. Finally, there is a major genetic risk for the development of premature coronary atherosclerosis and myocardial infarction in patients less than 45 years of age with a first-degree family member in whom an infarct occurred at a similar or earlier age, even in those individuals without marked hypercholesterolemia.

MECHANISMS

Acute myocardial infarction occurs primarily in patients with significant coronary arterial disease. The primary determinants of vulnerability to acute myocardial infarction include (1) prolonged increases in myocardial oxygen demand under conditions in which the necessary increases in oxygen delivery cannot occur because of significant coronary artery luminal narrowing, or marked increases in heart rate, contractility, and/or myocardial wall tension, or (2) primary decreases in oxygen delivery to the myocardium associated with (a) coronary arterial thrombosis, (b) progressive coronary atherosclerosis, (c) hemorrhage into an atherosclerotic plaque, and (d) systemic arterial hypotension.

Recent studies have shown a strong association between acute coronary arterial occlusion and regional myocardial infarcts, especially "Q wave" or transmural infarcts. However, patients with "non-Q wave" infarcts (nontransmural infarcts) generally have multivessel coronary arterial stenoses and a "low-flow" perfusion state; approximately one-third of such patients have complete coronary arterial occlusion by thrombus. In addition, there is a frequent association of coronary thrombi with focal arterial lesions, including plaque rupture or hemorrhage. Coronary thrombosis may also develop without plaque disruption in severely stenotic coronary arteries. In this circumstance, platelet aggregation at the site of a severe coronary arterial narrowing and release of vasoactive substances, including thromboxane A_2 and serotonin, may cause local decreases in coronary blood flow and increases in coronary vascular resistance leading to further platelet aggregation and additional mechanical obstruction of a coronary artery and/or an increase in local coronary vascular resistance and a further reduction in coronary blood flow.

DIFFERENTIAL DIAGNOSIS

The coronary heart disease syndromes listed in Table 1 are included in the differential diagnosis of acute myocardial infarction. In general, angina pectoris occurs in patients with at least one coronary artery with a significant luminal diameter narrowing of 50 percent or more. In such patients, angina may occur when myocardial oxygen demand is increased, as with exercise, with emotional stress, and following heavy meals. Unstable angina pectoris, variant angina pectoris (Prinzmetal's angina), and acute myocardial infarction occur in association with primary reductions in coronary blood flow and myocardial oxygen delivery. Unstable angina pectoris may be caused by any process that results in progressive narrowing of the coronary artery so that coronary blood flow at rest

TABLE 1 Coronary Heart Disease Syndromes

Stable angina pectoris
Unstable angina pectoris
Variant angina (Prinzmetal's angina)
Acute myocardial infarction

394

declines. Variant angina is caused by coronary arterial spasm, usually involving a large epicardial coronary artery. Acute myocardial infarction is caused by coronary arterial thrombosis and/or multivessel coronary stenoses and a low-flow state.

The history is of the utmost importance in distinguishing the various coronary heart disease syndromes. In the patient with acute myocardial infarction, chest pain is usually severe and lasts until the patient receives analgesic medication. The chest pain is ordinarily described as being substernal or left precordial "heaviness," "tightness," or "like a weight on my chest," and it is often associated with nausea and diaphoresis. The chest pain may radiate to the back, the neck, the jaw, or the left arm, particularly down its ulnar aspect. Occasionally, the pain is present only in the back, the jaw, the left arm, or the neck. Many patients with acute myocardial infarcts have unstable angina pectoris for hours to days prior to their acute myocardial infarction. However, "silent" (i.e., painless) infarcts also occur, especially in patients with diabetes mellitus.

The differential diagnosis of acute myocardial infarction includes all other causes of chest pain, such as primary pulmonary abnormalities, musculoskeletal abnormalities, dissecting aortic aneurysm, hematologic neoplasms that cause a packing of the bone marrow with neoplastic cells, esophageal spasm, hiatal hernia, and intra-abdominal abnormalities that result in pain referred to the chest, especially peptic ulcer disease, cholecystitis, and pancreatitis. A careful history generally allows one to make the correct diagnosis.

Laboratory Tests Useful in the Initial Four Hours

Electrocardiogram. The electrocardiogram (ECG) provides an excellent means for the recognition of "Q wave" myocardial infarcts. The characteristic sequence of ECG alterations with Q wave infarction is as follows: (1) initial development of prominent peaked T waves in the leads representing sites of epicardial or transmural injury, (2) the development of hyperacute S-T segment elevation, (3) the development of significant Q waves, i.e., 0.04 seconds in duration, and/or reduction of 50 percent or more in the amplitude of the R wave, and (4) T wave inversion. The rate of evolution of these ECG changes is variable; they may occur in minutes or be delayed for hours. Problems in using the ECG to identify acute myocardial infarction accurately include some of the following: (1) in patients with left bundle branch block, acute anterior myocardial infarcts are not accurately recognized by the ECG; (2) in patients with previous extensive transmural ("Q wave") infarction, recognition of new injury may be difficult; and (3) in individuals in whom rapid ECG evolution occurs, it may not be possible to differentiate old from new infarction. S-T segment elevation also occurs with normal early repolarization, transient myocardial ischemia as with "Prinzmetal's" or variant angina pectoris, new ischemia in an area of previous myocardial infarction, chronic ventricular aneurysm, transiently following electrical cardioversion, left bundle branch block, left ventricular hypertrophy, and hyperkalemia.

In contrast, the ECG is of little value in the recognition of "non-Q wave" (subendocardial) myocardial infarcts. In these patients, the ECG demonstrates S-T segment depression and T wave inversion, and the only evolution is a return to baseline patterns. Occasionally, R wave loss and/or Q waves develop; however, in these instances there generally is some progression of the myocardial necrosis toward the epicardium. Unfortunately, subendocardial ischemia, ventricular hypertrophy, rapid heart rates, severe emotional stress, electrolyte alterations, and the use of certain medications including cardiac glycosides may result in the same ECG changes. In particular, bizarre T wave alterations occur in patients with intracerebral hemorrhage. Thus, the ECG changes occurring with "non-Q wave" infarcts may be consistent with subendocardial infarction, but they never suffice by themselves to document infarction with certainty.

Serum Enzyme Values. The diagnosis of myocardial infarction may be substantiated or excluded by the serial measurement of cardiac enzymes, especially the measurement of creatine kinase (CK), and the "myocardial specific" CK-MB isoenzyme, which should be measured by spectrophotometric, fluorometric, or radioimmunoassay methods. CK-MB increases in the sera of patients approximately 2 hours after myocardial infarction, may peak at 10 to 12 hours, and returns to normal within 24 hours with small and/or reperfused infarcts. However, it peaks at 18 to 24 hours and returns to control values within 24 to 36 hours with larger and nonreperfused infarcts. Thus, measurements of CK-MB at 8-hour intervals for the first 24 hours are useful in the detection of acute myocardial infarction. A single normal CK-MB value in the early hours after the onset of symptoms cannot exclude the diagnosis, and attempting to do so in the emergency department can lead to dangerous errors.

THERAPY

Immediate Treatment

Patients with suspected or proven acute myocardial infarcts should be admitted to a coronary care unit, where their heart rate and rhythm are monitored continuously. The most important aspects of initial treatment are (1) the relief of chest pain which is ordinarily severe and requires opiates and (2) immediate and continuous monitoring of heart rate and rhythm. Typically, either intravenous morphine (1 to 5 mg) or meperidine (25 to 50 mg) given repeatedly as necessary to relieve pain is utilized for this purpose. Oral, topical, or intravenous nitrates usually are not recommended in the first few hours after infarction unless chest pain is unresponsive to narcotics. Complete bed rest is initiated immediately as is oxygen therapy, 5 to 7 liters by either face mask or nasal prongs. Reassurance is provided, and continuous electrocardiographic monitoring is begun for the purpose of identifying and promptly treating important arrhythmias. More than 90 percent of patients with acute myocardial infarction have ventricular ectopic beats, which often require pharmacologic suppression. A prophylactic intravenous infusion of lidocaine, 1 to 2 mg per minute, may be administered for the initial 24 hours after myocardial infarction, although the impact of this prophylactic usage on mortality is unclear, and infusion of lidocaine is not without complications. However, patients with complex ventricular ectopic beats, defined as those occuring with a frequency of 7 per minute or more, coupled ventricular ectopic beats, short runs of ventricular tachycardia, and ventricular ectopic beats occurring on or close to the apex of the T wave ("R on T phenomenon") require an antiarrhythmic agent. Typically, lidocaine given as a bolus of 0.5 to 2 mg per kilogram body weight, followed by a sustained intravenous infusion of 1 to 4 mg per minute, is used to suppress complex ventricular ectopy. In most instances, adequate suppression of ventricular ectopic beats is achieved in this manner. However, lidocaine is metabolized in the liver, and relatively smaller doses of lidocaine should be administered to patients with underlying liver disease as well as to those with important congestive heart failure and to aged individuals. Patients with congestive heart failure and those who are aged have altered lidocaine clearance and metabolism so that they may develop lidocaine toxicity when normal doses of this agent are utilized. Evidence of lidocaine toxicity includes confusion, agitation, seizures, tremor, restlessness, and even sudden respiratory and/or cardiac arrest. If the suggested doses of lidocaine do not adequately control complex ventricular ectopy, one may add another antiarrhythmic agent, such as procainamide as a loading dose of 500 mg intravenously, followed by a sustained infusion of 1 to 4 mg per minute, carefully monitoring the Q-T and QRS intervals so as not to prolong either by 30 percent or more.

Thus, oxygen administration, pain relief, immediate bed rest, and careful surveillance and prompt treatment of complex ventricular ectopy are the cornerstones of the initial treatment of the patient with acute myocardial infarction. Frequent atrial premature beats generally are not treated, although one attempts to improve oxygenation and correct electrolyte abnormalities if they are present. Atrial arrhythmias are treated as necessary, including the administration of a cardiac glycoside to the patient with atrial fibrillation, usually digoxin in 0.25-mg increments given intravenously and repeated every few hours until the ventricular rate is controlled at approximately 90 to 100 beats per minute. Atrial flutter is generally associated with hypoxia; therefore, oxygen administration and relief of bronchospasm may help to convert this arrhythmia to sinus rhythm. Alternatively, low-level cardioversion or brief bursts of rapid atrial pacing may be used to convert atrial flutter to sinus rhythm. Irrespective of the etiology of a tachyarrhythmia, high-level cardioversion should be used to correct a tachycardia in the patient in whom an ectopic atrial or ventricular tachyarrhythmia causes cardiovascular collapse.

Patients developing second-degree heart block of the Mobitz II type or complete heart block should have temporary ventricular pacemakers inserted. Patients with Mobitz I heart block (Wenckebach block) require a pacemaker only if the ventricular rate is slow enough to result in hemodynamic instability, as reflected by dizziness or syncope, hypotension, heart failure, or angina pectoris.

Thrombolytic Therapy

In animals with an experimentally-created coronary arterial occlusion, release of a coronary occlusion or lysis of a clot with thrombolytic therapy, such as intracoronary or intravenous streptokinase, urokinase, or tissue plasminogen activating (TPA) factor, may reduce the size of the infarct and preserve regional ventricular function. However, thrombolytic therapy needs to be provided within the first 2 hours after coronary artery occlusion in order to salvage ischemic myocardium and provide important protection of regional ventricular function in experimental animal models, and probably in patients. Patients with acute transmural ("Q wave") myocardial infarcts usually have an occluding coronary thrombus in the infarct-related artery. However, it is not yet clear whether thrombolytic therapy given to patients with acute transmural myocardial infarcts also reduces infarct size and protects segmental ventricular function. There are recent data suggesting that mortality is reduced and segmental left ventricular function preserved when thrombolytic therapy is initiated within the first 2 to 3 hours after symptoms suggestive of myocardial infarction. However, other studies have failed to show a reduction in mortality or preservation of regional ventricular function with thrombolytic therapy. Multicenter randomized trials have recently demonstrated the advantages of thrombolytic therapy with TPA, especially when administered early after symptoms suggestive of myocardial infarction. When thrombolytic therapy is given and is successful, it is necessary to administer either an anticoagulant (usually heparin initially followed later by coumadin) or platelet-active agents (aspirin and Persantine) subsequently as an attempt to maintain patency of the infarct-related coronary artery. Alternatively, some investigators prefer to use transluminal coronary angioplasty (PTCA) in association with thrombolytic therapy acutely, arguing that once the occlusive thrombus is lysed, it is necessary to dilate the coronary artery to maintain patency of the infarct-related vessel. However, these approaches have not been proved as regards their efficacy in limiting infarct size, reducing mortality, and/or protecting segmental ventricular function, and it is necessary to await results of further studies to be absolutely certain of the clinical value of thrombolytic therapy with or without PTCA.

Other Interventions

There are also data to suggest that the acute administration of the beta-blocker, metoprolol, reduces mortality and limits infarct size in patients. However, other studies have failed to confirm the beneficial effect of beta-blockers when given acutely to patients with myocardial infarction. Other interventions, including selected calcium antagonists, intravenous nitroglycerin, and anticoagulants, have not been conclusively shown to reduce infarct size in patients. Thus, no specific pharmacologic regimen given for the purpose of reducing infarct size or mortality in the first few hours after myocardial infarction can be strongly recommended at present. There is convincing evidence that beta-blocker therapy (metoprolol, propranolol, or timolol) given to selected patients without contraindication in the days to weeks after the event reduces long-term mortality, including sudden cardiac death. Thus, one can recommend beta-blocker therapy chronically after myocardial infarction to patients presumed at risk for future ischemic events and without contraindication to such therapy.

Therapy in the First Eight Hours Following Myocardial Infarction

As already mentioned, during this time interval, the main concerns are relief of pain, careful monitoring to identify complex ventricular or supraventricular arrhythmias and heart block, and proper and prompt treatment of these events.

Specific Complications

Specific hemodynamic complications are treated as necessary, including the administration of cardiac glycosides (digoxin) and diuretics for patients with important congestive heart failure and the insertion of a flow-directed pulmonary artery catheter (Swan-Ganz catheter) in patients with systemic arterial hypotension, persistent sinus tachycardia, a new cardiac murmur thought to represent either ventricular septal defect or mitral insufficiency, and reduced urinary output. An arterial cannula should also be inserted for continuous measurement of systemic arterial pressure in the hypotensive patient. In patients with cardiogenic shock, the pulmonary capillary wedge pressure should be adjusted with either diuretics (in patients with severe heart failure) or with volume infusion (in patients with acute inferior myocardial infarcts in whom there is extensive right ventricular infarction) to an optimal value of 16 to 20 mm Hg. This level of left heart filling provides the idealized loading conditions for maximizing cardiac output in the patient with an acute myocardial infarction. Patients with cardiogenic shock based on extensive left ventricular infarction usually do not survive even if heroic measures, including intra-aortic balloon counterpulsation and/or emergency cardiac surgery, are undertaken. Such patients are candidates for thrombolytic therapy if they are identified within the first 1 to 2 hours of the event. On occasion, intra-aortic balloon counterpulsation, surgical revascularization, or thrombo-

lytic therapy results in survival of a patient with cardiogenic shock secondary to extensive left ventricular infarction. On the other hand, patients with acute inferior myocardial infarction and extensive right ventricular infarction usually survive if their shock is recognized and corrected promptly by the rapid administration of appropriate volume expanders.

New Systolic Murmurs

The development of a new systolic murmur and worsening congestive heart failure may indicate the development of an acute ventricular septal defect or acute mitral insufficiency. A pulmonary artery flow-directed catheter may help to distinguish between the two since with a significant ventricular septal defect there should be a step up in oxygen saturation in the right ventricle (7 percent or more) and with acute mitral insufficiency, prominent V waves usually develop (12 mm Hg or more above the mean pulmonary capillary wedge pressure). Mitral insufficiency associated with papillary muscle dysfunction generally improves with diuretic therapy, digoxin, and, when necessary, "unloading therapy" as provided by intravenous nitroprusside. However, acute mitral insufficiency caused by papillary muscle rupture generally causes fulminant heart failure, and the patient dies soon thereafter, unless surgical correction of the mitral insufficiency is accomplished emergently. The patient with a ventricular septal defect and a pulmonary-to-systemic shunt greater than 1.8:1 often develops heart failure and/or shock requiring intensive medical therapy, including unloading with the intra-aortic balloon or nitroprusside. Ideally, one wishes to wait 3 to 4 weeks after the myocardial infarct to correct the ventricular septal defect surgically since operative mortality risks are reduced. However, in a substantial number of patients with ventricular septal defects, progressive heart failure or progressive reduction in systolic blood pressure occurs despite intensive medical therapy, thus requiring immediate surgery to close the ventricular septal defect.

SUGGESTED READING

Buja LM, Willerson JT. Clinicopathologic findings in 100 episodes of acute ischemic heart disease (acute myocardial infarction or coronary insufficiency) in 83 patients. Am J Cardiol 1981; 47:343–356.

Willerson JT, Hillis LD, Buja LM. Ischemic heart disease—clinical and pathophysiological aspects. New York: Raven Press, 1982.

Willerson JT. Acute myocardial infarction. In: Wyngaarden JB, Smith LH Jr. eds. Cecil textbook of Medicine, 17th Ed. Philadelphia: WB Saunders, 1985: 284.

Willerson JT, Buja LM. Acute myocardial infarction, Clin Res 1983; 31:364–375.

PULMONARY EDEMA

SHIMON BRAUN, M.D.
BARRY M. MASSIE, M.D., F.A.C.C.

Pulmonary edema is a life-threatening illness, but if diagnosed rapidly and treated aggressively, it usually responds well to medical management.

PATHOPHYSIOLOGY

Pulmonary edema occurs when there is excessive fluid in the lungs, whether it be in the perialveolar lymphatic spaces or actually in the alveoli. The vast majority of patients with pulmonary edema have underlying heart disease with increased pulmonary capillary pressure secondary to pulmonary venous hypertension. This may be attributable to mitral stenosis (elevated left atrial pressure) or to left ventricular failure (elevated left ventricular filling pressure). Normally, the plasma oncotic pressure prevents excessive diffusion of intravascular fluid across the normal capillary membrane to the interstitial space. However, with increasing hydrostatic pressure in the pulmonary capillaries, the plasma oncotic pressure is exceeded, resulting in translocation of fluid first into the interstitial tissues and subsequently into the pulmonary alveoli themselves.

In contrast, noncardiac causes of pulmonary edema are characterized by either low or normal pulmonary capillary pressure. The common mechanisms in this setting are: decreased plasma oncotic pressure (hypoalbuminemia), increased negativity of interstitial pressure (rapid removal of pleural fluid), altered alveolar-capillary membrane permeability (adult respiratory distress syndrome, pneumonia, inhaled smoke or toxic gases), and other unknown or incompletely understood mechanisms (high-altitude pulmonary edema, narcotic overdose, increased intracranial pressure, pulmonary emboli). Table 1 summarizes the etiological causes of pulmonary edema.

CLINICAL PRESENTATION

The clinical presentation of pulmonary edema is often dramatic. Although some patients may give a history of a nonproductive cough and progressive dyspnea, others may suddenly become extremely breathless, terrified, agitated, and diaphoretic. A cough is usually present, and light pink frothy sputum may be expectorated. A history of chest pain may indicate a precipitating myocardial infarction, but it may also reflect ischemia secondary to hypoxia and the increased work of breathing or may be a nonspecific chest wall symptom. A history of previous congestive heart failure, with a change in medications, diet, or activity, points to the most common underlying etiology. Most noncardiogenic causes should be suspected

from the history, which should include questioning about drug exposure and central nervous system symptoms.

The clinical signs usually include tachycardia and, frequently, hypertension. A slight fever may be present. Cyanosis and diaphoresis are common. On auscultation of the lungs, moist rales are heard posteriorly over more than one-half of both lung fields. In some patients, only expiratory wheezing and rhonchi are present. Elevated jugular venous pressure may or may not be present. Cardiac auscultation may be difficult because of the widespread respiratory noise; however, an accentuated pulmonary second sound and an S_3 gallop rhythm are common. Careful auscultation of the heart is always important because the presence of murmurs may indicate underlying valvular disease or transient mitral regurgitation as the etiology for pulmonary edema. Hepatic congestion and edema suggest acute decompensation of chronic heart failure.

The chest roentgenogram may show a range of abnormalities, depending on the degree of interstitial and alveolar edema present and its duration. Cardiomegaly may or may not be present, but in cardiogenic pulmonary edema, distended upper lobe pulmonary veins (redistribution of flow) are usually apparent. The hilar regions show increased width and density, and the outlines of the central vessels are indistinct. The lung fields also appear indistinct because of the pulmonary congestion and the dilatation of the pulmonary vessels (ground glass appearance). An alveolar pattern extending from the hilum (butterfly pattern) is the classic finding. Pleural effusion and Kerley's B lines may be present. However, it should be remembered that the x-ray film findings often lag behind the clinical signs, in both appearance and resolution; thus the chest film may not be impressive.

There are no characteristic electrocardiogram, (ECG) changes associated with pulmonary edema, but an ECG should be obtained promptly, since it might provide evidence of acute myocardial infarction or cardiac arrhythmia. Electrocardiographic signs of left ventricular hypertrophy suggest antecedent systemic hypertension,

---

TABLE 1 Etiology of Acute Pulmonary Edema

Cardiac causes

    Left ventricular failure: acute myocardial infarction or ischemia, acute decompensation of chronic left ventricular failure, accelerated hypertension

    Valvular disease: acute mitral or aortic regurgitation, mitral or aortic stenosis

    Arrhythmias

Noncardiogenic causes

    Altered capillary permeability: inhalation of toxins or smoke, adult respiratory distress syndrome, drug hypersensitivity reaction, transfusion reaction

    Decrease plasma oncotic pressure

    Overhydration

    Incompletely understood mechanisms: narcotic overdose, neurogenic causes, high-altitude pulmonary edema, pulmonary emboli

---

cardiomyopathy, or a valvular lesion. The arterial blood gas invariably reveals severe hypoxia; often the P_{CO_2} is reduced owing to hyperventilation, but it may be high in the advanced stages, indicating alveolar hypoventilation. Metabolic acidosis may occur in severe cases and is an ominous sign of inadequate tissue perfusion or oxygenation.

The most difficult diagnostic problem in the acute setting is the differentiation of pulmonary edema from lung disease. The history should be helpful, since chronic pulmonary disease usually precedes acute exacerbations. However, many patients have both cardiac and pulmonary disease. The physical examination may not be helpful, but the roentgenogram often is. Nonetheless, widespread pulmonary infection, the adult respiratory distress syndrome, or other interstitial and alveolar processes may mimic cardiogenic pulmonary edema, and the latter may occasionally appear to be localized. Pulmonary edema may also present almost exclusively with bronchospasm and "cardiac asthma" and thus be misdiagnosed as pulmonary disease. In some patients, right heart catheterization or noninvasive assessments of left ventricular function may be required to make the distinction. Since these usually are time-consuming, the therapy instituted either should be appropriate for both cardiogenic pulmonary edema and lung disease or at least should not be deleterious to either. Such measures usually include positioning the patient upright, moderate supplementary O_2, diuretics, and aminophylline.

TREATMENT OF PULMONARY EDEMA

In general, the initial therapy of pulmonary edema is the same whether it is attributable to noncardiogenic or to cardiac disorders. In the treatment of pulmonary edema, a physician cannot usually work alone, since many simultaneous maneuvers are required. Therefore, as soon as time and logistics permit, the patient should be transferred to an intensive care unit. However, it must be emphasized that transfer to the hospital and institution of monitoring should not delay the initial treatment. Thus, acute treatment should take precedence over many diagnostic tests. Two goals should be kept in mind in the initial treatment of acute cardiac pulmonary edema: (1) improvement and maintenance of adequate tissue oxygenation and (2) reduction of the workload of the heart. The following measures are usually employed in the order listed.

Positioning

The patient should be placed in a sitting position with legs dependent, because this position increases lung volume and vital capacity, diminishes the work of respiration, and decreases venous return to the heart.

Oxygenation

Oxygen should be administered by means of a well-fitted face mask. When oxygen is administered at a flow rate of 5 to 6 L per minute, a concentration of 50 to 60 percent inspired oxygen can be attained; when 12 L per minute are given, a concentration of almost 100 percent oxygen can be delivered. When arterial oxygen tension cannot be maintained at PaO_2 of 60 mm Hg despite 100 percent oxygen delivery, or if there are signs of cerebral hypoxia or progressive hypocapnia, as evidenced by advancing lethargy or obtundation, immediate intubation and mechanical ventilation become necessary. Arterial blood gases should be obtained initially to assist in decision making to serially assess the efficacy of treatment.

Diuretics

Potent, rapidly acting loop diuretics, such as furosemide, have been the mainstay of emergency treatment of cardiogenic pulmonary edema. Furosemide has a biphasic action. It causes an immediate decrease in venous tone, and the resulting increase in venous capacitance may be responsible for the early fall in left ventricular filling pressure and symptomatic improvement. Subsequent improvement is related to the diuresis, which need not be massive to be effective.

The inital dose of furosemide should be 20 to 40 mg intravenously, unless the patient is receiving higher doses of oral diuretics. The onset of action is within 5 minutes, the peak of diuresis is at 30 to 60 minutes, and the duration of action is about 2 hours. If no diuretic effect is seen within 20 minutes, the dose given should be double that given initially. In patients with massive fluid retention and renal insufficiency, higher doses should be used initially. One must always be aware of the possibility of hypokalemia and hypovolemia, which can follow the diuresis introduced by furosemide.

Morphine Sulfate

Morphine remains a remarkably effective agent in acute pulmonary edema, and it should usually be part of the initial therapy. It works by a number of unrelated mechanisms. By dilating the capacitance vessels of the peripheral venous bed, morphine reduces venous return to the central circulation. This diminishes the preload of the heart. In addition, morphine has a sedative effect, decreasing musculoskeletal and respiratory activity, and it also has a mild arterial vasodilating effect.

Morphine should be administered in a dose of 4 to 8 mg intravenously, and subsequent doses can be given as needed, as soon as 30 minutes later. Consequent hypotension or respiratory depression may be reversed by the administration of naloxone hydrochloride, which should be readily available whenever morphine is ad-

TABLE 2 Drugs Used in the Initial Treatment of Pulmonary Edema

Drug	Dosage and Administration	Onset of Action	Precautions	Side Effects
Furosemide	20–40 mg IV; may be repeated	Venodilation in 5–10 min; diuresis 30–60 min	Hypokalemia; hyponatremia	Electrolyte depletion; hypovolemia
Morphine sulfate	4–8 mg IV; may be repeated	5–10 min	Lung disease; hypotension	Respiratory depression; nausea; vomiting; hypotension
Aminophylline	250 mg slow IV drip over 10–20 min; may be repeated once and/or followed by an infusion	15–30 min	Arrhythmia; ischemia	Ventricular and supra-ventricular arrhythmias; nausea; vomiting
Nitroglycerin	0.3–0.6 mg sublingually	5–10 min	Hypotension	Hypotension
Isosorbide dinitrate	2.5–10 mg sublingually	5–15 min	Hypotension	Hypotension

ministered. Morphine should be administered with caution when underlying pulmonary disease or CO_2 retention is present or when narcotic-induced pulmonary edema is a possibility.

Aminophylline

Aminophylline is indicated when pulmonary edema is resistant to the standard treatment and is associated with bronchospasm, with or without underlying pulmonary disease. Aminophylline improves dyspnea by its potent bronchodilating effect, but also by its preload- and afterload-reducing, diuretic, and positive inotropic actions, all of which are mild.

Aminophylline should be given in a dose of 250 mg by a slow intravenous drip over a period of 10 to 20 minutes; this may be repeated once and be followed by an infusion, but blood levels should be monitored during continuing treatment since the therapeutic range is narrow. Aminophylline should generally be avoided in the presence of supraventricular arrhythmias or sinus tachycardia in patients with ischemic heart disese.

Vasodilator Treatment

More recently, nitroglycerin and other vasodilators have been used successfully in the treatment of acute pulmonary edema. Some of these drugs are capable of reducing not only preload, but also afterload, thereby indirectly improving cardiac performance. The most useful vasodilators are nitroglycerin, isosorbide dinitrate, and sodium nitroprusside. Nitroglycerin and isosorbide dinitrate have a predominant effect on the venous capacitance vessels, whereas sodium nitroprusside produces a balanced effect,

significantly reducing both preload and afterload.

Nitroglycerin and isosorbide dinitrate should be considered early in the management of acute cardiogenic pulmonary edema if the patient has not responded to the initial measures or when the patient is either normotensive or hypertensive. Sublingual dosing produces a rapid and consistent effect, but oral or topical administration is less reliable in the acute setting. Intravenous nitroglycerin can be highly effective, especially in ischemic heart disease, but it should be given with continuous arterial pressure monitoring. Pertinent information relevant to the use of these drugs is given in Table 2.

Sodium nitroprusside is also effective, especially in accelerated hypertension, but it usually should be given with the aid of invasive monitoring. The recommended initial dosage of nitroprusside is 10 μg per kilogram per minute; this can be increased in increments of 10 μg per kilogram per minute every 5 minutes until pulmonary edema is relieved or until arterial systolic pressure falls excessively.

Digitalis and Inotropic Drugs

The role of digitalis in the management of acute cardiogenic pulmonary edema has been re-examined. In particular, the wisdom of directly increasing inotropy in the failing heart, wich its attendant increase in myocardial oxygen consumption, has been questioned. Digitalis is most useful in patients in whom rapid atrial fibrillation or another supraventricular tachycardia is the precipitating event, especially in the setting of mitral stenosis. Other parenteral agents that stimulate contractility such as dopamine, dobutamine, and amrinone are available. However, these usually are reserved for patients with combined pulmonary edema and hypotension.

Rotating Tourniquets

Recent studies failed to reveal any significant fall in pulmonary capillary pressure with the use of rotating tourniquets. Thus, this measure should be used only if the more standard therapy is unavailable or ineffective.

Phlebotomy

Phlebotomy may be helpful when other measures are ineffective. However, owing to excessive demand in time and the lack of advantage of phlebotomy over medications that increase venous capacitance, this form of preload reduction is seldom used today. Peritoneal dialysis or hemodialysis may be helpful in selected individuals.

Artificial Ventilation

If the patient does not respond to these measures or if he develops progressive hypercapnea and acidosis, endotracheal intubation should be performed. In patients with acute myocardial infarction or cardiac ischemia, early institution of artificial ventilation is often indicated. The institution of positive end expiratory pressure (PEEP) may accelerate the clearing of pulmonary edema and reduce the needed inspired O_2 concentration. The physician should be aware that these patients are at risk for the postintubation syndrome. Their high level of sympathetic nervous system discharge elevates their blood pressure. After intubation, this discharge decreases; in combination with the vasodilating effects of drugs and the reduced cardiac filling caused by PEEP, hypotension can rapidly develop.

Recognition and Treatment of Underlying Condition

A favorable response to therapy can be recognized by the decrease in dyspnea and work of breathing and improved oxygenation. These often occur before marked diuresis and may precede improvement in the chest examination or x-ray film findings by one or even several days. Once the primary goals of therapy have been achieved, a further diagnostic evaluation can proceed. All patients should be admitted, regardless of how quick and complete their recovery.

The history, physical examination, chest film, and electrocardiogram are of great value and should be reevaluated after the acute crisis has passed. An acute myocardial infarction should be excluded. The echocardiogram is probably the most helpful and readily available diagnostic test. It can help in the diagnosis of mitral or aortic valve disease and in characterizing congestive or hypertrophic cardiomyopathies. It can discriminate between primary pulmonary disease and heart disease. Coronary arteriography probably should be performed early in patients whose pulmonary edema is thought to effect ischemic left ventricular dysfunction. Radionuclide angiography might be helpful in revealing the status of left ventricular function.

SUGGESTED READING

Ingram RH, Braunwald E. Pulmonary edema: cardiogenic and noncardiogenic forms. In: Braunwald E, ed. Heart disease. Philadelphia: WB Saunders, 984:571–589.

Nowakowski JF. Acute alveolar edema. Emerg Med Clin North Am 1983; 2:313–343.

Pentle P, Benowitz N. Pharmacokinetic and pharmacodynamic consideration in drug therapy of cardiac emergencies. Clin Pharmakokinet 1984; 9:273–308.

THE PATIENT WITH S-T AND T WAVE CHANGES ON ELECTROCARDIOGRAPHY

G. THOMAS EVANS Jr., M.D.
MELVIN M. SCHEINMAN, M.D.

Since coronary heart disease (CHD) is the cause of at least 600,000 deaths per year and approximately 1.3 million cases of nonfatal myocardial infarction, it is the single most important health problem in our society. The electrocardiogram (ECG) is the simplest, quickest, and least expensive method of evaluating the possibility of acute infarction. The variety of ECG changes seen in myocardial ischemia or injury may include repolarization changes manifest by S-T segment elevation or depression and T wave changes producing tall upright T waves or inverted T waves. We will not discuss the pre-hospital phase of management, since standard single-channel ECG tracings acquired either in the ambulance or transmitted to a base station lack sufficient diagnostic specificity for meaningful S-T and T wave analysis.

If significant ECG changes and symptoms consistent with myocardial ischemia or injury are present, standard therapy for myocardial infarction should be promptly instituted (see chapter on *Myocardial Infarction*).

OBTAINING A 12-LEAD ECG IN THE EMERGENCY DEPARTMENT

The ECG has a significant role in the emergency department setting because of its noninvasive character, its relatively low cost, and its prompt availability and ease of acquisition. Computerized ECG analysis has the potential to aid significantly in diagnostic accuracy, but currently lacks sufficient specificity in diagnosis to be relied upon.

We will assume, for the purpose of this discussion, that a standard 12-lead ECG has been obtained to aid in the diagnostic assessment of patients with:

1. Typical or atypical chest or epigastric pain, possibly cardiac in origin
2. Acute pulmonary edema or congestive heart failure
3. Bradycardia, tachycardia, or irregular pulse
4. Syncope or cardiac arrest
5. Hypotension in an adult (either traumatic or non-traumatic)
6. Unexplained weakness
7. Coma, altered mental status, or cerebrovascular accident (CVA)
8. Blunt chest trauma with obvious precordial injury

A patient in whom an ECG is performed for the aforementioned causes and who is physiologically unstable or has a potential life-threatening condition should be placed in an acute management setting, receive oxygen, have an intravenous catheter placed, and have his or her cardiac rhythm monitored.

DIAGNOSTIC APPROACH TO THE ECG WITH S-T AND T WAVE CHANGES

Patients with recent onset of chest pain suggestive of myocardial origin and/or S-T and T wave changes compatible with acute ischemia and/or injury should be treated according to guidelines for acute myocardial infarction. These diagnoses cannot be ruled out by an initial normal ECG. It should be emphasized that any precipitating causes of these findings (e.g., dissecting aortic aneurysm, hypovolemic shock) should be diagnosed and treated accordingly.

Several entities mimic myocardial ischemia (see Tables 1 through 4 and Fig. 1 and 2). Before arriving at a diagnosis of ischemia; these mimics should be sought and eliminated as causes of S-T and T wave changes. When multiple factors that produce S-T and T wave changes coexist in the same patient, one should assume the most serious is present until it is proven otherwise. If these changes are new, the index of suspicion for myocardial ischemia should be high.

Categories Producing S-T and/or T Wave Changes

Five factors cause most S-T and T wave changes. These include:

1. Physiologic factors or normal variants
2. Ventricular enlargement
3. Altered ventricular depolarization and/or repolarization
4. Myocardial ischemia, injury, or infarction
5. Miscellaneous causes

Tables 1 and 2 list the differential diagnoses for major causes of S-T segment elevation or depression, along with the typical ECG pattern that accompanies each major entity. Note that some causes of S-T segment elevation or depression are best seen in either the right or left precordial leads, whereas other changes are more widespread.

Causes of S-T Segment Elevation

Nonischemic causes of S-T segment elevation include left ventricular hypertrophy and left bundle branch block. Less commonly, the early repolarization variant of the normal population, and rarely hyperkalemia, ventricular pre-excitation, hypothermia, acute cor pulmonale, and the CVA pattern of subarachnoid hemorrhage produce S-T segment elevation. Acute pericarditis represents an epicardial injury current. The most accurate criterion for this diagnosis is the ratio of the height of the S-T segment divided by the height of the T wave in lead V_6, which is usually more than 25 percent. (The baseline for the calculation is the P-Q segment.) Ischemic causes of S-T segment elevation include Prinzmetal's variant angina, ventricular aneurysm, and myocardial injury or infarction.

Causes of S-T Segment Depression

Common nonischemic causes of S-T segment depression include (1) depression of the P-Q segment attributable to the T_a or atrial repolarization wave, which impinges on and depresses the S-T segment (seen in some tachycardias), (2) right (RVH) and left (LVH) ventricular hypertrophy with the "strain" pattern, and (3) right (RBBB) or left (LBBB) bundle branch block. Hypokalemia and various drugs, such as digitalis and the type I antiarrhythmics, commonly produce S-T segment depression. Ventricular pre-excitation may produce S-T segment depression. Ischemic causes include Prinzmetal's angina, ischemia, and subendocardial injury.

Figures 1 and 2 depict an algorithmic approach to the analysis of S-T segment elevation and depression, respectively. This approach uses the worst case hypothesis, so that if insufficient clinical or historical information is available, myocardial ischemia should be strongly suspected, and ruled out by hospitalization.

Tables 3 and 4 list, according to the categories aforementioned, the major causes of tall T waves and marked T wave inversion, along with the typical ECG pattern that accompanies each major entity.

Causes of Tall T Waves

Common, nonischemic causes of tall T waves include LVH and LBBB, giving reciprocal changes in the right precordial leads. Early repolarization syndromes give predominantly tall T waves and some degree of S-T segment elevation. The ratio of the height of the S-T segment divided by the height of the T wave in lead V_6 in this syndrome is usually less than 25 percent. (The baseline for this calculation is the P-Q segment.) Hyperkalemia classically produces tall peaked T waves, but with increasing levels of potassium, the peaks may become more rounded. The CVA pattern secondary to central nervous system (CNS) injury may occasionally produce tall

T waves, as does the "diastolic overload" pattern of LVH. A rare cause for tall T waves is hemopericardium. Acute pericarditis, Prinzmetal's variant angina, and the hyperacute phase of acute myocardial injury or infarction may produce tall T waves.

Causes of Marked T Wave Inversion

Common nonischemic causes of marked T wave inversion include RVH and LVH with the "strain" pattern, and RBBB and LBBB with associated repolarization abnormalites. Less common or rare causes include the CVA pattern seen with subarachnoid hemorrhage, post-tachycardic changes, the mitral valve prolapse and Q-T prolongation syndromes and normal variants. Ischemic causes include acute myocardial ischemia, injury, or infarction.

EVOLUTIONARY ECG CHANGES IN VARIOUS CONDITIONS

The earliest changes of acute infarction involve S-T segment elevation with upright T waves. With evolution,

TABLE 1   Differential Diagnoses of S-T Segment Elevation

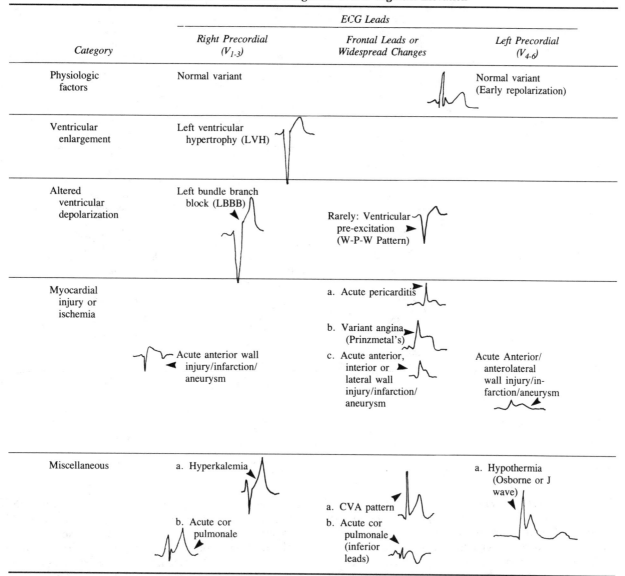

	ECG Leads		
Category	Right Precordial (V₁₋₃)	Frontal Leads or Widespread Changes	Left Precordial (V₄₋₆)
Physiologic factors	Normal variant		Normal variant (Early repolarization)
Ventricular enlargement	Left ventricular hypertrophy (LVH)		
Altered ventricular depolarization	Left bundle branch block (LBBB)	Rarely: Ventricular pre-excitation (W-P-W Pattern)	
Myocardial injury or ischemia	Acute anterior wall injury/infarction/ aneurysm	a. Acute pericarditis b. Variant angina (Prinzmetal's) c. Acute anterior, interior or lateral wall injury/infarction/ aneurysm	Acute Anterior/ anterolateral wall injury/in- farction/aneurysm
Miscellaneous	a. Hyperkalemia b. Acute cor pulmonale	a. CVA pattern b. Acute cor pulmonale (inferior leads)	a. Hypothermia (Osborne or J wave)

In the left hand column are listed the five major causative categories for S-T segment elevation. To the right of each category are listed the major entities that produce S-T segment elevation, along with their typical ECG patterns. Note that the entities are arranged according to which ECG leads most commonly contain these changes, e.g., LBBB produces S-T segment elevation in the right precordial leads (V₁₋₃), while the CVA pattern may be present in limb or precordial leads. This scheme applies also to Tables 2, 3 and 4.

TABLE 2   Differential Diagnoses of S–T Segment Depression

Category	ECG Leads		
	Right Precordial (V$_{1-3}$)	Frontal Leads or Widespread Changes	Left Precordial (V$_{4-6}$)
Physiologic factors		Tachycardia changes (increased T$_a$ waves)	Tachycardia changes (increased T$_a$ waves)
Ventricular enlargement	Right ventricular hypertrophy (RVH) with "strain" pattern	RVH and/or LVH with "strain" pattern	Left ventricular hypertrophy (LVH) with "strain" pattern
Altered ventricular depolarization	a. Right bundle branch block (RBBB) b. Ventricular preexcitation	a. LBBB b. Ventricular pre-excitation	a. Left bundle branch block (LBBB) b. Ventricular preexcitation
Myocardial injury or ischemia	a. Acute posterior injury b. Anterior ischemia or subendocardial injury	Anterior, inferior, or lateral ischemia or subendocardial injury	a. Lateral ischemia or subendocardial injury b. Acute myocarditis
Miscellaneous	a. Hypokalemia b. Nonspecific	a. Hypokalemia b. Drug effects (1) digitalis (2) + quinidine-like c. Nonspecific	a. Hypokalemia b. Drug effects (1) Digitalis (2) quinidine-like c. Nonspecific

the elevated convex upward S-T segment is accompanied by inverted T waves. The fully evolved infarction has pathologic Q waves, and isoelectric or slightly elevated convex upward S-T segment, and inverted T waves. Pericarditis in its early stages usually involves concomitant P-Q segment depression and convex downward S-T segment elevation. This elevation gradually subsides, and the T waves then become inverted, in contrast to those seen in infarction, in which the T wave becomes inverted at an early stage. Changes produced by electrolyte abnormalities or drugs are generally associated with widespread sagging or depression of the S-T segment and with lowering of the T wave, except in hyperkalemia. A more horizontal S-T segment depression is usually a manifestation of ischemia, which also produces a more acute proximal angle of the S-T and T wave junction, in contrast to the gradual angle produced by normal repolarization.

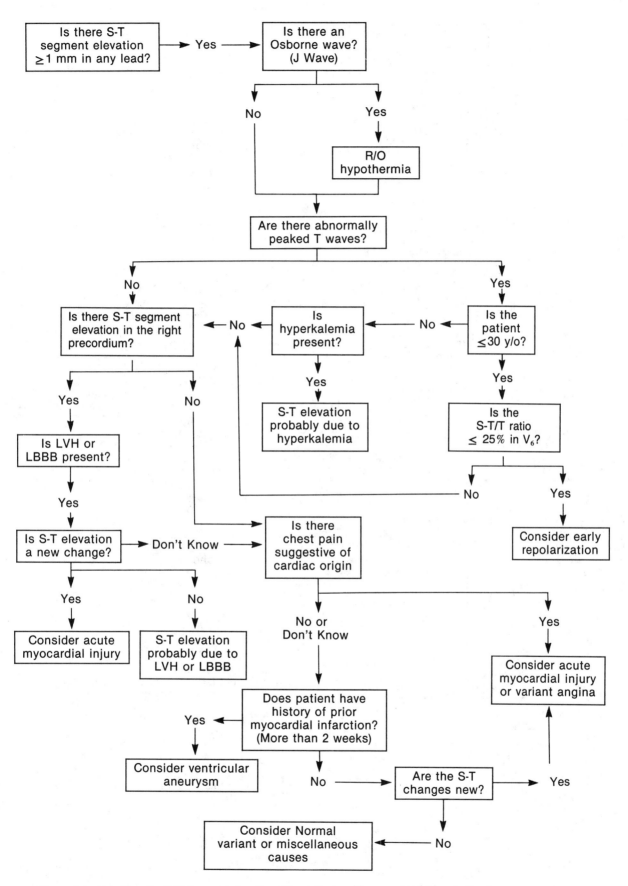

Figure 1   Algorithm for S-T Segment elevation: (for patients with supraventricular rhythms).

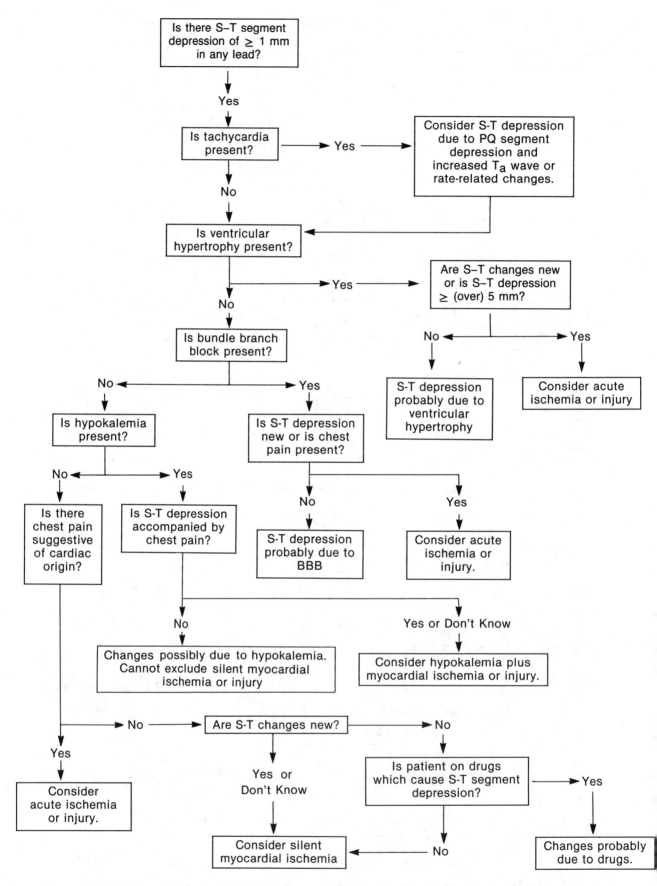

Figure 2 Algorithm for analysis of S-T Segment depression (for patients with supraventricular rhythms).

TABLE 3 Differential Diagnosis of Marked T Wave Inversion

Category	Right Precordial (V$_{1-3}$)	ECG Leads Frontal Leads or Widespread Changes	Left Precordial (V$_{4-6}$)
Physiologic factors	Normal variant (young women)		
Ventricular enlargement	Right Ventricular hypertrophy with "strain" pattern		Left ventricular hypertrophy with "strain" pattern
Altered ventricular depolarization	a. Right bundle branch block b. W-P-W pattern		a. Left bundle branch block b. W-P-W pattern
Myocardial injury or ischemia	Anterior wall ischemia/ infarction	Anterior lateral inferior ischemia/ infarction	Anterolateral/ wall ischemia/ infarction
Miscellaneous		a. Subarachnoid hemorrhage b. Post-tachycardia changes c. Mitral valve prolapse (inferior leads) d. Q-T prolongation syndrome	

TABLE 4 Differential Diagnosis of Tall T Waves

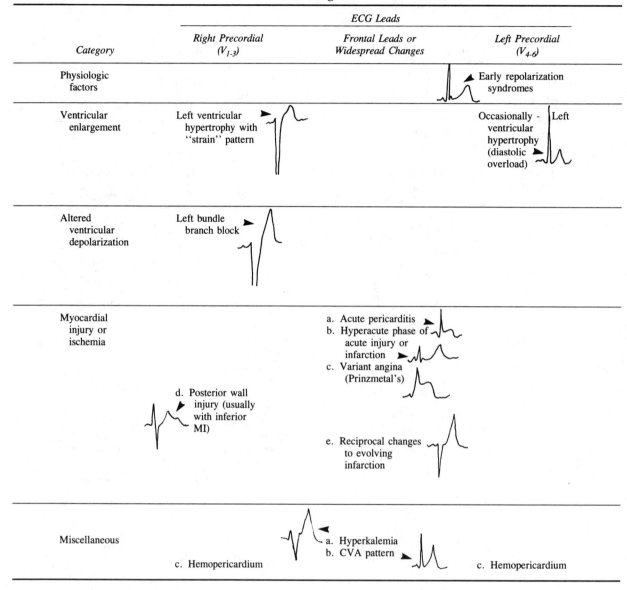

Category	ECG Leads		
	Right Precordial (V₁₋₃)	Frontal Leads or Widespread Changes	Left Precordial (V₄₋₆)
Physiologic factors			Early repolarization syndromes
Ventricular enlargement	Left ventricular hypertrophy with "strain" pattern		Occasionally - Left ventricular hypertrophy (diastolic overload)
Altered ventricular depolarization	Left bundle branch block		
Myocardial injury or ischemia	d. Posterior wall injury (usually with inferior MI)	a. Acute pericarditis b. Hyperacute phase of acute injury or infarction c. Variant angina (Prinzmetal's) e. Reciprocal changes to evolving infarction	
Miscellaneous	c. Hemopericardium	a. Hyperkalemia b. CVA pattern	c. Hemopericardium

In conclusion, one should acquire a fundamentally sound knowledge of electrocardiography in order to fully evaluate patients with S-T and/or T wave changes on the ECG. A problem-solving style should be developed which helps in the diagnosis of nonischemic causes for these changes and which keeps high the index of suspicion for myocardial ischemia, injury or infarction, whether overt or silent.

SUGGESTED READING

Goldberger AL. Myocardial infarction: electrocardiographic differential diagnosis. 3rd ed. St. Louis: CV Mosby, 1984.

Pozen MW, et al. A predictive instrument to improve coronary-care-unit admission practices in acute ischemic heart disease. N Engl J Med 1984; 310:1273.

Schamroth L. An introduction to electrocardiography. 6th ed. Oxford, England: Blackwell Scientific Publ, 1982.

NONTRAUMATIC CARDIAC TAMPONADE

NOBLE O. FOWLER, M.D.

Cardiac tamponade is characterized by impaired diastolic filling of the heart owing to a rise in intrapericardial pressure. The pressure rise is usually the result of the accumulation of intrapericardial liquid; rarely are air or other gases responsible. A discussion of the treatment of cardiac tamponade requires that consideration be given to its causes and its diagnosis.

PATHOGENESIS

Beck's acute cardiac compression triad described patients who underwent acute cardiac compression because of traumatic injury (penetrating gunshot or knife wounds) to the heart or who had suffered rupture of the intrapericardial aorta or the infarcted left ventricle. These events usually lead to the acute cardiac compression triad, that consists of increasing systemic venous pressure, falling arterial blood pressure, and small quiet heart. These signs are caused by rapid bleeding into the pericardial sac and the resulting quick increase of intrapericardial pressure.

In medical patients, the onset of tamponade is often more gradual; tamponade is often caused by neoplasm, infection, or uremia, with a more gradual fluid accumulation, rather than by intrapericardial bleeding with a more rapid increment of intrapericardial pressure. Hence, in some instances the medical patient with tamponade, in contrast to the surgical patient, might be expected to have a larger cardiopericardial silhouette on chest roentgenogram, a higher arterial blood pressure, and more readily audible heart sounds. We found these concepts to be true in our study of 56 medical service patients with cardiac tamponade (Circulation 1981; 64:633). Fifty-two patients had enlarged cardiopericardial silhouette on chest roentgenogram; most had arterial blood pressures in the normal range; only 11 had rapidly falling blood pressure. Heart sounds were considered to be normal in the majority (Table 1).

DIAGNOSIS

The diagnosis of cardiac tamponade may be made in five steps. The first step requires that this diagnosis be considered in every patient who has elevated venous pressure. In most such patients, the possibility of tamponade is dismissed after finding reasons for the more common alternative diagnosis, congestive heart failure.

The second step is careful study of the patient for paradoxical arterial pulse with a sphygmomanometer. A paradoxical pulse is considered present when systolic blood pressure falls more than 10 mm Hg during each inspiratory cycle. Almost all patients with cardiac tamponade have a paradoxical pulse. Absence of paradoxical arterial pulse, presence of cardiac valvular disease, evidence of dilated heart chambers, presence of S_3 gallop, and absence of pericardial fluid usually settle the issue rather simply in favor of congestive heart failure. When the patient is found to have both elevated systemic venous pressure and a paradoxical pulse, then a tentative diagnosis of cardiac tamponade is made.

The third step is to study the patient for evidence of pericardial effusion, unless the blood pressure is so low that immediate pericardiocentesis is required in an effort to improve the circulation and to save the patient's life. The usual method of determining the presence of pericardial fluid is echocardiogram. Angiocardiography and computer-assisted scanning are also sensitive and relatively specific methods, but are more expensive, requiring more time, and are slightly more hazardous. Two-dimensional (2-D) echocardiography has the advantage over M-mode echocardiography of better quantification of the fluid volume, and better localization in the event that this information is needed for pericardiocentesis later.

The fourth step involves checking for pericardial effusion. When pericardial fluid, in at least moderate amounts, is present, pericardial tamponade may be considered highly likely. Anterior effusion, as well as posterior effusion, is usually found. Small-to-moderate amounts of fluid may be found in as many as one-third of patients with severe congestive heart failure. In them, the cardiac chambers are usually dilated, but in cases of tamponade the chambers are usually below normal size. Further, paradoxical pulse is usually absent in congestive failure.

The fifth step entails proof of the diagnosis by pericardial fluid drainage. Pericardiocentesis should never be attempted in the emergency department (ED) on patients who are not rapidly deteriorating; the incidence of complications is fairly high, and they occur most frequently in those who have small or no effusions. When needle pericardiocentesis or surgical drainage of pericardial fluid is followed by a fall in systemic venous pressure toward normal and disappearance of paradoxical ar-

TABLE 1 Physical Findings in 56 Patients with Nontraumatic Cardiac Tamponade

Sign, Symptom	Present	Absent
Heart rate	43 (77%)	13 (23%)
≥ 100/min	36 (64%)	20 (36%)
Systolic blood pressure	6 (12%)	44 (88%)
≥ 100 mm Hg	27 (54%)	23 (46%)
≥ 40 mm Hg	41 (77%)	12 (23%)
Paradoxical pulse	16 (29%)	40 (71%)
≥20 mm Hg	19 (34%)	37 (66%)
Pericardial friction rub	45 (80%)	11 (20%)
Diminished heart sounds		
Respiratory rate ≥20 min (1 intubated)		

terial pulse, the diagnosis of cardiac tamponade may be considered to be proven.

If no or minimal pericardial fluid is demonstrated, an alternative cause of elevated systemic venous pressure and paradoxical arterial pulse must be sought. Among these alternative causes are chronic obstructive airway disease with cor pulmonale, large pulmonary embolism, right ventricular infarction, restrictive cardiomyopathy, and constrictive pericarditis.

ETIOLOGY

The continuing or follow-up treatment of cardiac tamponade depends, in part, on the etiology of the pericardial effusion. Thus, it is important to be familiar with the more common causes of cardiac tamponade. The causes to be expected depend in part on the activity of various services in the hospital concerned; these include oncology service, renal transplantation and dialysis programs, and cardiac surgical program. In our institution, metastatic neoplasm was the most common cause of cardiac tamponade (Table 2); other common causes were nonspecific (idiopathic) pericarditis, uremia, infections, and iatrogenic intrapericardial bleeding induced by anticoagulant therapy or invasive diagnostic procedures.

TREATMENT OF CARDIAC TAMPONADE

Drainage of Pericardial Fluid

Nearly all patients with cardiac tamponade require immediate or early drainage of pericardial fluid. In most

TABLE 2 Etiologies of Cardiac Tamponade in Medical Patients

Cause	Number
Malignant disease	20
Definite	(18)
Probable	(2)
Idiopathic pericarditis	9
Uremia	7
Anticoagulant therapy (cardiac infarction, cardiomyopathy)	6
Bacterial	6
Diagnostic procedures	4
Tuberculosis	3
Radiation	2
Dissecting aortic aneurysm	2
Myxedema	2
Systemic lupus erythematosus	2
Postpericardiotomy	1
Trauma	1
Total	65

patients, needle aspiration of the fluid suffices, but this procedure may be risky; laceration of a cardiac chamber (especially the right ventricle), laceration of a coronary artery, or a fatal ventricular arrhythmia may occur. The mortality rate may be 1 to 2 percent. If time permits, and a skilled thoracic surgeon is available, open drainage is probably safer; the procedure offers the advantage of better drainage. Further, a pericardial biopsy specimen may be obtained for microscopic and bacteriologic study.

Pericardiocentesis, except in cases of absolute emergency, should be done by an experienced cardiologist or thoracic surgeon. The localization of the fluid should have been studied by 2-D echocardiography. The procedure should be carried out under fluoroscopy, with a resuscitation team and equipment at hand. A thoracic surgeon should be available to repair cardiac laceration if necessary. A needle 8 inches in length is usually inserted at the left xiphicostal angle and is directed toward the upper thoracic spine, after appropriate local anesthesia. I monitor the cardiac rhythm with an oscilloscope, but do not use an electrode attached to the aspirating needle to guide the needle. In our first 56 cases, 40 of 46 in which needling was used were adequately treated initially with pericardiocentesis. However, the right ventricle was lacerated in three of the six failures, and two of these three died. No deaths have occurred since we have required that the procedure be done by cardiologists or thoracic surgeons. Although removal of 50 to 100 ml of pericardial fluid may relieve the urgent symptoms of tamponade and improve systemic blood pressure, it is preferable to remove fluid until systemic venous pressure is normal and pulsus paradoxus has disappeared. Some authorities believe that right atrial pulmonary wedge and intrapericardial pressures should be monitored during withdrawal of pericardial fluid. Right atrial pressure, pulmonary wedge pressure, and intrapericardial pressures should be at first equal and in the range of 13 to 32 mm Hg. Decline of intrapericardial pressure to zero or to normal subatmospheric levels gives reassurance that satisfactory relief has been obtained. In some cases, a plastic tube is inserted into the pericardial sac by the Seldinger technique and left in place for continued drainage for as long as 4 days. One may use for this purpose a 5 F, 25-cm catheter with mutliple holes near the tip.

Indications for Open Pericardial Drainage

The indications for open pericardial drainage are:

1. *Recurrence of cardiac tamponade after satisfactory relief by needle drainage.* In the case of cardiac laceration or perforation, the operation would include repair of the cardiac rent. In our 56 patients, 9 had pericardial resection because of reaccumulation of fluid following one or more pericardiocenteses.

2. *Purulent pericarditis.* Purulent pericarditis cannot be expected to respond to antibiotics alone. Open pericardial drainage is essential. In some cases, loculation of pus requires pericardial resection.

3. *Inability to obtain satisfactory needle drainage* and relief of tamponade or preference for surgical drainage

as the first procedure. This was done in seven of our first 56 patients with tamponade of the heart. Of our first 56 patients, 18 underwent pericardial resection. Of these, nine required surgical drainage because of recurrent tamponade after initial relief by needle pericardiocentesis; two required surgical repair of a lacerated right ventricle; in one pericardiocentesis was unsuccessful. In six others, surgical resection was done initially, and pericardiocentesis was not attempted.

4. *Need to obtain biopsy specimen* to establish an etiologic diagnosis.

The pericardial fluid should be sampled for bacteriologic culture, including acid-fast bacilli, anaerobic organisms, and fungi. The white cell count is made. Fluid specific gravity and protein content are determined. A study is made for tumor cells.

Circulatory Support and Monitoring

When there is delay in obtaining relief of cardiac tamponade by needle aspiration or by surgical drainage, one may wish to consider pharmacologic means of improving cardiac output and thus increasing blood flow to the liver, intestine, brain, kidney, and other vital organs. Plasma volume expansion, in experimental animals, may increase effective filling pressure of the cardiac ventricles and thus improve ventricular stroke volume and cardiac output. Dextran or dextrose solutions may be superior to whole blood and more quickly available. Positive cardiac inotropic agents that also decrease systemic resistance usually increase cardiac output in experimental tamponade; dopamine and isoproterenol have been effective. Hydralazine has also been useful. However, it must be cautioned that the use of these substances has been effective only in experimental animals. Limited studies in patients with tamponade have raised serious questions about their usefulness in the human disease. Hence, their use should not cause delay in seeking an effective pericardial drainage procedure. The dosages of isoproterenol or dopamine are similar to those used in treating cardiogenic shock. If these agents are used, their hemodynamic effects should be monitored; systemic blood pressure, cardiac output, and pulmonary wedge pressures should be observed in a coronary care unit or intensive care unit.

Monitoring. When cardiac tamponade is treated by needle aspiration or limited surgical drainage, recurrence of tamponade often takes place unless there is an effective treatment that can be directed toward the primary cause. Hence, it is essential that arterial blood pressure, right atrial pressure or pulmonary arterial wedge pressure, and degree of pulsus paradoxus be monitored, preferably in a coronary or intensive care unit, in anticipation of recurrent tamponade.

Treatment of Underlying Cause

The follow-up treatment of cardiac tamponade after pericardial drainage should take into consideration the cause of the pericardial disease.

1. *Anticoagulant therapy.* When tamponade is associated with excessive dosage of anticoagulants, or when it is attributable to therapeutic dosage in the presence of preexisting pericarditis (e.g., postinfarction pericarditis), the treatment should include withdrawal of the drug or diminishing its dosage. I prefer to stop all anticoagulants as a rule.

2. *Intrapericardial bleeding* owing to trauma or diagnostic procedure (e.g., Brock procedure, heart catheterization). Needle aspiration may be unsatisfactory owing to clotting. A small subxiphoid incision for rapid pericardial drainage may be necessary. As a rule, if tamponade recurs, a surgical procedure is used to relieve tamponade and/or to repair the rent in the cardiac chamber wall. However, a late recurrence of tamponade may be attributable to a postinjury syndrome rather than to bleeding. In this case, adrenal steroid therapy is usually effective.

3. *Reaction to certain drugs* (e.g., procainamide, Dilantin, hydralazine). Withdrawal of the drug is recommended, and at times adrenal steroid therapy is required.

4. *Infectious pericarditis.* The appropriate antibiotic is indicated. If there is purulent pericarditis, open pericardial drainage (and at times pericardial resection) is required.

5. *Uremic pericarditis.* A change in dialysis procedure may help, especially a change to peritoneal dialysis, which eliminates the need for heparin. Adrenal steroid therapy may be useful. If both measures fail, pericardial resection is probably indicated.

6. *Cardiac tamponade associated with connective tissue disease* (e.g., systemic lupus erythematosus, acute rheumatic fever, or rheumatoid arthritis) should probably be treated with adrenal steroids.

7. *Cardiac tamponade that recurs* in patients with idiopathic pericarditis, Dressler's syndrome, postcommissurotomy syndrome, or post-traumatic syndromes probably will respond to adrenal steroid therapy.

CONGESTIVE HEART FAILURE

KANU CHATTERJEE, M.B., F.R.C.P.

Congestive heart failure is a common clinical syndrome that may result from right or left ventricular dysfunction owing to various etiologies. The hemodynamic cause of the congestive signs and symptoms is systemic or pulmonary venous hypertension. Although reduced cardiac output and its clinical expressions frequently accompany elevated venous pressures, cardiac output may be normal or even higher than normal in congestive heart failure because of certain etiologies.

Chronic congestive heart failure may be caused by a variety of cardiovascular disorders, including chronic ischemic heart disease, valvular heart disease, primary myocardial disease, and pericardial disease. The important causes are summarized in Table 1.

SYMPTOMS

The major signs and symptoms of congestive heart failure are related to the severity of the hemodynamic abnormalities. *Dyspnea*, orthopnea, and paroxysmal nocturnal dyspnea result from increased pulmonary venous pressure, irrespective of its cause. In patients with mitral valve obstruction, pulmonary venous and left atrial pressures are elevated, but left ventricular diastolic pressure may be normal. Conditions that cause left ventricular hypertrophy and decreased left ventricular compliance (such as aortic stenosis, severe systemic hypertension, hypertrophic cardiomyopathy) cause increased left ventricular diastolic pressure, which is passively transmited to the left atrium and pulmonary veins. Marked elevation of pulmonary venous pressure may precipitate pulmonary edema with a pink, frothy sputum. This alarming symptom is not an infrequent cause for a visit to the emergency care unit. Severe pulmonary venous and arterial hypertension may cause profuse, frank *hemoptysis* (pulmonary apoplexy), which may require emergency care. Although this is a rare complication, congestive heart failure associated with pulmonary venous hypertension should be considered in the differential diagnosis of frank hemoptysis. It needs to be emphasized that many patients with chronic congestive heart failure are asymptomatic at rest and experience dyspnea only during physical activity.

Symptoms owing to systemic venous hypertension result in *peripheral edema, weight gain, and hepatic congestion*. Right upper quadrant and epigastric discomfort and pain may be caused by hepatic congestion and may lead to a mistaken diagnosis of hepatitis, gallbladder disease, or peptic ulcer. Severe congestive hepatopathy may be associated with jaundice, which may further confuse the diagnosis. Pulsation in the neck veins owing to tricuspid regurgitation occasionally produces an unpleasant throbbing sensation. Ascites and abdominal distention are infrequently observed, even in patients with severe congestive heart failure.

Fatigue, tiredness, and poor exercise tolerance are the major symptoms caused by low cardiac output. Marked muscular wasting (cardiac cachexia), occasionally observed in patients with severe chronic congestive heart failure, may be confused with cachexia of malignant disorders. *Syncope during exercise* may occur in some patients with aortic stenosis, idiopathic hypertrophic subaortic stenosis, and severe pulmonary hypertension. Lack of a significant increase in cardiac output during physical activity, which decreases systemic vascular resistance, induces hypotension and syncope in these conditions. However, spontaneous syncope, unrelated to exercise, can also occur and probably results from dysrhythmias. Syncope with change of position should arouse the suspicion of left atrial myxoma.

TABLE 1 Important Causes of Chronic Congestive Heart Failure in Adult Patients

Chronic atherosclerotic obstructive coronary artery disease (chronic ischemic heart disease)
Valvular heart disease: mitral valve obstruction (mitral stenosis, left atrial myxoma), primary mitral regurgitation, aortic stenosis, aortic regurgitation, tricuspid regurgitation
Primary myocardial disease: dilated cardiomyopathy, hypertrophic cardiomyopathy, restrictive cardiomyopathy
Pericardial disease: constrictive pericarditis, chronic pericardial effusion
Postoperative (after valve surgery or coronary artery bypass surgery) myocardial dysfunction
Precapillary pulmonary hypertension, long-standing systemic hypertension
High-output failure: thyrotoxicosis, beriberi, AV fistula

Angina may accompany other symptoms of congestive heart failure, not only in patients with ischemic cardiomyopathy, but also in patients with aortic valve disease, hypertrophic cardiomyopathy, primary dilated cardiomyopathy, and precapillary pulmonary hypertension.

Nonspecific symptoms of congestive heart failure include nonproductive cough, confusion, cold intolerance, insomnia or somnolence, nocturia, atypical chest pain, dryness of the mouth, and excessive thirst. Some of these symptoms result from associated metabolic derangements (hyponatremia, inappropriate arginine vasopressin release, elevated circulating catecholamines) and aggressive diuretic therapy.

PHYSICAL EXAMINATION

Diagnosis of congestive heart failure depends on the detection of evidence of systemic and pulmonary venous hypertension. Systemic *venous pressure* is estimated by determining the highest level of internal or external (preferably internal) jugular venous pulse above the sternal angle. Right atrial pressure is approximated by adding 5 cm to the height of the jugular venous pulse. It is assumed that the distance between the right atrium and the sternal angle is 5 cm. If the estimated venous pressure exceeds 7 to 10 cm H_2O, systemic venous hypertension should be diagnosed. Other manifestations of increased systemic venous pressure are dependent edema, hepatomegaly, and occasionally ascites. In the absence of superior vena cava obstruction, elevated jugular venous pressure indicates increased right atrial pressure. When tricuspid valve obstruction is excluded, elevated systemic venous pressure indicates increased right ventricular diastolic pressure. Right ventricular third heart sound and right ventricular presystolic (a′) wave also suggest elevated right ventricular diastolic pressure.

Clinical diagnosis of *pulmonary venous hypertension* is difficult in patients with congestive heart failure. Widespread pulmonary rales indicate significant elevation of pulmonary capillary wedge pressure; however, rales are nonspecific findings and are present in primary pulmonary disease. A palpable left ventricular presystolic wave (fourth heart sound) and third heart sound are usually associated with significant elevation of left ventricular diastolic pressure and, hence, passive increase in left atrial and pulmonary capillary wedge pressures. An audible discrete, sharp third heart sound or gallop rhythm is also suggestive of increased left ventricular end-diastolic pressure, usually exceeding 20 to 25 mm Hg. However, these findings are not present when the mitral valve is significantly obstructed (e.g., mitral stenosis).

The plain *chest roentgenogram* is useful in the diagnosis of pulmonary venous hypertension. Vascular redistribution, perihilar haziness, Kerley's B lines, and alveolar edema indicate increased pulmonary capillary wedge pressure. It needs to be emphasized, however, that in chronic dilated cardiomyopathy, significant elevation of pulmonary capillary wedge pressure may be present in the absence of these radiologic findings; thus, in these patients, the chest film cannot always be used to exclude pulmonary venous hypertension. However, radiologic examination is imperative to detect not only evidence of pulmonary venous hypertension, but also the possible etiology of chronic congestive heart failure. Massive cardiomegaly (pericardial effusion, multivalvular lesions, dilated cardiomyopathy), left atrial enlargement (mitral and aortic valve disease, dilated and hypertrophic cardiomyopathy, and hypertensive and coronary heart disease), pulmonary artery enlargement (pulmonary hypertension), valve calcification (aortic and mitral valve stenosis), left atrial calcification (mitral stenosis), and coronary artery calcification (severe coronary artery disease) can be detected, and these findings provide important clues in the diagnosis of the etiology of heart failure.

Assessment of cardiac output is difficult, if not impossible, by physical and radiologic examination. Tachycardia, thready pulse, and markedly reduced amplitude of the carotid pulse may suggest decreased cardiac output. Sustained and diffuse outward movement of the left ventricular apical impulse point of maximal impulse (PMI) is usually associated with decreased ejection fraction, except in the presence of severe left ventricular hypertrophy (severe chronic hypertension, aortic stenosis, and hypertrophic cardiomyopathy). Sustained systolic left parasternal impulse, in the absence of mitral regurgitation, usually indicates reduced right ventricular ejection fraction or right ventricular systolic hypertension. It needs to be emphasized that abnormal physical findings and radiologic signs only provide indirect information regarding the hemodynamic abnormalities and the pathophysiology of congestive heart failure.

In the emergency care unit, however, an assessment of a patient with congestive heart failure has to rely primarily on clinical evaluation. Chest film and electrocardiogram should also be routinely performed and may aid in the diagnosis of the etiology of congestive heart failure. If echocardiogram is available, its application may resolve the diagnosis in many instances. The suggested stepwise clinical approach in the diagnosis of chronic congestive heart failure is summarized in Tables 2 and 3. If the patient has an elevated venous pressure without pulsation, suspect superior vena cava obstruction. If pulsation is present in the patient with an elevated venous pressure, examine for precordial impulse (Table 2). In the case of normal venous pressure, examine for dilated heart size (by clinical and x-ray examination) and assess left ventricular systolic function (by clinical and echocardiographic examination) (Table 3). In patients with a history of episodic pulmonary edema, the differential diagnosis should include reversible myocardial ischemia, dysrhythmia, intermittent mitral valve obstruction or regurgitation, and stiff heart syndrome. Of all the potential causes of chronic congestive heart failure, ischemic dilated cardiomyopathy is the most common.

PRECIPITATING CAUSES

Deterioration of heart failure and exacerbation of symptoms frequently bring a patient with chronic congestive heart failure to the emergency care unit. Worsening heart failure in a patient who is otherwise stable may result from a number of causes (Table 4). These potential causes need to be carefully sought while evaluating a patient with accelerated heart failure, since often only by treating the cause can the failure be reversed.

Worsening heart failure should be suspected when there is exacerbation of symptoms, such as decreased effort tolerance, increased dyspnea or fatigue, and increasing peripheral edema, or when new symptoms are experienced, such as angina, palpitations, or dizziness. When secondary causes are suspected, evaluation of these causes should be considered (see Table 4). A chest film and an electrocardiogram should be obtained routinely and a careful physical examination should be performed. As coronary artery disease is the most common cause of chronic congestive heart failure, myocardial ischemia and/or *infarction* should always be considered as a potential cause for deterioration of heart failure, particularly in patients with known coronary artery disease. In patients with valvular heart disease, bacterial *endocarditis* and dysrhythmias should be excluded as the potential causes of sudden worsening of heart failure. Determination of blood gases is helpful to assess the presence and severity of hypoxia.

ADMISSION CRITERIA

The majority of patients with worsening or exacerbation of chronic heart failure do not require admission to the inpatient service. However, the following are criteria for admission of the patient to the hospital for further evaluation and treatment: (1) severe pulmonary edema, (2) unexplained severe hypotension (systemic blood pressure of 80 mm Hg or less), (3) a history of prolonged or crescendo angina, or evidence of myocardial ischemia or infarction on the electrocardiogram, (4) a history of syncope with electrocardiographic evidence of dysrhythmias, (5) marked electrolyte imbalance (severe hypokalemia or hyponatremia), (6) overt digitalis toxicity, (7) overt

TABLE 2   Clinical Diagnosis of the Etiology of Chronic Congestive Heart Failure in Patient with Elevated Venous Pressure, Pulsation Present: Examine for Precordial Impulse

Quiet Pericardium
(Severe COPD or obesity may dampen the precordial impulse)

Pericardial Effusion	Constrictive Pericarditis
Tachycardia	Tachycardia, atrial fibrillation
Pulsus paradoxus	Venous pulse (sharp 'y' descent-Kussmaul's sign)
Distant heart sounds, auscultatory alternans, no gallop sounds	Precordial knock
	Relatively fixed splitting of S_2
ECG: tachycardia, low voltage QRS, electrical alternans	P_2 is not markedly accentuated
Lungs: clear	Lungs: clear
Chest film: cardiomegaly	ECG: nonspecific
Echocardiogram (mandatory): pericardial effusion	Chest film: relatively normal heart size, absence of significant hypertension, pericardial calcification

Palpable Precordial and/or Epigastric Impulse
(Search for evidence of pulmonary arterial hypertension: loud P_2, pulmonary ejection sound, tricuspid regurgitation, pulmonary insufficiency, PA+ on chest film)

Pulmonary Hypertension Suspected

1. Exclude Primary Mitral Valve Disease

Obstruction	Regurgitation
Loud S_1, mid-diastolic murmur, opening snap	Pansystolic murmur, S_3, hyperdynamic LV
ECG: RVH	ECG: LVH
Chest film: PVH, LA+, mitral valve calcification, PA+	Chest film: LA+, PVH, PA+, cardiomegaly
Echocardiogram (mandatory): for confirmation of diagnosis and to exclude left atrial myxoma	Echocardiogram: dilated, normally contracting LV, LA+

2. Exclude Aortic Valve Disease

Obstruction	Regurgitation
Slow rising, diminished amplitude, delayed peak carotid pulse	Wide arterial pulse pressure, pulsus bisferins
Soft S_1 and A_2	High frequency decrescendo, early diastolic murmur
Ejection systolic murmur	Austin-Flint murmur (diastolic murmur heard at apex in aortic regurgitation)
Decreased pulse pressure	
Sustained LV impulse	Soft A_2
	Cardiomegaly
ECG: LVH, LA+	Hyperdynamic or sustained LV impulse
	ECG: LVH
Chest film: mild cardiomegaly; PVH, LA+, prominent ascending aorta	Chest film: cardiomegaly, PVH, LA+, aortic root dilatation
Echocardiogram: restricted AV movement, AV calcification, LVH normal or depressed LV function	Echocardiogram: mitral valve flutter, dilated and usually normally contracting LV

TABLE 2 Clinical Diagnosis of the Etiology of Chronic Congestive Hert Failure in Patient with Elevated Venous Pressure, Pulsation Present: Examine for Precordial Impulse-*Continued*

3. Exclude Cardiomyopathy

Hypertrophic Cardiomyopathy (IHSS)	Dilated Cardiomyopathy
Sharp carotid pulse upstroke with normal or increased pulse volume, pulsus bisferins	Displaced and sustained LV impulse
Ejection systolic murmur that increases in intensity following amyl nitrite or during Valsalva maneuver	No mitral valve disease
Sustained LV impulse with palpable 'a' wave	ECG: Pseudo-infarction, conduction disturbances, LVH, presence of myocardial infarction in ischemic cardiomyopathy
Pansystolic murmur along with paradoxical splitting of S_2 in the absence of LBBB	Chest film: cardiomegaly, PVH
Prominent S_4	Echocardiogram: dilated, poorly contracting left ventricle with little or no LVH
ECG: LVH, pseudo-infarction, LBBB	
Chest film: moderate cardiomegaly, LA+, PVH	
Echocardiogram: asymmetric LVH, SAM, normal or hypercontractile LV	

4. Exclude Eisenmenger's Syndrome
   Central cyanosis, clubbing and ASD (widely split S_2) or VSD (loud single S_2), patent ductus arteriosus (normal splitting of S_2, differential cyanosis)
   ECG: severe RVH
   Echocardiogram: right-to-left shunt

5. If Mitral and Aortic Valve Disease, cardiomyopathy and intracardiac shunt are excluded, precapillary pulmonary hypertension as the cause of congestive heart failure should be suspected.

Pulmonary Hypertension not Suspected

1. Exclude Tricuspid Stenosis
   'a' wave in JVP, mid-diastolic rumble along left sternal border, that increases in intensity during inspiration
   ECG: nonspecific
   Echocardiogram: RA +, tricuspid valve stenosis
2. Exclude Atrial Septal Defect
   Widely split and relatively fixed S_2
   ECG: rsr' in V_1
   Echocardiogram: dilated RA and RV with normal LV

3. Exclude Primary Tricuspid Regurgitation
   Pansystolic murmur along left sternal border, that increases in intensity during inspiration; P_2 is not markedly accentuated
   Chest film: cardiomegaly, no PVH
   ECG: nonspecific changes

4. Exclude Ebstein's Anomaly
   Cyanosis, clubbing, triscuspid regurgitation, "sail sounds"
   Chest film: cardiomegaly, no PVH
   ECG: RBBB, right atrial enlargement

RA, LA=right and left atrium; RA+ =right atrial enlargement; RV, LV=right and left ventricle; PVH=pulmonary venous hypertension; ASD, VSD=atrial, ventricular septal defect; JVP=jugular venous pulse; RVH, LVH=right, left ventricular hypertrophy; SAM=systolic anterior motion; PA+ =pulmonary artery enlargement.

TABLE 3 Clinical Diagnosis of the Etiology of Chronic Congestive Heart Failure in Patient with Normal Venous Pressure, Dilated Heart Size: Assess LV Systolic Function

Massive cardiomegaly and normal LV systolic function

   Exclude pericardial effusion
   Exclude mitral and aortic regurgitation
   Exclude high output failure

Marked cardiomegaly and depressed systolic function

   Exclude dilated cardiomyopathy

Little or no cardiomegaly and normal LV systolic function

   Exclude mitral valve obstruction
   Exclude aortic stenosis
   Exclude hypertrophic cardiomyopathy
   Exclude episodic myocardial ischemia

manifestations of bacterial endocarditis, (8) markedly reduced arterial blood Po_2, (9) altered consciousness (suspected very low cardiac output or metabolic derangement, and (10) suspected cardiac tamponade.

TREATMENT

The need for immediate therapy is dictated by the nature of the clinical problem in individual patients with worsening heart failure. In patients with exacerbation of dyspnea or obvious pulmonary edema, administration of sublingual *nitroglycerin* (0.4 mg, up to three doses at 5-minute intervals) can cause prompt and dramatic improvement. Sublingual nitroglycerin is preferred over intravenous diuretic (furosemide) or morphine therapy. Nitroglycerin is well tolerated by patients with dilated cardiomyopathy, aortic and mitral valve disease (including aortic and mitral stenosis), and hypertrophic cardiomyopathy with congestive symptoms. In patients with chronic obstructive lung disease, nitroglycerin and nitrates are safer than diuretics and narcotics; thus, administration of nitroglycerin, along with oxygen therapy, is preferable as initial therapy, even when the cause of dyspnea remains uncertain. In patients with obvious cardiac pulmonary edema, nitroglycerin administration may be followed by diuretic and morphine therapy.

When *myocardial ischemia* is suspected as the precipitating cause for worsening heart failure, *nitroglycerin and nitrates* should be considered as the initial treatment of choice. In patients who fail to respond to nitroglycerin, nifedipine (10-mg capsule), a calcium entry blocking agent, may be administered sublingually. For maintenance therapy, nitroglycerin ointment ($\frac{1}{2}$ to 2 inches) or oral isosorbide dinitrate (20 to 40 mg) is safer in patients with chronic heart failure before further evaluation can be accomplished.

If *hypotension* accompanies symptoms and signs of hypoperfusion, routine intravenous fluid administration, based on the assumption that hypotension is owing to hypovolemia, *must be avoided*. Hypotension in these patients usually results from low cardiac output; thus, the intravenous inotropic vasopressor agent, *dopamine*, should be used for initial therapy. Subsequent therapy should be decided after determining the etiology of heart failure and the precise mechanism of the hypotension. Hypotension may result from either low cardiac output or inappropriately low systemic vascular resistance, or may be attributable to both of these hemodynamic abnormalities. For identification of these mechanisms, and to provide appropriate therapy, admission to the intensive care facility with hemodynamic monitoring is required. When malignant *tachyarrhythmias* are recognized, patients should be admitted to the intensive care unit after initial intravenous antiarrhythmic therapy (e.g., intravenous lidocaine).

Increasing peripheral edema and weight gain or mild worsening in pulmonary congestion can be treated by increasing diuretic therapy and the addition of nitrates. These patients do not require immediate admission to the inpatient service, and subsequent outpatient evaluation is usually sufficient. However, digitalis therapy can be initiated in undigitalized patients.

In addition to digitalis and diuretic therapy, vasodilator drugs are often useful in the management of patients with chronic congestive heart failure. Drugs with combined arteriolar and venodilating effects (prazosin, captopril) or a combination of predominantly arteriolar dilators (hydralazine, minoxidil) and venodilators (nitrates) are frequently required for maintenance therapy of chronic refractory heart failure. However, initiation of vasodilator or inotropic therapy with newer cardiotonic agents (e.g., milrinone, enoximone) can be delayed until appropriate evaluation is made to assess the etiology and severity of chronic congestive heart failure.

For immediate therapy, *diuretic agents* can be administered intravenously (e.g., furosemide 40 to 80 mg), particularly in patients with overt pulmonary edema or peripheral edema. Adjustment of diuretic therapy can be made subsequently, depending on the severity of systemic and pulmonary congestion of systemic and pulmonary congestion, response to diuretic therapy and changes in electrolytes and renal function. Combination diuretic therapy (consisting of furosemide, metolazone, and aldactone) is occasionally required in patients with severe refractory heart failure. Intravenous furosemide can cause transient deterioration of hemodynamics (decrease in cardiac output and an increase in pulmonary capillary wedge pressure) in some patients, usually 20 to 30 minutes after its administration; thus, careful observation for this potential adverse response is recommended, particularly after administration of large doses (80 to 120 mg intravenously.)

The effectiveness of maintenance *digitalis therapy* for heart failure of patients in sinus rhythm has been challenged recently. However, it appears to exert beneficial hemodynamic and clinical effects in patients with moderately depressed left ventricular systolic function with S_3 gallop. Thus, digitalization is recommended in these patients. In patients with atrial fibrillation or flutter with rapid ventricular response and heart failure, digitalis produces salutary effects, and therefore rapid digitalization should be considered. Digoxin, 1 mg, can be infused intravenously over 15 to 20 minutes, followed by 0.125 to 0.25 mg orally every day for maintenance therapy. For slow digitalization, oral administration of 0.25 mg of digoxin daily for 5 to 7 days is usually sufficient. The maintenance digoxin dose should be adjusted according to the clinical response, serum digoxin level, and renal function. Even when rapid digitalization seems necessary, one should avoid rapid bolus injection of digoxin, as this mode of administration can induce a significant increase in systemic and coronary vascular resistance, and precipitate worsening heart failure and myocardial ischemia.

The principal rationale for *vasodilator therapy* in patients with heart failure is twofold: (1) to decrease systemic vascular resistance to improve cardiac output and (2) to decrease systemic venous tone to reduce systemic and pulmonary venous pressures. Some vasodilator agents are predominantly venodilators (e.g., nitrates), which tend to decrease pulmonary and systemic venous pressures con-

TABLE 4 Important Secondary Causes of Deterioration of Heart Failure

Cause	Evaluation
Myocardial ischemia or infarction	History, electrocardiogram
Dysrhythmias	History of palpitation or dizziness, physical examination, electrocardiogram
Alcohol abuse	History (particularly from relatives or friends), liver function tests
Electrolyte disturbances and deterioration of renal function	Measurement of serum concentration of electrolytes, BUN, creatinine
Intercurrent illness	History, physical examination, appropriate laboratory tests
Bacterial endocarditis in patients with valvular heart disease	History, physical examination, blood cultures, appropriate laboratory tests
Dietary indiscretion (increased sodium and fluid intake)	History, measurement of weight
Adverse drug effects: digitalis toxicity, negative inotropic agents, type I antiarrhythmic drugs (disopyramide, procainamide), nonsteroidal anti-inflammatory agents (indomethacin)	History, plasma drug concentration
Hypermetabolic states (thyrotoxicosis, fever)	History, physical examination, appropriate laboratory tests
Pulmonary emboli	History, physical examination, appropriate laboratory tests
Hypertension	Blood pressure recording

sistently with little or no increase in cardiac output. Arteriolar dilators (e.g., hydralazine), on the other hand, increase cardiac output significantly, and pulmonary and systemic venous pressures may remain unchanged. Drugs with combined venous and arterial dilating effects (e.g., captopril) decrease pulmonary and systemic venous pressures and also increase cardiac output. The expected hemodynamic effects and the usual doses of the commonly used vasodilators for treatment of chronic congestive heart failure are summarized in Table 5.

For treatment of an acute, severe exacerbation of chronic heart failure, intravenous vasodilator therapy (nitroprusside or nitroglycerin) is preferred with hemodynamic monitoring. However, in normotensive pa-

TABLE 5 Commonly Used Vasodilator Drugs for the Treatment of Chronic Congestive Heart Failure

Drug	Mechanism of Vasodilation	Major Hemodynamic Effects	Usual Dose	Major Adverse Effects
Nitroprusside	Direct (arterial, venous)	CO↑PCWP↓RAP↓ HR↔AP↓SVR↓	15-400 µg/min	Hypotension
Nitroglycerin	Direct (venous)	PCWP↓RAP↓CO↑↔ HR↔AP↓SVR↓↔	10–200 µg/min	Hypotension
Hydralazine	Direct (arterial)	CO↑PCWP↔RAP↔ HR↔↑AP↓↔SVR↓	50-100 mg/4 times daily	Hypotension, fluid retention, lupus
Isosorbide dinitrate	Direct (venous)	PCWP↓RAP↓CO↑↔ HR↔AP↓SVR↓↔	20-80 mg/PO 4-6 times daily	Hypotension, fluid retention, headache, tolerance
Nitroglycerin ointment (2%)	Direct (venous)	PCWP↓RAP↓CO↑↔ HR↔AP↓SVR↓↔	½-2 inches, 4-6 times daily	Hypotension, fluid retention, headache, tolerance
Prazosin	Alpha-adrenoreceptor blockade (arterial, venous)	PCWP↓RAP↓CO↑ HR↑↔AP↓SVR↓	2-5 mg, 3-4 times daily	Hypotension, tachyphylaxis, fluid retention
Captopril	Angiotensin-converting inhibitors (arterial, venous)	PCWP↓RAP↓CO↑ HR↔↓AP↓SVR↓	6.25-25 mg, 3 times daily	Hypotension, rarely skin rash, proteinuria, renal failure

Abbreviations: ↑=increase; ↓=decrease; ↔=no change; PCWP=pulmonary capillary wedge pressure; RAP=right atrial pressure; CO=cardiac output; HR=heart rate; AP=arterial pressure; SVR=systemic vascular resistance.

tients, particularly with dyspnea, sublingual administration of nitroglycerin (0.4 mg) or of isosorbide dinitrate (2.5 to 5 mg) can provide immediate benefit and does not require hemodynamic monitoring. Similarly, in hypertensive patients, nifedipine (10 mg) can be administered sublingually for the immediate treatment without hemodynamic monitoring. In hypotensive patients, vasodilator therapy should be avoided until further evaluation, and in these patients intravenous inotropic agents (dobutamine, 5 to 10 μg per kilogram per minute, or dopamine, 5 to 15 μg per kilogram per minute, or amrinone, 0.75 μg per kilogram bolus) should be considered for initial therapy.

For outpatient management of chronic heart failure, nonparenteral vasodilators should be considered in patients who remain symptomatic despite diuretic and digitalis therapy. Placebo-controlled studies have demonstrated sustained clinical benefit with angiotensin-converting enzyme inhibitors (captopril and enalapril) and nitrates (isosorbide dinitrate). No conclusive evidence exists for such benefits with other vasodilators. Thus, *captopril* and *nitrates* have emerged as the vasodilators of current choice for long-term therapy of heart failure. For initiation of captopril therapy, the starting dose should be low (6.25 mg) and the dose should be increased gradually to 12.5 and then to 25 mg, if required, monitoring changes in blood pressure. The dose that decreases blood pressure modestly (mean pressure by 10 mm Hg or less) should be used for maintenance therapy. The initial dose of oral isosorbide dinitrate is usually 20 mg; however, the majority of patients with severe heart failure require 40 to 80 mg, 4 to 6 times daily. In patients who are intolerant of captopril or in relatively hypotensive patients (systolic blood pressure less than 95 mm Hg), the combination of hydralazine and nitrates may provide benefit without causing significant hypotension. Prazosin, although effective for short-term therapy, has been proved to induce tachyphylaxis; furthermore, it also causes hypotension. Thus, it is not the preferred vasodilator agent for the majority of patients.

COR PULMONALE

HERBERT P. WIEDEMANN, M.D.
RICHARD A. MATTHAY, M.D.

Cor pulmonale is defined as enlargement of the right ventricle caused by pulmonary artery hypertension secondary to structural or functional abnormalities of the lungs. The right ventricular enlargement may take the form of hypertrophy or dilatation or both, depending on the degree and duration of the pulmonary artery hypertension. Cor pulmonale is not a single disease entity, but rather a state of cardiopulmonary dysfunction that may have several different pathophysiologic mechanisms. The clinical hallmarks are those that result from right ventricular hypertrophy and right ventricular failure. Although most of the diseases that cause cor pulmonale are chronic in nature and progress rather slowly, patients often present with acute, severe symptoms and life-threatening physiologic derangements. Such an abrupt decompensation occurs because the right ventricle is suddenly unable to compensate as further demands are placed on it; this is either the result of progression of the underlying disease or of a superimposed acute process such as pulmonary infection or left ventricular failure.

The most frequent underlying cause of cor pulmonale is chronic obstructive pulmonary disease (chronic bronchitis or emphysema or both). Anatomic evidence of cor pulmonale can be found at autopsy in about 40 percent of patients with bronchitis and emphysema. In the United States, cor pulmonale accounts for approximately 10 to 30 percent of the patients admitted to the hospital for congestive heart failure.

ETIOLOGY AND PATHOPHYSIOLOGY OF COR PULMONALE

Under normal conditions, the pulmonary circulation is a low-pressure, low-resistance system; the normal pulmonary vascular bed can accept increases of cardiac output approximately 2.5 times that of normal without any appreciable rise in pulmonary artery pressures. Thus the normal right ventricle rarely has to function against significant afterload stress.

Cor pulmonale results when pulmonary hypertension places a workload on the right ventricle that is significantly greater than normal. Among the pathogenetic mechanisms that can create elevations in pulmonary artery pressure, either individually or in combination, are increases in pulmonary vascular resistance, pulmonary blood flow, pulmonary blood volume, blood viscosity, and pulmonary venous pressure (Table 1). The most important cause of pulmonary artery hypertension is an increase in pulmonary vascular resistance owing to active vasoconstriction or fixed anatomic destruction of the vascular bed.

Pulmonary Vasoconstriction

Alveolar hypoxia is a potent activator of pulmonary vasoconstriction. It usually results from parenchymal lung diseases that lead to ventilation-perfusion abnormalities. These include chronic obstructive pulmonary disease and destructive interstitial diseases of the lung (e.g., sarcoidosis, idiopathic pulmonary fibrosis). Alveolar hypoxia

TABLE 1 Causes of Pulmonary Hypertension and Cor Pulmonale

Pulmonary vasoconstriction
    Alveolar hypoxia
        Parenchymal lung disease (COPD, cystic fibrosis,
            pulmonary fibrosis)
        Hypoventilation (sleep apnea, obesity-hypoventilation
            syndrome)
        Respiratory muscle weakness (myasthenia, ALS, scoliosis)
        High altitude
    Acidosis (respiratory or metabolic)
Anatomic reduction of pulmonary vascular bed
    COPD, pulmonary fibrosis
    Pulmonary emboli
    Pulmonary vasculitis
    Primary pulmonary hypertension
Left ventricular dysfunction
Increased blood viscosity (sickle-cell disease)

also may occur in diseases characterized by inadequate ventilatory drive and resultant hypoventilation (primary alveolar hypoventilation, obesity-hypoventilation syndromes, sleep apnea syndromes). Abnormalities of the neuromuscular apparatus or chest wall (e.g., myasthenia gravis, amyotrophic lateral sclerosis, and severe scoliosis) may also cause alveolar hypoxia and be associated with cor pulmonale. Exposure to high altitude produces alveolar hypoxia through a reduction in the ambient inspired oxygen tension. Sojourns to high-altitude areas may precipitate cor pulmonale in patients with underlying lung disease.

Plasma acidity also promotes pulmonary vasoconstriction. Therefore, any disorder associated with systemic acidosis, including respiratory acidosis seen with decompensated chronic obstructive pulmonary disease, may contribute to pulmonary vasoconstriction.

Anatomic Reduction of the Pulmonary Vascular Bed

Pulmonary hypertension at rest usually does not develop unless more than one-half of the cross-sectional area of the vascular bed is destroyed. However, such marked reduction in the pulmonary vascular bed can be seen in several lung diseases, including emphysema and the various forms of pulmonary fibrosis.

Disorders that primarily affect the lung vasculature can also contribute to pulmonary arterial hypertension. Among such diseases are primary pulmonary hypertension, pulmonary emboli, and vasculitis.

Left Ventricular Abnormalities

Left ventricular dysfunction and the resultant elevation in pulmonary venous pressure are frequent causes of pulmonary arterial hypertension. In fact, the most common cause of right ventricular failure may be left ventricular dysfunction. Technically, right ventricular failure that is caused solely by left-sided heart disease does not constitute cor pulmonale (defined as heart disease secondary to disease of the lung or its vasculature). Although it is worthwhile maintaining this distinction, it should be remembered that left-sided heart dysfunction frequently complicates cor pulmonale.

Cor pulmonale by itself does not necessarily seriously affect intrinsic left ventricular performance. However, right ventricular dysfunction may indirectly affect left ventricular performance because of a reduction in left ventricular diastolic filling. Reduced filling is secondary either to a reduced right ventricular stroke output or to a septal shift caused by a dilated right ventricular cavity. Of course, patients with cor pulmonale may have coexisting disease processes, such as coronary arteriosclerosis or valvular heart disease, which may affect left ventricular performance.

CLINICAL MANIFESTATIONS OF COR PULMONALE

Physical examination of patients with cor pulmonale characteristically reveals dyspnea, peripheral edema, and distended neck veins. Right ventricular hypertrophy is often suggested by a palpable parasternal or subxiphoid heave. Cardiac auscultation may reveal an S_3 gallop, a loud pulmonic second heart sound, and a murmur of tricuspid regurgitation (caused by right ventricular dilatation). However, the clinical signs may be quite variable, since they are influenced by several factors, including the intravascular volume status of the patient and the underlying disease process.

A *chest roentgenogram* is important to document the nature of the underlying lung disease or the possible presence of superimposed problems such as pneumonia. The *electrocardiogram* may show patterns suggestive of right ventricular strain or hypertrophy; however, these changes are not completely reliable for making the diagnosis. The electrocardiogram may be more important in detecting exacerbating conditions such as arrhythmias or myocardial infarction.

TREATMENT OF COR PULMONALE—ACUTE DECOMPENSATION

The fundamental goal of emergency therapy for cor pulmonale is the reduction of pulmonary arterial hypertension. Frequently, the history and clinical setting are characteristic enough that the diagnosis of decompensated cor pulmonale can be made quickly by physicians or trained paramedical personnel. Furthermore, the initial therapy consists of commonly available medications and equipment. Therefore, the emergent management of cor pulmonale often can be initiated in the home or ambulance before the patient arrives in the emergency department.

Oxygen

Supplemental oxygen constitutes important initial therapy for patients with acutely decompensated cor pulmonale. Oxygen administration serves the dual purpose of reversing that component of pulmonary hypertension that is attributable to hypoxic vasoconstriction and also of helping to relieve cerebral and myocardial hypoxia.

Oxygen therapy must be instituted with some care, especially in those patients who exhibit hypercapnia. High oxygen concentrations may occasionally worsen respiratory acidosis owing to depression of ventilation. The initial administration of oxygen should be conservative, perhaps at a level of about 24 to 30 percent. Such levels can be achieved either with nasal prongs (a typical low-flow system) or with a Venturi mask (a high-flow system). The Venturi mask allows greater control of the inspired fraction of oxygen but inhibits communication, intake of fluid and nutrients, coughing, and clearance of secretions. Nasal prongs provide less precise control of the inspired oxygen fraction but permit greater patient comfort.

Administration of oxygen should be monitored by observing ventilation and sampling arterial blood gases to check the adequacy of arterial oxygenation and to detect any increase in arterial carbon dioxide tension. Generally, an arterial oxygen tension of at least 60 mm Hg or an arterial oxygen saturation of at least 85 to 90 percent is adequate. If meeting these goals leads to excessive carbon dioxide elevation and acidosis, mechanical ventilation may be necessary.

Bronchodilators

In patients with reversible airway obstruction, pharmacologic therapy may be valuable in reducing the work of breathing and in decreasing dyspnea. Furthermore, by aiding pulmonary gas exchange, bronchodilators often lead to an improvement in arterial oxygenation and a decrease in hypercapnia. Bronchodilators may be delivered through aerosol inhalation or by systemic administration.

The *sympathomimetic amines* currently marketed in the United States for aerosol delivery include isoproterenol (Isuprel), isoetharine (Bronkosol), and metaproterenol (Alupent). The latter two agents are selective beta$_2$-agonists and are preferred over nonselective agents such as isoproterenol to limit the possibility of cardiovascular side effects such as arrhythmias. The suggested dose of metaproterenol is 0.2 to 0.3 ml diluted in 2 to 3 ml of normal saline; the nebulized aerosol is inhaled every 4 hours. The aerosol route is ideal initial therapy because of its rapid onset of action, high potency, and low toxicity. In severely affected patients, systemic administration (oral or subcutaneous) of terbutaline can be added cautiously if the front-line therapy of inhaled sympathomimetics, along with theophylline and corticosteroids (described below), proves inadequate. Terbutaline is given at 2.5 to 5.0 mg every 8 hours.

The *methylxanthines* provide bronchodilation through a pathway that is probably different from that of the sympathomimetic amines. Consequently, in patients who do not respond rapidly to inhaled aerosol therapy, intravenous administration of aminophylline is indicated. In the acutely ill adult, a 6 mg per kilogram loading dose should be followed by a continuous infusion of between 0.3 and 0.9 mg per kilogram per hour. In patients with heart failure or liver disease, theophylline clearance may be markedly reduced and an infusion rate at the low end of this range should be selected. If the patient has already been taking theophylline medication within the previous 24 hours, the loading dose should be reduced or entirely omitted. Assessment of theophylline blood levels is necessary to ensure that the selected dosing regimen provides a therapeutic level of 10 to 20 μg per milliliter. Seizures or severe tachyarrhythmias have occurred at levels above 40 μg per milliliter.

Theophylline and the sympathomimetic amines may have salutary effects not related to bronchodilation. These agents may improve myocardial contractility and provide pulmonary vasodilatation. Theophylline may also improve diaphragm endurance and enhance respiratory drive.

Anticholinergic agents may provide some bronchodilatation in patients who are refractory to adrenergic medications. Atropine sulfate may be administered by nebulized aerosol (up to 0.02 mg per kilogram in 2 to 3 ml of saline given every 6 hours). Side effects are usually tolerable, although patients should avoid letting the aerosol come in contact with their eyes and should wash their mouths out after use. Ipratropium bromide (Atrovent) is an atropine derivative with minimal systemic absorption when administered as an aerosol. Although this agent is not currently available in the United States, its release is expected soon.

Corticosteroids

Information from a recent double-blind randomized study suggests that the use of systemic corticosteroids can enhance the rate of improvement in the FEV$_1$ in patients with an acute decompensation of chronic obstructive pulmonary disease. The recommended dose is 0.5 mg per kilogram of methylprednisolone delivered intravenously every 6 hours for the first 3 days. Good information is not available on whether higher doses may have an even more favorable effect or perhaps be associated with adverse side effects.

Digitalis

Digitalis should be considered only in cases where it is specifically indicated as treatment for a supraventricular arrhythmia or coincident left-sided heart failure. In isolated right ventricular failure, digitalis appears to have no benefit and may in fact be associated with detrimental effects. Although digitalis does improve right ventricular contractility, it also may have a direct action on the pulmonary vasculature to increase pulmonary hypertension. The use of cardiac glycosides is associated with a higher risk of arrhythmias or other complications in decompensated patients with cor pulmonale attributable to hypoxemia, acidosis, and catecholamine excess.

Diuresis

Diuretic administration is indicated in the presence of left-sided heart dysfunction and pulmonary edema. Diuretics may also improve cardiovascular performance in a patient with isolated right ventricular dysfunction and extreme volume overload. If the right ventricular end-diastolic volume is markedly elevated, diuretic therapy might improve the function of both the right ventricle and the left ventricle (the latter effect being achieved as left ventricular diastolic filling is enhanced through a reduction in the dilatation of the right ventricle).

Excessive volume depletion must be avoided, however. If right ventricular filling volume and pressure are reduced too dramatically in the face of pulmonary hypertension, there may be a drop in cardiac output. Diuretics must therefore be administered with careful attention to the cardiovascular status of the patient rather than in an aggressive attempt to totally eliminate all peripheral edema or other signs of increased peripheral venous pressure.

Serum *electrolyte* levels must also be carefully monitored during diuretic administration. Hypokalemic metabolic alkalosis may result from excessive use of diuretics, and this condition diminishes the effect of the carbon dioxide stimulus to the respiratory centers and reduces ventilatory drive. Moreover, as potassium and chloride are depleted, renal excretion of bicarbonate is jeopardized, and this may hinder subsequent attempts to correct a compensated respiratory acidosis. (As hypercapnia is reversed, the desired subsequent reduction in serum bicarbonate may be difficult to achieve.) In such a situation, it is important to give adequate replacement of potassium and chloride.

Phlebotomy

In patients with severe erythrocythemia (hematocrit reading exceeding 55 to 60 percent) who have not responded to the initial therapy outlined above, phlebotomy can be considered. This usually achieves a significant drop in mean pulmonary arterial pressure and total vascular resistance. These effects may be produced by a decrease in total blood volume or a decrease in blood viscosity.

Phlebotomy probably has no role in the treatment of cor pulmonale in those patients who have only mild to moderate elevations in hematocrit values.

Antibiotics

In patients with pneumonia or purulent bronchitis, antibiotics should be considered. A Gram stain of sputum is helpful in the initial selection of a drug. In an outpatient without underlying immunosuppression, empiric therapy directed against *Haemophilus influenzae* or *Streptococcus pneumoniae* is generally used. Ampicillin, tetracycline, or a cephalosporin is frequently utilized. In the acutely ill patient, the antibiotics are usually delivered parenterally.

Vasodilator Medications

It is tempting to achieve pulmonary vasodilation and the acute relief of pulmonary hypertension through the use of vasodilator medications. Medications that have been suggested include hydralazine, nitroprusside, nitroglycerin, nifedipine, diazoxide, and phentolamine. However, these agents should be used with extreme caution and with frequent monitoring of the patient's cardiovascular status. Unfortunately, they are often associated with adverse physiologic effects. First, these agents may potentially worsen ventilation-perfusion relationships within the lung and thereby exacerbate arterial hypoxemia through an increase in physiologic shunt. Furthermore, use of these agents may be associated with a much more profound effect on the systemic arterial circulation than on the intended target of the pulmonary vasculature. This may lead to profound hypotension in patients with relatively fixed pulmonary hypertension. In addition to the obvious detrimental consequences, this systemic hypotension also limits right coronary artery blood flow and adversely affects right ventricular performance. This may initiate a vicious cycle of rapid cardiovascular collapse and may account for instances of death that have been attributed to use of these agents in patients with severe pulmonary hypertension.

These medications may be used when specifically indicated for coexisting problems such as angina or systemic hypertension, but should not be used in the initial therapy of otherwise uncomplicated cor pulmonale, especially if adequate means for cardiovascular monitoring are not in place.

SUGGESTED READING

Matthay RA. Cor pulmonale. Med Grand Rounds 1983; 2:197–207.

McFadden ER, Braunwald E. Cor pulmonale and pulmonary thromboembolism. In: Braunwald E, ed. Textbook of cardiovascular medicine. 2nd ed. Philadelphia: WB Saunders, 1984; p. 1572.

Wiedemann HP, Matthay RA. Acute right heart failure. Crit Care Clin 1985; 1:631–661.

PERICARDITIS

P. SUDHAKAR REDDY, M.D.

Inflammation of the pericardium, regardless of the cause, produces clinical syndromes characterized by pain or restriction of cardiac filling. Although pain is not usually present with constrictive pericarditis, pain and pericardial effusion and constriction can coexist.

The painful syndrome of pericarditis constitutes a true emergency only when it is associated with effusion significant enough to compromise cardiac filling. In patients without hemodynamically significant effusion, the treatment of pericarditis is directed toward the relief of pain, which is usually simple and straightforward. For the emergency physician it is more important to differentiate the painful syndrome of acute pericarditis from more ominous clinical conditions that require urgent and specific therapies.

DIFFERENTIAL DIAGNOSIS

Pericarditic pain has to be distinguished from the pain of acute myocardial infarction, pulmonary infarction, pleurisy with or without underlying pneumonia, acute pneumothorax, mediastinal emphysema due to rupture of the esophagus, and aortic dissection, as well as from the many other less severe causes of chest pain see the chapter *Chest Pain*.

In addition to certain features of the pain, the presence of a pericardial rub, characteristic electrocardiographic changes, and echocardiographic evidence of pericardial fluid distinguish pericarditic pain from other types of chest pain.

Pericarditic pain may or may not be of sudden onset. It is usually sharp and superficial rather than dull and deep as encountered in patients with acute myocardial infarction. The pain is usually localized to the precordium, but can radiate to the neck and left shoulder, mimicking closely the pain of an acute myocardial infarction. This pain may be aggravated by motion of the upper torso and by breathing, thus mimicking the pleuritic pain of pleurisy. Rarely, it may present as a vague discomfort throughout the precordium.

A pericardial rub is a pathognomonic sign of pericarditis. One should not lose sight of the fact, however, that pericarditis itself may be secondary to a more ominous underlying illness, such as acute myocardial infarction.

A pericardial rub is usually scratchy and superficial. Its intensity can vary with respiration, position, and varying pressure of the stethoscope. It can have one, two, or three components. When systolic and early diastolic components are present, they can be confused with a to-and-fro murmur. When only the systolic component is present,

it can be confused with a systolic murmur. The presence of a rub may also vary considerably with time and be transient in some patients, particularly those with an acute myocardial infarction. Some pericardial rubs may change considerably with respiration and are thus heard only in a particular phase of respiration. If there is associated pleurisy, a pericardial rub may coexist with a pleural rub and may be heard anywhere over the precordium. Occasionally, however, it may be heard only at the apex with the patient turned in the left lateral position.

Acute pericarditis is usually associated with electrocardiographic (ECG) changes, which may be confused with those of an acute myocardial infarction. The classic ECG finding of acute pericarditis is diffuse S-T segment elevation (except for aV_R, which shows depression) without abnormal Q waves. There is usually no reciprocal S-T segment depression (except for, in rare instances, leads III and aV_L). The absence of reciprocal S-T depression and Q waves helps distinguish acute pericarditis from acute myocardial infarction. The early repolarization pattern noted in some normal individuals can also be confused with the changes of acute pericarditis. Comparison with the prior ECG, if available, is most helpful in such situations.

Echocardiographic evidence of pericardial effusion lends support to the diagnosis of pericarditis. A segmental wall motion abnormality of the left ventricle would suggest an acute myocardial infarction. Thus, an echocardiogram performed in the emergency department may help to distinguish acute pericarditis from acute myocardial infarction in some doubtful cases.

A chest roentgenogram is frequently helpful in excluding pulmonary causes of chest pain. The presence of a pulmonary infiltrate or pleural effusion favors pleuropericarditis or pulmonary infarction. Air in the pleural cavity or mediastinum confirms pneumothorax or mediastinal emphysema, respectively.

In the absence of roentgenographic findings, a ventilation-perfusion scan of the lungs may be helpful in excluding the diagnosis of acute pulmonary embolism or infarction. In equivocal cases, a pulmonary angiogram is required for confirmation. Thallium or technetium pyrophosphate scanning of the heart may be useful to confirm the diagnosis of acute myocardial infarction in some cases.

MANAGEMENT OF ACUTE PERICARDITIS

The best approach to the treatment of acute pericarditis is not to miss the diagnosis of conditions that need lifesaving emergency treatment. Even when the clinical findings are highly suggestive of acute pericarditis, other serious conditions must be entertained and excluded. Emergency physicians must understand the subtle differences between acute myocardial infarction and pericarditis and the possible association of these two entities. If pericarditis cannot be excluded with reasonable certainty, and acute myocardial infarction remains a possibility, the patient should be subjected to cardiac catheterization or some other confirmatory test before the institution of thrombolytic therapy for myocardial infarction. Until intravenous thrombolytic therapy is proven efficacious either in improving survival or decreasing morbidity, it should be withheld when the distinction between acute myocardial infarction and pericarditis is uncertain.

The management of acute pericarditis involves two steps: treatment of pain, and investigation of any underlying systemic illness.

For severe pain, morphine sulfate 5 mg IV every 15 minutes to a maximum of 30 mg or meperidine hydrochloride 25 mg IV every 15 minutes to a maximum of 100 mg should be administered. Since respiratory depression is more likely to occur with morphine sulfate, my preference is for meperidine hydrochloride.

Simulaneously with the initiation of intravenous analgesia, aspirin should be administered orally as two tablets (650 mg) every 3 to 4 hours. The individual dose can be increased to four tablets every 3 to 4 hours if necessary. Morphine and meperidine may be omitted in the majority of patients who are not in acute distress.

If the patient does not respond to aspirin, indomethacin should be administered in doses of 25 to 75 mg 4 times daily. The dose may be tapered after 5 to 7 days of a symptom-free state.

Although pain is promptly relieved by prednisone, recurrences are common when the therapy is discontinued. Therefore, prednisone should be administered only if aspirin and indomethacin in full recommended doses fail to relieve the symptoms. The initial recommended dose is 60 mg daily and should be tapered after 5 to 7 days of symptom free state at the rate of 5 mg per week up to 30 mg per day and then 2.5 mg a week.

INVESTIGATION OF UNDERLYING SYSTEMIC ILLNESS

Although the idiopathic variety is the most common type of acute pericarditis, there are many other causes. Frequently, acute pericarditis is the first clue to an underlying systemic illness. Therefore, most patients with acute pericarditis should be admitted to the hospital, and careful and prompt follow-up should be arranged for those who are not admitted. A work-up of the various causes listed in Table 1 should be undertaken. If a specific diagnosis is established, therapy should be tailored to that cause.

CONSTRICTIVE PERICARDITIS

Constrictive pericarditis is rarely an acute emergency; however, misdiagnosis of this condition may result in costly errors. Recently, two patients with constrictive pericarditis were referred to our institution for liver transplantation. Since constrictive pericarditis is a curable condition, an emergency or outpatient physician should suspect the diagnosis in any patient with ascites or edema and elevated venous pressure, but without marked enlarge-

TABLE 1 Etiologic Classification of Pericardial Disease

Acute idiopathic or nonspecific pericarditis

Acute myocardial infarction

Postmyocardial infarction syndrome (Dressler's syndrome)

Post-traumatic pericarditis (penetrating or nonpenetrating)

Post-thoracotomy syndrome or postcardiotomy syndrome

Connective tissue diseases: rheumatoid disease; rheumatic fever; disseminated lupus erythematosus; scleroderma; Takayasu's arteritis

Specific infections
   Bacterial infections; infective endocarditis
   Tuberculosis
   Fungal infections: histoplasmosis, nocardiosis, blastomycosis
   Viral (Coxsackie B, influenza, ECHO)
   Amebiasis
   Toxoplasmosis
   Meningococcal disease
   Gonococcal disease

Primary or metastatic neoplasm, including lymphoma and leukemia

Postradiation pericarditis

Aortic aneurysm: rupture or leakage of dissecting or nondissecting aneurysm into the pericardial sac

Drugs: hydralazine; psicofuranine; procainamide; anticoagulant therapy; isonicotinic acid hydrazide; penicillin, minoxidil

Chylopericardium

Uremia, and in association with hemodialysis

Miscellaneous: sarcoidosis; myxedema; amyloid disease; multiple myeloma, scleroderma

Adapted from Fowler, Noble O. Etiology of pericarditis. In: Hurst JW, (ed). The heart 4th ed. New York: McGraw Hill, 1978:1643.

ment of the heart. Such a patient should be admitted electively for appropriate work-up. Many times the diagnosis is missed because of failure to recognize the elevated venous pressure. If one is not comfortable with the evaluation of venous pressure in a patient with edema and/or ascites, the patient should be referred to a cardiologist for further evaluation. An echocardiogram is helpful, but not diagnostic. A computed tomography scan of the chest may be useful for confirming the presence of a thickened pericardium. Cardiac catheterization is usually diagnostic except for its inability to distinguish constrictive pericarditis from restrictive cardiomyopathy, which can be diagnosed only by extracardiac manifestations or surgery. Rarely, myocardial biopsy is useful in such circumstances.

SUGGESTED READING

Fowler NO, ed. The pericardium in health and disease. Mount Kisco, NY: Futura Publishing Company, 1985.

Reddy PS, Leon DF, Shaver JA, eds. Pericardial disease. New York: Raven Press, 1982.

Shabetai R, ed. The pericardium. New york: Grune & Stratton, 1981.

VALVULAR HEART DISEASE

JOHN M. FIELD, M.D.

A CONCEPTUAL DIAGNOSTIC APPROACH

Although the incidence of rheumatic valvular heart disease is declining, valvular lesions often confront the emergency physician as primary problems and complicate the management or treatment plans for other cardiac and noncardiac emergencies. The physician must determine the significance of a valvular murmur and decide upon appropriate intervention or disposition. In this chapter, the common valvular abnormalities and their most frequent patterns of presentation to the emergency physician will be discussed.

A cardiac murmur does not always indicate a cardiac disorder, and the physician must be cautious not to create pathology where none exists. To the contrary, many cardiac murmurs merely reflect increased or mildly turbulent flow in the absence of serious cardiac pathologic changes. In fact, it has been estimated that between 50 and 75 percent of school-age children will exhibit a physiologic cardiac murmur at some time. Most physicians are familiar with the outflow tract murmur associated with aortic atherosclerosis and advancing age.

ETIOLOGY

While a detailed description of the causes of valvular heart disease is not indicated, knowledge of the common types of valvular heart disease encountered (nonrheumatic acute mitral regurgitation; rheumatic and nonrheumatic clinical mitral regurgitation; nonrheumatic aortic regurgitation; valvular aortic stenosis; mitral stenosis; and tricuspid regurgitation) will assist the emergency physician in framing the answers to several important questions. The treating physician needs to ascertain the "triage" answers to these key questions: First, is the murmur benign (innocent) or pathologic? Second, what is the hemodynamic significance of the murmur? Third, are pathophysiologic consequences of this particular valve lesion responsible for the present symptom complex? Fourth, what immediate or intermediate intervention is required, if any? Fifth, what disposition is appropriate for this particular valvular lesion? Sixth, does this patient have endocarditis or need endocarditis prophylaxis?

The critical initial decision is the differentiation of pathologic from benign or physiologic murmurs. Those qualities usually associated with a benign or physiologic murmur are mid-systolic in timing; localized to left sternal border; maximal intensity grade II–III/VI; normal second heart sound; no diastolic component; and no ejection or mid-systolic click. Much of the initial management, as well as subsequent referral and diagnostic tests, relies on the physician's index of suspicion and ability to differentiate the "benign from the malignant."

While complex and multiple valve lesions may and do coexist, many forms of valvular heart disease are common, typical, and specific for a given clinical set of presenting symptoms and signs. Moreover, the examining physician can anticipate abnormalities on physical examination, electrocardiogram (ECG), and chest roentgenogram based on the symptoms and predicted overload patterns of the disease process. These noninvasive tests are then often confirmatory.

Each valvular lesion will cause a combination of myocardial hypertrophy and cardiac dilation specific for its degree of pressure and/or volume overload. To a great degree, symptoms will be more or less well tolerated depending upon the chronicity or acuteness with which the hemodynamic stress develops or progresses. Also in this context, cardiac adaptive mechanisms may be obvious, or chronically and clinically silent to the patient and/or physician. A firm basic understanding of these relationships is crucial to diagnosis and management.

NONRHEUMATIC MITRAL REGURGITATION

The causes of nonrheumatic mitral regurgitation are many and varied. Coaptation of the mitral leaflets requires the orchestration of several components of the mitral apparatus, including the mitral leaflets, mitral annulus, left atrial wall, chordae tendineae, papillary muscles, and left ventricular wall. Any disorder that disrupts these relationships can cause acute or chronic mitral regurgitation. For practical purposes, however, these nonrheumatic causes can be divided into those related to mitral valve prolapse (floppy valve syndrome), ischemic mitral regurgitation, and degenerative-calcific mitral dysfunction. The first is discussed in the chapter *Mitral Valve Prolapse*.

Clinical Features

Ischemic mitral regurgitation can present as intermittent episodes or an acute event complicating severe myocardial ischemia or infarction. Intermittent episodes of ischemic mitral regurgitation are usually secondary to transient ischemia of the papillary muscle or the left ventricular free wall associated with the posteromedial papillary muscle. More ominous is the acute mitral regurgitation associated with myocardial infarction complicated by pulmonary edema. Rupture of the papillary muscle is life-threatening and is one of the clinical entities associated with cardiac rupture and abrupt electrical mechanical dissociation with sudden death. Isolated rupture of a chordae tendineae is better tolerated, but often presents with the acute onset of a new murmur and pulmonary edema in the setting of a recent or evolving myocardial infarction.

Pathophysiologic derangements relate to an acute volume overload of the left atrium and ventricle with transmission of increased filling pressures to the left atrium and pulmonary vasculature. These patients are clinically ill with tachycardia, tachypnea, dyspnea, and findings consistent with variable degrees of pulmonary vascular congestion. Many of these patients are also in cardiogenic shock. In a patient with an otherwise uncomplicated inferior wall infarct, the development of a new cardiac murmur and hemodynamic instability should suggest the possibility of this hemodynamic lesion.

Emergency department diagnosis requires identification of the mechanical lesion complicating myocardial infarction. The major differential diagnosis involves acute mitral regurgitation or rupture of the interventricular septum. Both of these events are associated with similar clinical findings. A holosystolic murmur develops with wide transmission. The localization of a holosystolic murmur to the lower left sternal border, and its association with a palpable thrill, are sometimes helpful. These clinical findings are usually reported with ventricular septal defects; however, they may be inconsistent and not specifically associated with a ventricular septal defect.

Management

Emergency management requires prompt recognition of the disorder. Standard treatment for congestive heart failure should be instituted immediately, but the diagnosis should be confirmed by cardiac catheterization and the hemodynamic severity of the acute event delineated. Many of these patients require pharmacologic intervention using a combination of dopamine or dobutamine and sodium nitroprusside together with afterload augmentation via an intra-aortic balloon pump. Early consultation and intervention by an invasive cardiologist and cardiothoracic surgical team is necessary. Quite often, coexisting coronary artery disease is present in other vascular beds, and an attempt at mitral valve repair and/or replacement combined with coronary revascularization is the only solution that offers some chance of survival for patients with this complicated and often fatal lesion.

RHEUMATIC AND NONRHEUMATIC CHRONIC MITRAL REGURGITATION

Chronic mitral regurgitation is usually much better tolerated owing to the compensatory and adaptive mechanisms that occur with time. The pathophysiologic volume overload of the left ventricle and the volume/pressure overload of the left atrium are compensated for by hypertrophy of the left ventricular myocardium, dilation of the left ventricular chamber, left atrial enlargement, and pulmonary artery hypertension.

The clinical symptom complex caused by these pathophysiologic changes includes exertional dyspnea, orthopnea, paroxysmal nocturnal dyspnea, palpitations (usually paroxysmal atrial tachyarrhythmias or atrial fibrillation), and fatigue. Acutely, these patients may decompensate and present with acute pulmonary edema. If these patients are in atrial fibrillation or experience episodes of sinus rhythm alternating with paroxysmal atrial fibrillation, embolic episodes may be the first signal of their valvular heart disease.

Physical examination of patients with hemodynamically significant mitral regurgitation is remarkable for accentuation of the left ventricular impulse with lateral displacement. The cardiac murmur is described as pansystolic and grade II–III/VI or louder at the lower left sternal border and cardiac apex, with radiation to the axilla and the infrascapular or interscapular area. In the absence of mitral stenosis, a third heart sound may exist in response to increased volume and to compliance changes in the left ventricle or may represent LV failure. As hemodynamic decompensation occurs, signs and symptoms of pulmonary artery hypertension and right ventricular dysfunction develop. Systemic and peripheral edema develop and tricuspid regurgitation may become prominent.

ECG findings, chest roentgenogram, and physical findings are related to specific cardiac chamber enlargement, pressure/volume overload of the left atrium, and increasing pulmonary artery hypertension with right ventricular pressure overload. The ECG often demonstrates atrial fibrillation, although if sinus rhythm is preserved, left atrial enlargement is present in the majority of patients. Left ventricular enlargement is demonstrated by noting criteria for left ventricular hypertrophy with repolarization abnormalities ("hypertrophy with strain"). As right ventricular failure becomes more pronounced a rightward shift in the patient's axis may be noted, although it may be interpreted as only a vertical axis shift by the electrocardiographer. Additionally, a right ventricular conduction delay (rSr) or right bundle branch block may develop as pulmonary hypertension and right ventricular hypertrophy and dilation progress. Diagnostic ECG criteria for right ventricular hypertrophy are often lacking because of the predominance of left ventricular forces. As occurs in mitral stenosis, obvious signs of an enlarged left atrium are present in advanced stages. The roentgenogram may reflect a double density along the right heart border, elevation of the left main stem bronchus, straightening of the left heart border, and cephalization of the pulmonary vasculature. In addition, the degree of left atrial enlargement is usually proportionally greater with the volume lesion of mitral regurgitation. In addition, the usually small left ventricle of mitral stenosis has greatly enlarged to accommodate the regurgitant volume of mitral regurgitation.

NONRHEUMATIC AORTIC REGURGITATION

Aortic regurgitation can occur acutely, subacutely, or chronically, and usually presents as an isolated valvular lesion. In this context, especially when it afflicts adults during middle age or beyond, it is generally regarded as a nonrheumatic disorder.

Aortic regurgitation may have diverse causes and may occur as a result of intrinsic valvular pathologic changes or because of abnormalities of the ascending aorta and diseases that involve this structure. These include aortic dissection and/or aneurysmal formation, connective tissue disorders, aortic dilatation secondary to hypertension and atheromatous disease, cystic medial necrosis, and other uncommon disorders such as syphilis, ankylosing spondylitis, and inherited connective tissue disorders.

Acute aortic insufficiency is a serious disorder and may result from disruption of the valvular leaflets or from destruction of valve tissue, as in infective endocarditis.

Particularly when a virulent organism—such as *Staphylococcus*—is involved, the lesion may be life-threatening.

Clinical Features

Acute aortic insufficiency usually manifests itself in a clinically ill patient with tachypnea, tachycardia, dyspnea, and usually incipient heart failure or pulmonary edema. Heart failure accompanying acute aortic regurgitation is an especially ominous sign, since most of these patients acutely decompensate and require emergency aortic valve replacement.

These patients are generally acutely ill. Examination of the peripheral arterial pulse reveals a wide pulse pressure with aortic diastolic pressures averaging 35 to 50 mm Hg. There may be varying degrees of jugular venous distention. The carotid pulsations are both hyperdynamic and hypervolemic, attesting to an increased cardiac output compensating for the regurgitant volume. The lungs are clear or demonstrate pulmonary rales consistent with the degree of heart failure. The point of maximal impulse is hyperdynamic and may contain a palpable third heart sound. A summation gallop is often present. A grade II–III/VI aortic systolic ejection murmur may be appreciated in the second right intercostal space. This often does not reflect coexisting aortic stenosis, but rather the volume flow requirements of an acute aortic regurgitant lesion. A grade II–III/VI murmur of aortic insufficiency is present along the left sternal border. While radiation of the diastolic murmur along the right sternal border has been noted in patients with nonrheumatic causes, this finding is inconsistent and of minimal clinical value. In acute aortic insufficiency, the murmur may be of short duration because of early equalization of left ventricular and aortic pressures.

In marked contrast, chronic aortic regurgitation may be *well tolerated* for years with a short diastolic murmur the only mark of its existence. However, when dyspnea or other cardiac symptoms combine with cardiomegaly, valve replacement is indicated. The optimal timing for surgical intervention in the asymptomatic, but hemodynamically compromised, or minimally symptomatic patient is currently being studied.

VALVULAR AORTIC STENOSIS

Isolated pure valvular aortic stenosis occurs primarily as a result of hemodynamic deterioration in patients with congenitally bicuspid aortic valve or degeneration and calcification of the valve apparatus. Such patients present to the emergency physician with angina pectoris, symptoms of left ventricular dysfunction, and presyncope or syncope. Correlation of these symptoms with the murmur of aortic stenosis is important, since the life span of patients developing symptoms is often less than 5 years.

The cardiac murmur typically is a loud, harsh, rough systolic ejection murmur that is crescendo-decrescendo and most intense in the second right intercostal space. This murmur is well transmitted into the neck, but may also be appreciated at the lower left sternal border and even the cardiac apex. Carotid pulsations typically have a slow up stroke and low volume. There may be a transmitted thrill into the right (or less commonly left) carotid artery. As the lesion becomes hemodynamically significant, the diamond-shaped murmur begins to peak later in systole and eventually obscures the second heart sound. During this period of time, the aortic component of the second heart sound typically diminishes, decreases, and finally disappears. Some mild degree of aortic insufficiency may accompany the hemodynamically significant lesion of aortic stenosis. A prominent fourth heart sound most often accompanies the compliance changes of aortic stenosis. Notably, these patients maintain sinus rhythm and a fourth heart sound long into the natural history of their disease process. A conversion to atrial fibrillation and the loss of atrial systole will often precipitate acute pulmonary edema.

The ECG is abnormal in 85 to 90 percent of the patients with aortic stenosis. The systolic pressure overload of the left ventricle and atrial compliance changes elicit the characteristic electrocardiographic pattern of left ventricular hypertrophy with repolarization abnormalities and left atrial enlargement. Some 10 to 15 percent of patients with critical aortic stenosis documented by cardiac catheterization do not have the typical electrocardiographic changes consistent with left ventricular hypertrophy.

The chest roentgenogram reveals "mild concentric hypertrophy/left ventricular predominance." These findings are consistent with the concentrically hypertrophied, but not dilated left ventricle of aortic outflow tract obstruction. Close inspection of the chest x-ray film will usually reveal prominence of the ascending aorta, consistent with post-stenotic dilatation of the ascending aorta.

Special attention should be paid to the symptom of *angina pectoris* or complicating myocardial infarction. More than 50 percent of patients with aortic stenosis have coexisting coronary artery disease, and the differentiation between ischemic pain of valvular origin and coronary artery obstruction is often difficult. Most frequently, it requires cardiac catheterization to exclude or define the extent and severity of coexisting coronary artery disease.

Emergency treatment calls for the usual measures to alleviate pain, whether from coronary artery disease or the "subendocardial ischemia" of a hypertrophied ventricle. Nitrates may be used, but with caution and in a lower dose. In patients with critical aortic stenosis, a fixed cardiac output may be compromised by vasodilation, but nitrates may be tolerated if used judiciously. I prefer to use initial doses of 0.15 mg of sublingual nitroglycerin (or at most 0.3 mg of sublingual nitroglycerin), and 10 to 25 μg of intravenous nitroglycerin. Topical nitrates should be avoided. Similarly, morphine should be used with caution and titrated, preferably in 2-mg increments. Should hypotension develop during treatment, particular attention should be paid to any preload condition that may have been altered.

Similar cautions apply to treatment of congestive heart failure if vasodilators are employed. While preload agents improve pulmonary vascular congestion, afterload reducing agents may complicate hypotension in the presence of a "fixed" afterload at the aortic valve.

If congestive heart failure does not respond to therapy, *urgent* valve replacement is necessary. During periods of decreased cardiac output and aortic flow, critical valve murmurs may be reduced in intensity.

MITRAL STENOSIS

In contrast to the valvular lesions presented above, valvular mitral stenosis is almost always the result of rheumatic heart disease, requiring decades of valvular degeneration to present a clinically symptomatic state. Exertional dyspnea is usually the presenting initial symptom. As the valvular orifice index decreases, progressive dyspnea and fatigue become prominent symptoms. At this time left atrial enlargement and hypertrophy frequently cause atrial arrhythmias, including premature atrial complexes, paroxysmal supraventricular tachycardias, and atrial fibrillation. Eventually symptoms of paroxysmal nocturnal dyspnea, orthopnea, and right ventricular dysfunction develop. Decreased cardiac output and peripheral cyanosis are prominent features of end-stage mitral valvular disease. With the onset of right heart failure, jugular venous distention, hepatosplenomegaly, and peripheral edema occur.

Should the patient develop sustained or paroxysmal episodes of *atrial fibrillation*, the threat of systemic embolization is ever present. Left atrial thrombus should be included in the differential diagnosis of any patient suspected of systemic embolization. An unexplained fever should alert the physician to the possibility of endocarditis, and antibiotics should be withheld while this possibility is excluded.

Clinical Features

Patients with mild to moderate mitral stenosis are asymptomatic until the normal mitral valve orifice area has been reduced by at least 50 percent. At this time, exertional dyspnea may be the initial presenting symptom. The general physical examination is usually quite unremarkable. However, on auscultation in patients with sinus rhythm, the classic "tetrad" of an accentuated first heart sound, opening snap, diastolic rumble, and presystolic accentuation can be appreciated. These findings may need to be elicited with the patient in the left lateral position.

As the left atrium enlarges in excess of 40 mm, the typical radiographic appearance of the heart is found on chest roentgenogram and includes a right heart border double density, elevation of the left main stem bronchus, straightening of the left heart border, and cephalization of the pulmonary vascular pattern. With fixed obstruction to left ventricular inflow, the left ventricle is normal to small in size. Initially, the ECG demonstrates features of left atrial hypertrophy and enlargement with a typical "P-mitrale pattern," a notched or diphasic P wave. Consistent with inflow tract obstruction, left ventricular voltage is normal. With the onset of pulmonary hypertension and right ventricular hypertrophy, right axis deviation or right ventricular hypertrophy may develop.

The emergency physician must maintain a high index of suspicion for rheumatic mitral stenosis in the appropriate clinical setting. Exertional dyspnea is a common symptom in women in the fourth and fifth decades of life. Careful auscultation for an opening snap and early diastolic rumble should be included in the physical examination of these individuals. Similarly, palpitations and paroxysmal supraventricular tachycardias should alert the physician to the possibility of structural organic mitral valve disease. Paroxysmal tachycardias are poorly tolerated by the patient with mitral stenosis, since diastolic filling time is abruptly shortened and left atrial pressure acutely elevated.

Emergency treatment should be directed at alleviating pulmonary edema caused by paroxysmal tachycardia and control of the ventricular rate. In patients with sustained or paroxysmal atrial fibrillation, oral anticoagulation with Coumadin is indicated as prophylaxis for systemic arterial emboli.

In contrast to aortic stenosis, symptoms of mitral stenosis can be treated medically until the patient develops symptoms of dyspnea and fatigue which limit or restrict their daily activity, or complications such as systemic embolization or recurrent pulmonary edema supervene. In younger patients without coexisting mitral regurgitation or calcification of the valve, annuloplasty and valve reconstruction may be attempted. In older patients, or in those with calcification of the valves, prosthetic valve replacement is required.

TRICUSPID REGURGITATION

As noted previously, in several of the valvular lesions, progressive disease leads to right ventricular hypertrophy, dilation, and failure. In addition, many pathologic states that progress to severe left heart failure eventually cause right heart failure.

As a result, the lesion of tricuspid regurgitation is rarely an isolated finding. Its symptoms are often those of the coexisting or predominant valvular lesion or myocardial process. Signs of tricuspid regurgitation include a holosytolic murmur best appreciated along the left sternal border, and jugular venous distention with a large V wave and rapid Y descent. In approximately one-half of the patients, inspiratory augmentation of the murmur can be appreciated. In many patients, concomitant valvular murmurs or coexisting mitral regurgitation often obscures the isolated findings of tricuspid insufficiency. In severe cases, pulsatile hepatomegaly, splenomegaly, ascites, and marked peripheral edema are present.

In the appropriate clinical setting, right-sided *endocarditis* with tricuspid regurgitation should be included in the differential diagnosis. A high index of suspicion for this lesion should be entertained when tricuspid insufficiency appears to be an isolated finding.

Treatment for tricuspid regurgitation is directed at the underlying cause. Symptomatic treatment for venous congestion consists of fluid and salt restriction, the judicious use of diuretics, and digoxin. In selected cases, afterload reduction of the left ventricle may improve right ventricular dysfunction when a reversible component secondary to pulmonary hypertension is present.

ENDOCARDITIS PROPHYLAXIS

Finally, a word about subacute bacterial endocarditis and its prophylaxis. First, the recognition of an organic heart murmur carries with it the obligation to obtain a definitive diagnosis and appropriate follow-up for the patient with valvular heart disease. Many of these patients will have long clinical histories and hemodynamic profiling of these patients is indicated. Second, in the presence of an organic heart murmur, it is necessary to instruct and emphasize the need for prophylaxis against endocardi-

tis. Recommendations for endocarditis prophylaxis and patient wallet cards can be obtained from the American Heart Association, which revises these recommendations on a regular basis. Third, the physician must maintain a high index of suspicion in a patient with valvular heart disease and the potential for subacute or acute endocarditis. This disease presents with numerous symptom complexes, often masquerading as many benign or confusing illnesses. In any patient with valvular heart disease and fever, blood cultures should be obtained and antibiotics withheld pending results in predisposed patients, except those with acute endocarditis. In emergency situations, procedures involving instruments and those associated with bacteremia require antibiotic prophylaxis. Quite often, endocarditis prophylaxis is omitted and forgotten while therapeutic efforts are directed toward other life-threatening or emergency situations.

MITRAL VALVE PROLAPSE

CHARLES F. WOOLEY, M.D.
HARISIOS BOUDOULAS, M.D.

At present, mitral valve prolapse and the mitral valve prolapse syndrome are widely used terms subject to continued redefinition and refinement (Figure 1). A consensus is gradually developing, but it would be a mistake to present a semi-fluid, gelatinous substrate in the solid, orderly, constructed terms that most physicians prefer.

We will consider mitral valve prolapse as the anatomic entity, and the mitral valve prolapse syndrome as anatomic mitral valve prolapse occurring in the presence

of a widely recognized symptom complex. Table 1 presents this classification in an outline form and provides the basis for a simplified approach to therapy.

ANATOMIC MITRAL VALVE PROLAPSE

Anatomic mitral valve prolapse has as its basis a common mitral valve abnormality, the result of a hereditable disorder of connective tissue resulting in collagen disruption within the valve substance, with the development of a floppy or redundant mitral (and at times, tricuspid) valve. There is a spectrum of valve abnormality ranging from overlap with the normal mitral valve at one end, to varying degrees of valve floppiness or redundancy at the other end. Mild degrees of chordal elongation or mitral valve prolapse serve as the basis for auscultatory systolic

TABLE 1 Spectrum of Mitral Valve Prolapse

Mitral Valve Prolapse (anatomic)	Mitral Valve Prolapse Syndrome (anatomic prolapse plus symptom complex)
Common mitral valve abnormality associated with a heritable disorder of connective tissue involving collagen disruption	Constitutional, neuroendocrine process in which the heart and cardiovascular system are target organs
Spectrum of valve abnormality ranges from mild to severe and is basis for: Systolic click Late systolic murmur Mild mitral regurgitation Progressive mitral regurgitation with atrial fibrillation and congestive failure Infective endocarditis Embolic phenomenon	Adrenergic/autonomic dysfunction may be basis for symptom complex of: Chest pain Tachycardia Fatigue Exercise intolerance Postural phenomenon Anxiety Arrhythmias
Conduction system involvement may lead to arrhythmias and conduction defects	Mitral valve prolapse may be a marker closely related to centrally mediated adrenergic/autonomic dysfunction
Therapy—major considerations: Infective endocarditis prophylaxis Management of arrhythmias Progressive mitral regurgitation Ruptured chordae Congestive heart failure Prevention of emboli	Therapy—major considerations: Careful explanation Remove stimulants Stress management Consider cardiac rehab program Great care with drugs

clicks and mid to late mitral systolic murmurs (the murmurs reflect minimal to mild mitral valvular regurgitation). At the far end of the spectrum we find progressive mitral regurgitation, ruptured chordae tendineae, left atrial enlargement, atrial fibrillation, and congestive heart failure as the late clinical manifestations increasing in frequency with age.

While the breadth of the spectrum has been defined, the frequency of the stages of involvement in the population at large has been the subject of wild speculation. In particular, those clinical characteristics that are indicators of stability or harbingers of progression are poorly understood. The incidence of clinically significant floppy mitral valves is quite high within populations of individuals with clinically recognizable hereditable disorders of connective tissue, such as the Marfan or Ehlers-Danlos syndromes. Within the general population, mitral valve prolapse is of clinical significance as illustrated by the occurrence of floppy mitral valves in 5 percent of a prospective necropsy study, by the fact that floppy mitral valves have been recognized as a frequent cause of symptomatic mitral regurgitation requiring mitral valve surgery, and by the gradual realization that mitral valve prolapse is a cause of symptomatic heart disease (chest pain, arrhythmia, congestive failure) in the elderly population as well.

In addition to progressive mitral regurgitation, left atrial enlargement, atrial fibrillation, and congestive heart failure, complications of the floppy mitral valve include infective endocarditis, embolic phenomena, chordal rupture, and conduction system involvement which may lead to arrhythmias or atrioventricular and interventricular conduction defects. Recognition of the spectrum of clinical expression, and awareness of complications and occurrences form the basis for a therapeutic approach to this problem.

Treatment

The major therapeutic concerns in patients with anatomic mitral valve prolapse include infective endocarditis prophylaxis, progressive mitral regurgitation which may occur with or without ruptured chordae tendineae, embolic events, and cardiac arrhythmias.

It is important to confirm the presence of a floppy mitral valve in order to define that portion of the spectrum to which the patient should be assigned. Clinical examination, chest roentgenogram, electrocardiogram (ECG), and echocardiography are usually sufficient for this definition in the younger patient; more detailed evaluation may be necessary in the older patient. Definition and categorization with a careful explanation to the patient and a program for follow-up are frequently sufficient at this stage.

The patients with isolated mitral systolic clicks probably have minor chordal abnormalities and/or mild mitral valve prolapse of limited clinical significance, and in all likelihood this will not be a progressive lesion. Prevention of infective endocarditis is the primary consideration here.

Patients with mitral systolic click or clicks, mid to late systolic murmurs, and increased valve annulus and surface area have mitral valve prolapse with mild to moderate mitral regurgitation, with a greater potential for progression. Therapeutic concerns in this group would be the prevention of, or recognition of, progressive mitral regurgitation, and the prevention of infective endocarditis.

At present, in our opinion, patients with mild to moderate mitral regurgitation should receive endocarditis prophylaxis at the time of dental extractions or procedures with predictable bacteremia. It should be understood that endocarditis prophylaxis in general, and in this group of patients in particular, is currently a matter of considerable debate and the subject of changing attitudes and recommendations.

Patients with long-term, mild to moderate mitral regurgitation and progressive left atrial enlargement with the recent onset of atrial fibrillation or atrial flutter require medical therapy for control of ventricular response, consideration of cardioversion, and maintenance in sinus rhythm with drug or electrical therapy. The addition of antiembolic therapy with anticoagulation therapy may be necessary if the atrial fibrillation cannot be reverted to sinus rhythm.

Patients with mitral valve prolapse may be at risk for embolic events, the embolic source presumably being the surface of the mitral valve. Women with mitral valve prolapse may be at increased risk for thromboembolic disease, and if reasonable, we think it best to avoid oral contraceptives. Individuals who have had clinical manifestations of retinal, cerebral, or peripheral emboli should discontinue oral contraceptives, and abstain from chronic cigarette smoking; treatment with antiplatelet aggregation therapy is reasonable.

Patients who are symptomatic on the basis of intermittent cardiac arrhythmias (without evidence of progressive mitral regurgitation) cannot be managed satisfactorily until the exact mechanism of the arrhythmias is determined. Ambulatory electrocardiographic monitoring, transtelephonic monitoring, exercise stress testing, or electrophysiologic testing may be necessary to define the nature of the arrhythmia before making a decision to withhold therapy or to consider the necessity of long-term antiarrhythmic therapy. Abstinence from caffeine, stimulants, and smoking may be effective therapeutic steps and allow us to avoid inappropriate antiarrhythmia therapy. Since the affected population contains numbers of young patients, long-term antiarrhythmia therapy may well be inappropriate. If drug therapy is necessary, we avoid drugs that prolong the Q-T interval, such as quinidine. Initial therapy with beta-blockers is monitored with ambulatory arrhythmia detection devices. If this is unsatisfactory, we proceed with electrophysiologic testing, and make a subsequent choice of antiarrhythmia drugs on this basis.

THE MITRAL VALVE PROLAPSE SYNDROME

Anatomic mitral valve prolapse may be accompanied by a constellation of symptoms including chest pain, palpitations, fatigue, asthenia, exercise intolerance, postural phenomena, and anxiety. Thus it is, in our opinion, a constitutional, neuroendocrine cardiovascular process in which the heart and cardiovascular system may be viewed as target organs, much as cardiovascular involvement occurs in thyrotoxicosis or pheochromocytoma. It is necessary to remove the focus of attention from the mitral valve and take a more global view in order to understand the possible mechanisms of underlying signs and symptoms here.

For at least a century, these patients have been subjected to a series of labels which came about partly as a result of our profound ignorance of neurochemistry, neurotransmitters and receptors, and partly because these individuals did not respond to the physical and emotional stresses of war time in the manner that the military-medical complex deemed appropriate. Thus, one can trace these labels from the United States Civil War: DaCosta's syndrome or irritable heart, through World War I: soldier's heart, the effort syndrome, and neurocirculatory asthenia, to World War II: anxiety neurosis. At present, the symptom complex noted above may be variously diagnosed as "nerves," anxiety syndromes, panic attacks, or if a systolic click is heard, as mitral valve prolapse syndrome—depending on the orientation of the involved physician.

There are those who doubt the existence of the mitral valve prolapse syndrome, and prefer to consider the matter as coexistence of a common cardiac process (mitral valve prolapse) with the equally common anxiety and autonomic dysfunction syndrome. In any case, these patients present themselves to physicians with this symptom complex and require help.

Treatment

The frequency with which the valve abnormality and constellation of symptoms occur together suggest to us that they are closely related or overlap phenomena. In our opinion, these patients manifest a constitutional, neuroendocrine-cardiovascular process that results from a close relationship between anatomic mitral valve prolapse and centrally or peripherally mediated adrenergic-autonomic dysfunction. The basis for the symptom complex is probably altered modulation of adrenergic and autonomic function; rational therapy in this group of individuals obviously is dependent upon better understanding of these adrenergic-autonomic mechanisms.

Although individuals with the mitral valve prolapse syndrome may recall palpitations, chest pain, or exercise intolerance dating from childhood or adolescence, most of the symptomatic patients who come to us seeking medical care are young adults, in their 20s and 30s, with a peak incidence at approximately 28 years. The age at presentation to the physician is important, since any therapeutic decision involving long-term drug therapy should answer the inevitable question: How long will I have to take this medicine?

Their symptoms frequently occur against a background of acute or gradual increases in the physical or emotional stresses of life, quite often with a precipitating event such as trauma, an operation, an illness, marital separation or divorce, a demanding or stressful job, working two jobs, impending job change or loss. When excessive use of caffeine, cigarettes, alcohol, chemical substances, over-the-counter or presciption drugs is added to the above stresses, the sum contributes to symptoms in susceptible individuals.

A concerned approach by the physician is important, since patient uncertainty, fear, and inability to understand these alterations of body function are the usual motivating factors for seeking medical help. In our opinion, the single most important noninvasive test and therapeutic step is a carefully taken medical history and properly performed physical examination. These patients are at risk for physician misinterpretation of history, physical findings, nonspecific ECG, stress test or echocardiographic changes, and borderline laboratory results, which in turn may lead to inappropriate, long-term drug therapy often without clear-cut goals regarding duration of treatment.

A careful explanation of the physician's findings, an explanation of what is known about the mechanism of symptoms, and the best possible answers to the anxious patient's list of questions constitute the cornerstone of long-term management.

Removal of catecholamine and cyclic adenosine monophosphate stimulation by abstinence from caffeine, cigarettes, alcohol, and prescribed or over-the-counter drugs containing epinephrine or ephedrine is an important initial step.

A common sense approach to stress modification, where possible and feasible, may seem too fundamental to the physician to even mention; however, such an approach may never have occurred to the patient who is wrapped up in attempts to meet demands well beyond his or her capabilities. Undue anxieties, phobias, or panic attacks may form the basis for consultation with an informed psychiatrist.

The question of physical activities, physical fitness, and exercise programs should be addressed. Fatigue and previous exercise intolerance may have resulted in avoidance of exercise or limited exercise attempts. If there are no serious exercise-induced abnormalities or arrhythmias, enrollment in a cardiac rehabilitation program for graduated aerobic conditioning may be accompanied by gratifying physical, physiological, and psychological benefits.

There are many potential mechanisms for chest pain in patients with the mitral valve prolapse syndrome. We believe that the chest pain is of cardiac origin in most circumstances, and that the pain may be catecholamine-related or -mediated. The management of mitral valve prolapse syndrome patients with severe or incapacitating chest pain may be a source of frustration for patient and physician alike. Certainly some individuals with chest pain may have pain associated with coronary artery disease, tachyarrhythmias, or myocardial abnormalities with alterations in myocardial perfusion or diastolic function; identification of this subset of individuals obviously leads to more specific therapy with cardioselective beta-

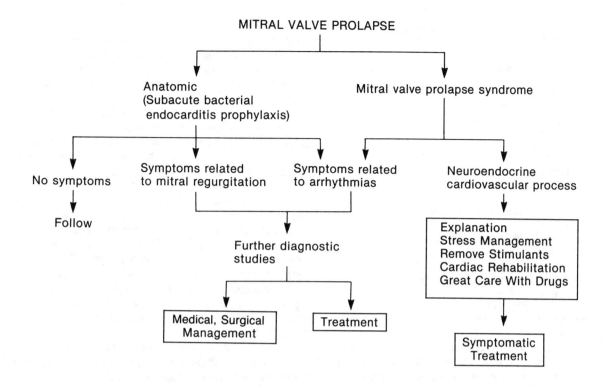

MITRAL VALVE PROLAPSE

Anatomic
(Subacute bacterial
endocarditis prophylaxis)

Mitral valve prolapse syndrome

No symptoms

Symptoms related
to mitral regurgitation

Symptoms related
to arrhythmias

Neuroendocrine
cardiovascular process

Follow

Further diagnostic
studies

Explanation
Stress Management
Remove Stimulants
Cardiac Rehabilitation
Great Care With Drugs

Medical, Surgical
Management

Treatment

Symptomatic
Treatment

Figure 1   Mitral valve prolapse: a therapeutic approach.

blockers, nitrates, or calcium antagonists. In individuals with incapacitating chest pain without a definable cause, (1) we believe the patient (i.e., we do not attempt to deny the patient's symptom), and (2) we recommend the nondrug approach outlined previously, before beginning what must be, given our present state of knowledge, a program of empiric therapy.

SUGGESTED READING

Boudoulas H, Reynolds JC, Mazzaferri E, Wooley CF. Mitral valve prolapse syndrome: the effect of adrenergic stimulation. Am Coll Cardiol 1983; 2:638–644.
Wooley CF. Where are the diseases of yesteryear? DaCosta's Syndrome, soldiers heart, the effort syndrome, neurocirculatory asthenia, and the mitral valve prolapse syndrome. Circulation 1976; 53:749–751.

INFECTIOUS ENDOCARDITIS

J. LOUISE GERBERDING, M.D.
MERLE A. SANDE, M.D.

Infective endocarditis is a localized infection of the heart valves or other cardiac endothelial surfaces which, if left untreated, has a mortality of 100 percent. Early recognition, correct bacteriologic diagnosis, and aggressive antibiotic, and sometimes surgical, treatment of this disorder are therefore essential.

PATHOPHYSIOLOGY

Structural lesions of the heart that produce turbulent blood flow and scarring cause fibrin and platelets to be deposited on the cardiac endothelial surfaces and provide an environment conducive to bacterial adhesion and further fibrin deposition. The resulting vegetation is protected from the host's phagocytic defense mechanisms and is the source of the continuous bacteremia and embolic phenomenon associated with this disease. Intracardiac lesions that produce turbulent blood flow, such as rheumatic valvular disease, congenital heart defects, degenerative heart diseases, and many iatrogenic factors, are preexisting conditions associated with an increased incidence of bacterial endocarditis (Table 1).

The organisms which cause endocarditis are those that most often produce bacteremia after trauma or manipulation of the oral, gastrointestinal and genitourinary mucosal surfaces. Streptococci, staphylococci, and, rarely, aerobic gram-negative bacilli are the usual pathogens (Table 2). The absolute number of circulating organisms and their ability to adhere to the fibrin-platelet lesion are the two most important factors in establishing infection.

CLINICAL MANIFESTATIONS

The clinical manifestations of endocarditis are a direct consequence of the continued propagation of the infected

TABLE 1 Predisposing Cardiac Lesions In Endocarditis

Rheumatic valvular disease

Congenital heart disease

    Ventricular septal defect
    Patent ductus arteriosus
    Tetralogy of Fallot
    Aortic coarctation
    Pulmonic stenosis
    Aortic stenosis
    Hypertrophic obstructive cardiomyopathy

Degenerative heart disease

    Marfan's syndrome
    Calcified mitral annulus
    Postinfarction intracardiac thrombus
    Luetic aortitis
    Mitral valve prolapse

Iatrogenic conditions

    Arterial shunts vigule fistula
    Intracardiac pacemaker
    Intracardiac catheters
    Prosthetic valve implantation

vegetation. Large friable vegetations mechanically interfere with the function of the cardiac valves and result in valvular insufficiency, outflow obstruction, cardiac murmurs, and congestive heart failure. The more virulent organisms such as *S. aureus* and *S. pneumoniae* can destroy the valve tissue directly and rapidly extend into the perivalvular tissue (ring abscess), conducting system (arrhythmias), myocardium (myocardial abscess or even cardiac rupture), and pericardium (purulent pericarditis).

The *extracardiac manifestations* of endocarditis are attributable to arterial embolization of the vegetations and to immune-complex deposition. Major embolic events occur in as many as one-third of patients and may be delayed until therapy is initiated or even completed. Embolization to the coronary vessels can result in myocardial infarction. Mesenteric artery occlusion may produce bowel infarction and acute abdominal pain. Metastatic abscesses in the kidney, bowel, and spleen are common with *S. aureus* endocarditis.

Cerebral emboli may produce focal neurologic findings such as stroke, diffuse cerebritis with altered mental status, seizures, or even coma. Mycotic aneurysms are produced when septic emboli invade the vascular endothelium or vasa vasorum and are especially common in the cerebral circulation. These aneurysms often go unsuspected until rupture occurs. Headache, meningeal signs, and neurologic deficits are clues to the diagnosis and should prompt immediate hospitalization and neurologic evaluation.

Many of the *cutaneous lesions* associated with endocarditis are attributable to small-vessel embolization and infarction although immune complex deposition may also play a role. Petechiae (small nonblanching lesions developing in crops on the mucous membranes and distal extremities), Osler's nodes (small painful nodular lesions on the pads of the digits), Janeway lesions (hemorrhagic

TABLE 2 Incidence of Endocarditis Due to Various Infectious Agents

Organism	Percentage with Natural Valve	Percentage with Prosthetic Valve
Streptococci	60—80	10—35
Viridans streptococci	30—40	3—23
S. sanguis		
S. mutans		
S. mitior		
Enterococcus	5—18	5—9
Other streptococci	15—25	1—4
Staphylococci	20—35	40—50
S. aureus	10—30	15—20
S. epidermidis	1—3	20—30
Gram-negative aerobic bacilli (Pseudomonas Enterobacteriaceae)	1.5—13	10—20
Diphtheroids	<10	4—10
Fungi (Aspergillus, Candida, Histoplasma)	2—4	5—15
Miscellaneous	<5	<1
Gonococcus		
Borrello		
Listeria		
Meningococcus		
Bacteroides		
Haemophilus		
Rickettsia (Coxiella burnetii)		
Psittacosis		
Cell defective bacteria		

From Sande MA, Gerberding JL. Infective endocarditis. In: Stein JH. Internal medicine. 2nd ed. Boston: Little Brown, 1986.

macular painless lesions on the palms and soles), Roth's spots (pale ovoid retinal lesions with a peripheral hemorrhagic halo), splinter hemorrhages (subungual red-brown streaks), and clubbing are found in as many as 50 percent of patients. Focal and diffuse glomerulonephritis may be directly related to immune complex deposition in the kidney and can progress to acute renal failure.

Fever and heart murmur are the hallmarks of endocarditis, but all too often the diagnosis is delayed or obscured by other findings (Table 3). The initial clinical presentation is determined in large part by the etiologic organism. *S. aureus* and encapsulated organisms such as *S. pneumoniae* and *N. gonnorhoea* usually produce an acute febrile illness with high fever, rapid valve destruction, and peripheral emboli. Mortality is high and congestive heart failure often develops. Immediate surgical intervention may be necessary, particularly with aortic valve involvement.

Subacute endocarditis is more common and is usually seen in patients with underlying cardiac conditions. Viridans streptococci and enterococci are by far the most common organisms producing this syndrome, and a history of dental or urogenital procedure predisposing to bacteremia with these organisms is often given. Nonspecific symptoms of low-grade fever, night sweats, anorexia, weight loss, myalgias, and arthralgias are common complaints. Since the duration of subacute endocarditis may be prolonged before diagnosis, the manifestations of peripheral embolic phenomenon including petechiae, Osler's nodes, and Janeway lesions occur in approximately 50 percent of patients in this setting. The presence of splenomegaly is also correlated with the duration of the disease and is found in over 60 percent of patients with subacute infection.

TABLE 3   Clinical Presentations of Endocarditis

Fever and heart murmur
Sepsis
Fever of unknown origin
Transient ischemic attacks or stroke
Meningitis
Subarachnoid hemorrhage
Peripheral arterial embolization
Myocardial infarction
Unexplained congestive heart failure
Pulmonary infarction, necrotizing pneumonia
Constitutional symptoms suggestive of
  Neoplasm
  Hematologic malignancy
  Collagen vascular disease
Musculoskeletal complaints suggestive of
  Polymyalgia rheumatica
  Acute rheumatic fever
  Rheumatoid arthritis
Anemia
Renal failure

From Sande MA, Gerberding JL. Infective endocarditis. In: Stein JH. Internal medicine. 2nd ed. Boston: Little Brown, 1986.

ENDOCARDITIS IN INTRAVENOUS DRUG USERS

Intravenous drug users are predisposed to endocarditis with *S. aureus*, although the course is generally less severe than in other patients infected with this organism. This may be attributable in part to the predilection for tricuspid valve involvement and the younger age of these patients. Fever and heart murmur in an intravenous drug user should be considered presumptive evidence of endocarditis unless an alternative source of fever is discovered. In urban medical centers, the incidence of endocarditis in this population when unexplained fever is documented is greater than 50 percent, and therefore fever alone, even in the absence of heart murmur, should prompt admission if no other source is identified. Tricuspid valve vegetations frequently embolize to the pulmonary arteries, and transient pulmonary infiltrates corresponding to areas of septic infarction are frequently seen on the chest film.

PROSTHETIC VALVE ENDOCARDITIS

Endocarditis is a common complication of prosthetic heart valve replacement. Unexplained fever in patients with prosthetic valves should also prompt hospitalization to exclude the diagnosis of endocarditis. Soon after valve replacement (within 2 months), nosocomial organisms such as *S. epidermidis, S. aureus, Pseudomonas aerugenosa*, Enterobacteriaceae, and rarely fungi are the predominant etiologic pathogens. Late prosthetic valve endocarditis resembles native valve endocarditis, with streptococci and staphylococci (including *S. epidermidis*) accounting for the majority of cases. The consequences of prosthetic valve infection are severe, and valve dehiscence as a result of ring abscess formation, outflow obstruction, and peripheral embolization is a well-known complication. Surgical replacement is nearly always necessary, and antimicrobial therapy should be instituted immediately after blood cultures are obtained when the diagnosis is suspected.

LABORATORY STUDIES

Bacteremia can be documented in over 95 percent of patients when three or more blood cultures are obtained at 20 to 30 minute intervals. The most common cause of culture-negative endocarditis is previous antibiotic administration, but in rare instances, nutritionally deficient (pyridoxal-dependent) variants of streptococci are implicated as well. Unusual organisms such as *Aspergillus, Candida, Histoplasma*, and *Brucella* should also be considered when cultures are persistently negative despite clinical evidence of the disease. Serologic tests including measurement of teichoic acid antibody with *S. aureus* infection and tests for fungal, *Coxiella burnettii*, and chlamydial antigens are occasionally helpful in this setting.

Normochromic normocytic anemia is often seen in the subacute form of endocarditis. Leukocytosis is more common with acute fulminant infection, although leukopenia has also been described. Thrombocytopenia and histiocytosis are other hematologic findings. The erythrocyte sedimentation rate is elevated in 90 to 100 percent of patients, but is by no means specific for endocarditis.

Immune complexes are also detected in over 90 percent of patients. Mixed cryoglobulins, rheumatoid factors, hypergammaglobulinemia, and hypocomplementemia are present in many patients as well. These serologic abnormalities reflect the immunologic response to the persistent antigenemia from continuous bacteremia, and their presence correlates with the duration of infection.

The urine sediment is abnormal in over 50 percent of patients. Proteinuria is the most common finding, although microscopic hematuria is also typical. Red cell casts are seen in patients with active glomerulonephritis and are detected in less than 15 percent of patients in most series.

An electrocardiogram should be performed in any patient suspected of endocarditis. Conduction defects such as first-degree AV block, junctional rhythms, advanced heart block, and bundle branch block are particularly ominous and suggest the possibility of suppurative involvement of the conduction system. Evidence of ischemia or pericarditis may also be detected. Patients with electrocardiographic abnormalities should be carefully monitored for evidence of progressive disease or congestive heart failure, and surgical consultation should be obtained.

A chest roentgenogram should also be obtained. Evidence of underlying valvular disease such as valvular calcification and chamber enlargement may be found. Signs of pulmonary vascular congestion, pleural effusion, or septic emboli should be noted.

Echocardiographic evidence of vegetations may be found in 38 to 83 percent of patients with documented endocarditis. The two-dimensional technique is more sensitive than M-mode in detecting small vegetations and vegetations on the tricuspid valve. A negative echocardiogram does *not* exclude the diagnosis of endocarditis. However, patients with documented vegetations do have a higher incidence of embolic complications, congestive heart failure, and need for surgical intervention. Echocardiography therefore provides important prognostic information and facilitates the diagnosis of lesions likely to require early surgical intervention.

TREATMENT

Bactericidal antibiotics, in dosages high enough to produce peak levels exceeding the minimum bactericidal concentration, are administered over prolonged periods to sterilize the endocardial vegetations. Bacteriostatic drugs should never be used. Correct bacteriologic diagnosis is essential to establish sensitivities to the antibiotic agents.

Empiric therapy should be directed toward the most likely pathogens in a given clinical setting. In acute endocarditis and in intravenous drug users, coverage for *S. aureus* should be included. A combination of a

penicillinase-resistant penicillin and an aminoglycoside should be adequate unless methicillin-resistant *S. aureus* or *S. epidermidis* is suspected. In such cases vancomycin should be substituted. In the subacute setting when *S. aureus* is unlikely, penicillin and an aminoglycoside usually suffice.

Antimicrobial therapy should be adjusted once the organism responsible for the infection is isolated. Susceptibilities should be determined by serial tube dilution methods in broth. Disc sensitivity testing is of little use in the management of endocarditis. Peak serum bactericidal activity should be checked at periodic intervals during therapy to ensure that good activity is present in vivo.

It is important to recognize the need for immediate surgical intervention. Since rapid valve destruction leads to early death, any patient with endocarditis, valvular insufficiency, or congestive heart failure should be evaluated promptly by a cardiologist and a cardiac surgeon. Immediate valve replacement may be lifesaving.

PROPHYLAXIS OF ENDOCARDITIS

Prophylaxis of endocarditis with bactericidal drugs is recommended for patients at high risk for acquiring the disease (Table 4) prior to procedures associated with a significant incidence of bacteremia. Drug regimens are designed to eradicate organisms associated with specific procedures (Tables 5 and 6). Viridans streptococci are likely to be isolated from the blood after dental or oral pharyngeal procedures. These organisms are usually sensitive to penicillin unless the patient is already taking penicillin, in which case erythromycin or a parenteral regimen should be employed. Bacteremia with group D strep-

---

TABLE 4 Cardiac Conditions and Endocarditis Prophylaxis*

Endocarditis prophylaxis recommended
  Prosthetic cardiac valves (including biosynthetic valves)
  Most congenital cardiac malformations
  Surgically constructed systemic-pulmonary shunts
  Rheumatic and other acquired valvular dysfunction
  Idiopathic hypertrophic subaortic stenosis (IHSS)
  Previous history of bacterial endocarditis[†]
  Mitral valve prolapse with insufficiency[†]

Endocarditis prophylaxis not recommended
  Isolated secundum atrial septal defect
  Secundum atrial septal defect repaired without a patch
    6 or more months earlier
  Patent ductus arteriosus ligated and divided 6 or more
    months earlier
  Postoperative coronary artery bypass graft (CABG) surgery

From Committee on Rheumatic Fever and Infective Endocarditis of the Council on Cardiovascular Disease in the Young. Special Report. Prevention of bacterial endocarditis. Circulation 1984; 70:1123A. By permission of the American Heart Association, Inc.

* This table lists common conditions, but is not meant to be all-inclusive.
† Definitive data to provide guidance in management of patients with mitral valve prolapse are particularly limited. It is clear that, in general, such patients are at low risk of development of endocarditis, but the risk-benefit ratio of prophylaxis in mitral valve prolapse is uncertain.

TABLE 5 Summary of Recommended Prophylactic Antibiotic Regimens for Dental and Respiratory Tract Procedures

Standard regimen*	
For dental procedures that cause gingival bleeding, and oral/respiratory tract surgery	Penicillin V 2.0 g orally 1 hour before, then 1.0 g 6 hours later. For patients unable to take oral medications, 2 million units of aqueous penicillin G IV or IM 30–60 minutes before a procedure and 1 million units 6 hours later may be substituted
Special regimens*	
Parenteral regimen for use when maximal protection desired (e.g., for patients with prosthetic valves)	Ampicillin, 1.0–2.0 g IM or IV, *plus* gentamicin, 1.5 mg/kg IM or IV, ½ hour before procedure, followed by 1.0 g oral penicillin V 6 hours later; alternatively, the parenteral regimen may be repeated once 8 hours later
Oral regimen for penicillin-allergic patients	Erythromycin, 1.0 g orally 1 hour before, then 500 mg 6 hours later
Parenteral regimen for penicillin-allergic patients	Vancomycin, 1.0 g IV *slowly* over 1 hour, starting 1 hour before; no repeat dose is necessary

From Committee on Rheumatic Fever and Infective Endocarditis of the Council on Cardiovascular Disease in the Young. Special Report. Prevention of bacterial endocarditis. Circulation 1984; 70:1123A. By permission of The American Heart Association, Inc.
* Pediatric doses: Ampicillin, 50 mg/kg per dose; erythromycin, 20 mg/kg for first dose, then 10 mg/kg; gentamicin, 2.0 mg/kg per dose; penicillin V, full adult dose if greater than 60 lb (27 kg), one-half adult dose if less than 60 lb (27 kg); aqueous penicillin G, 50,000 units/kg (25,000 units/kg for follow-up); vancomycin, 20 mg/kg per dose. The intervals between doses are the same as for adults. Total doses should not exceed adult doses.

TABLE 6 Summary of Recommended Prophylactic Antibiotic Regimens for Gastrointestinal-Genitourinary Procedures.

Standard regimen*	
For genitourinary-gastrointestinal tract procedures listed in the text	Ampicillin 2.0 g IM or IV *plus* gentamicin 1.5 mg/kg IM or IV, given ½ to 1 hour before procedure. One follow-up dose may be given 8 hours later
Special regimens*	
Oral regimen for minor or repetitive procedures in low-risk patients	Amoxicillin 3.0 g orally 1 hour before procedure and 1.5 g 6 hours later
For penicillin-allergic patients	Vancomycin 1.0 g IV *slowly* over 1 hour *plus* gentamicin 1.5 mg/kg IM or IV given 1 hour before procedure. May be repeated once 8–12 hours later

From Committee on Rheumatic Fever and Infective Endocarditis of the Council on Cardiovascular Disease in the Young. Special Report. Prevention of bacterial endocarditis. Circulation 1984; 70:1123A. By permission of the American Heart Association, Inc.
* Pediatric doses: Ampicillin, 50 mg/kg per dose; gentamicin, 2.0 mg/kg per dose; amoxicillin, 50 mg/kg per dose; vancomycin, 20 mg/kg per dose. The intervals between doses are the same as for adults. Total doses should not exceed adult doses.

tococci is caused by procedures involving the genitourinary and gastrointestinal tract such as catheterization of an infected bladder, cystoscopy, prostatic surgery, vaginal hysterectomy, gallbladder surgery, colonic surgery, colonoscopy, sclerotherapy,endoscopy with biopsy, and proctosigmoidoscopy with biopsy. Since these organisms are more resistant to penicillin than are other streptococci, penicillin and an aminoglycoside are necessary to achieve a bactericidal effect.

Procedures that do not require antibiotic prophylaxis include uncomplicated vaginal delivery, pelvic examination, dilation and curettage of the uterus, insertion and removal of an IUD, endoscopic procedures without biopsy, and barium enema. When infected tissue is manipulated, antibiotic selection should be adjusted to cover the organisms most likely to be present, i.e., drainage of cutaneous infections should be preceded by prophylactic treatment with a penicillinase-resistant penicillin with activity against *S. aureus* such as nafcillin.

SUGGESTED READING

Sande MA, Kaye D, Root RK, eds. Endocarditis. vol. 2, Contemporary issues in infectious diseases. New York: Churchill Livingstone, 1984.
Committee on Rheumatic Fever and Infective Endocarditis of the Council of Cardiovascular Diseases of the Young. Special report. Prevention of bacterial endocarditis. Circulation 1984; 70:1123A.
Sande MA, Gerberding JL. Infective endocarditis. In: Stein JH, ed. Internal medicine. 2nd ed. Boston: Little, Brown, 1986.
Scheld WM, Sande MA. Endocarditis and intravascular infections. In: Mandell GL, Douglas RG, Bennett JE, eds. Principles and practice of infectious diseases. 2nd ed. New York: Wiley & Sons, 1985.

VENTRICULAR TACHYCARDIA

FRED MORADY, M.D.

DIAGNOSIS

Rapid ventricular tachycardia or ventricular fibrillation associated with a cardiac arrest or shock rarely presents a problem in diagnosis. However, the diagnosis of ventricular tachycardia may be less clear-cut when the ventricular tachycardia takes the form of a wide-complex tachycardia in a patient who has little or no hemodynamic compromise during the tachycardia. A wide-complex tachycardia may be caused by ventricular tachycardia or by supraventricular tachycardia with aberrant ventricular activation. The aberrant ventricular activation may be caused by either an underlying bundle branch block, a rate-related functional bundle branch block, or an accessory pathway, as in the Wolff-Parkinson-White syndrome.

If the patient is hemodynamically stable upon presentation to the emergency department with a wide-complex tachycardia, it is important to obtain a 12-lead electrocardiogram (ECG). Although there are no ECG findings that are absolutely diagnostic of ventricular tachycardia, there may be several suggestive clues (Fig. 1). When the width of the QRS complexes is greater than 0.14 seconds in the absence of use of antiarrhythmic drugs that widen the QRS complex, this is suggestive of ventricular tachycardia. When the QRS axis during the tachycardia is superior, this also favors the diagnosis of ventricular tachycardia. Two very helpful clues are atrioventricular (AV) dissociation and fusion beats. It is important to keep in mind, however, that these clues are helpful only when present, i.e., the absence of AV dissociation or fusion beats does not make the possibility of ventricular tachycardia less likely. When the QRS complexes in all of the precordial leads have basically the same configuration, this favors the diagnosis of ventricular tachycardia. In regard to the specific configuration of the QRS complexes, when there is a right bundle branch block configuration and the R wave in lead V_1 is monophasic, this favors the diagnosis of ventricular tachycardia.

It should be emphasized that the patient's clinical status during a wide-complex tachycardia is not helpful in distinguishing ventricular tachycardia from supraventricular tachycardia with aberration. Although ventricular tachycardia is certainly often associated with hemodynamic collapse, this is not necessarily always the case. There appears to be a prevalent misconception that if a patient with a wide-complex tachycardia has a normal blood pressure and minimal symptoms, the tachycardia is much more likely to be supraventricular than ventricular in origin. This misconception often leads to inappropriate therapy. Depending on several factors, including the underlying cardiac function and the rate of the tachycardia, ventricular tachycardia may be associated with little or no hemodynamic compromise. The differentiation of ventricular tachycardia from supraventricular tachycardia with aberration should be based on the electrocardiographic findings and not on the severity of the patient's symptoms.

The physical examination may be helpful by revealing cannon waves in the jugular venous pulse. An irregular pattern of cannon waves would indicate the presence of AV dissociation, which would favor the diagnosis of ventricular tachycardia. If P waves are not apparent on the ECG, and if the patient is hemodynamically stable, it may be appropriate to insert an esophageal lead in the emergency department to look for the presence of AV dissociation. It should be kept in mind that the absence of AV dissociation is not of diagnostic value in differentiating ventricular from supraventricular tachycardia.

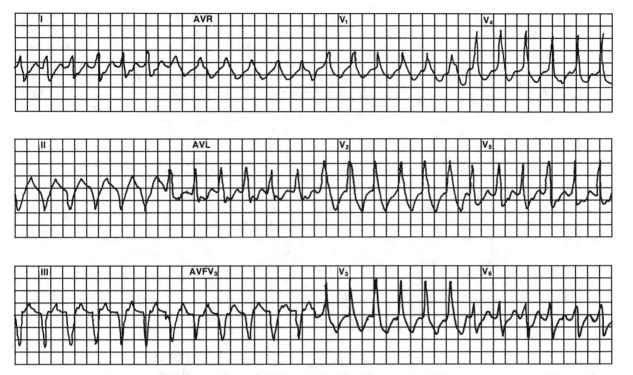

Figure 1 A 12-lead electrocardiographic recording of a wide-complex tachycardia in a 63-year-old man with a history of a myocardial infarction who presented to an emergency department complaining of rapid palpitations and mild lightheadedness. The rate of the tachycardia is 145 beats per minute. Although there are no findings diagnostic of ventricular tachycardia, the monophasic R wave in lead V_1, the superior axis, and the width of the QRS complex (0.16 seconds) are clues that suggest this is ventricular tachycardia rather than supraventricular tachycardia with aberrant ventricular activation. The mild nature of the patient's symptoms is of no diagnostic value in distinguishing ventricular tachycardia from supraventricular tachycardia with aberrant ventricular activation.

UNDERLYING CAUSES

The most common form of underlying heart disease in patients who present with ventricular tachycardia is coronary artery disease. Ventricular tachycardia may occur in the setting of an acute myocardial infarction, or it may be a consequence of cardiac ischemia without infarction. Ischemia may result not only from fixed atherosclerotic coronary disease, but also from coronary artery spasm. Often, ventricular tachycardia in patients with coronary artery disease is a primary arrhythmic problem related to chronically diseased myocardium rather than acute ischemia or acute infarction.

Ventricular tachycardia may be associated with all forms of cardiomyopathy, including the dilated cardiomyopathies, hypertrophic cardiomyopathies, and infiltrative cardiomyopathies. An acute myocarditis without chronic cardiomyopathy may also cause ventricular tachycardia.

The two most common types of valvular heart disease associated with ventricular tachycardia are aortic stenosis and mitral valve prolapse. Ventricular tachycardia may be associated with congenital heart disease, such as in patients who have undergone surgical repair of tetralogy of Fallot, or patients with arrhythmogenic right ventricular dysplasia. Arrhythmogenic right ventricular dysplasia should be suspected whenever the ventricular tachycardia has a left bundle branch block configuration and there is evidence of right ventricular dysfunction on a right ventricular angiogram or echocardiogram.

It is of the utmost importance to recognize when ventricular tachycardia is associated with a delayed repolarization syndrome, as manifested by a prolonged Q-T interval. When ventricular tachycardia is related to Q-T prolongation, it often takes the form of "*torsade de pointes*" (Fig. 2). This is an undulating pattern of ventricular tachycardia in which the QRS complexes alternate in a cyclic fashion between being upright and inverted. Q-T prolongation and ventricular tachycardia may be caused by electrolyte abnormalities such as hypokalemia or hypomagnesemia, or may be drug-induced. The drugs most often incriminated in causing ventricular tachycardia as an idiosyncratic reaction are quinidine, procainamide, disopyramide, and the phenothiazines and tricyclic antidepressants. Ventricular tachycardia and Q-T prolongation may be a part of the congenital long Q-T syndrome. Q-T prolongation and ventricular tachycardia may also be a result of severe bradyarrhythmias, e.g., complete AV block.

Ventricular tachycardia may be idiopathic. However, myocardial biopsies in patients with "idiopathic" ventricular tachycardia have demonstrated that some of these patients have histologic evidence of myocarditis or cardiomyopathy.

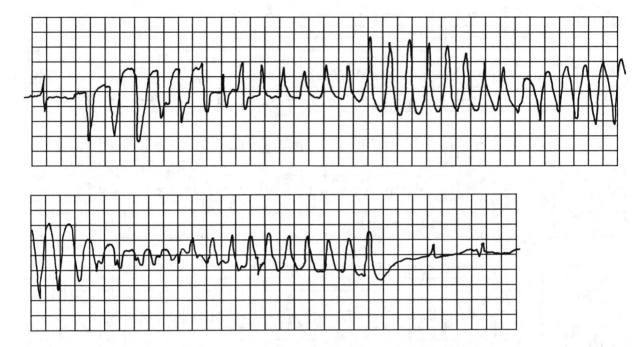

Figure 2 A continuous electrocardiographic recording of lead V_5 in a patient who experienced syncope 3 days after the initiation of treatment with quinidine for the suppression of ventricular premature depolarizations. The rhythm strip demonstrates "torsade de pointes" type of ventricular tachycardia. The QRS complexes alternate in a cyclic fashion between being upright and inverted. This type of ventricular tachycardia is associated with prolongation of the Q-T interval and in this patient was drug-induced.

PRE-HOSPITAL TREATMENT

When ventricular tachycardia is associated with severe hemodynamic compromise and loss of consciousness or a full cardiac arrest, the first form of treatment in addition to basic life support should be direct current countershock applied to the chest. In the setting of a cardiac arrest, it is appropriate to use an energy level of 300 J. If the ventricular tachycardia or fibrillation does not convert to sinus rhythm with direct current countershock, or if ventricular tachycardia or fibrillation recurs immediately after direct current countershock, this may be because of a severe metabolic abnormality that has occurred as a result of the cardiac arrest, e.g., acidosis or severe hypoxemia. Direct current countershock should be repeated after establishment of an airway to permit adequate ventilation, administration of sodium bicarbonate to correct acidosis, and administration of lidocaine. After venous access is established, lidocaine can be administered in a bolus of 100 mg IV. This dose can be repeated after 5 minutes if necessary. If the patient requires repeated direct current countershock for recurrent ventricular tachycardia or fibrillation after the administration of lidocaine, bretylium should then be given in a dose of 5 mg per kilogram of body weight IV. A dose of 5 to 10 mg per kilogram may be repeated if necessary if the rhythm has not been stabilized after 10 to 15 minutes. It should be noted that bretylium's predominant acute effect is to facilitate defibrillation; when used to treat ventricular tachycardia, its onset of action may be delayed for 20 to 30 minutes.

If the patient has ventricular tachycardia or a wide-complex tachycardia associated with little or no hemodynamic compromise, it is appropriate to transport the patient to an emergency department without immediate drug therapy or direct current countershock.

EMERGENCY DEPARTMENT TREATMENT

As is the case in the pre-hospital treatment of ventricular tachycardia, whenever ventricular tachycardia is associated with severe hemodynamic collapse and loss of consciousness, the first therapeutic modality in addition to basic life support should be direct current countershock with 300 J. During attempts at resuscitation, lidocaine and bretylium may be used as described above for the pre-hospital treatment of ventricular tachycardia.

In the patient with ventricular tachycardia who does not have severe hemodynamic compromise requiring immediate direct current countershock, the progression of drugs administered in an attempt to convert the ventricular tachycardia pharmacologically should be first lidocaine, then procainamide, then bretylium. Lidocaine should be given in a dose of 100 mg IV. Administration of this bolus over approximately 1 to 2 minutes decreases the incidence of central nervous system toxicity from the lidocaine. If the lidocaine is effective in converting the ventricular tachycardia, it is appropriate to maintain the patient on intravenous lidocaine. A continuous infusion of lidocaine can be started at a dose of 2 mg per minute. In addition, because lidocaine has a short therapeutic half-life in its distribution phase (8 minutes), two to three 50-mg boluses of lidocaine should be administered intravenously every 5 minutes after the first bolus.

If lidocaine is effective in terminating the ventricular tachycardia, a continuous infusion should be maintained and the infusion rate adjusted to maintain a serum level of 2 to 5 μg per milliliter. Dosage requirements are less in patients with congestive heart failure or liver disease. Manifestations of lidocaine toxicity include disorientation, dysarthria, nystagmus, drowsiness, and seizures. High serum levels of lidocaine may cause further myocardial depression in patients with underlying myocardial dysfunction.

If lidocaine is ineffective in converting ventricular tachycardia, procainamide can be administered intravenously at a rate 50 mg per minute, for a total dose of 1 g. The blood pressure should be monitored because procainamide may cause a fall in blood pressure. If procainamide is successful in converting the ventricular tachycardia, a continuous infusion of 2 to 4 mg per minute should be instituted. Therapeutic serum levels of procainamide range from 4 to 10 μg per milliliter. In the presence of renal insufficiency, the dosage required to maintain a therapeutic serum level of procainamide decreases.

If lidocaine and procainamide are unsuccessful in converting ventricular tachycardia to sinus rhythm, bretylium should be administered in a dose of 5 to 10 mg per kilogram IV over 5 to 10 minutes. This may be repeated if necessary after 1 hour. If the bretylium is effective, a continuous infusion of 2 mg per minute should be instituted. The principal adverse effect of bretylium is orthostatic hypotension.

In the patient who has the "torsade de pointes" type of ventricular tachycardia in association with a long Q-T interval, administration of antiarrhythmic drugs should be avoided, particularly type I drugs such as procainamide, because antiarrhythmic drugs may aggravate this problem. Potassium, magnesium, and calcium levels should be checked, and if a deficiency in any of these electrolytes is discovered, appropriate measures should be taken to correct the deficiency. The most effective immediate therapeutic maneuver for control of torsade de pointes is to increase the heart rate either by institution of temporary pacing, or with an infusion of isoproterenol. By increasing the heart rate, these maneuvers result in a decrease in dispersion of refractoriness. A temporary pacemaker is usually preferable to isoproterenol in this setting, because if the patient has coronary artery disease, isoproterenol may precipitate myocardial ischemia. In addition, if the patient's ventricular tachycardia is not related to a delayed repolarization syndrome, isoproterenol may aggravate the ventricular tachycardia. Temporary pacing in either the atrium or ventricle is effective in preventing torsade de pointes. Atrial pacing is preferred because placement of a temporary pacemaker lead in the right ventricle may cause ventricular irritability. A pacing rate of approximately 90 to 100 beats per minute is usually effective in preventing a recurrence of torsade de pointes.

Placement of a temporary pacemaker lead is also appropriate in the patient who has "bradycardia-dependent" ventricular tachycardia, e.g., ventricular tachycardia occurring in association with complete AV block.

In the patient who has recurring episodes of ventricular tachycardia that do not require immediate direct current countershock, placement of a temporary pacemaker in the right ventricle allows overdrive pacing to be used in an attempt to terminate the ventricular tachycardia. Ventricular tachycardia may be terminated by either a burst of rapid pacing at a rate exceeding the ventricular tachycardia rate, or by one or more premature stimuli introduced during the ventricular tachycardia. The use of pacing techniques to terminate ventricular tachycardia requires the availability of a programmable stimulator and a physician trained in the use of this technique.

In the patient who is having a wide-complex tachycardia and in whom there is diagnostic uncertainty as to whether it is ventricular or supraventricular in origin, if there is severe hemodynamic compromise, the immediate form of therapy should be direct current countershock. If the patient is hemodynamically stable, antiarrhythmic drugs should be administered. The two most appropriate drugs to use in this setting are lidocaine and procainamide. Lidocaine may be effective if the wide-complex tachycardia is ventricular in origin, and does not aggravate any form of supraventricular tachycardia. Procainamide may be effective if the wide-complex tachycardia is ventricular or supraventricular in origin. Although verapamil is highly effective in terminating paroxysmal supraventricular tachycardias, it should be avoided in the patient with a wide-complex tachycardia of unclear origin, because if the tachycardia is in fact ventricular in origin, verapamil often results in severe hypotension related to vasodilatation. In addition, if the patient has the Wolff-Parkinson-White syndrome with atrial fibrillation, the administration of intravenous verapamil (or digitalis or propranolol) may facilitate conduction through the accessory pathway and increase the ventricular rate to dangerous levels during atrial fibrillation.

There is one type of ventricular tachycardia in which the use of verapamil is appropriate. In many patients who have an idiopathic form of ventricular tachycardia that has a right bundle branch block and superior axis configuration, verapamil has been found to be effective in terminating the tachycardia. Verapamil can be administered in a dose of 5 to 10 mg IV.

LONG-TERM MANAGEMENT

In patients who have had an episode of sustained ventricular tachycardia or a wide-complex tachycardia of unclear origin, it is usually appropriate to consult with a cardiologist. Electrophysiologic testing is often of great value in the management of these patients, and because electrophysiologic studies may not be available in many community hospitals, referral to a university medical center is often appropriate.

In the patient who has had a wide-complex tachycardia, the tachycardia can often be reproduced during electrophysiologic testing and its mechanism determined with certainty. In the patient who has had ventricular tachycardia, electropharmacologic testing is performed to identify a drug regimen effective in suppressing the tachycardia. A drug regimen is selected for long-term therapy based on its ability to suppress the induction of ventricular tachycardia during electrophysiologic testing. Electrophysiologic testing is also helpful in evaluating potential forms of nonpharmacologic therapy in patients who have not been adequately controlled with antiarrhythmic drugs. Nonpharmacologic forms of management include an antitachycardia pacemaker, an automatic implanted defibrillator, cardiac electrosurgery, and transcatheter ablation of a ventricular tachycardia focus.

If a correctable cause of ventricular tachycardia can be identified, long-term management to prevent a recurrence should include measures directed toward the underlying cause, e.g., prevention of hypokalemia or myocardial ischemia.

SUGGESTED READING

Anderson JL, Harrison DC, Meffin PJ, et al. Antiarrhythmic drugs: clinical pharmacology and therapeutic uses. Drugs 1978;15:27.
Scheinman MM, Morady F, Shen EN. Invasive cardiac electrophysiologic testing: the current state of the art. Circulation 1983;67:1169.
Wellens HJJ, Bar FWHM, Lie KI. The value of the electrocardiogram in the differential diagnosis of tachycardia with a widened QRS complex. Am J Med 1978;6:27.

VENTRICULAR FIBRILLATION AND TORSADE DE POINTES

W. DOUGLAS WEAVER, M.D.

VENTRICULAR FIBRILLATION

Etiology

Several metabolic and anatomic abnormalities may initiate ventricular fibrillation. Acute myocardial *infarction* or acute *ischemia*, such as that evoked during stress or exercise in patients with coronary artery disease, are common precipitating conditions. The time of greatest risk for developing ventricular fibrillation during acute infarction is the first 6-hour period following onset of chest pain; however, there remains a substantial risk of serious arrhythmia throughout the first day. Ventricular fibrillation may also occur immediately following reperfusion of a thrombosed coronary artery, such as during thrombolytic therapy using streptokinase or tissue plasminogen activator. "Warning" ventricular arrhythmias (frequent or repetitive or R on T premature ventricular beats) are of little help in selecting patients with acute infarction for prophylactic antiarrhythmic drug treatment. Premature ventricular beats are present in only half the patients who develop fibrillation. Warning arrhythmias are also nonspecific events, occurring in the majority of patients with uncomplicated infarction. The value of prophylactic drug therapy has also been questioned. Therefore, preparations must be made primarily to allow for quick recognition and treatment of fibrillation should it occur.

Metabolic abnormalities that may initiate ventricular fibrillation include hypothermia ($\leq 30°$ C), hypokalemia, drug overdose with tricyclic antidepressants and phenothiazines, and treatment with antiarrhythmic drugs.

There is an overall 15 percent incidence of arrhythmias directly induced by almost any of the available antiarrhythmic agents. Ironically, simple ventricular arrhythmias may be changed to complex and serious arrhythmias following initiation of antiarrhythmic drug treatment.

Ventricular fibrillation also may occur in patients with the hereditary *prolonged Q-T interval syndromes* in which left and right sympathetic nervous imbalance exists. This condition results in a prolongation of the Q-T interval, a reduction in the ventricular fibrillation threshold, and an increase in ventricular ectopic activity. The *Wolff-Parkinson-White* syndrome may also be associated with ventricular fibrillation. Atrial fibrillation can be rapidly conducted through the bypass tract, leading to rapid ventricular rates of 270 beats per minute (bpm) or more. This rapid rate prevents adequate diastolic filling. Consequently, blood pressure and cardiac output fall; the ventricle becomes ischemic and ventricular fibrillation results.

Sudden arrhythmic death is usually the result of an unexpected collapse due to ventricular fibrillation. There are more than 300,000 deaths each year from this disorder. The immediate precipitating cause causing ventricular fibrillation is unknown in most cases. Most patients have underlying coronary heart disease, although aortic and mitral regurgitation, mitral valve prolapse, and hypertensive and hypertrophic heart disease are rare associated cardiac anatomic abnormalities. A minority of the coronary patients (25 percent) show evidence of acute coronary thrombosis or demonstrate clinical evidence of acute infarction following resuscitation from ventricular fibrillation. For this reason, complete diagnostic studies, including prolonged electrocardiogram (ECG) monitoring to assess ambient arrhythmias, echocardiography and cardiac catheterization to assess anatomy, plus programmed electrical stimulation to assess vulnerability are mandatory to better elucidate the likely cause. In addition, the frequency of ventricular ectopy, extent of coronary disease, left ventricular function and the results of programmed ventricular stimulation are helpful in assigning risk for a recurrent event, and in selecting protective therapy. The overall rate of recurrence is high in resuscitated patients; 20 percent die in the first year following resuscitation and 36 percent are dead at 2 years. Most deaths are due to another episode of cardiac arrest. When ventricular fibrillation occurs in the setting of acute infarction, prognosis is much better. One year mortality in this subset is less than 5 percent, presumably because the abnormality that initially caused fibrillation is no longer present.

Diagnosis

Although the ECG waveform may appear chaotic, in fact, ventricular fibrillation displays a characteristic sinusoidal shape with a fundamental frequency of 3.5 to 8 Hz. The wave front may also be directional. Thus, monitoring through one set of leads may show coarse fibrillatory waves, and through orthogonal leads the *ECG may appear almost isoelectric* and be mistaken for asystole. For this reason, initial evaluation of the ECG during cardiac arrest should assess the rhythm using either lead II or the typical defibrillation electrode pathway, and if asystole is apparent, the lead direction should be rotated 90 degrees (lead III or left shoulder and right body).

Defibrillation is the mainstay of treatment for ventricular fibrillation, and thus if asystole has been incorrectly diagnosed, correct and lifesaving therapy may be inadvertently withheld.

A second common error during ECG interpretation can be caused by *pacemaker spikes during ventricular fibrillation.* Demand permanent pacemakers may not sense the ventricular fibrillation waveform and therefore the generator will pace at the preselected rate. These high-amplitude electrical pulses (particularly those associated with unipolar pacemakers) combined with the attenuated frequency response of most defibrillator monitors may almost mask ventricular fibrillation (Fig. 1). The rhythm in a pacemaker patient must therefore be carefully scrutinized during cardiac arrest. If the underlying rhythm cannot be ascertained and the patient is unresponsive and pulseless, defibrillation should be carried out immediately.

The initial amplitude of the fibrillation waveform is an indicator of the duration from collapse until initiation of treatment. Fibrillation amplitude diminishes as the duration of arrest increases. The amplitude is also a prognostic indicator of resuscitation outcome. In a series of 394 patients, only four of 36 (11 percent) whose initial

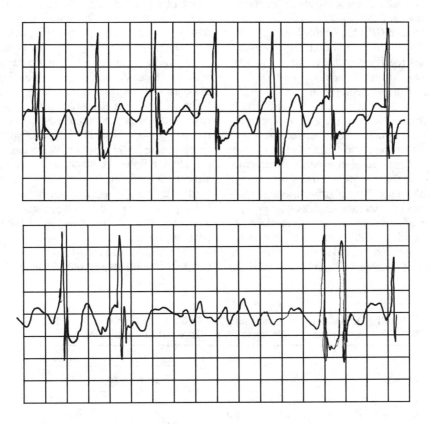

Figure 1 Ventricular fibrillation in a patient with a dual chamber pacemaker. The waveform is intermittently detected by the atrial and ventricular electrodes and sensing circuits. The rhythm shown on the top strip can be easily confused as representing a paced rhythm and the pacer spikes mask ventricular fibrillation. On the lower stirp, the fibrillation waves are seen during a pause in pacing. When pacer spikes are present the rhythm must be carefully assessed so that ventricular fibrillation will not be overlooked and defibrillation inadvertently withheld.

fibrillation amplitude was 0.2 mV or less survived compared with 117 (30 percent) of those patients whose initial fibrillation waveform amplitude was more than 0.2 mV.

Prehospital Treatment

Mobile paramedic systems have dramatically changed the outcome for patients who develop ventricular fibrillation outside the hosptial. Several communities have reported yearly survival rates (discharged alive from hospital) of 20 to 30 percent. The likelihood of survival is greatest in patients in whom collapse is witnessed and for whom defibrillation and basic life support can be rapidly provided. When advanced life support is not available until after the patient is brought to the hospital emergency department, survival rates of 5 percent are usual. Two major changes in prehospital medical care are currently in development and will likely further improve survival rates following cardiac arrest attributable to ventricular fibrillation. Several communities are now active in teaching cardiopulmonary resuscitation (CPR) techniques to laypersons. Such efforts can substantially affect one of the important time factors that influence survival: the delay from collapse until initiation of CPR. In several cities, layperson-initiated CPR has doubled the survival rate of patients suffering ventricular fibrillation; however, the proportion of cases receiving such treatment remains low (Table 1). A goal for this decade will be to target CPR training toward family members of patients with known cardiac diseases, instead of using an undirected approach. Seventy percent of cardiac arrests occur at home. Therefore, training family members of coronary patients is most important and could significantly increase the proportion of patients receiving early treatment. Promotional information about CPR training programs must be made available in hospital and office waiting areas as well as in pharmacies in order to reach this target group. Secondly, a number of communities are experimenting with the concept of teaching CPR over the telephone to bystanders. Such an approach could definitely reduce the delay until initiation of treatment. Telephone CPR has been shown to be feasible. Following initiation of telephone CPR in suburban King County, there was a trend toward improved survival rates in those patients who received CPR from a lay person directed by the emergency dispatcher.

Another major development in prehospital care will be the widespread implementation of "early" defibrillation delivered by minimally trained rescuers using automatic external defibrillators. These devices are in their technologic infancy, but essentially are capable of automatically assessing the ECG rhythm and delivering a limited number of shocks. They relieve the operator of the need for hours of initial training and maintaining ECG recognition skills. In Seattle, we have trained hundreds of firefighters and other laypersons using a 5-hour course in which persons learned to use the automatic defibrillator; CPR techniques were also refreshed or taught. Contrast this to the hundreds of hours required to train paramedics using conventional defibrillation monitors. Even teaching only the recognition of ventricular fibrillation requires 30 hours or more per year. The automatic defibrillator can substantially reduce the other time factor affecting survival from cardiac arrest: the delay until shock (Table 2). Because of the modest training requirements, automatic defibrillators can be used by first responders in tiered emergency systems, by ambulance personnel, and by police and other volunteer rescuers in communities or areas not having paramedic systems. In addition, these devices may be suitable for use by staff of coliseums, sporting arenas, large industries, and public buildings—virtually any place having organized security, safety or emergency personnel and a population at risk for cardiac arrest. The impact of such treatment could be enormous. When defibrillation can be delivered immediately following collapse with ventricular fibrillation, almost all such victims survive. There have been 25 cardiac arrests during an out-of-hospital cardiac rehabilitation program in Seattle. All victims were shocked within a minute by medical personnel in attendance, and 100 percent survived.

The widespread use of automatic external defibrillators will require substantial physician supervision to es-

---

TABLE 1 Influence of Shortening the Delay Until Initiation of CPR Through Bystander Participation on Survivial of Cardiac Arrest

Location	Rhythm	Witnessed	% Discharged (Total No. of Cases)	
			Bystander CPR	EMS CPR
Seattle	VF	All	47 (89)	21 (146)
Suburban King County	VF	All	37 (436)	29 (509)
Los Angeles	All	41%	22 (93)	5 (150)
Pittsburgh	VF/VT	Unknown	24 (25)	7 (59)
Vancouver	All	77%	21 (43)	6 (272)
Winnipeg	VF/VT	Unknown	25 (65)	5 (161)
Oslo	Unknown	Unknown	36 (75)	8 (556)
Reykjavik	All	Unknown	42 (38)	6 (84)

CPR = cardiopulmonary resuscitation; EMS CPR = initiation of CPR after arrival of emergency medical system; VF = ventricular fibrillation; VT = ventricular tachycardia.

TABLE 2 Effect of Delays Until Initiation of Treatment on Outcome of Cardiac Arrest—Witnessed Cases

Time to CPR (min)	Time to Shock (min)			
	≤10 No. (% discharged)	11–15 No. (% discharged)	>15 No. (% discharged)	Total No. (% discharged)
≤4	42 (56)	17 (38)	1 (9)	60 (46)[*]
>4	17 (41)	19 (36)	5 (18)	41 (34)[*]
Total	59 (51)[†]	36 (37)[†]	6 (16)[†]	

[*] p = 0.08
[†] p < 0.001

tablish adequate training programs and provide certification of rescuers. In addition, review of the recordings of the resuscitation attempt are necessary to make an assessment of user and device performance in order to provide appropriate feedback and guidance to users.

It seems possible that targeted CPR instruction and automatic external defibrillators may have an impact on survival from sudden cardiac arrest as great as that which paramedic systems achieved when first implemented in the early 1970s.

Hospital Management of Ventricular Fibrillation

Every witnessed case of cardiac arrest should be presumed to be ventricular fibrillation until proven otherwise. More than 95 percent of patients monitored within 4 minutes of collapse will have ventricular fibrillation as the initial recorded rhythm. The most important fact to keep in mind is that the only proven treatment for ventricular fibrillation is defibrillation. Secondly, the sooner defibrillation occurs, the better the likelihood of survival. Outcome of patients with all other rhythms associated with cardiac arrest is dismal and therefore treatment emphasis during resuscitation should be defibrillation. The person assuming charge must be aware of the well-intended but sometimes time-consuming efforts spent by others to initiate CPR, intubate the patient, and establish intravenous lines. These are all secondary measures and should not be done if a defibrillator is immediately available and ventricular fibrillation is present.

Up to three *initial shocks* should be delivered using 175 to 200 J of delivered energy. More than 75 percent of patients who will ultimately be resuscitated and survive hospitalization will require three or fewer shocks. This initial shock sequence is first aimed at causing defibrillation and ideally restoring an organized rhythm. More than 90 percent of patients will be at least transiently defibrillated by using up to three initial shocks. Initial use of maximum defibrillator energy levels is not necessary and possibly even harmful. Lower energy levels are equally effective in causing defibrillation as the maximum energy level used for initial shocks. As the amount of delivered energy increases, periods of ventricular asystole following the shock are longer, which in turn retard the return of spontaneous circulation and may increase the rate of refibrillation. If the initial lower energy levels prove to be adequate in achieving defibrillation, the energy level

setting also need not be increased for treating episodes of refibrillation.

In most patients, multiple shocks are not necessary for effecting initial defibrillation, but instead are used for treating recurrent episodes of ventricular fibrillation. Following return of spontaneous circulation, a profound metabolic imbalance is present and coronary reperfusion occurs. Both of these factors may cause marked ventricular irritability and recurrent episodes of fibrillation. There have been no clinical trials that support the superiority of one particular antiarrhythmic drug in this setting. Most animal studies raise serious doubt as to the effectiveness of any of the available antiarrhythmic drugs for treating reperfusion arrhythmias. Consequently, the pharmacologic approach should be simple. Following episodes of refibrillation or when ventricular fibrillation persists throughout the initial three shocks, 100 mg of lidocaine (1 mg per kilogram of body weight) should be administered and repeated after 5 minutes if the condition is not changed. Defibrillation should be attempted at least twice between each drug administration and CPR should be performed to circulate the drug. Arterial pH should be corrected using sodium bicarbonate only following measurement of the blood gases. The arterial pH is not abnormal early in the course of resuscitation and administration of excessive amounts of sodium bicarbonate may cause severe alkalosis, making defibrillation even more difficult. In addition, intracellular acidosis may worsen following sodium bicarbonate administration and possibly cause further insult to heart and brain. The mainstay of attempts to normalize the pH should be ventilation, and the use of sodium bicarbonate should be minimized.

Bretylium (500 mg) and procainamide (500 mg) are second line drugs and should be used only following unsuccessful repeated use of lidocaine. Epinephrine (1 mg) should be administered intravenously every 5 to 10 minutes during the resuscitation effort if CPR continues to be required. Epinephrine's major effect is in reducing arterial compliance. It augments aortic diastolic blood pressure and consequently improves myocardial and cerebral perfusion during CPR. The absorption of epinephrine following tracheal administration has been shown not to be predictable during cardiac arrest and therefore should be avoided if possible.

Episodes of refibrillation appear to be especially difficult to treat in the patient with acute myocardial infarction. Such patients often develop a transient pulse and blood pressure between shocks, but within 15 to 60 seconds lapse back into recurrent episodes of ventricular tachycardia or fibrillation. Antiarrhythmic drug therapy is often ineffective. Such patients can be kept alive, however, if they are rapidly defibrillated during each episode, although multiple shocks may be required. It is important to remain cognizant of this course of events, as such a prolonged intensive effort requires substantial resources and is a set-up for inappropriate and excessive drug therapy, which can be toxic and further reduce the likelihood of resuscitation. However, if these episodes of refibrillation are rapidly shocked and the patient is not made worse by drug therapy, the patient's rhythm usually stabilizes after 30 to 60 minutes.

Ventricular Fibrillation and Hypothermia

Both atrial and ventricular arrhythmias may accompany hypothermia. Ventricular fibrillation is of imminent concern when body temperature is less than 30° C. Cellular function is markedly depressed during hypothermia, and therefore survival is still possible even after prolonged periods of cardiac arrest. There is one report of survival following 3 hours and 40 minutes of continuous ventricular fibrillation. Several exceptions to standard resuscitation measures should be recalled in the treatment of patients with hypothermia. CPR should not be administered in the setting of hypotension and an organized rhythm because cardiac arrest is frequently precipitated by any mechanical stimulation of the heart. On the other hand, in the setting of cardiac arrest, CPR should be initiated and continued until the victim has been rewarmed and either been resuscitated or failed to respond to treatment. Methods to effect core rewarming should be considered if temperatures are less than 30° C. These include inhalation rewarming, peritoneal dialysis, extracorporeal blood rewarming, and hemodialysis. If available, open chest cardiac massage and rewarming should be strongly considered. Cardiac drug therapy for resuscitation should be withheld. Antiarrhythmic and cardiac stimulatory drugs are ineffective during hypothermia and complicate the condition following rewarming. Arterial blood gases should be adjusted for body temperature before treatment

with sodium bicarbonate is considered. Hemoconcentration is frequently associated with hypothermia, and fluid replacement using warmed saline should be done intravenously. The heart is relatively refractory to pacing and countershocks when temperature is below 28° C. An initial attempt at defibrillation is warranted, but if unsuccessful, rewarming should be initiated and defibrillation tried again after the core temperature has increased.

TORSADE DE POINTES

Etiology and Diagnosis

Ventricular tachycardia is usually characterized by a uniformity of QRS complexes. Additionally, there is an unusual type of ventricular tachycardia having differing QRS morphology and characterized by a changing QRS configuration and axis (Fig. 2). Torsade de pointes is accomplished by prolongation of the Q-T interval and therefore does not include every polymorphous ventricular tachycardia. Torsade de pointes occurs most frequently following therapy with quinidine, but may follow treatment with other types of antiarrhythmic drugs, phenothiazines, and even lidocaine. In addition, hypokalemia, hypomagnesemia, the hereditary Q-T prolongation syndrome, acute central nervous system damage, and myocardial ischemia may all be associated with this arrhythmia. The underlying common disorder is development of uneven ventricular repolarization, thus providing suitable conditions for the establishment of reentry arrhythmias. The tachycardia episodes are usually paroxysmal, lasting 3 to 20 beats and usually at rates of 150 to 300 bpm.

Treatment and Management

In the uncomplicated and asymptomatic case of torsade de pointes, withdrawal of the causative agent or correction of the underlying electrolyte abnormality may be all that is necessary for treatment. However, prolonged episodes may cause serious hemodynamic compromise and degenerate to ventricular fibrillation. Defibrillation

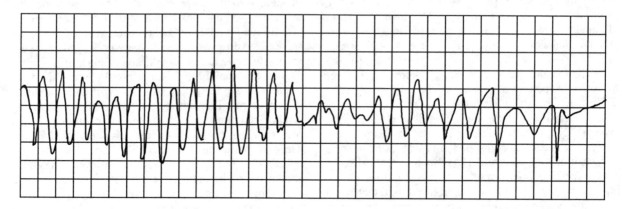

Figure 2 Torsade de pointes is characterized by a long Q-T interval during sinus rhythm and then tachycardia morphologic characteristics showing "twisting of the points."

or cardioversion is usually helpful only transiently, with frequent recurrence of the tachycardia. The use of conventional antiarrhythmic drugs such as lidocaine or procainamide is usually ineffective, and in fact these drugs may further aggravate the arrhythmia. Procainamide, quinidine, and disopyramide should not be administered in this setting, since they all may increase the repolarization delay and worsen the arrhythmia. The initial maneuver that may be simplest and frequently terminates the arrhythmia is to speed the heart rate and shorten the refractory period using isoproterenol. The drug should be diluted and given at a rate of 2 to 8 μg per minute, beginning at the smallest infusion rate and increasing by 1 μg per minute every 3 to 5 minutes. Serious side effects may occur with isoproterenol and patients should be monitored for these effects frequently. They include rapid sinus tachycardia, worsened arrhythmias, hypertension owing to increased cardiac contractility, and hypotension owing to the drug's effect on peripheral vasculature. The drug also markedly increases myocardial oxygen demand and should be avoided in patients with angina, acute myocardial infarction or hypertension.

Ventricular pacing is also effective and can be used for all patients, including those with ischemic heart disease. It is almost always effective. Following placement of a right ventricular transvenous catheter, the pacing rate should be increased to a rate of 10 bpm more than the baseline sinus rate and further increased up to 120 bpm to maintain ventricular capture. The overdrive technique usually prevents reentry and therefore rapidly terminates the tachycardia. Cardioversion may be necessary in addition to break the arrhythmia so that pacing can be initiated.

Magnesium sulfate (2 g in 25 percent solution) may also be infused as an intravenous bolus and has been shown to be effective in a limited number of cases. It can be given to patients with ongoing ischemia and can be applied while preparing for introduction of a temporary pacemaker catheter.

SUGGESTED READING

Cobb LA, Hallstrom AP. Community-based cardiopulmonary resuscitation. What have we learned? Ann NY Acad Sci 1982; 382:330–342.

Eisenberg MS, Copass MK, Hallstrom AP, Blake B, Bergner L, Short FA, Cobb LA. Treatment of out-of-hospital cardiac arrest with rapid defibrillation by emergency medical technicians. N Engl J Med 1980; 302:1379–1382.

Eisenberg MS, Hallstrom AP, Carter WB, Cummins RO, Berger L, Pierce J. Emergency CPR instruction via telephone. Am J Pub Health 1985; 75:47–50.

Smith WM, Gallagher JJ. "Les torsades de pointes": an unusual ventricular arrhythmia. Ann Intern Med 1980; 93:578–584.

Soffer J, Dreifus LS, Michelson EL. Polymorphous ventricular tachycardia associated with normal and long Q-T intervals. Am J Cardiol 1982; 49:2021–2029.

Weaver WD, Cobb LA, Copass MK, Hallstrom AP. Ventricular defibrillation—a comparative trial using 175-J and 320-J shock. N Engl J Med 1982; 307:1101–1106.

Weaver WD, Copass MK, Bufi D, Ray R, Hallstrom AP, Cobb LA. Improved neurologic recovery and survival after early defibrillation. Circulation 1984; 69:943–948.

Weaver WD, Copass MK, Hill DL, Fahienbruch C, Hallstrom AP, Cobb LA. Cardiac arrest with a new automatic external defibrillator by out-of-hospital first responders. Am J Cardiol 1986; 57: 1017–1021.

ELECTROMECHANICAL DISSOCIATION AND ASYSTOLE

HARLAN A. STUEVEN, M.D.

The primary cause of cardiac arrest is a rhythm disturbance. The three rhythms that are primarily associated with cardiac arrest are ventricular fibrillation, electromechanical dissociation (EMD), and asystole and/or fine ventricular fibrillation. The focus of this chapter is on reviewing the incidence, pathophysiology and treatment of EMD and asystole.

INCIDENCE AND MORTALITY

The reported incidence of asystole and/or EMD varies widely among emergency medical systems (EMS). This is most likely a phenomenon of "nonresuscitation bias." The nonresuscitation bias is the incidence with which resuscitation is not attempted, for whatever reason. The higher the rate of unattempted resuscitation, the more unrepresentative the reported incidence of the presenting rhythm. When reviewing the EMS rhythm incidence data, this factor must be kept in mind; unfortunately, most systems do not report their incidence of unattempted resuscitation. Ten years of experience with witnessed paramedic-resuscitated arrests have revealed a precipitating rhythm incidence of 31 percent for coarse ventricular fibrillation, 36 percent for EMD, and 33 percent for asystole.

The respective mortalities likewise vary with the nonresuscitation bias. A higher nonresuscitation bias yields a higher system hospital discharge rate (save rate), because poorly resuscitated patients are excluded. A review of our series of patients with paramedic-witnessed arrests shows a save rate of 8 percent for EMD and 12 percent for asystole. System save rates for both witnessed and unwitnessed cases approximate 6 percent for EMD and 4 percent for asystole.

ELECTROMECHANICAL DISSOCIATION

Pathogenesis

There have been no large autopsy studies investigating the causes of electromechanical dissociation. A review of cardiology textbooks fails to reveal a consensus on the definition of EMD, further confounding our understanding of pathogenesis and treatment. We define EMD as any organized electrical complex without a discernible pulse. (Since arterial pressure monitoring is not available, some of these patients obviously may have nonpalpable pressure pulses.) A number of causes of EMD have been implicated, including the following:

1. A severely depressed preload. Examples include exsanguinating hemorrhage from a rupture of the myocardium, tension pneumothorax, or an acute cardiac tamponade. All conditions reduce the amount of effective blood inflow to the heart.
2. Primary myocardial dysfunction. Examples of this include papillary muscle dysfunction, intraventricular septum rupture, parasympathetic stimulation, severe ischemia and hypoxia, severe electrolyte abnormalities, certain types of drug ingestions (especially type I antiarrhythmics), calcium phosphate pump dysfunction, and the administration of verapamil. All conditions decrease the heart's ability to contract effectively.
3. Outflow obstruction and/or markedly altered afterload. Examples include massive pulmonary embolism and hypertrophic cardiomyopathy. All conditions either decrease effective blood outflow or reduce effective blood pressure.

History and physical examination are of limited practical value in determining the cause of EMD, except to rule out obvious hemorrhage or tension pneumothorax. A tension pneumothorax may be suspected by tracheal deviation, increased tympany on the pneumothorax side, or reduced unilateral breath sounds, and can be confirmed by needle aspiration of the chest on the affected side.

Treatment

Since asphyxia and/or hypoxia may be primary precipitating causes of EMD, initial management must be directed toward intubation and airway control (Table 1). The institution of external cardiac compression has been shown to increase the save rate in patients with EMD. If hypovolemic EMD (decreased preload) is felt to be the cause, the application of military antishock trousers (MAST) or fluid challenge may be of value. MAST garments have been shown to increase survival when placed on patients with EMD. Volume loading during normovolemic cardiopulmonary resuscitation (CPR) has been shown experimentally to increase total cardiac output, but regional blood flow to heart and brain decreases significantly owing to shunting to other organs. This makes its clinical use questionable. If decreased afterload is thought to be the cause, interposed abdominal compression CPR may increase effective blood flow to the heart and brain. Because of the limited blood flow to the brain and vital organs associated with standard external compression CPR, consideration should be given to thoracotomy and manual compression of the heart in an otherwise viable patient.

TABLE 1 Treatment Approach to Electromechanical Dissociation

Intubation and airway control
External cardiac compression
MAST
Epinephrine, 1 mg 1:10,000 IV
Dopamine, > μg/kg/min
Sodium bicarbonate based upon degree of acidosis *
Atropine, 2 mg IV for bradycardia
Thoracotomy and manual heart compression

* Most recent ACLS guidelines suggest this should be avoided if possible.

Pharmacologic Intervention

No drugs have conclusively been shown to be effective in the management of EMD. The American Heart Association recommends epinephrine, and sodium bicarbonate when necessary, for EMD.

Epinephrine is recommended because of its alpha-adrenergic sympathetic effects (its beta-adrenergic effects do not contribute to resuscitation). Methoxamine is a pure alpha-adrenergic drug that has been reported effective in animal studies and may become the favored sympathomimetic, and is being studied in humans.

Sodium bicarbonate administration has not been studied nor has it been shown to be of any value in the treatment of EMD or asystole. Intuitively, the administration of sodium bicarbonate should be dependent upon the severity of the acidosis and the length of time of the arrest, but the exact role of bicarbonate in the treatment of acidosis is currently the subject of much scientific debate.

Calcium chloride has been studied in animals and humans and found to be of some value in resuscitating the heart. Two large human studies have shown that 11 to 16 percent of patients respond with a pulse after the administration of calcium and are successfully resuscitated and admitted to the hospital. Unfortunately, there are no data to show that calcium is associated with an increased hospital discharge and survival rate. Serious concern has been raised regarding the potential adverse effects of calcium in brain resuscitation, since calcium influx into cells is one of the major mechanisms of the brain damage that occurs in the hours after resuscitation. Calcium chloride has been deleted from the American Heart Association's guidelines.

Isoproterenol and dopamine have been advocated in the treatment of EMD; however, there have been no definitive studies outlining the value of these modalities. Both have significant beta-adrenergic activity, which dilates vessels, shunts blood flow away from the heart and brain, and lessens the chance of resuscitation in animal studies.

Although atropine sulfate has not been adequately evaluated in the management of EMD, it might be of value in patients with severe bradycardic rhythms, and has no direct harmful effects.

ASYSTOLE

Pathogenesis

There have been no extensive autopsy studies delineating the origins of asystole. The literature is confusing regarding its definition. Some authors define asystole as no spontaneous electrical activity for a duration of 5 seconds. We define asystole as the complete absence of electrical activity for at least 1 minute.

A number of factors have been implicated in the development of asystole. Increased parasympathetic tone as a result of vagal stimulation has been suggested as the primary cause. Right coronary artery occlusion and resultant sinus node dysfunction have been implicated. Asystole may be the end result of ventricular fibrillation or EMD or the result of electrical countershock defibrillation. History and physical examination are probably of limited value in determining the cause of asystole.

Treatment

As with EMD, attention must first be directed toward airway management and correction of asphyxia and/or hypoxia (Table 2). CPR is of limited value in resuscitating patients from asystole and/or maintaining patients in a state in which they can be resuscitated, but may be of value in enhancing medication flow during arrests.

Ventricular fibrillation has been shown to masquerade as asystole; therefore, the initial approach to the patient in asystole should include one countershock. Eight percent of patients respond to countershock with a rhythm and 5 percent are resuscitated. A number of studies have been reported using transcutaneous pacing fairly late in the treatment of asystolic patients. The survival rate for patients with bradyasystolic cardiac arrest has not been dramatically increased with pacing, but no large prehospital or early initiated pacing series has been reported.

Pharmacologic Interventions

The American Heart Association recommends epinephrine, atropine, and electrical pacing in the treatment of asystole. There are no data to support the use of epinephrine for asystole. Debate continues as to whether asystole represents a state of excess catecholamines. If such were the case, exogenous catecholamines would only exacerbate that state. Some authorities therefore recommend that catecholamines not be administered to the asystolic patient.

Atropine has been studied retrospectively. Fourteen percent of patients receiving it for asystole develop a rhythm and pulse. However, it has not been shown to increase survival rate. Calcium chloride has been studied retrospectively and prospectively and been shown not to be of value in resuscitating asystole. There are no data to support the use of isoproterenol.

Patients have been reported to survive prolonged asystole resulting from hypothermia and tricyclic antidepressant overdose. In these circumstances, consideration should be given to prolonged mechanical resuscitation or cardiac bypass.

SUGGESTED READING

Electromechanical Dissociation

Bircher N, Safar P. Manual open-chest cardiopulmonary resuscitation. Ann Emerg Med 1984; 13:770–773.
Friedman H. Diagnostic considerations in electromechanical dissociation. Am J Cardiology 1976; 38:268–269.
Harrison E, Amey B. Use of calcium in electromechanical dissociation. Ann Emerg Med 1984; 13:844–845.
Stueven H, Thompson B, Aprahamian C, Tonsfeldt D, Kastenson E. The effectiveness of calcium chloride in refractory electromechanical dissociation. Ann Emerg Med 1985; 14:626–629.
Stueven H, Troiano P, Thompson B, Mateer J, Kastenson E, Tonsfeldt D, Hargarten K, Kowalski R, Aprahamian C, Darin J. Bystander/first responder CPR: ten years experience in a paramedic system. Ann Emerg Med 1985; 14:510 (abstract).

Asystole

Hedges J, Syverud S, Dalsey W. Developments in transcutaneous and transthoracic pacing during bradyasystolic arrest. Ann Emerg Med 1984; 13:822–827.
Stueven H, Thompson B, Aprahamian C, Tonsfeldt D. Calcium chloride: reassessment of use in asystole. Ann Emerg Med 1984; 13:820–822.
Stueven H, Tonsfeldt D, Thompson B, Whitcomb J, Kastenson E, Aprahamian C. Atropine in asystole: human studies. Ann Emerg Med 1984; 13:815–817.
Thompson B, Brooks RC, Pionkowski R, Aprahamian C, Mateer J. Immediate countershock treatment of asystole. Ann Emerg Med 1984; 13:827–829.
Vassalle M, Caress D, Slovin A, Stuckey J. On the cause of ventricular asystole during vagal stimulation. Circulation 1967; 20:228–241.

TABLE 2 Treatment Approach to Asystole

Intubation and airway control
External cardiac compression
Countershock 360 w/sec × 2
Epinephrine, 1 mg 1:10,000 IV
Atropine, 2 mg IV
Transcutaneous pacing
Sodium bicarbonate based upon degree of acidosis *
Cardiac bypass or mechanical resuscitation in hypothermia
  or tricyclic antidepressant overdose

---

* Most recent ACLS guidelines suggest this should be avoided if possible.

WIDE-COMPLEX TACHYCARDIAS

JEROME R. HOFFMAN, M.D.

The unifying principle in the management of wide-complex tachycardias, as it is in every arrhythmia, is that treatment is based on the clinical condition of the patient, rather than on any electrocardiographic characteristics of the arrhythmia. While it is ultimately valuable to distinguish arrhythmias of various causes and origins from each other, the single most critical element in determining emergent treatment is the end-organ effect of the abnormal rhythm. Patients who are hemodynamically unstable require electrical cardioversion or defibrillation, while drug therapy can be undertaken in those patients who are tolerating their tachycardia without signs of end-organ hypoperfusion. (See the chapter *Narrow-Complex Tachycardia* for a brief discussion of the clinical indicators of end-organ hypoperfusion. In addition, the same comments regarding electrocardiogram [ECG] interpretation contained in that chapter are relevant here; while there will occasionally be a limited discussion regarding differentiation of various types of wide-complex tachycardias on the basis of surface ECG findings, for the most part such diagnostic considerations will be avoided).

While narrow-complex tachycardias are all generated from above the vertricles, wide-complex tachycardias can originate anywhere in the heart. This is because wide QRS complexes (QRS $\geq$ 0.12 sec) reflect abnormal depolarization of the ventricle; thus, cardiac depolarizations that are conducted abnormally, on a cell to cell basis, through the ventricles, regardless of their point of initiation, produce wide complexes. Ventricular tachycardia, which generally reflects a re-entrant arrhythmia originating in the ventricle, will indeed be represented by wide QRS complexes, as conduction through the ventricles will not occur rapidly down the normal conduction system pathways. On the other hand, wide QRS complexes will also be created in the presence of bundle branch blocks, and when a patient with a bundle branch block develops a tachycardia, this will appear with wide QRS complexes. Finally, tachycardias associated with Wolff-Parkinson-White (WPW) syndrome, in which impulses reach the ventricle via antegrade conduction down the accessory pathway, will also be conducted through the ventricles on a cell to cell basis, resulting in wide complexes (see discussion in the chapter *Narrow-Complex Tachycardias*). Wide complex tachycardias associated with WPW syndrome will be discussed later in this chapter.

A number of surface electrocardiographic criteria have been described which may help to distinguish between complexes originating in the ventricle and those originating in the atrium or atrioventricular (AV) node, but which also produce wide QRS complexes because of bundle branch block, (Table 1). Ultimately, these charac-teristics can only suggest the rhythm's origin, and it may actually be impossible in many cases to distinguish these entities definitively on the basis of surface electrocardiography. In the presence of tachycardias with wide QRS complexes this distinction may be even more difficult, but once again it is ultimately not of terrible importance to the emergency physician, since treatment of the patient is based on the hemodynamic effects of the tachycardia rather than on the precise nature of its origin. Unstable patients must be treated with cardioversion; in stable patients in whom there is any doubt about the origin of a wide-complex tachycardia, the emergency physician should proceed on the assumption that this may represent ventricular tachycardia.

VENTRICULAR TACHYCARDIA

Ventricular tachycardia (VT) is usually a life-threatening medical emergency when seen in an emergency department. There are patients who have intermittent asymptomatic runs of VT, usually comprising episodes of less than ten beats in a row, but occasionally consisting of episodes lasting significantly longer; the long-term diagnostic and therapeutic management of such patients is beyond the scope of this chapter. Any patient seen in an emergency department with what appears to be VT, in the absence of acute symptomatic heart disease, should be referred immediately for cardiologic consultation and work-up. Short runs of VT in patients with acute ischemic heart disease require prophylaxis with lidocaine, and hospitalization, even if there are no symptoms attributable to the brief bursts of tachycardia.

Sustained VT usually causes symptoms because the heart rate is too fast to allow adequate end-organ perfusion. Patients who have significant lightheadedness, chest pain, or pulmonary edema, as well as those with hypotension and frank alterations of mental status, require emergent cardioversion. Ventricular tachycardia is highly electrosensitive, and perhaps 90 percent of patients will respond to as little as 10 watts per second of delivered energy. Most clinicians elect to begin cardioversion, however, at levels of 20 or 50 watts per second, although there is probably little reason to use more than 20 watts per second as an initial dose, particularly in patients who are awake and alert. Subsequent increases in energy can be delivered if initial attempts are unsuccessful.

Cardioversion should be performed in the synchronized mode, as there would otherwise be a danger of producing ventricular fibrillation by delivering an electric current during the vulnerable period of the cardiac cycle. VT produces definable QRS complexes which the machine should have no trouble sensing.

Following successful initial conversion all patients require stabilization with anti-arrhythmic therapy. This topic is further discussed in the chapter, *Ventricular Tachycardia*.

PAROXYSMAL SUPRAVENTRICULAR TACHYCARDIA

In some instances patients have tachycardias with ven-

TABLE 1 Clues to the Differentiation of Ventricular Tachycardia vs. Supraventricular Tachycardia with Aberrancy

	Ventricular Tachycardia	Supraventricular Tachycardia With Aberrancy
Rate	130–170 up to 280 beats per minute	170–200 beats per minute
Irregularity (>.02 sec)	21%	6%
QRS Duration	.10 to >.20 sec	Rarely >.14 sec if no preexisting IVCD
QRS Morphology (valid only if no prior IVCD) Concordant V_1–V_6	Diagnostic but uncommon	Absent
RBBB axis	<−30° in 75%	<−30° in 4%
V_1		
V_6		
LBBB axis	<−30° in 57%	<−30° in 13%
V_6		
Atrial Activation	1:1 VA conduction in 33%	≥1:1 relationship between P and QRS in approximately 100% if P identifable
Fusion Beats	Diagnostic incidence 12%	Absent

IVCD = Intraventricular conduction defects   RBBB = Right bundle branch block   LBBB = Left bundle branch block

tricular response rates between 150 and 200, with wide QRS complexes whose durations are approximately 0.11 to 0.14 seconds. This may represent VT, with relatively slow ventricular rates, or it may represent paroxysmal supraventricular tachycardia (PSVT) with aberrant conduction. While most patients with PSVT present with narrow complexes, there may be rate-related bundle branch blocks, or this may represent PSVT with antegrade conduction through the bypass tract (see the chapter *Narrow-Complex Tachycardia*). Verapamil and digitalis are contraindicated in this circumstance for a number of reasons. In the first place, they will not be beneficial should the arrhythmia represent VT: Digitalis could well produce a deterioration to ventricular fibrillation, while verapamil would not be expected to affect the arrhythmia (in most cases) and would therefore be deleterious because its vasodilatory and negative ionotropic effects might well contribute to increasing hypotension and hemodynamic instability. If, on the other hand, this condition represented PSVT with antegrade conduction through the bypass tract, verapamil and digitalis would still be potentially dangerous: Neither drug would be expected to slow conduction through the bypass tract, and might in some circumstances speed such conduction.

The best treatment of wide-complex PSVT secondary to WPW syndrome is unclear. Lidocaine has long been deemed an excellent choice in this circumstance, since it was thought to slow conduction in the bypass tract and would be expected to positively affect VT as well, but a recent study has suggested that lidocaine may in fact speed conduction through the bypass tract, thus making it potentially dangerous. Procainamide, which also would

be useful should the arrhythmia prove to be VT, seems to have a therapeutic effect in this circumstance by slowing conduction through the bypass tract, and thus may ultimately be the drug of choice. A number of experimental agents also show promise in this situation, but are not currently available.

ATRIAL FIBRILLATION

While the vast majority of patients with atrial fibrillation (AF) present with narrow QRS complexes, wide-complex AF is occasionally seen. Probably the most common reason for this is underlying *bundle branch block*, which will be seen as well on ECGs taken during normal sinus rhythm. Rate-related bundle branch block can also occur, in which case complexes following longer R-R intervals may have prolonged duration, while those complexes following longer R-R intervals will be narrow. Treatment of wide-complex AF, when it is clearly caused by bundle branch block, is similar to treatment of routine narrow-complex AF (see the chapter *Narrow-Complex Tachycardia*).

In rare instances AF will present with intermittent wide complexes because of antegrade conduction down an accessory pathway in WPW syndrome. It is critical to recognize these instances because a variety of medicines used successfully in the treatment of narrow-complex AF could have catastrophic effects in this circumstance. When AF occurs in patients with WPW syndrome, some of the beats will be conducted through the AV node and will appear normal, with narrow QRS complexes. On the other hand, some of the impulses generated in the atrium will be conducted to the ventricle antegrade down the accessory pathways; these impulses will produce very wide and very bizarre QRS complexes. This is not only because there is cell to cell conduction from ventricular muscle activation when impulses are conducted down the accessory pathway, but also because the extremely rapid rate of AF made possible by antegrade conduction through the bypass tract causes many of the impulses to reach the ventricle when it is still relatively refractory from previous impulses; this further slows conduction through the ventricle, producing QRS complexes that are distinctly abnormal as well as very prolonged.

The treatment of wide-complex AF secondary to WPW syndrome is unique. Drugs that would normally slow conduction through the AV node are distinctly contraindicated, both because they may actually speed conduction through the bypass tract, thus increasing the ventricular response rate and the risk of hemodynamic instability, and because (even in the absence of increased conduction through the bypass tract) relative blockade of the AV node will cause a higher percentage of impulses to be conducted through the bypass tract, which will itself increase ventricular response. There have been a number of reports of death from refractory ventricular fibrillation in patients with WPW syndrome–related AF who received either verapamil or digitalis preparations. In any case of AF in a patient with known WPW syndrome, or any AF with wide and bizarre QRS complexes, or any patient with wide complexes during AF in which the cause cannot definitively be ascribed to bundle branch block, these drugs are specifically contraindicated. Cardioversion, as described in the chapter *Narrow-Complex Tachycardia*, is the treatment of choice; procainamide is the current pharmacologic agent of choice.

VENTRICULAR FIBRILLATION

Ventricular fibrillation is a terminal rhythm representing random reentry in the ventricular muscle, which cannot produce effective cardiac pumping. It is always important to check a patient's clinical status if ventricular fibrillation appears on a monitor, because the presence of pulses or intact mental status would clearly mean that the monitor is not functioning correctly. In the event of true cardiac arrest, of which ventricular fibrillation is the most common cause in adults, immediate defibrillation in the nonsynchronized mode is by far the most important treatment. When a defibrillator is immediately available no other activities should take precedence. This means that *no* time should be spent starting intravenous lines, securing an airway, performing CPR, or giving drugs, if this delays the performance of electrical defibrillation. Ventricular fibrillation is discussed in detail in a separate chapter.

SUGGESTED READING

Eisenberg MS, Hellstrom A, Bergner L. The ACLS score. JAMA 1981;246:50–52.

Eisenberg MS, Copass MK, Hallstrom AP, Blake B, et al. Treatment of out of hospital cardiac arrests with rapid defibrillation by emergency medical technicians. N Engl J Med 1980;302:1379–1383.

Gascho JA, Crampton RS, Cherwiek ML, Sipes JN, et al. Determinants of ventricular defibrillation in adults. Circulation 1979;60:231–240.

Haynes RE, Chinn TL, Copass MK, Cobb LA: Comparison of bretylium tosalate and lidocaine in management of out-of-hospital ventricular fibrillation: a randomized clinical trial. Am J Cardiol 1981;48:353–356.

Standards and Guidelines for Cardiopulmonary Resuscitation (CPR) and Emergency Cardiac Care (ECC). JAMA. 1980;244:453–509.

Waxman HL, Meyerburg RJ, Appel R, Sung RJ: Verapamil for control of ventricular rate in paroxysmal superventricular tachycardia and atrial fibrillation or flutter. A double-blind, randomized study. Ann Intern Med 1981;94:1–6.

Weaver WD, Cobb LA, Copass MK, Hallstrom AP: Ventricular defibrillation—a comparative trial using 175-J and 320-J shocks. N Engl J Med 1982;307:1101–1106.

NARROW-COMPLEX TACHYCARDIAS

JEROME R. HOFFMAN, M.D.

Although different underlying causes may be responsible for the development of different forms of tachyarrhythmia, and although specific arrhythmias themselves to some extent require different treatments, the basic approach to patients with tachyarrhythmias is relatively simple, and is essentially uniform regardless of the precise arrhythmia involved: Treat the patient, not the electrocardiogram! Although this may seem self-evident, it is truly the underlying principle of management of these patients, and failure to adhere to it is undoubtedly the greatest source of therapeutic errors encountered in this circumstance.

When a patient is brought in with a rapid heart rate, the first job for the emergency physician is to evaluate the patient's stability. Distinctions between wide- and narrow-complex tachycardia, and among the various types of each subgroup, are basically irrelevant, until the primary decision has been made regarding the immediate hemodynamic effect of the arrhythmia. With the exception of sinus tachycardia, a simple rule for all tachyarrhythmias is that patients who are hemodynamically unstable require cardioversion–defibrillation, although those who do not show signs of significant end-organ hypoperfusion may receive pharmacologic therapy, as appropriate. If the patient is in shock, it is truly irrelevant whether he has ventricular tachycardia, atrial flutter, or paroxysmal supraventricular tachycardia, because the treatment for each is identical, involving emergent conversion of the rhythm by electrical means. If and when it is determined that the patient is not hemodynamically unstable, attempts to distinguish the precise arrhythmia are usually (although not always) useful, and can help guide subsequent therapy.

SINUS TACHYCARDIA

Sinus tachycardia is somewhat different from other arrhythmias that are discussed subsequently, so it is dealt with briefly at this point. Sinus tachycardia is a manifestation of a variety of underlying causes, and its general treatment involves attention to and reversal of those underlying causes. By far the most common cause of sinus tachycardia requiring treatment in an emergency department is hypovolemia, and fluid repletion is the treatment of choice. In most instances this is accomplished with a crystalloid solution using relatively rapid infusion rates (300 to 500 ml per hour in a typical adult); bolus infusions of 200 to 500 ml which can be repeated as necessary, are often given. Far greater amounts are used if there is ongoing fluid depletion, as with continuing blood loss. Traumatized patients may require blood replacements as well, although adequate fluid repletion is the first priority, since lack of volume, rather than lack of oxygen carrying capacity, is the primary defect in most patients with traumatic shock. Children with hypovolemic shock should generally receive an initial bolus of 20 ml per kilogram of body weight, and elderly patients, particularly those who are frail and small, and those with underlying heart disease should have their rate of infusion somewhat diminished. There are no magic numbers regarding amounts of fluid required in the wide variety of circumstances that may occur, so the critical element in determination of fluid volumes infused is careful and ongoing monitoring of hemodynamic status.

Other relatively common causes of sinus tachycardia in an emergency department include high fevers, drug overdose, and anxiety. The latter rarely causes heart rates high enough to require any therapy. Adequate treatment of the cause of fever is almost always sufficient (sometimes in association with antipyretic measures), whereas the tachycardia associated with drug overdose is almost always related to venodilation, and thus relative hypovolemia; it should therefore be treated with fluid infusion as described above. The treatment of specific drug overdoses causing tachycardia is outside the scope of this chapter, but occasionally beta-blockade, often in conjunction with other therapy (such as alpha-blockade in amphetamine overdose), may be required. The same is true for patients with thyroid storm, beta-secreting pheochromocytomas,

and other rare conditions. Patients with moderate degrees of tachycardia during the acute evolution of a myocardial infarction may also be at increased risk because of increases in their heart rates (which raises myocardial oxygen consumption), and are also occasionally candidates for emergent beta-blockade. This can be accomplished in most instances with low doses of intravenous propranolol, given at a rate of 1 mg per minute to a total of 4 mg as necessary. It is nevertheless unusual for beta-blockade to be required for the treatment of sinus tachycardia in the emergency department, and when it is called for total dosage should be determined by the response of the patient rather than by any preselected end points.

Distinguishing among the other causes of supraventricular tachycardia on the basis of the electrocardiographic findings is most often, though not always, relatively simple. It is beyond the scope of this chapter to discuss the differences in appearance of the various narrow-complex tachycardias on electrocardiogram, but such a discussion can be found in any number of excellent texts dealing with the interpretation of electrocardiography. In cases in which distinction is extremely difficult, or even impossible, it is fortunate that treatment basically does not vary.

PAROXYSMAL SUPRAVENTRICULAR TACHYCARDIA

Paroxysmal supraventricular tachycardia (PSVT) is perhaps the most common narrow-complex tachycardia, other than sinus tachycardia, encountered in most emergency departments. Most PSVT is caused by reentry phenomena, usually involving two distinct pathways within the atrioventricular (AV) node. Reentry is also the mechanism responsible for PSVT in patients with the Wolff-Parkinson-White (WPW) syndrome, although in this instance one of the two pathways is the bundle of Kent, an accessory pathway that conducts atrial impulses directly to the ventricles, bypassing the AV node. A brief discussion of reentry is necessary to understand the genesis of these arrhythmias, as well as the approach to their treatment.

Three factors are required for the development of reentrant tachycardias: there must be two separate pathways that meet both proximally and distally; there must be differential refractoriness in these two pathways, such that one pathway is blocked while the other is capable of propagating an electrical impulse; and the rate of conduction down the more normal pathway must be slow enough such that the other pathway becomes unblocked, and thus capable of retrograde conduction, by the time the impulse has reached the distal point where the two pathways are joined (Fig. 1). In WPW syndrome, in the absence of PSVT, impulses are propagated antegrade down the bundle of Kent and reach the ventricle rapidly, thus producing a short P-R interval. This is followed by cell-to-cell conduction in the ventricles, prior to the impulse reaching the bundle branches, where normal rapid conduction takes place, and is represented on the electrocardiogram by a delta wave. This delta wave widens the QRS to the same degree that the P-R interval is narrowed.

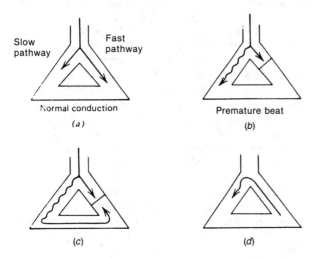

Figure 1 Requirements for reentry. (*a*) Two pathways with differing refractory and conduction patterns, linked by a common distal pathway. A normally conducted impulse enters both pathways and is conducted more rapidly down the fast pathway. (*b*) Disparity in the refractory periods of these pathways allows a premature beat to block in the fast pathway and conduct down the slow pathway. (*c*) Sufficiently slow conduction within the slow pathway allows the fast pathway to regain excitability. (*d*) Conduction of the impulse up the fast pathway. Continued propagation of the impulse in the circuit results in a sustained reentrant arrhythmia. (Reproduced with permission from Morady F, Scheinman, MM: Paroxysmal supraventricular tachycardia. I. Diagnosis. Mod Concepts Cardiovasc Dis 1982; 51:107.)

When a reentrant tachycardia of PSVT occurs in WPW syndrome, the shape of the QRS complexes is determined by the pathway through which impulses are conducted in an antegrade fashion. Thus, when the bundle of Kent is relatively blocked, and impulses are conducted antegrade through the AV node and then retrograde through the accessory pathway, conduction through the ventricle is along the normal portions of the conduction system, and a narrow-complex tachycardia is produced. This is the circumstance in most cases of PSVT associated with WPW syndrome. Much less frequently, antegrade conduction occurs down the accessory pathway, with retrograde conduction through the AV node. In these instances ventricular myocardium is stimulated directly, and propagation of the impulses occurs on a cell-to-cell basis, producing a wide-complex tachycardia, such as would be seen if the impulse initially developed in the ventricle, as in ventricular tachycardia. Indeed, one may not be able to differentiate this wide-complex tachycardia from ventricular tachycardia by surface electrocardiography. Treatment of wide-complex tachycardias is discussed in a separate chapter.

Emergency treatment of narrow-complex PSVT, like all other arrhythmias, is primarily dependent upon its hemodynamic effects. Patients who are hemodynamically unstable with this tachyarrhythmia, as with all other tachyarrhythmias (with the above noted exception of sinus tachycardia), require electrical cardioversion. In all

patients with narrow-complex tachycardias that are cardioverted, the machine should be set in the synchronized mode, such that QRS complexes are sensed, and the electrical current delivered is timed to coincide with these complexes, thus avoiding the possibility of R-on-T or R-on-P phenomena (which can produce ventricular tachycardia or ventricular fibrillation). The energy required for conversion of PSVT is generally small, and 90 percent of such patients can be converted to sinus rhythm with a delivered energy of 20 watt seconds. In those few instances in which such energy doses fail, repeat cardioversion can be attempted, with serial increases in dosage of 40 watt seconds, 80 watt seconds, 150 watt seconds, up to a maximum of 400 watt seconds if absolutely required. It would be extremely unusual for a patient to require more than 100 watt seconds for the conversion of any narrow-complex tachycardia. Patients with atrial flutter can often be converted with as little as 5 watt seconds, although most clinicians would probably use a similar initial dose of perhaps 20 watt seconds in these circumstances. In atrial fibrillation (AF) higher doses are generally needed, as this rhythm is somewhat more refractory to electrical stimulation. Most patients with AF respond to 100 watt seconds, and an initial dose of 50 watt seconds is probably reasonable. Should lower doses fail, 200 watt seconds, and rarely higher doses, may be attempted.

Cardioversion may be accomplished without any premedication if the patient is critically ill and cannot tolerate any delay or if the patient is obtunded. Most other patients with narrow-complex tachycardias, even those requiring emergent cardioversion, should be given a small dose of a sedating medicine prior to the procedure. Most emergency physicians are comfortable with using diazepam intravenously, and doses of 5 mg, repeated as necessary to produce light sedation, are appropriate. Short-acting barbiturates, such as methohexital (Brevital),1 to 2 mg per kilogram, may also be used with great success by physicians familiar with this drug.

When patients with narrow-complex tachycardias are hemodynamically stable, pharmacologic therapy is acceptable and generally appropriate. Hemodynamic stability requires the absence not only of shock, but also of impaired mental status, acute ischemic chest pain, pulmonary edema, and anuria. The last of these is generally not amenable to diagnosis in the emergency department, but the presence of any of the former should be considered indications for emergent therapy with cardioversion. Occasionally, patients have mild chest pain or mild congestive heart failure, signaling the need for rapid therapy, but not necessarily cardioversion. This remains a matter of judgment for the clinician, but it is worth emphasizing that patients with signs of tachycardia-related end-organ hypoperfusion are potentially critically ill, and should be cardioverted if there is significant doubt about their ability to withstand any delay in reversion to a normal cardiac rhythm.

In the past many agents were used to treat hemodynamically stable PSVT. Since the introduction of verapamil, which is effective in converting more than 95 percent of these patients, most other such therapies are rarely used. Although many patients with PSVT can be converted to sinus rhythm without any drugs by the use of vagal maneuvers (such as carotid sinus massage or Valsalva's maneuver), such patients have usually learned to perform these maneuvers themselves, and thus rarely present to an emergency department. Therefore patients who are seen in emergency departments with PSVT rarely respond to vagal maneuvers. These are nevertheless worth trying in most circumstances. Should they fail, therapy with verapamil, a calcium entry blocker, is almost always successful. Verapamil should be given at an initial dose of 5 to 10 mg IV, infused rapidly. A few patients convert virtually immediately, although most patients convert within 2 to 3 minutes. The verapamil dose may be repeated in 10 to 15 minutes if the initial dose does not produce conversions; the repeat dose should be 10 mg IV. Simultaneous use of vagal maneuvers may facilitate conversion, as may concomitant administration of Tensilon, a pharmacologic vagal agent, at a dose of 10 mg IV.

Verapamil is contraindicated in the presence of heart block or significant sinus node disease; it is also contraindicated in the presence of severe congestive heart failure or hypotension. With mild congestive failure, successful termination of the tachycardia in most cases reverses the heart failure, and thus verapamil therapy can be expected to be successful. If there is any question, however, other modalities should be employed. In the presence of hypotension that is hemodynamically significant, cardioversion should be used, as discussed above. With patients who have relatively low blood pressures but are obviously well perfused, use of verapamil may be relatively contraindicated, because its vasodilatory and negative inotropic effects could produce further drops in blood pressure with resultant significant hypotension. In this instance phenylephrine, a direct alpha-agonist, can be combined successfully with verapamil. A phenylephrine infusion, with 5 mg mixed in 50 ml of normal saline, can be begun, with the infusion titrated to produce elevations of systolic blood pressure of 30 to 40 mm Hg. This may sometimes be sufficient to terminate the tachycardia itself, because of reflex increase in vagal tone produced by the elevation in pressure sensed by the carotid body. If this increase in pressure does not produce conversion, further increases should not be attempted, as these may be dangerous; at this point, however, verapamil can be safely used, and should in almost all instances produce reversion to normal sinus rhythm.

In those few patients in whom verapamil cannot be used, and in whom cardioversion is not required, digitalis can be given intravenously for PSVT. Digitalis can be used in a dose of 0.25 mg, with repeat doses up to a total of 1 mg, every half hour. Intravenous digoxin should begin to have an effect in slowing the rate or producing conversion in approximately 20 to 45 minutes.

ATRIAL FIBRILLATION

Patients with AF can present in a wide variety of ways. Some patients with chronic AF, with a relatively well controlled heart rate (less than 100 beats per minute), do not require emergent treatment. Hemodynamically unstable patients with very rapid rates, in the presence of either acute or chronic AF, do require emergent therapy with electrocardioversion. Many patients fall between these two extremes.

Once again the approach to therapy depends on the clinical status of the patient. In general, patients with higher heart rates are more likely to suffer hemodynamic effects from their tachycardias. Patients with relatively rapid rates, but who are not compromised with regard to end-organ perfusion, should have expeditious attempts made to slow their rates. Digitalis, in the form of intravenous digoxin, is the drug most frequently used to accomplish this. Digoxin can be given in the manner described above, although an initial dose of 0.5 mg is not unreasonable in patients with significantly high ventricular responses to atrial fibrillation. In addition, higher total doses of digitalis may be given in this circumstance. Because digoxin does not exert an immediate effect on heart rate, it may be reasonable in some circumstances to treat a patient who is not hemodynamically unstable, but in whom a continued very rapid heart rate over a period of perhaps one-half hour would be considered potentially dangerous, with intravenous verapamil to slow the rate acutely, while simultaneously giving the first dose of intravenous digoxin. In this circumstance verapamil's effect will have worn off by the time the digoxin independently slows the heart rate. In the absence of other contraindications, digoxin and verapamil may be given simultaneously, intravenously, and with caution. Severe heart block is a contraindication to digitalis as well as to verapamil. In addition, intravenous digitalis should be avoided whenever possible in the presence of hypercalcemia, whereas digitalis toxicity is a contraindication to the use of verapamil. Digitalis may be given intravenously in combination with beta-blockade, unlike verapamil.

Patients with acute onset of AF generally respond to cardioversion, although initial energies as high as 100 watt seconds may be required. Patients are less likely to convert to normal sinus rhythm, or to remain in normal sinus rhythm if successfully converted, in the presence of enlarged left atria and/or chronic AF (of longer than 1 year's duration), which are suggested by small "a" waves on the electrocardiogram. Any patient with life-threatening hemodynamic instability should nevertheless have attempts at electrocardioversion, with the recognition that this may not be successful in producing and maintaining sinus rhythm in the presence of chronic AF. Patients with chronic AF who are hemodynamically stable should have their heart rate controlled, as described above, without extensive attempts to achieve normal sinus rhythm. Regardless of the duration of the arrhythmia, elective attempts to restore normal sinus rhythm should not be made without prior anticoagulation, and thus emergency department cardioversion is relatively contraindicated unless continued AF is clearly an acute danger to the patient.

AF of recent onset should generally be accompanied by a heart rate of at least 130 to 150 beats per minute, and lower heart rates, in the absence of digitalis therapy or beta-blockade, should generally be interpreted as indirect evidence of AV nodal disease. In any case, all instances of recent-onset AF require admission to the hospital, as does any tachyarrhythmia producing significant enough hemodynamic changes to require electrical cardioversion.

Wide-complex AF is discussed in the chapter *Wide-Complex Tachycardias*.

ATRIAL FLUTTER

Atrial flutter is so electrosensitive that cardioversion is the treatment of choice in almost all cases. As noted above, it can be successfully performed at extremely low delivered energies. Verapamil converts atrial flutter to sinus rhythm in perhaps 2 to 35 percent of cases and slows the ventricular response in perhaps another 50 percent; it is thus a conceivable alternative if rapid slowing of the rate is required, but cardioversion is for some reason contraindicated. Digitalis can also be used, at doses similar to those listed above, but once again is rarely necessary in the case of atrial flutter, where cardioversion can be easily accomplished in almost all cases. In some instances, however, cardioversion may produce AF, rather than sinus rhythm, and here digitalis can be extremely useful.

SUGGESTED READING

Epstein SE, Goldstein RE, Redwood DR, Kent KM, Smith ER. The early phase of acute myocardial infarction: pharmacologic aspects of therapy. Ann Intern Med 1973; 918–936.

Kuhn M. Verapamil in the treatment of PSVT. Ann Intern Med 1981; 10:538–544.

Lown BE. Electrical reversion of cardiac arrhythmias. Br Heart J 1967; 29:469–489.

Standards and Guidelines for Cardiopulmonary Resuscitation (CPR) and Emergency Cardiac Care (ECC). JAMA 1980; 244:453–509.

Stueven HA, Tonsfeldt DJ, Thompson BM, Whitecombe J, et al. Atropine in asystole: human studies. Ann Emerg Med 1984; 13:815–817.

Waxman HL, Meyerburg RJ, Appel R, Sung RJ. Verapamil for control of ventricular rate in paroxysmal superventricular tachycardia and atrial fibrillation or flutter. A double-blind, randomized study. Ann Intern Med 1981; 94:1–6.

Waxman MD, Sharma AD, Cameron DA, Huerta S, Wald RW. Reflex mechanisms responsible for early spontaneous termination of paroxysmal supraventricular tachycardia. Am J Cardio 1982; 49:259–271.

ATRIAL DYSRHYTHMIA

GERALD P. WHELAN, M.D., F.A.C.E.P.

For our purposes, atrial dysrhythmia refers to abnormalities of impulse generation confined to the atrium. Those generated or sustained by sites outside the atrium are addressed in the chapter on *Narrow-Complex Tachycardias*.

Insofar as ventricular function is not directly affected by atrial dysrhythmias, they are usually less critical than ventricular dysrhythmias. However, there are two circumstances in which they can compromise cardiac output. The first and most common is when an abnormality of atrial rate leads to a parallel ventricular rate producing either a bradycardia or a tachycardia profound enough to impair cardiac output. The second is in the patient with already compromised ventricular function in whom the loss of the atrial component of diastolic filling (the "atrial kick") may tip the balance and produce overt failure.

Atrial dysrhythmias are also unique in that they may appear transiently in normal hearts as a response to physiologic stress, drugs, or noncardiac disease and will often revert to normal when these problems are addressed.

ATRIAL DYSRHYTHMIAS CHARACTERIZED BY ABNORMALITIES OF RATE

Sinus Bradycardia

In sinus bradycardia the only abnormality is the slow rate at which the sinoatrial (SA) node generates impulses. Once the impulse is generated, it is normally conducted producing a systole that is normal except for its slow rate. Hence the P wave, P-R interval, and QRS complexes are all normal. Since cardiac output is a function of both rate and ventricular stroke volume, the output at any given rate depends on that stroke volume. A well-conditioned athlete may have an adequate output at a rate of 50, whereas, a patient with ventricular dysfunction may be profoundly hypotensive at the same rate.

Probably the most critical setting in which sinus bradycardia is encountered is that of acute myocardial infarction (MI), particularly inferior MI. Sinus bradycardia here must be carefully evaluated and therapy judiciously provided or withheld. Although mild bradycardia may be an appropriate physiologic cardiac response that is best left untreated, it may also be the earliest sign of impending and progressive SA or atrioventricular (AV) block or dysfunction.

In the absence of signs of hypoperfusion, such as hypotension or altered mental status, sinus bradycardia needs no treatment. If such signs are present, therapy is directed toward increasing the rate. Intravenous atropine, 0.5 mg, is the initial therapy and can be repeated every 3 to 5 minutes up to a total dose of 2.0 mg. Isoproterenol infusion (2 to 20 μg per minute) may be considered in the symptomatic patient who is refractory to atropine. However, because of its adverse effects on myocardial oxygen consumption and its effect of peripheral vasodilation, it should be used only as a temporizing measure if at all in the face of possible infarction. The definitive therapy is electrical pacing and can be instituted in the emergency department. The new generation of external transcutaneous pacemakers may prove particularly suitable in this setting, allowing insertion of transvenous pacers under much less hurried and harried conditions.

Sinus Tachycardia

To call sinus tachycardia a dysrhythmia is probably a misnomer, since it usually represents an appropriate response to any number of physiologic states in which increased heart rate is of benefit. Alternatively, it may be a response to pharmacologic or metabolic stimuli, but again the pathologic condition is not primarily cardiac.

As in sinus bradycardia, other than the rate of SA node discharge all other aspects of the cycle are normal, including P-wave morphology (although this may be buried in the preceding T wave at rapid rates), P-R interval, and QRS complexes. By definition sinus tachycardia is present at rates in excess of 100, and although some authors accept rates as high as 200, beyond 140 there should be suspicion of another mechanism. This rate cutoff is also significant in that it is unusual to see frank hypotension resulting exclusively from such relatively mild tachycardias. If it is present, a primary source of such hypotension, such as hypovolemia (e.g., hemorrhage, gastrointestinal loss) or ventricular dysfunction (acute MI), should be sought and the tachycardia recognized as compensatory.

Sinus tachycardia must be differentiated from other atrial tachycardias. Its regularity differentiates it from atrial fibrillation and many cases of atrial flutter. Carotid sinus massage (CSM) may be helpful by transiently slowing the rate, revealing discrete normal P waves conducted on a 1:1 basis, or by its failure to terminate the tachycardia, as might occur in paroxysmal atrial tachycardia.

Treatment of sinus tachycardia is always directed at the underlying cause. Hence volume deficits must be corrected, hemorrhage controlled, sympathomimetic drugs discontinued or decreased, infection treated, and metabolic disorders managed. When the tachycardia is compensatory for ventricular dysfunction, inotropic agents such as digoxin may be indicated, as may diuretics in the face of fluid overload.

Sinus Arrhythmia And Sick Sinus Syndrome

A third primary rate abnormality occurs when there is variation in the rate of sinus discharge. One example is sinus arrhythmia, in which the rate cyclically slows coincident with the inspiratory phase of the respiratory cycle. By definition the longest and shortest R-R cycles vary by at least 0.16 msec. This dysrhythmia occurs exclusively in children and young adults, is a purely physiologic variant, and needs no investigation or treatment.

However, in an older patient it may represent the earliest sign of the sick sinus syndrome, the extreme of which would be the so-called bradycardia-tachycardia syndrome. The tachycardic phase usually represents an atrial escape occurring in response to the failure of the SA node to either discharge or conduct its discharge out of the node, and it may take the form of any of the atrial dysrhythmias. In the absence of such escape, there may be syncopal episodes.

Diagnosis is dependent on identifying both phases of the disorder either on electrocardiogram (ECG) or by history. A major mistake would be the use of digoxin in the tachycardic phase, since reversion to the bradycardic phase after digoxin loading might result in worsening of the bradycardia via either SA or AV block. If such a condition is suspect, hospitalization for a temporary transvenous pacer is indicated prior to digitalization. Long-term therapy involves a permanent pacemaker and an appropriate atrial anti-arrhythmic such as quinidine.

All patients with sick sinus syndrome require hospital admission.

ATRIAL DYSRHYTHMIAS CHARACTERIZED BY ECTOPIC IMPULSE GENERATION

Premature Atrial Contractions

Premature atrial contractions (PACs) are complexes that originate from an atrial site outside the SA node and occur early in the cardiac cycle, prior to the next anticipated sinus discharge. Although this may be an abnormal finding, it may also occur in the normal heart in response to stimuli such as stress, caffeine, alcohol, nicotine, or other drugs, or it may occur idiopathically.

Since the impulse arises from an extranodal site and the path of depolarization through the atrium differs from the normal, the P wave displays a different morphology and the P-R interval also differs, usually being shorter. In most cases the PAC depolarizes the SA node and there is a noncompensatory pause before the next sinus beat, i.e., the interval from the P wave of the PAC to the P wave of the subsequent sinus beat is identical, or nearly so, to the previous regular P-P interval. Unless the PAC occurs so early as to find the AV node refractory, it is conducted normally. Absolute refractoriness would block the impulse altogether, resulting in a nonconducted P wave, whereas relative refractoriness would show a P wave with a prolonged P-R interval. Similarly, if the impulse emerging from the AV node finds the ventricular conduction system relatively refractory, aberrant conduction occurs, yielding a wide, bizarre QRS complex. Here it is essential to identify the early abnormal P wave to preclude the misdiagnosis of premature ventricular contraction (PVC), which has significantly different prognostic implications.

PACs usually require no specific therapy other than discontinuance of potential stimulants. However, if the frequency of PACs is sufficient to produce symptoms such as palpitations, or if PACs are implicated in the triggering of sustained narrow-complex tachycardias, suppression with quinidine, procainamide, or beta-blockers may be indicated. Such long-term therapy is best deferred or begun in consultation with the physician who will follow the patient; it rarely needs to be initiated in the emergency department.

Atrial Fibrillation

As the mean age of our population increases and with it the incidence of arteriosclerotic heart disease, atrial fibrillation (AF) is being seen more commonly in the emergency department. It is important to put this dysrhythmia in perspective, particularly in differentiating new-onset AF from chronic AF, since there are significant differences in potential causes and therapy.

Atrial fibrillation represents a random disorganized depolarization of multiple groups of atrial fibers, which pre-empts any dominant pacemaker site. It has two effects on cardiac function. The first is its failure to produce an effective atrial systole and thus any significant contribution to ventricular diastolic filling. The second is a continuous bombarding of the AV node with impulses. Depending on the ability of the AV node to conduct, this leads to a ventricular response that varies continually and may be so fast as to prevent effective ventricular function because of decreased diastolic filling time. The loss of the atrial contribution to diastolic filling is usually only significant if ventricular function is previously compromised for some other reason and can only be regained by conversion to sinus rhythm. However, the decreased diastolic filling can be significantly improved by slowing the ventricular response. This can most easily be accomplished by decreasing the rate of conduction through the AV node; this is the mainstay of therapy in most patients.

New or old, the hallmark of AF is an irregularly irregular ventricular response and an erratic fibrillatory baseline lacking any discrete P waves. With rapid AF it may be difficult to see the baseline, and here CSM can be useful in transiently slowing the tachycardia, allowing the baseline to be seen more easily. If the rapid ventricular response causes the ventricle to be in a sustained state of partial refractoriness or if there is coexisting bundle branch block (not uncommon), there may be confusion as to whether the rhythm is in fact ventricular tachycardia (VT). If the rate is not too fast, the irregularity of the rhythm may be a clue, since VT tends to be regular. Again, CSM may help in the differential diagnosis, as noted previously.

New-onset AF should raise the question of acute myocardial infarction (AMI), pulmonary embolus, or undiagnosed hyperthyroidism, and these require investigation. In an older patient, the bradycardia-tachycardia syndrome should also be considered. It is always desirable to convert patients back to sinus rhythm. Those with new-onset AF have the best prognosis for that by cardioversion, pharmacologically, or spontaneously.

In the patient on chronic AF therapy, there is less concern with conversion. There is, in fact, the danger in converting chronic AF of causing significant embolization, and prophylactic anticoagulation must be considered. More appropriate to the emergency setting is control of the ventricular response by decreasing AV nodal conduction. The drug of choice here continues to be digoxin, since in contrast to other classes of drugs that decrease AV conduction (such as calcium-channel blockers and beta-blockers) it has a positive inotropic effect on the ventricle, which is often failing in the face of rapid AF. Assessing for and correcting hypokalemia should always be a part of digoxin therapy. Digoxin 0.5 mg, can be given slowly intravenously to the nondigitalized patient, with additional 0.25 mg doses given at 2- to 4-hour intervals as response is monitored. Although it may take several hours for digoxin to manifest its inotropic effect, its effect on AV conduction can be seen in 20 to 40 minutes. The end point is a ventricular rate in the 80 to 100 range and not reversion to sinus rhythm.

If a patient presents in AF so rapid as to be the primary cause of *hypoperfusion*, with the associated signs and symptoms of significant hypotension, chest pain, pulmonary edema, and/or altered mentation, immediate termination of the tachycardia must be achieved. In this setting, electrical cardioversion is the only approach that provides immediate relief. Synchronization minimizes the chance of ventricular fibrillation and an initial setting of 25 to 50 joules may be tried, although most AF requires 100 joules for conversion. Pretreatment with an amnesic sedative such as intravenous diazepam, 10 mg, should be considered in the alert patient.

If such a patient presents who is already on digoxin, cardioversion can be safely attempted provided electrolyte imbalance is corrected and attempts are titrated beginning with low energy levels (10 watts per second). Noncompliance or subtherapeutic digoxin levels must always be considered since rapid ventricular rates are virtually never seen with adequate digitalization. Hence digoxin levels should be drawn before any additional digoxin is administered, although treatment cannot await the results. Other options include cautious cardioversion after pretreatment with lidocaine (1 mg per kilogram intravenously) or use of other agents to impede AV conduction such as verapamil, 5 to 10 mg intravenously, or propranolol, 1 to 2 mg intravenously. As noted previously, use of these agents carries a risk of worsening ventricular function. However if the tachycardia itself is the primary cause of cardiac failure, such therapy is logical.

Occasionally a patient with chronic AF who is receiving digoxin may present not with tachycardia, but with bradycardia in the range of 60 and with regular ventricular complexes. This is pathognomonic of digitoxicity with complete AV block and junctional escape. Treatment here is withholding of digoxin and hospital admission.

A special case of AF is that of paroxysmal atrial fibrillation (PAF) occurring in the patient with Wolff-

Parkinson-White syndrome. Again this is more extensively discussed in the chapter on *Narrow-Complex Tachycardias*, but it should be noted that in this setting the goal is not to block normal AV conduction, but rather to impede conduction over the accessory tract. Here a type I antiarrhythmic such as lidocaine (1 mg per kilogram intravenously) or procainamide would be most appropriate.

Atrial Flutter

Atrial flutter is a relatively rare dysrhythmia, and unlike any of the other atrial dysrhythmias, it generally occurs only in the presence of atrial distention caused by primary cardiac or pulmonary disease, although it can be seen in the setting of acute MI or as the tachycardic phase of the bradycardia-tachycardia syndrome. It also tends to be transient, either converting back to sinus rhythm or degenerating into atrial fibrillation before too long.

An ectopic atrial focus usurps pacemaker function by discharging at a rate of 280 to 300, thereby pre-empting any sinus or AV pacer sites. Unlike atrial fibrillation, atrial flutter is characterized by an orderly depolarization and contraction of the atrium, but because of its rapidity, the atrial contribution to ventricular diastolic filling is questionable.

Impulses are conducted through the AV node, and ventricular response becomes a function of the degree of AV conduction. Fortunately, in most cases there is a 2:1 AV block with a resultant ventricular rate of 140 to 150. In fact, a regular ventricular rate in this range should always raise the question of atrial flutter. If the AV block is in the 3:1 or 4:1 range, the resultant ventricular rate may be in a normal range of 70 to 100 and the patient may be asymptomatic. On the other hand, if there is no physiologic AV block and 1:1 conduction ensues, the ventricular rate becomes intolerable at 280 to 300, a rate too rapid to sustain a cardiac output. It is also possible to have varying degrees of AV block in either an orderly or random variance. Hence atrial flutter has the distinction of being the only dysrhythmia in which the ventricular response may be regular, regularly irregular, or irregularly irregular.

Critical to the identification of atrial flutter is the recognition of the saw-toothed F or flutter waves in the baseline. These may be poorly seen in the standard leads and may require special leads such as V_3R (Fig. 1). Response to CMS is similar to AF in that there is only transient slowing, eliminating paroxysmal atrial tachycardia from the diagnosis, but sometimes unmasking previously hidden flutter waves. Unless there is ventricular refractoriness or bundle branch block, the QRS complex is normal.

Since atrial flutter is uniquely sensitive to cardioversion, this is the first line of therapy. Flutter may convert with as little as 10 joules of synchronized countershock. Smaller doses may be dangerous, actually converting the flutter to fibrillation. Obviously if the patient is awake, pretreatment with 5 to 10 mg of intravenous diazepam or another sedative is indicated. Repeated attempts at cardioversion using increments of 10 joules may be at-tempted, but probably no more than six times nor beyond 100 joules. If this is unsuccessful, the patient may be digitalized. This sequence is considerably safer than cardioversion after digitalization. Digitalization can proceed as in AF, with 0.5 mg given slowly intravenously after checking potassium levels and repeated doses of 0.25 mg every 2 to 4 hours as needed. Slowing of the ventricular response can be expected as in AF, but unlike AF conversion to sinus rhythm is the expected end point.

Alternatively or in addition to digoxin, other drugs that slow AV conduction may be considered. Verapamil, 5 to 10 mg given slowly intravenously, will convert a small number of patients, but slow the ventricular rate (by A-V block) in most. Its rapid onset has made it more popular than the beta-blockers, which also slow AV conduction, but drugs such as intravenous propranolol, 1 to 2 mg given slowly, are still useful in slowing ventricular response. Beta-blockers do carry the risk of impairing ventricular contractility and worsening failure, as do calcium-channel blockers to a lesser degree. Hence they probably should not be used together, although either can be used in conjunction with digoxin.

The availability of calcium-channel blockers has probably all but eliminated the need to resort to the use of quinidine or procainamide in the termination phase (as opposed to the prophylaxis phase) of management of atrial flutter. However, if these agents are used it is essential to pretreat with one of the drugs that will increase AV block (digoxin, verapamil, or propranolol), since prior to the suppression of the ectopic flutter focus, quinidine or procainamide may first enhance AV conduction with a paradoxical increase in the ventricular rate and worsening of the clinical condition.

Multifocal Atrial Tachycardia

Multifocal atrial tachycardia (MAT) is a potentially fatal atrial dysrhythmia seen almost exclusively in the setting of decompensated chronic pulmonary disease.

It is characterized by the appearance of three or more morphologically different P-wave configurations (usually with differing P-R intervals as well) in a single ECG lead with a ventricular response in excess of 100 (Fig.2).

Despite its apparent similarity to atrial fibrillation, it is not responsive to digoxin, and aggressive treatment with digoxin could further compound the situation by inducing digitoxicity. Such patients are often on a number of medications that may have cardiac effects (e.g., beta-agonist bronchodilators and theophylline); it is difficult to elucidate a clear etiology, but in the vast majority of cases hypoxia appears to be a major factor, hence the appearance of this dysrhythmia concurrent with decompensation.

Since most treatments have been either ineffective (digoxin and cardioversion) or contraindicated (beta-blockers worsen bronchoconstriction), attention has been directed primarily to treating the hypoxia by means of brochodilators, ventilatory support, and antibiotic therapy of infections. While these should continue to be the mainstays of therapy, encouraging results using a single

LEAD 1

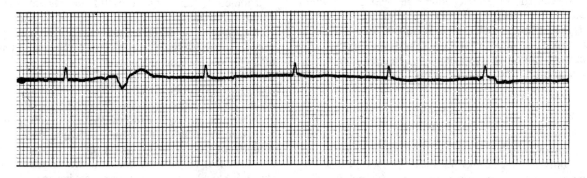

LEAD aVr

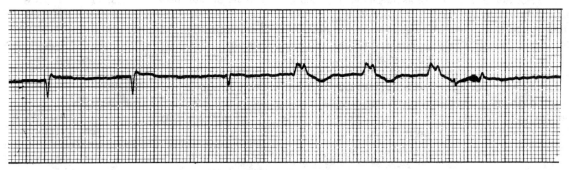

LEAD V₂

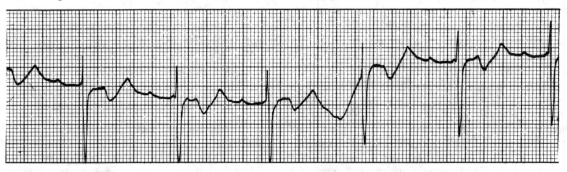

LEAD V₃R

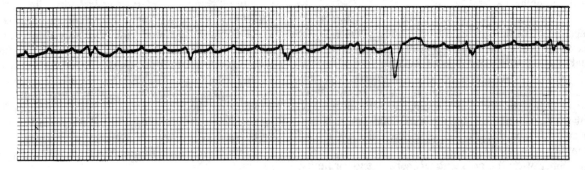

Figure 1 Atrial flutter poorly visible in leads I, aVr, and V₂ but clearly seen in lead V₃R.

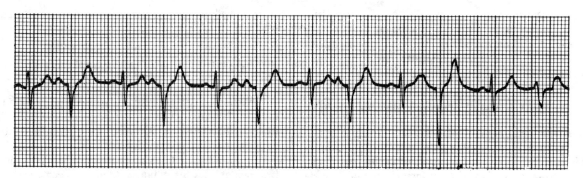

Figure 2. Multifocal atrial tachycardia showing multiple P-wave configurations in one lead.(From Instructors manual for advanced cardiac life support. Am Heart Assoc. 1982: 421.)

dose of 5 to 10 mg of verapamil intravenously have been obtained in rapidly terminating the tachycardia.

PRE-HOSPITAL CARE OF ATRIAL DYSRHYTHMIAS

Common to all of the atrial dysrhythmias and most relevant to the pre-hospital care (PHC) setting is their variable presentation, depending on the actual ventricular rates, the duration of the dysrhythmia, and prior ventricular function.

Thus such patients fall into one of two categories regardless of the specific underlying dysrhythmia, namely, those stable enough to transport without treatment in the field and those in whom acute decompensation warrants immediate intervention.

Symptomatic bradycardia can safely be treated using intravenous atropine in the doses already described and isoproterenol infusions in transit if absolutely needed. Pacemakers are generally not available in the PHC setting, although external pacers may change future PHC capabilities.

The tachycardic patient with a systolic blood pressure below 90 who is deteriorating in the field and who additionally manifests signs of cerebral hypoperfusion (unconsciousness or deteriorating mental status), pulmonary edema, or chest pain becomes a candidate for synchronized cardioversion without much time being spent elucidating the specific nature of the tachycardia. Patients

in this category should not need further sedation. The initial delivered charge should reflect the critical situation and begin with a higher than usual setting of 50 joules.

CSM may be tried as the defibrillator is being set up, but no time should be wasted with this maneuver. On the other hand, if the patient is relatively stable, CSM is contraindicated in the field because of the danger of induction of complete AV block with or without ventricular escape. Such complications are clearly better dealt with in the controlled environment of the emergency department.

The only drug likely to be effective in the pre-hospital treatment of tachyarrhythmias is a calcium-channel blocker such as verapamil. To date, experience with this drug in the PHC setting is too limited to make a recommendation regarding its use.

SUGGESTED READING

Ali N, et al. Titrated electrical cardioversion in patients on digoxin. Clin Cardiol 1982; 5:417–419.

Benditt DG, et al. Atrial flutter, atrial fibrillation, and other primary atrial tachycardias. Med Clin North Am 1984; 68:895–919.

Brashear RE. Arrhythmias in patients with chronic obstructive pulmonary disease. Med Clin North Am 1984; 68:969-981.

Levine JH, Michael JR, Guarnieri T. Treatment of multifocal atrial tachycardia with verapamil. N Engl J Med 1985; 312:21–25.

Swiryn S, McDonough T, Hueter DC. Sinus node function and dysfunction. Med Clin North Am 1984; 68:935-955.

PREMATURE VENTRICULAR BEATS

BERNARD TABATZNIK, M.D., F.R.C.P.

The ventricular ectopic beat (VEB) has been described as both a "trick of the healthy heart" (Evans) and a "harbinger of sudden death" (Lown). Finding a proper balance between overkill and underplay in the

treatment of the patient with extrasystoles requires a careful assessment of the importance of a particular ectopic rhythm in a particular individual, mature judgment, and a modicum of courage. Factors that determine the prognostic role of the VEB in an individual patient are first and foremost "the company it keeps" and also certain qualitative features of the ectopic activity. These, together with a critical appreciation of the efficacy and dangers of antiarrhythmic drug therapy, form a clinical tripod that determines treatment in a given patient. The association of ventricular ectopy with sudden death in myocardial infarction has led to an instinct to regard all ventricular ectopy as malignant, but this must be resisted. Although the emergency physician usually treats only life-threatening ectopy, it is necessary to be familiar with the full spectrum of drugs and management because patients often come to the emergency department for evaluation and reassurance.

VENTRICULAR ECTOPIC ACTIVITY: CLINICAL CONTEXT

A simplistic view of sudden death is that it results from an interaction between the "seed" (ventricular ectopic activity), the "soil" (the state of the myocardium), and "spring rains" (a variety of factors, including acute ischemia; central and automatic nervous system factors; and metabolic factors, such as hypokalemia, drug effects, anoxia, and extremes of heat and cold, which may render cardiac tissue abnormally excitable and act as the trigger mechanism for ventricular fibrillation). Thus, even highly complex ventricular ectopic activity, such as ventricular tachycardia, seldom progresses to ventricular fibrillation if the heart is structurally normal; bizarre ventricular arrhythmias in patients with mitral valve prolapse may be observed for long periods of time without leading to sudden death; and the risk of sudden death is seemingly lessened in the surgically revascularized patient even though ventricular ectopic activity has not been substantially reduced.

On the other hand, even minor ventricular ectopic activity may result in ventricular tachycardia or fibrillation in the patient with an acutely injured heart as, for example, in acute myocardial infarction or acute myocarditis. Between these categories are patients with VEBs in association with chronic ischemic heart disease, hypertrophic cardiomyopathy, and the concentrically hypertrophied hearts of hypertension and aortic valve stenosis, the dilated hearts of chronic rheumatic valvular disease and congestive cardiomyopathy, the long Q-T syndromes, and survivors of ventricular fibrillation, all with varying degrees of susceptibility to sudden death. Within the category of chronic ischemic disease itself, the risk varies appreciably from high risk in the first 6 months after infarction, particularly in patients with compromised left ventricular function, to a much lower risk in the long-term survivor with efficient myocardial function. In the high-risk groups, the most intensive measures needed to suppress ventricular ectopic activity are justified, whereas in low-risk groups, antiarrhythmic drug therapy should be undertaken only after due consideration of the total clinical picture.

It is therefore particularly relevant in emergency situations that the clinical context be accurately appraised in the patient who presents with ventricular ectopic activity. For example, if a patient seeks emergency department advice for palpitations due to ventricular bigeminy and is found to have a normal heart or mitral valve prolapse, reassurance and an early referral back to the primary physician usually suffices. Conversely, if ventricular ectopy is associated with an acute ischemic syndrome such as myocardial infarction or unstable angina, suppression of the ectopic activity with intravenous lidocaine and admission to a monitored area such as the coronary care unit is indicated.

PROGNOSTIC CHARACTERISTICS OF VENTRICULAR ECTOPY

Numerous studies have confirmed a prognostic role for complex ventricular ectopy in patients with chronic ischemic heart disease. Although there have been different definitions of complexity and much argument about the value and limitations of various grading systems for Holter-identified arrhythmias, there has been an association in most studies between complex ventricular ectopic rhythms and both sudden and nonsudden cardiac death. Some studies (including my own) have shown a near-linear association between complexity and sudden death; others have indicated a prognostic role for only the more severe grades of ectopy, such as ventricular tachycardia. Many studies have demonstrated a prognostic power for ventricular ectopy independent of other factors, such as myocardial dysfunction. Much of the confusion in this area has stemmed from the fact that left ventricular dysfunction is also an important predictor of mortality; it has been difficult to separate the respective prognostic roles of ventricular ectopy and ventricular dysfunction, particularly when the two conditions coexist. However, there is sufficient evidence indicating a prognostic role for ventricular ectopic activity over and above that which is seen in patients with severe left ventricular dysfunction to warrant a positive approach to the treatment of patients with frequent (20 per minute) VEBs, multiformity, pairs, runs, and the R-on-T phenomenon.

Ventricular parasystole may have a lower risk of ventricular fibrillation than have VEBs with a fixed coupling interval because it is an automatic rather than a re-entrant rhythm that is protected against a rapid discharge rate by the phenomenon of exit block. Parasystole can be recognized on the standard electrocardiogram (ECG) by the marked variation in coupling interval between the ectopic beat and the preceding sinus beat; paired beats and fusion beats are frequently seen. *Ventricular escape beats*, easily recognizable by their prolonged coupling intervals, are protective of cardiac output during bradycardia and should not be suppressed.

INITIAL MANAGEMENT OF PATIENTS WITH VEBs

For the patient presenting to the emergency department with ventricular ectopy, an initial evaluation must be made of the etiology and severity of the underlying cardiac condition. Qualitative features of the ectopic activity must be analyzed in order to assess the risk of deterioration toward ventricular tachycardia or fibrillation. Potential precipitating factors such as hypokalemia, hypomagnesemia, digitalis toxicity, and the use of arrhythmogenic substances must be explored, and historical information must be obtained regarding the presence and extent of preexisting arrhythmias. The patient whose rhythm strip shows unifocal VEBs, ventricular parasystole, ventricular bigeminy, or accelerated idioventricular rhythm requires less vigorous therapy than the patient with frequent multiform VEBs, couplets, or runs.

On the other hand, if the presenting clinical diagnosis is an acute cardiac ischemic syndrome or a cardiomyopathy with a high propensity for ventricular fibrillation, aggressive measures are indicated to suppress the ventricular ectopic activity. Treatment is generally initiated with intravenous lidocaine, given in a bolus of 50 to 100 mg over a period of 1 minute and repeated in 5 to 10 minutes in order to maintain an adequate serum level. Simultaneously, a constant intravenous infusion of 1 to 4 mg per minute is given, the dose depending on age, body weight, and most importantly the presence or absence of congestive heart failure because the drug is metabolized in the liver. Some patients are exquisitely sensitive to lidocaine and may develop mental confusion, hallucinations, or grand mal seizures after relatively small doses. Fortunately, a sensitivity to lidocaine does not portend a sensitivity to procainamide, which is a very effective alternative to lidocaine. The initial dose is 1 g given as a slow intravenous bolus over 15 to 20 minutes together with an intravenous maintenance dose of 2 to 5 mg per minute. Patients who have been selected for intravenous lidocaine or procainamide therapy are subsequently transferred to a monitored area such as a coronary or progressive care unit for stabilization of the arrhythmia.

When aggressive measures are not needed, the physician must make a judgment on the potential of the ventricular ectopic rhythm to adversely affect longevity. *Historical information* on possible precipitants requires an assessment of the effect of cigarette smoking, alcohol, caffeine intake, physical activity, rest, fatigue, and emotional stress on the frequency and severity of symptoms. An intimate inquiry regarding medications being used, particularly psychotropic drugs, agents containing ephedrine or epinephrine, appetite suppressants, thyroid replacement drugs, digitalis, and diuretics, may yield a remediable cause for the arrhythmia. Recently, hypomagnesemia has also been recognized as a potent cause of ventricular arrhythmia.

Physical examination is directed at determining clinical associations such as a normal heart, mitral valve prolapse, and other forms of valvular disease; chronic ischemic heart disease with or without ventricular aneurysm; and hypertrophic or dilated cardiomyopathy and at assessing the severity of the disease in view of the established correlation between ventricular ectopy, ventricular dysfunction, and mortality.

Laboratory studies are directed specifically at renal and electrolyte function with emphasis on both serum potassium and magnesium levels. For the patient with symptomatic ventricular ectopy and a normal heart or mitral valve prolapse, the patient should be reassured in unequivocal terms of the benign nature of the ectopic rhythm in his or her particular clinical context. In addition, the cyclic behavior of ectopic rhythms should be emphasized because the patient may wonder whether the "skipped-beats" rhythm will ever disappear. In contemporary clinical practice, the patient with mitral valve prolapse and ventricular ectopy is at greater risk of suffering intractable neuroticism than of dying of ventricular fibrillation. Only the patient who has massive prolapse as seen on the echocardiogram (ECG), associated with documented ventricular tachycardia or exercise-induced ventricular ectopy and repolarization abnormalities on the resting ECGs, should be singled out for treatment if he or she is asymptomatic.

Although it is the exception rather than the rule for ectopic rhythms to respond to the withdrawal of cigarettes, alcohol, and caffeine, an attempt to eliminate these cardiac stimulants should always be made. Greater success might be anticipated from the discontinuation of a medication that has arrhythmogenic properties or from the correction of an electrolyte abnormality.

DRUG THERAPY

The emergency physician should virtually never initiate drug therapy in patients not needing hospital admission, but he must be familiar with outpatient regimens. All patients on such therapy should be managed by a primary physician such as an internist. Pharmacologic therapy in the patient with VEBs must be considered within the following context:

1. No randomized study has yet demonstrated a reduction in sudden-death mortality in groups of patients on antiarrhythmic drug therapy. However, suppression of ventricular arrhythmias with intravenous lidocaine or procainamide reduces the frequency of ventricular fibrillation in the early phases of acute myocardial infarction.
2. The adage that "the treatment may be worse than the disease" is applicable. Membrane-stabilizing or type 1A agents, such as quinidine, procainamide, and disopyramide, may prolong the Q-T interval and lead to the polymorphic type of ventricular tachycardia known as "torsade de pointes." Even in the absence of Q-T prolongation, these agents may exacerbate the arrhythmia under treatment. The frequency with which these drugs aggravate or induce major arrhythmias is estimated at approximately 10 percent, with a somewhat greater frequency for quinidine.
3. There are no well-defined end points in the treatment of the asymptomatic patient, other than reduction in mortality. Whereas it is comforting to the physician to see a reduction of 70 percent to 90 percent in the frequency of VEBs or to eliminate the more complex forms, such as pairs or runs of ventricular ectopic activity, these may not necessarily result in a reduction in ventricular fibrillation and sudden death. Conversely, failure to reduce ventricular ectopic activity may not be synonymous with failure to prevent ventricular fibrillation. One recent study suggests that the end point of treatment should be a consistently maintained therapeutic drug level in the serum, regardless of the effect on the frequency or complexity of the ectopic activity. The management of ventricular arrhythmias

would be revolutionized should this theory be confirmed.

It is essential that the physician set realistic objectives when treating the patient with ventricular ectopy; it is seldom possible to eliminate the arrhythmia entirely. For the symptomatic patient, the prime goal should be the control of symptoms. For the asymptomatic patient with potentially dangerous arrhythmias, the goal should be a reduction of the higher grade of ectopy. If this cannot be achieved, one should aim at maintaining an adequate blood level of the drug. For all patients with ventricular ectopic activity short of ventricular tachycardia and fibrillation, the principle of treatment should be to treat "cheaply," that is, to strive for a defined therapeutic goal without inducing significant side effects.

Based on these principles, the initial antiarrhythmic drug of choice for the ambulant patient is a *beta-blocking agent* because these agents are far freer of side effects than the membrane-stabilizing drugs. Unfortunately, their efficacy in controlling ventricular ectopic activity is often less than that of quinidine, procainamide, and disopyramide. They are more likely to be effective when the resting heart rate is above 70 beats per minute, and they are particularly effective in exercise-induced ventricular ectopy. However, their use is limited in the presence of sinus bradycardia, and they are contraindicated in the patient with congestive heart failure (CHF). Differences between beta-blocking drugs in terms of their membrane-stabilizing activity are of little practical importance; all of the currently available agents have adequate antiarrhythmic activity in standard dosages. Their side effects and contraindications are well known.

The *type-1A antiarrhythmic agents* are generally effective, either alone or in combination with a beta-blocking drug, in controlling VEBs. However, the high incidence of side effects with all three agents of this type is a major limiting factor. *Quinidine* is the prototype antiarrhythmic drug; the gluconate and polygalacturonate forms produce fewer gastrointestinal side effects. The standard therapeutic dose is between 800 and 1,600 mg of quinidine per 24 hours. Immediate side effects are diarrhea and other gastrointestinal symptoms. These occur within 1 or 2 days of starting the drug and may affect as many as 25 percent of patients using quinidine. If a patient has previously been sensitized to quinidine, fever or other major side effects, such as thrombocytopenic purpura or agranulocytosis, may occur after a single dose. Symptoms of cinchonism may appear in sensitive persons. Quinidine augments serum digoxin levels and may induce toxicity in patients on a previously well-tolerated dose of digitalis. It prolongs appreciably the Q-T interval and may lead to torsade de pointes or "quinidine syncope." It is estimated that it may aggravate ventricular arrhythmias either through the mechanism of Q-T prolongation or through other mechanisms in 15 percent of patients. Hence, only about one-half of patients treated with quinidine are able to use the drug on a long-term basis.

The side effects of *procainamide* therapy are equally common. Although early gastrointestinal side effects and hypersensitivity are much less frequent than with quinidine, the late development of a positive antinuclear antibody (ANA) titer occurs in approximately 70 percent of patients and the clinical lupus erythematosus syndrome in over one-half of them. Prolongation of intraventricular conduction time (QRS duration) and Q-T interval occur with procainamide as well as with quinidine, and it is estimated that procainamide may be arrhythmogenic in approximately 10 percent of patients.

Disopyramide (Norpace) has an antiarrhythmic spectrum similar to that of quinidine and procainamide, but it is often effective when the latter has failed. Unfortunately, it has an even greater frequency of side effects than its counterparts. Anticholinergic side effects, including urinary hesitancy and retention, constipation, dryness of the mouth, and blurring of vision, limit its usefulness appreciably, particularly in older male populations with potential prostate problems. Furthermore, the unusually potent negative inotropic action of disopyramide contraindicates its use in the presence of impaired ventricular function. It prolongs the Q-T interval and has often been incriminated as a cause of torsade de pointes. Like quinidine, it can depress sinus node automaticity in patients with sinoatrial dysfunction. The effective daily dose is between 300 and 800 mg.

Lidocaine is the most widely used antiarrhythmic drug in emergency medical practice. It is classified as a type 1B antiarrhythmic agent, differing from the type 1A agent mainly in its effect on cellular repolarization. Because it shortens the Q-T interval, it is much less proarrhythmic than the type 1A agents. It has the further advantage of not depressing myocardial contractility and is therefore the drug of choice in patients with ventricular ectopy complicating congestive heart failure and acute ischemic states. It is available only in parenteral form and is generally administered as an intravenous bolus in conjunction with a constant intravenous infusion. The major side effects are neurologic and range from drowsiness and confusion to frank seizures.

Phenytoin sodium (Dilantin) has electrophysiologic effects similar to those of lidocaine. It is probably the least effective of currently available antiarrhythmic agents, except in the case of digitalis-induced atrial or ventricular arrhythmias. Its use in the management of patients with symptomatic or asymptomatic VEBs is generally confined to those who have either developed side effects or failed to respond to a combination of beta-blocker and a type 1A antiarrhythmic drug. It may be used in combination with other antiarrhythmics; however, it does reduce serum quinidine levels. The usual maintenance dose is between 300 and 400 mg a day; the most important side effects are neurologic (drowsiness, nystagmus, ataxia, and nausea) and generally correlate with elevated blood levels of the drug.

Although other drugs, such as digitalis, atropine, and isoproterenol, have been used for the treatment of ventricular ectopy in certain specific clinical settings, they are more likely to induce ectopy than to control it. Imipramine (Tofranil) has recently been shown to have antiarrhythmic properties, but it has not yet been approved for this indication. None of the calcium-channel blocking agents in current use has any direct effect on ventricular ectopy.

New Antiectopic Drugs

Tocainide HCl (Tonocard), another type 1B antiarrhythmic agent, may prove to be as effective as the type 1A agents, but it has the advantages of not prolonging the Q-T interval; not affecting sinus node function, AV conduction, or His-Purkinje conduction; and not depressing myocardial contractility. A response to intravenous lidocaine predicts a response to tocainide in the majority of cases. The daily dose is 1,200 to 1,800 mg in divided doses of either 400 or 600 mg tablets three times a day. The important side effects are neurologic (lightheadedness, parasthesia, and tremor), nausea, and rash.

Mexiletine (Mexitil) is yet another lidocaine-like oral drug recently approved for the suppression of VEBs. Apparently mexiletine is very similar to tocainide in efficacy and side effects. Overall experience with this drug is limited in the United States, although it has been used extensively in Europe for several years.

Flecainide and *encainide* are type 1C antiarrhythmic agents. They exert a greater depressant effect on phase 0 depolarization than do type 1A and 1B agents, suppress intracardiac conduction particularly of the His-Purkinje system, and have little effect on repolarization. Hence they might be expected to be more effective than type 1A and 1B agents in suppressing VEBs and less proarrhythmic than type 1A agents. Early clinical experience, particularly with flecainide, tends to confirm these expectations. Flecainide acetate (Tambocor) is highly effective against both atrial and ventricular ectopic rhythms. Its side effects (dizziness, blurred vision, headache, and nausea) occur in fewer than 20 percent of patients, tend to be dose related, and seldom require discontinuation of the drug. It prolongs the QRS duration and the P-R interval and must therefore be used with caution in patients with bundle branch block or with P-R intervals exceeding 0.28 seconds. It should not be used in patients with sinoatrial dysfunction, second degree AV block, or congestive heart failure, because it has a significant negative inotropic action (a property not shared by encainide). It is proarrhythmic in 7 to 10 percent of patients, but no serious proarrhythmic effects have been observed in patients with ventricular ectopy short of ventricular tachycardia. The usual therapeutic dose is 100 mg every 12 hours, and the total daily dose should not exceed 400 mg.

Amiodarone (Cordarone) is perhaps the most efficacious antiarrhythmic agent currently available for the suppression of ventricular ectopy. However, the side effects are serious enough to limit its use to strictly life-threatening situations such as recurrent ventricular tachycardia or ventricular fibrillation, a topic beyond the scope of this chapter. Similar considerations apply to the use of *bretylium*.

SUGGESTED READING

Evans W. Diseases of the heart and arteries. 1st ed. Baltimore: Williams & Wilkins, 1964.

Lown B, Wolf M. Approaches to sudden death from coronary heart disease. Circulation 1971; 44:130–142.

Myerburg RJ, Kessler KM, Kiem I, Peskarios KC, Conde CA, Cooper D, Castellonas A. Relationship between plasma levels of procainamide, suppression of premature ventricular complexes and prevention of recurrent ventricular tachycardia. Circulation 1981; 64:280–290.

Siddoway LA, Roden DM, Woosley RL. Clinical pharmacology of old and new antiarrhythmic drugs. In: Josephson ME, ed. Sudden cardiac death. In: 15/3 Cardiovasc Clin. Philadelphia: FA Davis, 1985:199.

Velebit V, Podrid PJ, Lown B, Cohen B, Graboys TB. Aggravation and provocation of ventricular arrhythmias by antiarrhythmic drugs. Circulation 1982; 65:885–894.

IMPLICATIONS AND PHARMACOLOGIC TREATMENT OF CARDIAC CONDUCTION BLOCK

SCOTT A. SYVERUD, M.D.

This chapter reviews the therapy and prognostic implications of cardiac conduction blocks, including sinoatrial block and first-, second-, and third-degree heart block.

SINOATRIAL BLOCK

Sinoatrial (SA) block refers to a condition in which sinus node impulses are not conducted to the atria and do not result in atrial contraction. Resulting dysrhythmias include sinus arrest and sinus bradycardia. SA block is one manifestation of "sick sinus syndrome" (SSS), which is characterized by episodes of bradycardia accompanied by evidence of impaired cerebral perfusion. The bradycardia may be a sinus bradycardia, sinus arrest, or an atrial bradycardia alternating with a regular or irregular atrial tachycardia (tachy-brady syndrome).

Patients with SA block or SSS frequently have intrinsic sinus node fibrosis and are at high risk of suffering an embolic event or life-threatening dysrhythmia. Diagnosis is based on a history of symptomatic dysrhythmias and on electrophysiologic testing. Placement of a permanent pacemaker is the definitive therapy.

SA block and SSS rarely require emergent therapy in the emergency department (ED). The key role of the emergency physician is to suspect the diagnosis and to arrange admission to a monitored bed and consultation for appropriate electrophysiologic testing. Rare patients with SSS require therapy in the ED for a persistent bradycardia that is hemodynamically compromising (to be discussed).

FIRST-DEGREE HEART BLOCK

With first-degree atrioventricular block there is a delay in the conduction of normal sinus node impulses from the atria to the ventricles. All impulses are conducted (each P wave is followed by a QRS complex), but the PR interval is longer than 0.20 seconds.

This rhythm, by itself, does not cause hemodynamic compromise and does not require treatment. The clinical setting in which it is diagnosed determines the course of further evaluation. First-degree block can be seen as a normal variant in healthy individuals without organic heart disease. When seen in association with acute myocardial infarction, the block may progress to a conduction abnormality of higher degree or be accompanied by significant sinus bradycardia. First-degree block associated with drug toxicity (e.g., digoxin) resolves with clearance of the drug.

SECOND-DEGREE HEART BLOCK

With second-degree atrioventricular block, some but not all sinus impulses are conducted to the ventricle. *Mobitz type I* second-degree heart block is characterized by progressive PR interval prolongation culminating in a nonconducted P wave (Wenckebach phenomenon). *Mobitz type II* second-degree heart block is characterized by intermittent nonconducted P waves in the absence of preceding PR interval prolongation.

Mobitz type I block is commonly associated with acute inferior wall myocardial infarction or drug toxicity and does not usually cause hemodynamic compromise. Atropine therapy alone is usually sufficient therapy for resulting symptomatic bradycardia. Mobitz type I block rarely progresses to third-degree heart block. In contrast, Mobitz type II block is commonly associated with acute anterior wall myocardial infarction. In this setting, patients are at high risk of progressing to third-degree heart block and death. Emergent prophylactic transvenous pacemaker insertion is indicated in these patients (see next chapter on *Emergency Pacemaker Insertion and Malfunction*).

THIRD-DEGREE HEART BLOCK

With third-degree atrioventricular block, no atrial impulses are conducted to the ventricle. This rhythm is usually seen in patients with Lev's disease (conduction system sclerosis) or in the setting of acute myocardial infarction. When associated with acute inferior wall infarction, the resulting ventricular escape rhythm is usually a junctional rhythm at a rate greater than 40. Hemodynamic compromise, if present, usually responds to drug therapy.

Third-degree heart block is much more ominous when seen in the setting of acute anterior infarction. In these cases the ventricular escape rhythm is usually idioventricular at a rate less than 40. Hemodynamic compromise is usually present and is frequently resistant to drug therapy. Third-degree heart block requires emergent pacing in any patient who is hemodynamically compromised or who has an acute anterior myocardial infarction.

THERAPY

Patients with hemodynamically compromising bradycardias require emergent therapy in the emergency department. Included in this category are patients with angina, pulmonary edema, refractory ectopy, evidence of decreased cerebral perfusion (stroke, altered mental status), or hypotension. Pacing is the definitive therapy for bradycardia in this setting and should be instituted as soon as possible. Drug therapy can be used as a temporizing measure to stabilize these patients for a short interval while preparations are made for transvenous pacemaker placement.

Atropine is the first-line drug therapy for bradycardia. If the response to atropine is inadequate, isoproterenol or vasopressors may be used. As noted subsequently, isoproterenol is associated with significant complications and should be used with extreme caution. Transcutaneous pacing, when available, may obviate the need for temporizing drug therapy.

Atropine

Atropine is an anticholinergic agent that increases heart rate due to a vagolytic effect. Subtherapeutic doses may result in a paradoxical bradycardic response due to a central vagotonic effect. Atropine has no effect on denervated hearts (heart transplant patients). Although the drug may be effective when administered endotracheally (1.0 mg), the intravenous route is preferred. In adults, an initial dose of 0.5 to 1.0 mg can be administered by rapid intravenous push and repeated in 5 to 10 minutes if no rate increase or hemodynamic improvement occurs. A dose of 2.0 mg is vagolytic in the vast majority of adults; if improvement has not occurred after this dosage, the clinician should move immediately to pacing or other drug therapy.

Isoproterenol

Isoproterenol is a beta-selective sympathomimetic with positive chronotropic and inotropic effects. When given intravenously, it results in an immediate increase in cardiac output and heart rate and an immediate decrease in peripheral vascular resistance. Isoproterenol can be prepared by diluting 1 mg in 250 milliliters of 5 percent dextrose in water (4 μg isoproterenol per milliliter) and is administered as a continuous intravenous infusion (2 to 10 μg per minute), which is titrated to the desired heart rate. At this dosage range, blood pressure usually remains unchanged or increases, as the effect of decreased peripheral vascular resistance is more than offset by the increase in heart rate and cardiac output.

Isoproterenol causes an increase in myocardial oxygen consumption and increased ventricular irritability. Because of these effects, *isoproterenol should be used with extreme caution in patients with acute myocardial infarction*. If such patients are unresponsive to atropine, some clinicians prefer to use a vasopressor such as dopamine to support blood pressure while preparing for emergent pacing. In addition, the beta-stimulation of isoproterenol causes significant vasodilation in many patients, resulting in decreased vascular resistance and dramatic drops in blood pressure. As a result, isoproterenol should always be used with great caution and with expectation of adverse consequences.

SUGGESTED READING

Braunwald E, ed. Heart disease. 2nd ed. Philadelphia: WB Saunders, 1984:691–694; 729–736.
Goodman LS, Gilman A, eds. The pharmacological basis of therapeutics. 7th ed. New York: Macmillan, 1985:131–143; 160–161.

EMERGENCY PACEMAKER INSERTION AND MALFUNCTION

JAMES R. ROBERTS, M.D.
SCOTT A. SYVERUD, M.D.

Currently, over 500,000 patients are living with an artificial pacer in place, and over 100,000 permanent pacers are implanted each year. With increasing frequency, the emergency physician is called upon not only to diagnose and appropriately treat permanent pacemaker malfunction, but also to institute temporary cardiac pacing on an emergency basis in the setting of bradyasystolic arrest or precariously unstable bradyarrhythmia. Newer, less invasive methods have made pre-hospital use of cardiac pacing available.

In this chapter, we will discuss the specifics of emergency pacing techniques, including transcutaneous, transvenous, transthoracic, and transesophageal pacing. In addition, the major categories of permanent pacemaker malfunction will be highlighted, with attention to diagnosis and emergent management.

INDICATIONS FOR EMERGENT AND

EMERGENCY PACING

The indications for "elective" placement of a cardiac pacemaker are numerous, and specific recommendations vary somewhat among different authors and institutions. There is a distinct difference between *emergent* and *emergency* pacemaker placement. Emergent pacing is required in individuals who are clinically stable but may decompensate or become unstable in the near future. If time and the clinical condition of the patient permit, all emergent cardiac pacing should be attempted in a controlled environment; it should be performed by the most experienced physician available and therefore should not be performed in the emergency department. Likewise, if the patient can be stabilized with drug therapy or is not in extremis, the standard pattern of referral and consultation is recommended. Table 1 summarizes the indications for emergent pacing.

Emergency pacing is required in unstable patients with cardiac arrest, hemodynamically unstable bradyarrhythmia, or recurrent malignant escape rhythms that require pacing immediately. Such patients cannot realistically be transported to the intensive care unit or radiology suite, and certainly their condition warrants immediate and definitive, not conservative, therapy. These patients cannot await the arrival of a consultant. The techniques and equipment required for truly emergency pacing are often unique to the emergency department (Table 2).

TRANSCUTANEOUS PACING

Transcutaneous pacing is a technique in which the heart is paced by externally applied electrodes, which produce an electrical impulse that is conducted across the intact chest wall to stimulate the myocardium. Although transcutaneous pacers were the first type of pacers developed, they saw little clinical use until the early 1980s. Recent refinements in electrode size and pulse characteristics have led to the reintroduction of transcutaneous pacing into clinical practice. At least two major manufacturers have incorporated transcutaneous pacing into their newer defibrillator models.

Recent studies have demonstrated improved survival in bradyasystolic arrest patients who received pacing within 5 minutes of arrest onset. This observation, combined with its relative ease of application, has led to the application of transcutaneous pacing in pre-hospital settings. This technique is useful for initial stabilization of the patient in the emergency department who requires emergency pacing while arrangements for transvenous pacemaker insertion are being made.

TABLE 1   Indications for Emergent Pacing

Indication	Timeframe
Stable bradycardias (BP > 80, no evidence of hemodynamic compromise as outlined in Table 2, or hemodynamic compromise responsive to initial drug therapy)	Coronary care unit (CCU)- with fluoroscopic guidance when available
Prophylactic pacing in setting of acute myocardial infarction Symptomatic sinus node dysfunction Mobitz II second-degree heart block Third-degree heart block Newly acquired: left bundle branch block (BBB), right BBB, alternating BBB, or bifascicular block	CCU- fluoroscopic guidance when available
Tachycardias	Hemodynamic compromise requires cardioversion. If stable, overdrive pacing may be used after failure or drug therapy (usually in CCU).

TABLE 2   Indications for Emergency Pacing

Indication	Timeframe	Contraindications
Bradyasystolic cardiac arrest	Pre-hospital, if available Early in emergency department (ED) course Ineffective if more than 20 minutes after arrest	Bradyasystolic arrest > 20 minutes duration Bradycardia resulting from hypothermia Note: Most bradycardia in *children* results from hypoxia or hypoventilation and responds to adequate airway intervention with or without drug therapy. Pacing is rarely required. Pacing does not benefit ventricular fibrillation.
Hemodynamically compromising Bradycardias* (BP < 80, mental status change, ischemia, angina, pulmonary edema, refractory ectopy)	After initial drug therapy (atropine, isoproterenol, pressors) Pre-hospital or ED	

*Include complete heart block, symptomatic second-degree heart block, symptomatic sick sinus syndrome, drug-induced bradycardias (i.e., digoxin, beta-blockers, calcium-channel blockers, procainamide), permanent pacemaker failure, idioventricular bradycardias, symptomatic atrial fibrillation with slow ventricular response, refractory bradycardia during resuscitation of hypovolemic shock, and bradyarrhythmias, with malignant ventricular escape mechanisms.

Transcutaneous pacers differ from standard pacers in several important ways. The pulse duration of the stimulating impulse is usually 20 milliseconds compared to 2 milliseconds for standard internal leads. This longer duration selectively stimulates cardiac muscle rather than the skeletal muscle that the stimulus must traverse to reach the heart. However, some muscle contraction (usually the chest wall or diaphragm) does occur, especially at higher outputs. The resultant muscle contraction results in a twitching or mild bucking activity that can make assessment of cardiac output by palpation of the radial, carotid, or femoral pulse unreliable during transcutaneous pacing. Higher current outputs are required to produce capture with transcutaneous pacing (50 to 200 milliamps compared to 2 to 20 milliamps for internal leads). These higher outputs make cardiac monitoring with standard electrocardio-gram monitors impossible owing to interference from the large amplitude pacing spike. Most transcutaneous pacing units come equipped with a monitor, which automatically filters the pacing spike so that simultaneous monitoring is possible.

The externally applied pacing electrodes are quickly and easily applied to the skin. Electrode placement is key when using this technique. The anterior electrode is placed as close as possible to the point of maximal impulse on the left anterior chest wall. These 8-cm diameter electrodes adhere to the skin and have a large surface area for electrical contact. The second electrode is placed directly posterior to the anterior electrode. Failure to capture may be due to misplacement of the electrodes, and failure to pace may be rectified with even a small change in anterior electrode position. Some physicians prefer to apply the posterior electrode prophylactically to all critically ill patients to facilitate immediate transcutaneous pacing should decompensation occur.

There is little risk of electrical injury to health care providers during transcutaneous pacing. Power delivered during each impulse is less than 0.001 of that delivered during defibrillation. Chest compressions (CPR) can be administered directly over the insulated electrodes while pacing. Inadvertent contact with the active pacing surface results only in a mild shock.

To initiate transcutaneous pacing, the electrodes are applied and the device activated. In the setting of bradyasystolic arrest, it is reasonable to turn the stimulating current to maximum output, then decrease the output if capture is achieved. In the setting of a patient with a hemodynamically compromising bradycardia (but not in cardiac arrest), the operator should slowly increase the output from the minimum setting until capture is achieved. Assessment of capture can be made by monitoring the electrocardiogram on the filtered monitor of the pacing unit. The hemodynamic response to pacing must also be assessed, either by blood pressure cuff or arterial catheter. Ideally, pacing should be continued at 1.25 times the threshold of initial electrial capture.

Failure to capture with trancutaneous pacing may be related to electrode placement or patient size. Patients with barrel-shaped chests and large amounts of intrathoracic air conduct electricity poorly and may prove refractory to capture. A large pericardial effusion or tamponade also increases the output required for capture. Failure to capture transcutaneously in these settings is an indication for immediate transvenous or transthoracic pacer placement.

Patients who are conscious or who regain consciousness during transcutaneous pacing experience discomfort attributable to muscle contraction. Analgesia with incremental doses of morphine (2 to 3 mg IV push) and/or sedation with a benzodiazepine (2 to 5 mg diazepam IV push) makes this discomfort tolerable until transvenous pacing can be instituted.

To be safe, studies in animals and in humans have shown transcutaneous pacing of as much as one hour's duration. Cardiac and tissue damage caused by pacing during this interval is clinically insignificant. Longer use of transcutaneous pacing has not been fully investigated. Certainly the potential for cardiac and cutaneous damage does exist with prolonged pacing at these higher output levels. For this reason, transcutaneous pacing should be used for temporary stabilization only and should always be followed as soon as is feasible by an internal pacing technique (usually transvenous). Theoretically one may induce ventricular fibrillation by stimulating the myocardium during an electrically vulnerable period, but this complication has not yet been encountered clinically.

Transcutaneous pacing is technically the fastest and easiest method of emergency pacing. The use of the equipment is readily mastered, and the procedure is fast and noninvasive. Refinements in the equipment have made transcutaneous pacing the procedure of choice in those centers where pacing is rarely performed or when physicians are uncomfortable or inexperienced with more invasive techniques of transthoracic or transvenous pacing.

TRANSVENOUS PACING

Transvenous pacing consists of endocardial stimulation of the right ventricle via an electrode introduced into a central vein. The major difficulties of transvenous pacing are venous access and proper placement of the stimulating electrode. Venous access routes most commonly used include the subclavian, internal or external jugular, femoral, and brachial. Transvenous pacing catheters can be inserted through a variety of venous introducers (Cordis, Arrow). A soft flexible semifloating bipolar catheter is preferred. This type of pacer is safest to use and takes advantage of any forward blood flow that may be present. Temporary transvenous pacing electrodes are available in several sizes and are manufactured by a number of manufacturers (Elecath, Cordis).

Placement of the catheter tip into the apex of the right ventricle is key to successful transvenous pacing. Several techniques can aid successful placement. Fluoroscopic guidance is the surest method of right ventricular placement. This technique requires familiarity with the fluoroscopic anatomy of the chest and the availability of a fluoroscope.

Electrocardiographic guidance is useful in patients with narrow complexes and/or P waves when fluoroscopy is unavailable. When using this technique, the standard limb leads of an ECG machine are attached to the patient. The V lead is connected via an alligator clip to the distal lead of the pacing catheter. The tip of the pacing catheter, as it is being inserted, thus becomes the sensing V lead of the ECG machine. With the ECG machine in the "V" position, the ECG complexes mirror the position of the tip of the pacing catheter. As the catheter approaches and enters the right atrium, the P wave and QRS complex sensed through this lead become larger. When the tip of the catheter reaches the ventricle, the P wave diminishes in size and the QRS complex becomes large; ST segment elevation signifies placement of the tip against the wall of the ventricle (the position desired for pacing). Once this position is achieved, the alligator clip is disconnected. The pacing catheter leads are then connected to the pulse generator box to initiate pacing. If QRS deflection or P waves become smaller during insertion, the tip is moving away from the heart, usually down the inferior vena cava or up a great vein in the neck (see our listing in Suggested Reading).

Balloon-tipped "floating" catheters may aid placement when used in conjunction with ECG and fluoroscopic guidance or when used alone. The balloon is inflated after catheter insertion into a central vein. Forward blood flow then directs the catheter tip toward the ventricle as the operator slowly advances the catheter. As with all balloon-tipped catheters, the balloon should always be deflated prior to withdrawal; the catheter should never be pulled back with the balloon inflated.

When patients have decreased or no forward blood

flow (including most circumstances in which transvenous pacing would be used in the emergency department), positioning of the pacer tip within the right ventricle is difficult. Fluoroscopy usually is not immediately available and electrocardiographic guidance only aids placement in the patient with narrow complexes and/or a discernible P wave. Ballon-tipped catheters are not much of an aid in placement during low- or no-flow states. In a true emergency, the pacemaker electrodes are connected to the power source and the catheter advanced blindly in hopes that the tip will encounter the endocardium of the right ventricle and that capture will result. In this setting, a right internal jugular venous access route should be used. From this approach, the catheter traverses a straight line into the right ventricle and rarely curls in the atrium or deflects into the inferior vena cava.

Pacer settings vary with the clinical situation. An initial rate of 80 to 100 per minute is appropriate in most patients. Asynchronous mode (sensitivity off) should be used initially in patients requiring emergency pacing for hemodynamically unstable bradycardias. Output should initially be set at maximum (usually 20 milliamps), then decreased after capture is achieved. With optimal tip position, capture should occur at less than 2 milliamps. Pacing should be continued at 1.5 to 2 times the threshold output required for capture. Subsequent rate and sensitivity settings should be adjusted as clinically indicated by the patient's hemodynamic status and underlying rhythm disturbance.

Chest roentgenograms (AP and lateral) should be obtained after patient stabilization to ensure proper tip placement and to evaluate the possiblity of pneumothorax after central venous line placement. Finally, care should be taken to firmly affix the pacing catheter to the insertion site prior to patient transfer.

Transvenous pacing is a technique that can be easily mastered and rapidly performed in an emergency situation. With experience (and a certain amount of luck), a transvenous pacer can be inserted into the right ventricle in 3 to 4 minutes. The most common problems are difficulties with venous access, inability to pass the catheter into the right ventricle, and intermittent capture or failure to capture. Transvenous pacing is best used in urgent situations in which there is adequate time to utilize fluoroscopy. In the setting of cardiac arrest, transcutaneous or transthoracic pacing is preferred. When there is a hemodynamically unstable bradycardia or lethal escape rhythms, but the patient is not in extremis or can be temporarily stabilized with medication, a transvenous pacer placed under ECG guidance or with careful blind advancement is a reasonable alternative to the transthoracic route. Transcutaneous pacing, if available, is also a reasonable alternative in this setting.

TRANSTHORACIC PACING

Transthoracic pacing involves the percutaneous placement of a bipolar pacing wire directly into the right ventricular cavity via a trocar. The technique is quicker than transvenous pacer insertion and is more likely to result in right ventricular placement in the setting of hemodynamically unstable bradycardias or cardiac arrest. The intracardiac trocar can be properly positioned by an experienced physician, with only a brief interruption of CPR, in 30 to 45 seconds. Because of the significant incidence of serious complications associated with the procedure (pericardial tamponade, major vessel injury, pneumothorax), it should not be used indiscriminately. It is not indicated in the stable patient or cases in which medication can buy time to pass a transvenous pacing catheter. Because of its rapidity and certainty of intracardiac placement, transthoracic pacing is preferable to transvenous pacing in unstable or arrested patients. If transcutaneous pacing is unavailable, or if it fails to produce electrical capture, transthoracic pacing is the technique of choice in these critical patients.

Various transthoracic pacing kits are commercially available (Elecath Co., Rahway, N.J.). In addition to the kit, an external pulse generator is required. A wide variety of external pulse generators, adaptable for either transvenous or transthoracic pacing, is available.

Several placement routes have been advocated for transthoracic pacing. These include using the left fifth intercostal space and directing the needle toward the right second costosternal junction, or using the subxiphoid approach and directing the needle toward the left or right shoulder. In our experience, the subxiphoid approach aiming toward the sternal notch, as used in pericardiocentesis, is the preferred route for introduction of the intracardiac trocar.

If chest compressions are in progress, these should be interrupted until intracardiac placement has been achieved to minimize the possibility of myocardial laceration by the sharp needle. The trocar needle is introduced into the left xiphocostal angle and directed at a 30- to 45-degree angle to the skin toward the sternal notch. After advancing the needle 8 to 12 cm, the trocar is removed. A free return of blood indicates intracardiac placement. Aspiration of blood with a syringe confirms position. If no blood is aspirated, the needle is withdrawn and reinserted. After the intracardiac position is confirmed, the pacing wire is inserted through the needle. The needle is then removed over the wire (keep one hand on the wire at all times during removal), and the wire is connected to the pulse generator box. Care must be taken not to exceed a 45 degree angle to the skin during insertion, as this increases the chance of missing the heart and puncturing the diaphragm, the stomach, and/or the liver.

After the pacing wire has been connected to the pulse generator, pacing is initiated with the same settings as were indicated for emergency transvenous pacing (asynchronous, maximum output, rate 80 to 100). The presence or absence of capture should then be assessed on the ECG rhythm strip or monitor. If no pacer spikes are evident, the connections of the wire to the pulse generator should be checked. If pacer spikes are evident, but no capture occurs, the wire should be gently manipulated to change its position within the ventricle. If capture is achieved and the patient's hemodynamic status stabilizes, the entire pacing apparatus should be securely taped to the chest while arrangements are made for placement of a transvenous pacing catheter. Chest roentgenograms (AP and lateral) should be obtained to confirm catheter position and rule out pneumothorax, which is sometimes induced during insertion. The transthoracic pacing catheter should be replaced by a transvenous pacemaker as soon as possible, although pacing can be accomplished with the transthoracic pacemaker for a number of days.

TRANSESOPHAGEAL PACING

Atrial pacing via esophageal electrodes has been used in emergent and diagnostic situations since the 1960s. The technique requires passage of an electrode-bearing oro- or nasogastric tube followed by positioning of the electrodes behind the heart. The proximity of the atrial to the esophagus allows atrial capture at relatively low currents, which produce minimal pain and muscle contraction. Ventricular capture requires higher outputs (10 to 80 milliamps), which may produce pain and muscle contraction. In some cases it may not be possible to achieve ventricular capture using the transesophageal route. The transesophageal approach is therefore best suited for atrial pacing, a condition that has little application in the emergency department.

Transesophageal pacing offers the advantage of being less invasive than tranvenous or transthoracic pacing. In the conscious patient, it may be better tolerated than transcutaneous pacing. Some investigators have advocated transesophageal pacing for pre-hospital and emergency department use. Most indications for emergent pacing require ventricular pacing, however, and it would usually be faster and less invasive to use transcutaneous pacing as the initial pacing modality.

Placement of a transesophageal pacing lead has shown promise as a prophylactic measure in the operating room during procedures that may produce bradycardia. Transesophageal pacing may also have a place in the treatment of refractory tachyarrhythmias by overdrive pacing, particularly in conscious, hemodynamically stable patients. Further development of the technique awaits Food and Drug Administration approval and the commercial availability of transesophageal pacing units.

EPICARDIAL PACING

Epicardial pacing refers to placement of pacing leads directly adjacent to or through the epicardium under direct visualization. In the emergent situation, this is used almost exclusively during open thoracotomy for resuscitation of the patient with penetrating trauma. Frequently, these patients develop refractory bradyarrhythmias after initial fluid resuscitation. Dramatic improvement has been reported following epicardial pacing in this situation.

If a thoracotomy has been performed and pacing is required, epicardial leads may be placed (sutured or screw-in wires are available) in the ventricular wall. Since the equipment for epicardial pacing usually is not stocked in the emergency department, preparation for the even-

tual use of such a device should be made in advance. A transthoracic pacing wire may be placed under direct visualization as an alternative to epicardial pacing during thoracotomy.

IMPLANTED PACEMAKER MALFUNCTION

It is rare for a permanent pacer malfunction to require emergent intervention. Recent improvements in pacemaker design have decreased both the incidence and the severity of most malfunctions. In most cases, once a malfunction is recognized, further evaluation and treatment can await consultation by a cardiologist or cardiac surgeon. The key role of the physician rendering emergency care is to accurately identify the patient in whom malfunction may be present in order to appropriately initiate further evaluation and treatment. The emergency physician must also be ready to intervene appropriately in the rare patient who presents with an unstable clinical picture resulting from pacemaker malfunction.

Types of Permanent Pacemaker

Recognition of abnormal function requires a thorough understanding of normal function. With more than 100 types of implanted pacers currently in use, it may be difficult to determine what a given patient's normal pacer function is. Fortunately, many patients carry a card that indicates the model, pacing mode, and other useful information regarding their own pacer. This information is also prominently entered in the medical record at the time of implantation. One standard system of pacer identification uses a three-letter code as follows:

1st letter=chamber paced (A, V, or D)
2nd letter=chamber sensed (A, V, or D)
3rd letter=mode (T, I, or O) where A=atrium, V=ventricle, D=double (both chambers), T=triggered, I=inhibited, O=not applicable.

The most common type of implanted pacer is a ventricular inhibited pacer (VVI). This type of unit paces and senses the ventricle; pacing spikes are inhibited by the unit if intrinsic ventricular complexes are sensed at a rate greater than that set for the pacing rate. Another type of unit now being implanted with increasing frequency is the atrioventricular sequential pacemaker (DDI). These pacers preserve the atrial contribution to cardiac filling by using dual leads to sequentially pace the heart. Since both chambers are sensed and activity in either chamber may inhibit stimulation, several types of normal operation may be seen on the electrocardiogram including atrial pacing, AV sequential pacing, no pacing, or atrial sensing with coupled ventricular pacing. Rarer today, but still in use, are ventricular fixed-rate pacers (VOO). These units have no sensing capability and pace the ventricle at a fixed rate regardless of underlying cardiac activity. Usually implanted in patients with third-degree atrioventricular block and a slow ventricular escape rhythm, these pacers have the potential to induce ventricular arrhythmias should the pacer spike fall during the vulnerable period of a spontaneous ventricular contraction.

An increasing number of pacers allow *external programming* of the rate, mode, or AV interval. Programmable or demand-mode pacers can be momentarily converted to fixed-rate mode or to a faster demand mode by used of a magnet. This technique allows evaluation of pacer function in patients whose underlying rhythm is faster than the preprogrammed rate. Magnets are available from the various manufacturers to suit their particular units; any one magnet may not work for a different manufacturer's unit. To use a magnet, it is placed in contact with the skin directly over the pacemaker. It should be oriented perpendicular to the axis formed by a line joining the head and feet. Pacemaker function should return to normal after magnet removal. Demand function can be rapidly evaluated using a magnet; this is especially helpful when pacer spikes are not seen initially.

Pacemaker power sources have undergone several changes in recent years. Older mercury batteries manifest failure in any of a number of ways (change in pacer spike width, decrease in rate, intermittent capture, or loss of sensing). Observation of any of these findings in a patient with a mercury battery-powered pacer may fortell complete battery failure in a matter of days. Further evaluation and possible pacemaker replacement are required in all such patients. Newer lithium and nuclear power sources manifest impending failure by a slowly progressive decrease in rate over weeks to months. Most manufacturers recommend replacement when rate has decreased by 10 percent; this can usually be scheduled electively and does not require emergent intervention.

The Symptomatic Patient with a Permanent Pacemaker

Syncope, palpitations, orthostasis, and sudden death may all result from pacer malfunction. As many as 25 percent of patients with permanent pacers have cardiac arrest in a 12-month period. Five-year survival in patients with a permanent pacer is only about 60 percent. The majority of these patients die owing to ventricular arrhythmias or other disease; rarely is pacer failure or malfunction a cause of death. Nevertheless, when a patient with a permanent pacemaker arrives in the emergency department complaining of a syncopal episode, pacer malfunction must be suspected. Unless a definitive diagnosis can be established, these patients require admission to a monitored bed for further evaluation of their pacemaker function.

Chest pain occurring in the patient with a pacer requires careful evaluation of the pacemaker function on the electrocardiogram. Failure to capture or oversensing may result in bradycardia and resultant ischemic chest pain. Myocardial infarction may lead to increased threshold and failure to capture, especially if the infarct involves the endocardium adjacent to the pacer lead. Pacer malfunction may therefore be a cause of, or a result of, myocardial ischemia.

When cardiac arrest occurs in the patient with a permanent pacer, initial support follows standard advanced cardiac life support (ACLS) guidelines. If pacer spikes are visible on the cardiogram, it must be assumed that the pacer is working and the arrest is from another cause. It is easy to mistake pacer spikes for normal QRS complexes at first glance; the underlying rhythm is frequently ventricular fibrillation with superimposed pacing spikes. These patients require defibrillation, taking care not to place the defibrillation electrodes over the pacemaker generator. Defibrillation directly over the pacemaker may result in damage to the pacer or to the endocardium adjacent to the pacemaker lead; the pacer may not capture or function properly post-defibrillation as a result. If no pacer spikes are visible in the cardiac arrest patient with a permanent pacer, malfunction of the pacer must be assumed. Emergency pacing, either transcutaneous or transthoracic, is indicated as soon as possible in these cases if bradyasystolic arrest is present.

Pacemaker malfunction can be divided into three broad categories: (1) failure to pace, (2) failure to capture, and (3) failure to sense. Failure to pace is diagnosed on the monitor strip by the absence of pacer spikes with a rhythm slower than the programmed pacer rate. With failure to capture, pacer spikes are present, but are not coupled with ventricular contractions. Failure to sense can present in the same way as failure to pace, as outlined previously, or with inappropriate delivery of pacer spikes during the patient's intrinsic cardiac rhythm. The differential diagnosis of each of these malfunctions is shown in Table 3.

Lead Failures

The vast majority of permanent pacemakers use right ventricular endocardial leads placed transvenously. Rarely, epicardial leads are placed via open thoracotomy, usually during bypass surgery. Lead position can be ascertained using ECG and chest roentgenograms. A right ventricular (RV) endocardial lead results in a paced left bundle branch block pattern. A left ventricular endocardial lead results in a right bundle branch block pattern. On the AP chest film, the lead should curve out toward the left heart border at the apex with RV placement. On the lateral film, it should curve anteriorly. Posterior placement on lateral projection suggests coronary sinus or atrial position. The lead tip should never extend beyond the heart border; this rare finding usually occurs within 72 hours of lead placement and suggests perforation of the myocardium by the pacer tip. Perforation is associated with a high incidence of tamponade and requires lead replacement as well as possible operative intervention.

After an endocardial lead is placed, fibrosis gradually occurs about the tip. This process, which occurs over weeks to months, firmly fixes the tip to the myocardium and may contribute to a gradual increase in threshold over time. Before extensive fibrosis occurs, especially in the first few weeks after placement, the lead is prone to displacement. Displaced leads may result in failure to capture or sense. If the tip of a displaced lead migrates in

TABLE 3 Causes of Permanent Pacemaker Malfunction

Failure to pace (no detectable pacer spike)

  ECG recording difficulties: lead fault, interference, inadequate gain setting, lead perpendicular to pacing spike axis

  Internal inhibition: appropriate sensing of faster intrinsic rhythm is a demand pacer, oversensing (inappropriate sensing) in a demand unit

  External inhibition: external inhibition of demand pacer due to sensing of external electrical interference (e.g., microwave, electrical equipment)

  Lead faults: disconnection or fracture

  Generator: battery or component failure

Failure to sense (inappropriate delivery of pacer spikes)
  Electrical interference
  Battery failure
  Asynchronous function (fixed rate pacer or magnet induced mode change)
  Lead faults: displacement, fracture, perforation, fibrosis around tip
  Decreased QRS amplitude: acute myocardial infarction, drugs, metabolic changes

Failure to capture (pacer spikes, but intermittent or no capture)

  Lead faults: displacement, disconnection, fracture, perforation

  Threshold change: increase with time, fibrosis of tip, acute myocardial infarction

  Generator: fluid leak, component failure
  Battery failure
  Drugs (e.g., lidocaine)
  Electrolyte abnormalities

the great veins, it may result in diaphragmatic (tip in inferior vena cava) or upper extremity (tip in subclavian vein) stimulation. This event can therefore mimic a focal seizure or a pulsatile abdominal mass.

Lead fracture or disconnection usually occurs months after placement owing to stress at the lead connection site to the generator. It may also occur as a result of blunt chest trauma. Careful examination of the lead on roentgenogram or during fluoroscopy may reveal the fault and should always be performed in the setting of pacemaker malfunction after trauma.

Runaway Pacemaker

Newer pacemakers exibit a gradual slowing of pacing rate over time as the battery fails. However, some older units may accelerate the pacing rate as the battery fails. Most units have circuits that prevent the rate from exceeding 130. Rarely, a paced rate of 200 or greater occurs with a unit that does not have such a circuit or if the circuit malfunctions. Runaway pacemaker is a true emergency in that the standard treatment of tachyarrhythmias usually does not result in clinical improvement. Once the diagnosis is made, the malfunctioning pacer must be disabled as soon as possible. This is accomplished by opening the pacer pouch (sterile incision) and disconnecting the leads as close to the generator as possible. If the patient's underlying rhythm after disconnection is hemodynamically inadequate, the permanent leads can be stripped and connected to a temporary pulse generator (as used for emergency transvenous or transthoracic pacing)

and pacing then reinstituted. Alternatively, drugs can be used to increase the intrinsic rate while arrangements are made for temporary pacing.

Infection

Like any foreign body, pacemaker leads and generators are prone to infection. Infections occurring shortly after lead placement are commonly associated with sepsis or bacteremia, usually caused by gram-negative organisms or *Staphylococcus aureus*. Late infections may involve either the lead or the generator pocket. The presence of fluctuance, erythema, and/or pain at the site of the generator requires aspiration and culture of the pocket, blood cultures, and drainage if pus is present. Local infection may be managed with these measures and antibiotics, but any sign of systemic involvement requires replacement of the pacemaker.

SUGGESTED READING

Hedges JR, Syverud SA, Dalsey WC. Developments in transcutaneous and transthoracic pacing in bradyasystolic cardiac arrest. Ann Emerg Med 1984; 13:822–827.

Roberts JR. Cardiac pacing in the emergency department. In: Greenburg MI, Gernerd MD, Roberts JR, eds. Advanced techniques in resuscitation. Baltimore: Williams and Wilkins, 1985; 45–61.

Roberts JR, Suverud SA. Transthoracic and transcutaneous cardiac pacing. In: Roberts JR, Hedges JR, eds., Clinical procedures in emergency medicine. Philadelphia: WB Saunders 1985; 170–207.

Smith ND, Pacemaker Dysfunction. In: Greenburg MI, Roberts JR, eds. Emergency medicine , A clinical approach to challenging problems. Philadelphia: Davis FA, 1981; 355–384.

MANAGEMENT OF THE VASCULAR SYSTEM

DISSECTING ANEURYSM OF THE AORTA

MICHAEL E. DeBAKEY, M.D.

Sporadic observations on the pathology, histoanatomy, and pathogenesis of dissection and dissecting aneurysm of the aorta have been made since the 16th century, but the pathogenesis of this disease remained poorly understood until the 20th century, when much of the confusion was clarified. Medial degeneration is generally considered to be the most important underlying cause of dissection.

Dissecting aneurysm of the aorta is a complex form of aneurysmal disease. It is, in fact, the most serious and difficult type of aortic disease to treat. It is rapidly fatal, the reported mortality rates for such patients not operated on being more than 50 percent within the first few weeks and about 90 percent within a few months after onset; only a few live more than a year. Medical treatment has had little effect on the eventual prognosis, but surgical treatment has greatly improved the expected survival rate.

Dissecting aneurysms may be classified into three major types according to site (Fig.1). In type I, the dissecting process involves the ascending aorta as well as the remaining portion. Although most of these patients have a transverse tear in the anterior wall of the ascending aorta, the dissection may also begin distally and propagate proximally. Intimal tears may also be multiple. This type of dissection is most prone to be associated with aortic insufficiency or cerebral ischemia due to interruption of innominate or left carotid perfusion. Rupture into the mediastinum with bleeding into the pericardium producing tamponade may cause early death. Coronary ostial dissection or dissection into the myocardium, usually of the septum, may also prove fatal.

Type II dissection is limited to the ascending aorta proximal to the origin of the innominate artery. It is usually associated with a transverse aortic tear and may leave intact part of the posterior wall of the ascending aorta. Type II aneurysms may also be associated with the fatal intrapericardial complications of type I aneurysms. They are often associated with aortic valvular incompetence and sometimes with Marfan's syndrome.

Type III dissecting aneurysms develop just distal to the left subclavian artery and extend distally for varying distances. There are two subtypes: type IIIa, which is limited to the thorax, and the more common type IIIb, which extends into the abdomen.

DIAGNOSIS

Pain is the most common symptom of all three types of dissecting aneurysm. Other manifestations depend on the type of dissecting aneurysm. For example, congestive heart failure due to aortic insufficiency is common in types I and II but rare in type III. Stroke occurs mainly in type I. Other clinical manifestations include rupture, paraparesis, history of renal failure, cough, claudication, peripheral ischemia, stroke, visceral ischemia, hoarseness, dysphagia, and hemoptysis.

In the patient with chest pain suspected of having a dissecting aneurysm, a roentgenogram of the chest should be obtained; it will often show changes such as widening of the mediastinum, blurring of the aortic contour, an apical pleural cap, pleural effusion, or elevation of the left

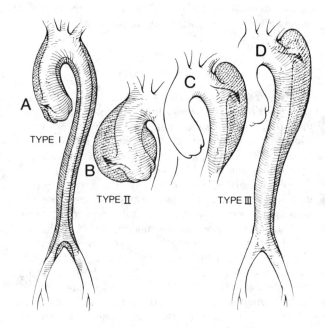

Figure 1 Classification of aortic dissections (arrows indicate site of intimal tear). (From DeBakey ME, McCollum CH, Crawford ES, et al. Dissection and dissecting aneurysms of the aorta. Surgery 1982; 92:1118–1125.

main stem bronchus. Ultrasonography can uncover complications of dissection, such as pericardial effusion and aortic incompetence, but this procedure has many false-positive and false-negative results for dissection itself. Computed tomography is useful but time-consuming. Aortography confirms the diagnosis and is essential to plan the surgical treatment. A cardiothoracic surgeon should be consulted immediately, however, before any such tests are ordered. Delays in diagnosis and treatment are often fatal.

Nonspecific electrocardiographic changes are often found in patients with dissection; electrocardiography is most helpful in ruling out the major differential diagnosis—myocardial infarction—in a patient with severe chest pain and evidence of peripheral hypoperfusion. The electrocardiogram cannot be solely relied on however, and if there is doubt, immediate consultation is advised.

TREATMENT

Patients with acute dissection should be placed in an intensive care unit for continuous monitoring of systemic arterial pressure, central venous pressure, and if cardiac function is impaired, of pulmonary artery wedge pressure with a Swan-Ganz catheter. Frequent examination of the patient to detect progression of symptoms or involvement of previously intact visceral branches is imperative. The patient should be typed and cross-matched for 6 to 10 units of blood and a cardiovascular surgeon notified immediately.

MEDICAL

Medical treatment for acute dissecting aneurysm should be directed toward reduction of the systemic blood pressure and myocardial contractility to the lowest levels compatible with maintenance of good cerebral and renal perfusion. The most commonly used pharmacologic agent is Nipride, 40 mg in 250 ml of 5 percent dextrose solution, titrated to the rate required to control the blood pressure by means of a mechanical infusion pump. Myocardial contractility is depressed, and control of hypertension is assisted by intravenous infusion of Inderal in increments of 0.5 mg to 1 mg, depending on the response of the heart rate and blood pressure. A maximum of 3 to 6 mg is given in this way in the first 6 to 12 hours. Then maintenance doses of 0.5 to 1 mg are given intravenously every 6 hours; this can be changed to an oral dosage of 40 to 80 mg every 6 hours. Rarely are intravenous infusions of Arfonad and reserpine needed. Small intravenous doses of morphine sulfate as required will keep the patient comfortable.

SURGICAL

Surgical treatment depends on the type of dissecting aneurysm visualized at arteriography and the clinical condition of the patient. For patients with chronic dissection, early elective operation should be planned. For those with acute dissection, a few hours to days of stabilization of the patient's condition allow for correct diagnosis and preparation of the patient for operation. Moreover, during the early stages of dissection, the aortic tissues are extremely friable and do not hold sutures well. Postponing the operation for this brief period permits the tissues to become less friable and to hold sutures better and therefore helps to reduce the surgical risk. It is more often feasible to delay operation with type III than with types I or II.

Emergency surgical treatment is indicated in patients with hypotension, evidence of imminent rupture, severe aortic valvular insufficiency with acute heart failure, cerebral ischemia with innominate or carotid arterial obstruction, progressive pericardial effusion, and occlusion of the coronary arteries and other vital aortic branches.

Patients with type I are operated on with use of cardiopulmonary bypass. In most of these patients, the ascending aorta is resected, the dissected wall is reapproximated distally, and the resected segment is replaced with a woven Dacron graft. Occasionally, it may be possible to approximate the inner and outer layers of the dissecting process proximally and distally by suture with the use of Dacron felt baffles and then to anastomose these sutured edges of the transected aorta end-to-end. In other patients, after the anterior dissected wall is removed, it may be possible to repair the defect by patch-graft angioplasty. Associated aortic valvular incompetence is usually produced by dilatation of the annulus or lack of support or fixation of the intimal attachment of the valves because of proximal extension of the dissecting process, which causes failure of the valves to meet properly in the closed position. Although valvular resuspension has proved satisfactory in some patients, we prefer aortic valvular replacement. If the dissecting process affects the origin of the coronary arteries, aortocoronary bypass may be performed or a button of the aortic wall around the coronary orifice may be sutured to an opening in the aortic graft.

Surgical treatment for type II consists in resection of the ascending aorta and dissecting process and replacement with a woven Dacron graft with use of cardiopulmonary bypass. Because the aortic valve is usually incompetent, particularly in the chronic form, in most cases it must be replaced. In the acute form, it may be possible to avoid this procedure by resuspension of the valves. Involvement of the coronary arteries may be repaired as described in the preceding paragraph.

Treatment for type III consists essentially in resection of the diseased segment and replacement with a woven Dacron graft through left lateral thoracotomy. Because the dissecting process rarely extends proximally beyond the origin of the left subclavian artery, the graft can usually be anastomosed proximally to the normal lumen. In type IIIa, the distal end of the graft can also be attached to the normal aortic wall after the entire dissecting process has been removed. In most patients with type IIIb, the false lumen tends to be smaller near the diaphragmatic hiatus. In these patients, the inner and outer walls of the dissection are first approximated by suture with a Dacron velour patch baffle, and the distal end of the graft is anastomosed to the normal lumen. In some patients, the procedure may be modified by extending the incision as for a thoraco abdominal approach with removal of all the dissecting process in the abdomen.

Our studies have shown that surgical treatment results in substantial improvement in survival. Better understanding of this condition and continuing refinements in surgical treatment have greatly improved the prognosis in these critically ill patients.

Supported in part by HEW research grant HL-17269, National Heart and Blood Vessel Research and Demonstration Center, Houston, Texas.

SUGGESTED READING

DeBakey ME, McCollum CH, Crawford ES, Morris GC Jr, Howell JF, Noon GP, Lawrie G: Dissection and dissecting aneurysms of the aorta: twenty-year follow-up of five hundred twenty-seven patients treated surgically. Surgery 1982, 92:1118–1134.

DeBakey ME, Lawrie GM, Crawford ES, Morris GC Jr, Howell JF, Noon GP, McCollum CH. Surgical treatment of dissecting aortic aneurysms: 28 years experience with 527 cases. Contemp Surg 1984; 25:13–23.

ABDOMINAL AORTIC ANEURYSM

RONALD J. STONEY, M.D.
JOSEPH H. RAPP, M.D.

Abdominal aortic aneurysm occurs in about 2 percent of the population. The abdomen is the most common site of aneurysmal disease. The incidence appears to be increasing, probably because an enlarging segment of our population is living to the 7th and 8th decades, when aneurysms are most likely to develop. In addition, the widespread use of new diagnostic techniques such as ultrasonography, computerized tomography (CT), and magnetic resonance imaging (MRI) may increase the number of asymptomatic aneurysms identified in this elderly population.

The presence of atherosclerotic changes in nearly all abdominal aortic aneurysms suggests that this process plays a prominent role in the weakening of the aortic wall. Structural changes in the medial layer, increased proteolytic enzyme activity, and arterial hypertension also may contribute to aortic dilation. Other causes of aneurysm, such as congenital abnormalities, mycotic processes, and trauma, account for less than 5 percent of cases. The text and accompanying algorithm (Fig. 1) outline the approach to diagnosis and treatment of patients with an abdominal aortic aneurysm.

DIAGNOSIS

A pulsatile abdominal epigastric mass can be readily palpated in over 75 percent of patients who harbor abdominal aortic aneurysms. In those patients in whom obesity or increased abdominal muscle tone precludes accurate palpation of aortic size, the diagnosis can be made by plain abdominal x-ray films, which will detect the calcified aortic rim in 70 percent of cases, or more reliably by ultrasonography. Other imaging techniques, such as CT and MRI, will also accurately record aortic size but at a considerably higher cost. Ultrasonography currently is the standard technique for routine assessment of abdominal aortic aneurysms. It is as accurate as CT and MRI except in the very obese patient or the patient with excessive bowel gas. Occasionally, a tortuous aorta or an abdominal tumor mass may suggest an aortic aneurysm. Careful bimanual palpation should determine that the tortuous aorta is mobile and has a width of less than 3 cm. A tumor mass can be differentiated from an aneurysm by determining that the structure in question is a solid mass and *transmits* the pulse rather than being the expansile aortic aneurysm wall itself.

Aortography is used to determine the dimension of the proximal aorta, the presence of coexisting occlusive disease, and the status of the adjacent renal and visceral aortic branches. It is rarely used for diagnostic purposes. Since the intraluminal thrombus present in most aneurysms reduces the true diameter of the aortic lumen, the aortogram will regularly underestimate both the size and configuration of the suspected aneurysm.

ASYMPTOMATIC PATIENTS WITH ANEURYSMS

Operative repair of aortic aneurysms falls into the classic schema of elective, urgent, and emergent. Elective repair is recommended in patients with aneurysms that are greater than 5 cm in diameter or those that have demonstrated a rapid rate of enlargement, i.e., greater than 0.5 cm in 6 months. Operative mortality for elective repair of infrarenal aneurysms is low (3 to 5 percent) in contrast to the 25 to 50 percent mortality for emergent repair of ruptured aneurysms.

Coexisting cardiac disease, impaired renal function, decreased pulmonary reserve, hypertension, and obesity have all been shown to increase perioperative morbidity and mortality. The decision to proceed with surgery must be individualized in these patients. However, with optimum preoperative preparation done in cooperation with the cardiology service, plus intraoperative monitoring with transesophageal 2-dimensional (2-D) echocardiography and pulmonary artery catheters, the risks of aneurysmectomy can be minimized even in patients with severe impairments of cardiac, pulmonary, and renal function. Careful postoperative care is also essential.

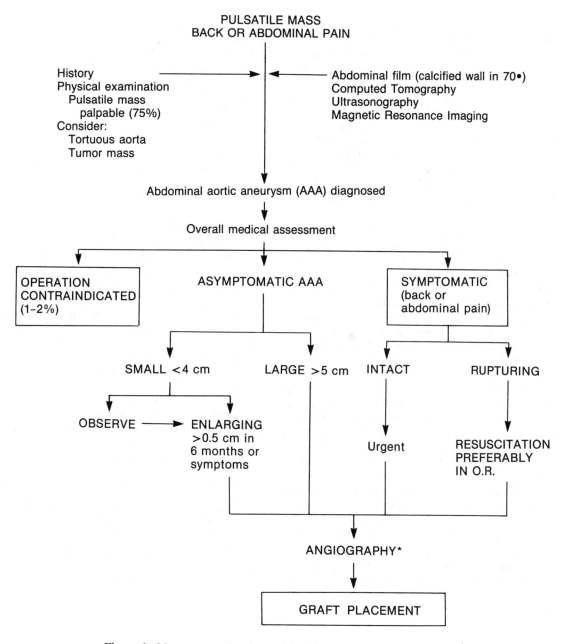

Figure 1 Management of patients with abdominal aortic aneurysm

* Applicable: if question of thoracic extension, renal or visceral artery stenosis, iliofemoral occlusive disease, or a horseshoe kidney.

Those patients who are at higher risk for elective aneurysm repair also have a much higher mortality if their aneurysms rupture. The primary predictors of rupture are size (transverse diameter) and the presence of hypertension. The 5-year risk of rupture for an aneurysm 4 cm in diameter or less is 10 to 15 percent, but it is 45 to 75 percent for an aneurysm 8 cm in diameter. Consequently, we recommend that serious consideration be given to graft replacement of large aneurysms in most high-risk patients.

SYMPTOMATIC PATIENTS WITH NONRUPTURED ANEURYSMS

Prior to rupture, some aneurysms may cause pain, presumably as a result of rapid expansion. These symptomatic aneurysms are unstable lesions. Thirty percent will rupture within 1 month and 80 percent within 1 year. Back or abdominal pain referable to a known aneurysm is an indication for urgent aneurysm repair.

Patients with a symptomatic aneurysm should be admitted to the hospital preferably to a monitored intensive care unit bed. Hypertension should be managed aggressively, and preparations should be made for aneurysmectomy. Aortography is usually recommended in this situation, as it is in preparation for an elective aneurysm repair. Absolute indications for aortography include suspected proximal extension of the aneurysm to or above the costal margin, hypertension that has been poorly controlled (suggesting a renovascular cause), symptoms suggesting visceral ischemia, signs or symptoms indicating coexisting occlusive disease, impaired renal function, a previous nephrectomy, or a suspected horseshoe kidney.

RUPTURED ANEURYSM

The diagnosis of a ruptured aneurysm is usually straightforward. The sudden onset of severe pain in the abdomen or back or both, with a pulsatile, tender epigastric mass and shock or hypotension, are the classic symptoms and can be found in the majority of cases. Rarely, a slowly leaking aneurysm may be confused with other causes of abdominal pain. If the patient's vital signs are stable, further work-up prior to surgery may be done. In this situation, ultrasonography has not ben found to be consistently useful because of frequent problems with visualization. However, an emergency CT scan may be performed that will detect even small extraluminal hematomas. Accurate preoperative diagnosis is desirable, but it should be emphasized that an unstable patient with abdominal pain and a pulsatile abdominal mass aneurysm requires an emergency laparotomy.

The most critical factor in patient survival is the time elapsed between rupture and repair. The initial hemorrhage from a ruptured aneurysm may be temporarily contained in the retroperitoneal space. These patients then have up to several hours before further expansion of the hematoma occurs; otherwise rupture into the free peritoneal cavity will cause severe hypovolemic shock and death. Interfacility transfer is not recommended but if it is necessary, the patient may be stabilized with the help of an external counterpressure gravity (G) suit for the abdomen and lower extremities. When the patient reaches the hospital, he or she should be transferred directly to the operating room for emergent resuscitation and operation.

Resuscitation and preparation for surgery must include at least two large-bore intravenous lines, with one preferably in a central vein, and at least 6 units of whole blood should be typed and cross-matched. Fluid resuscitation should be aimed at restoring the volume necessary to preserve myocardial, renal, and central nervous system flow.

The operative results for ruptured aortic aneurysm are improving as treatment and perioperative support have become more sophisticated. Currently, the size of the retroperitoneal hematoma, the degree of shock, and associated myocardial dysfunction at the time of surgery are the primary predictors of survival. As these factors primarily relate to the time elapsed from rupture to operation and the effectiveness of resuscitation, the goal for the treatment of the ruptured aneurysm patient should be rapid initiation of resuscitation in the emergency department and expeditious transfer to the operating room.

Supported in part by Pacific Vascular Research Foundation, 350 Parnossus Avenue, Suite 601, San Francisco, California.

SUGGESTED READING

Crawford ES, Saleh SA, Babb SW III, et al. Infrarenal abdominal aortic aneurysm: Factors influencing survival after operation performed over a 25 year period. Ann Surg 1981; 193:699–709.
Wakefield TW, Whitehorse WM Jr, Wa Shu Chen, et al. Abdominal aortic aneurysm rupture: Statistical analysis of factors affecting outcome of surgical treatment. Surgery 1982; 91:586–596.
Whittemore AD, Clowes AW, Hechtman HD, et al. Aortic aneurysm repair: Reduced operative mortality associated with maintenance of optimal cardiac performance. Ann Surg 1980; 192:414–421.

MESENTERIC VASCULAR OCCLUSION

JAMES GRENDELL, M.D.

ETIOLOGY

Arterial Causes

Occlusion of the major mesenteric arteries or their branches generally occurs owing to either thrombosis, usually as a result of advanced atherosclerotic disease or embolism from the heart (e.g., from mural thrombi, prosthetic valves, vegetations in endocarditis) or the aorta (e.g., from atherosclerotic plaques). Arterial occlusion may also occur owing to dissecting aortic aneurysm, fibromuscular hyperplasia, or systemic forms of vasculitis, and has been associated with use of oral contraceptives.

A similar clinical picture may be observed due to hypoperfusion of the small intestine or colon without demonstrable obstruction of arterial or venous flow (nonocclusive intestinal ischemia), usually in the setting of shock, hypoxia, myocardial infarction, or congestive heart failure. The use of alpha-adrenergic vasoconstrictors (and possibly digitalis glycosides) may also contribute to the development of nonocclusive intestinal ischemia.

Venous Causes

Thrombosis of a major mesenteric vein (almost always the superior mesenteric vein) may occur in the setting of stasis in the mesenteric venous bed (e.g., attributable to portal hypertension), abdominal neoplasms, intra-abdominal inflammation (e.g., peritonitis, abscess), abdominal surgery or trauma, or hypercoagulable states (e.g., antithrombin III deficiency, polycythemia vera). Oral contraceptive use has also been implicated. Occasionally there is no predisposing condition.

Occlusion of a mesenteric artery or vein or nonocclusive intestinal ischemia usually results in severe ischemia of the small intestine proceeding to infarction, perforation, and peritonitis, which carries a high mortality. Sometimes, however, the clinical syndrome may resolve spontaneously (especially in the case of ischemic colitis). In some of these patients, an ischemic stricture may later develop in the involved segment of bowel.

DIAGNOSIS

Patients usually present with severe abdominal pain which early in the course often is colicky in nature and periumbilical in location. At this stage, the severity of the pain reported by the patient often appears disproportionate to physical findings or laboratory studies. As ischemia progresses, pain tends to become more constant and poorly localized. Other commonly reported symptoms are nausea and vomiting as well as diarrhea which may be grossly bloody.

Physical examination may initially find only mild diffuse abdominal tenderness. Bowel sounds are usually present and may even be hyperactive. Gross or occult blood may be present in vomitus, stool, or nasogastric aspirate. As ischemia progresses, systemic manifestations such as tachycardia, hypotension, and fever may become prominent. At this stage signs of peritonitis (absence of bowel sounds, abdominal rigidity, rebound tenderness) may also be observed.

Initial laboratory studies commonly reveal hemoconcentration (elevated hematocrit) and a leukocytosis. The serum amylase concentration is often elevated. Late in the course metabolic acidosis may be observed. Abdominal roentgenograms usually show evidence of an ileus with distended, irregularly thick-walled loops of bowel (''thumbprinting'') and air-fluid levels. Gas in the intestinal wall or portal vein is a late finding and signifies a very poor prognosis. Paracentesis often shows a small amount of bloody ascites.

Major considerations in the differential diagnosis include a perforated viscus (e.g., perforated duodenal ulcer), acute pancreatitis, biliary sepsis, intestinal or colonic obstruction or ileus, and spontaneous bacterial peritonitis in the cirrhotic patient with ascites. Perforated viscus can usually be excluded by the absence of free air on upright or lateral decubitus abdominal x-ray films and by a negative Gastrografin upper gastrointestinal series or computed tomography (CT) with Gastrografin. Acute pancreatitis is best excluded by CT. Biliary sepsis is unlikely

without localization of symptoms and signs to the right upper abdominal quadrant, significant elevation of serum transaminase or alkaline phosphatase concentrations, and evidence of dilatation of the biliary tree on abdominal sonograpy or CT. Intestinal or colonic obstruction generally does not produce thick-walled loops of bowel or thumbprinting on abdominal x-ray films. Patients with an uncomplicated ileus do not generally have severe abdominal pain or systemic manifestations of a major acute intra-abdominal process (e.g., tachycardia, hypotension, metabolic acidosis). Spontaneous bacterial peritonitis does not usually produce bloody ascites or bowel-wall thickening on abdominal x-ray films.

Mesenteric ischemia or occlusion is unfortunately often not suspected or diagnosed until very late, since most of the findings are nonspecific. Early diagnosis helps determine outcome and can be achieved only with a very high index of suspicion.

THERAPY

Pre-hospital

Generally patients with mesenteric vascular occlusion require no specific prehospital therapy except for intravenous infusion of 0.9 percent sodium chloride if the patient is found to be hypotensive at the time of initial evaluation by emergency medical personnel.

Emergency Department

Initial therapy should be directed toward stabilization of the patient's condition by *replacement of fluid* and electrolyte deficiencies. This should be done by infusion, through a large bore (greater than or equal to 16-gauge) catheter, of 0.9 percent sodium chloride and supplemental potassium chloride if there is evidence of hypokalemia. Hemodynamic monitoring of central venous pressure or pulmonary artery wedge pressure may be necessary in some patients to prevent either under- or over-hydration. Fluids should be administered to maintain a systolic blood pressure of at least 100 mm Hg as well as adequate urine output. In the management of shock unresponsive to volume replacement, alpha-sympathomimetic amines should be avoided because of their adverse effects on intestinal perfusion. If a pressor agent is necessary, dopamine in doses of 2 to 10 μg per kilogram of body weight per minute should be the initial choice.

Other supportive measures include *nasogastric suction* to decompress the stomach and bowel and broad-spectrum *antibiotic coverage* for enteric Gram-negative and anaerobic bacteria after two or three blood cultures have been obtained. Appropriate antibiotic choices include an aminoglycoside (e.g., tobramycin 1.7 mg per kilogram intravenously every 8 hours) and either metronidazole (loading dose of 15 mg per kilogram intravenously over 1 hour, followed by 10 mg per kilogram intravenously over 1 hour every 8 hours) or clindamycin (10 mg per kilogram intravenously every 8 hours).

Initial laboratory studies should include a complete blood count with differential white blood count; urinalysis; serum electrolytes, blood urea nitrogen, and creatinine; serum transaminases, alkaline phosphatase, and bilirubin; serum amylase; and arterial blood gas determination. A supine abdominal reoentgenogram and either an upright or lateral decubitus abdominal roentgenogram should be obtained.

Consultation with an experienced abdominal surgeon should be obtained early in the patient's initial evaluation and management. If the patient has clear-cut findings of peritonitis, especially in the setting of hypotension and metabolic acidosis, then emergency exploratory laparotomy should be undertaken. Patients who are less severely ill or in whom the diagnosis is in doubt should undergo additional studies to confirm the diagnosis. In this setting computed tomography (CT) is especially valuable in excluding acute pancreatitis or biliary sepsis and in demonstrating the characteristic changes in the bowel wall and mesentery seen in mesenteric vascular occlusion. Thrombi or emboli in large mesenteric vessels may be identified by contrast-enhanced CT.

Emergency angiography is not always indicated in the early evaluation of patients with suspected mesenteric vascular occlusion. In patients in whom signs of peritonitis are already present, suggesting that perforation may have already occurred, the information to be gained by angiography does not justify the delay in surgery.

However, when signs of peritonitis are absent and especially when *embolization* to a mesenteric artery is suspected (based on younger age of patient, very sudden onset of symptoms, or associated cardiac disease), early angiography may be helpful in delineating the cause of mesenteric ischemia and permitting the performance of early surgical embolectomy or vascular reconstruction (or angiographic embolectomy) with potential salvage of involved bowel.

Disposition

Patients with suspected mesenteric vascular occlusion should be admitted to an intensive care unit for evaluation and treatment. Emergency surgical consultation should be obtained as part of the patient's initial evaluation. Patients who do not have evidence of peritonitis and who are hemodynamically stable may be transferred to another facility better equipped to diagnose or treat this problem.

SUGGESTED READING

Boley SJ. Acute mesenteric vascular occlusion. Contemp Surg 1983; 22:125–161.

Federle MP, Chun G, Jeffrey RB, Rayor R. Computed tomographic findings in bowel infarction. Am J Roentgenol 1984; 142:91–95.

Grendell JH, Ockner RK. Vascular diseases of the bowel. In: Sleisenger MH, Fordtran JS, eds. Gastrointestinal disease: pathophysiology, diagnosis, and treatment. 3rd ed. Philadelphia: WB Saunders, 1983: 1543.

HYPERTENSIVE CRISIS

CHRISTOPHER R. BURROW, M.D.

Malignant hypertension, accelerated hypertension, hypertensive encephalopathy, and hypertensive crisis are terms frequently applied to hypertensive patients found to have severely elevated blood pressures. In many instances, no true crisis exists and the administration of rapidly acting potent antihypertensive agents is not only unnecessary, but also ill-advised, given the potential complications that predictably follow overly rapid reduction of the blood pressure. In the comparatively rare situation in which rapid lowering of the blood pressure should be a major therapeutic goal, it is common to encounter an overly cautious approach in selecting appropriate antihypertensive drugs. The clinical treatment of severe hypertension is muddled by such excessive treatment of nonurgent cases and dilatory therapy of true hypertensive emergencies. Hypertensive encephalopathy, hypertensive pulmonary edema, crescendo angina with hypertension,

aortic dissection, and malignant hypertension with acute renal failure all represent commonly encountered hypertensive crises in which emergent therapy with rapidly acting antihypertensive agents is the number one therapeutic priority. Patients without such end-organ failure, but with a diastolic pressure of 125 mm Hg or more should have their blood pressure lowered less aggressively over a period of several hours with less potent agents.

The selection of the appropriate drugs for a given hypertensive crisis is facilitated by grouping the available agents into two main classes, as shown in Table 1. Class I agents are immediately effective, administered intravenously, and best restricted to patients hospitalized in an intensive care unit (ICU) where minute-by-minute intra-arterial blood pressure monitoring is available. Class II drugs are widely accepted as effective and reasonably prompt therapy for lesser degrees of hypertensive crisis when a reduction of blood pressure over 1 to 8 hours is the therapeutic goal.

The clinical presentation of the patient with a hypertensive crisis has considerable bearing on the selection of antihypertensive therapy and should serve as the starting point when considering drugs within individual classes. The commonly encountered hypertensive emergencies can be generally separated into two groups shown in Ta-

TABLE 1 Available Antihypertensive Medications: Pharmacologic Protocol

Drugs	Mode of Administration	Onset of Effect	Duration of Action	Dosage
Class I				
Sodium nitroprusside	IV	Seconds	3–5 min	0.25–8.0 μg/kg/min
Diazoxide	IV	1–5 min	1–24 hour	5 mg/kg, 15 mg/min/drip
Trimethaphan Camsylate	IV	1–5 min	5–10 min	0.5–5 mg/min
Class II				
Nifedipine	PO or SL	5–15 min	3–5 hour	10 mg
Clonidine	PO	½–2 hour	6–8 hour	0.2 mg loading, 0.1 mg/hour
Minoxidil*	PO	1–2 hour	24 hour	20 mg

* Administered in concert with 40 mg propranolol, 40 mg furosemide PO.

ble 2. The first group is made up of diseases in which severe hypertension is the primary etiology. Renovascular hypertension, pheochromocytoma, toxemia of pregnancy, acute glomerulonephritis, and chronic essential hypertension can all result in hypertensive encephalopathy, pulmonary edema, or acute renal failure. The second group of hypertensive crises is made up of clinical situations in which hypertension is a major secondary aggravating complication of a life-threatening disease that requires specific immediate treatment.

The patient with elevated blood pressure must be carefully examined for evidence of end-organ failure, which would make their situation a true emergency. Tests of mental status, neurologic examination, and retinal examination for such changes as papilledema and flame hemorrhages should be performed to assess the possibility of hypertensive encephalopathy. A careful cardiovascular examination to look for signs of congestive heart failure and pulmonary edema and an electrocardiogram to detect myocardial ischemia are mandatory. Renal function should be assessed by urinalysis, serum urea nitrogen (BUN), and creatinine determinations.

If the function of these organs is not affected, the urgent need to lower blood pressure is greatly diminished, regardless of numerical values. The history is often of paramount importance. In general, patients with recent-onset hypertension deserve an early evaluation and more deliberate, urgent therapy. Patients and their families need to be closely questioned about changes in mental status that may indicate hypertension encephalopathy in process. Taken together, the history and physical examination are essential elements in the interpretation of the blood pressure and provide the best means to plan appropriate medical care for the hypertensive patient.

ANTIHYPERTENSIVE DRUGS

Sodium Nitroprusside

This drug is a potent arterial and venous vasodilator, which causes a simultaneous reduction in peripheral vascular resistance and an increase in venous capacitance. It is often the best agent in the treatment of hypertensive crises, although it requires intravenous infusion and con-

TABLE 2 Common Hypertensive Crises Amenable to Antihypertensive Medications

Hypertensive crises in which severe hypertension is primary etiology of clinical findings:

Hypertensive encephalopathy
Hypertensive pulmonary edema
Malignant hypertension with secondary acute renal failure

Hypertensive crises in which hypertension is a major contributing pathophysiologic mechanism:

Crescendo angina, myocardial infarction with hypertension
Aortic dissection
Leaking aortic aneurysm or postoperative hemorrhage at a vascular suture line
Hypertensive cerebral hemorrhage

tinuous intra-arterial blood pressure monitoring during its administration. The onset of drug effect occurs within minutes, and the cessation of drug action is equally rapid due to rapid metabolism of the drug to thiocyanate. The transient and dose-dependent hypotensive effect of sodium nitroprusside can be used to great therapeutic advantage as it allows precise titration of blood pressure to a desired range.

Sodium nitroprusside is supplied in a vial containing 50 mg of lyophilized powder. The drug is reconstituted with 2 to 3 ml of 5 percent dextrose solution in water and then usually diluted in 500 ml of the same solution. As the compound is chemically unstable when exposed to light, the intravenous solution must be carefully shielded from light with aluminum foil during administration. The usual initial dose is 0.25 or 0.5 μg per kilogram per minute, using an infusion pump to ensure constant infusion rates. The infusion rate is then titrated upward every 3 to 5 minutes until the blood pressure begins to fall to the desired range. If the blood pressure falls too rapidly, the infusion can be stopped and then restarted at a lower dose after several minutes have passed and the blood pressure has begun to increase.

The major toxicity of nitroprusside is its potent hypotensive effect. As will be discussed subsequently, overly rapid reduction of the blood pressure can produce cerebral ischemia, myocardial ischemia, and hypoperfusion of other organ systems. Thus, careful nursing care is essential in administering this agent so that appropriate titration of the blood pressure to ensure vital organ blood flow can be made on the basis of clinical observations. Thiocyanate intoxication may occur with prolonged administration or if the rate of infusion is greater than 15 μg per kilogram per minute. For this reason, thiocyanate levels should be monitored if more prolonged infusions are going to be undertaken or if nitroprusside is to be used in significant dosages in patients with renal insufficiency. The maximum dosage of nitroprusside recommended is 8 μg per kilogram per minute. Given the potential for thiocyanate intoxication, orally active antihypertensive drugs should always be administered soon after the initiation of nitroprusside to allow its early discontinuation.

Nitroprusside is the drug of choice in *hypertensive encephalopathy*, which is a state of cerebral ischemia with microvascular lesions. Diazoxide is not acceptable because of its long duration of action, which increases the probability that prolonged cerebral hypoperfusion will occur as a complication of therapy. In hypertensive encephalopathy, the dosage of nitroprusside should be rapidly titrated upward to achieve an initial 25 percent reduction in the blood pressure. The blood pressure should not be reduced below 160/100 in patients initially presenting with severely elevated values because the cerebral vessels of such patients have lost their normal capability for autoregulation. Occasionally, patients demonstrate neurologic deterioration even when these precautions are taken and require an even more deliberate and cautious lowering of the blood pressure.

In combination with propranolol, nitroprusside is also a first-line agent in the treatment of *aortic dissection*. Trimethaphan camsylate has also proved acceptable, but has the disadvantage of tachyphylaxis and anticholinergic side effects of ganglionic blockade.

Nitroprusside is also useful in *pulmonary edema* related to primary severe hypertension that does not respond to parenteral nitroglycerin. In the presence of crescendo angina, nitroprusside may be especially useful in decreasing myocardial oxygen requirements by reducing ventricular filling pressures and afterload, although excessive hypotension can pose a risk of reducing coronary perfusion. In both hypertensive pulmonary edema and crescendo angina, nitroprusside offers the unique advantage of precise, reversible titration of ventricular preload and cardiac output. Parenteral nitrate therapy alone or in combination with nifedipine may be satisfactory in less severely ill patients, but should not be used instead of nitroprusside in stabilizing a critically ill patient.

Diazoxide

This drug is a potent direct arteriolar vasodilator which has no effect on the venous capacitance vessels. Its use is associated with reflex activation of the sympathetic nervous system, and tachycardia may result in symptomatic myocardial ischemia in the presence of coronary artery disease. When the drug was first introduced, it was recommended that 300 mg be administered as an intravenous bolus for severely hypertensive patients. When used in this fashion, the drug can produce signifi-

cant toxicity in the form of undesired and prolonged hypotension, resulting in cerebral or myocardial ischemia.

It is currently recommended that diazoxide be administered in a dosage of 5 mg per kilogram as a continuous intravenous infusion at a rate of 15 mg per minute. The infusion can then be discontinued if excessive hypotension is observed prior to administration of the full dose. With this protocol, potentially hazardous hypotension is said to be avoided with this drug. An alternative approach is to administer multiple small intravenous doses of 50 to 100 mg at 10- to 15-minute intervals until satisfactory lowering of the blood pressure is observed. Despite both of these more cautious drug administration schedules, the hypotensive effect of diazoxide is prolonged, lasting 2 to 12 hours. If excessive hypotension occurs, the effect is likely to be sufficiently prolonged to risk serious myocardial and cerebral complications.

Diazoxide is not the drug of choice for hypertensive encephalopathy and is *contraindicated* in the management of aortic dissection, hypertensive pulmonary edema, and angina secondary to severe hypertension. In malignant hypertension with acute renal failure, diazoxide probably still has a therapeutic niche, although nifedipine might be equally effective and easier to use. Certainly the use of oral minoxidil, nifedipine, or clonidine should be carefully considered in this setting before selecting parenteral diazoxide. Diazoxide causes sodium retention and thus furosemide is usually administered along with it.

Clonidine

This orally active antihypertensive agent is an alpha$_2$-agonist. It exerts its hypotensive effect by its cerebral effect of inhibiting the vasomotor centers and reducing peripheral sympathetic nerve norepinephrine release. The onset of drug action occurs within an hour of the first dose and has been correlated with a significant fall in the plasma norepinephrine concentration in treated patients. Clonidine produces controlled gradual reduction in the blood pressure in severe hypertension when administered in an initial oral dose of 0.2 mg followed by 0.1 mg hourly until a total dosage of 0.8 mg has been administered over a 7-hour titration period. Because of its relatively slower onset of action, it has been classified in Table 1 as a class II drug along with nifedipine and minoxidil. The major complications of this form of administration of clonidine are excessive sedation and the anticholinergic side effect of a dry mouth. Excessive sedation may complicate the evaluation of a change in mental status in a patient with early hypertensive encephalopathy, and for this reason clonidine is perhaps a less useful drug in this setting than alternative agents. If the patient fails to respond to clonidine during the titration phase, alternative antihypertensive drugs should be initiated.

Clonidine and other class II drugs are not indicated in the initial emergent management of severe hypertensive crises because it is not always effective, has a relatively slow onset of action, and may reduce cerebral bloodflow in hypertensive encephalopathy. Clonidine is exceptionally useful in asymptomatic patients with a diastolic blood pressure over 125 mm Hg, who require controlled blood pressure reduction over a 6- to 12-hour time frame. The drug can also be used to advantage early in nitroprusside therapy to allow early discontinuation of nitroprusside.

Nifedipine

Although not approved as an antihypertensive agent by the FDA, multiple recent publications attest to the potent antihypertensive effect of this drug when administered to patients with severe hypertension. The agent is a calcium-channel blocker which acts predominantly as a peripheral arteriolar vasodilator. The onset of drug effect is rapid, occurring within 15 to 60 minutes whether it is administered orally or sublingually. If an immediate antihypertensive effect is needed in hypertensive encephalopathy, nitroprusside should be preferred to sublingual nifedipine because a more controlled rate of blood pressure reduction can thereby be achieved. The duration of drug effect with nifedipine is 4 to 6 hours, and its usual elimination half-life is 2 hours. The initial dose is usually 10 mg orally or sublingually, which can be repeated in 1 to 2 hours if needed to a maximum of 30 mg. (The capsule can be multiply punctured and placed under the tongue, or chewed for sublingual administration.) The dosage of nifedipine can be consolidated and administered in four divided doses every 6 hours. Concurrent beta-blocker therapy is recommended to attenuate the usually mild drug-induced reflex tachycardia.

The ultimate place of nifedipine in hypertensive emergencies is not yet resolved. The drug can produce potentially harmful acute hypotension in severely hypertensive patients, and this may occur unexpectedly. The marked hypotensive potency of nifedipine holds forth the possibility of similar complications as those seen with diagoxide. It is a particular risk in the patient who is hypovolemic or on other vasodilators, such as nitrates. Once hypotension does occur, the drug effect persists for hours and this could lead to prolonged cerebral, renal, or myocardial ischemia. Early reports of its use in hypertensive emergencies have been optimistic and have not underscored the potential for uncontrolled hypotension. Until prospective trials become available that compare the safety and efficacy of the two drugs, prudent management of critically ill hypertensive patients requires nitroprusside, not nifedipine.

Captopril

This drug is an orally active angiotensin-converting enzyme inhibitor which merits special mention as an oral agent in the treatment of severe hypertension. If a patient is known to have *renovascular disease*, or is suspected to have this secondary form of hypertension on clinical grounds, initial oral therapy with captopril is warranted. For the severely hypertensive patient, a dosage of 25 mg orally is safe and can produce a rapid fall in blood pressure within 1 hour. The blood pressure should be carefully monitored in the first 60 minutes after administration. If the fall in blood pressure is excessive, intravenous saline is an effective antidote. Thereafter, the drug should be administered every 6 hours. The dose can be safely titrated upward to a maximum of 200 mg daily.

The major toxicities of captopril include allergic dermatitis, hyperkalemia in patients with renal insufficiency, and renal failure in bilateral renal artery stenosis or renal artery stenosis with a single kidney. The latter complication responds promptly to drug withdrawal. Captopril can be effective as adjunctive therapy to nitroprusside in patients with renin-dependent hypertension who merit emergent blood-pressure reduction with this intravenous agent. Caution should be exercised by first lowering the nitroprusside dosage somewhat to allow the blood pressure to increase before the initial test dose of captopril is given.

Minoxidil

This drug is a potent arteriolar vasodilator that produces maximal lowering of the blood pressure within 4 hours of oral administration. The plasma half-life of the drug is 4 hours, but its antihypertensive effect lasts at least 24 hours. In the treatment of severe hypertension, this drug can be administered in an initial dosage of 10 to 20 mg if the diastolic blood pressure exceeds 120 mm Hg. When minoxidil is used in this fashion, the patient should first receive 40 mg of propranolol orally, and it is wise to administer concurrently a dose of 40 mg of furosemide. The major side effects of minoxidil are reflex tachycardia and sodium retention. Thus, propranolol and furosemide are always indicated when this drug is administered. The reflex tachycardia produced by minoxidil can occur after propranolol administration and, if a patient has symptomatic coronary disease, minoxidil should not be the drug of choice as an oral agent in lowering the blood pressure. Minoxidil can be an invaluable orally active antihypertensive agent for patients who have failed to respond adequately to a conventional three-drug antihypertensive regimen. When used in the setting of severe hypertension, a booster dose of minoxidil can be administered 4 hours after the initial dose and can be expected to produce a percentage reduction in the blood pressure similar to that of the initial dose.

Minoxidil has not been a widely used drug in hypertensive crises as a first-line agent; this is justified by its relatively slow onset of action and its propensity for producing reflex tachycardia. Nifedipine will probably prove to be a more frequently used agent than minoxidil when a fast-acting potent vasodilator antihypertensive drug in severely hypertensive patients is needed. However, minoxidil is likely to be a more powerful vasodilator than nifedipine, and it can be an invaluable agent in patients who have failed conventional antihypertensive therapy.

Other Drugs

Other drugs still occasionally used in severe hypertension include guanethidine, hydralazine, intravenous alpha-methyldopa, prazosin, trimethaphan camsylate, and reserpine. For instance, hydralazine is commonly used in hypertension associated with toxemia of pregnancy, in which its potent ability to produce reflex tachycardia is not a significant risk factor in young women of childbearing age not likely to have coronary disease. Trimethaphan camsylate is occasionally used in hypertension associated with aortic dissection, although it is clearly not superior to nitroprusside and propranolol in this application.

THERAPEUTIC AND DIAGNOSTIC DECISIONS AFTER INITIAL THERAPY

Once the initial therapeutic decisions have been made concerning selection of appropriate antihypertensive therapy for the severely hypertensive patient, and a successful lowering of the blood pressure has been observed, management decisions must be made about interim and long-term antihypertensive therapy. For patients with *chronic essential hypertension*, this is usually not particularly difficult as their responses to conventional antihypertensive therapy often are evident from the medical history. In such instances, drugs found to be previously effective can be reinstituted and additional agents initiated as needed to achieve adequate long-term regulation of blood pressure.

For patients who present with *recent-onset hypertension*, it is crucial to proceed with an effective diagnostic evaluation to pursue treatable primary causes of hypertension. In particular, patients known to have atherosclerotic vascular disease and who provide a history of recent-onset of severe hypertension should be hospitalized and appropriately evaluated for the possibility of renovascular hypertension with angiography and renal vein renin sampling.

Other diseases that result in severe hypertension, such as pheochromocytoma, adrenal adenoma, glomerulonephritis, aortic coarctation, and Cushing's syndrome should not be missed at the time of the initial hypertensive crisis. This is possible only if appropriate care is taken to make an appropriate diagnostic evaluation in such patients after their acute hypertensive crisis has passed and before long-term antihypertensive therapy is begun.

The patient who presents with *acute renal failure* and severe hypertension may have a particularly difficult management problem. In such instances, it is well to keep in mind that the renal failure may be secondary to malignant hypertensive nephropathy or severe renovascular disease; alternatively, a primary parenchymal disease, such as glomerulonephritis, may be the cause of the renal failure and hypertension. If the diagnosis appears to be malignant hypertension as the primary etiology of the acute renal failure, emergent antihypertensive therapy is warranted. Nitroprusside is an acceptable initial agent although its potential for thiocyanate intoxication with renal failure should not be overlooked. If the patient does not have hypertensive encephalopathy, early institution of a class II agent, such as nifedipine or clonidine, can frequently reduce the blood pressure and allow prompt tapering of the nitroprusside. Again, excessive hypotension should be avoided because further aggravation of renal ischemia is undesirable. Such patients always need hospital admission and often early hemodialysis to reduce the extracellular fluid volume.

POSTEMERGENCY CARE OF HYPERTENSIVE PATIENTS

Apart from the patients with end-organ damage, or complicating medical conditions who require hospitalization, a sizable number of patients can be successfully treated in an emergency medicine center and safely discharged home after a satisfactory reduction in the blood pressure has been observed. It is especially important to ascertain that the patient has not developed orthostatic hypotension or neurologic deterioration with antihypertensive drug therapy. The still asymptomatic patient with an acceptable blood pressure should always be evaluated within 3 days by his primary physician. At this follow-up visit, further necessary adjustments in medication can be made and the hypertensive episode can be viewed in perspective with the patient's previous medical history. This will assure that the short term goal of blood pressure reduction does not obscure the need for judicious diagnostic evaluation of selected hypertensive patients after the crisis has passed.

ARTERIAL INSUFFICIENCY AND OCCLUSION

JONATHAN B. TOWNE, M.D.

Accurate evaluation of the acutely ischemic extremity is essential; it is necessary to distinguish acute limb threatening ischemia (a surgical emergency) from more chronic forms of ischemia that allow the luxury of time for complete evaluation. The *severity* of vascular insufficiency is primarily related to the time interval during which the occlusion develops, the extent of the blocked arterial segment, and the patient's inherent ability to develop collateral circulation around the obstruction. When the occlusion is acute and the vascular system has little time to develop collateral flow, the result is more severe ischemia than when the occlusion develops over a longer period of time. The patient who gradually develops an atherosclerotic occlusion of the distal aorta frequently manifests only mild intermittent claudication. In contrast, the patient who has acute distal aorta occlusion secondary to an embolus has urgent limb-threatening ischemia, which if not promptly corrected results in irreversible ischemic changes.

The extent of atherosclerotic occlusive disease, both proximal and distal to the site of occlusion, also profoundly affects the severity of resulting ischemia. The more extensive the occlusive disease, the longer the distance that the blood must traverse highly resistant collateral channels. The effect of several sequential areas of occlusion in the major inflow vessels of the foot has a cumulative effect with each occlusion, which results in increased resistance to flow and decreased arterial pressure and reduction in the volume of flow.

Because of the suddenness of onset, acute ischemia is likely to cause limb-threatening problems requiring urgent surgical intervention. The most common *causes* are arterial emboli, trauma, and vascular coagulation disorders. Occasionally patients with atherosclerotic occlusive disease may have an acute arterial ischemia, most often from extensive thrombosis in the presence of low cardiac output or from the propagation of thrombus into the distal circulation beyond a more proximal atherosclerotic occlusion.

ACUTE ISCHEMIA

Diagnosis

The diagnosis of acute ischemia of the extremity depends on a carefully performed *physical examination*. This examination quantitates the severity of the ischemia and locates the site of arterial obstruction. On inspection the extremity is pale, and occasionally cyanotic, with collapsed pedal veins and pale or blanched nail beds. When only one extremity is involved, comparisons of warmth and color between the uneffected extremity and the symptomatic extremity aids in diagnosis. The absence of hair on the extremity, the thinning of the skin, and the presence of ulcers or localized areas of gangrene indicate the presence of a chronic process such as arterial occlusive disease as a likely cause of ischemia rather than embolic disease. The interdigital spaces should be examined because these are sites of early gangrene, especially in diabetics. The presence of edema alerts the examiner to possible infection. The presence of ischemic rubor can be confusing. In the ischemic foot, vasodilation causes pooling of blood when the foot is in a dependent position, resulting in a characteristic cyanotic red color. This is easily distinguished from a normal extremity or one with venous insufficiency by elevation, which causes the color to disappear rapidly with the development of a pale, ischemic color characteristic of poor arterial inflow.

Palpation of pulses localizes the level of obstruction. The absence of a femoral pulse indicates involvement of the aortoiliac segment, and absence of popliteal pulses demonstrates involvement of the superficial femoral artery. Pulses always should be compared with those in the asymptomatic extremity. The warmth of the extremity should be ascertained by examination with the dorsum of the hand because the level and the degree of coolness are directly proportional to the severity of the ischemia. Comparison with the asymptomatic extremity aids in this determination. Capillary fill time is a good estimation of arterial flow and is measured by placing mild pressure on the skin and noting the time it takes the color to return. Normal value is less than 2 seconds. Evaluation of the status of the sensation in the affected extremity is important. Inability to detect touch and pain are important indicators of severe ischemia; the only exception is a patient with diabetes mellitus who has peripheral neuropathy. In the sensory and neurologic examination, muscular function of the involved extremities should also be tested. The intrinsic muscles of either the hand or foot should be tested by abducting the fingers or by asking the patient to wiggle his toes. The presence of anesthesia and muscle paralysis in the extremity indicates severe ischemia, which results in an irreversible ischemia and tissue loss if not corrected in a short period of time. Immediate vascular surgical consultation is mandatory.

The use of the *Doppler* pressures can help in making the diagnosis of acute arterial ischemia by aiding in the detection of pulses and measuring the arterial pressure in the foot. A patient with a pressure of less than 40 mm Hg at the ankle is in the limb-threatening category.

The principal *differential diagnoses* are embolic disease and acute thrombosis secondary to occlusive arterial disease. The origin of the embolus is often the left atrium in patients with atrial fibrillation and the left ventricle in patients with recent myocardial infarction. Emboli can also originate from ulcerated atheromatous plaques, most often seen in the infrarenal aorta and iliac arteries. Abdominal aortic and iliac aneurysms as well as femoral and popliteal aneurysms can also shower the distal circulation with emboli. Clinical findings that favor embolism as the cause of the ischemia include the involvement of only one leg with all of the pulses present in the unaffected extremity, absence of history of intermittent claudication, and no evidence of occlusive disease elsewhere in the body, which may be manifested by differential arm blood pressure or the presence of bruits anywhere in the vascular system. Once the diagnosis of embolism is made, the location is determined by examination of the pulses. Most often only one leg is affected; however, on occasion an aortic saddle embolus obstructs both iliac arteries, resulting in absence of both femoral pulses with profound ischemia in both legs.

Treatment

Patients with acute ischemia are immediately given 5,000 units of *heparin* intravenously. Patients with the absence of one or both femoral pulses who are producing adequate amounts of urine are immediately taken to the operating room for thromboembolectomy. If anuria is present, angiography is necessary to determine whether there is involvement of the renal arteries. In patients with acute ischemia who have palpable femoral pulses, angiography is likewise done because of the difficulty of distinguishing between thrombosis secondary to arterial occlusive disease from emboli. In this case angiography facilitates the operative procedure in directing the surgeon to the sites of problems. Operative intervention is required immediately because the time in which revascularization can be performed without having tissue loss is usually limited to a 4- to 8-hour time period.

ATHEROSCLEROTIC DISEASE

Another cause of acute arterial ischemia is occlusion secondary to atherosclerosis. The arterial disease that results in occlusive disease involves primarily the lower extremities and is only rarely seen in the upper extremities. Patients with occlusive disease are classified both by level of arterial involvement and by the degree of the resulting ischemia. There are three degrees of symptoms: the first is asymptomatic, which requires no treatment; the second is intermittent claudication, which is the mild manifestation of occlusive disease and classically involves the calf of the leg, but can involve the thigh, gluteal region, or foot; and the most severe is limb-saving ischemia, which implies that the patient is at significant risk for losing the extremity. Severe ischemia manifests as rest pain, which signifies that the arterial flow is unable to meet the resting metabolic needs of the foot. Ischemic rest pain worsens when the patient is supine and the legs are horizontal and improves when the legs are in a dependent position, when hydrostatic pressure augments arterial flow. Another presentation of limb-salvage ischemia is the presence of ischemic ulcers. In a nondiabetic, these are often in areas of trauma such as the anterior aspect of the tibia or the lateral aspect of the ankle or are the result of injury while trimming toenails. In these patients, although there is sufficient blood supply to maintain normal metabolic needs of the tissue, there is inability to augment the blood flow, which is required for healing. These patients are usually smokers, are more commonly men, and usually have a history of coronary artery disease and a high incidence of diabetes mellitus and hypertension.

Occlusive disease of the lower extremities can be divided into *four regions*: the aortoiliac segment, the femoral bifurcation including the superficial femoral and profunda femoris artery, the distal popliteal and tibial vessels, and the small vessels of the foot (which are usually involved only in diabetics). The severity of the symptoms depends both on the interval during which the occlusion develops and on the length of the blocked vessel. Occlusion that develops over long periods of time gives the vascular system optimal chance to develop collateral flow and results in milder symptoms than acute occlusions.

When the disease is limited to the *aortoiliac segment*, the patient presents with intermittent claudication at the calf, thigh, and occasionally buttock. Clinically there is a decreased groin pulse on the involved side. Distal pulses may be present at rest but disappear with exercise. In mild cases there is normal capillary filling time in the foot, but as the disease progresses capillary filling time becomes progressively prolonged. A definitive diagnosis can be made by obtaining Doppler blood pressure evaluations at the ankle, which document the decrease in arterial perfusion pressure.

When the occlusive disease involves the *femoral system*, it often extends into both the superficial femoral and profunda femoris arteries. These patients present with either intermittent claudication of the calf or limb-salvage ischemia, depending on the development of collateral circulation of the thigh and the extent of tibial occlusive disease. Occlusive disease in the *popliteal-tibial system* is often associated with superficial femoral obstruction, but it can present as isolated disease, especially in diabetics. These patients generally have advanced intermittent claudication or are in the limb-salvage category. Patients who present with rest pain, areas of cellulitis, and signs of acute ischemia require immediate hospitalization.

BUERGER'S DISEASE

Buerger's disease, or thromboangiitis obliterans, is an arterial disease that involves primarily the medium and small arteries of both the upper and lower extremities and almost always affects young men who smoke. These patients often have recurrent episodes of superficial thrombophlebitis. Angiography confirms the diagnosis with the classic finding of segmental arterial occlusion. Primary treatment of Buerger's disease is cessation of smoking. If the patient can abstain from tobacco use, amputation can often be avoided. Ulcerations of the tips of the digits is managed with debridement and antibiotics if local infection is present. If the patient continues to smoke, major bilateral amputation is ultimately required.

BLUE TOE SYNDROME

Another unusual and dramatic presentation of acute ischemia is the blue toe syndrome. The patient presents with excruciating pain, most often in one toe or several toes, accompanied by a cyanotic discoloration of the involved digits despite palpable pedal pulses. Atheroembolization from an ulcerated plaque proximal in the arterial system is the cause. The emboli that occlude digital arteries are usually too small to occlude more proximal, dorsal pedal or posterior tibial arteries. This results in ischemia of a solitary digit or two adjacent digits with normal flow to the rest of the foot. The syndrome should not be confused with gout or other arthritides. Treatment is symptomatic, with the addition of aspirin to cause inhibition of platelet aggregation. The toe gradually returns to normal in 2 to 3 weeks as collateral flow improves. On occasion, there can be tissue loss requiring amputation of a digit and portions of the forefoot. This syndrome is a harbinger of an ulcerative plaque in the proximal arterial system that should be evaluated by arteriography and repaired to prevent further episodes of embolization.

VASOSPASTIC DISEASES

Vasospastic diseases are relatively uncommon in clinical practice. The most common is *Raynaud's disease*, which consists of intermittent attacks of vasospasm aggravated by cold or anxiety. It is important to distinguish between a patient with Raynaud's phenomenon and a patient with Raynaud's disease, which is a diagnosis of exclusion. In *Raynaud's phenomenon*, symptoms of arterial vasospasm are common in both upper extremities and are secondary manifestations of other disease processes, notably collagen vascular diseases such as scleroderma, lupus erythematosus, rheumatoid arthritis, and dermatomyositis. The Raynaud's phenomenon is also seen in Buerger's disease, and can be associated with nerve injuries such as carpel tunnel syndrome, thoracic outlet syndrome, and traumatic nerve injury. Occasionally patients with cryoglobulinemia, macroglobulinemia, and cold agglutinins have Raynaud's phenomenon. In its end stage, there is necrosis of the fingertip from the prolonged vasospasm. *Evaluation* should include lupus erythematosus (LE) prep, ANA, complete platelet count, cold agglutinins, sedimentation rates, serum protein electrophoresis, and barium swallow. If the patient's symptoms are mild, he will do well by protecting his hands with gloves and avoiding smoking. If this is insufficient, he should be started on nifedipine, 10 mg orally three times a day. In an occasional patient who develops severe Raynaud's disease with necrosis of the fingertips, a dorsal sympathectomy is indicated.

Another vasospastic syndrome that should be considered is *ergotism*, which can present with marked vasospasm. The diagnosis is primarily obtained by the history of a patient taking ergot-type drugs who has significant vasospasm. Treatment is discontinuation of ergot-type drugs. If the ischemia is severe, heparin administration and intravenous administration of low-molecular-weight dextran is indicated. In the rare case of limb-threatening ischemia, intra-arterial tolazoline and intravenous papaverine are helpful.

COAGULATION PROBLEMS

Paradoxic *thrombotic complications of heparin* sodium therapy are an uncommon but potentially limb-threatening and occasionally fatal complication of heparin anticoagulant therapy, caused by a chemically induced immune thrombocytopenia. This complication usually occurs after several days of exposure to heparin. The earliest clinical evidence of this syndrome is a thrombocytopenia caused by a factor found in the plasma of afflicted patients that produces agglutination of normal platelets when heparin is added. The thrombosis can be arterial or venous and has been called the white clot syndrome because the clot, which is composed primarily of platelets and fibrin, is a white color. All patients who develop thrombotic complications while on heparin therapy should be evaluated for this syndrome, and all patients on heparin therapy should have platelet counts performed regularly. If thrombocytopenia is detected, platelet aggregation studies are indicated. When abnormal platelet aggregation is noted, heparin therapy should be reversed with protamine sulfate and the patient treated with lower-molecular-weight dextran and warfarin sodium.

Antithrombin deficiencies are another cause of acute arterial ischemia. Although initial cases were primarily limited to thrombosis of mesenteric and extremity veins, this problem can also be the cause of acute arterial occlusion. Antithrombin deficiency has also been implicated as the mechanism in which oral contraceptives make young women prone to thrombotic episodes. We have identified patients in whom this was a cause of acute arterial thrombosis involving the lower extremities. If this is not promptly recognized, major amputation may be necessary.

DIABETIC FOOT PROBLEMS

Diabetic patients, because of the unique combination of peripheral neuropathy and small-vessel involvement, are prone to develop foot infections. Patients with diabetic foot lesions are generally classified in two categories: those in whom ischemia or lack of arterial flow is a predominant factor in the formation of the ulcer, and those in whom infection is the major problem.

In the former group, *ischemia* is easily detectable. These patients lack pulses distal to the popliteal artery, and the skin has the classic findings of vascular insufficiencies such as skin atrophy, absence of hair, and abnormal nails. Frequently the lesion on the foot has an innocuous origin: a blister from tight-fitting shoes, injury to toes from cutting the toenails, or a minor abrasion or contusion from walking in bare feet. Minimal lesions progress because the patient has impaired pain sensation. *Treatment* consists primarily of revascularization if a graftable distal vessel is present. Otherwise, a below-knee amputation is necessary when the area of necrosis is too extensive.

Patients with diabetic foot *infections* in whom the infectious process is the overriding clinical factor often have palpable pedal pulses. They present with a purulent discharge from the wound and often have plantar or proximal fascia space infection. The patient's diabetes is often out of control, with marked hyperglycemia and ketoacidosis. Because of the high incidence of coronary artery disease, congestive heart failure often is present. *Treatment* consists of obtaining Gram's stains of the purulent discharge to determine the type of bacteria involved and appropriate intravenous antibiotics. Clinical experience has shown that most commonly these patients have mixed infections that require a broad spectrum of antibiotics.

Following 12 to 18 hours of intensive medical treatment with antibiotics, during which time medical control of the diabetes and any heart failure is obtained, the patient is taken to the operating room for *debridement*. All involved fascia spaces are widely opened and the necrotic material is excised. In occasional patients, the septic process is so extensive that a supermalleolar guillotine amputation is necessary to control the infective process. Following initial debridement, a patient takes one of two courses. If the blood supply is adequate and the bacterial infection is controlled, the patient promptly develops a cleanly granulating wound, which can be closed with a split-thickness skin graft. If a necrotizing infection progresses, it is necessary to proceed with a below-knee amputation.

TRAUMA

Evaluation of the trauma patient for extremity ischemia can be difficult because of coexisting hypovolemic shock, inability to give an adequate history because of altered levels of consciousness, and swelling of the extremity secondary to contusions. All patients with *long bone fractures* should be evaluated for vascular injury because the neurovascular bundle runs adjacent to the bones in both upper and lower extremities. In patients with only one involved extremity, comparison of the injured and uninjured limbs helps in the evaluation. With restoration of blood loss, the hypovolemic changes of vasoconstriction make the diagnosis of acute ischemia easier. Obtaining Doppler pressures at the ankle or wrist and comparing them with the values in the uninvolved extremity is often helpful. Pressure differential of more than 20 mm Hg in the nonatherosclerotic patient indicates an arterial injury. In patients with penetrating injury to the extremity, there are often other indications of vascular injury (e.g., hemorrhage, hematoma, and swelling). If doubt persists, angiography should be performed.

VASCULITIS

BRUCE C. GILLILAND, M.D.

The vasculitides comprise a number of clinical disorders requiring early recognition and appropriate management. The clinical manifestations are diverse, depending on the organ system involved and the severity of inflammation. Vasculitis may present as palpable purpura, painful subcutaneous nodules, glomerulonephritis, mononeuritis multiplex, or fever of unknown origin. Ischemia or infarction of an extremity, bowel, or cerebral vessel in a person unlikely to have atherosclerosis also raises the possibility of vasculitis.

The vasculitides can be separated into recognized clinical disorders based on the size and type of blood vessel involved, the histologic characteristics of the vascular lesion, and the anatomic predilection of the vasculitis. Four major groups of vasculitis can be distinguished using these criteria: hypersensitivity vasculitis, polyarteritis nodosa and related disorders, Wegener's granulomatosis, and giant cell arteritis (temporal arteritis and Takayasu's arteritis). Mucocutaneous lymph node syndrome (Kawasaki disease), Behçet's disease, erythema elevatum diutinum, and Cogan's syndrome are also described.

HYPERSENSITIVITY VASCULITIS

Definition, Etiology, and Pathogenesis

Hypersensitivity vasculitis (also referred to as allergic vasculitis or leukocytoclastic vasculitis) involves venules, capillaries, and arterioles. The mechanism for vessel damage is thought to be deposition of immune complexes in the wall of blood vessels. A variety of drugs and infections have been implicated in the etiology of hypersensitivity vasculitis. Hypersensitivity vasculitis is also associated with certain malignancies and connective tissue disorders.

Clinical Features

Palpable purpura is the most common presentation. Lesions are predominantly on the feet, ankles, and lower legs but also may be present on the arms, face, conjunctiva, or in the mouth. The lesions are approximately the same age and vary in size from a few millimeters to several centimeters. Other forms of vasculitic skin lesions reflecting small-vessel involvement are petechiae, vesicles, ulcers, urticaria, and erythema multiforme. Arthralgias or arthritis, myalgias, abdominal pain, gastrointestinal bleeding, hematuria, proteinuria, peripheral neuropathy, pulmonary infiltrates, and pleural effusions may be manifestations of vasculitis, and their association with one another and with skin lesions is highly variable.

*Henoch-Sch*önlein purpura is a syndrome occurring most often in children, but it can be seen in adults in a less complete form. The full syndrome consists of palpable purpura, abdominal pain, gastrointestinal bleeding, hematuria and proteinuria, and arthralgias and/or arthritis. An upper respiratory infection often antedates the onset of vasculitis.

Palpable purpura is seen in benign hypergammaglobulinemia purpura of Waldenström. Recurrent showers of lesions appear after prolonged periods of sitting or standing. Serum protein electrophoresis shows an elevated level of polyclonal IgG.

Chronic urticaria can be caused by a leukocytoclastic vasculitis. A vasculitis-induced urticarial lesion usually lasts longer than 12 hours, while a nonvasculitic one is faded. Patients with urticarial vasculitis and reduced levels of the early acting complement components fit into a syndrome referred to as hypocomplementemic urticarial vasculitis. These patients may also have arthralgias and/or arthritis, angioedema, abdominal pain, and glomerulonephritis.

Mixed cryoglobulinemia may also be associated with a small-vessel vasculitis. In some patients, hepatitis B antigen can be identified in serum or in the cryoprecipitate. Purpuric lesions appear predominantly on the lower extremities and are precipitated by standing or exposure to cold. Patients may also have arthralgias and/or arthritis and glomerulonephritis.

Evaluation and Management

A complete blood count including platelets, erythrocyte sedimentation rate (ESR), urinalysis, blood urea nitrogen (BUN), creatine, and cryoglobulins should be obtained. Adequate number of platelets excludes thrombocytopenia purpura, which can be confused with vasculitis. Blood culture should be drawn in patients suspected of having infective endocarditis, *Neisseria* infection, or other infections. Hepatitis screen and liver function tests are ordered even when hepatitis is not clinically evident. Chest film may show an infiltrate, effusion, or a malignancy that may be associated with the vasculitis. Patients with left atrial myxoma may have skin lesions resembling small-vessel vasculitis and an echocardiogram is indicated if a mitral murmur is present or if etiology of the vasculitis remains unclear.

The majority of patients with hypersensitivity vasculitis require admission for evaluation and initiation of appropriate treatment. Skin biopsy should be done as soon as possible to confirm the diagnosis. Suspect drugs are stopped and underlying infection is appropriately treated. Prednisone is indicated when symptoms are severe or when there is evidence of decreasing renal function. The initial dose is 40 mg per day, which usually can be tapered slowly based on clinical activity. The prognosis is very good for most patients with hypersensitivity vasculitis.

POLYARTERITIS NODOSUM

Definition, Etiology, and Pathogenesis

Polyarteritis nodosum (PAN) is a necrotizing vasculitis involving small to medium-sized arteries and affecting mainly middle-aged persons. The lesions are segmental, are at different stages of development, and have a predilection for branching points and bifurcations of arteries. Kidneys and other internal organs are involved with sparing of the lungs. An association with hepatitis B infection exists. Deposition of circulating immune complexes plays a role in the pathogenesis of the arteritis.

Clinical Features

Patients usually present with nonspecific symptoms of fever, malaise, weakness, myalgias, and weight loss. Tender skin nodules, palpable purpura, or digital gangrene may be present. Other symptoms include hypertension, leg pain, abdominal pain, and peripheral neuropathy. Patients may also present with myocardial infarction, bowel infarction, or cerebrovascular accident.

Evaluation and Management

The diagnosis of PAN should be considered when a patient presents with fever and weight loss in association with painful skin nodules or abdominal or leg pain. PAN should also be considered in a young to middle-aged patient who presents with a cerebrovascular accident, myocardial infarction, or peripheral vascular occlusive disease and who has little if any risk factors for these entities. The finding of infiltrates on chest film in a patient suspected of having PAN suggests the diagnosis of allergic angiitis and granulomatosis (Churg and Strauss), a rare disorder associated with asthma and a peripheral blood eosinophilia. PAN does not involve the lungs. Left atrial myxoma or nonbacterial thrombotic endocarditis can produce symptoms similar to those of PAN. Echocardiogram and biopsy of a skin lesion help to exclude these disorders.

Patients suspected of having PAN should be admitted to the hospital. Patients are often admitted with other diagnoses such as acute abdomen, myocardial infarction, or cerebrovascular accident, and the diagnosis of PAN should be considered in the inpatient work-up. Diagnosis is confirmed by muscle biopsy. Angiography of the renal or hepatic circulation may show microaneurysms. Treatment is usually begun with prednisone 60 mg per day and cyclophosphamide 2 mg per kilogram per day in proven cases of PAN.

WEGENER'S GRANULOMATOSIS

Wegener's granulomatosis is characterized by necrotizing and granulomatous vasculitis involving the upper and lower respiratory tracts and the kidneys. Etiology is unknown but the clinical presentation suggests that infectious agents and environmental antigens may be involved. There is evidence of hyperreactivity of the immune system.

Clinical Features

Patients usually present with sinusitis along with symptoms of lower respiratory disease such as cough, sputum production, hemoptysis, and shortness of breath. Microscopic hematuria and proteinuria may be present and usually indicate glomerulonephritis. Nonspecific symptoms such as myalgias, arthralgias, weight loss, and fever are often present. The diagnosis of Wegener's granulomatosis should be considered in any patient with pulmonary infiltrates and sinusitis, especially when the urinalysis shows hematuria, red cell casts, and proteinuria. Patients with Wegener's may also appear to have pneumonia or a sinus infection and indeed may have superimposed infection, which should be treated with antibiotics.

Evaluation and Management

The diagnosis of Wegener's granulomatosis should be entertained in a patient presenting with sinus or respiratory tract symptoms along with fever and weight loss.

Radiographs of the chest and sinuses should be immediately obtained. Chest film shows solitary or multiple infiltrates as well as cavities. The borders of these infiltrates are often ill defined. Radiographs of involved sinuses show cloudiness and air fluid levels. Urinalysis may show hematuria with or without red cell casts as well as proteinuria. A leukocytosis and elevated ESR are usually present. Palpable purpura, ulcerative lesions, or subcutaneous nodules may be present.

Wegener's granulomatosis may be confused with Goodpasture's syndrome; however, in the latter, sinusitis is not a predominant feature. Patients with Goodpasture's syndrome have antibodies to the glomerular basement membrane.

Lymphomatoid granulomatosis is a disease characterized by infiltration of vessels with atypical lymphoid and plasmacytoid cells and may be difficult to differentiate from Wegener's granulomatosis. Lymphomatoid granulomatosis, however, does not primarily involve the kidneys. Neoplastic disorders, tuberculosis, and other pulmonary granulomatous diseases are distinguished by the appropriate cultures and biopsies.

The mortality from untreated Wegener's granulomatosis is high. The drug of choice is cyclophosphamide in a dose of 1 to 2 mg per kilogram per day orally. Remissions have been reported in over 90 percent of patients treated with cyclophosphamide. Glucocorticoids are often given along with cyclophosphamide early in the treatment. Glucocorticoids alone are not adequate for the treatment. Patients require admission for evaluation and initiation of treatment.

TEMPORAL ARTERITIS

Temporal arteritis is a granulomatous vasculitis involving medium- to large-sized arteries and most often affects older patients. The disease is rare under the age of 50. Branches of the carotid artery are most frequently involved. Other medium-sized vessels can be affected but rarely lead to symptoms. Temporal arteritis rarely if ever directly involves intracranial arteries.

Clinical Features

Headache is the most common symptom and is described as being continuous with episodes of lancinating pain. The scalp may be very tender. Patients may have decreased or sudden loss of vision or diplopia. They may complain of jaw claudication. Polymyalgia rheumatica may be present and is characterized by aching pain, stiffness, and soreness of the proximal muscles of the hip and shoulder girdles and neck. Patients are often able to recall the exact date of the onset of symptoms. In addition, the patient may have nonspecific symptoms such as fever, weight loss, malaise, and arthralgias.

Evaluation and Management

A patient over 50 who presents with a recent onset of headache, transient or sudden loss of vision, or symptoms of polymyalgia rheumatica should be suspected of having temporal arteritis. The temporal artery may be tender to palpation as well as the scalp. An ESR should be immediately obtained and supports the diagnosis if above 50 mm per hour (Westergren method). If the diagnosis of temporal arteritis is highly suspected, the patient should be admitted for temporal artery biopsy even if the ESR is not elevated. High-dose prednisone treatment should be immediately started with the initial dose of prednisone being 60 mg per day in divided doses.

Patients who have only symptoms of polymyalgia rheumatica can be given a diagnostic trial of low-dose prednisone, 10 to 15 mg per day. Dramatic improvement of symptoms should be seen within 4 days. The patient should be seen in 1 week and, if he is not significantly better or if other symptoms of temporal arteritis are now present, temporal artery biopsy should be performed. Other causes of polymyalgia and ESR should be explored in patients who have a negative biopsy and absence of other symptoms of temporal arteritis.

TAKAYASU'S ARTERITIS

Takayasu's arteritis is a granulomatous arteritis of unknown etiology affecting large and intermediate-sized arteries. The aorta and its major branches are frequent sites of involvement. There is a female predominance.

Clinical Features

In the early phase of disease, patients experience fever, night sweats, weakness, myalgias, and arthralgias. Later, patients manifest symptoms of ischemia due to narrowing and occlusion of involved vessels. Symptoms of claudication may be experienced in both upper and lower extremities. Angina pectoris can occur. Renal artery involvement can cause hypertension leading to heart failure. The diagnosis should be considered in a young to middle-aged person presenting with ischemic symptoms in the arms, legs, or abdomen as well as unexplained hypertension.

Evaluation and Management

Patients should be admitted for further evaluation. Arteriography is an important diagnostic test and shows narrowing or occlusion of involved arteries. Aneurysms, both saccular and fusiform, may be seen in the aorta and its branches. Arteries commonly involved are the subclavian, renal, descending aorta, and carotid arteries. The pulmonary artery may also be involved. In an older person, the differential diagnosis should include atherosclerotic disease. Arteriogram and elevated ESR help to distinguish Takayasu's from arteriosclerotic peripheral vascular disease. Prednisone may help prevent long-term vascular complications. In patients with significant ischemic symptoms, a vascular surgeon should be consulted because reconstructive vascular surgery may be beneficial in selected patients.

MUCOCUTANEOUS LYMPH NODE SYNDROME (KAWASAKI DISEASE)

Mucocutaneous lymph node syndrome (MLNS) is an acute inflammatory disease affecting mostly infants and young children (mean age 4 years) and characterized by fever, conjunctivitis, erythematous lips and oral mucosa, exanthem, and enlargement of the cervical lymph nodes. The etiology is unknown. The disease is more common in patients of Japanese ancestry.

Clinical Features

Patients usually present with fever, redness of the hands and feet, and edema of the extremities. The skin of the hands and feet desquamates. A maculopapular rash develops on the third to fifth day and may become generalized. Conjunctivae are injected, and the lips and mucosa are erythematous and dry. Cervical adenopathy is present. Other manifestations include arthritis, aseptic meningitis, myocarditis, heart failure, and focal encephalopathy. Leukocytosis is usually present.

The diagnosis should be considered in a youngster presenting with fever, red hands and feet, a maculopapular rash, and lymphadenopathy. This disorder may mimic meningococcemia, systemic lupus erythematosus, Stevens-Johnson syndrome, or toxic shock syndrome. The latter is excluded by the absence of hypotension, azotemia, and thrombocytopenia.

Evaluation and Management

The patient should be admitted immediately to the hospital, and electrocardiogram and chest film obtained as soon as possible. The disease is usually self-limited unless cardiac complications ensue. The drug of choice is aspirin 30 mg per kilogram per day in divided doses.

BEHÇET'S DISEASE

Definition, Etiology, and Pathogenesis

Behçet's disease is characterized by recurrent episodes of oral ulcers, genital ulcers, and eye lesions and may be accompanied by thrombophlebitis, meningoencephalitis, arterial occlusions and aneurysms, arthritis, or colitis. Immunologic abnormalities include the presence of circulating immune complexes, immunoglobulins, and complement deposits within blood vessels, and increased chemotactic activity of polymorphonuclear cells. Small blood vessels are the primary site of vasculitis, with the vasa vasorum being the initial site of involvement in large vessels. Behçet's disease is most prevalent in Mediterranean countries and Japan and has a male predominance. In the United States the sex ratio is approximately equal.

Clinical Manifestations

Oral ulcers are usually the first sign of disease. These lesions are small, punched-out ulcerations that range in size from 2 to 10 mm and have erythematous margins and a yellowish base. They are indistinguishable from aphthous ulcers (canker sores) and appear throughout the oral cavity. Genital ulcers appear most commonly on the scrotum and vulva but may also be present in the vagina, in the perianal area, and on the penis. Iridocyclitis with a hypopyon is the most common eye lesion and lasts several days, leaving no significant residual effect. Posterior uveitis also occurs and can lead to blindness. Several types of skin lesions are seen including papules, pustules, furuncles, and erythema nodosum and are most often located on the lower extremities. A sterile pustule with surrounding erythema may develop at a site of a needle puncture. A nondeforming inflammatory arthritis involving only a few joints may be present. Hematuria and proteinuria may reflect glomerulonephritis. Gastrointestinal involvement includes nausea, vomiting, diarrhea, flatulence, and colitis, which can be complicated by bowel perforation. Thrombophlebitis of both the superficial and deep venous systems also occurs. Arterial occlusion leads to strokes, diminished or absent peripheral pulses, or renal hypertension. Neurologic manifestations include headaches, meningoencephalitis, mental changes, and cerebrovascular accidents and occur later in the disease. Death usually results from neurologic or vascular complications.

Evaluation and Management

The diagnosis of Behçet's disease is suspected when patients present with oral or genital ulcers in combination with any of the following: uveitis, skin lesions, arthritis, meningoencephalitis, or other neurologic abnormalities. Laboratory work may show a leukocytosis, elevated ESR, proteinuria, or hematuria. A decision for admission is based on the severity of the patient's symptoms and signs. The majority of patients require admission for both further evaluation and treatment. Treatment is usually only supportive; however, a variety of therapies have been reported to be beneficial in selected patients and include blood transfusions, transfer factor, azulfidine, phenformin, glucocorticoids, and immunosuppressive drugs.

ERYTHEMA ELEVATUM DIUTINUM

Erythema elevatum diutinum is a rare chronic disorder characterized by persistent brownish red to purple plaques or nodules located symmetrically on extensor surfaces of extremities, around joints, and on the dorsa of the hands and feet. The etiology is unknown. Histology shows a leukocytoclastic vasculitis involving primarily venules. The disorder affects mostly Caucasians, with onset in middle age. Skin lesions may be asymptomatic, painful, or pruritic. The rash is often resistant to treatment, but dapsone in a dose of 150 to 250 mg daily has improved some patients. Patients should be referred to a dermatologist.

COGAN'S SYNDROME

Cogan's syndrome consists of interstitial keratitis and audiovestibular symptoms. Some patients develop an aortitis, which may lead to aortic insufficiency. The disease affects mainly young adults. An upper respiratory tract infection often precedes the onset of disease. The onset of interstitial keratitis is abrupt and causes photophobia, lacrimation, and pain. Symptoms of audiovestibular involvement include nausea, vomiting, vertigo, and progressive hearing loss. There is a mild leukocytosis and elevated ESR. If symptoms are severe, the patient should be admitted and immediately examined by an ophthalmologist and otolaryngologist. Treatment is high-dose glucocorticoids, which improve both the eye and audiovestibular disease.

SUGGESTED READING

Cupps TR, Fauci AS. The vasculitides. Philadelphia: WB Saunders, 1981.
Haynes BF, Allen NB, Fauci AS. Diagnostic and therapeutic approach to the patient with vasculitis. Med Clin North Am 1986; 70:355–368.

THROMBOPHLEBITIS

MARVIN L. SACHS, M.D.

When deep venous thrombosis (DVT) is suspected, there always is a sense of urgency, because pulmonary embolism may occur. Even if this complication were not common and sometimes fatal, there would be concern about extension of clot, with damage to venous valves and production of a permanent and troublesome postphlebitic syndrome. Whether the setting be office, emergency department, or inpatient service, management of a patient with DVT should be prompt.

A physician unfamiliar with current knowledge of deep thrombophlebitis* will, on the basis of history and physical examination alone, likely be wrong in the diagnosis nearly half the time; an expert, using only information from the history and physical examination, might be wrong a quarter of the time. These are unacceptable rates of error when, on the one hand, there is a dangerous complication, and on the other hand, appropriate therapy can in itself be hazardous. Seeking help from objective tests has therefore become the accepted approach. Most of the time, noninvasive tests will be sufficient to clarify the situation. When they are not appropriate or not clarifying, contrast venography, the best diagnostic standard we now have, is usually done.

Since acceptably accurate diagnosis depends on objective tests, it might seem that judgment and experience are displaced, but this is by no means true. Clinical competence is crucial at the initial step in evaluation, when a decision must be made whether or not DVT is in the differential diagnosis. Is the patient suspected of having DVT? This is the question that is answered on the basis of history and physical examination. If the patient is not suspected of having DVT, he is free from further investigation of that diagnosis. If the patient is suspected of having DVT, the objective tests become relevant and the patient falls into a higher risk group.

HISTORY

There are two categories of historical information that must be elicited. The first consists of the symptoms of the present illness usually volunteered by the patient. The second comprises predisposing events of the present illness and predisposing background factors, which often must be sought out by the physician.

Symptoms

When the history of the present illness suggests DVT it is usually because the patient complains of pain, generally in a calf, or swelling of a leg. Occasionally other symptoms, such as local warmth or redness will be mentioned. Although there is no combination of symptoms that adequately supports a diagnosis of DVT, typical symptoms can make the patient a suspect (Table 1).

Predisposing Events and Background Factors

For more than a century it has been believed that venous thrombosis is triggered by endothelial injury, venous stasis, and an abnormal tendency to coagulation—the process not necessarily requiring all three. Commonly accepted *predisposing factors* are: trauma, immobilization of limb, inactivity, postoperative state, paralysis, infection, malignant disease, connective tissue disease, pregnancy and postpartum state, estrogens, hypercoagulopathy, advanced age, previous DVT, and previous pulmonary thromboembolism.

Inactivity is a strong predisposing factor, particularly prolonged bed rest, but it is not clear how frequently this is significant entirely on its own. Most people who are notably inactive are also ill, or were injured, or are in a postoperative state; and illness and trauma can be associated with hypercoagulability and with endothelial injury. *Underlying diseases* include some that are highly

---

* The terms thrombophlebitis, venous thrombosis and phlebitis are used interchangeably in this chapter.

predisposing, such as malignancies, specific coagulopathies, and some cases of connective tissue disorders. Advanced age is associated with increased incidence of DVT.

A *history of previous thrombophlebitis* is usually listed as a predisposing factor, but it is truly predisposing only if the diagnosis of the prior episode was correct and if the factors that led to that episode still exist. Many patients give histories of episodes of thrombophlebitis for which the diagnosis was never established.

SIGNS

Adding data from the physical examination can often be persuasive with respect to classifying the patient as a suspect, but absence of suspicious signs is in itself of little value in excluding the diagnosis.

Common signs are listed in Table 2. They correspond closely to symptoms, and they share, with one exception, the lack of specificity that is characteristic of the symptoms.

Tenderness is a notoriously misleading sign, since any number of conditions can produce it, including contusions, muscle sprain, and infection. A *palpable deep linear cord* is suggestive but not specific. *Swelling* is nonspecific. When bilateral, it suggests other conditions. When unilateral, it can still mislead; for example, in cases of unilateral venous valvular incompetence with superimposed early cardiac failure, edema may first be noticed in the limb with venous insufficiency. *Redness* is rarely a reliable sign of deep venous thrombosis, virtually never if the skin is bright red, as is sometimes seen with cellulitis or certain dermatitides. *Local warmth*, unless slight, again is usually a better indicator of infection than of thrombophlebitis. High *fever*, especially if associated with chills, is rarely due to thrombophlebitis, though in extreme cases of massive DVT involving an entire limb, fever may be relatively high. *Homans' sign*, as Homans himself noted, is entirely nonspecific and is of no use in distinguishing DVT from other causes of calf discomfort. The only sign that correlates relatively well with proved

TABLE 1   Symptoms Associated with Deep Venous Thrombosis

Symptoms	More Suggestive of DVT	Equally Suggestive of DVT and Other Diagnoses	More Suggestive of Other Diagnosis
Pain			
Severe			X
Moderate		X	
Slight		X	
Swelling			
Unilateral		X	
Bilateral			X
Chills			X
Fever			
High			X
Moderate		X	
Slight		X	

TABLE 2   Signs Associated with Deep Venous Thrombosis

Signs	More Suggestive of DVT	Equally Suggestive of DVT and Other Diagnoses	More Suggestive of Other Diagnoses
Tenderness		X	
Palpable cord		X	
Edema			
Unilateral		X	
Bilateral			X
Erythema			
Bright			X
Slight		X	
Local warmth			
Marked			X
Slight		X	
Fever			
High			X
Moderate or slight		X	
Homans' sign		X	
Dilated veins	X		

DVT is *dilatation of superficial veins*, which may be seen when the patient is supine, and is usually interpretable only in cases of unilateral DVT when comparison with the normal limb is possible. Though this is a good sign, it is subtle and so has less value than would be hoped.

SUPERFICIAL THROMBOPHLEBITIS

In the discussion so far, superficial thrombophlebitis has not been mentioned. The superficial veins of the lower extremities are the greater, or long, saphenous and the lesser, or short, saphenous. (Keep in mind that the superficial femoral vein is the main deep vein of the thigh [Fig. 1].) Superficial phlebitis usually is distal, and involves veins well toward the ankle. Occasionally the greater saphenous vein will be involved at higher levels, or the lesser saphenous high on the back of the leg. Superficial phlebitis rarely justifies concern about pulmonary embolism, but clot can extend into the deep system. There is therefore a weak indication for screening patients with noninvasive studies when superficial phlebitis is found. If superficial venous thrombosis approaches the popliteal space or the femoral triangle, however, a more serious view of it must be taken. Occasionally, superficial phlebitis in distal calf veins will be followed by extension

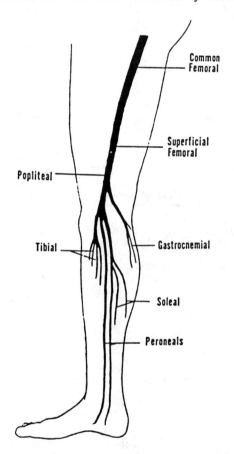

Figure 1 Major deep veins of the lower extremity, medial view. (Valves, communicating veins, and superficial veins are not shown.) Reproduced with permission from Friedman SA, ed. Vascular diseases. Boston: John Wright/PSG, 1982:133.

through perforators into the deep system, so if such distal phlebitis is not clearing well, noninvasive studies for deep venous obstruction should be done.

ESTABLISHING OR EXCLUDING THE DIAGNOSIS

From the historical and physical findings, the doctor must decide whether the patient should be evaluated further for DVT. If there is no evidence that DVT should be in the differential diagnosis, the matter is closed, with the recognition that persistence of marginal complaints or development of new ones might require a diagnostic review. When in doubt, pursue the evaluation.

It is important to have in mind whether the clinical suspicion of DVT is high or low or somewhere between. Such classification depends on experience and judgment.

For the suspects, *noninvasive testing* is usually the next step. The two kinds of noninvasive testing that have become established for prompt diagnosis are plethysmographic tests and Doppler ultrasound examination. Several instruments are available for doing plethysmographic tests, of which the most widely used and most firmly established is the impedance plethysmograph. Another extremely reliable instrument is the phleborheograph. Other instruments probably can be used successfully, but they are less well established. In experienced hands, a Doppler examination is reliable, but a novice can easily be fooled.

A major limitation of plethysmographic and Doppler tests must be recognized: Although they are reliable for detecting clot in the proximal deep veins (the popliteal vein and the veins proximal to it), they can miss clot, at least small clots, in the calf veins (soleal, gastrocnemial, tibial, and peroneal). Therefore, if localized calf vein thrombosis is suspected, normal noninvasive studies are only partly reassuring. There is little likelihood of major pulmonary embolism, and most small calf vein clots are not threatening. In these cases, it is reasonable to follow the noninvasive studies, or, if a diagnosis is needed promptly, to get a venogram. Some believe that small calf vein clots can be ignored, but the potential for extension is not predictable.

Special problems arise when venography itself is hazardous, which is particularly the case in patients with renal insufficiency and possibly most commonly in those who are also diabetic, in whom the dye load of venography can cause acute worsening of renal function. There is also a group of patients who have histories of allergic reactions to contrast dye, for whom preparation with steroids and antihistamines is appropriate if venography must be done. In some situations, such as pregnancy, the x-ray exposure is unwanted, and this forces greater reliance on noninvasive studies.

The algorithm in Figure 2 illustrates a strategy for working through the diagnosis. After a patient has been labeled a suspect and a level of suspicion has been assigned, a noninvasive study is done. The choice normally depends on what is available at a suitable level of skill at the time. Sometimes it is appropriate to do both a Doppler examination and a plethysmographic test, a combination that is likely to improve accuracy if both are done skillfully.

High Probability of DVT

If clinical suspicion is high and the noninvasive test is abnormal, the likelihood that the patient has deep venous obstruction is sufficiently high to justify treatment. In cases in which the use of anticoagulation would be dangerous, venography might be needed in addition to the noninvasive study (or it might have been selected in place of the noninvasive study).

Low Probability of DVT

In cases in which the clinical suspicion of DVT is low and the noninvasive study is normal, the situation can be considered resolved and the diagnosis dropped with the recognition that change in clinical status with time would require reevaluation.

Intermediate Probability of DVT

The cases with intermediate level of suspicion are more difficult. For this group it is appropriate to consider a clearly abnormal noninvasive test as indicative of DVT with the patient handled as noted above; and it is appropriate to consider a clearly normal noninvasive test as indicative of exclusion of the diagnosis. Difficulties arise when the noninvasive studies are equivocal or when, if more than one kind of study is done, they disagree. In

these cases, repeating the noninvasive study may be clarifying; if not, the resolution is usually reached by venography. If that is not available, then a decision has to be made either to treat for DVT or to follow the patient closely with repeated noninvasive studies, which may subsequently either be clearly normal or clearly abnormal.

While specific diagnostic tests are under way, other studies should be done, particularly blood counts, including platelet count, prothrombin time (PT) and activated partial thromboplastin time (APTT), serum creatinine, and blood urea nitrogen. It is desirable to know the creatinine level before venography is done and the hematologic test results before anticoagulation therapy is started.

THERAPY

Although some authorities feel that *fibrinolytic therapy* is appropriate for many cases of DVT, this usually is reserved for patients in whom massive amounts of clot have formed or large emboli have already reached the lungs (see the chapter *Pulmonary Embolism*).

The treatment regularly relied on is *anticoagulation with heparin*, started as soon as possible after the diagnosis has been established. It is necessary to give enough heparin to raise the APTT to at least twice the control and hold it there continuously for the first 2 days, then to 1.5 to 2 times control. To do this, an intravenous bolus of 5,000 to 10,000 units should be given, followed by continuous intravenous heparin, the dose established according to repeated APTTs. Intravenous therapy can also be given by injecting a bolus of heparin every 4 hours. The more clot present, the higher the dose of heparin needed.

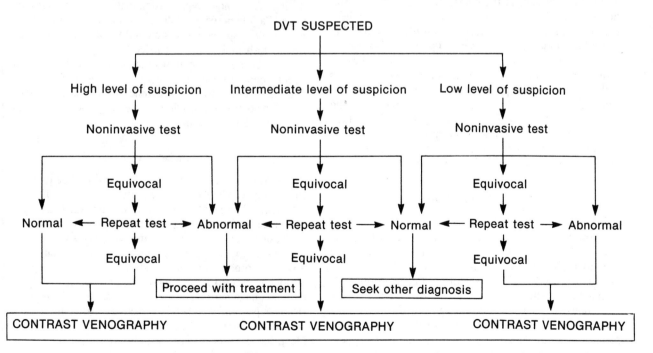

Figure 2 This algorithm assumes no unusual risk of venography or of anticoagulation. Where "Repeat test" appears, this is optional; sometimes venography will be chosen directly. DVT = deep venous thrombosis.

During the first 2 days of treatment, when bleeding complications are relatively uncommon, it is better to give too much than too little heparin.

It is not unusual to see a patient in circumstances where confirmatory noninvasive or invasive testing is not available for a day or more. If suspicion of DVT is high, and if there is no high risk of anticoagulation, heparin should be given in full doses until objective tests refute the diagnosis. In cases of intermediate-level suspicion, it is harder to know what to do while waiting for objective tests, and there are no rules. Where the level of suspicion is low, anticoagulation is inappropriate until an objective test indicates that DVT is highly likely or is definitely present.

Full anticoagulation with heparin is continued from 5 to 15 days or more, depending on severity of the thrombotic disease, but the usual duration is 7 to 10 days. The

---

* This assumes the use of rabit-brain thromboplastin in the PT test as in conventional in North America. The ratio of PT to control would be greater in those countries where a more sensitive thromboplastin is used.

incidence of recurrence of DVT is greatly reduced by providing full anticoagulation for 3 to 6 months, so it is usual to switch from heparin to an *oral medication*, Coumadin (warfarin) being the one commonly used. Loading doses of warfarin are not recommended. One should start with daily doses of 7.5 to 10 ml. Since it takes at least 4 or 5 days, possibly 7 days, for the full anticoagulant effect of warfarin to develop, even if the prothrombin time (PT) is in therapeutic range in 3 days, an overlap with heparin of 5 or 6 days is important. Although in the past it has been conventional to give enough warfarin to prolong the prothrombin time to 1.5 to 2 times control, this practice is associated with an unnecessarily high incidence of bleeding complications. Currently it is believed that prothrombin time prolongation of 1.3 to 1.6 times control will provide good protection against recurrent thrombosis and little likelihood of serious bleeding. Meticulous monitoring and regulation of therapy with warfarin or other oral anticoagulants is essential.

CHRONIC VENOUS INSUFFICIENCY AND ULCER

ERIC STIRLING, M.D.

Chronic venous insufficiency is an unexciting, generally tedious disease in the emergency setting. Recognition is generally easy, but therapeutic options are limited, both in number and effectiveness. This is unfortunate because the incidence approaches 0.5 percent of the population in the United States. In follow-up studies of iliofemoral thrombosis, more than 80 percent of patients had developed a venous ulcer within 10 years. An average of eight outpatient visits per year were required, and in 1977 over the preceding 10-year period, an average of $40,000 per patient was spent on the sequelae of the thrombotic episode. This is the "worst-case scenario," but nonetheless it illustrates the magnitude of the problem.

PATHOPHYSIOLOGY

There is a strong correlation between proximal deep vein thrombosis and subsequent venous insufficiency. Symptoms generally start within 30 months after the acute thrombotic episode, and the mean time for ulcer development is 7 years. Either nontreatment of acute thrombosis or standard treatment with heparin allows destruction of the venous valves in the affected segment. The key valves for venous insufficiency are those of the popliteal segment. If these are damaged, the subsequent venous hypertension causes reversal in the usual superficial to deep flow of blood, resulting in secondary varicose veins, edema, hemosiderin deposits, fibroblast proliferation, stasis dermatitis, and ulcers. Stasis dermatitis is the result of chronic

stasis with pruritus that leads to scratching and excoriation. Weeping, crusting, and inflammation follow. The inflammation is violaceous, with an underlying brownish hue due to hyperpigmentation from extravasated blood. Initially it is at the ankle level, but spreads to the foot and lower leg. Ulcers invariably follow.

Ulcers develop at the medial ankle area because of a unique anatomical feature. The perforating veins that drain the subcutaneous space in this area do not communicate with the superficial veins, unlike the remainder of the leg. The venous hypertension in the perforators results in capillary hyperpermeability, fibrinogen leakage into the pericapillary space, conversion of the fibrinogen to fibrin, minimal fibrinolysis, poor nutrient and gas exchange, and finally cell death. It follows that with this sequence of events, continuing even during the treatment of an ulcer, healing will be slow and recurrences frequent. Squamous cell carcinomas may develop in an ulcer present more than 5 years without healing.

PREVENTION

Although the rapidity of progression of venous insufficiency can be slowed, the disease is inexorable once established. Prevention can be accomplished only by preserving valvular competence during the acute thrombosis, or better yet, preventing the thrombosis itself. Current trends in acute-phase treatment are more and more toward thrombolytic therapy: streptokinase, tissue plasminogen activators, and combinations of thrombolytic therapy and heparin. The ideal prophylaxis in the highest risk groups—patients with hip fractures, pelvic malignancies or surgeries, and major trauma—has not yet been identified. Low-dose heparin studies for the general medical and surgical hospital populations are now in question because of the methodology and use of the fibrinogen scans. There will be many sequelae of acute thrombosis for some years to come.

DIAGNOSIS

The history and clinical examination should reliably differentiate between arterial and venous insufficiency, lymphedema, and edema of systemic disorders (see Table 1). Venous insufficiency presents with aching pain on standing, relief of pain on recumbency, complaints of pruritus, swelling, varicosities, and rarely venous claudication (aching pain on walking due to extensive deep venous obstruction, mimicking arterial insufficiency). On examination, the leg is seen to be swollen with pitting edema, hyperpigmentation, cyanosis on dependency, stasis dermatitis, and varicosities. Liposclerosis (stasis dermatitis with woody fibrotic changes) and ulcers are late findings. A "chemical" cellulitis (sterile) is especially confusing in the evaluation of exacerbations of venous insufficiency. Heat, redness and tenderness, fever, and leukocytosis result in many admissions for presumed bacterial cellulitis. With hospital bed rest, application of heat, and elevation, more rapid clinical improvement occurs than would be expected. There is no possible differentiation in the emergency department.

The *Trendelenburg test* helps confirm saphenous or communicating vein incompetence. The leg is elevated for 60 seconds, and then a tourniquet is applied to the midthigh and the leg is lowered. If the saphenous fills from above, it is incompetent. If rapid filling from below occurs, the communicating veins are incompetent. *Perthe's test* helps further to establish the patency of the deep veins. A tourniquet should be applied at midthigh while the patient is standing and the veins are full. He or she should then walk about for 5 minutes. If the superficial veins collapse below the tourniquet, the deep veins are patent and the communicators are competent. If the venous volume is unchanged, the communicators are incompetent. If the superficial veins become more distended and pain occurs, the deep veins are obstructed and the communicators are incompetent.

Laboratory tests available to help both in diagnosis and in guiding therapy include venous Doppler, real-time ultrasonography, plethysmography, and contrast phlebography (venography). A major stumbling block with all of these tests (including venography) is the poor sensitivity in diagnosing a new thrombotic event in the presence of chronic venous insufficiency. Laboratory investigation is mandatory if venous corrective surgery is planned.

TREATMENT

There is no cure for venous insufficiency, although the progression can be slowed. Only prevention of thrombosis or early lysis of formed clots prevents valvular damage. Deep obstruction and perforator incompetence without severe stasis or ulcers are treated by use of stockings, rest and elevation, and muscle-toning exercises. Simple compression stockings have not been shown to help. Fitted stockings (Jobst, Siggvarus) can reduce ambulatory venous pressures by as much as 30 mm Hg. Rest periods with elevation of the leg above heart level spaced throughout the day retard stasis complications. Muscle-toning exercises increase natural fibrinolysis as well as enhance blood return. Enhancement of fibrinolytic activity by chemical means has been studied with stanozolol (an anabolic steroid). Because of side effects (virilization, weight gain, liver toxicity), its use will probably be limited to those with severe liposclerosis if approved.

Weepy, crusted, inflamed areas must be treated with elevation and intermittent soaks (saline, aluminum acetate—Domeboro). Potent topical steroids (Lidex, Halog) can be applied after soaking if no infection is present. Lubricants (Eucerin, Lubriderm, Keri Lotion) should be used along with topical steroids once the weeping and crusting have resolved.

Venous ulcers are a trial for the patient and physician alike. Healing time is measured in months, recurrence is frequent, and satisfaction is poor. The most effective outpatient treatment is the medicated plaster bandage (Unna's boot). The leg should be cleaned and loose debris should be removed. The ulcer crater should then be filled with some material. Many have been proposed: Debrisan, Gelfoam, Polysporin, magnesium hydroxide (Maalox), Stomahesive, sugar, Vaseline or other petrolatum, Castellani's paint, silver nitrate, silver sulfadiazine (Silvadene), or Betadine ointment. Potent topical steroids can be applied to stasis areas before the boot is applied. The boot should be left on for 7 to 10 days, removed, the leg cleaned and debris removed, and the

TABLE 1 Differential Diagnosis of Venous Insufficiency

	Venous Insufficiency	Arterial Insufficiency	Lymphedema	Swelling of Systemic Disease
Edema	Asymmetric	Absent	Usually asymmetric	Symmetric
Varicosities	Extensive	Absent	Absent	Absent
Skin Appendages (hair, nails, sweat gland activity)	Decreased in stasis areas only	All decreased: hair, nails, sweating	No change	No change
Pain	On dependency, standing, better with walking or elevation	On walking, elevation better with dependency, rest	Painless	Painless unless marked
Skin Appearance	Cyanosis on dependency, stasis dermatitis, varicosities, medial ankle ulcers, liposclerosis	Pale, cool, thin skin, foot or toe ulcers, atrophic changes	Pale, doughy swelling	Pitting edema, occasionally brawny, or weepy
Pulses	Good	Poor	Good	Good

process repeated. Typically, 2 to 3 months of this modality is required to achieve healing or to prepare for grafting. Because the bandage is wrapped firmly, the patient must be compliant with elevation or a tourniquet effect will occur. With large ulcers, the goal with the boot is to achieve a clean ulcer base with decreased leg swelling in preparation for split-thickness grafting. Deep ulcers require full-thickness flaps or, in the case of surrounding fibrosis, wide excision and muscle flaps to provide a vascular bed.

SURGICAL TREATMENT

Subfascial ligation of the ankle perforating veins is now much less popular than in years past. If good selection is made, it may help to prevent high venous pressures from reaching the subcutaneous tissue. However, in the presence of gross deep venous incompetence, the failure rate is greater than 50 percent. Likewise, vein stripping procedures must be preceded by study of the deep and communicating systems. If deep venous obstruction is present, the procedure is bound to fail. There are many divergent views in this area. The middle ground is that subfascial ligation is helpful in those patients who have failed conservative therapy (with good compliance), who have demonstrable gross perforator incompetence, *and* who have an intact deep venous system. This must involve the laboratory in addition to the clinical evaluation.

Venous bypass surgery is a recent advance for a few highly selected patients who have proximal (usually iliac) obstruction and patent distal veins with good valves. Femorofemoral cross leg vein bypass using the greater saphenous vein has had a "success" rate of 75 percent. Many innovative surgical procedures have been recommended for those with valveless deep veins, including superficial femoral vein ligation, venous transposition of the superficial femoral to the deep saphenous or greater saphenous (whichever has the competent valves), valvuloplasty, or autograft of segments of intact vein (usually axillary). Long-term follow-up results are not yet available.

SUGGESTED READING

Barnes RW. Current status of non-invasive tests in the diagnosis of venous disease. Surg Clin North Am 1982; 62:489–500.
Browse NL, Clemenson G, Thomas M. Is the postphlebitic leg always postphlebitic? Br Med J 1980; 281:1167–1170.
Burnand KG, et al. Pericapillary fibrin in the ulcer bearing skin of the lower leg: the cause of lipodermatosclerosis and venous ulcerations. Br Med J 1982; 285:1071–1072.
Dale WA. Venous bypass surgery. Surg Clin North Am 1982; 62:391–398.
Hyde GL, et al. Long term results of subfascial vein ligation for venous stasis disease. Surg cynecol Obstet 1981; 153:683–686.
Immelman EJ, Jeffery PC. The postphlebitic syndrome: pathophysiology, prevention and management. Clin Chest Med 1984; 5:537–550.
Raju S. Venous insufficiency of the lower limb and stasis ulceration: changing concepts and management. Ann Surg 1983; 197:688–697.

VENOUS ACCESS

ROBERT H. DAILEY, M.D.

Establishment of a secure airway and rapid venous access remain the emergency physician's two most critical lifesaving skills. Yet the practical details of these techniques are seldom covered in depth in the literature. It is the purpose of this chapter to describe the establishment of reliable venous access, then focus on particular aspects of blood and crystalloid infusion. Central venous access and venous cutdown will be dealt with only briefly; the reader is referred to more extensive works.

INTRAVENOUS SITES

Although the body has many accessible veins, those in the arm have traditionally been the most used because of their usual visibility and adequate size, and for the technical ease of cannulation of these veins. Clearly the *preferred* arm vein is the cephalic vein at the wrist; it is straight and large, and the forearm stabilizes the site. The cephalic vein on the upper arm is also excellent; however,

because of the placement of the tourniquet, this vein is underutilized. In obese people, the veins of the hand are frequently used because they are seldom completely obscured by subcutaneous fat; cannulation here, however, is painful, the veins are tortuous, and the catheter site is difficult to stabilize. The antecubital fossa provides the large median basilic and median cephalic veins, but these sites are usually reserved for acute emergencies, since arm movement can deform or dislodge the catheters. Finally, blind brachial vein catheterization has recently been described. The brachial vein lies deep in the antecubital fossa, and is closely apposed to the brachial artery. Although the vein is large, not surprisingly, brachial artery puncture has been a frequent complication. Other superficial veins of the arm may also be used. In particular, the basilic vein on the posterior aspect of the forearm is often large, superficial, and straight; however, it is awkward to cannulate this vein and even more difficult to prevent contact with the gurney.

Leg veins have traditionally been avoided. In general, they are tortuous and difficult to cannulate, and cannulation is frequently complicated by superficial phlebitis. How often such superficial phlebitis extends to the deep veins is unknown, but this is frequently cited as a reason not to use leg veins. Still, the saphenous vein at the ankle has traditionally been used for venous cutdowns (see subsequently) and does not appear to be associated with an excessive incidence of deep vein thrombosis.

Use of the femoral vein is on the increase. This vein is one of the largest in the body, bears an extremely constant relationship to the femoral artery, and is easily cannulated, even in severely hypovolemic patients. It is worth reviewing the anatomy and technique used here (Fig. 1). The femoral vein lies at the inguinal ligament, approximately at the junction of the middle and median third of a line drawn from the symphysis pubis to the anterior superior iliac spine. It is also immediately medial to the femoral artery, which provides the traditional pulsatile landmark for cannulation. Extremely large (8-F) wire-guided catheters can be placed at this site with ease. However, one cannot emphasize too strongly that catheters placed in the femoral vein must be removed as soon as stabilization is accomplished and another intravenous site is established; thrombosis or infection can lead to fatal pulmonary embolization. Long catheters inserted through the femoral vein can be threaded into the right atrium and superior vena cava and then used for central venous monitoring.

The external jugular vein has become an increasingly popular and effective route for venous cannulation. This vein is generally very constant in locale, straight, and large; and with J-wire guides, catheters can be reliably threaded into the superior vena cava. This vein is particularly useful in intravenous drug abusers whose other veins are scarred. Because patients are often apprehensive about having neck veins cannulated, they should be reassured and instructed before an attempt is made. The patient should be shown how to make the Valsalva maneuver forcefully; this is the best method of distending the vein. The needle should be inserted next to and parallel to the vein with a quick penetration of the skin only. The needle is then redirected laterally against the vein, bowing it laterally until the needle enters the vein with a slight pop (if the needle is initially directed on top of the vein, it frequently penetrates both walls of the vein, causing cannulation failure). With the needle in the vein, the patient should be allowed to relax and breathe several times; then, during another Valsalva maneuver, the J-wire or

catheter should be advanced. Once the operator becomes familiar with these tips, the external jugular vein will become a favorite, providing fast and reliable access in almost all patients. The intravenous (IV) tubing should be looped about the ear before being secured with a loose circumferential dressing about the neck.

There is renewed interest and enthusiasm for intraosseous infusion in pediatric patients with difficult venous access. The distal femur or proximal tibia can be penetrated with a bone marrow needle. Crystalloid, blood, and drugs can be given by this route; with pressure infusion bags, entry into the central circulation is rapid. A voluminous literature from the 1950s describes infrequent complications: infection, thrombosis, fat emboli and marrow damage. Extremely hyperosmolar solutions (standard bicarbonate or 50 percent glucose) should be avoided.

TECHNIQUE

Poor preparation often results in cannulation failure or complications. Emergency departments should have IV trays with all the necessary materials. The potential IV site should be thoroughly cleansed with povidone-iodine by brisk skin rubbing. Shaving is not only unnecessary, but tiny nicks may even predispose to infection. Some authorities recommend application of topical or intracutaneous anesthesia before large catheters are inserted. If time does not permit a proper, sterile preparation, the catheter should be considered contaminated and removed within 12 to 24 hours; otherwise, septic thrombophlebitis will invariably occur.

Adequate venous dilatation must also be achieved. Although rubber tourniquets are customary, a standard blood pressure tourniquet, inflated to approximately diastolic pressure, achieves greater dilatation. Recently, an ingenious device was described that encloses the forearm in a cylinder to which vacuum is applied. This device produces better venodilatation than even the blood pressure tourniquet method. Standard adjuncts for venodilatation include (a) placing the arm in dependency, (b) applying hot, moist packs, and (c) tapping or lightly abrading the vein. Following successful insertion, a jot of Betadine ointment and sterile gauze should be applied, and the site should be secured by taping the looped IV tubing. If the patient is combative or uncooperative, a sturdy circumferential taping is necessary, even though it makes visualization of the IV site more difficult. Finally, it is also wise to write on the dressing the size of the intravenous catheter used.

EQUIPMENT

A high degree of sophistication has been achieved in modern IV equipment. The polyethylene intravenous fluid bag has replaced the glass bottle; it is easy to store, easy to use, unbreakable, convenient for paramedics, and allows pressure infusion devices to be used.

A wide variety of IV lines are available; many have not only large macroparticulate filters, but also on-line microparticulate filters (0.45 μ). There are also check-

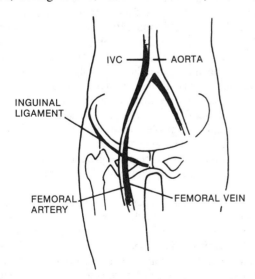

Figure 1 Femoral vein anatomy

flow valves that prevent retrograde flow. All these devices markedly inhibit flow rates and thus have no place on lines being used to resuscitate hypovolemic patients. Blood administration lines have recently been greatly enlarged.* These larger lines considerably enhance flow, even when catheter size remains constant.

Myriad IV catheters are flooding the market. Choice depends on ease of insertion, their flow rates, the degree of painlessness they provide, and cost. Most are quite satisfactory. There is little place any longer for naked steel needles because of their invariable infiltration, despite their demonstrated low infection rate. The catheter-over-needle device is the current standard in intravenous catheters. In adults, the standard 20-gauge catheter is perfectly adequate for administration of fluids and drugs to nonhypovolemic patients. However, no smaller than a 16-gauge catheter should be used for patients who need acute crystalloid or blood infusions. Although 12-, 10-, and even 8-gauge catheter-over-needle devices are commercially available, extreme pain and difficulty in use make them impractical. Instead, the *Seldinger (wire-guided) catheter* is now becoming the standard device for insertion of large-bore catheter sheaths. The technique and usage of these catheters has been well described in the emergency literature. Using the step-up capability of this technique, one can use needles as small as 18 or 20 gauge, in conjunction with wires to introduce catheters up to 14 F (internal diameter 3.2 mm).

A number of devices to deliver intravenous fluids under pressure have been devised. It has been shown that the most efficient of them is a pressure infusion bag enclosing the intravenous bag. Pressures as high as 600 mm Hg can be safely achieved without damaging equipment or veins. This equipment is more efficient than on-line, manually operated "squeeze" bulbs or on-line 50-ml syringes connected by a three-way stopcock. The use of such pressure infusion devices in conjunction with large-bore intravenous tubing and wire-guided large-bore catheters allows crystalloid flow rates greater than 3,000 ml per minute. The customary trauma team reflex of starting "IVs in all four (or even two) extremities" should be a thing of the past. Emergency physicians should also be well aware that volume overload is a real danger with such equipment; liberal use of central venous pressure (CVP) monitoring is advised.

Finally, many archaic intravenous devices are still on the shelves of emergency departments; they should be removed.

WARMING AND INFUSION OF INTRAVENOUS FLUIDS AND BLOOD

Recent developments in blood and fluid warming for the massively exsanguinated patient require special mention. Hypothermia secondary to delivery of large amounts of room-temperature fluids and refrigerator-cooled blood causes clotting problems and other complications. Yet, until recently, these problems had not been adequately ad-

* Medex Hi Flo Trauma Set, Hilliard, Ohio; Travenol IV Set No. 4C2194, Deerfield, Illinois.

dressed. Every department should keep five to ten 1-L bags of Ringer's lactate bath-warmed at 37 to 40 °C. Alternatively, fluids can be rapidly warmed in microwave ovens. Warming techniques must be standardized for each individual oven, however, and mixing must be performed to ensure uniformity of heat distribution.

Blood warming during massive transfusion is a greater problem. Microwaving blood is not possible, because of hemolysis of superheated cells at the periphery of the bag. Second, standard blood warmers do not function adequately when blood is given at high flow. Third, packed cells, the blood product of choice in trauma patients, are so viscous that unacceptably slow flow rates result. The solution to all these problems is remarkably simple: (a)saline preheated to 50 °C is placed on one limb of a Y blood administration set, the bag of packed cells on the other limb; (b)with the main IV line closed and both limbs of the Y open, 250 ml from the saline bag are expressed into the packed cells, diluting them to a hematocrit of about 30 percent and heating them to about 34 °C; (c)warmed and diluted blood is then ready for rapid transfusion with a pressure infusion bag compressing the blood bag. This technique has been proven effective without significant red cell hemolysis.

Finally, every emergency department must have a policy to obtain and deliver multiple units of packed cells prior to and during trauma surgery. A designated "blood runner" can accomplish this task; this person takes blood specimens to the laboratory and returns to the emergency department or operating room, first with 0-negative or type-specific and then with cross-matched blood.

VENOUS CUTDOWN

No discussion of intravenous access is complete without the mention of venous cutdown. This simple, time-honored procedure remains—by custom and logic—the standard by which all venous access techniques are measured. Every emergency physician must be able to perform it rapidly and with dexterity. Unfortunately, in inexperienced hands or in difficult sites (brachial, femoral) it can be both difficult and extremely time-consuming. The long saphenous vein at the ankle is the most commonly used vein; it runs constantly over the anterior margin of the medial malleolus. Occasionally, however, several small veins exist instead of a single large one. The basilic vein at the antecubital fossa is also readily available; it lies two fingerbreadths above and two fingerbreadths medial to the olecranon. Other veins to be considered are the long saphenous vein on the thigh, the cephalic vein at the deltopectoral groove, and the superficial femoral vein at its entry into the common femoral vein.

After appropriate preparation and local anesthetic infiltration, an incision is made through the skin and transverse to the vein. Then, using blunt dissection with mosquito clamps, subcutaneous tissue is separated to expose the vein. The clamp is then thrust beneath the vein for spreading and further vein exposure. A distal ligature is placed and, with gentle traction on that ligature, a small nick is made in the vein with a 15 scalpel blade. Insertion of a catheter should be followed by a proximal ligature to prevent leakage from the vein.

Polyethylene cutdown catheters and infant feeding tubes are obsolete. The wire-guided catheter is ideal as a cutdown catheter; the straight, floppy-tipped wire prevents intima stripping and allows insertion of the catheter with absolute certainty. Also, one need make only a small nick in the vein initially, then enlarging the opening as the catheter or venodilator obturator is gently inserted. It is possible to preserve the vein if the wire guide can be inserted through a needle placed in the vein under direct visualization. This is a preferable method with patients in whom the vein is likely to be needed again in the future.

CENTRAL VENOUS CANNULATION AND MONITORING

The use of central venous pressure monitoring has been of inestimable value to the emergency physician. Its use has been adequately chronicled over the last 20 years, and so it will be dealt with only briefly here. Shock, inaccessible peripheral veins, or the need for central venous pressure monitoring are indications for this technique. Peripheral sites are preferable, because they are neither blind nor invasive; therefore, they have lower complication rates. Such sites include the basilic (not the cephalic!) at the antecubital fossa, the femoral vein, and the external jugular vein, as mentioned previously. The invasive techniques at the root of the neck (internal jugular, subclavian) have relatively high complication rates, especially in hypovolemic or uncooperative patients. A thorough understanding of anatomy is necessary before one embarks on use of these techniques, and the reader is referred to the bibliography for detailed references. The wire-guided catheter has become the standard device for use in central venous lines, replacing now obsolete catheter-through-needle equipment. Emergency physicians should be capable and competent in the use of central venous lines from both peripheral and central insertion sites. No one is always successful with a single technique, so the operator must master several alternative techniques.

Every emergency department should have a CVP manometer set up, ready for monitoring. Although it has been shown that such setups remain sterile for days, it is probably wise to change them every 24 to 48 hours. Unfortunately, actual measurements of CVP are often forgotten. If this measurement is not made, or is made incorrectly, a major purpose of the placement has been neglected. A zero point must be drawn on the patient's chest wall a centimeter or two above the midaxillary line; this approximates the level of the right atrium. The manometer is then filled from the IV, its zero point is apposed to the zero point on the chest wall, and the manometer is opened into the CVP line to equilibrate. An accurate reading is obtained in relaxed end-expiration with the patient supine.

SUGGESTED READING

Dailey RH. Femoral vein cannulation: a review. J Emerg Med 1985; 2:367–372.

Dailey RH. Use of wire-guided catheters in the emergency department. Ann Emerg Med 1983; 8:489–492.

Dailey RH. Venous access. In: Tintinalli J, ed. Emergency medicine: a comprehensive study guide. New York: McGraw-Hill, 1985.

Dula DJ, Muller HA, Donovan JW. Flow rate variance of commonly used IV techniques. J Trauma 1981; 21(6):480–482.

Iserson KV, Reeter AK, Criss E. Comparison of flow rates for standard and large-bore blood tubing [Clinical Investigation]. West J Med 1985; 143:183–185.

Millikan JS, Cain TL, Hansbrough J. Rapid volume replacement for hypovolemic shock: a comparison of techniques and equipment. J Trauma 1984; 24(5):428–431.

Rosetti VA, et al Intraosseous infusion: an alternative route of pediatric intravascular access. Ann Emerg Med 1985; 14:885–888.

Schwartz AJ Intrathoracic vascular catheterization via the external jugular vein. Anesthesiology 1982; 56:400–402.

ORTHOSTATIC HYPOTENSION

TERRY M. WILLIAMS, M.D., F.A.C.E.P.

When normal individuals stand, complex homeostatic mechanisms compensate for the effects of gravity on the circulation in order to maintain systemic arterial pressure and cerebral perfusion. These responses include (1) baroreceptor-mediated arteriolar vasoconstriction, (2) venous constriction and increased muscle tone in the legs and abdomen to augment venous return, (3) sympathetic-mediated inotropic and chronotropic effects on the heart, and (4) activation of the renin-angiotensin-aldosterone system. These compensatory mechanisms preserve cerebral perfusion in the upright position with minimal changes in vital signs. On assuming the upright posture, there is normally a small increase in the pulse rate (13 beats per minute), no change or a small drop in the systolic blood pressure (up to 25 mm Hg), and either no change or a small rise in the diastolic blood pressure.

Orthostatic hypotension occurs when the normal compensatory responses to standing fail to preserve adequate cerebral perfusion in the upright position. Patients may complain of lightheadedness, tightness in the neck and shoulders, blurred vision, cold sweats, yawning, apprehension, unsteadiness, weakness, or syncope. Symptoms are brought on by assuming the upright position or after prolonged standing. Postural symptoms are aggravated in the morning, after a large meal, by exercise, or by high heat or humidity. Approximately half of the patients with orthostatic hypotension complain of postural syncope.

Usually, postural syncope results in a brief (seconds) loss of consciousness.

Obtaining orthostatic vital signs is indicated as part of the evaluation of any patient with known or suspected volume loss, a history of syncope, or the previous pattern of complaints. The patient's blood pressure and pulse are recorded in the supine position and after 1 minute of standing. If severe symptoms or syncope develops, the examiner should be prepared to immediately assist the patient to a supine position. Orthostatic vital signs should not be performed in patients with shock, severely altered mental status, in the setting of possible spinal injuries, or in patients with acute lower extremity fractures.

A clinical diagnosis of orthostatic hypotension is established when the supine to standing blood pressure consistently drops 30 mm Hg or more and symptoms are present. In the setting of hypovolemia, severe symptoms, or a pulse increase of 30 beats per minute from the supine to standing position most accurately predicts significant (1 liter) acute blood loss. However, if the orthostatic hypotension is caused by autonomic dysfunction, this postural tachycardia will often be absent. Beta-blocking drugs and factors increasing vagal cardiotonic activity may also blunt this reflex tachycardia. Such a "paradoxic bradycardia" has been reported in hypotensive women with ruptured ectopic pregnancies.

ETIOLOGY

The disorders of orthostatic blood pressure regulation have been divided into factors affecting postural adjustment, primary (or idiopathic) orthostatic hypotension, and secondary orthostatic hypotension (see Table 1). The emergency physician is primarily concerned with identifying the patient with orthostatic hypotension owing to hypovolemia. Other important secondary causes of orthostatic hypotension include diabetes, anemia, and drugs (see Table 2).

Idiopathic orthostatic hypotension occurs in patients who have no identifiable causative disease. Men are afflicted three to four times more often than women. Symptoms develop over a period of years and are heralded by complaints of lightheadedness or faintness on arising. Other autonomic complaints then surface, such as urinary retention or incontinence, decreased libido, impotence, and anhidrosis. Some patients develop neurologic manifestations (dysarthria, tremor, ocular palsies, ataxic gait, or parkinsonism) 2 to 5 years after the onset of the orthostatic hypotension. The combination of orthostatic hypotension and somatic neurologic symptoms is referred to as the Shy-Drager syndrome, which is felt to be attributable to a primary degeneration of the central nervous system.

The most important aspect of the evaluation of a patient with orthostatic hypotension is the identification of potentially *reversible causes*. The emergency physician is primarily concerned with any evidence of volume loss. The evaluation should focus on any possible causes of occult blood loss such as ectopic pregnancy, abdominal aortic aneurysm, splenic rupture, or gastrointestinal bleeding.

TABLE 1 Classification of Disorders of Postural Blood Pressure Regulation

Poor postural adjustment
  Tall, asthenic habitus
  Advanced age
  Physical exhaustion
  Prolonged recumbency
  Pregnancy
  Gastrectomy
Orthostatic hypotension
  Secondary orthostatic hypotension
    Endocrinologic-metabolic disorders
      Diabetes mellitus
      Primary amyloidosis
      Primary and secondary adrenal insufficiency
      Pheochromocytoma
      Primary aldosteronism with marked hypokalemia
      Porphyria
    Central and peripheral nervous system disorders
      Intracranial tumors (parasellar and posterior fossa)
      Idiopathic paralysis agitans
      Wernicke's encephalopathy
      Multiple cerebral infarcts
      Brain stem lesions
      Tabes dorsalis
      Syringomyelia
      Traumatic and inflammatory myelopathies
      Guillain-Barré syndrome
      Chronic inflammatory polyradiculoneuropathy
      Peripheral neuropathies
      Familial dysautonomia (Riley-Day syndrome)
    Miscellaneous disorders
      Hypovolemia
      Hypochromic anemia
      Electrolyte disturbance
      Psychotropic and antihypertensive drugs
      Extensive surgical sympathectomy
      Chronic hemodialysis
      Anorexia nervosa
      Hyperbradykininism
  Primary or idiopathic orthostatic hypotension
    Idiopathic orthostatic hypotension
    Idiopathic orthostatic hypotension with somatic neurologic deficit (Shy-Drager syndrome)

From Thomas JE, Schirger A, Fealey R D, et al. Orthostatic hypotension. Mayo Clin Proc 1981; 56: 117.

TABLE 2 Commonly used Drugs Causing Orthostatic Hypotension

Antihypertensives
  Diuretics
  Peripheral ganglionic blockers (guanethidine)
  Anti-adrenergic agents (prazosin hydrochloride, methyldopa, phentolamine)
  Ganglionic blockers (trimethaphan camsylate)
Psychotherapeutics
  Phenothiazines
  Tricyclic antidepressants
  Monoamine oxidase inhibitors
Vasodilators
  Nitrates
  Hydralazine
  Diazoxide
  Alcohol
Calcium-channel blockers
Levodopa
Methysergide maleate

A careful history of vomiting, diarrhea, melena, hematemesis, trauma, abdominal pain, and medications should be taken. Other medical problems known to be associated with orthostatic hypotension should be sought (see Table 1).

The pulse change in the patient with orthostatic hypotension will help to differentiate hypovolemia from autonomic dysfunction. If the orthostatic hypotension is caused by autonomic dysfunction, an increase in the standing pulse will usually be absent. In contrast, hypovolemic patients usually have a pronounced tachycardia (pulse rise of 30 beats per minute) on standing. More advanced evaluation of autonomic function is not appropriate in the emergency department. Patients who are felt to have autonomic dysfunction should be referred for further evaluation.

THERAPY

Most emergency department patients with acute onset of orthostatic hypotension are hypovolemic. Therapy should primarily be directed at correcting the underlying cause. Patients with occult blood loss require hospitalization. The initial evaluation and resuscitation should begin in the emergency department.

Some patients with *dehydration caused by gastroenteritis* can be rehydrated with intravenous fluid in the emergency department and discharged home to continue oral rehydration. Young, healthy patients can be given repeat boluses of isotonic crystalloid until the abnormal orthostatic vital signs correct. The elderly or patients with poor cardiac or renal function usually require slow rehydration with careful reassessment of volume status; therefore they are most appropriately cared for as inpatients. Hospital admission should also be considered for any patient who is not responding to rehydration in a reasonable time period (6 hours).

Other reversible causes of orthostatic hypotension can be identified and corrected. These include hypotension-inducing drugs (see Table 2) and *adrenal insufficiency*. The latter should be suspected in any steroid-dependent patient with infection or physiologic stress. Patients with poor postural adjustment (especially tall, asthenic individuals, the elderly, and pregnant women) may have difficulty standing after a prolonged period of being supine on a hospital gurney. This can be corrected simply by having the patient rest in a semirecumbent position and then gradually rise to the standing position. Providing a meal or oral fluids is often helpful. Orthostatic hypotension that is persistent and symptomatic may require admission for further evaluation and treatment.

If the cause of orthostatic hypotension is not reversible and the symptoms are chronic, then symptomatic treatment measures are employed. Patients can be instructed to sleep with the head of the bed elevated 8 to 12 inches. They should sit on the edge of the bed before standing and should postpone any exertion until they have been up for a while. Custom-fitted elasticized garments are available for selected patients.

Chronic drug therapy should be initiated by a physician who will be following the patient closely. Multiple agents have been tried with varying results. Volume expansion with a high sodium intake (at least 150 mEq per day) and 9α-fluorohydrocortisone (0.1 to 1.0 mg per day) can be used in patients who do not respond to mechanical measures. This treatment often produces hypertension in the supine position. Other agents such as vasoconstrictors (ephedrine, vasopressin, amphetamines, methylphenidate, and monoamine oxidase inhibitors with tyramine or amphetamines), indomethacin, clonidine, propranolol, and dihydroergotamine have been used in primary or secondary orthostatic hypotension. The severe forms of this disorder require a multifaceted approach with variable and sometimes poor results.

SUGGESTED READING

Thomas JE, Schirger A, Fealey RD, et al. Orthostatic hypotension. Mayo Clinic Proc 1981; 56:117.

Williams TM, Knopp R. The clinical use of orthostatic vital signs. In: Roberts JR, Hedges JR, eds. Clinical Procedures in Emergency Medicine. Philadelphia: WB Saunders, 1985:367.

MANAGEMENT OF THE GENITOURINARY SYSTEM

HEMATURIA

LYNNETTE A. DOAN, M.D., F.A.C.E.P.

DEFINITION

Hematuria is a commonly encountered problem that may result from a myriad of genitourinary and nonurologic conditions. Red cells may be found in the urine of healthy persons; the normal excretion of red blood cells per 12-hour period for healthy adults is up to 600,000. In clinical practice, hematuria is generally defined as five or more red blood cells per high-powered field on microscopic examination of urinary sediment. An Addis count of a 12-hour urine specimen is occasionally used to quantify the hematuria, in which case more than 500,000 to 1 million red cells is considered abnormal.

CAUSES OF HEMATURIA

The potential causes of hematuria are numerous; they can be divided into systemic (including hematologic disease), renal glomerular, renal nonglomerular, postrenal, and false hematuria. In adults, neoplasms, urinary tract infections, calculi, benign prostatic hypertrophy, urethritis, and urethrotrigonitis are important causes of hematuria. In patients over the age of 50 painless total hematuria is suggestive of a tumor of the urinary tract; at least 20 percent of people with this presenting symptom prove to have urinary tract neoplasm. In children, glomerulonephritis accounts for about half of the cases of hematuria, and urinary tract infection, although it occurs much less frequently, is the second most common cause. Hematologic abnormalities such as bleeding dyscrasias and sickling disorders, especially sickle cell trait, are important causes of hematuria and may be the etiology of up to 12 percent of unexplained hematuria in children. Vigorous exercise, lordotic posture, acute febrile illness, dehydration, and unbalanced dietary intake may produce microscopic hematuria in the absence of serious disease of the urinary tract. Urologic trauma must not be neglected as a significant cause of bleeding.

OTHER CAUSES OF RED URINE

Not all red urine contains blood; cell-free hemoglobin or myoglobin stains the urine red and gives a positive orthotoluidine test (Labstix) in the absence of red cells on microscopic analysis. Certain drugs—e.g., phenolphthalein, phenazopyridine (Pyridium), and nitrofurantoin—and dyes present in certain foods—e.g., carrots, rhubarb, and beets—may produce a red or brownish discoloration of the urine that resembles the presence of blood. Discoloration from pigments can be quickly recognized because they yield negative results with orthotoluidine tests and microscopic examination. In infants, uric acid crystals excreted in large amounts during the first few days of life may confer a pinkish color to the diaper, which may be mistaken for blood. Again the results of an orthotoluidine test or microscopic examination are negative, and uric acid crystals dissolve if the urine is heated or made alkaline in a test tube.

DIAGNOSIS

The diagnosis in patients with hematuria may be readily apparent during the first visit or may require referral for extensive laboratory and diagnostic investigation. In either case the first step of evaluation is a thorough history and physical examination and a few basic laboratory studies.

HISTORY

Initial or terminal gross hematuria suggests an origin in the urethra, bladder, or prostate. In total hematuria, the red cells are dispersed throughout the urinary stream; this suggests the kidney, ureter, or bladder as the source. Brownish urine is often seen with glomerulonephritis; clots in the urine usually indicate nonglomerular renal or lower urinary tract bleeding.

Particular attention should be given to a history of flank or abdominal pain, urinary symptoms, an abnormal tendency to bruising or bleeding and other complaints suggestive of systemic disease such as fever, rash, and arthralgias. A prior or family history of urinary stones is of particular importance in the diagnosis of urinary calculi.

A history of recent infection may be important not only in diagnosing hemorrhagic cystitis, but also in diagnosing glomerulonephritis or interstitial nephritis secondary to a wide variety of bacterial, viral, and parasitic diseases, including infectious mononucleosis and malaria. Episodes of gross hematuria following upper respiratory infection may indicate Berger disease and other mesangiopathic glomerulonephritides, the nephritic manifestations of Henoch-Schonlein purpura, rapidly progressive glomerulonephritis, and membranoproliferative glomerulonephritis.

Although drugs are not a common cause of hematuria, certain medications may cause a chemical cystitis, particularly the anticancer agents cyclophosphamide and mitotane; papillary necrosis may be caused by the chronic ingestion of phenacetin or other nonsteroidal anti-inflammatory agents. Hematuria, which occurs in 2 to 6 percent of patients on anticoagulant therapy, may be precipitated by an occult lesion such as a stone or tumor unmasked by anticoagulation. Pigmenturia may result from the excretion of certain highly colored drugs or their by-products in the urine.

PHYSICAL EXAMINATION

Signs of acute glomerulonephritis (hypertension and volume overload), edema suggestive of nephrotic syndrome, evidence of systemic disease (fever, rashes, lymphadenopathy, organomegaly, and cardiac murmurs), and the presence of abdominal, pelvic, or prostatic tenderness or masses should be particularly noted on physical examination. Inspection of the urethral meatus may reveal the source of bleeding, such as foreign bodies, infection, stenosis, or ulceration. If benign prostatic hypertrophy is found, it should not be considered the source of hematuria until other sources have been excluded.

INITIAL LABORATORY EXAMINATION

Initial laboratory studies should always include a complete urinalysis and urine culture; blood urea nitrogen, serum creatinine level, complete blood count, and clotting studies should be added when the diagnosis remains in doubt. Hemoglobin electrophoresis and/or a sickle cell preparation should be added in susceptible patients in the presence of anemia. Hematuria significant enough to cause anemia, particularly in older patients, should arouse the suspicion of renal or urothelial carcinoma and thus requires prompt urologic referral. Anemia may also accompany chronic renal failure. Serum electrolytes, calcium, phosphorus, and uric acid may be added to complete initial diagnostic work-up.

A dark urine without red cells on microscopic examination indicates pigmenturia as noted earlier. A positive orthotoluidine test indicates hemoglobinuria or myoglobinuria. Urinary tract infection is usually accompanied by pyuria and bacteriuria on microscopic examination of the sediment. A positive urine culture with a colony count of greater than 10^5 organisms per milliliter of urine from a clean catch specimen confirms the diagnosis. Smaller colony counts occurring in conjunction with symptoms of infection typically lead to the diagnosis of urethritis.

The presence of proteinuria or casts in the urine is presumptive evidence of a renal origin of the bleeding. In the presence of normal renal function, these patients should receive prompt referral for verification and quantification of the proteinuria through a 24-hour urine collection and subsequent intravenous pyelography. Serum complement levels, antistreptococcal enzyme titers, and antinuclear antibody testing may then be necessary. Patients with elevated blood urea nitrogen or serum creatinine levels should be dealt with as problems of renal insufficiency and often need to be hospitalized.

DISPOSITION AND MANAGEMENT

When the cause of an episode of gross hematuria is not apparent, immediate referral to a urologist is mandatory and further evaluation, preferably in an inpatient setting, should be carried out promptly. In most cases of microscopic hematuria, however, several repeated urinalyses to confirm the presence of hematuria are usually indicated before extensive evaluation is initiated to exclude those transient conditions that account for up to half of the cases of microscopic hematuria in children and for a smaller percentage of cases in adults. Hematuria persisting in several succesive urine specimens in adults requires a complete urologic evaluation no matter how few the number of red cells, because of the presence of serious but treatable conditions such as obstructive uropathy or carcinoma.

The evaluation of hematuria in children is modified by the finding that microscopic hematuria alone is usually not significant, is usually transient, and is rarely related to identifiable or treatable renal disease. Referral to the pediatrician is indicated, however, for repeated urinalysis, family screening for hematuria, and hemoglobin electrophoresis where appropriate. The treatment of children with gross hematuria is similar to that of adults, with urgent referral and extensive diagnostic evaluation.

FURTHER DIAGNOSTIC STUDIES

The classic diagnostic study used in the emergency department, particularly in trauma patients and those with suspected calculi, is the intravenous urogram (IVU). Typically, a preliminary plain x-ray study of the kidneys, ureter, and bladder is obtained, which may suggest the presence of a foreign body or stone in a small percentage of patients. Approximately 50 ml of an iodine-containing compound is then injected and films are taken at 5, 10, 15 and 25 minutes. When excretion is delayed, x-ray films are taken at longer intervals.

Major allergic reactions such as laryngeal spasm and hypotension are rare, occurring approximately once in every 100,000 examinations. Discomfort such as warmth, dizziness, and nausea are minor reactions and do not in themselves contraindicate subsequent dye injection. With patients at risk for allergic reactions—e.g., those with a history of prior reactions, asthmatics, and those with a history of drug reaction—intravenous urography should be performed with great care and only when absolutely indicated. Pretreatment with steroids may be necessary. Dehydrated patients (especially those with diabetes) with elevated creatinine may have renal failure precipitated by IVU and should be rehydrated before receiving it.

Ultrasonography has recently received attention as an accepted diagnostic modality in the emergent evaluation of patients with suspected renal disease, particularly calculi, and it may be the initial investigation of choice in pregnant patients and those with a history of major allergic reactions to IVU dye. Ultrasonography also provides an additional study for the evaluation of space-occupying lesions identified by urography.

Computerized tomography has similarly gained popularity in the evaluation of renal disease. In the acute setting its use is typically limited to the evaluation of trauma. For more extensive diagnostic evaluations its uses include distinguishing between solid and cystic lesions and evaluating renal, ureteral, and bladder tumors. Antegrade pyelography, cystourethroscopy, anteriography, and renal biopsy are among the more definite diagnostic studies under the domain of the urologist and uroradiologist.

SUGGESTED READING

Abuelo JG. Evaluation of hematuria. Urology 1983; 21:215–225.

Datta PK. The diagnosis of hematuria. Practitioner 1982; 226:1863–1870.

Mota-Hernandez F, Munoz-Arizpe R, Lunar OR. Hematuria in children. Paediatrician 1979; 8:270–286.

Ng RCK, Seto DSJ. Hematuria, a suggested workup strategy. Postgrad Med 1984; 75:139–145.

RENAL STONES AND URINARY OBSTRUCTION

JOHN R. BURNS, M.D.

Urolithiasis is a common medical problem in the United States. As many as 12 percent of people in this country may eventually form a urinary calculus. Urolithiasis normally begins in middle age, with the first calculus occurring between the ages of 30 and 50. Upper urinary calculi are unusual in both children and the elderly. Calculi are more common in males than females and are unusual in blacks of either sex. Urolithiasis is a chronic disease with a recurrence rate of 80 percent in patients followed for 20 years.

Urinary calculi form as a result of (1) excessive supersaturation of urinary stone salts (e.g., calcium oxalate, uric acid), and (2) insufficient concentration of crystallization inhibitors. In this country, the major types of urinary calculi are sterile calcium (calcium oxalate, calcium phosphate), 81 percent; magnesium ammonium phosphate (infection calculi), 11 percent; uric acid, 7 percent; and cystine, 1 percent.

The *symptoms and physical signs* caused by a urinary calculus vary according to its location. A renal calculus can grow to a large size and the patient may remain asymptomatic. In contrast, a 3-mm ureteral calculus can cause disabling pain. Renal colic usually begins abruptly. The pain originates in the flank and then courses laterally around the abdomen and radiates to the groin; it is often accompanied by nausea. As a ureteral calculus nears the bladder, urinary urgency may occur. The abrupt onset of symptoms limits the differential diagnosis. Vascular accidents to the kidney can mimic renal colic but this can be excluded with appropriate radiologic studies. Pyelonephritis causes flank pain but can usually be differentiated from colic by the absence of pain radiation, a more gradual onset of pain, and the presence of urinary infec-tion with associated fever. A right ureteral calculus may be mistaken for acute appendicitis. In the patient suspected of having appendicitis, a urinalysis is mandatory to exclude hematuria. If hematuria is present, radiologic studies of the urinary tract are indicated.

In addition to a detailed history, *laboratory* and radiologic studies are required in diagnosing an obstructing urinary calculus. Microscopic or gross hematuria occurs in about 80 percent of patients with a symptomatic urinary calculus. In patients with complete ureteral obstruction, however, hematuria may be absent. Pyuria often occurs without active infection, and mild proteinuria is common.

Radiologic studies are required both to confirm the diagnosis of a urinary calculus and to determine a proper treatment plan. A plain abdominal roentgenogram is often the first test ordered in a patient suspected of having a urinary calculus. This is a mistake for a number of reasons. It is often difficult to distinguish a calculus from extraurinary shadows such as a phlebolith, calcified costal cartilages, calcified mesenteric lymph nodes, or the increased density of the tip of a transverse process of a lumbar vertebra. A calculus may be missed if it overlies the bony pelvis. An additional problem is that not all urinary calculi are radiopaque. Calcium-containing calculi are highly radiopaque, magnesium ammonium phosphate and cystine calculi are of intermediate density, and uric acid calculi are radiolucent. For all these reasons, the emergency physician should order an *excretory urogram (EXU, IVP)* as the initial radiologic study in the patient with a suspected urinary calculus. Although the study results may not be perfect in the unprepped patient, a firm diagnosis will result in most cases.

The appearance of the EXU will depend on the degree of urinary obstruction present. It is not unusual for a large renal or ureteral calculus to cause no obstruction. In most cases of symptomatic calculi, however, some degree of obstruction is present. After the administration of intravenous contrast medium, an obstructive nephrogram often appears. The combination of decreased fluid flow and increased water reabsorption in the renal tubules causes increased contrast material in the tubules. This appears on the roentgenogram as opacification of the renal parenchyma. The collecting system opacifies later than the contralateral collecting system. When obstruction is severe, the collecting system may not visualize for many hours. Delayed films at 1, 2, and 4 hours are useful to determine both the degree and exact point of obstruction. In cases with severe obstruction, the collecting system may not visualize for 8 to 24 hours. Oblique films should be a part of every EXU to verify that a suspected calculus is really located in the urinary tract.

In the occasional patient with a history of severe contrast allergy, renal ultrasonography and retrograde pyelograms can be performed as inpatient procedures. When evaluating a pregnant woman with renal colic, an abbreviated EXU consisting of a scout and 20 minute film can be done. These films are usually sufficient to provide a diagnosis. In diabetics and other patients prone to renal insufficiency, a serum creatinine concentration should be measured before proceeding with the EXU. Although it is a topic of controversy, we feel that an outpatient EXU should not be performed if the creatinine level is ≥ 2.0, unless it can be lowered by hydration. If not, ultrasonography or retrograde pyelography under the direction of a urologist is preferred.

Two additional types of patients should be mentioned. The severity of pain caused by urinary calculi makes the complaint of renal colic popular with drug seekers. The physician should be wary of a patient with symptoms of renal colic plus a history of both previous uric acid calculi and allergy to contrast medium. The second type of patient is one with a classic history of renal colic, little or no hematuria, and a normal EXU. These patients are usually told that they do not have a calculus and are not given a diagnosis. However, the patient may pass a calculus the following day, since pain can occur even in the absence of significant radiologic findings. A patient may also pass a ureteral calculus into the bladder coincident with the injection of contrast medium, resulting in a normal EXU. Any patient felt to have a urinary calculus on clinical grounds should be treated for a calculus in spite of normal radiologic findings.

The *treatment* of an obstructing calculus depends on the answers to the following questions: (1) Will the calculus pass spontaneously? (2) What is the degree of obstruction? (3) Can the patient be managed with oral analgesics? (4) Can reliable follow-up be assured? (5) Is the patient febrile?

Spontaneous passage of a calculus depends primarily on its location and size. Approximately 80 percent of ureteral calculi are located in the lower third of the ureter at the time of presentation. These calculi are more likely to pass than calculi found in the kidney or upper ureter. The relationship between the size of a calculus and the chance of spontaneous passage has been well described. Calculi less than 4 mm in greatest diameter will pass in more than 90 percent of patients. If the calculus is 4 to 6 mm in diameter, the chance of its passing spontaneously is 50 percent. When the calculus exceeds 6 mm in diameter, spontaneous passage occurs in less than 10 percent of patients.

The degree of obstruction can be useful in determining patient management, especially with larger calculi. An afebrile patient with a calculus smaller than 4 mm can usually be managed as an outpatient despite the degree of obstruction. Management of the patient with a 6-mm calculus often depends on the degree of obstruction. If obstruction is minimal, several weeks of expectant treatment are justified. If the same patient is severely obstructed, hospital admission may be required.

A person with an obstructing urinary calculus and a temperature higher than 101 °F requires immediate hospital admission. The elevated temperature should be assumed to be secondary to urinary infection. Complete obstruction of an infected collecting system can result in rapid irreversible renal damage and septic shock. Febrile patients should be admitted to the urology service for the institution of antibiotics, close observation, and possible placement of a ureteral stent to relieve the obstruction.

Approximately 70 to 80 percent of patients with symptomatic obstructing urinary calculi can be treated as outpatients. A patient is discharged from the emergency department after being given oral analgesics and a urine strainer. Percodan or Dilaudid is usually necessary to provide adequate pain relief. Patients with nausea should be given a prescription for a suitable suppository (B&O, Compazine). The patient should be advised to strain all urine so that the recovered stone can be sent for analysis and appropriate long-term therapy can be started. A follow-up appointment to the urology department is scheduled for several days later. The patient should also be advised to seek prompt medical attention if either the pain worsens or fever develops.

Supported by the Veterans' Administration.

SUGGESTED READING

Burns JR, Finlayson B. Strategies for the medical management of patients with urinary stone disease. Monographs in Urology, Princeton, NJ: Custom Publishing Services, Inc., 1981.

Carstensen HE. Stones in the ureter. Acta Chem Scand 1973; 433:66–71.

EPIDIDYMITIS AND ORCHITIS

DAVID R. MELZER, D.O.
ANN HARWOOD-NUSS, M.D.

EPIDIDYMITIS

Although inflammation may occur in any of the intrascrotal contents, epididymitis is by far the most common clinical syndrome. It accounts for 600,000 physician visits in the United States annually and considerable morbidity in time lost from work. In the military, it is responsible for more days lost from work than any other disease and for 20 percent of urologic hospital admissions.

Epididymitis is generally a disease of adult men, occurring most frequently between the ages of 19 and 35 and only rarely affecting the prepubertal male. In the prepubertal and over 35 age groups, epididymitis is usually caused by coliforms and may be associated with structural abnormalities of the urinary tract.

Etiology

In the past, there has been controversy about the cause of acute epididymitis. Current evidence strongly favors an infectious etiology. Recent studies have resulted in identification of pathogenic organisms in over 80 percent of cases and have implicated *Chlamydia trachomatis* as a major etiologic agent.

In addition to the more common organisms, there are other etiologic agents that may cause inflammation of the epididymis. These include *Mycobacterium tuberculosis, Ureaplasma urealyticum, Trichomonas vaginalis, Blastomyces, Coccidiodes immitis, Wucheriria bancrofti, Neisseria meningitidis, Brucella, Streptococcus pneumoniae,* and *Treponema pallidum.*

Classification

Acute epididymitis may be divided into two major categories: (1) nonsexually transmitted epididymitis, and (2) sexually transmitted epididymitis. It has been demonstrated that in men under age 35, *Chlamydia* and *Neisseria gonorrhoeae* are the major pathogens (*Chlamydia* accounting for 66 to 80 percent). Typically, there is no associated structural urologic abnormality. In men over 35 as well as in prepubertal males, coliforms or *Pseudomonas* is the usual offending agent. In this group, structural urologic abnormalities may be found in a significant number of cases. It should be mentioned, however, that epididymitis is rare in prepubertal boys, and other causes of an acutely painful scrotum should be ruled out first.

Syphilitic epididymitis probably occurs more frequently than is generally believed. It may occur early in the second stage of the disease up to 9 years after onset. Diffuse thickening of the superior aspect of the epididymis and rubbery nodules may be palpable. The diagnosis is presumptive based on evidence of syphilis elsewhere.

Tuberculous epididymitis generally follows involvement of the prostate and seminal vesicles and may be the earliest indication of renal tuberculosis. It typically presents as a relatively painless mass that is most prominent in the globus minor, with development of bead-like swelling in the vas deferens and chronically draining sinuses. Urine sediment may show abacterial (sterile) pyuria. The diagnosis is confirmed by isolating *Mycobacterium tuberculosis* from the urine.

ESSENTIALS OF DIAGNOSIS

History

The patient with epididymitis usually complains of painful swelling in the scrotum, progressing in severity over a period of several hours to days. Associated dysuria or other irritative voiding symptoms are often present. One should inquire about any history of genitourinary tract disease or manipulation as well as sexual exposure.

Physical

There may be tenderness over the groin, lower abdomen, and scrotum. Painful swelling of the scrotum with erythema may be noted, primarily in the posterior aspect. If the patient is examined early in the course of the disease, the swelling may be localized to one portion of the epididymis. Later on, involvement of the testicle may be seen secondary to spread from the adjacent epididymis (epididymo-orchitis) or from passive congestion. Many patients will demonstrate a urethral discharge. If *Chlamydia* is the etiologic agent, it may be scant. Fever and generalized toxicity may be seen, especially in older patients.

Laboratory Studies

Initial studies should include a urinalysis, a Gram stain of the urinary sediment, and a urine culture. Urethral smear should be obtained for Gram stain and Neisseria gonorrhoeae culture. The presence of white blood cells on a urethral smear or in the first voided urine is strong presumptive evidence for the existence of urethritis and epididymitis. A complete blood count will often reveal leukocytosis (10,000 to 30,000 WBC per cubic millimeter).

Differential Diagnosis

Proper management of the patient with an acutely painful scrotum requires a rapid but thoughtful differential diagnosis. Two serious intrascrotal processes commonly confused with epididymitis are testicular torsion and testicular tumor. Torsion must be rapidly differentiated. In general, the younger the patient, the higher the likelihood of torsion. (Peak age is 14 years with 65 percent of cases occurring between the ages of 12 and 18). There may be considerable overlap, however, with the peak age range of epididymitis. Factors that aid in distinguishing torsion include a very sudden onset of pain, history of similar episodes in the past, presence of vomiting, lack of pyuria or irritative voiding symptoms, high-riding testicle position, and no signs of infection (e.g., fever, leukocytosis).

It should be stressed that torsion is the most common acute scrotal condition in pubertal boys and that epididymitis is unusual. Therefore, in the younger patient, diagnosis of epididymitis is one of exclusion. Doppler ultrasonography may aid in the diagnosis but has a high false-negative rate. Radionuclide scans differentiate torsion from epididymitis rapidly and accurately. Decreased activity occurs with torsion, whereas an increase in activity is seen in epididymitis. Scans are accurate and extremely useful adjuncts but should be utilized only if immediately available.

Diagnosis of a testicular tumor can be difficult. One-fourth of patients with testicular tumors present with pain in the scrotum. A discrete intratesticular mass should strongly suggest the presence of a tumor. The patient thought to have epididymitis who does not respond to antibiotic therapy should be referred and evaluated for a testicular tumor.

Management

The treatment of acute epididymitis consists of appropriate antibiotics and supportive measures such as bed rest, scrotal elevation, ice packs, and analgesics. The treatment of sexually transmitted epididymitis is amoxacillin, 3 g orally with 1 g of probenecid, followed by tetracycline, 500 mg 4 times a day, or doxycycline, 100 mg twice a day for 10 days. Erythromycin, 500 mg 4 times a day for 10 days, may be used alternatively to a tetracycline product. Treatment of epididymitis secondary to coliform or *Pseudomonas* infections should be guided by the results of a urinalysis and urine culture. Treatment may be accomplished with a variety of antimicrobials, including trimethoprim-sulfamethoxazole (TMP/SMZ), ampicillin, cephalosporins, and aminoglycosides. In sexually transmitted cases the partners should be treated. Structural abnormalities should be sought in prepubertal boys and those adults with nonsexually transmitted epididymitis. Appropriate referral should be made. If epididymitis is secondary to a systemic disease such as tuberculosis, treatment should be directed toward the primary condition as well

Complications of epididymitis include infertility (most common with the sexually transmitted form), abscess formation, and chronic epididymitis. All patients with epididymitis should have urologic follow-up examination.

Indications for Hospital Admission

Older patients with epididymitis should be treated very conservatively with close follow-up, especially if there is a history of recent urinary tract manipulation. Patients of any age with systemic signs of toxicity (fever, chills, nausea, vomiting) or complications of acute epididymitis should also be hospitalized for treatment with parenteral antibiotics. Scrotal abscesses should be referred for incision and drainage.

ORCHITIS

Etiology

Orchitis is an infection involving the testicles. It is less common than prostatitis or epididymitis because the testes possess a relatively high threshold of resistance to inflammation. The majority of cases of orchitis are secondary to direct extension from an infected epididymis (epididymo-orchitis). In addition, blood-borne dissemination is a major route of infection. Viruses are also significant etiologic agents.

Orchitis may be classified according to etiology into (1) viral (mumps most commonly, but also infection caused by coxsackie B virus and other diseases such as varicella, mononucleosis, and dengue fever); (2) bacterial pyogenic (usually from contiguous spread of epididymitis), and (3) granulomatous (syphilis, mycobacterial infection, actinomycosis, and fungal diseases).

Essentials of Diagnosis

Mumps rarely cause orchitis in prepubertal boys but may occur in 20 percent of postpubertal patients. Typically, testicular pain and swelling begin 4 to 6 days after the onset of parotitis but may occur without parotid involvement. These symptoms occur unilaterally in 70 percent of cases but may occur on the contralateral side 1 to 9 days after involvement of the first testicle. The clinical picture varies from mild swelling of the testicle to marked swelling with generalized toxicity (nausea, vomiting, and fever).

The patient with pyogenic orchitis usually appears acutely ill, with swelling of the testicle and epididymis and marked discomfort radiating to the inguinal canal. Nausea and vomiting are common. On examination, there is often an acute reactive hydrocele. The scrotal skin is generally erythematous and edematous. When both the epididymis and testicle are involved, the condition is called epididymo-orchitis

Granulomatous orchitis has a variable presentation, depending on the etiologic agent. In acquired syphilis, the testes are enlarged and rubbery in consistency, but the condition is painless. *Mycobacterium tuberculosis* usually involves only the epididymis, but *M. leprae* often involves the testes as well.

Patients with actinomycosis usually present with a firm, nontender testicle associated with draining scrotal sinuses. Orchitis secondary to systemic fungal diseases may resemble testicular carcinoma, with a firm mass palpable on examination. Diagnosis of granulomatous orchitis depends on specific cultures and histologic stains from surgical specimens.

Differential Diagnosis

The differential diagnosis of acute orchitis should include testicular torsion, scrotal trauma with hematoma, acute hydrocele, fat necrosis, and incarcerated hernia. A patient with a testicular tumor may also present with an acutely painful scrotum. All patients with epididymoorchitis should be followed until the induration has completely resolved. If the testicle remains abnormal, scrotal exploration is indicated to rule out tumor.

Management

The treatment of viral orchitis is supportive and includes bed rest, scrotal support, and analgesics. Mild cases of mumps orchitis resolve in 4 to 5 days, but more severe cases may take 3 to 4 weeks for resolution. About one-half of cases show testicular atrophy, but infertility occurs rarely.

Pyogenic bacterial orchitis should be treated with specific antibiotic therapy, directed toward the usual pathogens: *Escherichia coli, Klebsiella pneumoniae, Pseudomonas aeruginosa, Staphylococcus aureus,* or *Streptococcus.* Local scrotal measures are helpful. Hospital admission is required for those with systemic signs of toxicity. Granulomatous orchitis requires treatment for the underlying disease with specific anti-infective agents. Surgery is often necessary to treat the local complications of the infection.

SUGGESTED READING

Ireton RC, Berger RE. Prostatitis and epididymitis. Symposium on sexually transmitted diseases. Urol Clin North Am 1984; 11:83–94.
Krieger JN. Epididymitis, orchitis, and related conditions. Sex Transm Dis 1984; 11:173–181.
Sufrin G. Acute epididymitis. Sex Transm Dis 1981; 8:132–139.

TESTICULAR TORSION

BRUCE E. HAYNES, M.D.

All physicians seeing patients with acute scrotal swelling should be able to make a rapid, accurate diagnosis to avoid what British authors term "castration by neglect" resulting from misdiagnosis of testicular torsion. Diagnosis appears to be improving over the past, when mistaken diagnosis and testicular loss were common. Despite this, the potential for misdiagnosis, resulting in testicular atrophy and impaired fertility, is a very real concern.

Most cases of torsion result from an overly capacious tunica vaginalis—the so-called bell-clapper deformity. This high investment of the tunica vaginalis interferes with the testicle's posterior attachment to the gubernaculum and creates instability that may lead to twisting of the testicle and occlusion of the spermatic cord's vessels. Trauma sometimes plays a role in the initiating event, although most cases occur spontaneously.

DIAGNOSIS

Table 1 outlines characteristics of the history and physical examination that help distinguish between the two most common conditions considered in the differential diagnosis: epididymitis and torsion of the spermatic cord. The peak incidence of spermatic cord torsion occurs at about age 14 years, although more cases occur between ages 14 to 28 than birth to 14 years, clouding the usefulness of age as a distinctive feature. Patients with torsion frequently present with an acute onset of severe testicular pain that may radiate to the groin and abdomen. Intermittent torsion can be responsible for previous episodes of similar pain in as many as one third of patients.

The *physical examination* may disclose the affected testicle high in the scrotum after shortening from several twists in the cord, and the contralateral (unaffected) testicle may display a horizontal lie or horizontal position in the scrotum rather than the nearly vertical position of the normal testicle.

Several physical findings should raise the examiner's index of suspicion for torsion. Marked tenderness of the testicle is usually seen in epididymitis only if the testicle is involved in severe epididymo-orchitis. Edematous, thickened scrotal skin is often present with the severe inflammation accompanying torsion. In addition, unclear scrotal landmarks, which make it difficult for the examiner to distinguish scrotal contents, signify a significant pathologic process, either torsion or severe epididymitis.

Torsion of the testicular appendages occurs most frequently in children under the age of 16. The pain may begin in the appendage and then spread to the testis, but vomiting is uncommon and tenderness is usually localized to the appendage. A necrotic appendage may be visible through the scrotal skin, the so-called blue-dot sign found by stretching the scrotal skin over the area of the appendage.

Urinalysis is important in the evaluation of scrotal swelling, and pyuria (more than or equal to 5 white blood cells per high-power field) strongly supports the diagnosis of epididymitis. Unfortunately, only about one-half of men with epididymitis exhibit pyuria; occasional patients with torsion also have WBCs in their urine but rarely more than or equal to 5 per high-power field.

Beginning in the early 1970s, several noninvasive techniques allowing evaluation of testicular perfusion became available. The *nuclear scan* is performed by inject-

TABLE 1 Differential Diagnosis of Torsion

Characteristics	Torsion of Spermatic Cord	Epididymo-orchitis
Age (year)	<35	>16
Pain		
Onset	Acute	Gradual
History of similar pain	Common	Uncommon
Vomiting	Common	Uncommon
Dysuria, urethral discharge	Rare	Common
Fever	Unusual	Common (low grade)
Involved testis		
Position	High-riding	Dependent
Tenderness	Diffuse	Epididymal, becomes diffuse
Contralateral testis	Possible horizontal lie	Normal (vertical)
Ipsilateral spermatic cord	Normal	Thickened, tender
Pyuria	Unusual	Common
Blood flow (Doppler studies, technetium-99m scan)	Decreased	Increased

ing a small amount of ^{99m}Tc pertechnetate into a peripheral vein and recording dynamic and static images. Technetium scans are widely used, with investigators reporting a high degree of accuracy (about 95 percent). Errors are approximately equally divided between false-positive and false-negative examinations. False-positive scans indicating that torsion is present when it is not may result from hernias or hydroceles attenuating detection of tracer over the testicle. False-positive scans are not a major problem if they lead to unnecessary surgical exploration. False-negative examinations, on the other hand, are a serious concern. They can be seen if torsion has been present for a prolonged time, or they may occur in association with retractile scrotums in which the testicle is pulled up out of the scrotum. Partial torsion without vascular compromise or spontaneous detorsion may also lead to a false-negative examination or diagnosis.

Doppler ultrasound examination also has been advocated for the evaluation of testicular blood flow, and in many initial reports results were found to be accurate, although several case reports and more recent studies indicate that the number of false-negative examinations may be unacceptably high, especially if torsion has been present more than 8 to 12 hours. Proper examination technique is important with the Doppler method. A small probe should be used, and it should be held over the lower pole of the testicle to avoid confusing pulsations from the cord above the level of the twist with blood flow in the testicle itself. In addition, the *funicular compression test* must be employed to assure the examiner that the blood flow auscultated is actually from the testicle. Once pulsations are heard, the spermatic cord is compressed high in the scrotum; disappearance of the pulsations and their reappearance when the cord is released indicate that

the blood flow is from the testicle. Pulsations that continue during cord compression make the examination indeterminate. The Doppler's greatest role may be in rapid diagnosis of torsion. For example, if no pulsations are heard, it may be rapidly concluded that blood flow is impaired, since false-positive examinations are rare.

B-scale ultrasonography has been investigated for diagnosis of torsion, but in general it has been useful only in determining testicular infarction, and at this point in time it is probably not useful diagnosing early torsion with reversible ischemia.

THERAPY

Patients with a history and physical findings compatible with torsion must undergo immediate surgical exploration, since there is a direct correlation between ischemic time and testicular necrosis.

Patients with minimal scrotal swelling and definite enlargement and tenderness of the epididymis but little or no testicular tenderness can often be diagnosed confidently as having epididymitis, particularly if they also have pyuria. Scrotal swelling or marked tenderness can make the examination difficult and the findings less clear in many patients; in some, there is only a small amount of pyuria. Technetium scans are useful in these patients to confirm the clinical diagnosis of epididymitis.

In any patient in whom torsion is suspected who must wait for a prolonged period for a nuclear scan, surgical exploration should be carried out promptly; this is also true for any patient with a solitary testicle.

Manual detorsion of the torsed testicle has enjoyed a recent revival in popularity with some clinicians and may shorten ischemic time. Reduction is accomplished by twisting the testicle, usually toward the thigh, until there is relief of pain or return of blood flow is documented with the Doppler technique. This may be performed without anesthesia in order to document pain relief or with a spermatic cord block using the Doppler to confirm reperfusion. If pain worsens or blood flow is not reestablished, untwisting in the opposite direction may be attempted. Unfortunately, this technique does not guarantee that ischemia will be completely relieved or prevent recurrence of the torsion. For that reason, I believe that surgical exploration should be undertaken immediately after manual detorsion and not scheduled on an elective basis.

Spermatic cord blocks not only provide anesthesia during attempts at manual detorsion but also encourage spontaneous detorsion by relaxing the cremaster muscle. The block also relieves pain in epididymitis. The cord block is performed by raising a skin wheal in the superior portion of the scrotum with 1 percent plain lidocaine, and the cord is fixed, if possible, between the thumb and index finger. About 10 ml of lidocaine is injected in and around the cord high in the scrotum, aspirating before each injection and minimizing the number of cord punctures.

Since torsion followed by *spontaneous detorsion* may occur in as many as one third of patients who eventually experience sustained spermatic cord torsion, clinicians may see patients who complain of intermittent pain that resolves spontaneously. At surgical exploration many such patients have the bell-clapper deformity, and their symptoms are resolved by elective testicular fixation. Patients with a clinical diagnosis of intermittent torsion should be admitted to the hospital for prompt surgical fixation, although many physicians elect to perform fixation on an elective basis.

Patients with continuing symptoms after treatment for epididymitis or other conditions not requiring scrotal exploration must be managed with caution. *Missed torsion* can masquerade as presumed epididymitis responding poorly to antibiotic therapy, and the physician must make the diagnosis if loss of the contralateral testicle is to be avoided. Nuclear scans in missed torsion demonstrate a cold, avascular testicle with a surrounding ring of hyperemia; alternatively, surgical exploration may be undertaken. In occasional patients who respond poorly to therapy, the original pain was caused by hemorrhage into the necrotic portion of a *testicular tumor*. For this reason, all patients with scrotal swelling should be followed carefully or referred to a urologist. Scrotal ultrasonography may assist in evaluation of patients with continuing symptoms or abnormal physical examination by defining scrotal anatomy and disease. Alternatively, surgical exploration may be undertaken.

Testicular torsion is a surgical emergency. Loss of spermatogenic tissue may be complete in as short a time as 6 hours, with loss of hormone-producing Leydig's cells occurring shortly thereafter. Patients in whom torsion is suspected need *urgent surgical exploration* and should not be admitted to a ward to await a consultant's eventual arrival. In general, patients with torsion can be operated on most quickly at the hospital where they are initially evaluated and should only be transferred to another institution if that will result in more rapid surgical therapy.

The rapid diagnosis of torsion and testicular salvage require a high degree of suspicion on the part of clinicians examining males with acute scrotal swelling and appropriate use of noninvasive diagnostic techniques.

SUGGESTED READING

Haynes BE, Bessen HA, Haynes VE. The diagnosis of testicular torsion. JAMA 1983; 249:2522–2527.
Knight PJ, Vassy LE. The diagnosis and treatment of the acute scrotum in children and adolescents. Ann Surg 1984; 200:664–673.
Williamson RCN. Torsion of the testis and allied conditions. Br J Surg 1976; 63:465–476.

ACUTE RENAL FAILURE

DENNIS A. DIEDERICH, M.D.

When filtration in the glomeruli suddenly decreases, the kidneys lose the ability to excrete salt, water, and nitrogenous wastes (azotemia) and the clinical syndrome of acute renal failure ensues. Acute renal failure may arise from a wide variety of insults to the kidneys, such as shock, nephrotoxins, urinary obstruction, and multisystem diseases. In the vast majority of cases, the development of acute renal failure does not produce any telltale signs or symptoms in the patient. The clinician must detect its presence by documenting a decrease in urine flow rate (oliguria) or the presence of an elevated blood urea nitrogen and creatinine (azotemia).

Early recognition of acute renal failure is critical because a large percentage of cases of acute renal failure are rapidly reversible with prompt, appropriate correction of the underlying renal insult. Delays in correction of ongoing renal insults, especially states of underperfusion or of renal obstruction, lead to the development of renal vascular and tubular injury (intrinsic acute renal failure, referred to as "acute tubular necrosis" in older literature), which is no longer immediately reversible. The development of intrinsic acute renal failure continues to represent a very serious medical complication, exacting a mortality ranging from 10 to 90 percent. Thus, it is imperative that the clinician promptly recognize the presence of acute renal failure and immediately initiate measures to reverse the renal failure. Because of the wide variety of causes of acute renal failure, a systematic approach in considering the causes simplifies the diagnostic evaluation. A most useful approach, based on the pathophysiology, is to consider the causes of acute renal failure as *prerenal, renal,* and *postrenal* in origin (Fig. 1).

ETIOLOGY OF ACUTE RENAL FAILURE

Prerenal failure results from inadequate perfusion of the kidneys. The major causes of prerenal failure are hypovolemia, an impaired cardiac output, and vascular obstruction of the renal arteries (Table 1). *Postrenal* failure arises from obstruction to urine flow, and when two kidneys are present, it requires obstruction of both. The major causes of postrenal failure are ureteral and urethral obstruction (Table 2). *Renal* causes of acute renal failure include glomerular and other microvascular diseases, tubular diseases, and interstitial diseases (Table 3). In general, intrinsic renal insults producing acute renal failure are of two types: ischemic and nephrotoxic. With both types of insults, renal blood flow tends to decrease somewhat in response to the insult. Restoring the patient's blood volume or blood pressure during the early initiating phase will minimize further injury; however, once failure is established (the maintenance phase), volume expansion will no longer restore normal glomerular filtration. The term *acute tubular necrosis* was used to describe the clinical picture in older literature; we now recognize that evidence for cell death (necrosis) is often lacking and, thus, the terminology is misleading. It is perhaps more

TABLE 1 Prerenal Causes of Acute Renal Failure

Pathophysiology	*Clinical Setting*
Hypovolemia	Hemorrhage
	Gastrointestinal losses: diarrhea, vomiting
	Renal losses: diuretics, glycosuria
	Skin losses
	Sequestration ("third space" losses): burns, trauma, sepsis, ascites
Impaired cardiac output	Myocardial infarction, congestive heart failure, pericardial constriction
Vascular obstruction	Atherosclerosis of aorta and renal arteries, aneurysm

useful to conceptualize the intrarenal pathophysiology as arising from perfused but nonfiltering glomeruli.

IDENTIFYING THE CAUSE OF ACUTE RENAL FAILURE

The cause of acute renal failure can usually be identified promptly with the use of a few simple clinical tools: (1) a careful history, (2) assessment of physical findings, (3) a urinalysis with urinary sediment examination by the physician, and (4) urine-serum screening studies (urinary indices). When prerenal factors are suspected as the cause of acute renal failure, the response to a volume challenge is a very important component of the diagnostic evaluation. Similarly, bladder catheterization and possibly renal sonography should be considered integral components of the diagnostic evaluation for acute renal failure whenever urinary obstruction is suspected.

The History in Acute Renal Failure

Prerenal failure should be suspected in the patient who presents with a history of nausea, vomiting, diarrhea, fever, hemorrhage, or recent weight loss. Similarly, prerenal failure due to congestive heart failure is suggested by a history of orthopnea, progressive edema, paroxysmal dyspnea, or angina. Overdiuresis must be suspected particularly in the elderly patient (with some inherent renal insufficiency) who is taking potent diuretic agents. Oliguria in a patient who has sustained burns or recent trauma strongly suggests prerenal failure.

Postrenal failure, a consequence of obstruction to urine flow, must be pursued assiduously when the patient describes difficulty in voiding or sudden changes in urine flow (abrupt increases or decreases). A history of renal stones, blood clots in the urine, recent abdominal surgery, radiation therapy to the abdomen, or flank pain likewise should alert the physician to the presence of obstruction. Administration of drugs that interfere with urinary bladder emptying, such as anticholinergic agents or psychotropic agents, should be noted in the history.

Intrarenal causes of acute renal failure are much more likely when the history and clinical setting fails to suggest prerenal or postrenal failure. A history of fever, skin rash, and arthralgia may be the first clues of a drug-

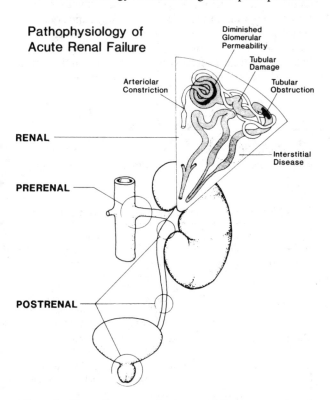

Pathophysiology of Acute Renal Failure

Figure 1 The major causes of acute renal failure may be viewed as being prerenal (underperfusion), postrenal (obstruction), or intrarenal in nature. Intrarenal insults may involve the microvasculature, the tubular epithelia, or the interstitium.

TABLE 2 Postrenal Causes of Acute Renal Failure

Pathophysiology	Clinical Setting
Ureteral obstruction	Bilateral stones, clots Retroperitoneal fibrosis Atonic, distended bladder
Bladder outlet obstruction or dysfunction	Prostatic enlargement or cancer Cervical cancer Anticholinergic drugs
Urethral obstruction	Strictures, foreign body Acute urethritis Meatal stenosis

induced acute interstitial nephritis. Similarly, a history of severe myalgia following a febrile illness should alert the clinician to the presence of myonecrosis with renal failure. The recent appearance of edema, hematuria, and hypertension raises the possibility of acute glomerulonephritis. A careful review of all medications taken by the patient, including nonprescription anti-inflammatory preparations, is essential in recognizing potential nephrotoxic agents. Accidental or deliberate ingestion of poisons constitute an important cause of acute renal failure in the emergency department setting and must be considered in the patient with unexplained acute renal failure.

The Physical Examination in Acute Renal Failure

A thoughtful physical examination can be most helpful in recognizing prerenal as well as postrenal causes of acute renal failure. The patient's general state of hydration is often reflected by the skin's general appearance, texture, and color. The findings of cool, pale extremities, absence of moisture in the axillae, and poor skin turgor with tenting all support dehydration. Similarly, collapsed veins in the neck and extremities and weak rapid peripheral arterial pulsations reflect poor peripheral circulation. A decrease in systolic blood pressure greater than 10 mm Hg, accompanied by an increase in heart rate from a supine to a sitting or standing position, supports a functionally significant (15 to 20 percent) decrease in effective intravascular volume. The patient may demonstrate such orthostatic hypotension even in the presence of edema or ascites. Noting a palpable or percussible urinary bladder, an enlarged prostate gland, or firm, fixed adnexa on pelvic examination strongly suggests bladder obstruction. A catheter should be inserted into the bladder to exclude lower urinary obstruction in this setting. Heart failure sufficient to produce acute renal failure must be severe. Presence of a gallop rhythm, distended neck veins, and evidence of pulmonary congestion would be expected.

Urinary Findings in Acute Renal Failure

Urine flow rate may be normal (nonoliguric) or decreased (oliguric, less than 20 ml per hour) in acute renal failure. Acute renal failure occurring in the setting of trauma, sepsis, nephrotoxic injury, and partial urinary obstruction is more commonly accompanied by a nonoliguric presentation.

As soon as renal failure is suspected, urine and blood samples should be sent to the laboratory for measurements of creatinine, urea, sodium, potassium, and glucose. A urinalysis to include specific gravity and urine osmolality should be obtained. Finally, the physician should examine the centrifuged urine sediment for casts. A tabulation of the findings expected in the various settings of acute renal failure is presented in Table 4. A concentrated urine, devoid of sodium and containing occasional hyaline casts, is most characteristic of prerenal azotemia. Similar findings can be observed during the first hours of acute obstruction and in the presence of intrinsic acute renal failure arising from intense renal cortical vasoconstriction (see Fig. 1). The presence of proteinuria and red cell casts signal the existence of glomerulonephritis; an increased number of leukocytes, particularly eosinophils, in the sediment suggests an acute interstitial nephritis.

A low fractional sodium excretion (urine-serum sodium divided by urine-serum creatinine ratio × 100), although classically seen with prerenal azotemia, is also observed with intrinsic renal failure arising in the clinical settings of radiocontrast injury, fulminant hepatic failure, severe burns, trauma, cardiopulmonary bypass, cyclosporine and amphotericin-B nephrotoxicity, and acute glomerulonephritis. Thus, findings from the urinary indices must be interpreted in conjunction with findings in the physical examination and with attention to the clinical presentation of the patient. Pathologic intrarenal arteriolar vasoconstriction can not only decrease the glomerular filtration rate, but also decrease the urine flow rate and sodium excretion to levels that closely mimic prerenal failure resulting from hypovolemia.

INITIAL MANAGEMENT OF ACUTE RENAL FAILURE

When the physician is presented with a patient with oliguria and decreasing kidney function, the initial goals

TABLE 3 Intrarenal Causes of Acute Renal Failure

Pathophysiology	Clinical Setting
Arteriolar constriction	Fulminant hepatic failure Iodinated radiocontrast agents Prostaglandin inhibitors Cyclosporine; other vasoconstrictors Accelerated hypertension, vasculitis, microangiopathy, hypercalcemia
Glomerular injury	Acute glomerulonephritis, preeclampsia
Tubular injury	Nephrotoxins: aminoglycoside anti- bodies, heavy metals, paraproteins
Intratubular obstruction	Ischemia, heme pigment, uric acid, oxalate, drug crystals
Interstitial inflammation	Acute transplant rejection, drug hypersensitivity, pyelonephritis

TABLE 4 Urine Findings in Acute Renal Failure

Index	Prerenal	Renal	Postrenal
Urine osmolality (mOsm/kg H_2O)	>500	<350	<350
Urine/serum creatinine	>40	<20	<20
Urine sodium (mEq/L)	<20	>40	>40
Fractional sodium excretion (%)	<1	>1	>1
Urinary casts	Occasional hyaline or fine granular	Brown granular tubular cell	Rare

of management are to identify and rapidly correct any reversible causes of the renal failure. Volume contraction and obstruction represent the two major concerns. Prompt correction of prerenal insults is critical to avoid the development of intrarenal injury and acute renal failure. Hypoperfusion of the kidneys and other vital organs resulting from hypovolemia must be aggressively corrected with intravascular volume expansion. When hypovolemia is sufficiently severe to produce supine hypotension, colloid infusions consisting of 5 percent human albumin with physiologic salt concentrations are most effective. In the event of hemorrhage, hypotension is ideally corrected with whole blood. Macromolecular dextran solutions are likewise effective in resuscitating a depleted intravascular volume. Infusions of crystalloid solutions generally suffice when volume deficits are less severe. One must recall that only 20 to 30 percent of the volume of crystalloid infused actually remains in the intravascular compartment; the bulk infused enters the interstitial (extravascular) compartment. Hence, 1,500 to 2,000 ml of saline is required to achieve the same acute *intravascular* volume expansion as that achieved by 500 ml of plasma protein solutions.

When uncertainty exists as to the adequacy of the patient's intravascular volume, a catheter should be inserted to monitor central venous pressure and pulmonary artery wedge pressure to provide a more reliable assessment of adequacy of the intravascular volume status. Diuretics have no place in the *initial* management of oliguria. If the patient remains oliguric in the face of a volume challenge and an adequate (i.e., 20 mm Hg) or elevated pulmonary artery wedge pressure, administration of a potent loop diuretic (furosemide, bumetanide, or ethacrynic acid) may be appropriate. Early diuretic administration by producing renal vasodilatation may convert oliguric to nonoliguric acute renal failure.

The axiom that every patient with acute renal failure is obstructed until proven otherwise, deserves reemphasis. The treatment of obstruction is relief of the obstruction. A renal sonogram should be obtained in every patient with unexplained renal failure. Administration of radiocontrast agents should be very judicious in the setting of acute renal failure to avoid an additional superimposed renal insult. Volume status should be corrected before radiocontrast agents are administered. Radionuclide scanning and renal ultrasound studies have largely replaced intravenous urography in screening for obstruction.

Patients presenting with oliguria and azotemia (acute renal failure) should be admitted to the hospital. Nephrology consultation ideally is initiated while the patient is in the emergency department. Baseline data that should be obtained there include weight, acid-base studies, a general chemistry profile, and accurate recording of intake, type of fluid, and urinary output; all are essential to the subsequent management of the patient. Patients presenting with acute renal failure in the setting of trauma, sepsis, burns, or other causes of multiorgan failure should be admitted to hospitals that can provide acute dialysis support.

Acute renal failure should be treated as a medical emergency. Every effort should be expended to promptly recognize and correct renal failure arising from underperfusion and obstruction of the kidneys. The most important goal in therapy is *prevention* of further renal insult.

SUGGESTED READING

Diederich DA. Oliguria and acute renal failure. In: Bone RC,ed. Critical care: a comprehensive approach. Park Ridge,IL:American College of Physicians, 1984; 126–141.
Rudnick MR, Bastl CP, Elfinbein IB, Narins RG. The differential diagnosis of acute renal failure. In: Brenner BM, Lazarus JM, eds. Acute renal failure. Philadelphia: WB Saunders, 1983:176–222.

PRIAPISM AND CUTANEOUS LESIONS OF THE PENIS AND SCROTUM

HABIB ANWAR, M.D., F.A.C.I.P.

The genitalia are subject to the same cutaneous lesions found on other parts of the body. Often the lesions are more pronounced in this location. The skin of the scrotum is unique in several ways. It is very sensitive to chemicals and medications. Acting as a temperature regulator of the testicles, it expands and contracts depending on temperature changes. In addition, it is very vascular and usually heals quickly, given the proper therapy. Some of the more common lesions are described in this chapter.

ALLERGIC CONTACT DERMATITIS

Diagnosis. This is an acute skin reaction with different degrees of reaction to different allergens. Reactions range from only redness to the full-blown picture of eczematoid dermatitis, with edema, erythema, itching, scaly eruptions, vesiculation, and weeping.

Any object or material can be an allergen, including douches, soaps, deodorants, clothing (nylon, dacron, etc.), plants (poison ivy and oak), and topical medications.

Treatment. Treatment consists of the removal of the allergen and any suspected material. The area should be washed with copious amounts of water and covered with cool, wet compresses. If the area is not infected, then topical corticosteroids (Hydrofluocinolone and betamethasone) should be applied. Oral antihistamine or oral prednisone may be given in addition to topical application, depending on the severity of the eruption.

DRUG ERUPTION

Diagnosis. Drugs such as sulfa, tetracycline, phenolphthalein, and barbiturates can cause fixed eruptions. These eruptions disappear spontanously, but recur with each exposure to the drug. The glans penis is usually affected.

Treatment. Treatment requires cessation of the drug. Symptomatic treatment is the same as for allergic contact dermatitis.

ERYTHEMA MULTIFORME

Diagnosis. These are acute, annular or iris-like, multicolor lesions that appear on the penis and scrotum as well as other areas such as palms, knees, oral cavity, and anal regions. In its severe form (Steven–Johnson syndrome), the mucous surfaces of orifices of the body are involved, and systemic symptoms such as fever, anorexia, and malaise are noted.

The cause of erythema multiforme is unknown in the majority of cases. Occasionally drugs and vaccinations, acute and chronic bacterial infections, viral infections (herpes simplex), and rheumatoid conditions are found to be causative or precipitating factors.

Treatment. Treatment consists of removal of the causative factors if they are known. Local treatment with steroids and systemic corticosteroids for a short time is adequate. Patients with Steven–Johnson syndrome should be hospitalized and parenteral steroids and antibiotics should be administered.

SEBORRHEIC DERMATITIS

Diagnosis. Scaly red patches involve the genitalia and inguinal folds as well as the face, axilla, anterior chest, around the ears, and the crease of the chin. They start as red scaling papules, then become larger and create an annular configuration. They can be confused with psoriasis, pityriasis rosea, or lichen planus. The cause is unknown.

Treatment. Topical steroids are very useful, as is an emulsion base of 3 percent sulfa and 1 percent salicylic acid applied twice daily. Vioform 2 percent may be used in addition to topical steroid.

PSORIASIS

Diagnosis. Silvery scales over moist red patches or plaques are characteristic of psoriasis. It is commonly seen in moist areas such as the groin, scrotum, and glans penis. The silvery scales may be minimal or absent. Pruritus may be intense.

Appearance of the lesions and presence of plaques in other areas, such as the scalp, elbow, and knee, will help in the diagnosis. Involvement of the nails with pitting is almost pathognomonic.

Treatment. Topical steroid ointment covered with a cellophane sheet, to increase absorption, is the most effective treatment. Systemic steroids are occasionally used and ultraviolet light is often effective. Dermatologic referral is appropriate.

CANDIDIASIS (MONILIASIS)

Diagnosis. The inguinal folds and genitalia are commonly involved with red, itchy confluent eruption, which characteristically includes a few pustules. Diagnosis is made by a culture or microscopic examination, demonstrating branching and budding mycelia.

Treatment. Any topical antifungal cream such as nystatin, miconazole, or clotrimazole will be effective.

TINEA CRURIS

Diagnosis. This is characterized by scaly, erythematous, itchy, sharply marginated eruptions, which involve the inguinal folds and the scrotum. The causative fungi are *Trichophyton* or *Epidermophyton*. Diabetes mellitus should be ruled out. Microscopic examination of skin scrapings treated with 10 percent potassium hydroxide reveal hyphae or fungal culture, which confirms the diagnosis.

Treatment. Topical antifungals, or a combination of 1 percent hydrocortisone and antifungal ointments, is the most effective treatment of choice. Oral griseofulvin is also effective, but is recommended only in very stubborn cases.

WARTS (CONDYLOMA ACCUMINATA)

Warts are caused specifically by Papova virus. The moist area of the external genitalia (under prepuce and the penile shaft) are commonly affected. The urethral meatus must be inspected. If the urethra is involved, dysuria and microscopic hematuria will be present. The number of warts varies from one to as many as hundreds. If meatal warts are present or if the patient has dysuria or microscopic hematuria, then a cystourethroscopy should be performed.

Treatment. A 25 percent podophyllum resin in compound tincture of benzoin carefully applied on the lesion only is the treatment of choice. Excision and fulguration (electrocautery) of warts is another effective treatment. Warts involving the urethra are best treated with 5 percent fluorouracil cream. Giant condyloma accuminata with a deeper invasion of the skin need surgical excision and fulguration, which are best carried out by a urologist.

HERPES SIMPLEX

This is an acute, localized, self-limited eruption consisting of shallow ulcers or grouped vesicles with an erythematous base. The disease is caused by *Herpes-virus hominis*, type II, and occasionally type I. Herpes simplex is contagious until the epidermis is completely healed. It is a recurrent disease that commonly appears on the penis; unilateral inguinal adenopathy is common. The individual's immune state is a major factor in determining the frequency and intervals of recurrences. Diagnosis is made by Tzank smear or viral culture; the latter is more practical and reliable.

Treatment. Patients should be educated as to the risks of sexual transmission. The best treatment is 5 percent acyclovir (Zovirax) ointment applied generously to cover all lesions. The applications should be repeated every four hours and continued for several days. Acyclovir capsules are used to treat any initial episode of the disease, 200-mg capsules should be taken every 4 hours, for a total of 5 capsules daily for 10 days. To prevent or reduce recurrences of herpes, one 200-mg capsule of acyclovir is given three times daily for up to 6 months.

PYODERMAS

Pyodermas of the external genitalia include impetigo, folliculitis, furunculosis, hydradenitis suppurativa, and infectious eczematoid dermatitis. Any part of the external genitalia may be involved. Staphylococci and streptococci are common causative agents.

Treatment. A penicillinase-resistant antibiotic such as sodium cloxacillin is required. Topical application of polymycin-bacitracin ointment and unroofing of the lesion expedite the response to treatment.

BALANOPOSTHITIS

Inflammation of the glans penis with its surrounding prepuce can occur at any age, but it is commonly found in debilitated patients, diabetics, and obese people with poor hygiene. Inflammation of glans and prepuce can occur as two separate entities, respectively known as balanitis and posthitis. Depending on the severity of the inflammation, symptoms vary from minor itching to severe dysuria, foul-smelling drainage, fever, tight phimosis, and inguinal adenopathy.

Treatment. Bathe the inflamed area with mild soap and water three to four times daily. The space between the glans and prepuce should be cleaned with Q-tips. The prepuce must be retracted and washed thoroughly, if phimosis is not present. Antibiotic ointments and steroid ointments, such as Kenalog or Mycolog, can be used topically.

For fever and pain, aspirin or Tylenol and rest should be prescribed. Systemic antibiotics may be required in addition to local applications. Meticulous hygiene should be exercised.

Occasionally the phimosis is so tight that the glans penis and the prepuce cannot be thoroughly cleaned. A dorsal slit must then be performed in the emergency department under local anesthesia. After injection of 2 percent lidocaine in the dorsal, lateral, and ventral aspects of the penile base, a straight clamp should be applied on the dorsal aspect of the prepuce in the axis of the shaft and left in place for at least two minutes. The incision is then done along the crushed part of the prepuce, to minimize the amount of bleeding. After completing the dorsal slit, the glans penis is exposed and washed adequately with povidone-iodine solution. The edge of the dorsal slit should be sutured with 3-0 chromic suture to prevent future bleeding (Fig. 1). An elective circumcision is usually required, and should be scheduled when balanoposthitis is completely resolved.

Meatitis and meatal stenosis associated with balanoposthitis are commonly seen in children. Voiding difficulties and severe dysuria are common symptoms. Meatal stenosis is usually corrected by a ventral meatotomy at the time of circumcision.

PHIMOSIS

Phimosis is the narrowing of the prepuce opening to the extent that it cannot be retracted over the glans penis. Cleaning under the prepuce is almost impossible. Smegma accumulates and balanoposthitis may develop. Occasionally it may be so tight that it causes voiding problems. Some of the voided urine may be retained inside the prepuce and secondary infection may develop. Dribbling is noted, and further blockage, especially in children, may cause bladder and upper tract overdistention and secondary infection.

Congenital phimosis is uncommon. During infancy, the foreskin normally adheres to the underlying glans penis and does not retract. If the prepuce can be retracted enough to visualize the meatus, then a congenital phimosis does not exist and the infant will void without difficulty. After one year of age, the prepuce should slide easily over the glans. Acquired phimosis usually occurs after recurrent bouts of infection such as balanoposthitis, dermatitis (especially in diabetic patients), trauma such as a forceful retraction of the prepuce, and inadequate circumcision.

Treatment. Advanced degrees of phimosis should be treated surgically and a circumcision should be performed before a balanoposthitis develops. If infection and inflammation have already started, circumcision should be postponed until balanoposthitis is completely treated. Although a local anesthesia is used for adults, circumcision in the pediatric age group requires general anesthesia.

PARAPHIMOSIS

Normally the foreskin slides over the glans penis without any difficulty. If some degree of phimosis exists and the foreskin is retracted proximal to the glans and left for a long time, a paraphimosis will develop. This occurs in children and in debilitated and senile people.

The retracted prepuce causes a ring-type constriction associated with pain, swelling, and discoloration of the glans. Superimposed infection follows further complicating the situation.

Treatment. Paraphimosis is an emergency and should be treated promptly. Manual reduction of paraphimosis is possible if it is not of long duration and swelling is absent or minimal. Adequate pain medication should be administered before manipulation. Compression over the glans penis reduces swelling and makes the reduction easier. Place both thumbs on the glans and two fingers of both hands on the retracted skin. Push the glans inside and pull the skin forward until the paraphimosis is reduced. Schedule the patient for elective circumcision when the foreskin appears healthy and inflammation has subsided. When paraphimosis cannot be reduced manually, a dorsal slit under local anesthesia should be performed immediately as described under the Balanoposthitis section. Make a longitudinal incision over the constricted area and close the incision with 3-0 chromic transversely. The dorsal slit will permit the foreskin to be reduced easily. Elective circumcision can be scheduled when the swelling and inflammation have subsided.

GANGRENE OF THE SCROTUM (FOURNIER'S DISEASE)

Scrotal gangrene is characterized by a sudden onset of infection with rapid evolution of necrosis associated with systemic symptoms. The scrotum is swollen, and discoloration is obvious. In general the patient is very sick, complaining of fever, anorexia, and pain. Different underlying causes will be associated with Fournier's disease, such as diabetes mellitus, alcoholism, ischiorectal abscess, balanoposthitis, urethritis, indwelling Foley catheter, etc. Different microorganisms have been blamed for the gangrene, but hemolytic and nonhemolytic streptococci have been commonly isolated. Other microorganisms alone or in combination with streptococci include *Staphylococcus*, *Escherichia coli*, *Proteus*, *Klebsiella* and anaerobics (e.g., *Bacteroids*). Prompt attention to the medical aspect as well as the surgical aspect of this devastating infection is essential, as it is a life-threatening emergency.

Dehydration and unbalanced electrolytes should be corrected. Broad-spectrum intravenous antibiotics should be administered to cover aerobic and anaerobic microorganisms. The combination of gentamycin and ampicillin is a good choice. After initial replacement of fluid and electrolytes, the patient must go to surgery because extensive debridement of all necrotic tissue is mandatory. Without this, resolution will not occur. Once the sepsis is controlled and adequate debridement is done, tissue regeneration is rapid; remnants of scrotal skin or skin grafts will cover the denuded area. Mortality varies between 7 and 30 percent depending on the general condition of the patient and promptness of treatment. When gangrene is secondary to anorectal pathology, mortality is very high.

PRIAPISM

Priapism is a prolonged pathologic erection of the penis that is associated with pain and is not necessarily related to sexual stimulation relieved by intercourse or masturbation. Only the corpora cavernosa are involved; they are filled with sludge-like blood while the corpora spongiosum (including the glans penis) remains soft.

The cause of priapism in most cases is unknown. Sickle-cell disease or trait, leukemia, trauma, polycythemia, and metastatic malignancies are known causative factors in 30 percent of cases. Occasionally paraplegic patients will develop priapism secondary to autonomic dysfunction. Rarley, prostatitis will cause priapism. Drugs are another cause; phenothiazines and heparin are known offenders. If it is not known if a patient has these conditions, a complete blood count (CBC), differential, and sickle test should be performed.

Treatment. Conservative measures should be tried first, but if this approach fails, then operative treatment should not be delayed further. Priapism is an emergency and the need for prompt treatment should be emphasized. Delay will increase the chance of impotency. Most patients will need parenteral narcotics for control of pain. Many treatments have been recommended; none is of proven value. Initial steps are application of ice packs to the penis and inhalation of amyl nitrite (a vasodilator) for 15 to 20 seconds. Ice-water enemas may reduce the erection in several hours. Others have recommended warm enemas. Any known precipitating cause should be treated. If detumescence has resulted previously with a particular regimen, it should be tried first. Spinal anesthesia to the level of T8 has occasionally been effective. Irrigation of the corpora cavernosa with saline is another choice. A 14-gauge butterfly needle is inserted into one corpora, and forceful irrigation is carried out until thin, bright red blood can be aspirated into the irrigation syringe. The technique can also be done with two needles, one for irrigation and one for aspiration. Nirtoprusside decreases the blood flow in the penis, not only by lowering systemic blood pressure but also by acting as a vasodilator. Its use requires careful monitoring with an arterial line, and it should not be done in the emergency department.

Surgical Treatment of Priapism. Not only is surgical treatment of the priapism the most effective approach, but in many cases (idiopathic) it should be considered first. The chances of impotence in this group of patients are very high because of secondary fibrosis. Medical treatment, if successful, should be continued for 5 to 6 days, at which time surgery should be considered.

If priapism is primary and idiopathic, then a surgical approach should be undertaken if detumescence does not occur with conservative measures in 48 hours. Delaying further causes more fibrosis and less satisfactory results, with more chances of impotence. Finally, all patients should be informed of the possibility of impotence, whether they are treated medically or surgically.

Disposition. Patients with priapism should be admitted to the hospital under the care of a urologist.

SUGGESTED READING

Epstein E. Controversies in dermatology. Philadelphia: WB Saunders, 1984.
Epstein E. Regional dermatology. Orlando: Grune & Stratton, 1984:290.
Stone J. Dermatologic immunology and allergy. St Louis: CV Mosby, 1985.

PROSTATITIS

MICHAEL W. BROWN, M.D.
DAVID F. PAULSON, M.D.

Acute bacterial prostatitis may produce symptoms of perineal or low back pain, fever, chills, hematuria, or irritative bladder symptoms such as dysuria and urinary frequency. In older men, its presence may often aggravate underlying obstructive voiding symptoms, thus causing the presenting symptom of urinary retention. Rectal examination usually reveals a boggy, tender prostate.

Patients with chronic bacterial prostatitis often present with less specific symptoms, including perineal or low back pain, painful ejaculation, or chronic irritative bladder symptoms. This diagnosis is established in the patient with such chronic symptoms by documenting recurrent bacteriuria between courses of appropriate antibiotics.

Both acute and chronic prostatitis should be documented with appropriate *cultures*. For patients with suspected acute bacterial prostatitis, prostatic massage is discouraged because of potential production of bacteremia or epididymitis. A clean-catch urine specimen is usually adequate for culture of the organism responsible for acute prostatitis. The causative agent for chronic bacterial prostatitis is more difficult to elucidate. Evaluation should include culture of the midstream urine sample followed by prostatic massage. The expressed prostatic secretions (EPS) are cultured and examined. Microscopic demonstration of oval fat bodies and greater than 12 white blood cells per high-power field in the EPS supports a diagnosis of prostatitis. Following prostatic massage, a second urine culture is sent for analysis. A tenfold increase of an organism in the postmassage urine culture

relative to the midstream voided urine specimen establishes the diagnosis of prostatitis.

Patients with nonbacterial prostatitis present with the same symptoms as those with chronic bacterial prostatitis. The EPS examination will be consistent with this diagnosis as well, but both EPS and postmassage urine cultures will be negative. The cause is frequently thought to be *Chlamydia* or T-strain *Mycoplasma*, but specific cultures are not usually productive. A further distinction is made in the patient with prostatodynia (i.e., symptoms consistent with chronic prostatitis) by both negative culture results and examination of the EPS.

THERAPY

Therapy should be initiated in the emergency department following examination and collection of an appropriate culture sample. Empiric antibiotic therapy should be initiated until culture results are available. Most patients with prostatitis can be managed as outpatients and provided with general support with hydration, analgesia, initial bed rest, and a stool softener. Severe irritative bladder symptoms may respond to topical urinary analgesics or anticholinergic agents, as discussed further on.

The presence of a high temperature or chills may require hospitalization to institute intravenous antibiotics. Rarely, the presence of urosepsis may require intensive care monitoring. If symptoms suggest significant obstruction to voiding, a postvoid urine specimen should be obtained with passage of a small (no. 14 French) catheter. If the residual urine is greater than 100 to 125 ml, temporary catheter drainage may be necessary to facilitate clearing the infection. Although we prefer initial placement of a small-caliber Foley catheter, this carries a risk of producing epididymitis, and suprapubic catheter drainage is therefore occasionally necessary.

TABLE 1 Antibiotic Regimens for Bacterial Prostatitis (in Approximate Order of Effectiveness)

Antibiotic	Dosage	Interval	Route	Comments
Trimethoprim-sulfamethoxazole	160 mg–dash 800 mg (double-strength tablet)	q12h	PO	Contraindicated in G-6-PD deficiency; may produce GI symptoms, occasional blood dyscrasias, and severe cutaneous reactions, including epidermal necrolysis
Tetracycline	250–500 mg	q6h	PO	Avoid dietary calcium; may produce photosensitivity, GI symptoms
Minocycline hydrochloride	200 mg initially, then 100 mg	q12h	PO	May produce GI symptoms, photosensitivity, or renal toxicity
Ampicillin	500 mg	q6h	PO	Contraindicated in patients with penicillin allergy
Cephradine	500 mg	q6h	PO	Dosage should be reduced for patients with renal failure; possible cross-reactivity with penicillin allergy

PREFERRED MANAGEMENT

Our initial management of acute prostatitis or a recurrent episode of chronic prostatitis begins with the empiric institution of one of the oral antibiotic regimens described in Table 1. For acute bacterial prostatitis, an appropriate regimen should be continued for 2 weeks. In chronic prostatitis, therapy should continue for 4 to 6 weeks. The ultimate eradication of prostatic infection is a complex problem of obtaining adequate levels of antimicrobial agents in the prostatic interstitium, ducts, and acini. Diffusion across the prostatic epithelium requires a high degree of lipid solubility and preferably a weak base to allow concentration in the prostatic fluid by ion-trapping. Our initial choice for the management of acute or chronic prostatitis is trimethoprim-sulfamethoxazole because of the unique characteristics of trimethoprim as a weak base that is lipid-soluble and only moderately bound to plasma protein. The potentiation of the antifolate mechanism of sulfamethoxazole by trimethoprim favors their combined use, although the acidic pKa of sulfamethoxazole prevents high prostatic concentrations despite its good lipid solubility. Although tetracycline and its derivatives are a good choice in the young male because of possible chlamydial etiology, protein binding of these agents limits their prostatic concentration.

If the need for hospitalization has been established, intravenous therapy is indicated. An aminoglycoside is begun such as gentamicin, 1 mg per kilogram intravenously every 8 hours. Neurotoxicity manifested as auditory or vestibular deficit may warrant the use of another aminoglycoside, i.e., tobramycin or amikacin. The potential renal toxicity of all these agents requires close monitoring of peak and trough levels as well as of serum creatinine. In combination with an aminoglycoside we generally initiate therapy with a second drug, usually ampicillin, 500 mg intravenously every 6 hours. In patients with penicillin allergy, we usually substitute with sodium cefazolin, 500 mg to 1 g intravenously every 8 hours.

Although it is rarely necessary, we prefer to treat irritable bladder symptoms with topical analgesics for the urinary tract. Phenazopyridine hydrochloride, 200 mg given orally three times daily, is usually effective, although it is contraindicated in renal insufficiency. More severe symptoms may require institution of anticholinergic agents. We usually start with oxybutynin chloride, 5 mg orally three times daily, or propantheline bromide, 15 mg orally four times daily. Both of these medications are contraindicated in patients with glaucoma, myasthenia gravis, or underlying obstructive uropathy. The patient should be forewarned about side effects of cardiac tachyarrhythmias, blurred vision, drying of salivary secretions, and urticarial reactions.

Nonbacterial prostatitis is usually responsive to a 2- to 4-week course of tetracycline or minocycline. If *Trichomonas vaginalis* is present in the urine or EPS, a 10-day course of metronidazole is recommended, 250 mg orally, four times daily. Simultaneous treatment of the patient's sexual partner is necessary, as is warning against the concurrent use of alcohol.

DISPOSITION

Clinical response to an oral regimen for treatment of acute bacterial prostatitis should be progressive over a 7- to 10-day period. Poor response is demonstrated by persistent fever, chills, perineal pain, or fluctuance on rectal examination. This should prompt urologic consultation to exclude the presence of a prostatic abscess that might require drainage. Our preference in such cases is transurethral drainage, although perineal drainage is required on rare occasions

The response of chronic bacterial prostatitis is less reliable. Prolonged and varied antibiotic regimens are often required. Surgical management is occasionally indicated in the face of infected prostatic calculi. Regular sexual activity is encouraged to provide emptying of engorged prostatic acini, although this may require regular prostatic massage (twice weekly for 2 weeks, then weekly for several weeks). Patients with chronic symptoms should be referred for urologic evaluation to exclude unusual etiologies of prostatitis (parasitic, tuberculous, or mycotic) or another disease that might produce obstructive or irritative voiding symptoms (e.g., carcinoma of the prostate, carcinoma in situ of the urinary bladder, neurogenic bladder, benign prostatic hyperplasia, urethral stricture, or interstitial cystitis).

SUGGESTED READING

Drach GW. Prostatitis: Man's hidden infection. Urol Clin North Am 1975; 2:499–520.
Stamey TA. Urinary infection in males. In: Pathogenesis and treatment of urinary tract infections. Baltimore: Williams & Wilkins, 1980:342.

URETHRITIS

WILLIAM R. BOWIE, M.D., F.R.C.P.(C)

Urethritis is virtually never an emergency for physical reasons, but because of its frequency and the attendant psychological distress, patients do present in emergency departments. However, most cases are seen in office practice or in special clinics. Once the possibility of urethritis is considered, the appropriate initial management is straightforward. Diagnosis of urethritis is usually made in males who present with symptoms of urethral discharge, burning on urination, or urethral itch. The classic sign is urethral discharge. The usual laboratory findings are an increased number of polymorphonuclear leukocytes in urethral material or a positive diagnostic test for *Neisseria gonorrhoeae* or *Chlamydia trachomatis* or both. Although urethritis arises in women, the clinical presentation is that of cystitis, and women should be medically managed as for cystitis.

ETIOLOGY

There are numerous causes of urethritis, but the vast majority of cases are caused by sexually transmitted pathogens. We will not discuss urethritis arising in catheterized men, or the rare presentation of urethritis arising because of urethral structural abnormalities, or urethritis produced by urethral foreign bodies. With respect to sexually transmitted pathogens, until the last few years the major clinical concern has been restricted to *N. gonorrhoeae*. This was exceedingly unfortunate, because the most frequent important cause of urethritis in heterosexual men is *C. trachomatis*, which is also present concurrently in 20 percent of those with gonorrhea. Single-dose penicillins do not reliably eradicate *C. trachomatis*, thus leaving infected individuals at risk for sequelae and failure to interrupt the chain of transmission. The newer treatment schedules discussed here have simplified management of urethritis because they recognize the need to eradicate both *N. gonorrhoeae* and *C. trachomatis*.

Clinically, urethritis has been divided into gonorrhea and nongonococcal urethritis (NGU). By definition, *N. gonorrhoeae* is present in those with gonorrhea, but urethral *C. trachomatis* is present in 20 percent of heterosexual men and 5 percent of homosexual men with gonorrhea. When urethritis is present but *N. gonorrhoeae* is not detected, NGU is diagnosed. For men with NGU who present with onset of symptoms within the past 1 to 2 months and have not received treatment in the past 3 months, *C. trachomatis* is recovered from 30 to 50 percent, and a genital mycoplasma, *Ureaplasma urealyticum*, is probably the cause in a further 30 to 40 percent. In 20 to 30 percent of men the cause is not apparent. Although *C. trachomatis* is readily eradicated by 1 week of tetracycline or erythromycin therapy, urethritis may persist or recur in 30 to 40 percent of men with NGU. When this occurs, *C. trachomatis* is almost never recovered unless the patient is not compliant in taking medications or has been reexposed to a new or untreated partner. *U. urealyticum* is recovered from only 20 to 30 percent of these men with persistent or recurrent urethritis, so that in the vast majority the etiology is not known. A variant of NGU is postgonococcal urethritis, which is diagnosed when men with gonorrhea are treated with a regimen that eradicates *N. gonorrhoeae*, but urethritis persists or recurs. The etiology of postgonococcal urethritis is similar to that of NGU, except that *C. trachomatis* is recovered slightly more frequently.

DIAGNOSIS

One of the errors in the management of urethritis is the impression that one can clinically differentiate between gonorrhea and NGU without laboratory examination. Although the presentation is often highly suggestive, mistakes can be made in this judgment. There is definitely no clinical way of identifying *C. trachomatis* in those men who have gonorrhea. Gonorrhea tends to be more acute and florid than NGU, but *N. gonorrhoeae*, *C. trachomatis*, and NGU can be present without any symptoms or discharge, and both bacteria can be present without a polymorphonuclear leukocyte response. These patients are unlikely to present to an emergency department because of urethritis, but they could present because of complications such as disseminated gonococcal infection, Reiter's syndrome, or epididymitis.

Many men with urethritis are initially misdiagnosed because they do not receive a proper urethral examination or because they have recently voided prior to the examination. When urethral discharge is not present spontaneously, the urethra needs to be milked from the base to the glans three or four times. If a male has voided within the last 3 to 4 hours, the discharge can be missed. In this situation, he should be seen again the next morning prior to voiding or at least after an interval of 4 or more hours without voiding. Depending upon the availability of diagnostic tests for *N. gonorrhoeae* or *trachomatis*, different tests may be indicated. In all cases, however, a Gram stain should be prepared on exudate if present, or on endourethral material obtained with an endourethral swab inserted 3 to 4 cm into the urethra. A properly prepared Gram stain interpreted by an experienced microscopist can usually readily differentiate gonorrhea from NGU within minutes. Results of cultures for *N. gonorrhoeae* and *C. trachomatis* are not available soon enough to help in initial management. Some newer nonculture techniques for these organisms will provide results more quickly than cultures, but again treatment is usually initiated before the results are available.

When a patient with suspected urethritis is first seen, it is important to question him about symptoms indicative of other diseases. Complaints of frequency and urgency of urination, nocturia of recent onset, hematuria, a problem with the urinary flow, including strangury, perineal pain, scrotal masses, or chills and fever are not typical of urethritis. If any of these are present, then classic urinary tract infections, acute prostatitis, a flare-up of chronic prostatitis, or acute epididymitis or orchitis needs to be considered. The presence of inguinal lymphadenopathy with or without pain or a genital rash should prompt consideration of diseases like herpes simplex virus, syphilis, or chancroid. A history of conjunctivitis, arthralgias and arthritis, or prior diarrhea suggests the possibility of Reiter's syndrome.

Although they are not necessary for initial management, diagnostic tests should usually be performed for *N. gonorrhoeae*. The author prefers a culture to a nonculture technique because of the increasing prevalence of isolates resistant to penicillin. When an isolate is available, the sensitivity to penicillin (or other antimicrobials) can be evaluated. However, nonculture techniques have some advantages, especially when there may be a problem maintaining the viability of a culture in transit. If treatment regimens for urethritis are used that will eradicate *C. trachomatis*, the need to specifically diagnose it is minimal in most circumstances unless there are special factors that make it important to know the specific result (e.g., the man's partner is pregnant). When diagnostic tests are performed, either exudate or endourethral material can be used for culture of *N. gonorrhoeae*, but endourethral material must be used for *C. trachomatis*. Urethral discharge at the meatus is not an appropriate specimen for a culture for *C. trachomatis*.

THERAPY

The first goal of management is to eradicate pathogens from the index case. However, an equally important goal is to ensure that the partners are treated so that they are placed at less risk of developing sequelae. Lasting physical sequelae for the male are exceedingly infrequent, even if treatment is delayed for long periods, whereas irreversible sequelae can arise within days in females. These reasons, and the need to interrupt transmission to others, necessitate early treatment before microbiologic results are available.

Men with uncomplicated urethritis do not need hospitalization. There are several choices for treatment, depending upon whether *N. gonorrhoeae* is present. Patients fall into three categories: (1) those with urethral gonorrhea, (2) those with NGU, and (3) those with undifferentiated urethritis where gonorrhea has not been excluded or cannot be excluded. Table 1 indicates the in vivo activity against *N. gonorrhoeae*, *C. trachomatis*, and *U. urealyticum* of currently available antimicrobials used for treatment of genital infections. The activity against *N. gonorrhoeae* is shown according to the site of infection (i.e., urethra, rectum, or pharynx) and type of strain according to susceptibility to penicillin (penicillin-sensitive, and penicillin-resistant). Isolates can have decreased sensitivity on the basis of plasmid or chromosomally mediated resistance. Penicillinase-producing *N. gonorrhoeae* isolates are resistant to penicillin on the basis of a plasmid and show absolute resistance. Gonococci acquired in Africa or South Asia should always be considered to be penicillinase-producing strains, as should all *N. gonorrhoeae* treatment failures. Penicillinase-producing strains of *N. gonorrhoeae* can, however, be present with no history of travel or contact with someone who has traveled. Chromosomally mediated resistance of *N. gonorrhoeae* tends to produce lower degrees of resistance but is still clinically significant. In these cases, a history of travel is very infrequent, and the problem is usually only noted when a standard penicillin treatment regimen fails or isolates are tested for susceptibility to penicillin.

The treatment of NGU is the least controversial (Fig. 1). The regimens of choice are 7 days of tetracycline, 500 mg orally 4 times daily, or doxycycline, 100 mg twice daily orally. The only significant advantage of tetracycline is decreased cost. Doxycycline is much more expensive but is better tolerated, can be taken with food, requires fewer pills, has greater in vitro activity, better tissue penetration, and a long half-life, so that a missed capsule would probably not result in a marked fall in serum levels. When tetracycline cannot be used, erythromycin, 500 mg 4 times daily for 7 days, is indicated.

Opinion is divided on the best treatment of men with gonorrhea. The causes for the differences include the need to eradicate *N. gonorrhoeae* at different sites, the preva-

TABLE 1 In Vivo Efficacy of Selected Antimicrobials Against Genital Pathogens

	Neisseria gonorrhoeae				Chlamydia trachomatis (%)	Ureaplasma urealyticum (%)
	Penicillin-Sensitive (%)			Penicillin-Resistant (%)		
Antimicrobial	Urethra	Rectum	Pharynx			
Tetracycline	95	70	95	50	95–100	80–90
Doxycycline	95	?70	?95	50	95–100	90–95
Aqueous procaine penicillin	97	95	90–95	0	20	0
Ampicillin/amoxicillin	95	80	50	0	20	0
Ceftriaxone	100	100	100	100	0	0
Spectinomycin	100	100	40	98	0	70
Erythromycin	75	?	?	?40	90–95	80–90
Trimethoprim-sulfamethoxazole	90	?	?	90	90–95	0
Metronidazole	0	0	0	0	0	0

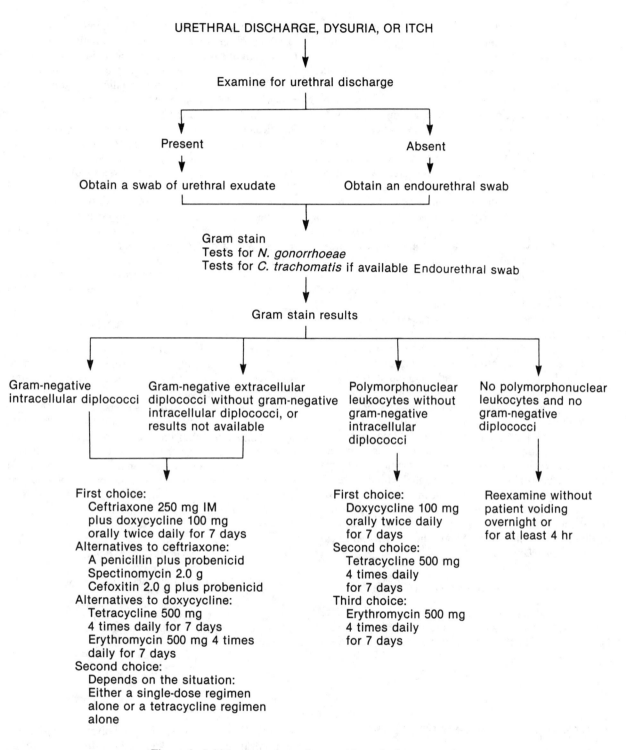

URETHRAL DISCHARGE, DYSURIA, OR ITCH

Examine for urethral discharge

Present

Absent

Obtain a swab of urethral exudate

Obtain an endourethral swab

Gram stain
Tests for *N. gonorrhoeae*
Tests for *C. trachomatis* if available Endourethral swab

Gram stain results

Gram-negative intracellular diplococci

Gram-negative extracellular diplococci without gram-negative intracellular diplococci, or results not available

Polymorphonuclear leukocytes without gram-negative intracellular diplococci

No polymorphonuclear leukocytes and no gram-negative diplococci

First choice:
  Ceftriaxone 250 mg IM
  plus doxycycline 100 mg
  orally twice daily for 7 days
Alternatives to ceftriaxone:
  A penicillin plus probenicid
  Spectinomycin 2.0 g
  Cefoxitin 2.0 g plus probenicid
Alternatives to doxycycline:
  Tetracycline 500 mg
  4 times daily for 7 days
  Erythromycin 500 mg 4 times
  daily for 7 days
Second choice:
  Depends on the situation:
  Either a single-dose regimen
  alone or a tetracycline regimen
  alone

First choice:
  Doxycycline 100 mg
  orally twice daily
  for 7 days
Second choice:
  Tetracycline 500 mg
  4 times daily
  for 7 days
Third choice:
  Erythromycin 500 mg
  4 times daily
  for 7 days

Reexamine without patient voiding overnight or for at least 4 hr

Figure 1 Initial management of men with urethral symptoms.

lence of isolates with decreased sensitivity to penicillins, the desire to use a single-dose regimen that will eradicate *N. gonorrhoeae*, and the importance of coexisting *C. trachomatis* infection. None of the single dose regimens will eradicate *C. trachomatis*. The best regimen to accomplish all four goals is ceftriaxone, 250 mg intramuscularly once in conjunction with doxycycline, 100 mg orally twice

daily for 7 days (Fig. 1). The use of spectinomycin, 2.0 g intramuscularly, or cefoxitin, 2.0 g intramuscularly plus 1.0 g of probenicid orally instead of ceftriaxone, will produce good but marginally less effective results against *N. gonorrhoeae*. For treatment of urethral gonorrhea in heterosexual men in an area where increased reistance to penicillin is infrequent, 1.0 g probenicid plus 4.8 million units of aqueous procaine penicillin G, 3.0 g of amoxicillin orally, or 3.5 g of ampicillin orally could be substituted for ceftriaxone.

Men with undifferentiated urethritis should be treated as if they have both gonorrhea and NGU (see Fig. 1). In many parts of North America, this can be adequately managed with 7 days of doxycycline, 100 mg orally twice daily, or tetracycline, 500 mg orally 4 times daily. A single-dose anti-*N. gonorrhoeae* regimen is also indicated in conjunction with a course of tetracycline if there is a concern about patient compliance and in areas where there is increased resistance of *N. gonorrhoeae* to tetracyclines.

Single-dose penicillin regimens and week-long regimens of tetracycline, doxycycline, or erythromycin are probably all adequate for incubating syphilis, although data are not extensive for the latter three regimens. Spectinomycin does not eradicate *Treponema pallidum*. Few data are available for ceftriaxone.

Appropriate management of the male requires management of the female or male partners, both for the sake of the partner and of the index case. Unless the partner is pregnant, treatment regimens are usually the same as in the male. During pregnancy, tetracyclines are contraindicated, and erythromycin, 500 mg orally 4 times daily for 7 days or 250 mg orally 4 times daily for 14 days, can be substituted for tetracycline for activity against *C. trachomatis*. When gonorrhea is suspected or proved, one of the single-dose regimens is needed as well.

In general, presenting features in children are similar except that children may present with more vague or nonspecific symptoms such as eneuresis, unwillingness to urinate, or behavioral symptoms associated with the overall syndrome of sexual abuse. Diagnostic tests are similar. Treatment regimens are altered for weight and are similar except that tetracyclines are contraindicated before age 8; therefore, erythromycin should be used for eradication of *C. trachomatis*.

FOLLOW-UP EXAMINATION

Ideally, all patients treated for urethritis should have a follow-up examination to ensure that pathogens have been eradicated and that the index case has not been reexposed to an untreated partner. In patients with urethritis in whom *N. gonorrhoeae* was not initially present, and *C. trachomatis* was either absent or could not be screened for because of a lack of diagnostic tests, follow-up care is less necessary but certainly is indicated if the male has persistent or recurrent symptoms. When *N. gonorrhoeae* or *C. trachomatis* is initially detected, a follow-up visit is indicated for a test of cure studies. For *N. gonorrhoeae*, this is best performed approximately 7 days after treatment. For *C. trachomatis*, if only a single follow-up visit is performed, it is best done 3 to 4 weeks after treatment. *N. gonorrhoeae* treatment failures should be treated with ceftriaxone, spectinomycin, or cefoxitin. *C. trachomatis* treatment failures are almost always caused by noncompliance or reexposure to an inadequately treated, untreated, or new partner and can be retreated with a tetracycline regimen. Persistence or recurrence of NGU after a tetracycline course is best treated with erythromycin, 500 mg 4 times daily for 14 days, if no cause is found.

ADVERSE REACTIONS

With the exception of the well-known anaphylactic or accelerated reactions to penicillins and procaine reactions when aqueous procaine penicillin G is used, most reactions are a nuisance. Cephalosporins are much less likely than penicillins to produce anaphylaxis. Tetracycline, and to a greater extent erythromycin, are frequently accompanied by gastrointestinal side effects that may necessitate decreasing the dose or occasionally ceasing treatment. However, life-threatening complications are infrequent. Doxycycline tends to be better tolerated. Its major potentially serious side effect is photosensitivity, which is preventable.

SUGGESTED READING

Bowie WR. Nongonococcal urethritis. Urol Clin North Am 1984; 11:55–64.
Centers for Disease Control. Sexually transmitted diseases treatment guidelines. MMWR 1985; 34 (5): 75S–108S.
Washington AE. Update on treatment recommendations for gonococcal infections. Rev Infect Dis 1982; 4:S758–S771.

URINARY OBSTRUCTION AND RETENTION

NORMAN E. PETERSON, M.D.

A discussion of urinary retention is best begun by defining terms. *Anuria* is a cessation of urine production or delivery to the bladder; this implies a parenchymal, vascular, or obstructive process involving the kidneys or upper drainage system, either bilaterally or unilaterally in the case of a single functioning kidney. *Urinary retention* is an inability to void, with the expected result of bladder distention. Not all cases of urinary retention are acute, nor is anuria always present.

ESTABLISHING PROMPT BLADDER DRAINAGE

Draining the bladder has the dual purposes of achieving acute relief of obstruction and maintaining urinary drainage until diagnostic measures and therapeutic remedies can be instituted. Drainage can be done perineally, suprapubically (percutaneous or operative), or transurethrally (manual or endoscopic). Several of the available methods should only be done by urologists and may require formal operative facilities. If doubt exists regarding the nature of obstruction or the advisability of nonurologic management and if circumstances permit, intervention should await urologic consultation.

Most urinary retention episodes can be treated by urethral catheterization. A well-lubricated No. 12 to 16 caliber catheter is comfortably tolerated. A straight Robinson catheter is adequate for simple decompression, whereas a balloon-retention (Foley) catheter is employed for sustained drainage. Although it has traditionally been taught that rapid drainage of large volumes can cause hematuria and cardiovascular collapse, a recent large study did not support this dictum.

Mechanical obstructions to successful catheterization include urethral stricture (from prior trauma, instrumentation, or infection), urethral false passage (from prior or concurrent instrumentation),vesical outlet contracture, benign or malignant prostatic or urethral obstruction, or extrinsic compression from local nonurologic processes.

Obstruction of the vesical outlet or prostatic urethra is commonly accompanied by a posterior (ventral) elevation that obstructs straight-catheter passage; such obstructions are usually easily traversed by an angulated coudé catheter. An alternative maneuver employs a malleable semirigid mandrin inserted within the catheter and then molded into a suitable configuration for manipulation as with a urethral sound. The mandrin technique should be restricted to experienced personnel.

Urethral strictures and false passages frequently coexist and are often resistant to attempts at routine catheterization. Isolated false passages (without accompanying stricture) may be bypassed by the mandrin catheter technique. An alternative maneuver, particularly suited to urethral stricture disease with or without false passage, employs flexible filiform guides, available in a variety of sizes and configurations, which are maneuvered across obstructions and false passages into the bladder, and to which are then attached any of a series of progressively larger follower catheters that may then be employed to dilate as well as drain. Follower catheters do not incorporate balloon retention and therefore must be replaced by a Foley catheter or otherwise secured. The mandrin and filiform-follower maneuvers require experienced personnel.

Failure of these maneuvers warrants urologic consultation, with endoscopic procedures likely to yield successful access to the bladder. An alternative approach for consideration in the setting of impassable pendulous urethral pathology is catheterization through a surgical perineal urethrostomy. A formal surgical suprapubic cystostomy is the final option when all lesser maneuvers have failed.

Suprapubic percutaneous cystotomy permits introduction of a small catheter for drainage. Intravenous Intracath sets are ideally suited to this maneuver, although specific Cystocath and larger trocar sets are commercially available. The small-caliber Intracath tubing is vulnerable to obstruction and therefore requires protection from kinking and periodic flushing. Effectiveness is only temporary, but this is an ideal maneuver for providing relief while awaiting urologic consultation. The bladder must be palpable and there must be no indication of prior suprapubic surgery. If there is doubt as to whether the bladder is distended, as in the obese patient, sonographic confirmation is advisable. The procedure consists of a simple midline needle puncture one finger breadth above the symphysis pubis, directed slightly caudally and advanced until urine is returned. The catheter is then advanced, the needle is withdrawn, and the catheter is secured in position and connected to drainage.

The urethra should not be immediately catheterized in the trauma patient. Such patients may have posterior urethral injury accompanying pelvic fracture, prostatic displacement at rectal examination, or blood at the urethral meatus. Traumatic forces may produce incomplete urethral injury or total avulsion. Catheterization is contraindicated with the former and not possible with the latter. More importantly, catheterization may convert an innocuous incomplete injury into a potentially devastating complete lesion. Suspected urethral trauma should be investigated initially by a retrograde urethrogram. Injury is indicated by local extravasation. Either injury necessitates emergency operative suprapubic cystostomy.

After urinary retention is relieved, a decision must be made as to immediate catheter withdrawal versus continued drainage. The suspected cause of the retention is important; urologic, gynecologic, pediatric, or neurologic consultation may be needed to make the decision. Also significant is whether the presenting episode represents an isolated event or is part of a chronic process. Acute urinary retention (usually approximately 500 ml) may be acutely decompressed with secure expectations of resuming preretention voiding. In contrast, the chronically overdistended patient with overflow incontinence (who lacks the writhing discomfort characterizing the former patient) will require sustained bladder drainage and formal urologic management. Chronic retention volumes commonly exceed 1,000 ml. Concern regarding pathologic postobstructive diuresis, hematuria, or cardiovascular collapse is generally exaggerated, as these events are very rare.

ADULT MALE URINARY RETENTION

Nontraumatic urinary retention is encountered most often because of obstruction at the level of the vesical outlet or posterior urethra, usually caused by benign prostatic hypertrophy or prostatic carcinoma.

The typical presentation of benign prostatic hypertrophy is of insidious progressive onset in the late 6th decade of life or later, with nocturia being the most reliable clinical indicator. Hesitancy, dribbling following voiding, a sensation of incomplete emptying, diminution in size and force of the voided stream, and occasional hematuria are other clinical features. Digital rectal examination of the prostate will usually reveal a symmetric, firm enlargement of homogeneous consistency. No reliable correlation exists between estimated size on palpation and the degree of symptomatic obstruction. In contrast is the malignant prostate which, in the setting of obstruction, is typically represented by diffuse or extensive stony, nodular indurations.

Symptoms of benign prostatic hypertrophy occurring in younger patients (prior to the early 6th decade) are commonly the result of fibromuscular obstruction at the bladder outlet (median bar). Clinical features may include a history of enuresis, epididymitis, or nocturia. The physical nature of the obstruction may defeat straight catheterization and require coudé or mandrin techniques. A patient in the same relative age group who abruptly develops isolated symptoms of outlet obstruction must be considered to have prostatic carcinoma until this can be ruled out by biopsy.

Infectious obstructions to urinary drainage most commonly include urethritis and prostatitis; normal voiding is usually restored following appropriate antibiotic therapy during interval catheter drainage.

Urinary retention has also been reported in homosexual men after intense anal intercourse, due to stimulation of reflex nerve arcs. Treatment consists of an indwelling Foley catheter and administration of bethanechol and phenoxybenzamine.

ADULT FEMALE URINARY RETENTION

Urinary retention in adult women has frequently been attributed to psychogenic factors, a presumption derived from reported absence of objective organic or obstructive disease, dismal results of surgical intervention, and incrimination of conversion hysteria and schizophrenia among potential psychogenic diagnoses.

However, a series of female patients with urinary retention from atypical lumbar disk syndromes has provoked a less prejudicial diagnostic approach, which has been given further impetus by urodynamic advancements. One report documented complete or incomplete urinary retention in otherwise healthy young females secondary to urethral sphincter or pelvic floor spasticity, confirmed by urodynamic improvement after bilateral lidocaine pudendal block. Another study of adult female urinary retention attributed causation to psychogenic (30 percent), myelitis (19 percent), other neurologic (11 percent), diabetes mellitus (11 percent), postoperative (15 percent), and idiopathic (15 percent) factors. Therefore, although psychogenic retention predominates, evidence of neurologic disease or drug ingestion should be sought. When ignored, isolated or intermittent retention episodes may evolve into chronic vesical overdistention with myotonic detrusor degeneration.

Basic evaluation should include a check of anal sphincter tone and ability to voluntarily contract the anal sphincter, integrity of perianal sensation, bulbocavernosus reflex (evocation of anal contraction by clitoral stimulation), and lower extremity sensorimotor, gait, and reflex abnormalities. More sophisticated analysis may include a voiding cystourethrogram, cystometrogram (supine and

erect), bethanechol supersensitivity testing, urethral pressure profilometry, uroflowmetry, postvoid residual urine measurement, pelvic floor electromyography, pudendal neurolysis, myelography, and psychiatric examination. Obviously the majority of these studies are inappropriate in the emergency setting.

Therapy varies with etiology. In the absence of organic disorder, simple decompression suffices. In the setting of chronic myogenic detrusor degeneration, intermittent self-catheterization with or without adjunctive pharmacologic medication may be necessary on a temporary or permanent basis.

PEDIATRIC URINARY RETENTION

Congenital anatomic abnormalities underlie the majority of pediatric retention syndromes, and specialty consultation is advisable regarding both initial and later management. Congenital urologic anomalies often coexist with others—both urologic and nonurologic—and the latter often are more important. Moreover, the renal consequences of congenital urologic disorders range in significance from mild to cataclysmic, mandating prompt and comprehensive appraisal and treatment. Some disorders are restricted to male or female patients: obstructing posterior urethral valves in males and hydrocolpos resulting from vaginal atresia or imperforate hymen in females.

Occurring in both sexes (but more common to females) is the *ureterocele* formed by urinary distention of redundant intravesical ureteral mucosa. The most common consequence is obstruction of the ureter, but large ureteroceles may prolapse across or into the urethral orifice, resulting in bladder obstruction. An uncommon variant (cecoureterocele) dissects along the urethral lumen, with significant urethral obstruction.

Congenital neurologic disorders resulting in pediatric urinary retention syndromes include lumbosacral myelomeningocele and sacral agenesis. Disorders in older children are often functional and include the primary megacystis syndrome and external sphincter hyperactivity. Both of these disorders are considered to be learned phenomena. The former is the consequence of infrequent voiding, culminating in chronic vesical overdistention and potential permanent myogenic damage; the latter may result from deliberate avoidance of painful voiding during infection or from efforts to prevent incontinence during uninhibited detrusor contractions. Urodynamic evaluation is diagnostic.

Common examples of *neurologic disorders* resulting in inefficient micturition or urinary retention include spinal cord trauma or myelodysplasia at or below the level of the motor nuclei governing detrusor and sphincteric activity (spinal segments S2 to S4; vertebral level L2) and therefore interrupting the spinal reflex arc, producing an areflexic (flaccid) bladder. One review of urodynamic data from patients with urinary retention syndromes described detrusor areflexia in 22 percent. Such lesions may be transitory and fully restored spontaneously after variable intervals (spinal shock), during which intermittent catheterization is adequate as management. Other examples may be reversible upon correction of the causative process. Recovery in the remainder may be incomplete or irreversible and require permanent adjunctive therapeutic measures (surgical, pharmacologic, self-catheterization).

Alternatively, lesions located above the spinal micturition center commonly produce a reflex or spastic voiding pattern, often with detrusor-sphincter dysfunction (in which the hypertonic external sphincter fails to relax normally during detrusor contraction). High voiding pressures contribute to potentially calamitous ureteral reflux and detrusor damage and to residual bladder urine volumes vulnerable to infection, stone formation, and urinary retention. Treatment may include self-catheterization and biofeedback techniques for cases of lesser severity; more extreme cases may require attempted pharmacologic external sphincter relaxation intermediate to surgical sphincterotomy.

Multiple sclerosis should be considered in cases of otherwise idiopathic urinary retention. An estimated 90 percent of all patients with multiple sclerosis develop lower urinary tract symptoms at some time during the illness; approximately 50 percent demonstrate voiding problems with increased residual urine volumes, 25 percent have detrusor areflexia, and 25 percent experience detrusor instability with urgency and incontinence. Correlations are observed between limb spasticity, impaired vibration sensation, and bladder symptoms, and worsening of bladder symptoms often parallels a progression of the neuropathology. Management is symptomatic, including self-catheterization.

The urologic consequences of *Landry-Guillain-Barré* syndrome are present in up to 30 percent of involved patients and appear as a motor paralytic bladder with urinary retention. The syndrome may be provoked by viral infection, vaccination, surgery, or other infections, and clinical manifestations reflect predominantly areflexic motor neuropathy with minimal sensory loss. There is afebrile symmetric motor weakness or paralysis progressing proximally, so that voiding difficulties are frequently a secondary complaint. Symptoms peak at 4 weeks in 90 percent of patients, and functional recovery is typically final at 6 months, although occasionally it is incomplete. Urologic management is usually limited to intermittent self-catheterization.

More commonly encountered is temporary vesical motor paralysis from *herpes simplex and herpes zoster infections*, with risk of infection increasing with numbers of sexual partners and with immunosuppressant medication (activating latent infection). Incubation ranges from 7 to 21 days, and clinical manifestations include fever, malaise, and pain over the involved dermatome (usually unilateral) for 2 to 4 days prior to appearance of erythema, papules, and vesicles. Infection can traverse both visceral and somatic nerves and therefore produce either skin eruption or bladder atonia or both. Neuropathy may be bilateral despite unilateral cutaneous manifestations, and neuropathy rather than cystitis is the more likely source of the retention syndrome. Isolated visceral nerve

TABLE 1 Drugs Contributing to Urinary Retention

Beta-adrenergic stimulation (detrusor relaxation)
  Isoproterenol (Isuprel)
  Progesterone
  Atropine

Alpha-adrenergic stimulation (vesical outlet contraction)
  Ephedrine sulfate
  Pseudoephedrine HCl (Sudafed)
  Phenylephrine HCl (Neo-Synephrine)
  Phenylpropanolamine HCl (Ornade; appetite suppressants)
  Imipramine HCl (Tofranil)
  Estrogen, estradiol
  Levodopa, dopamine, epinephrine
  Antihistamines
  Bromocriptine (Parlodel)
  Mercurial diuretics
  Nortriptyline HCl (Aventyl; Nortylin)
  Phenothiazines
  Testosterone
  Amphetamines
  Amitriptyline HCl (Elavil, Triavil)
  Benztropine mesylate (Cogentin)
  Hydralazine (Apresoline)
  Isoniazid
  Morphine sulfate

Musculotropic detrusor relaxation
  Propantheline (Pro-Banthine)
  Methantheline (Banthine)
  Belladonna
  Oxybutynin HCl (Ditropan)
  Flavoxate HCl (Urispas)
  Dicyclomine HCl (Bentyl)
  Hyoscyamine sulfate (Cystospaz)
  Imipramine HCl (Tofranil)
  Estrogen
  Emepronium bromide
  Diazepam (Valium)
  Terbutaline
  Indomethacin
  Nifedipine

involvement may produce retention without cutaneous or other manifestations. Reversibility is prompt and complete, and interval therapy requires only intermittent self-catheterization.

PHARMACOLOGIC URINARY RETENTION

Many drugs have effects on the bladder. Table 1 provides a comprehensive listing of the commonly encountered urotropic agents. Treatment consists of intermittent or sustained catheterization and drug withdrawal (or tapering).

SUGGESTED READING

Peterson NE. Urinary retention. In: Wolfson A, Harwood-Nuss A, eds. Emergency urology. New York: Churchill Livingstone. In press.

Smith DR. Psychogenic urinary problems, including urinary retention. In: Kaufman JJ, ed. Current urologic therapy. Philadelphia: WB Saunders, 1980:452.

Wein AJ. Drug therapy for neurogenic and non-neurogenic bladder dysfunction. In: Kaufman JJ, ed. Current urologic therapy. Philadelphia: WB Saunders, 1980.

CYSTITIS AND PYELONEPHRITIS

JOHN B. McCABE, M.D., F.A.C.E.P.

Urinary tract infection is common and occurs in all age groups and both sexes. Most commonly it affects the adult female patient because of the shorter urethra.

Infection of the urinary tract may involve any of a number of structures. Cystitis describes the symptom complex of dysuria, frequency and urgency of urination, and suprapubic tenderness. Anatomically, the term refers to infection limited to the urinary bladder. Pyelonephritis describes the symptom complex characterized by flank pain, fever, nausea, and vomiting in addition to the typical symptoms of cystitis. Anatomically, pyelonephritis represents an infection of renal parenchyma. Bacteriuria refers to the presence of bacteria in the urine, without specification of the site of infection.

The typical presentations of cystitis and acute pyelonephritis are easily recognized. However, the most common cause of dysuria in the adult female is vaginitis, and it is the most frequently found other diagnosis for the patient with urinary tract symptoms. Other renal abnormalities, gynecologic problems, and gastrointestinal problems may also be confused with urinary tract infection.

Although urinary tract infection may arise by ascending infection, hematogenous bacterial spread, or lymphatic pathway spread, ascending infection is the most common. Normal urine is sterile. Perineal and periurethral colonization, along with alteration in intrinsic host resistance, may allow ascending spread of bacteria with subsequent colonization of bladder urine and possible renal infection. Factors that increase the risk of infection include obstruction, calculi, altered vaginal pH, abnormality in normal bladder emptying, instrumentation, and local trauma. Local trauma, particularly related to sexual activity, is the most common factor in subsequent development of urinary tract infection.

Most urinary tract infections are caused by gram-negative bacilli normally found in the gastrointestinal tract. The predominant pathogen is *Escherichia coli*, followed in order of frequency by *Klebsiella, Proteus, Enterobacter,* and *Pseudomonas. Staphlyococcus* is an infrequent pathogen, but may be especially important in nosocomial infections.

Urinary tract infection may often be suggested by the patient's symptoms. However, diagnosis and localization of the infection based on symptoms alone are unreliable. Half of the female patients with urinary tract symptoms may have vaginitis. Up to 50 percent of patients with typical cystitis symptoms may have sterile urine. Preliminary diagnosis can be made utilizing examination of the urine. Definitive diagnosis rests with urine culture.

The diagnostic accuracy of the microscopic examination of the urine depends upon the quality of the specimen obtained. In the neonate, suprapubic aspiration is the procedure of choice for obtaining a urine specimen. In older children, a sterile midstream urine specimen can usually be collected. If it is not possible to obtain such a specimen free of epithelial contamination, suprapubic aspiration is indicated. Adult males can usually provide a clean midstream urine specimen that is acceptable for analysis. Controversy exists regarding the most appropriate specimen collection technique in the adult female patient. In some series, up to 50 percent of women with sterile bladder urine have significant bacteriuria in the midstream clean-catch specimen. Other studies have demonstrated little correlation between the technique of collection and the ultimate culture result. Most adult females can reliably obtain a midstream clean-catch urine specimen. If not, urinary catheterization should be performed. Adequacy of the urinary specimen can be ascertained by the presence or absence of significant numbers of epithelial cells. As the ratio of leukocytes to epithelial cells decreases in the specimen, the more likely it is that the leukocytes are simply vaginal contaminants.

The patient with urinary tract infection has *pyuria*. Pyuria is generally accepted as the presence of more than ten white blood cells per high power field in a microscopic examination of centrifuged urinary sediment. The number of white blood cells varies, depending upon severity of infection, fluid intake, time of day, and method of urine collection. Pyuria alone is nonspecific, and diagnosis utilizing pyuria alone is not reliable.

The single most useful finding for presumptive diagnosis of urinary tract infection is the presence of *bacteria in the urine*. The presence of at least one bacteria per high-power field in a midstream clean-catch Gram-stained unspun urine specimen correlates well with a culture result of more than 100,000 bacteria colony–forming units per milliliter. The absence of bacteria is a reliable indicator of absence of urinary tract infection.

The combination of pyuria and bacteriuria on microscopic examination of the urine correlates well with urinary tract infection. Diagnostic accuracy of 75 to 85 percent (both from a negative and positive predictive value point of view) can be reached utilizing these criteria.

Although clinical symptoms are unreliable in differentiating cystitis from *pyelonephritis* (Table 1), a subgroup of patients exist who are more likely to have infection involving the kidney. These are patients with classic upper urinary tract symptoms and such signs of systemic toxicity as severe fever, rigors, nausea, and vomiting. Such patients must be presumed to have acute pyelonephritis.

Patients with pyelonephritis may require analgesics, antipyretics, and intravenous fluid administration to correct dehydration. Emergency department evaluation should include urinalysis and urine culture. Blood cultures should be obtained. Tests of renal function should be performed, especially if parenteral antibiotics are to be administered. Intravenous pyelography should be performed if there is any suspicion of an obstructing renal calculus.

Hospital admission is indicated for patients who are unable to maintain a normal state of hydration because of persistent nausea and vomiting. Patients with severe systemic symptoms, complicating medical conditions,

TABLE 1 Acute Urinary Tract Infection: Correlation with Infection (%)

Symptoms	Sterile Urine or Insignificant Bacteriuria	Renal Bacteriuria	Bladder Bacteriuria
Symptoms suggesting lower tract			
Frequency	95	98	70
Burning	70	68	70
Suprapubic pain	70	68	51
Symptoms suggesting upper tract			
Flank pain	50	48	19
Fever	35	44	4
Rigors	15	32	15
Nausea and vomiting	25	24	8
Hematuria	25	30	12

From Fairley KF, Carson NE, Gutch RC, et al. Site of infection in acute urinary tract infection in general practice. Lancet 1971; 1:616.

known urinary tract anatomic abnormalities, at the extremes of age, and all male patients with significant systemic symptoms should be admitted.

Once initial laboratory evaluation has been performed in the emergency department, *antibiotic therapy* can be started. Appropriate initial therapy would include gentamicin 1.5 mg per kilogram every 8 hours, and ampicillin, 1 g intravenously every 6 hours. The dosage must be adjusted if renal function is decreased. A second- or third-generation cephalosporin such as cefamandole or intravenous trimethoprim-sulfamethoxazole would be an acceptable alternative. An occasional patient with mild to moderate systemic symptoms may be treated over a 6- to 8-hour period in the emergency department with intravenous fluid administration and antibiotic therapy. After appropriate response, discharge from the emergency department is warranted. However, most patients with significant signs of systemic toxicity should be admitted for parenteral antibiotic therapy.

Most patients with pyelonephritis will respond to treatment within 8 to 12 hours. If this does not occur, further investigation is warranted to exclude complicating factors such as obstruction, papillary necrosis, or a drug-resistant organism.

The remaining patients who have urinary tract symptoms, but no systemic symptoms may be treated as *outpatients*. This group includes patients with both cystitis and relatively asymptomatic pyelonephritis. Goals of therapy in this group include:

1. Rapid cure of patients with simple cystitis.
2. Identification of patients with true renal infections.
3. Treatment with minimal cost and minimal side effects.
4. Prevention of complications of incompletely treated infections.

Two forms of therapy are available, single-dose antibiotic therapy and multiple-dose therapy. A single dose of antibiotics cures simple bacterial cystitis in 85 to 90 percent of cases. At the same time, it identifies a group

TABLE 2 Oral Antibiotics for Outpatient Treatment of Urinary Tract Infection

Single Dose

  Ampicillin, 3.5 g
  Amoxicillin, 3.0 g
  TMP/SMZ*, 3 double-strength tablets

Multidose (10–14 days)

  Ampicillin, 250–500 mg 4 times a day
  TMP/SMZ*, 1 double-strength tablet twice a day
  Sulfisoxazole, 1 g 4 times a day
  Nitrofurantoin, 100 mg 4 times a day

* Trimethoprim-sulfamethoxazole (double-strength tablet = 160 mg trimethoprim, 800 mg sulfamethoxazole)

of patients with renal infection, since cure in this group is uncommon. Cost and complications are minimal. Single-dose therapy is indicated for patients with a low likelihood of renal infection. This includes acutely symptomatic adult female patients without pregnancy or complicating disease states. Males, children, and adult females with prolonged symptoms (more than 3 to 5 days) or other complicating conditions (diabetes, chronic renal disease, pregnancy) should be treated with 10- to 14-day therapy to ensure eradication of renal infection, if it exists. Only patients with a good chance of follow-up examination should be treated with single-dose therapy. If follow-up is neglected, asymptomatic renal bacteriuria may persist and progress to chronic renal failure.

Prior to therapy, urinalysis and urine culture should be performed. The cost effectiveness of culture in uncomplicated urinary tract infection is open to debate. However, useful information is obtained from the culture for patients who do not respond to initial therapy. Assessment of the patient's past medical history, acuteness of illness, and ability to follow up determines the choice of therapy. Many medication schemes are available (Table 2). All patients should be reassessed in 48 to 72 hours to determine if symptoms have abated. However, clinical response to treatment does not ensure negative urine culture results.

Follow-up urine cultures should be obtained upon completion of therapy.

The pregnant patient should always be treated with prolonged therapy. Any indication of systemic symptoms mandates hospital admission. Patients with hemorrhagic cystitis probably require prolonged therapy. Single-dose therapy in this group has not been studied.

Patients should be advised to maintain normal fluid intake. Pyridium (100 mg three times a day) may reduce the symptoms of dysuria. It should be given for 2 to 3 days.

Adult patients with pyelonephritis may be referred to primary care physicians. Urologic consultation is indicated if the patient does not respond to initial inpatient therapy. Adult patients with cystitis can be referred to primary care physicians. Infants and children should be referred for eventual urologic evaluation to rule out the presence of anatomic abnormalities of the urinary tract.

SUGGESTED READING

McCabe JB, Hamilton GC. Single dose antibiotic therapy of urinary tract infection: Is it appropriate in the emergency department? Ann Emer Med 1984; 13:432.

Ogra PL, Faden HS. Urinary tract infections in childhood: An update. J Pediatr 1985; 106:1023.

Ronald AR. Current concepts in the management of urinary tract infections in adults. Med Clin North Am 1984; 68:335.

EMERGENCIES IN PATIENTS WITH RENAL TRANSPLANTS

WILLIAM J. C. AMEND Jr., M.D.

Transplant emergencies may be subdivided into emergencies involving the transplanted kidney itself, emergencies arising in transplant patients because of immunosuppression, and emergencies owing to the transplant patient's underlying medical conditions. Kidney transplant patients usually have a good idea of their past medical history and current medical status, but often the present medical history must be obtained from relatives or friends (who often have a similar good understanding of the background of the patient's medical condition). Many transplant patients have Medi-alert bracelets or some other suitable reference material so that their primary transplant institution (and that facility's physicians and surgeons) can be rapidly contacted.

EMERGENCIES INVOLVING THE KIDNEY TRANSPLANT ITSELF

A common chief complaint is kidney pain. Renal transplants are extraperitoneal in adults and intraperitoneal in children, and have no instrinsic nerve supply. Therefore, pain near the kidney is a reflection of perinephric irritation and reaction rather than reaction within the kidney itself (or within the transplanted ureter).

If this pain occurs in a transplanted patient with a transplant in place less than 6 months, the differential diagnosis includes possible acute transplant rejection, acute pyelonephritis, traumatic perinephric hematoma, lymphocele, or diseases of other intra-abdominal organs that are structurally located near the transplant, such as appendicitis or ovarian cyst rupture. A careful examination and system review should be obtained to assess whether it is the kidney or one of the perinephric possibilities mentioned. For all transplant emergencies, and particularly this symptom complex, a urinalysis, serum blood urea nitrogen (BUN), and serum creatinine should be obtained to assess whether there has been primary transplant renal dysfunction. A urinalysis is also recommended for all patients, including methylene blue staining for the presence of bacteria in the urine.

An ultrasound study is often important in differentiating parenchymal processes such as pyelonephritis or rejection from perinephric processes such as hematoma and lymphocele. Should pyelonephritis be likely, a loading dose of 2 mg per kilogram of an aminoglycoside (gentamicin, tobramycin) is recommended following blood and urine cultures. If the patient is stable and the symptoms occur shortly after transplant, it is recommended that the primary transplant service be contacted and the patient be transferred to that service when stable. This is to allow observation for the potential worsening of renal function over the next 2 to 3 days (if the renal function has not already shown some change prior to the patient's arrival in the emergency room).

Transplant pain that occurs later than 6 months after transplantation, usually reflects acute pyelonephritis or some other intra-abdominal process. It is highly unusual for acute rejection to present with pain over the kidney so long after transplantation unless the patient has abruptly stopped his medication. The diagnostic and therapeutic approach to acute pyelonephritis in the transplant has been described previously. An ultrasound examination, when possible, is helpful to exclude the possibility of obstructive uropathy. The aminoglycoside antibiotics must be adjusted for creatinine clearance following their initial loading dose. The antibiotic may also have to be changed after the results of the urine culture and sensitivities are known.

A second common chief complaint is *leg swelling* (ipsilateral to the transplanted kidney). The differential diagnosis includes either a post-transplant lymphocele (fluid located extraperitoneally and usually medial to the transplant from nonligated, severed lymphatics); or a distal thrombophlebitis that may or may not coexist with a lymphocele. A careful physical examination usually demonstrates evidence of either thrombophlebitis or perinephric fluid collection. If thrombophlebitis is present, inpatient treatment with heparin is necessary along with bed rest and leg elevation. After admission, an ultrasound examination should be routinely ordered to rule out the possibility of a coexisting lymphocele. Should this be present, referral to the primary transplant surgical service is indicated.

A third complaint related to the transplant is *gross hematuria*. This could be related to either acute transplant rejection, painless renal or ureteral calculus disease, native kidney source (particularly if the patient had native polycystic kidney disease), other bladder and/or renal etiologies (which need later nonemergent evaluation), and finally (but unlikely) acute de novo glomerulonephritis.

If renal function has worsened, an ultrasound examination is necessary to rule out obstructive ureteral disease secondary to a painless calculus. If this study is negative for obstruction, treatment with high-dose steroids, 5 to 8 mg per kilogram of either prednisolone phosphate intravenously or Solumedrol, is indicated for presumed rejection. Admission to the hospital or close outpatient management is warranted. Finally, it is important to ascertain whether the patient is on Cytoxan (cyclophosphamide). This immunosuppressant can be associated with hemorrhagic cystitis after chronic usage. Even while taking Cytoxan, however, a patient may still have hematuria from other causes. A fourth transplant emergency related to the kidney itself is that of *decreased urine output*. There may not be actual oliguria, particularly if the patient's original native kidney urine output was substantial prior to the transplant. The differential diagnosis includes acute transplant rejection, obstruction in the kidney (either arterial or venous thrombosis), obstruction from urologic conditions such as ureteral, calculus, or bladder neck obstructive disease, and finally, the usual forms of prerenal, dehydrated states.

It is important always to rule out dehydration by checking for orthostatic hypotension and other signs. If noted, this should be treated with boluses of 300 to 500 ml of intravenous normal saline. Sometimes the analysis of the fractional excretion of sodium in the urine is helpful, but the transplanted kidney may not show a clear delineation between intrinsic and prerenal forms of oliguric renal failure. An ultrasound examination or a radioisotope scan can be important to differentiate various obstructive etiologies. While these studies are being performed, it is imperative to call the primary transplant service's attending surgeon to discuss the possibility of potential, pending vascular occlusive disease.

Another emergent condition, in which the patient complains of *too much urine output*, is the polyuric post-transplant renal disorder. The differential etiologic diagnosis includes (1) steroid-induced hyperglycemia with an associated osmotic diuresis, and (2) partial obstructive renal disease. The latter causes reduced urine-

concentrating ability in the transplanted kidney. It is important to get urine and blood sugar analyses as well as a serum calcium (although acute hypercalcemic - hypercalciuric processes are rare in the post-transplant setting). Should the cause be hyperglycemia, an initial dose of intravenous insulin (5 to 10 units of regular insulin) and initiation of an insulin drip are indicated (providing anywhere from 0.5 to 2 units per hour of regular insulin). If these metabolic etiologies are not present, examination by ultrasound or other uroradiographic techniques is indicated to rule out partial obstructive renal disease. Nonemergent readmission to the transplant service of record would be indicated.

Rare instances of *severe cardiovascular collapse*, with or without transplant pain, have been reported. One must consider the possibility (particularly in the early postoperative period) of an anastomotic or aneurysmal leak from the renal transplant artery. Hemodynamic stabilization and resuscitative efforts are as for any other acute hemorrhagic event. Rapid surgical treatment is indicated, with the treating surgeons in close phone contact with the primary transplant surgeon if at all possible.

EMERGENCIES OF IMMUNOSUPPRESSION

Glucocorticoids are routinely given to transplant patients and, at the doses employed (prednisone less than 30 mg per day), rarely prevent febrile or leukocytic responses, *but* reduce inflammation so that abdominal and other signs of infection may not be present.

It is important to review compliance with the immunosuppressive regimen with the patient and family, particularly when there has been a recent adjustment in drug dose. If immunosuppressive doses have been increased recently, owing to a recent rejection episode, the patient is at risk for "immunocompromised" complications. It is important to also treat the possibility of insufficient steroids to deal with "stress" and to administer supplemental glucocorticoids (an initial intravenous 50 to 200 mg of hydrocortisone or its equivalent). This is not initial treatment for rejection, but is given because the patient has a potentially inadequate endogenous steroid reserve.

Fever is due to infection, with or without localizing signs. If the infectious process is acute, 75 percent are of respiratory origin, 20 percent of genitourinary origin, and the remainder from central nervous system (CNS), ear, nose, and throat (ENT), or other origins. The infection may have a more prolonged or "subacute" course, coming from the same sources. When the pre-hospital course is subacute, fungal or protozoal etiologies must be considered. An infection is initally much more dangerous than rejection. Urinalysis with methylene blue staining is mandatory. A genitourinary infection should especially be sought if there has been a previous history of urinary tract infection, pre- and/or post-transplant, and if there has been a previous history of additional urologic surgery. A chest film is usually recommended and often demonstrates disease despite negative auscultatory findings. If the patient has a primary respiratory or wound infection, it is important to admit him or her to a room where isolation techniques can be practiced, particularly against contact with other immunosuppressed patients.

Gastrointestinal problems are myriad and include peptic or infectious esophagitis (all immunosuppressive drugs cause this; it may represent an esophageal monilial or herpetic infection); peptic ulcer disease and gastritis (often related to high-dose steroids); pancreatitis and pancreatic pseudocysts (related to azathioprine); cholelithiasis (not secondary to medications directly, but there is an increased incidence of cholesterol and bilirubinate stones in these patients); hepatitis (secondary to azathioprine and cyclosporine, or to infectious etiologies); colitis, with or without perforation; and diverticulosis (often related to prolonged or high-dose prednisone usage). If the patient is unstable hemodynamically, concern for prompt hydration and ''stress'' steroid management should be considered. Frequently, these patients show severe third spacing and require large amounts of intravenous saline for resuscitation purposes. As previously mentioned, intra-abdominal catastrophes may occur with little or no physical findings. The usual ''board-like'' abdomen may not be present despite intestinal perforation, a fact that must never be forgotten in dealing with abdominal pain in all transplant patients. Antibiotic coverage for gram-negative and/or anaerobic infections must be provided for the more severe forms of gastrointestinal emergent conditions (See Chapter on *Sepsis in Adults*).

Acute central nervous system changes may represent infection or metabolic abnormality associated with the immunosuppressive medications. Steroid-induced hyperglycemia or the metabolic abnormalities of hypercalcemia or hypophosphatemia may present with acute neurologic manifestations. In addition, although not medication-related, there may be hypertensive encephalopathy and/or ruptured Berry aneurysm, often seen with previous history of hypertension and/or associated with the polycystic kidney disease state.

If the CNS changes are more the subacute or chronic type, one must consider a subacute or chronic infection that is related to immunosuppressive use or consider a primary central nervous system lymphoma (seen in the immunosuppressed host). Emergency lumbar puncture testing should be delayed until a computed tomography (CT) scan is performed. Finally, *seizures and tremors* can be seen with structural, infectious, or metabolic etiologies. In addition, these findings occasionally can be related to cyclosporine, in which case there are usually high cyclosporine blood levels. It is important to rule out the structural, metabolic, and infectious processes before assuming that the changes are owing to medication. The usual antiepileptic therapy should be given, as is prescribed for other patients with seizures.

Musculoskeletal complaints also are common. Osteopenia and osteoporosis secondary to prolonged steroid use may occur with or without secondary hyperparathyroidism. This may predispose these patients to spontaneous vertebral fractures and/or rib fractures after relatively minor strain. These can be dealt with by prompt

roentgenographic diagnosis and symptomatic therapy. As the patient tapers his oral prednisone from higher doses (often after rejections), moderately severe *bilateral arthralgias* are frequently reported. This is not associated with arthritis findings and responds to analgesic use alone. In contrast, *monarticular arthralgias* and arthritis suggest the possibility of either gout or a pyogenic process (usually with associated leukocytosis and fever). In such cases, joint aspiration and culture are required with the initiation of anti-inflammatory or antibiotic therapy. The organism in such infected joints is frequently related to a previous infection (previous genitourinary infection, respiratory source, or the like). The antibiotic coverage should include both gram-negative and gram-positive organisms, and should be given parenterally on an inpatient basis.

Finally, *psychological emergencies* can occur in the form of steroid-induced psychosis. It is important *not* to label all such psychotic episodes as related to prednisone, however, and the patient needs a thorough evaluation (particularly if the symptoms are of an emergent nature) to rule out structural or infectious central nervous system processes.

EMERGENCIES ATTRIBUTABLE TO UNDERLYING SYSTEMIC DISEASE

Cardiovascular emergencies are common because there is a high incidence of atherosclerotic complications and venous thrombotic diseases in these patients, since many have significant pre-existing hypertension, hyperlipidemia, diabetes mellitus, or diabetic vasculopathy. Chest pain in these patients must be taken seriously, and a close evaluation for coronary insufficiency, myocardial infarction, or pulmonary vascular occlusive disease must be undertaken. The emergency approach is as given for other groups of patients (see other chapters). *Psychological emergencies* are also frequent. The patients have a longstanding history of stress and often worry ''about (my) kidney.'' They have an extensive familiarity with the health care system and often need careful, detailed evaluations before they accept reassurance. In addition, many transplant patients know more about themselves and their potential health risks than do health care providers in the communities. It is important to discuss the transplant patient during most emergency visits by phone consultation with the primary transplant center. The transplant patient needs a direct and thorough approach. Diagnostic testing must be more thorough than for a similar complaint in a nontransplant patient. If the condition is nonemergent, reassurance should be given, and follow-up with their primary physician advised.

SUGGESTED READING

Guttman RD. Renal transplantation. N Eng J Med 1979; 301:975–982; 1038–1048.
Strom TB. The improving utility of renal transplantation in the management of end-stage renal disease. Am J Med 1982; 73:105–124.

DIALYSIS EMERGENCIES

LAUST H. NIELSEN, M.D.
KARL D. NOLPH, M.D.

This chapter is divided into conditions in which dialysis is essential or helpful in initial management and conditions arising during dialysis treatment or shortly after a patient has completed dialysis. Important aspects of the initial evaluation of patients in preparation for admission or transportation to a dialysis facility are discussed and brief definitions of the techniques involved are given.

Details of the approach to dialysis emergencies are given for three separate groups of patients: *group 1*, patients with no previously known renal disease in whom acute renal failure is evolving and in whom initial attempts to stabilize, maintain, or improve renal function take priority; *group 2*, patients with known chronic renal disease in whom the functional reserve may be quite limited; and *group 3*, patients with end-stage renal disease (ESRD) who are already established on chronic maintenance dialysis.

BLOOD PURIFICATION AND FLUID REMOVAL

Definitions

Hemodialysis is a process whereby blood is passed from the circulation through an extracorporeal dialyzer before being returned to the patient's circulation. Small-solute removals from blood result mainly by diffusion across a synthetic membrane into dialysis solution. Efficiency of small-solute removal as well as water removal is very high. Urea clearances of more than 150 ml per minute are readily achieved. If fluid removal is the main goal, isolated ultrafiltration, that is, ultrafiltration without simultaneous dialysis, can remove several liters of fluid per hour.

Hemofiltration is a variant of hemodialysis using membranes with high hydraulic permeability and pore size. Small-solute removal is by ultrafiltration (convection). There is no dialysis solution; ultrafiltrate is replaced in part into the blood path. Efficiency of small solute and water removal is high.

Continuous arteriovenous hemofiltration (CAVH) is a low-efficiency system using a small filter and no mechanical pumps. The driving force is the patient's blood pressure. Net ultrafiltration is achieved by applying a positive net pressure on the blood side of the membrane or by decreasing the volume replaced during treatment.

Plasmapheresis can be carried out in much the same manner as hemodialysis. The filter has a high hydraulic permeability and the pore size allows plasma protein including immune complexes to escape and, thus, be removed from the circulation. There is no dialysis fluid on the other side of the membrane. Replacement with plasma or human albumin in Ringer's lactate is standard practice. No dialysis takes place during the treatment.

Hemoperfusion is much like hemodialysis, but instead of dialysis solution and a dialyzer, blood is passed through a path lined with either resin or coated charcoal particles. Here a number of toxic substances are nonspecifically absorbed and, thus, removed from the circulation. No ultrafiltration or dialysis takes place.

Peritoneal dialysis (PD) is an intracorporeal dialysis system. The dialysis solution electrolyte composition prevents depletion of essential substances from the body and facilitates correction of acidoses. High glucose concentrations remove fluid by osmotic pressure. Efficiency of small-solute removal is only a fraction of that achieved by hemodialysis. The dialysis solution is placed in the peritoneal cavity, and dialysis takes place across capillary walls and peritoneal mesothelium.

Intermittent PD uses repeated 24- to 36-hour courses of treatment at intervals as needed. Usually cycles of 2 L every one-half to 2 hours are used in adults.

Access for Hemodialysis, Hemofiltration, CAVH, Hemoperfusion, and Plasmapheresis

Arteriovenous fistulas are used for conventional subcutaneous access for chronic hemodialysis treatment, which is established by creating an anastomosis between an artery and a vein in close proximity. Through large-caliber needles inserted into the arterialized vein, blood can be circulated through the dialyzer at rates exceeding 200 ml per minute.

Arteriovenous grafts are used in patients with unsuitable veins. An artificial segment is introduced, for instance, in the form of a Gortex graft in order to anastomose artery to vein. The access still remains subcutaneous. Forearm, upper arm, or leg placements may be used.

A shunt is the classic external arteriovenous silicon rubber connection of plastic implants in an artery and a vein. This serves the same purpose as direct cannulation of, for instance, the femoral artery and vein, in that it provides excellent arterial blood flow. It is more stable and can be used for long periods of time, but it is more predisposed to clotting and infection than subcutaneous fistulas.

Direct venous access for acute hemodialysis with subclavian catheters provides quick access. Double-lumen catheters can be inserted at the bedside, allowing blood flows of 200 to 300 ml per minute. The single-lumen catheter is infrequently used and requires a different return site or a pulsating single-needle device. A chest roentgenogram is needed after placement or change to confirm position in the superior vena cava and to exclude complications such as pneumothorax or hemothorax.

The quickest way to gain access to the circulation for the purpose of dialysis is undoubtedly the double-lumen femoral vein catheter, which is a short version of the subclavian catheter. If good flow is obtained and no hematoma develops, it is a matter of only minutes to get dialysis started.

Access for Peritoneal Dialysis and Peritoneal Lavage

A chronic indwelling Silastic catheter exists in many versions. A soft, tissue-compatible catheter with one or more Dacron or felt cuffs is implanted through a subcutaneous tunnel into the peritoneal cavity. The current approach is usually surgical placement, but placement may be done at the bedside if urgent. Peritoneal dialysis may be established quickly using this approach. Even if dialysis is only anticipated to last a few days, this "permanent" access pays off in fewer complications, lower rates of infection, better flow, and thus higher efficiency as well as better patient tolerance and acceptance.

The acute temporary catheter is a 30-cm, stiff, plastic tube that may be inserted 2 cm below the umbilicus in the linea alba into the peritoneal cavity in a matter of minutes. However, complications are many, and the life span of the catheter is limited to 48 hours, with increasing risks of infection thereafter. It is useful for lavage and for urgent corrections of life-threatening acidosis when no other therapy is immediately available.

EMERGENCY PATIENTS WITHOUT KNOWN PREEXISTING RENAL DISEASE

The key to successful management in this group of patients is early suspicion, early referral, and early treatment. The vast majority of patients have hospital-acquired acute renal failure; this subject is dealt with in the chapter on *Acute Renal Failure*. The suspicion of renal functional impairment is often not aroused until the urine output drops or the serum creatinine rises. At this time it is important to ascertain that ventilation is adequate, cardiac function is optimal, offending toxins are discontinued or removed, circulating volume is optimal, and urine flow is unobstructed.

When dehydration is not present, a challenge with a diuretic may be considered, particularly with volume overload. Large doses are often used. Furosemide, 40 to 320 mg in 50 ml of normal saline, may be infused intravenously over 20 to 30 minutes. If diuresis does not ensue within a short period of time (1 to 2 hours) after high doses, further doses should be avoided. Diuretics should *not* be used prior to volume repletion because this may aggravate the situation by increasing the sodium and water deficit or aggravate shock by venous dilatation and pooling.

Hyperkalemia should be avoided by restricting potassium intake. If hyperkalemia is unavoidable, it may be treated with kayexalate, bicarbonate, calcium, or glucose-insulin infusions as discussed in the chapter on *Potassium Disorders*.

The aim of the previously mentioned therapies is to stabilize the patient's condition so that he may be moved to a facility for acute dialysis, which is the only option apart from return of renal function for control of hyperkalemia, acidemia, volume overload, or uremia refractory to the above maneuvers. If dialysis is available at the institution where the patient presents, these measures should be instituted first to minimize the risk until dialysis can be initiated.

Intoxications

It is extremely important to recognize the place of dialysis in the treatment of exogenous intoxications because it may not only prevent irreversible organ damage, but also be lifesaving. Again it must be emphasized that dialysis is part of the total treatment and not the only treatment.

Drugs that are water soluble are most readily dialyzed, whereas substances that are protein bound or liquid insoluble are harder to remove through an exogenous medium. For the latter, hemoperfusion may aid in the treatment, but only the most severe cases warrant treatment of this kind. The indication is often multi-organ failure that worsens with medical management. One of the blood purification modalities may be considered helpful, but no general agreement has been reached on this because of lack of clear documentation of the clinical efficacy. Dialysis, however, is of proven value in the treatment of intoxications with methanol, ethyleneglycol (antifreeze), salicylate, or lithium.

Other Indications

Acute pancreatitis may be regarded as a nonindication in that recent evidence does not promote the notion that the use of peritoneal dialysis is associated with a better outcome than medical management alone. If, however, dialysis becomes necessary because of associated acute renal failure, peritoneal dialysis may certainly be useful and is by no means contraindicated. Diagnostic lavage to facilitate diagnosis may be done, but no evidence is available to support the use of extended lavage in the clinical management of acute pancreatitis.

Hypothermia and hyperthermia respond well to peritoneal dialysis with warm (37 °C) or cold (20 °C) respectively. There is ample evidence that central core rewarming in this fashion may be of great benefit when resuscitating patients suffering from prolonged hypothermia. Acid-base and electrolyte disturbances are corrected simultaneously, and cardiac arrhythmias have been reported to be less frequent and less severe. The peritoneal dialysis technique employed should keep the dwell time short (5 to 10 minutes) in order to maximize the availability of heat calories. The demonstration of the efficacy of peritoneal dialysis in hyperthermia is much less satisfactory than in hypothermia, but rapid central core cooling is believed to facilitate dissipation of a large number of heat calories in addition to standard cooling measures.

Hypercalcemia, hyperphosphatemia, and hyperuricemia occur in a variety of settings. Standard medical management with natriuresis, phosphate binders, and allopurinol may correct most problems. If, however, the load becomes too high as is sometimes the case with lysis of massive tumor burdens or if renal function declines, dialysis may be of benefit in the management of these conditions. Hypercalcemia that does not respond adequately to medical management responds quickly to hemodialysis, especially against a calcium-free dialysis solution. Hemodialysis for this indication is temporary in nature, to relieve or prevent symptoms while the possibility of definitive therapy is being investigated.

Hyperphosphatemia alone is rarely ever an indication for dialysis. However, when the calcium-phosphorus product reaches a level of 75 to 100 and medical management fails to stabilize or improve the condition, dialysis should be considered to prevent widespread metastatic calcifications.

Hyperuricemia may cause acute renal failure in its own right, and uric acid is easily dialyzable. If allopurinol therapy does not keep levels below 15 mg per deciliter or renal function declines, dialysis may be considered.

PATIENTS WITH CHRONIC RENAL INSUFFICIENCY

This group of patients includes those with a spectrum of renal failure from mild chronic renal insufficiency to virtual ESRD. Dialysis is indicated promptly when a patient presents with one or more of the symptoms or signs below. Other measures may be contemplated, but dialysis should be commenced as soon as possible.

Symptomatic uremia may present in various ways. Encephalopathy should not be allowed to develop, but dialysate reverses the condition if instituted promptly. In the emergency department other forms of encephalopathy must be ruled out such as those owing to hypoxia, hyperglycemia or hypoglycemia, hypercapnia, hyponatremia or hypernatremia, and hepatic or hypothyroid encephalopathy.

Gastrointestinal bleeding may occur, originating anywhere from the gums to the anus, with increasing uremia. The patients have an increased bleeding tendency secondary to the many effects of uremia on the coagulation system (for instance, decreased platelet function despite normal number), and they are already anemic because of chronic disease (normochromic, normocytic). To compound matters, any gastrointestinal hemorrhage leads to increased gastrointestinal reabsorption of potassium, and dangerous hyperkalemia may ensue. Also, the blood urea nitrogen (BUN) may increase rapidly. Uremic gastrointestinal bleeding is therefore a reason for acute admission and prompt dialysis along with medical management, including blood transfusions as needed.

Uremic pericarditis is a relatively common presenting symptom in the emergency department. There is little doubt that dialysis should be started right away, but the question is whether any other therapy is needed. If there are signs of cardiac tamponade, pericardiectomy or a pericardial window should be the procedure of choice.

Hyperkalemia and acidosis may be handled as previously described. Dialysis treatment is acutely needed only if urine output is very low or rapidly diminishing despite the use of diuretics.

Hypertension is often volume dependent in this group of patients. Acute treatment includes diuretics and fluid restriction and, if necessary, other antihypertensive medications. If diuretics become ineffective, dialysis should be initiated. Volume control is easy and, if needed, can be achieved in a matter of 1 to 3 hours.

Pulmonary edema is an infrequent presentation in patients except those already on chronic intermittent dialysis. The symptoms are no different from those seen in other patients, nor is the treatment, as long as urine output is adequate or can be stimulated with diuretics. If urine output is minimal, the following recommendations should be implemented:

1. Patient should be sitting upright.
2. Oxygen should be given by mask to ensure adequate FIO_2.
3. Morphine should be given subcutaneously, intramuscularly, or rarely intravenously (IV) in standard doses. A narcotic antagonist should be immediately available if excessive respiratory depression occurs.
4. Give aminophylline 200 to 500 mg IV.
5. Furosemide 120 to 250 mg IV may be used even in the absence of diuresis, because it tends to cause venular dilation, thereby relieving some of the alveolar congestion.
6. Digoxin may be started if the patient is not already digitalized; 0.5 to 1.0 mg IV for an adult is an adequate starting dose. Loading may be completed as usual when the acute problem has been solved. Maintenance digoxin doses in the absence of renal function, however, are only about one-third of normal, or 0.125 mg 3 to 4 times per week. A serum concentration should be checked after a week of treatment.

If the previous measures are not sufficient to ensure safe transport of the patient to a dialysis facility, as evidenced by stable improving arterial blood gases, intubation and positive pressure ventilation with 100 percent oxygen may be required. Once ultrafiltration has relieved the pulmonary edema, the patient may be extubated, usually after only a few hours.

A chest x-ray examination should be performed after treatment to rule out infiltrates or other mass lesions. Chest x-ray films taken with florid pulmonary edema usually only confirm the obvious diagnosis, waste valuable time, and add to the total cost of the management. They rarely, if ever, change anything in the acute therapy. One should always suspect that the pulmonary edema may be secondary (for instance, to an acute infection) to another disorder that requires attention.

Patients Established on Chronic Dialysis

These patients have an attending nephrologist at their usual dialysis facility. When such a patient presents to an outside emergency department with a complaint, the nephrologist should be contacted promptly for background information on primary renal disease, treatment, medications, and so on, and advice and recommendations can be solicited simultaneously. This also ensures that the patient's regular attending physicians know about the acute problem, and that action can be taken to follow up next time he sees the patient. Pulmonary edema, volume-dependent hypertension, acidosis, and hyperkalemia may be treated on an outpatient basis, and these problems are usually corrected in a matter of hours. Precipitating factors should be looked for thoroughly in the history and physical examination before dismissing the problem as merely a dietary indiscretion. Admission for observation overnight should be readily available.

Pericarditis, or other acute symptoms of inadequate dialysis, should lead to immediate admission and inpatient dialysis until the condition is stabilized or improved. A number of problems may arise during or shortly after regular hemodialysis and the patient may present after a few hours to the local emergency department.

Fever is most often a symptom of the same pathology as in other patients. However, patients with chronic renal failure have decreased immune defense and thus otherwise trivial infections may develop into a disaster. Also, one should think of more unusual agents like cytomegalovirus, hepatitis B, HTLV-III/LAV, or *Pneumocystis* if the cause is obscure. Admission for a complete work-up is often necessary. Patients on hemodialysis may become infected in or through their access. This is often attributable to poor hygiene or technique. Organisms are most frequently gram positive. If an access infection is noted, blood cultures should be drawn and vancomycin 1 g given intravenously. This single dose covers the patient for 4 to 7 days and allows for transfer back to his dialysis facility for further work-up and management. If a temporary access is in place and infected, this should be removed after consultation with the patient's dialysis unit. The tip of the catheter should be cultured in addition to the other measures. Patients on hemodialysis now and then have transient fevers of less than 38.5 °C after their treatment. This often recurs every time a new dialyzer is used (as opposed to subsequent uses of the same dialyzer). The fever may be attributable to activation of the immune system by contact with substances in the dialyzer membranes. Pyrogens may be absorbed from dialysis solution. The condition is self-limiting and requires no treatment. Other potentially more serious problems should be ruled out by observation of the patient.

Arrhythmias are most often the result of the same organic heart disease as seen in nonrenal patients. Patients should therefore be worked up and treated in the same way, with consideration for drug dosing in the absence of renal function and the actual mode of dialysis employed in that particular patient. Predialysis hyperkalemia or postdialysis hypokalemia may induce transient arrhythmias, some of which may be quite serious. Hyperkalemia responds promptly to treatment as previously described (bicarbonate, calcium, glucose-insulin infusion) and is corrected by dialysis. Hypokalemia may require oral supplementation, and the need to increase potassium concentration in the dialysis fluid in the future should be considered.

The disequilibrium syndrome presents with symptoms of increased intracranial pressure including nausea and vomiting, headache, visual disturbances, stupor, and sometimes seizures. The syndrome, which develops during or shortly after dialysis, is caused by rapid removal of small solutes (urea) from the extracellular fluid space. The blood-brain barrier retards solute removal from brain tissue and cerebrospinal fluid, leaving it hyperosmolar. This in turn leads to water shifts into the brain, resulting in increased intracranial pressure. Often the patient presents immediately after hemodialysis with bizarre neurologic complaints. This picture is today usually associated only with acute hemodialysis in patients with severe azotemia. It is not usually reported for other than hemodialysis treatments. Symptomatic treatment usually suffices because the syndrome abates when the osmotic gradient over the blood-brain barrier dissipates. Infusion of a hyperosmolar compound like mannitol (25 to 50 g IV) may help to shorten the symptomatic period. Antiseizure medications may be useful for a short period of time as well. Temporary hyperventilation may also decrease intracranial pressure.

Seizures owing to accidental electrolyte disturbances such as hyponatremia or hypernatremia or hypokalemia after hemodialysis should be treated promptly with antiseizure medications until dialysis can be reinstituted to correct the problem. Initial treatment may also include appropriate electrolyte solutions, but this therapy is often limited by the decreased volume tolerance of this group of patients.

Nonfunctioning access for hemodialysis is a common presenting complaint. If the duration of the problem is short (a few hours) the patient should be admitted acutely for revision of the access. If the problem is longstanding (more than 6 to 12 hours) the access may well be lost, and plans should be made for placement of the new one electively. A nonfunctioning subclavian catheter may be changed over a guide wire if no infection is suspected in the area. The risk of a small pulmonary embolus is always present, but clinically apparent embolic phenomena have not been reported.

Bleeding after hemodialysis is usually attributable to a combination of uremic bleeding diatheses and excessive anticoagulation during treatment. The bleeding most often occurs at the access site. Local compression with a 4×4 for 15 to 30 minutes with the extremity elevated, if possible, usually suffices. Circular bandages are contraindicated because they may compromise distal circulation and lead to local thrombosis. They also prevent close inspection of the site for further bleeding. Neutralizing excess heparin with protamine sulfate intravenously can be done if needed. Because protamine sulfate has anticoagulating properties of its own, a dose to counteract no more than one-third to one-half of the total dose of heparin given during the treatment should be used.

Patients may need to be admitted overnight for observation. Hemoglobin and hematocrit should be checked, at least when the bleeding has subsided, because these patients often have marginal, if any, reserves.

Hypotension following dialysis is often the result of hypovolemia. Most often the blood pressure normalizes quickly after a few hours due to redistribution between fluid compartments and the body. Occasionally, extra oral fluid or, if symptoms are severe, a few hundred milliliters of normal saline intravenously may be needed. Reevaluation of total body water (TBW) should be carried out. Drug therapy of hypertension, if any, should be revised.

Fluid overload in patients on peritoneal dialysis may be treated in several ways. An increase in the number of daily continuous ambulatory peritoneal dialysis (CAPD) exchanges and thereby a shortened dwell time yields a greater ultrafiltration volume. If the congested heart failure is severe and ventilation borderline, admission for intermittent peritoneal dialysis with rapid cycling of hypertonic solutions is a safe alternative. Supplemental oxygen and digoxin should be used as needed. Reevaluation of the patient's individual dialysate and ultrafiltration needs should be performed to avoid repetition.

Peritonitis in patients treated with CAPD is unfortunately still a frequent complication in this group of patients. The diagnosis is made solely on the presence of any two of the following:

1. Cloudy drainage or 100 white blood cells per mm^3 with more than 50 percent neutrophils in the dialysate
2. Abdominal pain or tenderness
3. Positive culture from peritoneal drainage or microorganisms seen on Gram stain from peritoneal dialysate.

Once the diagnosis has been made, a decision to admit or to treat as an outpatient is made, based on the patient's general condition. Most peritonitis in patients on CAPD can be treated on an outpatient basis. Each center has its own protocol for treatment, which should be carried out in consultation with the nephrologist. The catheter exit site should be inspected to look for a tunnel infection (drainage, swelling, erythema, or tenderness).

There are several potential pitfalls that should be kept in mind when dealing with peritonitis in patients on chronic peritoneal dialysis: The presenting symptoms and signs may be owing to another pathologic process such as a gastric ulcer, pancreatitis, diverticulitis, or cholecystitis. The culture result will not be available for 24 to 48 hours. The patient should therefore stay in touch and report any deterioration in his condition promptly. Bleeding into the peritoneum may be due to menstruation in some women. This does not mean that they have peritonitis. It is a self-limiting process that requires only observation. True hemorrhage is exceedingly rare, but systemic anticoagulation for other reasons is a predisposing factor. Peritoneal dialysis can continue in almost all cases.

After being seen and treated in the emergency department, the patient should be referred back to his dialysis center for further management. This should preferably take place as soon as possible and no later than when culture results are available. Failure of peritonitis to respond in 48 to 72 hours may indicate a seeding source of bacteria in debris in the catheter or on the catheter surface. Catheter removal may be required.

SUGGESTED READING

Drukker W, Parsons FM, Maher JF, eds. Replacement of renal function by dialysis. 2nd ed. Dordrecht: Martinus-Nijhoff, 1983.

Nolph KD, ed. Peritoneal dialysis. 2nd ed. Dordrecht: Martinus-Nijhoff, 1985.

Twardowski ZJ, et al. Blood purification in acute renal failure. Ann Intern Med 1984; 100:447–449.

MANAGEMENT OF THE ABDOMINAL AND GASTROINTESTINAL SYSTEM

APPROACH TO ACUTE ABDOMINAL PAIN

STEVEN J. DAVIDSON, M.D., F.A.C.E.P.
DAVID K. WAGNER, M.D., F.A.C.S., F.A.A.P.

UNDIFFERENTIATED PROBLEM PRESENTATION

Acute abdominal pain is a frequent presenting complaint in an emergency unit. Because patients commonly present with an undifferentiated pain pattern rather than the differentiated disease of a known organ system, the role of the emergency physician involves early differentiation of pain patterns, often without the benefit of sequential evaluation or extensive laboratory data.

In differentiating abdominal pain, one must distinguish between impulses of somatic origin and those of visceral origin. Somatic sensory impulses originate from parietal peritoneum or the root of the mesentary, travel via myelineated fibers to the dorsal root ganglia, and thence into the posterior horn of the spinal cord (Fig. 1). Because myelinated nerve fibers are capable of clear transmission of impulses, somatic pain is perceived by the patient as sharp or knife-like.

Visceral impulses generally originate from points within the wall of an organ (e.g., intestine, gallbladder), and travel along the sympathetics to the dorsal root ganglia. From the dorsal root ganglia these fibers follow in company with somatic neurons into the posterior horn of the spinal cord (see Fig. 1). Because afferent visceral neurons are mainly unmyelinated, they usually produce a diffuse, poorly localized, dull, aching pain.

Pain experienced at a site other than that of primary noxious stimulation, but in structures supplied by the same or adjacent neurosegments, is called referred pain. Both visceral and deep somatic structures are capable of producing referred pain. In general, referred pain indicates an intensification of stimulation or a lowering of the pain threshold by a disease process. Abdominal muscle guarding, when localized to a spinal nerve root, provides a typical example of referred somatic pain (from the peritoneum). The subscapular pain of acute cholecystitis is typical of referred visceral pain and is followed by the acute, localized, somatic pain of peritoneal involvement

as the disease process extends through the wall of the gallbladder to involve the peritoneum. Table 1 shows the common sequence of abdominal pain and the neurologic paths of that progression.

HISTORY

There is no substitute for an accurate history as well as an understanding of the natural history of disease processes. Although the emergency physician sees a higher percentage of the acute aspects of disease process, he or she must continually be aware that the presentation of acute symptoms can occur at any point in the course of the disease causing the pain. Therefore, a detailed history to the point of presentation assumes even greater importance for the emergency physician who does not see the patient on continuing basis.

In taking a history from a patient with acute abdominal pain, the physician should keep two facts in mind. First, although there are many extra-abdominal sources of abdominal pain, pain that is localized to the abdomen is usually caused by intra-abdominal disease. Second, severe abdominal pain that persists for 6 hours or longer in a previously well individual usually requires surgical intervention. With these thoughts in mind, the approach to the history involves attention to six specific points.

Onset

Pain that begins suddenly and is associated with episodes of colic usually indicates a process associated with complete or partial visceral obstruction and/or devascularization (e.g., pancreatitis, cholecystitis, or diverticulitis). With sudden perforation or devascularization, pain is acute and severe in onset and persists with the same or increased intensity.

Pain that is gradual in onset and maximizes slowly is usually associated with an inflammatory process without visceral obstruction or devascularization (e.g., pelvic inflammatory disease, ulcerative colitis).

The patient should be asked what was occurrring at the time the pain developed. For example, increased pressure in the pelvic cavity caused by such activities as defecation or lifting may cause torsion or rupture of an ovarian cyst, or rupture of an isolated colonic diverticulum.

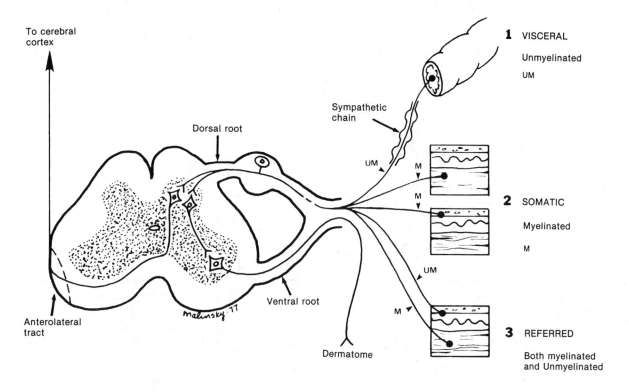

Figure 1 Pathways of abdominal pain.

TABLE 1 Types of Abdominal Pain

Type	Location	Intensity	Conduction	Examples
Visceral	Primary organ	Diffuse Dull Aching	Unmyelinated via sympathetics	Early cholecystitis without peritoneal involvement
Referred	Neural segment	Sharp Localized	Afferent nerve roots	Cholecystitis with early peritoneal involvement
Somatic	Peritoneum Root of mesentery	Intense Sharp	Myelinated via nerve roots	Cholecystitis with intense peritoneal involvement

Location

Certain viscera provide reasonably good localization of pain while others afford little reliable information in this regard. Typically, the gallbladder, appendix, stomach, and duodenum tend to be specific in their location of pain whereas the small intestine and pancreas have less accurate pain localization. Pain that persists in a given quadrant suggests specific entities (Fig. 2). Localized pain that becomes generalized throughout the abdomen usually indicates perforation and dissemination of contaminated material.

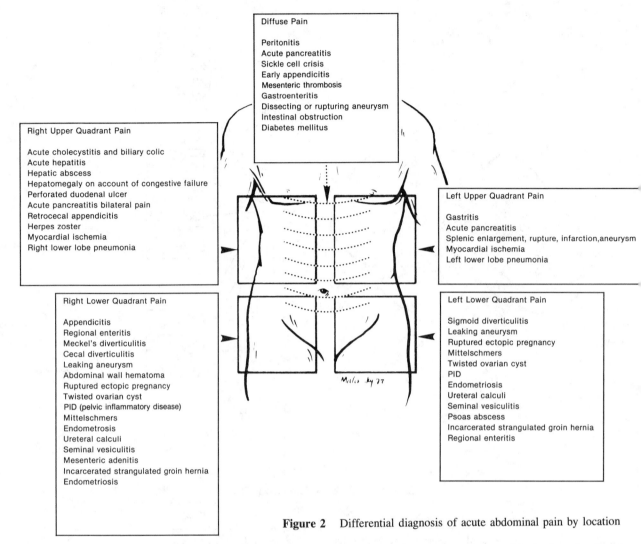

Diffuse Pain

Peritonitis
Acute pancreatitis
Sickle cell crisis
Early appendicitis
Mesenteric thrombosis
Gastroenteritis
Dissecting or rupturing aneurysm
Intestinal obstruction
Diabetes mellitus

Right Upper Quadrant Pain

Acute cholecystitis and biliary colic
Acute hepatitis
Hepatic abscess
Hepatomegaly on account of congestive failure
Perforated duodenal ulcer
Acute pancreatitis bilateral pain
Retrocecal appendicitis
Herpes zoster
Myocardial ischemia
Right lower lobe pneumonia

Left Upper Quadrant Pain

Gastritis
Acute pancreatitis
Splenic enlargement, rupture, infarction,aneurysm
Myocardial ischemia
Left lower lobe pneumonia

Right Lower Quadrant Pain

Appendicitis
Regional enteritis
Meckel's diverticulitis
Cecal diverticulitis
Leaking aneurysm
Abdominal wall hematoma
Ruptured ectopic pregnancy
Twisted ovarian cyst
PID (pelvic inflammatory disease)
Mittelschmers
Endometrosis
Ureteral calculi
Seminal vesiculitis
Mesenteric adenitis
Incarcerated strangulated groin hernia
Endometriosis

Left Lower Quadrant Pain

Sigmoid diverticulitis
Leaking aneurysm
Ruptured ectopic pregnancy
Mittelschmers
Twisted ovarian cyst
PID
Endometriosis
Ureteral calculi
Seminal vesiculitis
Psoas abscess
Incarcerated strangulated groin hernia
Regional enteritis

Figure 2   Differential diagnosis of acute abdominal pain by location

Character

Pain severe enough to interfere with normal activities is likely to represent a significant disease entity. Collapse or fainting with the onset of abdominal pain testifies to its severity and is commonly associated with dissecting aneurysm, hemorrhagic pancreatitis, or ruptured ectopic pregnancy. Colic is the result of smooth muscle contraction against resistance and is compatible with luminal obstruction whether in the intestine, biliary tract, or urinary tract.

It is often difficult to quantitate severity of pain. In these instances, comparison with previous episodes of pain is useful. For example, women who have borne children may compare the presenting pain to that of delivery. Others may compare the pain to previous episodes of pain of known etiology. The patient's reaction to mild sedation may also be of use in determining the severity of the pain.

Radiation or Referral

Typical patterns of pain radiation may be virtually diagnostic. The well-known patterns of subscapular radiation with biliary disease, genitalia pain with renal colic, and low back referral with uterine and rectal disease are best understood with knowledge of the basic referral pathways described above (see Fig. 1). Ruptured or leaking aneurysm often gives pain in the lumbosacral area and the proximal thigh. Collections of blood or pus under the posterior diaphragm causes pain referred to the lateral aspect of the shoulder, whereas subclavicular pain occurs when the anterior diaphragm is irritated. Epigastric pain that radiates straight through to the back usually indicates pancreatitis or an ulcer penetrating into the pancreas.

Alteration of Pain

The physician should determine what, if anything, has influenced the pain pattern. Position may be of particular importance. For example, recumbency exacerbates the pain of reflux esophagitis and pancreatitis. The use of food or alkali may improve the patient with peptic ulcer diasthesis, but increases the discomfort of a patient with pyloric channel ulcer. Pain that is exacerbated with cough or movement indicates somatic peritoneal irritation.

Associated Symptomatology

The vomiting of bile-stained material in the child or feculant material in the adult indicates mechanical obstruction as the source of gastrointestinal dysfunction until proved otherwise. Diarrhea associated with vomiting is typical of inflammatory diseases of the bowel, both specific (e.g., ulcerative colitis) and nonspecific (e.g., viral gastroenteritis). Chills and fever characterize pelvic phlebitis and bacteremia. Persistance of a low-grade nonspiking fever is consistent with nondisseminated, localized inflammatory process (Fig. 3).

PHYSICAL EXAMINATION

A concise systematic approach to the physical assessment of the patient with abdominal pain is essential. Four component parts should be emphasized.

General Appearance

Does the patient "look sick"? The facies, position in bed, and whether the patient is motionless or writhes in pain may be assessed in a matter of seconds. Spasm of the ileopsoas muscle by a retrocecal inflammatory process causes the patient to flex the right hip in an attempt to relieve the spasm. Patients with peritoneal irritation lie immobile whereas patients with colicky obstruction, in the absence of peritoneal irritation, tend to writhe with discomfort. Abdominal distension alerts one to early compromise of normal bowel motility.

Palpation and Percussion

Palpation is the most important aspect of the physical examination. All quadrants of the abdomen should be examined with both hands to assess tenderness, spasm, and the presence of masses. The judicious use of narcotic analgesics in the agitated patient often enhances this critical aspect of the examination. The presence of asymmetrical rectus muscle spasm is always a significant objective finding, usually indicating an inflammatory process localized to that side. Rebound tenderness means peritonitis is present. This may vary from the mild peritoneal irritation of a severe gastroenteritis to the severe inflammation produced by bacterial or chemical contamination of the peritoneal lining. The finding of rebound tenderness elicited by palpation should always be confirmed by having the patient cough while the abdominal wall in the area of previously elicited rebound tenderness is supported.

Auscultation

Bowel sounds vary in three parameters: frequency, intensity, and pitch. To auscult the abdomen adequately a minimum of 5 minutes should be allowed. Three variations in bowel sounds provide important data:

1. Absence of bowel sounds (for 5 minutes) indicates intestinal atony (ileus) associated with peritonitis.
2. High-pitched crescendo sounds coincidental with colicy abdominal pain and separated by periods of silence indicate intestinal obstruction.
3. Continuous hyperactive bowel sounds in the patient with diffuse, mild peritoneal irritation is consistent with gastroenteritis.

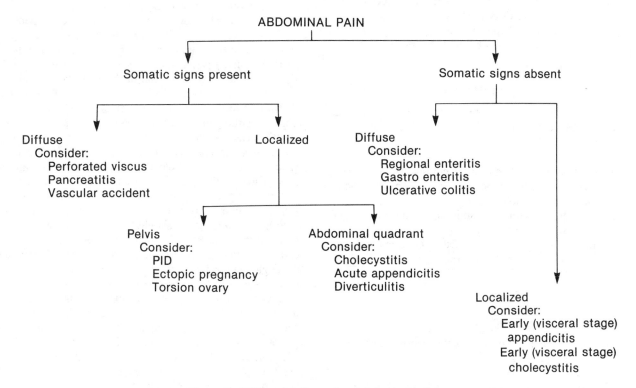

Figure 3 Differential diagnosis of abdominal pain.

Rectal Examination

The examination of the abdomen is not complete without a rectal examination, noting whether the ampulla is full or empty, whether lateralizing tenderness is present, and whether prostatic or cervical pressure produces discomfort. A sample of stool, when present, is obtained for color, consistency, and evaluation for occult blood.

The rectal and pelvic examination is of most use in assessing point tenderness, such as in pelvic appendicitis with minimal abdominal signs or tenderness in the adrexa in ectopic pregnancy or salpingitis, and in determining the degree of discomfort produced by uterine motion.

DIAGNOSTIC PROCEDURES

Four fundamental laboratory procedures should receive initial consideration in all patients presenting for emergency care.

Complete Blood Count

The CBC is most useful in the following instances:

1. To provide a baseline hematocrit in the patient suspected of bleeding. (An initially normal hematocrit may be misleading, since it may not reflect acute blood loss for several hours.)
2. To reveal polymorphonuclear leukocytosis consistent with bacterial infection.
3. To reveal the leukopenia [3,000 to 5,000 white blood cells (WBC) per mm³] with relative lymphocytosis suggestive of viral disease.
4. To reveal the leukopenia (<3,000 WBC per mm³) associated with sepsis or blood dyscrasia.

Urinalysis

Urinalysis may be helpful in delineating acute abdominal pain. The most directly useful findings are the following:

1. Glycosuria—both diabetic acidosis and pancreatitis may cause acute abdominal pain. Glycosuria points to one of these etiologies.
2. Hematuria—with acute abdominal pain, this strongly suggests renal calculus.
3. Bacteriuria, pyuria—with acute abdominal pain, this strongly suggests urinary tract infection.

Radiology

The abdominal "flat plate" (anteroposterior view of abdomen), though of limited value, is most useful in revealing the following:

1. Radiopacity, especially renal and biliary calculi.
2. Baseline air pattern against which subsequent changes may be measured.

3. Occasional pathognomonic changes of large bowel obstruction, small bowel obstruction, or volvulus.
4. Free intraperitoneal air. Because free air takes up to 20 minutes to rise within the peritoneal cavity, the patient should be upright for that period of time before the x-ray film is taken. Alternatively, the patient may be placed in the lateral supine position and a cross table x-ray study obtained.

Electrocardiography

An electrocardiogram (ECG) should be done routinely in the patient over 40 years old with abdominal pain, since myocardial infarction may be present with referred abdominal pain.

Ultrasonography

Ultrasonography is becoming increasingly widespread. It may be particularly helpful in revealing the following:

1. Biliary calculi.
2. Ectopic pregnancy.
3. Aneurysmal dilation of the abdominal aorta.
4. Something of the character of any palpated mass.

Initial Management

Obviously, specific therapy depends on reaching a specific diagnosis. However, in the emergency unit, this is often not possible. Simply recognizing that the patient's illness may require hospitalization or surgery or perhaps can be managed on an outpatient basis, helps clarify the issue. For many patients, the key to the ultimate diagnosis is subsequent reevaluation of the physical examination. The entire process of evaluation through history, physical, and further diagnostic studies can be aided by improving the patient's comfort and certain simple therapeutic measures. When abdominal pain presents with evidence of gastrointestinal tract dysfunction, resting the gastrointestinal tract is clearly a major part of therapy. Nasogastric intubation and suction are often helpful not just in the diagnostic sense, but also for therapeutic reasons, even in patients with simple gastroenteritis. Patients with a nasogastric tube should have intravenous hydration to prevent further dehydration often produced by concomitant vomiting and diarrhea. Young people with severe acute gastroenteritis often respond marvelously to 1 to 3 hours of nasogastric tube suction and vigorous rehydration with isotonic fluids intravenously. I routinely rehydrate these patients with 1,000 to 2,000 cc of saline solution, or at least until they pass a urine of low specific gravity. This ensures that even if they are unable to take adequate oral intake for a brief additional period, they are still not likely to return dehydrated.

For the patient with severe pain continuing during the duration of evaluation despite nasogastric intubation and intravenous hydration, the judicious use of intravenous narcotics may be of great value. Classic surgical teaching points out the great difficulty of evaluating patients for peritoneal irritation when they are so sedated with narcotics that they are unresponsive. This derives from an era when typical doses of intramuscular narcotics ranged from a quarter to a half grain (15 to 30 mg) of morphine sulfate intramuscularly. Titration of small, intravenous doses of morphine can be most effective in relieving some of the patient's apprehension and, thus, voluntary guarding, permitting the skilled examiner to more clearly recognize intra-abdominal mass and localized findings. This does not confound the physical examination, but rather may contribute to its accuracy. We routinely use morphine intravenously in an initial aliquot of 2 to 4 mg followed by subsequent dosing at 5- to 10-minute intervals, up to a maximum of 8 to 10 mg. Of course, the use of this approach in diagnosing the patient's pain almost invariably mandates admission to the hospital.

Consultation for further evaluation and admission varies with local circumstances, but in general suspicion of acute vascular compromise or any evidence of instability of vital signs, mandates urgent consultation with the appropriate surgical or gynecologic specialist. Routine follow-up care for less urgent conditions may also be most effectively rendered by a gastroenterologist or surgical specialist, and an appropriate referral should be offered to all patients.

The patient with acute abdominal pain presents an undifferentiated problem, one of the many that emergency physicians must confront. Determination of the specific cause may be difficult, despite the availability of a full history, a careful physical examination, and ancillary diagnostic studies. The emergency physician frequently is reduced to simply deciding whether or not the patient's abdominal symptoms require further consultation, hospitalization, or simply discharge to outpatient follow-up. Nonetheless, a systematic approach usually elucidates the magnitude of the problem, leading to an appropriate therapy and disposition.

SUGGESTED READING

Silen W, ed. Cope's early diagnosis of the acute abdomen. New York: Oxford University Press, 1983.

Sabiston DC Jr. Textbook of surgery. 12th ed. Philadelphia: WB Saunders, 1981.

UNCOMMON CAUSES OF ABDOMINAL PAIN

HOWARD A. WERMAN, MD.

Acute appendicitis, renal colic, cholecystitis, pancreatitis, intestinal obstruction, diverticulitis, pelvic inflammatory disease, perforated ulcer, and ruptured ovarian cysts have been identified in many series as the most common causes of the acute surgical abdomen. However, many nonsurgical diseases may result in abdominal pain that mimics a surgical abdomen. One must recognize these diseases so that unnecessary surgery is avoided and appropriate therapy is instituted. It is the purpose of this chapter to discuss unusual nonsurgical causes of acute abdominal pain and their diagnosis.

DIABETIC KETOACIDOSIS

Ketoacidosis is a common complication of diabetes. Nausea and vomiting are commonly seen; significant abdominal pain and tenderness are reported in approximately 25 percent of adults and up to 80 percent of children. Abdominal pain is often accompanied by fever, absent bowel sounds, and leukocytosis. Diabetics who present with these findings are difficult to distinguish from patients with a surgical abdomen.

In addition, certain causes of abdominal diseases such as pancreatitis and cholethiasis are more common in diabetic patients than in the general population. This confuses the diagnosis of abdominal pain in diabetic ketoacidosis.

Diagnosis. The diagnosis of diabetic ketoacidosis can be rapidly made using Dextrostix and Acetest. The Dextrostix demonstrates elevated levels of serum glucose whereas Acetest is positive for serum ketones. Additional supportive evidence is provided by the presence of glucosuria and ketonuria on urinalysis. Acidosis and decreased serum bicarbonate are noted on arterial blood gas samples.

A history of prior diabetes mellitus or recent polyuria, polydypsia, and malaise should suggest a diagnosis of diabetic ketoacidosis. On physical examination, findings such as dehydration, mental status changes, fruity odor to the breath and Kussmaul respirations also support the diagnosis. The diagnosis is confirmed by laboratory measurements. If the patient is older than 40 years or the serum bicarbonate is more than 10 mEq per L causes of acute abdominal pain other than ketoacidosis should be sought. Therapy of the ketoacidosis with volume repletion and insulin should relieve the abdominal pain.

SICKLE CELL DISEASE

Sickle cell anemia is a genetically inherited disease characterized by abnormal betaglobulin synthesis, which is most common in black persons of African origin. This results in the production of abnormal erythrocytes, which tend to aggregate in the presence of hypoxia, dehydration, and acidosis. Clinically, patients that are homozygous for the gene (sickle cell disease) are subject to painful vaso-occlusive crises. Patients who are heterozygous for the gene (sickle cell trait) do not manifest clinical symptoms unless exposed to hypoxic stress such as in air travel or at high altitudes.

Vaso-occlusive crises that result in splenic autoinfarction give rise to painful abdominal episodes that may mimic an acute abdomen. This is generally seen in younger patients with sickle cell disease or in adults with sickle cell trait. Abdominal crises are rare in adults with sickle cell disease because of the small size of the spleen after repeated episodes of infarction. These episodes result in sudden onset of severe left upper quadrant pain with anorexia and vomiting. The abdomen may be found rigid on examination. Fever and a significant leukocytosis often accompany the onset of symptoms. Patients with sickle cell disease often have a chronic leukocytosis of 15,000 or so. Patients with sickle cell disease are particularly prone to gallstones, which can predispose to cholethiasis and cholecystitis.

Diagnosis. The definitive diagnosis of sickle cell syndromes is made by either hemoglobin electrophoresis or by means of a "sickle cell preparation" of a peripheral smear. Neither of these tests is generally available for immediate diagnosis on an emergency basis. Also, no test currently exists to determine if a patient with sickle cell syndrome is in acute crisis. Historical information including a positive history of sickle cell disease, a prior history of sickle cell crises, or a history of similar painful episodes in the abdomen and joints suggests acute abdominal crisis. On physical examination, splenomegaly and a splenic friction rub may be seen. Laboratory findings that are consistent with the diagnosis include anemia, an increased reticuloyte count, and the presence of sickled cells on a peripheral smear.

Any of the above findings plus the presence of normal bowel sounds support the diagnosis of abdominal crisis. Shaking chills, a leukocyte count greater than 30,000, and a history of atypical pain should raise the possibility of another cause for the abdominal pain.

Therapy. See the chapter on *Sickle Cell Anemia* for details of therapy. Patients who do not get relief within a few hours or in whom other abdominal conditions such as cholecystitis are suspected should be admitted to the hospital for evaluation.

BLACK WIDOW SPIDER BITES

The bite of the black widow spider, or *Latrodectus mactans*, sometimes produces a symptom complex that has been confused with a surgical abdomen. This spider produces a web in dark protected places. Although the spider used to be found more often in rural areas, black widow spiders are now more commonly seen in urban centers. The spider produces a neurotoxin that apears to act at the neuromuscular junction.

The initial bite is usually painless. Occasionally, an area of erythema may surround the wound. Severe muscle cramping develops 30 minutes to 3 hours after the initial bite. If the lower extremities are involved, the pain is most prominent in the abdominal musculature. The pain is crampy and is associated with abdominal wall rigidity. The pain usually resolves after 24 to 48 hours. Seizures,

shock, and respiratory depression occasionally complicate significant envenomation.

Diagnosis. The only certain method of diagnosing a black widow spider envenomation is by obtaining a specimen of the spider responsible for the bite. These spiders are generally about 1½ inches long, with a characteristic red or yellow hourglass marking on their ventral surface. If a specimen cannot be obtained, the diagnosis is usually obtained on the basis of the characteristic clinical and historical picture. No laboratory test is currently available to establish the diagnosis.

Although victims of black widow spider bite experience severe abdominal pain, there is usually little tenderness on manual palpation. The patient also tends to be more comfortable changing positions whereas the patient with peritonitis is more comfortable remaining still. Finally, other symptoms such as headache, conjunctivitis, skin rash, pruritus, profuse sweating, and weakness are not seen with other causes of the acute abdomen.

Treatment. Calcium gluconate can be used to treat abdominal cramping. The usual dosage is 10 ml of 10 percent solution given intravenously over 15 to 20 minutes. This dose can be repeated up to three times during the first few hours, but cardiac monitoring is required. Muscle relaxants have also been used to relieve the symptoms of a black widow spider bite. Methocarbamol, 1 g is administered intravenously over 10 minutes followed by 0.5 to 1.0 g in 250 to 500 cc of D5W over 3 to 4 hours. For children, the dosage is 60 mg per kilogram given in four divided doses every 6 hours. Valium, 5 to 10 mg given intravenously, has also been used. The dosage is 0.2 to 0.5 mg per kilogram intravenously in children given every 2 minutes up to a dosage of 5 mg. Finally, supplementation with parenteral narcotics such as meperidine may be required. Antivenin can also be given.

Patients who receive black widow spider antivenom as well as those who do not show clinical improvement within several hours of therapy should be admitted to the hospital for observation.

ACUTE INTERMITTENT PORPHYRIA

Acute intermittent porphyria is an autosomal dominant inherited defect of heme biosynthesis that results in accumulation of excess porphyrin precursors. The disease is caused by a defect in the enzyme uroporphyrinogen I synthetase, which results in the accumulation of delta-aminolevulinic acid and porphobilinogen. The disease is most common in patients of Swedish or Irish ancestory and is slightly more common in women. Clinical manifestations of the disease include abdominal pain, constipation, and nervous system derangements including seizures, autonomic neuropathy, the syndrome of inappropriate antidiuretic hormone secretion (SIADH), and psychosis.

The abdominal pain associated with acute intermittent porphyria tends to be colicky. There is often diffuse abdominal tenderness. Associated findings include a low-grade fever, nausea, vomiting, tachycardia, and leukocytosis.

Diagnosis. The most specific tests used to diagnose acute intermittent porphyria (including erythrocyte uroporphyrinogen I synthetase assay or urinary delta-aminolevulinic and porphobilinogen levels) are not readily available to the emergency physician. The most specific readily available test is the Watson-Schwartz test. A sample of the patient's urine is mixed with Ehrlich's reagent to yield a cherry-red color in positive cases. Alternatively, a sample of urine can be exposed to sunlight. In cases of acute disease, the urine turns burgundy red.

Information such as a family history of the disease or a history of recurrent attacks should make one suspicious of acute intermittent porphyria as a cause of abdominal pain. Associated symptoms such as seizures, hallucinations, or peripheral neuropathy also make the diagnosis more likely. Finally, although there is diffuse abdominal tenderness, the patient with acute intermittent porphyria often has no rebound tenderness and has normal bowel sounds.

Treatment. The first goal of therapy in acute intermittent porphyria is to establish the proper diagnosis and avoid unnecessary surgery. This is particularly important in porphyria because several anesthetic agents have been shown to exacerbate the disease.

Several drugs provide symptomatic relief for abdominal pain and associated symptoms. Meperidine, 50 to 100 mg intramuscularly every 3 to 4 hours, or morphine sulfate, 2 to 4 mg intravenously every 3 to 4 hours, is safe and effective. Chlorpromazine, 25 to 50 mg intramuscular every 6 to 8 hours, has been used for mild abdominal pain and psychosis.

Two specific therapies have been shown to decrease the severity of the acute attack. The first is a high glucose diet in which 450 to 500 g is administered daily by oral intake and by intravenous infusion. Recently, hematin in dosages of 3 to 4 mg per kilogram, given in two divided doses daily by intravenous infusion, has been shown to be effective if administered early in therapy. Complications of the drug include renal insufficiency and coagulopathy.

Finally, an important aspect of therapy includes the prevention of further attacks of acute intermittent porphyria. Certain drugs that increase the production of porphyrin precursors should be avoided (Table 1).

LEAD INTOXICATION

Lead poisoning remains a major public health problem in the United States. Lead is derived from many sources including battery casings, gasoline additives, and pain and plumbing in older buildings.

The clinical manifestations of lead poisoning are related to the rise in lead concentrations in the soft tissues of the body, such as bone marrow, the central nervous system, kidney, and gastrointestinal tract. Abdominal pain is a common finding in patients with lead poisoning. Patients experience colicky abdominal pain, which is accompanied by anorexia, nausea, vomiting, diarrhea, or constipation and guarding on examination.

Diagnosis. The diagnosis of lead poisoning is made

TABLE 1 Drug Use in Acute Intermittent Porphyria

Unsafe Drugs	Safe Drugs
Alpha-methyldopa	Acetazolamide
Barbiturates	Allopurinol
Cimetidine	Aspirin
Clonidine	Atropine
Dimenhydrinate	Beta-blockers
Erythromycin	Bromides
Furosemide	Bupivacaine
Glutethimide	Cephalosporins
Griseofulvin	Chloral hydrate
Hydantoins	Chlorpheniramine
Lidocaine	Chlorpromazine
Meprobamate	Codeine
Metoclopramide	Colchicine
Metronidazole	Diazoxide
Pentazocine	Digitalis
Phenylbutazone	Diphenhydramine
Sulfonamides	Epinephrine
Theophylline	Guanethidine
	Heparin
	Ibuprofen
	Indomethacin
	Insulin
	Labetalol
	Lorazepam
	Meclozine
	Morphine
	Naproxen
	Nitrous oxide
	Penicillins
	Prochlorperazine
	Propoxyphene
	Reserpine
	Thyroxine

on the basis of serum lead levels above 60 μg per milliliter and free erythrocyte protoporphyrin (FEP) levels greater than 250 μg per deciliter. These tests may not be available to the emergency physician on an urgent basis.

The diagnosis is difficult to establish on clinical grounds alone because the symptoms complex is nonspecific. Historical information that is helpful includes a family history of lead intoxication, a prodrome of fatigue, malaise, weakness, and irritability, or a history of exposure to lead products. Laboratory findings such as a microcytic anemia and lead lines at the ends of growing bones are seen in lead poisoning.

Abdominal pain from lead intoxication can be distinguished from other causes of the acute abdomen by the absence of true rebound tenderness and the presence of normal bowel sounds. In addition, the presence of other nonspecific findings such as headache, insomnia, peripheral neuropathy, fatigue, and a metallic taste can be used in distinguishing lead poisoning from other causes of abdominal pain. Patients with these symptoms should be admitted for chelation therapy.

ACUTE MESENTERIC ISCHEMIA

Acute mesenteric ischemia is an uncommon cause of severe abdominal pain that represents a true surgical emergency. It is briefly mentioned here because it may mimic nonsurgical causes of abdominal pain. Further discussion is found in the chapter on *Mesenteric Vascular Occlusion.*

Acute mesenteric ischemia is most common in patients older than 50 years. Several predisposing factors have been identified, including underlying atherosclerotic heart disease, atrial fibrillation, rheumatic heart disease, hypercoagulation states, sepsis, and hypotension.

The onset of symptoms varies from sudden with mesenteric arterial emboli to insidious with mesenteric venous thrombosis. The absence of physical findings often leads to a delay in proper diagnosis, contributing to the high mortality.

Diagnosis. The diagnosis of acute mesenteric ischemia is confirmed only by selective angiography or surgical exploration. Because of the high mortality, this entity should be suspected in any patient over the age of 50 with a history of atherosclerotic heart disease, atrial fibrillation, rheumatic heart disease, or a predisposition to coagulation abnormalities.

Differentiation of acute mesenteric ischemia from other conditions is difficult because of the paucity of physical findings and the indistinct nature of the laboratory data. As such, this disease is not often recognized as a true surgical emergency and is confused with many nonsurgical causes of abdominal pain.

HEREDITARY ANGIOEDEMA

Hereditary angioedema is the result of a genetically inherited deficiency of C1 esterase inhibitor. The disease is characterized by recurrent attacks of abdominal pain along with edema of the extremities, face, and larynx. Larngeal edema is responsible for reported mortality rates of up to 33 percent.

Diffuse abdominal tenderness is reported in more than 50 percent of acute attacks of hereditary angioedema. It is often accompanied by nausea, vomiting, and watery diarrhea. Because of sequestration of fluid, shock and hypotension have been reported. Leukocytosis and fever are often noted.

Diagnosis. Hereditary angioedema is diagnosed by specific complement assays that show decrease C1 esterase inhibitor and C4 levels. These tests are not available in the emergency department.

The emergency physician must rely on the clinical history of recurrent attacks, findings of edema of the face and extremities, and a positive family history to make the diagnosis. Abdominal radiographs show a classic "stacked coin" appearance and "thumbprinting" of bowel because of mucosal edema. This distinguishes the disease from other conditions causing acute abdominal pain. In addition, rebound tenderness is absent and bowel sounds are normal in these patients.

Treatment. Emergency department management of abdominal pain in patients with hereditary angioedema involves the exclusion of other causes of abdominal pain. Careful attention must be given to signs of airway obstruction such as hoarseness and stridor. There is no specific therapy; these attacks are generally self-limited and last for 24 to 72 hours.

Tabes Dorsalis. Tabes dorsalis is a late complication of untreated syphilis. The disease is characterized by ataxia, lightning pains in the extremities, pupillary find-

OTHER CONDITIONS MIMICKING THE ACUTE ABDOMEN

ings, and tabetic crises. Painful contraction of the gut smooth muscle results in severe abdominal pain.

The disease is diagnosed using specific serologic tests (fluorescent treponemal antibody absorption [FTA-Abs] and treponemal pallidum immobilization [TPI]) and by examining the cerebrospinal fluid. Findings of elevated protein, normal glucose, and elevated immunoglobulins confirm the diagnosis. The treatment of tabes dorsalis is aqueous penicillin G, 2 to 4 million units IV every 4 hours for 10 days.

Familial Mediterranean Fever. This disease is characterized by recurrent attacks of peritonitis, pleuritis, and arthritis in patients of Middle Eastern background. Attacks can occur once or twice a month and usually last 1 to 2 days. The most severe attacks result in abdominal tenderness, distension, and rebound tenderness. Nausea, vomiting, and fever are common. Abdominal radiographs can show air-fluid levels and bowel edema.

The disease is distinguished from other conditions by its recurrent nature and associated pleuritis and arthritis. Treatment is generally supportive, including nasogastric suction and intravenous fluids. Colchicine, 0.6 mg given orally every hour for 4 hours and then tapered, has been effective early in acute attacks.

Thyrotoxicosis. Abdominal pain has been reported to occur in both the hyperkinetic and apathetic forms of thyrotoxicosis. The abdomen is usually diffusely tender with active bowel sounds. Nausea, vomiting, fever, and leukocytosis are often noted. Rebound tenderness is absent.

The disease is distinguished from other conditions causing acute abdominal pain by observing associated findings such as exophthalmos, skin changes, arrhythmias, and an enlarged thyroid gland. The diagnosis is made by measuring thyroxine and triiodothyronine (T_4, T_3) and calculating the free thyroxine index. Relief of abdominal pain is obtained by treating the underlying condition.

Other Diseases. Several other medical diseases can give rise to severe abdominal pain. Despite the fact that patients with these conditions may complain primarily of significant abdominal pain, physical findings such as rigidity, guarding, and rebound tenderness are absent. Acute myocardial infarction, basal pneumonias, and acute pulmonary emboli have often presented as severe abdominal pain. Historical information, physical findings, and laboratory data are all useful in establishing the correct diagnosis.

Uremia may also present with significant abdominal discomfort. Findings such as deteriorating mental status, peripheral edema, bleeding diatheses as well as characteristic laboratory findings confirm the diagnosis.

Hyperparathyroidism and familial hyperlipidemias may result in acute abdomen by producing an acute pancreatitis. Involvement of the mesenteric arteries gives rise to a high incidence of abdominal pain in patients with polyarteritis nodosum. Abdominal epilepsy and causalgia are neurogenic causes that result in severe abdominal pain. Acute glaucoma presents with nausea and vomiting and, rarely, referred abominal pain that can lead to a mistaken abdominal diagnosis. Finally, Henoch–Schönlein purpura can produce severe abdominal pain in children. This can be distinguished from other causes of acute abdominal pain by the characteristic purpuric rash, involvement of the joints, and laboratory findings suggesting renal impairment.

SUGGESTED READING

Campbell IW, Duncan LJ, Innes JA, et al Abdominal pain in diabetic decompensation: clinical significance. JAMA 1975; 233:166–168.

Gordon NC, Brown S, Khosla VM, Hansen LS. Lead poisoning: a comprehensive review and report of a case. Oral Surg 1979; 47:500–512.

Kobernick M. Black widow spider bite. Am Fam Phys 1984; 29(5):241–245.

Marenah CB, Quiney JR. C1 esterase inhibitor deficiency as a cause of abdominal pain. Br Med J 1983; 286:786–787.

Silen W. Abdominal pain. In: Thorn GW, Adams RD, Braunwald E, Isselbacher KJ, Petersdorf RG, eds.Principles of internal medicine. 9th ed. New York: McGraw-Hill, 1980.

Trubowitz S. The management of sickle cell disease. Med Clin North Am 1976; 60:933–944.

Vavra JD, Avioli LV. Intermittent acute porphyria. Arch Intern Med 1982; 142:1527–1529.

HERNIA

JOHN H. MORTON, M.D.

ETIOLOGY AND PRESENTATION TO THE EMERGENCY DEPARTMENT

A patient may present to the emergency department with an acute problem associated with a hernia either in the groin or in the abdominal wall.

There are three types of hernias in the groin—indirect, direct, and femoral. Although a patient with any type of groin hernia may present in the emergency department, this is unusual for an individual with a direct hernia.

Children

The most common groin hernia is the indirect variety; almost all groin hernias in children are of this type. The childhood indirect hernia is a congenital defect with a persistent peritoneal sac entering the groin through the internal inguinal ring. Although the hernia is present from birth, it is not usually diagnosed until some intraperitoneal structure enters the hernia sac and a mass is evident in the groin. In an infant, an unexpected groin mass is the most common emergency department presentation for an indirect hernia. This mass may be a loop of intestine, although an ovary is a frequent finding in female infants with indirect hernias. Usually the mass can be reduced easily into the abdominal cavity. Under these circumstances the parent can be reassured, and surgical referral can be made for elective hernia repair.

When the mass cannot be reduced by gentle pressure, an emergency exists. The contents of the sac may occlude the internal inguinal ring, interfering with its own blood supply. Gangrene of the bowel or the ovary may result unless the contents of the sac can be successfully reduced either by manipulation or by emergency operation.

Occasionally an infant is seen with a scrotal swelling discovered by a parent during a diaper change. If the swelling is above the testicle, is smooth and nontender, a narrow light beam should be directed across the scrotum. If the mass transilluminates, it is a scrotal hydrocele. In a youngster, the presence of a scrotal hydrocele implies an indirect inguinal hernia, and the patient should be referred for elective herniorrhaphy. In an adult, however, a scrotal hydrocele may occur without a hernia. An asymptomatic scrotal hydrocele in an adult requires operative correction only when an associated hernia is evident.

Teenager and Young Adult

In the teenager and the young adult, a groin hernia is usually of the indirect variety, and the patient may present to the emergency department in one of three ways: (1) with an unexpected but asymptomatic groin mass, (2) with a painful mass incarcerated or strangulated in the hernia, or (3) with pain in the groin in the absence of a mass.

The unexpected asymptomatic groin mass is probably a congenital hernia that did not become obvious at an earlier age because a narrow internal inguinal ring inhibited entry of abdominal contents into the hernia sac. It is possible but less likely that the hernia developed de novo following vigorous exercise or heavy work, a situation justifying the term *rupture* which is sometimes applied to a hernia. The unexpected groin mass, if it is nontender and reduces readily, can be managed in the emergency department with reassurance and appropriate surgical referral.

A testicular tumor usually presents as an asymptomatic scrotal mass. It may be mistaken for a scrotal hydrocele or a large indirect hernia. Careful palpation should indicate that the mass is within the testicle. Testicular malignancies are characteristically found in young adult males, but any patient with a suspicious testicular mass should be referred promptly to a urologist.

A mass in the groin that does not reduce may represent a strangulated hernia, which requires emergency operation. In an adult strangulation usually involves a loop of small bowel or a portion of the omentum. Consideration must be given in differential diagnosis, however, to the possibility of an enlarged inguinal lymph node. Usually more than one enlarged node is present in the groin. Nodes may be present at other sites. There may be evidence of some underlying cause such as infection or tumor in the draining area (most frequently the lower extremity, the scrotum, or the perianal region). Presence of symptoms and signs such as malaise and fever suggest a more generalized process.

A young male who presents with a painful scrotal

mass must be carefully evaluated to rule out testicular torsion. The testicle is usually tender and enlarged when torsion is present. The fact that there is no associated swelling in the inguinal canal rules out an incarcerated hernia. At any rate, emergency exploration is the appropriate therapy.

The patient with no visible mass who presents with groin pain after physical exertion should be examined for the presence of a hernia. This must be done with the patient in the upright position. Whether or not a hernia can be detected in this manner, it is appropriate to give the patient a prescription for a mild analgesic and to refer him or her to a physician for follow-up evaluation in a few days. It is important to realize that a hernia with a narrow neck may not be found even on careful physical examination once the contents of the sac have reduced. Therefore, when the history suggests the possibility of a hernia, the examination should be repeated after an interval.

Adult Males

In the older male a hernia is more likely to be of the direct variety. These hernias may or may not be secondary to trauma. They frequently present in men involved in heavy work, but they may occur without any convincing history of injury. Since the direct hernia protrudes through a weakness in the medial inguinal canal floor behind the spermatic cord, it is unlikely to extend with the cord through the external ring into the scrotum. Also, the hernia is likely to protrude through a larger defect than the indirect hernia; for this reason incarceration or strangulation is unusual. The patient who presents to the emergency department with a direct hernia usually requires only reassurance and referral to a surgeon for elective repair. A truss has never been a valuable form of therapy for control of a groin hernia, and the use of trusses should be discouraged. In the rare circumstance in which an acute incarceration is present, the patient should be prepared for emergency herniorrhaphy.

Adult Women

Although the common hernia in the adult woman is of the indirect variety, most femoral hernias occur in women. The femoral hernia enters the thigh underneath the inguinal ligament between the medial wall of the femoral vein and the pubic tubercle. Because this is a very small ring with rigid walls, it is not unusual for the patient to present in the emergency department following the abrupt appearance of a painful mass in the upper thigh. Once a hernia of this variety strangulates, it is almost impossible to reduce it through the narrow ring, and no effort should be made to do so. The patient should be prepared immediately for emergency surgical repair.

It is easy to mistake acute groin lymphadenopathy for a strangulated femoral hernia. Nodes are frequently matted rather than discrete. In an older woman an unwary physician may mistake the lymphadenopathy of acute lymphoma for an incarcerated or strangulated femoral hernia. In the differential diagnosis it is helpful to remember the location of the inguinal ligament, which runs between the anterior superior iliac spine and the pubic tubercle. These landmarks can be identified even in an obese individual, and the femoral hernia should lie below this line whereas enlarged lymph nodes may be palpable both above and below the inguinal ligament.

Abdominal Wall Hernias

Hernias of the abdominal wall occur most frequently at the umbilicus or at the site of a previous surgical incision. Umbilical hernias are common in infants, especially in black children. Most of them close spontaneously before the child reaches school age, and they are rarely symptomatic. A parent who is bothered by an umbilical hernia in a youngster should be reassured and the probability of spontaneous closure should be explained. The use of external support over the umbilicus—a popular home remedy—is of no value and an unnecessary nuisance.

In older adults, especially women who have borne children, an umbilical hernia may become symptomatic. Elective repair should be carried out unless the patient presents with bowel or omentum strangulated in the sac. Under these circumstances emergency herniorrhaphy should be undertaken.

A postoperative incisional hernia is most apt to occur when the initial operation was carried out through a vertical incision and a postoperative wound infection was present. These hernias are not easy to repair, and the recurrence rate is high. The physician who examines a patient with an uncomplicated ventral incisional hernia in the emergency department should leave the decision about management to the patient's surgeon. When acute incarceration or strangulation is present, the patient requires preparation for emergency reduction of the strangulated contents. At the time of the emergency reduction, repair of the hernia should be done if feasible. These individuals are frequently obese, and complications from heart disease or diabetes mellitus are not unusual. Any medical problem that can be addressed should be managed expeditiously in preparation for emergency reduction of the strangulation and attempted repair of the abdominal wall defect.

THERAPY

For the patient with mild groin pain or a reducible hernia, no therapy is required in the emergency department other than an explanation of the problem, reassurance, the prescription of an appropriate analgesic and referral for further care.

Occasionally a patient is seen with an irreducible hernia that has been present for some time. This patient may have no symptoms other than the presence of an unsightly swelling. A chronic incarceration that is not painful is not an emergency, and no attempt should be made to reduce the contents of the sac. The patient should be referred to a surgeon for elective repair.

When the patient presents to the emergency department with an acutely incarcerated or strangulated hernia, it is rational under most circumstances to attempt reduction of the hernia. For this to be successful the patient must be properly prepared. He or she should be recumbent, and an ice bag should be applied to the area. The patient should receive an appropriate subcutaneous dose of morphine. No effort should be made to reduce the hernia until this medication has a chance to take effect; for this reason the patient should be left undisturbed for 30 to 45 minutes after the opiate is administered. With these guidelines, a single effort at reduction is appropriate. Gentle pressure should be applied to the apex of the strangulated tissue, and it should be directed toward the neck of the hernia—laterally across the groin for an indirect hernia or directly posteriorly for an abdominal wall hernia. If the attempted reduction is successful, the physician will frequently be aware of a gurgle as gas and fluid move inside an entrapped hollow viscus. Once this happens a hernia that appeared firmly fixed may reduce into the abdominal cavity with surprising ease and rapidity. It is important not to be confused by partial reduction—only complete disappearance of the contents of the sac from the groin or the abdominal incision is acceptable. If the hernia is reduced successfully, the patient should be admitted to the hospital. Unless there are compelling medical reasons for withholding operation, the hernia should be repaired 2 to 3 days later. This short delay is justified because a better surgical repair can be carried out if local tissue edema subsides preoperatively. Longer delay is unwise because the hernia may strangulate a second time.

Under the following two circumstances no effort should be made to reduce an acutely incarcerated hernia, and emergency operation should be done. (1)Because the ring through which a femoral hernia enters the thigh is narrow and has rigid walls, efforts at reduction of a strangulated femoral hernia are unlikely to be successful and may injure edematous strangulated bowel. (2)If the patient has signs of critical injury to entrapped bowel—fever, significant tachycardia, marked local tenderness, leukocytosis—reduction is contraindicated. The risk of reducing bowel with compromised viability into the abdomen, resulting in peritonitis, is too great.

When attempted reduction of an acutely incarcerated hernia is unwise or unsuccessful, preparations for *emergency operation* should be instituted immediately. Intravenous fluids should be started, lactated Ringer's solution being the appropriate choice for most patients. A nasogastric tube and a urethral catheter should be inserted. Appropriate preoperative medication such as subcutaneous morphine and atropine should be administered. Corrective steps should be undertaken for any associated medical problems such as congestive heart failure or uncontrolled diabetes mellitus. There is no consensus about the use of preoperative antibiotics in these patients. Some surgeons believe that any patient undergoing an emergency operation should receive preoperative antibiotic therapy. However, this precaution seems unnecessary and expensive unless there are symptoms and signs that suggest the presence of necrotic bowel. Under these circumstances an intravenous broad-spectrum antibiotic such as cefazolin should be instituted preoperatively. If no abnormal bowel is encountered during the procedure, the antibiotic can be discontinued after 24 hours. If necrotic bowel is present, the agent should be continued for a full 10-day therapeutic course. With any evidence of peritonitis an aminoglycoside such as tobramycin should be added.

Significant changes have occurred in the routine management of groin hernias in recent years; the use of local anesthesia and performance of the herniorrhaphy on an outpatient basis are two examples. These approaches are not appropriate when an emergency operation is required. Because of the risk of peritonitis from necrotic bowel, an emergency hernia repair should be done under optimal circumstances. This requires hospital admission (although the hospital stay may last only 3 to 4 days if there are no complications). The operation should be performed under general or spinal anesthesia. With appropriate preoperative and postoperative care, most patients tolerate emergency herniorrhaphy satisfactorily.

SUGGESTED READING

Condon RD, Nyhus LM. Complications of groin hernia. In: Nyhus LM, Condon RE, eds. Hernia, 2nd ed. Philadelphia: JB Lippincott, 1978: 264.

Dennis C, Enquist IF. Strangulating external hernias. In: Nyhus LM, Condon RE, eds. Hernia, 2nd ed. Philadelphia: JB Lippincott, 1978: 279.

Morton JH. Ventral incisional hernias. Infect Surg 1985; 4:212–217.

Ponka JL. Diagnosis of hernia. In: Hernias of the abdominal wall. Philadelphia: WB Saunders, 1980: 40.

ABDOMINAL MASS

FRANK L. WEAKLEY, M.D., F.A.C.S.

NORMAL ORGAN

An abdominal mass can be produced by a normal organ, an abnormal organ, or an abnormal collection of fluid.

Any physician carrying out a physical examination must be able to differentiate a normal organ from an abnormal mass. Tenderness, fever, elevated white count, and a reliable history from the patient attesting to a recent appearance of the mass alerts the examiner to a possible pathologic diagnosis. Slender patients and those who obtain full muscular relaxation are the ones in whom normal organs can often be palpated. The muscular sigmoid colon or stool in any portion of the colon might be palpable in a patient who is easy to examine. A normal kidney or liver might also be easily felt in such a person, and a stomach or bladder full of normal contents can be mistaken for an abnormal mass.

If a mass cannot easily be diagnosed on the basis of the history and findings readily available to the emergency personnel, simple measures available in the emergency room setting can be utilized helpfully. An extensive, time-consuming work-up to identify a normal organ is not necessary. A stomach that is distended because of downstream obstruction should be treated by addressing the cause of the obstruction after placement of a nasogastric tube. A urinary bladder that is full enough to be palpated because of retention, despite attempts at voiding, can be relieved by the insertion of a urinary catheter. A palpable normal kidney or liver can be confirmed by plain abdominal and pelvic roentgenograms with the addition of pyelography or cholecystography studies.

ABNORMAL ORGAN

Diagnosis

The abnormal liver produced by congestive heart failure or hepatitis or the liver of increased size owing to metastatic cancer often can be palpated, even in the obese patient. Clues to the category in which the abnormality falls can be obtained by the presence or absence of other signs of congestive heart failure, such as evidence of pulmonary edema, distended peripheral veins, weak and thready pulse, arrhythmias, or an abnormally wide heart contour on chest film. In the patient with hepatitis the liver will be tender, and etiologic clues will be reflected in blood tests of liver function. Metastatic liver cancer is associated with characteristic hardness and nodularity and usually an appropriate history suggesting the primary cancer site. The cirrhotic liver is less tender and usually is associated with a history of prior hepatitis or alcoholism. Cholelithiasis and cholecystitis usually can be differentiated by local tenderness and the history of prior attacks, which supports the diagnosis of cholecystitis.

Abnormal lymph nodes reflecting lymphoma can be differentiated from acute masses by their history and their usual lack of tenderness. Diagnosis is not necessary on an emergency basis, and confirmation of their true nature can be determined by computed tomography (CT) scan or by sonography.

Small and large bowel neoplasms are often more mobile than retroperitoneal lymph node abnormalities. Diagnosis by palpation should not be attempted, but large and/or small bowel barium roentgenography or fiberoptic endoscopy should be used. An obstructing neoplasm is better diagnosed by retrograde, transanal barium roentgenography than by oral, anterograde barium studies. A mass caused by a polyp is usually the mass of the intussuscepted bowel caused by the polyp rather than the polyp itself. It is accompanied by signs and symptoms of intermittent intestinal obstruction. Obstruction from malignancy usually causes progressive signs and symptoms, and

the patient is usually in a more depleted nutritional state than the patient with intussusception from a polyp.

Masses caused by Crohn's disease, ulcerative colitis, or radiation enteritis can be differentiated by similar intestinal barium studies in the nonacute phases or by history and plain abdominal films in the presence of acute findings of perforation or distention. Ischemic bowel masses may be difficult to differentiate from radiation or Crohn's disease masses. In acute, emergency situations, the need for surgical treatment is urgent and there is no specific diagnostic test or pattern. In less urgent cases, arteriography is diagnostic.

Problems of the spleen do not usually represent an emergency situation, but an enlarged spleen can be palpable in the presence of portal hypertension, lymphoma, hypersplenism, infectious mononucleosis, and following trauma when a subcapsular hemorrhage is present. The last condition may require urgent treatment and can be differentiated from the others by ultrasonography. The history of trauma is not mandatory for hemorrhage to occur as the spleen can be ruptured in some medical conditions such as infectious mononucleosis.

If the stomach is palpable as a mass in the absence of its distention or fullness, carcinoma or lymphoma should be considered. Fiberoptic examination is decisive.

A palpable midabdominal mass that pulsates may represent an aortic aneurysm. If it is rupturing, acute signs are present, often causing unequal lower extremity pulses, back pain, and signs of general circulatory compromise or collapse. In the absence of these signs, ultrasonography and plain abdominal films can confirm the diagnosis and indicate the size of the aneurysm.

The abnormal appendix with appendicitis or neoplasm can be differentiated by associated inflammatory signs and, in their absence, by contrast-medium roentgenography.

In the abnormal kidney, uterus, and ovaries benign conditions usually need to be differentiated from malignant ones. Benign kidney enlargement is usually cystic. Cystic ovaries can be benign or malignant, but a tender tubo-ovarian abscess or tubal ectopic pregnancy needs immediate further diagnosis and surgical treatment. Uterine myomata are usually benign. Abruptio placentae presents as a painful mass in a pregnant woman; immediate obstetric attention is needed.

The most important job for the emergency physician is to determine whether the mass requires surgery within the next hour or does not require surgery until an accurate diagnosis is made. Examples of the latter are neoplasms, polyps of the intestinal tract, and lymphomas. In the absence of other illnesses, such patients can be referred to the appropriate specialist for a work-up.

Toxic dilatation of the colon resulting from Crohn's disease or mucosal ulcerative colitis requires surgery within a few hours of diagnosis. Walled-off perforative masses such as may be found in Crohn's disease, radiation enteritis, and diverticulitis should be dealt with after consultation with a colorectal or general surgeon. Patients who have suffered attacks of diverticulitis often need only bowel rest and antimicrobial treatment if gross perfora-

TABLE 1 Abdominal Masses: Abnormal Organ

Organ	Condition	Treatment
Liver	Congestive heart failure	Digitalization, diuresis
	Hepatitis	Rest, nutritional support
	Metastatic cancer	Chemotherapy
Gallbladder	Cholelithiasis	Cholecystectomy, if symptomatic
	Cholecystitis	Cholecystectomy
Lymph node(s)	Lymphoma	Chemotherapy
Small bowel	Polyp	Radiotherapy polypectomy
	Carcinoma	Resection and anastomosis
	Lymphoma	Chemotherapy
		Radiotherapy
		Resection and anastomosis
	Crohn's disease, radiation enteritis	Surgical treatment if medical treatment is unsuccessful
Colon	Polyp	Colonoscopic polypectomy
		Colotomy and polypectomy
		Resection and anastomosis
	Carcinoma	Resection and anastomosis
	Lymphoma	Chemotherapy
		Radiotherapy resection and anastomosis
	Crohn's disease, ulcerative colitis	Surgical treatment if medical treatment is unsuccessful
	Diverticulitis	Surgical treatment when diagnosis is made with certainty and if surgical risk to patient is not greater than risk of the disease
	Ischemia	Surgical treatment
Spleen	Portal hypertension	No treatment
		Varices surgery
		Portal bypass surgery
	Lymphoma	Chemotherapy
		Radiotherapy
		Splenectomy
	Hypersplenism	Splenectomy
	Subcapsular hemorrhage	Surgery
Stomach	Carcinoma	Gastrectomy
	Lymphoma	Chemotherapy
		Radiotherapy
		Gastrectomy
Aorta	Aneurysm	Surgery
Appendix	Appendicitis	Appendectomy
Kidney	Cyst	Aspiration
		No treatment
	Neoplasm	Nephrectomy
Uterus	Myomata	Myomectomy
		Hysterectomy
		No treatment
Ovaries	Cyst	Laparoscopy
		Oophorectomy
		Cystectomy

tion is not present. Resection is preferable after inflammation has subsided (about 6 weeks). The patient's surgical risk must always be measured against the risk of the disease state.

Patients with ischemic bowel may need urgent resection, but if so, associated signs of tenderness, toxicity, increased white count, metabolic acidosis, and perhaps fever usually are present.

Renal cysts usually can be differentiated from renal malignancy by sonography, intravenous pyelography, and renal tomograms. Aspiration for malignant cells should be left to an experienced urologic surgeon.

TABLE 2 Abdominal Masses: Abnormal Fluid Collection

Collection	Treatment
Pus	Aspiration, tube drainage, laparotomy and drainage
Blood	Surgical treatment for active bleeding. Blood replacement and rest if bleeding has stopped.
Cystic fluid	Aspiration, tube drainage, laparotomy and drainage.
Enteric contents, extraluminal	Laparotomy and drainage, and resection of the offending organ (usually colon or small bowel)

TABLE 3 Initial Treatment of Abdominal Masses

In presence of circulatory decompensation:

Intravenous crystalloids immediately

Intravenous whole blood when available

Urinary bladder catheter for monitoring and evaluation

If mass is increasing in size, or if initial fluid therapy does not reverse signs of circulatory decompensation (low BP; tachycardia; weak pulse), call vascular surgeon, especially in the presence of back pain and absent or unequal inguinal or lower extremity pulses

In presence of toxic signs (fever, tachycardia, elevated WBCs):

Intravenous cephalosporin or ampicillin 500 mg–1 g. Specimens should be obtained for Gram stain and culture and sensitivity determinations before antimicrobial therapy is started; if this cannot be done, the lab should be notified to use the appropriate suppressors to prevent the antimicrobials from affecting culture results.

Urinary bladder catheter for monitoring and evaluation

Call colorectal or general surgeon in consultation

In absence of circulatory decompensation or toxicity signs:

Get kidney, ureter, bladder, and chest films in prone and erect positions

Get complete blood count, urinalysis, and SMA-18 determinations

Start intravenous crystalloids, pass nasogastric tube if patient is nauseated or vomiting, insert urinary bladder catheter, allow the patient nothing by mouth

ABNORMAL FLUID COLLECTION

Sometimes the principal constituent of an abdominal mass is pus, blood, cystic fluid, or extraluminal enteric contents. In all of these instances, plain abdominal films, sonography, CT scan, and radiopacification of adjacent organs help in differentiation.

Aspiration may help in diagnosis and even in treating the patient's condition, but it is best carried out with collaborative assistance of the appropriate specialist. Circulatory support and restoration should be used early, and laparotomy and drainage or definitive surgery may be required in the early hours.

SUGGESTED READING

Conn H, Conn RB. Current diagnosis 5. Philadelphia: WB Saunders, 1977.

Harvey AM, Bordley J III. Differential diagnosis. 2nd ed. Philadelphia: WB Saunders, 1970.

CONSTIPATION AND IMPACTION

FRANCIS J. OWENS Sr., M.D.

Constipation is a disturbance of bowel function in which the stool is abnormally hardened and/or delayed. The normal stool holds its shape, but is passed readily as often as several times daily (usually after meals), or as infrequently as several times weekly.

Constipation may be acute or chronic, but in each case it represents a change from a previous habit, except in lifelong constipation. In that case, comparison with the norm stated above is the basis of the definition.

DIAGNOSIS

The diagnosis of acute constipation is made in the patient who fits the definition given previously. A delay of a day or two in the usual frequency of bowel movements may be considered acute—although mild—constipation at that point.

Pain is seldom a complaint in acute constipation. However, the patient is uncomfortable with lower abdominal fullness or vague distress in the rectal or sacral area. Symptoms more severe than these may herald the onset of the irritable bowel syndrome, which I and many other authors think is different from constipation as such.

Occasionally malaise or headache is ascribed to constipation; these are probably due to rectal distention. The same symptoms have been elicited by inserting cotton in the rectum.

Any pain greater than mild, or any other gastrointestinal symptoms such as nausea or vomiting may indicate an inflammatory process. This should be cause for an intensive work-up either in the emergency department or as an inpatient.

The initial examination of the patient may suggest the cause of constipation: bed-ridden, apathetic, disturbed, dehydrated, and febrile patients are often constipated. The examination is directed largely to the gastrointestinal tract in those whose appearance or complaints do not suggest generalized or severe disorders.

The digital rectal examination is the sine qua non of diagnosis and may be the first step—no procedure is more obvious or has been more neglected. Examination of the abdomen follows. Distention of the abdomen, although a common subjective complaint, is infrequently evident. Only in a chronic condition such as megacolon is this likely to be present. Tenderness may be present and rebound tenderness in the area of palpation is simply an exaggeration of sensitivity. If it is more than minimal, a special search for an inflammatory lesion is needed. Palpable masses may indicate obstructing lesions, including an impaction. Percussion, except as it helps outline solid organs or masses, is simply a means of eliciting tenderness. Auscultation lends little information except in the acute abdomen.

X-ray study in acute constipation is primarily for the exclusion of bowel obstruction. The plain abdominal or lateral rectal film usually shows any accumulation of feces because of the air margins around the fecal masses. A diameter of greater than 5 cm in the rectum, left colon, or transverse colon or greater than 8 cm in the right colon is abnormal and may be dangerous.

ACUTE IMPACTION

This refers to a sudden blockage of the bowel by a large localized mass of feces. This is usually located in the distal rectum but may occur more proximally, particularly at a lesion or stricture. The diagnosis is made from the history of sudden cessation of bowel movements or passage of only small fragments. The patient may have mild-to-moderate distress associated with bearing down sensations, but more severe distress warrants consideration of perforation from a stercoral ulcer. In such cases intensive study is needed, usually requiring hospitalization.

The digital rectal examination discloses the rectum full of feces, preventing the examining finger from probing the walls. If the accumulation is higher up, it may be palpable on abdominal examination and may measure 4 to 5 cm in diameter. Minimal tenderness may be present, but greater tenderness or guarding raises the question of perforation of a stercoral ulcer.

The x-ray study in acute impaction serves to exclude bowel obstruction. A plain x-ray film of the abdomen and a lateral film of the rectum serve to delineate the extent of the impaction and alert the examiner regarding the risk of perforation (more than 5 cm in diameter on the left and more than 8 cm on the right). A barium enema may occasionally be needed to delineate a high impaction, although it may be evident on the plain film. Iodinated contrast media (e.g., Gastrografin, Hypaque, MD-Gastroview) are not as useful because of limited contrast, although if perforation is a possibility, such an absorbable medium should be used. Ultrasonography may also show an impaction, but intestinal gas usually limits its application. Computerized tomography (CT) has recently been cited for special use in the differential diagnosis of acute diverticulitis. Endoscopy can differentiate an impaction from a tumor. Thorough x-ray and endoscopic studies are obvious modalities in the patient with chronic constipation, a subject beyond the scope of this chapter.

ACUTE AND CHRONIC IMPACTION

This condition is encountered among the bed-ridden, especially in nursing homes and chronic care hospitals. The patients have a gradual accumulation of feces, but eventually may present as emergencies because of sudden complete cessation of bowel movements. The colon may be stuffed with huge amounts of feces; more than 30 lb have been recorded.

The patients' complaints vary with their mental and

physical status. Usually pain is not severe, except with perforation. Examination discloses the rectum as in acute impaction. The abdominal examination may disclose numerous masses of feces 4 to 5 cm in diameter or even a long cast of stool. Tenderness varies, but must be sought to rule out perforation.

The plain x-ray film of the abdomen and rectum in acute and chronic impaction may show a large accumulation of feces. The diameter of the cecum may be up to 12 cm, and that of other portions of the colon may be up to 8 cm. However, in any such instance perforation may be imminent (see under x-ray studies of acute impaction).

TREATMENT

Acute Impaction

Disimpaction using the gloved finger is the simplest approach. A topical anesthetic such as 1 percent dibucaine may be needed for anal hypersensitivity. Initial softening of the stool with a mineral oil enema is useful, but time-consuming. However, if it is successful the discomfort of digital disimpaction may be avoided. The enema tip often embeds in the stool, hence gentle manipulation is needed to get it alongside the impaction so that the oil can be spread over the surface of the stool. Alternatively, a large rubber tube may be gently passed into the mass, either directly or through a proctoscope, and water or enema solution instilled into it. A combination of equal parts of cottonseed oil and 1 percent docusate sodium may be used (1,000 ml of that combination may be used as a cleansing enema).

Acute Constipation

Without impaction, this may be treated with a glycerin suppository (3 g) or, that failing, with a bisacodyl suppository (10 mg). Alternatives are a tap water enema or a sodium phosphate enema (120 ml). Soapsuds and hydrogen peroxide solutions are known causes of colitis and are no longer acceptable.

If a painful anal lesion is present, a saline laxative such as milk of magnesia (12 to 30 ml) or sodium phosphates oral solution (10 to 20 ml diluted) produces a liquid stool, as does lactulose (20 to 30 g), but not as quickly. Lactulose must not be used in complete bowel obstruction.

Alternatives are phenolphthalein (100 mg), cascara (2 ml of the aromatic fluid extracts), or bisacodyl (5 to 10 mg). Danthron has become more popular recently, but not because of any special advantage. Castor oil (30 to 60 ml) is much stronger and is reserved for problems resistant to less potent agents. It should be emphasized that repeated usage of any medicinal agents may result in a laxative dependency. The management of chronic constipation is briefly considered at the end of the treatment section.

TABLE 1 Emergency Conditions Frequently Causing Constipation

Acute diverticulitis
Anal lesions and rectal prolapse
Dehydration and/or electrolyte imbalance
Fecal impaction, special aspects:
  Celiac sprue
  Chronic invalidism
  Psychiatric syndromes including "giant megacolon
    of the insane"
Hypercalcemia syndromes
Incarcerated hernia
Injuries and tumors of the spinal cord and cauda equina
Medications and poisons:
  Anesthetics and muscle paralyzers
  Antacids
  Anticholinergics
  Antihypertensives
  Bismuth
  Calcium-channel blockers
  Iron
  Metallic poisons
  Neuropsychiatric therapeutic drugs
  Opiates
Multiple sclerosis
Traveler's constipation
Volvulus
X-ray studies with barium sulfate

Acute and Chronic Impaction

Digital disimpaction is the first step, but disimpaction even under anesthesia may be needed. Oil retention enemas followed by warm-water or saline enemas are next. Mineral oil (30 to 60 ml) by mouth may be used if the patient is alert and the prevention of aspiration is ensured.

Polyethylene glycol (PEG) electrolyte gastrointestinal lavage solution is a convenient, effective new treatment modality. Actual obstruction anywhere in the gastrointestinal tract or any acute process is a contraindication. The solution is prepared from a special combination of polyethylene glycol, sodium and potassium chlorides, and sodium sulfate and bicarbonate, available with specific instructions from Braintree Laboratories as Golytely and from Reed and Carnrick as Colyte. The material is reputed to cause no change in water or electrolyte balance, but close observation of patients with any significant disabilities is appropriate as the 3 to 4 L are to be administered over 2 to 3 hours. Metoclopramide (Reglan), 10 mg, is usually given before the solution. A diuretic may be needed. Admission or transfer of such a patient to an acute care hospital may be necessary.

Chronic constipation is not the subject of this chapter. However, a few points should be emphasized. After adequate exclusion of lesions and diseases, the treatment consists primarily of reeducation and use of bran; either wheat or oat bran is suggested, but wheat bran is more available. The re-education is vital in that faulty habits as well as inadequate fiber are the principal causes of constipation.

SUGGESTED READING

Earnest DL. Fecal impaction. In: Sleisenger MH, Fordtran JS. Gastrointestinal disease 3rd ed. Philadelphia: WB Saunders, 1983: 1316.

Haubrich WS. Constipation. In: Berk JW, ed. Bockus gastroenterology 4th ed. Philadelphia: WB Saunders, 1985: 111.

Owens FJ. Constipation. In: Farmer RG, Achkar E, Fleshler B, eds. Clinical gastroenterology 1st ed. New York: Raven Press, 1983:61.

FUNCTIONAL BOWEL PROBLEMS

MARTIN BROTMAN, B.Sc.(Med), M.Sc., M.D.

The various functional bowel disorders are among the commonest problems seen by the primary care physician. They account for up to 70 percent of the referrals for outpatient gastrointestinal consultations, and, although usually chronic and recurrent, they may be sufficiently acute, severe, or disabling to prompt emergency evaluation. Despite their "benign" nature, this group of disorders is an important cause of work disability, impaired productivity, social incapacity, and family disruption.

The etiology of these disorders is unknown. There are no convincing objective correlations between physiologic abnormalities of the gut and symptoms. Semantic confusion continues (Table 1), and therapy is largely empiric. We do not yet know whether these are psychosomatic disorders, motility disorders, or a form of stress response. Nevertheless, patients presenting with functional-type bowel complaints require careful evaluation to rule out underlying organic disease and can be treated successfully.

HISTORY

The presenting complaint may be abdominal pain, altered bowel habits (diarrhea, constipation, or both), abdominal distention, excess gas (eructation or flatulence), anorexia, nausea, or any combination of these.

The pain is most commonly infraumbilical, diffuse rather than localized to either lower quadrant, and varies from dull aching to agonizing cramping. The pain often precedes bowel movements and may increase after defecation—distinguishing this pain from that caused by colon-obstructing lesions. Although infraumbilical distribution is most typical, the pain may be epigastric, generalized, or radiate to the back and even the chest. The epigastric component may mimic peptic ulcer disease but may lack the seasonal variation, nocturnal occurrence, and food and antacid relief features of ulcer disease.

The abnormal bowel habit includes a history of chronic constipation, often with hard "rabbit-pellet" stools and laxative abuse, or of diarrhea, without blood but often with mucus, or cycles of these. A history of hematochezia or nocturnal awakening by diarrhea strongly suggests an organic rather than a functional etiology. The patient will often describe a history of "cycles," beginning with a period of constipation with progressive malaise, sensations of abdominal bloating, borborygmus, and increasing lower abdominal pain, followed by the passage of hard and then increasingly explosive liquid stool.

The abdominal distention is more often felt by the patient than observable by the examiner. The patient often relaxes the abdominal muscles and increases the lumbar lordosis, "pouching out" the abdomen in the absence of distended intra-abdominal organs.

A history of associated excessive eructation is almost invariably associated with aerophagia. Flatulence most commonly is related to dietary factors, particularly lactose and poorly digestable oligosaccharides such as flatleafed vegetables (lettuce, cabbage, spinach) and beans with skins.

The patient who presents to the emergency department with functional bowel disorder may be seeking relief of chronic symptoms, having finally become intolerant of them, or may have had an acute exacerbation of these chronic disorders leading to severe distress. The physician must be aware of the major importance of the history, particularly in the elderly patient. It is extremely rare for functional bowel problems to present for the first time in patients over the age of 55. In these cases the absence of history of the bowel as a "target organ" strongly suggests organic disease.

PHYSICAL EXAMINATION

Examination rarely reveals significant abnormality and is conspicuously "benign" compared with the severity of patient complaints and the frequent appearance of

TABLE 1 Terms Used Interchangeably with Functional Bowel Syndrome

Adaptive colitis	Membranous catarrh of
Chronic catarrhal colitis	the intestine
Chronic spasmodic affections	Membranous enteritis
Colica mucosa	Mucomembranous colic
Colon neurosis	Mucous colitis
Colonic enterospasm	Myxoneurosis
Dyskinesia of the colon	Nervous diarrhea
Dyssynergia of the colon	Neurogenic mucous colitis
Functional enterocolonopathy	Nonspecific diarrhea
Functional diarrhea	Spasmodic stricture
Glarry enteritis	Spastic colon
Glutinous diarrhea	Tubular diarrhea
Intestinal croup	Unhappy colon
Irritable colon syndrome	Unstable colon
Irritable gut syndrome	Vegetative neurosis
Lienteric diarrhea	

marked anxiety and agitation. Vital signs are normal, sometimes with sinus tachycardia. Abdominal inspection is usually normal, although the "pseudocyesis" mentioned before may be observed. There may be generalized guarding, but this is invariably voluntary and often disappears with repeated examination or when assessed by firm pressure on the stethoscope diaphragm while auscultating the abdomen. There may be direct tenderness, sometimes marked, over the distribution of the colon, particularly the sigmoid colon, but rebound tenderness is not observed. Bowel sounds are often hyperactive but nonobstructive.

DIFFERENTIAL DIAGNOSIS

The differential diagnosis is extensive in view of the varied presenting complaints. Table 2 lists organic diagnoses frequently missed in patients with chronic gastrointestinal symptoms. The physician in the emergency department should consider these possibilities in determining the extent of testing to be ordered.

EVALUATION

The history and normal findings on examination often convince the physician of the functional nature of the complaints. If the patient is already under care for this dis-

TABLE 2 Differential Diagnosis of Functional Bowel Syndrome

Pain prominent
    Early Crohn's disease
    Missed peptic ulcer disease
    Recurrent partial obstruction
        Volvulus
        Internal hernia
        Adhesions

Abdominal distention prominent
    Gas producers
    Small bowel obstruction

Constipation prominent
    Hollow visceral myopathy
        Scleroderma 50%
        Idiopathic 40%
        Miscellaneous 10%

    Anorexia nervosa

    Drugs

Diarrhea prominent
    Lactase deficiency
    Sorbitol intolerance
    Fructose intolerance

    Giardiasis or other infectious diarrheas

    Mild nontropical sprue

    Collagenous colitis

    Drugs
    Idiosyncratic reaction
    Factitious diarrhea

    Cholereic diarrhea

order, discussion with the patient's primary care physician and arrangement for follow-up care without further evaluation may be sufficient (see treatment discussion to follow).

In the absence of such history, when symptoms of relatively recent onset are presented, or when there is any suggestion of organic disease, further evaluation is indicated. This includes:

1. Complete blood count.
2. Fecal tests for occult blood.
3. Stool smear for leukocytes.
4. Flat and upright films of the abdomen (it is particularly important that these be done during an attack of pain or distention or both).
5. Stool studies for ova and parasites and stool culture for pathogens (if not previously done in patients with disease in which diarrhea is prominent).

Other diagnostic studies that may be required to confirm the functional nature of the diagnosis should be deferred to the outpatient setting under the guidance of the patient's primary care physician. These may include proctosigmoidoscopic or colonoscopic examination, abdominal ultrasonography, contrast studies of the upper and lower gastrointestinal tract, a lactose tolerance test, a qualitative or quantitative fecal fat determination, and duodenal aspiration for microscopy, depending on the presenting complaint.

MANAGEMENT

The successful treatment of functional bowel disorders requires long-term commitment by patient and physician and thus is largely the responsibility of the primary care physician, gastroenterologist, or occasionally psychiatrist. The major responsibility of the physician in the emergency department is to exclude organic disease (as already described), to relieve anxiety by reassurring the patient of the absence of life-threatening disease, and to relieve acute symptoms. Since there is frequently associated psychopathology, including anxiety-tension states, hypochondriasis, obsessive-compulsive traits, and depression, little can be done in the emergency department to influence the long-term course of the disease. Discussion with the patient and family may reveal recent stress that precipitated the acute event; counseling may relieve some of the resulting anxiety. The physician should take the time to explain the nature of the disorder to the patient and must avoid trivializing the symptoms when no organic disease is found. The patient's fear of being labeled neurotic and being told "its all in your mind" may contribute significantly to the severity of symptoms, the refractoriness to therapy, and the hostility toward physicians. The patient must be told that the disorder is real and that a multifaceted treatment approach in a compassionate therapeutic relationship is essential to recovery.

It is very important that an appropriate and prompt follow-up visit (within 3 days) in a stable patient-physician relationship be arranged at the time of the patient's discharge from the emergency department.

The following may be helpful for symptomatic relief:

1. Glucagon, 1 mg IV, or atropine, 0.4 mg subcutaneously, may relieve acute pain, presumably by relieving severe colonic spasm. Although the duration of action of glucagon is very brief, the patient may experience relief of much longer duration. The patient should be cautioned regarding the possible development of nausea with glucagon and dry mouth or blurred vision with atropine.
2. Compazine, 10 mg orally or IM, or 25 mg by suppository for nausea.
3. Anxiolytics (diazepam, 5 or 10 mg by mouth every 6 hours, or chlordiazepoxide in similar doses) may relieve anxiety. If utilized, only a small number of pills should be given to the patient, sufficient only for the acute episode. Patients should be cautioned regarding the sedative potential of these agents.
4. Narcotic analgesics may be required for severe pain that is not relieved by the modalities listed.
5. Anxiolytic-anticholinergic combinations such as Librax, Donnatal, and Combid are best reserved for use by the physician responsible for long-term management.
6. Antidiarrheals such as loperamide should be avoided in the emergency setting. Their judicious use for temporary symptom control in selected social situations should be the responsibility of the physician responsible for long-term care. Similar caution applies to the use of antidepressant medications such as amitriptyline, which appear to be beneficial in low doses for symptomatic control of functional bowel symptoms.
7. Instructions for modification of diet may be helpful, restricting gas-forming and high-bulk foods such as raw fruits, leafy vegetables, beans, and dairy products. The patient should be advised that this is only a short-term dietary modification and that long-term diet instruction will be given by the primary care physician.
8. The patient should be observed in the emergency department for a sufficient period of time to rule out organic diagnoses, to observe response to treatment, and to arrange appropriate follow-up care by a primary care physician or consulting gastroenterologist. Admission to the hospital is rarely, if ever, necessary, unless the associated psychopathology is sufficiently severe to mandate psychiatric inpatient management.
9. The importance of follow-up care has been described. With appropriate long-term management, the vast majority of patients with functional bowel disorders may be relieved of symptoms and enjoy a much improved quality of life.

SUGGESTED READING

Kirsner JD. The irritable bowel syndrome. Arch Int Med 1981; 141:635–639.
Thompson WG. The irritable bowel. Gut 1984; 25:305–320.

ADULT INFECTIOUS DIARRHEA

GEORGE A. PANKEY, M.D.
SANDRA M. ABADIE, M.D.

Diarrhea is a frequent complaint among patients seeking care in emergency departments in the United States. It is usually self-limited and not life-threatening; however, in debilitated and elderly patients, diarrhea may be associated with dehydration, electrolyte disturbances, mental status changes, and hypotension.

Diarrhea can be defined as an increased volume of fecal material (more than 250 ml in 24 hours) and increased frequency of bowel movements. Large volumes of stool result from an inability of the intestine to absorb ingested fluids, food, and endocrine secretions, or the excessive secretion of fluids from the small bowel and colon under various stimuli, which include enterotoxins from bacteria, viral enteritis, malabsorption, intestinal peptides secreted by tumors.

The pathophysiology of diarrhea involves four mechanisms:

1. *Secretory diarrhea* is characterized by increased amounts of water and electrolytes secreted from the mucosa into the lumen. Vibrio cholera is the prototype, but this may result from other enterotoxins, malabsorption of bile acids following ileal resection, and Crohn's disease.
2. *Osmotic diarrhea* results from materials present in the intestine that are not well absorbed, as in patients with lactose intolerance who eat ice cream.
3. *Exudative diarrhea* results from inflammation of the mucosa, with exudation of red and white blood cells and mucus.
4. *Disorders of motility* are responsible for diarrhea in irritable bowel syndromes, diabetes mellitus, and scleroderma.

Diarrhea can be further categorized according to etiologic agent. Acute diarrhea is usually infectious, and the Norwalk virus is the most common viral offender in adults. It is usually mild and self-limited, and it completely resolves after 2 to 3 days. Rotavirus is more common in children. A number of other microorganisms may cause acute diarrhea. These include *Salmonella, Shigella, Vibrio* species, *Campylobacter jejuni, Clostridium difficile* and *perfringens, E. coli, Yersinia enterocolitica, Bacillus cereus, Giardia lamblia, Entamoeba histolytica, Strongyloides,* and *Cryptosporidium. Staphylococcus aureus* "food poisoning" is primarily associated with nausea and vomiting, although occasionally diarrhea is prominent. Chemical intoxicants have the shortest incubation periods, which can begin minutes after ingestion of the contaminated water or food. Heavy metals, mushroom poisons, fish poisons (ciguatoxin, scombrotoxin), and shellfish poisons, which include a paralytic shellfish toxin and neurotoxic shellfish toxins, may cause acute vomiting and diarrhea. Diarrhea may also be a symptom of botulism.

Enterotoxin (both heat-stable and heat-labile) producing *E. coli* is the most common cause of traveler's diarrhea. *Salmonella* gastroenteritis occurs world-wide and is the most common cause of outbreaks of food-associated diarrhea. *Campylobacter* is a leading cause of bacterial diarrhea in the United States. *Vibrio parahaemolyticus* may cause diarrhea through ingestion of raw or poorly cooked seafood.

HISTORY AND PHYSICAL EXAMINATION

The initial evaluation in the emergency department should emphasize the history (Table 1). The duration of symptoms is helpful in distinguishing acute (0 to 10 days) from chronic diarrhea. Acute diarrhea is usually associated with ingestion of an infectious agent or a toxic substance, whereas chronic diarrhea may be a manifestation of a serious systemic process or may be functional in origin.

The presence of blood mixed with stool is another historical point that may be helpful in evaluating patients with diarrhea. Blood may represent an inflammatory process associated with infectious diarrhea or with chronic inflammatory or neoplastic bowel disease.

Fever, anorexia, and malaise can accompany both acute and chronic diarrheal illness. In acute diarrhea, the symptoms are of short duration; persistence of systemic symptoms and weight loss may indicate that a systemic

disease is responsible (such as Crohn's disease or chronic ulcerative colitis).

A food and drink history should be obtained, with particular attention to recent food and water ingestion or consumption of new, unusual, or earlier prepared foods, and whether any other members of the family or community have been affected with the same symptoms.

The travel history is of utmost importance when evaluating patients with diarrhea; 30 to 80 percent of travelers get diarrhea and nearly half of them become ill during the first 2 weeks of travel. Some patients become ill shortly after returning home if the trip has been short. Patients should be asked not only about travel to exotic foreign places, but also about out-of-state trips or about drinking from natural streams. For example, *Giardia* is prevalent in clear Rocky Mountain streams.

The volume of stool should be quantitated. Large volumes usually indicate small bowel disease; frequent smaller diarrheal stools are seen with left colon and rectal problems.

Because many drugs can cause diarrhea, all of the patient's medicines should be reviewed. Laxative abuse often results in acute or chronic diarrhea by causing local irritation. Pseudomembranous enterocolitis caused by *Clostridium difficile* is related to antibiotic treatment within the previous 3 to 4 weeks. Antihypertensive drugs (including methyldopa and propranolol), thyroid preparations, digitalis, quinidine, antimetabolites, colchicine, potassium supplements, anticoagulants, radiation therapy, and ethyl alchohol consumption may all produce diarrhea.

If the etiology is still unclear, the possibility of emotional stress may be discussed. All other causes should be excluded before acute diarrheal disease is attributed to emotional factors.

Neurological symptoms suggest a poison or toxin is involved. If the patient is immunosuppressed, the diarrhea may be due to many causes. However, some are unique, such as adenovirus in patients who have received bone marrow transplants, and cryptosporidia in patients with AIDS.

The physical examination is not usually helpful in establishing an etiologic factor, but can offer assistance in patient management. Signs of dehydration such as postural hypotension, tachycardia, poor skin turgor, dry mucous membranes, and mental lethargy (which may be a manifestation of an electrolyte imbalance) should all be assessed and documented. Fever and abdominal tenderness are nonspecific findings and can occur with acute or chronic diarrhea. A rectal examination should always be performed to determine if blood or tumor is present.

DIAGNOSTIC TESTS

Most patients with acute diarrhea do not seek medical care. If a patient has had diarrhea for more than 24 hours, has fever, or is dehydrated, or if a common source outbreak is suggested, laboratory investigation is needed (Table 2).

The most useful diagnostic test is the fecal leukocyte stain. This is performed by placing a fresh stool speci-

TABLE 1 Elements of History of Patients with Adult Infectious Diarrhea

Duration of symptoms

Presence of blood

Association with systemic symptoms

Food intake

Family/community outbreak

Travel away from home

Drug history

Neurologic symptoms

Association with emotional stress

Immunosuppressed states

TABLE 2 Diagnostic Tests for Patients with Adult Infectious Diarrhea

Stool examinations for
  Leukocytosis
  Blood
  Culture
  Ova, cysts, parasites
  C. difficile toxin
Blood studies
  CBC
  Electrolytes
  Creatinine/BUN

men or rectal swab onto a glass slide and staining one minute with methylene blue. The presence of polymorphonuclear cells indicates inflammation of the mucosal surfaces by invasive bacteria, *C. difficile* toxin, parasites, or an inflammatory systemic disease. The fecal leukocyte prep, in conjunction with the establishment of the duration of the illness, is helpful in diagnosis (Fig. 1). If the fecal leukocyte prep is positive, the stool should be cultured for *Salmonella, Shigella,* and *Campylobacter* and examined for parasites. Tests for *C. difficile* toxin should be performed if the patient has received antibiotic therapy within 3 weeks of onset of diarrhea.

The presence of blood in the stool also indicates an inflammatory process; however, it is also nonspecific and can be caused by gastrointestinal neoplasms, ischemic

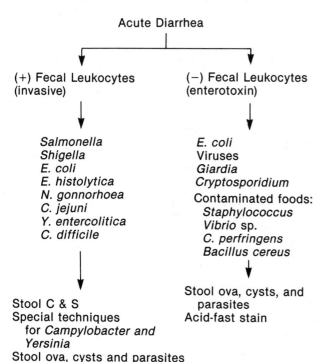

Acute Diarrhea

(+) Fecal Leukocytes (invasive)

(−) Fecal Leukocytes (enterotoxin)

Salmonella
Shigella
E. coli
E. histolytica
N. gonnorhoea
C. jejuni
Y. entercolitica
C. difficile

E. coli
Viruses
Giardia
Cryptosporidium
Contaminated foods:
  Staphylococcus
  Vibrio sp.
  C. perfringens
  Bacillus cereus

Stool C & S
Special techniques for *Campylobacter* and *Yersinia*
Stool ova, cysts and parasites
C. difficile toxins

Stool ova, cysts, and parasites
Acid-fast stain

Figure 1 Diagnosis of acute diarrhea.

damage, and heavy metal poisoning. Blood can be detected by guaiac. Viruses and toxin-mediated diarrheal disease are not characterized by bloody stools and should not be included in the differential diagnosis of causative agents. It is often helpful if these patients are further classified according to the presence of systemic illness (Table 3).

A complete blood count usually is not necessary in uncomplicated cases, but should be done if the patient is ill enough to require emergency care. Eosinophilia suggests *Strongyloides* or allergy as a cause of the diarrhea.

A standard electrolyte and renal function profile is helpful in the treatment of patients with dehydration, lethargy, or mental status changes.

MANAGEMENT

The mainstays of therapy are fluid replacement and symptomatic relief. Some patients require specific antibiotic therapy, but most have spontaneous resolution of their symptoms with rehydration alone.

Fluids are the most important aspect of therapy for all types of diarrhea, and patients should be instructed to force fluids. Liquids with salt added, soft drinks, tea, citrus juices, and commercial preparations such as Gatorade are helpful in the replacement of NaC1 and water. Oral glucose-saline solutions may be needed in more severely ill patients (Table 4). In patients who are markedly dehydrated, intravenous replacement with lactated Ringer's solution or its equivalent is required.

The antisecretory agent bismuth subsalicylate (Pepto-Bismol) has been shown to decrease the number of stools and other symptoms. The recommended dose is 30 ml every 30 minutes for 8 doses or until diarrhea stops. Patients should be forewarned that the stools will turn black and that this is harmless. The more convenient tablet form is also available. The popular kaolin and pectate mix-

TABLE 3 Presence of Blood in Stool

Systemically Ill
  Shigella
  Ulcerative colitis
  Amebiasis
  Ischemic bowel
Nonsystemically Ill
  Ulcerative proctitis
  Diverticulosis
  Polyps
  Carcinoma
  Coagulative disorders
  Campylobacter
  Yersinia

TABLE 4 Suggested Replacement Solutions

8 oz water with ¼ teaspoon bicarbonate of soda
8 oz fruit juice with ½ teaspoon honey or corn syrup and pinch of table salt
World Health Organization recommends 90 mEq/liter sodium, 20 mEq/liter potassium, and 110 mEq/liter glucose

tures (Kaopectate) produce a more formed stool, but do not significantly ameliorate infectious diarrhea.

Opiates are commonly prescribed to patients with diarrhea. However, all attemps to avoid these drugs should be made. Diphenoxylate (Lomotil) and loperamide (Imodium) delay intestinal motility and decrease stool frequency; however, they should not be used in patients with suspected *Shigella, Salmonella,* or *C. difficile* diarrhea because there is evidence that they lengthen the duration of illness and that toxic megacolon may result. Loperamide but not diphenoxylate is useful in treating traveler's diarrhea.

SPECIFIC TREATMENT

Antimicrobial treatment should be avoided for acute diarrhea unless the etiologic agent is *Giardia, E. histolytica,* or a severe case of presumed *Shigella* or *Salmonella*. Immunocompromised patients are more likely to benefit from antibiotic treatment for *Salmonella, Shigella,* and *Campylobacter* diarrheas.

Empiric antimicrobial therapy may be instituted in patients with diarrhea and fecal leukocytes who are immunocompromised or who have fever or leukocytosis. Certain invasive bacterial and parasitic diseases should also be treated if the etiologic agent has been demonstrated (Table 5).

Shigellosis should be treated with trimethoprim-sulfamethoxazole unless the patient is glucose 6-phosphate dehydrogenase (G6PD) deficient or is allergic to either agent. Doxycycline is an alternative. *Campylobacter* diarrhea has been successfully treated with erythromycin. Doxycycline is an alternative. The treatment of Salmonella enteritis is usually supportive only, but trimethoprim-sulfamethoxazole or amoxicillin may be used.

Giardia should be treated with quinacrine hydrochloride (Atabrine) or metronidazole. *Entamoebae histolytica* dysentery is treated with metronidazole. The emergence of *cryptosporidia* as an enteric pathogen has led to attempts at treatment with spiramycin in immunocompromised hosts, especially those with AIDS, but this has not benefited most patients.

TABLE 5   Treatment of Diarrhea Based on Etiologic Agent

Agent	Treatment
Salmonella	None or Trimethoprim–sulfamethoxazole, 1 double strength tablet PO every 12 hours for 5 days or Amoxicillin, 500 mg PO every 8 hours for 5 days
Shigella	Trimethoprim–sulfamethoxazole, 1 double strength tablet PO every 12 hours or Doxycycline, 100 mg PO every 12 hours for 5 days
Campylobacter	None or Erythromycin, 500 mg PO every 6 hours for 5 days or Doxycycline, 100 mg PO every 12 hours for 5 days
C. difficile	Metronidazole, 250 mg PO every 8 hours for 10 days or Vancomycin, 125 mg PO every 6 hours for 10 days
Giardia	Quinacrine hydrochloride (Atabrine), 100 mg PO every 8 hours for 7 days or Metronidazole, 250 mg PO every 8 hours for 10 days
E. histolytica	Metronidazole, 750 mg PO every 8 hours for 10 days Extraintestinal: Metronidazole 750 mg PO every 8 hours for 10 days
Strongyloides stercoralis	Thiabendazole, 25 mg/kg PO b.i.d. for 2 days
Cryptosporidium	Spiramycin, 1 g PO t.i.d. for 21 days

Patients who have developed antibiotic-associated diarrhea or pseudomembranous enterocolitis should no longer receive the initial antibiotic and should be treated with metronidazole. Patients should be warned of the possibility of a disulfiram (Antabuse-like) effect.

Most immunocompetent patients respond well to supportive care and under appropriate circumstances antibiotics with resolution of diarrhea and systemic symptoms.

Patients with diarrhea who usually require hospitalization for at least 24 hours include those with the problems listed in Table 6.

DISPOSITION

Most patients respond well to supportive care and antibiotics if needed, and can be managed well as outpatients. The indications for hospitalization are listed in Table 6.

Patient follow-up may be accomplished by telephone if cultures identify a pathogen. Following antimicrobial therapy, test of cure cultures or examination for ova, cysts, and parasites should be obtained by the patient's local physician. Local public health authorities should be informed if a food or waterborne outbreak is suspected.

TABLE 6 Indications for Hospitalization of Patients With Diarrhea

Advanced age, debilitation, or dehydration

Insulin-dependent diabetes

Chronic renal failure

Significant cardiac arrhythmias

Signs of systemic involvement and inflammation (increased peripheral WBC with increased immature forms)

Large volume of rectal bleeding

Immunocompromised state

Poor home situation where adequate fluid replacement and observation are not possible

SUGGESTED READING

NIH Consensus Development Conference Statement. Traveler's diarrhea. U.S. Department of Health and Human Services, Bethesda, Maryland, Vol. 5, No. 8, 1985.

Fekety R. Recent advances in management of bacterial diarrhea. Rev Infect Dis 1983, 5(2):246–257.

Hailey FJ, Newsom JH. Evaluation of bismuth subsalicylate in relieving symptoms of indigestion. Arch Intern Med 1984, 144:269–272.

Harres JG, Dupont AC, Hornick RB. Fecal leukocytes in diarrheal illness. Ann Intern Med 1972, 76:697–703.

Radetsky M. Laboratory evaluation of acute diarrhea. Pediatr Infect Dis 1986, 5(2):230–238.

BILIARY TRACT DISEASE

RICHARD A. CRASS, M.D.

The vast majority of cases of biliary tract disease are caused by gallstones. Approximately 75 percent of gallstones are predominantly cholesterol stones and 25 percent are relatively pure pigment stones. Pigment stones are frequently found in patients with increased pigment load in the bile, such as in patients with one of the hemolytic anemias or with intrahepatic stasis of bile. Since a large number of upper gastrointestinal inflammatory conditions can mimic the signs and symptoms of biliary tract disease and only approximately 15 percent of stones are radiopaque on plain abdominal films, special imaging studies are usually indicated to rule out the presence of biliary tract disease.

CHOLELITHIASIS

Gallstones in the gallbladder are most frequently asymptomatic, but they can result in two general symptom complexes, biliary colic and acute cholecystitis, Biliary colic is caused by the gallbladder's contracting after a meal against a partially obstructing gallstone, resulting in stretch of the gallbladder wall and visceral pain.

This pain, either mild or severe, usually occurs in the right upper quadrant or epigastrium. Acute cholecystitis is generally a febrile illness with signs of right upper quadrant peritonitis or right upper quadrant inflammation on physical examination, coupled with leukocytosis and frequent nausea and vomiting. In both presentations the differential diagnosis includes pancreatitis, peptic ulcer disease, hepatitis, gastroenteritis, and reflux esophagitis. If diagnosis of biliary tract disease is made on clinical grounds alone, at least a 50 percent error rate will result. The only time that an unequivocal diagnosis of acute cholecystitis can be made on clinical grounds alone is in the unusual case in which a tender gallbladder is palpable.

As outlined in Table 1, the most useful study for evaluation of a patient with suspected biliary colic is either *ultrasonography* or an *oral cholecystogram*. The oral cholecystogram shows positive findings if the gallbladder is visualized and the stones are outlined, or if there is nonvisualization of the gallbladder on repeat dose. Nonvisualization suggests chronic cholecystitis with inflammation of the gallbladder wall, which prevents the normal concentration of the dye in the gallbladder. In patients with mild to moderate pain and a typical history of biliary colic, these studies can be obtained on an outpatient basis.

The two studies most useful in making the diagnosis of acute cholecystitis are *ultrasonography* and the *TcHIDA radionuclide scan*. The TcHIDA scan is positive if the liver, bile duct, and duodenum are imaged but there is no visualization of the gallbladder, indicating cystic duct

TABLE 1 Biliary Diseases Accurately Detected by Various Imaging Tests

Imaging Study	Acute Cholecystitis	Biliary Colic	Ductal Dilatation	Hepatic Lesions	Specialized Anatomic Information
Oral cholecystogram		X			
Sonogram	X	X	X	X	
TcHIDA scan	X			X	
Intravenous cholangiogram*	X				X
Endoscopic retrograde cholangiopancreatography					X
Transhepatic cholangiogram					X

*Seldom indicated because of frequent hypersensitivity reactions.

obstruction, which is present in almost all cases of acute cholecystitis. The same information is available on intravenous cholangiograms, which were previously frequently performed but are seldom indicated currently in view of the high rate of hypersensitivity reactions to the intravenous contrast material.

Laboratory studies helpful in the patient with biliary colic or acute cholecystitis are a complete blood count, liver function studies, and a serum amylase concentration. Acute cholecystitis can cause a slight increase in the serum bilirubin level along with slight transaminase elevations.

Treatment of biliary colic in any patient who is considered a reasonable surgical risk consists of cholecystectomy. Concerns about the necessity of taking long-term medication, along with the risk of toxicity, limit the role of gallstone *dissolution therapy* with chenodeoxycholic acid to very few patients.

Patients with acute cholecystitis typically are ill enough to warrant hospitalization. Aside from the patient with extremely toxic symptoms, it is best to withhold antibiotics at first until other differential diagnoses are excluded. Treatment of acute cholecystitis consists of cholecystectomy at the earliest convenient time. Generally such patients are treated perioperatively with an antibiotic covering gram-negative organisms (cefamandole nafate, 1 g every 6 hours, and cefoxitin sodium, 2 g every 6 hours intravenously, two reasonable choices). In the patient who is a prohibitive operative risk, treatment with antibiotics alone will frequently get the patient over the acute cholecystitis, so that the decision to operate can be deferred. In the operative risk patient who does not respond to antibiotics, cholecystostomy under local anesthesia is an option.

CHOLEDOCHOLITHIASIS

Most stones that pass through the cystic duct into the common duct or that form primarily in the bile ducts pass through the ampulla of Vater into the small bowel without incident. Stones can, however, lodge at the ampulla, causing biliary obstruction. This will be indicated either by uncomplicated obstructive jaundice or, if bacteria are present in the bile, by cholangitis. Additionally, stones either passing through, lodging at the ampulla, or lodging in and dislodging from the ampulla can result in gallstone pancreatitis. In any patient presenting with *jaundice*, obstruction of the bile duct must be ruled out. In addition to full liver function tests, the best initial study to obtain in such patients is a sonogram. Sonography is extremely sensitive in demonstrating dilatation of intrahepatic ducts, and with more modern equipment the common bile duct is almost always imaged. Every patient with obstructive jaundice has dilatation of the intrahepatic ducts drugs, unless there is fibrosis of the liver preventing such dilatation. Since any patient with recent onset of jaundice is at risk for development of cholangitis (a very serious infection), admission and work-up studies in the hospital are appropriate.

If bacteria are present in the bile, and the bile duct is obstructed, *cholangitis* ensues. The majority (75 percent) of patients with cholangitis present with all three elements of Charcot's triad, namely, jaundice, fever, and right upper quadrant pain. All such patients should be started on antibiotics and intravenous fluids. The spectrum of severity of cholangitis ranges from a mild form all the way to suppurative cholangitis, which is diagnosed by the presence of overwhelming systemic sepsis with hypotension and, usually, mental confusion. Suppurative cholangitis is a bona fide surgical emergency, and many patients cannot be stabilized until the bile duct is surgically drained. Blood for cultures should be drawn, and early surgical consultation should be obtained in any patient suspected of having cholangitis. Urgent sonograms should be obtained to document the presence or absence of dilated intrahepatic ducts. In the milder forms of cholangitis, treatment with antibiotics and work-up studies of the biliary tree at a more leisurely pace, including perhaps endoscopic retrograde cholangiopancreatography or transhepatic cholangiography or both, with a possible addition of computed tomographic scanning, are appropriate.

The presentation of patients with *gallstone pancreatitis* is similar to that of patients with the more common alcoholic pancreatitis. Any patient with first-time pancreatitis who presents with typical upper gastric pain radiating into the back and elevated serum amylase levels should have a sonogram at some point during hospitalization to exclude the possibility of gallstones being present in the gallbladder. In addition to the usual supportive treatment for pancreatitis, patients with gallstones and pancreatitis should have cholecystectomy during their hospitalization to decrease the risk of recurrent bouts of gallstone pancreatitis, which runs as high as 40 percent.

MISCELLANEOUS BILIARY CONDITIONS

In addition to the more common gallstone-related cholelithiasis and choledocholithiasis, other conditions can cause presenting symptoms of abdominal pain, cholangitis, and jaundice not involving gallstones. These conditions include oriental cholangitis, tumors of the pancreas and biliary tree, congenital conditions, sclerosing cholangitis, and parasitic infections of the biliary tree. Using the same approach as outlined for gallstone-related biliary tract disease, these conditions sort themselves out during the patient's hospitalization. A special case in the differential diagnosis that deserves comment is amebic abscess of the liver. These patients present very similarly to those with acute cholecystitis but on the sonogram or TcHIDA scan, they are found to have a filling defect in the liver. Appropriate management of such patients entails documentation of extraluminal amebic disease by amebic precipitins, and while this is pending, treatment with metronidazole hydrochloride (loading dose 15 mg per kilogram infused over 1 hour intravenously, followed by 7.5 mg per kilogram infused over 1 hour every 6 hours intravenously).

SUGGESTED READING

Blumgart LH. The biliary tract. New York: Churchill Livingstone Inc, 1982.

Cohen S, Soloway RD. Gallstones. New York: Churchill Livingstone, 1985.

Matolo NM. Symposium on biliary tract disease. Surg Clin North Am 1981; 61:763.

Way LW: Biliary tract. In: Way LW, ed. Current surgical diagnosis and treatment. Los Altos, California: Lange, 1985.

HEPATITIS

SHALOM Z. HIRSCHMAN, M.D.

For the purposes of this discussion, hepatitis is defined as the sudden onset of malaise, weakness, anorexia, intermittent nausea and vomiting, and vague dull right upper quadrant abdominal pain, usually followed within 1 week by the onset of jaundice or dark urine or both. While this definition may describe a typical case of viral hepatitis, it must be appreciated that it represents the minority of cases of viral hepatitis. Indeed, viral hepatitis is best characterized by the variability of the clinical manifestations. Icteric cases probably represent no more than 20 to 50 percent of hepatitis virus infections; many infections are subclinical. Therefore, the spectrum of viral hepatitis includes the subclinical or inapparent, anicteric but symptomatic, icteric, and fulminant. Liver dysfunction may also be a manifestation of bacteremia, such as with *Bacteroides* species, local infections such as hepatic abscess or cholangitis, the effects of hepatotoxins such as alcohol, chloroform, and carbon tetrachloride, reactions to drugs such as isoniazid, congestive heart failure, especially right ventricular failure, and acute hemolytic anemia. Autoimmune hepatitis, seen especially in young women, can manifest with findings of acute hepatitis, hyperglobulinemia, and hemolytic anemia. Therefore, the most important requisite for proper therapy is to establish the cause of the liver dysfunction (Table 1).

THE HEPATOTROPIC VIRUSES

The most frequent cause of acute hepatic dysfunction is infection with hepatotropic viruses. Although many viruses (including the Epstein-Barr virus, cytomegalovirus, and herpes simplex virus) can infect the liver, it is the three classes of hepatotropic viruses that are of main concern as causes of acute hepatitis (Table 2). These include the hepatitis A virus (HAV), the cause of infectious or short incubation period hepatitis, the hepatitis B virus (HBV) the cause of serum or long incubation hepatitis, and the non-A, non-B hepatitis viruses that at present are the major causes of post-transfusion hepatitis in the United States.

The hepatitis A virus is an enterovirus, related to the picorna-viruses, that is usually transmitted by the fecal-oral route. HAV is the most common cause of acute hepatitis, responsible for 38 percent of reported cases in the United States. Outbreaks of food and water-borne cases of hepatitis are caused by HAV. Recent HAV infection can be diagnosed by finding IgM antibodies to HAV in serum.

The hepatitis B virus is usually transmitted parenterally via blood inoculation. Groups at high risk of infection include intravenous drug abusers, homosexuals, patients and staff in renal dialysis and oncology units, heterosexual contacts of patients with active viral infection, and neonates born to mothers with active infections. A characteristic prodrome of a serum sickness-like syndrome consisting of an urticarial rash, arthralgias and rarely arthritis, and fever may precede the onset of acute hepatitis B, especially in adults; papular acrodermatitis at the onset of symptoms is seen more commonly in children.

TABLE 1 Representative Causes of Hepatitis

Infection or Other Cause	Agent	Diagnosis	Therapy
Viral	Hepatitis A virus	Serologic	Supportive
	Hepatitis B virus	Serologic	
	Non-A, non-B	By exclusion	
	Cytomegalovirus	Serologic, virus isolation	
	Epstein-Barr virus	Serologic, heterophil antibody	
	Rubeola (in adults)	Serologic	
Coxiella	Coxiella burnetii (Q fever)	Serologic	Tetracycline
Spirochetal	Treponema pallidum (Syphilis)	Serologic	Penicillin (tetracycline if penicillin-allergic)
	Leptospira interrogans, serovar, ictero-haemorrhagiae	Serologic	
Bacterial	Salmonella, Brucella,	Isolation from cultures	Antimicrobial therapy
	Listeria monocytogenes	Serologic	
	Mycobacterium tuberculosis		
Parasitic	Schistosoma (schistosomeasis)	Eggs in feces	Chemotherapy
	Leishmania donovani (kalazar)	Liver biopsy, rectal biopsy (schistosomes)	
	Clonorchis sinensis (liver fluke)		
Autoimmune	Unknown	Hyperglobulinemia, antinuclear antibody, hemolytic anemia, liver biopsy	Corticosteroids
Hypersensitivity reactions	Sulfonamides, phenylbutazone	History, rechallenge	Supportive, remove drug, give corticosteroids if severe
Toxic reactions	Isoniazid, phosphorus carbon tetrachloride, ethanol	History	Supportive, remove toxic agent

TABLE 2 The Hepatotropic Viruses

Characteristics	Hepatitis A	Hepatitis B	Non-A, Non-B
Virus	(Infectious, epidemic) RNA genome, 27-nm particle	(Serum) DNA genome, 42-nm particle with 27-nm nucleocapsid	Not known
Transmission	Fecal-oral	Via patient's blood, sexual contact, maternal-fetal	Via patient's blood
Incubation period	15–45 days	60–180 days	40–60 days
Clinical onset	Acute	Insidious	Insidious
Chronic infection	No	About 10%	About 10%
Acute delta virus infection	No	Yes	No

Acute infection with HBV can be followed by a chronic phase often resulting in cirrhosis. Serologic tests used for the diagnosis of HBV infection as listed in Table 3. In areas of the world where HBV infection is endemic and contracted at an early age, hepatocellular carcinoma is an important complication. HBV infection can also be complicated by immune-complex deposition manifested by glomerulonephritis and polyarteritis nodosa.

Hepatitis delta virus (HDV), is an RNA-containing virus that requires the hepatitis B virus for replication.

TABLE 3 Patterns of Serologic Markers in Hepatitis B Virus Infection

Phase of Infection	Serologic Markers					
	HBsAg	HBcAg	HBeAg	anti-HBs	anti-HBc	anti-HBe
Presymptomatic or early acute hepatitis B	+	−	−	−	−	−
Early symptomatic acute hepatitis B	+	±	±	−	−	−
Symptomatic acute hepatitis B	+	±	±	−	+(IgM)	±
Recovery (window period)	−	−	−	−	+(IgM)	−
Recovery from infection	−	−	−	+	+(IgG)	±
Chronic hepatitis B	+	±	±	±	+(IgG;IgM)	±
Chronic hepatitis B (low level carrier state)	−	−	−	−	+(IgG)	−
Long after recovery or after immunization with vaccine	−	−	−	+	−	−

Key: HBsAG, hepatitis B surface antigen; HBcAg, hepatitis B core antigen; HBeAg, hepatitis B e antigen; anti-HBs, antibody to HBsAg; anti-HBc, antibody to HBcAg; anti-HBe, antibody to HBeAg.

+ = present; − = absent; ± = may or may not be present.

Delta virus infection can occur concomitantly with acute HBV infection or may complicate chronic hepatitis B infection, resulting in acute hepatic manifestations in the patient with chronic hepatitis. HBV is endemic in the Mediterranean countries, such as Italy and Greece, but has been reported increasingly in the United States in recent years, especially among intravenous drug abusers and homosexual males.

The non-A, non-B hepatitis viruses have not been well characterized. These viruses now account for 95 percent of post-transfusion hepatitis in the United States. The manifestations of infection with these viruses are more like those of hepatitis B than hepatitis A; chronic infection does occur.

Generally, hepatitis A virus infection is mild and followed by complete recovery; the mortality rate is lower than 0.5 percent. Hepatitis B virus and non-A, non-B hepatitis infections are more severe diseases with a mortality rate of 1 to 3 percent. Acute non-A, non-B hepatitis can become chronic and lead to chronic active hepatitis and cirrhosis. Acute hepatitis B infection can lead to fulminant hepatitis. Chronic infection ensues in 10 percent of cases, half of which develop chronic active hepatitis that may result in cirrhosis. Chronic hepatitis B infection also can be complicated by the immune complex-mediated diseases mentioned previously.

THERAPEUTIC APPROACHES

The approach to therapy of the patient with manifestations of hepatitis depends on the causative factors (Table 4). The history is most important and should include questions aimed to determine exposure to hepatotoxic chemicals in the home or the work place; the use of hepatotoxic drugs; exposure to *Entamoeba histolytica* in travel or restaurants; a history of cholelithiasis that may point to cholangitis; factors that may point to bacteremia such as

a history of diverticulitis; a history of heart disease that may point to congestive heart failure; or cough that may point to legionnaire's disease. When there is any doubt as to the diagnosis of acute viral hepatitis and the patient is febrile, blood should be drawn for cultures. A sonogram or computed tomographic scan of the abdomen may be helpful in pointing to the presence of hepatic abscess. It is important to try to determine whether there is a history of ethanol ingestion. It is imperative to establish whether immediately treatable causes of hepatitis are present.

There is no specific *therapy* for acute viral hepatitis. Indeed, most patients do not require hospitalization. During the symptomatic period, bed rest may be required because of patient fatigue and malaise. The amount of activity should be tailored to the patient's feelings of well being and physical ability. It appears advisable to prohibit alcohol intake during the acute phase. The diet should be well balanced and nutritious. Patients may be anorectic, and frequent small feedings of a low-fat, high carbohydrate diet may be helpful. If feedings cannot be tolerated, intravenous replacement of fluid, electrolytes, and glucose may be necessary. The patient's normal diet may be resumed when the anorexia abates.

TABLE 4 Clinical Appraisal of Patient with Hepatitis

Gather evidence of liver infection: fever, jaundice, hepatomegaly, and right upper quadrant abdominal pain are cardinal features.

Plan diagnostic investigation to determine presence of gallbladder and biliary tract infection.

Determine cause of liver injury so as to provide appropriate therapy and prevention.

Differentiate between acute and chronic hepatitis.

Determine presence of infiltrative disease.

Differentiate between abscess and tumor in space-occupying lesion.

There has been no demonstrated beneficial effect of corticosteroids, antimicrobial agents, or immune globulin in the treatment of acute viral hepatitis. Corticosteroids appear to be deleterious when given to patients with acute hepatitis B infection.

The hazardous complication of greatest concern in acute viral hepatitis is that of *fulminant viral infection with liver failure*. In some patients the progression of fulminant hepatitis is rapid, with only a few days intervening between the onset of symptoms of acute hepatitis and the deepening of jaundice followed by hepatic coma. On the other hand, the appearance of fulminant hepatitis may be insidious, with a slow worsening of anorexia, nausea, and jaundice, followed by a week of gradual clinical deterioration before onset of coma. Fulminant viral hepatitis leads to hypoprothrombinemia and hepatic encephalopathy (Tables 5 and 6). The prothrombin time may be prolonged in patients with even mild acute viral hepatitis. Vitamin K in doses of 1 to 5 mg may be administered intramuscularly. In patients with fulminant viral hepatitis, coagulation disorders require the use of fresh frozen plasma for correction. It is important to monitor such patients for gastrointestinal bleeding. Antacid therapy or cimetidine at a dose of 300 to 500 mg intravenously every 6 hours may help prevent upper gastrointestinal bleeding.

The often subtle signs and symptoms of incipient hepatic encephalopathy must be recognized. The patient may be restless, may show slight changes in personality, and may complain of nightmares. Some patients become physically aggressive. The major objective of therapy is to reduce the amount of nitrogenous products entering the portal circulation; these products produce cerebral dysfunction because they are not detoxified and removed by the failing liver. Hepatic coma is usually preceded by rapid clinical deterioration, elevated prothrombin time, rising arterial blood ammonia concentrations, leukocytosis, and a shrinking liver. The management of impending coma caused by hepatic encephalopathy includes a low-protein diet (15 to 30 g per day), oral laxatives such as Milk of Magnesia or castor oil or enemas to clean the bowel and remove nitrogenous wastes, and the use of oral neomycin, 1 to 1.5 g every 6 hours, to suppress intestinal bacterial proliferation (Table 7). In the patient with coma, protein intake is eliminated. High-colonic enemas with tap water or saline solutions are administered every 4 to 6 hours, being careful to monitor fluid and electrolyte balance. In order to achieve cleansing of the entire colon, including the cecum, it is useful to first place the patient in the left lateral decubitus position to allow the

TABLE 5 Therapeutic Approach to the Patient with Viral Hepatitis

Maintain fluid and electrolyte balance.
Maintain nutritional needs, including daily vitamin requirements.
Correct bleeding disorders.
Monitor for signs of encephalopathy.
If encephalopathy is present, cleanse bowel and reduce protein intake.

TABLE 6 Management of Acute Hepatitis

Diet	When, anorectic with frequent vomiting, give IV fluids. Frequent small feedings of high-carbohydrate diet when anorectic; otherwise normal diet.
Activity	Bed rest during acute symptoms, otherwise activity ad libitum.
Hospitalization	Reserved for very ill patient with bilirubin level >10 mg per 100 ml and alanine aminotransferase (SGOT) >2,000 Karmen units
Bleeding	Vitamin K IM (1–5 mg), cimetidine 300 to 500 mg PO or IV q6h antacids.

enema fluid to reach the splenic flexure, and then to roll the patient to the right lateral decubitus position, with the head and shoulders slightly elevated to allow irrigation of the right side of the colon. If the patient cannot swallow, or if a nasogastric tube is not in place, neomycin can be included in colonic irrigation fluid at concentrations of 1 g per liter; under these conditions, the total dose of neomycin should not be higher than 4 g per day.

In recent years, lactulose in an oral dose of 20 to 30 g 3 to 4 times per day has been used for the treatment of hepatic encephalopathy. Lactulose is a cathartic but may have other beneficial actions in the treatment of hepatic encephalopathy, such as acidification of the stool, thus pulling ammonia and other toxic bioamines from the blood into the lumen of the bowel.

In addition to the specific measures just outlined, it is important to pay careful attention to fluid and electrolyte balance, acid-base disturbances, respiratory function, and skin care in these patients. They also should be monitored carefully for signs of supervening infection in blood, urine, or lungs.

There is no good evidence that corticosteroids, arginine, glutamic acid, exchange transfusion, or L-dopa is useful in the treatment of hepatic coma.

PREVENTION

Another aspect of the treatment of viral hepatitis is the prevention of spread to the family and contacts of the patient. The highest concentration of HAV in feces occurs late in the incubation period and early in the prodromal phase and decreases rapidly once jaundice ap-

TABLE 7 Management of Fulminant Hepatitis with Liver Failure

Condition	Management
Bleeding	Vitamin K IM, fresh frozen plasma
Impending coma	Low protein diet (15–30 g/day), neomycin 1–1.5 g PO q6h, lactulose (30–60 ml in sorbitol q2–6h to achieve diarrhea)
Coma	Restrict protein intake, IV glucose for hypoglycemia, high colonic enemas (with neomycin 1 g/L, up to 4 g/day), maintain airway, monitor fluid and electrolyte balance

pears. Thus the patient is most infectious during the 2-week period before the onset of jaundice. Immune globulin (IG) administered before exposure or during the incubation period is protective against clinical illness with HAV. It is most effective when given early in the incubation period. Household and sexual contacts of patients with HAV infection should receive IG; the dose is 0.02 ml per kilogram intramuscularly. Depending upon the epidemiologic circumstances, IG administration may be considered for close contacts of the patient in classrooms and institutions for custodial care, in offices and factories, and in common source exposure from a food handler. The protection afforded by injection of IG should last for approximately 3 months.

Hepatitis B immune globulin (HBIG) is recommended for close family contacts, such as children and others sharing the same living quarters, and sexual contacts of patients with acute HBV infection. HBIG is administered at a dose of 5 ml intramuscularly and again 1 month later. This should be accompanied by administration of hepatitis B vaccine at a dose of 20 μg intramuscularly (given preferably in the deltoid areas) and repeated 1 month and 6 months later. The hepatitis B vaccine appears to be 90 percent effective. It has proved to be a safe vaccine with only minor side effects. Recent studies have shown that there is no risk of transmission of acquired immunodeficiency syndrome (AIDS) with either HBIG or the hepatitis B vaccine.

SUGGESTED READING

Centers for Disease Control. Immune globulins for protection against viral hepatitis. MMWR 1981; 30:423–428, 433–435.
Centers for Disease Control. Inactivated hepatitis B virus vaccine. MMWR 1982; 31:317–322, 327–328.
Hirschman SZ. Virologic, immunologic and clinical correlations in viral hepatitis. In: Weinstein L, Fields B, eds. Seminars in infectious diseases. Vol. II. Stratton New York: Intercontinental Medical Book Corp., 1979:48.
Hoofnagle JH. Acute hepatitis. In: Mandell GL, Douglas RG, Bennett JE, eds. Principles and practice of infectious diseases. New York: John Wiley and Sons, 1985:772.
Krugman S, Gocke DJ. Viral hepatitis. In: Smith LH, ed. Major problems in internal medicine. Philadelphia: WB Saunders, 1978:1.

ALCOHOLIC LIVER DISEASE

CHARLES S. LIEBER, M.D.
THERESA M. WORNER, M.D.

There are up to 15 million alcoholics in the United States. In addition, approximately two-thirds of the adult population uses alcohol on occasion, and about 12 percent can be defined as "heavy drinkers." Among the medical problems associated with alcoholism, hepatic disorders are at the forefront. The spectrum of alcoholic liver injury involves hepatic steatosis (fatty liver), early fibrosis (perivenular and perisinusoidal fibrosis), alcoholic hepatitis, and cirrhosis. Of all medical deaths attributable to alcoholism, 75 percent are the result of cirrhosis of the liver. In the United States, cirrhosis has overtaken diabetes as the fifth cause of death; in large urban areas, it has become the third cause of all deaths in the active group of 25 to 65 years. Early recognition of the alcoholic nature of many patients' complaints may lead to intervention at the initial stages of the disease prior to the medical or social disintegration of the patient and prior to the development of irreversible cirrhosis.

ALCOHOLISM

Essential of Diagnosis and Early Recognition of Alcoholism

The skid row alcoholic represents only 3 to 5 percent of the alcoholic population; the average alcoholic is a middle-class, blue-collar, or white-collar worker or housewife who comes for medical help for any of a variety of problems. He or she is likely to appear in a sober state, neatly dressed, and may be treated with an assortment of drugs aimed at controlling various symptoms, such as abdominal pain, "liver abnormalities," or "nervousness."

Using fairly stringent criteria for alcoholism (outlined below), this disorder is seen in 3 to 5 percent of the female and 5 to 10 percent of the adult male population. These should be distinguished from the percentage of people who are drinkers (90 percent of adults drink at some time during their lives with 65 percent or more drinking currently) and even from those individuals who have relatively isolated and temporary minor alcohol-related problems (e.g., arguments with friends or absence from work); such temporary problems are seen in up to 40 percent of males by the age of 40, the majority of whom do not go on to develop persistent alcoholism. The rate of alcoholism and alcohol-related problems is even higher in medical and surgical patients, with between 20 and 35 percent of them meeting the criteria for alcoholism.

To warrant a diagnosis of alcoholism, the individual must have developed physical dependence (as indicated by withdrawal symptoms) or psychological dependence (progression from the early warning signs to more severe and persistent alcohol-related difficulties) (Table 1). An individual is also labeled alcoholic if he or she has demonstrated a significant alcohol-related life problem, including a marital separation or divorce, multiple arrests, evidence that alcohol has harmed health, or a job loss or layoff related to drinking. The average sober, well-groomed, and functional alcoholic can present with any of a variety of psychological or physical complaints. None of these are diagnostic of alcoholism, but many are seen

TABLE 1 Diagnosis and Treatment of Alcoholism

	Alcoholism	*Alcohol Withdrawal*
Clinical signs	Alcohol on breath during examination, hepatomegaly	Tremulousness Anxiety Seizures Delirium tremens
Laboratory parameters	Blood alcohol 300 mg/dl Blood alcohol 150 mg/dl in nonintoxicated patient Unexplained MCV, GGTP increases	No specific abnormalities
Therapy	Abstinence Support groups (e.g., AA)	Benzodiazepines (PO or IV) Thiamine, parenteral Hydration for delirium tremens Phenothiazines contraindicated

at such an elevated rate in alcoholics that they must be viewed with suspicion.

The alcoholic may be recognized by the medical community when a pattern of mild abnormalities emerges. The early recognition of heavy drinking enables the detection and treatment of alcoholism prior to the onset of irreversible organ damage and severe social consequences. At present no test has been found that has optimal sensitivity and specificity, but several commonly available tests may alert the physician to the possibility of latent heavy drinking.

Perhaps the most obvious test for heavy drinking is the measurement of blood alcohol. Although it provides incontrovertible evidence of recent intake, it does not distinguish acute from chronic alcohol consumption. Furthermore, alcohol is rapidly metabolized and cleared from the blood over a period of several hours. Therefore, the level at any given time depends upon the amount consumed, the rate of absorption, the rate of metabolism, and the duration of abstinence. Unless an observed level is high or is present at an unusual time (see below), little can be inferred from this test with certainty.

A level of 300 mg per deciliter of ethanol (three times the level generally considered as evidence for driving while intoxicated) in the blood at any time is used as one definite criterion for the diagnosis of alcoholism. A level of 150 mg per deciliter in the absence of any gross signs of intoxication is also used as a criterion, since this indicates that tolerance has developed. The presence of alcohol on the breath on physical examination, a blood level of 100 mg per deciliter at the time of any medical appointment, and evidence of drinking in the morning have also been used as criteria of heavy drinking.

An increase in mean red blood cell volume may occur in the alcoholic through a variety of possible mechanisms, including folate deficiency, liver disease, and reticulocytosis. In addition, in many instances the macrocytosis is attributed to a possible "direct" effect of ethanol. An increase in MCV is observed frequently in populations of alcoholics; its ease of measurement by Coulter Counter has made its use routine. Following cessation of drinking, the MCV returns to normal only gradu-

ally, despite folate supplementation and institution of a nutritious diet. In fact, the changes persist beyond the life span of the average red blood cell. Furthermore, in patients who relapse, the MCV increases only slowly. Thus, it is not a good test for monitoring treatment success or relapse following treatment for alcoholism.

An increase in serum gamma glutamyl transpeptidase (GGTP) is regularly observed in more than 50 percent and in some studies in up to 80 to 90 percent of chronic heavy drinkers. This enzyme appears to be increased to a greater extent than other "liver" enzymes such as SGOT and GDH (glutamic dehydrogenase) by chronic alcohol consumption. The increase requires several weeks of heavy ethanol consumption and occurs progressively during this time period. GGTP, like other liver enzymes, may be increased by liver injury due to alcohol as well as other causes. In alcoholic populations the highest levels of GGTP are found among subjects who both actively consume alcohol and have severe liver injury. However, very high levels may be observed in patients with acute and chronic liver disease unrelated to alcohol. Thus, in populations with a high incidence of liver damage, such as drug addicts and general hospital populations, GGTP measurements are of limited value as a screening test.

Chronic alcohol consumption of even moderate proportions leads to an elevation in plasma high-density lipoproteins (HDL). Interest in this observation has been heightened by the fact that elevations in plasma HDL may be protective against coronary artery disease. However, other factors may modify HDL as well, including sex (females have higher levels), medications, exercise, genetics, and diet. Thus, variability of levels in different populations may be very large. Incidence of elevated HDL levels in alcoholics ranges from 20 to 66 percent.

Measurement of hemoglobin A_1 is now used extensively for the monitoring of average blood glucose in diabetics to assess degree of control of diabetes. It has recently been observed that alcoholics may also have elevated A_1 hemoglobin levels even in the absence of glucose intolerance. The elevation occurs over a period of weeks and is reversible within weeks following cessation of drinking. At present, the lack of specificity and sensitivity of the test makes its clinical application limited.

Alpha-amino-n-butyric acid (AANB) is a nonessential amino acid that was first observed to be increased in the plasma following chronic alcohol consumption in subhuman primates. Subsequently, it was demonstrated in humans that an increase in this amino acid occurs after chronic but not after acute ethanol administration. As with GGTP, AANB levels increase over a period of several weeks of drinking and decrease over approximately 1 week following abstinence. The increase in AANB produced by chronic alcohol consumption has been confirmed by several groups in animal models, but studies in human alcoholics have been less consistent, perhaps because of the many uncontrolled variables that may affect amino acids, such as nutritional and endocrine factors.

Alcoholism is sometimes suspected because of complications such as gastritis and pancreatitis. Psychiatric and emotional problems likely to be seen in the alcoholic include insomnia (since alcohol fragments the sleep and results in a restless night), impotence (related to both psychological factors and the direct effects of ethanol on the testes and hypothalamus), interpersonal problems, and depression. The psychological symptoms cannot be adequately treated or even properly evaluated while the patient continues to drink heavily. The usual alcoholic may present with a variety of nonspecific symptoms, and the underlying diagnosis of alcoholism must be made in order for the problems to be properly treated.

The most common diagnostic error is failure to consider the diagnosis. A history of alcohol consumption should be obtained in every patient. The major differential considerations of the early withdrawal syndrome are essential or familial tremor and early hepatic encephalopathy. Likewise, it is important to recognize that withdrawal signs may be present despite a positive blood alcohol test. The familial tremor usually begins in childhood and persists, despite prolonged abstinence. This tremor responds to treatment with propranolol. In early hepatic encephalopathy, additional findings may include drowsiness and asterixis. However, both an alcohol withdrawal tremor and early encephalopathy may be present in the same patient.

Therapy of Alcoholism

Pre-hospital

The main goal in the management of the alcoholic is the withdrawal of alcohol. Detoxification is most conveniently accomplished in an inpatient setting. Dealing with the alcoholism issue is often frustrating, but even limited success can have a major impact on the morbidity and mortality of the heavy drinkers. To that effect, the practicing physician should avail himself of the services of the various specialized units and self-help groups (for instance, AA) willing to tackle the root of the problem and to provide the patient with the support and follow-up needed to avoid relapses.

Detoxification

Withdrawal from alcohol may be manifest in a wide range of symptoms, and is further discussed in the chapter on *Alcohol Intoxication and Withdrawal*.

Fluid losses and correction of nutritional deficiencies when present should not be neglected. Treatment should be administered orally when possible. However, in the patient with frank delirium tremens, there may be extensive fluid losses (secondary to fever, agitation, or vomiting) that may require parenteral replacement with 5 to 6 L of fluid per day. Thiamine (100 mg) given intravenously or intramuscularly is recommended empirically, since severe thiamine deficiency can be precipitated by administration of intravenous glucose and may cause irreversible brain damage if uncorrected, and since thiamine administration is innocuous. Multivitamins, folate, and vitamin B_{12} are not needed unless there is clinical or biochemical evidence of a deficiency state, but because of their lack of toxicity, they can be given liberally. The same does not pertain to lipid-soluble vitamins such as vitamin A. Although depletion of hepatic levels of vitamin A is common in the alcoholic and may contribute to the liver damage, replenishment is complicated by enhanced susceptibility to the hepatic toxicity of vitamin A. Therefore, it is now recommended not to exceed a daily dose of 2,000 IU. Routine administration of magnesium is not recommended. Although alcohol withdrawal is frequently associated with low levels of serum magnesium, the decrease is usually transient, with a return to normal levels within 1 to 2 days of the withdrawal period.

ALCOHOL-DRUG INTERACTIONS

In addition to the minor transquilizers useful in the period of withdrawal, alcoholics may of course require treatment with various other drugs. Drug use in the alcoholic, however, is complicated by hepatic alterations of drug metabolism resulting from the microsomal induction following chronic ethanol consumption, the nonspecific effects of liver injury, or the acute interaction of ethanol with the metabolism of various drugs. Alcoholics, when sober, may display an increased tolerance to a variety of drugs, including commonly used sedatives, tranquilizers, anticoagulants, and hypoglycemic agents. To offset this effect, the dosage of the drug has to be increased. However, when liver damage is severe, reversal to normal or even decreased dosage is possible.

These patterns also pertain when ethanol is still present. Ethanol may compete with the metabolism of some drugs, thereby slowing their degradation and prolonging and enhancing their effects. The acute ingestion of ethanol in conjunction with administration of phenothiazines may result in competitive inhibition with decreased clearance of one or both drugs and enhanced sedative effects. Phenothiazines may also lower the threshold for post-withdrawal convulsions. In addition, hypotension, a side effet of these drugs, can be exacerbated by alcohol. Use of phenothiazines to control alcohol withdrawal can thus be hazardous. Tricyclic antidepressants also increase susceptibility to convulsions and should be administered cautiously during alcohol withdrawal. The tricyclic antidepressants are either synergistic or antagonistic to ethanol according to their ratio of sedative-stimulant activity. Since these drugs produce hypotension, they should be prescribed only for alcoholics who can be carefully monitored. The combination of these drugs with alcohol adversely affects motor skills, particularly driving.

The interaction of ethanol with barbiturates represents a particular danger. The lethal dose for barbiturates is nearly 50 percent lower in the presence of alcohol than it is when the drug is used alone. Blood levels of secobarbital or pentobarbital as low as 0.5 mg per deciliter combined with blood alcohol levels of 0.1 g per deciliter can cause death from respiratory depression. Thus, barbiturates should not be used in the treatment of alcoholism.

Acute intoxication does not solely affect drugs acting on the central nervous system. For instance, it reduces the metabolism of warfarin, leading to increased anticoagulant effects and the danger of hemorrhage. The combination causes blood warfarin levels to be higher than expected from a given dose. Chronic alcohol abuse, however, can enhance enzyme activity, leading to decreased anticoagulant effects (vide supra). Because the effects on prothrombin time can change with varying intake of alcohol, physicians need to monitor prothrombin times closely.

Thus, an alcoholic's previous history of alcohol abuse can be a key factor in prescribing decisions, because alcoholics, when sober, need doses higher than those required by nondrinkers to achieve therapeutic levels of certain drugs, such as warfarin, phenytoin, and tolbutamide, whereas the opposite pertains if an episode of acute drinking is superimposed upon chronic intake or if severe liver damage is present.

ALCOHOLIC LIVER DISEASE

Diagnosis of Alcoholic Liver Disease

Fatty Liver and Early Fibrosis. Alcoholic steatosis is completely reversible in most cases. In some extremely severe cases, alcoholic fatty liver may have a fatal outcome, but as a rule even those cases needing hospitalization improve within a few days or weeks after cessation of alcohol consumption. The clinical spectrum of alcoholic fatty liver may extend from silent nonsymptomatic hepatomegaly to severe hepatocellular failure with cholestasis and portal hypertension. However, most patients with pure fatty liver are virtually asymptomatic. Hepatomegaly is the commonest clinical sign. In contrast to what occurs in alcoholic hepatitis, abnormal laboratory values rapidly return to normal levels, and hepatomegaly decreases in the absence of further alcohol intake.

Alcoholic Hepatitis and Cirrhosis. Alcoholic hepatitis is a *histologic* diagnosis characterized by ballooning and disarray of the hepatocytes associated with polymorphonuclear cell inflammation. Thus, it is essential to perform a liver biopsy to document this lesion. Differential diagnosis consist of alcoholic fatty liver, cirrhosis, nonalcoholic liver disease; and rarely, extrahepatic obstruction. Diagnostic errors occur when traditional liver tests are used to predict histology, since the correlation between enzymes and histology is poor in a given patient. Glutamic acid dehydrogenase level is a more reliable predictor of alcoholic hepatitis in subjects without underlying cardiac, muscle, or pancreatic disease.

Cautions. The patient with alcoholic hepatitis or cirrhosis is likely to have additional medical problems, such as nutritional deficiencies (anemia, folate deficiency, Wernicke's encephalopathy, Korsakoff's psychosis), peripheral neuropathies, portal hypertension, gastritis, esophageal varices with bleeding, ascites, hepatorenal syndrome, and multitudinous infections, including tuberculosis. All of these should be sought out and aggressively treated.

Similarly, cirrhosis is a histologic diagnosis, defined as the presence of nodular regeneration on liver biopsy. The diagnosis may be suspected clinically when the patient manifests typical stigmata such as spider angiomata and gynecomastia in the presence of hepatosplenomegaly or ascites or both.

Hepatic encephalopathy, a metabolic disorder of the nervous system, may occur in the presence of severe liver disease. Manifestations include confusion, waxing and waning of consciousness, and asterixis (flapping tremor). This neurologic picture is nonspecific and must be differentiated from uremia, underlying psychiatric disorder, ventilatory failure, and hypoglycemia. Fetor hepaticus (musty odor) in the presence of stigmata of chronic liver disease helps distinguish this condition from other metabolic encephalopathies. The electroencephalogram has a typical high-voltage, slow-wave pattern. The diagnosis and treatment of alcoholic liver disease is outlined in Table 2.

Therapy of the Alcoholic with Liver Disease

Fatty Liver and Early Fibrosis. Other than treatment of alcohol withdrawal, continued abstinence, and the provision of a diet with sufficient calories, vitamins, and protein, no other treatment is generally needed. It should be noted, however, that there is a growing body of evidence in the recent literature that suggests that the alcoholic fatty liver may not be as benign a condition as was formerly thought. These patients have early fibrotic changes, and it is of practical importance to recognize at an early, still reversible stage, those individuals whose disease is prone to progress to cirrhosis. Therefore, the histologic confirmation of alcoholic liver injury by liver biopsy is highly desirable, and liver biopsy is indicated in patients who are hospitalized with signs of alcoholic liver disease and in ambulatory subjects when results from laboratory tests have continued to be abnormal for more than 3 months.

Alcoholic Hepatitis and Cirrhosis. The reported mortality rate for acute alcoholic hepatitis depends on the

TABLE 2 Diagnosis and Treatment of Alcoholic Liver Disease

Diagnosis	Fatty Liver/Early Fibrosis	Alcoholic Hepatitis	Cirrhosis
Clinical signs			
Hepatomegaly	+	+	+
Fever	Rare	+	Rare
Jaundice	Rare	+	+
Portal hypertension	Rare	+	+
Encephalopathy	Rare	+	+
Laboratory parameters			
Transaminases	↑		↑
Alkaline phosphatase	Normal	↑	↑
Glutamic acid dehydrogenase	Normal	↑ ↑	Normal
Bilirubin	Normal	↑	
Liver biopsy	Fat in hepatocytes ±fibrosis (perivenular and perisinusoidal)	Polymorphonuclear cell infiltration, ballooning and necrosis of hepatocytes	Fibrotic nodules
Therapy			
Alcohol	Abstinence	Abstinence	Abstinence
Nutrition	Normal diet	Parenteral alimentation in severe cases	Dietary protein restriction with encephalopathy
Drugs	None	Experimental	Lactulose for encephalopathy

material selected. A mortality of from 1.5 to 8 percent in individuals with alcoholic hepatitis ill enough to require hospitalization but well enough to permit liver biopsy has been found. The survival of patients with alcoholic hepatitis is dramatically improved by the discontinuation or reduction of alcohol consumption.

Clinical and pathologic signs of alcoholic hepatitis regress within weeks or months in most cases. A poorer short-term prognosis can be expected in patients with a prolonged prothrombin time and ascites.

In contrast to the well-compensated subject, those patients with jaundice or evidence of portal hypertension (esophageal varices, ascites, splenomegaly) require immediate hospitalization. All patients should be assessed for occult gastrointestinal bleeding. In addition, those presenting with such bleeding require urgent attention, including large-bore intravenous lines for fluid administration. In the actively bleeding patient, urgent diagnostic studies (CBC, SMA-6, creatinine, prothrombin time (PT), blood type and crossmatch) should be performed to exclude a coagulopathy and establish baseline parameters. Vitamin K (10 mg subcutaneously) must be administered if the prothrombin time is prolonged. Although thrombocytopenia may be present, platelet transfusion, in the absence of severe bleeding, is not necessary. Gastrointestinal consultation should be obtained without delay to document the source of bleeding. If esophageal varices are confirmed as the source of bleeding, peripheral intravenous vasopressin (0.4 U per milliliter) should be started immediately. For those patients in whom vasopressin is contraindicated (e.g., patients with coronary artery disease) or unsuccessful, balloon tamponade or sclerotherapy should be used. (See chapter on *Upper Gastrointestinal Bleeding.*)

In addition to bleeding, infection is another major cause of increased morbidity and mortality in these im-

munocompromised hosts. In particular, alcoholics have increased susceptibility to pneumonias, with an increased mortality rate. Thus, hospitalization is mandatory for the majority of these patients.

The general treatment for the majority of patients with alcoholic hepatitis is the same as for alcoholic steatosis. Although daily infusion of 70 to 85 g of amino acids has been reported to decrease mortality in alcoholic hepatitis, encephalopathy must be considered a potential risk of such treatment, and therefore this form of therapy cannot be advocated on a routine basis.

Expeditious work-up of the decompensated patient is essential. Although ascites may be transudative secondary to severe liver disease, it is incumbent to exclude other etiologies such as sepsis, pancreatitis, and tumor. Thus, diagnostic paracentesis is urgently required.

Icteric patients require evaluation to exclude extrahepatic causes of jaundice, particularly biliary, pancreatic, or hematologic etiologies. When such causes have been excluded, a diagnostic biopsy should be performed to document the underlying alcoholic liver disease. A particularly severe and usually fatal complication in the jaundiced cirrhotic alcoholic is the hepatorenal syndrome. Typically, as liver function deteriorates, urine volume and sodium concentration fall, with a concomitant increase in blood urea nitrogen and creatinine levels. Since this syndrome is difficult to differentiate from prerenal azotemia, current therapeutic recommendations include cessation of diuretics with simultaneous judicious volume expansion. At the present time, no other therapeutic measures have shown clinical value. However, in selected cases, the insertion of a peritoneojugular shunt has been reported to reverse the oliguria.

Encephalopathy (mental clouding, hepatic fetor, and asterixis) may be associated with any of the above complications of liver disease or may be precipitated by therapeutic measures, particularly the use of minor tranquilizers for management of alcohol withdrawal or the institution of a relatively high-protein diet. Contributory factors such as hypokalemia, gastrointestinal bleeding, and infection should be searched for and treated. It may be necessary to restrict protein to 40 g daily or even less and institute lactulose therapy (30 ml four times a day). It is particularly important to anticipate the complications and to institute treatment prophylactically.

Several pharmacologic agents have been utilized in the treatment of alcoholic hepatitis. The compounds most extensively tested have been corticosteroids, with at least 10 randomized double-blind trials since 1971. Results were conflicting. Furthermore, in one of the controlled studies, an increased risk of fungal infection associated with corticosteroid therapy was reported. Therefore, we do not recommend routine corticosteroid treatment for acute alcoholic hepatitis, although selected cases might be helped. Anabolic steroids (oxandrolone) have also been claimed to have beneficial effects on long-term survival; confirmatory studies are being awaited before this treatment can be adopted for routine use.

Propylthiouracil (PTU) has also been suggested for the treatment of alcoholic hepatitis. However, before this drug can be recommended for widespread use, further studies are indicated in view of a lack of beneficial therapeutic effect recorded by some. Colchicine, which inhibits collagen synthesis and procollagen secretion, may provide a new approach for the treatment of alcoholic liver injury, but further results of controlled trials are needed before this treatment can be recommended.

Disposition. Any jaundiced alcoholic requires immediate hospital admission for diagnostic evaluation, including gastrointestinal consultation. Nonemergency surgical procedures should be deferred until the hepatitis has resolved.

SUGGESTED READING

Lieber CS. Alcohol and the liver: 1984 update. Hepatology 1984; 4:1243–1260.
Lieber CS. A public health approach for the control of the disease of alcoholism. Alcoholism 1982; 6:171–177.
Lieber CS. Medical disorders of alcoholism: pathogenesis and treatment. Philadelphia: WB Saunders, 1982.

PANCREATITIS

JAMES E. POINTER, M.D.

Pancreatitis is an inflammatory condition of many presentations with a wide range of severity. The distinction between acute and chronic pancreatitis is somewhat ill defined and artificial. Acute pancreatitis has numerous causes, a mortality rate of 10 percent, and myriad treatments, most of which have not been proved efficacious in clinical trials. Ethanol abuse accounts for almost all cases of chronic pancreatitis and for a smaller majority of cases of acute pancreatitis. Patients who continue to drink may be mildly symptomatic on a daily basis, with intermittent attacks of the acute form. Chronic pancreatitis is relatively benign and its emergency treatment is essentially limited to relief of pain and vomiting.

Alcohol has several effects that contribute to the development of acute pancreatitis: increase in ductal permeability; hyperlipidemia, which results in sludging of small vessels; and ductal obstruction from duodenal edema. Biliary tract disease is the most common cause of acute pancreatitis in nondrinkers. Trauma, posterior penetrating peptic ulcer, infections (such as mumps and coxsackie virus), various metabolic disorders (Table 1), drugs and medications (Table 2), and connective tissue disease also can be responsible. Pancreatitis is very unusual in the pediatric population. In children, abdominal trauma, ingestion of certain drugs, and idiopathic factors each cause approximately 30 percent of cases of acute pancreatitis.

The emergency physician must consider acute pancreatitis when considering many other diagnoses. Lower lobe pneumonia, myocardial infarction, pulmonary embolus, peptic ulcer disease, cholecystitis, peritonitis, gastrointestinal bleeding, shock or coma of any cause, or kidney or liver infection or failure can mimic pancreatitis.

ASSESSMENT

About one-quarter of patients with acute pancreatitis develop a major complication. It is useful to distinguish these severe cases from the more common mild ones. Patients with the severe disease require admission to the hospital and intensive care; those with the milder forms can safely be managed as outpatients. Identification of severe cases also ensures that more aggressive, expensive therapy be reserved for those who need it. The physical examination usually is of little help in selecting patients with a poor prognosis. Table 3 lists the common clinical findings for acute pancreatitis. Abdominal pain, weight

TABLE 1   Metabolic Causes of Acute Pancreatitis

Diabetes mellitus
Hyperlipidemia (Fredrickson types I, IV, and V)
  (triglycerides $\geq 1,000$ mg/dl)
Hypercalcemia (hyperparathyroidism, sarcoidosis,
  metastatic breast carcinoma)
Hemochromatosis
Uremia
Vitamin A or D deficiency
Glycogen storage disease (type I)
Cystic fibrosis
Scorpion bites

TABLE 2 Drugs and Medications Associated with Acute Pancreatitis

Corticosteroids	Alcohols
Oral contraceptives	Tetracyclines
Estrogens	Rifampin
Phenformin	Isoniazid
Thiazide diuretics	Valproic acid
Furosemide	Cimetidine
Ethacrynic acid	Paracetamol
Warfarin	Salicylates
Calcium	Indomethacin
Azathioprine	Dextropropoxyphene
L–Asparaginase	

TABLE 4 Clinical Factors Useful in Identifying Severe Cases of Acute Pancreatitis

Signs of shock or sepsis

Laboratory factors

Three or more factors must be present in the patient with suspected pancreatitis:

Upon Admission	Within 48 Hours
Age >55 years	Hematocrit fall >10%
WBC >15,000 cu mm	BUN rise >5 mg/dl
Blood glucose >200 mg/dl	Serum calcium <8 mg/dl
Serum LDH >350 IU/L	Arterial Po_2 <60 mm Hg
Serum SGOT >250 IU/dl	Serum albumin <32 g/L
	Base deficit >4 mEq/L
	Fluid sequestration >6 L

(Adapted from Blamey SL, et al. Gut 1984; 25:1340–1346.)

loss, and diarrhea are the most common complaints in patients with chronic pancreatitis.

The laboratory is invaluable in assisting the emergency physician in selecting those patients with severe disease and the poorer prognosis. Clinical factor scoring lists are helpful (see Table 4). Of course, patients with clinical signs of shock or sepsis also have the severe disease.

The *laboratory* is less helpful in establishing the diagnosis of acute pancreatitis. Nonetheless, the serum or urine amylase level remains the mainstay of diagnosis in spite of severe limitations. The patient with acute pancreatitis may have a high, normal, or low serum amylase concentration, and the amylase level does not correlate with the severity of disease. The fallopian tubes, breast, ovaries, lungs, salivary glands, kidneys, heart, liver, and small intestine can produce a high amylase level on the basis of nonpancreatic isoenzyme. Amylase isoenzyme fractionation is not commonly available, although a quick method does exist. When isoenzymes are tested, the majority of patients with alcohol-induced pancreatitis with elevated serum amylase levels have a nonpancreatic source for the elevation. Patients with acute pancreatitis may have a normal or low pancreatic amylase isoenzyme level for two reasons. First, renal clearance for the enzyme may be rapid. The 2-hour urinary amylase level may be elevated in these cases. Second, the pancreas of patients with chronic disease may have "burned out" and not contain sufficient enzyme levels to result in elevated levels. Serum lipase levels are usually elevated in acute pancreatitis as well as by those other conditions that elevate amylase. However, the test is not specific enough and also is not commonly available. The amylase-creatinine clearance ratio (amylase clearance (percent) ÷ creatinine clearance (percent) = (urine amylase ÷ serum amylase) ×

(serum creatinine ÷ urine creatinine) × 100) has been extensively studied. It probably adds no information not provided by the amylase alone. Its sensitivity has been questioned, and in diabetic ketoacidosis and renal failure it is elevated to the same levels (higher than 5 percent) as in pancreatitis. Its clinical use has been largely abandoned.

Any intra-abdominal or retroperitoneal bleeding, including acute pancreatitis, can result in detectable serum methalbumin, another laboratory study with limited application in the diagnosis of pancreatitis. *Radiologic studies* also are not of much help in diagnosing pancreatitis. The presence of a duodenal air bubble, dilatation of the first jejunal segment (sentinel loop), and pancreatic calcification are common but not pathognomonic findings. Ultrasonography and computed tomography are best reserved for cases in which the diagnosis is in doubt or for complications.

THERAPEUTIC REGIMEN

Because the diagnosis of pancreatitis is beyond the scope of pre-hospital personnel, treatment is based on assessment of signs of shock. Rescuers should attend to the patient's airway and circulation, administer high-flow oxygen, initiate intravenous crystalloid fluids, and rapidly transport the patient in shock with suspected pancreatitis.

The emergency physician must tailor the treatment to the severity of the disease. The laboratory is essential not only to support the diagnosis but also to recognize severe cases. Serum and urine amylase levels, a complete blood count, a metabolic panel, a coagulation panel, serum calcium concentration, a liver panel, and arterial blood gas readings are baseline studies for patients with the acute disease.

The patient with *mild acute pancreatitis* usually requires only pain relief, limited intravenous hydration, and antiemetics. Meperidine hydrochloride, 50 to 150 mg intramuscularly, every 3 to 4 hours, is the parenteral narcotic analgesic of choice, as it does not cause spasm of the sphincter of Oddi, which would elevate biliary pres-

TABLE 3 Clinical Findings of Acute Pancreatitis

Abdominal pain (epigastric area with radiation
  straight through to back)
Nausea
Vomiting
Abdominal distention (ileus)
Dehydration
Jaundice
Shock
Gastrointestinal bleeding
Prior history

sure. Intravenous crystalloid fluids should be used for hydration of the volume-depleted patient. Nasogastric suction is not effective or necessary. Prochlorperazine, 5 to 10 mg, intramuscularly every 3 to 4 hours, or hydroxyzine hydrochloride, 25 to 100 mg intramuscularly every 4 to 6 hours, is useful in controlling vomiting and nausea once the diagnosis is established. Patients should be able to take clear fluids by mouth as a requisite to discharge home. Even if the patient does not meet the clinical criteria for severe disease, hospital admission is necessary for patients who are unable to tolerate oral fluids, have intractable pain, or are immunocompromised.

Severe acute pancreatitis requires aggressive supportive therapy and careful monitoring. Admission to an intensive care unit and consultation with an internist or gastroenterologist are essential. These patients require rapid volume replacement and electrolyte repletion. Shock patients with respiratory or cardiac disease need central venous pressure monitoring. Severely ill patients should receive nasogastric suction, particularly if abdominal distention and ileus are present. As in patients with the milder forms, pain relief is important. Antibiotics have no place unless there is sepsis or biliary tract disease. Anticholinergics, glucagon, cimetidine, calcitonin, and heparin have not proved effective in controlled clinical trials. Patients with pancreatitic ascites, renal failure, or who are refractory to standard treatment should receive a course of peritoneal dialysis. It is important to restrict dialysate volume to under 1.0 L to prevent respiratory compromise. The emergency physician must carefully monitor physiologic and laboratory parameters during the management of acute pancreatitis. Blood pressure and pulse should be assessed every 15 minutes in the nonshock patient and constantly in the patient with shock. Urine output requires hourly monitoring. Temperature, and levels of serum glucose, hematocrit, and serum electrolytes, as well as arterial blood gas analysis require monitoring every 2 to 3 hours. The physical examination should be repeated every 3 to 4 hours. Tests of the serum amylase and calcium levels and the white blood cell count are repeated every 6 to 12 hours in the acutely ill patient. Other laboratory parameters need monitoring every 24 hours.

The emergency physician can usually manage patients with *chronic pancreatitis* as outpatients with oral analgesics and antiemetics and occasionally antispasmodics. Acetaminophen, 1,000 mg every 4 to 6 hours, is sufficient for many patients. Acetaminophen, 325 mg with codeine, 30 mg, or acetaminophen, 500 mg with hydrocodone bitartrate, 5 mg, may occasionally be required. It is important to restrict the chronic use of narcotics in this

TABLE 5 Management of Pancreatitis

Acute Pancreatitis

Severe	Mild
Assess and treat airway, breathing, cardiac status	Order pancreatic function tests
Assess and treat shock	Order other metabolic tests if appropriate
Give IV crystalloids (Ringer's lactate or normal saline) wide open	Give intravenous fluids if necessary
Order CBC, arterial blood gases, electrolytes, glucose, coagulation panel, calcium, liver, and renal function tests, serum amylase	Administer analgesics and antiemetics, if appropriate
	Test for oral fluids, inderdict alcohol
Administer analgesics if appropriate	Admit patients with intractable pain or unable to tolerate oral fluids
Insert nasogastric tube	Arrange for outpatient follow-up examinations for other patients
Dialyze if appropriate	
Consult internist or gastroenterologist	
Admit to intensive care unit	

Chronic Pancreatitis

Confirm diagnosis
Administer analgesics and antiemetics, if appropriate
Refer for follow-up study

and other chronic pain syndromes. The emergency physician should avoid salicylic acid acetate or the nonsteroidal anti-inflammatory agents because of their well-known gastrointestinal side effects. Prochlorperazine, 5 to 10 mg by mouth, 3 to 4 times daily, or promethazine hydrochloride, 25 mg every 4 to 6 hours, is useful for nausea. Both medications are available in rectal suppositories. Dicyclomine hydrochloride, 20 to 40 mg every 6 hours for 2 to 3 days, may abate a particularly painful episode. Admission to the hospital is usually not required. Cessation of drinking and follow-up examination are important but unlikely outcomes in the noncompliant patient. Recalcitrant cases may require celiac nerve block, surgery, or pancreatic enzyme replacement. Table 5 outlines emergency department treatment of pancreatitis.

SUGGESTED READING

Blamey SL, Imrie CW, O'Neill J, et al. Prognostic factors in acute pancreatitis. Gut 1984; 25:1340–1346.
Ranson JHC. Acute pancreatitis: pathogenesis, outcome, and treatment. Clin Gastroenterol 1984; 13:843–863.
Worning H. Chronic pancreatitis: pathogenesis, natural history, and conservative treatment. Clin Gastroenterol 1984; 13:871–894.

GASTRITIS AND ULCER DISEASE

RONALD L. KROME, M.D., F.A.C.S.

Both gastritis and peptic ulcer disease, regardless of etiology, result from either (1) an excess of acid in relation to mucosal protection mechanisms, or (2) a defect in the mucosal protection mechanism of the stomach or the duodenum. Treatment, both acute and chronic, is aimed at reducing the total acidity of the stomach in relation to the patient's protective mechanisms. This holds true even if surgical intervention is indicated.

Gastric ulcers are frequently associated with prolonged emptying times of the stomach, which is not the case in duodenal ulcer disease. Gastritis is most often associated with the ingestion of drugs or foods that "irritate" the gastric mucosa. They produce an increase in relative acidity in relation to the mucosal protective system. In some traumatic stress situations, such as with extensive burns or massive trauma, the mucosal protective systems are impaired. Prolonged nasogastric tube drainage may also be associated with gastritis and esophagitis. Alcohol and aspirin are probably the two most common causes of gastritis.

PRE-HOSPITAL THERAPY

When these patients call on the emergency medical system (EMS), their principal complaints are abdominal pain, vomiting, and hematemesis. Initial paramedic evaluation (Table 1) requires a careful history of precipitating causes and a search for drug usage, especially the use of aspirin and corticosteroids, or the ingestion of alcohol. Vital signs, including the temperature, should be taken, and a general patient inspection should be conducted. A history of hematemesis and melena should be sought.

If the vital signs are consistent with hypovolemia (which may result from either prolonged vomiting or hematemesis and/or melena), then an intravenous line should be established, with a balanced electrolyte solution as the fluid of choice. Fluids should be given at a volume sufficient to maintain vital signs, if possible. Military anti-shock trousers (MAST) has not been shown to be beneficial in this circumstance; in fact, it may produce vomiting in the patient with abdominal distention if the abdominal portion is inflated. Oxygen should be administered at high flow rates (10 to 12 L) because the oxygen-carrying capacity of patients with blood loss is already limited by a lack of hemoglobin.

During transport, the patient should be placed on his or her side, to minimize the possibility of aspiration, should vomiting occur. If the patient is over 50 years of age, if there is a history of angina or coronary artery dis-

ease, or if he or she has chest pain (a low hemoglobin may precipitate angina), the patient should be monitored. If the hemoglobin is low enough, congestive failure may occur. In this case, treatment is aimed at maintaining the patient's oxygen-carrying capacity as close as possible to normal.

EMERGENCY DEPARTMENT MANAGEMENT

Unless the patient is in frank shock, the history and physical examination should be completed before therapy is initiated.

History

Patients with peptic ulcer disease commonly complain of pain between meals and, on occasion, pain in the middle of the night, which wakes them from sleep. The pain, usually burning in character, occurs when acid increases in the stomach—hence, the pain between meals and during the night. If the ulcer is posteriorly located, or if perforation occurs posteriorly, then the patient may complain of pain through to the back, similar to the pain of acute pancreatitis. The pain of perforation is sudden and severe, occasionally causing the patient to double up. It can often be timed because of its suddenness.

The pain of gastritis, on the other hand, usually occurs with meals, as does the pain of a gastric ulcer. That is, the ingestion of food, or other known gastrin stimulants, exacerbates the pain. This pain, too, may go through to the back. Although both of these descriptions are the classic presentation, the pain pattern should not be relied on to establish the diagnosis. Other helpful factors in the history are a history of frequent aspirin ingestion, alcohol abuse, heavy smoking, and the frequent ingestion of caffeine-containing fluids.

Differential Diagnosis

The differential diagnosis includes biliary disease, pancreatitis, and other bowel disease. The Zollinger–

TABLE 1 Prehospital Care

Initial History
  Drug use
  Alcohol ingestion
  Hematemesis
  Melena
  Pain pattern

Initial Physical Examination
  Signs of shock
  Presence of vomitus
  Color/character of vomitus

Initial Therapy
  Place on side to minimize aspiration
  Balanced electrolyte solution
  High flow oxygen

Ellison syndrome, a rarity, is difficult to diagnose even after an extensive work-up. It should be entertained in the patient with a past history of peptic ulcer disease, especially one who has had surgery for ulcer disease, who also has a history of chronic diarrhea, and who resists aggressive medical therapy. The literature suggests that cimetidine may be of some help in treating ulcers occurring in this syndrome.

Physical Examination

Physical examination should include both a rectal examination and the insertion of a nasogastric tube. The nasogastric tube need be placed only if the patient has a history of hematemesis, melena, or consistent vomiting. In this fashion, acute bleeding can be assessed, and the volume of gastric return can be estimated. If the patient denies any history of melena or hematemesis, but melena or guiac-positive stool is found on rectal examination, then a nasogastric tube should still be inserted.

The nasogastric tube is both diagnostic and therapeutic. The presence of constant nasogastric suction serves to decrease gastric stimulation and to empty the stomach of excess acid. Gastric distention stimulates gastrin secretion and increases gastric and duodenal acidity.

If no blood is found when nasogastric suction is started, then the nasogastric tube can be removed; assuming there is no sign of an acute abdomen, and the patient has no significant vomiting by history, feeding should be begun then, since an empty stomach also stimulates gastrin secretion.

The presence of tenderness indicates some element of visceral irritation, but is an extremely nonspecific finding. If there is rebound tenderness, or board-like rigidity, then an acute abdominal condition, such as perforation, may be present. The finding of a tender mass in the right upper quadrant is suggestive of acute gallbladder disease, such as biliary stones with acute cholecystitis. Pancreatitis is often difficult to distinguish from both peptic ulcer disease and gastritis, especially because the antecedent factors may be the same in each of these.

The presence of melena or bloody nasogastric return is unlikely with either pancreatitis or biliary disease. It is possible to have either, however, when ischemic bowel is present. In the latter, the nasogastric return is more likely to be feculent, or at least, what blood is present is not massive.

Gastric carcinoma can present in an identical fashion to either gastric ulcer disease or gastritis, although it does tend to be more insidious. Endoscopic examination is key to establishing the diagnosis.

Laboratory Evaluation

Laboratory studies should include a hemogram to assess blood loss, although acute blood loss may not be reflected in the hemoglobin level in the first few hours. An elevated white blood cell count may indicate an inflammatory or infectious process but is very nonspecific. Serum amylase, classically elevated in acute pancreatitis, may also be elevated in biliary disease or ischemic bowel disease, especially if perforation has occurred. The serum bilirubin can also be elevated in biliary disease or if the acute pancreatitis involves the head of the pancreas, functionally obstructing the common bile duct. Type and cross-matching of blood is indicated if blood loss is present or expected. Serum electrolytes are helpful in treating patients with vomiting, pancreatitis, or ischemic bowel disease, and should also be obtained if prolonged fluid replacement is anticipated. The serum calcium and a blood sugar may be helpful in assessing the severity of pancreatitis, if that is the diagnosis. Other laboratory studies should be done as indicated by the differential diagnosis and the past medical history of the patient.

Radiography

Routine x-ray studies of the abdomen may be helpful in at least ruling out other causes of acute abdominal pain. In any acute abdominal series either an upright chest x-ray film, to demonstrate free air under the diaphragm, or a left lateral decubitus should be done. Gallstones, renal stones, and calcifications in the pancreas should be sought. Air in the biliary tract may be present if a common duct stone has eroded into the duodenum. Air in the bowel wall, thickening of the bowel wall, and the presence of air fluid levels can be helpful in detecting significant bowel problems, such as ischemic bowel diseases.

Because not all patients with perforations demonstrate free air, the absence of free air does not rule out a perforated ulcer. Those that do perforate frequently do not have a history of ulcer disease. Sitting the patient upright for 10 to 15 mintues after air is instilled in the stomach through a preexisting nasogastric tube may help. When this is done, the nasogastric tube must be clamped; a Salem tube cannot be used.

An emergency upper gastrointestinal series is of very limited value. Subsequent to the emergency visit, patients suspected of having peptic ulcer disease or gastritis should have both an endoscopic examination and an upper gastrointestinal series. An emergency endoscopic examination is helpful when the diagnosis is in doubt, or if therapy for bleeding is mandatory.

Treatment

The treatment of the patient who is actively bleeding is discussed in the chapter *Upper Gastrointestinal Bleeding*.

If the patient has signs of volume depletion—most often the result of blood loss or loss of large volumes of gastric contents from vomiting—*volume should be replaced* using a balanced electrolyte solution, either Ringer's lactate or normal saline, in volumes sufficient to maintain the patient's vital signs or to correct orthostatic changes. When volume replacement does not correct vital signs, or if the patient develops angina, then blood transfusion is usually necessary.

When there is bloody return from the nasogastric

tube, gastric lavage is indicated using iced saline. Whether iced fluids are better than non-iced gastric lavage has not been clearly documented, but experience suggests they are. In patients with gastritis, gastric lavage will usually be sufficient to stop gastric bleeding; it is not always sufficient in patients with bleeding from peptic ulcer disease.

Antacids instilled through the nasogastric tube have been of some help in stopping bleeding. This may be done intermittently, or as a milk-antacid drip. If it is done intermittently, the nasogastric tube must be clamped for 30 to 45 minutes and returned to suction after that. Cimetidine in a dose of 300 mg inserted through the nasogastric tube has also been shown to be of some benefit. In a dose of 200 to 300 mg intravenously every 6 hours, cimetidine stops bleeding in both peptic ulcer disease and gastritis. Rebleeding, however, is not uncommon.

If instead of a bloody return, the return is clear and colorless, then gastric outlet obstruction should be suspected. Usually these patients will give a history of large-volume vomiting, and when the nasogastric tube is first inserted the return may exceed 800 cc. The absence of the usual green or yellow color from the nasogastric return may indicate that the obstruction is present and the normal bile return cannot enter the stomach through the obstructed pylorus.

Surgical therapy is indicated when complications occur or medical therapy fails. The accepted indications for surgical intervention are uncontrolled bleeding, gastric outlet obstruction, perforation, and complete failure of medical therapy. Because gastritis is an extensive disease, involving the entire gastric mucosa, when surgery is indicated, it is usually extensive.

If there is no indication for surgical intervention, and the patient appears able to tolerate it, a trial at outpatient therapy is indicated. After the nasogastric tube is removed, feeding should consist of antacids. Most antacids only reduce gastric acidity for 45 to 60 minutes. Therefore, if the classic antacids, Maalox or Mylanta, are given, they must be repeated every 1 to 2 hours, alternating with skim milk, both in a volume of 30 cc. Patients with suspected gastritis should refrain from ingesting the offending agent. Antacids are helpful. They should be given with meals and at bedtime. If there is no contraindication in the patient's medical history, then the patient may select from any inexpensive over-the-counter antacid taken regularly (Table 2). An anticholinergic, such as Donnatal, may also be given, usually half-hour before meals and at bedtime, although the usefulness of these agents is controversial.

In patients with suspected peptic ulcer disease, the antacids should be given between meals, 2 hours after eating, and at bedtime. The anticholinergics should still be administered half-hour before eating.

Cimetidine, 400 mg twice a day, is an easy regimen for the patient to follow, and it is of some benefit in the short-term healing of peptic ulcer disease. Like the other H_2-antagonist, ranitidine, it blocks the histamine receptor on the parietal cell and also blocks pariental cell acid

TABLE 2 Neutralizing Capacity, Sodium Content, and Cost-Effectiveness of Antacids

Antacid	Composition	Acid Neutralizing Capacity (mEq/ml)	Volume Containing 140 mEq (ml)	Sodium Content (mg/5 ml)	Monthly* Cost of Therapy ($)
Maalox TC	Aluminum hydroxide, magnesium hydroxide	4.2	33	1.2	44
Titralac	Calcium carbonate, glycine	4.2	33	11.0	35
Delcid	Aluminum hydroxide, magnesium hydroxide	4.1	34	1.5	57
Mylanta II	Aluminum hydroxide, magnesium hydroxide, simethicone	3.6	39	1.1	63
Camalox	Aluminum hydroxide, magnesium hydroxide, calcium carbonate	3.2	44	2.5	55
Gelusil II	Aluminum hydroxide, magnesium hydroxide, simethicone	3.0	47	1.3	74
Basaljel ES	Aluminum carbonate	2.9	48	23.0	101
Maalox Plus	Aluminum hydroxide, magnesium hydroxide, simethicone	2.3	61	2.5	68
Gelusil	Aluminum hydroxide, magnesium hydroxide, simethicone	2.2	64	0.7	80
Riopan Plus	Aluminum hydroxide, magnesium hydroxide, simethicone	1.8	78	0.7	78
Amphojel	Aluminum hydroxide	1.4	100	7.0	114
Phosphajel	Aluminum phosphate	0.3	466	12.5	498

From Hollander D. Duodenal ulcer. In: Current therapy in internal medicine. Toronto: BC Decker, 1984:579.
* Wholesale costs, 1971.

secretion by gastrin or acetylcholine. Recent evidence shows, however, that there is no statistical support of an advantage of cimetidine over vigorous antacid therapy. In fact, studies comparing ranitidine and cimetidine and ranitidine and antacids have failed to demonstrate any such significant difference in long-term healing or the recurrence of bleeding. The H_2-antagonists do possess side effects, although these are rare and cause mild elevation of serum glutamic-oxaloacetic transaminase and glutamic-pyruvic transaminase (SGOT and SGPT). Mild muscle weakness and slight impairment of clarity of thinking may occur. There may also be reactions with other drugs the patient is taking, so they should be used judiciously. However, the H_2-antagonists are particularly effective at reducing acid secretion at night, when few patients take antacids, and compliance in taking them is higher than with antacids.

Antacids, on the other hand, are inexpensive, over-the-counter drugs. Their use is relatively free of problems, except in those patients with chronic renal disease, and unlikely to produce difficulty unless taken in exceptionally large volumes. However, they can cause diarrhea (aluminum-magnesium types) and interfere with absorption and renal clearance of other drugs.

Sucralfate is a new drug that adheres to and protects gastric mucosa, preventing pepsin activity by adsorbing it directly, binding bile acids, and promoting gastric secretion of mucus. Side effects are very rare, since the drug is not absorbed. It is as effective as cimetidine or antacids, and its advantage is its absence of side effects, ease of administration, and better compliance. Dosage is a 1 g tablet four times a day.

The benefits of a bland diet are in question. Probably what is best for the patient, and least difficult to adhere to, is a diet free of known gastric stimulants such as alcohol, tea, coffee, and tobacco. Eating frequently may be more important than a bland diet.

The mainstay of therapy in patients with peptic ulcer disease, or with gastritis, remains antacids, anticholinergics, diet, and limitation of smoking and alcohol ingestion.

DISPOSITION

Patients who are discharged on any of the above regimens will probably do well and resolve their acute episode. The usefulness of these regimens in prevention of recurrences is less well known, and for long-term follow-up and confirmation of diagnosis, referral to a primary physician is advised.

SUGGESTED READING

Bezuidenhout DJ. A comparison of 4-week peptic ulcer healing rates following treatment with antacids and ranitidine. S Afr Med J 1984; 65:1007–1009.

Krome RL. Peptic ulcer disease. In: Tintinalli JE, Rothstein RJ, Krome RL eds. Emergency medicine: A comprehensive study guide. New York:McGraw-Hill Book Co., 1985.

Morris DL. Optimal timing of operation for bleeding peptic ulcer: prospective randomized trial. Br Med J 1984; 288:1277–1280.

Thomson AB, Maguire T, Wensel RH, Sherbaniuk RW, Bailey RJ, Kideikis P. Ranitidine versus cimetidine in the management of acute upper gastrointestinal tract bleeding. J Clin Gastroenterol 1984; 6:295–299.

Thompson JC, Walker JP. Indications for parental H_2 receptor antagonists. Am J Med 1984 77;111—115.

Walan A. Antacids and anticholinergics in the treatment of duodenal ulcer. Clin Gastroenterol 1984; 13:473–499.

UPPER GASTROINTESTINAL BLEEDING

DAVID J. SCHNEIDERMAN, M.D.
JOHN P. CELLO, M.D.

Acute upper gastrointestinal tract hemorrhage is usually manifested by signs and symptoms that are easily noted by both patient and physician. Hematemesis and melenemesis ("coffee ground" emesis) are startling events for most patients and usually prompt them to seek immediate medical attention. However, some patients delay seeking medical care until the fatigue, lightheadedness, or frank syncope of blood loss anemia occur.

Despite the fact that nearly 80 percent of upper gastrointestinal hemorrhages are self-limited (i.e., requiring no surgery) it is the duty of the physician first encountering the patient to determine the presence or absence of active bleeding, to provide hemodynamic stabilization and to make an intelligent decision of patient disposition, i.e., whether admission to the hospital is warranted (and if so, whether intensive care monitoring is necessary), and if surgical consultation is urgently needed.

ESSENTIALS OF EARLY MANAGEMENT

With rare exception, the patient who notes passage of bloody or coffee-ground emesis, melena, or hematochezia should receive prompt evaluation, preferably in an emergency facility. Reliance on the patient alone to quantitate blood loss is invariably fraught with inaccuracies, since *any* blood in the emesis is abnormal and as little as 10 ml of blood colors the toilet water red.

Whether to transport a patient to the emergency facility by ambulance or paramedic service or to allow prompt travel with a friend or relative is a difficult decision to make after a brief encounter with a patient on the telephone. Erring on the side of caution and assuming the worst possible circumstances is the most reasonable judgment. Patients who are transported by ambulance should have their vital signs monitored and a large-bore (16- or 18-gauge) intravenous catheter with normal saline infusion introduced, the rate dependent on the stability of the particular patient. Low-flow oxygen supplementation via nasal cannula is suggested, especially for the elderly.

Once the patient has reached the emergency facility, *assessment of hemodynamic status* is the first priority. Tachycardia and hypotension in the supine patient indicate, at the least, an acute 20 percent loss of circulating intravascular volume. If pulse and blood pressure permit, determination of postural changes in vital signs with the patient sitting with legs dangling or standing erect provides additional information regarding hypovolemia. An upright pulse rise of more than 15 beats per minute or a blood pressure fall of more than 15 mm Hg indicates substantial acute volume loss (at least 10 to 15 percent). Supine or postural hypotension on presentation to the emergency facility demands insertion of two large-bore (16- or 18-gauge) catheters with infusions of saline or lactated Ringer's solution while further evaluation is carried out. For the patient in hemorrhagic shock, type-specific blood should be transfused immediately. Again, supplemental oxygen may avoid cardiovascular or cerebrovascular catastrophes.

An appropriate blood sample should be sent to the laboratory for determination of hematocrit, platelet count, coagulation profile (prothrombin time, partial thromboplastin time), and blood typing and screening. For patients who arrive in shock, at least 6 to 10 units of packed red blood cells should be crossmatched. Patients with postural hypotension or tachycardia should have at least 4 to 6 units of blood urgently crossmatched, whereas lesser amounts should be requested for patients without evidence of acute volume loss.

HISTORY AND PHYSICAL EXAMINATION

Most patients with acute upper gastrointestinal hemorrhage note bright red (or maroon) emesis, "coffee-ground" emesis, and/or passage of melenic stools. Dark brown or black flocculated blood, best described as "coffee ground" emesis, is older blood; likewise, *melena* is blood that has traversed the gastrointestinal tract, with its hemoglobin oxidized to hematin or other hematochromes, which blacken the stool. In greater than 90 percent of patients, melena represents hemorrhage from an upper gastrointestinal source, proximal to the ligament of Treitz (the duodenal-jejunal junction), although small intestinal bleeding more distally, or even right-sided colonic bleeding if transit is sluggish, may allow sufficient time for oxidation of heme. In rare instances, patients with bleeding from the nasopharynx, tracheobronchial tree, or pancreaticobiliary systems develop melena. However, melena should be regarded primarily as a manifestation of upper gastrointestinal tract bleeding until proved otherwise.

The passage of bright red or maroon blood per rectum in the patient with signs of acute hypovolemia should likewise alert the physician to the possibility of hemorrhage from the upper gastrointestinal tract (as well as the more likely possibility of colonic bleeding) since this presentation occurs in about 5 to 10 percent of all upper tract hemorrhages. Usually, massive bleeding from an ulcer crater with an eroded large vessel is responsible for this presentation. Blood itself is a powerful stimulant of intestinal peristalsis and may promote its own rapid transit through the bowel before oxidation of heme can be accomplished. The patient with partial resection of large or small bowel is especially prone to develop hematochezia from a briskly bleeding upper gastrointestinal source. Therefore, the primary physician must *always* eliminate a proximal site of bleeding in the patient presenting with red or maroon blood per rectum by passing a nasogastric tube and lavaging with at least a liter of fluid. The return of bile-stained, nonbloody effluent almost certainly excludes bleeding proximal to the descending duodenum.

A history of abdominal pain may reflect the presence of duodenal or gastric ulcer disease. Classically, the pain pattern of duodenal ulcer disease is one of mid-epigastric burning, occurring while fasting (particularly in the early morning) and relieved promptly by food or antacids, whereas gastric ulcer pain may be exacerbated by food and associated with vomiting after some time has elapsed after meals, especially when edema and ulceration create a relative gastric outlet obstruction. A considerable overlap of symptoms can occur between these two diseases, however, and mislead even the most astute clinician. Moreover, pain and vomiting may also be seen with the diffuse mucosal lesions of gastritis, although the emesis associated with gastritis occurs shortly after food is ingested. A history of acid reflux, particularly substernal burning and acid regurgitation, may likewise suggest esophagitis as the etiology for the acute upper gastrointestinal hemorrhage.

Antecedent retching, vomiting, or paroxysmal coughing may produce linear *Mallory-Weiss tears* of the gastroesophageal junction, although approximately 40 percent of these tears are not associated with a history of forceful straining. Hemorrhage from esophageal or gastric varices is not associated with abdominal pain unless the patient has concomitant gastritis, pancreatitis, or alcoholic hepatitis. Although most patients bleeding from varices have established parenchymal liver disease, some may develop variceal hemorrhage as the first manifestation of unsuspected cirrhosis and portal hypertension.

Alcohol and nonsteroidal anti-inflammatory medications are the main offending agents in producing severe erosive gastritis, and a careful history of their use should be sought. Hundreds of over-the-counter preparations (e.g., Excedrin, Anacin, Alka Seltzer) contain salicylates, and ibuprofen (Nuprin, Advil) has become an easily accessible nonprescription analgesic over the past year. Ingestion of bismuth, iron, and licorice should not be overlooked as a cause of guaiac-negative black stools when other evidence for acute gastrointestinal hemorrhage is lacking.

Physical assessment of the hemorrhaging patient should be focused initially on volume status, as noted earlier. Findings of diaphoresis, ashen or pale hue to the skin, or cool, clammy extremities often accompany hypotension. Spider angiomata, icterus, hepatosplenomegaly, ascites, and asterixis provide clues suggesting cirrhosis and portal hypertension. An abdominal scar representing previous ulcer surgery or an aortic graft raise possibilities of recurrent or anastomotic ulcers or aortoenteric fistulas, respectively. Digital examination of the rectum may yield melena or red blood, supporting the diagnosis of acute hemorrhage.

DIFFERENTIAL DIAGNOSIS

Although the bleeding lesions are diverse in cause, hemodynamically significant bleeding episodes originate one-third each in the esophagus, stomach, and duodenum (Table 1). The most frequent sources from each location are esophageal varices and esophagitis; gastric ulcer and erosive gastritis; and duodenal ulcer. It is rare for gastric or esophageal carcinomas to hemorrhage briskly, although chronic blood loss anemia is common.

Diagnostic and Therapeutic Options

A large-bore (16 or 18 F) Salem sump *nasogastric tube* should be passed initially with the patient in the left decubitus position to avoid aspiration. Local anesthetic usually is not necessary, although some physicians administer lidocaine jelly or intranasal cocaine (5 to 10 percent solution). The presence of blood in the stomach is conclusive evidence for acute upper gastrointestinal hemorrhage, but in its absence, bile-stained drainage must be obtained to ensure that duodenal contents have been adequately sampled. Prepyloric or duodenal ulcerations occasionally provoke intense pylorospasm and edema, preventing reflux of blood into the stomach. A briskly bleeding duodenal ulcer may occasionally be overlooked in this setting.

Occult blood testing of nonbloody or "non-coffee-ground" gastric aspirates is of little use. False-positives and false-negatives are well documented, and the nasopharyngeal trauma induced by tube passage is inevitable. Flecks of red blood that accompany intubation generally can be ignored.

TABLE 1 Cause of substantial upper gastrointestinal tract hemorrhage (One hundred consecutive patients admitted to San Francisco General Hospital)

Source of Hemorrhage*	Number of Patients	
Esophagitis	7	
Esophageal cancer	1	
Esophageal varices	16	36 - esophagus
Mallory-Weiss tears	12	
Gastric ulcer	18	
Gastric cancer	2	
Gastritis	11	37 - stomach
Pyloric ulcer	5	
Cystogastrostomy site	1	
Duodenal ulcer	21	
Duodenitis†	6	27 - duodenum
	100	

*Site determined by endoscopy or surgery
†Multiple superficial erosions in duodenum

Gastric lavage through the tube is a time-honored practice. Whereas clearing the stomach of food and old blood is helpful for future endoscopy, determining the activity of bleeding is the most useful gain from this procedure. Instilling aliquots of fluid (100 to 200 ml) and then removing the infusate by gravity or gentle suction drainage provides evidence of active bleeding if pink or red effluent persists after 1 to 2 liters. Although temporary cessation of bleeding is common after lavage, the physician must not thereby conclude that the hemorrhage has stopped permanently.

The choice and temperature of fluids used probably are not so important as once postulated. Most emergency departments stock sterile saline, which is usually iced and utilized for gastric lavage. Since the majority of fluid instilled is removed, saline or water lavage does not precipitate congestive heart failure or hyponatremia. Moreover, sterile saline and sterile water are costly and not obligatory in an already contaminated lumen. Whereas iced fluids were purported in the past to cause local vasoconstriction and hence decrease bleeding, the cold temperatures may impair local clotting factors and contribute to continued hemorrhage. The best choice overall is probably room-temperature tap water lavage.

The addition of the vasoconstrictor *levarterenol* (Levophed or norepinephrine) or the antifibrinolytic tranexamic acid to lavage solution appears to provide no added benefit.

If bleeding persists despite vigorous lavage and the hematocrit is low, transfusions may be required. Since in the early acute bleed the hematocrit may be normal, a repeat hematocrit *must* be obtained after *each* 1 to 2 liters of crystalloid is infused intravenously. The need for transfusion is patient-dependent, and possible viral contamination of blood products makes most physicians justifiably hesitant about transfusing in borderline situations. Factors to be considered are the age of the patient (as the elderly are more susceptible to changes in oxygen-carrying capacity), the presence of ongoing bleeding, and underlying cardiopulmonary disease. In general, a hematocrit less than 25 percent in the patient who is 60 years old or less, and less than 30 percent in patients older than 60 years should necessitate transfusions. Transfusions of packed red blood cells dilute the absolute number of platelets and plasma clotting factors, and therefore, empiric administration of 1 to 2 units of fresh frozen plasma and 10 units of platelets is warranted after administration of 3 to 4 units and 10 units of red cell transfusions respectively.

There is no evidence to date that either commercially available histamine H_2-receptor antagonists (*cimetidine* or *ranitidine*) or *antacids*, or a combination of both, arrests acute upper gastrointestinal bleeding. Yet, their use for treating underlying acid peptic disease is well supported. Therefore, treatment with either regimen (cimetidine, 300 mg intravenously every 6 hours, ranitidine 50 mg intravenously every 6 hours, or antacids 30 to 60 ml via nasogastric tube every 1 to 2 hours to maintain gastric pH at 4.0 or above) may be instituted early to inactivate pepsin, promote coagulation, and heal ulcerations, all of which are effected by the raising of gastric pH. Once again the physician should not expect this early anti-ulcer therapy to play a major role in the cessation of bleeding. If early endoscopy is needed, antacids must be withheld so that the mucosal view is not obscured.

If active esophageal varix hemorrhage is suspected, *vasopressin*, a powerful but nonselective peripheral vasoconstrictor, is sometimes effective in decreasing blood loss or temporizing until more definitive therapy (injection sclerotherapy or portosystemic shunt) can be carried out. An intravenous infusion at 0.2 to 0.4 units per minute can be administered. However, caution should be exhibited in the elderly, who are more prone to myocardial, intestinal, or cerebral ischemia. Bolus infusions of vasopressin or its continuous intravenous infusion outside an intensive care monitoring situation is both unsafe and unwise.

The *Sengstaken-Blakemore or Minnesota tubes* have gastric and esophageal balloons which, when inflated, may tamponade actively bleeding varices. They can cause life-threatening complications; they must not be passed by the inexperienced; and their use necessitates endoscopic documentation of variceal bleeding prior to their insertion. These tubes therefore are of limited use early in the treatment of gastrointestinal hemorrhage.

Other Diagnostic Tests

Early emergency endoscopy in the actively bleeding but stabilized patient serves a diagnostic and therapeutic role. Localization of the bleeding site can be achieved in more than 95 percent of patients. Injection sclerotherapy of esophageal varices and electrocoagulation or photocoagulation of eroded vessels in ulcer craters and angiodysplastic lesions are available to halt bleeding. Use of the Argon or Neodymium-YAG laser, monopolar and bipolar electrocautery, and heater probe has been reserved for patients who have been at high surgical risk in the past, but is being employed more often as an alternative to surgery in a wider spectrum of patients. Controlled trials comparing endoscopic coagulation with surgery for active upper gastrointestinal hemorrhage are ongoing at this time.

With the exception of persistent hemorrhage, however, there appears to be no advantage to emergency endoscopy in reducing mortality, transfusion requirement, or length of hospitalization. Moreover, urgent endoscopy in these situations may have added complications when the patient is hemodynamically unstable. The responsibility falls on the attending physician to ensure adequate resuscitation in the acute setting and be cognizant that in the stable patient, satisfactory endoscopic visualization of the bleeding site can be delayed for up to 24 to 48 hours. Whether early or late in the hospital course, most patients who require hospitalization should have definitive endoscopic verification of the site of hemorrhage. The only possible exception to this rule would be the young nonalcoholic patient with a hemodynamically insignificant hemorrhage who is discharged from the emergency department. An outpatient double-contrast upper gastrointestinal series is an appropriate examination in this setting since the majority of these patients are hemorrhaging from peptic ulcers.

Generally, *barium studies* are not recommended for patients with brisk upper gastrointestinal tract hemorrhage. Esophageal varices, Mallory-Weiss tears, and superficial mucosal lesions are especially difficult to visualize when hemorrhage is brisk. Moreover, in the patient with more than one potential site of blood loss (e.g., varices and peptic ulceration), clear-cut evidence localizing the site of hemorrhage (visible vessel, overlying clot, or active oozing) is accurately assessed only by endoscopy.

DISPOSITION AND CONSULTATION

Bleeding that persists in spite of the foregoing measures clearly warrants admission to an intensive care unit. However, patients who have had minor hemorrhages should be admitted to a less intense hospital service. Along the continuum lie patients who are elderly, but have ceased bleeding, and younger patients who bleed only intermittently or slowly. Proper disposition for these patients is dictated by the judgment of the physician. A hemodynamically insignificant bleed in a young reliable patient can be managed, after initial assessment, on an outpatient basis.

A consultation with a gastroenterologist and general surgeon on an emergency basis is essential for patients with severe persistent bleeding.

SUGGESTED READING

Cello JP, Thoeni RF. Gastrointestinal hemorrhage—comparative values of double-contrast upper gastrointestinal radiology and endoscopy. JAMA 1980; 243:685.

Peterson WL, Barnett CC, Smith JH, et al. Routine early endoscopy in upper-gastrointestinal-tract bleeding. Engl J Med 1981; 304:925.

Zuckerman G, Welch R, Douglas A, et al. Controlled trial of medical therapy for active upper gastrointestinal bleeding and prevention of rebleeding. Am J Med 1984; 76:361.

LOWER GASTROINTESTINAL BLEEDING

GARY A. NEWMAN, M.D.
HOWARD M. SPIRO, M.D.

INITIAL EVALUATION

Management of the patient with acute rectal bleeding depends first on the assessment of the rapidity and severity of blood loss. The initial consideration in massive bleeding is resuscitation and stabilization of the patient's hemodynamic state. Clinical signs of shock, postural hypotension, tachycardia, and pallor require rapid recognition and the placement of large-bore catheters for volume repletion. Monitoring is advisable. Blood should be drawn at once for complete blood count, coagulation values, electrolyte and blood urea nitrogen levels, and for cross-matching.

A brief but careful *history* is then elicited, with attention to the duration of bleeding and the character of the blood loss (i.e., red, maroon, black). The relationship of the bleeding to bowel movements, cramps, and abdominal pains helps distinguish between painless gastrointestinal (GI) bleeding, which is more likely to stem from diverticular disease, angiodysplasia, colonic polyps, malignancy, or hemorrhoids, and painful GI bleeding with abdominal cramps, which at least initially suggests infection, inflammatory bowel disease, or ischemia. Dizziness, syncope, or fecal incontinence suggests massive or rapid bleeding. In patients with chronic lower GI bleeding, such symptoms as weight loss, change in bowel habits, abdominal distention, and anorexia point to a malignancy. It is always important to ask about drugs, especially salicylates, alcohol, or nonsteroidal anti-inflammatory agents, all of which are associated with gastrointestinal bleeding (Table 1).

The initial *physical examination* should be brief and direct. Once the patient's hemodynamic status has been considered, the patient should be examined for signs pointing to the source of bleeding. Cutaneous clues to chronic liver disease, such as spider telangiectasias and palmar erythema, are helpful. A significant murmur of aortic stenosis, particularly in the elderly, has been associated with colonic angiodysplasia. Obviously, the abdomen must be carefully examined for localized tenderness, masses, guarding, or other signs of peritoneal inflammation. Active bowel sounds point to upper GI bleeding with volume distention of the small intestine, whereas infrequent peristalsis supports a lower GI source.

The *rectal examination* is especially important. External and internal hemorrhoids can be seen, anal fissures or fistulas may be detected, and rectal masses can be felt. While black stools usually suggest a slow-bleeding upper tract source, tarry stools can also come from the right colon if colonic transit is slow. Small amounts of bright red blood suggest an anal, rectal, or sigmoid lesion, as does blood-streaking of brown stool. Bloody stools mixed with mucus may indicate infections with organisms such as *Salmonella*, *Shigella*, or *Campylobacter*, inflammatory bowel disease, or ischemia, especially in elderly people with known vascular disease. Massive amounts of maroon clots or bright red blood suggest a rapidly bleeding upper GI source and mandates at least nasogastric aspiration, seeking blood. Remember that the commonest cause of massive rectal bleeding is upper GI bleeding.

INITIAL TREATMENT (SEE FIGURE 1)

In patients with minimal blood loss, anoscopy and sigmoidoscopy can be carried out in the emergency department. While hemorrhoids and anal fissures can be treated with stool softeners, local suppositories, and sitz baths, the detection of an anal fistula or rectal neoplasm requires appropriate referral. If an inflamed, friable rectal mucosa is seen, stool samples must be sent for routine culture, ova and parasite evaluation, and *Clostridium difficile* toxin.

If no local disease is found, patients with evidence of minimal blood loss can be worked up electively and will not be discussed further here. Needless to say, the decision to accept bleeding hemorrhoids as the sole cause of rectal bleeding depends on clinical judgement, the age of the patient, and other considerations. The decision to admit a patient depends on the degree of bleeding and overall medical status. Colonoscopy is the appropriate procedure to rule out lower tract lesions and has replaced barium enema, which is still ordered too often.

TABLE 1 Causes of Rectal Bleeding

Colonic source
  More common
    Diverticular disease ⎤ major sources in
    Angiodysplasia   ⎦ patients >60 years old
    Polyp
    Malignancy
    Inflammatory bowel disease
  Less common
    Ischemic colitis
    Infectious colitis (*Salmonella*, *Shigella*, *Campylobacter*)
    Radiation colitis
  Least common
    Endometriosis
    Colonic varices
Local anal pathology
  Hemorrhoids
  Anal fissures

Small bowel source
  Crohn's disease
  Small bowel neoplasm
  Meckel's diverticulum (in infants, children, and adolescents)
  Angiodysplasia

Upper GI source
  Peptic ulcer disease
  Gastritis/stress ulcer
  Esophagitis
  Esophageal varices/gastric varices
  Mallory-Weiss tear
  Malignancy

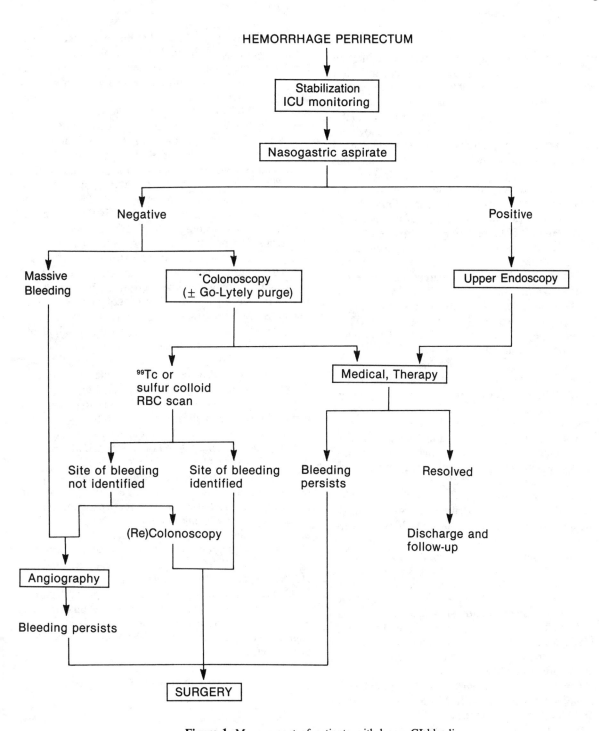

Figure 1 Management of patients with lower GI bleeding.

* In patients with massive bleeding, colonoscopy is unlikely to be helpful. The patient should be taken directly to angiography or surgery. In patients who have stopped bleeding, as 70 to 90 percent will, *elective* colonoscopy is suggested as the initial procedure.

Our major discussion will focus on the patient with massive, active bleeding. As already noted, standard resuscitation and stabilization of the patient's hemodynamic status are key. Saline or colloid can be used for volume repletion until blood is available. Pressors may be required. Non-cross-matched blood can be used if the patient has had a massive blood loss, but is obviously less optimal than appropriately cross-matched transfusions. Aiming for a hematocrit of 30 ml per deciliter is reasonable in most cases. Any coagulation abnormalities require correction with fresh frozen plasma and should prompt consideration of their cause.

DIAGNOSTIC WORK-UP

First, in any patient with copious rectal bleeding, an upper GI source should always be considered. Insertion of a number 16 to 18 F nasogastric tube should be carried out immediately after the initial physical examination. The absence of blood and the presence of bile in the aspirate virtually exclude a source of bleeding above the ligament of Treitz. For practical purposes a clear, non-bilious aspirate eliminates active or recent bleeding from the stomach or esophagus but does not totally rule out an upper tract source. Fiberoptic scrutiny of the upper tract may still be necessary, particularly if the patient's history *strongly* suggests an upper GI origin of the bleeding. Some gastroenterologists, realizing that 3 percent of patients with negative nasogastric aspirates still have upper GI bleeding, will choose to perform endoscopy on the upper GI tract of all patients with apparent massive lower GI bleeding. We do not recommend this approach but prefer to be more selective in our diagnostic testing.

Next in order is a careful *fiberoptic* study of the colon. Sigmoidoscopy has been the most utilized and in the emergency department makes good sense. We prefer an attempt at full colonoscopy, if possible, advancing the scope as far as is necessary to detect the bleeding source. The unprepared colon full of blood is difficult to navigate, but rectal lavage with enemas can often clean out much of the left colon and allow a bleeding site to be directly visualized or at least located. Oral saline lavage (e.g., Go-Lytely) in patients with active bleeding has led to adequate preparation of the colon without apparently stirring up bleeding. As soon as the anal effluent is clear or pink, colonoscopy can be carried out. Good visualization with insertion of the scope to the cecum is usually obtained. Inflammatory bowel disease, neoplasm, ischemia, diverticular disease, and particularly angiodysplasia can be detected. Equally important is that diagnostic biopsies be obtained and therapy with multipolar electrocautery, laser photocoagulation, or polypectomy be carried out. Contraindications to early colonoscopy include massive bleeding with rapid deterioration in clinical status and recent surgical anastomosis. A relative contraindication is a strong suspicion of mesenteric ischemia, but such considerations are the province of the consultant.

It is important to stress that *barium studies* play *no* role in the management of patients with acute rectal bleeding. Barium studies are insensitive in detecting sources of lower GI bleeding and coat the bowel wall, precluding subsequent angiography or colonoscopy.

If colonoscopy supplies no diagnosis, and if the patient remains fairly stable with careful support, a ^{99m}TC sulfur colloid or tagged *red blood cell scan* is necessary. The sulfur colloid scan can be performed rapidly, but requires ongoing bleeding. It is excellent in detecting lower GI bleeding, but accumulation of colloid in the liver and spleen makes detection of bleeding at the splenic and hepatic flexures difficult. Moreover, the half-life of the radionuclide tracer is only 2 to 2.5 minutes, so that intermittent bleeding may be missed. The ^{99m}TC-tagged RBC scan requires about 30 to 40 minutes of preparation to incubate and tag the red blood cells, but it displays bleeding from the upper tract much more precisely, since it is not selectively taken up by the liver and spleen. Moreover, tagged red blood cells remain in the circulation so that the patient can be scanned several times over the next 24 to 48 hours to find the source of intermittent bleeding. Although both scans are reported to detect bleeding in the 0.05 to 0.10 ml per minute range, studies in less dedicated centers have not been as rewarding.

A positive radionuclide scan should be followed at once by selective angiography. The positive scan helps direct catheter placement in order to lessen the dye load needed to find a bleeding site. The angiographer can find the source in patients bleeding at a rate faster than the 0.5 ml per minute range; thus, there is little chance of finding ongoing bleeding if the ^{99m}TC scan is negative. If the scans are negative, active bleeding has probably stopped, and colonoscopy can be (re)attempted.

The angiographer has two therapeutic maneuvers to try to stem ongoing bleeding. Selective *vasopressin infusion* stops bleeding in 70 to 90 percent of patients. If bleeding stops, the angiographic catheter is positioned so that its tip remains in the artery supplying the bleeding site. A continuous infusion of vasopressin is maintained at a rate of 0.2 to 0.4 U per minute, the dose being tapered at 36 to 48 hours. Problems include cardiac, visceral, and peripheral ischemia, arrhythmias, pulmonary edema, hypertension, bronchospasm, oliguria, hyponatremia, catheter-related complications, and a rebleeding rate of *30 percent*. Embolization of colonic bleeding sites has been reported, but the possibility of ischemic injury makes this a risky procedure.

In patients with massive bleeding, colonoscopy is impossible and radionuclide scanning, offering little therapeutic benefit, is unnecessary. In these cases, the patient should go directly to angiography or to surgery. This is, of course, a clinical decision, based on the patient's overall medical state, degree of bleeding, and availability of diagnostic testing. While the type of surgery performed obviously depends on the operative findings, in some patients no source of bleeding is found at exploratory laparotomy. Then a right hemicolectomy or even a subtotal colectomy is often carried out for presumed bleeding from angiodysplasic lesions, a decision beyond the scope of our discussion.

SUGGESTED READING

Brandt LJ, Boley SJ. The role of colonoscopy in the diagnosis and management of lower intestinal bleeding. Scand J Gastroenteral 1984; 19 Suppl 102:61–70.

Eckstein MR, Athanasoulis CA. Gastrointestinal bleeding: an angiographic perspective. Surg Clin North Am 1984; 64:37–51.

Pingleton SK. Gastrointestinal hemorrhage. Med Clin North Am 1983; 67:1215.

Shinya H, Cwesn M, Wolf G. Colonoscopic diagnosis and management of rectal bleeding. Surg Clin North Am 1982; 62:897–903.

Smith JL. Approaches to the problem of lower gastrointestinal bleeding. Compr Ther 1984; 10:43–48.

Steer ML, Silen W. Current concepts: diagnostic procedures in gastrointestinal hemorrhage. N Engl J Med 1983; 309:646–650.

Tedesco FJ, Gottfried EB, Corless JK, Brownstein RE. Prospective evaluation of hospitalized patients with nonactive lower intestinal bleeding—timing and role of barium enema and colonoscopy. Gastrointest Endosc 1984; 30:281.

Waye JD. A diagnostic approach to colon bleeding. Mt. Sinai J Med 1984; 51:591–595.

FOREIGN BODY INGESTION

COREY M. SLOVIS, M.D.

Foreign body ingestion (FBI) is not a rare event. Most ingestions are accidental and often go unnoticed; thus the exact incidence is unknown. More than 90 percent of all ingested objects, regardless of size, shape, or type, pass through the gastrointestinal tract without causing significant morbidity. This chapter will deal only with FBI that progresses beyond the gastroesophageal junction. See chapter on *Esophageal Trauma, Foreign Bodies, and Perforation* for the therapy of objects that become lodged in the esophagus.

ETIOLOGY

The most common categories of patients who ingest foreign bodies are listed in Table 1. Accidental ingestions are the most common, especially in children who swallow rounded objects such as coins, buttons, disk batteries, and rings or slender objects such as pins, nails, and pencils. Although open safety-pin ingestions still occur, the popularity of disposable diapers with self-adhesive closures has markedly decreased the frequency of this FBI. Adult accidental ingestions most often occur in the elderly who wear dentures that decrease their gingival sensitivity. Other adult risk factors include ethanol use, senility, and mental impairment.

Psychotic or suicidal patients or those trying to manipulate their situation, such as prisoners, may deliberately ingest single or multiple objects. These types of patients are prone to ingest sharp objects such as razor blades, broken glass, or knives. This group of patients is more likely to develop acute complications, to require surgical intervention more often, to ingest larger and multiple objects, and to be repeat offenders.

The final group of ingestors are those who use internal transport as a method of attempting to smuggle illicit drugs past customs agents. These people are known as body packers, or mules, and they usually carry high-grade cocaine or heroin, commonly in tied-off condoms.

THERAPY

Conservative therapy is the treatment of choice for the vast majority of patients with FBI. If there is no im-

TABLE 1 Categories of Foreign Body Ingestion

Accidental ingestion
  Childhood
  Adult

Intentional ingestion
  Psychotic
  Suicidal
  Manipulative
  Body packer

pedance to passage, most objects will pass in less than 5 days, usually within the first 3.

Pre-hospital Therapy

There is little definitive pre-hospital treatment for patients who have ingested foreign objects. Parents should be advised to check and clear if necessary the oropharynx of infants and children. Broken glass or other sharp fragmented objects should be carefully removed from the child's mouth. During transport the patient should be kept sitting or in a semi-Fowler's position. This is to avoid the potential for a gastric or esophageal object's being vomited or gagged upward and subsequently aspirated. Parents and emergency medical technicians (EMT) should be cautioned to be especially alert for evidence of airway obstruction and be prepared and educated for appropriate and immediate therapy. Some experts feel that partially digested strands of asparagus may wrap around ingested broken glass fragments in the stomach. This therapy may be advised if readily available. If transport is not significantly delayed, it is certainly not harmful and may have a calming effect on the parent.

All patients should be evaluated by physical examination and x-ray film studies. Even with potentially dangerous esophageal lodgement, most patients will be asymptomatic. Physicians shouald never advise careful, at-home observation in asymptomatic patients over the phone.

Ipecac, forced gagging, and cathartics are absolutely contraindicated in the pre-hospital setting. Not only are the former two rarely successful but they increase the danger of aspiration of the foreign object into the tracheobronchial tree.

First 8 Hours

A protocol for the step-wise management of FBI appears in Table 2. Once a patient has arrived in the emergency department with a secure airway, the type and time of ingestion, number of ingested objects, and reasons for the FBI must be established. A history with attention to FBI-induced complications should be taken (Table 3). The

TABLE 2 Step-wise Management of Foreign Body Ingestion

Rule out airway compromise.
Perform history and physical examination (see Table 3).
Perform x-ray evaluation to rule out esophageal lodgement and document diagnosis.
Evaluate need for hospital admission (see Table 4).
Educate patient or parents on symptoms and complications.
Encourage high-fiber diet for sharp objects or mild daily cathartics for rounded objects.
Patient's stools should be checked for elimination of object.
Discharge from hospital with concurrence of patient's physician.
Repeat x-ray study in 4–7* days if object is not observed in stool.
Avoid ipecac, activated charcoal, extensive laboratory testing, and hospital admission in all asymptomatic patients if the object is beyond the esophagus.

* Forty-eight hours in 20–23 mm-diameter button batteries.

**TABLE 3   Historical Facts to be Elicited and Symptoms
to be Monitored at Home in FBI**

Fever, cyanosis, drooling, refusal to eat.

Pain or discomfort on swallowing or breathing.

Gagging, vomiting, or choking.

Throat, neck, chest, or abdominal pain.

Hematemesis, hemoptysis, melena, or hematochezia.

Modified from Binder L, Anderson WA. Pediatric gastrointestinal foreign body
ingestions. Ann Emerg Med 1984; 13:112–117.

physical examination findings are almost always negative,
but the throat should be evaluated for trauma, the chest
listened to for wheezing, and the abdomen carefully evaluated. A stool guaiac test is mandatory.

It is incumbent upon clinicians to confirm or rule out
suspected FBI by x-ray evaluation. Most patients will
present without symptoms and thus radiologic studies are
mandatory to (1) establish the diagnosis, and (2) determine the ingested object's location.

In neonates, usually a single anteroposterior chest film
is all that is required, while in adults, chest films may
need to be supplemented by supine and upright views of
the abdomen. If these films are nondiagnostic, a lateral
cervical spine film with attention to soft-tissue detail is
required to confirm an esophageal location and rule out
tracheobronchial involvement. In some cases of FBI, patients present with signs or symptoms that are the complications of an inadvertent ingestion (e.g., a swallowed
toothpick presenting as a duodenal perforation) and diagnosis is only made interoperatively. Some objects, especially those composed of plastic, glass, or wood, may
be difficult to see on routine x-rays films. Those that are
large enough to cause obstruction are either visible on
plain films or may be outlined with the aid of swallowed
barium-soaked cottonballs. Xeroradiographs are sometimes helpful with wooden objects if contrast study results
are equivocal.

Once an object has passed the gastroesophageal
sphincter, its likelihood of eventual passage is above 90
percent and the risk of perforation less than 1 percent.
Earlier literature often recommended forced removal of
potentially dangerous objects. Ipecac rarely is effective;
in one study, no successes were observed in 15 cases in
which it was used for button battery ingestions. Based on
its high failure rate, side effects of continued nausea and
vomiting, and the potential for a patient to subsequently
aspirate the foreign object, there is no indication for the
use of ipecac in FBI. Although earlier touted as the appropriate aggressive form of therapy, *endoscopy* with
polypectomy snare or basket is successful in less than one-
third of cases once an object has passed into the stomach
or duodenum. Because of its expense, invasiveness, the
need for anesthesia, and the high failure rate, endoscopy
is not recommended in nonesophageal FBI. Activated
charcoal should not be administered. It is of no proven
benefit and may obscure the diagnosis of gastrointestinal
hemorrhage once the patient is discharged for conservative, at-home management.

Disposition

Most asymptomatic patients may be discharged with
appropriate education and follow-up instructions. If the
object is sharp, such as broken glass, a high-fiber diet
may be recommended. For rounded objects, such as coins
or batteries, daily cathartics (e.g., Milk of Magnesia) may
be advocated. Patients or parents should be told that the
diet and cathartic are empiric and not of proven value.
In cases of sharp object ingestion, the incidence of perforation may be increased by giving cathartics. The types
of patients requiring hospital admission are listed in
Table 4.

PATIENTS REQUIRING HOSPITAL ADMISSION

Ingestions Causing Symptoms

Hospital admission is required for any patient who
is symptomatic secondary to FBI. Obstruction, perforation, and gastrointestinal hemorrhage are the three major
complications of FBI and require immediate hospital admission and operative intervention. Patients should be
stabilized, typed and cross-matched for appropriate quantities of blood, and a pediatric or general surgical consultation obtained immediately. When there is evidence
of shock or significant hemorrhage, an intensive care unit
bed is mandatory if the patient is not going immediately
to the operating room. Transfer to another facility is only
appropriate if the referring hospital or clinic does not have
the ability to perform surgery rapidly.

Patients who are symptomatic because the contents
of their foreign body are leaking require immediate medical and surgical intervention. In the case of ruptured disk
batteries, patients may have perforation, gastrointestinal
hemorrhage, obstruction, or potential mercury poisoning.
In the first three instances, standard supportive preoperative resuscitation is required, while mercury poisoning
will require penicillamine therapy. In patients who are
transporting illicit drugs by body packing, leakage is often

TABLE 4   Indications for Admission in Nonesophageal FBI

Symptomatic object

   Evidence of obstruction

   Evidence of perforation

   Evidence of gastrointestinal hemorrhage

   Contents of object leaking

High-risk foreign body

   Body packer

   Object larger than 6.5 cm

   Multiple objects

   Lack of adequate or reliable home observation

   Attempted suicidal ingestion in still suicidal patient

Lack of progression according to follow-up x-ray films

   (Note: normally 4–7 days but 48 hours in 20–23 mm-button battery
   ingestions.)

a preterminal event. If possible, high-dose naloxone or propranolol should be used for heroin- and cocaine-related symptoms, respectively. Dosage should be titrated to individual patients and will be far in excess of the clinician's previous experience. Immediate surgical intervention is required for these patients.

High-Risk Foreign Body Ingestions

Those asymptomatic patients who have ingested packets or condoms containing illicit drugs require hospital admission. These patients are usually under police guard and should be admitted to an acute care area for monitoring. Because of the high potential for condom rupture, attempts at endoscopic removal are contraindicated.

Those patients who have ingested objects larger than 6.5 cm are unlikely to pass them spontaneously. They should be transferred to either a gastroenterologist or a general surgeon, depending on the radiologic location of the FBI.

Patients who ingest multiple objects, especially sharp or large objects, are at high risk for complications. This group is generally composed of psychotic patients or incarcerated individuals who desire to manipulate their confinement. The incidence of obstruction, perforation, and hemorrhage is highest in this group and may approach 25 percent.

Almost all asymptomatic children can be discharged with appropriate follow-up care and a second x-ray study if necessary by their pediatrician. If there is inadequate at-home supervision, then children who have swallowed a high-risk object, such as an alkaline disk battery or a long, pointed object, should be admitted to the hospital for observation.

Any still suicidal patient who presents with FBI should be admitted to a psychiatric treatment facility or area under a psychiatrist's care. Suicide precautions must be enforced while the patient is in the emergency department. Care must be taken to rule out concomitant occult methods of suicide along with the FBI. If any additional ingestion is suspected, a toxin screen is advised, with specific testing for acetaminophen and tricyclic antidepressants. A screening electrocardiogram with attention to rate, QRS duration, and Q-T interval should be performed while the patient is still in the emergency department.

Lack of Progress

The final category of patients requiring admission are those who return to the emergency department following FBI and demonstrate failure of the object to progress. Elongated, slender, foreign bodies such as pencils, pens, bobby pins, nails, and chicken bones have the highest failure of passage. The usual repeat x-ray film is performed 4 to 7 days after ingestion. Those patients with known gastrointestinal motility disturbances, anatomic abnormalities (e.g., strictures, diverticula) or 20 to 23 mm

battery ingestions should be advised by their physician to return sooner for follow-up films.

BATTERY INGESTION

There is considerable controversy surrounding the management of ingested batteries.

Alkaline disk or button batteries are easily swallowed and have the potential to cause death if they become impacted in the gastrointestinal tract and begin leaking their contents. The danger is based on (1) high alkaline content (usually highly concentrated potassium hydroxide), (2) potential to cause low voltage burns, (3) ability to "hang up" in the gastrointestinal tract and cause pressure necrosis, and (4) potential for some to cause mercury poisoning. Some authors recommend endoscopic removal if possible or immediate surgery in asymptomatic patients if endoscopy either failed or was not possible.

Litovitz has recently published the recommendations of the National Button Battery Ingestion Study, which is based on 125 cases of battery ingestion. In this ongoing study, 90 percent of all button battery ingestions were passed without complication using a conservative approach. Of the 10 percent of patients who became symptomatic, all but one had minor complications. The general treatment protocol in Table 2 incorporates the recommendations of the study. Physicians should note the difference in plans for x-ray follow-up studies when dealing with a 20 to 23 mm-diameter camera battery as compared with the more common 11.6 mm- and 7.9 mm-diameter batteries. Physicians are advised to call the 24-hour emergency number at 202-625-3333 both to report a battery ingestion and for additional treatment advice.

DISCHARGE INSTRUCTIONS

At the time of hospital discharge, patients or their parents should be knowledgeable in the signs and symptoms of perforation, obstruction, and gastrointestinal blood loss. They should be told unequivocally to return if any of the signs and symptoms listed in Table 2 appear. The patient's stool should be checked for the presence of the ingested object. If the object is not passed within a predetermined number of days, the patient should consult his private physician or return to the emergency care facility. Four to 7 days are usually allowed for gastrointestinal transit (48 hours in large disk batteries). The patient's private physician should be contacted and be in agreement with all plans.

SUGGESTED READING

Binder L, Anderson WA. Pediatric gastrointestinal foreign body ingestions. Ann Emerg Med 1984;13:112–117.

Garcia C, Frey CF, Bodai BI. Diagnostic and management of ingested foreign bodies: a ten year experience. Ann Emerg Med 1984; 13:30–34.

Litovitz TL. Battery ingestion: product accessibility and clinical course. Pediatrics 1985;75:469–476.

CAUSTIC AND CORROSIVE INGESTION

ROBERT S. PETERS, M.D., F.A.C.P.

Strong alkalis and acids and, in rare instances, some medications in pill form are only a small part of the list of substances that may cause injury to the mucosa of the gastrointestinal tract when intentionally or accidentally ingested (Table 1). Medications in pill form cause esophageal injury with symptoms of odynophagia, hemorrhage, and late strictures on very rare occasions (Table 2). The number and character of such chemicals and medications continue to grow as new materials are added and the formulas of existing ones are changed. The severity of the damage and its consequences vary with the agent, the details of ingestion, the ability of the esophagus to empty, and the contents of the stomach at the time. Independent evaluation of each patient, including complete identification of the contents of the ingestant and its potential for injury, is required.

Ingestions of 5 ml or more of particulate alkali or suspended alkali (e.g., most liquid drain cleaners) or concentrated acids (e.g., swimming pool acid) almost always results in some injury to the mouth, esophagus, or stomach. The action of such strong corrosives is essentially complete in less than 5 minutes, and neutralization or removal attempts are more likely to create more injury than provide aid. Traditionally, acids that form an eschar in their early action as opposed to the liquefaction necrosis of the alkalis were thought to spare the esophagus and do more damage to the stomach. However, the current suspensions of alkalis often cause severe gastric damage, including perforation, and up to 50 percent of strong acid ingestions produce esophageal burns leading to stricture or perforation.

Accidental ingestion very often involves storage in unusual containers, such as soft drink bottles, canning jars, and drinking glasses, or storage in unusual places, such as kitchen cupboards or refrigerators. Intentional ingestions may be preceded by ingestions of sedatives, alcohol, or other drugs. In any case, people on the scene should be instructed to bring in any container of any type present in the area, since even those without labels may be identified as strong or weak acids or alkalis by pH testing in the laboratory or with the use of pH paper. Alkaline solutions with a pH of less than 12.0 are not associated with injury.

DIAGNOSIS

Most patients present with their own or an accompanying observer's history of ingestion. Determining the nature of the ingested substance as corrosive, hydrocarbon, or other may at times not be clear. If any doubt exists as to whether or not an ingestant was a corrosive, it is usually wise to assume this as a possibility and to search for oropharyngeal injury. Finding burns or mucositis establishes the ingestant as a corrosive. In those in whom such signs are not found, the possibility of esophageal or gastric injury cannot be ruled out, and the pursuit of the identity and characteristics of the material must continue while studying the patient for other toxicologic reactions. When no information or specimens can otherwise be obtained, cautious passage of the nasogastric tube or gastroscopic aspiration from the stomach, using a Lukens trap in the suction line of the instrument, may provide an analyzable specimen. The endoscopic approach appears the most conservative, if available, as it provides a concurrent estimate of the presence or absence of gastroesophageal damage.

TABLE 1 A Partial List of Chemicals and Other Agents Associated with Severe Esophageal or Gastric Injury When Ingested

Alkalis
  Lye: Sodium or potassium hydroxide in any form
  Ammonia solutions

Acids
  Hydrochloric or muriatic acid
  Sulfuric acid
  Lactic acid
  Phosphoric acid
  Acetic acid

Disinfectants
  Phenol
  Lysol
  Potassium permanganate
  Iodine
  Hydrogen peroxide
  Mercuric chloride

Detergents
  Automatic dishwasher
  Laundry

Household cleaners
  Toilet bowl cleaners
  Drain cleaners
  Tile cleaners
  Oven cleaners

Reference to a complete source, such as Poisindex, to a Poison Control Center, to a text such as Gosselin RE, Hodge HC, Smith RP, Gleason MN. Clinical toxicology of commercial products, 5th ed. Baltimore: Williams & Wilkins, 1984, or the manufacturer for complete contents and specific references is advised.

TABLE 2 Medications That May Cause Esophageal Injury*

Doxycycline
Tetracycline and minocycline
Clindamycin-lincomycin
Potassium chloride†
Ferrous sulfate†
Quinidine†
Indomethacin†
Aspirin-containing drugs

---

* These are rare and often represent single case reports. In most instances, patients will present with transient odynophagia or dysphagia.
† Hemorrhage, perforation, and late stricture formation have been reported, and endoscopy and/or follow-up examination is indicated.

CLINICAL PRESENTATION

Up to one-half of all cases present with no external evidence of mouth, tongue, or pharyngeal burns or pain. The lesions and symptoms that can be seen are listed in Table 3. These are almost always seen in patients with more severe injuries. The presence or absence of esophageal and gastric injuries does not correlate directly with the presence or absence of symptoms. Those cases with more extensive symptoms or signs or both must be considered to have perforation or be in danger of perforation and should be evaluated immediately for this complication.

DIFFERENTIAL DIAGNOSIS

Failure to consider corrosive ingestion as a cause of symptoms and to look for mouth and pharyngeal signs is much more likely than is confusion with another diagnosis. The following situations have been observed in this context.

1. The accompanying vomiting may produce sufficient bleeding to create an initial impression of a Mallory-Weiss tear as the cause.
2. Chest pain may be sufficiently severe, particularly when accompanied by some hypotension, to create an initial assessment of the case as myocardial infarction or Boerhaave's syndrome.
3. With laryngeal aspiration or severe pharyngeal edema, stridor and respiratory distress may suggest asthma or epiglottitis.

TABLE 3 Symptoms and Signs of Corrosive Ingestion in the Acute Phase*

Symptoms
   Persistent salivation
   Inability to swallow
   Dysphagia
   Odynophagia
   Epigastric pain
   Retching
   Vomiting
   Blood-streaked vomitus
   Hematemesis, frank or coffee grounds
   Emesis of tissue or eschar
   Hoarseness
   Tachypnea
   Dyspnea
   Stridor
   Shock
Signs
   Redness and swelling of the lips and tongue
   Edema of the uvula and faucial pillars
   Easy bleeding of mucosa
   Lip and mouth eschars
   White membranes on the oral mucosa
   Mediastinal crunch
   Crepitus
   Epigastric tenderness
   Abdominal rigidity, ileus

* As many as one-half of the patients with a history of ingestion may have no symptoms or signs. There is no good correlation between symptoms and injury.

Perhaps the most overlooked issue in the concern surrounding a severe case in which there are often major mouth burns and pain is that of coexisting ingestion of alcohol, acetaminophen, salicylic acid acetate, benzodiazepines, and tricyclic antidepressants. These may often precede the corrosive in intentional cases and require concurrent study in every such case. In a rare instance such a combined ingestion (including corrosives) may be incidentally found in an unresponsive patient who presents in the emergency department without information. In such a case, mouth and pharyngeal burns may provide the necessary information; if a corrosive container is also recovered, this must be considered to have been a part of the ingestion until otherwise established. A caution is also in order regarding the possibility of overlooking coexisting conditions such as diabetes, coronary artery disease, and hypertension in the activity that often surrounds a more severe case.

DIAGNOSTIC PROCEDURES

Radiologic

In the severely ill patient with evidence of burns or a solid history of ingestion of a known strong corrosive, prompt chest and abdominal films are in order to observe for aspiration, pneumonitis, and mediastinal and subdiaphragmatic air collections. In the event that free air is observed or suspected, films utilizing contrast media are taken with the patient in the supine position while swallowing; after a wait, they are then repeated with the patient in the upright or sitting position. Swallowing while supine requires muscular action of the esophagus and is at least theoretically more likely to reveal a perforation than upright swallows, which may move more rapidly. Similarly, antral perforations may become more obvious in the upright position, since the supine position favors pooling primarily in the fundus.

Serologic

In all significant cases and any with depressed responses, a complete screen for additional common ingestants is conducted. These should include alcohol, acetaminophen, salicylic acid acetate, benzodiazepines, and tricyclic antidepressants at a minimum. Complete blood count, determination of electrolyte levels and typing and cross-matching of blood may be called for according to the clinical condition.

Endoscopic

As previously noted, the extent of esophageal and gastric injury in almost any corrosive ingestion patient correlates poorly with the oral mucosal and general symptoms. They vary with the ingestant, its physical and chemical state, concentration, and physiologic factors. A patient with delayed esophageal motility or stricture could receive a severe burn from a small amount of a dilute alkali, whereas a stomach full of food might dilute a significant amount of an acid material. Conversely, the material may have caused mouth burns, but the amount actually swallowed may have been insufficient to cause significant injury. Accordingly, almost all patients require endoscopic evaluation. A recently appreciated special exception is in patients who have ingested common liquid laundry bleach, 3 percent hypochlorite, which has not been associated with serious esophageal injury. Endoscopy is not performed in favor of follow-up studies as outlined below when this can be established as the agent with certainty.

In those patients with any chest film changes suggestive of aspiration or symptoms of hoarseness or stridor, *bronchoscopy* is usually performed simultaneously with the gastrointestinal examination. The modern fiberoptic bronchoscopes make a satisfactory instrument for examining small infants and can be used in the adult esophagus as well. This may be convenient in patients with severe mouth and pharyngeal burns, allowing a nasopharyngeal approach and both examinations with one instrument if the lung study is indicated. Technically, this requires the addition of an air source via the oxygen channel for the esophageal examination.

TREATMENT

Immediate, On Site

Damage to the mucosa of the gastrointestinal tract for most ingestants is rapid and completed in seconds in the case of strong alkalis and acids and estimated to be within 1 to 2 minutes or at least less than 5 minutes for most others. Antidotes, emetics, and other home remedies are probably of little or no value and in some instances may cause injury through vomiting, re-exposure of the tissues, or aspiration. The majority opinion at present is that the most effective, immediate therapy is to gather all containers, including any alcohol or medication packages, and to take the patient to the nearest hospital emergency facility.

Paramedics and Ambulance Transport

In cases in which vomiting and severe symptoms occur, intravenous fluid support with lactated Ringer's solution and maintenance of a patient airway are the major steps.

Emergency Department

The role of the emergency department is essentially limited to diagnosis, physiologic support, and organization of diagnostic and definitive care activities. The diagnostic issues and steps are listed above. The patient should be given nothing by mouth and kept under observation. When vomiting occurs, it should be controlled with intramuscular or intravenous Compazine, 5 to 15 mg, as needed. Pain relief, most often intravenous morphine, is needed in the more severe cases. Other suport may require (1) fluid replacement and maintenance, (2) blood transfusion, (3) oxygen therapy, and (4) endotracheal intubation, depending on the severity of injury and the presence of hemorrhage, pulmonary involvement, glottic or subglottic edema, or perforation.

The role of prophylactic antibiotics is currently debated, and most authorities feel that they should be reserved for specific therapy of an established infection. Accordingly, they should not be initiated routinely in the emergency department. Similarly, the efficacy of prophylactic steroids has not been conclusively established, and they should not be initiated automatically by emergency department personnel.

Disposition by the Emergency Department

Gastroenterologists or endoscopically trained surgeons interested in this field should be consulted. In the more severe cases, they should be informed of the presence of hemorrhage, suspicion of or presence of perforation or glottic and tracheal injury, and the possible need for surgery. According to the extent of injury, emergency surgery could be limited or could involve total esophagogastrectomy with pharyngostomy and jejunostomy.

Essentially all patients who have ingested significant corrosive substances (with the exception of proven 3 percent hypochlorite and those alkaline solutions of less than pH 12.0) require endoscopy and follow-up care. As a general rule, those patients with symptoms or mouth burns should be examined immediately. Those patients who are asymptomatic but clearly have ingested a potentially injurious or unknown substance can often reasonably be examined at a convenient time within the next 24 hours.

There remains a group of asymptomatic children and adults who have ingested unknown amounts of an unknown substance most often described as "bad-tasting." In these cases, judgment must be exercised with respect to the need for endoscopic examination, and it may often appear reasonable to simply inform the patients that if they develop painful or difficult swallowing, prompt medical attention is advised. Table 4 summarizes the essentials of treatment.

DEFINITIVE CARE

Significant corrosive injury to the gastrointestinal tract progresses in three stages: (1) acute necrosis and inflammation in 4 to 7 days, (2) removal of injured tissue and repair with formation of collagen in 7 to 14 days, and (3) consolidation and contraction of fibrous tissue in 14 to 180 days. Perforation and acute hemorrhage are most likely in stage 1 and to a lesser extent in stage 2. Stricture formation and gastric outlet obstruction occur in stage 3. Definitive care varies according to the severity of in-

TABLE 4 Essentials of Treatment

Initial contact prior to arrival at emergency department

Do not attempt to neutralize (NPO)
Search for and bring any containers found (includes manufacturers and/or any secondary containers such as Coke bottles or Mason jars and any alcohol or medication containers)
Prompt transport to the emergency department

Pre-hospital care

If hemodynamic instability, start large-bore IV catheter with lactated Ringer's solution
If vomiting occurs, position the patient to prevent aspiration
Oxygen if respiratory distress
Pain relief as ordered
Maintain airway if pharyngeal or oral burns

Presentation in emergency department

Asymptomatic (up to one-half of patients)
Mouth eschars or burns
Pharyngeal burns and edema
Odynophagia, dysphagia, and chest pain
Stridor and respiratory distress
Abdominal pain and/or rigidity
Shock

Diagnosis

History from patient or relatives
If containers or substance identification does not accompany patient, send someone for all available (as above)
Physical examination for mouth or pharyngeal burns
Evaluation of accompanying containers
Endoscopic examination and collection of specimens

Cautions

Other ingestants
Overlooking coexisting diseases early in severe cases
Overlooking corrosive ingestion in patients found unresponsive responsive

Differential considerations

May appear to be Mallory-Weiss syndrome with hematemesis
May simulate myocardial infarction or Boerhaave's syndrome if chest pain predominant
May appear as asthma or epiglottitis when major symptoms are stridor and respiratory distress

Laboratory and radiologic examinations to be considered

PA and lateral chest views, with attention to mediastinal air
Upright abdominal series
Blood studies for alcohol, salicylic acid acetate, acetaminophen, benzodiazepines, and tricyclic antidepressants
Complete blood count, urinalysis, and electrolyte levels
Type and crossmatch for packed red blood cells if patient is bleeding

Disposition and definitive care

Gastroenterologist or surgeon with endoscopic experience; pulmonologist may also be indicated if lung involvement suspected
Endoscopic studies:
Upper gastrointestinal
Bronchoscopy if suspect aspiration
If perforation suspected or established:
Surgeon with thoracic and chest experience on an emergency basis for possible esophagogastrectomy with pharyngostomy and jejunostomy as lifesaving measures for later reconstruction
Certain asymptomatic children and adults who have ingested unknown materials or 3 percent hypochlorite may not be endoscoped but referred for follow-up study
Follow-up examination
Patient should be instructed to observe for pain or difficulty in swallowing and to report signs promptly
Follow-up barium studies by a physician if any suspicion appears warranted at 8, 12, and 16 weeks

---

TABLE 5 Definitive and Late Treatments Utilized in Gastrointestinal Corrosive Injury

Observation and follow-up studies
Prophylactic and/or directed antibiotics
Corticosteroids for up to 90 days
Total parenteral nutrition
Oral or soft nasogastric tube liquid nutrition maintenance
Prophylactic bougienage
Bougienage: Prophylactic, or wait for early stricture formation
Pharyngostomy and ileostomy for perforation or massive destruction
Colon interposition
Late hemigastrectomy for antral scarring and gastric retention
Appropriate surgical reconstruction in patients requiring initial surgical resections

---

jury and the concepts of the physician in charge. The approaches most commonly reported and employed alone or in combination are listed in Table 5.

FOLLOW-UP CARE

Patients found at endoscopy to have no apparent lesions or in whom endoscopy is not elected should be discharged and a follow-up visit scheduled. Although they are very unlikely to occur, late strictures have been reported. Follow-up visits at 8 and 12 and 16 weeks appear to be most appropriate. These usually involve barium studies to identify potential stricture development.

SUGGESTED READING

Castell DO. Esophageal function in health and disease. New York: Elsevier Biomedical, 1983:255.
Gosselin RE, et al. Clinical toxicology of commercial products. 5th ed. Baltimore; William & Wilkins, 1984:1900.
Sleisenger MH, Fordtran JS. Gastrointestinal disease. 3rd ed. Philadelphia: WB Saunders, 1983:148.

APPENDICITIS AND DIVERTICULITIS

KENNETH ENG, M.D.

APPENDICITIS

Although the incidence of appendicitis has declined in the past decade, it remains a major cause of acute abdominal emergencies. When the clinical picture is typical, even the layman can make the diagnosis; however, the atypical case may tax the judgment of the most experienced clinician. The diagnosis may be especially obscure in infants and the elderly. Delay in diagnosis results in increased morbidity and may lead to death.

The emergency physician or primary care physician is in a unique position to affect the course of the disease by prompt diagnosis and initiation of treatment. He must decide which of the many patients with abdominal pain are to be sent home, admitted to hospital, or referred for surgical consultation. Because the progression of acute appendicitis may be subtle, a patient should be sent home only when the diagnosis is extremely unlikely. A follow-up phone call or visit within 12 hours is essential. In doubtful cases the safest course is to admit the patient to the hospital or to a holding area of the emergency department for close observation. This is particularly helpful for appendicitis in the early stages, with little or no inflammation. Progression of the illness is detected by frequent abdominal examination or by following the temperature and white blood cell count.

Surgical consultation and emergency surgery, of course, follows in the patient with probable diagnosis of appendicitis, but the surgeon should also be called early to evaluate the doubtful case. A puzzling clinical picture is puzzling to the surgeon as well, and only by serial observation is he or she able to arrive at the appropriate diagnosis.

Differential Diagnosis

In the typical patient with acute appendicitis, the initial symptom is a vague or colicky central abdominal pain due to obstruction of the appendiceal lumen. This visceral pain is usually associated with anorexia, and is sometimes followed by nausea and vomiting. As the appendix becomes infected, pain appears in the right lower quadrant due to peritoneal inflammation. Fever and leukocytosis appear, and tenderness and rigidity of the overlying muscle is noted.

Plain and upright x-ray films of the abdomen may support the diagnosis if a fecalith, localized ileus, or loss of normal fat shadows are seen. Adjunctive examinations should be reserved for ruling out appendicitis when the diagnosis is highly unlikely (barium enema), or to support another diagnosis such as ureteral stone (intravenous

pyelography), ovarian cyst (pelvic sonography), or diverticulitis (computerized tomography). Some variants of acute appendicitis are discussed in the following sections.

Vomiting

With high-grade obstruction of the appendiceal lumen, the patient may present with repeated vomiting, which could divert attention from lower abdominal signs and symptoms and suggest upper gastrointestinal obstruction or gastroenteritis. Right lower quadrant tenderness and the absence of obstruction on abdominal x-ray film help to establish the diagnosis of appendicitis. Early perforation is most likely in these patients.

Flank Pain

Retrocecal appendicitis produces flank pain and tenderness and may be confused with a ureteral stone. An inflamed appendix resting on the ureter may even produce some red and white cells in the urine, but the presence of numerous cells should raise the suspicion of urinary tract disease. An intravenous pyelogram may be diagnostic.

Diarrhea and Tenesmus

An inflamed appendix lying in the pelvis or behind the ileum produces no abdominal wall peritoneal signs. Moreover, local irritation of the rectum may produce diarrhea and tenesmus that mimic infectious enteritis. Rectal examination may reveal the true diagnosis, but when the appendix lies beyond the examining finger, the diagnosis may be obscure. A barium enema, songram, or computerized tomogram may be helpful.

Peritonitis

Perforated appendix with lower abdominal peritonitis may be indistinguishable from peritonitis from other etiologies. A characteristic history or obvious finding on computerized tomography may indicate the source of the peritonitis. Otherwise exploratory laparotomy is necessary.

Pelvic Mass

Perforation of the appendix may result instead in an appendix mass. With no systemic toxicity and no spreading peritonitis, a precise diagnosis may be sought. Diagnosis may be aided by one or more techniques of the following sequence: sonography, computerized tomography, barium enema, and upper gastrointestinal series.

Common Diagnostic Errors

Systemic medical diseases such as ketoacidosis, leukemia, or Henoch-Schönlein purpura with abdominal pain may be mistaken for appendicitis. Right lower lobe pneumonia with diaphragmatic pleurisy may also present with abdominal pain. Laparotomy in these instances would be a disservice to the patient.

Misdiagnosis of intra-abdominal diseases that require

surgery, such as leaking duodenal ulcer or inflamed Meckel's diverticulum, presents no problem provided the true pathology is recognized at laparotomy. In other intra-abdominal conditions such as hepatitis, pancreatitis, and uncomplicated Crohn's disease, surgery should be avoided whenever possible.

The most serious error in acute appendicitis, however, is in failure to make the diagnosis. For this reason, removal of a small percentage (5 to 10 percent) of normal appendices is still considered to be good practice. A delay in diagnosis of appendicitis, leading to perforation or gangrene increases morbidity. Even more serious is continued treatment of a perforated appendix as a medically treatable disease, such as pelvic inflammatory disease or diverticular abscess, until septic shock intervenes. Such an error may be fatal. Diagnosis is especially difficult in infants, because of a lack of history, and in the aged, who often have minimal abdominal signs. Optimal treatment of the patient with acute abdominal pain requires thorough evaluation of the whole patient, a prompt diagnosis, and continued reevaluation of that diagnosis during the course of treatment.

DIVERTICULITIS

Major advances in the understanding of diverticular disease have been achieved in the past two decades. Technical advances such as colonoscopy, ultrasonography, and computerized tomography have improved the diagnostic armamentarium. New knowledge of the pathophysiology has improved both medical and surgical management of diverticular disease and its complications.

Epidemiologic studies suggest dietary fiber deficiency as the cause for the prevalence and increasing frequency of diverticular disease in Western society. The most consistent pathologic abnormality is narrowing of the colon due to muscular hypertrophy. Motility studies reveal abnormally high intraluminal pressures in patients with symptomatic diverticular disease. Correlation of motility studies and cineradiography showed that abdominal pain, high intraluminal pressure, and herniation of mucosa are all associated with segmentation of the lumen by adjacent rings of muscular contraction. Although the precise role of fiber in the development of diverticula and their complications is problematic, a high-fiber diet does prevent segmentation, lower intraluminal pressure, and relieve pain. Most emergency visits and admissions are occasioned by one of the complications of diverticular disease, particularly perforation.

Acute Diverticulitis

Acute diverticulitis is caused by erosion of a mucosal sac by a fecalith at the neck of a diverticulum. This may lead to peridiverticulitis with the characteristic phlegmon involving the colon wall and adjacent structures. Perforation with abscess walled off by the leaves of the mesocolon, small bowel, bladder, abdominal wall, omentum, or retroperitoneal structures is common. When the infection is present for a long time, the abscess may drain into an adjacent viscus to form a fistula. Rarely, perforation is free into the peritoneal cavity, producing fecal peritonitis; or an enlarging abscess may rupture into the peritoneal cavity and produce purulent peritonitis.

Therefore, a patient with diverticular perforation may present with a illness varying from mild fever and left lower quadrant pain and tenderness to severe collapse and generalized peritonitis. Rational management depends on the physician's judgment as to whether a phlegmon, an abscess, or free perforation has occurred. The management may be further modified by the development of obstruction of the colon or small bowel.

Many patients with mild acute diverticulitis with continued bowel function have been treated successfully as outpatients using oral antibiotics. Although most respond to medical management, there is a danger of misdiagnosis of a different surgical emergency, and free perforation may be overlooked. In most instances it is best to hospitalize the patient for intravenous antibiotic therapy and serial abdominal examination. The diagnosis is primarily a clinical one and rests on the finding of local peritonitis in the left lower quadrant. A tender mass may be palpable by abdominal, pelvic, or rectal examination. If the diagnosis is in doubt, or there is evidence of spreading peritonitis, emergency operation is indicated. The surgeon must be prepared to make this choice at any time in the patient's course. Among the conditions confused with diverticulitis are appendicitis and intestinal ischemia.

Most patients respond to nonoperative management. A nasogastric tube is inserted for ileus or intestinal obstruction. A broad-spectrum antibiotic such as ampicillin (2 g every 6 hours) is administered intravenously. Antibiotics are changed as dictated by clinical response and cultures. Generally the patient should show some evidence of improvement in 48 to 72 hours. Fever and leukocytosis should diminish. Pain, tenderness, and abdominal masses should decrease. Return of bowel function, as evidenced by decreased distension and the passage of stool and flatus, should ensue. When the patient responds to these measures, no other treatment is necessary, although this regimen may have to be continued for 7 to 10 days. Following recovery, it is necessary to obtain a barium enema to confirm the diagnosis. This study may be obtained in the hospital or deferred until after discharge.

Diverticular Abscess

A diverticular abscess may be apparent as a tender abdominal or pelvic mass. More presumptive evidence for diverticular abscess is the failure of abdominal signs, fever, or leukocytosis to respond to antibiotic therapy. Sonography or computerized tomography may be helpful in confirming the diagnosis, but if surgery is considered to be necessary a contrast study of the colon should be obtained. The radiologist should be warned of the possibility of colonic peforation. The examination is performed without laxative preparation and using only water-soluble contrast. The study should at least show diverticula. Positive evidence for diverticular perforation, such as extraluminal accumulation of contrast and/or extrinsic compression of the lumen is helpful, but therapeutic decisions are still based on clinical signs. At this time a decision must be reached for continued medical management, immediate operation, or preparation for elective operation.

Resection of the perforated segment has evolved as the most reliable alternative in the emergency management of diverticular abscess. Drainage of the abscess and exteriorization of the proximal and distal bowel as an end colostomy and mucous fistula ensure control of peritoneal soilage. Formal resection of the diseased colon and restoration of intestinal continuity are performed as a second stage. Another alternative for diverticular abscess is resection and anastomosis in one stage. One-stage resection is considered only if inflammation is localized and the return of bowel function permits bowel preparation.

Free Perforation and Generalized Peritonitis

In some cases, free perforation of a diverticulum or rupture of an enlarging abscess produces generalized peritonitis. Patients with diffuse peritoneal signs should be prepared for emergency operation without delay. Volume deficits are replaced rapidly with appropriate monitoring of urinary output and cardiac filling pressures. Clindamycin (300 to 600 mg every 6 hours) or cefoxitin (1 g every 6 hours) and gentamycin (1 to 1.5 mg per kilogram every 8 hours, adjusting for serum creatinine) are given intravenously to provide broad coverage of aerobic and anaerobic intestinal microorganisms.

Control of peritoneal contamination is the most urgent consideration in patients with free diverticular perforation. Emergency resection with temporary colostomy and mucous fistula controls peritoneal contamination.

Fistula

A fistula may involve any adjacent viscus, but the urinary bladder, small intestine, and vagina are the most common sites. Emergency surgery is indicated only in the unusual colovesical or colo-ureteral fistula with ascending urinary tract infection. This is particularly true in the presence of urinary obstruction and impending pyonephrosis. More commonly a patient with mild chronic or episodic diverticulitis will develop pneumaturia. Most fistulas may be treated by elective one-stage resection with colon anastomosis and closure of the communicating viscus.

Obstruction

Acute sigmoid diverticulitis produces some degree of colonic obstruction in most cases. This may be because of local peritonitis, spasm, and edema or encroachment on the lumen by abscess. Fibrous stricture is far less common, and complete obstruction is unusual. Most often bowel function returns and distention improves with nasogastric decompression and intravenous antibiotics. However, serial abdominal examination and x-ray studies are necessary, and if progressive cecal distention develops, emergency colostomy will be necessary. The large bowel is decompressed and later resected.

Small bowel obstruction resulting from entrapment by diverticular abscess or inflammation should be suspected if crampy abdominal pain, nausea, and vomiting are prominent. Nasogastric decompression may be attempted, but if symptoms do not improve promptly, emergency operation will be necessary. Small bowel adhesions are lysed, the perforated segment of colon is resected, and the anastomosis is deferred.

Elective Operation

With improved dietary management, elective operations for symptomatic diverticular disease or recurrent attacks of diverticulitis have decreased in frequency. Primary resection and anastomosis can be carried out with minimal morbidity and mortality under elective conditions. A patient who recovers from a complication of diverticular disease may be a candidate for elective operation, particularly if he is 50 years old or younger. Following a single episode of acute diverticulitis, operation should be considered for persistent mass, urinary symptoms suggestive of impending fistula, and radiologic demonstration of fixed narrowing or extraluminal barium. Resection is mandatory if carcinoma cannot be excluded.

SUGGESTED READING

Silen W. Cope's early diagnosis of the acute abdomen, 16th ed. New York: Oxford University Press, 1983.

Smith AN. Diverticular disease. In: Clinics in gastroenterology. Vol 4. London: WB Saunders, 1975.

BOWEL OBSTRUCTION

GEORGE L. STERNBACH, M.D., F.A.C.E.P.

Bowel obstruction is the occlusion of the intestinal lumen which results in blocking of normal flow of intestinal contents. Small bowel obstruction is more commonly seen than is obstruction of the colon. More than 80 percent of all bowel obstruction is caused by adhesions, hernia, or neoplasm.

SMALL INTESTINE

Small intestinal obstruction is most commonly secondary to entrapment of a portion of intestine by postoperative adhesions or incarceration in a hernia. Other causes of small bowel obstruction—volvulus, intussusception, neoplasm, and gallstone ileus—are encountered less frequently.

Abdominal pain, distention, vomiting, and constipation are characteristic features of small bowel obstruction. The nature and predominance of each of these depends on the level of involvement. Some features may be minimal or absent. Frequently several stools are passed in the first hours after obstruction as a result of the initial increased peristalsis. A proximal obstruction usually produces profuse vomiting with variable discomfort. Obstruction of the mid intestine generally produces a more classic crescendo-decrescendo pain. In distal obstruction, vomiting may appear late in the course of the illness, and may become feculent. Distention is more pronounced in distal than in proximal obstruction.

Vital signs may be normal early, but with progression of the process they reflect the development of dehydration. Volume deficit results from a number of factors: (1) vomiting, (2) sequestration of secreted intraluminal fluid proximal to the site of obstruction, (3) decreased intestinal absorption distal to this area, and (4) diminished flux of fluid from intestinal lumen into tissue spaces. If the intestine becomes strangulated, loss of blood or plasma from the involved intestinal segment may occur. *Strangulation*—impairment of the blood supply to the obstructed loop—is an ominous consequence of intestinal obstruction, the recognition of which mandates emergency surgery. Unfortunately, the purportedly classic findings of vascular compromise—fever, tachycardia, leukocytosis, and peritoneal signs—have been found to be unreliable as indicators of strangulation. In fact, no parameter, including experienced clinical judgment, proves to be consistent in this regard.

Plain abdominal x-ray film is the mainstay of diagnosis. Taken in the supine and, most important, the upright and decubitus positions, x-ray studies may reveal air—fluid levels and dilated loops of small bowel in a ladder-like pattern, diagnostic of obstruction.

The differential diagnosis includes acute gastroenteritis, pancreatitis, appendicitis, and perforated peptic ul-

cer. Clinical and x-ray evaluations, as well as the serum amylase level, should serve to distinguish small bowel obstruction from these entities. A more difficult differentiation is that from *paralytic ileus* secondary to an intraperitoneal inflammatory process, intestinal ischemia, metabolic disturbance, medications, or ureteral colic.

The radiographic and clinical pictures produced by obstruction and *adynamic ileus* may be quite similar. The characteristic presentation of ileus includes the early appearance of abdominal distention, diffuse mild continuous pain, and diminished or absent bowel sounds. In mechanical obstruction, abdominal distention frequently is not pronounced until late in the course of the illness. The pain tends to be colicky, although it may become steady, especially if strangulation ensues. Bowel sounds are high-pitched, last at least a second, and have a characteristic gurgling quality.

Treatment

Pre-hospital

Unless the evaluation of vital signs, skin turgor, and mucous membranes indicates the presence of dehydration, the requirement for field intervention is minimal. If dehydration is present, infusion of lactated Ringer's solution should be instituted at a rate of administration commensurate with the degree of dehydration.

Emergency Department

The most pressing therapeutic demand is to restore the fluid and electrolyte balance. Fluid losses that result from small intestinal obstruction are isotonic. The patient may be dehydrated by as much as several liters. A central venous pressure monitor and Foley catheter should be inserted for monitoring purposes, and the rapidity of intravenous rehydration should be guided by the clinical appearance of the patient. In many cases, the administration of 2 to 3 L over the first 4 hours is required. If emergency surgery is required, this is generally safe when three-quarters of estimated fluid deficit has been replaced and urinary output exceeds 35 to 50 ml per hour.

Hypokalemia may result from small bowel obstruction, small intestinal fluid being rich in potassium. Replacement should be dictated by serum potassium levels. However, intravenous potassium should not be administered until adequate renal function is established on the basis of urinary output. Repeated serum electrolyte levels should be obtained as treatment proceeds, since total body potassium deficit is not reflected in initial serum levels.

Arterial blood gases should be used to determine the presence of metabolic disturbances. This most commonly consists of alkalosis if the obstruction is proximal and of acidosis resulting from bicarbonate depletion if it is more distal. Intravenous replacement of bicarbonate, however, is rarely required.

Gastrointestinal decompression should be instituted in all patients with suspected intestinal obstruction. Whether this should be accomplished by means of a nasogastric tube or a long intestinal tube is a matter of considerable disagreement. Some clinicians have strong preferences for one of these methods over the other. However, no clear superiority for either type of tube has been objectively demonstrated.

Antibiotics should be administered only in cases of suspected strangulated obstruction. Cefoxitin, 2 g, or clindamycin, 300 mg intravenously every 6 hours, are recommended, in addition to gentamicin. The latter should be administered to a total of 5 mg per kilogram per day intravenously or intramuscularly, with a 2 mg per kilogram loading dose. This dosage may be reduced to 3 mg per kilogram per day as soon as clinically indicated.

Surgical consultation should be obtained in cases of suspected intestinal obstruction. Urgent surgical intervention is required in cases of strangulated or complete obstruction. As noted, however, it is often difficult to identify the patient with strangulation early in the course of the process. Accurate delineation of the patient with partial obstruction—who may sometimes be managed nonoperatively with hydration and nasogastric suction—is also difficult, because the clinical features of partial and complete intestinal obstruction are similar.

In certain specific instances of bowel obstruction early operative intervention is not indicated. Obstruction produced by an acute episode of Crohn's ileitis, for example, will frequently resolve with 24 to 48 hours of treatment with parenteral corticosteroids. Initial intravenous administration of hydrocortisone sodium succinate, 200 to 400 mg, is recommended.

LARGE INTESTINE

Colonic obstruction is produced by primary intestinal carcinoma in more than half of all cases. Diverticulitis and volvulus cause the majority of the remainder, with a variety of causes accounting for the balance.

Acute obstruction of the large bowel usually presents with abdominal pain, constipation, and abdominal distention. The onset of symptoms is typically insidious. Although most patients complain of constipation or obstipation, some experience diarrhea. This represents either the passage of liquid stool beyond an incomplete obstruction or mucous discharge from an intestinal carcinoma. Vomiting, an infrequent presenting complaint, is either minimal or absent.

The most consistent physical finding is abdominal distention. Diffuse tenderness to palpation may also be present. High-pitched bowel sounds during peristaltic rushes may be audible. The diagnosis is confirmed on abdominal x-ray studies performed in the supine and upright positions. Such studies will reveal distention of the colon and possibly the small intestine as well. If perforation has occurred, free air may be in evidence. Sigmoid volvulus appears radiographically as a markedly distended loop of bowel emerging from the pelvis, which may reach to the diaphragm and have a "bent inner tube" or "beak-like" appearance. In cecal volvulus the dilated loop is generally located in the epigastrium or left upper quadrant, having a "kidney bean" shape. Both forms of obstruction are most common in the elderly. Dilated loops of small intestine may be present as well. A cecal fluid level may be visible on upright x-ray films.

Differential Diagnosis

The radiographic appearance of large intestinal obstruction may be mistaken for small bowel obstruction or adynamic ileus. The clinical picture may mimic gastroenteritis. In addition, an entity known as *pseudo-obstruction* produces characteristic signs, symptoms, and radiologic findings of colonic obstruction without a mechanical cause. Pseudo-obstruction is most commonly encountered in elderly patients with chronic illness, such as congestive heart failure, myxedema, or chronic renal failure. Barium enema may be required to distinguish this condition from mechanical obstruction. This procedure is also useful in localizing the site of obstruction and planning a surgical procedure.

Treatment

Pre-hospital

Specific pre-hospital treatment of colonic obstruction is rarely feasible. Patients are usually older than those suffering small intestinal obstruction, so they should be monitored for cardiovascular complications of dehydration and systemic illness. Fluid and electrolyte losses are not generally as severe as those produced by small bowel obstruction. However, fluid may be lost into the intestinal lumen to the extent that dehydration results. Intravenous infusion of lactated Ringer's solution or normal saline should be initiated at an infusion rate controlled in accordance with the magnitude of vital sign abnormality.

Emergency Department

Treatment should be continued with respect to monitoring and intravenous fluid. The amount of fluid and electrolytes administered should be guided by the patient's vital signs and serum electrolyte determination.

A nasogastric tube should be inserted. However, this reduces the accumulation of gas and fluid only in the proximal gastrointestinal tract; it does not effect any large bowel decompression per se. The patient will require surgery, the type and timing of which will depend on associated factors. Immediate surgical consultation is imperative. Antibiotic coverage should be initiated with cefoxitin or clindamycin and gentamicin in the doses described for small bowel obstruction.

The initial management of sigmoid volvulus differs from that of other forms of colonic obstruction. In this instance, reduction may be achieved by entry of the twisted loop by a sigmoidoscope. A rectal tube should be placed through the sigmoidoscope and left in place following derotation. Elective surgical intervention may then follow. The role for nonoperative management of cecal volvulus is small. Although some success has been reported with colonoscopic decompression, this technique must be considered investigational.

Patients with acute colonic obstruction (with the exception of that caused by sigmoid volvulus as noted above) generally require emergency surgical intervention. Those with uncomplicated obstruction will require urgent decompression by means of a colostomy as soon as they are stable. Carcinoma resection may be carried out at this time, or by means of a second procedure.

The nature and the timing of surgery does, however, depend on a variety of factors, including the competency of the ileocecal valve. In the event of an incompetent ileocecal valve, colonic gas will regurgitate proximally and fill a portion of the small intestine. If the valve is competent, however, a closed-loop obstruction is produced. The colon may become substantially dilated, producing the risk of perforation. Such perforation most commonly occurs through the cecum, whose walls are thinner than those of the adjacent colon. Distention of the cecum, as seen on a plain x-ray film, to a diameter exceeding 10 cm has traditionally been viewed as a sign portending rupture. Although distention in excess of this size is occasionally tolerated, this degree of cecal dilation should be an indication for emergency surgical decompression, generally by means of cecostomy or proximal colostomy.

If colonic perforation has occurred, physical signs of peritoneal irritation may be present, as well as radiographic evidence of pneumoperitoneum. The prognosis for such patients is poor, and acute surgical intervention is indicated as soon as volume deficit and electrolyte imbalance have been corrected.

SUGGESTED READING

Greenlee HB. Acute large bowel obstruction: an update. Surg Annu 1982; 14:253–276.

Sarr MG, Bulkley GB, Zuidema GD. Preoperative recognition of intestinal strangulation obstruction. AM J Surg 1983; 145:176–182.

Turner DM, Croom RD III. Acute adhesive obstruction of the small intestine. Am Surg 1983; 49:126–130.

INTESTINAL PARASITES

DANIEL S. BLUMENTHAL, M.D., M.P.H.

There are literally dozens of intestinal parasites that may infect humans. The following are considered in this chapter:

1. *Giardia lamblia*, probably the most common intestinal parasite in the United States.
2. *Enterobius vermicularis*, the pinworm, also very common.
3. The major intestinal nematodes *Ascaris*, hookworm, *Trichuris*, and *Strongyloides*.
4. *Trichinella spiralis*, an intestinal parasite that may cause serious disease when its larvae invade the tissues.
5. Intestinal nematodes of dogs and cats that sometimes infect humans and cause visceral larva migrans.

Infection with intestinal parasites rarely causes a true emergency. Nonetheless, parasitic infection often causes acute illness that may be seen in the emergency department. The practitioner should remember that, in addition to the parasites listed above, many others may occur in immigrants, especially refugees, from tropical countries. The physician practicing in a community that includes many such immigrants should keep a textbook of tropical medicine at hand.

GIARDIASIS

Etiology and Diagnosis

Giardia lamblia is probably the most common pathogenic intestinal parasite in the United States, and several large water-borne municipal outbreaks have been reported. It is particularly common among backpackers in the Rocky Mountains, children in day-care centers, and tourists returning from abroad. It presents as subacute or recurrent diarrhea, often accompanied by bloating, flatulence, and steatorrhea. The diagnosis is made by finding cysts or trophozoites in the stool, which should be examined fresh or preserved in polyvinyl alcohol as well as 10 percent formalin. Several stool examinations may be necessary, and sometimes the diagnosis can only be made with the use of a string test (Enterotest) or even an intestinal biopsy. In an epidemic situation (as in a day-care center), a presumptive diagnosis can be made on clinical grounds.

Treatment

Quinacrine (Atabrine) is usually considered the treatment of choice (Table 1). Metronidazole (Flagyl) is also effective, but has been shown to be mutagenic in bacterial test systems and carcinogenic in rats. It is considered experimental for this condition by the U.S. Food and Drug Administration. It is contraindicated for patients in the first trimester of pregnancy. A third drug, furazolidone (Furoxone), is somewhat less effective but has the advantage of availability in a liquid formulation for pediatric use. It has also been implicated in producing neoplasia in rats. It should not be used in infants younger than 1 month old or in patients taking monoamine oxidase inhibitors.

PINWORM INFECTION

Etiology and Diagnosis

Enterobius vermicularis is the most common intestinal nematode in this country and is found in all strata of society. This organism most often infects children, particularly those housed in institutional settings, but it may also infect adults. Many (perhaps most) infections are asymptomatic; however, perianal itching is a common complaint.

The adult pinworm inhabits the large intestine and cecum. Females emerge from the anus while the host sleeps and deposit their eggs around the anus. When the host scratches the site of deposition, the eggs adhere to the fingers and are thence transmitted to playmates and family members. The infection is acquired when the eggs are ingested. If worms migrate into the vagina or urethra, vaginitis or urinary tract infection may result.

Eggs are found infrequently on stool examination. The diagnosis is made by performing a cellophane tape test: the gummed side of a piece of transparent cellophane tape ("Magic Tape" is not suitable) is dabbed on the anus and surrounding skin and then applied to a glass slide. When examined under the microscope, the ova are readily seen. The test should be performed shortly after the patient has awakened and before bathing. Three tests, performed on different mornings, are necessary to obtain a sensitivity of 90 percent.

Treatment

Several drugs are effective in the treatment of enterobiasis (see Table 1): mebendazole (Vermox), pyrantel pamoate (Antiminth), and pyrvinium pamoate (Povan) all offer single-dose therapy. Treatment should be repeated in 1 week. None of these drugs should be given to pregnant women. Since the infection is readily transmitted within households, all members of the family should be treated simultaneously. At the time of treatment, bedding should be changed and nightclothes washed; however, ex-

treme measures (such as disinfecting the entire house) should be discouraged. Follow-up tape tests may be obtained to assure cure.

MAJOR NEMATODE INFECTIONS

Etiology and Diagnosis

Four major nematode species infect humans in the United States: *Ascaris lumbricoides* (large roundworm), *Trichuris trichiura* (whipworm), *Necator americanus** (hookworm), and *Strongyloides stercoralis*.

In the United States, these infections are most common among rural residents of the Southeast and migrant farm workers. They are generally more common among children than adults. Their greatest prevalence, of course, is among residents of tropical countries.

The infections may be transmitted when stools of an infected individual are deposited on the ground. *Ascaris* and *Trichuris* are transmitted when persons playing or working on the ground inadvertently ingest the ova that have been passed with the stool. In the case of *Necator* and *Strongyloides*, infective larvae penetrate the skin, usually of bare feet.

These infections are often asymptomatic. When symptoms are present, they are usually nonspecific gastrointestinal complaints, such as diarrhea, abdominal pain, or loss of appetite. However, there are occasional serious complications. A bolus of *Ascaris* organisms may cause an intestinal obstruction. Rarely, an ascarid may

---

* *Ancylostoma duodenale* is the prevalent species of hookworm in many tropical countries. Its ova are indistinguishable from those of *Necator*.

TABLE 1 Treatment of Intestinal Parasites

Parasite	Drug	Adult Dose (mg)	Pediatric Dose (mg/kg)	Treatment Duration	Common Side Effects
Giardia	Quinacrine	100 t.i.d.	2 t.i.d.	5 days	Dizziness, headache, vomiting
	Metronidazole†	250 t.i.d.	5 t.i.d.	5 days	Nausea, headache, dry mouth, Antabuse effect
	Furazolidone	100 q.i.d.	1.25 q.i.d.	7 days	—
Enterobius	Mebendazole	200	100*	Once;	—
	Pyrantel pamoate	11/kg	11	repeat in 1 wk	—
Ascaris	Mebendazole	100 b.i.d.	100 b.i.d.*	3 days	—
	Pyrantel pamoate	11/kg	11	Once	—
	Piperazine citrate	75/kg q.d.	75 q.d.	2 days	—
Trichuris	Mebendazole	100 b.i.d.	100 b.i.d.*	3 days	—
Hookworm	Mebendazole	100 b.i.d.	100 b.i.d.*	3 days	—
	Pyrantel pamoate†	11/kg	11	Once	—
Strongyloides	Thiabendazole	25/kg b.i.d.	25 b.i.d.	2 days	Vomiting, vertigo
Toxocara	Thiabendazole†	25/kg b.i.d.	25 b.i.d.	5 days	Vomiting, vertigo

* 100 mg per dose, not based on body weight.
† Considered experimental for this condition by FDA.

migrate into the common bile duct or pancreatic duct, perforate the wall of the intestine, or be regurgitated and aspirated. A heavy infection with *Trichuris* may cause a rectal prolapse. Heavy hookworm infections cause severe anemia and hypoproteinemia. *Strongyloides* infection in an immunosuppressed or malnourished individual may result in the hyperinfection syndrome in which larvae migrate throughout the body thereby causing sepsis and death.

Diagnosis of these infections is made by the discovery of ova on stool examination. A single examination is usually sufficient to diagnose *Ascaris*, hookworm, or *Trichuris*. In the case of *Strongyloides*, larvae rather than ova are found, and multiple examinations, or even a string test, may be necessary.

Treatment

Effective and relatively safe drugs are available for the treatment of uncomplicated infections. These include mebendazole (Vermox), pyrantel pamoate (Antiminth), and piperazine citrate (Antepar) for *Ascaris*; mebendazole for whipworm; mebendazole and pyrantel pamoate for hookworm; and thiabendazole (Mintezol) for *Strongyloides* (see Table 1).

Follow-up stool examinations should be obtained to assure cure, and stool samples should be obtained for examination from other household members, since multiple infections in the same household are likely. Reinfection is also likely unless environmental sanitary conditions are improved; patient education on proper disposal of excrement may be helpful.

Intestinal obstruction caused by a bolus of ascarids should be treated in the hospital by giving the patient nothing by mouth, administering appropriate intravenous fluids, and giving an anthelmintic through a nasogastric tube. Surgery is rarely necessary.

Rectal prolapse caused by a heavy *Trichuris* infection may be reduced with a tissue paper-covered finger. The tissue remains after the finger is withdrawn and is expelled later. The buttocks should be taped together for 2 or 3 days.

Transfusions may be necessary in severe hookworm disease.

The hyperinfection syndrome in strongyloidiasis is treated with the same dose of thiabendazole used for ordinary *Strongyloides* infection, but treatment should be continued for at least 5 days. Appropriate antibiotics should also be given for sepsis and other supportive therapy administered as necessary.

TRICHINOSIS

Etiology and Diagnosis

Trichinosis is acquired by eating undercooked pork (or bear or walrus meat) that contains encysted larvae of *Trichinella spiralis*. Annually, 100 to 200 cases are reported. An estimated 200,000 new infections occur each year, but most are asymptomatic. The larvae excyst in the intestine and a gastroenteritis-like illness may follow. The typical trichinosis syndrome follows 1 to 3 weeks later, after the ingested larvae mature and produce new larvae that penetrate the host's tissues. The larvae invade skeletal muscle, and they may also attack the heart and the central nervous system.

Symptoms and signs include fever, muscle pain and tenderness, periorbital edema, and petechial hemorrhages of the subungual skin, conjunctivae, and mucous membranes. Laboratory findings include a moderate leukocytosis with accompanying eosinophilia (5 to 50 percent) and positive serologic studies, including counterimmunoelectrophoresis and bentonite flocculation tests. A definitive diagnosis can be made with a muscle biopsy, usually from the deltoid or gastrocnemius muscle.

Treatment

Effective therapy can be offered if the diagnosis is suspected during the enteric phase of the infection, before the larvae begin to penetrate host tissues. In this case, mebendazole (Vermox) should be given in a dose of 200 mg daily for 4 days. An alternative is pyrantel pamoate, 10 mg per kilogram (maximum 1 g). Unfortunately, the diagnosis is rarely considered at this stage.

Once larval migration has begun and systemic symptoms have occurred, no specific therapy is available. Antipyretics may be given for fever. Prednisone (60 mg per day) or other steroids, given for 2 weeks, may lessen the symptoms.

VISCERAL LARVA MIGRANS

Visceral larva migrans results from ingestion of ova of the dog ascarid, *Toxocara canis* or, less often, the cat ascarid, *Toxocara cati*. The larvae of these species migrate aberrantly in the human body, thereby causing either a visceral syndrome of fever, cough, and hepatosplenomegaly or an ocular syndrome in which involvement is limited to the eyes, particularly the retina, and may be mistaken for retinoblastoma. Cases of toxocariasis occur most commonly in children under 5 who have a dog (especially a puppy) in the home. The ocular form tends to occur in older children, and the visceral form, in younger children.

Diagnosis is based on history and physical findings, a high eosinophil count (up to 70 percent), and serologic tests. The enzyme-linked immunosorbent assay is the most specific serologic test available, but sensitivity is only about 78 percent and is lower in ocular cases.

Treatment

Thiabendazole (25 mg per kilogram twice a day for 5 days) may be given as treatment, but evidence for its effectiveness is controversial. Steroids may help suppress the acute symptoms and may limit eye damage in the ocular form. Children with the ocular form should be seen by an ophthalmologist. Household pets should, of course, be examined by a veterinarian for nematode infection and treated as necessary.

SUGGESTED READING

Blumenthal DS. Intestinal nematodes in the United States. N Engl J Med 1977; 297:1437–1439.

Campbell WC, ed. Trichinella and trichinosis. New York: Plenum Press, 1983.

Drugs for parasitic infections. Med Lett Drugs Ther 1984; 26:27–34.

Glockman LT, Schantz PM. Epidemiology and pathogenesis of zoonotic toxocariasis. Epidemol Rev 1981; 3:230–239.

Wolfe MS. Giardiasis. N Engl J Med 1978; 298:319–320.

INFLAMMATORY BOWEL DISEASE

JOHN V. CARBONE, M.D.

CROHN'S DISEASE

Crohn's disease (regional enteritis, ileocolitis) is a subacute or chronic inflammation of any part of the gastrointestinal tract. The ileum is most frequently involved, either alone or with involvement of the colon or jejunum. The involvement may be confined to a single isolated area or to multiple areas of bowel with "skipping." The disease also has been described in skin, muscle, and synovial tissue.

Etiology

The etiology of Crohn's disease is unknown. Current theories invoke infectious, genetic, and immunologic factors. The infectious etiology of Crohn's disease is suggested by the clinical and morphologic similarity to known infectious diseases of the bowel (*Yersinia*, tuberculosis). Various authors have reported viral, chlamydial, cell wall defective *Pseudomonas*, and mycobacterial isolates from tissue in Crohn's disease. The familial incidence of Crohn's disease (15 to 40 percent), including monozygotic twins and the association with ankylosing spondylitis, suggests a genetic role in the causation. However, just as in idiopathic ulcerative colitis, the disease is not classically a genetically transmitted disease, and no conclusive histocompatibility markers have been found in Crohn's disease. The association with immunologically mediated complications, histologic evidence (granuloma formation, lymphocytic and plasmocytic inflammation), and the response to immunosuppressive drugs (such as azathioprine and adrenal corticosteroids) suggest that an altered immunologic mechanism may play a role in the etiology and pathogenesis of Crohn's disease.

Diagnosis

Inflammation, ulceration, and stricture of the intestine can result from many causes (Table 1). The differential diagnosis of an intestinal disease that may involve any segment of the intestine as a single lesion or as multiple lesions, or that may present with extraintestinal complaints with fever or no gastrointestinal complaints, can be difficult. The average duration of complaints from the onset to the diagnosis of Crohn's disease is approximately 3 years.

Diagnostic criteria for Crohn's disease include an insidious onset; intermittent diarrhea, fever, abdominal cramping, and weight loss; right lower quadrant pain or tenderness; and characteristic radiologic abnormalities. There is no laboratory test that allows a diagnosis of Crohn's disease or defines the level of activity of the disease. Infection must be ruled out by stool cultures and stool examination for ova and parasites. Urinalysis is important to evaluate the possibility of infection and enteric contamination of the urinary tract. The diagnosis is confirmed by the characteristic radiologic abnormalities in most instances.

Characteristic radiologic findings in the small intestine include nonstenotic changes (thickening of mucosal folds and narrowing of the lumen owing to spasm), stenotic changes (narrowing of the bowel with proximal dilation), and rigidity and thickening of the bowel wall with separation of bowel loops.

Characteristic radiologic changes on contrast study of the colon include aphthoid ulcers 1 to 3 mm in diameter surrounded by a radiolucent halo, nodules, deep ulcers, longitudinal and transverse ulcers, strictures, thickened bowel wall, fistulas, and pseudopolyps.

Treatment

The treatment of Crohn's disease is dependent upon the extent and severity of the disease and the presence and severity of complications. Fulminant Crohn's disease with toxic megacolon is treated as discussed under ulcerative colitis. The treatment of other complications is described in Table 2.

TABLE 1 Differential Diagnosis of Crohn's Disease

Infection
M. tuberculosis
Yersinia enterocolitica
E. histolytica
Miscellaneous
Acute appendicitis
Mesenteric adenitis
Lymphoma
Carcinoid

TABLE 2 Treatment of Specific Complications of Crohn's Disease

Intestinal obstruction
    Intestinal decompression
    Correction of fluid and electrolyte deficits
    Hospitalize until obstruction is relieved or
      surgical decompression is accomplished

Intra-abdominal or psoas abscess
    Confirmation by ultrasonography or CT scan
    Hospitalize for surgical drainage

Enteroenteric fistula
    Confirm by x-ray film
    Hospitalize for definitive surgical therapy

Ocular inflammation
    Ophthalmologic consultation to rule out
      uveitis or ocular candidiasis

Massive hemorrhage
    Correct acute blood loss
    Hospitalize for definitive diagnosis:
      colonoscopy;
      upper gastrointestinal series with
        small bowel study
      upper gastrointestinal tract endoscopy

Outpatient management of Crohn's disease is dependent upon the extent and severity of the disease and the presence and severity of complications. The presence of major complications precludes outpatient management. These complications include fulminant Crohn's colitis, intestinal obstruction, intra-abdominal abscess, enteroenteric fistulas, and massive hemorrhage.

The acute inflammatory intestinal lesion responds best to prednisone, 20 mg to 60 mg daily. Prednisone is most useful in terminating the acute attack of Crohn's disease. It is less useful in prolonging clinical remission.

Sulfasalazine has been shown to be useful in the acute phase of Crohn's disease in a dosage of 2.0 to 4.0 gm per day. Metronidazole, 250 mg four times daily, has been shown to be effective in Crohn's colitis. This drug may prove useful particularly when the patient with Crohn's colitis fails to respond to sulfasalazine.

Azathioprine, 2 mg per kilogram per day by mouth, may prove useful in allowing a reduction of prednisone dosage in patients requiring high dose prednisone therapy (greater than 30 mg per day) to remain in a clinically acceptable state. There is evidence to suggest that azathioprine may prolong remissions. However, the effectiveness of azathioprine requires long term therapy. These patients must be followed closely to monitor bone marrow, pancreatic, and hepatic function.

If small bowel disease predominates, a low residue diet is often symptomatically of benefit. Milk restriction may be of symptomatic benefit. The diet should be palatable. Supplements of iron, vitamin B_{12}, folic acid, and calcium may be necessary.

Treatment in the mild or moderate form of the disease should not be initiated until stool examinations for bacterial pathogens, ova, and parasites and mucosal biopsy have ruled out infectious colitis. The use of antispasmodics or opiates could be hazardous in infectious colitis and may precipitate dilation of the colon if the disease proves to be severe or fulminant. Although diet has not been shown to be a major factor in precipitating or aggravating inflammatory bowel disease, restriction of milk products and ingestion of only cooked foods can be symptomatically beneficial. In instances of chronic stable disease, judicious use of diphenoxylate (2.5 mg) and loperamide, 2 mg, may prove helpful in decreasing the frequency of defecation.

ULCERATIVE COLITIS

Ulcerative colitis is a chronic inflammatory disease involving the rectal or colonic mucosa. The disease most commonly involves the rectum and left colon. However, it can involve any or all segments of the large bowel and on occasion may extend into the mucosa of the terminal ileum. The disease may occur at any age but occurs most commonly between the ages of 15 and 40, being rare in infancy and infrequent in old age.

Ulcerative colitis presents with one or more of the following: bloody rectal discharges, abdominal pain and cramping, abdominal tenderness, weight loss, fever, anemia, extraintestinal complications (uveitis, arthritis, pyoderma), and colonic mucosal abnormalties revealed by endoscopy or a barium enema.

The course of the disease is characterized by chronicity, exacerbations, and remissions. Most attacks of the disease are mild to moderate in intensity. However, severe or fulminant attacks may lead to toxic megacolon, massive hemorrhage, sepsis, or death.

Etiology

The etiology and pathogenesis of ulcerative colitis are unknown. Current theories include infectious, genetic, and immunologic factors. Infectious causes were suggested by the similarities of infectious colitis attributable to various bacterial, viral, and protozoal agents to idiopathic ulcerative proctocolitis. Genetic factors are suggested by the familial incidence of the disease. However, ulcerative colitis is not classically genetically transmitted, and no enzymatic, metabolic, or chromosomal abnormalities have been demonstrated as yet in this disease.

Immunologic factors are suggested by the chronic relapsing course, the association with diseases linked to immunologic mechanisms (e.g., autoimmune hemolytic anemia, cholestatic liver disease, uveitis) and the beneficial effects from immunosuppressive drugs (azathioprine, adrenal corticosteroids).

Diagnosis

The differential diagnosis can be difficult, since inflammation and ulceration of the colon can result from many etiologies (Table 3). The clinical picture may be identical to that of idiopathic ulcerative proctocolitis. Infections must be ruled out in every instance of suspected idiopathic ulcerative colitis. Stool cultures, stool specimens for ova and parasites, and serologic studies to rule out syphilis, amebiasis, and lymphogranuloma may be necessary. The distinction of idiopathic proctocolitis from

TABLE 3   Differential Diagnosis of Ulcerative Colitis

Infection
  Bacterial
    Salmonella
    Shigella
    Campylobacter jejuni
    N. Gonorrhoeae
    T. pallidum
    C. trachomatis
    Aeromonas hydrophila

  Protozoal
    E. histolytica

Miscellaneous
  Radiation proctitis
  Ischemic colitis
  Behçet's syndrome
  Lymphoma

Crohn's colitis

Crohn's colitis may be difficult. The clinical presentations may be identical. However, rectal bleeding, toxicity, and a diffusely friable, superficially ulcerated mucosa favor the diagnosis of ulcerative colitis. Diarrhea, perianal disease, discreet ulcerations with normal intervening mucosa, and lack of systemic toxicity favor Crohn's colitis.

The diagnostic characteristics of idiopathic ulcerative colitis include a history of bloody rectal discharges with abdominal pain and cramping; physical examination revealing abdominal tenderness, evidence of weight loss, and fever; laboratory data documenting anemia and leukocytosis, with no fecal pathogens demonstrated by culture, microscopic examination of fresh stool specimens, or serologic studies; colonic abnormalities demonstrated by endoscopy and by barium enema; and mucosal biopsy with crypt abscesses, superficial ulceration, and intramucosal hemorrhage.

The mucosa in idiopathic ulcerative colitis is characterized macroscopically by involvement with a continuous symmetrical inflammatory process characterized by hyperemia, hemorrhage, friability edema, and ulceration. The mucosal vascular pattern is absent, and there are varying amounts of necrotic mucosal surface debris. With severe involvement, extensive ulceration can occur. The mucosa may be denuded in varying degree with remnants of mucosa "pseudopolyps."

The mucosa in idiopathic ulcerative colitis is characterized microscopically by depletion of goblet cell mucin and a reduction in the number of goblet cells. Inflammatory cells accumulate in the crypts (crypt abscesses). Vascular congestion, dilation of the capillaries, and intramucosal hemorrhages are noted. Lymphocytes and plasma cells accumulate in the lamina propria. Ulceration remains superficial, except with toxic megacolon.

Treatment

The therapy of the patient with ulcerative colitis is dependent upon the extent and severity of the disease.

The initial efforts in the management of patients with complaints consistent with ulcerative colitis should include correction of fluid, electrolyte, and blood volume deficits,

determination of the extent and severity of the disease process (mild, moderate, severe-fulminant), and differentiation from other disease processes that may mimic idiopathic ulcerative proctocolitis. Patients with mild to moderate disease are best referred to an internist or gastroenterologist for long term care.

However, the patient with severe or fulminant disease requires a careful and timely evaluation to determine the extent and severity of the disease process and to exclude the possibilities of perforation, megacolon, peritonitis, and sepsis. Initial evaluation should include a complete blood count, blood cultures, and blood chemistry and serum electrolyte determinations. The initial treatment is directed toward correction of fluid and electrolyte deficits and anemia. The fulminant course of ulcerative colitis is often complicated by toxic megacolon or perforation. As soon as is feasible, flat and upright films of the abdomen are obtained. Free air in the abdominal cavity necessitates immediate surgical consultation for a colectomy.

The presence of a dilated colon (larger than 6 cm), a temperature higher than 101°, leukocytosis higher than 12,000 per mm³, and serum albumin less than 3.0 gm per deciliter defines toxic megacolon. This complication occurs in the presence of severe ulceration of the colon, inappropriate use of opiates and anticholinergic drugs, and electrolyte depletion.

The treatment consists of intestinal decompression by a long tube, correction of fluid and electrolyte deficits and anemia, discontinuation of opiates and anticholinergic drugs, intravenous administration of adrenocortical steroids (hydrocortisone, 100 mg every 8 hours or methylprednisolone, 16 mg every 8 hours); and broad spectrum antibiotics. Patients with toxic megacolon are at immediate risk for perforation and sepsis, and broad spectrum antibiotics should be utilized.

Triple antibiotic therapy should include ampicillin, 1 to 2 gm intravenously every 4 hours; metronidazole, 500 mg intravenously every 8 hours; and aminoglycosides (tobramycin or gentamycin), 2.0 mg per kilogram as a loading dose and 1.5 mg per kilogram every 8 hours intravenously. Alternative broad spectrum antibiotic therapy includes cefoxitin, 2.0 gm every 6 hours, or cefotaxime, 2.0 g every 4 to 6 hours.

Patients with toxic megacolon should be hospitalized, preferably in an intensive care unit under the care of both a gastroenterologist and a surgeon. If the colon does not decompress and the toxicity does not begin to subside in 24 to 48 hours, colectomy is indicated.

Fulminant ulcerative colitis and toxic megacolon may be caused by infection (amebiasis, shigellosis, cholera), ischemia, and Crohn's colitis. Stool examination for ova and parasites, cultures for pathogens, and rectal mucosal biopsy may prevent an unnecessary colectomy.

SUGGESTED READING

Kirsner JB, Shorter RG. Inflammatory bowel diseases. 2nd ed. Philadelphia,: Lea & Fehiger, 1980.
Schacter H, Kirsner JB. Crohn's disease of the gastrointestinal Tract. New York: John Wiley & Sons, 1980.
Winship DH, ed. Symposium on inflammatory bowel disease Med Clin North Am 1980; 64:1021-1031.

NONINFECTIOUS COLITIS

ERIC Z. SILFEN, M.D., F.A.C.P., F.A.C.E.P.

Inflammatory and infectious diseases of the colon and rectum span a wide range of diagnostic possibilities. Presenting signs and symptoms include visceral or colicky lower abdominal pain, rectal pain, tenesmus, alterations in usual bowel habits, watery or bloody diarrhea, rectal bleeding, fever, and weight loss.

Differential diagnosis consists of inflammatory bowel disease (IBD); illness related to trauma and foreign body injury induced by medication, environment, and radiation; neuroendocrine disorders; infectious agents of bacterial, viral, chlamydial, protozoal, helminthic, and fungal origin; vascular and ischemic bowel disease; disorders of colon function; and tumor (Table 1).

HISTORY

Points of importance include the acuteness or chronicity of the symptoms (infectious processes tend to be of acute origin whereas inflammatory processes may be of longstanding duration); the presence or absence of nocturnal symptoms (absence of symptoms during sleep implicates a functional process as opposed to an organic process); the presence or absence of bloating and the passage of flatus (bloating and flatus point to an infectious process and away from an obstructive process); the presence or absence of diarrhea, how often the diarrhea occurs, and whether or not the diarrhea is associated with blood, pus, or mucous (diarrhea implies an abnormal intestinal osmotic load, abnormal intestinal wall metabolism, or violation of the normal intestinal wall architecture); the underlying past medical or surgical history (an exacerbation of a chronic problem may be revealed as well as a complication from that problem or from therapy); the use of medications (opiates for diarrhea, laxatives for constipation); the therapy for an underlying illness (chemotherapy or radiation therapy); a change in bowel habits (an early clue to the development of carcinoma); tenesmus (indicating rectal carcinoma, proctitis); emotional stress (may activate a quiescent inflammatory process or be a clue to a functional or factitious illness); and travel, occupational, traumatic, environmental, and sexual history (implicates a host of related traumatic and infectious causes).

PHYSICAL EXAMINATION

Signs to be examined and explored include the age of the patient (colon cancer occurs with greatest frequency among those who are 50 to 60 years of age); abnormal vital signs (fever, tachycardia, tachypnea all signify an acute process that requires rapid evaluation); weight loss (may indicate a chronic illness such as carcinoma or acquired immunodeficiency syndrome); the presence of dehydration (indicates a severe or longstanding process); systemic toxicity (may indicate violation of the bowel wall with bacteremia, abscess formation, or perforation); evidence of other organ system involvement (tuberculosis, acquired immunodeficiency syndrome); evidence of an exanthem (implicates an acute infectious process); visceral or colicky generalized abdominal pain (indicates bowel hyperfunction with distention, the presence of mass material, or the presence of diarrheal material); somatic or localized pain with guarding and referred pain (indicates a localized inflammatory or infectious process such as a diverticular abscess or a colonic microperforation); the presence or absence of bowel sounds (absence indicates bowel paralysis attributable to peritonitis or mechanical obstruction); the findings on rectal examination (may reveal carcinoma, occult blood, or fecal impaction with a stercoral ulcer); fecal blood (blood coating a formed stool indicates an anal or rectal lesion; blood admixed with stool indicates bleeding from above the rectum; bloody diarrhea indicates destruction of the normal colonic mucosa; hematochezia represents vascular hemorrhage); palpable abdominal masses, hepatomegaly, or splenomegaly (indicates a pathologic process of longstanding duration, chronic infectious illness, or underlying medical illness); and percussive abdominal signs (hepatic tympany may imply a ruptured viscus; distention with tympany may indicate a mechanical obstruction or toxic megacolon).

ABDOMINAL ROENTGENOGRAPHY

Abdominal roentgenography includes a supine or prone AP film and an erect film of the abdomen. Cross-table lateral and decubitus views are specialized views used to confirm selected diagnostic possibilities and are not routine views. Barium contrast studies are not emergency studies and should not be utilized in making a diagnosis until the patient is stable, a surgical abdomen has been excluded, and the possibility of creating a surgical or morbid situation from the procedure is minimal. Radionuclide and angiographic procedures may be utilized in an emergency evaluation if a diagnostic possibility indicates the need.

Helpful roentgenographic findings include an ileus pattern, which, though nonspecific, does indicate bowel motility dysfunction; step-wise air and fluid levels of bowel obstruction; transverse colonic dilatation of megacolon syndromes; radiopaque foreign objects; subdiaphragmatic air seen in a perforated viscus; portal vein gas and gas in the intestinal wall thus indicating bowel necrosis; thickened colonic mucosa and mucosal "thumb printing" seen in chronic infiltrative and inflammatory bowel disease; evidence of prior surgery such as clips and grafts; and evidence of underlying medical illness such as hepatomegaly in protozoal disease or lymphangiogram dye from a staging for lymphoma.

PROCTOSIGMOIDOSCOPY

This procedure should be performed on patients in whom inflammatory or infectious proctocolitis is sus-

TABLE 1 Differential Diagnosis of Inflammatory and Infectious Diseases of the Colon and Rectum

Inflammatory bowel disease
  Ulcerative colitis
  Crohn's disease: granulomatous colitis, granulomatous proctitis
  Diverticulitis
  Fecal impaction, stercoral ulcer
  Solitary rectal ulcer, colitis cystica profunda
  Anorectal disease: fistula, fissure, abscess, rectal prolapse/procidentia

Tumor
  Carcinoma
  Lymphoma

Trauma, foreign objects, and factitious illness
  Sexual practices
  Child abuse

Environmental effects, ionizing radiation, and medication-related injury

  Ionizing radiation: natural sources of both external and internal irradiation, diagnostic and therapeutic x-irradiation and
    radiopharmaceuticals, nuclear reactions, and industrial x-irradiation
  Heavy metal intoxication
  Plant intoxication: glycosides, amanita, narcissine
  Hypothermia
  Medication: medicinals, lotions, potions; bowel ischemia (from digoxin, birth control pills, propranolol); laxative abuse; cancer
    chemotherapeutic agents; antiobiotic therapy (pseudomembranous enterocolitis, sulfonamide reactions)

Malnutrition
  Vitamin deficiency

Disorders of colon function
  Irritable bowel syndrome
  Megacolon syndromes: congenital (Hirschsprung's disease) or acquired (idiopathic, psychogenic, medication induced, mechanical
    obstruction, neurologic disease) metabolic disease, rectal pain
  Toxic megacolon

Neuroendocrine disorders
  Amyloidosis
  Thyroid disease: hypothyroidism, hyperthyroidism
  Diabetic enteropathy

Bowel ischemia
  Trauma
  Medication
  Vasculitis
  Mesenteric thrombosis
  Mesenteric embolus
  Atherosclerotic disease
  Dissecting aortic aneurysm
  Postoperative vascular graft complications

Immunologic dysfunction
  Acquired immunodeficiency syndrome
  Graft-versus-host reaction

Infectious agents
  Bacterial agents: streptococci (streptococcal proctitis*), T. hominis (mycoplasma proctitis*), E. coli sp. (enterotoxigenic enterocolitis,
    enteropathogenic enterocolitis), Salmonella (enterocolitis*, typhoid fever), Shigella (bacillary dysentery*), Neisseria sp. (gonorrheal
    proctitis,* meningococcal proctitis*), Chlamydia sp. (lymphogranuloma venereum*), Yersinia (enterocolitis), Clostridium sp.
    (Necrotizing enterocolitis [NEC], pseudomembranous enterocolitis), Treponema pallidum (syphilitic proctitis*), Spirillum (Spirillar
    dysentery), Vibrio sp. (enterocolitis), Mycobacterium sp. (tuberculosis, atypical mycobacteria*), Campylobacter sp. (enterocolitis*),
    H. ducryei (chancroid proctitis*), Calymmatobacterium granulomatis (donovanosis proctitis*)

  Viral agents: herpes simplex virus (types I and II proctitis*) cytomegalovirus (enterocolitis*), papilloma virus (Condyloma acuminata*)

  Protozoal agents: Entamoeba sp. (amebic colitis*), Balantidium coli (ciliary dysentery*), Giardia lamblia (Giardiasis*— not strictly a colitis
    but a jejunitis; however, the disease often enters the differential diagnosis due to its association with nonspecific abdominal pain,
    bloating, and diarrhea; sexually transmitted illness and travel related illness); Cryptosporidium (cryptosporidiosis*), Isospora (coccidiosis), T. cruzi
    (SA trypanosomiasis/Chaga's disease)

  Fungal agents: Paracoccidoides brasiliensis (SA blastomycosis enterocolitis), Histoplasma capsulatum (enterocolitis), Candida sp.
    (proctitis*), Phycomycetes (mucor enterocolitis)
  Helminths

  Roundworm: Trichinella spiralis (trichinosis enterocolitis), Ascaris lumbricoides (ascariasis), hookworm, Enterobius vermicularis
    (''pin worms''*), Strongyloides stercoralis (strongyloidiasis*), Trichuris trichura (''whip worm''), Capillaria philippinensis (capillariasis)

  Tapeworms: Taenia sp., Diphyllobothrium latum, Hymenolepsis nana

  Flukes: Schistosoma sp. (schistosomiasis), Fasciolopsis sp. (fasciolopsiasis), Clonorchis sinensis (clonorchiasis)

*Associated with the ''gay bowel syndrome'' (constellation of infectious and traumatic enterocolitides found to occur in homosexual males).

pected. The procedure may be performed in the emergency department on the patient who has stable vital signs and in whom a surgical abdominal process has been excluded. Otherwise, flexible sigmoidoscopy or straight sigmoidoscopy may be performed in the gastroenterology laboratory or in the operating room in order to confirm a diagnosis. The procedure should be performed without any cleansing enema or bowel prep so as not to distend and distort the normal rectal mucosa and wash out any plaques or exudate. During the procedure, the mucosa should be examined for friability, petechiae, ulcers, and exudate (all seen with inflammatory bowel disease); diffuse versus discrete ulcers (ulcerative colitis versus amebic colitis, herpes simplex proctitis); mucosal polyps and pseudopolyps (granulomatous colitis); bacterial proctocolitis (stool-free mucosal cultures should be plated on the appropriate media); mucosal pseudomembranes (pseudomembranous enterocolitis); melanosis coli (indicates the use of anthracen cathartics); parasites (stool specimens should be obtained for evaluation); pus cells on mucosal smears (indicating an invasive inflammatory or infectious disorder as opposed to a functional bowel syndrome). Rectal biopsy using colonoscopy forceps may detect amyloidosis, mild granulomatous colitis, or chronic schistosomiasis while minimizing the chance of rectal perforation. Examination of the stool from the end of the sigmoidoscope and comparing it with that from the anal area for blood, either occult or gross, determines whether the site of bleeding is the anal area or the sigmoid.

LABORATORY EVALUATION

Laboratory evaluation should include a complete blood count (decreased hematocrit indicates blood loss; an increased white blood cell count indicates an acute infectious or inflammatory process; increased "band" forms are seen in shigellosis; increased lymphocytes are seen in salmonellosis; an elevated eosinophil count indicates chronic parasitic infection); urinalysis (increased specific gravity indicates dehydration; oxalate crystals indicate abnormal terminal ileal function in active Crohn's disease); erythrocyte sedimentation rate (elevation occurs in active inflammatory disease); serologic tests for ameba and chlamydia, lymphogranuloma venereum-type (LGV).

Stool examination should include a Wright stain for pus cells (the presence of pus cells implicates an active inflammatory or infectious process as opposed to a functional bowel syndrome); a Gram stain (a modified Gram stain using carbolfuchsin as a counter-stain may be useful in identifying the "gull-winged" organisms of *Campylobacter* sp.; cresyl violet from a Gram stain identifies the "coconut" shaped budding yeast forms of Candida sp.); an evaluation for parasites (*Entamoeba* sp.) and ova (*Strongyloides* sp.; "pinworms"); an evaluation for occult and gross blood; Sudan III stain for fat (seen with malabsorption syndromes); an evaluation for pseudomembranes; determination of alkalinization of the stool (indicates phenolphthalein ingestion with self-induced chronic diarrhea owing to laxative abuse); *Clostridium difficile*

toxin titer (establishes the diagnosis of antibiotic-induced pseudomembranous enterocolitis); a culture for enteric and fungal pathogens (using special media.)

SYMPTOMATIC THERAPY

Symptomatic therapy includes (1) prevention of dehydration (2) treatment of visceral, colicky abdominal pain (3) alleviation of rectal burning and pain (4) slowing of the diarrheal process and (5) alleviation of fever, with acetaminophen.

Prevention of Dehydration

In an adult, intravenous rehydration includes the use of lactated Ringer's solution, containing appropriate amounts of added bicarbonate and potassium, to match fluid loss. Initial infusions may be given at a "wide open" rate for 1 or 2 liters, followed by a rate appropriate for urinary output and volume of diarrhea. Oral rehydration may consist of soup, water, cola, or Gatorade, but it must be noted that the electrolyte composition of any of these fluids is not physiologic (even Gatorade is relatively potassium-deficient). An alternate oral solution (a modified WHO cholera mixture) composed of 4 level tablespoons of sugar, 3/4 teaspoon of salt, 1 teaspoon of sodium bicarbonate in 1 cup of juice to make up 1 quart of water provides physiologic amounts of glucose and electrolytes for replacement in cases of severe diarrhea. In children, intravenous rehydration may be initiated with lactated Ringer's solution, 20 ml per kilogram given in a bolus over 1 hour followed by an appropriate electrolyte solution calculated from the percent estimated dehydration, the maintenance fluid requirements, and the serum sodium. Oral rehydration may consist of the use of Pedialyte, juice and crackers, cola, or soup, again with the understanding that none of these solutions is physiologic. Oral fluids should be given in small frequent doses in order to allow maximal intestinal absorption and to decrease the risk of the gastric distention and vomiting seen with larger doses.

Alleviation of Rectal Burning and Pain

Rectal burning and pain may be treated with sitz baths for 20 minutes, four times per day; by gentle wiping of the inflamed area with witch hazel pads (Tucks) after each bowel movement and as needed; and by gentle massage of the area with hydrocortisone, 1 percent cream four times per day, and lidocaine, 2 percent jelly or 5 percent ointment four times per day. Hydrocortisone enemas (Proctofoam-HC) can be added four times per day. Hydrocortisone rectal suppositories are not used because the coating action of the medication is not consistent.

Treatment of Colicky Abdominal Pain and Diarrhea

Opiates and anticholinergic medications, with or without atropine, relieve colicky pain and retard diarrhea.

TABLE 2 Treatment of Colicky Abdominal Pain and Diarrhea

Codeine
    Adult: 30 mg PO q6h
    Child: 1 mg/kg/day in divided doses
Diphenoxylate with atropine (Lomotil)
    Adult: 1–2 tablets q.i.d.
    Child: liquid, 0.3 mg/kg/day in four doses
Loperamide (Imodium)
    Adult: 2 mg after each diarrheal movement not to exceed 16 mg per day
All medications should have their dosages reduced as soon as symptoms subside.

They decrease stool frequency, stool volume, and the urge to defecate, thus alleviating the diarrhea, and they alter intestinal motility, thus decreasing the pain. (Table 2).

These medications should be used with care in any abdominal process because they may mask symptoms of catastrophe (perforation, toxemia), allow a chronic process to take an acute turn for the worse (ulcerative colitis developing toxic megacolon) or initiate a complication (diverticulitis developing a diverticular abscess) (see also chapters on *Adult Infectious Diarrhea* and specific disease states).

In adults, high fiber diets and Metamucil (1 packet in 8 ounces of juice every 6 hours) may be utilized to control the symptoms in patients with inflammatory bowel disease. If infection is believed to be the cause of symptoms, bismuth subsalicylate (Pepto-Bismol, 60 cc every 30 minutes for eight doses) or Kaolin and pectin (Kaopectate, four to six times per day) may be given to control symptoms. These agents can make the results of diagnostic procedures (barium enema) and stool collections (ova and parasites) difficult to accurately interpret.

SPECIFIC THERAPY

Trauma, Foreign Objects, and Factitious Illness

Besides symptomatic therapy and desisting from the offending practices, no further therapy is necessary. In the case of factitious illness, counseling is advised if the patient is amenable. In children in whom child abuse is suspected, the appropriate authorities must be contacted, and appropriate arrangements must be made for the care and protection of the child.

Environmental Agents, Ionizing Radiation, and Medication-Related Injury

Injury from ionizing radiation, hypothermia, and cancer chemotherapeutic agents is treated with supportive therapy until the bowel mucosa has been allowed to regenerate. The offending agents must be removed or halted. In the case of ionizing radiation, steroid retention enemas or sulfasalazine may be utilized.

Injury from medicines, lotions, and potions requires that usage be discontinued. Heavy metal intoxication requires removal from exposure, supportive care, and specific antidotes if available. Plant intoxication requires supportive care, gastric emptying, and the use of specific antidotes. Laxative abuse is treated by behavior modification and referral for counseling. Sulfonamide reactions (Azulfidine) during therapy for inflammatory bowel dis-

ease requires discontinuance of the medication and switching to alternative modes of therapy such as corticosteroids, azathioprine, and surgery. Such changes in regimen should not be made without consulting the primary physician caring for the patient.

Pseudomembranous enterocolitis is an acute inflammatory disease characterized by greyish-yellow, exudative, mucosal plaques, most often seen in patients who have been receiving antibiotic therapy (Table 3). The illness is caused by a *Clostridium difficile* enterotoxin, but without invasion of the intestinal mucosa. The disease spectrum ranges from mild diarrhea to bloody diarrhea with systemic toxicity. Treatment includes supportive care; discontinuance of the inciting antibiotic therapy; refraining from the use of antiperistaltic medications; and either vancomycin, metronidazole, or cholestyramine by mouth (Table 4). Severely ill patients require immediate hospitalization.

Toxic megacolon represents the final common pathway of colon dysfunction and inflammation. It is defined as the acute dilatation of all or part of the colon to a diameter greater than 6 cm, associated with systemic toxi-

Disorders of Colon Functions

city. There is widespread inflammation of all layers of the colon with loss of muscle tone, microperforation, and microabscess formation. Treatment consists of aggressive fluid therapy to maintain intravascular volume and to correct for electrolyte losses (especially potassium). Methylprednisolone (Solu-Medrol), 125 mg IV every 6 hours, should be given in order to ameliorate the inflammatory process. Nasogastric suction or intestinal intubation with a Kanter tube is useful in reducing air and fluid passage into the colon. Opiate and anticholinergic medication

TABLE 3 Causes of Pseudomembranous Colitis

Antibiotics
    Clindamycin
    Lincomycin
    Ampicillin (and other penicillins)
    Chloramphenicol
    Tetracycline
    Cephalosporins
Systemic illness
    Staphylococcal infection
    Uremia
    Congestive heart failure
    Ischemic bowel
    Shock

TABLE 4 **Treatment of Pseudomembranous Enterocolitis**

Cholestyramine:	1 packet (4g) orally t.i.d. for 5 days for mild disease
Metronidazole:	500 mg orally t.i.d. for 5–10 days for mild or recurrent disease
Vancomycin:	500 mg PO q.i.d. for 7–14 days for serious disease

should be withheld. Immediate admission is indicated. Broad-spectrum triple antibiotic therapy should be initiated with intravenous ampicillin, 1 g every 4 hours; tobramycin 3 to 5 mg per kilogram per day (further adjustments for decreased renal function); and clindamycin, 600 mg every 6 to 8 hours. Colonic perforation, hemorrhage, and abscess formation require emergency surgical intervention.

Acquired Immunodeficiency Syndrome

Acquired immunodeficiency syndrome is associated with an enteropathy that affects both the small intestine and the colon. Colorectal abnormalities include a specific pathologic process in the lamina propria that shows intranuclear viral inclusions, mast cell infiltration, and crypt degeneration. At present, therapy is supportive including fluid and blood replacement as necessary and enteral or parenteral hyperalimentation in an attempt to compensate for the malabsorptive and diarrheal process. Definitive therapy for the illness is at present unknown.

Infectious Agents

Treatment of infectious agents is determined by the chronicity of the illness and the patient's toxicity. If possible, outpatient therapy is preferred. Supportive therapy is aimed at preventing dehydration and decreasing abdominal discomfort. Definitive therapy is discussed in the chapter on *Adult Infectious Diarrhea*.

Inflammatory Bowel Disease

Ulcerative colitis and the forms of Crohn's disease are chronic problems that may be treated initially in the emergency department, but require long-term follow-up. Initial therapy may consist of sulfasalazine (Azulfidine),

4 g per day (1 g per 15 kilograms per day) for mild-to-moderate symptoms. Concomitant use of oral prednisone, beginning with 60 mg per day (0.5 mg per kilogram per day) may be initiated to control inflammatory symptoms. Loperamide, 2 mg every 6 hours to control diarrhea and abdominal cramps, may be utilized if toxic signs are absent. Patients should be advised to maintain good hydration and nutrition (see chapter on *Inflammatory Bowel Disease*).

ADMISSION CRITERIA

Criteria for admitting a patient to the hospital include (1) development of an acute surgical condition, (2) systemic toxicity and dehydration requiring intravenous rehydration and intravenous and/or parenteral medication, (3) a condition requiring an acute radionuclide, radiographic contrast, endoscopic, echographic, computed axial tomographic, or angioinvasive procedure to guide further therapy based on the outcome and findings, and (4) development of toxic megacolon. Other patients may be discharged, depending on the physician's confidence in the discharge diagnosis, and the patient's ability to follow the therapeutic plan.

INSTRUCTIONS TO THE DISCHARGED PATIENT

The initial presentation of inflammatory or infectious colitis or proctitis may be nonspecific, and the final diagnosis may not be evident for 12, 24, or 72 hours. Therefore, initial therapy must be tempered with caution and the patient given clear advice as to the therapeutic plan, expectations for the therapy, and possible complications.

Discharge plans should include specific recommendations for diet and fluids, medications, further diagnostic testing, further outpatient therapy, and appropriate referral. All patients should be advised that if their condition worsens, pain increases, diarrhea worsens, nausea and vomiting ensues with an inability to retain fluids and/or medication, and if there is uncontrollable fever and chills, or any questions arise, they are to contact their private physician or the emergency department, and if necessary they are to return for a reevaluation. A prearranged follow-up for the patient is always in the patient's best interest and serves to promote good quality and continuity of care.

SEXUALLY TRANSMITTED ENTERIC INFECTIONS

THOMAS C. QUINN, M.S., M.D.

Intestinal infections have become a major health problem among homosexually active men and to a limited degree, among heterosexual women. Although these infections are frequently referred to as "the gay bowel syndrome," homosexuality itself is not necessarily a risk factor for intestinal infections, which may occur in persons with a wide variety of life-styles. Sexually transmitted intestinal infections typically occur among promiscuous individuals who engage in sexual activities that allow fecal contamination. Specifically, sexual practices that include anal intercourse, oral–anal sex (anilingus), or fellatio following anal intercouse can result in person-to-person transmission of highly infectious pathogens. Thus, it is important when examining a patient with intestinal complaints to obtain an extensive sexual history to determine whether any of these risk factors may be responsible for an intestinal infection.

ETIOLOGY

The etiology of intestinal infections in high-risk populations is polymicrobial and requires a careful diagnostic evaluation. Recent studies within the past decade have demonstrated a high incidence of enteric pathogens, including *Shigella, Salmonella, Campylobacter, Giardia lamblia,* and *Entamoeba histolytica,* among homosexually active men. These infections have now been added to the long list of traditional venereal pathogens that have been shown to cause anorectal disease in both homosexual and heterosexual individuals, including *Neisseria gonorrhoeae, Chlamydia trachomatis, Treponema pallidum,* herpes simplex virus, and human papillomavirus. More recently, intestinal disorders in homosexual men have become even more complex with the recognition of opportunistic infections within the gastrointestinal tract of patients with acquired immunodeficiency syndrome (AIDS). Prominent among these infections are *Candida albicans, Cryptosporidia, Isospora belli, Mycobacterium avium-intracellulare* and cytomegalovirus. In addition, patients with AIDS have also been noted to have an increased incidence in gastrointestinal malignancies such as Kaposi's sarcoma, B-cell lymphoma, and squamous cell carcinoma. Consequently, these intestinal infections and malignancies represent a formidable array of disorders responsible for intestinal disease in homosexual men and a challenge to the clinician whose goal is to provide adequate diagnostic and therapeutic care for his or her patients.

GENERAL APPROACH

The spectrum of disease associated with each of these infections and tumors depends on a variety of factors including immunologic competence of the individual, the pathogenicity of the microbe, the duration of infection, the presence of more than one infectious agent, and prior exposure to the infecting pathogen. Many of these infections induce a chronic asymptomatic carrier state that represents the human reservoir for the majority of these infections. The persistent, unrecognized transmission of intestinal infections from asymptomatic individuals to other sexual partners through anal intercourse or oral–anal sex explains the continued epidemic of these infections within the gay community and among heterosexual women. Furthermore, the problem of secondary transmission from infected individuals to the general community through traditional means of transmission such as food contamination extends this problem of intestinal infection to the entire community.

Most of the intestinal pathogens or malignancies may also induce a symptomatic state, which may range from mild to severe. Due to the long list of possible etiologies, the diagnostic approach must be comprehensive, including an extensive history and physical examination with anoscopy or sigmoidoscopy, followed by a full microbiologic evaluation based on symptoms and signs of disease. In some cases an assessment of the immunocompetence of the patient may be required if one suspects infection with human T-cell lymphotropic virus-III (HTLV-III), the causative agent of AIDS. Because most of these infections have a predilection for certain segments of the gastrointestinal tract, a practical approach has been to divide symptomatic disease into several distinct syndromes that are associated with particular infectious agents. Thus, the medical history should attempt to differentiate between clinical syndromes of proctitis, proctocolitis, enteritis, and esophagitis and assess for the constellation of symptoms that might suggest one or another etiologic infectious agents. A list of infectious agents frequently associated with these intestinal syndromes is shown in Table 1.

Examination should include inspection of the perianal area and anal canal, including digital rectal examination and anoscopy to identify mucosal abnormalities, such as friability, exudates, discrete polyps, ulcerations, or fissures, from which culture and biopsy should be obtained, if appropriate. Initial screening laboratory tests on all patients with intestinal symptoms should include a rectal Gram stain for the evaluation of polymorphonuclear leukocytes and intracellular gram-negative bacilli indicating infection with *N. gonorrhoeae* or leukocytes alone indicating invasive inflammatory or infectious disease. Serologic tests for syphilis and a darkfield examination of any external ulcerations should be performed. Routine cultures of the pharynx, rectum, and urethra of men or cervix of women should be performed for *N. gonorrhoeae.* Specific therapy may be instituted based on initial clinical evidence of infection due to *N. gonorrhoeae,* herpes, syphilis, or condyloma acuminatum (Table 2).

DISPOSITION AND FOLLOW-UP

If initial screening tests are negative, a more extensive microbiologic evaluation based on clinical syndromes

606

TABLE 1 Enteric Infections and Clinical Intestinal Syndromes in Homosexual Men

Esophagitis
  Candida albicans
  Herpes simplex virus
  Cytomegalovirus
Enteritis
  Giardia lamblia
  Cryptosporidia
  Isospora belli
  Microsporidia
  Mycobacterium avium-intracellulare
  Cytomegalovirus
Enterocolitis-Proctocolitis
  Shigella
  Campylobacter
  Salmonella
  Clostridium difficile
  Entamoeba histolytica
  Chlamydia trachomatis (LGV strains)
  Cytomegalovirus
Proctitis
  Neisseria gonorrhoeae
  Chlamydia trachomatis (non-LGV strains)
  Treponema pallidum
  Herpes simplex virus
  Cytomegalovirus
  Condyloma acuminatum

described below will need to be obtained before discharge from the emergency department. Hospitalization is rarely required for these infections, unless the patient has marked evidence of dehydration due to chronic diarrhea or evidence of systemic infection manifested by fever of several days' duration, leukocytosis, hypotension, or evidence of an acute abdomen. Otherwise, cultures may be obtained and the patient discharged with follow-up within 2 to 3 days for results of culture. If symptoms persist and initial cultures remain negative, a more extensive examination including sigmoidoscopy, rectal biopsy, and endoscopy may be required, necessitating hospitalization. If a specific agent is identified and treated with antimicrobial agents, follow-up examination is recommended in all cases approximately 1 week following treatment for test of cure or for evaluation of other pathogens. Sexual contacts of these patients should be examined for the presence of the same infection.

DIFFERENTIATION OF CLINICAL SYNDROMES

Proctitis

Symptoms of proctitis frequently include constipation, tenesmus, rectal discomfort or pain, hematochezia, and a mucopurulent discharge. On anoscopy, inflammation of the lower 5 to 10 cm of the rectum is evident depending on the infecting agent. When the presence of proctitis is suggested on anoscopy and leukocytes are present on rectal Gram stain, rectal cultures for non–lymphogranuloma venereum (non-LGV) strains of *C. trachomatis* and herpes simplex virus should be obtained

in addition to *N. gonorrhoeae. N. gonorrhoeae* and *C. trachomatis* may coexist, frequently inducing a mild proctitis associated with erythematous mucosa with mucopus at the anorectal junction near the anal crypts and columns of Morgagni. Empiric therapy for such infections, pending culture results, might include a combined antimicrobial regimen that is active against both rectal gonorrhea (procaine penicillin G 4.8 million units IM, plus 1.0 g of oral probenecid) and rectal chlamydial infection (tetracycline 500 mg 4 times a day for 7 days).

If perianal or rectal ulcers are found in association with proctitis, rectal syphilis or herpes simplex virus infection should be suspected. Rectal mass lesions or mucosal induration suggests secondary syphilis, which may be accompanied by other manifestations of secondary syphilis such as generalized lymphadenopathy or a maculopapular rash. Darkfield microscopic examination of suspicious lesions and an immediate rapid plasma reagent test should be performed for syphilis. If these tests are negative, repeat serologic tests for syphilis are still indicated within the next several weeks. Herpes simplex virus proctitis is frequently a distinctive syndrome with severe anorectal pain, often with multiple perianal ulcers, focal or diffuse rectal ulceration, fever, inguinal lymphadenopathy, difficulty with micturition, impotence, and parasthesias in the S4 to S5 distribution. Lymphogranuloma venereum (LGV) of *C. trachomatis* can also produce severe proctitis, perianal or rectal ulceration, fever, and inguinal lymphadenopathy, and consequently mimic herpetic proctitis. However, LGV is not associated with neurologic symptoms and it causes proctocolitis more frequently than proctitis.

New rapid diagnostic tests may be helpful in differentiation between *N. gonorrhoeae,* herpes, *C. trachomatis,* and syphilis. Most of these tests are monoclonal antibody specific for an infectious agent. Swabs are obtained of the rectal mucosa or the genital ulcerations and are applied directly to a slide. With the use of an immunofluorescent monoclonal antibody that is applied to the slide, the presence of one of the above infectious agents can be identified by use of an immunofluorescent microscope. These tests, as well as enzyme-linked immunosorbent assays (ELISA), have aided the clinician in establishing a definitive diagnosis within a relatively short period of time, resulting in specific therapy.

Anal warts may be evident on perianal examination and anoscopy. It is important to differentiate between condyloma acuminatum and condyloma latum of secondary syphilis. Condylomata acuminatum is caused by human papilloma viruses, and they have a raised cauliflower appearance. Condylomata latum are moist flat papules of secondary syphilis, scrapings of which are positive by darkfield microscopy. The treatment of condyloma acuminatum within the emergency setting consists of cryotherapy with liquid nitrogen applied directly onto the wart or repeated daily applications of topical podophyllin. Condylomata latum are treated according to guidelines for secondary syphilis (see Table 2) and do not require any local therapy.

TABLE 2 Treatment of Sexually Transmitted Enteric Infections

Pathogen	Recommended Treatment	Alternative
Neisseria gonorrhoeae Neisseria meningitidis	Aqueous procaine penicillin G, 4.8 million units IM + probenecid 1.0 g orally	Ceftriaxone 250 mg IM, or Spectinomycin HCI 2.0 g IM, or Tetracycline HCI, 500 mg orally q.i.d. for 7 days (alternative only for pharyngeal gonorrhea)
Chlamydia trachomatis	Tetracycline, 500 mg orally q.i.d. for 1 week (3 weeks for LGV infection)	Erythromycin, 500 mg orally q.i.d. for 1 week (3 weeks for LGV infection)
Herpes simplex virus	Supportive, analgesics, stool softeners, sitz baths	Acyclovir, 200 mg orally 5 times daily for 14 days
Treponema pallidum 1°, 2°, early latent (<1 yr)	Benzathine penicillin 2.4 million units IM	Tetracycline, 500 mg orally q.i.d. for 15 days
Latent syphilis (>1 yr)	Benzathine penicillin, 2.4 million units IM once a week for 3 weeks	Tetracycline or erythromycin as above, but for 30 days
Neurosyphilis	Aqueous penicillin G, 12-24 million units IV for 10 days followed by benzathine penicillin G 2.4 million units IM weekly for 3 doses	Aqueous procaine penicillin G 2.4 million units daily + probenecid, 500 mg q.i.d. for 10 days, followed by benzathine G, 2.4 million units once a week for 3 weeks
Shigella sp.	Trimethoprim–sulfamethoxazone, 160-180 mg orally twice daily for 7 days	Ampicillin, 500 mg q6h for 7 days
Campylobacter sp.	Erythromycin, 500 mg q6h for 7 days	Tetracycline, 500 mg q6h for 7 days
Salmonella	Chloramphenicol, 500 mg IV q6h for 10 days; or ampicillin, 1 g IV q5h for 10 days; or trimethoprin–sulfamethoxazole, 2 tabs q12h for 10 days	
Giardia lamblia	Metronidazole (Flagyl), 250 mg t.i.d. for 7 days	Quinacrine, 100 mg t.i.d. for 7 days
Entamoeba histolytica	Metronidazole 750 mg orally t.i.d. for 10 days + diiodohydroxyquine, 650 mg orally t.i.d. for 20 days	Diiodohydroxyquine, 650 mg t.i.d. for 20 days, or diloxanide furoate, 500 mg t.i.d. for 10 days, or paromomycin 25-30 mg/kg/day in 3 divided doses for 7 days (luminal amebicides) recommended by some if patient is asymptomatic cyst passer)
Strongyloides stercoralis	Thiabendazole 25 mg/kg orally for 2 days	
Enterobius vermicularis (pinworm)	Mebendazole, 100 mg orally for 1 day	Pyrantel pamoate, 11 mg/kg orally for 1 day
Cryptosporidia	Supportive fluid replacement	
Condyloma acuminatum	Podophyllin, 10%, daily as a topical application	Cryosurgery (liquid nitrogen), electro surgery, or surgical removal

Proctocolitis

Evidence of proctocolitis is frequently confirmed in a person with lower abdominal cramps and diarrhea, which may be bloody, by the sigmoidoscopic observation of abnormal mucosa extending beyond 10 to 15 cm. The presence of proctocolitis should lead to rectal cultures for LGV strains of *C. trachomatis;* stool cultures for *Shigella, Salmonella,* and *Campylobacter;* and stool examination for ova and parasites including *E. histolytica* and cryptosporidia. Systemic symptoms of fever, chills, myalgias associated with a history of diarrhea, nausea, and cramps are frequently present. Sigmoidoscopy or colonoscopy may reveal discrete ulcerations and mucopus. Rectal biopsies frequently reveal nonspecific inflammation with polymorphonuclear leukocyte infiltration of the lamina propria and occasionally cryptitis and giant cells. Granulomas are rarely present except in LGV infection, which helps to differentiate LGV from the other bacterial pathogens, but which frequently causes a misdiagnosis of Crohn's disease. A history of recent antibiotic use should suggest the need for evaluation for *Clostridium difficile* infection. It is nearly impossible to differentiate between these bacterial and parasitic infections at the time of examination except in the case of *E. histolytica.* This parasite can be diagnosed by a wet-prep examination of mucus obtained during anoscopy or sigmoidoscopy. Otherwise, therapeutic options for proctocolitis are varied and are influenced by the cause and by local differences in the prevalence of enteric pathogens and in the patterns of antimicrobial susceptibility of these pathogens. Therefore, it is mandatory that stool cultures for enteric pathogens and for ova and parasite examination be obtained in addition to cultures for *N. gonorrhoeae* and *C. trachomatis.*

Enteritis

Enteritis is frequently suspected in individuals who have symptomatic complaints of diarrhea, upper abdominal cramps, bloating, and nausea and who have no evidence of inflammation on sigmoidoscopy or anoscopy. *G. lamblia* is most frequently associated with enteritis, but the bacterial enteric pathogens of *Shigella, Salmonella,* and *Campylobacter* may initially present with enteritis before becoming more fully manifest as proctocolitis. In patients with AIDS, cryptosporidia, *Isospora*, cytomegalovirus, and *M. avium-intracellulare* have also been found to cause a diffuse enteritis. Specific evaluation of stool for ova and parasites and culture for enteric pathogens is required to help differentiate between these infectious agents. Multiple stool examinations are frequently necessary to document infection with *G. lamblia*. When stool examinations have been negative, sampling of jejunal mucus by the enterotest or small bowel biopsy is necessary to confirm the diagnosis. Recently the development of an ELISA for the detection of *Giardia* antigen in the stool has facilitated a rapid diagnosis of this infection. Specific cultures and acid-fast stains are required for identification of *M. avium-intracellulare* in AIDS patients with gastrointestinal symptoms. This organism takes several weeks to grow in the laboratory and the symptoms may frequently be misdiagnosed as Whipple's disease based on small bowel biopsy that reveals foamy intestinal macrophages with PAS-positive staining organisms. *M. avium-intracellulare* is also acid-fast positive, and this helps to differentiate this infection from Whipple's disease, in which the putative agent is acid-fast negative. Likewise, special laboratory procedures must be employed to identify cryptosporidia and *Isospora* on ova and parasite examination. Both of these organisms are also acid-fast positive, and this helps the microbiologist to identify these within the stool. Cytomegalovirus enteric infection is confirmed by small bowel biopsy.

Esophagitis

Oral-esophageal infections among homosexual men are most commonly caused by *N. gonorrhoeae*, *C. trachomatis,* herpes simplex virus, and in the immunocompromised, *C. albicans*. Pharyngeal infection with *N. gonorrhoeae* is one of the most common infections found in homosexual men, although it is frequently asymptomatic. Rarely, pharyngeal gonorrhea is associated with a mild pharyngitis. Diagnosis is dependent on recovery of the organism on routine cultures for *N. gonorrhoeae*. *C. trachomatis* rarely induces a symptomatic pharyngitis, and its presence can be detected only by routine culture. The presence of oral candidiasis or thrush in a homosexual male is indicative of an underlying immunosuppression and is highly predictive of HTLV-III infection. Oral candidiasis has a poor prognosis in these patients, usually leading to oroesophageal candidiasis, confirming a diagnosis of AIDS. The predominant symptoms of invasive *Candida* esophagitis is odynophagia. The clinical appearance of *Candida* esophagitis is rather characteristic with dilatation and abnormal motility of the esophagus with presence of cottage cheese exudates on endoscopy. Deep esophageal ulcerations may be associated with *Candida* but may be caused by herpes simplex virus or cytomegalovirus infection. In esophageal candidiasis, biopsies of the esophagus typically reveal invasive hyphae through the mucosa and submucosa.

SPECIFIC TREATMENT GUIDELINES

Neisseria Gonorrhoeae

Suspicion of anorectal or pharyngeal gonorrhea based on a positive gram stain, history and physical examination, culture, or even history of sexual contact with another individual with documented gonorrhea should result in immediate treatment for gonorrhea. Treatment of gonococcal infection typically consists of administration of aqueous procaine penicillin G 4.8 million units IM with 1 g of probenecid orally. In penicillin-allergic patients, spectinomycin hydrochloride, 2 g IM is recommended for anorectal gonorrhea. Tetracycline hydrochloride 500 mg orally 4 times a day for 7 days is recommended for pharyngeal gonorrhea in penicillin-allergic patients, because spectinomycin is not highly effective against pharyngeal gonorrhea. Treatment with oral tetracycline or oral ampicillin has been less effective for the treatment of anorectal gonorrhea and should not be used. Careful follow-up with post-treatment cultures 10 days after therapy is essential.

Penicillinase-producing *N. gonorrhoeae* (PPNG) may be responsible for drug failure in some patients and therapy for PPNG should include either ceftriaxone 250 mg IM or spectinomycin 2 grams IM. Because drug resistance to spectinomycin is now being reported in some areas, alternative therapeutic regimens, particularly if a patient remains culture positive after spectinomycin, include ceftriaxone 250 mg IM cefoxitin 2 g IM plus probenecid 1 g orally, or cefotaxime without probenecid. A daily single dose of 9 tablets of trimethoprim–sulfamethoxazole (80 mg to 400 mg) tablet for 5 days or ceftriaxone 250 mg IM should be used to treat pharyngeal gonococcal infection due to PPNG because spectinomycin appears to be less effective in pharyngeal infection. Other possible causes of persistent infection due to *N. gonorrhoeae* include poor compliance if an oral medication has been prescribed and reinfection through an untreated sexual partner.

Chlamydia Trachomatis

Treatment of suspected or proven *Chlamydia* infections consists of tetracycline 500 mg 4 times daily for 7 days for non-LGV rectal infections. For more severe systemic LGV infections, treatment should be extended for 3 to 4 weeks. Frequently patients with suspected or confirmed gonococcal infections are treated with penicillin followed by a 1-week course of tetracycline because co-infection with these two pathogens is so frequent in this population. Patients should be followed carefully with repeat sigmoidoscopy or anoscopy, particularly when there is a question about the differential diagnosis of LGV and inflammatory bowel disease.

Anorectal Herpes Simplex Virus Infection

The clinical course of initial primary anorectal herpes is usually self-limited, resolving in 3 weeks. Recurrences are frequently seen but are less symptomatic and shorter in duration. Treatment has typically been supportive, consisting of sitz baths, stool softeners, and analgesics. Recently acyclovir, a new antiherpes drug has been developed for the treatment of primary and recurrent herpes infection, and it is available in intravenous, ointment, and oral forms. For severe primary herpes infection of the gastrointestinal tract, intravenous acyclovir may be given at 5 mg per kg every 8 hours for 7 days. The ointment is ineffective in treatment of intestinal infection and is therefore not recommended. However, oral treatment with acyclovir can be instituted at 200 mg 5 times daily for 14 days for primary or severe recurrent disease. Recent studies have also indicated that suppressive therapy of acyclovir at 200 mg 2 to 3 times a day is also effective in suppressing herpetic recurrences. Suppressive therapy should be recommended in immunocompromised individuals, or individuals having frequent recurrences (4 or more per year). Suppressive dosages of acyclovir have been shown to be effective in preventing recurrences in up to 80 percent of individuals known to have frequent recurrences prior to institution of therapy.

Intestinal Syphilis

The recommended treatment of early syphilis, which includes primary, secondary, and early latent syphilis of less than 1 year's duration, is benzathine penicillin G 2.4 million units IM. Tetracycline hydorchloride or erythromycin 500 mg 4 times per day for 15 days may be used for patients who are allergic to penicillin. For patients with syphilis of more than 1 year's duration, (except neurosyphilis), benzathine penicillin G 2.4 million units IM once per week for 3 weeks should be administered. Tetracycline or erythromycin should be used in penicillin-allergic patients for a duration of 30 days. Cerebrospinal fluid (CSF) examination should be done in patients with clinical symptoms consistent with neurosyphilis. It is perhaps desirable to exclude asymptomatic neurosyphilis in patients with syphilis of unknown duration or in those with greater than 1 year's duration by performing a lumbar puncture. If a CSF pleocytosis is present with a positive CSF serology for syphilis, a diagnosis of neurosyphilis should be made and treated with aqueous crystalline penicillin G, 12 or 24 million units IV in 4 to 6 divided doses per day for 10 days followed by benzathine penicillin G 2.4 million units IM weekly for 3 weeks. Aqueous procaine penicillin 2.4 million units IM daily plus probenecid 500 mg 4 times a day for 10 days, followed by benzathine G 2.4 million units for 3 weeks is an alternative treatment regimen. Careful serologic follow-up and reexamination of intestinal lesions at regular intervals are necessary to document eradication of the infection. Case reporting and treatment of recent sexual contacts is also required.

Enteric Bacterial Pathogens

The treatment of enteritis or proctocolitis due to bacterial pathogens such as Shigella, Salmonella, and Campylobacter is usually supportive and does not require antimicrobial therapy. Fluid replacement is recommended in cases of dehydration, and antibiotic treatment is recommended only in severe prolonged cases. The choice of antibiotics is often based on the sensitivity of the identified pathogen because the susceptibility to different antibiotics varies in different parts of the country. In general, shigellosis should be treated with trimethoprim-sulfamethoxazole 2 tablets every 12 hours for 7 days. Alternatively, ampicillin 500 mg 4 times a day for 7 days may be used, but resistance to ampicillin has been widely documented. Patients with prolonged symptoms associated with Campylobacter infection should be treated with erythromycin, 500 mg 4 times a day for 7 days. Tetracycline 500 mg four times a day for 7 days is an alternative antibiotic. Salmonella, infection probably should not be treated, because antibiotics prolong the carrier state of Salmonella. Exceptions to this rule can be made when there is evidence of sepsis or bacteremia. If the isolate is susceptible, ampicillin 1 g IV every 4 hours for 10 days, or trimethoprim–sulfamethoxazole 2 tablets orally twice a day for 10 days, should be used. If there is antibiotic resistance or if antibiotic susceptibilities are not known, treatment with chloramphenicol 500 mg IV every 6 hours for 10 days is warranted until antibiotic sensitivities are known. If there is a remote possibility of sexual transmission of these pathogens, tracing of sexual partners of infected individuals is important, because asymptomatic carriers of these infections exist and pose a potential hazard to the general community, particularly if an asymptomatic carrier is employed as a food handler.

Parasitic Infections

Following identification of E. histolytica, treatment with metronidazole 750 mg orally 3 times a day for 10 days, with or without the addition of either diiodohydroxyquin 650 mg orally 3 times a day for 20 days or diloxanide furoate 500 mg orally 3 times a day for 10 days, are recommended. More recently, a study has shown that treatment with paromomycin at a dose of 25 to 35 mg per kg per day in 3 divided doses for 7 days is effective in producing long-term eradication of intestinal E. histolytica infection in 92 percent of evaluated men, which is comparable to the above treatment regimen. Paromomycin is a luminal amebicide that is well tolerated with minor side effects. However, it should not be used if there is evidence of systemic amebiasis such as hepatic abscess because the drug is not absorbed systemically.

The treatment of G. lamblia infection also consists of metronidazole 250 mg orally 3 times a day for 7 days or quinacrine 100 mg orally 3 times a day for 7 days. If a patient is infected with both Giardia and E. histolytica, metronidazole at a higher dose of 750 mg 3 times a day for 10 days should be recommended. Both of these drugs are associated with a 10 to 15 percent failure rate, and a follow-up stool examination is required following treatment.

Infection with cryptosporidia and Isospora has been recently recognized in animals and both immunocompetent and immunocompromised patients. In an immunocompetent individual, cryptosporidia and Isospora both induce a self-limited diarrheal illness for about 2 weeks. However, in immunosuppressed individuals such as those with AIDS, the illness is manifested by a chronic profuse watery diarrhea that may persist for several months. Very little is known about therapy except that many drugs have been used and shown to be ineffective. In limited studies, spiromycin and dimethyl sulfoxide (DMSO) have been shown to be anecdotally effective in several AIDS patients with cryptosporidia. Unfortunately, there are no well-controlled studies documenting this efficacy.

Another gastrointestinal infection frequently seen in AIDS patients is *M. avium-intracellulare* infection. As with cryptosporidia and *Isospora*, no single effective therapy has been identified as efficacious against this infection. Consequently, it is not uncommon that three to six antimyocobacterial drugs may be used in these patients, usually unsuccessfully. These infections tend to disseminate and eventually result in death of the patient within several months after diagnosis.

Oroesophageal Candidiasis

Oral candidiasis is often well controlled with oral nystatin, 300,000 units (swish and swallow) 4 times a day. Persistent oral candidiasis or *Candida* esophagitis should be treated with ketoconazole, 200 mg twice a day until effective clearance of oroesophageal lesions is documented. The patient can then be switched to nystatin for a prolonged period of time as suppressive therapy. Hepatotoxicity has been associated with ketoconazole, and liver enzymes should be obtained periodically while the person is maintained on ketoconazole. In severe cases of oroesophageal candidiasis, treatment may be required with intravenous amphotericin B up to a maximum total dose of 200 to 400 mg. Following intravenous therapy the patient may be placed on either oral ketoconazole or nystatin. The rationale for aggressive therapy of esophageal candidiasis is to help prevent intractable esophageal ulcerations that may develop. Periodic endoscopy should be done because the disappearance of esophageal symptoms does not reliably indicate that fungal plaques have been fully eradicated or that esophageal ulcerations have disappeared.

Condyloma Acuminatum

The modes of treatment of anal warts are incorporated into six categories: cryotherapy, surgery, treatment with caustic agents, treatment with antimetabolites, immunotherapy, and other approaches. Cryotherapy (freezing with liquid nitrogen) has been used for genital and external anal warts, and when applicable this therapy is recommended because it does not require general or local anesthesia and is not associated with formation of surgical scars. Standard procedure for cryotherapy is to apply liquid nitrogen to a wart with a cotton-tipped applicator for a period of 10 to 30 seconds. This treatment is then repeated weekly for 3 weeks. Another alternative therapy is topical podophyllin in a 10 percent compound of tincture of benzoin. The treated area is washed by the patient 4 to 6 hours later and then, the treatment repeated on a daily basis for 2 to 3 weeks. For internal rectal warts, podophyllin is not recommended because it is toxic to the normal mucosa. Use of podophyllin is also contraindicated in pregnant women because of its antimycotic effects. Surgical techniques which include excision, blunt dissection, curettage, and electrocauterization, have been used if "standard" topical therapeutic regimens have not been effective. Treatment with antimetabolites and immunotherapy are under evaluation and are not recommended at this time.

Anorectal Trauma

The complications of anal intercourse include prolapsed hemorrhoids, fissures, rectal ulcers, rectal tears, and retained foreign bodies. Patients with anorectal trauma frequently present with acute onset of rectal bleeding or with signs of acute abdomen if rectal perforation has occurred above the peritoneal reflelection. Management of these cases is based on clinical history, evidence of acute abdomen, the degree of rectal trauma, and the type of retained object. If an object is present, digital and radiographic examination should confirm the position of the object. The object may then be removed by a proctoscope and biopsy forceps or a Foley catheter. Occasionally, local or general anesthesia may be required to remove the foreign body manually or with obstetric forceps.

SUGGESTED READING

Centers for Disease Control. 1985 STD treatment guidelines. MMWR 1985; 34:Suppl:15–355.

Quinn TC, Stamm WE, Goodell SE, et al. The polymicrobial origin of intestinal infections in homosexual men. N Engl J Med 1983; 309:576–582.

Washington AE, Schultz MG, Cohen ML, Juranek DD, Owen RL. Treatment of sexually transmitted bacterial and protozoal enteric infections. Rev Infect Dis 1982; 4:Suppl:864–876.

PERIRECTAL INFECTION AND ABSCESS

THOMAS R. RUSSELL, M.D., F.A.C.S.

Perirectal infection and abscesses are commonly missed in the emergency setting, and this diagnosis must *always* be considered when a patient has severe unremitting perianal pain. Constant pain is the hallmark of this condition, and there is no position of comfort; often sleep is interrupted. Such activities as bowel movements, coughing, sneezing, and sitting exacerbate the painful condition.

The most common cause of perianal infection is a small perforation of an anal gland at the anorectal junction. This allows bacteria from the rectum to gain access to the perirectal tissue, the result being inflammation and abscess formation. Depending on the site of perforation, the eventual abscess may be superficial (perianal and ischiorectal) or deep (intramuscular or supralevator) (Fig. 1). Other potential causes of perianal sepsis and abscess include folliculitis, hidradenitis suppurativa, infected sebaceous cyst, infected pilonidal cyst, infected Bartholin's cyst, infected hemorrhoid after banding, and trauma. The exact cause of infection may be difficult to establish initially, but drainage of all abscesses is crucial to treatment.

Diagnosis can frequently be established on the basis of the history and physical examination. Temperature elevation, leukocytosis, and systemic signs of sepsis may exist. Inspection of the perianal area often reveals swelling with redness, induration, and fluctuance when the abscess is superficial, in which case no further examination is needed. Deeper abscesses of the perianal area are more difficult to accurately assess and are the type that are neglected and misdiagnosed. After a careful inspection and palpation of the perianal area, and if an abscess is not evident, digital rectal examination is performed. This should be done carefully, even though often painful. Bidigital palpation (index finger in rectum and thumb outside) of the perirectal tissues may reveal induration, a mass, and tenderness when the area involved is felt. Particular attention must be directed to the posterior midline, where a small abscess may exist in the postanal space and only be palpable on bidigital examination. Further diagnostic measures such as anoscopy and proctoscopy generally are not needed in the acute setting, but are useful to assess the epithelium of the anal canal and rectal mucosa if the diagnosis remains uncertain.

Abscesses are frequently *misdiagnosed*; patients are told that they have hemorrhoids and are subsequently discharged and instructed to take sitz baths and use suppositories. It must be stressed that only external hemorrhoidal thrombosis (perianal hematoma) is exquisitely tender, and this should be readily apparent on inspection alone. Internal hemorrhoids are *not* painful unless thrombosis and prolapse exist. This also is apparent on inspection. Internal hemorrhoids, when symptomatic, bleed or occasionally prolapse, but do not create the intense deep pain of an abscess. A fissure (ulcer) of the anal canal is a common condition, but is generally painful during and immediately after defecation. This lesion can frequently be noted on inspection and has an accompanying skin tag. Other conditions in the differential diagnosis of perianal pain include pruritus ani, venereal infection of the perianal and rectal area, and anal carcinoma. Rectal disease generally is not painful, owing to a lack of somatic nerve fibers.

THERAPY

Once the diagnosis of perianal abscess is made, the needed treatment is incision and drainage. The use of antibiotics is limited and reserved for patients with valvular heart disease or for the immunocompromised patient. Sitz baths, topical creams, and suppositories are of little benefit and only delay needed drainage. One need not wait for fluctuance to occur prior to drainage.

The majority of otherwise healthy, reliable patients with superficial abscesses (perianal, ischiorectal) may safely and effectively undergo a drainage procedure on an outpatient basis. Patients must be instructed to expect moderate discomfort for a brief period during drainage, but relief of pain and pressure follows the drainage of an abscess. Also, they should be informed that further studies and additional surgery may be required after resolution of the acute infection.

Local anesthesia (1 percent lidocaine) should be infiltrated into the skin overlying the most tender or fluctuant area and into the abscess. This allows a curvilinear or cruciate-type incision over the most tender or fluctuant area. The incision must be adequate to allow egress of purulent drainage. Cultures for aerobic and anaerobic bacteria may be obtained. Further probing and packing

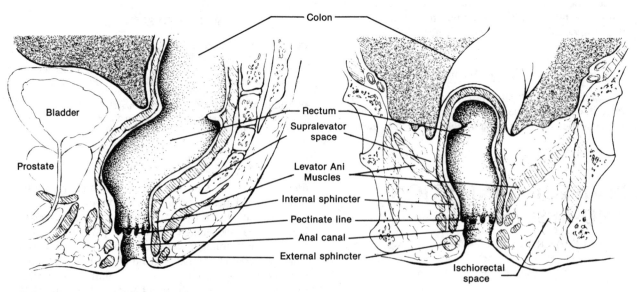

Figure 1 Anatomy of the rectum and perianal region. (From Simon R, Brenner B. Procedures and techniques in emergency medicine. Baltimore: Williams & Wilkins, 1982.)

are generally unnecessary once purulent drainage is observed. Frequent sitz baths or showers facilitate further drainage, keep the site open, and increase local perfusion of the tissue. Follow-up after drainage is mandatory and must be arranged by the physician performing the procedure.

Abscesses occurring in the immunocompromised patient (e.g., with diabetes, leukemia, lymphoma) or deep abscesses must be treated in the hospital. Intravenous antibiotics are useful, and drainage is best accomplished in the operating room under general or regional anesthesia by a trained general surgeon or colorectal surgeon. The patient who presents to the emergency department with severe rectal pain and who cannot be adequately diagnosed as an outpatient should be admitted to the hospital and examined under anesthesia in the operating room. Many such patients are found to have a deep, occult abscess that requires drainage.

Following drainage, whether on an outpatient or an inpatient basis, care consists in frequent baths to promote drainage and comfort. Follow-up is needed to assess adequacy of drainage. Persistent pain suggests inadequacy of the procedure and may necessitate further drainage, generally in the operating room. After resolution of pain and tissue reaction, a more thorough examination is needed to ascertain whether a communication with the lumen of the rectum exists, i.e., fistula in ano (see chapter on *Hemorrhoids, Anal Fissure, and Anal Fistula*), in which case a fistulectomy or unroofing of the tract will be required to allow complete healing.

However, if no rectal communication is shown, other causes, such as cysts or foreign bodies, are sought to explain the infection and appropriately treated surgically.

SUGGESTED READING

Chrabot CM, Prasad MI, Abcarian H. Recurrent anorectal abscesses. Dis Colon Rectum 1983; 26:105–108.

Read DR, Abcarian H. A prospective survey of 474 patients with anorectal abscesses. Dis Colon Rectum 1979; 22:566–568.

Vasilevsky C, Gordon PH. The incidence of recurrent abscesses on fistula in ano following anorectal suppuration. Dis Colon Rectum 1984; 27:126–130.

ANAL FISSURE, ANAL FISTULA, AND HEMORRHOIDS

STANLEY M. GOLDBERG, M.D., F.A.C.S.
CHRISTOPHER M. LAHR, M.D.

The healthy anal canal is required to maintain an airtight valve that intermittently and on command must relax to allow the passage of gas, liquid, and solid rectal contents of various calibers and consistencies. Diarrhea, hard stools, or chronic straining can result in disorders involving anal canal components (mucosa, skin, connective tissue, blood vessels, and muscle) that present with pain, bleeding, and discharge. Four common benign nonseptic lesions must be sought out in the evaluation of anal complaints: external hemorrhoid thrombosis, bleeding or prolapsing internal hemorrhoids, anal fissure, and anal fistula.

The profusely innervated skin of the anal canal (anoderm) meets the insensitive anal mucosa at the dentate line. Hemorrhoidal tissue consisting of blood vessels and loose connective tissue is present in all healthy individuals. Thrombosis of a hemorrhoidal vessel under the skin of the anal canal (anoderm) results in inflammation, edema, and unrelenting pain. Mucosal lesions proximal to the dentate line present with painless rectal bleeding. Once thought to be varices, internal hemorrhoids are actually composed of edematous redundant mucosa and underlying connective tissue that can prolapse into the anal canal, where repeated fecal traction and abrasion result in ulceration and bleeding.

Anal fissure is a linear radial tear in the skin of the anus where the skin passes over the distal sphincter muscle and into the anal canal. It usually causes pain on defecation that may be excruciating and bright red rectal bleeding, most often on toilet paper or into the toilet bowl water.

Fistula in ano is an enterocutaneous fistula with its enteric opening in the anal canal usually at or near the dentate line and with its cutaneous opening anywhere on the perineum. It is thought to be caused by linear extension of a localized septic focus beginning in the anal crypts at the dentate line.

HISTORY AND EXAMINATION

Pain indicates either the presence of a cutaneous lesion distal to the dentate line or infection. Thrombosed external hemorrhoids produce a rapid but not sudden onset of pain. The pain is continuous, but not excruciating, and it is not necessarily related to defecation. The pain of an anal fissure may be sudden in onset and is often associated with passage of a singularly hard bowel movement. It may be severe and stabbing when acute or deep and burning when chronic. Anal fistulas are associated with pain only if infection is present. Internal hemorrhoids do not characteristically produce pain unless necrosis, ischemia, or infection is present. A large prolapsing hemorrhoidal mass present in the anal canal may, however, cause discomfort, as can the pruritus ani that occurs when prolapsing hemorrhoids or skin tags make good anal hygiene difficult. Dull aching pain can also be caused by pelvic, rectal, or perirectal tumors that may be obvious on examination.

All anal or rectal pain warrants early circumanal digital rectal examination to rule out abscess. No combination of responses in the history can rule out abscess. Sometimes examination under anesthesia is required if severe pain precludes an adequate, complete examination. *Bleeding* from anal lesions is commonly bright red and first seen on toilet paper or in toilet bowl water. It is usually quite limited in amount (to a tablespoon), but on occasion it can be massive. Patients with thrombosed external hemorrhoids do not present with bleeding, and those with fistulas only rarely. In the later case there more often is drainage or the pain of associated infection.

The presence of perianal drainage may be attributable to an anal fistula; soilage can also be related to prolapsing internal hemorrhoids. Diarrhea may cause or exacerbate anal disorders and may indicate the presence of inflammatory bowel disease. Constipation is also related to the cause of some anal lesions and, in the presence of fissures, can initiate a vicious cycle of constipation, defecation, pain, avoidance of defecation, constipation, and finally defecation with increased pain. Diarrhea may be a sign of partial bowel obstruction, as may constipation. The presence of diarrhea, constipation, dark or persistent bleeding, or pain resistant to adequate treatment of local benign anal lesions should always prompt further evaluation of the proximal gastrointestinal tract.

Anorectal physical examination is performed either with the patient in a prone kneeling position with hips and knees flexed or with the patient lying on his side. Inspection may reveal the presence of skin tags, prolapsing internal hemorrhoids, or thrombosed external hemorrhoids. Anal fissures are the most commonly missed lesions because they lie just inside the anal canal, concealed by overlying skin folds. To avoid missing anal fissures, the gluteal cheeks must be firmly retracted laterally, and using the examiner's gloved fingertips and a gauze sponge for traction, the distal anoderm must be drawn outward and visualized. If excruciating pain is elicited on digital examination, the examiner should be alerted to the need for a more thorough inspection. Fissures are most common in the midline and are much more often posterior than anterior. The finding of a lateral fissure should alert the physician to the presence of Crohn's disease or some other systemic disorder.

Having the patient strain while squatting over a toilet often reveals gross rectal prolapse or procidentia. The presence of a protuberant and puckered or fishmouth anus is evidence of an occult rectal prolapse that can cause rectal ulcers, bleeding, and difficulty with evacuation. Finally, inspection may reveal the presence of external fistula openings and of perianal infections.

Digital examination is performed to rule out masses and to evaluate anal sphincter tone and caliber. Anal stenosis predisposes to fissures. Fecal impactions can be identified, as can the presence of hard constipated stool in the rectal vault. Most critical is the use of digital examination to identify and localize induration, mass, and tenderness of a perianal or perirectal abscess. A spastic and excruciatingly tender levator muscle (left side worse than right) may indicate levator muscle syndrome, which is simply chronic spasm of this striated muscle; this can be very painful. The levator ani muscle runs from an anterior to posterior direction along the right and left sides of the top of the anal canal and can be felt as a firm horizontal band when the patient voluntarily squeezes his sphincter around the examiner's finger.

Anoscopy using a short, open-ended, slightly coned anoscope is required after inspection and digital examination. It is possible to visualize the anal mucosa and also to judge the degree of hemorrhoidal redundancy and prolapse. Some hemorrhoidal tissue is normally present and can be seen bulging slightly into the slotted end of the anoscope. Hemorrhoids that fill the slotted end of the anoscope or prolapse through the anal canal are called prolapsed internal hemorrhoids and are graded I, II, or III. Grade I hemorrhoids protrude through the anal canal, but reduce spontaneously. Grade II hemorrhoids require manual reduction, and grade III hemorrhoids have come to rest outside the anal verge and cannot be reduced. The surface of the hemorrhoids is friable and granular if they are the cause of chronic rectal bleeding.

Rigid proctoscopy or flexible sigmoidoscopy should be performed on all patients with anorectal complaints; however, it need not necessarily be done on the first visit, especially if there is an identifiable anal lesion present that would cause the examination to be unusually painful, such as an abscess or fissure. Proctoscopy can identify proctitis.

The need for further examinations such as colonoscopy and barium enema must be based upon the clinician's degree of suspicion of proximal lesions. This suspicion should be aroused by persistent rectal bleeding, melena, constipation, diarrhea, abdominal pain or distention, age over 60, associated gynecologic cancer, or family history of colon cancer.

PROLAPSED INTERNAL HEMORRHOIDS

Once the diagnosis of prolapsed internal hemorrhoids has been made, the therapy must be chosen. The advent of fiber stool softeners and rubber–band ligation of internal hemorrhoids has drastically reduced the necessity for surgical hemorrhoidal excision, which was once the mainstay of treatment. All patients with anorectal disorders benefit from bulk or fiber stool softeners such as bran, Metamucil, Hydrocil, and others. Patients should be placed on a dose adequate to produce one or two large soft bowel movements a day that pass through the anal canal easily, without straining. The patient should be warned that some abdominal cramping may occur during the first few weeks of therapy, but that this will resolve. He should also be aware that stool softeners do not have an instantaneous effect upon symptoms, and several days or more may elapse before symptomatic relief is noted. Long-term use may be required to prevent recurrence, but is not associated with laxative dependence. Usual starting doses are one tablespoon of bran in liquid or on cereal or fruit once a day or one tablespoon of Metamucil Per Diem Plain (without senna), or Hydrocil with any liquid once a day. The dosage and frequency may need to be adjusted to obtain the proper stool consistency. If bleeding is minimal initially and resolves, and if prolapse is minimal and reduces spontaneously, the fiber stool softeners may be all that is required. When deciding upon the best therapy, the amount of prolapse can be more objectively measured by gently grasping the hemorrhoidal tissue with forceps while the anoscope is in place and retracting the tissue into the canal to see how far it goes.

BANDING INTERNAL HEMORRHOIDS

Recent studies have produced a new understanding of prolapsed internal hemorrhoids. We now believe that chronic traction results in loss of the normal mucosal attachments to underlying muscle. With subsequent chronic trauma exacerbated by the prolapse, edema, inflammation, connective tissue proliferation, and fibrosis develop. Early in their course, when findings are limited to mucosal prolapse and bleeding, the treatment of choice is rubberband ligation, which removes redundant mucosa and causes fibrosis, which firmly reattaches the mucosa to the underlying muscle. The procedure can be performed in the office without anesthesia and with minimal pain. Results are equal to those obtained previously with surgery, and ligation can be repeated if necessary. The banding is not generally performed in the presence of fissure, fistula, or anal Crohn's disease.

The banding can be performed with the patient in a knee to chest position on his side or kneeling on the proctoscopy examining table. No anesthesia is required. The anoscope is inserted into the anal canal with the end slot pointing toward the quadrant to be banded. While the assistant holds the anoscope, an alligator forceps passed through the loaded barrel of the Barron ligator instrument is used to grasp the redundant mucosa high in the anal canal above the actual level of the hemorrhoidal tissue. It is not critical to include the entire hemorrhoid or even a large portion of it in order for the banding to be successful. Once the site is chosen and grasped with the alligator forceps, the forceps are withdrawn, pulling the redundant mucosa through the barrel of the ligator. The rubber band is then released around the base of the redundant mucosa that is inside the barrel. We generally do only one quadrant or occasionally two at one sitting, because though pain is usually not significant, some patients do note a visceral discomfort that increases with the number of bands placed.

If the band is placed too close to the dentate line and includes anoderm, the patient will probably experience immediate severe pain. When this occurs, the tissue around the base of the banding can be infiltrated with local anesthetic and the band removed with a scalpel blade. The banding can then be performed more proximally. Another potential complication is bleeding, which may occur 7 to 10 days after banding when the necrotic banded tissue falls off, leaving a raw incompletely healed base. Bleeding can usually be controlled with electrocoagulation, repeat band ligation, or suture ligation. Aspirin, Coumadin, and hemodialysis are *not* absolute contraindications to banding. External hemorrhoid thrombosis sometimes follows banding and is treated just like spontaneous thrombosis, discussed further on.

Finally, infection can complicate banding, although in our experience this has rarely occurred, and it responds well to early treatment. It must be mentioned, however, that several deaths caused by fulminating sepsis have been reported to follow hemorrhoidal banding. Whether or not this occurred in patients who might have had occult immune deficiency is unknown. Although it is not a standard procedure now, in the future it may be wise to obtain signed consent for banding.

OTHER TREATMENTS OF INTERNAL HEMORRHOIDS

Though some authors recommend injection therapy, cryotherapy, or infrared hyperthermic coagulation therapy, we do not recommend any of these. We have seen severe complications from mucosal sloughing and anal stricture following use of these treatments. The size of the necrotic area produced cannot be precisely controlled, as it can with band ligation.

Surgical hemorrhoidectomy is required if mucosal prolapse has become associated with significant connective tissue proliferation and fibrosis resulting in a large prolapsed hemorrhoid that may or may not reduce easily. Associated conditions such as large external skin tags, fissure, fistula, or anal stenosis may make surgery the preferred initial therapy.

Grade II or grade III hemorrhoidal prolapse that is associated with necrosis or gangrene requires immediate surgical hemorrhoidectomy to prevent infection. The surgical procedure differs only in the amount of tissue excised. This is one of the few indications for hospitalization for nonseptic benign anal lesions.

THROMBOSED EXTERNAL HEMORRHOIDS

Thrombosis of one or more of the veins under the densely innervated skin of the distal anal canal distal to the dentate line (anoderm) can result in swelling and pain. The thrombosis presents as a swollen, tender, palpable mass at the anal verge. The natural history of thrombosed external hemorrhoids is rapidly increasing anal pain that may be quite severe, reaching its peak 2 to 3 days after thrombosis and then gradually resolving over the next 6 to 10 days. Treatment is therefore based upon the duration of the thrombosis at the time of presentation. If the thrombosis is acute and pain is moderately severe or worsening, then immediate excision under local anesthesia is indicated. If thrombosis has been present for 3 to 4 days and seems to be resolving, then only bulk stool softeners are indicated, since excision would only replace the resolving pain at thrombosis with postoperative incisional pain.

Surgical excision can be carried out in the office or emergency department. After subcutaneous injection of local anesthetic (0.25 percent Marcaine plus epinephrine 1:200,000 will result in prolonged pain relief and decreased local bleeding), the boundary of the thrombosed external hemorrhoid is incised in a radial elliptic pattern. Traction is placed on the hemorrhoid with forceps, lifting it away from the surrounding skin, and the entire hemorrhoid is excised with scissors. Hemostasis is obtained with electrocoagulation, although excision can often be performed through a bloodless plane with minimal or no bleeding. Though the wound can be closed with sutures this is not necessary, since surrounding folds of skin fill in the wound, which quickly heals secondarily. Relief of pain after excision is immediate and often dramatic. Bulk stool softeners are recommended in all patients.

We do not perform incision of the hemorrhoid with evacuation of the clot, since all of the multiple intravascular clots may not be removed, pain is incompletely relieved, bleeding may be difficult to control, redundant skin is likely to form skin tags, and it is not significantly less invasive a procedure than excision. Hospitalization is not generally required.

Multiple areas of thrombosis, recurrent episodes of thrombosis, and external hemorrhoids associated with symptomatic internal hemorrhoids may be indications for formal surgical hemorrhoidectomy, sometimes on an emergency basis.

FISTULA IN ANO

The development of fistulas is caused by perianal infection of some type, usually infection of the anal glands or crypts. Other factors that can predispose to fistulas include inflammatory bowel disease, granulomatous infections, foreign body trauma, and radiation. These must be ruled out in the investigation of fistulas. Once fistulas form, epithelialization of the tract may result in their persistence.

Patients with chronic fistulas present with a persistent discharge from a small fistula, which may be causing skin excoriation and pruritus. There may be pain or bleeding on defecation or both. Patients with acute fistulas have continuous throbbing pain aggravated by defecation that is owing to the causative fistula abscess.

History and physical findings are based upon the magnitude of the associated infection. Acute fistulas with abscess show redness, heat, swelling, and tenderness, sometimes with pus exuding from a crypt. More chronic fistulas manifest a firm fibrous subcutaneous cord associated with absent or limited signs of infection or inflammation. Diligent search for abscesses must accompany the investigation of all anal fistulas, since these must be quickly dealt with and often dictate the management of associated lesions. The treatment of anal infections is covered elsewhere in this volume (see chapter on *Perirectal Infection and Abscess*, and here we will confine ourselves to a discussion of fistulas alone. Treatment of fistulas not associated with infection generally does not require hospitalization. Surgical treatment of fistulas should be carried out by an anorectal surgeon.

Postoperative bleeding following any anorectal surgery should never be treated by packing or by the variety of tamponade devices (Foley balloon catheter) that have been described. These are not only painful but also ineffective. If bleeding is real and not merely the passage of clotted operative blood from the rectum, then the patient should be returned to the operating room where, with the patient in the prone position, bleeding is usually easily controlled, often with a single stitch,

Postoperative treatment for anal fistulas includes bulk stool softeners, warm baths, local anesthetic ointment, and a regular diet. Special dressings, solutions, diets, enemas, and dilatations are unnecessary and detrimental. Some patients may experience transient incontinence that will resolve if the external sphincter ring is intact. Healing will occur anywhere from 1 to 4 months later, depending upon the complexity of the fistula and the size of the wounds.

Antibiotics are not routinely used in the treatment of fistula in ano. Even the presence of an associated perianal abscess should be treated not by antibiotics but by adequate surgical drainage. Antibiotics should be used only in immunosuppressed patients requiring antibiotics for other reasons, such as cardiac valvular disease, internal prosthetic device, or associated cellulitis.

ANAL FISSURES

Anal fissures can be acute or chronic, superficial or deep. All acute uncomplicated fissures should be treated initially with bulk stool softeners, unless the pain is excruciating. Hospitalization is not required. Hydrocortisone suppositories have never been proved to be effective despite their widespread use. If the fissure is deep and chronic, associated with a sentinel pile, hypertrophied papillae or anal stenosis, or if it does not respond to medical therapy, then surgery is indicated.

ANAL SPASM

A nonsurgical cause of severe anal pain is spasm of either the external anal sphincter or of the levator ani muscle. These can be detected when palpation reveals a tender, firm, or spastic sphincter levator ani muscle. Treatment is primarily by massage sometimes augmented by anesthetic injection.

FECAL IMPACTION

The presence of a hard fecal mass in the distal rectum that is too large to pass through the anal canal can cause pain that the patient may feel in the lower abdomen, pelvis, or anus. Sometimes associated with constipation, chronic laxative use, or prolonged immobility, it can present as a distal bowel obstruction. It is readily diagnosed on digital examination and is best treated with repeated water enemas with minimal instrumentation. Oil enemas should be avoided

SUGGESTED READING

Goldberg SM, Buls JG. Perianal disease and rectal prolapse. In: Moody FG, ed. Surgical treatment of digestive disease. Chicago: Year Book Medical Publishers, 1985.

Goldberg SM, Nivatrongs S. Anorectal disease. In: Berk JE, ed. Bockus gastroenterology. 4th ed. Philadelphia: WB Saunders, 1985.

Goldberg SM, Nivatrongs S. Rectum and anus. In: Schwartz SI, ed. Principles of surgery. 4th ed. New York: McGraw-Hill, 1984.

Goldberg SM, Gordon PH, Nivatrongs S. Essentials of anorectal surgery. Philadelphia: JB Lippincott, 1980.

OBSTETRIC AND GYNECOLOGIC EMERGENCIES

DIAGNOSIS AND COURSE OF NORMAL PREGNANCY

RALPH W. HALE, M.D., F.A.C.O.G.

Pregnancy is one of the most common "conditions" found in women from the onset of puberty until the menopause. Although it is frequently planned, it may be unplanned and unsuspected. As a result, the patient may attribute her complaints to other systems. As pregnancy advances, it has an effect on every body system. These changes can mask or alter the symptoms and patterns of other diseases, leading to confusion of the physician. For these reasons, it is important for any physician who takes care of women to have a knowledge and understanding of pregnancy.

DIAGNOSIS

The most common and prominent *symptom* of pregnancy is amenorrhea. Any woman of reproductive age should always be asked when her last normal period occurred, and the date should be documented. If it has been more than 3 weeks since the period and she is not on contraceptives or sterilized, pregnancy must be part of the differential diagnosis.

Another common symptom of early pregnancy is nausea with or without vomiting. The cause is high levels of circulating estrogen that occur suddenly in early pregnancy. This condition is usually referred to as "morning sickness", but this is a misnomer. The sensation may occur at any time and persist throughout the day or night. Sharp smells such as diesel fumes or cooking odors may cause an acute exacerbation.

Other symptoms that may occur because of the changes in early pregnancy include mastodynia, as the breasts enlarge, and bladder symptoms. As the uterus enlarges, it is not unusual to develop urgency and frequency. This occurs as the enlarging uterus fills the pelvic cavity and displaces the bladder. The symptoms may be indistinguishable from the frequency and urgency associated with a urinary tract infection. Constipation, lethargy, and fatigue may also occur and should increase the physician's suspicion of pregnancy.

Most of the early *signs of pregnancy* are nonspecific and nondiagnostic. They represent the response to elevated levels of estrogen, progesterone, and human chorionic gonadotropin (hCG) (Fig. 1). The earliest of these signs is a persistent elevation of the basal body temperature. The level may attain 99.4 to 99.6 °F and can lead the unsuspecting physician to diagnose a low-grade fever when all that is present is a thermogenic response to progesterone. As pregnancy advances, changes in skin pigmentation occur. The patient notices a darkening of the breast areola and development of a midline abdominal line from the pubis to the umbilicus and occasionally the xiphoid, called a linea nigra. These pigmentation changes occur earlier and are more pronounced with each subsequent pregnancy. In some women a change in the pigment of the nose and cheeks occurs in a butterfly pattern called chloasma. Other changes include telangiectasia of the skin.

The major signs of pregnancy are found in the pelvic organs. As the blood supply to these organs increases, their appearance alters. The vagina and cervix change from a deep pink to a blue and then a purplish color. At the same time, the cervix begins to soften and may even be compressible in some women. *Uterine size* will start to increase at this time, although it may be difficult to appreciate in early pregnancy. As the uterus continues to grow,, the rapid increase in size is a good indication of pregnancy (Fig. 2). After 10 weeks, the fetal heart tones may be heard by use of a Doppler-type fetoscope.

In most cases, the diagnosis of pregnancy can be confirmed in the laboratory. In the past, *x-ray studies* were used as a tool for this purpose. For many years, we have recognized the potential teratogenic effects of the x-ray,

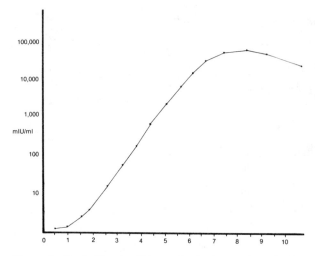

Figure 1 Typical levels of human chorionic gonadotropin during pregnancy.

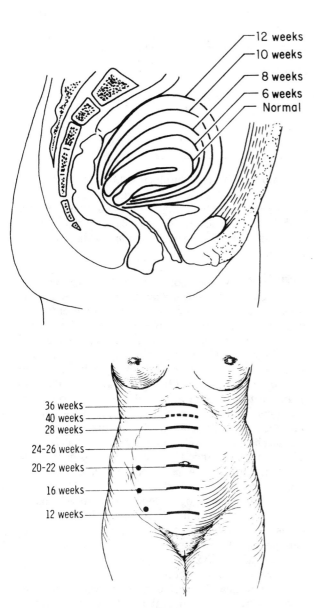

Figure 2 Uterine size at different stages of pregnancy. (Reproduced by permission from Benson R, ed. Current obstetric and gynecologic diagnosis and treatment. 2nd ed. Los Altos, California: Lange Medical Publishers, 1978:47.)

and it is not recommended. Unfortunately, however, x-ray film is used for many of the conditions that occur in women and may show an unsuspected pregnancy. The American College of Obstetrics and Gynecology and the American College of Radiology both recommend that pregnancy be ruled out before x-ray films of the pelvis are taken in any women in the reproductive age group. In an emergency situation, it is not always practical or possible to determine pregnancy before ordering x-ray studies, however, the physician can ask about menses, contraception, and sterilization. When in doubt, it is preferable to place a lead apron over the pelvic area unless it is imperative that an x-ray view of the region be taken.

Ultrasonography has rapidly become the tool of choice in evaluating the pelvis for and during early preg-

nancy. With ultrasonography the uterine cavity can be identified and the intrauterine contents can be seen, as well as possible extrauterine pathology. As pregnancy advances, the actual growth of the fetus can be measured and calibrated. If it is available, ultrasonography should be used to evaluate any problem in the lower abdomen or pelvis of the female. This gives a safe evaluation of the area that can rule out pregnancy or pelvic lesions. After this scan, x-ray films can be ordered as needed.

Pregnancy tests are still the most common means of verifying pregnancy in its early stages. Most common pregnancy tests use an immunologic assay to hCG. By mixing a suspected urine with the test solution, the presence or absence of hCG is determined. These tests have varying degrees of sensitivity and can take 2 minutes to 2 hours to complete (Table 1). When they are positive, the physician is 90 to 95 percent sure that a pregnancy is present. Unfortunately, the degree of accuracy is less when the test is negative. Other conditions such as proteinuria may also alter the sensitivity. The home pregnancy test kits are based on this principle and can be subject to the same inaccuracies. When the physician doubts the validity of a result from a home pregnancy test kit, the test should be repeated.

The most accurate of the pregnancy tests is the radioimmunioassay of the beta unit of hCG. This unit is specific to pregnancy and has essentially no crossover with the pituitary gonadotropins that have the same base unit. When beta-hCG is present, the physician can be virtually certain that viable trophoblastic tissue is present. The test can be qualitative or quantitative. For most purposes, the qualitative test will suffice.

More recently a new type of test, the monoclonal antibody, was released. This immunologic type of test is more sophisticated and more accurate than were the older tests. Its accuracy approaches that of the radioimmunioassay of beta-hCG when performed correctly.

DIFFERENTIAL DIAGNOSIS

Because many of the signs and symptoms of pregnancy are nonspecific, they may also occur in a wide variety of other diseases. There are a number of diagnoses that should be considered. Obviously, if the beta-HCG or ultrasonography are available, the diagnosis of pregnancy can be established. On the other hand, these tools are not always available, and the physician must be aware of other conditions.

Amenorrhea may be associated with a number of other medical problems. Emotional problems and stress can and do delay the onset of menses. They may even lead to prolonged amenorrhea. Endocrinopathies are frequently associated with menstrual changes. When these are obvious, it is easy to recognize the association, but most early stages are not obvious. For example, an elevated prolactin from a microadenoma of the pituitary may have no other symptoms; early hypothyroid disease may begin with amenorrhea. Systemic disease, metabolic disease, and infections can also alter the menstrual pattern. Finally, the physician should carefully inquire about medications. Women on hormone pills for birth control or other conditions can experience amenorrhea.

TABLE 1 Sensitivity of Common Urine and Serum Pregnancy Tests

Pregnancy Test Type	Reported Sensitivity (mIU/ml)	Days from LNMP to Positive Test
Slide	500–4,000	30
Tube	200–2,000	25
Enzyme immunoassay	50	21
Radioimmunoassay	1–5	14

Nausea and vomiting may result from a large number of diseases. Almost all gastrointestinal disorders will result in nausea. Infections and chronic illness can do the same, as well as medications for these diseases. Although the sudden onset of nausea and vomiting could make one suspicious of pregnancy, it should never be used to confirm a diagnosis.

Urinary tract symptoms are also very common. When they occur, the physician should always evaluate the urinary tract first. In the absence of other etiology, pregnancy may be the cause, however, it is a diagnosis of exclusion.

Many of the changes in the pelvic organs seen during pregnancy can be the result of other conditions. Ovarian cysts and leukorrhea are just two of the common ones that mimic pregnancy. Ultrasonography can help establish the diagnosis. Pregnancy-related conditions such as ectopic pregnancy and spontaneous abortions should also be considered; these are covered in more detail in other chapters of this book. A pregnancy-related condition that must always be considered is hydatidiform mole. This aberration of a pregnancy is indistinguishable in its early stages from a normal pregnancy. As the pregnancy progresses, however, there is a more rapid increase in uterine size; bleeding occurs frequently; and hypertension in the 16th to 18th week is not unusual. The diagnosis is made by ultrasonography or passage of grape-like molar tissue.

PROGRESS OF PREGNANCY

A human gestation lasts approximately 270 days with a variability of plus or minus 2 weeks. We still do not know what initiates labor in most patients or prevents its occurrence in others. As a result, we use the same methods of calculation for everyone. This formula, Nägele's rule, is simply the first day of the last normal menstrual period (LMP) minus 3 months and plus 7 days (expected date of confinement [EDC] = LMP − 3m + 7d).

Each time the patient is seen following the initial diagnosis, the physician should measure the size of the uterus, listen for fetal heart tones, determine the presence of edema, measure the blood pressure, and check the urine for protein and sugar. When there is any question about the growth or status of the pregnancy, an ultrasound determination should be made. By use of ultrasonography early in pregnancy, prolonged gestations can be prevented; this is especially important in a patient with irregular menses or an unreliable history, in whom the EDC is uncertain.

As the pregnancy progresses, a number of changes take place that may result in patient complaints or may be confused with other problems. Many of these complaints are listed below with the etiology and a recommended therapy. Obviously, no list could be complete, so the reader must refer to a standard textbook on obstetrics for details. These common conditions are as follows:

Heartburn. The etiology is related to relaxation of the muscles of the diaphragm at the distal end of the esophagus and the reflex of gastric acid. Treatment usually consists of antacid therapy. In extreme cases, the patient should sleep with the head of the bed slightly elevated.

Nausea and Vomiting. This is a very common complaint. Initial treatment consists of frequent small feedings and crackers at the bedside. Currently, there are no medications recommended for use, owing to possible teratogenicity. In its extreme form, hyperemesis gravidarum, the patient is unable to take any fluid or food, and she must be hospitalized to prevent dehydration and metabolic changes. Most nausea and vomiting is gone by the end of the third month of pregnancy, although it may recur in the last 3 to 4 weeks.

Constipation. Progesterone has a smooth muscle relaxant effect. When it is combined with the enlarging uterus and iron therapy, the patient frequently develops constipation. The usual treatment is stool softeners. These are preferable to laxatives and stimulants. In extreme cases, enemas may be necessary.

Leukorrhea. Normal pregnancy results in an increased secretion of vaginal fluids. These are nonirritating and require no treatment. However, the pregnant woman is also susceptible to infections, especially *Candidia Albicans* (*Monilia* or yeast). Her first symptom will be itching and, if untreated, the itchy sensation will progress to edema and secondary infection. Treatment consists of topical steroids to relieve the irritation and intravaginal suppositories containing a fungicidal agent such as miconazole (Monistat) or clotrimazole (Mycelex). Depending on the severity of the infection, the therapy should last 3 to 7 days and be repeated as needed.

Hemorrhoid. Increased venous stasis in the hemorrhoidal veins as well as constipation will lead to symptoms of hemorrhoids. These should be treated, if symptomatic, with rectal suppositories. In the occasional woman, the hemorrhoid will thrombose. When this occurs, it should be treated the same as in nonpregnant women.

Vasicose Veins. Increased distention of the veins of the lower extremities is common in pregnancy. This occurs as the uterine size increases and causes pressure on the iliac veins and the vena cava. Depending on the severity, the patient should be instructed in daily leg elevations and the use of panty or support hose. Careful evaluation is necessary to diagnosis thrombosis.

Headache. Headache is a common complaint during pregnancy. This is partially attributable to the changes in vascular volume, but it is not completely understood. If the headache is severe, it will usually require therapy with an analgesic. The patient should be monitored for development of pregnancy-induced hypertension, since that may be the cause of severe headaches. Migraine headaches may occur during pregnancy. Ergot alkaloids should not be used in treatment of these patients, because they may have a direct effect on the uterine muscle as well.

Orthopaedic Complaints. As pregnancy progresses, the levels of progesterone cause relaxation of the ligaments and joints. This results in instability and complaints of joint aches and backache. In later pregnancy, a marked lordosis occurs, which further increases these symptoms. There is very little treatment other than support and rest. In some women, the pubic symphysis develops excessive separation and, rarely, rupture. This causes severe pain and instability. Treatment consists of a pelvic corset and rest. Other women may develop symptoms of spinal disk protrusion during pregnancy. Again, conservative therapy is all that can be offered until delivery.

Other Conditions. Many other complaints may occur as pregnancy progresses. These include excessive salivation (ptyalism), abnormal food craving and eating habits (pica), frequency of urination, mastodynia, leg cramps, an elevated white blood cell count, Bartholin gland enlargement, vulvar varicosities, and others. Two of these need special attention. Leukocytosis may be the result of an early infection or the pregnancy. In general, a white blood cell count of lower than 14,000 to 16,000 is considered normal and should be observed. A higher count may also be normal, but warrants some investigation. Leg cramps are usually attributable to a deficiency of calcuim, although they can also be due to venous stasis and poor posture. Calcium supplementation should be tried first. Milk is not a good source because it also contain phosphorus, and the ratio of these two minerals may be as important as the absolute amount of calcium.

In addition to these conditions that may present as abnormal symptoms, there are several conditions that may be precipitated by the normal progress of pregnancy.

Patients with cardiac disease need to be followed carefully during pregnancy. The blood volume of the patient gradually increases until the 28th to 32nd week of pregnancy, when it hits its peak. At this time, the patient may be at risk for cardiac decompensation.

As the uterus enlarges during pregnancy, it can cause compression of the vena cava. This usually occurs while the patient is lying on her back. The compression reduces venous return, producing subsequent hypotension. The condition, called supine hypotension syndrome, is treated by turning the patient to her left side or having her sit up or stand.

Sickle cell anemia is another condition that may be acutely exacerbated during pregnancy. The patient has severe limb and abdominal pain and is easily misdiagnosed unless the physician is alert to the possibility.

Finally, many medical and surgical problems may develop concurrently with pregnancy. When they do, the diagnosis may be delayed or missed because of the masking symptoms of pregnancy or the alterations of classic symptoms that pregnancy causes. For example, appendicitis is a diagnosis that is frequently missed during pregnancy because the enlarging uterus displaces the appendix cephalad. In addition, there may already be gastrointestinal symptoms, such as constipation or anorexia, and an elevation of the white blood count. Therefore, the physician who sees women must always be alert to the effect that pregnancy has on symptom complexes.

It is important for the physician to remember that during pregnancy, all medications are suspect. Many drugs that are perfectly safe in the nonpregnant woman have potential teratogenic effects on the fetus and/or adverse effects on the mother. Prior to prescribing any medication, the physician should check on the safety of the medication.

SUGGESTED READING

Warkentin DL. From A to hCG in pregnancy testing. Diagnostic Med 1984; 4:35:
Weingold A. Surgical disease in pregnancy, Clin Obstet Gynecol 1983; 26:193.

ECTOPIC PREGNANCY

GAIL V. ANDERSON, M.D., F.A.C.S., F.A.C.O.G.

EMERGENCY CONSIDERATIONS

One in 100 pregnancies occurs in an abnormal location. These ectopic pregnancies cause two-thirds of the deaths in the first trimester of pregnancy and one-tenth of all deaths related to pregnancy. The occurrence of symptoms usually means rupture and may be fatal. The emergency physician often is the first physician responsible to make the diagnosis.

Ectopic pregnancy should be a prime consideration in any female with abdominal pain during the reproductive years. If the patient with genital bleeding has a delay or variation in the last menstrual period and unexplained abdominal pain, the diagnosis is ectopic pregnancy until proven otherwise. Complaints of abdominal pain starting in the first and lasting into the third trimester should be considered suggestive of abdominal pregnancy if no other cause of pain is found.

CLINICAL CONSIDERATIONS

Pregnancies implanted at a site other than the fundal area of the uterus can and often do lead to life-threatening hemorrhage. The fertilized ovum can implant in rare locations such as the ovary or cervical stump following subtotal hysterectomy, but the most common site of ectopic implantation, as would be expected, is in the oviduct at the point where the infundibulum narrows to the isthmic portion. Although the entire oviduct distal to the uterus is the most common location of ectopic gestation (Fig.1), tubal rupture usually occurs before 6 weeks and the initial hemorrhage usually does not result in death. However, a gestation location in the cornual (uterine) position of the oviduct usually advances beyond 6 weeks, and rupture often results in the patient's death because of serious hemorrhage associated with tearing through a major (uterine) artery. Cervical pregnancy, though rare, also carries significant threat because it is more advanced and, again, is in the region of the uterus where the uterine arteries and veins are located.

Tubal abortion and secondary implantation in the peritoneal cavity posterior to the uterus or on the bowel results in the so-called abdominal pregnancy, which may advance to term but usually ruptures prior to term and often leads to catastrophic hemorrhage.

MEDICOLEGAL FEATURES

Failure to recognize ectopic pregnancy has resulted in significant successful malpractice action against emergency physicians. More important is the unnecessary death of a patient because the physician did not consider the possibility of ectopic pregnancy in the differential diagnosis. All female patients in the reproductive age (12 to 50 years) should be asked about their menstrual history and the date of the last menstrual period (LMP), and it should be recorded on the chart.

ETIOLOGY

It is well established that prior tubal infection, infertility in a nulliparous patient, previous ectopic pregnancy, use of an intrauterine device, recent currettage, and previous plastic tubal surgery or tubal sterilization are predisposing factors and increase the incidence of ectopic pregnancy (Table 1). Intraluminal synechiae as a residual of primary infection or infection secondary to a recent currettage or an intrauterine device obstruct the migration of the fertilized ovum and result in oviductal implantation.

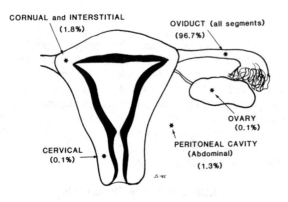

Figure 1 Location of ectopic pregnancy.

TABLE 1 Factors Predisposing to Ectopic Pregnancy

IUD
Prior salpingitis
Tuboplasty
Progesterone (only) contraceptive
Previous ectopic pregnancy
Tubal ligation

Although oviductal plastic surgery may reestablish patency, the normal cilial action and peristalsis are not necessarily restored, so the fertilized ovum matures to the blastocyst stage before it reaches the uterine cavity, which again results in oviductal implantation.

The "simple loop" type of tubal ligation for sterilization is associated with a high incidence of ectopic gestation but any type of tubal sterilization must be considered as a predisposition for ectopic gestation. The theory that an intrauterine device creates excessive peristalsis of the oviduct and thereby "traps" the fertilized ovum, permitting the more mature blastocyst to implant in the tube, is debatable but a definite possibility.

DIAGNOSIS

The history of missed menstrual bleeding is variable in the literature. However, if the physician goes into some detail relative to the last menstrual period, almost all patients will remember some aberration or difference in the last "menstruation." It will usually have been a few days late or early, shorter, longer, lighter, or heavier than the previous menses.

Pain is usually what causes the patient to seek medical help. The pain is usually abdominal, occurring in the lower portion of the abdominal cavity; however, it may be anywhere. Pain may radiate to the back and shoulders if extensive bleeding has occurred. Abdominal pain usually indicates rupture of the ectopic pregnancy; this is why pain in the reproductive age must be considered a potentially life-threatening event.

Syncope indicates hypovolemia in this situation, and if the patient gives a history of menstrual aberration, abdominal pain, and syncope, the diagnosis is certainly ectopic pregnancy until this is ruled out. If the rupture occurs when the patient is sleeping and she is awakened by abdominal pain, experiences shoulder pain, has the urge to defecate, and subsequently has syncope on the toilet stool, the patient should be taken promptly to surgery for laparotomy. Intra-abdominal blood loss has been sufficient to cause diaphragmatic irritation and early hypovolemic shock.

Five to 10 percent of patients will bring a *uterine cast* to the physician; this is a decidual cast of the uterus and always indicates ectopic gestation. It also indicates that the pregnancy has terminated either by rupture or the spontaneous death of the conceptus in situ.

The abdominal findings may or may not be helpful. By the time findings of peritoneal irritation occur, there is significant abdominal distention, due to encroachment of bleeding from the ruptured ectopic pregnancy into the peritoneal cavity. Thus, rebound tenderness usually indicates that hypovolemic shock is impending. Findings of peritoneal irritation are present only 55 percent of the time.

Pelvic examinations usually reveal an enlarged uterus in ectopic pregnancy, because of the effect of hormones. If, in a suspected case, an adnexal mass is present as well as fullness in the cul-de-sac, the diagnosis is more certain. Tenderness on palpation of the uterus and adnexa is usually present, but the patient usually tolerates pelvic examination more readily than when inflammatory disease is present.

Hypotension and tachycardia or bradycardia may be present and indicate significant hypovolemia and deterioration of the patient, and at this time the diagnosis should be obvious. However, relative hypovolemia often becomes apparent with a decrease in blood pressure (10 to 20 mm Hg) when the patient is placed in the sitting position with normal readings in the supine position. This so-called "tilt test" should be part of the evaluation of all patients when ectopic pregnancy is considered in the presence of normal vital signs. Obviously patients with signs of hypovolemia (hypotension) should not be placed in the sitting position, because this will cause rapid deterioration of a compensating vascular system.

Culdocentesis, pregnancy testing, and ultrasonography, if available, are the more valuable tests for the diagnosis of ectopic pregnancy. Because culdocentesis is positive in 85 to 90 percent of ruptured ectopic pregnancies and pregnancy tests are positive in 80 to 85 percent, the diagnosis is virtually a certainty if both are positive. Consequently these tests will be given special consideration below.

Laboratory tests such as complete blood count (CBC), hematocrit (HCT), serum electrolytes, and chemistries are of little value in the emergency evaluation of ectopic pregnancy. As with radiologic findings of the abdomen and pelvis, only at the time of serious deterioration do consistent abnormal findings exist.

CULDOCENTESIS

When the history is vague and the pelvic and abdominal findings are not certain, the single most valuable diagnostic procedure is culdocentesis. False negatives (absence of nonclotting blood) are usually due to lack of familiarity with the procedure and the anatomy involved. Unawareness of a retroflexed or retroverted uterus (due to inadequate bimanual examination) results in the insertion of the needle into the posterior aspect of the uterus. The so-called false-negative culdocentesis is most often due to nonpenetration of the posterior cul-de-sac (Fig. 2). If blood is present, it can be aspirated because it is liquid (fibrin removed) and is located in the most dependent part of the peritoneal cavity with the patient in the lithotomy position.

The equipment necessary for culdocentesis is listed in Table 2. However, success is determined by the confidence and security the physician inspires in the patient. This will be enhanced by shielding the patient from viewing the instruments, the appropriate use of analgesia, and

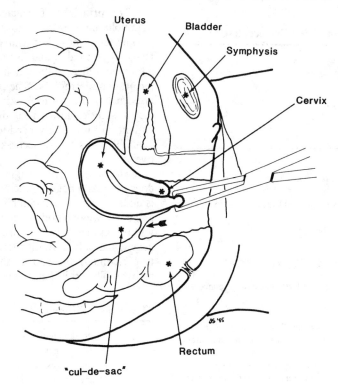

Figure 2 Culdocentesis. Needle entry occurs at location indicated by arrows.

the use of lidocaine on the cervix and in the posterior fornix (topical) areas 3 to 5 minutes prior to instrumentation (Table 3). Traction on the posterior lip of the cervix is necessary to align the uterus along the axis of the body and to demonstrate the bulging posterior cul-de-sac.

PREGNANCY TESTS

Laboratory tests for pregnancy are based on the presence of human chorionic gonadotropic (hCG) hormone in the serum and urine. Radioimmunoassay of serum using antibodies to the beta subunit of hCG has lowered the sensitivity from 100 mIU per milliliter (urine tube tests) to the detection of 5 mIU per milliliter (serum). Though useful, the 24- to 28-hour "turnaround time" of the ectopic pregnancy test inhibits the early diagnosis of ectopic pregnancy by the emergency physician. The B-Neocept and the UCG Beta Stat are beta-hCG-specific tests on the urine and have a turnaround time of 1 to 2 hours. They are sensitive to 150 mIU per milliliter and 200 mIU respectively, so are useful in the emergency department in the diagnosis of ectopic pregnancy, since beta-hCG in this condition are typically below this level.

Ultrasonography should be used if the beta-hCG is below 500 mIU with an equivocal history, physical findings, and culdocentesis (see Fig. 2). The absence of an intrauterine sac and the presence of peritoneal fluid and a mass in the cul-de-sac usually confirm ectopic pregnancy. However, the physician must be aware of the coexistence of an extrauterine and intrauterine pregnancy concurrently, which can be a challenge in diagnosis.

TABLE 2 Equipment for Culdocentesis

Bivalve speculum
Tenaculum (single tooth)
Sponge forceps
No. 20 spinal needle (sharp)
10-cc syringe
2% lidocaine

TABLE 3 Technique for Culdocentesis

1. Place patient in the lithotomy position (shields patients from instruments and procedure)
2. Perform pelvic examination (bimanual)
3. Insert warmed speculum
4. Prep cervix and posterior fornix with antiseptic solution using sponge and forceps
5. Apply 2% lidocaine to cervix and posterior fornix with sponge stick (topically)
6. Wait 3 to 5 minutes
7. Place single tooth tenaculum on posterior lip of cervix (anteroposterior plane). Elevate cervix, align uterus, and demonstrate bulging cul-de-sac
8. Insert No. 18 sharp spinal needle with quick motion 1 cm posterior to cervicovaginal junction in the midline to a depth of 2 cm
9. Aspirate initially and while withdrawing needle
10. If no fluid is aspirated, may repeat one time

Laparoscopy can rule out ectopic pregnancy at this point, but if it is present, then laparotomy is indicated.

DIFFERENTIAL DIAGNOSIS

Salpingitis (PID) may predispose or present with the same clinical picture as ectopic pregnancy, such as pain, vaginal bleeding, and an adnexal mass (tubo-ovarian abscess or hydrosalpinx) (Table 4). However, fever, leukocytosis, and more intense abdominal and pelvic tenderness make inflammation disease a more probable diagnosis. Purulent or cloudy peritoneal fluid on culdocentesis indicates pelvic infection. Threatened and incomplete abortion with an intact corpus luteum (adnexal mass) can produce all of the classic features of ectopic pregnancy. Here the beta subunit test of hCG rules out ectopic pregnancy if negative, particularly if the culdocentesis is also negative (see Fig. 1).

Rupture or torsion of an ovarian cyst can mimic ectopic pregnancy; however, the beta-hCG test and culdocentesis will be negative. Culdocentesis of fluid from a ruptured ectopic pregnancy usually has an HCT above 15 percent while straw-colored fluid or blood-tinged fluid with a lower HCT will be aspirated from ruptured cyst fluid. Acute appendicitis may also mimic ectopic pregnancy; however, patients with appendicitis usually have a low-grade fever, leukocytosis, and more obvious gastrointestinal findings (Fig. 3).

MANAGEMENT

The principle of management of any patient with hypovolemia from blood loss is the same in patients with ectopic pregnancy. The main difference is that the hemorrhage is concealed and most patients compensate up to a point and then, if the blood volume is not restored, deteriorate quite rapidly. The patient should be typed and crossmatched for 4 to 6 units of whole blood. Ringer's lactate solution infused rapidly can "buy time," but the patient will ultimately need whole blood as soon as it is available. It is rarely necessary to give type O Rh negative blood.

The patient hemorrhaging from an ectopic pregnancy does not really begin to recover until the bleeding source is under control. The administration of intravenous fluids and even whole blood are only temporizing measures and will not in themselves ensure the patient's survival. Surgery is the only definitive treatment, and the sooner this is performed, the sooner the patient really begins to recover. The critical and essential factor in improving sur-

TABLE 4 Differential Diagnosis of Ectopic Pregnancy

Acute salpingitis
Acute appendicitis
Endometriosis
Ovarian cyst, ruptured or twisted
Gastroenteritis
Threatened incomplete abortion

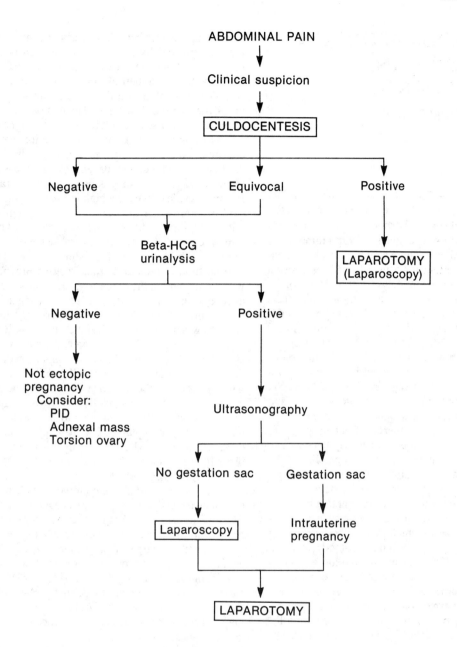

Figure 3 Diagnosis of ectopic pregnancy.

vival from ectopic pregnancy is early recognition and diagnosis, because most patients who have ruptured ectopic pregnancies have visited a physician a few days before the rupture. Surgery is usually performed promptly once the diagnosis is made. The emergency physician will always make the diagnosis if he or she has a high "index of suspicion" and uses the appropriate combination of history, physical examination, laboratory (including beta-hCG tests), culdocentesis, ultrasonography, and in some cases laparoscopy.

SUGGESTED READING

Breen JL. A 21 year survey of 654 ectopic pregnancies. Am J Obstet Gynecol 1970; 106:1004–1019.

Brenner PF, et al. Ectopic pregnancy: a study of 300 consecutive surgically treated cases. JAMA 1980; 243:673–676.

Freeman J, Goldberg L. Ectopic pregnancy. Ann Emerg Med 1984; 13:339–342.

Hayes H, et al. Intrauterine and ruptured tubal ectopic pregnancy: a diagnostic challenge. Ann Emerg Med 1984; 13(5):355–358.

Kaunitz AM, et al. Causes of maternal mortality in the United States. Obstet Gynecol 1985; 65:605–612.

Mishell D, Brenner P. Management of common problems in obstetrics gynecology. Medec Books, 1983; 237–240.

Queenan J. Managing OB/GYN emergencies, 2nd ed. Oradell, NJ: Medec Books, 1983:2–7.

Roberts M, et al. Diagnosis of ruptured ectopic pregnancy with peritoneal lavage. Ann Emerg Med 1982; 11:556–558.

Romero J, et al. Value of culdocentesis in the diagnosis of ectopic pregnancy. Obstet Gynecol 1985; 65:519–522.

SPONTANEOUS ABORTION AND BLEEDING IN EARLY PREGNANCY

RAPHAEL B. DURFEE, M.D.

Abortions are classified as threatened, inevitable, incomplete, complete, missed, and induced (incomplete). The etiology of spontaneous abortion is shown in Table 1.

Threatened abortion is associated with cramping or bleeding and rarely both. There is no cervical dilation, but there may be spotting for a few days. This is not a disease entity, but approximately 40 percent go on to abort. In complete abortion there is cramping, bleeding, cervical dilation, and the passage of blood clots and tissue, with loss of all the products of conception. An incomplete abortion is diagnosed when the conception products are not completely passed. There is dilation of the cervix, which can be determined by feeling with a finger tip or can be judged using a graduated dilator. Six to 10 mm will permit the passage of a suction curet and is evidence of dilation. Tissue may be seen extruding through the external os, and there is frequently severe bleeding with large blood clots, which may become life threatening. Infection may be present and complicates the course and treatment of condition. The presence of incompletely removed tissues at the time of induced abortion is similar to incomplete abortion except that infection is much more frequent and must always be suspected. Inevitable abortion is one in which there is both cramping and bleeding with passage of fluid or blood clots and progressive dilation of the cervix. A missed abortion is diagnosed when there are disappearing signs of pregnancy, a negative pregnancy test, and continued uterine enlargement not compatible with gestational dates (being smaller). There may be a brownish discharge with a little blood and small dark clots without evidence of cramping or bright bleeding.

DIFFERENTIAL DIAGNOSIS

The most common cause of first trimester bleeding is spontaneous abortion. A differential diagnosis must be done at once to identify other problems that may cause such bleeding. The most important of these is ectopic pregnancy, which is frequently missed and which may cause critical intra-abdominal bleeding as well. Other diagnoses to consider include products of conception incompletely removed by induced abortion, an endocervical polyp, an intracavitary pedunculated myoma that is being expelled, endometrial polyps, an extensive area of columnar epithelium on the vaginal surface of the cervix, hydatid mole, low lying placental tissue near the internal cervical os, and rarely cervical pregnancy.

Most important is the differentiation between the abortion states and ectopic pregnancy or hydatid mole. A diagnosis of ectopic pregnancy in a case of first trimester vaginal bleeding depends upon several criteria. It is most critical to have a high index of suspicion in any case of vaginal bleeding and a positive pregnancy test. Ultrasonography will establish the presence of a tubal ectopic pregnancy by indicating an absence of intrauterine tissue and the presence of an adnexal mass. There may also be fluid in the cul de sac. Positive pregnancy tests will aid in making the diagnosis; urine tests are not quite as reliable as serum because of rare occasional false negative results but are valuable in the emergency department. A falling serum beta-HcG level may indicate dying trophoblastic tissues in spontaneous abortion. Culdocentesis using a long 20 or 22 gauge spinal needle inserted through the posterior vaginal wall into the cul de sac frequently indicates the presence of blood in the peritoneal cavity. It is not always positive, however, especially if the cul de sac is filled with a solid blood clot, or if the tubal ectopic is unruptured. Laparoscopy is frequently the most valuable procedure in making this diagnosis but ordinarily is not done in the emergency department. (See also *Ectopic Pregnancy*.)

The diagnosis of a hydatid mole is made by observation of an exceedingly high titer of beta HcG in the blood. The patient may have exaggerated symptoms of pregnancy, including hyperemesis, extremely tender, enlarged breasts, a uterus larger than gestation dates, bilateral adnexal cysts, and symptoms of toxemia of pregnancy. The physician looks for the presence of one or several small clear cysts in the vaginal blood; such a ''grape'' is positive in the diagnosis of a hydatid mole. Ultrasonography may indicate a characteristic appearance of cystic intrauterine tissues.

TREATMENT

The treatment of an incomplete abortion requires total evacuation of the uterus. This can be accomplished easily in the emergency department by lifting out the tissue extruded through the external os and judicious use of a suction curet. Six to 10 mm of cervical dilation is needed for this purpose. Administration of either pitocin, 20 IU, or Methergine, 0.2 mg either intramuscularly or intravenously, prior to removal of conception products reduces bleeding and lessens the possibility of uterine perforation. Anesthesia, when necessary, can readily be accomplished using 1 percent Carbocaine solution (total dose, about 10 cc), which is injected directly into the cervix at the 3 and 9 o'clock positions in doses up to 5 cc each, by means of a long 20 or 22 gauge spinal needle. A sharp curet and an ovum forceps are then used to in-

TABLE 1 Causes of Spontaneous Abortion

37%	unknown cause
23%	corpus luteum endocrine factors
15%	maternal müllerian system defects
13%	maldevelopment of embryo
12%	ovular factors, trauma, hydropic degeneration, chromosomal anomalies

sure removal of all tissue. Care should be taken not to overcuret because of the potential for producing intrauterine adhesions.

In the case of complete abortion or threatened abortion usually only observation in the emergency department is needed. Both situations usually resolve in a brief period of time. In threatened abortion it is important to inform the patient of the potential for pregnancy loss and to encourage her not to have intercourse until all symptoms have subsided and also not to engage in extensive exercise, hard work, vaginal douching, or to use harsh laxation. In inevitable abortion the pregnancy can be terminated in the emergency department, or the patient can be admitted to the hospital, depending upon her wishes. In missed abortion, if a hydatid mole is not suspected, the patient should be referred to a gynecologist for further management rather than to try to terminate the pregnancy in the emergency department. Warn the patient of potential infection and the dangers of procrastination for treatment.

When it is suspected that incomplete removal of tissue at a previous induced abortion is the problem, some degree of triage is recommended. It must be determined when the operation was done and where. Infection must be suspected and investigated thoroughly, (e.g., the presence of fever, local or abdominal pain, the presence of bloody purulent vaginal discharge, elevated leukocyte count, and elevated sedimentation rate). If the patient is in shock and has signs of peritonitis or hemorrhage, suspect uterine perforation. In any of these complications, admit to hospital at once. One g of ampicillin, penicillin, or Ancef should be given intravenously immediately, and a culture should be taken from the vagina and cervix as well as the blood. The patient should be advised of the importance of completion of the abortion and of the possibilities of complications and what they may be.

DISPOSITION

Patients with vaginal bleeding in the first trimester should always be observed for 2 or more hours, especially after an operative procedure or if there is a questionable diagnosis. They may have some other gynecologic problem that requires care, or if bleeding persists (especially with abdominal pain), she should be admitted. The patient with an ectopic pregnancy should always be admitted. Rapid preliminary diagnostic and therapeutic measures may be carried out in the emergency department prior to such admission, and these include the establishment of an intravenous line with an 18 gauge needle, preliminary complete blood count and hematocrit, serum beta-HcG determination, coagulation studies, and urine specimen. If vaginal bleeding persists after drainage and curettage, repeat the curettage.

Most patients can be discharged when bleeding has stopped or slowed to very little, and there are no obvious complications. A prescription for Methergine, 0.2 mg, to be taken orally, may be given and, if possible, written advice sent home with the patient. This should include the following: use no tampons or douches, no intercourse, no swimming or bathtub bathing (shower only), and call the physician for a follow-up appointment or if there is any recurrence of bleeding, cramps, abdominal pain, fever, or malaise.

SUGGESTED READING

Stock R, Nelson K. Ectopic pregnancy subsequent to sterilization: histologic evaluation and clinical implications. Fertil Steril 1984; 42:211–214.
Weckstein LN. Current perspective on ectopic pregnancy. Obstet Gynecol 1985; 40:259–272.

ABDOMINAL PAIN AND VAGINAL BLEEDING IN LATE PREGNANCY

MARSHALL W. CARPENTER, B.S., M.D.

The gravida in late pregnancy may seek emergency care unexpectedly for problems other than labor. Complaints that most often result in an emergency visit include recent trauma (see chapter on *Trauma in Pregnancy*), abdominal pain, vaginal bleeding, decrease in fetal movement, and questions about possible labor. This chapter addresses two of the more serious complaints: abdominal pain and vaginal bleeding in the third trimester.

ABDOMINAL PAIN

Abdominal pain in the third trimester of pregnancy may be the result of distention, inflammation, or ischemia of any of the abdominal viscera. The presence of an enlarged uterus and the physiologic state of pregnancy may change presenting symptoms and signs. In addition, the presence of a fetus limits diagnostic evaluation and changes therapeutic intervention.

History

Obtaining the medical history is essential. If abdominal trauma has been the precipitating event, damage to the uterus or its contents is a prime consideration. Abruptio placentae and uterine rupture are common sequelae to severe, blunt trauma to the abdomen. In addition, spleen or liver damage may be present. Any of these events may result in rapid hypovolemia. The young, pregnant woman usually remains well perfused, despite significant hypovolemia, until homeostatic compensation is exhausted. Because of the abruptio-related release of thromboplastin-like material into the maternal circulation and shock-related peripheral hypoperfusion, clinically significant coagulation defects are common in these cases. (See chapter on *Trauma in Pregnancy*).

When trauma is not noted, other historical features may be important. A prior vertical cesarean section places the patient at risk for uterine rupture, even before the onset of labor. A history of prior abruptio placentae, chronic hypertension, or early vaginal bleeding in the present pregnancy is associated with an increased risk for abruptio placentae. Abruptio placentae may present as signs consistent with labor. In its more obvious manifestations, it causes the uterus to be constantly painful and tender and show lack of relaxation between uterine contractions. Uterine rupture is usually a cataclysmic event with hypotension and constant pain.

Gastrointestinal symptoms are largely nonspecific, although the nature of onset and character may point to a diagnosis. Nausea and vomiting may occur in the early stages of normal labor as well as be associated with appendicitis and pyelitis. Vomiting associated with the torsion of an adnexal mass tends to be acute and temporally related to the occurrence of localized colic.

When located in the flank, colic may be difficult to ascribe to a particular organ. Ovarian torsion, partial ureteric obstruction from infection or stone, and distention of the colon secondary to constipation may present similarly. Hemorrhage into a uterine leiomyoma or ischemia of such a tumor may present as colicky pain, which may be difficult to differentiate from other sources of colic, depending on its position in the uterus.

Most causes of abdominal pain in late pregnancy present with episodic recurrences every few minutes or hours. Exceptions to this include hepatitis or hepatic swelling due to preeclampsia and appendicitis associated with peritonitis. The pain associated with appendicitis is also influenced by the duration of the pregnancy. As the uterus enlarges in the second half of pregnancy, the point of maximum symptoms rises cephalad and rotates to the flank as the appendix is displaced in this direction by the growing uterus. Focal pain may not be related to McBurney's point, therefore, and may be located virtually anywhere from the right groin to the costovertebral angle.

Abdominal pregnancy may present with pain that is usually most prominent in the lower abdominal quadrants. Gastrointestinal symptoms such as nausea, vomiting, flatulence, diarrhea, and constipation may be prominent. Intraperitoneal bleeding or suppuration may present with acute local or systemic symptoms.

Physical Examination

Changes in vital signs may indicate preeclampsia, sepsis, or hypovolemia. Even small elevations in blood pressure may indicate a significant rise compared with recent blood pressure readings, suggesting vasospasm associated with preeclampsia; this requires comparison with previous records. On the other hand, blood pressures of 100/60 are common in late pregnancy. Blood pressures should always be measured with the patient in the lateral recumbent position.

The patient in the third trimester should not be left in a supine position because of resulting aortic and vena caval obstruction by the uterus. *Fetal evaluation* begins with monitoring of the fetal heart rate. Signs of fetal distress may result from abruptio placentae, uterine rupture, sepsis, or even normal labor when uterine perfusion or placental function is compromised.

Physical examination may show the generalized or regional tenderness characteristic of esophagitis, appendicitis, or upper urinary tract infection. Abdominal catastrophes, such as uterine rupture or rupture of a necrotic adnexal mass, may yield generalized peritonitis. Focal tenderness is more characteristic of the liver of preeclampsia or hepatitis, cholecystitis, pyelitis, or ischemic uterine leiomyoma. The presence of uterine contractions reduces the list of differential diagnoses to those involving the uterus or its contents and adjacent inflammatory or infectious processes. Abdominal rigidity, which serves well during pregnancy as a marker for peritonitis, should be distinguished from a rigid, tender uterus, which may be markedly enlarged, pushing other abdominal viscera to the flanks and back. Such a tense and tender uterus may result from distention due to polyhydramnios (frequently associated with fetal anomalies), chorioamnionitis, or abruptio placentae. With a chronic abdominal pregnancy and with uterine rupture, fetal parts may be easily palpable just within the abdominal wall. Such findings in the stable patient suggest the need for sonographic examination.

Laboratory Evaluation

Initial laboratory tests aid in limiting the differential diagnosis and providing needed information in preparation for potential surgery or parturition. These include hematocrit and hemoglobin, white cell count and differential, serum creatinine, uric acid, and electrolytes. Elevated leukocyte counts (15,000 to 20,000 per mm³) and mild shift to the left are commonly associated with labor. Serum transaminase levels may be elevated in syndromes of hepatitis, whether viral in origin or ischemic in nature due to preeclampsia. Alkaline phosphatase levels may be markedly elevated during a normal pregnancy because of the heat-stable fraction derived from the placenta. A urinalysis may show proteinuria, possibly related to preeclampsia. Pyuria may be present both in urinary tract infection and with appendicitis. The presence of pyuria with no bacteriuria occasionally is due to the inflamed appendix lying next to the ureter. In cases of suspected abruptio placentae, or with unexplained sustained fetal tachycardia, a Kleihauer-Betke stain for fetal red cells in the maternal circulation helps quantitate the amount of fetal-maternal hemorrhage.

Ultrasound examination of the abdomen may be very helpful. It shows the location of the pregnancy in utero, indicates fetal position, and yields approximate gestational age based on fetal dimensions. In severe abruptio placentae, it may show a retroplacental or retromembranous clot within the uterus. In addition, abdominal ultrasound may show the presence of adnexal masses, abscesses, hydronephrosis, and free peritoneal fluid. The nature of fluid (whether blood, pus, or ascites) may be difficult to distinguish. Paracentesis or culdocentesis is not contraindicated by third-trimester pregnancy but may be technically more difficult. Amniocentesis may serve to differentiate chorioamnionitis from abruptio placentae and idiopathic preterm labor. Amniotic fluid analysis also aids in identifying fetal pulmonic maturity.

BLEEDING IN THE THIRD TRIMESTER

Diagnosis

Vaginal bleeding in the third trimester may be the result of intrauterine or other genital or urinary lesions. Uterine events, which usually account for more substantial vaginal bleeding, include placenta previa and abruptio placentae. The former is a random event that holds little predictive value for subsequent pregnancies. Abruptio placentae tends to be recurrent from pregnancy to pregnancy with increasing risk with each preceding affected pregnancy. Bleeding may also result from the rupture of a fetal blood vessel, which may be stretched across the internal os. These vasa praevias are most usually found with low-lying placentas and placentas complicated by a succenturiate lobe. In addition to uterine events, cervicitis or other cervical lesions, vaginal or vulvar trauma, and urinary tract bleeding may present as vaginal bleeding in the third trimester of pregnancy.

Upon arrival, patients with significant amounts of vaginal bleeding should have a large-caliber intravenous catheter inserted and be given, initially, a liter or more of crystalloid solution, such as normal saline. Large volumes of fluids are well tolerated by the young, pregnant woman who is physiologically vasodilated.

Diagnostic studies include physical examination, history (include history of fetal movement), sonographic imaging, fetal heart rate monitoring, and blood studies. Vaginal examination should be avoided until placenta previa can be adequately ruled out by ultrasound. In the event of placenta previa, a digital examination of the cervix should not be carried out unless the physician is able to proceed immediately with delivery. In the event of abruptio placentae or vasa praevia, in which there is a need to determine the status of cervical dilatation and sample vaginal blood for fetal red blood cells, cautious speculum examination is appropriate.

Abdominal ultrasound examination accurately locates the site of placental implantation. It is important to exclude the possibility of a succenturiate lobe in the event that the placenta is located distant from the internal cervical os. Ensuring that the maternal bladder is filled with urine or with water via a Foley catheter aids in diagnosis. Ultrasound also provides information about fetal position and provides confirmatory information about gestational age.

Fetal heart rate monitoring should be obtained via a Doppler transducer. This provides a continuous heart rate tracing necessary to evaluate fetal oxygenation. Normally, the fetal heart rate is between 120 and 180 beats per minute. There is usually a short-term variability of five or more beats per minute every 10 to 15 seconds. If there is very little short-term variability and this persists for longer than 20 to 30 minutes, fetal asphyxia may be present. The recent use of narcotics, tranquilizers, barbiturates, or other depressant drugs may also cause this pattern, however. Short periods of decreased short-term variability are physiologic, indicating fetal sleep. Fetal tachycardia (above 180 beats per minute) may be a result of fetal bleeding, increased sympathetic tone, or maternal fever. Decelerations or bradycardia (heart rate below 120 beats per minute) may be associated with fetal asphyxia. Decelerations of abrupt descent and ascent lasting less than 1 minute with variable timing relative to uterine contractions are usually benign. The vagally mediated "variable decelerations" are the result of a baroreceptor response frequently due to umbilical cord compression. Unless prolonged or associated with a slow ascending return to baseline heart rate, these are generally not associated with asphyxia. Bleeding may be associated with uterine contractions. Heart rate decelerations that uniformly follow contractions and return slowly to a baseline heart rate strongly suggest the presence of fetal asphyxia. This is particularly true if they are associated with poor short-term variability.

Occasionally, in the preterm pregnancy complicated by uterine bleeding, significant concern about the presence of fetal asphyxia may exist. The nonstress test documents fetal heart rate acceleration in response to fetal movement. If accelerations of 15 beats per minute of 15 seconds' duration can be documented twice in a 20-minute observation, fetal asphyxia *at that time* can be reliably excluded. If, over a period of 1 to 2 hours, there is no fetal movement, this may be an indication of asphyxia, especially in a suspicious clinical context.

Preoperative Assessment

Cases of profound maternal hemorrhage in the third trimester necessitate preparation for surgery. Two issues need to be addressed before surgery can be safely performed. *First*, coagulation status should be assessed. In the event of fetal distress or massive maternal bleeding, an untreated tube of blood can be observed for clot formation. If a firm clot forms within 7 to 8 minutes, surgery can be performed while other coagulation studies are processed, providing the patient is otherwise an appropriate candidate. In the case of abruptio placentae, fibrin degradation products are increased coincident with decreased fibrinogen concentration. If the fibrinogen level is below 100 mg per deciliter, replacement should be undertaken before surgical intervention. Thrombocytopenia is also commonly found in these circumstances. Fibrinogen replacement by means of cryoprecipitate or fresh frozen plasma is usually begun before surgery. Unless coagulopathy is clinically problematic, platelet transfusions are usually reserved for the intraoperative period. With massive blood loss and transfusion with multiple units of banked blood, deficiencies in coagulant enzymes may manifest as a prolongation of the activated partial thromboplastin time or prothrombin time. *Second*, the patient's circulating blood volume should be adequate before surgery is performed. Average blood loss during cesarean section is 1,000 cc. Postural hypotension and prerenal oliguria should be evaluated and treated prior to surgery.

The in-hospital management of the pregnant woman with significant vaginal bleeding is complex. Factors that influence the timing of delivery include maternal status, the presence or absence of fetal distress, and gestational age. If the fetus has an advanced gestational age and has been shown to have a mature pulmonary status, then the presence of vaginal bleeding or labor in the mother usually occasions delivery. If the fetus is extremely premature and the rate of maternal bleeding is modest, then blood replacement may offer significant advantages over early delivery. In these circumstances, it is important to document that there is no evidence of fetal asphyxia. The effectiveness of tocolysis in premature labor with either placenta previa or abruptio placentae is unproved. If tocolysis is used, it requires the intensive monitoring of both mother and fetus and the commitment to effect delivery if the rate of bleeding or fetal status worsens.

Rarely, patients who present with third-trimester bleeding have primarily cervical bleeding. Cervical epithelial erosion may cause spotting but not hemodynamically significant bleeding. Cervical varicosities may occasionally result in notable bleeding. Undiagnosed cervical neoplasia may result in significant blood loss acutely. This diagnosis, although rare, should always be kept in mind for the patient with absent or incomplete antenatal care.

If no abdominal complaints are present, the patient gives a history of nothing more than vaginal "spotting," and active bleeding can be seen on the visible aspect of the cervix on speculum examination, then the diagnoses of abruptio placentae and placenta previa can be reasonably excluded. These criteria are only occasionally met, however, and few patients with bleeding in late pregnancy have trivial causes. Most patients will require hospitalization for observation to exclude significant abruptio placentae. If a patient bleeds from a placenta previa beyond 24 to 26 weeks, most obstetricians follow the patient until delivery in the hospital. In these circumstances, obstetric consultation is mandatory.

SUGGESTED READING

Berkowitz RL, ed. Critical care of the obstetric patient. New York: Churchill Livingstone, 1983.

Iffy L, Kaminetzky HA, eds. Principles and practice of obstetrics and perinatology. New York: John Wiley & Sons, 1981.

ECLAMPSIA AND PREECLAMPSIA

ARTHUR B. SANDERS, M.D., F.A.C.E.P., F.A.C.P.

The syndrome of preeclampsia is characterized by a combination of signs, symptoms, and abnormal laboratory test results during the latter half of pregnancy (Table 1). The presence of one or more of these symptoms in a woman who is more than 20 weeks pregnant should alert the physician to suspect a diagnosis of preeclampsia.

Eclampsia is marked by the presence of seizures in addition to one or more of the symptoms mentioned in Table 1.

The cause of the eclampsia-preeclampsia syndrome is unknown. However, the common thread to this symptom complex is that it occurs in the latter half of pregnancy and resolves completely after the delivery of the fetus.

DIAGNOSIS

The diagnosis of the eclampsia-preeclampsia syndrome can often be obscure. The classic findings of markedly elevated blood pressure, gross proteinuria, and peripheral edema, need not be present. The patient may present with vague symptoms such as mild epigastric or right upper quadrant pain. Only when appropriate laboratory tests are done (blood smear, platelet count, liver function tests, urine analysis) are findings consistent with this syndrome discovered.

The diagnosis of the preeclampsia syndrome is ultimately based on clinical grounds, and there is controversy in the literature on exact diagnostic criteria. Each one of these signs, symptoms, or abnormal laboratory tests by itself has a differential diagnosis that includes preeclampsia. Thus, if only one finding is present (proteinurea, mild hypertension, thrombocytopenia, etc.), the patient needs to be evaluated for other possible causes of that symptom. Particularly if only mild hypertension is found, or mild proteinuria (see Table 1), it may not be clear whether preeclampsia is even present. In view of this uncertainty, it is best always to consult an obstetrician before discharging any patient who meets any of the diagnostic criteria. If discharge is recommended by the consultant, the pa-

TABLE 1 Signs and Symptoms in Preeclampsia

Pregnancy-induced hypertension. This may be marked by blood pressure readings above 140/90 on several readings hours apart. Alternatively, a rise in systolic pressure of 30 mm Hg or diastolic pressure of 15 mm Hg from previous blood pressure readings may be indicative of this syndrome

Proteinuria >1+ on the standard urine dipstick on two separate urine specimens

Thrombocytopenia

Abnormal liver function tests

Microangiopathic hemolytic anemia

Oliguria

Cerebral or visual disturbances

Pulmonary edema

tient should be followed-up closely and carefully for the development of new symptoms.

THERAPY

Pre-hospital Care

The diagnosis of the eclampsia-preeclampsia syndrome is generally made in the emergency department. However, women in the latter half of pregnancy who present with seizures, hypertension, abdominal pain, central nervous system disturbances, or pulmonary edema should be suspected of having this syndrome. Calm reassurance, a quiet environment, and prompt transport to an appropriate hospital are the mainstays of treatment. An intravenous catheter should be placed with 5 percent glucose to be available for pharmacologic treatment as needed. Nasal oxygen should be provided if there are any respiratory difficulties. If seizures occur, the administration of diazepam is recommended. Magnesium sulfate and hydralazine are generally not part of the pharmacologic therapy available to paramedics in the field. Therefore, transport to an appropriate facility for stabilization and definitive treatment is of utmost importance.

Emergency Department

The appropriate treatment of patients with the eclampsia-preeclampsia syndrome over the first 8 hours is highly important to avoiding maternal and fetal morbidity and mortality. The definitive treatment is delivery of the fetus. Risks associated with the induction of labor or cesarean section must be balanced by the maturity of the fetus and severity of the syndrome. Thus, obstetric consultants must be involved early in the care of these patients. If eclampsia-preeclampsia syndrome is diagnosed, treatment with magnesium sulfate is appropriate to prevent seizures. The patient should be closely followed for magnesium toxicity as described subsequently. If seizures occur before therapeutic levels of magnesium can be obtained, diazepam should be used. Diastolic blood pressures greater than 110 mm Hg should be treated with

intravenous hydralazine. Close monitoring of these patients' neurologic, respiratory, and cardiovascular status is essential.

The inpatient management of patients with eclampsia–preeclampsia is aimed toward achieving the following therapeutic goals: (1) safe delivery of the fetus, (2) prevention or control of convulsions, and (3) control of blood pressure.

Admission to a High-Risk Obstetrical Service. The eclampsia-preeclampsia syndrome is a major cause of maternal and fetal mortality. Once the diagnosis is suspected, prompt obstetrical consultation should be initiated. Ultimately, delivery of the fetus is the only definitive treatment for this syndrome. These patients should all be admitted to a high-risk obstetric service for careful observation, even when symptoms appear to be mild.

Prevention or Control of Convulsions. General measures include bed rest in a quiet environment with little external stimuli. The treatment of choice for eclampsia-preeclampsia syndrome is *magnesium sulfate*. Although controversy exists in the literature, magnesium sulfate is generally regarded as the safest drug to use and has a long history of effective use. It reduces neuromuscular irritability and improves uterine blood flow without producing central nervous system depression in either the mother or the fetus. There is much less clinical experience with traditional anticonvulsants such as phenytoin, diazepam, and phenobarbital. These drugs are effective, but may produce undesirable side effects such as central nervous system depression of both the mother and fetus.

The loading dose is 4 g of magnesium sulfate intravenously slowly, over at least 4 minutes. This may be prepared by mixing 8 ml of the 50 percent magnesium sulfate solution with 12 ml of sterile water. The resulting solution will be 20 ml of 20 percent magnesium sulfate solution (4 g).

The maintenance dose may be given intravenously or intramuscularly. Studies have shown that when magnesium sulfate was given at the rate of 3 g per hour intravenously, therapeutic levels of magnesium were consistently obtained. Alternatively, intramuscular injections may be given according to the Parkland Hospital protocol. Immediately following the initial 4-g loading dose of magnesium sulfate, 10 g are given intramuscularly. Five grams of a 50 percent solution of magnesium sulfate (10 ml) is deeply injected into each buttock with a 3-inch 20-gauge needle. Lidocaine (1 ml of a 2 percent solution) may be added to the syringe to lessen the discomfort from the intramuscular injections. This is then followed by an injection of 5 g of magnesium sulfate every 4 hours intramuscularly (10 ml of a 50 percent magnesium sulfate solution).

The patient should be observed closely for signs of *magnesium toxicity*. These include absence of reflexes, oliguria, depressed respirations, and finally cardiac arrest. Prior to the administration of the maintenance doses, a clinical examination must be done to ensure that (1) the patellar reflexes are present, (2) respirations are not depressed, and (3) a urine output of at least 25 ml per hour has been maintained. Therapeutic serum magnesium levels range from 3 to 8 mg per deciliter. If serum magnesium levels can be obtained quickly, they may be useful in following the patient. Unfortunately, many laboratories are unable to provide stat magnesium levels, and the clinical examination must be used to follow the patient for magnesium toxicity. Loss of the patellar reflexes is thought to occur at a magnesium level of about 10 mg per deciliter. Thus, ideally one would strive to keep the reflexes at the 1+ response level.

Magnesium sulfate toxicity may be treated with supportive care such as assisted ventilation and calcium gluconate. Ten milliliters of a 10 percent calcium gluconate solution may be given intravenously over 5 minutes to reverse the effects of magnesium toxicity.

The administration of magnesium sulfate and the attainment of therapeutic blood levels will control and prevent seizures in the vast majority of patients. If the patient is experiencing active seizures, especially in the pre-hospital care environment, treatment with diazepam (1 to 5 mg intravenously) is appropriate. Diazepam, however, may depress the fetus, and its use increases the need for prompt fetal monitoring and obstetrical intervention.

Control of Blood Pressure. In the eclampsia-preeclampsia syndrome, placental blood flow is often decreased. It is thought that some elevation in blood pressure may represent a physiologic response of the body to maintain placental perfusion pressure. Aggressive antihypertensive treatment to lower the pressure to normotensive levels may be detrimental to placental perfusion. On the other hand, severe acute hypertension increases the maternal risk of intracranial hemorrhage. It is recommended, therefore, that the blood pressure be treated with antihypertensive agents only when the diastolic pressure exceeds 110 mm Hg. When the diastolic pressure does exceed 110 mm Hg, antihypertensive drugs should be used to lower the diastolic pressure to 100 mm Hg.

Hydralazine is the drug of choice for the treatment of hypertension associated with the eclampsia-preeclampsia syndrome. Five milligrams are administered intravenously, and the blood pressure is monitored at least every 5 minutes for 20 minutes. Another 5 to 10 mg of hydralazine may be administered every 20 minutes in attempts to keep the diastolic pressure at about 100 mm Hg.

It is important to remember that antihypertensive drugs do not affect the underlying mechanism of disease or increase fetal survival. Delivery of the fetus must be accomplished as soon as the situation is stabilized.

SUGGESTED READING

Cunningham FG, Pritchard JA. How should hypertension during pregnancy be managed? Experience at Parkland Memorial Hospital. Med Clin North Am 1984; 68:505–527.
Ferris TF. How should hypertension during pregnancy be managed? An internist's approach. Med Clin North Am 1984; 68:491–503.
Sibai BM, Lipshitz J, Anderson GD, Dilts PV. Reassessment of intravenous MgSO4 therapy in preeclampsia–eclampsia. Obstet Gynecol 1981; 57:199–202.
Weinstein L. Syndrome of hemolysis, elevated liver enzymes and low platelet count: a severe consequence of hypertension in pregnancy. Am J Obstet Gynecol 1982; 142:159–167.

INFECTION IN PREGNANCY

STEPHEN C. SCHOENBAUM, M.D., M.P.H.

ANTIBIOTICS IN PREGNANCY

Selection of an antimicrobial in pregnancy or the postpartum period requires more than the usual general considerations of benefits, cost, and risks. There are the special considerations of the effects of antimicrobials on the pregnant woman, the fetus, or the newborn. Almost all antimicrobials cross the placenta and almost all can appear in breast milk. The relative concentrations achieved in the fetus or in a breast-feeding neonate vary widely.

Penicillins, cephalosporins, erythromycin, and nitrofurantoin have low toxicities in general and are not associated with any special problems in pregnancy or the puerperium. These drugs plus sulfonamides should be useful in treating virtually all common bacterial infection problems associated with pregnancy that occur prior to the third trimester.

Sulfonamides do pose a special problem in late pregnancy. They cross the placenta readily and become highly bound to fetal proteins, thus displacing bilirubin from albumin binding sites. Fetal and neonatal livers do not have mature enzymatic systems for conjugating free bilirubin. Babies whose mothers were treated with sulfonamides shortly before delivery can have increased problems with neonatal jaundice, and long-acting sulfonamides must not be considered in pregnancy.

Clindamycin and chloramphenicol have an anaerobic spectrum that can be beneficial in treating postpartum infections. Owing to their general toxicity they should be used only when the benefit clearly outweighs the risk, even though they pose no special problems in pregnancy or the postpartum period. Chloramphenicol should not be used in newborns without the availability of direct monitoring of serum levels, since the neonatal liver cannot detoxify it well and toxic concentrations rapidly build up. Clindamycin-induced pseudomembranous colitis, should it occur, can be treated in pregnancy or the puerperium with oral vancomycin, which is nonabsorbable from the gut and thus poses no special additional risk.

The general toxicity of aminoglycosides dictates that their use be reserved for serious infections. Though questions have been raised about their potential ototoxicity for the developing fetus, such ototoxicity appears to occur infrequently. The use of metronidazole and trimethoprim should be avoided in pregnancy if at all possible because of their known effects in animal models. Metronidazole is oncogenic for mice and mutagenic for bacteria. For these reasons, the United States Food and Drug Administration has cautioned against its use in pregnancy. Trimethoprim is teratogenic for rodents and related to amethopterin, a known human teratogen. There are no specific data implicating or absolving trimethoprim with regard to adverse effects on human pregnancy. Nevertheless, there usually are suitable alternative drugs, and when sulfonamides are given to women in early pregnancy they should be given alone, not in combination with trimethoprim.

Finally, tetracyclines, though widely used in pregnancy in the past, can cause a variety of special problems ranging from staining of developing teeth, even after small doses, to severe maternal hepatic necrosis when large doses are given. Accordingly, tetracyclines are considered hazardous for pregnant women and should not be used.

URINARY TRACT INFECTIONS

If routine urine cultures are obtained early in pregnancy, approximately 5 percent of women are found to have asymptomatic bacteriuria. This does not differ from the percentage of nonpregnant women who have asymptomatic bacteriuria, but if it is untreated, about one-third of pregnant women with asymptomatic bacteriuria develop symptomatic urinary infections, often pyelonephritis, during the course of the pregnancy. This may be a result of pregnancy-associated structural changes in the urinary tract, especially ureteral dilatation. Treatment of pregnant women with asymptomatic bacteriuria has been shown to decrease the subsequent frequency of symptomatic infection five- to sixfold. Treatment has also been shown to decrease the frequency of anemia and low birth weight in newborns. Accordingly, I favor obtaining a urine culture from all pregnant women at the first prenatal visit and then treating those with asymptomatic bacteriuria. Their community-acquired organisms tend to be sensitive to a variety of antibiotics that are safe to use in early pregnancy, including amoxicillin, nitrofurantoin, and sulfonamides. If pyelonephritis does develop in a pregnant woman, it must be treated promptly. This often involves hospitalization and the use of intravenous antibiotics such as a cephalosporin or a combination of ampicillin and an aminoglycoside.

INFECTIONS WITH TERATOGENIC POTENTIAL

Many infections with teratogenic potential are not clinically apparent during pregnancy, including most cytomegalovirus, many *Toxoplasma*, and some rubella infections. I do not favor routine repeated serologic screenings to detect asymptomatic infections unless there has been a well-documented exposure. Even if the maternal infection is clinically apparent, the agent may not necessarily reach the fetus. Nevertheless, a sufficient percentage of first-trimester rubella and first- and mid-trimester *Toxoplasma* infections do reach the fetus to warrant considering termination of pregnancy when maternal infection has been documented.

When the exposure is documented or a mother develops a compatible clinical picture, a diagnosis of toxoplasmosis or rubella can usually be made by serology, either by the demonstration of a rise in titer or by demonstration of a high specific IgM titer. This requires that when the patient is initially seen, blood be drawn for titers for later comparison. Some cases of toxoplasmosis present as lymphadenopathy, and node biopsy leads to the discovery of characteristic *Toxoplasma* pathology.

A small percentage (about 4 percent) of offspring of women who have varicella in the first trimester develop a malformation syndrome consisting of burnlike scars on the skin, corneal opacities, and congenital glaucoma. This risk appears to be low enough so that interruption of pregnancy is not advocated routinely for mothers who develop varicella early in pregnancy. The efficiency of globulin in preventing viremia and congenital infection has not been established. Therefore, it is not generally recommended for women who are exposed to varicella during pregnancy.

It is most important to remember that congenital rubella infection is entirely preventable by assuring that women of childbearing age are no longer susceptible to rubella. Young adult women who have never had rubella vaccine must be identified and vaccinated. Women should not be given rubella vaccine intentionally when they are, or might be pregnant. Nevertheless, it is increasingly apparent that rubella vaccine is not teratogenic and that inadvertent rubella vaccination during pregnancy does not mandate termination of pregnancy. Rubella vaccine can also be given to women safely during the immediate postpartum period. It is recommended for women who were found to be susceptible during pregnancy so that they will enter the next pregnancy immune.

INFECTIONS AROUND THE TIME OF DELIVERY

Endometritis is the most common infection occurring in the puerperium. It sometimes occurs after prolonged rupture of membranes, but much more commonly after cesarean section. The incidence of endometritis varies from hospital to hospital, but is at least 15 to 20 percent after cesarean section. The diagnosis of endometritis is made purely on clinical grounds based on the presence of fever and a more tender uterus than would normally be expected. On occasion the lochia is purulent or foul-smelling. The organisms cultured from patients with endometritis include all the normal vaginal flora. Thus the flora is usually a combination of gram-positive and gram-negative organisms, aerobes and anaerobes. A remarkable percentage of these organisms, however, is sensitive to a single drug such as ampicillin, and ampicillin has been effective in treating about 70 percent of cases. Use of cefoxitin as a single drug, or a two-drug combination such as clindamycin and gentamicin, leads to prompt resolution of signs and symptoms in over 90 percent of cases. If a narrow spectrum agent is used and fever persists, then the regimen must quickly be broadened to cover additional organisms. The duration of treatment can be short. Once the patient has defervesced convincingly (for 1 or 2 days), the infection can be assumed to be under control and antibiotics can be discontinued.

About 5 to 10 percent of normal women have staphylococcal vaginal colonization. When these women develop endometritis, they may have associated staphylococcal bacteremia. Though I am always concerned about the possibility of metastatic staphylococcal infection, I have treated these young, otherwise healthy women for not longer than 2 weeks and then followed them carefully off antibiotics rather than taking the most conservative approach to staphylococcal bacteremia and treating for 4 to 6 weeks.

Most fevers following a vaginal delivery are of short duration and self-limited. Though studies have shown that many of these fevers are associated with mycoplasmal bacteremia, no specific antimicrobial treatment is needed in most cases.

When the newborn is healthy, I encourage the pediatricians to permit early breast-feeding for most mothers receiving antimicrobials. Exceptions at this time would be mothers receiving sulfonamides or metronidazole.

DRUGS IN PREGNANCY

ROBERT R. WHIPKEY, M.D.
PAUL M. PARIS, M.D., F.A.C.E.P.

This chapter will outline many of the most commonly prescribed medications in clinical practice, along with special considerations for their use in pregnant women.

Relatively few drugs have been proven to harm the fetus directly. However, to reduce any risks, a few general principles should be followed:

1. Decrease the exposure by giving the minimum effective dose for the shortest time possible.
2. Prescribe oral forms when possible.
3. Choose well-known preparations over newer drugs about which less is known.
4. Be aware of multiple components of many formulations.

ANTIBIOTICS

The *penicillins*, including the semi-synthetic forms, are safe for use in the nonallergic pregnant patient. Based on widespread use and extensive experience, the penicillins cross the placenta readily without teratogenicity, decreased efficacy, or adverse effects on the mother allowing simultaneous and effective treatment of infection in both mother and fetus. The newer synthetic compounds, such as mezlocillin and azlocillin, generally should not be used unless they are indicated by serious infections (owing to lack of clinical experience). For patients with immediate-type sensitivity to penicillin, erythromycin base is the preferred alternative therapy. For nonanaphylactic reactions, cephalosporins are the preferred alternative therapy.

Erythromycin base is effective and safe for use during pregnancy, especially in the treatment of community-acquired pneumonias and in the management of syphilis in patients with penicillin sensitivity. The estolate form of erythromycin should not be used because of an increased risk of cholestatic hepatitis in the mother. After 4 months gestational age, intravenous erythhromycin is needed to achieve therapeutic levels in fetal serum.

Cephalosporins have had no reported teratogenicity, decreased efficacy, or adverse metabolic effects in the fetus and no reported cases of problems in their history.

Chloramphenicol appears to be safe without increased incidence of adverse side effects on the fetus or mother when used during pregnancy. Of special interest during pregnancy is the association with a severe, rare idiosyncratic toxic reaction seen especially in premature infants. Fetal cardiovascular collapse after chloramphenicol therapy in neonates was first observed in 1959 and labeled the "gray syndrome." Onset is usually 3 to 4 days into therapy, beginning with vomiting, irregular and rapid respirations, and abdominal distention. This progresses to flaccidity, ashen gray cyanosis, and decreased body temperature. Approximately 40 percent survive if this drug is discontinued. The incidence of this reaction is extremely low and should not deter the use of chloramphenicol when indicated in pregnant females or neonates, but close attention must be paid to serum levels.

The *aminoglycosides* cross the placenta poorly, but still expose the fetus to the risk of ototoxicity. They are suggested in pregnancy as backup therapy for organisms resistant to chloramphenicol. Overall, the use of aminoglycosides in pregnancy has been too infrequent to allow their unqualified recommendation.

The *sulfonamides*, including those in combination preparations, such as Bactrim, should be avoided in the third trimester. The use of sulfonamides during the third trimester is associated with an increased risk of kernicterus in the newborn. There is also theoretical concern for adverse effects on fetal development during the first trimester because of the antifolate activity of the sulfonamides, although this has not been proved. It may be prudent to use other antibiotics in this period if possible, but treatment should not be withheld on this basis alone when no alternative treatments exist.

During pregnancy, changes in the vaginal environment occasionally allow overgrowth of organisms, including *Trichomonas vaginalis* and *Candida albicans. Candida* is a normal component of vaginal flora and requires no treatment unless bothersome symptoms exist. *Candida* infections in normal newborns can be treated easily should they arise. *Clotrimazole* is safe for use during pregnancy in those women with the findings of symptomatic *Candida vaginitis. Trichomonas* is found in from 3 to 15 percent of asymptomatic women at gynecology clincs and from 20 to 50 percent of women at sexually transmitted disease clinics. The more alkaline environment of the vagina during pregnancy favors the growth of *Trichomonas. Trichomonas vaginitis* during pregnancy does not seem to harm the fetus. When symptoms exist, the initial therapy should be directed toward symptomatic relief with tub baths twice daily and biweekly douches with a weak vinegar and water solution. In cases in which these forms of therapy fail, clotrimazole has been shown to be effective occasionally against *Trichomonas. Metronidazole* use in pregnancy is controversial because of possible teratogenic effects, with studies showing it to be carcinogenic in rodents and mutagenic in bacteria. As a result of these studies, metronidazole should be used only in cases that remain symptomatic with the other therapies outlined, and then only during the second half of pregnancy.

Tetracycline is contraindicated during pregnancy because of its effects on both the fetus and the mother. The risk of hepatotoxicity in the mother is greater in pregnancy. The higher risk in pregnancy may be the result of altered renal clearance owing to the hemodynamic effects discussed earlier, with further alteration in pyelonephritis, resulting in higher than therapeutic levels. The chelating property of tetracycline results in tetracycline–calcium orthophosphate complexes. This poses a risk of discoloration of the teeth in the offspring of pregnant women treated with tetracycline. The period of greatest damage seems to be after the fourth month of gestation. This same chelating property can also result in deposition in bones with depression of bone growth.

Little is known about the side effects of *spectinomycin* in pregnancy. However, it is recommended as an alternative therapy to penicillin for uncomplicated gonorrhea during pregnancy.

GASTROINTESTINAL MEDICATIONS

Heartburn is a frequent complaint during pregnancy, the cause being controversial. In general, *antacid preparations* are well tolerated in the usual doses during pregnancy. Sodium bicarbonate is contraindicated because it is absorbed in greater proportion than other antacids, which may alter the pH of the mother and fetus with effects on enzyme function oxygen–hemoglobin dissociation, and many other sensitive metabolic processes in the fetus. One study associates antacid use early in pregnancy with an increased occurrence of a group of heterogene-

ous anomalies. It should be emphasized that these anomalies are heterogeneous, no causality can be inferred, and no supporting data have followed.

Hemorrhoids are best treated by using dietary fiber and/or one of the bulk-forming fiber preparations to avoid constipation. Anal analgesia may also help, either with sitz baths or one of the nonsteroidal soothing ointments or suppositories, such as Anusol.

The standard initial treatment for nausea and vomiting associated with pregnancy is reassurance that it is a transient problem and the avoidance of factors associated with the onset of symptoms. For vomiting associated with disease states, it is customary to rest the gastrointestinal (GI) tract for several hours and then slowly advance the diet, beginning with clear liquids. When such conservative modalities fail, many alternatives exist. There is a strong concern in the general public over pharmacologic treatment of nausea in pregnancy, initially stemming from the severe limb deformities associated with thalidomide use during pregnancy. The fertility and Maternal Health Advisory Committee of the U.S. Food and Drug Administration (FDA) reviewed both published and unpublished data on *Bendectin* and was unable to demonstrate a direct increase in birth defects with its use. However, Bendectin was recently removed from the market because of lingering doubt concerning its teratogenicity.

An alternative antinauseant is *trimethobenzamide* (Tigan), which is also safe. *Prochlorperazine* (Compazine), a phenothiazine, is also probably safe. However, with the small risk of maternal hypotension with the phenothiazines and resultant placental insufficiency, the former drug should be used as second-line therapy after nonpharmaceutical treatment.

Anticonvulsant Drugs

One study showed seizure frequency during pregnancy increased in 45 percent, decreased in 5 percent, and unchanged in 50 percent of women.

There is no current evidence to contraindicate the rapid intravenous use of standard drugs to control status epilepticus, though the shorter-acting preparations may be preferred to shorten the exposure time.

If teratogenic potential exists for anticonvulsants, it appears to be very small. The only drug to be avoided is *trimethadione*, which is strongly associated with fetal malformation and mental retardation in a high proportion of those exposed.

Antiasthmatic Drugs

The major concern in pregnant asthmatics is the maintenance of fetal oxygenation. A combination of maternal hypoxemia and respiratory alkalemia, as in acute airway obstruction, can be greatly detrimental to the fetus. Maternal hyperventilation has been shown to decrease fetal oxygenation.

Theoretically, *beta-adrenergic drugs* should be avoided in pregnancy because the peripheral vasodilatation may shunt blood from the fetus as the uterine vessels constrict, but the true significance of this effect is unknown. The Perinatal Collaborative Project found a statistically significant increase in malformations in a group of mother-child pairs exposed to epinephrine in the first 4 lunar months of pregnancy. However, since epinephrine is used only in severe attacks, it is not clear if the severity of the asthma itself or the epinephrine was at fault. When possible, epinephrine should be avoided during pregnancy if other modalities will suffice.

Isoproterenol, and ephedrine have not been well studied in pregnancy. Clinical review of ephedrine has failed to associate its use with an increased risk of malformation. With the availability of other, more preferred treatments, isoproterenol and ephedrine should not be used in pregnancy unless the clinical situation warrants the potential though unknown risk.

Terbutaline, has never been studied in a controlled fashion, but no reports of adverse effects have been found in humans. Terbutaline and the other beta-2 stimulants, are also given by continuous infusion to arrest premature labor through inhibition of uterine activity. Theoretically, beta-2 stimulants near term could prolong labor, though this seems unlikely with the dosages used to treat asthma. Terbutaline should be reserved for situations in which other forms of therapy fail.

Neither the aerosol nor the oral forms of *metaproterenol*, are known to have had adverse effects in human fetuses in their 20 years of clinical use or an increased incidence of side effects in pregnant females.

The Perinatal Collaborative Project failed to demonstrate any increased risks with the use of aminophylline or theophylline.

Cromolyn sodium has not been studied to any great extent, and its safety has not been established unequivocally. Clinical observations over its long clinical history have failed to demonstrate damage to the fetus.

Many combination products used in asthmatics contain phenobarbital. There is no evidence to suggest its use results in undue risk to the mother or fetus. However, the value of phenobarbital in asthma therapy has not been shown.

Oral *glucocorticoids* are highly effective in the treatment of severe asthma. A retrospective study evaluated three groups of mothers, including those using prednisone for short-course therapy, daily prednisone initiated during pregnancy, and those continued on daily prednisone initiated before pregnancy. The study failed to reveal any adverse effects in the offspring during the first 2 years of life. Conticosteroids should not be withheld when indicated during pregnancy, but the lower dosages with the aerosol forms are preferred.

Decongestants may also be indicated in certain conditions during pregnancy. Pseudoephedrine has not been studied prospectively or retrospectively and cannot be condoned for use during pregnancy. The cautious use of phenylephrine seems safe in pregnancy.

Antihistamines may be needed to treat various conditions including urticaria, angioedema, drug reactions, and allergic and vasomotor rhinitis. Histamine is found in high concentrations in fetal tissue. With one exception,

no increased incidence of teratogenesis has been associated with the use of antihistamines. The relative risk of *brompheniramine* use shows a statistically significant correlation with malformed offspring. A study suggests diphenhydramine use causes cleft palate. Such an association has not been supported prospectively, and current data suggest its safety. In conclusion, the commonly prescribed antihistamines, with the exception of brompheniramine, are probably safe for use during pregnancy.

Analgesics

Alternatives to the pharmacolgic treatment of pain should be strongly considered in pregnant patients. Modalities such as heat therapy, cryotherapy, massage, transcutaneous nerve stimulation, and hypnosis may be the preferred treatments for pain during pregnancy. However, cases in which these methods are not practical are common.

The analgesic and antipyretic of choice in pregnancy is *acetaminophen*. Though it crosses the placenta readily, there appears to be no teratogenic effects when taken in the usual doses.

The second-line analgesic–antipyretics are the *salicylates*. Salicylates readily cross the placenta and are more slowly eliminated by the fetus because of the immaturity of the glucuronidation and renal excretory pathways. Numerous retrospective studies have shown a relationship between salicylate use and congenital problems of decreased birth weight, cleft lip and palate, and bleeding disorders. On the other hand, others have shown no such relationship. A prospective study in 1976 of 50,000 mother–child pairs failed to show a higher incidence of malformations in heavy and occasional salicylate users compared with nonusers.

Prostaglandins are known to initiate uterine contractions and labor. One of the effects of aspirin products and *nonsteriodal anti-inflammatory medications* is to inhibit prostaglandin synthesis. As would be expected with such inhibition, both animal and human studies of aspirin use show an increase in average length of gestation, increased frequency of postmaturity, and increased mean duration of spontaneous labor. Of theoretical concern is premature closure of the ductus arteriosus as a result of prostaglandin inhibition. After review of the available data, the FDA Panel on Over the Counter Medications concluded *aspirin* to be a potentially hazardous medication in pregnancy. Hemostasis is adversely effected by aspirin's antiplatelet activity. Bleeding tendencies are of clinical concern only rarely, with only one reported severe fetal hemorrhage in infants of aspirin users. The panel recommended that all labels of aspirin-containing products include the warning "Do not take this product during the last 3 months of pregnancy except under the advice and supervision of a physician."

Narcotic use during pregnancy can affect the fetus and neonate in two ways—first, by causing fetal hypoxia and acidosis attributable to maternal respiratory depression and second by direct fetal or neonatal depression once the narcotic has crossed the placental barrier. Narcotics readily cross because of their lipid solubility, poor ionization in blood, and low molecular weight. Narcotics may remain in the fetal circulation for prolonged periods, probably because of underdeveloped degradation pathways. Meperidine, for example, has a half-life of 18 hours in the neonate compared with 4 hours in adults. Most conclusions on narcotic effects during pregnancy are based on observation of narcotic addicted mothers. These retrospective studies show higher incidences of meconium-stained amniotic fluid, anemia, low birth weight, and stillbirth. To minimize the effects of narcotics on the fetus or neonate, several guidelines should be followed:

1. Avoid prolonged use of narcotics during pregnancy.
2. Avoid acute detoxification, as with naloxone in suspected or known narcotic addicts because of possible deleterious effects on the fetus.
3. Approach deliveries in narcotic-addicted mothers as high risk for potential serious neonatal problems.
4. Administer intravenous medications for pain control in labor only during uterine contractions. Placental blood flow from the maternal side ceases as uterine intramural pressure rises during contractions, thus decreasing the bolus reaching the fetus.

Based on years of clinical experience and research, several narcotics appear safe for short-term use during pregnancy or labor. *Meperidine* has no known teratogenic effects. The major concern with its use is the possibility of neonatal respiratory depression when used during labor. There is some evidence that different metabolic patterns exist, with some people forming the metabolites responsible for respiratory depression more quickly. Though no statistical analysis was done, the authors suggest safety from respiratory depression if meperidine is given more than 6 hours or less than 60 minutes prior to delivery, because lower levels of active metabolite reach fetal circulation when it is given at these points. *Morphine sulfate* is also probably safe to use cautiously, though it has a greater effect on the carbon dioxide (CO_2) response curve than does meperidine. *Alphaprodine* (Nisentil) may also be used safely with the advantage of a shorter duration of action (seldom longer than 2 hours) and a low incidence of nausea and vomiting. Studies suggest a 0.9 percent incidence of neonatal depression when the total dose is limited to 40 mg, and the dosage given less than 45 minutes prior to delivery resulted in no depression.

Nitrous oxide is frequently used as an analgesic in the pre-hospital setting. The usual method of use is patient titrated analgesia using a mixture of 50 percent oxygen and 50 percent nitrous oxide. Such use has also been employed during labor. The babies of mothers receiving continuous nasal nitrous oxide with supplemental nitrous oxide during contractions had no significant differences in mean Apgar scores at 1 and 5 minutes, with neither group showing any significant neonatal depression. This suggests that nitrous oxide does not impair adjustment to early life or have apparent ill effects on the infant during late pregnancy. Nitrous oxide has been shown to be fetotoxic in pregnant rats when they were exposed to a 70 to 75 percent nitrous oxide concentration for 24 hours on day 9 of gestation. Other studies have shown that continuous exposure of pregnant rats to low concentration of nitrous oxide for the first 19 days of gestation resulted in a higher incidence of adverse effects compared with that in controls. Exposure to low levels by health care personnel has also been implicated in causing an increase in the incidence of spontaneous abortion and fetal malformations. As a result, the FDA warns health professionals who may become pregnant that chronic occupational exposure to nitrous oxide may pose a risk to the fetus and that such a risk may also exist for pregnant patients when nitrous oxide is used as an anesthetic agent. However, no evicence to date implicates the short-term intermittent use of a 50:50 nitrous oxide and oxygen mixture in causing adverse effects during pregnancy.

Local anesthetics are weak bases and, as with narcotics, are subject to ion trapping on the fetal side. Local anesthetics have been shown to be myocardial depressants, with an even greater negative inotropic effect when combined with acidemia. Therefore, prolonged exposure to local anesthetics during labor, as with epidural blocks, should be avoided, especially when signs of fetal distress are present. Perivaginal and paracervical blocks with *mepivacaine* result in a rapid rise in maternal plasma anesthetic levels. Direct diffusion across vascular walls from the site of anesthetic deposit seems plausible with these blocks. This direct diffusion can result in higher levels in the fetal serum than in maternal serum. In a study of 17 fetuses treated with 200 mg of paracervical blocks, seven had episodes of significant bradycardia. Those with bradycardia had a mean mepivacaine level of 4 μg per milliliter, whereas those with levels below 3 μg per milliliter showed no adverse effects. Similarly, a 3 μg per milliliter threshold was found for lidocaine. Low-dose intermittent lidocaine for peridural anesthesia, as outlined by Zador et al, successfully kept umbilical vein lidocaine levels below 0.6 μg per milliliter. Other research showed that the addition of epinephrine (1:400,000) to bupivacaine halved the maternal levels and decreased the fetal level by 30 percent.

Outpatient use of *lidocaine* for local infiltration appears to be safe during pregnancy following the recommended usage guidelines. Using a 1 percent solution generally results in a total dosage of less than 5 mg of lidocaine. Nearly complete absorption from a subcutaneous site occurs over a 4-hour period. Interestingly, subcutaneous intercostal nerve blocks with 400 mg of lidocaine resulted in a mean peak level of 2.0 μg per miligram.

SUGGESTED READING

Berkowitz RL, Coustan DR, Michizuki TK, eds. Handbook for prescribing medications during pregnancy. Boston: Little, Brown, 1981.

Ledger WJ, ed. Antibiotics in obstetrics and gynecology. Boston: Martinus Nijhoff, 1982.

Ledward RS, Hawkins DF. Drug treatment in obstetrics. London: Chapman and Hall, 1983.

Quilligan EF, ed. Current therapy in obstetrics and gynecology 2. Philadelphia: WB Saunders, 1983.

Rayburn WF, Zuspan FP, eds. Drug therapy in obstetrics and gynecology. Norwalk, CN: Appleton-Century-Crofts, 1982.

NORMAL DELIVERY

RUSSELL K. LAROS Jr., M.D.

When the emergency physician is presented with a woman who believes that she is in labor, several critical questions must be asked and answered: Is this patient really in active labor? What is the status of the membranes? What is the presentation? What is the status of the fetus? Is delivery imminent?

EVALUATION OF LABOR

Labor is defined as regular, painful uterine contractions, occurring every 3 to 5 minutes, that lead to changes in the cervix. Clearly, all episodes of uterine contractions are not true labor, because the cervix does not always change. Unfortunately, one needs to have a prior examination against which to compare current findings or to examine the cervix serially in order to be able to document changes confidently. Often this is not possible in the emergency setting. At one extreme is a patient in whom the initial vaginal examination reveals a cervix that is soft and dilated 3 to 4 cm. It is best to assume that this patient is in labor. At the other extreme is a patient with regular, painful contractions who is found to have a cervix that is long, firm, and undilated. This patient may or may not be in early labor; only serial observations allow a definitive diagnosis. Because the latent phase of labor is usually 4 to 6 hours in length, there is ample time for serial observations either in the emergency department or in another setting.

NORMAL LABOR PATTERNS

Progress in labor is determined by evaluating cervical dilatation and station of the presenting part. Table 1 presents norms for the latent and active phases of the first stage of labor and for the second stage of labor. The latent phase lasts from the onset of painful, regular contractions until rapid cervical dilatation begins (usually 4 cm). The active phase is from 4 cm to full cervical dilatation.

STATUS OF THE MEMBRANES

The membranes usually rupture during the first part of labor, and most women can give an accurate history of when rupture occurred. If there is a question as to the status of the membranes, a sterile speculum examination should be performed. The posterior vaginal fornix is inspected for the presence of pooling. If doubt still exists, a specimen should be taken for testing with nitrazine paper and microscopic examination. Normal amniotic fluid is alkaline, and thus turns nitrazine paper a dark blue color.

TABLE 1 Patterns of Labor

Stage of Labor	Mean Duration	
	Primigravida	Multigravida
Latent phase (hrs)	6.4	4.8
Active phase (hrs)	4.6	2.4
Maximum slope (cm/hr)	3.0	5.7
Second stage (hrs)	1.1	0.4

When allowed to dry on a glass slide it forms a fern-like pattern, which is easily observed using the low-power objective of a microscope.

DETERMINING PRESENTATION

A reasonable diagnosis of presentation can be made during a careful abdominal examination. First one should determine which fetal pole occupies the fundus of the uterus. The head is round, hard, and smooth and can be balloted between the examining hands. The fetal back is located by feeling for a smooth, convex surface. This contrasts with the fetal belly, which is concave, soft, and irregular. The fetal pole overlying the pelvic inlet should then be palpated. Fetal presentation can then be confirmed by vaginal examination.

EVALUATION OF FETAL STATUS

The fetal heart rate (FHR) should be determined. This can be accomplished either by auscultation with a fetoscope or by listening with a Doppler device. The FHR should be observed during and just after a contraction, and both the baseline rate and changes in relationship to the contractions should be noted. If bradycardia (a baseline rate less than 120 beats per minute) or deep decelerations (decrease of more than 20 beats per minute during and after a contraction) are noted, the fetus should be considered to be in distress.

TREATMENT OF FETAL DISTRESS

Emergency treatment of presumed fetal distress includes measures aimed at improving maternal oxygenation and uterine blood flow and at decreasing cord compression should it exist. The mother is given oxygen by mask and turned on her left side. If bradycardia persists, she should be placed in the knee-chest position in a further attempt to relieve pressure on a frank or occult prolapse of the umbilical cord. If a frank prolapse of the cord is detected, the fetal head should be manually elevated with the vaginal examining finger and the elevation maintained until cesarean section is performed.

TRANSPORT

Once it is clear that a woman is not going to deliver imminently, she can be transported to the labor and delivery area of the hospital or to another facility. The deci-

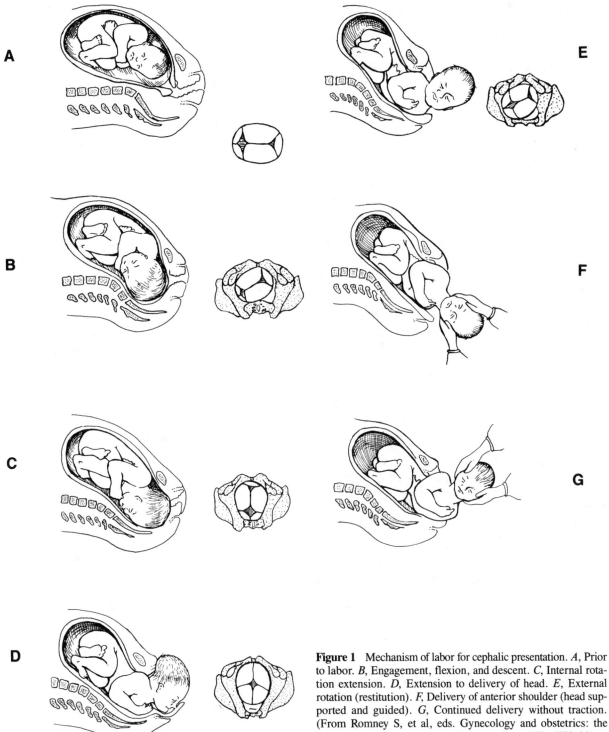

Figure 1 Mechanism of labor for cephalic presentation. *A*, Prior to labor. *B*, Engagement, flexion, and descent. *C*, Internal rotation extension. *D*, Extension to delivery of head. *E*, External rotation (restitution). *F*, Delivery of anterior shoulder (head supported and guided). *G*, Continued delivery without traction. (From Romney S, et al, eds. Gynecology and obstetrics: the health care of women. New York: McGraw-Hill, 1975:661.)

sion to transport is predicated on evaluation of the progression of labor versus the time required to get the mother to a delivery area. It is better to conduct delivery under controlled circumstances in the emergency department than in the cramped quarters of an elevator or an ambulance.

Under no circumstances should measures be taken to forestall delivery by holding a woman's legs together.

However, in selected cases it may be appropriate to begin *tocolysis* with a beta-adrenergic sympathomimetic to slow the progress of labor and allow transport to another facility. Agents available include terbutaline and ritodrine. Terbutaline can be given subcutaneously in a dose of 0.25 mg every 2 to 4 hours or as a continuous intravenous infusion starting at a dose of 10 to 20 μg per minute. Ritodrine is administered as a continuous intravenous infusion starting at a dose of 100 to 150 μg per minute. Toxic reactions to these agents include tachycardia, tachyarrhythmias, anxiety, hypotension, hyperglycemia, hypokalemia, ileus, and urinary retention. Beta-adrenergic sympathomimetic therapy usually should not be started if the cervix is dilated more than 5 cm.

SPONTANEOUS VAGINAL DELIVERY

When delivery is imminent, the patient should be placed in the dorsal lithotomy or lateral Sims' position. Use of the lateral position places less stress on the perineum and reduces the risk of laceration. With each push, more of the presenting part becomes visible, and the head extends under the pubis. Delivery of the head is aided by applying gentle upward pressure with the thumb and forefinger through the distended perineum while preventing overextension by applying downward pressure with the fingers of the other hand.

As soon as the head is delivered, the physician should check for a cord around the neck. If the cord is present and loose, it should be slipped over the anterior shoulder. If there are several tight loops of cord present, it may be impossible to slip them over the shoulder. Under these circumstances, the cord is doubly clamped and cut before the shoulders are delivered.

After the head has been delivered, the anterior shoulder rotates under the pubis and is delivered by gentle traction. The remainder of the infant is then delivered by continued gentle traction coupled with maternal pushing. Following delivery, the infant can be placed on the maternal abdomen while the cord is doubly clamped and cut. The newborn should be dried off promptly to prevent excessive cooling, and the nasopharynx should be suctioned with a bulb syringe if excessive secretions are present.

If the amniotic fluid is heavily stained with meconium, special precautions must be taken to prevent meconium aspiration. Following delivery of the head, the nasopharynx is thoroughly suctioned using a fine-gauge catheter and a DeLee suction trap. After delivery of the infant, the cords are inspected, and the trachea suctioned with an endotracheal tube. If meconium is aspirated from below the cords, the tube is reinserted and suction repeated until no more meconium is retrieved.

When the fetus is in a *breech presentation*, spontaneous delivery to the umbilicus should be allowed. The body is then pulled gently downward with the back toward the maternal pubis. When the scapula becomes visible under the pubis, two fingers are introduced beneath the pubic arch to a position in front of the fetal humerus, and the arm of the fetus is wiped down over its chest. The body is then lifted upward and the posterior arm delivered in a similar manner. The head can then be delivered by maintaining flexion with a finger in the fetal mouth while gentle upward traction is placed on the fetal trunk and shoulders.

RESUSCITATION OF THE NEWBORN

If the infant has not respired spontaneously by 1 minute after birth, resuscitation should be begun. The most important factor in treating neonatal apnea is thorough clearing of the airway. The infant's nasopharynx is cleared by suction, an oxygen mask is placed over the nose and mouth, and the physician or nurse stimulates the infant by rubbing its back and slapping its feet. If spontaneous respirations are not immediately forthcoming, positive pressure oxygen is given using pressures of 25 to 35 cm of water at a rate of 35 to 40 per minute. If the infant's respiration is severely depressed, consideration should be given to endotracheal intubation. A 2.0 to 3.5-mm tube is inserted under direct laryngoscopic view. The tube should go about 2 cm past the cords. Skill at neonatal intubation can be maintained by practicing on stillborn infants or on anesthetized cats.

OBSTETRIC LACERATIONS

Perineal lacerations are divided into four types depending on their depth. First-degree lacerations extend through the skin and the superficial tissues above the muscles. Second-degree lacerations involve the perineal muscles but not the rectal sphincter. Third-degree lacerations extend through the sphincter. Fourth-degree lacerations extend into the rectum itself. First and second-degree perineal lacerations should be repaired promptly with 3–0 chromic suture. Third-and fourth-degree lacerations require meticulous repair if anal function is to be maintained without fistula formation. Such repairs should usually be carried out by a physician familiar with the techniques of the repair.

Vaginal and cervical lacerations are rare in the absence of an instrument delivery. However, they can occur spontaneously and bleed profusely. When identified, they should be repaired with 3–0 chromic suture. Exposure can be difficult and may require the assistance of another physician or technician.

PLACENTAL DELIVERY

The third stage of labor usually lasts for 15 to 30 minutes. Signs of placental separation include a show of blood, advancement of the cord, a rising of the fundus, and a change in the shape of the uterus from discoid to globular. As the fundus becomes globular, placental delivery can be aided by downward pressure on the uterus with the palm of the hand. As the placenta enters the vagina, the uterus is pushed upward with the finger tips. Following delivery of the placenta, uterine contraction can be assured by the administration of 10 units of oxytocin intramuscularly.

POSTPARTUM HEMORRHAGE

Postpartum hemorrhage can be caused by retained placenta, placenta accreta, genital-tract lacerations, uterine inversion, and, most commonly, uterine atony. Whatever the cause, an intravenous infusion should be started through a large-bore catheter, blood should be crossmatched, and consultation should be obtained. If uterine atony is believed to be the cause based on a normal-appearing placenta, the absence of genital-tract lacerations, and the presence of a soft, boggy uterus, a uterotonic agent is begun. A rapid intravenous infusion of oxytocin (20 to 40 units in 1,000 ml of 5 percent dextrose in Ringer's lactate) is an appropriate first step. If atony persists, the patient is given 0.2 mg of methylergonovine by IV push. If this also fails, a prostaglandin preparation should be tried. One to 2 mg of prostaglandin F_2 alpha can be injected directly into the myometrium transabdominally. Alternatively, 250 to 500 μg of prostaglandin F_2 alpha-15-methyl is injected intramuscularly. The side effects of both prostaglandins include nausea, vomiting, diarrhea, hyperpyrexia, flushing, and bronchospasm in asthmatic individuals.

SUGGESTED READING

Oxorn H, Foote WR. Human labor and birth. New York: Appleton-Century-Crofts, 1975.

Pritchard JA, MacDonald PC, eds. Williams obstetrics. New York: Appleton-Century-Crofts, 1980.

PROBLEM DELIVERIES

ALAN J. MARGOLIS, M.D.

GENERAL PRINCIPLES

All the normal precautions and complications of childbirth must be sought in any delivery (see chapter on *Normal Delivery*). However, certain deliveries are particularly high risk or carry their own special complications. In any case in which a difficult or complicated labor is suspected, the mother should be given supplemental oxygen, 6 to 8 L per minute, by nasal prongs, a history of the last time fetal movement was felt should be elicited, and uterine contractions should be palpated and timed for frequency and duration. Fetal heart monitoring should be carried out (ideally with a Doppler monitor) continuously or at very frequent intervals. Normal fetal heart rate is 120 to 160 beats per minute; this may decrease by 20 to 40 beats per minute during a contraction with return to the normal baseline as the contraction ends (early deceleration, attributed to fetal head compression). If the decrease in fetal heart rate begins later in the contraction and persists after the contraction ends—late deceleration—there is evidence of uteroplacental insufficiency and possible fetal hypoxia. Decelerations which are inconsistently related to contractions in time and are changeable in rate (variable deceleration) are evidence of cord compression. Vaginal examination to rule out cord prolapse is indicated and changes in maternal position are required (Fig. 1). A rate of 90 beats per minute or less documents severe fetal distress.

An obstetric delivery pack and infant resuscitation equipment should be made ready (see chapter on *Complications of Late Pregnancy*), and the obstetrician and pediatrician should be called immediately. The emergency physician must monitor mother and fetus closely until their arrival and be prepared to deliver the infant immediately if fetal distress becomes severe.

IMPENDING DELIVERY OF A PREMATURE INFANT

The delivery of a premature infant with the vertex as the presenting part requires careful control of the delivery of the head to prevent rapid decompression changes in the cerebral vasculature. This may require a small episiotomy.

Intact membranes minimize pressure on the presenting part and also slow delivery, allowing maximal stretching of the cervix. Membranes should not be artificially ruptured until delivery is imminent. A premature infant may require immediate resuscitation after delivery, and appropriate equipment and additional personnel should be available to assist in newborn ventilation, possible intubation, and maintenance of circulation. The prevention of hypothermia can be accomplished by immediate drying of the infant and wrapping him or her with blankets.

Breech deliveries are more frequent in premature labors and may be difficult mechanically because the aftercoming head is significantly larger than the body and shoulders. Cervical dilation sufficient to deliver the baby's body may be insufficient to allow the shoulders and head to deliver easily. Allow as much of the breech as possible to deliver spontaneously; the lower extremities and body will usually do so unaided (Fig. 2). Avoid cord tension or traction after the umbilicus appears. Gentle downward traction on the baby's hips and rotation will deliver the scapulae. The fetal arms are easily swept across the front of the body. With body lying over the forearm and the hands in the vagina, a finger can be placed in the baby's mouth. With this maneuver, flexion of the head can be accomplished, thus minimizing the dimensions of the head that pass through the cervix (Fig. 3).

Dührssen's incisions into the cervix at 10, 2 and 6 o'clock can be used to increase cervical dilation in the presence of a *trapped head*. Incisions are made entirely through the cervix to the vaginal-cervical junction. Oxygen should be administered to the mother continuously and constant Doppler (or fetal heart sound) monitoring of the fetus carried out. This heroic procedure is only warranted in the presence of an obviously viable fetus when simpler maneuvers to deliver the aftercoming head have failed. If used, it should be done in a timely fashion before profound fetal distress occurs, not as a delayed final resort. If the obstetrician is not physically present to perform it, simpler maneuvers have failed, and fetal distress is present, the procedure should be performed immediately by the available physician.

Compound presentations are more common in premature births before 28 weeks. A foot can be distinguished from a hand by searching for the obvious prominence of the heel. Hand-vertex presenting parts offer no problems and usually evolve spontaneously. Hand-foot presentations occur with transverse lie and are sometimes associated with cord prolapse. Operative delivery with anesthesia is often necessary and will minimize maternal injury in the face of uncertain fetal survival. Immediate transfer of patients with compound presentation fetuses to the delivery area is imperative.

PRECIPITATE DELIVERIES

Short first stages of labor and rapid deliveries are often associated with degrees of fetal asphyxia. Very frequent contractions may have threatened uterine circulation and fetal gas exchange. This must be sought for in the neonate and treated.

RETAINED PLACENTA

In the absence of heavy vaginal bleeding, retention of the placenta after delivery of the child can be managed expectantly. Intravenous infusion of dilute oxytocin (10 U in 1,000 ml of lactated Ringer's solution) will increase uterine contractility and allow spontaneous passage of the placenta into the vagina. Vaginal examination to confirm the presence of the placenta in the vagina is more advisable than cord traction.

In the absence of heavy bleeding, a placenta remaining in situ for over 30 minutes should be removed manually. This can be performed effectively in a delivery unit under appropriate general anesthesia.

PROLAPSE OF THE UMBILICAL CORD

The presence in the vagina or at the vulva of a pulsating umbilical cord requires immediate attempts to relieve cord pressure and minimize chilling, which would cause umbilical artery spasm. The possibility of an immediate delivery should be ruled out by vaginal examination. Then the patient should be placed in the knee-chest position, high-flow oxygen administered, and if possible, the cord replaced in the vagina to minimize temperature change. Transfer to the delivery room for immediate cesarean section is mandatory. The patient can be transported in the knee-chest position with the appropriate attendants to aid in relieving pressure of the presenting part on the prolapsed umbilical cord.

In the presence of a pulseless cord and obvious fetal death, a vaginal delivery can be expected unless cephalopelvic disproportion or abnormal presentation (transverse lie) precludes it. Further evaluation by ultrasonography and follow-up examination in the delivery areas are indicated.

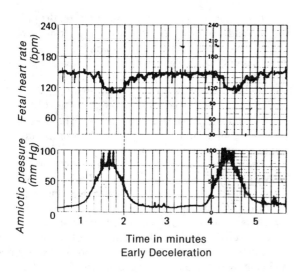

Time in minutes
Early Deceleration

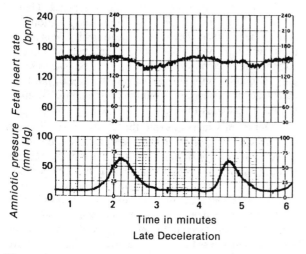

Time in minutes
Late Deceleration

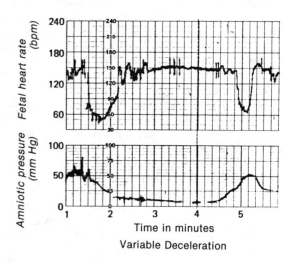

Time in minutes
Variable Deceleration

Figure 1   The relationship of fetal heart rate decelerations to uterine contractions. (From Benson R, ed. Current obstetric and gynecologic diagnosis and treatment. Los Altos, California: Lange Medical Publishers, 1978.)

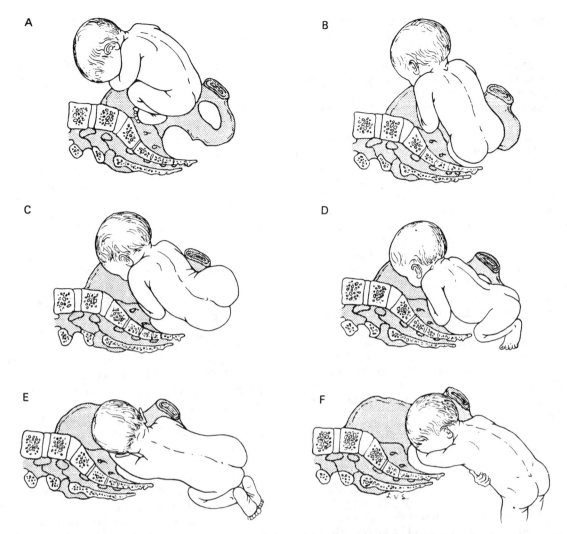

Figure 2 Mechanism of labor for breech presentation. *A*, Prior to labor. *B*, Engagement of the buttocks, internal rotation. *C*, Lateral flexion of the trunk, delivery of the buttocks. *D*, External rotation of the buttocks, engagement of the shoulders. *E*, Internal rotation of the shoulders, delivery of the posterior shoulder. *F*, Lateral flexion of the trunk, delivery of the anterior shoulder. (From Benson R, ed. Current obstetric and gynecologic diagnosis and treatment. Los Altos, California: Lange Medical Publishers, 1978:406–407)

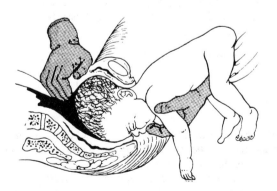

Figure 3 Delivery of head in breech presentation: fingers inserted in mouth help flex the neck and deliver the occiput. (From Benson R, ed. Current obstetric and gynecologic diagnosis and treatment. Los Altos, California: Lange Medical Publishers, 1978:408.)

MULTIPLE BIRTHS

Premature labor often occurs in women with multiple fetuses. Immediate assessment to ascertain whether fetal membranes are intact and whether dilation of the cervix is 4 cm or less is important. Women in early pre-term labor (20 to 34 weeks) are candidates for suppression of contractions. Immediate transfer to the labor area is indicated for intravenous administration of ritodrine (Yutopar) or other tocolytic agents. If the delivery of the first of multiple births is at hand or has been accomplished, assessment of the remaining fetuses is indicated. Depending on size, position, and fetal heart stability, there is usually time for transfer to the delivery area for further treatment.

THE LABORING PATIENT IN SHOCK WITHOUT EXTERNAL BLEEDING

After immediate maternal resuscitative efforts with large-bore intravenous lines and crystalloid infusion and verification of fetal heart rate, concealed hemorrhage or uterine rupture must be ruled out. Vaginal examination is indicated to assess whether delivery is imminent. Severe concealed hemorrhage from a premature separation of the normally implanted placenta (abruptio placentae) is associated with marked abdominal pain and a tense tetanic uterus. Disseminated intravascular coagulation may have occurred, and blood should be drawn for assessment of clotting factors (platelets, prothrombin time, partial prothrombin time, fibrinogen, and fibrin split products). Transfer to the delivery area for immediate termination of pregnancy and for further therapy is indicated.

Ruptured uterus is a consideration in patients with prior uterine surgery (myomectomy or cesarean section) or multiparas with long labors and possible cephalopelvic disproportion. Some patients report a sense of 'tearing' as the uterus separates. Subsequently there is increased abdominal pain as peritoneal surfaces are irritated. Uterine contractions cease. Physical examination confirms lack of uterine contractions and may detect a more clearly defined fetal outline if the separation is large enough to allow escape of the fetus. Localized tenderness can be observed if the uterine rupture is small or within the lower uterine segment, which is extraperitoneal below the vesicouterine fold of peritoneum. Intraperitoneal bleeding can occur from the placental site, uterine wall, or uterine vessels. Immediate transfer to the delivery area is indicated.

THE LABORING PATIENT WITH SHOCK AND EXTERNAL BLEEDING

Significant premature separation of the normally implanted placenta or placenta previa is most likely. In either case, prompt attention to maternal vital signs with initiation of intravenous support should be followed by transfer to the delivery area for more specific therapy. Vaginal examinations are contraindicated, as they may accelerate bleeding from a placenta previa.

MECONIUM IN THE AMNIOTIC FLUID

Because of the possibility of meconium aspiration at the onset of respiration after delivery, the nares and pharynx of the newborn should be aspirated as the head delivers. A DeLee trap is especially useful because it frees the attendant's hands for delivery. A direct laryngoscopy and suction below the vocal cords further ensure minimal meconium inhalation into the alveoli of the lungs.

SHOULDER DYSTOCIA

Following delivery of the fetal head, the shoulders generally follow with ease. With the patient in the lithotomy position, downward traction on the fetal head assists the delivery of the anterior shoulder, and the posterior shoulder follows promptly with upward traction.

If this classic maneuver is unsuccessful, shoulder impaction should be suspected. Immediately, a hand should be placed in the vagina along the baby's back to attempt rotation of the anterior shoulder into the oblique position, which allows more room for passage of the shoulder into the pelvis.

If the anterior shoulder does not pass into the pelvis with this maneuver, the posterior arm should be sought, quickly changing examining hands to allow easy palpation of the ventral surface of the child. The humerus should be identified, and the posterior forearm brought down. With arm traction the posterior shoulder should deliver into the pelvis and allow the anterior shoulder to follow.

Brachial plexus injuries occur due to prolonged, repetitive attempts to deliver the anterior shoulder, during which the neck is stretched while the shoulder is immobilized at the pelvic inlet. Accidental fracture of the humerus or clavicle can occur during attempts to deliver the shoulders by intravaginal maneuvers. These fractures generally heal without difficulty and present no problem of chronic disability, unlike a brachial plexus injury.

SUGGESTED READING

Pritchard JA, MacDonald PC, Gant NF. Williams Obstetrics. 17th ed. Connecticut: Norwalk, Appleton-Century-Crofts, 1985.

PUERPERAL AND POSTABORTAL INFECTION

ROBERT KIWI, M.D., M.R.C.O.G., F.A.C.O.G.

Puerperal infection includes all infections of the genital tract (and extragenital) following delivery (or abortion), characterized by a fever of 38 °C or more on two occasions after the first 24 hours and within 10 days postpartum or following abortion.

The most commonly seen puerperal infections are (1) endometritis, often with extension resulting in pelvic peritonitis and in severe instances in a pelvic abscess; (2) further extension of this infective process may result in septic pelvic thrombophlebitis; (3) urinary tract infections; (4) breast infections, and (5) cesarean section wound infections (Table 1).

TABLE 1 Sites of Puerperal Infection

Genital
    Salpingitis
    Endometritis
    Parametritis
    Peritonitis (pelvic abscess)

Extragenital
    Urinary tract infection
    Breast infection
    Septic thrombophlebitis
    Wound infection
        Abdominal (following cesarean section)
        Episiotomy

PREDISPOSING CAUSES

The most frequent predisposing cause of puerperal infection in current obstetric practice is probably operative delivery, e.g., cesarean section or forceps delivery associated with intrauterine manipulation. Other factors include prolonged rupture of the membranes and prolonged labor. Premature rupture of the membranes and chorioamnionitis also are associated with postpartum endometritis. Retained products of conception in the post abortal group is the most frequent cause of endometritis.

Patients in the lower socio-economic groups are predisposed to infection, especially if associated with prolonged rupture of membranes or cesarean section.

POSTPARTUM ENDOMETRITIS

Patients presenting in the emergency department following delivery frequently complain of fever and abdominal pain. A thorough history should be taken. This should include the type of delivery, duration of labor and ruptured membranes, and immediate postpartum course.

Examination should include a general physical examination with emphasis on abdominal and pelvic examination. Uterine tenderness is a significant feature of postpartum endometritis. Uterine enlargement (or failure of involution) is often present. Pelvic examination shows the presence of profuse, foul-smelling vaginal discharge. The cervix is open and often is tender on movement.

Evaluation

1. Complete blood count with differential.
2. Blood cultures (if temperature is higher than 39 °C).
3. Urine culture.
4. Endometrial culture (transcervical), aerobic and anaerobic.

Initial Management

At the time of pelvic examination, confirm that the uterus is draining adequately. If doubt exists, then the passage of a ring forceps into the uterus to open the cervix and allow free drainage may be of value.

Ultrasound evaluation to exclude the diagnosis of retained products of conception is occasionally necessary.

Ergotrate maleate, 0.2 mg orally 2 to 4 times per day, given to stimulate uterine contraction is often helpful to expel retained blood and necrotic debris.

Antibiotic therapy should be instituted without waiting for culture results. The majority of pathogenic organisms respond to a broad-spectrum antibiotic combination, e.g., ampicillin and gentamicin or the newer cephalosporins.

Patients with mild symptoms may be evaluated and outpatient treatment initiated in the emergency department. Follow-up should be in 1 to 2 days to determine response. Initial treatment with ampicillin, 500 mg 4 times a day, or tetracycline, 500 mg 4 times a day. When the physician is suspicious of gram-negative anaerobic organisms, Flagyl, 250 mg 3 times a day, may be added to the treatment.

Patients with severe symptoms or illness with nausea or vomiting are admitted and given intravenous antibiotic therapy, intravenous ampicillin, 1 to 2 g every 6 hours, and gentamicin, 60 to 80 mg, every 8 hours. When a strong suspicion of gram-negative anaerobic organisms (*Bacteroides fragilis*) exists, then the addition of clindamycin, 600 mg every 8 hours, is suggested. Use of the cephalosporins, e.g., Mefoxin, may eliminate multiple antibiotic therapy in the initial therapy.

Additional in-hospital procedures may include curettage to remove retained products of conception, if fairly rapid response to antibiotic therapy is not noted or ultrasonography suggests the presence of retained products of conception.

PELVIC ABSCESS

Pelvic abscess is usually seen in association with endometritis or parametritis that has failed to respond to antibiotics, or in the patient who presents after the infectious process is well established. Patients present to the emergency department with fever, abdominal pain, abdominal swelling, or nausea and vomiting and with either constipation or diarrhea.

Examination may be difficult if the patient has had a cesarean section or if significant abdominal swelling is present. If a pelvic abscess is suspected but not confirmed on clinical examination, ultrasonography will be helpful to outline the mass.

Evaluation in the emergency department should include

1. Complete blood count with differential.
2. X-ray films of the abdomen in the supine and erect positions.
3. Urine and blood endometrial cultures.
4. Ultrasonography.
5. Blood for electrolyte levels and renal and hepatic function studies.

Management in the emergency department should start with intravenous fluids and broad-spectrum antibiotics given intravenously once material for cultures has been obtained.

Gynecologic consultation should be obtained, as these patients need admission to the hosptial.

Management in the hospital consists of intravenously administered antibiotics, intravenous fluids, and gastrointestinal rest by not allowing the patient anything by mouth. Nursing in a modified Fowlers position will help to localize the abscess to the cul-de-sac to aid in drainage. Once the abscess points either to the posterior fornix or abdominally, then drainage will be necessary. This generally results in rapid resolution.

SEPTIC PELVIC THROMBOPHLEBITIS

The patient who has postpartum endometritis and who is not responding to adequate therapy either requires a change of antibiotic based on available bacteriologic information or further evaluation, which may reveal the presence of a pelvic abscess. In some cases neither of these complications may exist and the diagnosis of septic thrombophlebitis should be considered.

Patients with septic thrombophlebitis have abdominal tenderness, and on pelvic examination a subinvoluted tender uterus is felt. Tenderness over the hypogastric vessels is noted bilaterally along with tachycardia. Occasionally, chest pain or bloody sputum or both suggest that embolization has already occurred.

When the diagnosis of septic pelvic thrombophlebitis is suspected, urine, blood, and endometrial cultures should be obtained. Chest films, ECG, and a lung scan (^{125}I) also should be obtained.

Management that should be initiated in the emergency department, if possible, includes broad-spectrum intravenous antibiotics. Heparinization should be begun once the diagnosis is confirmed.

Further in-hospital procedures may include laparotomy with inferior vena caval ligation and, in certain circumstances, removal of all septic foci. This may require hysterectomy with or without bilateral salpingo-oophorectomy. Antibiotics and heparin should be continued for 10 days and prolonged anti-coagulation therapy continued when pulmonary embolization has been confirmed.

BREAST INFECTION (PUERPERAL MASTITIS)

Puerperal mastitis is a bacterial inflammatory disease of nursing mothers. It is usually unilateral and can rapidly convert to a breast abscess if therapy is not instituted. Breast infections commonly occur in the second or third week postpartum.

Patients present with breast tenderness and enlargement. The breast shows cutaneous erythema; fever with chills is often present. Breast engorgement should not be confused with this condition; it is mostly bilateral and is also associated with a slight fever. The breast(s) show marked distention but no localized tenderness or redness.

Antibiotics should be started immediately. The most frequent choice of antibiotic is ampicillin, 2 g per day in divided doses continuously for 5 days. Alternative drugs include dicloxacillin or cephalosporin or erythromycin in the penicillin-allergic patient. This topic is also discussed in the chapter on *Lactation Disorders and Mastitis*.

BREAST ABSCESS

In those instances where there is a delay in diagnosis and treatment, a breast abscess may develop. The abscess is obvious on examination; the patient is in much pain, with significant swelling and superficial edema and redness of the breast. The abscess may be evident as a fluctuant mass. Surgical drainage and antibiotic therapy are needed (chapter on *Lactation Disorders and Mastitis*).

PUERPERAL URINARY TRACT INFECTION

Urinary tract infections are the next most common cause of puerperal pyrexia after endometritis. *Escherichia coli* is the infective organism in the vast majority of cases.

During pregnancy, urinary tract infections are more common because of urinary stasis, dilation of the ureter, and ureteric reflux. In the postpartum patient the predisposing factors include catheterization during labor, prolonged labor, and difficult or traumatic delivery.

Patients present with symptoms of acute cystitis and on occasion urinary retention leading to cystitis. Cystitis may be complicated by ascending infection leading to pyelonephritis.

Evaluation should include urinalysis and a clean-catch urine specimen for culture and sensitivity testing. Spun deposits will show the presence of white and red blood cells. The presence of nitrites and tests for leukocytes on the urine dipstix assist in the diagnosis.

Patients should be advised to take additional oral fluids. In patients who have urinary retention or in those who have had significant trauma a Foley catheter should be placed for from 24 to 48 hours, to allow edema to resolve. These patients most often require hospitalization. Trimethoprim (160 mg) and sulfisoxazole (800 mg), twice a day, or ampicillin, 250 mg every 6 hours, is given orally for 10 days for complete treatment. Following cessation of treatment, a repeat urine culture should be obtained and the patient retreated if the infection is not cleared completely.

PUERPERAL WOUND INFECTIONS

Abdominal incisions may become infected and patients may present occasionally after being discharged from the hospital with significant fever, swelling, and redness of the incision. The incision may be fluctuant in a particular area, and in such cases opening the incision, taking a culture sample, and allowing free drainage of the pus or infected hematoma are indicated. Use of a broad-spectrum antibiotic often aids in the resolution; however, continued drainage and irrigation are required. Patients should have frequent follow-up examination to assess adequacy of treatment until it is clear that the wound is healing appropriately. Secondary closure of incisions is occasionally required.

Occasionally patients present with fever and perineal pain, and examination reveals an infected episiotomy. Drainage of the stitch abscess or ischiorectal abscess (with large mediolateral episiotomies) is required. Frequent sitz baths are necessary, and use of broad-spectrum antibiotics is recommended.

POSTABORTAL INFECTION

Induced abortion is a frequent procedure in freestanding clinics. Following the abortion, patients are mostly given follow-up advice. Occasionally, patients present in the emergency department following an induced abortion complaining of fever and abdominal pain. They may also have a varying amount of vaginal bleeding. Most frequently the diagnosis of retained products of conception associated with infection can be made clinically by finding fever, abdominal tenderness, pelvic tenderness, and an enlarged tender uterus with an open cervix. Products of conception may or may not be evident in the cervix or vagina or both.

Included in the differential diagnosis is ectopic pregnancy, although these patients are usually not febrile, but have abdominal pain and persistent vaginal bleeding.

Careful evaluation is required and gynecologic consultation is necessary, as these patients most often require admission. Intravenous broad-spectrum antibiotics (e.g., Mefoxin) should be used preoperatively with intravenous Pitocin (or Ergotrate) to aid uterine contractions and promote expulsion of products of conception and blood clots. This should be started in the emergency department once the diagnosis has been confirmed. Ultrasonography may be necessary in cases where ectopic pregnancy cannot be ruled out. This will reveal intrauterine echoes and dilation of the endometrial canal with no adnexal masses in cases of incomplete abortion with sepsis.

Following hospitalization, repeat curettage is necessary under antibiotic cover. A rapid response is usually seen.

SUGGESTED READING

Cavanagh D, Woods RE, O'Connor TCF, Knuppel RA. Obstetric emergencies. 3rd ed. Philadelphia: Harper and Row, 1982:81.

Monif GRG. Infectious diseases in obstetrics and gynecology. 2nd ed. Philadelphia: Harper and Row, 1982:377.

Pritchard JA. Williams Obstetrics. 17th ed. New York: Appleton-Century-Crofts, 1984:719.

LACTATION DISORDERS AND MASTITIS

MAX BORTEN, M.D.

Early discharge from the hospital following delivery is currently the norm. In most instances, mothers are sent home before lactation is well established. The opportunity to teach about and observe problems that appear in the immediate postpartum period is thus foreshortened. Patients must be encouraged to communicate symptoms of breast disease to their physicians as they appear. These include sore nipples, painful breasts, localized inflammation or swelling or both, and fever or chills.

BREAST ENGORGEMENT

Breast engorgement is a common occurrence during the early puerperium. It usually begins during the second or third postpartum day. The breasts become full, hard, warm, and tender to palpation. The patient complains of throbbing and aching pain that is only relieved when she is lying on her back.

Initially, breast engorgement is produced by the increased vascularity and lymphatic distention that precede lactation. Manual expression or mechanical pumping is not productive and may be traumatic. At this early stage, the mother should be advised to wear a well-fitting brassiere 24 hours a day. If left alone, the engorgement will subside as the milk begins to flow. The breast becomes progressively softer thereafter.

Accumulation of milk within the lacteals and lactiferous ducts as a result of poor emptying may lead to severe engorgement. The breasts become much fuller and very tender. The areola becomes engorged, obliterating the nipple. The axillary region is extremely painful as a result of tension on Cooper's ligament.

Therapy is essentially symptomatic. The mother should be encouraged to continue breast-feeding to relieve the distention owing to the accumulation of milk. Manual expression or mechanical pumping is helpful. This permits manual compression of the areola so that the nipples regain their original shape. Breast massage in a radial fashion (from the periphery to the areola) will soften the peripheral lobules.

Emptying the gland is the appropriate treatment. Mild analgesics (e.g., codeine) provide temporary relief. Cold packs are said to help some patients during the early stages of engorgement by reducing vascularity. Warm packs or a warm shower may be helpful at a later stage. A tight brassiere provides relief by supporting the engorged breasts. The patient may require hypnotic medication to obtain some rest.

Breast engorgement can also be seen when breast-feeding is abruptly halted. Its presentation is similar to that which occurs in the immediate postpartum period.

Treatment is symptomatic. Support of the breasts by a tight binder and cold packs has proved effective.

SORE NIPPLES

Some nipple tenderness is common during the first days of nursing. Its persistence or progression requires measures to avoid cracking the nipple. Painful nipples are frequently given as the reason for mothers to abandon breast-feeding during the first few postpartum days.

Breast-feeding can be successfully continued in most instances. Steps to be taken to improve and prevent recurrence of nipple soreness include the following. (1) Prolonged nursing should be avoided. Manual initiation of milk flow hastens the let-down reflex and shortens feeding time. Initiation of feeding at the healthy breast also facilitates the let-down reflex, reducing the force exerted on the nipple by the infant to extract milk. (2) Nipples should be exposed to air for 15 to 20 minutes after each feeding. Anhydrous lanolin cream or vitamin A and D ointment applied to the irritated area between feedings promotes healing. (3) Nipples should be rinsed with plain water. Washing the breasts with soap and water before feedings dries the skin and may cause sore nipples. Nursing brassieres ought to be rinsed thoroughly to eliminate any residue of detergent that will irritate the nipple between feedings. (4) A soft, clean cloth can be used to cover the nipples between feedings. (5) Breast engorgement must be avoided because it flattens the nipple. This makes sucking more difficult and the infant tends to irritate the nipple further.

CRACKED NIPPLES

A nursing woman complaining of sore nipples must be evaluated for the presence of nipple fissures, which can be exquisitely painful. Nipple cracks can be circular on the nipple-areolar junction or vertical on its long axis.

Treatment consists of (1) discontinuing feedings from the affected breast for 24 to 48 hours. (2) To prevent engorgement, the breast should be manually expressed or pumped. (3) Gently apply a small amount of breast milk over the injured nipple and allow it to air dry. (4) Analgesics, when required, must be short-acting (e.g., codeine) and given immediately after nursing. (5) Lanolin cream or vitamin A and D ointment or both are useful. Use small amounts to avoid the need for removal of the remnant before the next feeding. (6) If nursing with the affected breast is continued, the use of a nipple shield is required to prevent further irritation to the cracked nipple.

GALACTOCELE

Galactoceles, also known as milk-retention cysts, are usually the result of the occlusion of the lactiferous duct. They may affect one or more lobules. The patient presents with a painful breast in which a lump or cyst can be easily identified. The cyst and surrounding tissue are sensitive to touch but show no sign of inflammation. Pain is usually caused by pressure on the contiguous glandular tissue.

The content of the cyst is at first pure milk. The mass is ordinarily fluctuant on palpation. Compression of the cyst may result in milk secretion. Spontaneous resolution is not unusual. If the cystic enlargement does not subside within 24 to 48 hours, aspiration is indicated. The patient should refrain from massaging the breast.

Because the lactating woman is not immune to breast cancer, ultrasonographic evaluation should be done. It will generally confirm the cystic nature of the mass. Aspiration of the fluid-filled cyst can be performed under local anesthesia. Breast-feeding does not have to be discontinued. Infection rarely ensues.

PUERPERAL MASTITIS

At present, infection of the lactating breast is a sporadic event. It is commonly seen between the second and third postpartum weeks. A moderate degree of breast engorgement routinely precedes the appearance of puerperal mastitis. The mother relates progressive breast discomfort between feedings. Increased unilateral mammary pain differentiates a bacterial inflammatory process from functional breast engorgement.

The lactating woman complains of pain localized over a segment of the affected breast. Intralobular involvement produces a wedge-shaped area of cellulitis. This portion of gland feels hard on palpation. Breast discomfort may become exaggerated during nursing. A low-grade fever of 24 to 48 hours' duration may be reported preceding the appearance of chills and temperature spikes to 40° C (104° F). The breast becomes progressively hard and reddened. Generalized malaise is not uncommon.

Staphylococcus aureus is the organism most commonly found in patients with puerperal mastitis. The mother is usually infected by her newborn infant, who has been colonized within the nursery by a nosocomial coagulase-positive penicillin-resistant *Staphylococcus*. The infant may be totally asymptomatic. It is unclear if the presence of nipple cracks is essential for bacterial invasion to occur. The offending organism may gain access to the gland through its lactiferous ducts.

Complete resolution within 36 to 48 hours accompanies prompt diagnosis and treatment. Culture of the expressed milk is indicated before therapy is initiated. The choice of antibiotics is influenced by the prevalent type of staphylococcal organism in the hospital in which the woman delivered (the nursery in particular).

Initial therapy consists of the following measures. (1) Give oral antibiotics, e.g., a penicillinase-resistant penicillin such as dicloxacillin, 125 to 250 mg every 6 hours for 10 days. Cephalosporins and erythromycin have also proved effective. (2) Nursing from the affected breast must be discontinued. (3) A tightly fitted brassiere provides adequate support. (4) Cold packs and mild analgesics are useful measures for symptomatic relief. Nursing from the inflamed breast may be resumed after the mother has remained afebrile for 24 hours.

BREAST ABSCESS

Suppuration with abscess formation may complicate puerperal mastitis. Persistence of fever and chills beyond 48 hours after therapy has been initiated alerts the physician to this possibility. Delayed initiation of therapy for puerperal mastitis is usually contributory.

A segment of breast appears inflamed, hardened, and tender on palpation. Fluctuation can sometimes be observed. Persistent mastitis despite appropriate therapy may indicate a deeply located abscess even in the absence of the aforementioned clinical signs.

Treatment of a breast abscess is surgical, by drainage. Antibiotic therapy alone is not sufficient. Evacuation of the purulent material can be accomplished by repeated aspiration with a large-bore needle. When more than one lobe is involved, multiple abscess cavities are to be expected. Incision and drainage of all loculations are the appropriate therapy. This is best performed under general anesthesia. Antibiotic therapy must be continued until healing is completed. It is prudent to discontinue nursing.

SUGGESTED READING

Lawrence RA. Breastfeeding. A guide for the medical profession, 2nd ed. St. Louis: C.V. Mosby Company, 1985.

Marshall BR, Hepper JK, Zirbel CC. Sporadic puerperal mastitis. An infection that need not interrupt lactation. JAMA 1975; 233:1377.

Thomsen AC, Hansen KB, Moller BR. Leukocyte counts and microbiologic cultivation in the diagnosis of puerperal mastitis. Am J Obstet Gynecol 1983; 146:938.

Tyson JE, Zacur HA. Diagnosis and treatment of abnormal lactation. Clin Obstet Gynecol 1975; 18:65.

RAPE

G. RICHARD BRAEN, M.D., F.A.C.E.P.

The number of reported rapes in the United States has increased dramatically over the past 10 years, and it is now estimated that about one in six adult females will be the victim of either rape or attempted rape. More of these victims currently seek care on their own at emergency departments or are brought there by police for evaluation than in the past, and emergency physicians and nurses are being asked to provide evaluation and care for them. Unfortunately, these victims often arrive at times when either the patient load is great or the staffing is low. Rapes occur most frequently between 8 PM and 2 AM, on weekends, and during warm weather months. Fortunately, there is an increased understanding of the unique needs of rape victims by hospital personnel, and their care has improved significantly over the past few years. Some emergency departments have been designated as "rape evaluation" centers, particularly in urban areas, but any emergency department may at some time be called upon to evaluate and care for a victim of rape, and each department should be adequately prepared to provide appropriate, timely care.

PREPARATION

Few types of emergencies require as much preparation for management as rape cases. This preparation extends not only to the hospital and its staff but also to the community and to all the resources available for the psychological, legal, and medical support that is needed.

Preparations by the emergency staff includes cooperative educational meetings with the police, prosecuting attorneys, crime laboratory representatives, hospital laboratory representatives, rape crisis center volunteers, ambulance personnel, nurses, and physicians. From these meetings, protocols for total medical-psychological and legal care can be generated so that no aspect will be overlooked. Each step, from the initial contact, through the emergency department visit, through the police investigation, and through a potential court case and beyond should be analyzed so that it can be complete and achieved within a minimal time frame and without confusion or indecision.

At a minimum, preparation within the hospital should include the establishment of a sexual assault protocol, the assembly of appropriate forms, and the collection of all necessary equipment into a "rape evaluation kit" (Table 1). Provisions should also be planned for patient privacy, utilizing a separate area in or near the emergency department if possible.

PRE-HOSPITAL CARE

There are three primary principles of pre-hospital care for rape victims: (1) preservation of life or limb, (2) reassurance to the victim of safety without being condemnatory, and (3) preservation of evidence. Occasionally, rape victims are severely injured, sometimes with bodily parts mutilated or amputated, and the first priority for their pre-hospital care is the preservation of life and limb. This extremely simple, routine step may be overlooked during the confusion and anxiety generated by a "rape case." Usually, injuries are not this severe, and the major job in the pre-hospital phase is to assure the victim that she is safe and to listen to her in an empathetic, noncondemning manner. This initial compassion frequently sets the psychological stage for the further evaluation and treatment of the victim.

It is also important that the pre-hospital personnel avoid the inadvertent destruction of evidence that may be

TABLE 1 Basic Rape Examination Kit

Contents	Purpose
Paper bags	Clothing collection
Two urine containers	Urine for pregnancy test and drug screen
Fingernail file and envelope	Fingernail scrapings
Forceps, scissors, envelope	Pubic hair trimming
Plastic comb, large paper towel, envelope	Pubic hair combing
Vaginal speculum, aspiration pipette, red-topped test tube and stopper	Aspiration of vaginal contents
Two glass slides (one frosted at one end), two cotton-tipped swabs, red-topped test tube and stopper, pencil for marking slide	Swabbing of vagina
10 ml of saline, aspiration pipette and bulb, test tube	Vaginal washing
Cervical scraper, slides, Pap smear fixative	Pap smear
Thayer-Martin plates or Transgrow media, cotton-tipped swabs	Gonorrhea culture
Three cotton-tipped swabs and a test tube or an envelope	Saliva for secretor status
Three red-topped test tubes, tourniquet, nonalcohol swab to prepare skin, syringe, and needle	Blood samples
Appropriate laboratory forms, rape examination forms, labels for samples, camera and film (optional)	
5 ml of toluidine blue dye	Vaginal laceration examination

(From Braen GR. Sexual assault. In: Rosen P, et al, eds. Emergency medicine, concepts and clinical practice. St. Louis: CV Mosby, 1983.)

vital to the case. The scene of the crime should not be disturbed, and no physical evidence should be altered. If it is necessary to partially disrobe a victim to start intravenous lines or apply traction or compression dressings, clothing should be carefully cut along the seams so that potential damage to the clothing from the sexual assault itself is not altered. A carefully documented report should be generated for inclusion in the medical record, in the event that the case comes to court.

MANAGEMENT IN THE EMERGENCY DEPARTMENT

In the following discussion, assume that the patient does not have life- or limb-threatening injuries. If these were present, they would take priority and would need to be brought under control before further evaluation for the rape itself was conducted.

As soon as a rape victim arrives in the emergency department, she should be escorted to a private area and should not be left alone. Here, in private, *consent* for evaluation, treatment, and release of information to the police should be obtained. It should be remembered that the victim has the right to refuse evaluation and release of information to the police. She may, for example, choose to be evaluated purely medically, but she should be made fully

aware that unless the evidence is collected in a timely fashion, it may be lost for future use if she later decides to prosecute the assailant. Witnessed, written, informed consent should be obtained before proceeding. Obtaining consent, however, should not take absolute precedence over the assurance to the patient that she is safe and that you care about her condition.

The history of the rape and of pertinent medical conditions may be obtained by a trained nurse (and then confirmed by a physician) or by a physician. The medical history is divided into two parts: general medical and gynecologic. The history of the rape should not be the exhaustive type that will later be obtained by the police, since the chances that two extensive histories (police and hospital) will contain discrepancies are great, and these discrepancies may weaken a case. The history obtained by the physician or nurse should concentrate on those elements that direct the examining physician toward areas that might produce the most evidence or that allow the physician to best treat the patient medically. Questions regarding color of the assailant's hair or the type of his car are better left to the police, who routinely obtain this type of information and are appropriately trained.

The history of the event should include the following: time, date, and place of the rape, a description of the use of force or threats of force, and the type of assault. Knowledge of the place where the rape occurred (such as on a beach or in the woods) may lead the examiner to look for bits of sand, leaves, or other residue on the clothing or body of the victim. The assault itself may have simply involved fondling, but may also have involved vaginal, oral, or anal penetration, ejaculation on or in the victim, use of a condom, or insertion of a foreign body such as a knife, a stick, or a bottle into the vagina or anus. A history should also be obtained regarding other injuries, use of alcohol or drugs, and any loss of consciousness. The goal of this portion of the history is to establish a basis from which a physical examination will further evaluate the use of force, restraint, alcohol or drugs, and the type of sexual assault that occurred.

A basic gynecologic history should be obtained to help plan for medical treatment of the patient should therapy be needed. This history includes the use of birth control measures, last normal menstrual period, last voluntary intercourse, gravidity and parity, recent gynecologic therapy, and recent venereal disease. This information is for medical purposes only and may be suppressed by a judge if the case is litigated.

Further medical history includes the current use of both prescription and over-the-counter medications, tetanus immunization status, and allergies. It should be noted whether or not, following the assault, the victim changed clothing, bathed, douched, defecated, urinated, used a mouthwash, or brushed her teeth (the last two are important if oral sodomy occurred.)

PHYSICAL EXAMINATION

The purpose of the physical examination is twofold: medical and legal. Medically, the examination aids in the establishment of a data base for treatment of injuries or concomitant medical problems, and the prevention of pregnancy and venereal disease. The "legal" portion of the physical examination will help the examiner determine if the victim was capable of consenting to intercourse, if force or restraints were used, if vulvar, anal, or oral penetration occurred, and if there is collectible physical evidence from the scene or from the rapist either in or on the body and clothing of the victim.

A determination of the victim's ability to consent to intercourse is important. The common defense of rapists today is that the victim agreed to voluntary intercourse. If the victim was unable to give her consent because of intoxication, loss of consciousness, mental retardation, then the intercourse may be found to have been against her will—an important factor in the basic definition of rape in most jurisdictions.

If the patient is wearing the clothing in which she was assaulted, the examiner may choose to examine it for signs of violence or restraint. Photographs may be taken, or abnormalities may be indicated on a whole-body chart. If photographs are taken, a special consent form should be signed by the victim. The victim should then remove her own clothing, placing each article in a separate, labeled paper bag (not plastic, which may promote mold growth), and then she should gown. The examiner should investigate all areas of the skin and hair for foreign material (collected in separate, labeled envelopes) and signs of violence. Up to 30 percent of victims show signs of having experienced violence, and certain nonpelvic areas should be given attention: the back, breasts, thighs, neck, wrists, and ankles. If stains are found on the body that are felt to be seminal in origin, they should be removed with a saline-moistened swab that is then air-dried and placed in a labeled envelope. Fingernail scrapings should routinely be obtained from the rape victim because these scrapings may contain bits of the assailant's skin, hair, or blood or other evidence from the crime scene.

Before performing a pelvic examination, the perineal area should be inspected for foreign matter and seminal stains. If present, this evidence should be preserved. Combing of pubic hair onto a paper towel (folded along with the comb, placed in an envelope, and labeled) should be done because some of the assailant's hair or other evidence may be found in the victim's pubic hair. Pubic hair comparisons may later type the rapist but will not pinpoint him.

The pelvic examination begins with inspection of the vulva and introitus for signs of trauma, which are more common in the sexually inexperienced. Any evidence found should be collected, labeled, and saved. The hymen should be inspected and a note made on the type of hymen:

1. present, intact, free of evidence of trauma
2. present, intact, shows old scarring
3. present, recently ruptured
4. absent

A hymen that has been ruptured recently will show signs of active bleeding or fresh clots.

The vaginal vault should be inspected for lacerations (especially the right posterior fornix) and foreign bodies or material. Any foreign bodies or material should be collected, preserved, and labeled. The cervix should be inspected for signs of pregnancy, menstruation, trauma, and preexisting infection. Vaginal swabs or washings (if there are no pooled secretions) should be obtained. The examiner may choose to prepare a saline mount for microscopic examination for motile sperm. Vaginal swabs should be air-dried, placed in paper envelopes, and labeled. These swabs will later be tested for sperm (Table 2) and acid phosphatase. Often a Papanicolaou smear yields sperm that might otherwise be missed.

Cervical, rectal, and oral material should be obtained for *Neisseria gonorrhoeae* cultures. Each of these should be appropriately labeled. A bimanual examination should be performed to determine uterine size, tenderness, and any adnexal abnormalities. Following this, the anorectal area should be examined for foreign material and trauma. An anorectal swab for acid phosphatase and sperm testing may be obtained, but an anorectal washing using a plastic catheter and 10 ml of saline may be more productive. The washing can be examined for motile sperm, and slides or swabs may be made, dried, placed in envelopes, and labeled for nonmotile sperm and acid phosphatase.

If oral sodomy occurred, inspect the mouth (especially the frenula) for trauma. If oral ejaculation occurred, swab between the teeth and preserve the swabs appropriately. An acid phosphatase test is rarely positive in such material, but spermatozoa have been found in swabs from the teeth for up to 6 hours after being deposited, despite brushing and use of mouthwashes.

Other tests from rape victims include saliva samples for secretor status (80 percent of people secrete blood group antigens in saliva and semen) obtained on swabs that are then air-dried, blood for drug and alcohol testing, blood typing, serologic testing for syphilis, and, if available, a beta subunit of human chorionic gonadotropin as a definitive pregnancy test. Urine drug screens and pregnancy testing may also be performed. Each sample must be labeled with the patient's name, the date and time of collection, the type of specimen, the place it was collected from, and the collector's name. Some samples may go to the police crime laboratory and some to the hospital laboratory, but each sample must be accompanied by a "chain of evidence" form that contains the signature or initials of each providing authority and each accepting authority. If this "chain" is broken, the evidence that was so carefully collected may become worthless in court.

TREATMENT

Treatment of rape victim involves providing for venereal disease prevention, pregnancy prevention, prevention of additional psychological stress, and follow-up care. The incidence of gonorrhea in rape victims is 1 in 30 (*Chlamydia* infection may be higher); of syphilis 1 in 1,000; and of pregnancy is 1 in 100. All victims suffer psychological distress. Therapy for gonorrhea, pregnancy,

TABLE 2 Survival Time of Spermatozoa

Source	Motile Sperm	Nonmotile Sperm
Pharyngeal	Up to 6 hours	Unknown
Rectal	Undetermined	Up to 24 hours
Cervix	Up to 5 days	Up to 17 days
Vagina	Up to 8 hours	Up to 48 hours

and psychological distress should be *offered* to each victim, but it is her choice whether to accept or not.

Gonorrhea is best treated with a regimen approved by the Centers for Disease Control for anyone considered to be a contact of a known case of gonorrhea. I prefer oral ampicillin (3.5 g) and probenecid (1.0 g), feeling that the use of intramuscular injections adds unnecessary pain to a patient who is already in significant psychological distress. If *Chlamydia* is of concern, this regimen can be followed by oral tetracycline. However, follow-up cultures and syphilis testing should be planned. Most drugs for the treatment of gonorrhea will also treat incubating syphilis, with the exception of spectinomycin.

Pregnancy prevention may be of tremendous concern to a victim. If a beta human chorionic gonadotrophin test is used on the initial visit (within a few hours of the rape), it would be expected to be negative. If results are positive, the patient was already pregnant when raped. If initially negative and then positive at a 2-week follow-up test, the patient can be referred for suction and curettage (this could mean treatment for only 1 percent of rape victims or less). Several "morning-after" pill regimens are also available, and one with a very high success rate and a low incidence of side effects is norgestrel and ethinyl estradiol (Ovral), two tablets every 12 hours for two doses. All patients should have 2- and 6-week medical follow-up visits for reevaluation of venereal disease, pregnancy (if appropriate), and psychological status. These are minimal follow-up requirements.

The emergency department's psychological care of a rape victim entails some basic concepts. First, the examiner should introduce himself or herself and immediately assure the patient that she is now safe. Listening to the patient in an empathetic manner will support the development of a "safe" feeling. In addition, involve the patient in procedures and decision making by allowing her to determine the rate of questioning, by requesting permission for examination and treatment, and by requesting assistance in decisions regarding contacting and giving information to a husband, boyfriend, or family. Then, briefly discuss the psychological sequelae of rape with the patient or provide contact with someone trained in rape crisis intervention. Follow-up visits should be arranged.

SUGGESTED READING

Braen GR. Examination of the female rape victim. In: Roberts JR, Hedges JR, eds. Clinical procedures in emergency medicine. Philadelphia: WB Saunders, 1985.
Martin CA, Warfield MC, Braen GR. Physician's management of the psychological aspects of rape. JAMA 1983; 249:501–503.

ACUTE SALPINGITIS

GILLES R. G. MONIF, M.D.

The term *pelvic inflammatory disease* (PID) traditionally has been applied to the infectious inflammatory process involving the uterus, the fallopian tubes, or both. Although PID is a convenient categoric term, it does little to describe the pathology in a given patient. Endometritis and parametritis in the immediate postpartum period differ bacteriologically and mechanistically from endometritis and salpingitis with or without peritonitis observed in a nongravida. To negate the ambiguities inherent in the term PID (alias "pretty inadequate diagnosis"), the presumed site of bacterial replication should be used to designate the process.

ETIOLOGY

Acute salpingitis is the end point for a number of agents, the principal ones being *Neisseria gonorrhoeae* and *Chlamydia trachomatis*. The alterations induced by these organisms initiate the anaerobic progression and recruit participation by other bacteria within the vaginal flora environment. The consequence of this process is the induction not of a monomicrobial state but of a polymicrobial infection.

DIAGNOSIS

The principal disease entities in the differential diagnosis are ruptured appendix with peritonitis, intrauterine device (IUD)-associated chronic anaerobic endometritis with either superimposed sexually transmitted disease or unilateral adnexal involvement, acute pancreatitis, bilateral pyelonephritis, infected ectopic pregnancy, or a ruptured viscus.

The patient's entry into the health care system is usually caused by bilateral, crampy lower *abdominal pain.* The pain tends to be aggravated by any jarring movement, particularly in the presence of peritonitis. The pelvic examination characteristically demonstrates exudate issuing from the endocervix, marked uterine and adnexal tenderness, and exquisite cervical tenderness to motion. Rebound tenderness is consistent with the presence of peritonitis. These findings, along with an elevated temperature and elevated white blood cell count (WBC), produce the stereotypic picture of acute salpingitis. The absence of fever or an elevated WBC does not exclude the diagnosis. Fever is not a sensitive measure of pelvic infection. Up to one-third of patients with acute salpingitis confirmed by laparoscopy may have a temperature equal to or lower than 38° C.

A diagnostic procedure often neglected in the differential diagnosis of acute abdomen is that of taking *serial temperatures* immediately before and every 10 minutes after doing a bimanual examination, for a total of 30 minutes. Patients with acute salpingitis often exhibit a transient, spiking elevation of the temperature with manipulation of the genital tract. This strongly correlates with the presence of infection involving the area of manipulation.

Diagnostic Work-up

Useful diagnostic tests include (1) a Gram stain of cervical exudate, looking for the presence or absence of white blood cells and gram-negative intracellular diplococci; (2) a culture of the endocervix for *N. gonorrhoeae* on modified Thayer-Martin medium to document not the actual infection but causation; (3) monoclonal antibody test for *C. trachomatis*; and (4) beta-human chorionic gonadotropin determination. The recovery of *N. gonorrhoeae* has therapeutic implications for the patient's sex partners. Unless ruptured tubo-ovarian abscess is thought to be present or the patient's condition is thought to be septic, blood cultures rarely contribute to the management of the case. In the absence of a markedly elevated erythrocyte sedimentation rate (ESR) or the finding of an adnexal pelvic mass, it is my policy not to obtain blood cultures, because they are not cost effective.

One procedure that is strongly recommended is that of obtaining the *ESR.* If the ESR is moderately elevated, it has little diagnostic significance. However, an ESR in excess of 60 mm suggests the probability of tubal occlusion or the presence of tubo-ovarian abscess, and it may be a significant aid in staging acute salpingitis.

THERAPY

Antibiotic selection is governed by the need to treat polymicrobial infection and superinfection and the penicillinase-producing strains of *N. gonorrhoeae*, when possible, with a single therapeutic regimen. Because the ultimate goal of the therapy of acute salpingitis is preservation of fallopian tube structure and function, one should not start one regimen and later correct it if the anticipat-

ed therapeutic response does not materialize. In terms of preserving fallopian tube structure and function, the game is won or lost within the first 24 hours.

The critical issue is not the treatment of disease caused by one organism, but rather of bacterial superinfection and its ensuing polymicrobial peritonitis. Temperature, WBC, and physical findings have been proposed as quantitatable titration points against which the adequacy of therapy can be judged. Any one parameter by itself is inadequate. Patients with single-organism gonococcal salpingitis have an anticipated therapeutic response of being afebrile in 36 hours, having marked amelioration of physical findings in 48 hours, and having a normal WBC in 48 hours.

THE GAINESVILLE STAGING OF ACUTE SALPINGITIS

The intent of nomenclature or classification is to increase clarity of diagnosis. The term PID, even when restricted to that spectrum of disease attributable to bacterial agents, prevents understanding of the different stages of involvement, each of which requires its own therapeutic regimen. The consequences for women have been unwanted secondary infertility, ectopic pregnancies, augmented occurrence of tubo-ovarian complexes, and possible surgical removal of the genital organs. Each stage of the Gainesville staging of acute salpingitis is based on the need for different therapeutic approaches (Table 1).

Stage I: Acute Salpingitis Without Peritonitis

Patients with acute salpingitis and no peritonitis are those typically seen in office practice who have bilateral lower abdominal pain, cervical or adnexal tenderness to motion, and at least one of the following: increased vaginal discharge, temperature above 37.8° C, and WBC greater than 10,000 mm³.

If an *IUD* is in place, we recommend that the patient be moved up one stage and treated as if she has stage II disease because of the potential for accelerated or antecedent anaerobic infection. Stage II disease is an indication for hospitalization. Removal of the IUD is part of the therapy after antibiotics have been started. My drug choice is doxycycline, 200 mg loading dose, then 100 mg every 12 hours, given intravenously until improvement occurs, followed by 50 mg orally 2 times a day to complete 5 to 10 days of therapy. The first-day dosage exceeds that commonly recommended by the Food and Drug Administration. Frequently we administer oral metronidazole 500 mg every 6 hours for 2 days.

Stage II: Acute Salpingitis With Peritonitis

Clinically, patients with acute salpingitis and peritonitis have more advanced disease and bilateral rebound tenderness is demonstrable. Once peritonitis is diagnosed either by clinical examination or by culdocentesis, the patient should be treated as having a polymicrobial infection. Polymicrobial infection requires the traditional

TABLE 1 Gainesville Staging of Acute Salpingitis

Stage I: Acute Salpingitis without peritonitis

Therapeutic goal: Eradication of symptoms and infections
Therapy: Doxycycline, 200 mg loading dose, then 100 mg every 12 hours, given IV
until improvement occurs, followed by 50 mg orally two times a day to complete 5
to 10 days of therapy

Stage II: Acute salpingitis with peritonitis

Therapeutic goal: Preservation of fallopian tube structure and function
Therapy: Doxycycline, 200 mg loading dose, then 100 mg every 12 hours given IV.
Once clinical amelioration is achieved, conversion to oral cefoxitin, 2 g loading dose,
then 2 g every 6 hours. Once anticipated therapeutic response is achieved, parenteral
drug administration can be discontinued. When administering a bacteriostatic–
bactericidal antibiotic combination, the bactericidal antibiotic should be administered
½ hour before the bacteriostatic drug.

Stage III: Acute salpingitis with evidence of tubal occlusion or ruptured tubo-ovarian
complex

Primary therapeutic goal: Preservation of ovarian function
Therapy: Penicillin G, 5 million units every 6 hours, given IV; clindamycin, 600 mg every
6 hours, given IV; gentamicin or tobramycin, dosage adjusted to body weight.

Stage IV: Ruptured tubo-ovarian complex

Primary therapeutic goal: Preservation of life
Therapy: Triple therapy as Stage III and surgical removal of diseased organ

---

four-category coverage of the Gainesville classification. In addition, there has to be adequate coverage for principal venereal pathogens, namely *N. gonorrhoeae*, penicillinase-producing strains of *N. gonorrhoeae*, and *C. trachomatis*. The rationale for this selection of an antibiotic combination is to achieve best coverage for the maximum number of the seven organisms. The combination of cefoxitin and doxycycline covers the principal venereal pathogens and is additive in stage II and, to a relatively minor degree, in stage IV. Seventy percent of cefoxitin-resistant *Bacteroidaceae* are responsive to doxycycline. The shortcoming of this drug combination is its lack of coverage for enterococci; however, the significance of those organisms in pelvic infection is not known.

My recommended therapy is doxycycline, 200 mg loading dose, then 100 mg every 12 hours given intravenously. Once clinical amelioration is achieved, conversion to the oral route should be implemented and therapy continued long enough (10 days total) to ensure eradication of *C. trachomatis*. Once the anticipated therapeutic response is achieved, parenteral drug administration can be discontinued in favor of oral cefoxitin, 2 g loading dose, then 2 g every 6 hours.

When administering a bacteriostatic-bactericidal antibiotic combination, it is prudent to administer the bactericidal antibiotic at least one-half hour before beginning the bacteriostatic drug.

Stage III: Acute Salpingitis With Evidence of Tubal Occlusion or Ruptured Tubo-Ovarian Complex

Stage III indicates advanced disease. The probability of preserving fallopian tube function is diminished. The major goal becomes preservation of ovarian function by eliminating the need for surgical intervention. Triple antibiotic therapy is given, consisting of penicillin G, 5 million units every 6 hours, given intravenously; clindamycin, 600 mg every 6 hours, given intravenously; and *gentamicin* or *tobramycin* in appropriate dosage (mg per kilogram of body weight) intravenously. Its major focus is eradication of the anaerobic progression.

With triple therapy the signs of peritoneal irritation should disappear within hours. Persistence of such signs should alert the clinician to the possibility of a ruptured tubo-ovarian complex.

Stage IV: Ruptured Tubo-Ovarian Complex

The goal of therapy for a ruptured tubo-ovarian complex is no longer preserving ovarian function but saving the patient's life. Combinations of antibiotics, including penicillin, an aminoglycoside, and either clindamycin or metronidazole, can be used to prevent metastatic bacterial complications. If the patient fails to respond to therapy or deteriorates, definitive therapy is achieved by surgical removal of the diseased organ and by peritoneal lavage.

DURATION OF ANTIMICROBIAL THERAPY FOR ACUTE SALPINGITIS

In the absence of complicating factors such as the presence of an IUD, significant prior structural damage, or tubal ligations, successful treatment of single-organism disease has a predictable anticipated therapeutic response. The parameters used are (1) the patient's sense of well-being, (2) serial WBCs, (3) abdominal and pelvic physical findings, and (4) temperature. These parameters permit the establishment of a therapeutic end point for stage I, II, and III disease. Stage III disease carries with it an additional parameter that influences the duration of therapy: the ESR. The ESR should be clearly dropping before discontinuation of triple therapy. Once the therapeutic end points have been documented, my policy is to continue parenteral antimicrobial therapy for 24 hours, after which the patient is discharged on oral medication.

Outpatient therapy for stages I and II disease is that required to complete eradication of *C. trachomatis* (10 to 14 days). My drug of choice is doxycycline.

Outpatient therapy of stage III acute salpingitis involves the administration of metronidazole and doxycycline. The duration of doxycycline therapy is again governed by the time of administration required to eradicate *C. trachomatis* (10 to 14 days). The duration of metronidazole therapy is based on the ESR.

SUGGESTED READING

Monif GRG. Significance of polymicrobial bacterial superinfection in the therapy of gonococcal endometritis-salpingitis-peritonitis. Obstet Gynecol 1980; 55:154s.

Monif GRG. Choice of antibiotics and length of therapy in the treatment of acute salpingitis. Am J Med 1985; 78:188.

Monif GRG, Welkos SL, Baer H. Clinical response of patients with gonococcal endocervicitis and endometritis-salpingitis-peritonitis and gonococcal endocervicitis to doxycycline. Am J Obstet Gynecol 1977; 129:614.

VAGINITIS AND CERVICITIS

MICHAEL S. POLICAR, M.D., M.P.H.

Vaginal discharge is one of the most common complaints reported by women of reproductive age to their physicians. The presence of a vaginal discharge does not necessarily indicate a vaginal infection, because cervical infections and noninfectious vaginal conditions may also present with this symptom (Table 1). Because most of the agents that cause vaginal and cervical infections are sexually transmitted, simultaneous infection of the cervix and the vagina is frequently encountered, and the possibility of mixed infection must be considered and evaluated. Pelvic examination with systematic examination of cervical and vaginal discharge is mandatory for appropriate diagnosis and therapy.

DIAGNOSIS

Vaginal Infection

The most common cause of vaginal infection is bacterial vaginosis, previously referred to as *Gardnerella vaginalis* vaginitis, *Haemophilus vaginalis* vaginitis, or nonspecific vaginitis. The etiology of this condition is vaginal colonization with *G. vaginalis* accompanied by a quantitative overgrowth of a number of anaerobic bacteria. Most cases are sexually transmitted, although conversion from asymptomatic colonization to the symptomatic condition may occur after a long latent period. The primary symptom is a copious white or gray homogenous vaginal discharge with an objectionable fishy odor, especially after intercourse. Vaginal and vulvar irritative symptoms are absent or minimal. Examination shows the characteristic discharge with minimal inflammatory findings. The amine test consists of alkalinizing the discharge found on the posterior blade of the speculum with two

---

Table 1   Causes of Vaginal Discharge

Vaginal discharge of cervical origin
   Infectious cervicitis (gonorrhea, chlamydia, herpes)
   Endocervical polyps
   Cervical neoplasms

Vaginal epithelial irritation
   Vaginal contraceptive products: spermicidal creams and jellies, contraceptive sponge
   Medicated or perfumed douche products
   Foreign bodies, especially retained tampons

Physiologic vaginal discharge
   Increased cervical mucus in preovulatory period
   Increased epithelial cell turnover owing to pregnancy or use of oral contraceptives

Atrophic vaginitis

Infectious vaginitis
   Bacterial vaginosis
   Trichomonal vaginitis
   Monilial vaginitis

to three drops of 10 percent potassium hydroxide. Production of the characteristic fishy odor is considered a positive test and is highly correlated with the diagnosis of bacterial vaginosis. A fresh saline suspension of the vaginal discharge shows characteristic "clue cells," which are epithelial cells coated with *Gardnerella*, causing a granular stippled appearance and a ragged cell border. Additional microscopic findings include a relative decrease in both white blood cells (WBCs) and lactobacilli.

Trichomonal vaginitis is caused by a flagellated protozoan and is the most widely and deeply invasive of the vaginitides, frequently involving the endocervix, urethra, and bladder. Transmission is virtually always sexual, although an asymptomatic carrier state exists in both men and women. Symptoms include a moderate to profuse malodorous watery yellow, green, or white vaginal discharge that is associated with variable degrees of vaginal and vulvar irritation and dysuria. Examination may show minimal to severe epithelial erythema, and in longstanding cases, a "strawberry cervix" may be present. A fresh saline suspension of the discharge shows motile trichomonads with large numbers of WBCs. Treatment is necessarily systemic because of the potential of infection beyond the reach of topical vaginal preparations.

Monilial vulvovaginitis is mainly attributable to infection with *Candida albicans*, with approximately 5 percent of cases attributed to *Candida glabrata*. Autoinoculation of the fungus from the gastrointestinal tract to the vagina is the most common source of introduction, although genital and oral sexual transmission also occur frequently. Predisposing factors to infection include use of broad-spectrum antibiotics; pregnancy; and relative immunosuppression, particularly owing to diabetes, corticosteroid use, or chronic disease. The characteristic symptoms are vaginal and usually vulvar itching and burning associated with a nonmalodorous white vaginal discharge and, occasionally, meatal dysuria. Examination reveals mild to severe vulvar and vaginal erythema and a vaginal discharge that is classically "curdy" but may also appear as an unremarkable white floccular discharge. A suspension of the discharge in 10 percent potassium hydroxide usually shows characteristic monilial pseudohyphae but less commonly contains only fungal spores or buds.

Cervicitis

The term *cervicitis* is confusing because of its variable use to describe morphologic, microbiologic, and histopathologic findings. Terms such as *chronic cervicitis* and *cervical erosion* should be abandoned because they are nonspecific and inaccurate. Additionally, the finding of a "red cervix" should not be equated with a cervical infection, because the differential diagnosis of this clinical finding includes benign ectropion, "true" erosion (a rare condition), cervical neoplasm, and cervical infection. If a woman with a red cervix and cervical friability (easy cervical bleeding) is found not to have a cervical infection, referral to a gynecologist for further evaluation should be considered, especially for women over 30 years of age.

Infectious cervicitis is most commonly attributable to endocervical *Chlamydia trachomatis* or *Neisseria gonorrhoeae*, although herpetic ectocervicitis, trichomonal cervicitis, and mycoplasmal or viral infections may also cause this condition. Endocervicitis owing to chlamydia or gonorrhea may present symptomatically as a vaginal discharge, may be found on examination as a mucopurulent cervicitis, or may be diagnosed as the result of chlamydia or gonorrhea screening in an asymptomatic woman. Mucopurulent cervicitis is a recently described clinical syndrome consisting of three findings: a green or yellow cervical discharge (called mucopus), WBC in the cervical mucus, and a clinical "cervicitis" associated with a hypertrophic ectropion, friability, and erythema. In women with mucopurulent cervicitis, 40 to 60 percent have endocervical chlamydia; the remainder have gonorrhea or other causes of infectious cervicitis. If all three findings of mucopurulent cervicitis are present, chlamydial or gonorrheal infection should be assumed and the patient should be treated empirically depending upon history of gonorrhea contact and cervical Gram stain findings. This is necessary primarily to prevent ascending infection and resultant acute salpingitis, but it is also desirable so that spread to other partners can be avoided. The presence of mucopus, friability, or cervical erythema alone is not sufficiently specific for empiric treatment, but tests for gonorrhea and chlamydia should be performed if available.

The role of *C. trachomatis* as an important cause of infectious cervicitis has been widely accepted. The risks of untreated cervical chlamydia include endometritis, salpingitis (with further risk of tubal infertility and ectopic pregnancy), female urethral syndrome, and Curtis-Fitz-Hugh syndrome. Furthermore, newborns delivered through a cervix infected with *C. trachomatis* have a 50 percent chance of acquiring chlamydial conjunctivitis or pneumonia. The prevalence of cervical chlamydia in sexually active women is 3 to 10 percent, although in high-risk groups such as women younger than 24 years old, those with multiple sexual partners, users of nonbarrier contraceptives, and women with mucopurulent cervicitis, the prevalence is significantly higher. Confirmation of the presence of chlamydia was previously confined to culture, but recently, less expensive screening tests such as enzyme immunoassay and direct fluorescent antibody tests have become available. When resources for screening are limited, first priority should be given to high-risk women not empirically treated, with second priority given to empirically treated women who are tested mainly for confirmation of diagnosis and to allow test of cure for those found to be positive on initial testing.

EVALUATION

In addition to routine information, the medical history should include a discussion of sexual habits, contraceptive use, medications, menstrual history, and pregnancy symptoms. If pregnancy is suspected, a high-sensitivity pregnancy test should be ordered before systemic medications are begun.

Pelvic examination should begin with observation of the vulva for evidence of lesions, vulvitis, and discharge. After introduction of a warm, water-moistened speculum, the cervix is evaluated for ulceration, edema, hypertrophic ectropion, and leukoplakia. Cervical friability may be tested with a Pap spatula or swab, and then the "swab test" for mucopus is performed by the placement of a cotton-tipped swab into the endocervical canal. A positive swab test reveals yellow, green, or opaque white pus; a negative test shows cloudy or clear mucus. The same swab may then be used to inoculate a culture plate or transport media for *N. gonorrhoeae*. A second swab is then introduced if a chlamydia test is to be performed, and a third swab is used to apply cervical mucus to a slide for a Gram stain for estimation of WBC count and for observation of gram-negative intracellular diplococci, which are presumptive evidence of gonorrhea. Other culture and sensitivity studies of the cervix are not indicated.

Evaluation of the vaginal discharge begins with vigorous swabbing of the vaginal sidewalls with a cotton-tipped applicator. The accumulated material is first mixed with a few drops of saline previously placed on a microscope slide; then the remaining discharge is mixed with a few drops of potassium hydroxide on a second slide and cover slips applied. When the speculum has been removed, the amine test is performed by adding three to four drops of potassium hydroxide to the residual discharge on the posterior blade of the speculum with observation for the characteristic odor of bacterial vaginosis. Another helpful test in women of reproductive age is an evaluation of the vaginal pH with nitrazine paper. An acidic pH (below 5) is consistent with a normal discharge or a fungal infection; a pH above 5 is found with either trichomonal vaginitis or bacterial vaginosis. Vaginal cultures are not indicated except in resistant cases.

TREATMENT

Vaginal Infection

Bacterial vaginosis is most effectively treated with metronidazole, 500 mg twice a day for 7 days. Secondary drugs of choice include ampicillin, 500 mg four times a day, and oral cephalosporins used in the same manner for 7 days. Tetracycline and vaginal sulfa preparations are not effective in treating this condition. Metronidazole is not recommended in pregnancy, so ampicillin can be used. Vaginal acidification with vinegar douches or an acidic vaginal jelly may give symptomatic relief. Treatment of male partners is controversial. Although this condition is sexually transmitted, treatment of male partners has not significantly reduced recurrences in treated women. Therefore, partner treatment is optional at the time of a woman's primary treatment, but it should be attempted if infections recur. Condoms should be used during the treatment period. Treatment of male contacts is the same as for women with bacterial vaginosis.

Trichomonal vaginitis is treated with metronidazole, 2 g orally, given as a single dose for both men and women. Trichomonal infections during the first half of pregnancy should be treated symptomatically with vaginal acidification (as described for bacterial vaginosis); severe cases in the second half of pregnancy may be treated with metronidazole. Male partners should be treated routinely with the regimen already described.

Monilial vaginitis is treated with a fungicidal medication such as miconazole or clotrimazole given as a cream, suppository, or tablet. One-, 3-, and 7-day preparations are available. The use of nystatin is discouraged because it has a lower cure rate and requires a longer course, which decreases compliance. Monilial vulvitis should be treated with topical clotrimazole or miconazole with or without 0.5 percent hydrocortisone cream. A combination of triamcinolone-nystatin (Mycolog) is not appropriate for most infectious vulvitis, because fluorinated steroids may cause vulvar atrophy. Each of the preceding fungicides may be used in pregnancy. If there is a failure of therapy with one of the fungicides, the other should be used. Recurrent monilial vaginitis may be managed with early antifungal therapy started with the onset of symptoms or used prophylactically when systemic antibiotic therapy is given.

Cervicitis

Treatment of Mucopurulent Cervicitis or a Patient with a Positive Cervical Chlamydia Test. Treatment for chlamydial endocervicitis consists of doxycycline 100 mg orally twice a day for 7 days or tetracycline HCl 500 mg four times a day for 7 days. The second drug of choice (and primary choice during pregnancy) is erythromycin ethylsuccinate 800 mg orally four times a day for 7 days or 400 mg orally four times a day for 14 days. If there is any history of contact with gonorrhea or if there is evidence of gonorrhea on cervical Gram's stain, then initial empiric treatment should begin with treatment for gonorrhea, followed immediately by treatment for chlamydia (Table 2). Neither of these regimens constitutes adequate outpatient therapy for pelvic inflammatory disease (see chapter on *Acute Salpingitis*).

Treatment of a Patient with a Positive Cervical Gonorrhea Culture. Because of the high likelihood that a woman with endocervical gonorrhea also has endocervical chlamydia, women with a positive cervical gonorrhea culture should be treated for both gonorrhea and chlamydia (see Table 2). If a woman who was initially treated empirically for chlamydia with tetracycline or doxycycline is later found to have a positive gonorrhea culture, it is recommended that she return for definitive gonorrhea treatment. Alternatively, she may complete the 7-day course of tetracycline or doxycycline and return for a cervical culture for test of cure of gonorrhea and, if available, chlamydia.

All women treated for mucopurulent cervicitis or found to have a positive gonorrhea or chlamydia test must be advised to inform their sexual partners of the diagnosis so that they may seek evaluation and treatment. Con-

TABLE 2 Combination Treatment of Endocervical Gonorrhea and Chlamydia

Single Dose Treatment for Gonorrhea

Ampicillin 3.5 g PO *or*
Amoxicillin 3.0 g PO *or*
Aqueous Procaine Penicillin G 4.8 million units IM

Plus Probenecid 1 g PO *or*
Ceftriaxone 250 mg IM

Followed by Treatment for Chlamydia

Doxycycline 100 mg PO twice a day for 7 days *or*
Tetracycline HC1 500 mg PO four times a day for 7 days

or

if allergic to tetracycline or pregnant:

Erythromycin ethylsuccinate 800 mg PO 4 times a day for 7 days *or*
Erythromycin ethylsuccinate 400 mg PO 4 times a day for 14 days *or*
Erythromycin base or stearate 500 mg PO 4 times a day for 7 days

doms should be used until both partners complete the prescribed course of treatment. The use of barrier methods of contraception may prevent recurrences.

SUGGESTED READING

Brunham RC et al. Mucopurulent cervicitis: the ignored counterpart in women of urethritis in men. N Engl J Med 1984; 311:1–6.
Centers for Disease Control. 1985 Sexually transmitted disease treatment guidelines. MMWR 1985; 34 Suppl 4:75–108
Centers for Disease Control. *Chlamydia trachomatis* infections: Policy guidelines for prevention and control. MMWR 1985; 34 Suppl 3:53–74.
Friedrich EG. Vaginitis. Am, Obstet Gynecol 1985; 152:247–251.
Handsfield HH et al. Criteria for selective screening for *Chlamydia trachomatis* infection in women attending family planning clinics. JAMA 1986; 255:1730–1734.
Rice RJ, Thompson SE. Treatment of uncomplicated infections due to *Neisseria gonorrhoeae*. JAMA 1986; 255:1739–1746.
Sanders LL et al. Treatment of sexually transmitted chlamydial infections. JAMA 1986; 255:1750–1756.

VAGINAL TRAUMA AND FOREIGN BODY

JAMES R. DINGFELDER, M.D.

Most vaginal trauma is easily recognized after careful examination based on the patient's chief complaint and history. Usually this involves assessment of abnormal vaginal bleeding, discharge, or pain. Rarely, significant vaginal trauma remains undetected for a time because the clinician fails to perform a thorough vaginal examination when the patient is young, anxious, intoxicated, or obstreperous, or when visible external evidence of injury is minimal or absent. Embarrassing or even life-threatening diagnostic lapses must be avoided by performing a vaginal examination in *every* instance in which there has been a history of trauma to the perineum or lower abdomen.

Most patients are symptomatic, although the cause of their vaginal bleeding, discharge, or pain may not be clear at first, and the cause or agent denied or disbelieved by the patient (as in the case of foreign bodies). Children are always the most complex cases in this regard, and ordinary paper is the most common offending agent.

In our litigious age, meticulous documentation of a thorough evaluation is imperative for the protection of the accident or assault victim as well as the examining physician.

EXTERNAL TRAUMA

All patients with external vulvar and perineal trauma must be assumed to have vaginal trauma until proven otherwise. Similarly, all patients with perforating vaginal injuries must be assumed to have a retained intra-abdominal foreign body until proven otherwise (by abdominal roentgenogram, lack of peritoneal air, or by laparoscopy or laparotomy if necessary).

It is not unusual to find concurrent vaginal injuries of the "blowout" type when blunt abdominal trauma (frequently seen in automobile accidents) ruptures the urinary bladder. In the pediatric age group such impact frequently causes a vesicovaginal fistula, which can be overlooked during evaluation and treatment of other significant injuries such as pelvic fractures. Straddle injuries in children can be accompanied by penetrating vaginal injury subsequently concealed by vulvar contusions, ecchymoses, and sometimes massive hematomas. Even without bleeding, such injuries require examination to rule out concurrent vaginal trauma and prevent infectious damage to the reproductive tract. Such trauma is more common in active younger patients, who may resist appropriate vaginal examination. Nevertheless, it must be performed, under general anesthesia if necessary. Administration of a commonly used pediatric "cocktail" may obviate the need for general anesthesia (Table 1).

Straddle-type "picket-fence" impalement injuries invariably involve dirty, contaminated objects and will require broad-spectrum antibiotic coverage and hospital admission to prevent gas gangrene and toxic effects of clostridial infections.

Traumatic perforation of the vaginal vault as well as partial avulsion of the cervix have been seen secondary to forceful introduction of water into the vagina during water skiing (rectal mucosal perforation may occur via a similar mechanism in both sexes). A similar type of water injury was reported in an intoxicated woman who sat on a park water fountain jet in a playfully futile attempt to stop the flow of water. This resulted in an 8-cm vaginal laceration with a more than 2,000-ml blood loss that necessitated laparotomy and hypogastric artery ligation for final hemostatic control.

Evisceration of the small bowel into the vagina is not unusual as a result of coital injuries as well as traumatic openings through the upper vagina into the abdomen. Obviously, all such cases demand immediate hospitalization for operative repair. In the past, mortality rates up to 10 percent were reported, most of them secondary to postoperative thromboembolic events.

COITAL INJURY

It is not uncommon for coitus, forceful or not, to precipitate a rupture of the postoperative vaginal apex (which may be foreshortened after hysterectomy). Such vault ruptures may be bloodless. Consequently, patients may delay seeking help for hours or days until peritonitis symptoms ensue.

Pneumoperitoneum has also been reported secondary to forceful oral introduction of air into the vagina, which led to partial disruption of the vaginal incision line. In one case of a patient complaining of abdominal and shoulder pain, careful vaginal examination revealed only a 5-mm rent in the incision line, which could have easily been overlooked during a more casual examination. A roentgenogram showing free abdominal air led to a correct diagnosis after more extensive questioning of the patient. Perforation of the posterior fornix by forceful intercourse or by foreign bodies in a normal patient with

an intact uterus has also been reported and deserves similar meticulous evaluation and concern.

Hymenal lacerations associated with normal intercourse may present with a dramatic amount of bleeding from a very superficial tear. A simple hemostatic suture will usually suffice to quell bleeding from such lesions, usually located at the 4 and 8 o'clock aspects of the hymenal ring. It may be preferable to leave very superficial tears open, as long as hemostasis is secured, since tight closure of tears with sutures may result in scar formation and subsequent dyspareunia.

VAGINAL LACERATIONS

External and coital trauma, as well as foreign bodies, can cause lacerations. In recent years a new type of inadvertent self-induced vaginal laceration secondary to a plastic tampon inserter has been reported. One university student health service gynecologist reported six similar cases of vaginal bleeding caused by the Playtex tampon inserter lacerating the vaginal mucosa. Bleeding in some cases lasted up to 10 weeks before the persistent menorrhagia prompted a diagnostic vaginal examination. Only a few patients require hemostatic sutures (although one patient experienced near-fatal hemorrhage). The remainder had persistent oozing from the necrotic base of the laceration, aggravated by continuous tampon use to control the same bleeding, which promptly healed after discontinuation of tampon use.

VAGINAL FOREIGN BODIES

Retained vaginal foreign bodies rarely present as emergency bleeding. Rather, a chronic offensive vaginal discharge is the usual presenting complaint. On occasion, chronic infection and ulceration of the vaginal tissue eventuate in vaginal bleeding as the initial symptom. Unfortunately, because of embarrassment or altered consciousness secondary to alcohol or other drugs, trauma caused by foreign bodies can never be ruled out by history or patient recollection.

The premenstrual pediatric patient is the most common victim, with retained paper or toilet tissue the most frequent offender. A purulent discharge in the pediatric age group is never normal and nearly always secondary to a foreign body or sexually transmitted pathogen. Administration of antibiotics without a thorough vaginal examination serves only to delay the correct diagnosis. Appropriate sedation (see Table 1) or even general anesthesia may be necessary and should be employed without hesitation.

A variety of diagnostic instruments are available to aid in diagnosis. Pediatric vaginoscopes are generally available. The air cystoscope is a suitable substitute and may help to distend the vagina for improved visibility. Bayonet forceps will aid in removal of foreign bodies, usually paper fragments, seeds and nuts, plastic beads, pencil and crayon fragments, and small game pieces. Microscopic examination of vaginal secretion is imperative to rule out sexually transmissible pathogens, such as

TABLE 1 Pediatric Analgesic Cocktail

Meperidine (Demerol) 50 mg	1	ml
Chlorpromazine HCL (Thorazine) 12.5 mg	0.5	ml
Promethazine HCL (Phenergan) 12.5 mg	0.5	ml
Give 1 ml per 20 lb of body weight;		
maximum dose =	2	ml

TABLE 2 Features of Toxic Shock Syndrome

Early:
Fever—often as high as 103–106 °F
Diarrhea—often profuse
Rash—erythematous, macular, or
confluent like diffuse sunburn

Subsequently:
Vomiting—may lead to volume depletion
Headache
Myalgia
Pharyngeal soreness and hyperemia
Syncope, hypotension, orthostatic dizziness
Desquamation—soles and palms after
1 to 2 weeks

Laboratory findings:
Elevated WBC
Hypocalcemia
Severe acidosis
Thrombocytopenia
Elevated liver function studies
Elevated BUN, creatinine, CPK, bilirubin

Trichomonas vaginalis and *Gardnerella* organisms, but a culture must also be obtained to rule out *Neisseria gonorrhoeae*. Ampicillin or cephalosporin antibiotics will usually eliminate the discharge, which is commonly due to a mixed bacterial infection initiated by the foreign body.

The list of foreign bodies discovered (but often denied) in the adult vagina is remarkable and ranges from salt shakers, pill boxes and vials, gourds, and condoms to dentures, diaphragms, cervical caps, fitting rings, and forgotten tampons. A profuse, foul vaginal discharge is the usual presenting complaint. The longer the object has been retained the more likely that a chronic vaginal mucosal ulceration has occurred. Nearly all objects can be removed in the emergency department (and promptly enclosed inside an inverted examination glove for odor control). A rare patient may require general anesthesia for foreign body removal, especially larger glass objects and those with sharp edges.

Recently the *toxic shock syndrome* has garnered publicity and public awareness. Although usually associated with super-absorbent tampon use, it has also been reported with diaphragm use and in association with the new vaginal contraceptive sponge, particularly when difficult insertion or removal has caused trauma. The pathologic characteristics involve microulcerations of the vaginal mucosa which allow the toxins produced by *Staphylococcus aureus* (found in 10 percent of all normal vaginas) to gain systemic access. The usual presenting and ensuing symptoms of toxin-induced septic shock are outlined in (Table 2).

SUGGESTED READING

Christiansen WC, Danzl DF, McGee HJ. Pneumoperitoneum following vaginal insufflation and coitus. Ann Emerg Med 1980; 9:480–482.
Druzin ML, Gottesfeld SA. Management of serious vaginal injury. J Reprod Med 1986; 31:151–153.
Gray MJ, Norton P, Treadwell K. Tampon-induced injuries. Obstet Gynecol 1981; 58:667–668.
Merchant WC, Gibbons MD, Gonzales ET. Trauma to the bladder neck, trigone and vagina in children. J Urol 1984; 747–750.
Wilson F, Swartz DP. Coital injuries of the vagina. Obstet Gynecol 1972; 39:182–184.

VULVAR DISEASE

RAYMOND H. KAUFMAN, M.D.
DALE BROWN Jr., M.D.

Vulvar disorders rarely necessitate emergency treatment. However, occasionally one encounters acute emergencies involving the vulva. Most often, this is related to trauma, acute infection, hemorrhage, and allergic and irritant vulvitis.

TRAUMA

The subject of rape is discussed elsewhere. Because of its protected location, the vulva is seldom injured accidentally. Those injuries most commonly seen occur in prepubertal girls as a result of traumatic straddling of such objects as fence rails, gymnasium equipment, bicycle frames, edges of chairs, bath and toilet seats, and occasionally from splinters acquired from boards on which the youngsters slide. Traumatic injuries of the genitalia are also seen following automobile and motorcycle accidents. The latter are usually associated with trauma elsewhere on the body. Injuries to the vulva are manifested by development of hematomata and lacerations.

Hematomata

Hematomata are seldom serious, although the ecchymosis may be alarming. The lesion is manifested by swelling and tenderness and, if the hematoma is large, it may be quite painful. In most instances, the hematoma is small and localized. On rare occasions, blood loss into the tissue spaces may be sufficiently severe to produce shock. Significant edema may develop in the vulvar area following severe trauma.

Management. Small hematomata require the use of analgesics and careful observation for evidence of continued enlargement. A large fluctuant collection of blood should be incised and evacuated and, if feasible, any active bleeding source should be identified and occluded by clamping and ligation. Extensive exploration for obscure vessels, however, is not advisable. If there is considerable generalized oozing, the cavity of the hematoma should be carefully packed; or, if it appears dry, a drain should be inserted and left in place for at least 24 hours.

If the hematoma is not unusually large or increasing in size, it is advisable not to treat it surgically. Rather, ice packs should be applied to the vulva soon after the injury and for at least the next 8 to 12 hours.

Lacerations

Laceration of the vulva is likely to occur after a violent fall on a slender object, such as a stake or picket fence, or bicycle handlebars. The injury may occasionally extend through the vagina and even continue on into the rectum, bladder, or urethra.

When multiple severe lacerations are also found in the vagina, a foreign body should be suspected as the cause.

Treatment. Bleeding vessels should be ligated and tissue edges carefully approximated. Large, traumatized areas should be thoroughly irrigated with sterile saline, and necrotic tissue debrided. Adjacent organs such as the bladder and rectum should be examined for evidence of damage. In most instances, if the lacerations are extensive and extend into adjacent organs such as the rectum, the patient will require stabilization with fluids and blood in the emergency department before transfer to surgery for repair under anesthesia.

Treatment of children involves special consideration. Forcible examination of a child should never be attempted. In the presence of pain, bleeding, or evidence of laceration, she should be examined under anesthesia. Lacerations should be repaired by careful approximation of the tissue edges with small instruments, taking small bites of tissue.

Counseling of the parents following traumatic injury to the child is quite important. If the injury will not result in permanent structural changes or impaired normal reproduction, the patient and her parents should be reassured about this. Likewise, the patient or her parents should be informed if the injury will result in impairment of reproductive function.

Hemorrhage

Varicosities

These large tumors of the vulva are rarely encountered apart from pregnancy. Whereas 2 percent of pregnant women have vulvar varicosities, thrombus and hemorrhage requiring emergency treatment or hospitalization are rare. Clinically, these tumors have a bluish purple cast and appear worm-like below the surface of the skin. They may be confused with epidermal cysts, but on palpation are soft and reducible.

In cases of bleeding, pressure should be applied, and the use of ice packs may be an adjunct. For significant bleeding of large and progressive varicosities, hospitali-

zation is needed for ligation of the veins. A specially designed support for vulvar varicosities is available from Ortho-Vascular Products Co., Yonkers, New York. When varicosities complicate pregnancy, it is best to delay any major definitive therapy for 4 to 6 months postpartum.

Cancer

Occasionally, a patient may present bleeding from a neoplasm of the vulva. Control of bleeding may be accomplished by the usual supportive measures of pressure, ice pack, and Monsel's solution (a hemostatic caustic solution of ferric subsulfate). Acetone or silver nitrate may be used as chemical cauterizers. Definitive therapy requires hospital admisison.

INFECTIONS

Bartholin Abscess

Most Bartholin abscesses, especially if recurrent, develop as the consequence of infection of the fluid content of Bartholin's duct cysts. Today, abscesses are rarely found to be secondary to gonorrheal infection. The chief symptoms of a Bartholin abscess are pain and tenderness over the infected gland. The rapidity of development and the extent of involvement depend on the size of the infected cyst and the virulence of the infectious agent. Some abscesses develop slowly and give rise to mild symptoms. Usually, however, Bartholin abscesses develop rapidly within 2 to 3 days and are associated with acute pain and tenderness. They may rupture spontaneously within 72 hours. The objective signs include unilateral swelling over the site of the infected gland, redness of the overlying skin, and edema of the labia. This frequently results in marked enlargement and distortion of the labia on the affected side. The abscess is palpable as a tender, fluctuant mass. The differential diagnosis from other acute inflammatory processes of the vulva must be considered. Usually, however, correct diagnosis of Bartholin abscess is easily made. If one carefully examines the mass, one notes that the labia minora, even though distorted by edema, tends to bisect the swelling longitudinally.

Treatment. Occasionally, the early treatment of an obvious bartholinitis with broad-spectrum antibiotics prevents abscess formation. In most instances, however, the patient presents with an intact abscess, as already described. The appropriate treatment is incision and drainage of the contents of the abscess cavity. This is done easily by infiltrating the site of pointing with a small amount of 1 percent lidocaine. Ethyl chloride spray can be used over the planned puncture site. A small stab incision is made into the cavity, and the purulent contents are expressed. Cultures for aerobic and anaerobic organisms should be obtained. A wick of iodoform gauze should be inserted into the cavity and left in place for 1 to 2 days. Continued applications of heat accelerates resolution and healing.

The Word catheter has been successfully used in treating Bartholin abscesses and in allowing for marsupialization of the abscess cavity. This is a small closed catheter with a small bag at its distal end (a Foley catheter is too large for this purpose). After the contents are drained, the catheter is inserted into the cavity and the balloon inflated with 2 cc of saline. The incision should not be made too large or the catheter slips out. The distal end of the catheter is then tucked into the vagina. The catheter should be left in place for 4 to 6 weeks before it is removed.

Herpes Genitalis

Primary genital herpes virus infections can be very severe. Lower abdominal pain secondary to pelvic lymphadenopathy is frequently present. The patients often have systemic symptoms including temperature elevation, headache, malaise, and chills. A profuse watery discharge is frequently associated with herpetic cervicitis. Many individuals with initial disease develop urinary retention secondary to herpetic involvement of the urethra and bladder.

The differential diagnosis includes any vesicular ulcerative disease involving the vulva—herpes zoster, chancroid, multiple chancres of syphilis, lesions of Behet's syndrome, and vaccinia. Excoriations from any cause, such as candidiasis, may also be suggestive of herpes.

The diagnosis is made on the basis of clinical history and physical findings. A Tzanck smear, in which a direct smear preparation is taken from the ulcers and stained using paregon multiple stains, may be helpful in confirming the diagnosis. Characteristic multinucleated giant cells are highly suggestive of a herpetic infection.

Management. Cultures should be taken from the vulvar lesions and cervix. The virus can be isolated from sterile cotton-tipped swab specimens taken from ulcers or recently ruptured vesicles. The swab should be placed in Eagle's medium containing 10 percent fetal bovine serum and antibiotics. The specimens must be rapidly transported to the virology laboratory, where the virus is isolated in tissue culture. If immediate transportation is not possible, the culture tube should be immediately placed in a refrigerator but *not* freezer.

Hospitalization is required if the patient is having severe vulvar pain and is unable to urinate. Immediate treatment should consist of administration of systemic analgesics to control the pain; insertion of either a suprapubic cystocath or Foley catheter for drainage of the bladder; and the institution of treatment with intravenous acyclovir. Five mg per kilogram of body weight every 8 hours should be given intravenously for a period of 5 days. This shortens the duration of clinical symptoms and viral shedding. If hospitalization is not required, the patient should be started on oral acyclovir, 200 mg 5 times a day for 5 to 7 days. Warm sitz baths and oral analgesics are usually necessary to relieve the patient's discomfort.

On rare occasions, disseminated infection follows primary herpes virus genital infection. Rarely, meningitis and encephalitis are associated with the primary infection. In the presence of severe headache and nuchal rigidity, one should consider the possibility of meningitis and obtain a spinal tap for viral culture and white count.

Pyodermas

Pyodermas involving the vulva may be seen as infection of hair follicles, including folliculitis, furuncles, and carbuncles; infection of apocrine glands (hidradenitis suppurativa); periclitoral abscesses; pyogenic ulcers; and infection such as erysipelas and cellulitis. The most likely infections to require emergency treatment are carbuncles and periclitoral abscess.

Pain and tenderness are common features of the follicular pyodermas, with the pain increasing in proportion to the depth and extent of the lesions.

In the presence of a furuncle, a red, tender nodule with a purulent apex is seen. A carbuncle may have multiple openings onto the surface of the skin, with thickening and induration of surrounding tissues. The periclitoral abscess usually presents as a painful, fluctuant swelling in the region of the clitoris. The lesions are unilateral and located on one side of the clitoris.

Treatment of all of the above pyodermas is accomplished by draining the lesion and starting the patient on appropriate antibiotics, such as ampicillin, 500 mg 4 times daily for a period of 5 days. Hot sitz baths several times daily for a few days accelerates resolution of infection.

ALLERGIES AND IRRITANT REACTIONS

Most vulvar reactions are contact dermatitis caused by substances intentionally applied for therapeutic or hygienic purposes. Individuals who may incite an inflammatory reaction from a topical agent are often considered to be allergic to that agent when, in reality, such reactions are usually caused by a hypersensitivity.

Primary Irritant Reactions

Such corrosive chemicals as concentrated acids applied to the skin or certain base carrier substances used in other topical medications may produce an irritant response in a person on first exposure. Some irritants produce responses only after repeated contacts or in the presence of moisture or occlusiveness. Irritant responses that occur after prolonged exposure are called accumulative primary irritations.

Allergic Reactions

Allergic contact dermatitis, also called eczematous or allergic eczema, is an eruption that has arisen from contact in susceptible individuals to substances to which they are allergic. For an allergic reaction to occur, the patient must have been previously sensitized to the allergenic substance. Subsequent topical or systemic reactions to contact may follow administration of the allergen; however, some of these reactions are not clinically evident until several days or weeks after contact.

Clinical Features. Irritant and allergenic responses are so similar that it is often difficult for any expert clinician to make the differential diagnosis. With the exception of lesions caused by strong corrosive substances, the two varieties of contacts are clinically identical, consisting of erythema, edema, eruption of vesicles or bullae, and weeping. Vesiculation and ulceration are more often induced by primary irritants used in strong concentrations or prolonged contact. The severity of the reaction is influenced by the sensitivity of the affected person as well as the site of contact.

Symptoms may consist of varying degrees of tenderness, pain, burning, and, most commonly, pruritus. Urinary retention is not unusual with severe reactions, and painful adenitis similar to that seen with acute primary herpes may be experienced.

Diagnosis. Careful inquiry regarding possible contacts is helpful in detecting the responsible agent. Many times, reactions to primary agents are easily recognized by the patients. Such specific contactants as feminine hygiene sprays, perfume present in toilet tissue, and even insect bites may present similarly.

Treatment. Severe painful reactions require immediate external treatment after the diagnosis of any infectious disease has been eliminated. The use of wet compresses of aluminum acetate (Burow's solution, 1:20) or concentrated boric acid solution may afford considerable relief. Because preparations with a cream base do not usually adhere to moist surfaces, initial treatment of eczematoid eruptions are accomplished better with wet compresses. Topical applications of an appropriate corticosteroid preparation, such as fluocinolone acetonide (Synalar) cream or ointment, hydrocortisone acetate (Cortef), or triamcinolone acetonide (Aristocort) cream, often promptly relieve the patient's symptoms. Systemic antihistamines leave much to be desired in effectiveness. Topical use of antihistamines or anesthetic-type medications may involve a risk of inducing an allergic reaction to the therapeutic agent itself. Systemic corticorsteroids may be effective for severe allergic reactions.

Specific Contactants

Any organic or inorganic chemical agent has the potential to cause an allergenic or irritant reaction. An effective candidacidal agent used on the vulva that has been known to cause marked irritant reactions is gentian violet, usually applied in a 1 or 2 percent aqueous solution. Topical fluorouracil, used in the treatment of intraepithelial vulvar carcinoma, vulvar dysplasia, and condyloma acuminata, is known usually to cause a moderate to severe irritative reaction, with superficial ulcerations found at the site of application.

Poison Oak and Poison Ivy

The oleoresins produced by poison oak and poison ivy when transmitted to the vulvar tissue by contaminated hands, causes redness and wheals with vesicular formation at the point of contact.

Miscellaneous Agents

Colored toilet tissue, dyes in underwear, detergents, and perfumes are known to cause marked vulvar vesiculation.

INSECT BITES

Pediculosis Pubis

Pediculosis pubis is an infestation of the hairy area of the vulva by the crab louse. Itching is the common symptom, and scratching may induce secondary lesions of the skin with small excoriations and pyodermas. Pediculosis should be suspected when the patient has pruritus of the hairy area of the lower trunk, especially the mons pubis. Diagnosis can be made by the discovery of nits and parasites at the bases of the hairs, and this may be facilitated by the use of a magnifying glass. Pediculosis may be confused with scabies; however, lesions of scabies are usually spread over the body, including nonhairy areas. Treatment is application of gamma benzene hexachloride (Kwell), which has a low irritation rate. Kwell, in shampoo, cream, or lotion form, contains 1 percent of the active ingredient, lindane.

Chigger

Chigger bites are acquired in the summer months in the southern part of the United States. The bite gives rise to intense pruritus, and the typical lesion is a small, erythematous papule. A shake lotion with hydrocortisone is helpful in controlling pruritus, and 3 percent sulfa added to the lotion kills the chiggers.

Bed Bugs

The lesion produced may be a wheal, papule, or blister; the lesions are usually found in groups or in a straight line. Relief can be obtained by the use of antihistamines.

Ticks

Whereas the skin lesion is *usually* a minor inflammatory reaction, if the head of the tick is left embedded in the skin (as a result of attempted mechanical removal of the tick), its presence may give rise to a longstanding pruritic papule. If an individual presents with a tick on the vulva, the tick may be smothered and induced to drop off by application of an oily substance, such as petrolatum or fingernail polish. Excision of the site where the head is embedded may be necessary if the embedded head cannot be extracted. Small lesions usually occur as small wheals; however, in a hypersensitive patient, giant wheals or blisters may devleop. Treatment should be administration of an antihistamine and supportive therapy.

SUGGESTED READING

Gardner HL, Kaufman RH. Benign diseases of the vulva and vagina. 2nd ed. Boston: GK Hall Medical Publishers, 1981.

ABNORMAL UTERINE BLEEDING

ALAN B. LITTLE, M.D., F.R.C.S.(C)
MARK E. BOYD, M.D., F.R.C.S.(C)

Abnormal uterine bleeding is the most common of all gynecologic problems and accounts for the majority of gynecologic emergencies. The patient herself defines the bleeding as abnormal by describing a change from her previous menstrual pattern, but she may be unable to quantitate accurately the amount of blood lost, either underestimating or overestimating it.

MANAGEMENT

Management of abnormal uterine bleeding is based on the general cause of bleeding.

Abnormal Pregnancy

A diagnosis of incomplete abortion or threatened abortion is made for a large proportion of the patients seen. Diagnosis is not difficult. Dilatation of the cervix and a history of passage of placental tissue are central to the differentiation of threatened and incomplete abortion. Treatment recommendations are clear: the uterus must be emptied for inevitable abortion or incomplete abortion. The choice of menstrual extraction or curettage is moot. In cases in which threatened abortion is diagnosed, the history being vaginal bleeding associated with abdominal cramps, observation is the initial management and diagnostic pelvic ultrasonography is the primary investigation. The diagnosis of ectopic pregnancy, except in instances of obvious rupture, is often difficult. Delay in therapy may be dangerous. All women seen in an emergency with abnormal bleeding should be screened with a quantitative beta-human chorionic gonadotropin (beta-HCG) pregnancy test (Hybritech, Tadem Icon). This test is remarkably sensitive, inexpensive, and invaluable in this setting. Using the beta-HCG pregnancy test almost completely removes the critical danger of missing an ectopic pregnancy. The combined use of diagnostic ultrasonography and the quantitative beta-HCG subunit test frequently permits the determination of the exact site and nature of the pregnancy including diagnosis of early unruptured tubal ectopic pregnancy.

Bleeding Associated with Contraceptive Use

Intermenstrual bleeding and oligomenorrhea often result from the use of oral contraceptives. The pathophysiologic cause of this bleeding is variable and is frequently inadequate estrogen stimulus of the endometrium. Reassurance that the patient is not pregnant, confirmed by testing, and explanation of the basis for the complaint are all that is necessary in most instances. If the bleeding is persistent, conjugated estrogen (Premarin) 1.25 mg or 2.5 mg daily may be taken in conjunction with the oral contraceptive that the patient is using for the first 10 days of each of the next two cycles.

Patients with an intrauterine device (IUD) often develop abnormal uterine bleeding. The IUD itself must be considered to contribute to the problem. If the bleeding is sufficiently disturbing, the IUD should be removed; it is unlikely that the bleeding will abate with it in place. Unless the string is not visible, IUDs should also be removed if the patient is found to be pregnant. This will decrease the chances of abortion and sepsis.

Bleeding at Extremes of Age (Menopause and Menarche)

When abnormal bleeding occurs at menarche or menopause, the first objective is to rule out complex pathology or pathophysiology. The postmenopausal patient rarely presents with a gynecologic emergency. If she is seen with a complaint of postmenopausal bleeding, it is essential to rule out endometrial cancer. The patient should be referred to a gynecologist for an endometrial biopsy.

The teenager who has heavy bleeding with her first menses or who has had heavy bleeding in the first years following the menarche may present with a particularly acute problem. The bleeding may be so severe that the patient is rendered hypovolemic. In most instances, the bleeding is anovulatory and dysfunctional in nature, but in some cases there is a bleeding disorder. Management of the dysfunctional bleeding is discussed in detail in the following paragraphs, but a hematologic screen of prothrombin time (PT), partial thromboplastin time (PTT), platelet count, and bleeding time is necessary because of the frequency with which bleeding diatheses occur in this age group in this setting.

FINAL TRIAGE

A majority of patients are not pregnant, are not using oral contraceptives or IUDs, and are between the ages of 20 and 50. Most patients do not present at the extremes of gynecologic age when anovulation is more common. The clinical working diagnosis should be that the abnormal bleeding is due to a nonspecified disturbance of hormone function, so-called dysfunctional uterine bleeding. The disturbance of hormonal function will be reflected by the endometrial histology, but histology cannot be predicted on the basis of menstrual history alone. Although the pattern of the endometrium in cases of acute vaginal hemorrhage is more likely to demonstrate an anovulatory pattern than in the nonacute cases, it is possible to find menstrual, secretory, or atrophic endometrium, decidua or pseudodecidua, or endometritis. To manipulate the hormonal milieu in order to correct the abnormal bleeding, therapy is needed that is equally effective for all types of endometrium.

The diagnosis of dysfunctional bleeding is confirmed only when organic disease is excluded. Although history and physical examination give immediate clues about the presence or absence of benign or malignant disease, it must be recognized that special investigations such as endometrial biopsy, cytology, bacteriologic studies, endocrine studies, and endoscopic techniques may be necessary for definitive diagnosis in selected patients.

It is difficult to separate immediately patients with dysfunctional uterine bleeding from those with organic disease. Even in cases in which the diagnosis of organic disease is obvious (e.g., fibroids) the bleeding may be dysfunctional. The guiding principle is that the distinction between dysfunctional uterine bleeding and organic disease should become clearer as a result of the therapeutic response. Dysfunctional uterine bleeding responds to proper hormonal manipulation; organic disease does not. A gratifying therapeutic response demonstrates that the disorder was indeed functional; a failure to respond mandates further investigation. Before embarking on a costly and sometimes inefficient investigation to prove the absence or presence of organic disease, it is almost always worthwhile to use a therapeutic trial of hormone therapy. An exception to this delay in investigation is cervical culture for gonorrhea. Gonorrhea is frequently cultured from women on emergency admissions, and gonorrhea is frequently associated with irregular uterine bleeding. Endocervical culture for gonorrhea should be considered for all women admitted to the emergency department with abnormal uterine bleeding.

THE NEED FOR IMMEDIATE TREATMENT

Objective evidence must be obtained as to the amount of blood loss. The pulse rate, blood pressure, pallor, the amount of blood found in the vagina, and the hematocrit give the emergency physician the first indication of this and the need for immediate crossmatching, intravenous fluids, or transfusion. In many instances, only a short period of observation (during which time pad counts and degrees of saturation are recorded) is necessary to permit a decision to be made as to the urgency of the situation. A suggested scale of the pad saturation during this time is 1+ (soaking of a portion of the pad), 2+ (soaking of entire pad), and 3+ (soaking the pad and the surrounding area). If the bleeding is acute, (hematocrit drop, orthostatic hypotension, or more than one 3+ pad per hour), admission to hospital is advised.

Surgical Treatment (Curettage)

In recent years the practice of curettage has been criticized. It is reassuring to know, however, that this simple surgical procedure almost always stops acute bleeding, although long-term benefit is not always assured. It also allows time for further investigation and treatment.

Medical Treatment

In cases in which the indications for surgery are not strong, e.g., juveniles, patients who have had a previous curettage and whose endometrial histology is known, or patients whose medical condition does not permit an operative procedure, the accepted therapy is hormonal.

Intravenous Premarin may be used as immediate therapy in the patient with acute bleeding. The treatment is empiric. There are few studies that demonstrate Premarin's efficacy in this regard. The hemostatic effect is apparently due to a nonspecific change in coagulation factors rather than a direct effect on the endometrium. The recommended dose is 25 mg intravenously every 4 hours for a maximum of 6 doses. At the same time, 4 tablets per day of Ortho-Novum 1/50 (norethindrone 1 mg and mestranol 50 μg is prescribed. After 2 days this dosage is reduced to 2 tablets a day, this dosage is continued for the following 21 days. Following a withdrawal bleed, Ortho-Novum 1/50, at a conventional dosage is continued for 3 months, at 1 tablet per day.

LESS ACUTE HEMORRHAGE

In most cases the hemorrhage does not constitute an immediate danger to the patient's well-being. The bleeding will have abated over the period of observation and is clearly not immediately threatening. In many instances, reassuring the patient, asking her to record any further blood loss, and providing for later follow-up and possible investigation constitute the most appropriate management. If medical treatment is required, the choice is whether to use progestational agents, antiprostaglandins, or combined hormonal therapy (oral contraceptive equivalent).

Progestational Agents

Progestational agents cause withdrawal bleeding and therefore will not stop the bleeding immediately. Their effect is to create secretory endometrium in the presence of an adequately estrogen-stimulated endometrium. Over a long period of administration, progestins cause atrophy and decidualization of the endometrium. Progesterone or a progestin is most worthwhile in those cases in which the patient is anovulatory. Anovulatory endometrium may be proven by endometrial biopsy. Because they offer no immediate benefit and there is often no demonstrable need for them, progestational agents are infrequently used in the emergency treatment of abnormal uterine bleeding.

Antiprostaglandins

Antiprostaglandins are prescribed in some instances to reduce the amount of blood loss without altering the pattern of bleeding. They are valuable for patients who complain of heavy regular menstrual cycles. The antiprostaglandin mefenamic acid (Ponstel) in a dosage of 500 mg three times daily has been shown to reduce bleeding by as much as 40 percent. Side effects are few, and immediate results can be gratifying.

Oral Contraceptives

In most instances, bleeding of a dysfunctional nature responds best to oral contraceptives. This medication will be effective in the presence of all types of endometrium, and the reduction of blood loss is on the order of 75 percent. The medication may be prescribed to most patients; a flexible attitude is advised. Contraindications such as a history of phlebitis or active liver disease are infrequently encountered. Patients who are over 30 years of age who smoke should not be regarded as being prohibited from using oral contraceptives. Any risk of administration is generally balanced by the need for treatment.

Other Regimens

Other medical regimens have included the use of danazol or LH analogues. Both produce medical menopause, they are expensive, and their side effects make them difficult to tolerate. Their use is not normally considered in an emergency setting. The simultaneous use of Micronor (norethindrone 350 μg) and Premarin has been suggested as a means of producing an atrophic endometrium in older women without causing menopausal symptoms. This combination may well be prescribed for the older patient with a previously normal endometrium who continues to have abnormal uterine bleeding.

SUGGESTED READING

Claessens EA, Cowell CA. Acute adolescent menorrhagia. AM J Obstet Gynecol 1981;139:277–280.
DeVore GR, Owens O, Kase N. Use of intravenous premarin in the treatment of dysfunctional uterine bleeding—a double-blind randomized control study. Obstet Gynecol 1982;59:285–291.
MacKenzie IZ, Bibby JG. Critical assessment of dilatation and curettage in 1,029 women. Lancet 1978;2:566–268.
Magos AL, Brincat M, Studd JWW, et al. Amenorrhea and endometrial atrophy with continuous oral estrogen and progestogen therapy in postmenopausal women. Obstet Gynecol 1985;65:496–499.

PREMENSTRUAL SYNDROME AND CRAMPS

CAROL J. JESSOP, M.D.

PREMENSTRUAL SYNDROME

Diagnosis

Sometime during their reproductive lives, many women will experience some change in their well-being specifically related to the hormonal changes that occur 1 to 10 days before the onset of their menstrual cycle. Although most of these women will not be seriously affected, others may experience physical and/or behavioral changes that are quite severe and cause recurrent, cyclical disability. If this is the case, the diagnosis of premenstrual syndrome (PMS) is made.

The symptoms of PMS may vary significantly from one patient to another, yet each woman tends to recognize her own symptom complex. Most commonly reported physical symptoms are headache, breast swelling and tenderness, generalized bloating and weight gain, constipation, acne, backache, tinnitus, and increased craving for sweets and salty foods. Behavioral changes may be very prominent and include agitation, insomnia, irritability, fatigue, emotional lability, depression, and suicidal ideation.

At present, no laboratory tests are available to document the diagnosis. Physical examination is important to rule out other medical, especially endocrine, disorders. To make this clinical diagnosis, one must establish a premenstrual cyclical pattern to the symptoms, in that they occur from 1 to 10 days before the menses and end with the onset of bleeding. The most common error in diagnosis is mistaking endogenous depression for PMS. Endogenous depression is manifested by many of the same behavioral changes and can be *exacerbated* by premenstrual hormonal changes, but the symptoms do not resolve with the onset of menses. PMS is sometimes confused with painful menstrual cramping or dysmenorrhea. It is possible to have PMS symptoms followed by dysmenorrhea, but the two are considered *separate* conditions and have *different* therapies.

The etiology of PMS is still unclear. Recent research has focused on the hormonal imbalance of estrogen-progesterone levels in most patients, which may secondarily cause central nervous system (CNS) neurotransmitters to fluctuate abnormally. The symptoms of PMS are thought to result from such changes in these neurotransmitters; however, some believe that stressful life changes and poor eating habits may be the actual precipitant to the hormonal changes.

Treatment

With the exception of patients with severe agitation or depression, few women with PMS actually present with life-emergent situations. These patients should be assessed for suicidal ideation, and hospitalized for supportive care and observation if the risk of suicide is present. Antidepressants and tranquilizers are usually not indicated unless the patient has an underlying psychiatric disorder or fails to improve once menses begins. Referral to an appropriate health care provider with experience and sensitivity towards patients with PMS is then indicated once the patient is discharged.

Many patients with PMS will respond to reassurance and patient education about this disorder. Therapy, in most cases, should begin with conservative, noninvasive, and nonpharmacologic means. A careful review of the patient's diet and life stresses should be made. Suggestions for modifying the diet are eventually helpful, but it may take 3 to 6 months to achieve noticeable results. Restrict foods that contain chocolate, caffeine, black tea, nicotine, refined sugar, and large amounts of salt. In addition, patients should be told to limit alcoholic beverages because tolerance for alcohol decreases during the premenstrual phase.

Administration of vitamin B_6 is beneficial in many patients, especially those who are under 40 years of age and experiencing water retention and bloating. The vitamin should be taken in doses of 200 to 500 mg a day throughout the cycle for several months. Many nutritionists suggest taking it along with a daily multivitamin as well.) Since B_6 is a necessary co-factor in the synthesis of dopamine, its diuretic action is thought to be a result of increased dopaminergic activity. Although there have been rare reports of peripheral neuropathy occurring in patients taking B_6, the doses in these patients were generally greater than 4000 mg a day for an extended period of time. More commonly noted side effects are nausea, headache, and recollection of one's dreams. If no benefit is noted after 4 to 6 months, then the vitamin should be discontinued.

If the patient's main complaint is related to water retention and breast tenderness—and vitamin B_6 has not helped—then the addition of vitamin E 400 IU a day, and avoidance of caffeine should help. A trial of potassium-sparing diuretics is indicated only if these options fail. They should be used for only 3 to 5 days prior to menses.

Progesterone supplementation is often helpful in women who are 30 years or older and in those women who develop PMS subsequent to tubal ligation with the cauterization method. This population of women is more likely to have decreased progesterone levels and may experience some relief with administration of progesterone suppositories during the premenstrual phase. Suppositories usually contain 200 to 400 mg of natural progesterone and are administered either rectally or vaginally in doses of 200 to 1600 mg daily. The progesterone can be mixed with three different suppository bases (polyethylene glycol, glycogelatin, and cocoa butter), but it has been demonstrated that the peak circulating levels obtained with polyethylene glycol suppositories were significantly higher than with the other two bases.

Individualization of therapy is very important, and the use of a menstrual diary often aids the patient in knowing when to begin using the suppositories. The progesterone should be started after ovulation and before the symptoms begin. It should be stopped when the menses is anticipated, or it may prolong the cycle. The rate of absorption, utilization, and metabolism of progesterone varies with each woman. Oral forms of progesterone are rapidly absorbed into the portal circulation and rapidly metabolized to inactive metabolites.

Progesterone administered by vaginal or rectal suppository reaches its peak blood level within 4 to 8 hours, with the return to baseline occurring within 12 to 24 hours.

Consequently, a patient may require several administrations each day to maintain adequate blood levels. Side effects have not been a problem, and many women have used progesterone for several years without any apparent increase in malignancies. Although some providers have tried to use synthetic progestagens (available in oral preparations) instead of the natural progesterone suppositories, many women have noted worsening of their symptoms with these agents.

Birth control pills have also been used in the treatment of PMS, and, again, they may worsen symptoms in some patients. Presumably, this is due to the suppression of natural progesterone levels and the increase in estrogen level. If oral contraceptives are tried, a progestin-dominant pill should be selected, because evidence suggests that this type of oral contraceptive is more effective for PMS treatment.

Bromocriptine (Parlodel) has been recommended for the treatment of PMS patients who have higher than normal prolactin levels and whose main symptom is breast engorgement. The drug is administered in a dosage of 2.5 mg twice daily. However, the incidence of side effects and the rate of discontinuance with this medication have been very high, outweighing any benefit to the great majority of women.

Recently, PMS patients with severe emotional instability have been treated successfully with Catapres (*clonidine*). Doses of 0.1 to 0.3 mg a day were used, with drowsiness and orthostatic hypotension being noted in only a few patients. Again, this medication should be used only during the symptomatic period, and after other therapeutic measures have failed.

CRAMPS

Dysmenorrhea (or cramps) is the term used to describe painful lower pelvic pain that accompanies the onset of menstruation. It has been found that approximately 50 percent of menstruating women experience dysmenorrhea during their reproductive lives; 10 to 15 percent of these women are incapacitated by their pain for 1 to 2 days each month. Indeed, menstrual cramps has been found to be the most common cause of lost working hours and school days among young women, thus being a loss to the community as well as the individual patient.

Dysmenorrhea must be classified as *primary* or *secondary* before it is possible to evaluate and treat the patient adequately.

Primary dysmenorrhea is unrelated to a specific organic pelvic condition. It is likely to first present 1 to 2 years after menarche, and is commonly associated with nausea, vomiting, low back pain, presyncope, and diarrhea. The patient is most commonly nulliparous and ovulating and not taking birth control pills. The etiology is almost always increased production of prostaglandins (particularly PGF2a), which results in an increase in the frequency and strength of uterine contractions. The diagnosis of primary dysmenorrhea is generally made by a clinical history, as the *pelvic examination should be entirely normal*. Other diagnoses that could have similar presen-

TABLE 1 Nonsteroidal Anti-Inflammatory Agents

Generic Name	Dose (mg)	Intervals (hours)	Comments
Naproxen sodium	275	8–12	Rapid onset
Naproxen	250, 375, 500	12	Long action
Ibuprofen	200, 400, 600	4–6	Available over the counter Inexpensive
Indomethacin	25 or 50	6–8	More side effects
Mefenamic acid	250	6	Side effects common (dizziness, headache)

tations to primary dysmenorrhea include (1) pelvic inflammatory disease in a young adolescent, which may cause pelvic pain on the first day of the cycle, and (2) nonspecific pelvic pain in an adolescent girl who has been sexually traumatized as a child.

Secondary dysmenorrhea is usually seen in women in their 20s to 50s and is most often caused by specific pelvic pathologic conditions such as salpingitis, recurrent ovarian cysts, intrauterine devices (IUDs) causing a bacterial infection, endometriosis, cervical stenosis, intrauterine synecchiae (Asherman's syndrome), foreign bodies of the pelvic tract, or uterine anomalies. The patient may have a history of primary dysmenorrhea, but generally reports that this pain is different. Diagnostic evaluation for a patient with secondary dysmenorrhea may include a complete blood count (CBC), urinalysis, sedimentation rate, bacterial culture of vaginal discharge, pelvic ultrasonography, and/or laparoscopy. Pelvic examination is usually abnormal and may disclose a pelvic mass, pelvic infection, evidence of endometriosis, or a stenosed cervix. Special attention should be paid to vaginal discharge, ovarian size and tenderness, the uterosacral ligaments (commonly found to have endometrial implants), and the appearance of the cervix.

Therapy

The treatment of *primary dysmenorrhea* is rather straightforward in the majority of women. Nonsteroidal anti-inflammatory compounds are active inhibitors of prostaglandin synthesis and can be given at the onset of menses with fairly rapid resolution of pain (Table 1). There is no one compound that is really superior to the others, although a patient might prefer one agent over another because of features specific for that agent (i.e., rapidity of onset, duration of action, cost, incidence of side effects, or just individual response to an agent). Therefore, it is important to try three or four agents before abandoning this form of therapy.

Secondary dysmenorrhea, of course, is treated by eliminating the precipitating condition.

SUGGESTED READING

Abraham G, Hargrove J. Effect of vitamin B$_6$ supplement on premenstrual syndrome. Infertility 1980; 3(2):155–165.

Akerlund M, Andersson KE, Ingemarsson I. Effects of terbutaline on myometrial activity, endometrial flow, and lower abdominal pain in women with primary dysmenorrhea. Br J Obstet Gynaecol 1976; 83:673–678.

Dingerfelder JR. Primary dysmenorrhea: treatment with prostaglandin inhibitors: a review. Am J Obstet Gynecol 1981; 140:874–879.

Norris RV. Progesterone for premenstrual tension. J Reprod Med 1983; 28(8):509–515.

Reid RL, Yen SSC. Premenstrual syndrome. Am J Obstet Gynecol 1981; 139:85–104.

Sandahl B, Ulmsten U, Anderson KE. Trial of the calcium antagonist nifedipine in the treatment of primary dysmenorrhea. Arch Gynecol 1979; 227:147–151.

BREAST DISORDERS

RICHARD A. CURRIE, M.D., C.M., F.A.C.S.

Breast disorders in clinical practice largely involve adult females. Rather few males are included, and these are mostly young men with gynecomastia. The presenting complaints of most patients with breast disease include one or more of the following: a breast lump, localized pain and tenderness, nipple discharge or erosion, and skin changes such as erythema, edema, dimpling, or ulceration. As the result of screening programs an increasing number of patients are now encountered with mammographic abnormalities not associated with other signs or symptoms of disease. Finally a few patients with advanced breast cancer still present initially with regional lymph node enlargements, arm swelling, satellite skin nodules, or evidence of distant metastases.

Physicians dealing with breast disorders need to be skilled in the art of thorough history taking and of breast examination, which goes a long way in the establishment of an accurate diagnosis. The recording of pertinent findings in a simple diagram or sketch is recommended. Needle aspiration of cysts and solid tumors, low-dose mammography or xeromammography, and preparation of Pap smears from nipple secretions are often useful in the initial assessment of breast complaints. Despite the fact that the majority of breast disorders are benign, experience dictates that a pathologic diagnosis often must first be obtained before treatment can be confidently begun. This clearly requires that all suspicious masses and mammographic abnormalities be promptly referred to a surgeon for consideration of biopsy. "Late" diagnosis of breast cancer is a claim now being made with increasing frequency in the litigation of malpractice cases.

There are few emergencies encountered in patients with breast disorders, but many are seen at short notice and in a state of considerable anxiety caused by concern about possible malignancy. Physicians caring for adult female patients with breast complaints should be aware of this apprehension and try to minimize delay in seeing these patients for an initial evaluation.

The examination of adults for unrelated illnesses is an opportunity to perform a careful breast examination which may lead to serendipitous discovery of potentially important findings. It may also offer a chance to teach a woman breast self-examination, to advise her about other pertinent surveillance measures such as mammography, or to identify individual risk factors that enhance the possible ocurrence of breast cancer.

MASTITIS AND ABSCESS

Mastitis most commonly occurs in nursing mothers within 6 weeks of delivery. It also may arise in the last few weeks of pregnancy or at the time of weaning. Less frequently a fulminating case may be seen in the early postpartum period in conjunction with an infection in the baby or in the setting of a newborn nursery epidemic.

Lactational mastitis is usually caused by stasis attributable to inadequate emptying of the milk ducts in one sector of the breast. The portal of entry of infection is the nipple and the lactiferous sinuses, although bacteria may also penetrate into the breast stroma through fissures or excoriations in the nipple or areola.

Diagnosis is made based on the presence of pain, tenderness, erythema, and induration in the affected segment of the breast. The epidemic type in post partum women may be more often associated with bilateral signs, and with fever and toxicity.

Treatment consists of use of the breast pump to empty the affected breast, a temporary pause in nursing for that breast, and the systemic administration of an antibiotic effective against penicillinase-producing staphylococci. Other useful measures include the application of moist heat, provision of a comfortable supporting bandage, analgesics and, in a home setting, help so that the patient can obtain proper rest and supportive care.

Abscess formation is heralded by appearance of a localized fluctuant mass within the involved sector.

Preliminary needle aspiration is carried out through a wheal of local anesthetic to obtain pus for confirmation of the diagnosis and for culture. Early surgical referral for incision and drainage should be arranged. The drainage operation involves a circumareolar incision, done under local anesthesia. Small soft rubber drains are inserted into the abscess cavity and sewn to the edges of the incision. Postoperative care includes the use of local heat, breast support, and frequent changes of saline compresses. Systemic antibiotics are administered until the inflammation subsides. Lactation is suppressed by having the patient stop all nursing, and by binding both breasts with a soft, snug bandage for 48 to 72 hours. Cold applications to the normal breast and oral analgesics may be necessary for control of pain.

Breast abscess may also occur in nonlactating nonpregnant women because of invasion of bacteria through the nipple or through open skin lesions. Fine needle aspiration may be helpful in cytologic diagnosis as well as in obtaining material for culture of bacteria. There is a frequent association of such abscesses with underlying disorders such as duct ectasia and carcinoma, so open biopsy of the abscess wall is done routinely at the time of incision and drainage.

Subareolar abscess is a chronic and recurring type of infection seen most often in young nonlactating women. It is an abscess located under the nipple with a lactiferous sinus leading into it which is dilated and plugged with keratotic debris from squamous metaplasia in its lining epithelium. There is often a sinus tract connecting the abscess and the skin surface of the areola near the base of the nipple. Definitive surgical treatment requires that the abscess and its ducts and sinuses be excised completely.

Breast abscess in newborn infants occurs in a breast that is engorged and hypertrophied by hormonal influences. Signs are swelling, tenderness, and erythema about the nipple. Early surgical drainage through a small circumareolar incision is recommended to avoid the skin necrosis and possible permanent injury to the breast bud which are seen in neglected infections.

DISORDERS OF NIPPLE AND AREOLA

Nipple Retraction

Flattening, deviation, or inward retraction of the nipple may be a sign of an underlying cancer which, with its accompanying fibrosis, has shortened the main ducts under the nipple. It is commonly accompanied by a palpable mass in the central part of the breast and a suspicous mammographic finding. Retraction of the nipple and areola is also sometimes seen in benign conditions such as duct ectasia and traumatic fat necrosis. It should not be confused with long standing nipple inversion, which is a developmental abnormality usually dating from puberty.

Nipple Erosion

Erosion of the surface of the nipple is often associated with crusting and a serosanguineous discharge. It represents Paget's disease of the nipple, an intraductal carcinoma of the breast. A mass may or may not be felt within the central portion of the breast. Mammography should be obtained, and the patient referred to a surgeon for open biopsy of the lesion.

Nipple Discharge

Spontaneous single or multiple duct discharges in nonpregnant and nonlactating women require explanation. Breast examination, mammography, and Pap smears of the discharge are routine studies.

Multiple duct discharges, frequently milky in appearance and from both breasts, may be caused by use of oral contraceptives, or by the ingestion of drugs such as the phenothiazines, methyldopa, and rauwolfia alkaloids. They are also frequently seen in nulliparous women at the time of menopause. Milky discharges may be seen in some endocrine disorders associated with amenorrhea and with high circulating levels of prolactin. Prolactin assays, and in some cases, skull roentgenograms and computed tomography scans should be obtained if galactorrhea suggests the possibility of a pituitary tumor.

The single duct discharge is most often caused by an intraductal papilloma which is usually not large enough to be palpable, but may be visible in the mammogram. Other underlying causes are ductal papillomatosis, duct ectasia, and carcinoma. The ectasias and ductal carcinomas are usually seen in menopausal or older women. Rather few patients with breast cancer will be found to have a nipple discharge without a palpable mass or a detectable mammographic abnormality.

The patients who require duct exploration are all those with single duct discharges and those with multiple duct discharges with an accompanying mass or a visible mammographic lesion. Exceptions might be made in postmenopausal women, in whom surgical exploration will be routine for any otherwise unexplained nipple dischage.

The bloody discharge of single or multiple ducts during the last trimester of pregnancy is attributable to sloughing of the ductal epithelium. It is a physiologic effect that is usually transitory and requires only that the patient be reassured concerning its benign nature.

BREAST MASSES

Fibroadenoma

Fibroadenoma is a benign painless tumor of young women which is multiple in about 15 percent of cases and bilateral in about the same number. It is felt as a smooth, rubbery mass that may be lobular in shape, but is both well demarcated and movable within the surrounding breast. It is treated in most instances by surgical excision with local anesthesia. In the case of small fibroadenomas in teenage girls, delay in surgical removal may be acceptable, particularly if fine needle biopsy can be used for confirmation of diagnosis.

Gynecomastia

Asymptomatic enlargement of the male breast is very common at puberty, and affects nearly two-thirds of boys ages 12 to 15 years. It is usually unilateral and regresses spontaneously in a year or two. Another common type of gynecomastia is seen in aged men, where it is usually bilateral.

The cause of gynecomastia lies in a change in the balance between the effects of circulating estrogens and androgens on the breast as an end-organ. Breast enlargement may be produced either by an estrogen excess or by a relative lack of androgens. It is seen in conditions involving hypogonadism such as cryptorchidism and testicular atropy. Klinefelter's syndrome is usually associated with gynecomastia, and is the only example of this disorder in which there is an increased risk of breast cancer. Neoplasms that can cause gynecomastia include adrenocortical tumors, testicular tumors (Leydig and germinal cell types), nontesticular tumors producing human chorionic gonadotropin (hCG), and certain lung cancers. In addition, many drugs can initiate breast enlargement or increase the size of an existing one, including digitalis, cimetidine, methyldopa, phenothiazines, reserpine, and several chemotherapeutic agents.

Investigation of gynecomastia as a symptom of underlying disease should be restricted to adult patients with a history of recent onset. Breast cancer can be excluded by its occurrence in older men in the form of a painless nodule with an eccentric location under the nipple, often in association with ulceration and an ipsilateral axillary lymph node enlargement. Biopsy of the lesion may be necessary to exclude neoplasia. Drug ingestion, primary hypogonadism, and underlying disorders such as hyperthyroidism, nutritional disturbances, and chronic liver disease should be considered in the diagnostic work-up. The testes should be palpated for nodules. A number of screening tests for endocrine disorders may be required to exclude testicular and adrenal tumors and other neoplasms (serum levels of estrogen, testosterone, hCG, gonadotropins and prolactin, and urinary 17-ketosteroids).

Mammary Dysplasia

Formerly called "fibrocystic disease," this condition is extremely common in women in the age range from 25 years to the menopause. Its cause is not well understood, but is clearly related to a cyclic interplay between the circulating ovarian hormones and the breast. The most consistent hormonal finding is an elevated level of estradiol in the luteal phase of the cycle.

The most common clinical manifestation of dysplasia is "physiologic nodularity," which gives the breast consistency a characteristic lumpiness. Clinical features usually involve premenstrual pain and tenderness in local areas of one or both breasts. Nodularity is the most common objective finding, but discrete lumps are frequently discovered, some of which prove to be cystic. A small subset of patients with biopsy-proven dysplasia are believed to have an enhanced risk of developing breast cancer. The management of mammary dysplasia requires patient education with simple explanations concerning the nature of the process, stressing its benign nature and its status as a condition rather than a disease. Instruction in breast self-examination and regular visits to a primary care physician for follow-up should be arranged. A baseline mammography is recommended for all patients with lumpy breasts at age 35 years or older.

When a discrete or dominant mass is discovered, aspiration should be carried out with a syringe and a 22-gauge needle. This allows prompt identification and elimination of cysts. The fluid is withdrawn completely, and if the mass disappears completely and the fluid is not bloody, it is discarded. If the mass persists or if the fluid is bloody, the fluid is sent in a nutrient medium for cytologic examination.

Breast pain of varying degrees is common in mammary dysplasia. Reassurance to the patient concerning its benign and usually self-limited nature is most helpful. Comfortable support of the breast with a padded bra, the use of analgesics, local application of heat, and rest of the upper extremities are useful measures. For intractable cases, a trial of the mildly androgenic drug danazol (Danocrine) may be instituted. The recommended oral dosage is 100 to 400 mg per day for periods of 4 to 6 months. This antigonadotrophic drug may have side effects such as amenorrhea and hot flashes. Surgical excision of a persistently painful and tender area of localized dysplasia can be considered as appropriate treatment for relief of symptoms and for confirmation of diagnosis.

Carcinoma

The main risk factors of carcinoma are a family history, a previous breast cancer, and a proliferative mammary dysplasia with atypia. A history of premenopausal occurrence of or bilateral occurrence in a mother or sister is particularly significant. Other factors include menarche before age 12 years, menopause after 50 years, first childbirth after age 35 years, and nulliparity.

This very common cancer usually presents as a painless breast lump that has been discovered by the patient herself. Abnormal mammography is an increasingly frequent method of discovering primary breast cancer. Nipple discharge, nipple erosions, axillary node enlargement, or the finding of a distant metastasis are other more unusual modes of presentation.

In the case of solid, discrete breast masses, those that are accessible should be aspirated with a fine needle for the purpose of rapid diagnosis. The technique is simple and not painful in most cases if a 21- or 22-gauge needle is passed in different directions through the mass with suction applied to the attached 20-ml syringe. Suction is released prior to withdrawal of the needle from the mass, and the specimen is expelled into a tube or bottle containing nutrient medium. Alternatively, slides may be prepared immediately by the standard Papanicolaou methods. Further investigation of solid breast tumors includes low-dose mammography or xeromammography. Open breast biopsy by a surgeon will usually follow.

Breast lumps detected during pregnancy or lactation should be managed as they would be in other circumstances although without recourse to mammography, i.e., with diagnosis by needle aspiration and, if necessary, open biopsy.

Preliminary outpatient assessment of the patient with a suspicious breast mass includes biopsy and clinical staging. The patient should be promptly referred to a surgeon. Mammography should always be obtained for study of the opposite breast and to provide a point of reference for follow-up studies after treatment.

An unusual type of locally advanced breast cancer is one that has features of inflammation suggestive of mastitis or breast abscess. The distinctive signs of inflammatory carcinoma are erythema and edema of the skin and an underlying breast mass. The process involves an extensive blockage of dermal lymphatics by tumor. Fever and leukocytosis are lacking. Skin biopsy is diagnostic.

When distant metastases are suspected in patients with a history of a proven primary malignant breast tumor, the usual screening examinations are helpful. Biopsy of metastatic lesions should be done if feasible to obtain diagnostic proof and new hormone receptor assays.

SUGGESTED READING

Henderson IC, Canellos GP. Cancer of the breast: the past decade. N Engl J Med 1980; 302:17–90.
Kopans DB, Meyer JE, Sadowsky N. Breast imaging. N Engl J Med 1984; 310:960–967.
Love SM, Gelman RS, Silen W. Fibrocystic "disease" of the breast—a nondisease? N Engl J Med 1982; 307:1010–1014.
Sommers RG, Young GP Kaplan MJ, et al. Fine-needle aspiration biopsy in the management of solid breast tumors. Arch Surg 1985; 120:673–677.

CONTRACEPTIVE PROBLEMS

JAN SCHNEIDER, M.D., M.P.H., F.R.C.S.(C)
MARY O. GABRIELSON, M.D., M.P.H.

Although great strides in pregnancy prevention have been made in the past 25 years since introduction of the combined oral contraceptive, the ideal method of birth control is yet to be devised. This is evident from the fact that 55 percent of all pregnancies occurring in the United States are still unplanned. Furthermore, all methods, including sterilization, carry some risks—risk of failure, risk of side effects, and risk of serious medical complications. Not surprisingly, some of the most effective methods, i.e., the oral contraceptive and the intrauterine device (IUD), carry the greatest risks of serious complications. Ultimately the final choice of contraceptive method must be a very personal one, based on the perceived need for protection against pregnancy, the appeal of a particular method, moral or ethical considerations, and a balancing of concerns about risks and side effects.

The effectiveness of a method of contraception is measured by the Pearl formula, which states the number of pregnancies per 100 years of exposure, or more practically stated, the number of pregnancies occuring per 100 women using the method in any given year. If no method is used the pregnancy rate is in the range of 85 to 90 percent. The most effective method is sterilization, with a failure rate in women of 0.2 to 0.5 percent. Sterilization is also the most widely used method in this country today; 35 percent of all couples who use contraception rely on sterilization. The pill is second both in effectiveness and in popularity. With a failure rate of less than 1 percent, it is used by 30 percent of women who practice contraception, or about 10 million individuals. No other drug is as successful in doing what it was designed to do as is the combined oral contraceptive. No other drug has been more extensively studied.

The condom follows the pill in popularity. About 14 percent use this barrier method, which has a failure rate of about 10 percent. Seven percent use the IUD, the method third in effectiveness after the pill with a failure rate of 0.5 to 5 percent. The remainder rely on barrier methods such as the diaphragm, foam, suppositories, and the recently introduced Today Sponge, or on withdrawal or the so-called natural methods including rhythm and fertility awareness.

All methods have a degree of risk. Those associated with the pill and the IUD will be considered in detail. Sterilization procedures all carry some risk, as is inevitable with any surgical procedure. This risk varies with the magnitude of the operation: no fatalities have been described with vasectomy in developed countries, whereas the mortality rate for women in recent United States studies is 3 to 4 per 100,000. The barrier methods rarely cause serious problems. A few cases of toxic shock syndrome have been described in diaphragm and sponge users. Use of the latter is not recommended during menses and it is important that it be removed after 24 hours of continuous use. Foams or jellies may cause irritation to one or both partners. Occasionally the diaphragm or sponge may be forgotten, and this results in a very malodorous discharge. A woman may also consult a physician because of inability to remove her diaphragm or sponge.

Beyond question the most serious complication of the barrier methods is failure either of the method itself or of the couple in their motivation to use it. No method of contraception, including sterilization, completely precludes the possibility of pregnancy, so complications of pregnancy, including life-threatening ectopic gestation, must *always* be entertained when a woman of childbearing age presents with signs and symptoms that may be attributable to pregnancy.

ORAL CONTRACEPTIVES

Minor side effects and complications of oral contraception include nausea, weight gain, fluid retention, mastalgia, breakthrough bleeding, and amenorrhea. Major complications include thromboembolic disease, intracranial vascular catastrophes, hypertension, hepatocellular adenoma, and post-pill amenorrhea.

Minor side effects, though widely publicized and accounting for many instances of pill discontinuation, are mainly of nuisance value. With the exception of breakthrough bleeding and amenorrhea, their incidence has declined with the reduction in dosage of both the estrogenic and progestational components of the pill.

Nausea is a common side effect, and perhaps the most frequent cause of pill discontinuation. Presumably it is caused by the estrogen in the pill. It usually abates within the first few cycles of pill use. Taking the pill with food or lowering the estrogen content may reduce or eliminate nausea.

Fluid retention and weight gain are not generally problems with the new low-dose pills. Weight gain may occur as a result of the anabolic effects of the synthetic progestins, which are derived from testosterone. Mastalgia, resulting from both estrogen and progestin effects on breast tissue, is a fairly common complaint.

Breakthrough bleeding or intermenstrual spotting is more likely to occur with the new low-dose pills. In this instance the low levels of both estrogen and progestin may fail to stimulate the endometrium sufficiently to maintain it for a full 21 days, and bleeding occurs prior to hormone withdrawal. This is not a serious problem and may be handled either by a switch to a more progestational pill or by adding exogenous estrogen—2.5 mg of Premarin or 20 μg of ethinyl estradiol daily for 7 days when the bleeding is present. Usually one or at most two courses of additional estrogen correct the problem. A similar approach (i.e., additional estrogen) may be employed in women who experience amenorrhea on the pill, provided one is certain that the amenorrhea is not the result of pregnancy.

Major Complications

Cardiovascular Disease

The most widely publicized and serious complications of oral contraceptives are cardiovascular, i.e., venous thromboembolic disease, myocardial infarction, and stroke. These risks have been well established by many case control and prospective studies, primarily in the United States and Great Britain. Risk of venous thrombosis and pulmonary embolism appears to be about four times greater for women on the pill than for women who do not take oral contraceptives. An estimate of one case per thousand women per year is a fair assessment of risk. The risk is dose-related and may well be lower with the newer low-dose pills. The incidence of thromboembolism increases with age and other risk factors, particularly conditions requiring prolonged immobilization. Women who suffer fractures or other injuries requiring casting or immobilization should be taken off the pill until full mobility has returned.

Women who use the pill are three to four times more likely to develop myocardial infarction than are nonusers. The risk of myocardial infarction increases dramatically with age and the presence of other contributory factors, particularly smoking. Additional risk factors include hypertension, diabetes, and familial hyperlipoproteinemia.

Risks of thrombotic or hemorrhagic stroke are also increased in oral contraceptive users by a factor of four to nine. Deaths have been ascribed to subarachnoid hemorrhage and again have been concentrated among older, smoking women. With the use of the newer low-dose pills containing 30 to 35 μg of estrogen and a much lower total progestin dose, the risk of myocardial infarction and stroke may be substantially decreased. Women who suffer stroke often complain of symptoms preceding the event, and those complaining of migraine headaches or other severe headaches that do not respond to the usual analgesics should be taken off the pill.

Hypertension

Oral contraceptives cause an elevation of blood pressure in most women. Usually the effect is small—1 to 2 mm diastolic and 5 mm systolic. However, about 1 to 5 percent of women on the pill develop hypertension, and in rare instances an acute onset, either with or without headache, may occur. Pill discontinuation usually results in return of blood pressure to premedication levels within 1 to 3 months. Periodic blood pressure check of the woman on the pill is probably more important than the routine pelvic examination.

Hepatocellular Adenoma

Hepatocellular adenoma is a rare tumor with an incidence of about one per million women of child-bearing age. Women who have been on oral contraceptives for more than 2 years appear to be at a substantially increased risk of developing this tumor, although even in long-term users only about 3 cases per 100,000 women have been described. Although benign, the tumor is extremely vascular. Approximately 50 percent of women present with bleeding either in the tumor or intraperitoneally if there is capsular rupture. Women with intraperitoneal bleeding almost always present with acute pain and/or circulatory collapse. The mortality rate is about 8 percent. In one large case control study 47 percent of the women were aware of an abdominal mass, whereas 19 percent had complained of vague abdominal pains. Those women who were pregnant or within 6 weeks of delivery had the highest mortality. Incidence of the tumor was found to increase with length of pill use, estrogen potency, and age.

Post-Pill Amenorrhea

Although there is no long-term impact on fertility in patients who use oral contraceptives, between 0.2 and 0.8 percent of patients who discontinue the pill report delay in resumption of menses. Amenorrhea is more likely to occur in women with a history of menstrual irregularity before starting the pill. Patients with a history suggestive of anovulation should not be given oral contraceptives until the nature of the ovulatory dysfunction has been defined. By the same token any woman who presents with 6 months or more of amenorrhea, with or without galactorrhea, merits an evaluation to exclude pituitary microadenoma, polycystic ovary disease, premature ovarian failure, or other endocrine abnormality. Usually post-pill amenorrhea is self-limited, with spontaneous resumption of normal cycles. The only emergency problem may be that of evaluating gestational age in a patient who becomes pregnant prior to the onset of what would have been the first post-pill menstrual period.

INTRAUTERINE CONTRACEPTIVE DEVICES

The intrauterine contraceptive device (IUD) has the advantage of providing reliable contraception over a long period of time without the continual motivation and planning required by pills or barrier methods. Although a highly effective method, it has been associated with serious complications, and probably accounts for more emergency visits than any other method of contraception. Complications associated with IUD use include expulsion, perforation, bleeding, intrauterine pregnancy, ectopic pregnancy, and infection and infertility.

Expulsion

Between 5 and 15 percent of patients have spontaneous expulsion of an IUD within a year of insertion. The incidence of expulsion is greater in patients who have never been pregnant and in younger patients. The highest expulsion rate occurs when the device is inserted soon after pregnancy. Insertion after a first trimester abortion does not, however, appear to carry a higher expulsion risk. The usual first evidence that a device has been expelled is the patient noticing that the string can no longer be palpated. On occasion the device is incompletely expelled with the end protruding from the cervical os. This may result in cramping or in discomfort for the partner during intercourse. When a patient presents with the complaint of being unable to find her IUD string there are three possibilities: the string may have been drawn up into the uterus, the device may have been expelled, or perforation may have occurred.

Perforation

Most IUD perforations occur at the time of insertion and are the result of faulty insertion technique. Occasionally fundal perforation by the uterine sound or introducer are recognized immediately, usually with minimal discomfort to the patient. At other times nothing is noted at the time of insertion, and perforation is suspected only when the string can no longer be palpated or visualized. Perforation of the uterus by an IUD at a time subsequent to insertion may occur, but again may well be the result of improper placement of the IUD within the uterine cavity. The risk of perforation is thus increased in those models requiring frequent replacement. One type of perforation seen with straight-stemmed devices, such as the SafeT Coil, CU7, or Tatum T, involves protrusion of the stem through the wall of the cervix. This may appear as a bulge in the cervix, or the stem may be seen actually protruding through the cervical wall. In this situation the device should *not* be pulled out through the cervical defect. The stem must be grasped within the uterus by an instrument inserted through the cervical os and the device backed up and then removed.

A patient who presents with a lost IUD must be assessed as to whether it remains in the uterus, has perforated, or has been expelled. On pelvic examination the string can occasionally be seen even though the patient was unable to palpate it. If the string is not visible, the cervical canal may be probed gently with a swab or dressing forceps in an attempt to bring down the string. Failing this, either radiologic studies or ultrasound should be performed. Ultrasound has the advantage of localizing the IUD within the uterus, and it is also the method that should be employed if there is any suspicion of pregnancy. It requires a skilled ultrasonographer to make an accurate diagnosis. Since all currently used IUDs are radiopaque, a roentgenogram will establish the presence or absence of an IUD. To localize the IUD, however, it is necessary to insert a metal sound into the uterus and take anteroposterior and lateral views to assess the location of the IUD. Another approach is to insert a second IUD, preferably of another type, and judge the distance between the two.

If the IUD is within the uterine cavity and removal is desired, this can usually be accomplished with a hook or alligator forceps. Paracervical block is used if necessary. Hysteroscopy or D&C should rarely be required.

When perforation of the uterus has occurred, most authorities agree the IUD should be removed from the peritoneal cavity. Older closed devices such as the Birnberg Bow carry the risk of intestinal strangulation. Copper bearing devices elicit a rapid and intense inflammatory response. Bowel perforation has been described with the Lippes Loop. Removal may be achieved by laparoscopy or colpotomy, although laparotomy is usually required for removal of copper devices because of the rapid dense adhesion formation.

Bleeding

Studies have shown that an IUD increases the amount of blood loss with each menstrual period by 50 to 100 percent. The progesterone IUD causes a reduction in the amount of blood loss with concomitant increase in duration of flow. Intermenstrual bleeding and spotting are also common. When a device has remained in utero for several years, a deposition of calcific salts may cause the once-smooth surface to become rough and saw-like, causing further endometrial erosion and spotting. From 5 to 15 percent of women have an IUD removed because of bleeding problems.

Pregnancy

Intrauterine pregnancy occurs in 0.5 to 5 percent of IUD users each year. Such pregnancies may coexist with an IUD; however, there is a significant risk of spontaneous abortion. The incidence of abortion may be as high as 50 percent. This is particularly dangerous because abortion in the presence of a foreign body is associated with a significant incidence of sepsis. A number of deaths have been reported in mid-trimester of pregnancy in association with sepsis and IUD use. Therefore an IUD should be removed immediately when pregnancy is diagnosed unless the strings have been drawn up into the uterus. The removal of the IUD may itself precipitate pregnancy loss, but this risk is considerably less than the 50 percent risk that would occur if the IUD were left in place.

Ectopic Pregnancy

The relative incidence of ectopic pregnancy in the presence of an IUD is significantly increased. About 3 to 4 percent of pregnancies among IUD users are extrauterine. Whether the absolute risk of ectopic gestation is increased in IUD users continues to be debated. Most important, women with an IUD who present with pain, bleeding, or any other symptoms of ectopic pregnancy must be evaluated with particular care.

Infection and Infertility

There no longer is any question that use of an IUD increases the risk of pelvic infection. This risk is particularly high in the young nulligravid patient. Upper genital tract infection is two to seven times more common among IUD users, with additional risk factors including number of sexual partners and history of previous pelvic infection. In addition to the gonococcus, *Chlamydia trachomatis* and a variety of aerobic and anaerobic organisms have been isolated. In the presence of infection the IUD should be removed. Antibiotics should be selected to cover both gonococcal and chlamydial infection. In cases of severe infection, high-dose antibiotics should be given prior to IUD removal to reduce the risk of bacteremia when the device is manipulated. Infection may progress to chronic changes and tubo-ovarian abscess formation. Such patients can be extremely ill, and it is imperative that they be accurately diagnosed and aggressively treated. Pelvic actinomycosis has also been described with prolonged IUD use. These organisms may be recognized on the Pap smear. If present, symptoms may range from abnormal bleeding and vague abdominal pain to those of severe infection with abscess formation.

Recent reports have substantiated fears that IUD use, even in the absence of overt infection, may result in infertility. Risk of infertility was greatest with the now-discontinued Dalkon Shield, followed by the other non-medicated devices. The lowest risk was associated with copper devices. The American College of Obstetricians and Gynecologists has recently recommended that IUDs not be used by young women who contemplate future child-bearing. Even more recently, several manufacturers in the United States have discontinued the sale of these devices because of the increasing number of lawsuits which their complications are generating.

SUGGESTED READING

Hatcher RA, Stewart GK, Stewart F, Guest F, Josephs N, Dale J. Contraceptive technology 1986–1987. New York: Irvington Publishers, Inc

Meade TW, Greenberg G, Thompson SG. Progestogens and cardiovascular reactions associated with oral contraceptives and a comparison of the safety of 50 and 30 μg oestrogen preparations. Br Med J 1980; 280:1157.

Ory HW, Forrest JD, Lincoln R. Making choices: evaluating the health risks and benefits of birth control methods. New York: The Alan Guttmacher Institute, 1983.

Stadel B. Oral contraceptives and cardiovascular risk. N Engl J Med 1981; 305:612–618; 672–677.

MANAGEMENT OF THE HEMOPOIETIC SYSTEM

ANEMIA

STEPHEN J. McPHEE, M.D.

Anemia is a common problem in emergency medical practice. Faced with an anemic patient, the emergency physician must not only classify the anemia, begin a diagnostic evaluation, and institute appropriate therapy, but carefully consider its underlying cause and decide whether it warrants hospital admission or specialty referral. The physician may be aided by answering several questions. First, how severe is the anemia? Second, how is the patient tolerating the anemia? Third, is there active bleeding or hemolysis? And finally, how can the anemia be classified?

HOW SEVERE IS THE ANEMIA?

Anemia is usually defined by reference to standard hematocrit and hemoglobin levels. For an adult man at sea level, the normal hematocrit is 47 percent (range, 42 to 52 percent) and the normal hemoglobin is 16 g per deciliter (range, 14 to 18 g per deciliter). For an adult woman, the normal hematocrit is 42 percent (range, 37 to 47 percent) and the normal hemoglobin is 14 g per deciliter (range 12 to 16 g per deciliter). Normal values for black patients are somewhat lower than for whites. At higher altitudes, normal hematocrit and hemoglobin values are somewhat higher, increasing roughly in proportion to the elevation above sea level.

Severe anemia is usually defined as one in which there is a hemoglobin deficit of more than 50 percent. For an adult man, this would mean a hemoglobin of less than 8 g per deciliter; for a woman, a hemoglobin less than 7 g per deciliter. In assessing the severity of the anemia, however, the clinician must take into account more than the absolute level of the hematocrit or hemoglobin for several reasons. First, in acute hemorrhage or dehydration, the hematocrit or hemoglobin may be spuriously high; only with time or rehydration does the hematocrit or hemoglobin level more accurately reflect the patient's true oxygen carrying capacity. Even then, the physician may be misled in some situations (e.g., carbon monoxide poisoning). Second, the symptoms of the anemia often depend more on the age of the patient, the presence of other disorders limiting cardiopulmonary compensation, the rate of development of the anemia, and the underlying cause, than on the level of the hematocrit or hemoglobin. Finally, anemias associated with pancytopenia are usually due to more serious illness, such as aplastic or myelophthisic anemias.

HOW IS THE PATIENT TOLERATING THE ANEMIA?

The history, physical examination, and simple laboratory tests can tell the physician a great deal about how the patient is tolerating the anemia. In general, a chronic anemia is better tolerated than an acute one. Symptoms of respiratory and circulatory decompensation (weakness, dyspnea on exertion, palpitations, faintness on arising from a sitting or lying position, and marked fatigue) suggest an acute or severe anemia. Measurement of orthostatic changes in the vital signs allows rapid assessment of the patient's blood volume; the physician finding orthostatic changes must exclude active hemorrhage. In addition, examination for signs of shock, congestive heart failure, myocardial infarction, or cerebrovascular insufficiency helps to determine the patient's response to the anemia, and may suggest the need for urgent transfusion.

IS THERE ACTIVE BLEEDING OR HEMOLYSIS?

Whether the patient is actively bleeding can usually be determined by examination of the skin, oronasopharynx, abdomen, vagina, and rectum, along with testing samples of the stool, urine, and in some cases nasogastric aspirate or peritoneal lavage fluid for blood. In addition, the emergency physician must be especially careful to exclude hemorrhage whenever anemia is found in certain patient groups. These are: (1) trauma victims, especially those with bony fractures, blunt trauma, and penetrating wounds; (2) elderly patients, particularly those ingesting aspirin and nonsteroidal anti-inflammatory agents; (3) chronic alcoholics, particularly those with cirrhosis; (4) patients with bleeding dyscrasias; (5) hypertensive patients at risk for or patients known to have, aortic aneurysm; and (6) pregnant women at risk for placenta previa or ruptured ectopic pregnancy. Such patients may require urgent transfusion in the emergency department.

Hemolysis is suggested by polychromatophilia, spherocytes, poikilocytes, sickle cells, or schistocytes on a smear of the peripheral blood, or by reticulocytosis. The diagnosis becomes more certain if there is an elevated indirect serum bilirubin or lactic dehydrogenase, a decreased serum haptoglobin, an increased plasma free hemoglobin, or free hemoglobin or hemosiderin in the urine. Patients at special risk for hemolytic anemia include (1) blacks, in whom sickle cell anemia, glucose-6-phosphate dehydrogenase deficiency, and thalassemia occur frequently; (2) patients with liver disease, uremia, or certain infections (e.g., *Mycoplasma*); (3) patients with prosthetic heart valves, systemic lupus erythematosus, chronic lymphocytic leukemia, or lymphosarcoma; (4) patients treated with certain drugs known to precipitate hemolysis (e.g., quinidine, alphamethyldopa, and penicillin); and (5) patients with a family history of anemia (see the chapters *Hemorrhagic Coagulopathy, Hemophilia and von Willebrand's Disease*, and *Sickle Cell Disease*).

HOW CAN THE ANEMIA BE CLASSIFIED?

The basic laboratory evaluation of the patient discovered to be anemic includes a complete blood count, including hematocrit, hemoglobin, white blood cell count, red cell indices, and platelet count or estimate; a smear of peripheral blood, stained with Wright's stain; and a reticulocyte count. The physician should then attempt to classify the anemia according to the red cell morphology, using the peripheral smear and red cell indices. Every anemia should fit one of three categories: (1) microcytic, hypochromic anemias, (2) macrocytic anemias, or (3) normocytic, normochromic anemias. Table 1 lists the common causes of anemia according to this classification. Further laboratory studies depend upon this initial classification (Table 2). Based upon these findings, the physician may then decide to undertake empiric therapy. Suggestions for treatment of the most common types of anemia seen by the emergency physician are given below.

IRON DEFICIENCY ANEMIA

The diagnosis of iron deficiency is suggested by red blood cell indices of mean corpuscular volume (MCV) less than 80 μm^3 and mean corpuscular hemoglobin concentration (MCHC) less than 30 g per deciliter and by hypochromic, microcytic red cells on peripheral blood smear. The reticulocyte count is normal or decreased. The diagnosis is confirmed by findings of decreased serum ferritin (less than 12 μg per liter), decreased transferrin saturation (serum iron/transferrin less than 16 percent), free erythrocyte protoporphyrin greater than 3 μg per gram hemoglobin (greater than 100 μg per deciliter packed red cells), or absent stainable iron in the bone marrow.

Patients requiring treatment for iron deficiency anemia include (1) infants aged 6 to 24 months (especially those of low birth weight), children, and adolescents undergoing rapid growth; (2) menstruating or pregnant women; (3) adults with abnormal blood loss (epistaxis, gastrointestinal bleeding, blood donation, trauma); (4) patients with anatomic reasons for poor iron absorption (e.g., postgastrectomy); and (5) uncommonly, malnourished adults (alcoholics, elderly).

TABLE 1 Classification of Anemia by Red Cell Morphology

Microcytic, Hypochromic Anemias
  (MCV less than 80 μm^3, MCHC less than 31 g/dl)
    Iron deficiency
    Sideroblastic anemia
    Thalassemia
    Hemoglobinopathy
    Chronic disease (some)

Macrocytic Anemias
  (MCV greater than 100 μm^3, MCHC 32–36 g/dl)
    Megaloblastic
      Vitamin B$_{12}$ deficiency (pernicious anemia)
      Folate deficiency
      Drug-induced
    Nonmegaloblastic
      Marked reticulocytosis
        Acute hemorrhage
        Acute hemolysis
      Increased red cell membrane surface area
        Chronic liver disease
        Postsplenectomy
      Myxedema (some)
      Marrow infiltration or failure (some)

Normocytic, Normochromic Anemias
  (MCV 80–100, μm^3, MCHC 31–34 g/dl)
    Acute hemorrhage
    Acute hemolysis
    Chronic disease (most)
      Chronic inflammation
      Chronic infections
      Chronic metabolic disorders
      Neoplasms
    Marrow infiltration or failure
    Pregnancy

MCV = mean corpuscular volume; MCHC = mean corpuscular hemoglobin concentration.

TABLE 2 Further Diagnostic Tests in the Evaluation of Anemia

Microcytic, Hypochromic Anemias
  Serum iron and transferrin, transferrin saturation
    or
  Serum ferritin
    or
  Free erythrocyte protoporphyrin
  Hemoglobin electrophoresis
  Sickle cell preparation
  Glucose-6-phosphate dehydrogenase assay
  Bone marrow aspirate

Macrocytic Anemias
  Serum vitamin B$_{12}$
  Red cell folate
  Schilling test
  Bone marrow aspirate or biopsy

Normocytic, Normochromic Anemias
  Serum iron and transferrin, transferrin saturation
    or
  Serum ferritin
    or
  Free erythrocyte protoporphyrin
  Serum vitamin B$_{12}$
    or
  Red cell folate
  Pregnancy test
  Bone marrow aspirate or biopsy

Before instituting therapy, the physician suspecting iron deficiency should obtain serum for an iron and transferrin saturation, ferritin, or red cell protoporphyrin determination.

If the patient is stable, therapy with oral iron is simplest. The amount of iron required for treatment depends upon the severity of the anemia, the rate of recovery desired, the presence of continuing blood loss, and the ability of the patient to tolerate iron. In an iron deficient patient, about 50 to 100 mg of iron can be made into hemoglobin each day. The normal person absorbs about 6 percent of the daily iron intake; in iron deficiency, absorption of iron increases to as much as 25 percent of intake. To correct the anemia most rapidly, therapeutic doses of oral iron must supply at least 200 mg of elemental iron (200 mg of ferrous iron × 25 percent absorption = 50 mg of elemental iron available per day). The physician can supply this amount by prescribing ferrous sulfate, 325 mg (65 mg elemental iron) in a dose of 3 tablets daily, ferrous gluconate, 320 mg (39 mg iron) in a dose of 5 tablets daily, or ferrous fumarate, 200 mg (66 mg iron) in a dose of 3 tablets daily. If blood loss continues, however, administration of more than 500 mg of ferrous iron per day may be required.

Although iron is two to three times better absorbed on an empty stomach than if given with food, gastrointestinal upset may be minimized by administering the iron with meals. Patient tolerance for iron may be improved by beginning therapy with 1 tablet daily and gradually increasing to three or more tablets daily. Alternatively, patients unable to tolerate large doses of iron may be given smaller doses (even 1 tablet per day) for longer periods. Provided that blood loss is not continuing, this results in complete, if slower, correction of the anemia and repletion of the marrow iron stores. Finally, hydrochloric acid in the stomach enhances oral iron absorption, and achlorhydria diminishes iron absorption. After gastrectomy, liquid iron may be preferable to pill forms to prevent iron malabsorption (ferrous sulfate elixir 220 mg per 5 ml supplies 44 mg of elemental iron).

Oral iron therapy should be continued for at least 3 to 5 months after the hemoglobin level has returned to normal in order to replete marrow iron stores. If bleeding continues, longer therapy may be required. Women with abnormally large menstrual blood losses may benefit from intermittent therapy (1 week per month); patients with continuing gastrointestinal blood loss (e.g., hereditary hemorrhagic telangiectasia) may require lifelong daily iron therapy. Patients given oral iron should be warned about its side effects particularly gastrointestinal upset, constipation, and darkening of the stool.

Patients may not respond to oral iron therapy for several reasons. The diagnosis of iron deficiency may be wrong (e.g., consider thalassemia minor). Side effects or forgetfulness may lead to noncompliance. Continuing blood loss may exceed red cell synthesis, or there may be an accompanying chronic illness preventing proper absorption of iron or synthesis of red cells. Parenteral iron is indicated for patients who do not adhere to or tolerate oral iron therapy, and for patients with rapid blood loss or malabsorption. Patients given parenteral iron must be informed about the risk of anaphylaxis. Failure to respond to parenteral iron therapy suggests either wrong diagnosis or continued bleeding.

Response to iron therapy is rapid. The serum iron level increases within hours of beginning iron, the reticulocyte count increases within 5 to 10 days, and the hemoglobin level increases by at least 2 g per deciliter within 3 weeks. To monitor the adequacy of treatment, the reticulocyte count may be determined at 1 week after beginning iron; the increase in reticulocytes is directly proportional to the severity of the anemia. Alternatively, the physician may determine the hemoglobin level at 3 weeks.

Most patients discovered to have iron deficiency anemia in the emergency department can be treated with oral iron and sent home. They should be instructed to schedule a follow-up appointment with their physician to determine the source of the iron deficiency and to monitor its correction. However, severely anemic patients who are actively bleeding or manifesting unstable angina or congestive heart failure should be admitted for transfusion therapy.

SIDEROBLASTIC ANEMIA

The diagnosis of sideroblastic anemia is suggested by finding anemia with normal or low red blood cell indices and a dimorphic population of red cells (both normochromic, normocytic and hypochromic, microcytic cells) on peripheral smear in a high-risk patient. The reticulocyte count is usually normal, but may be slightly increased. Free erythrocyte protoporphyrin levels are almost always moderately increased. The diagnosis is confirmed by increased serum iron concentration and transferrin saturation (greater than 16 percent) and is most firmly established by finding ringed sideroblasts in the marrow.

Therapy consists of: (1) withdrawal of agents known to cause sideroblastic anemia (isoniazid, cycloserine, pyrazinamide, ethanol, lead, chloramphenicol, antineoplastic chemotherapeutic agents); (2) treatment of associated underlying illness (myeloma, lymphoma, rheumatoid arthritis, myxedema, uremia); and (3) the administration of pyridoxine (vitamin B_6), folate, or androgens, or transfusion therapy.

Pyridoxine (vitamin B_6) should be prescribed in a dose of 50 to 200 mg orally daily; folate, 1 mg orally daily, should also be given if folate deficiency is present. Response is assessed by repeated measurement of the reticulocyte count or hemoglobin level; generally, the anemia does not respond completely, but response may be sufficient for symptoms to resolve.

Because of the risk of iron overload in patients with sideroblastic anemia, transfusions are contraindicated unless the patient has severe, symptomatic anemia. The patient should also be instructed to avoid iron or iron-containing vitamin preparations.

MEGALOBLASTIC ANEMIAS

The diagnosis of megaloblastic anemia is suggested by red blood cell indices of MCV greater than 100 μm^3 and MCHC 32 to 36 g per deciliter, and by peripheral smear findings of oval macrocytes and hypersegmented polymorphonuclear neutrophils (strictly defined, more than 5 percent of polymorphonuclear neutrophils with more than five lobes to the nucleus). Diagnosis is confirmed by finding megaloblasts, enlarged red cell precursors with excess cytoplasm and immature nuclei, in the bone marrow.

Vitamin B_{12} deficiency and folate deficiency megaloblastic anemias can usually be differentiated by red cell folate and serum vitamin B_{12} levels; a red cell folate level below 150 ng per milliliter is abnormal, and a serum B_{12} level below 200 pg per milliliter is abnormal. A two-stage or dual-labeled Schilling test confirms the diagnosis of vitamin B_{12} deficiency. Drug-induced megaloblastosis is usually suggested by a careful drug history. The physician should inquire about exposure to drugs that interfere with DNA synthesis (including methotrexate, 6-mercaptopurine, cytosine arabinoside, cyclophosphamide, and 5-fluorouracil), or that act as folate antagonists (pentamidine, pyrimethamine, triamterene, and trimethoprim), or that lead to folate deficiency (phenytoin, primidone, phenobarbital, and oral contraceptives).

Before beginning therapy, the physician suspecting megaloblastic anemia should obtain specimens for serum vitamin B_{12} and red cell folate levels. Because severe B_{12} or folate deficiency may cause gastrointestinal megaloblastosis and malabsorption interfering with its performance, the Schilling test is best delayed until several weeks after therapy has begun.

Patients requiring treatment for megaloblastic anemia due to vitamin B_{12} deficiency include: (1) older adults with pernicious anemia; (2) patients after total (and sometimes subtotal) gastrectomy; (3) patients with resection or disease of the terminal ileum (regional enteritis, tuberculosis, sprue); (4) patients with the fish tapeworm *Diphyllobothrium latum* infestation; (5) patients with malabsorption due to bacterial overgrowth; and (6) strict vegetarians (rarely). Normally, dietary vitamin B_{12} binds to intrinsic factor produced in the antrum of the stomach; the B_{12}-intrinsic factor complex is then absorbed in the terminal ileum.

Treatment of megaloblastic anemia due to B_{12} deficiency consists of vitamin B_{12}, 100 μg IM monthly. Acutely, however, some experts recommend slow reversal of megaloblastosis with much smaller doses (less than 15 μg daily for 2 to 3 days) to prevent potentially serious complications of hypokalemia and thrombotic or embolic episodes. Patients with B_{12} deficiency must be instructed that they require lifelong monthly therapy.

A brisk reticulocytosis is noted beginning 4 days, and peaking at 6 to 10 days, following parenteral B_{12} therapy. The hemoglobin will return to normal within 6 weeks. Hypokalemia, when it occurs, accompanies the brisk reticulocytosis during the first several days of therapy.

Patients at risk for folate deficiency include (1) pregnant or lactating women; (2) malnourished infants or adults (alcoholics, elderly, inadequate diets); (3) patients receiving anticonvulsant or contraceptive therapy; (4) some patients with chronic hemolytic (sickle cell) anemia; and (5) patients with folate malabsorption (sprue, extensive regional enteritis), abnormal losses (psoriasis, renal dialysis), or diminished hepatic stores (chronic liver disease).

Because folate is readily absorbed, treatment of megaloblastic anemia due to folate deficiency usually consists of folic acid, 1 mg orally daily. If the diagnosis of folate deficiency is uncertain, it can be established by a therapeutic trial of low doses of folate (200 μg per day orally), with careful monitoring of the reticulocyte count for a response. Higher doses (more than 1 mg per day) are not recommended in this situation because the diagnosis of pernicious anemia might be masked by a nonspecific reticulocytosis. High-dose folate therapy might correct the anemia but not provide the vitamin B_{12} essential to prevent progressive degeneration of the nervous system.

In general, treatment with folate, 1 mg orally daily, should be continued until the reason for the deficiency is corrected. Patients with chronic liver disease, renal dialysis, sickle cell anemia, or malabsorption may require lifelong daily folate therapy. Rarely, patients with severe malabsorption require parenteral therapy initially, but can usually be maintained on oral folic acid. Folic acid solution (5 mg per milliliter) is available for intramuscular use. Monitoring the reticulocyte count at 5 to 10 days or the hemoglobin level at 1 to 2 months allows assessment of the response to folate therapy.

Therapy for drug-induced megaloblastic anemia consists of withdrawing the offending agent if possible. If anticonvulsant or oral contraceptive therapy is required, administration of folic acid, 1 mg orally daily, promptly reverses the anemia. Once the anemia has resolved, folate therapy can usually be discontinued without relapse.

Elderly patients with severe megaloblastic anemia generally should be admitted to the hospital for treatment under close observation. Transfusion should be avoided if the patient is clinically stable, regardless of the severity of the anemia, because of the risk of death from acute pulmonary edema. If severe anemia is accompanied by angina pectoris or congestive heart failure, the patient should be put on bed rest, given oxygen, and treated with nitrates or diuretics. Only if symptoms persist despite these measures should transfusion be considered. If the decision is made to transfuse, the physician should undertake exchange transfusion, usually of no more than 1 unit of packed red cells, slowly over 4 to 6 hours with careful monitoring of the central venous pressure.

ANEMIAS ASSOCIATED WITH CHRONIC ILLNESS

In the anemias of chronic disease, the red cells are normocytic (MCV 80 to 100 μm^3) and normochromic (MCHC 31 to 34 g per deciliter); occasionally, they may be slightly hypochromic. Both the serum iron and transferrin levels are decreased, resulting in a normal or elevated transferrin saturation. The serum ferritin is generally increased to greater than 300 ng per milliliter. Free erythrocyte protoporphyrin levels are increased. The reticulocyte count is generally low or normal. Bone marrow examination reveals increased iron stores.

Patients at risk for this type of anemia are those with (1) chronic inflammatory disorders (e.g., rheumatoid arthritis); (2) chronic infectious diseases (e.g., tuberculosis); (3) chronic metabolic disorders (e.g., chronic renal failure, myxedema, cirrhosis); and (4) neoplastic diseases (e.g., pancreatic cancer).

Before beginning therapy, the physician should obtain serum for determination of iron and transferrin, ferritin, or red cell protoporphyrin levels. In addition, red cell folate or serum vitamin B_{12} levels may be indicated depending upon the underlying disorder.

Therapy for the anemias of chronic disease consists of treatment of the underlying condition, and exclusion of associated deficiencies of iron, folate, or vitamin B_{12}.

Treatment of the underlying condition is essential. Anti-inflammatory therapy for chronic inflammatory disorders may lead to gradual, though often incomplete, improvement of the anemia. Successful antibiotic therapy for infections or hormonal replacement for metabolic disorders gradually leads to total resolution of the anemia, usually over a period of 2 to 3 months.

Such therapy may be unsuccessful in correcting the anemia, however, if there are associated iron, folate, or vitamin B_{12} deficiencies. Patients with chronic inflammatory disorders (e.g., rheumatoid arthritis) are often treated with aspirin or nonsteroidal anti-inflammatory agents, and are therefore prone to iron deficiency from occult gastrointestinal blood loss. Folate deficiency may result from chronic oral contraceptive therapy for endometriosis. Methotrexate therapy for psoriasis is often complicated by drug-induced megaloblastic anemia.

Treatment of chronic infectious diseases with antimicrobial agents may entail risk of folate antagonism (trimethoprim or pentamidine therapy for *Pneumocystis carinii* pneumonia) or sideroblastic anemia (isoniazid, cycloserine, or pyrazinamide therapy for tuberculosis).

Similarly, chronic metabolic disorders may be complicated by vitamin or mineral deficiencies. Hypothyroidism may cause menorrhagia and iron deficiency; patients with myxedema from autoimmune (Hashimoto's) thyroiditis may develop antiparietal cell antibodies and pernicious anemia from vitamin B_{12} malabsorption. Cirrhosis is frequently complicated by folate deficiency (due to diminished hepatic stores) and iron deficiency (from gastrointestinal bleeding). Chronic renal failure may lead to folate deficiency from anorexia or iron deficiency from dialysis losses or bleeding.

Anorexia and malnutrition associated with malignancy may lead to folate deficiency. Drug-induced megaloblastosis can be caused by antineoplastic chemotherapy with cyclophosphamide, methotrexate, 6-mercaptopurine, 5-fluorouracil, and cytosine arabinoside.

Appropriate treatment with iron, folic acid, or vitamin B_{12} enables the anemic patient to recover fully.

APLASTIC ANEMIA

The diagnosis of aplastic anemia is suggested by finding pancytopenia (or occasionally selective depression of red cells, white cells, or platelets) in a patient with a history of exposure to a drug or toxic agent. Peripheral smear shows red cells to be slightly macrocytic; the reticulocyte count is generally depressed. The diagnosis is confirmed by finding marked hypocellularity and fatty infiltration of the bone marrow. Agents known to be associated with the development of aplastic anemia include chloramphenicol, phenylbutazone, mephenytoin, quinacrine, gold compounds, cytotoxic agents, estrogens, potassium perchlorate, benzene, arsenic, insecticides, and x-irradiation. In addition, patients with viral hepatitis, eosinophilic fasciitis, and the acquired immunodeficiency syndrome (AIDS) are at risk for aplastic anemia.

Patients discovered to have aplastic anemia (or pancytopenia of indeterminate cause) should generally be admitted to the hospital; immediate consultation with a hematologist is advisable. Treatment of aplastic anemia consists of (1) attempting to discover and avoid further toxic exposure; (2) performing allogeneic bone marrow transplantation; and (3) providing supportive measures, including red cell or platelet transfusions, antibiotics for complicating infections, and androgen or lithium therapy.

A careful history detailing medications, occupational and avocational exposures, recent illnesses, and sexual habits is essential; however, fewer than half the patients with aplastic anemia can identify a precipitating agent.

To avoid sensitization to transplant antigens, the patient must not be transfused with blood products from potentially histocompatible relatives. Transfusions with washed, frozen packed red cells from random donors is indicated only for severely anemic, symptomatic patients because of the risks associated with repeated transfusions (hepatitis, AIDS, iron overload, development of leukoagglutinins, and sensitization to red cell and transplant antigens).

Because of the risk of death from overwhelming infection, patients with aplastic anemia who present in the emergency department with fever and leukopenia should be pancultured and treated immediately with intravenous, broad-spectrum antibiotic therapy (including an antipseudomonal aminoglycoside, e.g., tobramycin, and an antipseudomonal beta-lactamase-susceptible synthetic penicillin, e.g., ticarcillin). Similarly, patients with aplastic anemia who present with hemorrhage secondary to thrombocytopenia should have a platelet count drawn and be given platelet transfusion. Corticosteroids (e.g., oral prednisone, 1 mg per kilogram of body weight per day) are sometimes administered to severely thrombocytopenic patients who are actively bleeding.

Treatment with androgenic steroids (such as oxymetholone or fluoxymesterone) is reserved for patients for whom marrow transplantation is not indicated or available. Lithium carbonate, 300 mg orally three times daily, may be given in an attempt to increase the granulocyte count. Side effects include tremor, polyuria, thirst, and nausea; more serious toxicity may be avoided by monitoring serum lithium levels (therapeutic range, 0.6 to 1.2 mEq per liter). Leukocyte transfusion should be reserved for the granulocytopenic patient with overwhelming sepsis.

HEMOLYTIC ANEMIA

The treatment of hemolytic anemia and sickle cell anemia are outlined in the chapters *Sickle Cell Anemia* and *Hemorrhagic Coagulopathy*.

SUGGESTED READING

Camitta BM, Storb R, Thomas ED. Aplastic anemia: pathogenesis, diagnosis, treatment, and prognosis. N Engl J Med 1982; 306:645–652, 712–718.
Chanarin I. The megaloblastic anemias. 2nd ed. Oxford: Blackwell Scientific Publishing, 1979.
Dallman PR. Iron deficiency: diagnosis and treatment. West J Med 1981; 134:496–505.
Hines JD. The normochromic-normocytic anemias. Drug Therapy 1984; 14:77–83.
Kushner JP, Cartwright GE. Sideroblastic anemia. In: Stollerman GH, et al, eds. Advances in internal medicine, Vol 22. Chicago: Year Bood Medical Publishers, 1977: 229.
McPhee SJ. The evaluation of anemia. West J Med 1982; 137:253–256.
Wallerstein RO. Role of the laboratory in the diagnosis of anemia. JAMA 1976; 236:490–493.

HEMORRHAGIC COAGULOPATHY

LAURENCE CORASH, M.D.

The spectrum of hemorrhagic coagulopathies seen in the emergency department encompasses hereditary and acquired syndromes affecting both the fluid and cellular phases of hemostasis. Abnormalities in either of these systems may present as a primary disorder or a secondary manifestation of another disease. Recognition of abnormal hemostasis and determination of its cause are essential to successful management of trauma, infection, chronic degenerative disease, neoplasia, and surgical emergencies.

ETIOLOGY AND PATHOPHYSIOLOGY

Quantitative Platelet Disorder

The etiology of the hemorrhagic coagulopathies can be divided into defects of the cellular and fluid phases of coagulation. Both platelets and endothelial cells are included within the cellular phase, although endothelial cell disorders are extremely rare. Platelet disorders may be either quantitative or qualitative in nature (Table 1), and they typically present with mucocutaneous bleeding manifested by petechiae and bleeding from the gastrointestinal, respiratory, or genitourinary tracts.

The most frequent causes of acute thrombocytopenia are the immune-mediated thrombocytopenic syndromes, which include autoimmune thrombocytopenia (idiopathic thrombocytopenic purpura, ITP), alloimmune neonatal thrombocytopenia, alloimmune post-transfusion purpura (PTP), and drug-induced thrombocytopenia. Isolated *ITP* is thought to be caused by autoantibodies directed against specific platelet proteins. In contrast, ITP associated with the collagen-vascular diseases is thought to be due to the nonspecific deposition of immune complexes on platelets. Patients with *PTP* lack the PL-Al antigen and after transfusion exposure produce antibodies directed against the missing antigen but also continue to destroy autologous platelets by an unknown process. Neonatal thrombocytopenia may be due to either concomitant maternal ITP with transplacental passage of IgG or to a maternal response against a foreign paternal antigen shared by the fetus. It is thought that drug-induced thrombocytopenia may be caused by an immune response directed against platelet-bound drug or by nonspecific deposition

TABLE 1 Platelet Disorders Associated with Hemorrhagic Coagulopathy

Quantitative Disorders	*Qualitative Disorders*
Drug-associated thrombocytopenia	Pharmacologically induced dysfunction
Autoimmune thrombocytopenia	Immune-mediated dysfunction
Neonatal thrombocytopenia	Activation-induced dysfunction
Post-transfusion purpura	Uremia
Hemolytic-uremic syndrome	Myeloproliferative syndromes
Thrombotic thrombocytopenic purpura	Malignant dysproteinemia
Preeclampsia	Bernard-Soulier syndrome
Sepsis	Glanzmann's thrombasthenia
Disseminated intravascular coagulation	Absent alpha granules
Bone marrow hypoplasia or aplasia	Absent dense bodies

on platelets of immune complexes composed of antibodies and drug–protein complexes. All of these immune-mediated platelet disorders are thought to end in a final common process in which macrophage Fc receptors bind and clear antibody-coated platelets.

Thrombocytopenia may also arise because of pharmacologically induced bone marrow failure with either generalized hypoplasia of all cell lines or isolated megakaryocyte toxicity. Bone marrow failure may occur spontaneously, in the course of severe infection, or as a complication of neoplasia or chemotherapy.

Thrombotic thrombocytopenic purpura (TTP) is characterized by severe thrombocytopenia, red cell fragmentation, fluctuating neurologic signs, and fever. The hemolytic-uremic syndrome (HUS) is clinically similar to TTP but is associated with glomerular thrombosis and renal failure. Preeclampsia may present with profound thrombocytopenia and hemorrhage. Recent studies point to evidence of platelet activation by a process independent of disseminated intravascular coagulation (DIC), and other studies suggest that immune-mediated platelet destruction may be important. DIC is often associated with marked thrombocytopenia, hemorrhage, consumption of coagulation factors, and excessive plasmin activation. DIC is the result of inappropriate thrombin-mediated activation of the coagulation system in a variety of disease states including sepsis, neoplasia, and obstetric complications.

Qualitative Platelet Disorder

Rarely, hemorrhagic coagulopathy may occur as the result of qualitative platelet disorders with a normal platelet level (Table 1), for example, via immune mechanisms that do not cause platelet destruction. Qualitative platelet defects may arise as the result of pharmacologic inhibition of platelet function. Generally these agents, (e.g., aspirin), cause only laboratory evidence of platelet dysfunction and do not produce clinically significant bleeding. However, in the presence of impairment of the plasma phase of the coagulation system or another bleeding diathesis, these agents may contribute to hemorrhage.

Acquired platelet dysfunction due to the production of dysplastic platelets has been observed in the course of the *myeloproliferative syndromes*: polycythemia vera, myelofibrosis, essential thrombocythemia, and chronic myelogenous leukemia. Toxic metabolites of uremia are reported to impair platelet function and produce bleeding. This was more common prior to agressive dialysis regimens, and presently the numbers of uremic patients with this complication are limited. A hemorrhagic diathesis has also been observed in patients with malignant dysproteinemic disorders: Waldenström's macroglobulinemia, multiple myeloma, and malignant lymphoma. Reduction in the level of the paraprotein frequently ameliorates the coagulopathy. Qualitative platelet dysfunction may also be seen with the rare hereditary syndromes in which a specific platelet membrane protein or subcellular organelle is deficient: the Bernard-Soulier syndrome, Glanzmann's thrombasthenia, and the absence of alpha granules or dense bodies.

Endothelial Cell Disorders

Hemorrhagic coagulopathy has been associated with endothelial cell disorders (Table 2). These syndromes are very rare and should be considered only after the platelet-related disorders have been eliminated. They are listed here for completeness only.

Hereditary Disorders of Coagulation Factors

Hemorrhagic coagulopathy may also arise because of congenital defects in the fluid phase of coagulation (Table 3). Hemophilia A, hemophilia B, and von Willebrand's disease are discussed in the chapter on *Hemophilia and von Willebrand's Disease*. The hereditary disorders of fibrinogen (afibrinogenemia, hypofibrinogenemia, and dysfibrinogenemia) are the most common hereditary coagulopathies after hemophilia A and B and von Willebrand's disease. Hypofibrinogenemia and dysfibrinogenemia are mild disorders that are frequently quiescent until the advent of trauma, surgical challenge, or childbirth. Afibrinogenemia is a rare but severe disorder.

Factor XI deficiency is an autosomal recessive disorder in which the homozygous patient generally presents with significant hemorrhage only after surgical intervention or trauma. The incidence among the general population is approximately 1 in 100,000 but is increased among persons of Jewish descent. There is no correlation between the magnitude of the deficiency and the severity of the clinical syndrome, and the degree of bleeding after sur-

TABLE 2 Endothelial and Vascular Disorders Associated with Hemorrhagic Coagulopathy

Hereditary telangiectasia
Cavernous hemangioma
Angiodysplasia
Kaposi's hemorrhagic sarcoma
Ascorbic acid deficiency
Ehlers-Danlos syndrome
Pseudoxanthoma elasticum
Osteogenesis imperfecta
Amyloidosis
Cryoglobulinemic purpura
Benign hyperglobulinemic purpura

TABLE 3 Hereditary Coagulation Factor Disorders Associated with Hemorrhage

Factor VIII deficiency (hemophilia A)
Factor IX deficiency (hemophilia B)
Von Willebrand's syndrome
Afibrinogenemia
Hypofibrinogenemia
Dysfibrinogenemia
Factor XI deficiency
Factor X deficiency
Factor VII deficiency
Factor V deficiency
Factor II deficiency
Factor XIII deficiency

gical challenge may be variable within the same individual. Isolated deficiencies of Factors X, V, and VII occur in fewer than 1 in 500,000 persons. Deficiency of Factor II (Prothrombin) is extremely rare. Congenital Factor XIII deficiency, a rare disorder, is associated with a severe hemorrhagic diathesis in which the typical bleeding pattern is characterized by umbilical hemorrhage, poor wound healing, moderate mucocutaneous and musculoskeletal hemorrhage, and fatal intracranial hemorrhage after minor trauma.

Acquired Disorders of Coagulation Factors: Deficiency States

Acquired defects in coagulation are more common than hereditary lesions and may be subclassified into acquired deficiency states and inhibitors of coagulation (Table 4). Hepatic dysfunction due to a variety of diseases may result in hemorrhagic coagulopathy secondary to depressed synthesis of vitamin K–dependent factors (II, VII, IX, X) and fibrinogen or low-grade DIC with defective hepatic clearance of activated coagulation factors. Overdosage with the vitamin K antagonists, 4-hydroxycoumarin derivatives, may occur voluntarily or as a complication of therapeutic anticoagulant regulation. The result is prolongation of the prothrombin time (PT), primarily as the result of Factor VII depression, and perhaps of the activated partial thromboplastin time (APTT) if the dose is adequate. Salicylates have also been reported to inhibit synthesis of the vitamin K–dependent clotting proteins. Antibiotics, most notably the synthetic cephalosporins such as cephamandole, also cause a profound depression of the vitamin K–dependent factors by a mechanism that acts more rapidly than the antibiotic-induced alteration of the intestinal flora. Snakebite due to the western diamondback rattlesnake may cause afibrinogenemia owing to marked fibrinolysis (see chapter on *Snake Bites*).

Acquired Disorders of Coagulation Factors: Circulating Anticoagulants

Hemorrhagic coagulopathy may also be associated with circulating anticoagulants, substances that inhibit the normal coagulation process. The most common circulating anticoagulants are *fibrin degradation products of DIC* which inhibit platelet aggregation and fibrin polymeriza-

tion. However, the other aspects of DIC are those that usually cause hemorrhage. Spontaneous Factor VIII inhibitors, immunoglobulins with anti-Factor VIII specificity, may rarely develop in nonhemophiliac patients and produce serious hemorrhage. These antibodies may develop after pregnancy, after exposure to high doses of penicillin, or as a secondary complication of connective tissue disorders. Frequently, no associated disease is present. The lupus anticoagulant commonly causes prolongation of the APTT, but only rarely does it cause significant hemorrhage. When it does cause hemorrhage, complicating thrombocytopenia and prothrombin deficiency are generally present. Specific immunoglobulin inhibitors directed against other factors, most commonly Factors IX and XI, have also been noted with connective tissue disorders. Hemorrhagic coagulopathy may also be seen as a consequence of surreptitious heparin administration or, more rarely, acquired circulating heparinoid factors. The latter are proteoglycans that arise as the result of neoplastic disorders. The dysproteinemic disorders cause hemorrhage by interference with the action of thrombin or fibrin polymerization. Acquired dysfibrinogenemia has been reported in the course of neoplastic disease and hepatic failure, although the latter usually does not produce significant hemorrhage.

DIFFERENTIAL DIAGNOSIS

Recognition of abnormal hemostasis is an important factor in the diagnosis of hemorrhagic coagulopathy. This may be a simple task when the patient's history is available, but it is complex when the defect is undiagnosed or the patient's history is unavailable. When an obvious primary cause for bleeding exists, the physician may fail to consider abnormal hemostasis as a significant factor. Clinical suspicion of abnormal hemostasis should be raised by a variety of physical findings (Table 5).

The first goal is to determine whether the hemostatic abnormality is congenital or acquired and whether it is present in the cellular or the fluid phase of hemostasis. Evaluation (Table 6) to ascertain which phase is affected can be carried out within 30 minutes, and blood samples should be obtained prior to any therapy, both to avoid altering laboratory data owing to partial treatment and to provide a therapeutic baseline. A careful history focused on bleeding should discriminate between the hereditary and acquired defects. Inspection of the peripheral smear, the platelet count, and the initial coagulation studies (PT and APTT) should discriminate between the common defects in the cellular phase and the fluid phase of hemostasis. Because it is not possible to perform a bone

TABLE 4 Acquired Coagulation Disorders Associated with Hemorrhage

Circulating Anticoagulants	Deficiency States
Spontaneous factor VIII inhibitors	Warfarin overdose
Other spontaneous factor inhibitors	Acute salicylate
Lupus anticoagulants	intoxication
Disseminated intravascular coagulation	Hepatic dysfunction
Surreptitious heparin administration	Vitamin K deficiency
Heparinoid inhibitors	Snakebite
Dysfibrinogenemias	afibrinogenemia
Dysproteinemic disorders	

TABLE 5 Physical Signs Suggestive of Abnormal Hemostasis

Purpura or petechiae unassociated with trauma
Spontaneous hematoma formation
Spontaneous mucocutaneous, respiratory, gastrointestinal, or genitourinary hemorrhage
Inability to obtain hemostasis during surgical procedures
Anemia/unexplained decrease in hematocrit

marrow examination in the emergency setting, measurement of the mean platelet volume (MPV), a readily available test, will help to distinguish between disorders of increased platelet destruction and disorders of decreased platelet production. The MPV is generally elevated in the platelet-destructive disorders and within the normal range in the production-failure disorders. Normal fluid-phase coagulation tests with a normal platelet count should suggest a qualitative platelet defect, an endothelial cell abnormality, or deficient Factor XIII activity (since the latter is not tested in the routine coagulation assays).

The differential diagnosis of hemorrhagic coagulopathy encompasses the disorders listed in Tables 1 through 4. A combined defect is suggested by laboratory abnormalities in both phases, and first consideration should be given to DIC with a search for inciting factors. An assay for fibrin degradation products (FDP) may be added to support the diagnosis of DIC. If all of the initial tests are normal, then consideration must be given to qualitative platelet defects or to von Willebrand's disease. Diagnosis of these disorders requires measurement of the bleeding time. The endothelial cell and vascular disorders should present with normal coagulation tests unless complicating DIC or the rare form of von Willebrand's disease associated with angiodysplasia is present. The differential diagnosis of these disorders (see Table 2) relies on the presence of physical findings or complicating diseases. The hereditary coagulopathies (see Table 3) and the acquired deficiency states (see Table 4) present with abnormalities in either the intrinsic (APTT) or the extrinsic (PT) pathways, and perhaps in both, depending on the location of the defect. The presence of a deficiency can be rapidly confirmed by performance of a mixing assay in which normal plasma is mixed with patient plasma. Complete correction of the clotting test (PT or APTT) should be observed in either the intrinsic (APTT) or the extrinsic (PT) pathways, and perhaps in both, depending on the location of the defect. Failure to correct completely, or prolongation with incubation of the mixture at 37° C for 60 minutes suggests the presence of an inhibitor (see Table 4). The lupus-type anticoagulant generally demonstrates immediate prolongation of the mixing study with little time-dependent potentiation, in contrast to the factor-specific inhibitors, which show time-dependent potentiation. The lupus anticoagulant is also evident in the diluted

Russell's viper venom test; factor-specific inhibitors above Factor X are not active. On occasion it may be necessary to prolong the mixing study to 4 hours in order to demonstrate the presence of weak Factor VIII inhibitors. Unfortunately, the strength of the inhibitor in the in vitro laboratory tests does not correlate well with the severity of hemorrhage.

Surreptitious use of heparin or the heparinoid inhibitors produces prolongation of the thrombin time, which corrects with the addition of toluidine blue. These inhibitors can also be confirmed by the presence of a normal reptilase time test. The dysfibrinogenemias and the dysproteinemic states also cause prolongation of the thrombin time and the reptilase time. These disorders should be distinguishable by the presence of a paraprotein. Hepatic dysfunction, a common cause of hemorrhage, presents with accompanying physical and laboratory evidence of liver disease.

MANAGEMENT

Emergency Stabilization

With major coagulopathy and blood loss (internal or external), initial management requires stabilization of vital signs, blood volume, and red cell mass by transfusion of either whole blood or packed red cells with an appropriate volume expander. If possible, a platelet count, PT, and aPTT should be performed to direct the emergency therapy. In the absence of an exact diagnosis, emergency management may be temporarily directed according to the type and severity of hemorrhage until a specific diagnosis is available (Table 7). Emphasis should be placed on obtaining pretherapy laboratory studies as rapidly as possible to direct subsequent therapy.

Rarely, immediate emergency tracheostomy may be required in the presence of an acute hemorrhagic diathesis before any diagnostic details are known. This may demand the empiric use of either whole blood, fresh frozen plasma, cryoprecipitate, or platelets, depending on the suspected defect.

Acute Management of Platelet Disorders

Acute hemorrhage with a suspected diagnosis of immune-mediated thrombocytopenia may require the infusion of platelets. Although platelet transfusion in these disorders usually does not result in improvement of the platelet level, hemostasis may be transiently improved. One unit of platelets should produce an approximate increment of 15,000 platelets per microliter per square meter of body surface area. Usually a platelet count above 20,000 per microliter provides adequate protection against spontaneous hemorrhage, but in the presence of an active bleeding site a level of over 50,000 per microliter is required. Adults generally require a minimum of four platelet units as an initial therapeutic trial. Post-transfusion platelet counts are useful to determine the efficacy and future frequency of transfusion.

TABLE 6   Initial Evaluation of Abnormal Hemostasis

> Hemostasis history
> Quantitative platelet count
> Peripheral blood smear review: platelet,
>   leukocyte, erythrocyte morphology
> Prothrombin time
> Activated partial thromboplastin time
> Thrombin time
> Fibrinogen
> Fibrin degradation products*
> Bleeding time†

---

* To be performed if DIC is suspected
† To be performed if von Willebrand's disease or a qualitative platelet
   defect is suspected

TABLE 7 Emergency Management of Hemorrhage Associated with Coagulopathy

Clinical Condition	Suggested Management
Minor hemorrhage* Mucocutaneous bleeding Stable vital signs Neurologic stability	PT, aPTT, PC; await laboratory results
Minor hemorrhage Deep tissue bleeding Stable vital signs Neurologic stability	PT, aPTT, PC; transfuse with whole blood to maintain HCT
Minor hemorrhage Neurologic instability Stable vital signs	PT, aPTT, PC; transfuse with 5 units FFP, 10 units CPT, 4 units platelets. Obtain post-transfusion PT, aPTT, PC.
Minor hemorrhage Respiratory tract bleeding Stable vital signs	PT, aPTT, PC; transfuse with 5 units FFP, 10 units CPT, 4 units platelets. Obtain post-transfusion PT, aPTT, PC.
Major hemorrhage† Mucocutaneous, GI, GU, deep tissue bleeding Stable vital signs	PT, aPTT, PC; transfuse with whole blood to maintain HCT
Major hemorrhage Unstable vital signs or neurologic instability	PT, aPTT, PC; transfuse with whole blood, 5 units FFP, 10 units CPT, 4 units platelets. Obtain post-transfusion PT, aPTT, PC.
Major hemorrhage Unresponsive to previous measures Persistently abnormal coagulation tests	Continue support with whole blood, FFP, CPT, platelets and add APX 50 units/kg body weight

* Blood loss <500 ml in 12 hours and/or HCT of less than 42% but greater than 37% in males and less than 36% but greater than 31% in females

† Blood loss >500 ml in 12 hours and/or HCT less than 37% in males and less than 31% in females

PT = prothrombin time, aPTT = activated partial thromboplastin time, PC = platelet count, HCT = hematocrit, FFP = fresh frozen plasma, CPT = cryoprecipitate, APX = activated prothrombin complex

Another approach is the infusion of gammaglobulin (400 mg per kilogram per day) to induce reticuloendothelial blockade and prolongation of autologous platelet survival or improved response to subsequent platelet support. It should be emphasized that these maneuvers are temporizing measures in the face of life threatening hemorrhage, and that they are not part of the general therapeutic approach to treatment of immune mediated thrombocytopenia. Corticosteroids, prednisone 1 to 2 mg per kilogram per day, are important first line therapy in the immune thrombocytopenias. Although the effect may be delayed for several days, in the face of hemorrhage, both corticosteroids and gammaglobulin may be followed by a trial of platelet transfusion to achieve a platelet level increment. If the thrombocytopenia is due to bone marrow hypoplasia, platelet transfusion will be efficacious.

Active bleeding due to qualitative platelet disorders also requires transfusion to at least 50,000 normal platelets per microliter. TTP and HUS respond best to plasmapheresis, although temporizing measures such as plasma infusion, steroids, low-molecular-weight dextran, and platelet inhibitory agents may be tried. PTP also responds to plasmapheresis. The usual procedure in both of these disorders is to perform a daily 4-liter exchange with plasma replacement for TTP and HUS and albumin replacement for PTP. Hemorrhage due to uremia has been reported to respond to intensive dialysis; failing adequate control with dialysis, transfusion with cryoprecipitate (10 units) has provided hemostatic control and transient bleeding time correction in some patients. Qualitative platelet disorders that cannot be treated by random donor platelet transfusion because of prior alloimmunization may respond to low-dose prednisone (10 mg, three times daily). This maneuver appears to cause a nonspecific improvement in platelet function, but it is of limited value during severe bleeding. Ultimately, patients will require support with HLA-matched platelets. Infusion with desmopressin (DDAVP), 10 μg per square meter or 0.3 to 0.5 μg per kilogram in 30 ml of normal saline infused over 5 minutes may produce temporary shortening of the bleeding time in some qualitative platelet disorders; however, its use to treat significant bleeding has not been adequately evaluated.

Acute Management of Endothelial Cell and Vascular Disorders

Treatment of the coagulopathy associated with cavernous hemangioma may respond to a DIC treatment regimen of heparin infusion (500 to 750 units per hour) or to the infusion of epsilon-aminocaproic acid (EACA) 0.1 g per kilogram loading dose and then 1.0 g per hour. Infusion of cryoprecipitate (10 units) may be added to this regimen in order to raise the fibrinogen level and potentiate thrombosis of the vascular lesion with reduction of the consumptive process. Platelet inhibitory agents (aspirin 0.5 g per day and dipyridamole 0.15 g 3 times daily) have also been reported to be useful in some cases. Vascular disorders secondary to other disease processes should be treated by treating the primary disease or with general supportive measures when no specific therapy is available.

Acute Management of Hereditary Coagulopathy

Hereditary disorders of coagulation factors (Table 3) are treated by infusion of appropriate replacement products that contain the missing factor. Recommended initial dosages for each deficient factor are provided, and the required level of each factor for effective hemostasis in either minor or major hemorrhage is shown (Table 8). The average normal level of the coagulation factors is arbitrarily defined as 100 percent (1.0 unit per milliliter) except for fibrinogen, which is expressed as milligrams per deciliter. The dosages are calculated on the basis of body weight. These dosages are approximations, and the required level of replacement depends on the anatomic bleeding site, the general metabolic state, and the volume of current blood loss. Each therapeutic maneuver should be evaluated by the effect on bleeding and by follow-up coagulation assays. For immediate monitoring, either the

TABLE 8 Replacement Therapy of Plasma Coagulation Factors

Defect	Minor Hemorrhage*	Major Hemorrhage*	Product	Dosage†	Recovery
Factor I‡	50–100 mg/dl	100 mg/dl	CPT	2 bags§	50%
Factor II	15%	40%	FFP	20 U	50%
Factor II	15%	40%	PCX	40 U	50%
Factor V	15%	25%	FFP	25 U	50%
Factor VII	10%	20%	FFP	10 U	100%
Factor VII	10%	20%	PCX	10 U	100%
Factor X	10%	20%	FFP	15 U	75%
Factor X	10%	20%	PCX	15 U	75%
Factor XI	15%	25%	FFP	20 U	90%
Factor XIII	1%	5%	FFP	3U	50%
Factor VIII inhibitor#	20%	50%	AHG	50 U	70%
Factor VIII inhibitor#	20%	50%	APX	50 U	70%

* Effective level suggested for hemostasis
† Dosage per kg of body weight for initial therapy
‡ Fibrinogen
§ Dosage per 10 kg of body weight; 1 bag = 1 unit of CPT
# Acquired Factor VIII inhibitor in nonhemophiliac

CPT = cryoprecipitate, FFP = fresh frozen plasma, PCX = prothrombin complex, AHG = antihemophilic globulin, APX = activated prothrombin complex

PT or the APTT may be used, because these assays are readily available; but the therapeutic response should be confirmed by assaying the specific factor. Long-term management is not discussed here.

The factor deficiencies other than the fibrinogen disorders may be treated initially with fresh frozen plasma to increase the missing factor level to the 30 to 50 percent level depending on the nature of the bleeding diathesis (see Table 8). Failure to achieve required levels with this regimen for deficiencies of Factor II, VII, or X may call for the use of more specialized products such as the prothrombin complex concentrates, which contain increased concentrations of the missing factors. Volume overload may be avoided by the use of prothrombin complex concentrates, although there is a greater risk for the development of hepatitis because these products are derived from large donor pools.

Initial Management of Acquired Coagulopathy

Initial management of the acquired coagulopathies may require infusion with fresh frozen plasma for therapy of vitamin K deficiency, warfarin intoxication, or acute salicylate poisoning. The same dosage schedules apply as for the congenital disorders (see Table 8). Spontaneous factor inhibitors require treatment with antihemophilic globulin (AHG), fresh frozen plasma, or prothrombin complex concentrates depending on the inhibitor type, strength, and level of bleeding. The strength of the inhibitor, expressed as the titer in Bethesda units, may not be available on an emergency basis. Generally, the degree

of APTT prolongation does not correlate well with the measured inhibitor titer level. Thus, the initial therapy must be empiric. Management of nonhemophilic Factor VIII inhibitors can be initiated with the infusion of AHG (50 units per kilogram); the APTT should be measured for improvement, and the degree of bleeding should be reassessed. Further management is not discussed here and should be supervised by a hematologist.

Heparinoid inhibitors and heparin toxicity may be treated with a trial of protamine infusion. One g of protamine neutralizes 100 units of heparin. The approximate heparin level may be calculated from the thrombin time assay using a heparin sensitivity curve. Hemorrhage due to malignant dysproteinemias should be managed with plasmapheresis and plasma replacement, with at least a 4-liter exchange. Acute hemorrhage due to DIC requires treatment of the primary inciting disorder; serious hemorrhage requires the addition of heparin (500 to 700 units per hour) by continuous infusion with replacement of platelets and fibrinogen for hemostatic stabilization.

SUGGESTED READING

Aster RH. Thrombocytopenia due to enhanced platelet destruction. In: Williams WJ, Beutler E, Erslev AJ, Lichtman MA, eds. Hematology. 3rd ed. New York: McGraw-Hill Book Company, 1983: 1299.

Colman RW, Robboy SJ, Minna JD. Disseminated intravascular coagulation: a reappraisal. Ann Rev Med 1979; 30:359–380.

Feinstein DI. Acquired inhibitors against factor VIII and other clotting proteins. In: Colman RW, Hirsh J, Marder VJ, Salzman EW, eds. Hemostasis and thrombosis. Philadelphia: JB Lippincott, 1982: 563.

Mammen EF. Congenital coagulation disorders. Semin Throm Hemost 1982; 9:1–24.

HEMOPHILIA AND VON WILLEBRAND'S DISEASE

MARC A. SHUMAN, M.D.

MANAGEMENT OF HEMOPHILIA

The term "hemophilia" generally refers to two genetic disorders, Factor VIII:antihemophilic factor (AHF), and Factor IX deficiency. These are rare disorders, with an incidence of one in 10,000 for Factor VIII deficiency and approximately one in 40,000 for Factor IX deficiency. Because these are X-linked recessively transmitted diseases, they are seen in males, with extremely rare exceptions. Patients with Factor VIII and Factor IX deficiency have virtually identical histories, physical examinations, and laboratory tests, with the exception of specific assays for these factors. The disorders are otherwise indistinguishable.

Many patients do not know what type of hemophilia they have. When the patient presents without a known diagnosis, the essential historical features that should raise the possibility of a diagnosis of hemophilia are a family history of hemophilia with only male members being affected, and episodic hemarthrosis (joint bleeding). The physical examination frequently reveals evidence of previous hemarthrosis with synovial thickening and joint deformity, most commonly in the knees, ankles, and elbows. The best diagnostic screening test for either Factor VIII or Factor IX deficiency is the activated partial thromboplastin time (APTT). This is always prolonged in moderate to severe hemophilia, but may be normal in mild hemophilia. In the latter case, patients do not bleed unless exposed to severe trauma, whereas patients with more severe hemophilia frequently bleed with little or no trauma. If there are other abnormalities in coagulation tests, such as a prolonged prothrombin time or thrombocytopenia, other diagnoses must be considered. von Willebrand's disease, which may also have a prolonged APTT, may be confused with Factor VIII deficiency. The distinguishing features of this disorder is discussed in greater detail in a later section.

Since Factor VIII deficiency is approximately four times more common than Factor IX deficiency, a Factor VIII level should be obtained first in evaluating the patient for hemophilia. If this is normal, then Factor IX level should be measured. Generally, the Factor VIII or IX level does not fluctuate to a significant extent, so it is unnecessary to repeat either the APTT or the factor level if these are known from previous evaluation.

Treatment of Bleeding Episodes in Hemophilia

A hemophiliac bleeding episode should be treated as quickly as possible, since the longer the bleeding persists, the more difficult it is to treat and the more factor replacement is required. In addition, prolonged bleeding can result in serious morbidity and irreversible injury.

Joint and Muscle Hemorrhages

Such hemorrhages should be treated quickly before visible objective findings appear. If this is done, only small amounts of replacement therapy are necessary. Usually pain and stiffness are the first symptoms of bleeding. Because of the recurrent nature of joint and muscle bleeding in hemophilia, the patients can tell early on when they are bleeding. With small joint or muscle hemorrhages, one dose of replacement therapy raising the Factor VIII or IX level approximately 25 percent is sufficient. (Details of calculating dosage and specific plasma product are discussed below.)

With more extensive bleeding, the patient usually has obvious hemorrhage associated with considerable pain. A larger amount of replacement therapy is generally indicated, raising levels of factor to 40 to 50 percent of normal. Repeat dosage may be necessary, depending on the response to therapy. If there is considerable pain associated with large hemarthroses, relief can be promptly obtained by joint aspiration. This should be done immediately after infusion of replacement therapy. Joint aspiration is not necessary for small hemorrhages. Exterior splints of affected joints are usually helpful, but should be discontinued when pain has subsided to the point where the patient can comfortably use the joint. Similarly, with hemarthrosis involving the lower extremity, nonweight bearing of the affected extremity is recommended until the joint can be used without excessive pain. Prolonged immobilization results in muscle atrophy and loss of joint motion.

In general, joint and muscle hemorrhages do not require hospitalization. Hemorrhages into the hip joint do usually require hospitalization with complete bed rest and intensive factor replacement for 1 to 2 weeks. Similarly, bleeding into the iliopsoas muscle requires hospitalization, complete bed rest, and intensive replacement therapy. These patients usually present with pain in the groin or lower abdomen. Frequently, the hip is maintained in a flexed position. In contrast to hemorrhage into the hip joint, which is associated with pain on rotation of the joint, bleeding into the iliopsoas muscle is usually associated with pain on extension of the hip to a much greater extent than on rotation. Another situation that usually requires hospitalization is when soft tissue bleeding results in compression of a nerve with impaired sensory or motor function. Under these circumstances, intensive replacement therapy is necessary and this is usually best accomplished in the hospital.

Central Nervous System Hemorrhage

Central nervous system (CNS) hemorrhage is potentially the most dangerous type of bleeding seen in hemophiliac patients, with a mortality of 30 percent. Characteristically, symptoms and signs of CNS bleeding are delayed following trauma; thus, a patient with hemophilia who presents with a history of significant head trauma, although asymptomatic, should be treated with replacement therapy with the goal of achieving a factor level of 100 percent. The patient should be hospitalized and observed for at least 24 hours. Patients who have CNS symptoms, such as unexplained headache, should receive replacement therapy and be admitted for observation.

Oropharyngeal Bleeding and Epistaxis

Hemorrhage in the mouth or anterior portion of the pharynx can be managed with factor replacement therapy and antifibrinolytic agents. Generally, raising the Factor VIII level 20 to 30 percent and oral administration of epsilon-aminocaproid acid (Amicar) is sufficient. The Amicar should be given in a dosage of 4 to 6 g 4 times daily in patients weighing more than 100 lb. The liquid suspension of Amicar is preferable to the tablets. Posterior pharyngeal bleeding or bleeding under the tongue is potentially dangerous because of the possibility of airway obstruction with extension of the hemorrhage. Under these circumstances, a higher level of Factor VIII should be achieved by replacement therapy, aiming for a 70 to 80 percent concentration. In addition, the patient should be hospitalized to receive regular replacement therapy and to be observed.

Urinary Tract Bleeding

Hematuria is common in hemophilia; it frequently follows minor trauma. Usually this can be managed on an outpatient basis. A level of approximately 50 percent factor should be achieved by replacement therapy. Amicar is contraindicated in these situations because of the danger of clot formation in the urinary tract with obstruction of the ureter. Structural lesions are not usually found with extensive evaluation of the urinary tract, although if an older patient with new onset of hematuria has not been previously evaluated, it is recommended that an anatomic basis for the lesion be sought.

Gastrointestinal Hemorrhage

Patients presenting with melena, hematochezia, or hematemesis should be immediately transfused, with replacement therapy aiming for a level of factor of approximately 100 percent, and they should be admitted to the hospital for further evaluation. In addition, if the patient has not been recently evaluated for a structural lesion, work-up of the gastrointestinal tract is indicated. Relatively minor causes of bleeding, such as hemorrhoids or fissures, can usually be managed with one infusion of factor replacement on an outpatient basis.

Calculation of Factor VIII and Factor IX Dosage

One unit of Factor VIII or Factor IX is defined as the amount of activity present in 1 ml of normal plasma. Patients with hemophilia who have a level of 5 percent, therefore have 0.05 units per milliliter. To calculate the amount of Factor VIII or Factor IX necessary to achieve a desired level, one must know the patient's usual factor level and decide on the desired level. For example, a patient who has a Factor IX level of 1 percent who requires a factor level of approximately 30 percent for a joint bleed would require replacement therapy of 0.29 unit per milliliter of plasma. There are several methods for determining how many units of replacement therapy are necessary in a given patient.

One technique for calculating the dosage is to first determine the patient's plasma volume. Assuming a blood volume of 70 ml per kilogram, this can be determined once the patient's weight and hematocrit have been ascertained. For example, a 70-kg patient with a hematocrit of 40 percent would have a plasma volume of approximately 3,000 ml. Therefore, raising the factor concentration 0.29 unit per milliliter would require a total dosage of 870 units. Because of additional considerations such as extravascular distribution, this amount must be multiplied by 1.5 for Factor VIII and 2.0 for Factor IX. If the patient had Factor VIII deficiency, therefore, the total dose infused would be 1,300 units.

A simplified method for calculating the dosage required is to infuse 1 unit of Factor VIII per kilogram of body weight for every 2 percentage point increase desired. For Factor IX deficiency the patient is infused with 1 unit per kilogram for every 1 percentage unit desired.

Choice of Replacement Therapy

There are several considerations when deciding on the type of factor replacement for bleeding episodes. These include the extent and severity of bleeding, the severity of the factor deficiency, whether or not the patient has previously had hepatitis, and the patient's cardiovascular status.

Plasma

Plasma may be used to replace Factor VIII or Factor IX in patients with hemophilia. In the case of Factor VIII deficiency the plasma must be either fresh-frozen or fresh, since Factor VIII activity declines in stored plasma. The risk of hepatitis is lowest with plasma therapy, since it involves the fewest donors. The limiting consideration in plasma therapy is that one cannot achieve increases of either Factor VIII or Factor IX greater than 20 percent owing to volume restrictions. In patients with compromised cardiovascular status, this becomes an even less desirable form of therapy. Plasma therapy may be used in patients who have relatively mild hemophilia with mild-to-moderate bleeding, if the patient has not previously had hepatitis and bleeding can be controlled with only a modest increase in the factor concentration. In patients who have had recurrent transfusions and have already had an episode of hepatitis, plasma therapy is not practical.

Cryoprecipitate

When plasma is frozen, then thawed at 4 °C, Factor VIII remains a precipitate; cryoprecipitate does not contain Factor IX. Cryoprecipitate is prepared in plastic bags containing approximately 100 units of Factor VIII in a volume of approximately 20 ml. Each bag of cryoprecipitate also contains approximately 250 mg of fibrinogen. The Factor VIII concentration can be raised to 100 percent with cryoprecipitate therapy, and therefore it can be used for severe bleeding. Each bag of cryoprecipitate represents plasma that has been processed from one donor, so that if multiple bags of cryoprecipitate are given, the risk of hepatitis is significantly higher than with plasma therapy. With both plasma and cryoprecipitate replacement therapy, allergic reactions to plasma proteins may occur, and these are best treated with antihistamines.

Factor VIII and Factor IX Concentrate

Highly purified preparations of Factor VIII and Factor IX concentrate are the treatment of choice for patients with severe hemophilia who require frequent treatment for recurrent bleeding episodes. Under these circumstances, there is no advantage to either plasma or cryoprecipitate therapy. One can easily achieve levels of factor of 100 percent, transfusing small volumes of the concentrate. Each vial has a predetermined amount of Factor VIII or Factor IX printed on the label, usually approximately 250, 500, 750 or 1,000 units, and multiples of these are given for replacement. The risk of hepatitis is highest with concentrates, as each bottle represents material purified from several thousand donors. Because of the recurrent need for transfusion in severe hemophilia, cryoprecipitate eventually offers no advantage over concentrate, since the patient will be exposed to multiple donors with both treatments. In some cases, when the patients are small children, designated family members have been used to prepare cryoprecipitate which is then stored specifically for the patient.

A small percentage of patients with hemophilia have developed the acquired immunodeficiency syndrome (AIDS) secondary to contamination of the Factor VIII concentrates with the AIDS-related virus. As a result of this, manufacturers of Factor VIII and Factor IX have developed a heat-treatment process that appears to inactivate the virus totally. These heat-treated products have now replaced the standard Factor VIII and IX concentrates. It remains to be proved, however, whether this will totally eradicate the risk of AIDS. There also appears to be a decreased risk of hepatitis with the heat-treated product, but this also requires further evaluation.

D-Desaminoarginine Vasopressin

D-Desaminoarginine vasopressin (DDAVP) is a synthetic analogue of vasopressin which has minimal pressor effects. DDAVP stimulates the release of Factor VIII and von Willebrand factor by an as yet uncharacterized mechanism. The advantage of this form of treatment for Factor VIII deficiency is that it does not involve the risk of transfusion therapy and attendant infectious complications. It generally is effective only in patients with mild hemophilia (Factor VIII deficiency) or von Willebrand's disease. Patients who have Factor VIII concentrations of 10 percent or more have the best response to DDAVP. Patients with levels between 5 and 10 percent have a variable response, and patients with levels below 5 percent generally do not respond. DDAVP stimulates only release of Factor VIII and does not stimulate synthesis. The response to DDAVP varies, with some patients achieving normal levels of Factor VIII while others have only a modest increase in the Factor VIII concentration. The dosage is 0.3 μg per kilogram of body weight infused intravenously over approximately 15 minutes. There is an immediate rise in the Factor VIII level with a decline over approximately 10 hours, as is the case with transfused Factor VIII. The general indication for DDAVP is mild-to-moderate bleeding episodes in patients who have not had hepatitis previously.

Management of Bleeding Episodes in Hemophilia Patients with Inhibitors

Approximately 10 to 15 percent of patients with Factor VIII deficiency and approximately 3 percent of patients with Factor IX deficiency develop antibodies against the transfused factor. Approximately 90 percent of these patients have severe hemophilia. Clinically, this manifests as refractoriness to replacement therapy. Management of this complication is extremely difficult and requires the expertise of a physician who specializes in the treatment of hemophilia. In patients with low titer inhibitors, the inhibitor may be overcome by transfusing large amounts of the factor concentrates. The disadvantage of this approach is that it usually stimulates synthesis of the antibody, making the patient even more refractory to replacement therapy. In patients with high titer Factor VIII inhibitors, Factor IX concentrates are partially successful. This appears to be due to the presence of small amounts of activated factors in the preparation. Also available are Factor IX concentrates that have been intentionally activated (Autoplex), specifically for management of patients with inhibitors to Factor VIII. The dosage is 75 units per kilogram of body weight. These, however, are quite expensive; the cost of one treatment is several thousand dollars.

MANAGEMENT OF von WILLEBRAND'S DISEASE

In contrast to hemophilia, von Willebrand's disease is an autosomal dominant disorder affecting both males and females. The pattern of bleeding also differs in von Willebrand's disease compared with hemophilia, in that joint hemorrhages are rare and present only in patients with severe von Willebrand's disease. The general pattern of bleeding in this disorder is mucocutaneous. The most common manifestation in childhood is epistaxis. Excessive vaginal bleeding is quite common in menstruating women. The primary deficiency in von Willebrand's disease is decreased amounts of von Willebrand factor, also termed Factor VIII:vWF. This plasma protein is necessary for normal platelet function; it promotes platelet adhesion to the subendothelium of injured blood vessels. There is a variable deficiency of Factor VIII:anti-hemophilic factor in this disorder as well. Most patients have either normal levels or a mild deficiency of Factor VIII:AHF. It is only in severe von Willebrand's disease that low levels of Factor VIII:AHF are seen. In von Willebrand's disease, the bleeding time is generally prolonged, whereas it is normal in hemophilia. Thus, in a patient in whom the diagnosis is uncertain, a template bleeding time should be helpful. When there is antihemophilic factor deficiency the APTT may be prolonged, but with mild deficiency the APTT may be normal, as discussed in the preceding section. The specific diagnosis of von Willebrand's disease requires measurement of von Willebrand factor. These tests usually take several hours and an answer cannot be readily obtained when the patient is being evaluated for a bleeding episode. Von Willebrand factor is measured by a functional assay in which the ability of the patient's plasma to support agglutination of normal platelets by ristocetin is measured (ristocetin co-factor assay). Von Willebrand factor is also measured immunologically (Factor VIII:vWF Ag).

Treatment

Management of bleeding episodes in von Willebrand's disease is more complicated than in hemophilia, owing to the possibility of deficiency of two factors—marked variability in the response to replacement therapy, and the lack of a readily available test to quantify the response to transfusion. In addition, there is only a fair correlation, at best, between the results of in vitro tests and the patient's response to replacement therapy. For these reasons, replacement therapy in von Willebrand's disease is somewhat arbitrary.

Two blood products are used primarily to manage bleeding episodes: plasma and cryoprecipitate. Although Factor VIII concentrates contain von Willebrand factor, it is present in markedly reduced amounts. Therefore, although the antihemophilic factor level can be adequately treated with concentrates, there is a suboptimal response to replacement of von Willebrand factor. For mild-to-moderate bleeding, one bag of cryoprecipitate per 10 kg, or fresh-frozen plasma, 10 ml per kilogram, is usually adequate therapy. The decision whether to hospitalize or discharge the patient depends on the location of the bleeding, as in hemophilia. With major bleeding episodes, cryoprecipitate is the only effective form of therapy, and 1½ to two bags of cryoprecipitate per kilogram should be used with a maximum of approximately 15 bags. If the patient's response to replacement therapy has not been previously evaluated, repeat of the bleeding time following the administration of cryoprecipitate may be helpful in determining the effectiveness of this therapy.

Patients with von Willebrand's disease who are also deficient in antihemophilic factor frequently respond differently to Factor VIII infusion than patients with hemophilia. For unknown reasons, a higher plasma level of factor VIII is obtained in many patients with von Willebrand's disease than is actually present in the transfused material. Therefore, it is usually unnecessary to administer an amount of Factor VIII more than that which would result in a calculated level of 60 percent.

DDAVP is also beneficial in managing bleeding episodes in patients with mild-to-moderate von Willebrand's disease, but not all patients respond. Patients who have a decrease in a structurally normal von Willebrand factor (type I von Willebrand's disease) generally have a beneficial response to DDAVP. Patients who have a structurally abnormal von Willebrand factor (type II von Willebrand's disease) usually do not have an adequate response to DDAVP and may in some cases have deleterious side effects.

As is the case in patients with hemophilia, epsilon-aminocaproic acid is helpful in managing bleeding episodes in the mouth and epistaxis as well as excessive vaginal bleeding associated with menses.

SUGGESTED READING

Bloom A, ed. The hemophilias. Edinburgh; Churchill-Livingstone, 1982.
Hilgartner MW, ed. Hemophilia in the child and adult. New York; Masson, 1982.

SICKLE CELL ANEMIA

STEPHEN H. EMBURY, M.D.
WILLIAM C. MENTZER, M.D.

Sickle cell anemia is an inherited disease in which the poor solubility and tendency to polymerize of deoxygenated sickle hemoglobin (Hb S) results in chronic hemolytic anemia, episodic pain, chronic and acute organ dysfunction, frequent infections, and shortened life expectancy. The sickling syndromes are classified as *sickle cell disease*, which is associated with anemia and painful episodes, and *sickle cell trait* (Hb AS), which is clinically benign (although the potential for renal and splenic infarction does exist). Sickle cell disease includes homozygous sickle cell anemia (Hb SS) and the compound heterozygous conditions Hb SC disease and beta-thalassemia.

The standard *diagnostic test* for each of these syndromes is hemoglobin electrophoresis, but the results of this test are usually not available on an emergency basis. It reveals nearly 100 percent Hb S in Hb SS and beta$_0$-thalassemia, approximately 80 percent Hb S and 20 percent Hb A in beta$_+$-thalassemia, 50 percent Hb S and 50 percent Hb C in Hb SC disease, and usually about 60 percent Hb A and 40 percent Hb S in sickle cell trait. A diagnostic test that is more rapidly available on an emergency basis is the *hemoglobin solubility test*. It is positive in all sickling syndromes in which Hb S is present, including the sickle cell diseases and sickle cell trait. It may be falsely negative in transfused patients and in the newborn. The most readily available test on an emergency basis is review of the peripheral smear for sickled red blood cells. This test distinguishes sickle cell trait from the sickle cell diseases in that sickle forms are present only in the latter.

All genotypic varieties of sickle cell disease are subject to the complications that are subsequently discussed.

VASO-OCCLUSIVE CRISIS

The clinical course of sickle cell anemia is punctuated by unpredictable episodes of localized vaso-occlusion because of intricately intertwined tangles of sickled erythrocytes. These episodes are often referred to as painful crises and may follow exposure to altitude or other forms of hypoxia, cold stress, infections, or they may have no obvious precipitating cause. The musculoskeletal system is the site of most painful crises, but internal organs may also be involved. Pain is usually relatively constant and often can be recognized by the patient as having a quality characteristic of previous painful crises. The duration of pain varies from hours to several weeks. More than one region of the body may be affected. Painful crises involving the abdomen may simulate an acute abdomen and require careful serial clinical observations for accurate diagnosis.

The location of a painful crisis is in part determined by the age of the patient. Sickle dactylitis, or *hand-foot syndrome*, is the result of vaso-occlusive events in the bone marrow in the extremities of an infant. This particular type of crisis is rare after the age of 5 because active marrow is found only in more central regions of the body after that age. In contrast, aseptic necrosis of the femoral or humeral head is a relatively common vaso-occlusive complication of sickling in late adolescence or adulthood, but is rare in younger children.

Symptoms attributed to vaso-occlusive crises must often be distinguished from those caused by infection. Painful crises are often accompanied by an acute inflammatory reaction with low-grade fever and leukocytosis. A temperature of above 102 °F or an absolute band count greater than 3,000 per mm³ is more likely to be associated with infection than with infarction.

The first step in evaluating a painful crisis in a patient with sickle cell anemia is to eliminate other causes of pain such as infection, ruptured viscus, or acute cholecystitis. With a diagnosis of sickle vaso-occlusive crisis established, appropriate therapy should be initiated. The three cornerstones of therapy are hydration, oxygenation, and adequate analgesia. These patients are usually dehydrated as a result of poor intake, loss of the ability to produce hyperosmotic urine, and fever (if present). Mild episodes are often managed at home; more severe ones may sometimes be treated successfully in the emergency department, but the most severe painful episodes often require hospitalization for more vigorous therapy. Prompt *fluid administration* at a level one and one-half to two times the usual maintenance should be begun immediately. Intravenous fluid administration is preferred, because oral intake in the presence of severe pain and administration of narcotics is likely to be poor. Serum electrolytes and measures of renal function should be drawn to provide a baseline for intravenous fluid therapy.

Supplemental oxygen is administered in the presence of impaired cardiopulmonary function as documented by arterial hypoxemia. Although oxygen therapy is often instituted even when the arterial oxygen tension is normal or unknown, its benefit in such a setting has not been clearly established. Although short-term oxygen therapy is unlikely to be harmful, prolonged treatment over a period of 4 to 5 days may suppress erythropoiesis.

It is important to appreciate the severity of pain associated with sickle vaso-occlusive crises and to provide prompt adequate analgesia. Narcotics are often required. We generally employ morphine sulfate (0.1 to 0.2 mg per kilogram body weight per 2 to 4 hours). Meperidine is relatively contraindicated because its repeated use has been associated with seizures caused by its metabolite, normeperidine. Initially, vigorous efforts should be made to suppress pain, after which maintenance analgesia should be titrated on a regular schedule rather than as needed. Excessive sedation should be avoided because suppression of respiration and the resultant hypoxemia represent a particular hazard for the patient with sickle cell anemia. Less severe pain can be treated effectively with oral acetaminophen plus codeine.

ANEMIC CRISIS

Anemia is a central feature of sickling hemoglobinopathies. The average hemoglobin level in sickle cell anemia is approximately 8 g per deciliter, whereas in hemoglobin SC disease and beta$_+$-thalassemia hemoglobin values are closer to normal. The values in any given patient occasionally fall slightly during vaso-occlusive crises, but usually remain relatively constant over long periods of time. Occasionally, there may be a dramatic and even life-threatening fall in the hemoglobin level. The most common cause of such anemic crises is a transient depression of erythropoiesis by *infection*. Often the organism implicated is the parvovirus, but a variety of other viruses and bacteria are also capable of suppressing red cell production. The period of aplasia usually lasts between a few days and several weeks. Even a brief period of aplasia, however, represents a hazard to an individual with hemolytic anemia, whose mean red cell life span may only be 2 to 4 weeks instead of the normal 4 months.

Another major cause of life-threatening anemia is the splenic sequestration crisis. Here, the spleen suddenly, often within hours, becomes engorged with red cells, creating a deficiency of circulating red cells, which may be severe enough to result in cardiovascular collapse and death. Splenomegaly is often striking. The condition is seen only in infants and young children with homozygous sickle cell anemia because infarction of the spleen prevents its occurrence in later life. On the other hand, splenic sequestration can occur in older children or adults with hemoglobin SC disease and beta-thalassemia because in these conditions the spleen does not ordinarily undergo autoinfarction. In this setting, anemia is not likely to be life threatening, although transfusion may be required.

Exacerbation of hemolysis is not common in sickle cell anemia and if encountered, it suggests the presence of an additional complication such as glucose-6-phosphate dehydrogenase (G6PD) deficiency or autoimmune hemolytic anemia. Severe megaloblastic anemia may develop in sickle cell anemia patients with a poor diet because folate requirements are increased on account of active erythropoiesis. This complication is rare in the United States.

The laboratory evaluation of individuals with anemic crisis should include an assessment of erythrocyte production. Examination of the peripheral blood smear for the presence of polychromatophilic erythrocytes rapidly establishes whether reticulocytes are present. A reticulocyte count provides the necessary quantitative confirmation of reticulocyte number. It is very important to know the steady-state reticulocyte count (which is usually above normal)of the individual under evaluation because even an elevated reticulocyte count, if it is well below the customary value for the patient, may indicate the presence of some degree of suppression of erythropoiesis. An elevated reticulocyte count may be seen during recovery from an episode of erythroid aplasia or during a hemolytic crisis.

If accelerated *hemolysis* is suspected, a direct antiglobulin (Coombs) test and other studies to reveal the cause of hemolysis are indicated. G6PD deficiency occurs in approximately 10 percent of males with sickle cell anemia, and in the setting of infection or exposure to oxidant drugs it may be the cause of accelerated hemolysis. Diagnosis of the African variant of G6PD deficiency is difficult in the presence of reticulocytosis, because high levels of enzyme activity in reticulocytes may mask deficiency in older cells.

Megaloblastic anemia should be suspected if the peripheral blood smear contains hypersegmented neutrophils or macrocytosis beyond levels customary for the patient. A bone marrow examination may provide rapid confirmation of the diagnosis, but does not distinguish between folic and vitamin B_{12} deficiency. Therefore, serum folate and B_{12} levels should be obtained.

The diagnosis of an anemic crisis is an indication for hospitalization. These patients require careful observation and transfusion. Transfusion of packed red cells (up to 10 cc per kilogram in children) to restore oxygen-carrying capacity is the recommended treatment for severe aplastic episodes. In patients whose cardiovascular function is compromised, partial exchange transfusion to avoid any major changes in blood volume is preferred. Another approach is to combine the vigorous use of diuretics with direct, rather than exchange, transfusion. For splenic sequestration crises both oxygen-carrying capacity and intravascular volume must be replaced by red cell transfusion and fluid resuscitation, respectively.

PULMONARY EVENTS

Both children and adults experience the "acute chest syndrome," a life-threatening event comprising chest pain, dyspnea, fever, leukocytosis, pulmonary infiltrates, and hypoxemia. Among different patients these clinical features occur with variable overlap, independent of etiology. Generally, in children, the acute chest syndrome is most likely because of an infectious process; in adults, it is more often caused by vaso-occlusion. It has been suggested that infection can be distinguished from vaso-occlusion on the basis of higher sedimentation rate, greater absolute numbers of bands, and increased leukocyte alkaline phosphatase scores. When the etiology of this complication is uncertain, the patient should be treated for both vaso-occlusive and infectious processes because of the risk associated with progressive hypoxemia due to inadequate therapy.

Sickle cell patients experience pulmonary embolism with no greater frequency than control populations. Because of their much higher frequency of pneumonia and pulmonary vascular occlusion compared to nonsickle patients, we recommend that the diagnosis of pulmonary embolus be entertained only when there are compelling clinical indications (e.g., evidence of deep venous thrombosis). One particular situation in which pulmonary embolism must be considered is in the patient who has no pulmonary infiltrate despite having chest pain, dyspnea, or hypoxemia. Because of the difficulty in interpreting ventilation-perfusion scans in adult patients with the unevenly distributed pulmonary blood flow of chronic pulmonary disease, a pulmonary arteriogram is the procedure of choice when the diagnosis of pulmonary embolus is under consideration. A partial exchange transfusion should be performed prior to pulmonary arteriography in order to protect patients from the possible induction of cellular sickling and vaso-occlusion by the hypertonic radiographic contrast material.

The diagnosis of the acute chest syndrome is an indication for hospitalization and careful blood gas monitoring. All sickle cell patients who have pulmonary infiltrates, dyspnea, or tachypnea should have arterial blood gas assessment. General therapeutic measures for all patients with the acute chest syndrome fall into the categories of hydration, analgesia, antibiotics, and oxygenation. In an attempt to disrupt the sickled cells obstructing the microvasculature, we recommend vigorous hydration with intravenous fluids (in adults at the rate of approximately 200 cc per hour). The appropriate level of analgesia for each patient is an individual matter, but especially in this situation, care must be taken not to suppress respiration. Antibiotic therapy is discussed under *Infection*, but especially in children, penicillin therapy should be given because of the threat of *Streptococcus pneumoniae* infection. The risk of progressive hypoxemia in patients with sickle cell disease is of vital importance, and inhaled oxygen must be used to maintain adequate arterial oxygen tension. If arterial oxygen tension cannot be maintained at levels greater than 65 mm Hg, partial exchange transfusion must be performed to protect the patient from the danger of widespread sickling.

INFECTION

As a result of functional hyposplenia or asplenia and impaired opsonization of bacteria, children with sickle cell disease have a greatly increased susceptibility to sudden overwhelming bacterial sepsis. The greatest frequency of septicemia is in the first 5 years of life, before natural humoral immunity is established. However, sporadic cases of overwhelming sepsis have been reported in older children and adults as well. The organism most frequently isolated is *S. pneumoniae*. Less commonly *Neisseria meningitidis, Escherichia coli*, or, particularly in children, *Haemophilus influenzae* is responsible. The onset of overwhelming sepsis may appear with devastating suddenness. The patient may be well one moment, develop a high fever (which is sometimes accompanied by diarrhea), and within less than 24 hours be dead. The need for rapid accurate evaluation and treatment is obvious.

Unfortunately, the signs and symptoms are nonspecific and therefore most physicians feel that any unexplained high fever in a child with sickle cell anemia or Hb SC disease should be treated with prompt intravenous antibiotic therapy and hospitalization. The choice of antibiotic depends on local factors such as the frequency of beta-lactamase-positive *H. influenzae* in the community. IV cefuroxime (100 mg per kilogram per 24 hours) or ampicillin (pediatric dose of 200 to 250 mg per kilogram per 24 hours) is widely used. It is difficult to establish a threshold temperature, but certainly any fever greater than 102 °F should be considered to represent possible bacterial sepsis unless a clear alternate diagnosis is discovered.

Distinguishing a localized infection from a vaso-occlusive episode is often difficult in patients with sickle cell anemia. Both can produce pain, swelling, and local signs of inflammation and tissue necrosis as well as fever and leukocytosis. Both may occur; areas of pneumonic consolidation in the lung may be poorly ventilated and hypoxic, factors that promote sickling and eventually infarction in the region. Laboratory results that suggest the presence of bacterial infection include an absolute band count greater than 3,000 mm³ or an elevated leukocyte alkaline phosphatase score. In contrast, striking elevation of serum lactate dehydrogenase (LDH) isoenzymes sometimes follow infarction. The sedimentation rate is an unreliable screening measure for infection because it may be normal in infected sickle cell patients. However, if elevated, it may be helpful in diagnosis. Nuclear medicine scans have been of little value in distinguishing infection from infarction, and the usefulness of newer imaging modalities such as nuclear magnetic resonance has not yet been assessed. The traditional approach to suspected infection remains the best one, namely, careful monitoring of the clinical course, frequent obtainment of appropriate samples for culture, and, when indicated, empiric antibiotic therapy.

Other general aspects of infection in sickle cell patients include the high frequency of urinary tract infection (in pregnant women with sickle trait), a tendency for *Mycoplasma pneumoniae* to run an unusually severe course, a somewhat higher than usual frequency of osteomyelitis (and a peculiar susceptibility to *Salmonella* etiology), and a close association between parvovirus infection and episodes of erythroid aplasia and severe anemia.

CENTRAL NERVOUS SYSTEM MANIFESTATIONS

Vaso-occlusive events that involve the central nervous system are a relatively common occurrence in sickle cell anemia. Thromboses with subsequent brain infarction predominate during childhood, and cerebral hemorrhage becomes increasingly frequent during adult life. Any of the cerebral vessels can be involved, resulting in a broad range of symptomatology that can include seizures, hemiparesis or other localizing neurologic findings, unexplained coma, headaches, visual changes, or syncope. Transient ischemic episodes can occur. Children who have experienced a neurologic event appear to be at increased risk for subsequent events.

Sickle cell patients with the recent onset of neurologic symptoms should be hospitalized for observation and evaluation. Suspected episodes of cerebral infarction or hemorrhage should be evaluated clinically and, if required, by noninvasive imaging procedures such as computed tomography (CT) or magnetic resonance imaging. The usual supportive measures, up to and including intensive care, should be used for such patients.

ABDOMINAL COMPLICATIONS

Complications of sickle cell disease that affect the abdomen include acute painful episodes, splenic infarction, and hepatobiliary disorders. The clinical features of these events often overlap, so their distinction may be difficult.

Tissues of the abdomen are frequent targets of painful vaso-occlusion (see the earlier section on *Vaso-occlusive Crisis*). Patients with abdominal pain, in addition to receiving appropriate analgesia, must have thorough evaluation for non-sickle-related causes of pain and careful observation for morbid complications associated with abdominal pain. Severe abdominal pain is an indication for hospitalization in sickle cell patients.

Patients with abdominal pain who do not have symptoms referable to their chest or respiratory system may nevertheless subsequently develop the acute chest syndrome as a result of widespread vaso-occlusion. Observation for the development of this life-threatening complication is important (see *Pulmonary Events*, earlier in this chapter).

The spleen is a particularly vulnerable target for painful vaso-occlusion because of its uniquely tortuous, acidemic, hypoxemic circulation. Homozygous Hb SS patients are vulnerable to *splenic infarction* only during childhood, as thereafter their spleens have autoinfarcted. Subjects with Hb SC disease and beta-thalassemia, however, are at risk even as adults. Uncomplicated splenic infarction results in left upper quadrant abdominal pain, often with fever and leukocytosis. The use of CT scanning in the evaluation of abdominal pain has permitted the documentation of splenic infarction and has also revealed that this clinical complex may be associated with subcapsular splenic hemorrhage. Progressive peritoneal signs may reveal that the infarcted spleen has ruptured. Falling hematocrit and hemoglobin levels, sometimes associated with hypotension, indicate the occurrence of splenic sequestration.

Uncomplicated splenic infarction is treated symptomatically with analgesia and observation. Splenic rupture is treated surgically. Splenic sequestration is treated with transfusion and fluid resuscitation, especially in children, in whom it may represent a life-threatening emergency.

The increased bile pigment load presented to the liver as a result of chronic hemolysis results in a high incidence of *gallstones*. Pigment stones occur in at least 70 percent of adult patients with sickle cell disease. The potential confusion between the pain of cholecystitis and an abdominal painful episode has led some to suggest that the mere detection of stones is an indication for cholecystectomy. Others require that stones be symptomatic before they recommend surgery. The use of cholescintigraphy may distinguish between asymptomatic gallstones and the dysfunctional gallbladder of cholecystitis. The risks of ascending cholangitis secondary to gallstones must be considered in surgical decision making.

So-called *sickle hepatopathy* encompasses three basic clinical syndromes. Chronic hepatopathy refers to persistent hepatomegaly, hyperbilirubinemia beyond that of chronic hemolysis, and transaminasemia. The etiologic roles of such factors as chronic viral hepatitis, hepatic ischemia, cholestasis because of bile sludge within biliary ductules, and toxic exposures (e.g., acetaminophen) have not been determined. This entity does not constitute an emergency.

Two distinct types of acute hepatic episodes may punctuate the course of sickle cell disease. It is important to distinguish these from one another and from acute viral hepatitis and acute acetaminophen toxicity because the clinical approaches to these entities are entirely different. Benign hyperbilirubinemia is a syndrome of extreme cholestasis with total bilirubin levels approaching and sometimes exceeding 100 mg per deciliter but without abdominal pain, fever, leukocytosis, transaminasemia, coagulopathy, or encephalopathy. It is probably a consequence of intrahepatic cholestasis from bile sludge. The episode resolves spontaneously, but patients should be observed carefully to be certain that the more morbid variety of acute hepatic crisis does not ensue. This latter entity consists of severe hyperbilirubinemia usually associated with abdominal pain, hepatic tenderness, fever, leukocytosis, extreme transaminasemia, and progressive coagulopathy and encephalopathy. This syndrome is probably related to compromised hepatic blood flow and is a medical emergency. The only patient reported to survive such an episode was treated vigorously with exchange transfusion and plasma exchange.

GENITOURINARY COMPLICATIONS

The renal complications of sickle cell disease are legion, but seldom do they result in true medical emergencies. Exceptions requiring more immediate medical attention or unique considerations exist, however, and are subsequently discussed.

The basis of many renal abnormalities is compromised blood flow in the vasa recta caused by sickling in the hypertonic, acidemia, hypoxemic environment of the renal medulla. The results of this deficit include inability to concentrate the urine and excessive obligatory water loss, diminished excretion of acid and potassium, hematuria, and renal papillary necrosis. Other complications occurring with increased frequency are mesangioproliferative glomerulonephritis, proteinuria, urinary tract infection, hyperuricemia, and chronic renal failure. Most of these complications are nonemergent and are managed as in nonsickle patients.

Because of obligatory excess water loss, patients tend to become dehydrated, especially during hot weather and exertion. Attention to hydration is essential. Occasionally the urinary acidification defect results in overt metabolic acidosis requiring bicarbonate therapy, but usually this lesion is subclinical. Similarly, the potassium excretion defect is usually subclinical but may result in overt hyperkalemia, particularly with the onset of chronic renal insufficiency. This event may require treatment with kaliuretic agents such as furosemide or even with Kayexelate. However, it must be remembered that serum potassium levels obtained from sickle blood samples may be artifactually elevated because of the vast potassium losses that accompany hypoxic storage of sickle cells even for brief periods. This is not necessarily associated with in vitro hemolysis, and collecting sickle blood in vacuum tubes is sufficient to cause it. Before sickle cell patients are treated for hyperkalemia, a stat plasma potassium measurement should be obtained on a fresh blood sample not exposed to a vacuum.

Hematuria may result in renal colic due to clots or necrosed papillae in the renal pelvis or ureters, and attention must be given to the presence of hydronephrosis and obstructive renal failure. Sickle cell patients with hematuria should be evaluated for the same etiologies of bleeding as nonsickle cell patients, keeping in mind their inherent potential for hematuria.

Urinary tract infections, hyperuricemia, glomerulonephritis, and chronic renal failure are managed the same way in sickle cell patients as in others. Chronic renal failure may result in extreme levels of anemia that are tolerated surprisingly well. Hemodialysis and renal transplantation have been used as successful therapy in sickle cell patients.

Priapism is defined as an unwanted painful erection. Its incidence is increased in sickle cell patients, and it may result in impotence. Unfortunately, the management of this complication is unsatisfactory, and no single treatment has proven to be satisfactory. Our recommendation for managing this problem is to hospitalize all patients who have had priapism lasting over 24 hours and perform partial exchange transfusion. For patients who do not respond to this therapy, urologic surgery including shunting between the corpora spongiosum and the corpora cavernosa (Winter procedure) or irrigation of the corpora cavernosa should be considered.

CARDIAC COMPLICATIONS

A major adaptation to the chronic anemia of sickle cell disease is increased stroke volume and cardiac output. Usually, patients with sickle cell disease have persistently elevated high cardiac output without congestive heart failure. Eventually (as late as in the third decade), they become susceptible to episodes of heart failure. Generally, diminished cardiac reserve is discovered at a time when cardiac performance is challenged by an episode of decreased oxygen-carrying capacity associated with an anemic crisis or by fluid overload with intravenous fluids, transfusion, or the postpartum condition. Patients who have experienced congestive heart failure under such circumstances should be managed subsequently so that fluid overload is avoided.

Cor pulmonale secondary to recurrent pulmonary insults is not uncommon among adult patients but does not usually result in medical emergencies.

One of the more common life-threatening events among adults is cardiorenal failure. The combination of congestive heart failure and prerenal failure results in a difficult therapeutic dilemma. The heart failure is usually caused by an anemic crisis that requires red cell transfusion to restore the oxygen-carrying capacity, but this therapy is precluded by the overloaded circulatory status of these patients. These patients must be hospitalized and managed by either vigorous diuresis prior to transfusion or exchange transfusion. Ultimately, restoring oxygen-carrying capacity with red cell transfusion is necessary to reduce cardiac demands and restore renal blood flow.

OCULAR COMPLICATIONS

Abnormal blood vessels in the conjunctiva are usual in sickle cell patients but constitute no danger to health or vision. On the contrary, retinal vascular disease poses the same problems to sickle cell patients as it does to diabetics. Compared with that in diabetics, vascular occlusion in sickle cell patients occurs more laterally within the globe and is difficult to see with an ophthalmoscope. Optimal management of these patients includes routine surveillance by a retinal specialist.

Threats to the vision that result from the vascular occlusion of sickle retinopathy include vascular proliferation with its attendant risks of fibrosis and intraocular hemorrhage, retinal infarct, and retinal detachment. These emergencies should be referred to a retinal specialist immediately.

Blunt trauma to the eye may result in bleeding into the anterior chamber (hyphema), and in sickle patients this often leads to increased intraocular pressure. These patients should receive medical or surgical therapy from an ophthalmology consultant immediately.

Preoperative partial exchange transfusion should be employed to reduce the incidence of anterior segment ischemia.

SUGGESTED READING

Charache S. Treatment of sickle cell anemia. Ann Rev Med 1981; 32:195–206.
Charache S, Lubin B, Reid CD. Management and therapy of sickle cell disease. NIH Publication No. 84-2117, Sept 1984.
Serjeant GR. Sickle cell disease. Oxford: Oxford University Press, 1985.

ONCOLOGIC EMERGENCIES

EDWIN C. CADMAN, M.D.

Cancer is diagnosed in nearly 1 million individuals annually. It is important to appreciate that cancer is a treatable illness and can often be cured. Therefore, when cancer presents in a life-threatening manner, the patient must be considered as having a potentially curable cancer; certainly a treatable cancer. The common oncologic emergencies are categorized in Table 1.

SUPERIOR VENA CAVA SYNDROME

Superior vena cava (SVC) syndrome occurs in nearly 4 to 5 percent of patients with lymphoma and lung cancer. The symptoms often occur insidiously and may go unrecognized for weeks until the late stages of obstruction become obvious. The superior vena cava is located within the right anterosuperior mediastinum behind the sternum and adjacent to the right main stem bronchus. The lymph drainage of the right thoracic cavity goes to the lymph nodes that completely surround this great vessel. In addition, the right anterior mediastinal nodes are above and the right paratracheal nodes below this vulnerable vein. Therefore, SVC syndrome is more often associated with lung cancer, usually small cell or squamous cell, that arises in the right chest. Nearly all the cases of

TABLE 1 Types of Oncologic Emergencies

Superior vena cava obstruction
Pericardial tamponade
Central nervous system
  Spinal cord compression
  Brain tumor
  Carcinomatous meningitis

Organ obstruction
  Bowel
  Bladder
  Airway

Bleeding
  Clotting factors
  Platelets
  Vessels

Metabolic
  Calcium
  Electrolytes
  Uric acid
  Tumor lysis

Infection

TABLE 2 Signs of Superior Vena Cava Syndrome

Observation	%
Chest vein enlargement	67
Neck vein enlargement	59
Facial edema	56
Tachypnea	40
Red face	19
Cyanosis	15
Arm swelling	10
Vocal cord paralysis	4
Horner's syndrome	2

SVC syndrome are attributable to malignancy, although benign conditions produce it in about 3 percent of cases.

The signs and symptoms of SVC syndrome (Table 2) can be dramatic in the late stages of this complication. However, a gradual and nearly complete obstruction can occur so insidiously that the signs and symptoms may be unappreciated. Any large mediastinal mass should be considered as having the potential for causing obstruction of the SVC.

DIAGNOSIS

The first goal is to document the problem. Chest roentgenogram shows a mass in 97 percent of cases (75 percent on the right side) and a pleural effusion in 25 percent. It is advisable to obtain a computed tomographic (CT) scan, which should delineate the extent of compression. Venograms are not necessary, add no new information, and can result in persistent bleeding owing to increased venous pressure when performed from the arm or neck veins.

It is extremely important to biopsy the tumor, since it could be curable. Unless the exact variety of cancer is known, it is unlikely that the patient will be given the best, and possibly curative, therapy. For example, Hodgkin's disease is curable with a certain combination of drugs that are not useful for the treatment of most other cancers. If it is determined that the patient cannot tolerate a biopsy and that treatment must be instituted immediately, a biopsy should be done as soon as the patient is capable of tolerating the procedure. This must be done before the mass disappears—and many do disappear quickly after radiation therapy (lymphomas, small cell cancers of the lung, and mediastinal germ cell tumors). Cytology tests of sputum or pleural effusion are extremely helpful for diagnosis.

Treatment

There are two basic treatment choices: radiation therapy or drugs. Radiation is generally effective regardless of the histologic findings. A small percentage decrease in the tumor mass can often result in marked improvement in blood flow owing to the resultant minimal increase in the size of the SVC. Occasionally, however, thrombosis of the SVC may have occurred and the clinical signs and symptoms may not improve dramatically in spite of a marked resolution of the tumor mass. In 90 percent of the patients treated with radiation there is objective improvement within 2 weeks of beginning the therapy.

Chemotherapy is also effective for the appropriate tumors. Dramatic tumor reduction can occur within a few days if the patient has small cell cancer of the lung or lymphoma. These treatments can be curative if the patient has a lymphoma, but only if the correct drug combination is given. The large cell lymphomas (diffuse histiocytic) are curative, but not with the drug combination that is curative for Hodgkin's disease. Therefore a histologic diagnosis is important and must be obtained.

Other treatments are useful while waiting for the definitive treatment to have an effect. Steroids are often given with the hope of reducing swelling. It is unclear whether this is beneficial, although short-term use of steroids is probably not a hazard to the patient. Respiratory support is important. Some patients may have a reduced tracheal airway. Occasionally patients have stridor and are gasping. The location of tracheal compression deep in the chest makes ordinary measures for airway occlusion useless. A mixture of helium and oxygen (Heliox) can be extremely beneficial. Because the density of helium is much less than nitrogen the turbulence of this gas mixture is reduced. Therefore its resistance is less than the normal oxygen-nitrogen mixture and allows increased airflow and thus greater delivery of oxygen into the lungs. Furthermore, helium enhances the delivery of oxygen even when compared with 100 percent oxygen because of the reduced resistance of the mixture compared with oxygen alone.

PERICARDIAL EFFUSION AND CARDIAC TAMPONADE

The involvement of the pericardial sac by malignancy is moderately common. Autopsy studies have documented tumor involving this space or the heart directly in up to 20 percent of patients. The major tumors associated with this problem are located in the chest and include lung and esophagus malignancies. In addition, breast cancer, lymphoma, and leukemia can often metastasize to this region and result in this clinical problem. Pericardial effusion occurs more frequently than one might expect. The general malaise, weakness, and anorexia that are commonly associated with malignancy can be attributable to the compromised cardiac output, the consequence of cardiac tamponade.

Diagnosis

Because the production of pericardial fluid can occur rapidly, the clinical signs and symptoms of cardiac tamponade appear quickly. The rapid fluid accumulation can exceed the capacity of the pericardium to stretch in response to the increased pressure. This can then result in dramatic symptoms with only a mild to moderate enlarged cardiac shadow on chest roentgenogram. If the tumor has resulted in pericardial thickening, there may be no observable cardiac enlargement. An echo examination should be done immediately upon considering the possibility of cardiac tamponade. Do not let a report of only moderate fluid collection allay your suspicion. In patients with only a moderate amount of fluid, there may be a thickened or fibrotic pericardial surface or even cardiac involvement by tumor causing clinical tamponade. Only 50 percent of cancer patients with this problem have a characteristic chest x-ray film which shows an enlarged heart and mediastinal widening. Electrocardiographic findings are generally nonspecific. If doubt remains after the ECG evaluation, then a right heart catheterization is warranted. A CT or magnetic resonance imaging scan may be helpful in showing thickened pericardium or tumor encasing the heart.

Management

Ultimately pericardiocentesis is needed. Symptomatic relief generally is transient; the fluid usually reaccumulates within 48 hours. Therefore a more definitive therapeutic approach is needed. There are several options, depending upon the general condition of the patient and the extent of tumor elsewhere within the patient: indwelling catheter in the pericardial space, intrapericardial tetracycline, pericardial stripping, pericardial window, radiation therapy, or chemotherapy.

Catheters can be left to drain in the pericardial space. In some patients the instillation of tetracycline to sclerose the visceral and parietal surfaces together has been successful. This could lead to cardiac constriction in a few months, however, and should be used only in patients who have a limited life expectancy. Surgical removal of the pericardium is perhaps the best long-term management choice. Local radiation therapy should also be given following the surgical procedure. Chemotherapy should not be expected to be beneficial unless the patient has a tumor for which this treatment has not been given and the tumor

is of a histologic variety for which a response would be anticipated (lymphoma, small cell carcinoma, or germ cell tumor). Pericardial windows— holes to allow the fluid to drain into the pleural space—often close and are not very effective.

CENTRAL NERVOUS SYSTEM

Spinal Cord Compression

This is perhaps the most common neurologic difficulty that can afflict a cancer patient. The cause of the spinal cord compression is almost always a metastatic tumor that has encroached extradurally onto the spinal cord. Prompt diagnosis and therapy are crucial to prevent permanent neurologic impairment.

The symptoms of this disorder may be present for months before catastrophe occurs. They can be categorized into four broad areas: pain, weakness, autonomic dysfunction, and sensory loss (Table 3). Two-thirds of the tumors causing compression are located in the thoracic spinal region. The other one-third are evenly divided between the cervical and lumbar regions.

The pain is of two varieties. It can radiate as if it were radicular in nature and in this way can be confused with a routine herniated intervertebral disc. A few features are different, however. The pain may be worse on lying down or at night and relieved by sitting. The other variety of pain is a local ache, probably owing to the local effects of the metastatic tumor. Generally tumors that involve the vertebrae cause pain. These tumors are also often the ones that encroach into the extradural space to cause the obstruction. Therefore, spinal x-ray films are of considerable importance in evaluating the pain. However, not all spinal cord compression is associated with local bone involvement; for example, lymphomas or other tumors that have metastasized to retroperitoneal lymph nodes can squeeze between the vertebral bodies and result in spinal cord compression also. Any cancer patient with back pain must be considered as possibly having an impending cord compression. Once paraplegia occurs it is nearly always irreversible (Table 4).

The diagnosis can be established only from a myelogram. If a block in the flow of the dye is noted from a lumbar injection site, a cisternal injection must also be performed to outline the extent of the block. CT scans are often done and perhaps in the near future will be the preferred alternative to myelography. However, if the CT scan is negative, a myelogram should be obtained. The cerebrospinal fluid should be examined for malignant

TABLE 3 Presenting Symptoms of Spinal Cord Compression

Symptom	%
Pain	96
Weakness	75
Autonomic dysfunction	50
Sensory loss	50

TABLE 4 Relationship of Presenting Symptoms and Outcome Following Therapy

Presenting Symptom	Status Following Treatment (%)		
	Walking	Weak	Paralyzed
Walking	60	27	13
Weak	35	43	22
Paralyzed	7	13	80

cells. Carcinomatous meningitis can present similarly to spinal cord compression, and its treatment is different from that used for cord compression. The cauda equina can be compressed by tumor also. Since the intradural space does not extend into this region, the myelogram is of no value in evaluating a tumor in this region and CT should be used instead.

Treatment used to be emergency surgery but now is immediate radiation therapy. The results have been shown to be equivalent, with between 50 and 80 percent of patients receiving some benefit from the therapy. Once the diagnosis of spinal cord compression is suspected, dexamethasone should be given 4 mg every 4 hours IV. This can be increased to a total of 100 mg a day if necessary.

Brain Tumor

Cancer patients who present with central nervous system findings consistent with a brain metastasis should be considered as being potentially treatable. Nearly 50 percent of patients with lung and breast cancer have cancer involving the brain when they succumb to their disease. An autopsy study from Memorial Sloan Kettering Hospital has demonstrated that 40 percent of these brain metastases are, in fact, single isolated lesions. Therefore, if a patient is not otherwise deteriorating from systemic cancer and presents with brain metastases, a thorough evaluation of the brain is indicated. Surgical removal of the brain lesion can result in amelioration of symptoms, and often the patient lives for several more years. There are many patients who have lived useful lives 2 to 5 years and more following the surgical removal of a metastatic brain lesion.

Patients with cancer who present acutely with the clinical evidence of brain metastases should be treated emergently unless surgical therapy is not an option. Medical management is as follows: maintain airway; begin dexamethasone, 8 mg IV; give mannitol, 50 g IV bolus or a 20 percent solution; and Lasix, 40 mg IV. The mannitol results in a reduction of intracranial pressure within 15 to 30 minutes. However, by 4 to 6 hours there may be a rebound increase in intracranial pressure because of equilibration of fluid across the blood-brain barrier. Therefore it is important to keep the patient dehydrated if the blood pressure is not excessively low. A definitive treatment plan must be made during the first hours of medical treatment because of these fluid shifts and predictable clinical deterioration.

Carcinomatous Meningitis

Carcinomatous meningitis can present in three basic patterns: cerebral alterations (altered mental status and ataxia), cranial nerve deficits, and spinal nerve pain and weakness. This form of metastatic spread of cancer is seen in breast cancer, lung cancer, and the lymphomas. It is also commonly observed in the hematologic malignancies. The median survival after diagnosis is 2 months, although an occasional patient does quite well with therapy and survives extended periods of time free of difficulty.

The evaluation is similar to that for suspected spinal cord compression. A CT scan is done initially to determine if a brain mass exists. If not, then cerebrospinal fluid cytologic studies are done. The lumbar puncture may need to be repeated several times before the cancer cells are actually detected. It is unusual (less than 5 percent of the time) that the cerebrospinal fluid protein, glucose, and cell count are normal when carcinomatous meningitis is present.

Treatment is the instillation of chemotherapeutic agents into the cerebrospinal fluid: either methotrexate or cytosine arabinoside. This is generally best achieved with an Omhya reservoir that is placed in the lateral ventricle. The drug instilled into the intrathecal space of the spinal column seldom gets to the surface of the brain or enters the ventricles. Radiation therapy is generally administered to the entire brain and steroids are also given as previously described.

ORGAN OBSTRUCTION

Bowel

If the patient presents with an isolated obstruction, independent of extensive disease elsewhere, consideration should be given to bypassing this obstruction. This is less of an emergency than SVC syndrome, but it is an urgent situation. If the obstruction is not recognized or dealt with properly, the patient's condition can deteriorate, making surgical correction impossible.

Bladder and Ureter

Obstruction of the renal system can be difficult. Dialysis, stents, and bypasses can resolve many of the problems that result from cancer. However, with few exceptions, the renal failure is accompanied by extensive tumor elsewhere. In these circumstances, resolution of the problem is not warranted for humanitarian considerations. The exceptions are if (1) this is the first time the patient is known to have cancer; (2) the tumor is locally recurrent, such as pelvic or retroperitoneal tumor; or (3) the renal failure is the consequence of hypercalcemia or tumor lysis syndrome. In the latter situation the tumor is in fact responding quickly to aggressive therapy.

Airway Obstruction

The most common causes of airway obstruction owing to malignancy are head and neck cancers. These cancers are generally extremely sensitive to radiation therapy and chemotherapy. If the patient has never received therapy, all measures should be taken to maintain an airway. A tracheostomy is generally required. Airway obstruction from mediastinal tumors is unusual, but it can occur and is discussed in the section Superior Vena Cava Syndrome.

BLEEDING

Vessels

Erosion of tumors into blood vessels can require immediate attention. There may be little time to consider all the alternatives. Therefore, in a situation in which vessel erosion is theoretically possible, careful discussion should precede the event. Head and neck cancers can erode into the great vessels in the neck, thus resulting in exsanguination. Gastric neoplasms can erode into gastric or nearby vessels, resulting in persistent intra-abdominal hemorrhage. A similar situation can occur with bowel tumors; palliative resection may be appropriate. Evaluation consists of an upper gastrointestinal contrast study, possibly a CT scan, and an arteriogram if surgery is a realistic consideration. Radiolabeled platelets are occasionally given to patients with suspected gastrointestinal bleeding. If blood does leak into the bowel, a radionuclide scan may demonstrate radioactivity in the region of the bleeding.

Occasionally there can be profuse bleeding from the rectal mucosa as a consequence of radiation enteritis following the local radiation treatment of a pelvic or bladder tumor. This may require emergency bowel resection.

Patients who have received cyclophosphamide can develop hematuria. The blood emanates from the bladder, which has become eroded by the metabolites of this agent. There have been patients who have required emergency removal of the bladder to prevent exsanguination. More conservative measures are often helpful, and these include bladder irrigation and direct instillation of epsilon-aminocaproic acid, which inhibits the activation of plasminogen to plasmin, the enzyme that degrades fibrin, thereby resulting in the destruction of blood clots. Since the urine contains concentrated quantities of plasminogen activators (urokinase), eroded bladder mucosa may not be capable of coagulating the bleeding sites. Therefore this medicinal approach is sometimes successful.

Platelets

Platelet reduction because of malignancy is generally the result of marrow replacement or the consequence of cytotoxic therapy. The latter is the most common cause of platelet reduction. Generally, bleeding owing to thrombocytopenia does not occur until the concentration of platelets is below 20,000 per cubic millimeter. Platelet transfusions are recommended when the platelet count falls below this level. Ten units of platelets are expected to result in approximately a 100,000 per cubic millimeter rise in the platelet count. There often is a gradual reduction in this level over 5 or 6 days to equilibration with the patient's own platelet level. A standard approach is to withhold platelet transfusions unless bleeding is present. Most patients have petechiae or mucosal bleeding as an initial clinical manifestation of thrombocytopenia. These patients should receive platelet transfusion. Those patients who show no signs of bleeding can be observed, but not ignored.

Other causes of thrombocytopenia are immunologic (ITP) and widely disseminated intravascular clotting (DIC). It is unusual for a cancer patient to have ITP as a result of malignancy. When ITP is present it is commonly in association with lymphoma. The platelet counts are generally between 1,000 and 2,000 to 10,000 per cubic millimeter. If the mechanism of thrombocytopenia is immunologic, platelet transfusions are not indicated unless bleeding is observed, and even then it has not been shown to be useful. A post-transfusion platelet count is routinely not increased above the platelet count obtained prior to transfusion.

Thrombocytopenia from DIC is also not effectively treated with platelet transfusions. In fact, DIC in cancer patients has not been effectively treated with any agents. Patients whose malignancy is associated with DIC have an average survival of a few weeks. DIC is extremely common in promyelocytic leukemia. It has been proposed that, as a consequence of the rapid lysis of these leukemic cells, the internal contents trigger the systemic clotting cascade, resulting in an overwhelming DIC. Heparin in this isolated situation is helpful.

Clotting Factors

Generally when the lack of clotting factors is the cause of a bleeding problem in a cancer patient it is because the liver is replaced by tumor and unable to make sufficient quantities of these needed factors. Replacement therapy in this clinical setting is therefore appropriate. Vitamin K should be given, although it must be appreciated that vitamin K is ineffectual in patients with severe liver damage. In this situation fresh frozen plasma would be the choice. However, if the patient has no metastasis to the liver and the prothrombin time, bleeding time, or partial thromboplastin time is prolonged, then the patient most likely is found to have DIC. Rarely there may be circulating clotting factor inhibitors. If this is suspected, appropriate factor therapy may be beneficial.

METABOLIC EMERGENCIES

There are many different metabolic derangements that can occur in a patient with a malignancy. Some of these problems are attributable to the tumor or the effects of the tumor (hypercalcemia, hypoglycemia, hyponatremia, hyperuricemia, or lactic acidosis), while others are the result of treatment (tumor lysis syndrome, hyponatremia, hyperuricemia).

Hypercalcemia

Hypercalcemia is perhaps the most common metabolic problem associated with malignancy. Nearly 10 percent of all cancer patients develop hypercalcemia. The majority of cancers associated with hypercalcemia metastasize to the bones, and the cause of the hypercalcemia is considered a result of the rapid bone resorption owing to the tumor. Tumors of breast, lung, kidney, and head and neck are the most common offenders. Approximately 20 percent of hypercalcemia cases, however, are not associated with the presence of bone metastasis. Hypercalcemia may be caused by: parathyroid hormone, humoral hypercalcemia factor, osteoclastic activating factor, prostaglandins (PGE2), and local bone resorption. The symptoms and treatment of hypercalcemia are listed in Tables 5, 6, and 7, and also discussed in the chapter *Hypercalcemia and Hypocalcemia*.

Electrolytes

The major electrolyte problem in cancer patients is hyponatremia from the inappropriate secretion of antidiuretic hormone, almost always from small cell lung cancer. A patient with this malignancy should be carefully monitored for the manifestation of this problem. If the hyponatremia is indeed attributable to antidiuretic hormone, then fluid restriction is needed. The use of hypertonic saline does not resolve the electrolyte imbalance for more than a few hours, since the kidney rapidly excretes the excess sodium. Therefore, saline or hypertonic saline should be used only if the patient is seizing or in a coma. Diuretics to remove free water may also be necessary.

TABLE 5 Symptoms from Hypercalcemia

General
  Fatigue
  Confusion
  Weakness
  Stupor
  Coma

Specific
  Renal: Polyuria, polydipsia
  Gastrointestinal: Anorexia, nausea, vomiting,
    constipation, abdominal pain
  Heart: Arrythmias

TABLE 6 Treatment of Hypercalcemia

Increased excretion
  Saline diuresis
Inhibit resorption
  Mithramycin
  Calcitonin
  Prostaglandin inhibitors
  Diphosphonates
  Steroids
Treat tumor

Careful monitoring of renal electrolyte and volume is needed to guide therapy.

Hypokalemia is occasionally seen in patients with malignancy, almost always from diuretics. Occasionally in a leukemic patient who has a white blood count between 50,000 and 100,000 per cubic millimeter, a low potassium concentration is observed owing to continued intracellular accumulation of potassium after blood has been drawn. Immediate separation of plasma from the blood cells gives a more accurate value. Metabolic inhibitors, such as sodium fluoride, can be placed in the tube to prevent further metabolism of the leukemic cells, thus eliminating the potassium accumulation within these cells.

Uric Acid

Uric acid in an untreated cancer patient is an indicator of a rapidly proliferating tumor. The only tumors that divide quickly enough to result in the rapid breakdown of purines into uric acid are the hematologic malignancies or the lymphomas. If elevated uric acid level is seen in patients with other tumors, it is most likely the result of renal failure and not the cause of renal impairment. Treatment is directed at two areas: reducing the production and increasing the renal excretion of uric acid.

The major problem of hyperuricemia is the resultant renal failure. Uric acid crystals precipitate in the distal nephron, primarily the collecting ducts. The pK'a of uric acid is 5.4; therefore, in an acid urine with a pH of 5, the predominant form of uric acid is un-ionized and therefore less soluble. The blood, with a pH of 7.4, has primarily the ionic form of uric acid and therefore it does not precipitate in this compartment. In addition, the urine is more concentrated in the collecting duct, and this favors uric acid crystal formation. Therefore it is important to maintain a high urine flow which is both dilute and at a pH of near 7.

Allopurinol, which is a competitive inhibitor of xanthine oxidase, prevents the formation of uric acid. Since allopurinol is a competitive inhibitor of this enzyme, this means that the more purine breakdown products that reach the enzyme xanthine oxidase, the less effective the inhibition of allopurinol will be; it competes with these purine products for the active site on the enzyme. Therefore, if there are high levels of uric acid or you anticipate the release of lots of purines subsequent to cancer treatment, give the patient more allopurinol. A patient can be given 900 or 1,200 mg of allopurinol daily if necessary. The 300-mg dose is used for high uric acid excretors—a chronic problem. In this setting more allopurinol is not necessary. Once the tumor responds to treatment the allopurinol should be discontinued.

TABLE 7 Recommended Drug Treatments

Drug	Dose	Time to Response (hr)	Side Effects
Mithramycin	25 µg/kg IV, repeat 2–6 days	24–48	Nausea, vomiting, thrombocytopenia, liver necrosis, reduced clotting factors
Calcitonin	4 units/kg SC, q 12 hr	2–8	Tachyphylaxis in a few days

TABLE 8 Intracellular Contents Released by Cells Which Result in the Tumor Lysis Syndrome

Intracellular Agent	Immediate Result in Blood	Clinical Consequences of Serum Abnormalities	
Phosphate	Increased PO_4^- and reduced CA^{++}	Increased $PO_4 =$	Renal obstruction
Potassium	Increased K^+	Decreased Ca^{++}	Muscle irritability, tetanus, weakness, confusion, convulsion
Purines	Increased uric acid	Increased K^+	Arrhythmias
		Uric acid	Renal obstruction

If a patient is expected to have a rapid tumor response to a new therapy and elevated uric acid levels are expected, then an alkaline diuresis in addition to the allopurinol should be instituted prior to the onset of therapy. Generally 2 to 12 hours is sufficient time for pretreatment.

Uric acid nephrolithiasis is the result of chronic hyperuricemia and is different from acute hyperuricemic nephropathy. The uric acid precipitates in the renal pelvis in this setting, forming the nidus of what can ultimately become large stones and ureteral obstruction.

Tumor Lysis Syndrome

This term refers to all that happens as the consequence of effective therapy. When billions of cancer cells are destroyed simultaneously, the released intracellular contents result in a myriad of clinical problems. These biochemical alterations can result in the death of the patient and therefore are indeed a true emergency. The difficulty is that these problems are less well treated than they are prevented. Three major intracellular constituents result in the syndrome (Table 8).

Once renal failure occurs, and it can be sudden, the electrolyte problems become even more complex and difficult to treat. In fact, if renal failure does occur, urgent dialysis is required. The criteria for hemodialysis in the tumor lysis syndrome are: phosphate greater than 10 mg per deciliter; K^+ greater than 6 mEq per liter; creatinine greater than 10 mg per deciliter; uric acid greater than 10 mg per deciliter; pH less than 7.2; and oliguria or anuria.

Medical treatment should be directed at the metabolic problems. Reduce the phosphate by improving renal excretion. Hyperkalemia should be treated with increased intracellular levels of bicarbonate, glucose, and insulin, and increased excretion via Kayexalate. Calcium supplementation may be needed and uric acid is reduced by giving allopurinol and improving excretion, alkalinizing urine, and increasing flow. General guidelines for treatment of tumor lysis syndrome are: (1) maintain alkaline diuresis at 200 to 300 ml per hour; (2) allopurinol, 900 to 1,200 mg daily; (3) Kayexalate enemas; and (4) glucose and insulin (only if potassium concentration is greater than 6 mEq per liter. Do (1) and (2) as pretreatment. Begin (3) and (4) if the potassium concentration increases and renal failure ensues.

INFECTION

Infections are common in the leukemic patient and are often seen in patients who are pancytopenic (white

TABLE 9 Recommendations for Treating the Pancytopenic Cancer Patient with a Fever

Broad-spectrum antibiotics
  Aminoglycoside + beta-lactam

Continue until:
  White count recovers *or* clinical response + 4 to 8 days

Stop if:
  No clinical response after 4 days

Restart if persistently febrile:
  After 24 hours off therapy with different antibiotics

Beta-lactam antibiotics are the penicillins and cephalosporins.

blood cell count less than 500 cells per cubic millimeter) following chemotherapy. Regardless of the cause of the presumed infection, all patients must be treated with a broad spectrum of antimicrobial agents. It is well established that broad antibiotic coverage of patients who are presumed to be septic is beneficial to the patient. The pancytopenic patient generally has no focal signs or symptoms of an infectious site. The only indication that a serious infection may be present is malaise and a fever.

Less than 50 percent of the time is an organism found to be responsible for what looks like clinical sepsis. Therefore, patients should be treated with the recommendations in Table 9. All possible sites should be cultured, including blood, and all patients admitted to the hospital.

If the leukemic patient is persistently febrile, has been receiving multiple antibiotics, and has remained pancytopenic for more than 2 weeks, consider the possibility of a fungal infection. Amphotericin B should be started. Cultures may not be positive during the initial phases of the infection.

Any patient considered to have any of the afore described oncologic emergencies should be admitted to the hospital.

SUGGESTED READING

Colman RW, Robboy SJ, Minna JD. Disseminated intravascular coagulation: a reappraisal. Ann Rev Med 1979; 30:359–374.

Gilbert RW, Kim JH, Posner JB. Epidural spinal cord compression from metastatic tumor: diagnosis and treatment. Ann Neurol 1978; 3:40–51.

Glass JP, Shapiro WR, Posner JB. Treatment of leptomeningeal metastases. Neurology 1978; 28:351.

Mundy GR, Martin TJ. The hypercalcemia of malignancy: pathogenesis and management. Metabolism 1982; 31(12):1247–1277.

Perez CA, Presant CA, Amburg AL. Management of superior vena cava syndrome. Semin Oncol 1978; 5:123–134.

Sise JG, Crichlow RW. Obstruction due to malignant tumors. Semin Oncol 1978; 5:213–224.

Theologides A. Neoplastic cardiac tamponade. Semin Oncol 1978; 5:181–192.

Winston KR, Walsh JW, Fischer EG. Results of operative management of intracranial metastatic tumors. Cancer 1980; 45:2639.

Young LS. Use of aminoglycosides in immunocompromised patients. Am J Med 1985; 79(Suppl 1A):21–27.

BLOOD COMPONENT THERAPY

MEYER R. HEYMAN, M.D.

Modern blood banking practices have made an array of blood components available to the clinician. The choice of an appropriate blood component depends on the underlying pathophysiologic disturbance for which the component is to be administered. Examples include the use of packed red cells for patients who have a deficit in oxygen-carrying capacity, but no disturbance of coagulation or evidence of plasma volume depletion. Alternatively, the patient with evidence of volume contraction may be more in need of volume correction with plasma protein fractions or albumin than with red cells. The use of appropriate blood components in lieu of whole blood is more specific, more efficient, and in many instances, safer. A knowledge of the properties of these various components is necessary to make a rational choice in a given clinical situation.

The use of specific blood components for the management of specific heritable coagulation distrubances, disseminated intravascular coagulation (DIC), thrombocytopenia, and hemorrhagic shock are discussed elsewhere in this text. Therefore, these situations are not discussed in detail here.

WHOLE BLOOD

A unit of whole blood contains about 500 ml of anticoagulated blood, approximately 50 cc of which is a citrate-based anticoagulant (citrate phosphate dextrose [CPD] or citrate phosphate dextrose adenine [CPD-A]). Whole blood stored for more than 24 hours is essentially devoid of viable platelets, and after 48 hours of storage it can be considered to be deficient in Factor VIII. Factor V levels may also fall below hematostatic levels after continued storage. Although whole blood can be used in patients who have a deficit in both oxygen-carrying capacity and volume, the use of whole blood is rarely justified, since the use of packed red cells along with crystalloids (0.9 percent normal saline, Ringer's lactate), plasma protein fraction, or albumin solutions will suffice in the majority of patients. Most blood banks do not store blood in its unfractionated form, so that a request for whole blood requires the suspension of packed cells in compatible plasma, a procedure that is unnecessary because these products can be administered separately. Although "fresh whole blood" has been suggested for use in massive transfusion following trauma or surgery, there is little convincing evidence that this practice is superior to the use of components such as packed red blood cells, fresh frozen plasma, and platelet concentrates in terms of patient outcome.

RED BLOOD CELL COMPONENTS

Packed Red Blood Cells

Packed red blood cells are prepared by centrifugation, which removes about 80 percent of the plasma. The resultant packed cells have an hematocrit of 65 to 80 percent in a total volume of approximately 300 ml. The plasma removed from these units is used to prepare cryoprecipitate, fresh frozen plasma, plasma protein fraction, albumin, and specfic factor concentrates. Packed red cells are suspended in citrate-based anticoagulant preservative solutions and have a shelf life, when stored at 4 °C, equivalent to that of whole blood (presently up to 40 days, depending on the additives and anticoagulant used). Although packed red cells obviously contribute to the maintenance of blood volume, the usual indication for packed cells is to increase oxygen-carrying capacity. Packed red cells should not be used in patients in whom volume expansion with saline or plasma protein fraction will suffice to restore tissue perfusion.

Leukocyte-Poor Red Blood Cells

Leukocytes can be removed from packed cells by inverted centrifugation, filtration, sedimentation, perfusion through microaggregate filters, and mechanical washing to provide concentrated red cell components relatively free of leukocytes. The extent of leukocyte removal varies between 70 to 90 percent depending on the technique used. Washed red cells are the most free of leukocyte and platelet contamination, but like other leukocyte-poor products, they must be used within 24 hours of preparation. Depending on the method used for preparation, there is a variable loss of red cells. This may result in a less than expected increase in hematocrit in patients transfused with a leukocyte-poor red cell preparation. Leukocyte-poor red cell transfusions are reserved for those patients in whom there is a previous history of febrile transfusion reactions related to leukocyte and platelet antigens. In the previously untransfused patient presenting in the emergency department, leukocyte-poor red cell replacement is unnecessary and should be avoided.

Frozen Red Cells

Frozen red blood cells are red cell concentrates that have undergone controlled freezing using glycerol as a cryoprotective agent. Red cells may be maintained in the frozen state for years. These cells must be thawed and washed several times to free them of the cryoprotective agent before they can be administered. Because of the multiple washes involved in the deglycerolization process, frozen washed cells are the most free of platelet, white cell, and plasma contamination. The cost of preservation and administration of frozen red cells, is approximately two to three times that of conventional red cells. The freezing of red blood cells allows the long-term maintenance of compatible blood for patients with rare blood types or for autologous transfusion of patients who have blood group antibodies that cannot be defined by appropriate serologic techniques. The latter patients may be phlebotomized and the units frozen so that autologous transfusion can be carried out if necessary at a later date. Such a maneuver may be lifesaving in patients liable to experience recurrent episodes of bleeding. Other than in the special situations mentioned above, the use of frozen red cells is unjustified. Since the time required for deglycerolization necessitates a delay in availability, frozen red cells should be considered in emergent situations only when they are likely to be the only source of compatible blood.

PLATELET CONCENTRATES

Platelet concentrates are made by separation of platelets from a single unit of whole blood by differential centrifugation. The platelets are usually suspended in approximately 50 to 70 cc of plasma. A unit of platelet concentrate usually contains in excess of 5.5×10^{10} platelets and can be stored for up to 7 days at 22 °C without significant loss of viability.

Platelet concentrates are contaminated with leukocytes and small amounts of red blood cells, allowing for alloimmunization to occur against platelet, leukocyte and red cell antigens. A unit of platelets increases the platelet count of a 70-kg adult by approximately 5,000 to 10,000 per cubic millimeter. A poor response to platelet administration can be expected with known platelet antibody, fever, sepsis, disseminated intravascular coagulation, or splenomegaly. In all of these situations, the platelets are rapidly consumed or sequestered. The transfusion of platelet concentrate is usually indicated in patients with significant thrombocytopenia (fewer than 50,000 per cubic millimeter) who are actively bleeding and in whom no surgically correctable or other cause of bleeding (coagulation factor deficiency) is demonstrable. Prophylactic administration of platelets to increase the count above 50,000 per cubic millimeter is warranted in patients who are to undergo invasive diagnostic or surgical procedures in which uncontrolled bleeding could be catastrophic (lumbar puncture, intracranial surgery, liver biopsy). The intraoperative administration of platelets to thrombocytopenic individuals should be guided not only by frequent platelet counts, but also by the surgeon's judgment concerning the adequacy of hemostasis. Platelet transfusion is also justified in selected patients with platelet counts below 20,000 in whom the risk for spontaneous bleeding is high and in selected patients with qualitative platelet abnormalities who are actively bleeding. In thrombotic thrombocytopenic purpura and idiopathic thrombocytopenic purpura, platelet transfusion is probably best avoided unless the patient has life-threatening hemorrhage. The decision to transfuse platelets should be made in consultation with the hematologist whenever possible.

PLASMA COMPONENTS

Fresh Frozen Plasma

Fresh frozen plasma is prepared by separating plasma from fresh whole blood and freezing it immediately after collection. Because fresh frozen plasma contains all of the plasma proteins including the coagulation factors, its use is indicated in bleeding patients in whom the simultaneous correction of volume depletion and decreased coagulation factors is required. Plasma separated from red cells of the same ABO group as the recipient should be used to avoid potential hemolysis induced by anti-A and anti-B isoagglutinins. Fresh frozen plasma should not be used purely as a volume expander in the absence of any coagulation disturbances because alternative volume expanders such as albumin and plasma protein fraction are available. Likewise, administration of fresh frozen plasma should be avoided in coagulation disturbances that can be corrected by the administration of specific factor concentrates such as cryoprecipitate or Factor VIII concentrate. The use of fresh frozen plasma in such situations is not only wasteful, but dangerous because the large amount of plasma needed to correct specific factor deficiency can result in serious volume overload.

Cryoprecipitate

Cryoprecipitate is the cold insoluble material that precipitates from a unit of fresh frozen plasma when it is thawed at 4 °C. The cryoprecipitate is then refrozen in a volume of approximately 15 ml. Cryoprecipitate is rich in Factor VIII (approximately 80 units of Factor VIII per unit) and fibrinogen (approximately 150 mg of fibrinogen per unit). Cryoprecipitate is indicated in coagulation disturbances attributable to a deficiency of the Factor VIII complex such as hemophilia A and von Willebrand's disease. Cryoprecipitate is also useful in states of severe hypofibrinogenemia (less than 100 mg percent) in which volume considerations preclude the administration of adequate amounts of fresh frozen plasma to correct fibrinogen deficiency such as in DIC. As with fresh frozen plasma, ABO-compatible cryoprecipitate is also preferred to avoid hemolytic reactions. This is less likely to be clinically significant however, with the smaller volumes employed.

Factor Concentrates

Concentrates of Factor VIII and Factor IX from multiple pooled donors are available. The indication and use of this material is discussed elsewhere in the text.

Plasma Protein Fractions

Albumin solutions and the less concentrated plasma protein fractions are colloids, which are indicated for plasma volume expansion. Neither of these products is suitable for replacement of labile clotting factors. Both solutions are prepared in concentrations of 5 g per deciliter, so that 250 cc (12.5 g of albumin) of such a solution is the osmotic equivalent of a unit of plasma (250 cc). Paradoxical hypotension secondary to Hageman factor activation of prekallikrein has been reported with rapid administration of large amounts of plasma protein fraction. These products are indicated whenever there is a need for volume expansion without the need for correction of any clotting factor deficiency.

Plasma Substitutes

Dextran and Hydroxyethyl Starch have been used as plasma volume expanders. Unfortunately, both of these substances have been associated with impairment of coagulation, although the precise mechanisms remain obscure. Dextran has also been associated with immediate hypersensitivity reactions. Because of these difficulties, the use of albumin-containing preparations as volume expanders is preferred.

INDICATIONS FOR TRANSFUSION: GENERAL CONSIDERATIONS

The decision to transfuse should not be taken lightly. All blood components, with the exception of heat-treated plasma protein fractions, can transmit hepatitis. Although products obtained from multiple pooled donors carry the greatest risk of transmitting hepatitis, hepatitis can be acquired even from a single unit of packed cells or fresh frozen plasma. Although the exclusion of paid donors and the screening of donor blood for the presence of hepatitis B surface antigen has markedly reduced the incidence of viral hepatitis related to this pathogen, the overwhelming majority of cases of transfusion-related hepatitis are now known to be attributable to the non-A non-B hepatitis agent. At present no routine screening method is available to detect the presence of this pathogen in donor blood products. Although the majority of cases of transfusion-related hepatitis are acute and self-limited, the occurrence of chronic active hepatitis with subsequent cirrhosis is not to be discounted in making the decision to transfuse blood products. Moreover, the human T cell lymphotrophic virus-III (HTLV-III virus) causative of acquired immunodeficiency syndrome (AIDS) has been transmitted through transfusion of blood products. The exclusion of donors in high risk groups for AIDS and the discarding of all donor units positive for HTLV-III antibody should, however, effectively prevent such transmission.

The transfusion of red cells as well as platelets and plasma products that are contaminated with small amounts of red cells may result in the subsequent development of alloantibodies against donor red cell antigens. These alloantibodies may make it extremely difficult, if not impossible, to find compatible blood in a potentially urgent situation in the future. This is a particularly cogent reason to avoid indiscriminant transfusion. Table 1 lists potential complications of transfusion.

TRANSFUSION INDICATIONS IN THE CHRONICALLY ANEMIC PATIENT

Many patients with slowly developing chronic anemia will be encountered in the emergency setting. The anemia may be attributable to a primary hematologic disorder or may be secondary to another underlying illness, such as peptic ulcer disease with chronic occult blood loss, chronic alcoholism, or renal failure. These patients may seek emergency room evaluation because of the symptoms of either their anemia or the underlying disease process. In the absence of superimposed acute blood loss, chronically anemic patients have relatively normal total blood volumes. Such patients compensate for their decreased oxygen-carrying capacity by an increase in cardiac output (primarily by an increase in stroke volume), as well as by a decrease in the oxygen affinity of hemoglobin

TABLE 1 Potential Complications of Transfusion*

Immunologic
　Febrile transfusion reaction (leukoagglutinins)
　Immediate hemolysis (ABO mismatch)
　Delayed hemolysis (alloantibody-induced)
　Urticaria (secondary to plasma proteins)
　Anaphylaxis (anti-IgA antibodies)
　Pulmonary leukostasis (transfusion of leukoagglutinins)
　Graft versus host disease

Infectious
　Septic transfusion reactions (bacterial contamination)
　Hepatitis (A, B, non-A, non-B)
　Cytomegalovirus (interstitial pneumonitis)
　Epstein-Barr virus
　Malaria
　Syphilis
　HTLV-III (AIDS)

Cardiovascular
　Air embolism
　Noncardiogenic pulmonary edema (? microaggregate-induced)
　Cardiogenic pulmonary edema (volume overload)

Metabolic (massive transfusion)
　Hyperkalemia
　Hypocalcemia (citrate-induced)
　Acidosis
　Hypothermia

* With the exception of febrile transfusion reactions, urticaria, and hepatitis, most of these complications are uncommon although potentially serious and not to be ignored when considering transfusion.

brought about by an increase in red blood cell 2,3-diphosphoglycerate.

The large majority of patients with chronic anemia with hemoglobins of 7 g or greater are relatively asymptomatic at rest. Even more severe anemia may be tolerated remarkably well. In the well-compensated patient, urgent transfusion in the emergency department is unnecessary and best avoided. It is far more prudent to admit the patient and search for a medically correctable cause such as folate, iron, or vitamin B_{12} deficiency rather than obligate the patient to a potentially hazardous transfusion. There can be no justification for transfusing a chronically anemic patient with adequate cardiovascular compensation in whom simple medical therapy such as iron or vitamin B_{12} administration will result in correction of the anemic process.

The chronically anemic patient with unstable angina at rest, incipient congestive heart failure, or overt pulmonary edema may require urgent transfusion, especially when he or she fails to respond to appropriate medical management. The development of cardiac symptoms at hemoglobins of 7 g or greater usually implies underlying coronary, hypertensive, or valvular heart disease. In the patient with incipient or mild congestive heart failure, transfusion should be carried out only with packed cells at slow infusion rates. The administration of diuretics prior to or concomitant with blood transfusion may be helpful in avoiding volume overload and worsening congestive heart failure. On rare occasions, it may be helpful to remove 250 to 500 cc of whole blood with the simultaneous transfusion of a unit of packed cells. The blood that is removed can be centrifuged, the plasma discarded, and the packed cells returned to the patient, thereby increasing the hematocrit without increasing total blood volume. These patients should be assessed clinically after each unit of transfusion to determine the response so that only the minimum amount of blood required for compensation is given. Indeed, in patients with marked peripheral edema and ascites owing to congestive heart failure, the transfusion of as little as a single unit of packed cells may result in a profound and continued diuresis. One should not forget that the usual measures such as administration of digitalis, diuretics, and antianginal agents are as important in these patients as in those without anemia.

THE USE OF NONCROSSMATCHED BLOOD FOR EMERGENCY TRANSFUSION

Occasionally, bleeding can be massive and exsanguination imminent. In this situation, the transfusion of noncrossmatched blood may sometimes be justified. The use of noncrossmatched blood may be necessary in patients with bleeding, such as occurs in ruptured abdominal aortic aneurysms, gastrointestinal bleeding (esophageal varices), or severe trauma. If the use of noncrossmatched blood is deemed necessary, Type O Rh-negative blood should be used. Units known to be low in titer of anti-A and anti-B are preferred to avoid hemolytic reactions. However, the use of packed cells with a minimum amount of plasma will help to avoid this problem when low anti-A

and anti-B titers cannot be assured. Although Rh positive blood can be given to Rh negative individuals in the acute situation, it should be remembered that anti-Rh antibodies are likely to develop and result in the delayed destruction of the Rh-positive cells. The risk of sensitizing Rh-negative women in the child-bearing age groups with Rh-positive blood must also be considered.

If a delay of 5 to 15 minutes is permissible, group- and type-specific blood can usually be provided and is preferred. Even in the absence of formal crossmatching, the recipient serum can be screened for atypical antibodies against multiple blood group antigens in a period of only 15 to 30 minutes. The administration of group- and type-specific blood to a patient with a negative serum antibody screen is effectively as safe as the transfusion of otherwise routinely crossmatched blood.

Certainly the use of noncrossmatched or universal donor blood should be strictly avoided in patients in whom volume expansion with appropriate crystalloids or colloids will restore adequate perfusion and oxygenation long enough to allow for appropriate blood typing, antibody screening, or formal crossmatching.

TRANSFUSION OF THE PATIENT WITH AUTOIMMUNE HEMOLYTIC ANEMIA

Autoimmune hemolytic anemia most frequently occurs in the elderly, who often have underlying cardiorespiratory problems that may be aggravated in the presence of severe anemia. Thus, the severely embarrassed patient with autoimmune hemolytic anemia may be in need of urgent transfusion. These patients may present themselves to emergency departments with established diagnoses, or the diagnosis may first become apparent on examination of the peripheral smear or with attempted crossmatching. The presence of jaundice and splenomegaly may also provide clinical clues.

Autoimmune hemolytic anemias may be of the warm or cold type, depending on the temperature at which the antibody is most reactive with red cells. The autoantibodies in these immunohemolytic states are panagglutinins. Thus, these antibodies react with the red cells of virtually all potential donors, making the procurement of truly compatible blood impossible. Moreover, the presence of these autoantibodies in the serum of patients with autoimmune hemolytic anemia may hide the presence of significant alloantibodies against donor red cell antigens, which could result in significant hemolytic transfusion reactions. In patients who have never previously been transfused and who have never been pregnant, the likelihood of preexistent alloantibodies is nil.

If necessary, transfusion of patients with autoimmune hemolytic anemia can be carried out safely, assuming that alloantibodies can be excluded by appropriate crossmatching technique. The transfused cells should be destroyed no more rapidly than the patient's own cells. Despite the decreased survival of these transfused cells, the transfusion of even small amounts of red cells in patients with autoimmune hemolytic anemia may have salutary results.

Unfortunately, techniques for the exclusion of alloantibodies in the serum of patients with autoimmune hemolytic anemia are time-consuming and may not be possible in the patient who is in need of immediate transfusion. If noncrossmatched blood needs to be given to such a patient, it must be given slowly and in small aliquots with extremely close observation for any evidence of an immediate hemolytic transfusion reaction. Because such reactions can be catastrophic and even fatal, the transfusion of noncrossmatched blood, especially to patients at risk of having alloantibodies, should be reserved for lifesaving emergencies. Hematologic consultation in such situations is imperative.

TRANSFUSION OF THE PATIENT WITH APLASTIC ANEMIA

The development of alloantibodies against donor human leukocyte antigens (HLA) and platelet-specific antigens is clinically unimportant unless long-term platelet support is necessary, such as in patients with aplastic anemia or acute leukemia. In these patients, the development of alloantibodies against HLA and platelet-specific antigens may make subsequent successful platelet transfusion difficult, if not impossible. For this reason, platelet transfusion therapy should be undertaken in patients with aplastic anemia only for major bleeding episodes. Often, minor bleeding can be controlled conservatively with other measures (local pressure, topical thrombin, Amicar). The transfusion of blood products to patients with aplastic anemia may result in sensitization to antigens that increase their risk of marrow graft rejection if bone marrow transplantation is attempted. Thus, in aplastic patients who are not bleeding and who have tolerable symptoms of anemia, transfusion is best avoided until it becomes absolutely necessary. If only red cell support is required, the use of washed red cells may be helpful in avoiding alloimmunization against antigens present on contaminating leukocytes and platelets.

THE PROBLEM OF MASSIVE TRANSFUSION

Although definitions vary, the patient who receives a volume of blood greater than his or her total blood volume can be considered to have been massively transfused. The effects of massive transfusion depend not only on the total volume replaced, but also on the rate at which it has been administered. The type and severity of the complications of massive transfusion also depend on which components are selected for blood replacement. The potential complications of massive transfusions include metabolic disturbances (hypocalcemia, hyperkalemia, acidosis), coagulation disorders, hypothermia, and pulmonary insufficiency. It should be remembered that the condition that necessitated the massive transfusion in the first place may be responsible for many of the abnormalities that may be inappropriately attributed to transfusion. For instance, persistent severe acidosis is more frequently related to inadequate treatment of the shock state than to the administration of lactate that has accumulated in stored blood.

Hypothermia

The rapid administration of large volumes of blood stored at 4 °C may result in significant hypothermia. This can be associated with life-threatening cardiac arrhythmias. In patients receiving large volumes rapidly, the blood may be warmed by an in-line mechanical blood warmer. The uncontrolled warming of blood in water baths and microwaves is dangerous and best avoided.

Citrate Toxicity (Hypocalcemia)

The rapid infusion of blood products anticoagulated with citrate may result in a decrease in the serum ionized calcium. There is, however, no convincing evidence that this decrease results in significant myocardial functional impairment or interference with the coagulation mechanism. Although symptomatic hypocalcemia (paresthesias and carpopedal spasm) have been noted in pheresis donors receiving citrated blood at rates of 70 to 80 cc per minute, such rates are rarely reached in massive transfusion, and if they are, they are unlikely to be sustained for any prolonged period of time. The routine prophylactic administration of calcium salts intravenously may result in transient but sharp rises in both the total and the serum ionized calcium. Indeed, the prophylactic administration of calcium salts may increase the risk of fatal arrhythmia in massively transfused patients. Apparently, some of the cardiac deaths previously attributed to citrate were actually the result of hypothermia resulting from the rapid transfusion of cold blood. The routine use of prophylactic intravenous calcium cannot be recommended. Moreover, one should be aware that the administration of calcium salts into the blood storage bag or into the intravenous (IV) line used for transfusion may result in clotting of the blood requiring its disposal.

Acidosis

Massive transfusion of stored blood presents the patient with an acid load secondary to the anticoagulant preservative solution and the accumulation of lactate as a result of blood storage. Although presented with an acid load initially, the metabolism of citrate to bicarbonate ultimately results in a state of alkalosis. Although some have recommended the routine administration of sodium bicarbonate (50 mEq per 5 units of blood), the administration of sodium bicarbonate is better guided by frequent determination of blood gases. The failure to reverse the shock state and provide adequate tissue perfusion will result in continued anaerobic glycolysis and lactic acidosis independent of the acid load initially resulting from transfusion.

Hyperkalemia

Because of the efflux of potassium from red cells into the plasma during storage, the potential for hyperkalemia exists as the result of the transfusion of several units of stored blood (two to three times the total blood volume).

This potential, however, is offset by the movement of potassium back into the red cells at the time of their recirculation, the ultimate metabolic alkalosis resulting from the metabolism of citrate, and renal excretion. Indeed, many studies have revealed that hypokalemia more frequently ensues as a result of massive transfusion. Still, the potential for hyperkalemia exists in patients with persistent shock, acidosis, and inadequate renal perfusion. The administration of bicarbonate, as guided by arterial blood gas monitoring, is appropriate in these situations.

Decreased Red Cell 2,3-Diphosphoglycerate (2,3-DPG) and Increased Hemoglobin Oxygen Affinity

The 2,3-DPG levels of stored blood begin to fall significantly after a week of storage. This fall in 2,3-DPG results in an increased affinity of hemoglobin for oxygen. Theoretically, the transfusion of large amounts of 2,3-DPG-depleted blood could result in decreased oxygen release at the tissue level. Despite this theoretic concern, there is no convincing evidence that the use of 2,3-DPG-depleted blood significantly impairs oxygen delivery in massively transfused patients. Furthermore, 2,3-DPG levels of stored blood are repleted very rapidly, so that by 24 hours after transfusion, 2,3-DPG levels have returned to normal. As long as anemia is corrected by the appropriate administration of packed cells, the increased oxygen affinity can be compensated for by increasing the cardiac output.

Microaggregates and Pulmonary Insufficiency

Microaggregates composed of fibrin, platelets, and white cells accumulate in blood with increasing length of storage. These microaggregates are not removed by the filters in standard blood administration sets that filter particles 170 to 260 mμ in size. Microaggregates have been implicated in the development of pulmonary insufficiency owing to adult respiratory distress syndrome (ARDS-shock lung). Considerable controversy exists as to whether or not these microaggregates play a role in the development of ARDS and whether or not the employment of microaggregate filters will lessen the incidence of this complication. Microaggregate filters with 40-μ pores allow the passage of platelets and remove most of the microaggregates except for those in the 10 to 40-μ range. A decreased frequency of pulmonary insufficiency in massively transfused trauma patients has been reported using this filter.

HEMOSTATIC ABNORMALITIES

Thrombocytopenia

As mentioned previously, blood stored for more that 24 hours at 4°C has essentially no viable platelets. Therefore, the administration of large amounts of blood will result in a dilutional thrombocytopenia. Significant thrombocytopenia (< 100,000 per cubic millimeter) rarely ensues until after a large number of red cell units (> 15) have been transfused, although consumption of platelets such as might result from disseminated intravascular coagulation (DIC), may result in severe thrombocytopenia much earlier in the course of massive transfusion.

Diffuse capillary oozing should alert the clinician to the possibility of significant thrombocytopenia. Although spontaneous bleeding rarely occurs at platelet counts substantially below 50,000 per cubic millimeter, significant bleeding secondary to thrombocytopenia may occur at higher platelet counts in patients with massive trauma. In adult patients with diffuse capillary oozing, an empiric trial of 4 to 6 units of platelet concentrate is warranted. The determination of the bleeding time is a time-consuming and awkward test, which is difficult to perform in an emergent situation such as that associated with massive trauma. Moreover, it has been well demonstrated that prolongation of the bleeding time does not always correlate with the presence of clinical bleeding. With the advent of whole blood counters, platelet counts can be obtained virtually instantaneously and can be used as a useful guide to appropriate platelet administration. Prophylactic transfusion of platelets (after several units of banked blood have been administered) has been advocated, but is probably unnecessary in a patient with no clinical evidence of diffuse bleeding and in whom a platelet count can be obtained rapidly to guide therapy.

Coagulation Factor Depletion

In the massively bleeding patient, restoration of plasma volume in addition to red blood cell replacement will obviously be necessary. The risk of depletion of coagulation factors depends on the amount and type of component used for volume replacement. Most often, volume is replaced initially with electrolyte solutions such as normal saline or Ringer's lactate. Maintenance of blood volume with crystalloids requires the infusion of approximately three times the volume of blood lost, since crystalloids rapidly equilibrate with the extravascular space. Blood loss in excess of 15 to 20 percent of the total blood volume will require the administration of colloids. Although both plasma protein fraction and albumin are adequate volume expanders, the use of large amounts of these products can result in dilution of the coagulation factors because these products do not contain the coagulation factors present in fresh frozen plasma. One suggested method in the patient who is having packed cell and colloid replacement such as albumin and plasma protein fraction is to administer 2 units of group-specific fresh frozen plasma for every 8 to 10 units of packed red cells. The administration of fresh frozen plasma, however, is best guided by the presence or absence of clinical bleeding and the laboratory evaluation of coagulation including the prothrombin time (PT), partial thromboplastin time (PTT), and fibrinogen. The PT and PTT, however, often do not correlate with the presence of a significant hemorrhagic diathesis unless they are markedly prolonged. In patients with hypofibrinogenemia unresponsive to fresh frozen plasma, cryoprecipitate may be used in amounts adequate to restore the fibrinogen to 100 mg percent or greater. This should rarely be necessary except in the patient with DIC. One should remember that bleeding from a site of operation or trauma is not always indicative of defective hemostasis, and in these situations surgical control of bleeding is crucial.

Only Factors V and VIII are labile in whole blood stored at 4 °C. Within 24 hours, the Factor VIII level has fallen below 50 percent. Factor V is considerably less labile, with levels of greater than 50 percent often being maintained for greater than 2 weeks. Thus, with the exception of Factor VIII and possibly Factor V, all of the other coagulation factors are maintained at hemostatic levels in blood stored for 21 days. In the rare patient who is replaced mainly with whole or modified whole blood (blood from which cryoprecipitate and platelets have been removed) the routine use of supplemental fresh frozen plasma is inappropriate since Factor V levels often do not fall below hemostatic levels in stored blood, and there is a large endogenous pool of Factor VIII that can be mobilized during periods of stress.

In considering the need for plasma replacement in patients with massive transfusion, the concomitant administration of platelet concentrate must be considered because this includes a significant amount of plasma (500 to 700 cc per 10 units of platelets) rich in coagulation factors.

The decision to transfuse should be made only after appropriate indications have been clearly defined and the risk/benefit ratio has been thoughtfully considered. Once this decision is reached, only those components required to correct the particular deficits are administered. Careful and continuous clinical and laboratory monitoring is required so that only the minimal amount of blood product required for maximum benefit is administered. Only in this manner can blood products be transfused effectively, efficiently, and safely.

SUGGESTED READING

Circular of information for the use of human blood components. American Association of Blood Banks, American Red Cross, Council of Community Blood Centers, 1985.

Counts RB, Haisch T, et al. Hemostasis in massively transfused trauma patients. Ann Surg 1979; 190:91–99.

Holland PV. Other adverse effects of transfusion. In: Petz LD, Swisher SN, eds. Clinical practice of blood transfusion. New York: Churchill Livingstone, 1981:783.

Howland WS. Anesthesiologic perspectives of blood transfusion. In: Petz LD, Swisher SN, eds. Clinical practice of blood transfusion. New York: Churchill Livingstone, 1981:471.

Masouredis SP. Preservation and clinical use of blood and blood components. In: Williams J, Beutler E, et al, eds. Hematology. New York: McGraw-Hill, 1983:1529.

Nusbacher JN. Transfusion of red blood cell products. In: Petz LD, Swisher SN, eds. Clinical practice of blood transfusion. New York: Churchill Livingstone, 1981:289.

Perkins HA. Strategies for massive transfusion. In: Petz LD, Swisher SN, eds. Clinical practice of blood transfusion. New York: Churchill Livingstone, 1981:485.

Swisher SN, Petz LD. Transfusion therapy of chronic anemic states. In: Petz LD, Swisher SN, eds. Clinical practice of blood transfusion. New York: Churchill Livingstone, 1981:603.

Wintrobe MM, et al, eds. Transfusion of blood and blood components. In: Clinical hematology. Philadelphia: Lea & Febiger, 1981:491.

MANAGEMENT OF THE ENDOCRINE SYSTEM

ANAPHYLAXIS AND SERUM SICKNESS

WILLIAM G. BARSAN, M.D.
JAMES C. HUNTER, M.D.

ANAPHYLAXIS

Anaphylaxis is a clinical syndrome caused by an immediate type I immunologic hypersensitivity reaction (Table 1). It first involves the exposure of the subject to an antigen, resulting in formation of specific IgE antibodies. These antibodies subsequently bind with mast cells and basophils, which sensitizes an individual to a specific antigen. With later exposure to the antigen, crosslinking or bridging of the IgE antibodies occurs and the mast cells and basophils form and release numerous vasoactive mediators via a complex series of intermembrane and intracellar events. These mediators include histamine (H), eosinophil chemotactic factor of anaphylaxis (ECF-A), platelet activating factor (PAF), and slow-reacting substance of anaphylaxis (SRS-A), which now is thought to be more specifically the leukotrienes C4 and D1. These and other mediators are continually being defined, and their relative importance in anaphylaxis is still under considerable research.

Histamine is known to promote increased vascular permeability, relaxation of vascular smooth muscle, constriction of bronchial smooth muscle, edema of the airways and larynx, and stimulation of smooth muscle in the gastrointestinal tract. These actions cause tenesmus, diarrhea, vomiting, and breakdown of cutaneous vascular integrity resulting in flushing, urticaria, and angioedema. SRS-A acts by altering bronchial smooth muscle tone and enhances the effect of histamine on target organs. PAF enhances the degeneration of platelets and release of histamine and serotonin. ECF-A selectively attracts eosinophils to the areas of activity. The eosinophils have a neutralizing effect on the mediators. The substances released by eosinophils can not independently reverse the situation.

Anaphylactoid reactions are clinically very similar to anaphylactic reactions and can be treated the same. They result from non-antibody–antigen complex–mediated release of vasoactive mediators from mast cells and basophils. Iodinated contrast agents, aspirin, and nonsteroidal anti-inflammatory drugs (NSAIDs) are among the most common agents implicated in anaphylactoid reactions and require no prior sensitization.

The clinical manifestations of anaphylaxis are extremely variable and can range from mild generalized pruritus to profound shock. Symptoms arise from the respiratory tract, the cardiovascular system, the eye, the skin, or the gastrointestinal tract, singly or in any combination. The most common manifestations are cutaneous and respiratory. In severe reactions, laryngeal edema and cardiovascular collapse are most prominent.

Early recognition and treatment may prevent progression to more severe symptomatology. Manifestation of symptoms may occur from minutes to hours from antigen exposure. Reactions to parenteral injections usually occur within 30 minutes. Laryngeal edema may be manifested by a lump in the throat, hoarseness, or, if severe, stridor. Bronchospasm is manifested by cough, wheezing, chest tightness and variable degrees of respiratory distress. Cutaneous manifestations are typically pruritic urticarial lesions that may be localized or diffuse with well-circumscribed, discrete cutaneous wheals with

TABLE 1 Hypersensitivity Reactions

Type	Mechanism	Example
I: Anaphylactic	Antigen-antibody reaction at the surface of mast cells and basophils	Systemic anaphylaxis
II: Cytotactic	Antibody binding with antigens on the surface of the cells	Hemolytic anemia
III: Complex mediated	Immunocomplex formation by antigen-antibody	Serum sickness
IV: Cell mediated	Direct interaction of antigen with sensitized T-lymphocytes	Contact dermatitis

erythematous, raised, serpiginous borders and blanched centers. Angioedema may also be present and represents a deeper edematous process that is frequently nonpruritic, is asymmetric, and involves an extremity or the perioral or orbital region. Cardiovascular reactions vary from tachycardia and mild hypotension to profound shock and cardiac arrest. Arrhythmias reported include atrial fibrillation, nodal rhythms, and ventricular fibrillation or asystole. There is little evidence of direct myocardial depression in anaphylaxis. The cardiac effect is believed to be secondary to hypoxia or decreased filling pressure from a precipitous drop in peripheral vascular resistance with massive venous pooling. Some animal studies have shown significant increases in pulmonary vascular resistance with right heart strain and failure. Gastrointestinal symptomatology includes nausea, vomiting, crampy abdominal pain, and bloody diarrhea. Conjunctivitis and increased lacrimation may be present with ocular pruritus.

The varied and broad symptom complex of anaphylaxis does not usually affect clinical recognition. There is most often a history of recent antigen exposure and a typical cutaneous and respiratory reaction present. The more severe manifestations of anaphylaxis may not present so clearly, and anaphylaxis must be included in the differential diagnosis of respiratory failure, shock, and cardiovascular collapse.

Treatment

The primary manifestations of anaphylaxis may occur singly or in combination. For cutaneous urticaria or angioedema alone, 0.3 to 0.5 ml of aqueous epinephrine (1:1,000) may be given subcutaneously (0.01 ml per kilogram in children). Diphenhydramine (Benadryl), 25 to 50 mg intramuscularly, should be given also to prevent further release of histamine.

The *pulmonary manifestations* of anaphylaxis are usually laryngeal and pharyngeal edema or bronchospasm. In the patient with airway obstruction and apnea, endotracheal intubation or cricothyroidotomy should be performed immediately, followed by pharmacologic therapy. When laryngeal edema or bronchospasm is present without apnea, 0.3 to 0.5 ml of 1:1,000 aqueous epinephrine should be given subcutaneously. If there is intense peripheral vasoconstriction, it may be necessary to give the epinephrine intramuscularly or intravenously for laryngeal edema (dosages follow). In patients with bronchospasm primarily, epinephrine therapy should be followed by treatment with aerosolized metaproterenol or isoetharine (0.3 ml in 2.5 cc saline). The epinephrine dose may be repeated every 15 to 20 minutes up to three times if needed. Intravenous aminophylline (5.5 mg per kilogram loading dose) may be helpful in refractory cases.

Patients presenting with circulatory shock should be given 1 to 2 ml of aqueous epinephrine in 1:10,000 dilution (i.e., 0.1 to 0.2 mg) over 2 to 3 minutes intravenously. Extreme care is advised because intravenous epinephrine will increase myocardial oxygen demand and is arrhythmogenic, particularly in patients with preexist-ing coronary artery disease. The rate of infusion of the epinephrine is a critical factor in avoidance of severe complications. At lower doses and with lower infusion rates it has been shown that the beta-adrenergic receptors are more affected than the alpha sites, producing bronchodilatation and moderate increases in systolic blood pressure without the more toxic effects seen with predominant alpha-adrenergic stimulation. Patients should have continuous cardiac monitoring during epinephrine treatment. Volume expansion with crystalloid or colloid solution (10 to 20 cc per kilogram) should be started concomitantly with epinephrine therapy. In refractory cases, an epinephrine infusion in a 1:100,000 dilution should be used. This can be done by using 1.0 mg epinephrine in 100 cc D5W and adjusting the flow from 6 to 30 cc per hour for a dosage range of 1 to 5 μg per minute. The infusion rate should be titrated to the blood pressure response or the production of arrhythmias. If hypotension is refractory to fluid and epinephrine infusion, antishock trouser inflation may be useful.

Diphenhydramine is usually given to patients with pulmonary and circulatory manifestations of anaphylaxis and may prevent further histamine release. It is a secondary treatment and should not take precedence over epinephrine therapy. The use of H_2 blockers such as cimetidine has not gained acceptance. Corticosteroids should also be given to patients with anaphylaxis (methylprednisolone 1 to 2 mg per kilogram). Although there are no studies demonstrating the effectiveness of this treatment, it is felt that the membrane-stabilizing effect of corticosteroids may be beneficial.

With certain reactions, most commonly to insect venom, local measures to reduce the antigen exposure are helpful. A tourniquet applied proximal to injection site can be used. It should not occlude arterial inflow and should be loosened every 15 to 20 minutes. The use of 0.1 to 0.2 ml 1:1,000 aqueous epinephrine infiltrated about the injection site may decrease the immediate antigen load. This method should not be used on any digits or areas of terminal arterial supply.

Disposition of patients with anaphylactic reactions depends on the severity of the presentation. Any patient with a reaction requiring advanced treatment modalities should be admitted to a monitored bed in the intensive care unit, where progress can be watched closely. Relapses are uncommon, but observation is necessary, especially in cases in which there may be further antigenic exposure from delayed absorption (as from ingested substances or long-acting parenteral preparations) and to monitor for complications of necessary aggressive therapy. The patients with more common mild reactions can usually be discharged if proper follow-up is arranged. It is customary to use a slow-release epinephrine solution (Sus-Phrine) in a dosage of 0.005 ml per kilogram to a maximum of 0.2 ml subcutaneously at discharge. The patient should be given at least 48 hours of Benadryl, 25 to 50 mg orally every 6 hours (1 mg per kilogram per dose for children).

Prevention is the most successful treatment of anaphylaxis, and the emergency physician is the first provider of this most important aspect. The patient should be advised of the possible agents that precipitated the reaction and the various compounds or methods of potential future exposure. If insect venom is the cause, consideration should be given to prescribing a self-injectable epinephrine pen or "bee-sting kit." The patient should be referred to an allergist for evaluation and potential desensitization treatment.

SERUM SICKNESS

Serum sickness is a type III hypersensitivity reaction (see Table 1) and is a systemic allergic reaction. Soluble circulating antigen–antibody immune complexes result in tissue injury by deposition in blood vessel walls and activation of the complement system. Most of the symptoms are thought to be mediated by IgE and possibly IgM complexes, although IgE-mediated release is believed to be responsible for the urticarial lesions through histamine release. IgE-mediated release may also enhance deposition of the complexes at the endothelial or basement membrane surfaces. In the past, serum sickness was described in relation to foreign serum reactions. Today, the most frequent cause is drugs. The most common agent involved is penicillin, but sulfonamides, streptomycin, phenytoin, and the thiouracils are frequently implicated.

The syndrome is manifested by an urticarial or maculopapular rash accompanied by fever, myalgia, arthritis, edema, and lymphadenopathy. Onset is usually 7 to 12 days after initial drug exposure, but this may vary. Skin lesions are the most consistent finding. Urticaria at the site of drug injection may be the initial manifestation.

The arthritis and arthralgias are commonly polymigratory, with the large joints involved most often. Lymphadenopathy is common and occurs in most patients. It may be mild or restricted to only those nodes draining a drug injection site. Some degree of malaise, anorexia, headache, and myalgia is also present in most patients. There is rare cardiac and neurologic involvement, including neuritis, meningoencephalitis, angina pectoris, and acute myocardial infarction. There are no laboratory findings helpful in the diagnosis of serum sickness. The illness is usually minor and self-limited to 2 to 3 weeks' duration.

Treatment

The treatment of serum sickness is far less urgent than that of anaphylaxis. Treatment consists of removing the patient from any further contact with the offending agent and alleviating bothersome symptomatology. Subcutaneous epinephrine, 0.3 to 0.5 ml of 1:1,000 dilution (.01 ml per kilogram in children), or Sus-Phrine 0.2 ml (0.005 ml per kilogram in children), is effective in affording relief from the pruritus and urticaria. Benadryl, 25 to 50 mg orally (1 mg per kilogram per dose in children), provides more prolonged relief of the urticaria. Fever, myalgia, and arthralgia are usually controlled with aspirin, 325 to 650 mg orally every 4 hours. In severe cases, corticosteroids can be used with a 2-week taper, beginning with 60 mg of prednisone daily. It is an unusual patient who could not be discharged home with the above management instituted, education given, and routine follow-up provided.

HYPOGLYCEMIA

MATTHEW C. RIDDLE, M.D.

Glucose is a major fuel for human energy metabolism. Certain tissues, notably the central nervous system (CNS), are almost entirely dependent on glucose. Since the CNS cannot function for even several minutes without an adequate supply of glucose, a complex mechanism opposes interruption of this supply. Glucose mobilization and hyperglycemia are favored acutely by epinephrine and glucagon, and subacutely by growth hormone and cortisol. When this hormonal system fails, declining plasma glucose leads to the clinical syndrome of hypoglycemia. This syndrome has two components: *sympathetic symptoms* and *CNS symptoms*. The sympathetically mediated events usually come first, and include hunger, sweating, tremor, palpitations and

tachycardia, anxiety, and restlessness. The CNS events that follow may include headache, personality change, confusion, stupor, coma, and seizures.

Several factors increase the *risk* of developing the hypoglycemic syndrome. Young children and elderly adults are vulnerable by virtue of their high ratio of CNS to lean tissue mass; gluconeogenetic substrates may be insufficient when the mass of muscle is small. Chronic malnutrition at any age also reduces muscle mass and favors hypoglycemia. Recent fasting favors hypoglycemia by reducing hepatic glycogen stores. Exercise enhances uptake of glucose by tissues.

DIAGNOSIS

The diagnosis of hypoglycemia is based on recognizing the clinical syndrome and confirming that the concentration of glucose in plasma is low. The typical sympathetically mediated symptoms and signs described before may not be present in persons with neuropathy or in those who are taking sympathetic blocking drugs. In such patients, additional clues may be sought. For example, the history of repeated headaches, nightmares, nocturnal sweating, and morning nausea or abdominal distress all suggest repeated prior hypoglycemia. Occasionally, hypoglycemia causes localized *neurologic findings*, especially in persons with prior cerebrovascular or other neurologic disease; these may be sensory, motor, perceptual, or expressive. Confirmation of the diagnosis rests on demonstration of plasma glucose less than 50 mg per deciliter (45 mg per deciliter whole blood glucose) in the presence of symptoms or signs and disappearance of these findings on restoration of normal glucose concentration. This basic definition must be amended by a cautionary note. Both the prior mean glucose concentration and the rate of decline of plasma glucose affect the threshold for symptoms. Thus, chronically hyperglycemic diabetic persons with rapidly falling plasma glucose may experience hypoglycemic symptoms at concentrations well above 50 mg per deciliter. Similarly, chronically overtreated diabetic persons or those with insulin-secreting tumors may have negligible symptoms when the concentration of glucose is 40 mg per deciliter or less.

Now that reliable *glucose-oxidose reagent strips* (e.g., Chemstrips BG, Visidex) for measuring capillary blood glucose are available, direct testing for hypoglycemia can be done anywhere. For the person who is able to use these strips, the traditional practice of giving intravenous dextrose to all persons suspected of being hypoglycemic is no longer appropriate.

CLASSIFICATION AND DIFFERENTIAL DIAGNOSIS

Nonhypoglycemia

Many patients (and some physicians) attribute a variety of sympathetically mediated symptoms due to other causes, usually emotional, to hypoglycemia.

Physiologic Hypoglycemia

Hypoglycemia may occur in entirely healthy persons under the right conditions. For example, persons exercising vigorously when fasting and pregnant women waking in the middle of the night craving food may both have low plasma glucose concentrations.

Inborn Errors of Metabolism

Infants and young children occasionally present with significant fasting or nonfasting hypoglycemia owing to inborn metabolic deficiencies. These may be serious and demand categorization by pediatric metabolic specialists.

Reactive Hypoglycemia

There are three subtypes of hypoglycemia provoked by meals. *Alimentary* hypoglycemia usually occurs 1 to 3 hours after a meal. This disorder is most common in patients with prior gastric surgery. *Early diabetic* hypoglycemia usually occurs 3 to 5 hours following a meal and seems to result from abnormal insulin secretion in early type II diabetes. *Idiopathic* hypoglycemia usually occurs 2 to 4 hours after a meal and, by definition, is poorly understood. All types of reactive hypoglycemia are generally benign and rarely require emergency medical attention.

Fasting Hypoglycemia

Hypoglycemia occurring 6 or more hours after a meal is often severe enough to require emergency services. There are many possible causes, including pituitary or adrenal insufficiency, overproduction of insulin by islet cell tumors, production of other hypoglycemic factors by other tumors, and rarely, hepatic necrosis (as in fulminant hepatitis). However, most cases of severe fasting hypoglycemia encountered in the emergency department fall into three categories, which require specific comment.

Hypoglycemia Secondary to Treatment of Diabetes. About 5 percent of American adults have diabetes and many of these people take insulin or sulfonylureas. Nearly all who use insulin eventually experience significant hypoglycemia. The most powerful sulfonylureas are chlorpropamide (Diabinese), tolazamide (Tolinase), glipizide (Glucotrol), and glyburide (Micronase, DiaBeta). All can cause severe hypoglycemia, especially in malnourished elderly persons. Hypoglycemia of this kind can occur at any time of day or night, often between 0200 and 0600 hours. Persons who have diabetic neuropathy may be unaware that glucose is falling, and those who have had diabetes longer than 10 years usually have decreased responses of glucagon and epinephrine to hypoglycemia, so that their protective mechanisms are impaired. Drugs that block sympathetic nervous function to treat hypertension or angina are often used by diabetic patients; these drugs further blunt symptoms and signs of hypoglycemia.

Drug-Induced and Factitious Hypoglycemia. Patients other than diabetics may have hypoglycemia secondary to drugs. Salicylate overdose and beta-blockers are occasional causes of hypoglycemia, but a surprising number of cases of severe hypoglycemia result from surreptitious use of insulin or sulfonylureas. Nondiabetic persons who inappropriately take hypoglycemic agents are usually medical personnel or relatives of diabetic patients. In rare instances, these agents are maliciously given by another person to an unknowing victim. Cases of this sort are difficult to distinguish from insulin-secreting tumors; they may be suspected when hypoglycemia is unusually sudden, unpredictable, and severe.

Alcoholic Hypoglycemia. Intoxicated persons, who are commonplace in emergency facilities, are at risk for hypoglycemia for several reasons. Ethanol itself impairs hepatic gluconeogenesis, and acute and chronic malnutrition are common among alcoholic patients. Alcoholic pancreatitis may lead to diabetes requiring insulin or sulfonylureas, both risky treatments for persons with erratic lives. Alcoholic neuropathy may obscure symptoms and signs of hypoglycemia. Obtaining a medical history may be difficult, and often the possibility of nutritional encephalopathy or head trauma as causes of altered mental status diverts attention from the possibility of hypoglycemia. Hypoglycemia secondary to alcohol ingestion develops slowly, at least a day after the last ingestion of food and up to a day after the last intake of alcohol. The incidence of alcoholic hypoglycemia is unknown, and it may be low. The diagnosis should nevertheless be kept in mind, since serious brain injury may ensue.

TREATMENT

Food

Once the diagnosis has been established, a conscious patient may begin therapy immediately by ingesting carbohydrate-containing food or liquid. This should not be attempted when the patient is stuporous or nauseated. Liquids containing little besides sugars (e.g., fruit juices, soft drinks, syrups) are most rapidly absorbed. Beverages or foods containing complex carbohydrates, proteins, and fats (e.g., milk, crackers, sandwiches) act more slowly, but have more prolonged effects. An item from the first group usually should be given first; 12 ounces of juice or a soft drink (about 20 grams of dextrose) is generally enough. One or more items from the second group should follow.

Glucagon

Subcutaneous or intramuscular injection of 1 mg of glucagon (freshly mixed in buffer) is appropriate early therapy for some persons who are too obtunded or nauseated to eat or drink, especially those who are taking insulin or sulfonylureas. Its advantage lies in ease of administration by a friend or family member at home or en route to the hospital. Its disadvantages are (1) dependence on the presence of hepatic glycogen stores, and (2) the tendency to cause gastric atony associated with nausea and delaying absorption of simultaneously ingested carbohydrate. When effective, glucagon usually increases plasma glucose within 20 minutes; its action persists for 1 to 2 hours.

Intravenous Dextrose

The standard initial therapy for serious hypoglycemia that is not treatable by oral carbohydrate is injection of 50 cc of 50 percent dextrose over 1 to 3 minutes. When necessary, this treatment can be repeated or followed by a continuous infusion of 1,000 cc of 5 percent dextrose over 1 to 2 hours. When hypoglycemia is unresponsive to these measures, or quickly recurs, infusion of 10 percent dextrose may be initiated. When glucose is given rapidly to malnourished individuals, serum potassium and phosphate may fall, and so these electrolytes should be monitored in serious cases.

Ancillary Drug Treatment

Other drugs sometimes used to treat serious hypoglycemia include corticosteroids, phenytoin, and diazoxide. In general, these should be reserved for selected chronic situations, such as inoperable insulin-secreting tumors. A notable exception is hypoglycemia suspected to be attributable to untreated primary or secondary adrenal insufficiency. In this case, 100 mg of hydrocortisone succinate (SoluCortef) may be given intravenously immediately, followed by an equivalent amount of corticosteroid orally or intravenously over the subsequent 24 hours.

MONITORING OF THE RESPONSE TO THERAPY AND DISPOSITION

The first priority after diagnosis is restoration of normal or supranormal plasma glucose. This may be documented by measurement of capillary blood glucose by glucose-oxidase reagent strips read visually or with a meter by competent personnel, or by laboratory measurement of plasma glucose. Glucose is usually returned to and maintained at normal levels without difficulty by the standard treatment in the first hour. When this occurs, and the reason for the hypoglycemic event is known and recurrence seems unlikely, routine ambulatory follow-up can be arranged. However, when normal glycemic levels cannot quickly be achieved, when significant hypoglycemia recurs despite adequate treatment, or when the cause of significant hypoglycemia remains obscure, hospital admission for further observation or treatment should be considered. Another indication for admission is known overdose with long-acting insulin of such magnitude that subsequent severe hypoglycemia is probable, even when it has not yet occurred.

When the pathogenesis of hypoglycemia is in doubt, plasma from initial blood collections should always be saved for possible future analysis for sulfonylureas, insulin, anti-insulin antibodies, C-peptide, or other substances. Prolonged severe hypoglycemia refractory to initial treatment usually proves to be attributable to long-acting insulin or sulfonylurea ingestion. Consultation with an endocrinologist who is experienced in the management of hypoglycemic disorders is desirable for such patients.

Once adequate plasma glucose levels are achieved, normal mental function usually follows within minutes. A small proportion of patients recover slowly, usually over 1 to 6 hours. A few remain severely impaired longer, some permanently. Patients who are not largely recovered an hour after normoglycemia is restored should be admitted to the hospital for observation. Those who show little improvement after an hour of treatment not only must be admitted, but also are possible candidates for mannitol and perhaps dexamethasone therapy. Neither procedure has been proved helpful, but both seem reasonable since cerebral edema is presumed to be present in most cases of prolonged coma following hypoglycemia. Mannitol is usually given as 100 to 200 cc of a 20 percent solution intravenously over 20 minutes, and dexamethasone, 8 mg, is also given by intravenous injection.

SUGGESTED READING

MacCuish AC, Munro JF, Duncan LJP. Treatment of hypoglycemic coma with glucagon, intravenous dextrose, and mannitol infusion in a hundred diabetics. Lancet 1970; 2:946–949.

Rotwein PS, Giddings SJ, Permutt A. Diagnosis and management of hypoglycemic disorders in adults. Spec Top Endocrinol Metab 1982; 3:87–115.

Williams HE. Alcoholic hypoglycemia and ketoacidosis. Med Clin North Am 1984; 68:33–38.

DIABETIC KETOACIDOSIS

ELLIOT J. RAYFIELD, M.D.
EDMUND W. GIEGERICH, M.D.

Diabetic ketoacidosis accounts for 14 percent of all diabetic hospital admissions in the United States. The high morbidity and mortality rates that still exist despite recent advances in therapy make diabetic ketoacidosis a medical emergency necessitating prompt diagnosis and treatment. Prevention of the development of ketoacidosis requires both patient education and physician awareness of potential problems facing the diabetic patient. This discussion outlines the evaluation and treatment of the patient with diabetic ketoacidosis.

CAUSES

The onset of diabetes mellitus may be heralded by ketoacidosis in a patient in whom insulin deficiency is severe and unrecognized. The main precipitating factors in a patient with known diabetes are infection, inappropriate insulin therapy by patient or physician, trauma, myocardial infarction, and emotional stress. The evaluation of the patient is incomplete if these factors are not actively sought. Despite a thorough evaluation, up to 20 percent of patients may have no obvious cause.

With the widespread use of home monitoring of blood glucose, the occurrence of ketoacidosis during the diabetic pregnancy is unusual. The high risk of fetal loss during ketoacidosis makes early diagnosis and therapy imperative, and fetal monitoring is recommended during therapy. Otherwise, the treatment for pregnant women is the same as presented in this chapter.

DIAGNOSIS

The initial diagnosis of ketoacidosis can usually be made by a combination of history, clinical examination, and simple diagnostic testing. Treatment should be instituted rapidly without waiting for extensive laboratory assessment. The hallmarks of diabetic ketoacidosis are dehydration in the presence of hyperglycemia and metabolic acidosis attributable to ketone bodies. The use of glucose oxidase reagent strips—Chemstrip bG (Bio-Dynamics, Inc.) by visual inspection, or Dextrostix (Ames) with a glucometer gives a close approximation of blood glucose concentrations in minutes. A semiquantitative estimation of plasma and urine ketone bodies can be made by using reagent tablets. The presence of dehydration, hyperglycemia, and ketonemia or large ketonuria on these screening tests is sufficient indication for the initiation of therapy.

The initial laboratory assessment in a patient thought to have diabetic ketoacidosis should include arterial blood gas measurements (pH, Po_2, Pco_2), a complete blood count, urinalysis, and serum determinations of glucose, ketones, electrolytes, urea nitrogen, creatinine, calcium, and phosphorus concentrations. Microbial cultures should be obtained when there is no obvious cause for ketoacidosis, especially in patients who are hypotensive, severely ill, or elderly. An electrocardiogram and chest film are also recommended.

TREATMENT

The consequences of insulin deficiency are hyperglycemia, metabolic acidosis, and osmotic diuresis with concomitant fluid and electrolyte depletion. The objective of treatment is to correct these abnormalities simultaneously by providing insulin and appropriate fluid and electrolyte therapy, as well as to evaluate and treat the precipitating cause. Although therapy should be initiated promptly, treatment should be controlled to prevent iatrogenic complications related to too rapid replacement of insulin, fluids, or electrolytes. (Refer to Table 1 for an outline of treatment.)

Insulin

The aim of insulin therapy is to correct the metabolic abnormalities with minimum risk to the patient. The major change in the treatment of ketoacidosis in the last decade has been the trend toward administering insulin in lower doses either by continuous intravenous infusion or by intermittent intramuscular injection. The high-dose insulin regimen used widely before the early 1970s required large doses of regular insulin given intravenously and subcutaneously and resulted in wide fluctuations of plasma insulin levels. The problems with this form of therapy in-

TABLE 1 Management of Diabetic Ketoacidosis

1. Rapid clinical examination with special attention to (a) mental status, (b) cardiovascular status, (c) state of hydration, (d) source of infection

2. Confirm diagnosis rapidly using blood glucose reagent strips (Chemstrip bG or Dextrostix) and blood/urine screen for acetone. STAT laboratory assessment: glucose, pH and arterial blood gases, serum electrolytes, BUN, creatinine, calcium, phosphorus, CBC, and urinalysis. Microbial cultures, ECG, and chest x-ray film as indicated

3. Diagnosis DKA confirmed; initiate therapy as follows:
   A. Insulin
      1) Intravenous regimen: Priming bolus of 6 units IV followed by a continuous IV infusion of 6 units/hour (pediatric age group 0.1 U/kg/hr). 12 units/hour recommended for patients with infection. Dose adjusted on basis of hourly blood glucose determinations. When blood glucose level reaches 250 mg/dl, insulin infusion should be decreased to 1-2 units/hour to maintain blood glucose at 150–200 mg/dl.
      2) Intramuscular regimen: Loading dose of 10–20 units IM with subsequent doses of 6 units IM per hour. Monitoring as for IV regimen. If no change in 2 hours, switch to IV regimen.
   B. Fluids and Electrolytes
      1) Fluids: Isotonic saline (0.9 percent NaCl) is the fluid of choice to restore blood volume. Initial rate 1 L/hr and subsequent fluid therapy 100–500 ml/hr based on clinical response. If serum Na rises > 145 mEq/L switch to 0.45 percent NaCl. When blood glucose reaches 250 mg/dl, add 5 percent dextrose to IV fluid at a rate of 100 ml/hr.
      2) Potassium: Withhold therapy until K^+ level is known. Initial rate of 20–30 mEq/hr adjusted to serial serum measurements; if $K^+ < 3.5$ mEq/L infuse K^+ at 40 mEq/L and if $K^+ > 5.5$ mEq/L no potassium. Potassium in the form of chloride salt and 10 mM/hour as phosphate salt (if renal failure present, omit phosphate).
      3) Serial glucose and electrolyte measurements hourly until glucose level reaches 250 mg/dl, then every 2 to 4 hours.
      4) Bicarbonate is given for pH $\leq 7.0–7.1$ in the form of an infusion of 44 mEq $NaHCO_3$ added to 1 L of 0.45 percent NaCl with 20 mEq/L KCl over 1 hour. Goal of therapy is to raise pH to 7.2.

4. Ancillary measures: Antibiotics, O_2 for $Po_2 < 80$ mm Hg, volume expanders for persistent hypotension, and central venous monitoring for patients with cardiovascular and renal disease.

clude a higher incidence of late hypoglycemia and hypokalemia. Also of concern is the possibility of osmotic disequilibrium syndrome caused by too rapid a shift in blood glucose concentration, and resulting in possible cerebral edema. Insulin given subcutaneously in DKA has an unpredictable absorption when the patient is initially hypovolemic, thus resulting in a potential depot for later absorption of insulin with fluid administration.

The favored route of administration at present is continuous "low-dose" intravenous insulin infusion. When insulin is administered as an intravenous bolus it has a circulating half-life of approximately 5 minutes. By contrast, intravenous insulin given as a continuous infusion has the advantage of achieving a relatively constant concentration after steady state is reached by 30 minutes. In steady state studies of intravenous insulin administration, for each unit of insulin infused per hour there is an increase of plasma insulin concentration of approximately 20 μU per milliliter.

The question of how much insulin is necessary to treat diabetic ketoacidosis is controversial. Although a priming bolus of insulin is not necessary, it does provide an immediate therapeutic level; the recommended dose is the same as for the initial infusion rate. The insulin should be administered by continuous intravenous infusion at a rate of 6 units per hour for adults or 0.1 units per kilogram per hour for children. Two points are relevant to the issue of how much insulin needs to be administered continuously per hour. First, it has been demonstrated in several insulin-sensitive tissues, including isolated adipocytes, that maximum stimulation of glucose transport from the periphery into the cell requires only 10 percent of the insulin receptors to be occupied. A greater increase in insulin levels will not result in a further enhancement of biologic response because the rate limiting step(s) are distal to membrane receptors. Second, there are relative sensitivities of the effects of insulin on different cellular functions. For example, lipolysis, glycogenolysis, and gluconeogenesis can be inhibited by insulin levels of 10 to 20 μU per milliliter. Insulin levels of 100 μU per milliliter are necessary to inhibit hepatic ketogenesis, while concentrations of up to 200 μU per milliliter are required for maximal stimulation of peripheral glucose uptake. Thus the rate of insulin infusion suggested here (6 units per hour) achieves an average plasma insulin level of 120 μU per milliliter, which is sufficient to inhibit lipolysis, ketone body formation, and hepatic glucose production. For any patient with evidence of infection at the time of presentation, an infusion rate of 12 units per hour is suggested because of the resistance to insulin action that accompanies infections.

Although insulin adsorbs to plastic and glass, it is unnecessary to add albumin to the infusion. However, flushing the solution through the intravenous lines to saturate adsorption sites is recommended. Insulin can be administered by an infusion pump inserted into a separate vein or "piggybacked" onto the intravenous line delivering rehydration fluids. Insulin should not be added to the fluid used for rehydration. One has more control over the treatment regimen when the rates of insulin and fluid delivery can be monitored independently of each other.

Insulin infusion should continue until both hyperglycemia and metabolic acidosis are corrected. The progess of therapy is assessed initially by serum glucose, ketone, and electrolyte determinations done hourly until the blood glucose reaches a level of 250 mg per deciliter, and then every 2 to 4 hours until the patient is restarted on his daily insulin dose. A glucose reflectance meter or glucose oxidase reagent strip should be used to avoid unnecessary delay in laboratory reporting and to facilitate therapeutic decisions. Assuming adequate rehydration, blood glucose levels usually fall at a rate of 75 to 100 mg per deciliter per hour. If no change in glucose level has occurred in 2 hours of therapy, the rate of insulin infusion should be doubled. At this point, the patient's rehydration status as well as the possibility of an occult infection should be reconsidered. Since hyperglycemia typically resolves prior to the acidosis, insulin therapy must be continued without inducing hypoglycemia. If acidosis or ketone bodies are present when the glucose level has fallen to 250 mg per deciliter, a glucose infusion (5 percent) should be administered at 100 cc per hour. The insulin infusion rate should be decreased to 1 to 2 units per hour to maintain blood sugar in the 150 to 200 mg per deciliter range until the patient is ready to eat.

A simple alternative to continuous intravenous infusion therapy is to administer insulin as intermittent intramuscular injections. The advantages and therapeutic responses are similar to those noted with continuous intravenous infusion. The simplicity and safety of intramuscular insulin injection make it advantageous in a hospital without available house staff or nurse clinicians. This modality is not recommended for the hypotensive or inadequately hydrated patient. A loading dose of 10 to 20 units given intramuscularly is required, and subsequent doses of 6 units per hour IM are given. Monitoring is the same as for intravenous therapy and lack of response in the presence of adequate hydration should prompt a change to an intravenous infusion.

Some patients with ketoacidosis may manifest insulin resistance as a consequence of concurrent infection or high titers of IgG anti-insulin antibodies. Such patients may require 20 or more units of insulin per hour by continuous infusion to decrease blood glucose levels at an acceptable rate (75 to 100 mg per deciliter per hour) and the physician should empirically double the insulin infusion rate every 2 hours until an appropriate fall in blood glucose level is observed. This patient should also be treated with a single component, highly purified pork regular insulin (e.g., Novo or Nordisk). The use of corticosteroids (as may sometimes be employed in treating insulin resistance attributable to IgG anti-insulin antibodies in the absence of ketoacidosis) is not recommended.

Other patients with ketoacidosis may have a current history of systemic insulin allergy, that is, diffuse urticaria usually within a half-hour of insulin administration. In this type of patient fluid and electrolyte replacement as well as treatment of the acidosis with bicarbonate (if pH is less than 7.2) should be carried out concomitantly with skin tests using both beef and pork insulin at a dilution of 1:1,000,000 (Lilly test kit). Since beef insulin is more allergenic than pork insulin, if the patient has a positive skin test to both beef and pork or beef insulin alone, he should be rapidly desensitized to pork insulin by the administration of serial dilutions of insulin (first intracutaneously, and then subcutaneously) every 20 minutes as tolerated. If the allergy is to pork insulin, the patient should be treated with beef insulin. Desensitization can be accomplished with either the Lilly test kit or the physician's own serial dilutions of a highly purified single-component pork insulin (Novo or Nordisk) in an isotonic saline vehicle. The usual precautions for anaphylactic shock should be taken. Once desensitization is accomplished, the ketoacidosis should be treated in the manner previously outlined, but the patient should receive a highly purified single-component pork insulin (Novo or Nordisk).

Fluid and Electrolyte Therapy of Diabetic Ketoacidosis

The osmotic diuresis that occurs in diabetic ketoacidosis results in profound deficits in total body water and electrolytes. Estimates from balance studies indicate average deficits: water, 5 to 10 liters; sodium, 500 mM; potassium, 300 to 1,000 mM; phosphorus, 67 mM; and magnesium, 37 mM. The marked dehydration is a result of a loss of water in excess of sodium. Attention must be paid to true hyponatremia on admission, since such patients may be at risk for the development of cerebral edema. The serum sodium level may be misleadingly decreased 1.6 mEq per liter for every 100 mg per deciliter elevation in blood glucose level, and this should be accounted for in assessing the laboratory data. Pseudohyponatremia may also result from hypertriglyceridemia.

Isotonic saline (0.9 percent or 154 mM NaCl) is the fluid of choice because it restores circulating blood volume and tissue perfusion and prevents a rapid reversal of osmotic gradients as blood glucose levels fall with treatment. Volume expansion should be at an initial rate of 1 L per hour and a patient in shock should be given saline and volume expanders at an even more rapid rate. Saline infusion should be slowed as volume is restored and changed to 0.45 percent sodium chloride (77 mM) if serum sodium level rises above 145 mEq per liter. The use of isotonic saline may be associated with the development of hyperchloremic metabolic acidosis following successful therapy of diabetic ketoacidosis. The bicarbonate deficit is of no consequence to the patient when there is no primary renal defect. The renal excretion of ammonium chloride during the next 24 to 48 hours corrects the bicarbonate deficit.

In the case of hypernatremia on presentation, the fluid of choice is 0.45 percent sodium chloride after circulating blood volume has been normalized. The patient with mild dehydration may be treated with 0.45 percent sodium chloride. Right- or left-sided heart venous pressure should be monitored closely in patients with conditions that are susceptible to volume overload (cardiac disease and chronic renal failure). A recent report has noted that volume loading with large amounts of crystalloid solution (0.45 percent sodium chloride) during the treatment of diabetic ketoacidosis may produce an acute hypooncotic state resulting in subclinical pulmonary and cerebral edema in otherwise healthy diabetic patients. This observation underscores the need for careful monitoring of the clinical course of patients with complicating medical illness for cardiovascular and central nervous system abnormalities that may result from treatment.

The total body deficits of potassium are large despite normal or high potassium levels on admission. With treatment of diabetic ketoacidosis, rehydration and insulin therapy cause a marked lowering of plasma potassium levels, which may result in life-threatening hypokalemia. Low-dose insulin therapy is associated with less precipitous declines in potassium levels. Since the total body potassium deficit is great and, owing to urinary losses only 50 percent of administered potassium in 24 hours is retained, total body replacement takes days to achieve. The major concern, therefore, is the prevention of hypokalemia. Potassium therapy is withheld until the serum level is known, and in most cases replacement therapy is begun when the concentration is at the upper half of the normal range. The patient who presents with a low serum potassium level should have vigorous replacement from the start of therapy and electrocardiographic monitoring until the potassium levels reach the normal range. Potassium therapy in all patients should be assessed on the basis of serum levels. An initial rate of 20 to 30 mEq per hour of potassium can be adjusted based on subsequent serum

measurements. Potassium infusion at a rate greater than 40 mEq per hour is rarely indicated and should be done with caution. The predominant form should be potassium chloride salt and the remainder as potassium phosphate. Care must be taken in oliguric patients or those with renal failure, who may need potassium replacement if serum levels fall. Since the usual urinary losses of administered potassium (approximately 50 percent) are not present, replacement should be in the form of potassium chloride at a reduced rate.

Total body phosphorus depletion has long been known to be a component of diabetic ketoacidosis, and there has been recent interest in adding phosphorus replacement to the treatment regimen. Phosphorus depletion theoretically may limit oxygen delivery to tissues by virtue of decreased 2-3DPG levels (which increase hemoglobin oxygen affinity) in addition to limiting phosphorus availability for high energy phosphate bonds. Severe hypophosphatemia may result in hemolysis, rhabdomyolysis, and cardiorespiratory and central nervous system dysfunction. In all series reported to date in which phosphorus repletion has been compared with standard therapy, there have been no changes in morbidity or mortality rates. In most patients, phosphorus levels are normal or high on presentation and fall with insulin and fluid therapy in a manner similar to potassium, since phosphorus is an intracellular anion. The patient with hypophosphatemia on presentation is at greatest risk for developing consequences of phosphorus deficiency. Current recommendations are to provide approximately 10 mM of phosphate per hour as a potassium solution (K 4.4 mEq per liter, PO_4 3.0 mM per milliliter, Abbott) with careful monitoring of phosphorus, and calcium every 4 to 6 hours, since hyperphosphatemia may cause hypocalcemia with tetany. Phosphorus therapy is contraindicated in patients with renal insufficiency.

The use of bicarbonate therapy in cases of diabetic ketacidosis is controversial. The rationale for bicarbonate therapy is simply to counteract the deleterious effects of acidosis in the short term, since appropriate insulin therapy increases ketone body utilization and decreases ketone body production. However, the administration of bicarbonate may cause a paradoxic fall of cerebrospinal fluid pH, which could alter the patient's mental status. Also, bicarbonate therapy may reverse acidosis relatively quickly with the occurrence of hypokalemia. The circumstances under which bicarbonate therapy should be considered are severe acidosis (pH 7.0 to 7.1 or less), the presence of shock unresponsive to volume expansion, and concomitant lactic acidosis. Bicarbonate therapy should never be given in the form of an intravenous bolus, but 1 ampule of sodium bicarbonate (44 mEq Na and 44 mEq HCO_3) should be added to 1 liter 0.45 percent NaCl with 20 mEq per liter of potassium chloride and infused over a 1-hour period. The goal of therapy is to raise pH to 7.2 or the serum bicarbonate level to 12 mEq per liter. Care should be taken to avoid fluid overload, which may occur with the administration of large amounts of sodium ion with the bicarbonate.

PREVENTION

The prevention of diabetic ketoacidosis requires prompt treatment of the precipitating cause as well as intensive therapy for the patient who suddenly begins to develop poor glucose control. Patients should be instructed to maintain fluid intake and, if the normal diet cannot be taken, nutrients should be in the form of carbohydrate containing fluids (juice or nondiet beverages). The patient should continue insulin therapy even though dietary intake is decreased to offset factors that worsen control. Urine testing and finger-stick blood glucose determinations with glucose oxidase strips every 4 to 6 hours should guide supplemental insulin therapy. The physician should keep in close contact with such a patient as well as provide the patient with a sliding scale of how much additional rapid acting insulin (regular, Actrapid) should be given. An example of such a sliding scale based on home glucose monitoring in a patient taking a total of 40 units of insulin daily would be as follows: blood glucose 150 to 200 mg per deciliter, 4 units regular insulin; 200 to 300 mg per deciliter, 8 units regular insulin; 300 to 400 mg per deciliter, 12 units regular insulin. If vomiting and dehydration exist, the patient should be advised to seek early admission to the hospital.

THYROID DISORDERS

RALPH R. CAVALIERI, M.D.

HYPOTHYROIDISM

The presenting signs and symptoms of hypothyroidism in the adult are often nonspecific and insidious in onset, so that the diagnosis of this condition presents a challenge. This is particularly true in the elderly, in whom the manifestation of hypothyroidism can be easily mistaken for senility. Because therapy is so often successful and the results gratifying to all concerned, the physician ought to maintain a high index of suspicion when faced with any patient presenting with dementia, stupor, coma, or any of the other manifestations of myxedema.

The most common cause of hypothyroidism is primary thyroid failure attributable to atrophic autoimmune thyroiditis. Other common causes include destructive therapy (radioiodine treatment or surgical resection) for Graves' disease and total removal of the thyroid for thyroid carcinoma. Radiation therapy for nonthyroid tumors of the head and neck can also lead to delayed hypothyroidism. In certain susceptible individuals, exposure to excess iodine (such as iodide or drugs containing iodine) or administration of lithium can cause myxedema. In contrast to the primary form of the disease, hypothyroidism due to pituitary or hypothalamic dysfunction (i.e., central hypothyroidism) is rare, accounting for no more than 5 percent of all cases of hypothyroidism.

Clinical Presentation

The presenting clinical features, for the most part, involve two organ systems: the skin and the nervous system. The skin is dry, hyperkeratotic, thickened, and cool. The face appears pale and puffy. The hair is often coarse and brittle. The patient seems dull-witted and depressed. Brain dysfunction runs the gamut from mild memory impairment to dementia, psychosis (myxedema madness), seizure, stupor, and, finally, coma. In milder forms the patient may be alert and even display a sarcastic humor (myxedema wit). Other central nervous system (CNS) manifestations that have been described include ataxia, neural deafness, loss of taste and smell, and paresthesias. In any patient with untreated hypothyroidism, the occurrence of somnolence ought to be considered a particularly worrisome sign, as this may quickly progress to stupor and coma, the most serious complication of this disorder. Obviously, CNS depressants should not be administered to hypothyroid patients.

Other clinical manifestations include delayed return of deep tendon reflexes, stiff muscles, slow heart rate, enlarged cardiac silhouette (usually due to a small pericardial effusion), low ECG voltage, slowed peristalsis, (ileus mimicking obstruction may occur), ascites, bleeding diathesis, and anemia (either normocytic hypochromic or macrocytic). Pernicious anemia coexists with primary thyroid failure more often than would be predicted by chance. An important clue to severe hypothyroidism is hypothermia. (Infection may raise the body temperature to normal in such patients.) The presence of exophthalmos or a thyroidectomy scar, of course, should raise the question of thyroid dysfunction in any patient.

Hypothyroid Coma

The term "hypothyroid coma" is preferred to "myxedema coma" because this extremely serious complication may overtake a hypothyroid patient who does not exhibit the full-blown picture of myxedema. The most useful clinical clues to the diagnosis of hypothyroidism as the cause, or a contributing cause, of coma are a history of thyroid disease, particularly previous radioiodine therapy or thyroidectomy, skin manifestations (described previously), hypothermia, hyponatremia, carbon dioxide (CO_2) retention, anoxemia, low ECG voltage, protein-rich effusions, and elevated cerebrospinal fluid (CSF) protein (Figure 1).

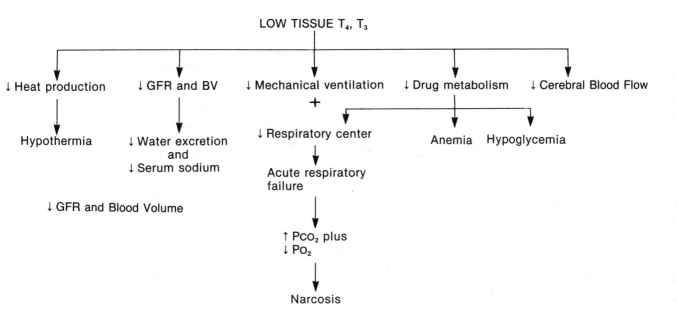

Figure 1 Myxedema coma—pathophysiology

It is important, however, to bear in mind that coma in a hypothyroid patient may be due to causes other than the hypothyroidism. Thus, overwhelming sepsis, encephalitis, cerebrovascular events, head trauma, CO_2 narcosis due to respiratory failure, intoxication by alcohol or other CNS depressants, hyperosmolar state, or hypoglycemia all may be direct causes of coma in a patient who is also hypothyroid. Some of these conditions are reversible with prompt and appropriate therapy, even if the thyroid deficiency is not immediately corrected. For example, mechanical ventilation may rapidly reverse coma due to CO_2 retention even before thyroid hormone replacement takes effect. In some cases, no cause of coma other than hypothyroidism can be found. The prognosis depends as much on the associated or precipitating condition as on the degree of hypothyroidism. Obviously, treatment must be directed at all of the contributing factors.

The elderly hypothyroid patient is at greater risk, particularly because cerebrovascular disease and chronic pulmonary disease are more common in this group. Untreated hypothyroidism at any age renders the patient more susceptible to CNS depressants, including alcohol. Two other points worth emphasizing: one of the most useful telltale signs of infection–namely, fever–may be absent in these cases, and relative or absolute adrenal cortical deficiency may coexist with hypothyroidism.

The initial dose of thyroid hormone given to the patient with hypothyroid coma is larger than that given to the hypothyroid patient who is not comatose, because the former condition is a medical emergency. The T_4-deficit can be calculated from the serum T_4 concentration, as-suming a T_4-distribution volume of 15 percent of body weight. However, thyroid hormone replacement should not be withheld merely because the serum T_4 result is not available. Most authorities recommend giving intravenous L-thyroxine (as the sodium salt) in an initial (loading) dose of 400 to 500 μg (to an average-size adult), followed by 50 to 75 μg IV at 24 hour intervals. The parenteral route is recommended because gastrointestinal absorption is incomplete and unpredictable, especially in severely hypothyroid patients.

Laboratory Diagnosis

The laboratory diagnosis of hypothyroidism rests on two parameters: serum free thyroxine (FT_4) and thyroid-stimulating hormone (TSH) levels. In the absence of a reliable measurement of FT_4, the total T_4 concentration can be used, but it is less specific than FT_4. The finding of a low FT_4 and an elevated TSH is virtual proof of primary hypothyroidism. A clearly normal FT_4 practically rules out clinically significant thyroid failure. Of course, mild cases may present with a low-normal or borderline FT_4 and a high TSH. The latter is an extremely sensitive indicator of mild or incipient primary hypothyroidism. The rare case of central hypothyroidism will usually show a normal or low TSH level and a low FT_4 level; such patients are usually diagnosed by finding evidence of failure of other endocrines (gonads, adrenal) and radiologic signs of pituitary or hypothalamic mass lesions. The laboratory evaluation of thyroid function in the patient with severe nonthyroid illness is discussed at the end of this section.

THYROID STORM

Thyroid crisis, or storm, is a serious complication of thyrotoxicosis characterized by fever, exaggerated manifestations of the hypermetabolic state (tachycardia, tremor, gastrointestinal hypermobility), and CNS dysfunction ranging from agitation, confusion, delerium, psychosis, eventually to coma. Fortunately, thyroid storm as a result of subtotal thyroidectomy occurs very rarely nowadays, thanks to the usually thorough preoperative preparation of the hyperthyroid patient. However, this complication can overtake any untreated or partially treated patient with hyperthyroidism who is exposed to serious intracurrent illness or stress (serious infection, diabetic ketocidosis, trauma, or nonthyroid surgery). The diagnosis of storm in such a patient rests entirely on clinical grounds; the laboratory findings are no different from those in any patient with moderate or severe thyrotoxicosis

Once the diagnosis is made, treatment must be begun immediately. The aims of therapy are (a) to reduce as quickly as possible the output of thyroid hormone from the gland, (b) to blunt the effects of excess thyroid hormone on critical organs (heart, brain, etc.), (c) to discover and treat the associated or precipitating condition (infection, diabetic acidosis, trauma, etc.), and (d) to provide essential nutrients and render supportive care. To accomplish these therapeutic goals, the following measures are taken:

a. High dosages of antithyroid drugs of the thionamide type are given, as well as iodide. Prophylthiouracil (PTU), 300 to 400 mg every 8 hours, is administered orally or by gastric tube. (PTU is not soluble in aqueous solutions.) As an alternative drug, methimazole can be dissolved in water and administered rectally, 40 mg every 8 hours. Within 1 hour after starting PTU or methimazole, iodides ought to be given to stop the secretion of preformed hormone from the gland: Lugol's iodine, 10 drops or potassium iodide (ssKI), 5 drops, orally, or sodium iodide, 0.5 g IV, every 8 hours. The reason for beginning therapy with a thionamide is to prevent the synthesis of more hormone from the iodide administered.

b. Many of the metabolic effects of excess thyroid hormone are attenuated by beta-blocking drugs. Propranolol is given intravenously, if necessary, 1 mg as a test dose injected slowly intravenously, repeated at 5-minute intervals until a drop in heart rate occurs, followed by an infusion of 5 to 10 mg per hour. In less urgent cases, oral propranolol, 40 mg every 6 hours, is recommended to start; the dose is then doubled every 12 hours until a response occurs. It is essential to monitor patients closely for signs of heart failure, which is a risk in the use of beta-blockers. Also, bronchospasm or a history of asthma is a contraindication to the use of these agents.

c. The precipitating condition is usually quite apparent, but infection can be overlooked and must be searched for diligently and treated promptly.

d. Replacement of fluids and electrolytes is important. The hypermetabolic state and the fever that often accompany this condition result in large fluid losses. No less important is the need for calories and vitamins. (Glucose is used at a rapid rate.) Other supportive measures include cooling blankets to reduce fever, pyschotropic drugs to treat agitation, and chlorpromazine, 25 to 50 mg every 4 to 6 hours or even larger doses in the severely agitated or pyschotic patient. Some have advocated use of corticosteroids in the management of thyroid storm and even in patients with severe thyrotoxicosis without overt storm. High dosages of corticosteroids (e.g., dexamethasone 2 mg every 6 hours) provide several benefits: the direct effect on the hyperfunctioning thyroid gland reduces hormone secretion, conversion of T_4 to triiodothyronine T_3 in body tissues is inhibited, and the possible "relative" adrenal insufficiency is treated.

HYPERTHYROIDISM

Most patients with hyperthyroidism present with a clinical picture of a milder degree than storm. The manifestations typically include evidence of hypermetabolism (heat intolerance, warm moist skin, weight loss in spite of normal or increased caloric intake), irritability, emotional lability, proximal muscle weakness, fine tremor, stare with or without proptosis, and cardiac symptoms (tachycardia even at rest, arrhythmias, congestive heart failure). The cardiac manifestations may be the predominant ones in the elderly patient with this disorder. Of course, thyromegaly, when present, is an important diagnostic finding, but the gland is not enlarged on examination in about one-third of elderly patients with hyperthyroid Graves' disease. The laboratory diagnosis of hyperthyroidism depends on finding an elevation of serum free T_4 and/or free T_3 and an increase in radioiodine uptake (RAIU) by the gland. In a minority of these cases the RAIU is normal (again, more often in the elderly). In some forms of thyrotoxicosis (subacute thyroiditis and thyrotoxicosis factitia), the RAIU is low. When serum free T_4 and T_3 levels are only minimally elevated, the thyroid-releasing hormone (TRH)-stimulation test may be helpful, because even slightly raised thyroid hormone levels will block the release of TSH from the pituitary. In all cases of suspected thyrotoxicosis, except those with thyroid storm, antithyroid drugs ought to be withheld until the diagnostic work-up is complete. However, when clinically indicatd, beta-blockers can be begun before RAIU or TRH-testing is done.

THYROID FUNCTION TESTING IN PATIENTS WITH ACUTE NONTHYROID ILLNESS

The problem of detecting thyroid dysfunction in patients with severe non-thyroid-related illness who present to an emergency department is a common one. All types of thyroid functional abnormalities have been described in such patients; yet the vast majority, after extensive testing and follow-up, do not have intrinsic thyroid dysfunction of the type requiring specific therapy. Since the frequency of abnormal laboratory findings increases with the number of tests done, it is generally recognized that the most cost-effective approach is to obtain *one test* that provides the highest possible sensitivity and specificity in those cases in which a *clinical* suspicion of disease is present. In the area of thyroid dysfunction, the single test that meets these criteria is the FT_4. A *normal* FT_4, performed by an appropriate assay, rules out thyrotoxicosis with 95 percent confidence and excludes overt hypothyroidism with nearly 99 percent certainty. A significant minority of severely ill euthyroid patients will exhibit abnormal FT_4 levels, ranging from 10 to 20 percent, depending on the type of assay used. In these "euthyroid-sick" cases, if clinically indicated, additional testing may be necessary–serum TSH if FT_4 is low and serum triiodothyronine if FT_4 is high. The predictive value of an *ab-normal* FT_4 in this population of patients is not very great. Nevertheless, a *normal* FT_4 level is reassuring and has diagnostic utility in the patient with nonthyroid illness.

SUGGESTED READING

Cavalieri RR. Laboratory evaluation of thyroid status. In: Current endocrinology: thyroid. Green WL, ed. New York: Elsevier Science Publishing, in press.

Kaplan MM, Larsen PR, Crantz FR, Dzau VJ, Rossing TH, Haddow JE. Prevalence of abnormal thyroid function test results in patients with acute medical illness. Am J Med 1982; 72:9–16.

Nicoloff JT. Thyroid storm and myxedema coma. Med Clin North Am 1985; 69:1005–1017.

ACUTE ADRENOCORTICAL INSUFFICIENCY

TERENCE D. WINGERT, M.D.
PATRICK J. MULROW, M.D.

Primary adrenocortical insufficiency, or Addison's disease, is attributable to adrenal gland lesions that result in reduced cortisol, aldosterone, and adrenal androgen production. The causes of primary adrenal insufficiency include idiopathic atrophy (probably autoimmune in etiology); granulomatous infections, such as tuberculosis or histoplasmosis; destruction by hemorrhage, tumor, or iron deposition; and adrenalectomy.

Lesions of the hypothalamus or anterior pituitary with decreased adrenocorticotropin (ACTH) production result in secondary adrenal insufficiency. Cortisol and adrenal androgen secretion are reduced, but aldosterone is normal. Diseases of the anterior pituitary that cause secondary adrenal insufficiency include neoplasms, infarction, granuloma, trauma, hypophysectomy, and, rarely, infection.

Suppression of the hypothalamic-pituitary-adrenal axis by administration of supraphysiologic doses of glucocorticoids for nonendocrine diseases can also result in secondary adrenal insufficiency and is the most common cause today. When supraphysiologic doses of glucocorticoid are administered, inhibition of the adrenal gland's ability to respond to ACTH occurs early, within days. Suppression of the hypothalamic-pituitary axis occurs with more prolonged therapy (weeks). Recovery from prolonged supraphysiologic glucocorticoid therapy occurs in the reverse order, with the return of hypothalamic-pituitary responsiveness preceding adrenal recovery. The risk of suppressing the hypothalamic-pituitary-adrenal axis varies widely with the dosage and duration of therapy as well as probable individual varia-bility. Potential suppression of the axis is minimized by alternate-day glucocorticoid therapy. There is little agreement as to when the patient should be considered to be at risk for impaired adrenal reserve. A conservative approach is recommended even though many patients may receive treatment during severe stress who do not require it. As a general rule, patients who have been on daily glucocorticoid therapy for longer than 2 weeks should be considered to have adrenal insufficiency. Glucocorticoids should be administered during stressful situations if endocrine testing has not been performed to document an intact axis. Complete recovery of the pituitary-adrenal axis may take up to 12 months in patients who have been on prolonged glucocorticoid therapy.

DIAGNOSIS

The diagnosis of adrenal crisis is based on the clinical presentation and is a medical emergency. The clinical presentation depends on whether the process is primary or secondary. In primary adrenal insufficiency there is a deficiency in glucocorticoids and mineralocorticoids, as well as adrenal androgens, with a concomitant increase in ACTH from the anterior pituitary. In secondary adrenal insufficiency, the basic deficit is in glucocorticoid production, since ACTH is not the main determinant of mineralocorticoid secretion. In both primary and secondary adrenal insufficiency, the presenting signs and symptoms may be subtle in the unstressed patient (Table 1), and a high index of suspicion is required to make the diagnosis.

When adrenal insufficiency is manifested as the life-threatening disorder of adrenal crisis, it usually presents as a syndrome of weakness, fever, and hypotension. Since many individuals may have enough circulating adrenocorticoids to accommodate normal demands, acute adrenal insufficiency may only occur with additional stress, and a precipitating event, such as infection or trauma, is often present. Thus, acute adrenal insufficiency can be difficult to differentiate from septic shock or hemorrhage. Less severe cases present with nonspecific signs and symptoms. These include anorexia, nausea and vomiting, abdomi-

TABLE 1 Symptoms and Signs of Acute Adrenal Insufficiency

Symptoms
  Weakness and fatigue
  Anorexia
  Nausea and vomiting
  Abdominal pain
  Diarrhea
  Dizziness
  Musculoskeletal complaints

Signs
  Pigmentation (primary adrenal insufficiency)
  Hypotension
  Dehydration (primary adrenal insufficiency)
  Tachycardia
  Fever
  Lethargy and confusion
  Weight loss

nal pain, fatigue, dizziness, and dehydration. The findings can often be confused with a "flu syndrome" or "gastroenteritis."

In a patient who is receiving anticoagulant therapy, acute back or flank pain along with the symptoms just described may signify adrenal hemorrhage. On careful questioning, patients usually admit to symptoms of a chronic illness, unless the etiology of the acute adrenal insufficiency is pituitary or bilateral adrenal hemorrhage or infarction. A history of autoimmune involvement of other glandular or nonglandular tissues (hypoparathyroidism, diabetes mellitus, pernicious anemia, hypogonadism, alopecia, vitiligo, and autoimmune thyroid disease) may occur as well. Regrettably, many cases occur in patients known to have adrenal insufficiency who have not been educated to their need for additional glucocorticoids during times of stress. Also, in a patient with known adrenal insufficiency, a crisis can be precipitated by certain drugs that increase the metabolism of glucocorticoids, such as phenobarbital, diphenylhydantoin, and rifampin.

Genetic abnormalities resulting in enzymatic defects in steroid synthesis (congenital adrenal hyperplasias) are typically the etiology of adrenal insufficiency in infancy.

The physical examination confirms intravascular volume depletion, but the only unique sign of adrenal insufficiency is pigmentation. If present, it indicates primary adrenal insufficiency and would call attention to the correct diagnosis. The pigmentation occurs in the sun-shielded as well as sun-exposed areas, in mucosal surfaces, and, most prominently, in friction areas, flexion creases, and new scars.

In *primary adrenal insufficiency*, laboratory findings are nonspecific, but a low serum sodium level, increased serum potassium level, and an elevated blood urea nitrogen (BUN) suggest the diagnosis. Hypoglycemia and mild metabolic acidosis may also be seen. A complete blood count (CBC) often shows a normochromic, normocytic anemia with a normal or elevated white blood count (WBC) and increased eosinophilia. Hypercalcemia is sometimes seen secondary to volume depletion. If urinary electrolytes are measured, urinary sodium losses are inappropriately high for the intravascular volume depletion. The plasma cortisol measurement can be of some help, but usually the result is available well after the crisis is over. If, in a critically ill patient, the plasma cortisol level is less than 10 μg per deciliter, one can strongly suspect adrenal insufficiency.

In *secondary adrenal insufficiency*, increased pigmentation is not observed. There are usually associated symptoms and signs of failure of other endocrine glands that are also regulated by pituitary hormones. Although vascular collapse may be present owing to a deficiency of cortisol secretion, dehydration generally is not seen since aldosterone secretion remains normal. The BUN and serum potassium are normal, but the serum sodium concentration is frequently low owing to dilutional hyponatremia.

The key to making the diagnosis of adrenal crisis is to have a high index of suspicion for the disorder. Treatment should not be withheld to establish the diagnosis if adrenal crisis is suspected. ACTH testing can be done at a later date while the patient is on maintenance steroid therapy, usually with dexamethasone since it does not interfere with the usual steroid measurement, to confirm the diagnosis.

TREATMENT

Whatever the underlying disease process, the management principles for adrenal insufficiency are basically the same. Once the diagnosis is suspected, treatment should be initiated after a blood specimen for cortisol measurement is drawn, but without awaiting the result. Treatment consists of glucocorticoid replacement and volume expansion (Table 2).

During the crisis, replacement of fluids and electrolytes is as important as hormonal replacement and can be initiated at home or in the ambulance. These patients have volume depletion with severe sodium and water deficits. Volume deficits are generally considerable in primary, but only slight in secondary adrenal insufficiency. Initial

TABLE 2 Treatment of Acute Adrenal Insufficiency

Major stress
  Glucocorticoid: 100 mg IV (bolus) hydrocortisone (Solu-Cortef), immediately followed by 100 mg intravenously continuously every 8 hours until stable
  Intravenous fluids and electrolytes: normal saline and 5 percent dextrose until intravascular volume is stabilized
  Identify and treat precipitating cause

Minor stress
  Glucocorticoid: double dose until illness improves (usually less than 5 days)
  Fluids and electrolytes: high salt and fluid intake
  Educate patient and family members about symptoms and signs that should prompt them to seek further medical attention

therapy should consist of intravenous normal saline and dextrose at a rate determined by the degree of dehydration. The first liter should be given over a period of one hour in adults. Dextrose is necessary to treat the hypoglycemia that may occur in adrenal crisis. Careful monitoring of the blood pressure or, occasionally, central venous pressure is necessary to guide fluid treatment. It is sometimes necessary to give several liters of normal saline in the first 24 hours to maintain adequate blood pressure, and urine output and to replace extracellular volume deficits. Hypertonic saline should not be used; its administration would exaggerate the dehydration of the intracellular space. The hyperkalemia and metabolic acidosis usually respond to volume expansion and hormonal replacement and need no specific therapy. Vasopressors for vascular collapse or bicarbonate for acidosis is rarely needed. If severe hyponatremia is present, frequent measurement of serum sodium concentration is necessary. Rapid normalization of severe, sustained hyponatremia should be avoided to prevent the rare complication of central pontine myelinolysis. Subsequently, body weight and serum electrolytes should be monitored daily to assess response to treatment.

Once the patient is in the emergency department, hydrocortisone should be given parenterally and is available as a water-soluble hemisuccinate or phosphate ester preparation. Steroids with minimal mineralocorticoid activity, such as dexamethasone, should not be used as initial therapy for adrenal crisis. Since maximal glucocorticoid secretion approximates 300 mg per day, this is the dose we recommend. One hundred milligrams should be given as an intravenous bolus, followed by 100 mg every 8 hours as a continuous intravenous infusion. We do not use intramuscular cortisone acetate because of concerns about variable absorption in these gravely ill patients who may be in shock. Three hundred milligrams of hydrocortisone provides sufficient mineralocorticoid activity to render mineralocorticoid replacement unnecessary. Once the patient's condition is stable, the dosage can be reduced daily by approximately one-third until a maintenance dosage of 20 to 40 mg is achieved, usually within 7 days. More than twice replacement doses for prolonged periods should be avoided to prevent side effects from excess glucocorticoids. Specific and effective steroid therapy is available for adrenocortical insufficiency. The more common steroid hormones and their relative potencies are listed in Table 3. When the dosage is less than 100 mg daily, mineralocorticoid replacement is usually needed, and fludrocortisone acetate therapy should be initiated.

The treatment of *precipitating factors* is crucial. We do not give antibiotic therapy routinely, but rather make this determination in each individual case based on clinical and laboratory evidence of infection.

All patients with adrenal crisis need to be hospitalized. The type of hospital bed is determined individually. It is safer to admit these patients to an intensive care unit bed for the first 12 to 24 hours. If the patient is not known to have adrenal insufficiency prior to presentation in adrenal crisis, urgent endocrinologic consultation is

TABLE 3 Relative Potencies of Some Common Steroid Compounds

Steroid	Glucocorticoid Activity	Sodium Retaining Potency
Short-acting steroids		
Cortisol (hydrocortisone)	1	1
Cortisone	0.8	0.8
Intermediate-acting steroids		
Prednisolone	4	0.8
Prednisone	3.5	0.8
Triamcinolone	3-5	0
Long-acting steroids		
Dexamethasone	25-30	0
Fludrocortisone (Florinef)	10	400
11-Deoxycorticosterone	0	20
Aldosterone	0.1	400

desirable. Any other patient who does not promptly improve with therapy should have subspecialty consultation to review management. The patient's condition generally improves within a few hours if the diagnosis of adrenal crisis is correct.

PREVENTION

Anticipation and education of the patient to the need for additional glucocorticoid replacement during periods of stress in individuals with established adrenal insufficiency can prevent adrenal crisis in many cases.

For treatment of minor stress, such as upper respiratory tract infections, fever above 100 °F, or dental extraction, the dosage of glucocorticoid should be doubled until the stress or illness has resolved. Rarely should this increase be necessary for more than 4 to 5 days. If there is no improvement within this time period, the patient should see his physician. If the patient is seriously ill or if vomiting prevents administration of oral medication, the patient should be hospitalized.

Major stress such as a surgical procedure, myocardial infarction, serious injury, and sepsis requires 300 mg of parenteral hydrocortisone daily. If the major stress is a planned event, such as surgery, we recommend that hydrocortisone administration be started the day before or at least a few hours before the stress. This is because there is a slight delay in the effect of glucocorticoids after administration. For example, we give 100 mg intravenously continuously on the night before surgery and every 8 hours until the patient is stable postoperatively. The glucocorticoid therapy should be tapered to the replacement dosage as rapidly as recovery allows.

There is no need to increase mineralocorticoid therapy for stress, as the high levels of glucocorticoids provide adequate mineralocorticoid activity. At times of severe stress when high doses of glucocorticoids are being administered, it may be best to omit the mineralocorticoid therapy temporarily.

Patient education is part of the treatment for individuals with chronic adrenal insufficiency. They must know that they will need to increase their dosage of glucocorticoids for minor stress, recognize symptoms of worsening adrenal insufficiency and report this to their physician, inform all medical professionals that they are steroid-dependent, and carry on their person a card or a "Medic-Alert" bracelet stating that they are steroid-dependent. A kit containing dexamethasone phosphate for intramuscular use is a good idea for patients who do extensive traveling where medical care might not be readily available.

The patient and physician should avoid increasing the replacement dosage of glucocorticoids without objective indication of stress or indication of inadequate replacement. The patient may report subjective improvement in well-being on higher doses of glucocorticoid, but supraphysiologic doses can be hazardous. Acutely (within hours to days), excess glucocorticoids cause increased catabolism of muscle and increased urinary excretion of potassium, calcium, and phosphorus, with decreased excretion of sodium and subsequent fluid retention. Impaired glucose tolerance and suppressed cellular immunity with an increased risk of infection also occur. Chronic (over a period of weeks) excess glucocorticoid therapy elevates blood pressure and causes truncal obesity, osteoporosis, muscle and cutaneous atrophy, vascular fragility, and poor wound healing.

SUGGESTED READING

Norenberg MD, Leslie KO, Robertson AS. Association between rise in serum sodium and central pontine myelinolysis. Ann Neurol 1982; 11:128–135.

Schimke RN. Adrenal insufficiency. Crit Care Q 1980; 3:19–27.

Tzagournis M. Acute adrenal insufficiency. Heart Lung 1978; 7:603–609.

Wingert TD, Mulrow PJ. Chronic adrenal insufficiency. In: Conn RB, ed. Current Diagnosis 7. Philadelphia: WB Saunders, 1985:860–863.

Wingert TD, Mulrow PJ. Adrenocortical insufficiency. In: Bayless TM, Brian MC, Cherniak RM, eds. Current therapy in internal medicine. Toronto and Philadelphia: BC Decker, 1984–1985:439–443.

STARVATION AND DIET-INDUCED EMERGENCIES

NYDA WILLIAMS BROWN, M.D., F.A.G.P.A.

Anorexia nervosa and bulimia, both psychiatric disorders, are characterized by disturbed eating habits. Anorexia nervosa is characterized by a weight loss of 25 percent of the normal weight for the patient's size, with the patient refusing to eat. A family history may indicate concerns over eating habits and amenorrhea. In bulimia, often perceived as the second-stage progression of anorexia nervosa, the patient binges large quantities of food and follows this by vomiting, laxative abuse, overexercising, or taking diet pills or diuretics. There is also a distinct group of women who are bulimic and have never been anorexic. Most of these patients state unequivocally that they are fat, and some do weigh 2 to 20 pounds more than the desired weight for their height. Both bulimic and anorexic patients have a distorted body image, complaining of "being fat," "having fat thighs," or "having cellulite on their bodies." Although anorexia nervosa and bulimia are listed as separate diagnostic entities in the Diagnostic and Statistical Manual (DMS-III), there is a lot of overlap.

Conservative estimates place the incidence of eating disorders at approximately 20 percent of women between the ages of 19 and 24. The mortality rate for "death by starvation" has been reported as high as 24 percent of the anorectic population.

DIAGNOSIS

The most common misdiagnosis is malabsorption syndrome, if the patient is a binge eater and her doctor doesn't know that she purges. Malignancy, hyperthyroidism, amphetamine or cocaine abuse, and diabetes mellitus or insipidus should be ruled out. Many of these can be excluded by the very fact that the patient with an eating disorder insists that she is fat, despite the objective evidence that she is clearly not obese. Patients with these other disorders know that they are thin and are concerned about it.

Bulimics frequently use phrases like "I got sick" to refer to induced vomiting. The physician generally interprets this to mean the patient is nauseated and does not realize that the patient also has an eating disorder. Specific questions must be directed to eating and purging habits. Many of the patients with these diseases are ballet dancers, flight attendants, models, cheerleaders, runners, gymnasts, or waitresses. Most of the patients are female.

Clinical Findings

Clinical findings of these diseases include bradycardia, hypotension, infarction and perforation of the stomach after acute dilatation, mesenteric artery occlusion, aspiration, injury or rupture of the esophagus, severe rectal bleeding from laxative abuse (which can cause anemia), hypokalemic nephropathy, salivary gland enlargement, diabetes mellitus, bleeding gastric ulcer, depressive disorders secondary to starvation, and severe erosion of the enamel of the teeth (Table 1). On electrocardiograms, a starved anorectic or bulimic patient may have S-T and T wave changes, low voltage, a prolonged Q-T interval (which predisposes to ventricular arrhythmias),

TABLE 1   Complications of Fasting

Anemia	Headache
Nausea	Abdominal pain
Orthostatic hypotension	Cramps
Gout	Edema
Renal insufficiency and failure	Oliguria
Amenorrhea	Parotitis
Polyneuritis	Ventricular arrhythmias
Small bowel obstruction	Lactic acidosis

a U wave due to hypokalemia, and various arrhythmias. As the starvation continues, the heart begins to slow; patients have been seen with a heart rate as low as 25 beats per minute. A decrease in the heart size due to atrophy and degeneration may be seen either on chest x-ray films or at autopsy. Because the body's metabolic rate has slowed down, it is not rare to find a body temperature of 96 °F (35.6 °C) or lower. These patients are constantly cold; their blood pressure may be quite low and their pulse slow. Congestive heart failure is not an uncommon consequence of rehydration. Depression, accompanied by withdrawal and decrease of libido, occurs in both male and female patients. The starvation also produces a great deal of weakness and fatigue.

If laxative abuse is suspected because of recurrent diarrhea, a stool sample should be checked for phenolphthalein. Five grams of stool can be sent to National Medical Services (Test #3642) to obtain this information. Furosemide is a favorite diuretic among bulimic patients. A toxicology screen for metabolites of common diuretics may be useful. Vomiting patients should be questioned strongly about whether their vomiting is self-induced. Direct questioning should be done about the use of Ipecac, since one of its active ingredients, emetine, is cardiotoxic and has resulted in the death of bulimic patients when ingested in large quantities.

The anorectic patient brought to the emergency department has usually fainted secondary to low blood pressure or is so weak that she or he can no longer stand and is carried in by parents or friends. Other anorectic patients may present with a bleeding ulcer, diabetes mellitus, or a mesenteric artery occlusion.

A bulimic patient who has abused laxatives may present with severe diarrhea and bloody stools. A bulimic patient who vomits may have throat lacerations secondary to clawing the back of the throat with fingers or other foreign objects to induce vomiting. Bulimic patients who

abuse diuretics present with severe fatigue and dehydration.

Bulimic patients may present with acute gastric dilatation and a rupture of the stomach. Repeated vomiting is associated with parotid enlargement, dental enamel erosion, esophagitis, Mallory-Weiss syndrome, and esophageal tearing or rupture. Vomiting during a state of decreased consciousness, as with concomitant alcohol or drug abuse, may cause aspiration, and many bulimic patients have required mechanical ventilation because of aspiration pneumonia.

EMERGENCY TREATMENT

Initial evaluation includes history, physical examination, electrocardiography, and laboratory work (Table 2). If an anorectic patient shows arrhythmias or prolonged Q-T interval, a potassium level below 3 mEq per liter, a body temperature below 96 °F, low blood pressure, and a heart rate below 30 beats per minute, a *hospital admission* is mandated in order to begin to restore some physical normality to the body and to obtain a psychiatric consultation for continuing treatment. *Toxicology panels* should be obtained on bulimic patients because of their tendency to abuse laxatives, diuretics, and diet pills. A bulimic patient with severe electrolyte abnormalities whose toxicology panel shows the presence of diet pills, diuretics, or laxatives should of necessity have a psychiatric consultation. If this patient has tried on an outpatient basis to stop any of the bulimic behavior and has not succeeded, hospitalization is mandated in order for the patient to break the habit long enough to have a chance at recovery. It is not uncommon to see a bulimic patient who has overdosed on as many as 40 nonprescription diet pills, 15 diuretics tablets, and 60 laxative tablets. With such an overdose, this patient should be admitted to an intensive care unit until she or he can be rehydrated and the electrolyte balance returned to normal.

If the patient is severely dehydrated or is having cardiac arrhythmias secondary to hypokalemia, an intravenous potassium should be started immediately at an appropriate dosage titrated for the patient's electrolyte balance.

Tricyclic antidepressants and monoamine oxidase inhibitors (MAO) have been used with some success with these patients. However, giving either of these drugs to a patient seen only in the emergency department is not advisable because the tricyclics may have adverse effects

TABLE 2   Useful Laboratory Studies in the Fasting/Purging Patient*

CBC—anemia

Electolytes—hypokalemia
Liver function tests—abnormal

LH (luteinizing hormone) and FSH (follicle-stimulating hormone) document degree of starvation by decreasing proportional to weight loss

Growth hormone and thyroid function—usually normal except low T_3

Chest x-ray examination—normal

* Not all are needed in every patient.

on cardiac functioning, and the anorectic patient is unlikely to comply with taking the medication. An MAO inhibitor may be dangerous for a bulimic patient, who will not stay on a prescribed dietary regimen, an absolute must if one is to take these very potent drugs in a safe way. Because bulimic patients who take diet pills, laxatives, or diuretics usually take large quantities of these pills, they tend to treat their antidepressants in the same way and may take an overdose of the pills.

Bulimic patients in particular should be given a routine drug screen because many of them abuse other drugs. They should be questioned about suicidal intent. An involuntary hold for evaluation should be undertaken if the patient is assessed to be a suicidal risk.

SUGGESTED READING

Garfinkel PE, Garnel DM. Anorexia nervosa: a multidimensional perspective. New York: Brunner/Mazel Publishers, 1982.
Herzog DB, Copeland PM. Eating disorders. N Engl J Med 1985; 313:295–303.
Minuchin S, Rosman BL, Baker L. Psychosomatic families: anorexia nervosa in context. Cambridge, Massachusetts: Harvard University Press, 1978.

POTASSIUM DISORDERS

DAVID G. WARNOCK, M.D.

The normal serum potassium (K^+) concentration is 3.8 to 5.0 mEq per liter. While the amount of K^+ in the extracellular compartment (50 to 100 mEq) is only 2 percent of the total body K^+ stores, the daily dietary K^+ intake is equal to this amount. Nearly all of the dietary K^+ load is absorbed and excreted by the kidneys in the steady state. Less than 10 percent of the dietary K^+ load is excreted in the feces and in sweat under normal conditions.

Clinically significant hypokalemia is a chronic process that results from inadequate dietary intake and/or increased excretion of K^+ in the urine (e.g., diuretic-induced renal K^+ wasting) or feces (e.g., malabsorption, diarrhea) (Tables 1 and 2). Hyperkalemia is a more immediate threat to the patient because of its detrimental cardiovascular effects, but it can also be viewed as the result of acute or chronic processes. Acute hyperkalemia represents a failure in the normal rapid regulation of serum K^+ by insulin or beta$_2$-selective catecholamines. Causes include acidosis (a decrease in pH of 0.1 unit will increase K^+ roughly 0.6 mEq per liter), renal failure, potassium-retaining diuretics, severe and extensive tissue injury (crush injuries, electrical injuries, rhabdomyoly-

sis, burns), and rarely, potassium salt ingestion (Table 3). Chronic hyperkalemia represents a failure of the renal K^+ secretory systems. Simultaneous measurement of serum and urine K^+ concentrations will give important insight into the pathogenesis of *chronic* disturbances in K^+ balance.

HYPOKALEMIA

Manifestations

Clinical manifestations depend on the degree of hypokalemia as well as the rate of decline in the serum K^+. Neuromuscular abnormalities (weakness, decreased reflexes, paresthesias, flaccid paralysis with respiratory arrest, tetany) are associated with severe K^+ deficits and serum K^+ levels well below 3.0 mEq per liter. The severity of the neuromuscular manifestations reflects the magnitude of the K^+ deficit. The cardiovascular manifestations of hypokalemia include dysrhythmias, electrocardiogram (ECG) changes (flattened or inverted T waves, U waves, and S-T segment depression) (Fig. 1), and potentiation of digitalis toxicity. Magnesium depletion often parallels K^+ depletion and potentiates the adverse cardiovascular effects of K^+ depletion. Other manifestations of K^+ deficiency include a defect in urinary concentration and dilution, central nervous system (CNS) irritability and polydipsia, nausea and ileus, and

TABLE 1 Etiology of Chronic Disturbances in K+ Balance

Serum K+	Urine K+	Etiology
<3.5 mEq/L	>40 mEq/L	Renal K+ wasting
	<30 mEq/L	Dietary K+ deficiency
		Extrarenal K+ loss (usually GI tract)
>5.0 mEq/L	>40 mEq/L	K+ loading or release by hemolysis, tissue breakdown, etc.
	<40 mEq/L	Renal K+ secretory defect

TABLE 2 Causes of Hypokalemia

Decreased input

Extrarenal K$^+$ loss:
   Cutaneous (burns)
   GI tract (diarrhea, villous adenoma)

Increased renal K$^+$ secretion:
   Diuretics
   Mineralocorticoid excess syndromes
   Renal tubular acidosis
   Magnesium deficiency
   Bartter's syndrome
   Miscellaneous (post-ATN*, obstruction)

Abnormal potassium distribution:
   Alkalemia
   Insulin
   Barium poisoning
   Rapid cell growth (malignancy)
   Catecholamines
   Periodic paralysis

*ATN = acute tubular necrosis

TABLE 3 Causes of Hyperkalemia

Increased input:
   Diet, salt substitutes
   Hemolysis, GI bleeding, crush injuries, catabolism

Decreased renal K$^+$ secretion:
   Inadequate distal delivery of Na$^+$ and fluid
   Impaired renin-aldosterone axis
     Addison's disease, enzyme deficiencies, hypoaldosteronism,
      hyporeninism, drug-induced impairment (heparin, beta-blockers,
      NSAIA*, captopril)
   Aldosterone antagonists (spironolactones, triamterine, amiloride)
   Primary secretory defects
     Sickle cell disease, systemic lupus erythematosus, post-transplant
      defects, obstructive uropathy, interstitial nephritis, amyloidosis,
      congenital defects, familial defects

Abnormal potassium distribution:
   Acidosis
   Hypertonicity
   Beta-blockers
   Periodic paralysis
   Succinylcholine
   Insulin deficiency
   Aldosterone deficiency
   Exercise
   Tissue damage
   Digitalis

*NSAIA = non-steroidal anti-inflammatory agents

impaired carbohydrate tolerance because of blunted insulin release. Metabolic alkalosis is often associated with hypokalemia and may worsen the K$^+$ deficit by increasing renal K$^+$ excretion while bicarbonate is being excreted in the urine.

Treatment

Hypokalemia is not generally as life threatening as hyperkalemia. Therapy is directed at replacing the total body K$^+$ stores to a normal level (Table 4). In most instances, oral K$^+$ replacement therapy is adequate. Potassium chloride (KCl) is the preferred form, except when treating conditions associated with bicarbonate loss (e.g., renal tubular acidosis with hypokalemia, or diarrhea with increased losses of K$^+$ and bicarbonate in the feces). Increasing dietary K$^+$ intake may not be as satisfactory a treatment as oral KCl because most of the K$^+$ in foodstuffs (citrus fruits, tomatoes, potatoes) is accompanied by anions other than chloride. If intravenous K$^+$ replacement therapy is used, then ECG monitoring should be continuous, checking for peaking of the T waves. Serum K$^+$ levels should be monitored every several hours and therapy curtailed if the urine flow rate is less than 20 ml per hour. Coexisting electrolyte disturbances (Mg^{++} depletion, metabolic acidosis, etc.) may have to be treated at the same time as K$^+$ depletion. K$^+$ should not be infused as a bolus, or through any central line because of major life-threatening adverse cardiovascular effects.

Other Considerations

Chronic diuretic therapy is an extremely common cause of K$^+$ deficiency. Reductions in the diuretic dosage or in the dietary sodium chloride (NaCl) intake may decrease diuretic-induced renal K$^+$ wasting. If these maneuvers are not successful, then K$^+$-sparing diuretics (amiloride, spironolactone, triamterene) should be considered.

Disposition

Patients with K$^+$ of less than 2.5 mEq per liter should be hospitalized; those with lesser degrees of hypokalemia can be discharged, but need follow-up within 7 to 10 days.

TABLE 4 K$^+$ Replacement Therapy

Serum K$^+$ (mEq/L)	K$^+$ Deficit (%)	Therapy
3.0–3.5	10	40–60 mEq/day KCl (10% solution, 20 mEq per tsp, or Slow-K tablets, 8 mEq/tablets)
		or
		40 mEq/L in saline, infused over 60–120 min if oral intake is limited by nausea, vomiting, etc.
2.0–2.5	15–20	0.8 mEq/kg/hour IV
2.0	25	1–1.3 mEq/kg/hour IV (use two different peripheral IVs)

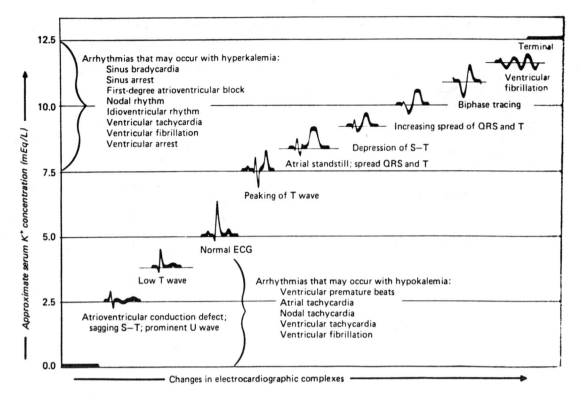

Figure 1 ECG changes in potassium disorders. (Reproduced with permission from Knepp MA, Chatton MJ, eds. Current medical diagnosis and treatment 1974. Los Altos, CA: Large Publishers, 1974.)

TABLE 5 Therapy of Hyperkalemia

Agent	Dosage/Route	Effect
Calcium gluconate	10–20 ml 10% solution IV over 2 min; may be repeated if no response seen after 10 min	Immediate effect, antagonizes K^+ at the membrane level, lasts 30–60 min; use with extreme caution if patient is taking digitalis
Sodium bicarbonate	1 ampule (44 mEq) IV over 5 min; may be repeated if no response seen after 15 min	Immediate effect, promotes K^+ uptake by cells, lasts 60–120 min; volume overload and hypernatremia may be a problem
Insulin and glucose	10–20 units regular insulin with 500 ml D_{10} weight IV over 30–60 min	Promotes K^+ uptake into cells, onset in 30 min, lasts 4–6 hours; watch out for hypoglycemia
Cation exchange resins (Kayexalate)	25 g PO or as a retention enema; also give sorbitol (15 ml of 70% solution) every 30 min to induce diarrhea	Slow onset of action (2 hours), but lasts 4–6 hours; the sodium load may cause worsening of congestive heart failure
Furosemide + saline	40 mg IV with normal saline infused at 100 ml/hour; repeat furosemide dosing to maintain urine flow rate and adjust saline infusion rate accordingly	Slow onset of action, and may cause loss of other electrolytes (e.g., Mg^{++})
Dialysis	Use low K baths with high flow rates	Hemodialysis much more efficient than peritoneal dialysis

HYPERKALEMIA

Manifestations

The cardiovascular complications of severe hyperkalemia (>6.5 mEq per liter) may be life-threatening; they include ventricular fibrillation and even asystole. The severity of the cardiovascular manifestations reflects the severity of the hyperkalemia: tall peaked T waves, depressed S-T segments, decreased R waves, prolonged P-R interval, atrial asystole, widened QRS complexes, and an agonal sine wave pattern (see Fig. 1). ECG monitoring should be instituted whenever hyperkalemia is suspected, and therapy should be instituted on the basis of the ECG findings, even before laboratory confirmation.

The neuromuscular manifestations of hyperkalemia are very similar to those of hypokalemia; these include weakness-diminished reflexes, paresthesias, and paralysis with respiratory arrest.

Therapy

Acute therapy is directed primarily at increasing K^+ uptake into nonrenal cells by use of the stimulatory effects of insulin and "membrane stabilization," with calcium and bicarbonate (Table 5). Decreasing the total body K^+ stores (gastrointestinal losses, decreased intake, increased renal excretion) is an important adjunct in the acute setting and the treatment of choice for chronic hyperkalemia. Significant acidosis, if present, may account for hyperkalemia and should be corrected also.

Other Considerations

Chronic hyperkalemia is usually attributable to defects in renal K^+ secretion (e.g., hyporeninemic hypoaldosteronism). These conditions will usually respond to a liberal NaCl diet plus oral diuretics (furosemide or thiazides). Some patients require mineralocorticoid replacement therapy or may even require pharmacologic amounts of mineralocorticoids. It is imperative to rule out iatrogenic causes of hypokalemia in the setting of mild to moderate renal insufficiency with hypoaldosteronism. Hyperkalemia is very commonly caused in this setting by oral K^+-sparing diuretics (amiloride, spironolactone, triamterene), beta-blockers, nonsteroidal anti-inflammatory agents, and converting enzyme inhibitors. Continued oral KCl replacement therapy in patients with mild to moderate renal insufficiency can cause serious hyperkalemia.

SUGGESTED READING

Alvo M, Warnock DG. Hyperkalemia—medical staff conference. Western J Med 1984; 141:666–671.
Sebastian A, Hernandez RE, Schambelan M. Disorders of renal handling of potassium. In: Brenner BM, Rector FC Jr, eds. The kidney. Vol I. 3rd ed. Philadelphia: WB Saunders, 1986: 619.
Smith JD, Bia MJ, DeFronzo RA. Clinical disorders of potassium metabolism. In: Arieff AI, DeFronzo RA, eds. Fluid, electrolyte and acid-base disorders. Vol I. New York: Churchill-Livingstone, 1985: 413.

HYPERCALCEMIA AND HYPOCALCEMIA

MICHAEL KLEEREKOPER, M.B., B.S., F.A.C.P.
D. SUDHAKHER RAO, M.B., B.S., F.A.C.P.

HYPERCALCEMIA

Hypercalcemia is common but only rarely does it threaten life and require emergency therapy. The clinical features of acute, symptomatic hypercalcemia include dehydration with postural hypotension, nausea, vomiting, lethargy, drowsiness, and if severe enough, coma. No specific features clearly distinguish acute hypercalcemia from other acute metabolic or toxic encephalopathies. Acute symptomatic hypercalcemia is most often a complication of malignant disease. Thus, one must also consider cerebral metastases in the differential diagnosis, and the index of suspicion of hypercalcemia should be high in patients with known malignant disease, particularly if skeletal metastases are known to be present or if the patient has symptoms of skeletal pain or tenderness. The absence of certain clinical findings (e.g., normal or only minimally elevated blood glucose on Chemstix testing, jaundice, or overt signs of uremia) should also alert the physician to the possibility of acute hypercalcemia.

With few, if any, exceptions, patients with acute symptomatic hypercalcemia are markedly dehydrated, and the mainstay of initial therapy during the first several hours is rapid rehydration with intravenous normal saline at a rate of at least 200 ml per hour. It is therefore inappropriate to withhold this treatment while awaiting biochemical confirmation of hypercalcemia in any patient in whom this diagnosis is being considered.

Most patients with hypercalcemia are not acutely ill and do not require urgent medical therapy. In general, the more severe the hypercalcemia and the more rapid the rise in serum calcium, the more likely that symptoms and signs are present, but patient tolerance of hypercalcemia varies considerably. One patient might be acutely ill with a serum calcium of only 13 to 14 mg per deciliter, whereas the next patient is relatively asymptomatic with a serum calcium of 16 mg per deciliter. This is a clinical situation in which one must treat the patient and not necessarily the serum calcium level.

Pathogenesis of Hypercalcemia

The various clinical entities that can cause hypercalcemia are listed in Table 1. The table also includes the relative frequency with which these diseases are associated with acute, symptomatic hypercalcemia and a brief description of the principal mechanism that results in hypercalcemia. In all cases of acute hypercalcemia there is an initial increase in the filtered load of calcium delivered to the kidney. As long as the glomerular filtration rate (GFR) is normal, the kidney can handle this increased filtered load of calcium; this results in progressive hypercalciuria without hypercalcemia. If there is a marked increase in the rate of bone resorption (i.e., growth of metastases) or a decrease in GFR, the kidney loses its ability to handle the increased filtered load of calcium, and hypercalcemia rapidly ensues. As hypercalcemia develops, several factors that further reduce GFR complicate the clinical picture and aggravate the hypercalcemia. An elevated serum calcium does, per se, decrease GFR. The patient also develops polyuria and polydipsia, largely as a result of an osmotic diuresis; maintaining adequate oral intake thus becomes increasingly difficult. As serum calcium rises further, nausea with or without vomiting occurs, further reducing the GFR and the ability to maintain fluid balance by the oral route. If serum calcium rises to a level at which mental function is impaired, the fluid balance falls even further behind and a life-threatening emergency develops.

Therapy of Acute Hypercalcemia

Initial Therapy

Because all patients with acute symptomatic hypercalcemia are clinically dehydrated at presentation, immediate therapy must begin with rehydration. The fluid of choice is normal saline at a rate of at least 200 ml per hour. Although it may not always be possible to restore normocalcemia with intravenous saline, this therapy alone is often sufficient to ameliorate the acute symptoms. Early in the course of therapy a, central venous pressure (CVP) monitoring system should be established and the patient given sufficient intravenous fluid replacement to restore CVP to normal without overshooting. Congestive cardiac failure so frequently complicates the initial fluid replacement phase of therapy for hypercalcemia when the patient is inadequately monitored that it has become almost standard practice to administer the diuretic furosemide in conjunction with the intravenous saline. This practice should be discouraged! There is no convincing evidence that calcium diuresis is enhanced by this diuretic in

dosages of less than 80 to 100 mg furosemide every hour. In fact, too often the reverse occurs—a sufficient amount of furosemide is given to reduce GFR, thereby aggravating hypercalcemia, without enough being provided to enhance a calcium diuresis. Hypokalemia often accompanies acute hypercalcemia. This may not be apparent initially while the patient is dehydrated, but may be detected only during rehydration. This is another reason for avoiding furosemide. The serum potassium must be monitored regularly during the initial therapy for hypercalcemia and potassium replacement provided as needed. Because the action of digitalis is potentiated by hypercalcemia, this drug must be discontinued in all acutely hypercalcemic patients.

Subsequent Therapy

The goal of the emergent therapy for hypercalcemia is to lower the serum calcium to a level at which the symptoms are substantially ameliorated. This does not mean that all patients need to be given emergency treatment until normocalcemia is achieved. There is generally no need to give any other therapy until rehydration is complete. By that time most patients have been transferred out of the emergency department to an intensive care unit or an oncology unit equipped to handle this syndrome. In patients whose clinical picture is not sufficiently alleviated by rehydration with normal saline, the next approach should be to administer synthetic salmon calcitonin (Calcimar), 100 MRC (Medical Research Council) units, subcutaneously every 8 hours. This is a very safe agent with few side effects. The only worrisome side effect is a possible anaphylactic reaction to the foreign protein; therefore, a skin test should be performed on each patient before this drug is used. This can be achieved with 0.10 ml of a 1:10 dilution (1 MRC unit) given subcutaneously; the patient should be observed for the development of a wheal and flair reaction at the injection site.

A significant reduction in serum calcium should be apparent within 12 to 24 hours if the calcitonin is going to be effective. Unfortunately, the response to calcitonin is unpredictable. The response is often potentiated by concomitant use of corticosteroids, e.g., hydrocortisone ace-

TABLE 1 Causes of Acute Hypercalcemia

Disease	Frequency	Mechanism for Hypercalcemia
Skeletal metastases Primary in thyroid, lung, breast, kidney, ovary	Most common	Widespread skeletal destruction
Squamous carcinoma without metastases Most commonly lung, but can occur with any solid tissue malignancy	Common	Humoral hypercalcemia of malignancy (HHM) with production of bone resorbing agents (lymphokines and monokines) by the tumor
Multiple myeloma	Common	HHM with widespread marrow infiltration
Primary hyperparathyroidism	Uncommon	Excess parathyroid hormone secretion
Vitamin D intoxication; granulomatous disease (TB, sarcoid)	Rare	Excess administration or production of 1–25 dihydroxycholecalciferol
Thiazide diuretic	Rare	Decreased renal excretion of calcium
Milk alkali syndrome	Rare	Increased intestinal absorption of calcium
Hyperthyroidism (endogenous and exogenous)	Rare	Increased bone resorption
Addison's disease	Rare	Unknown

tate 100 mg IV every 8 hours. This drug is also relatively free of side effects when given at this dosage for a short period of time (less than 1 week), so many clinicians who frequently treat acute hypercalcemia have adopted the practice of routinely administering calcitonin and steroids.

An alternative therapy is mithramycin, administered intravenously over 4 hours in a dosage of 25 μg per kilogram per body weight. This drug is more predictably effective than calcitonin and/or steroids, but has a delayed onset of action, and no fall in the serum calcium may be seen inside 24 to 48 hours. We therefore prefer to initiate second-line therapy with calcitonin and steroids. Mithramycin is an antimitotic agent with significant potential for bone marrow, liver, and kidney toxicity. These complications are dose and duration dependent and should not complicate therapy with one or two courses of mithramycin given in the above dosage. However, many patients who develop acute symptomatic hypercalcemia have recently been given therapy with other antineoplastic drugs, so it is essential to check for marrow suppression and hepatic and renal dysfunction before administering mithramycin. In common with many other antimitotic drugs, nausea is a frequent side effect of mithramycin therapy; thus, an antinausea agent should be administered with each infusion of this drug. Because the onset of action of mithramycin is delayed and its effectiveness may not peak until 72 hours after a single infusion, mithramycin therapy should not be repeated more often than once every 72 hours. There is no documented advantage to using a dose higher than 25 μg per kilogram of body weight for the treatment of hypercalcemia.

In rare circumstances the above approaches either do not control the hypercalcemia or are contraindicated. Other effective therapeutic modalities must be mentioned for completeness, but their use is rarely required by the emergency physician. In the anuric patient in whom a diuresis cannot be induced by intravenous saline replacement, acute hemodialysis against a zero or low (1 mEq per liter) calcium dialysate rapidly lowers the serum calcium. This effect is transient and the serum calcium rises toward predialysis levels within hours after dialysis has been completed. When necessary, the dialysis may be repeated. Intravenous phosphate (100 mmol IV over 6 hours) or intravenous trisodium ethylenediaminetetraacetic acid (EDTA) (3 g IV over 20 to 60 minutes) will both rapidly lower the serum calcium, usually within 1 to 4 hours. However, the potential for toxicity (local tissue necrosis if the fluid extravasates out of the vein, deposition of calcium phosphate in blood vessels, soft tissue, and kidneys) is so great it precludes the use of these drugs in most circumstances.

HYPOCALCEMIA

In contrast with hypercalcemia, clinically significant hypocalcemia is relatively uncommon, usually chronic, and most commonly due either to deficiency of parathyroid hormone (PTH) or some factor that impairs PTH action on its target organs (kidney, bone, and intestine).

Acute hypocalcemia is also uncommon; it is almost always caused by some iatrogenic factor such as that following neck surgery for hyperthyroidism or hyperparathyroidism or that following an aggressive therapy for hypercalcemia. The majority of patients seen in the emergency department have acute hypocalcemia. From both the diagnostic and therapeutic points of view it is convenient to consider chronic hypocalcemia under two general categories (Table 2).

Clinical Features of Hypocalcemia

Symptoms of hypocalcemia depend not only on the cause of hypocalcemia (PTH versus calciferol deficiency), but also on how rapidly it develops (acute versus chronic). Acute hypocalcemia, by definition, is almost always symptomatic, whereas chronic hypocalcemia may be seen without overt clinical manifestations. The earliest symptoms include tingling and numbness in hands and feet and circumoral paresthesias. Later, frank tetany may develop. Tetany, either latent or overt, results from increased neuromuscular excitability and can occur not only in hypocalcemia, but also in hypokalemia, hypomagnesemia, and alkalosis. In severe cases generalized seizures, similar to those of idiopathic epilepsy, may occur. Since calcium is an important trophic agent for skin and its appendages, chronic infections of the nail and nailbed may be seen. Enamel hypoplasia and pitting, staining, or fracture of the teeth may occur in young patients with chronic hypocalcemia. Cataracts, the most frequent complication of chronic hypocalcemia, is usually seen in PTH-deficiency hypocalcemia, but cataracts can also occur in any form of hypocalcemia of greater than 6 months duration. Less frequent complications include soft tissue and basal ganglion calcifications, cardiac arrhythmias, and increased intracranial pressure.

Skeletal symptoms or signs such as bone pain, fracture, or deformity are almost always seen in calciferol-deficiency hypocalcemia and are rarely if ever seen in PTH-deficiency hypocalcemia.

Treatment

It is necessary to distinguish between acute hypocalcemia, in which alleviation of symptoms is the main object, and chronic hypocalcemia, in which normalization of serum calcium is important even in the absence of symptoms.

Acute Hypocalcemia

The agent of choice for treatment of acute symptomatic hypocalcemia is intravenous calcium gluconate. It is available as a 10 percent solution and should be infused slowly over a period of about 10 to 15 minutes; this is to avoid potential cardiac arrhythmias. An alternative preparation is calcium chloride, but because of the hazards of local tissue necrosis at the site of injection, it is best avoided if possible. Depending on the clinical response and serum clacium level during the first 24

TABLE 2 Comparison of the Distinguishing Features of the Two Types of Hypocalcemia

Presenting Features	PTH Deficiency	Calciferol Deficiency
Clinical		
Major symptom	Neuromuscular	Skeletal
Cataracts	Common	Rare
Soft tissue or basal ganglion calcifications	Common	Rare
Biochemical (serum)		
Calcium	Low	Low
Phosphate	High	Low
Alkaline phosphatase	Normal	High
Immunoreative PTH	Low or high	High
Roentgenographic	Normal	Rickets or osteomalacia

hours, therapy with calciferol or its newer metabolites is usually needed in most patients. A reliable plan of treatment for a newly diagnosed hypoparathyroidism is to begin therapy with calcidiol (Calderol), in the following dosage schedule: administer 200 μg of calcidiol daily for 2 days, 100 μg daily for the next 2 days, and then 50 to 75 μg daily with future adjustments as necessary. The corresponding dosage schedule for calcitriol (Rocaltrol) will be 2.0 μg for 2 days, 1.0 μg for the next 2 days, and then 0.5 μg to 1.0 μg daily. This is somewhat analogous to administering digitalis and should normalize serum calcium within a week. Intravenous calcium can be discontinued within 48 hours after oral calcium has been initiated. Further adjustments should be made depending on the clinical and biochemical response (see below).

Chronic Hypocalcemia

Treatment of this type of hypocalcemia is exemplified in the long-term management of hypoparathyroidism, since this is the most common cause of chronic hypocalcemia. All patients require life-long therapy with some form of calciferol or its metabolites. Supplemental oral calcium is also needed in most patients. Magnesium deficiency is frequently seen in these individuals and may be responsible for failure of serum calcium to return to normal.

Other causes of inadequate response include use of deteriorated calciferol preparations, associated intestinal malabsorption, or anticonvulsant therapy.

Calciferol intoxication is a constant problem during therapy of hypoparathyroidism. Thiazide diuretic therapy may potentiate the effect of calciferol and thus lead to the development of hypercalcemia in a previously stable patient. Because requirements may change from time to time, patients need to be closely monitored. Treatment of calciferol intoxication is discussed in the previous section. Hypercalcemia resulting from calciferol toxicity is predictably responsive to corticosteroid therapy.

SUGGESTED READING

Binstock ML, Mundy Gr. Effect of calcitonin and glucocorticoids in combination on the hypercalcemia of malignancy. Ann Intern Med 1980; 93:269–272.
Heath DA. The emergency management of disorders of calcium and magnesium. In: Sönksken P, Lowy C, eds. Clinics in endocrinology and metabolism Vol 9. London: WB Saunders, 1980:487.
Mundy GR, Ibbotson KJ, D'Souza SM, Simpson EL, Jacobs JW, Martin TJ. The hypercalcemia of cancer. Clinical implications and pathogenic mechanism. N Engl J Med 1984; 310:1718–1727.
Rao DS. Disorders of divalent ion metabolism. In: Stein JH, et al, eds. Internal medicine systematic approach. Boston: Little, Brown, 1983:1836.

MAGNESIUM DISORDERS

FAITH T. FITZGERALD, M.D.
CONNIE WHITESIDE YIM, M.D.

HYPOMAGNESEMIA

Magnesium is the fourth most abundant cation in the human body and the second most abundant in the cells.

Total body magnesium averages 24 g, of which 60 percent resides in bone and 20 percent in skeletal muscle. Less than 1 percent is extracellular. Approximately one-third of plasma magnesium is protein bound. Normal serum levels in most laboratories are 1.6 to 2.1 mEq per liter.

Magnesium is an essential activator of numerous enzyme systems including those involving adenosine triphosphate. Thus it is important in oxidative phosphorylation, cell membrane permeability, neuromuscular excitability, muscle contraction, protein nucleic acid and fat synthesis, and stabilization of nuclear proteins.

The average daily U.S. diet contains 20 to 40 mEq of magnesium, obtained primarily from green vegetables. The daily intake required for positive magnesium balance is 0.30 mEq per kilogram (2 to 3 mEq per day for a 70-kg person). Its major absorptive site is the small bowel. The kidneys play a major role in the conservation and excretion of magnesium. Magnesium deficiency occurs when intake is inadequate, when requirement is markedly increased (as in growing children or pregnant or lactating women), when there is a deficit in absorption, or when there are increased losses. Table 1 provides a list of common causes of hypomagnesemia.

Manifestations

The effects of hypomagnesemia are difficult to differentiate from those due to associated metabolic abnormalities or underlying disorders. Magnesium deficiency perpetuates other electrolyte losses, commonly leading to hypokalemia, hypophosphatemia, and hypocalcemia. The major abnormalities noted in association with low serum magnesium levels involve the neuromuscular and cardiovascular systems. Early manifestations include anorexia, nausea, vomiting, diarrhea, personality changes, and intellectual defects. More profound magnesium deficits lead to neurologic hyperirritability manifesting as muscular fibrillation, tremors, ataxia, weakness, hyperreflexia, and vertical nystagmus. Tetany can occur (in the presence of normal serum calcium) and responds to magnesium replacement. Psychosis is occasionally seen and is attributed to interference with thiamine utilization by magnesium deficiency. Although the role of magnesium in adult seizure disorders is not established, neonatal hypomagnesemia may cause convulsions in infants who require exchange transfusions, who are born of mothers with hypomagnesemia, or who have magnesium malabsorption.

Cardiovascular effects primarily are arrhythmias including paroxysmal supraventricular tachycardia, ventricular extrasystoles, ventricular tachycardia, and ventricular fibrillation. Magnesium affects both calcium and potassium metabolism in the cardiovascular system. Be-

TABLE 1 Causes of Hypomagnesemia

Acute and chronic alcoholism

Gastrointestinal disease

    Malabsorption
    Short bowel syndromes
    Severe diarrhea
    Nasogastric suction
    Biliary, pancreatic, or fecal fistulae
    Laxative abuse

Renal loss

    Diuretics (including osmotic diuretics)
    Tubular abnormalities (amphotericin, cisplatinum, carbenicillin, aminoglycoside toxicity)
    Diuretic phase of acute tubular necrosis
    Hormonal–tubular effects (renal tubular acidosis, hypercalcemic states, hyperaldosteronism)
    Familial hypomagnesemia (rare)
    Renal disease: pyelonephritis, glomerulonephritis, chronic renal failure with magnesium wasting

Endocrine disease

    Hypoparathyroidism
    Hyperparathyroidism
    Primary or secondary hyperaldosteronism
    Hyperthyroidism
    Diabetic ketoacidosis, during and following treatment

Decreased intake

    Starvation
    Hyperalimentation with magnesium–poor solutions
    Protein–calorie malnutrition

Miscellaneous

    Acute pancreatitis
    Multiple transfusions with citrated blood
    Cardiopulmonary bypass
    Neonate of hypomagnesemic mother

cause magnesium is essential for activating Na-K-ATPase, deficiency causes cardiac cells to lose potassium, which alters the resting membrane potential, conductivity, and repolarization. Because magnesium is also a calcium inhibitor, insufficient magnesium increases slow calcium-mediated currents and increases the risk of arrhythmias. It has been demonstrated in animal studies that magnesium deficiency significantly lowers the dose of digoxin necessary to induce malignant ventricular arrhythmias.

A serum magnesium level should be obtained in the presence of: suggestive clinical features; conditions known to cause magnesium depletion; or unexplained hypokalemia, hypophosphatemia, hypocalcemia, or hyponatremia. Because serum magnesium varies with changes in acid-base status, serum albumin, and other factors, a normal value may not rule out total body magnesium deficiency. A low level, however (below 1.5 mEq per liter) in the presence of suggestive clinical signs or risk factors, mandates therapy. Measuring urine magnesium after magnesium administration is a useful confirmatory test if the diagnosis is equivocal. Thirty millimoles of magnesium sulfate in 500 cc D5W is infused over 12 hours. Twenty-four-hour urine is collected from the beginning of the infusion. This should not be performed in patients with renal insufficiency, cardiac conduction defects, or respiratory insufficiency. In magnesium deficiency, usually more than 50 percent of magnesium administered is retained. A retention of less than 30 percent indicates that magnesium deficiency is unlikely.

Therapy

The route of therapy of magnesium deficiency depends on the severity of the illness of the patient (Table 2). In a patient who has no clinical signs or symptoms and no defect of intestinal magnesium absorption, adequate diet and supplementary oral magnesium are sufficient. Various preparations of magnesium salts can be given, using aluminum hydroxide gel to prevent diarrhea. Magnesium levels should be followed as the percent of oral magnesium absorbed is variable.

In patients who cannot tolerate or absorb magnesium orally, replacement can be given parenterally. In chronic hypomagnesemia the deficit is estimated to be 1 to 2 mEq per kilogram. Because the kidneys excrete up to 50 percent of parenteral magnesium, 2 to 4 mEq per kilogram should be given over 5 days. A safe intramuscular regimen consists of 2 g (16.3 mEq) intramuscularly every 4 hours in 5 doses on day 1, followed by 1 g (8.1 mEq) every 6 hours on days 2 through 5. If the intramuscular route cannot be used, a 10 percent solution of magnesium sulfate can be given intravenously. On day 1, give 10 g (82 mEq) in 2 L of fluid with 5 g (41 mEq) per liter. On days 2 through 5 give a total of 6 grams (49 mEq) per day distributed evenly in intravenous fluids.

For life-threatening states such as seizures, coma, or arrhythmias, 2 g of magnesium sulfate (10 ml of a 20 percent solution) may be given intravenously over 1 minute followed by 5 g of magnesium sulfate in 500 cc D5W over 5 to 6 hours. The patient should receive treatment over

TABLE 2 Therapy of Magnesium Deficiency

Adults

  Oral

    Milk of Magnesia: 1 tsp 4 times daily

    Magnesium hydroxide tablets: 300 mg 4 times daily

    Magnesium acetate: (9.35 mEq/g of a 10% solution) 10 ml in water 4 times daily as tolerated

  Intramuscular (Magnesium sulfate, 50% solution)

    Day 1: 2.0 g (16.3 mEq) every 4 hours × 5 doses

    Day 2–5: 1.0 g (8.1 mEq) every 6 hours

  Intravenous (Magnesium sulfate, 10% solution)

    Day 1: 10 g (82 mEq) in 2 L fluid

    Day 2–5: 6 g (49 mEq) distributed equally in fluid

  Emergency Intravenous Treatment (Magnesium Sulfate, 20% solution)

    Day 1: 2 g (16.3 mEq) given over 1 minute followed by 5 g (40.5 mEq) in 500 ml solution over 5–6 hours

    Day 2–5: Follow above intramuscular or intravenous schedule.

Infants

  Oral

    Milk of magnesia (2.7 mEq/ml): 1–2 ml 3 times daily

    Magnesium sulfate, 50% solution: 0.5–2.0 mEq/kg (0.125–0.5 ml/kg) in divided doses. Dilute to 12.5–25% solution before use.

  Intramuscular (Magnesium sulfate, 50% solution) 0.4–1.0 mEq/kg (0.1–0.25 ml/kg) × 3–4 doses. In very small infants use a 12.5–25% solution.

  Intravenous (Magnesium sulfate, 1% solution) 0.5–1.0 mEq diluted in 6–10 ml given at a rate not to exceed 1 ml/min

Older Children

  Treat as for infants. If chronic malabsorption is present, may require up to 20–30 mEq daily.

the next 5 days following one of the parenteral recommendations above. Transient hypotension may develop with rapid intravenous replacement due, in part, to cutaneous vasodilatation, so the patient should be supine. When giving intravenous magnesium, calcium chloride (5 cc of a 10 percent solution) should be available for intravenous injection over 30 seconds in case of magnesium overdose (hypotension, respiratory insufficiency, muscle paralysis).

Hypomagnesemia in infants is often detected by hypocalcemia resistant to calcium replacement, hyperirritability, or convulsions. The asymptomatic patient can be treated orally with magnesium sulfate in a dose of 3 mEq per kilogram per day, using a 12.5 to 25 percent solution to prevent diarrhea. Parenteral administration is indicated when the infant is symptomatic or when gastrointestinal absorption may be insufficient. Intramuscular injection is the preferred route, using a dose of 0.4 to 1.0 mEq per kilogram (0.1 to 0.25 ml per kilogram) of a 50 percent solution of magnesium sulfate every 12 hours for 3 to 4 doses. Because magnesium is an irritant, it should be given deep into the muscle of the mid-thigh. In very small infants a more dilute solution (12.5 to 25 percent) is preferable. Intravenous injection is indicated

TABLE 3 Manifestations of Magnesium Excess

Approximate Magnesium Level	Signs and Symptoms
3–5 mEq/L	Bradycardia, cutaneous vasodilatation, nausea, vomiting, loss of deep tendon reflexes, hypotension
5–10 mEq/L	Drowsiness, stupor, ECG changes (increased P-R, QRS, Q-T intervals)
10–15 mEq/L	Muscle paralysis, respiratory depression, narcosis
15 mEq/L or greater	Complete heart block, asystole

if there are continuous seizures or the other routes can not be used. One-half to one milliequivalent of a 1 percent solution of magnesium sulfate can be given in 6 to 10 ml at a rate not to exceed 1 ml per minute. The electrocardigram (ECG) should be monitored and the blood pressure obtained during and after administration, because magnesium can have cardiac effects similar to those of calcium and can cause hypotension. In older children, treatment regimens are similar unless chronic malabsorption is present. These patients require larger quantities, up to 20 to 30 mEq daily.

HYPERMAGNESEMIA

Magnesium excess is an uncommon but potentially life-threatening problem occurring usually as a result of magnesium administration. It is seen most commonly in patients with acute or chronic renal failure whose glomerular filtration rate (GFR) is less than 10 to 30 ml per minute, especially if there is concurrent use of magnesium-containing antacids, enemas, infusions, or excessive dialysate magnesium. In normal individuals hypermagnesemia from oral administration is rare, but it has been reported after use of magnesium-containing enemas. Rapid intravenous therapy for toxemia of pregnancy or magnesium deficiency can lead to severe toxicity. Hypermagnesemia has been reported in neonates of mothers treated for toxemia. Administration of magnesium solutions to patients with megacolon, inflammatory bowel disease, or perforated viscus can also lead to toxic levels. Uncommon causes of mild to moderate magnesium excess include lithium ingestion, hypothyroidism, viral hepatitis, mild-alkali syndrome, acute diabetic ketoacidosis, and Addison's disease.

Patients with hypermagnesemia are usually asymptomatic until the serum level exceeds 3 mEq per liter. Above this level toxicity manifests itself primarily in the neuromuscular, cardiovascular, and gastrointestinal systems (see Table 1). Magnesium levels should be monitored in patients with acute or chronic renal failure whose GFR is less than 30 ml per minute. Serum magnesium levels should be obtained in the setting of acute deterioration of renal function, hypotension or acidemia, unexplained low anion gap, or symptoms or signs that suggest hypermagnesemia.

Therapy of magnesium excess in adults is determined by clinical signs and the serum level. In patients who are asymptomatic with levels less than 5 mEq per liter, treatment can be limited to correcting the underlying cause and limiting magnesium ingestion. Symptomatic patients with serum levels greater than 5 mEq per liter and any patients with levels greater than 8 mEq per liter should be actively treated. Calcium chloride (5 ml of a 10 percent solution) given over 30 seconds transiently reverses symptoms. If improvement is not seen in 2 minutes, this can be repeated. Further doses may be indicated in life-threatening situations. Peritoneal dialysis or hemodialysis rapidly lowers serum magnesium levels. Cardiac and respiratory support may be required. Hypokalemia, if present, should be treated.

In children who have minimal symptoms and normal renal function, serum magnesium may be lowered by increasing fluid intake. If respiratory insufficiency, weakness, or neurologic or ECG changes are present, exchange transfusion or dialysis is indicated depending on the age of the child. Cardiac and respiratory support may be required. A 10 percent solution of calcium gluconate (0.1 ml per kilogram) given intravenously over 2 minutes is useful acutely to counteract the effects of magnesium on the heart. If no response is obtained in 2 to 3 minutes, the dose may be repeated.

SUGGESTED READING

Flink EB. Nutritional aspects of magnesium metabolism. West J Med 1980; 1239:304–312.

Rude RK, Singer FR. Magnesium deficiency and excess. Ann Rev Med 1981; 32:245–259.

PHOSPHATE DISORDERS

FAITH T. FITZGERALD, M.D.
CONNIE WHITESIDE YIM, M.D.

HYPOPHOSPHATEMIA

The adult human body contains 500 to 700 gm of phosphate, of which 80 to 85 percent is in bone. The majority of remaining phosphorus is intracellular, where it is the primary anionic buffer. Normal serum levels range from 3 to 4.5 mg per deciliter in adults and 5 to 7 mg per deciliter in young children. These normal values may vary slightly with diet, time of day, respiratory rate, and hormonal status. Serum phosphorus levels, like serum levels of other primarily cellular ions, may not accurately reflect total body stores.

Phosphorus is an important constituent of cellular structure, nuclear proteins, and aderosine triphosphate (ATP). In addition it influences serum calcium levels, helps to regulate the rate of glycolysis, and (as a constituent of 2, 3-diphosphoglycerate) participates in the delivery of oxygen to body tissues.

Dietary intake varies enormously, but it is rarely deficient, because phosphorous is abundant in ordinary foods and readily absorbed by the normal intestine. The kidney is the principal excretory route.

The individual physician's chances of encountering clinically significant hypophosphatemia depends on the nature of the practice: those who care for alcoholics, diabetics, patients with severe bowel disease, and patients in intensive care units are more likely to encounter this problem. In one Australian general hospital survey, two of every 100 patients had a phosphorus level below 2 mg per deciliter. Although symptoms attributable to hypophosphatemia have been described when the serum phosphorous levels fall to less than 2 mg per deciliter, life-threatening complications occur only at levels less than 1 mg per deciliter.

Causes

Hypophosphatemia results from three basic mechanisms: increased intracellular shift of phosphate, intestinal losses, and increased renal clearance. The administration of carbohydrate lowers serum phosphorus as phosphorus moves with glucose into cells. This is most marked in patients who receive parenteral glucose, particularly if they are malnourished. It has also been described with rapid oral feeding of patients after prolonged starvation. The practical consideration here is that serum phosphorus measured on admission may be higher than after carbohydrate is administered. Starving, malnourished, and diabetic patients should have serial phosphorus levels measured rather than the more usual single admission value. Other causes of intracellular phosphorus shifts include respiratory alkalosis, sepsis, liver failure, the ad-

ministration of epinephrine, and the use of androgens in patients with catabolic illness.

Chronic ingestion of phosphate-binding antacids such as magnesium or aluminum hydroxide or aluminum carbonate may lead to phosphate depletion and hypophosphatemia. This becomes clinically significant only if dietary phosphate is also limited. Patients with severe protein-calorie malnutrition, malabsorption, or chronic vomiting may also develop hypophosphatemia.

Any form of renal tubular phosphate leak may lead to hypophosphatemia, including therapeutic diuresis and osmotic diuretics (as in the glycosuria of uncontrolled diabetes mellitus). Hypokalemia and hypomagnesemia impair renal conservation of phosphorus. Acidemia depresses phosphorylation and elevates serum phosphorus levels, which increases renal phosphorus excretion. Acute or chronic extracellular fluid excess can lead to moderate hypophosphatemia by increasing renal phosphorus clearance. Hemodialysis using a phosphate-poor dialysate can rapidly lead to hypophosphatemia in the renal failure patient, who may also be malnourished and taking phosphate-binding antacids. Patients recovering from profound hypothermia, as in open heart surgery, may become hypophosphatemic with inappropriately high phosphaturia. Rarely, a tumor, through mechanisms not yet known (but possibly hormonal), may cause renal tubular phosphate wasting.

In many patients mixed mechanisms are involved. The alcoholic patient may be starving, vomiting, or malabsorbing. He frequently has concurrent hypokalemia and hypomagnesemia. The catecholamine excess of alcohol withdrawal, respiratory alkalosis, liver disease, and frequent treatment with antacids and intravenous carbohydrates compound the risk of low phosphorus in the alcoholic. Similarly the diabetic patient in ketoacidosis who is vomiting and anorexic may have significant phosphaturia from glycosuria, hypokalemia, and acidemia. Following treatment with insulin glucose, and bicarbonate, phosphorus moves intracellularly, often causing significant hypophosphatemia. The patient with hyperparathyroidism loses phosphate through the kidneys, through the action of both parathyroid hormone and diuretic therapy for hypercalcemia, may not eat, and may be on antacids for hypercalcemia-induced ulcer disease. Severe hypophosphatemia can rarely develop in patients with extensive third-degree burns; respiratory alkalosis occurs early, forcing phosphorus intracellularly. As healing begins patients become anabolic, taking phosphorus into cells, and begin to diurese retained salt and water which causes phosphaturia. Causes of hypophosphatemia are outline in Table 1.

Manifestations

Severe hypophosphatemia is associated with dysfunction of several organ systems as outlined in Table 2. Weakness, bone pain, joint stiffness, and intention tremors have been described with serum phosphorus levels of 2 mg per deciliter or less. More profound hypophos-

TABLE 1 Major Causes of Severe Hypophosphatemia

Alcoholism
Phosphate–binding antacids
Hyperalimentation with phosphate–poor solution
Refeeding after prolonged starvation
Severe burns in diuretic phase
Diabetic ketoacidosis in recovery phase
Respiratory alkalosis

TABLE 2 Reported Manifestations of Hypophosphatemia

Neuromuscular
  Rhabdomyolysis
  Muscle weakness
  Intention tremor
  Paresthesias
  Coma
  Convulsions
  Anisocoria
  Ballismus
  Hyporeflexia
  Ataxia
  Death
Skeletal
  Osteomalacia
  Arthritis
Hematologic
  Red Cells
    Hemolytic anemia
    Decreased oxygen release
  White cells
    Decreased chemotaxis
    Decreased phagocytosis
    Decreased killing
  Platelets
    Decreased clot retraction
    Decreased survival in vivo
Renal
    Metabolic acidosis
Hepatic
  Hypoxia

phatemia has apparently resulted in marked disturbances of neuromuscular function including anisocoria, seizures, coma, paralysis, and death. Chronic phosphorus deficiency may lead to osteomalacia. Rhabdomyolysis, one of the most common manifestations of severe hypophosphatemia, occurs in patients who are alcoholic, receiving phosphorus-poor total parenteral nutrition (TPN), or, rarely, recovering from diabetic ketoacidosis. It is usually detected by elevated muscle enzymes in patients with minimal symptoms, but can lead to significant weakness, tenderness, and edema of muscles with myoglobinuria, which places the patient at risk of renal failure.

The hematologic consequences of hypophosphatemia involve the three major cell lines. Red blood cell ATP and 2, 3-diphosphoglycerate (2, 3-DPG) both decline in hypophosphatemic states. Decreased levels of 2, 3-DPG cause a leftward shift of the oxyhemoglobin association curve and decrease oxygen delivery to body tissues. Red blood cell membranes require phospholipids for structural integrity. In addition, when red cell ATP levels fall to less than 15 percent of normal, the membrane becomes more rigid. Severe hemolytic anemias have been documented in patients with serum phosphorus levels of 0.2 mg per deciliter and below whose red blood cell ATP was 11 percent of normal. Hyperalimented hypophosphatemic dogs show severe compromise in leukocyte chemotaxis, phagocytosis, and killing, which reverses with phosphorus repletion. Presumably this results from depleted white cell ATP, which provides energy for pseudopod and vacuole formation. This phenomenon may contribute to the known predisposition to infection of diabetics, alcoholics, and others who have a tendency toward hypophosphatemia. Platelet abnormalities have been described in hypophosphatemic dogs, including thrombocytopenia, impaired clot retraction and decreased platelet survival. It is possible that hypophosphatemia may compound the thrombopathy of alcoholism or uremia and may contribute to the increased tendency toward epistaxis and gastrointestinal bleeding described in phosphorus-depleted patients.

Metabolic acidosis may occur in hypophosphatemic patients. When phosphate depletion becomes advanced, phosphorus disappears from the urine, which prevents hydrogen excretion and titratable acid. Hypophosphatemia is also believed to decrease ammonia (NH_3) synthesis and thus impair the kidney's ability to excrete acid as ammonium (NH_4). Severe metabolic acidosis only rarely occurs due to the acid buffering effect of carbonate that is released from the bone of hypophosphatemic patients.

The role of phosphorus in hepatic decompensation remains conjectural. It is proposed that hypophosphatemia might blunt the compensatory rise in red blood cell 2, 3-DPG seen in liver disease and so worsen hepatic hypoxia.

Therapy

The vigor of treatment should, as with any disorder, depend on the severity of the patient's disease rather than on a laboratory determination. It is often difficult for the clinician to distinguish between the manifestations of hypophosphatemia (anemia, confusion, weakness) and those of the concurrent medical condition that induced it (starvation, diabetes, alcoholism). In the majority of patients who are either without symptoms or mildly symptomatic, the best treatment lies in discontinuation or avoidance of those things known to induce hypophosphatemia. The serum phosphorus then spontaneously elevates to normal levels over the next several days. Phosphorus replacement is indicated for patients with symptomatic hypophosphatemia, patients with serum phosphorus levels below 1 mg per deciliter, and patients predisposed to further phosphorus depletion. The majority of patients can be treated with oral phosphorus (Table 3). If the patient is able to eat and is not lactose intolerant, dairy products are advantageous in that they also supply absorbable calcium, avoiding the hypocalcemia that supplementation of phosphorus alone may induce. It is important to realize that large oral doses of phosphorus are poorly absorbed and can produce an osmotic diarrhea. Phosphorus preparations contain sodium or potassium, which can lead to volume overload or hyperkalemia in the predisposed patient.

Intravenous phosphorus replacement is indicated for patients with profound hypophosphatemia (below 1 mg per deciliter) with hemolytic anemia, coma, seizures, or paralysis, and as a supplement for patients on TPN. Because the total body phosphorus deficit can not be determined from the serum phosphorus, response to treatment varies considerably as do the dosage recommendations. Administration of 18 mmol of phosphorus (KH_2PO_4) per day for 2 days as a continuous infusion has recently been demonstrated to be safe and effective. An alternative recommended starting dose is 32 mmol per day as a constant intravenous infusion over 24 hours. The patient's clinical and laboratory responses determine further treatment. There is no evidence to support the contention that intravenous phosphorus replacement is required until normal serum levels are obtained. Patients on TPN have been found to require 10 to 15 mmol for each liter of D_{25} TPN.

Phosphorus therapy in infants is usually directed toward routine maintenance or treatment of associated calcium disorders, because phosphorus-depletion syndromes are rare in this age group. A recommended calcium-to-phosphorus ratio (1:5 to 2:1) in the diet of neonates is supplied by most current formula preparations. The precise phosphorus requirements of infants receiving TPN are not known, but recommended intakes for full-term neonates range from 0.5 to 2.0 mmol phosphorus per kilogram per day. Premature infants growing at intrauterine rates may have much higher needs. Current preparations of TPN allow up to 55 mg phosphorus per kilogram per day to be given. Phosphorus should routinely be added to TPN of infants to minimize the risk of poor bone mineralization. These patients should be monitored for the development of rickets by obtaining serum calcium, phosphorus, alkaline phosphatase, and radiographic bone studies.

Phosphate therapy can lead to hyperkalemia, hypocalcemia, hyperphosphatemia, and soft-tissue deposition of calcium phosphate, and it is dangerous in patients with hypercalcemia or renal dysfunction. During administration of phosphorus, serum calcium, potassium, and phosphorus levels should be obtained every 12 to 24 hours. Because hypomagnesemia occurs frequently with hypophosphatemia, serum magnesium levels should be measured routinely, with replacement if indicated. Phosphorus solutions contain both monobasic and dibasic phosphorus, whose ratio depends on pH. Therefore, the millequivalent of phosphorus for a given weight of phosphate varies, and different phosphorus preparations have different ratios of millequivalent to milligram of phosphate. To avoid dosing errors, phosphorus should always be ordered as milligrams or millimoles of elemental phosphorus.

HYPERPHOSPHATEMIA

Hyperphosphatemia (above 4.5 mg per deciliter in adults) develops most commonly as a result of decreased renal excretion, but can also result from movement of phosphorus extracellularly due to tissue breakdown, or (rarely) increased intake. By far the most common cause is severe renal failure. Serum phosphorus begins to rise at a GFR of less than 25 ml per minute. Hypoparathyroidism or pseudohypoparathyroidism (end-organ resistance to parathyroid hormone) increases the renal transport maximum (T_m) for phosphate, and serum phosphate levels may rise to 6 to 8 mg per deciliter. Patients with acromegaly may have hyperphosphatemia, possibly related to the ability of growth hormone to increase renal tubular reabsorption of phosphorus. It is postulated that the higher serum concentration of phosphorus normally seen in children (normal levels 5 to 8 mg per deciliter) is due in part to increased levels of growth hormone.

Any condition that leads to increased tissue breakdown with release of intracellular phosphorus, such as severe infection or rhabdomyolysis, may raise serum phosphate levels. Hyperphosphatemia may also develop in patients with myeloproliferative disease, owing primarily to the destruction of lymphoblasts, which contain four times the amount of phosphorus as normal lymphocytes. The administration of the vitamin D compound 1, 25, dihydroxycholecalciferol has been reported to lead to hyperphosphatemia in patients with renal failure, presumably by mobilizing phosphate from bone.

Although increased ingestion of phosphorus in adults rarely causes hyperphosphatemia, neonates fed exclu-

TABLE 3 Treatment of Hypophosphatemia in Adults

Product	mg P	mmol P	mEq Na+	mEq K+
Oral				
Skim milk, 1 qt	1000	32	24	40
Neutra-Phos capsules	250	8	7.1	7.1
Fleet's Phosphosoda (10 ml)	1200	39	54	0

Recommended starting doses: 2–3 g (65–97 mmol) per day in divided doses
Intravenous (Recommended starting dose)

1. K_2PO_4 18 mmol/day for 2 days as continuous infusion
2. K_2PO_4 32 mmol/day for 1 day as continuous infusion

sively cow's milk may develop hypocalcemia and hyperphosphatemia and present with neonatal tetany. Both adults and infants may become hyperphosphatemia after phosphate enemas. Use of intravenous phosphate to treat hypercalcemia has led to tetany and death in some patients.

Severe hyperphosphatemia (above 10 mEq per liter) in patients with renal disease may stimulate secondary hyperparathyroidism. When the "calcium precipitation product" (calcium × phosphorus = 70) is reached, microcrystalline calcium phosphate deposits in tissue may occur. This is most commonly seen around the joints, but may also affect blood vessels, causing ischemia. The "red eyes of renal failure" may occur from the bulbar conjunctival deposition of calcium-phosphorus microcrystals. Skin deposits of calcium-phosphorus salts may in part cause the puritus of uremia.

Treatment consists primarily of dietary phosphorus restriction and decrease in phosphorus absorption in the gut by phosphate binders. A suggested starting regimen is 30 to 45 ml of an aluminum hydroxide or aluminum carbonate gel 4 times daily. Intravenous fluids increase renal phosphate clearance in patients with volume depletion. In extreme cases, hemodialysis may be required.

SUGGESTED READING

Fitzgerald F. Clinical hypophosphatemia. Ann Rev Med 1978; 29:177–189.
Knochel JP. Hypophosphatemia. West J Med 1981; 134:15–26.
Ritz E. Acute hypophosphatemia. Kidney Int 1982; 22:84–94.
Slatopolsky E, Rutherford WE, Rosenbaum R, et al. Hyperphosphatemia. Clin Nephrol 1977; 7:138–146.
Vannatta JB, Whang R, Papper S. Efficacy of intravenous phosphorus therapy in the severely hypophosphatemic patient. Arch Int Med 1981; 141:885–887.

HYPONATREMIA AND HYPERNATREMIA

CATHERINE S. THOMPSON, M.D.
THOMAS E. ANDREOLI, M.D.

The osmolality of body fluids is regulated tightly in the range of 285 to 295 mOsm per kilogram H_2O regardless of daily variation in the intake of water and solute. Any change in body fluid osmolality triggers rapid compensatory responses designed to restore the osmolality to its set point. Disturbances of body fluid osmolality can occur when the normal homeostatic responses are impaired. These conditions of hyper- or hypo-osmolality often require prompt attention to diagnosis and treatment if adverse sequelae (to be described) are to be prevented.

Total body water constitutes about 60 percent of body weight and is divided into intracellular and extracellular fluid compartments. The osmolalities of the intracellular and extracellular compartments are equivalent, and are maintained so by the free flux of water across cells. Sodium is the major solute that determines the osmolality of extracellular fluid. True alterations of the serum sodium concentration, therefore, affect the osmolality of all body fluids. With few exceptions, the serum sodium concentrations can be used as a marker of body fluid tonicity.

The major consequence of a change in the serum sodium concentration is due to an effect on bulk water movement into or out of the intracellular space as osmotic equilibration across body fluid compartments occurs. Cell swelling occurs in hypotonic disorders and cell shrinkage in hypertonic states. These changes in cell volume are manifest clinically by central nervous system symptoms and signs. Acute, severe disturbances in the serum sodium concentration can induce profound and potentially lethal changes in brain cell volume. Changes that occur in the serum sodium concentration over days allow for compensatory responses that restore cell volume to nearly normal and protect against the more severe manifestations of disturbances of osmolality. The intent of this chapter is to outline a diagnostic and therapeutic approach to the patient with a disturbance of body fluid osmolality as manifested by either hyponatremia or hypernatremia.

HYPONATREMIC DISORDERS

Hyponatremia is defined as a reduction in the serum concentration of sodium to less than 135 mEq per liter. Hyponatremia signifies a decrease in the ratio of total body solute to water. It does not reflect total body sodium content, however, which may be normal, increased, or decreased, depending on the etiology of the hyponatremia. Hyponatremia may be mild (125 to 135 mEq per liter), moderate (115 to 125 mEq per liter), or severe (< 115 mEq per liter) and may develop slowly over days to weeks or acutely over several hours.

Hyponatremia is the hallmark of the hypotonic syndrome. However, not all hyponatremic conditions are hypotonic. It is important to identify those conditions in which hyponatremia is associated with a normal or elevated plasma osmolality (Table 1). "Pseudohyponatremia" may occur when the concentration of lipids or proteins is significantly increased in the blood. In this setting, the laboratory measures a falsely low sodium concentration because the fraction of plasma water used in the assay is reduced owing to the elevated lipid or protein content. There is no true disturbance of body fluid tonicity in these

TABLE 1 Hyponatremia: Relation to Serum Osmolality

	Measured Na+	Measured Osmolarity
Pseudohyponatremia Hyperlipidemia Hyperproteinemia	Low	Normal
Increased ECF solutes Hyperglycemia Mannitol	Low	High (>295 mOsm/kg)
Hypotonic hyponatremia	Low	Low (<285 mOsm/kg)

conditions since the serum osmolality is normal. Fortunately, newer technology, which employs a sodium electrode to measure the serum sodium concentration, negates the effect of elevated lipids or proteins in most laboratory assays in use today. Hyponatremia also occurs in association with certain hypertonic syndromes. An increase in extracellular fluid solute, as in severe hyperglycemia or excessive mannitol administration, obligates the movement of water from the intracellular fluid compartment into the extracellular space to maintain osmotic equilibrium. A dilutional hyponatremia develops. In general, the serum sodium concentration falls by 1.2 to 1.4 mEq per liter for each increment rise of 100 mg per deciliter in the serum glucose level above about 100 mg per deciliter.

Differential Diagnosis of Hypotonic Hyponatremia

True hypotonic hyponatremia, regardless of the underlying cause, can be viewed as the inability of the kidney to excrete a free water excess. The pathophysiology may involve (1) a decreased delivery of glomerular filtrate to the diluting segment of the nephron (thick ascending limb of the loop of Henle), (2) a functionally impaired diluting segment, (3) an antidiuretic hormone (ADH) effect on the collecting duct of the nephron, or (4) some combination of the aforementioned.

Clinically, hypotonic hyponatremic disorders fall into one of three categories that can be distinguished on the basis of the history, physical examination, and a few simple laboratory tests (Table 2). Hypovolemic disorders are characterized by both sodium and water depletion, with a larger deficit of sodium relative to water. These losses may be renal or nonrenal, the latter usually of gut or cutaneous origin. Hypervolemic disorders are associated with an excess of total body sodium and water as in advanced liver disease with ascites or congestive heart failure. Edema formation is a significant feature of these conditions. The third category encompasses individuals with an excess of free water, such as those with the syndrome of inappropriate antidiuretic hormone secretion (SIADH) or psychogenic polydipsia. These individuals have modest volume expansion, but are not edematous. The common causes of excess or inappropriate antidiuretic hormone release are outlined in Table 3.

TABLE 2 Classification of Hypotonic Hyponatremia

Hypovolemic hyponatremia: larger deficit of Na+ than water and associated with continued ingestion of water
  Renal losses: diuretics, salt-losing nephritis (interstitial renal disease or Addison's disease)
  Nonrenal losses: gastrointestinal, third-space losses (burns, muscle, retroperitoneal)
  Starvation
Hypervolemic hyponatremia: excess total body Na+ and water and associated with edema formation
  Advanced liver disease/ascites, congestive heart failure, nephrosis
  Acute or chronic renal failure
Excess total body water: nonedematous
  Syndrome of inappropriate antidiuretic hormone secretion (SIADH)
  Psychogenic polydipsia

Approach to the Patient with Hyponatremia

The institution of appropriate therapy for hyponatremic conditions requires (1) establishing the etiology of the disorder and (2) assessing the severity of the associated symptoms and signs. In conjunction with the history and physical examination, a few simple urine and blood tests aid in the differential diagnosis of hyponatremia (Table 4). The severity of hyponatremia is referable not only to the absolute level of the serum sodium concentration, but also to the rapidity of its decline. Patients with a decline in serum sodium to values as low as 120 mEq per liter over the course of days may have no symptoms or only mild lethargy or confusion. In contrast, patients with more severe hyponatremia, particularly if acute in onset, typically manifest significant central nervous system signs ranging from somnolence and confusion to frank coma, often with seizures. Brain cell swelling is the common denominator of all acute hypotonic disorders. If the process occurs gradually, however, compensatory processes can restore brain cell volume to near normal by the extrusion of intracellular solute.

TABLE 3 Nonosmotic Antidiuretic Hormone Release as a Cause of Hyponatremia*

Extracellular volume depletion (at least 10%)
Drugs

  Cyclophosphamide
  Vincristine
  Clofibrate
  Chlorpropamide
  Morphine sulfate
  Barbiturates

Syndrome of inappropriate ADH release (SIADH)
  Malignancies: lung, gastric, pancreatic, prostate
  Pulmonary disorders: pneumonia, lung abscess, tuberculosis
  Cerebral disorders: head trauma, meningitis/encephalitis, tumor, cerebral hemorrhage
  Miscellaneous: myxedema, severe hypokalemia, porphyria

* All disorders require the continued ingestion of water

TABLE 4 Laboratory Tests in Hypotonic Hyponatremia

	Urine Na+ (mEq/L)	FeNa	Urine Osm	Uric Acid	BUN
SIADH	>20 usually >40	> 1%	Inappropriately high†	Low	Normal to low
Hypovolemic hyponatremia (nonrenal)	< 20 *	< 1%	> serum osmolality	Normal to high	High
Hypovolemia hyponatremia (renal origin)	> 20	> 1%	Usually equal to serum osmolality	Normal to high	High
Hypervolemic hyponatremia	< 20 * often <10	< 1%	> serum osmolality	Normal to high	Normal to high

FeNa=fractional excretion of sodium (fraction of filtered Na+ that is excreted in urine). It is calculated as:

Urine Na+ × serum creatinine / serum Na+ × urine creatinine multiplied × 100.

SIADH=Syndrome of Inappropriate Secretion of Antidiuretic Hormone
† In SIADH, the urine osmolality usually exceeds serum osmolality but may be less. However, the urine osmolality is almost never maximally dilute (60–80 mOsm/kg)
* Diuretics may lead to urine Na+ > 20 and FeNa > 1%

Treatment of Hyponatremia

The goal of treatment in hyponatremic disorders is to restore body fluid osmolality to near normal. However, the specific therapeutic approach depends on the severity of the hyponatremia and its underlying cause. Severe, symptomatic hyponatremia (usually < 120 mEq per liter) demands immediate attention. It should be emphasized that overaggressive correction of hyponatremia is potentially dangerous. If the extracellular fluid tonicity rises rapidly, brain cell shrinkage and intracerebral hemorrhage may occur. Another potential risk of vigorous correction of hyponatremia is the development of central pontine myelinolysis, a rare but often lethal demyelinating condition of the midbrain. Therefore, the aim of treatment should be to raise the serum sodium concentration to no more than 125 mEq per liter over the first 6 to 12 hours. Complete correction to a serum sodium concentration of 135 to 140 mEq per liter should occur more slowly over the next 24 to 48 hours.

Table 5 outlines an approach to the emergent management of the severely hyponatremic patient (< 120 mEq per liter). The amount of sodium required to correct the serum sodium concentration to 125 mEq per liter can be calculated and the appropriate intravenous fluid replacement started, depending on the underlying cause of the hyponatremia (Table 6). The patient with hypovolemic hyponatremia can be treated with 0.9 percent or hypertonic 3 percent saline solution. The individual with hypervolemic, edematous hyponatremia should be treated with 0.9 percent saline solution in combination with a potent intravenous diuretic. The diuretic reduces the risk of further extracellular fluid volume expansion, and the dose should be titrated to keep urine output in excess of fluid intake. Hemodialysis should be considered as an alternative treatment in the hyponatremic patient with volume expansion, particularly when the risks of worsening the state of volume expansion are significant. Hypertonic sa-

line solutions should *not* be administered to these patients because of the risk of inducing pulmonary edema. The patient with nonedematous free water excess, as in SIADH, occasionally develops profound, symptomatic hyponatremia. The administration of 0.9 percent saline solution in combination with a potent diuretic forces the excretion of free water and the serum sodium concentration rises. The use of 0.9 percent saline solution without a diuretic rarely corrects the hyponatremia of SIADH since the sodium is excreted rapidly in the urine. Hemodialysis can also be considered for severely symptomatic patients with SIADH.

Patients with less severe hyponatremia (> 120 mEq per liter) generally manifest only mild symptoms and do not require aggressive treatment in the emergency department. The hypovolemic patient is most appropriately managed with isotonic saline solution. Individuals with hypervolemic disorders should have sodium and free water restricted and should be given diuretics. Patients with SIADH should have free water restricted to less than one liter of fluid per day. The use of oral demeclocycline, which antagonizes the effect of antidiuretic hormone on the renal collecting duct, may be beneficial when the hyponatremia is mild.

HYPERNATREMIC DISORDERS

Hypernatremia is defined as a hypertonic syndrome characterized by an elevation of serum sodium above 145 mEq per liter. Hypernatremia reflects an increase in the solute-to-water ratio in body fluids while total body sodium content may be normal, increased, or decreased, depending on the cause of the disorder. Hypernatremia is most often the result of inadequate water intake in the face of excessive free water losses by either renal or nonrenal routes. Affected individuals have either a blunted thirst response or an inability to gain access to water. Hypernatremia may also occur in the setting of salt poisoning,

TABLE 5 Emergency Treatment of Severe, Symptomatic Hyponatremia

Calculate amount of Na+ needed to correct serum Na+ to 125 mEq/L

$(125 - 105) \times 0.6$ (70kg)=mEq Na+ required to raise Na+ to 125

Correct Na+ to 125 mEq/L over about 6 hours

Use 0.9% NaCl (154 mEq/L Na+) in most instances, or
    3% NaCl (514 mEq/L Na+) only in volume-contracted states

Hypertonic saline should not be used in the treatment of hyponatremia associated with hypervolemia

Furosemide should be combined with saline replacement in the treatment of hypervolemic disorders or SIADH

Example: 70-kg male with hypovolemic hyponatremia Na+ = 105 mEq/L

$(125-105) \times 0.6$(70 kg)=mEq Na+ required to raise Na+ to 125

$(20) \times 42 = 840$ mEq Na+ required

Therefore: give 5.4 L 0.9% NaCl or
    1.6 L   3% NaCl

over 6-12 hours. Frequent assessment of volume status and electrolytes is critical

TABLE 6 Treatment of Hyponatremia

Hypovolemic hyponatremia	Na+ > 120 mEq/L:	0.9% saline
	Na+ < 120 mEq/L:	0.9% saline or 3% saline to correct Na+ to 125 mEq/L over first 6-12 hours
Hypervolemic, edematous hyponatremia	Na+ > 120 mEq/L:	salt and free water restriction with oral or intravenous loop diuretic
	Na+ < 120 mEq/L:	free water restriction combined with 0.9% saline and intravenous loop diuretic titrated to keep hourly urine output > input; hemodialysis if not effective
Nonedematous free water excess hyponatremia (SIADH)	Na+ > 120 mEq/L:	free water restriction to 750-1,000 ml fluid per day
	Na+ < 120 mEq/L:	free water restriction combined with 0.9% saline and intravenous loop diuretic titrated to match hourly urine output with intake; hemodialysis if not effective

Note: The division at serum Na+ = 120 mEq/L is somewhat arbitrary. There may be patients who are severely symptomatic at levels >120 mEq/L and who require more aggressive management.

which is almost exclusively an iatrogenic disorder. The causes of hypernatremia are outlined in Table 7. A careful history and physical examination are usually all that is required to determine the etiology of hypernatremia in any given individual. However, ancillary laboratory testing to include determinations of urine sodium, osmolality, and glucose can be helpful (Table 8).

Hypernatremic disorders increase the osmolality of extracellular fluid and obligate movement of water out of the intracellular compartment until osmotic equilibrium is achieved. The resultant cell shrinkage is recognized clinically by central nervous system signs such as lethargy, confusion, or coma. Intracerebral hemorrhage is the most ominous potential complication. The severity of the syndrome depends on both the magnitude of the hypernatremia and the rapidity of its development. Hypernatremia associated with a serum osmolality of less than 350 mOsm per kilogram is usually well tolerated, whereas a serum osmolality greater than 400 mOsm per kilogram

TABLE 7 Major Causes of Hypernatremia*

Excess free water loss

Mucocutaneous: fever, hyperventilation,
    hypercatabolic states

Renal: central diabetes insipidus,
    nephrogenic diabetes insipidus

Combined water and sodium losses

Mucocutaneous: sweating

Gastrointestinal

Renal: Osmotic diuresis due to hyperglycemia, mannitol
    administration, or postobstructive diuresis

Excess sodium intake

Intravenous: administration of excess sodium bicarbonate
during cardiopulmonary resuscitation

Oral salt poisoning: improper preparation of infant
formulas, hypertonic tube feedings, kayexalate
administration for hyperkalemia

* All hypernatremic disorders are associated with an inability to ingest sufficient amounts of free water.

TABLE 8 Laboratory Features of Hypernatremic Disorders

	Urine Na+	Urine Osmolality	Urine Glucose
Diabetes insipidus	<20	Dilute, usually less than 150 mOsm	Negative
Osmotic diuresis	>20	Isotonic or hypertonic relative to serum osmolality	Positive if caused by hyperglycemia
Excess non-renal water and Na+ loss	<20	Hypertonic relative to serum osmolality	Negative
Salt poisoning	>20	Hypertonic relative to serum osmolality	Negative

is almost always lethal, even if treated. As in hyponatremic disorders, compensatory mechanisms designed to restore cell volume to nearly normal are activated in hypernatremic syndromes. Specifically, the accumulation of intracellular solute, termed "idiogenic osmoles," returns cell volume toward normal in chronic hypernatremia of several days' duration.

Treatment of Hypernatremia

The therapeutic approach to the hypernatremic patient depends on the underlying disorder. The goal is to correct the serum sodium to normal, but it should be accomplished cautiously, particularly in cases of chronic hypernatremia in which compensatory responses have been activated. If hypotonic fluids are given too rapidly, cerebral edema may occur. Cautious correction dictates that the serum sodium fall only 1 mEq per liter per 2 hours. In some cases, complete correction may not be accomplished for several days. For acute rises in serum sodium, more vigorous correction may be pursued. The free water deficit can be estimated, as outlined in Table 9, and the rate of fluid replacement calculated.

Individuals with central or nephrogenic diabetes insipidus may have massive urinary losses of free water, but are typically able to osmoregulate by the ingestion of sufficient water to prevent the development of hypernatremia. If these persons become acutely ill or develop altered mental status, they may be unable to meet these free water demands. Appropriate management consists of free water replacement intravenously combined with aqueous vasopressin given intramuscularly in the case of central diabetes insipidus. The use of sodium-free dextrose solutions (5 percent dextrose in water) should be used with caution in these individuals. Rapid infusion of dextrose solutions (>500 ml per hour) may induce hyperglycemia and glycosuria and these aggravate urinary water losses. A safe practice is to alternate intravenous infusion of 5 percent dextrose in water with one-half normal saline solution (0.45 percent saline solution). This provides a final replacement solution of dextrose, 2.5 percent, and one-fourth normal saline, a formula that is unlikely to cause significant glycosuria, even at high rates of infu-

TABLE 9 Treatment of Hypernatremia

Simple free water losses
 Calculate free water deficit=0.6 (body wt kg) minus 140/actual Na+ ×0.6 (body wt kg)

Replace with hypotonic fluids

Alternating liters of D5% water with ½ normal saline provides final replacement solution of D2.5% ¼ normal saline and minimizes risk of hyperglycemia/osmotic diuresis.

Calculate hourly replacement rate to lower sodium by 1 mEq/L/2 hours; or 12 mEq/L fall in serum sodium concentration over 24 hours.
 Central diabetes insipidus: For emergent treatment, combine free water replacement with aqueous vasopressin—5-10 units IM every 4-6 hours

Combined water and sodium losses
 Calculate free water deficit as outlined above. These disorders also require electrolyte replacement.

Hypotonic fluids—½ normal saline most physiologic

Correct hyperglycemia if present

Salt poisoning
 Intravenous furosemide with free water replacement to keep urine output > fluid input if patient is hypervolemic; if normovolemic, fluid input to equal urine output; if hypovolemic, fluid input to exceed urine output

Hemodialysis

sion. As a precautionary measure, the urine should be tested for glucose routinely. Insulin may be required to control hyperglycemia in some individuals.

Hypernatremic disorders associated with a combined deficit of sodium and water, as with hyperosmolar nonketotic coma, are best managed by the administration of hypotonic saline solutions such as one-half normal saline (0.45 percent saline solution). The associated hyperglycemia should be corrected with insulin to reduce the ongoing water losses resulting from the osmotic diuresis.

Salt-poisoned individuals with a severe increase in total body sodium content and extracellular fluid volume are best managed with free water replacement coupled with a brisk saline diuresis. Intravenous loop diuretics are usually necessary. If this is not effective, hemodialysis should be instituted.

SUGGESTED READING

Andreoli TE. Osmolality disturbances. In: Wyngaarden JB, Smith LH, eds. Cecil Textbook of Medicine. 17th Ed. Philadelphia: WB Saunders, 1984:523–529.

Arieff A, Schmidt RW. Fluid and electrolyte disorders and the central nervous system. In: Maxwell MH, Kleeman CR, eds. Clinical disorders of fluid and electrolyte metabolism. 3rd Ed. New York: McGraw-Hill, 1980:1409–1480.

Ayus JC, Olivero JJ, Frommer JP. Rapid correction of severe hyponatremia with intravenous hypertonic saline solution. Am J Med 1982; 72:43.

DeFronzo RA, Thier SO. Pathophysiologic approach to hyponatremia. Arch Intern Med 1980; 140:897.

Narins RJ, Jones ER, Strom MC, Rudnick MR, Bastl CP. Diagnostic strategies in disorders of fluid, electrolyte, and acid-base homeostasis. Am J Med 1982; 72:496.

Robertson GL, Shelton RL, Athar S. The osmoregulation of vasopressin. Kidney Int 1976; 10:25.

METABOLIC ACIDOSIS AND ALKALOSIS

KATHLEEN DELANEY, M.D.
LEWIS R. GOLDFRANK, M.D.

METABOLIC ACIDOSIS

The patient with primary metabolic acidosis represents a critical diagnostic challenge in the emergency department, because appropriate intervention requires understanding of the etiology of the metabolic disorder. Metabolic acidosis is detected by finding an abnormal pH on arterial blood gas determination or an elevated anion gap noted on electrolyte studies. Simple metabolic acidosis causes "acidemia," manifested by a blood pH less than 7.35. The patient with primary metabolic acidosis who has superimposed respiratory or metabolic alkalosis has a normal or elevated pH and is "acidotic," but not "acidemic." Respiratory compensation in uncomplicated primary metabolic acidosis never raises the pH to normal. Pitfalls in diagnosis lie in the failure to detect metabolic acidosis when there is associated respiratory alkalosis (as may be seen in sepsis, hepatic failure, or salicylate toxicity) or in mistaking the low bicarbonate and elevated anion gap of compensated respiratory alkalosis for primary metabolic acidosis. Both pitfalls are readily avoided by the use of an acid-base nomogram (Fig. 1).

The history often suggests the diagnosis (Fig. 2). A diabetic patient who complains of increasing polyuria and polydipsia gives straightforward clues to the diagnosis of diabetic ketoacidosis. Similarly, the alcoholic patient who reports several days of vomiting and malaise suggests alcoholic ketoacidosis. Patients intent on suicide who become acidemic or acidotic may have ingested ethylene glycol, methanol, iron, isoniazid, or aspirin.

In the frequent absence of a reliable history, the physician who is confronted by a patient with metabolic acidosis can arrive at a reasonable diagnosis and initiate correct management by taking the following steps: The physical examination usually suggests the possibility (and sometimes the etiology) of metabolic acidosis. Deep regular breathing is associated with respiratory compensation for metabolic acidosis and mandates a determination of blood gas levels. The hydration status of the patient should be evaluated by assessment of the pulse and blood pressure (with orthostatic tests if possible) as well as examination of mucous membranes and skin turgor. Characteristic odors, such as acetone, ammonia, and paraldehyde, must be sought. The skin should be examined for uremic frost. Funduscopic examination is important in detecting diabetic retinopathy or the optic nerve hyperemia seen in methanol toxicity. One looks for stigmata of alcohol abuse or liver disease and sources of infection.

In emergent or urgent patients, treatment begins with intravenous infusion of at least 50 cc of D50W (or D20W in a child), thiamine, 100 mg, and normal saline to correct intravascular volume. D50W is given for two reasons: metabolic disturbances leading to acidosis are often associated with malnutrition and hypoglycemia (the patient with diabetic ketoacidosis [DKA] will not be harmed by the relatively small increase in blood glucose caused by administration of D50 prior to the diagnostic manuevers discussed below), and the diabetic, alcoholic, or cirrhotic patient who is comatose because of *hypo*glycemia will be harmed if empirical treatment is withheld.

The next step is the evaluation of the blood urea nitrogen (BUN) and serum electrolytes. The BUN helps to exclude uremia as the cause of the acidosis. The electrolytes allow for the calculation of the anion gap. The anion gap (AG) is estimated by the formula in millequivalents (Na + K) − (Cl + HCO₃). Since the serum potassium level is small and relatively constant, most practitioners leave it out of the equation, which becomes Na − (Cl + HCO₃). The normal AG is 12 mEq per liter with a 90 percent confidence range of 8 to 16 mEq per liter. The term AG is in actuality a misnomer, as the laws of electroneutrality dictate that the number of anions and cations in a solution be equal. AG refers to *unmeasured* anions. In normal plasma, the total of "unmeasured" anions (albumin + PO₄ + SO₄ + organic acids) is 23 mEq per liter, whereas the total amount of "unmeasured" cations (K

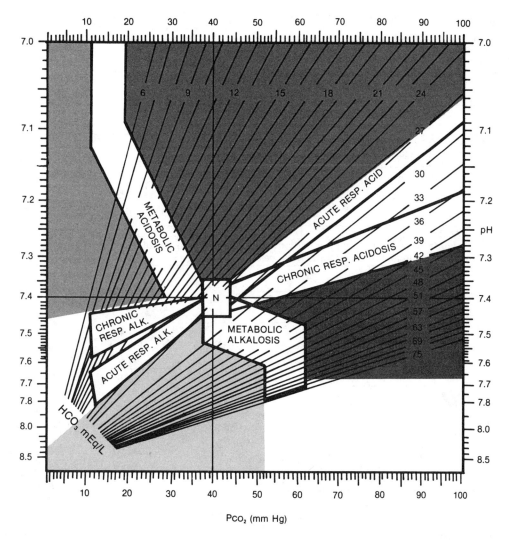

The significance bands for the various simple disorders are labeled on the map. Probably interpretations for points falling in the colored areas between
are:

▓ mixed respiratory and metabolic acidosis

▒ mixed metabolic acidosis and respiratory
  alkalosis

☐ mixed respiratory and metabolic alkalosis

■ mixed respiratory acidosis and metabolic
  alkalosis

The lines that fan diagonally from the lower left hand
corner represent serum bicarbonates corresponding
to the values given across the top and down the right
side within the diagram.

Figure 1 Acid-base map. (Adapted from Goldberg M, Green SB, Moss ML, et al. Computer based
instruction and diagnosis of acid-base disorders. JAMA 1973; 223:269–275.)

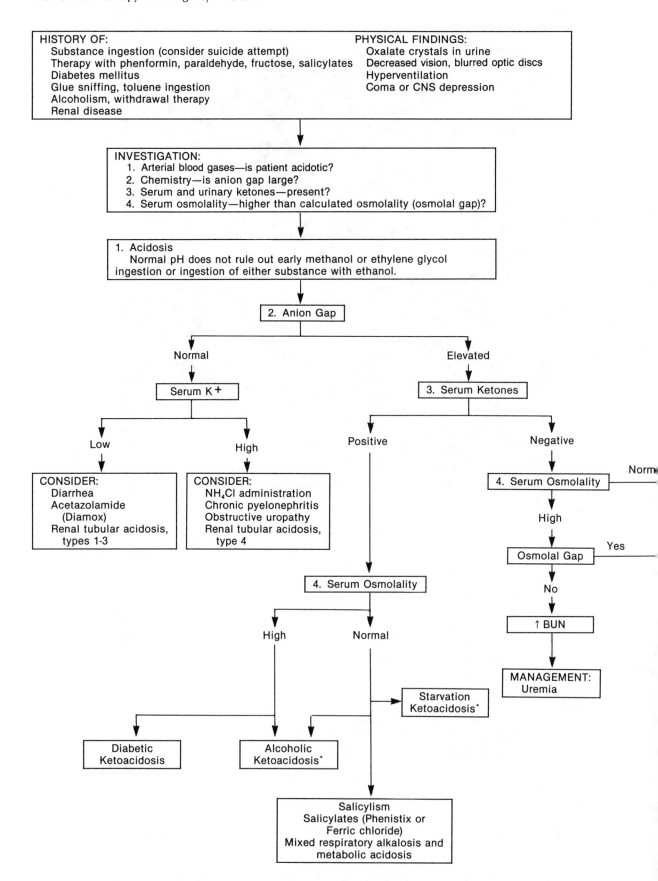

HISTORY OF:
  Substance ingestion (consider suicide attempt)
  Therapy with phenformin, paraldehyde, fructose, salicylates
  Diabetes mellitus
  Glue sniffing, toluene ingestion
  Alcoholism, withdrawal therapy
  Renal disease

PHYSICAL FINDINGS:
  Oxalate crystals in urine
  Decreased vision, blurred optic discs
  Hyperventilation
  Coma or CNS depression

INVESTIGATION:
  1. Arterial blood gases—is patient acidotic?
  2. Chemistry—is anion gap large?
  3. Serum and urinary ketones—present?
  4. Serum osmolality—higher than calculated osmolality (osmolal gap)?

1. Acidosis
   Normal pH does not rule out early methanol or ethylene glycol ingestion or ingestion of either substance with ethanol.

2. Anion Gap

Normal

Elevated

Serum K +

3. Serum Ketones

Low

High

Positive

Negative

CONSIDER:
  Diarrhea
  Acetazolamide
    (Diamox)
  Renal tubular acidosis,
    types 1-3

CONSIDER:
  NH_4Cl administration
  Chronic pyelonephritis
  Obstructive uropathy
  Renal tubular acidosis,
    type 4

4. Serum Osmolality

Norm

High

Osmolal Gap

Yes

No

↑ BUN

MANAGEMENT:
Uremia

4. Serum Osmolality

High

Normal

Starvation
Ketoacidosis*

Diabetic
Ketoacidosis

Alcoholic
Ketoacidosis*

Salicylism
Salicylates (Phenistix or
  Ferric chloride)
Mixed respiratory alkalosis and
  metabolic acidosis

Figure 2 Summary of approach to metabolic acidosis. (From Goldfrank L, et al. Methanol and ethylene glycol. In: Goldfrank's toxicologic emergencies. A problem solving approach to clinical toxicology. Norwalk: Appleton-Century-Crofts, 1986.)

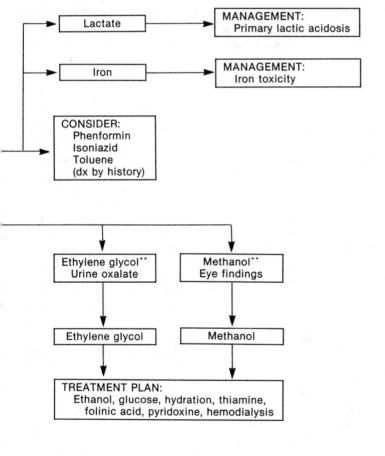

NOTES:
* In alcoholic and starvation ketoacidosis, the strength of the positive acetest determination is milder than would be expected from the degree of acidosis seen on ABGs. Isopropyl alcohol produces ketosis *without* metabolic acidosis.
** Start ethanol at once, even if toxicology results are not yet available.

+ Mg + Ca) is 11 mEq per liter. The total serum cations must equal the total serum anions; therefore, unmeasured cations (UC) plus sodium equal unmeasured anions (UA) plus chloride and bicarbonate, which can be expressed as $Na - (Cl + HCO_3) = UA - UC =$ the anion gap.

Metabolic acidosis is produced by loss of bicarbonate (through the gastrointestinal tract or renal tubules) or by gain of an acid. When the acidosis is caused by bicarbonate loss, there is no net gain of unmeasured anion, and chloride is retained to maintain electroneutrality. This results in a "nonanion gap hyperchloremic metabolic acidosis." The treatment in the case of metabolic acidosis due to gastrointestinal loss of bicarbonate is the adequate replacement of sodium, chloride, potassium, and fluids. In the stable patient without substantial potassium deficit or volume depletion, renal bicarbonate losses are treated with oral alkali regimens (sodium citrate, lactate, or bicarbonate), which are titrated to a near normal pH. Classic or distal renal tubular acidosis (type I RTA) requires 1 to 3 mEq per kilogram per day, whereas proximal (type II) RTA requires much greater supplementation. Patients with renal tubular acidosis are usually stable and do not require emergency treatment. These patients should be referred for specialist evaluation. An exception to this is the toluene abusing patient who may present with severe RTA, hypophosphatemia, and hypokalemia, requiring massive KCl, KH_2PO_4, and $NaHCO_3$ replacement.

When endogenous organic acids (ketoacids, lactic acid) or exogenous acids (salicylates, formic acid from methanol catabolism) are added to serum, they titrate the plasma buffer systems, primarily bicarbonate, causing release of CO_2 and adding an "unmeasured anion." It is these processes that lead to an increased anion gap acidosis that are of greatest concern to the emergency physician.

Once this "anion gap" acidosis is detected, the next step in the emergency department is the measurement of serum ketones. The presence of serum ketones in a patient with metabolic acidosis narrows the differential diagnosis to alcoholic, diabetic, or starvation ketoacidosis, or salicylate poisoning.

Initially hydration with normal saline is always appropriate. Insulin should never be given to the diabetic until a serum glucose level is available. The patient with alcoholic ketoacidosis (AKA), starvation ketoacidosis, or salicylate poisoning requires continuous infusion of glucose (initially D5 normal saline). The patient with DKA should receive insulin supplementation, as an intravenous bolus of 10 units of regular insulin, followed by a drip of 2 to 6 units per hour of regular insulin, with repeat boluses and an increase in the drip rate as required.

Although potassium is markedly depleted in these disorders, it is best to wait for the initial serum level, which is often elevated owing to the acidosis. When the potassium level is less than 5.0 mEq and a good urine output is established, potassium should be supplemented at 20 to 40 mEq per hour.

The use of phosphate in the treatment of DKA stirs mild controversy among experts. Although patients with DKA are often phosphate depleted, their levels may be elevated during the first 4 to 8 hours of treatment, and excessive empirical correction may lead to symptomatic hypocalcemia and hypomagnesemia, especially in pediatric patients. Because of the relatively acute nature of DKA, these patients rarely manifest complications of severe phosphate depletion (myoglobinuric renal failure or cardiac failure) as are seen in chronic phosphate depletion. If phosphate is given prior to the availability of a serum level, only small amounts (up to 45 millimoles over 10 hours) should be used.

Although sodium bicarbonate is one of the hallmarks of treatment of salicylate overdose, it is rarely given in AKA or DKA. The administration of insulin (or glucose and thiamine in AKA or starvation ketoacidosis) prevents further generation of ketoacids, while hydration improves tissue blood flow, decreasing lactic acid production by muscle tissue and increasing its metabolism via improved hepatic perfusion. This improvement is further aided by hepatic conversion of lactate and ketones to bicarbonate during recovery. If bicarbonate is administered during resuscitation, recovery may be complicated by significant metabolic alkalosis. In addition, increasing the pH shifts the hemoglobin oxygen dissociation curve to the left, further compromising tissue oxygen delivery and increasing lactic acid production.

A theoretical concern, probably of little clinical significance, is the possibility of central nervous system acidosis due to the more rapid transfer of carbon dioxide and the slower equilibration of bicarbonate across the blood-brain barrier. The most dangerous consequence of the rapid change in pH caused by bicarbonate administration is the potential for precipitation of life-threatening hypokalemia or hypocalcemia. In patients with severe metabolic acidosis who need bicarbonate, an electocardiogram is helpful in assessing the rare need for empirical calcium or potassium administration.

With these precautions in mind, we usually reserve bicarbonate use for patients with a measured (or calculated) serum bicarbonate level of less than 7 mEq per liter, or a pH less than 7.1. The goal is to raise the serum bicarbonate level to more than 7 mEq per liter, or the pH to 7.1. The frequency of supplementation depends on the cause of the acidosis and frequent blood gas monitoring. A patient with *severe* acidosis from DKA usually needs only one supplementation, whereas treatment of lactic acidosis from sepsis may require the institution of a bicarbonate infusion.

By alkalinizing the urine, sodium bicarbonate increases renal excretion of salicylates and is given freely in the treatment of salicylate poisoning. Salicylate poisoning may be suspected when respiratory alkalosis is superimposed on the metabolic acidosis, or when the patient complains of tinnitus, nausea, or vomiting. Fever and hypoglycemia may also be present. A ferric chloride test of the urine establishes the presence of salicylates and necessitates a quantitative serum salicylate level. In urgent cases, treatment should be initiated while waiting for the level. Sufficient sodium bicarbonate is given to raise the urine pH to more than 7.5. This may be accomplished by administration of 1 liter of D5 0.45 saline with 88 mEq of sodium bicarbonate over the first hour followed by 44 mEq with 500 cc of D5 0.45 saline per hour. Since urinary alkalinization cannot be achieved in the hypokalemic state, the serum potassium and urine pH levels must be monitored hourly and potassium and bicarbonate supplementation adjusted accordingly. Severe cases of salicylate toxicity are often mistaken for bacterial sepsis or organic mental syndrome when the diagnosis is not considered. Patients with severe salicylate poisoning may develop noncardiogenic pulmonary edema, may require hemodialysis, and should be managed in the intensive care unit of a hospital capable of hemodialysis.

If the serum ketones are negative, one of three problems is present. An anion gap metabolic acidosis is seen in uremia when there is failure of both glomerular filtration *and* renal tubular acid secretion. (Failure of only the latter results in a nonanion gap renal tubular acidosis.) Demonstration of a creatinine level above 8 mg per deciliter with an anion gap in the range of 20 to 25 mEq per liter can be attributed to failure of a uremic patient to clear the normal acidic products of metabolism. A higher anion gap should suggest a complicating disorder. Unlike the patient with a relatively acute process, the patient with chronic renal failure has little intracellular or extracellular buffering capacity and will need more extensive bicarbonate supplementation while awaiting emergency dialysis. Hyperkalemia is improved by this therapy, and metabolic alkalosis should not develop if blood gas levels are monitored frequently. Hypocalcemia and fluid overload are potential complications of $NaHCO_3$ supplementation. The uremic patient should be admitted to an institution capable of emergency peritoneal or hemodialysis.

When the patient is not uremic and the serum ketone tests are negative, either lactic acidosis or the acid metabolites of a toxin are present. Lactic acidosis is caused by states of low tissue oxygen delivery (cardiogenic or hypovolemic shock, hypoxia, severe anemia) and by toxins that interfere with cellular respiration (bacterial endotoxin, carbon monoxide, cyanide, iron). The commonest causes of acidosis seen in the emergency department are increased lactate production during seizures and in states of shock. The treatment of lactic acidosis is treatment of the underlying disorder. Sodium bicarbonate is not required for readily reversible problems (seizures), but severe continuing production of lactate may require frequent supplementation, using the guidelines already discussed.

If the history and physical examination are not strongly suggestive of a primary cause of lactic acidosis, the next diagnostic step should be the calculation of the osmolal gap. The serum osmolality is accurately approximated by the contributions of the serum sodium, glucose, and BUN levels. Serum osmolality can be estimated using the following formula: $2 (Na) + BUN/2.8 + glucose/18$. The normal serum osmolality is 280 to 290 mOsm. A measured osmolality of 10 mOsm more than the calculated osmolality suggests the presence of small osmotically active molecules, such as ethanol, methanol,

isopropyl alcohol, or ethylene glycol, and some of their metabolites. Of these, only methanol and ethylene glycol directly cause metabolic acidosis. A diagnosis of methanol ingestion, prior to obtaining a serum level, would be supported by the finding of hyperemia of the optic disc. Similarly, the diagnosis of ethylene glycol toxicity would be supported by the finding of calcium oxalate crystals in the urine or the demonstration of hypocalcemia. Neither of these toxic alcohols has a characteristic odor, although they are often consumed concomitantly with ethanol, so that the "odor of alcohol" may be misleading. Both these ingestions are treated with hydration, thiamine, folinic acid (methanol) and pyridoxine (ethylene glycol), glucose, and the administration of ethanol to block the toxins' conversion by alcohol dehydrogenase to their toxic metabolites. Any patient with metabolic acidosis due to methanol or ethylene glycol ingestion must be admitted to an ICU in a hospital capable of hemodialysis.

If the osmolal gap is normal, think of another toxic ingestion. Iron, phenformin (now off the market), and isoniazid can lead to severe metabolic acidosis. (A handy mnemonic for the assessment of anion gap acidosis is illustrated in Table 1.) Any patient with significant metabolic acidosis (pH less than 7.2) that is continuing needs observation in an ICU setting, where the electrocardiogram fluid balance, and electrolyte and blood gas levels can be closely monitored.

METABOLIC ALKALOSIS

Metabolic alkalosis is the most common acid-base disorder seen in the emergency department. In most cases (70 percent) it is simple and associated with alkalemia, a pH higher than 7.45, and a serum bicarbonate level higher than 27 mEq per liter. Thirty percent of the pa-

TABLE 1   Etiologies of Metabolic Acidosis[†]

Normal anion gap[*]	Elevated anion gap (MUDPIES)
Low serum K+	
Diarrhea	
Carbonic anhydrase inhibitor (i.e., Diamox)	M Methanol ingestion
Renal tubular acidosis types 1 to 3	U Uremia
High serum K+	D Diabetes (ketoacidosis)
Ammonium chloride administration	P Paraldehyde of phenoformin ingestion
Chronic pyelonephritis	I "Idiopathic lactic acidosis" or acidosis due to hemorrhage, septic, or myocardial shock, etc; or iron or isoniazid
Obstructive uropathy	
Renal tubular acidosis type 4	
	E Ethanol ketoacidosis or ethylene glycol ingestion
	S Salicylates or solvents (e.g., toluene)
	Others: liver disease, hereditary forms of lactic acidosis or lactic acidosis related to thiamine deficiency, leukemia, pancreatitis, fructose or epinephrine infusion, etc.

[*] Anion gap = $Na—HCO_3—Cl$; Normal = 12–16 mEq/L
[†] From Goldfrank L, et al. The liquid time bomb. Hosp Phys 1982; 18(2).

TABLE 2 Differential Diagnosis of Metabolic Alkalosis[*]

Sodium chloride-responsive ($U_{Cl}^- < 10$ mmoles per liter)
  Gastrointestinal disorders:
    Vomiting
    Gastric drainage
    Villous adenoma of the colon
    Chloride diarrhea
  Diuretic therapy
  Rapid correction of chronic hypercapnia
  Cystic fibrosis

Sodium chloride-resistant ($U_{Cl}^- > 20$ mmoles per liter)
  Excess mineralocorticoid activity:
    Hyperaldosteronism
    Cushing's syndrome
    Bartter's syndrome
    Excess licorice intake
  Profound potassium depletion

Unclassified
  Alkali administration
  Milk-alkali syndrome
  Nonparathyroid hypercalcemia

---

[*] From Kaehny WD. In: Schrier R. Pathogenesis and management of metabolic acidosis and alkalosis in renal and electrolyte disorders. Boston: Little, Brown and Company, 1976.

tients with metabolic alkalosis have associated respiratory acidosis or alkalosis. A normovolemic patient without an endocrine abnormality will rapidly excrete a bicarbonate load and will not become alkalotic. Thus, the maintenance of a metabolic alkalosis requires two factors: a source of bicarbonate, either endogenous (vomiting, renal tubules) or exogenous (commonly sodium bicarbonate, Ringer's lactate, sodium citrate) *and* a stimulus to the renal tubules to reabsorb bicarbonate and secrete hydrogen ion.

The latter stimulus is supplied most commonly by contraction of the extracellular fluid space and secondary stimulation of aldosterone secretion in the volume-depleted patient, or (much rarer) stimulation of renal H^+ secretion and bicarbonate retention in the normovolemic patient with endogenous or exogenous excess of adrenocorticoids. The commonest causes of metabolic alkalosis seen in the emergency department are persistent vomiting and diuretic use. The treatment is simple volume replacement with normal saline. Potassium is usually low and should be supplemented. If the history and physical examination are insufficient, the measurement of a random urinary chloride specimen helps to distinguish the patient with metabolic alkalosis due to volume depletion from the patient with mineralocorticoid excess. Metabolic alkalosis in the normovolemic patient with Cushing's syndrome, for example, is associated with a urinary chloride concentration greater than 10 mEq per liter, whereas it is less than 10 mEq per liter in the volume-depleted patient, unless a diuretic is still acting on the renal tubules. A complete list of the causes of primary alkalosis is given in Table 2.

SUGGESTED READING

Goldfrank L, Flomenbaum N, Lewin N, Howland MA. The liquid time bomb. Hos Phys 1982; 18:38–60.

Kaehny WD. Pathogenesis and management of metabolic acidosis and alkalosis. In: Schrier R, ed. Renal and electrolyte disorders. Boston: Little, Brown and Company, 1976:79–115.

Narins RG, Emmet M. Simple and mixed acid-base disorders: a practical approach. Medicine 1980; 59:161–87.

Oh MS, Carroll HJ. The anion gap. N Engl J Med 1977; 297:814–817.

MANAGEMENT OF THE SKIN

APPROACH TO SKIN DISEASE

EVAN R. FARMER, M.D.

The emphasis of this chapter is to present an approach for the nondermatologist to use in the evaluation of the patient with skin disease during the initial examination. The objectives are to establish the diagnosis or diagnostic category, to initiate therapy, to make appropriate referrals, and to determine when inpatient care is indicated.

EVALUATION OF CUTANEOUS DISEASE

There are three general principles to be followed in the evaluation of cutaneous disease; omission of any one increases the probability of misdiagnosis. *First*, the diagnosis of a skin disease is based on the patient's history in conjunction with the clinical appearance of the lesions. It is true that in some cases an experienced dermatologist can make an accurate diagnosis by clinical examination alone, but only a history may provide the necessary information to make an association of the skin lesions with drug ingestion, environmental exposure, genetic conditions, or abnormalities in other organ systems. *Second*, the entire skin surface including the oral, ocular, and genital mucous membranes should be examined. Only a thorough examination provides information on distribution and the variable morphology of the lesions. The diagnostic criteria in dermatology are based on the ap-

pearance and distribution of the primary lesion and then on its subsequent evolution. *Third*, the use of adequate light is very important. Sunlight through an open window and incandescent light give the best color rendition in contrast to fluorescent light. Side lighting of the lesions with an incandescent lamp directed tangential to the skin surface accentuates slight elevations or depressions. A hand magnifying lens is an invaluable aid in conjunction with adequate light.

History

Because a good history is the initial and best foundation on which to base the diagnosis, I recommend that the following information be obtained:

1. *Duration of disease.* This should be noted from the onset of the earliest symptom but in many cases is vague, such as several weeks, months, or years.
2. *Initial body site(s) involved.*
3. *Description of the earliest lesion.* What did the lesion look like before it evolved or was scratched, treated (e.g., pustule, vesicle)?
4. *Distribution of the lesions.*
5. *Recurrences.* Are the lesions part of a cyclical phenomenon with lesion-free intervals?
6. *Cutaneous symptoms.* Pain and itching may be helpful in the differential diagnosis but are subjective and may be misleading. Therefore, this information should be used only as soft data and not as a major differentiating feature.
7. *Prior therapy.* This information is very important because skin lesions tend to be easily modified in their appearance by treatment. Also, a new or second skin disease may develop from irritating forms of therapy and obscure the initial skin disease.
8. *Associated symptoms.* Are there coexistent systemic symptoms such as fever, arthritis, or diarrhea?
9. *Current and recent systemic medications*: These include both prescription and nonprescription drugs because medications are a frequent cause of cutaneous eruptions.

I cannot overemphasize the importance of examining the entire skin surface and the mucous membranes. The purpose of the examination is to determine the primary skin lesion, its distribution, and its subsequent evolution (see Table 1 for definitions). A general physical examination is also helpful, particularly with atten-

TABLE 1 Definitions

Macule—an area of altered skin color

Papule—a small, solid elevation of skin

Plaque—a flat, raised, solid area of skin

Nodule—a solid lesion measuring >10 mm in diameter

Vesicle—an elevated, fluid-filled cavity

Pustule—a fluid-filled cavity containing neutrophils

Wheal—a transient, localized area of edema

Ulcer—a localized area of loss of the epidermis

Scale—a dry flake on the skin surface

Crust—dried serum on the surface of a lesion

tion to the presence or absence of fever, lymphadenopathy, and hepatosplenomegaly.

Diagnostic Tests

Simple tests may be performed on the skin, such as a potassium hydroxide examination of scales for the presence of hyphae or spores and a Tzanck smear for the presence of viral-altered cells. These tests can be performed quickly, simply, and reliably. Skin biopsies in the emergency department should be performed only for acute, serious diseases such as infections of a life-threatening nature, vasculitis with potential systemic involvement, and blistering diseases for which there may be several treatment options, e.g., staphylococcal scalded skin syndrome versus toxic epidermal necrolysis. Part of the biopsy should be processed for frozen sections for an immediate answer, and part should be processed in a suitable fixative such as 10 percent formalin for permanent sections. Special stains and some antibody preparations are now available that can provide a quick and relatively definitive diagnosis of some of the serious infections. In addition to these tests, other tests such as blood tests may be helpful in the evaluation of systemic disease: complete blood count, serology for syphilis, liver function tests, urinalysis, and so forth.

Once the initial evaluation is completed, the patients can be categorized into those who have acute, potentially serious diseases and those who have less serious diseases that may be managed in a clinic or office setting rather than an emergency department (Fig. 1). I recommend a 14-day duration as the divisor for determining acute from chronic. This time span includes most of the serious infectious diseases, serious bullous diseases, and rapidly progressing connective tissue diseases in the acute category. Patients with acute skin lesions without evidence of systemic disease may be safely managed on an outpatient basis with follow-up in a clinic or referral to a dermatologist unless there is a potential for serious complications. Risk factors for these complications include widespread lesions with loss of the epidermal barrier in very young or elderly patients, extreme pruritus or pain in patients with suicide potential, and rapidly evolving lesions in patients with other underlying serious diseases.

DIAGNOSTIC CATEGORY

Serious Infection

Acute skin lesions in association with systemic disease constitute the potentially most serious category. This category encompasses the serious systemic infections, e.g., disseminated meningococcemia, Rocky Mountain spotted fever, and hepatitis. Systemic vasculitis with its potential for renal and central nervous system dysfunction also fits into this group. The acute bullous diseases such as staphylococcal scalded skin syndrome, erythema multiforme with mucous membrane lesions (Stevens-Johnson syndrome), and toxic epidermal necrolysis are all generally associated with constitutional systems and have the potential for significant morbidity and mortality. Therefore, these patients should be considered for inpatient care with consultation by a dermatologist. (See the chapter on *Inpatient Therapy in Skin Disease*.)

Chronic Skin Disease

Patients with chronic skin diseases may also be stratified into those with cutaneous involvement alone and those with associated systemic disease. The former includes such disorders as lichen planus, psoriasis (in the absence of arthritis), and atopic dermatitis (eczema). The chronic skin disease category with systemic disease includes such disorders as systemic lupus erythematosus (SLE), dermatomyositis, and necrobiosis lipoidica diabeticorum. Most patients in both categories have slowly evolving disease and seek emergency care for exacerbations of their skin lesions or for secondary changes such as a sunburn in the example of SLE or subsequent cutaneous bacterial infection in the case of atopic dermatitis. These cases generally do not require admission, but they do need a thorough evaluation for resolution of the problem and prevention of further complications. Sometimes there is an exacerbation of the skin disease in conjunction with an exacerbation of the associated systemic disorder. An example of this situation is again SLE with sunburn, in which there may be an associated flare of renal disease, central nervous system symptoms, or arthritis. The history and physical examination, along with basic laboratory studies, should quickly help to assess these patients and to determine the severity of their current status. These patients may require inpatient care.

NEOPLASIA AND INFLAMMATION

For treatment purposes, most skin disease seen in the emergency setting can also be divided into the two large categories of neoplasia and inflammation. Neoplasia of the skin, except for the complications of bleeding and infection, does not need same-day treatment and is not further considered at this point. Bleeding is managed surgically and infection is managed with antibiotics, preferably systemic rather than local. Penicillin, dicloxacillin, and erythromycin are good choices since *Staphylococcus* is the most common bacterium in these skin lesions.

The inflammatory skin disorders can be divided into those caused by microorganisms and those without an infectious agent. The diseases caused by infection, whether bacterial, fungal, or viral, should be treated with appropriate antibiotics. Anti-inflammatory therapy such as cool water compresses and topical drying agents are generally helpful. Therapy of specific diseases is discussed elsewhere in the text.

Noninfectious Inflammatory Disease

Noninfectious inflammatory skin diseases generally respond to conservative measures depending on extent and

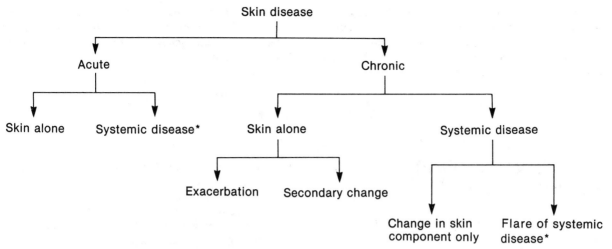

* Patients most likely requiring inpatient care.

Figure 1   Schema to triage patients in the emergency department.

type of disease. Cool water compresses, with or without additives such as sodium chloride or aluminum acetate, can be applied to any inflammatory skin disease without fear of harm using a soft cloth for 10 to 20 minutes several times a day. The evaporation of the solution and the gentle debridement, if the cloth is removed before completely drying, is quite soothing. Topical corticosteroids may then be applied to the lesions once the compresses have been removed. The strength of the corticosteroid and the type of vehicle carrying the medication depend on the specific disease and the body site involved. My general philosophy is to use a potent topical corticosteroid for a short duration in acute diseases and less potent preparations for longer-term use.

Pruritus

Other than cosmetic disfigurement, pruritus is the most common symptom of skin disease and is a major reason for visits to the emergency department. Pruritus, or itching, may be defined as the unpleasant cutaneous sensation that provokes the response of scratching. It is a feature of many cutaneous disorders, as well as some systemic diseases, and its severity may range from the very mild to totally incapacitating. The initial approach to the patient with pruritus is to categorize the most likely cause: (1) cutaneous disease, (2) systemic disease, (3) an adverse drug effect, and (4) idiopathic. Many cases are due to allergy, either systemic (food, drugs, contrast media, etc.) or topical (chemicals, detergents, cosmetics, clothing, etc.). The former is usually diagnosed by history, the latter by the distribution of the skin lesion on the body. Patients with allergic reactions severe enough to compromise circulation or respiration are discussed in the chapter on *Anaphylaxis and Serum Sickness*. Therapy

directed at the underlying cause has the best long-term effect.

Therapy.   Therapy of pruritus can be divided into the topical and systemic. Dry, xerotic skin seems to be more susceptible to the itch sensation. Therefore, cool water compresses as outlined above or cool baths or showers followed by emollients on damp hydrated skin help to alleviate the dryness and thus the itching. The addition of 0.25 percent menthol or 0.5 percent phenol to the emollient adds to the cooling antipruritic effect. Emollients range from petrolatum jelly to a wide variety of elegant nonprescription preparations. I prefer to use topical corticosteroids only if an active dermatitis is present.

The H_1-blocker antihistamines have been used for a number of years in the treatment of pruritus. Hydroxyzine seems to be slightly more effective than the other H_1 antihistamines in my experience, but there is a great deal of variation in patient response. I have found two approaches in the management of pruritus to be helpful. For the adult patient with severe, disabling pruritus, antihistamines such as hydroxyzine, 25 to 50 mg, may be given up to 4 times per day. Because many patients are bothered by pruritus primarily at night, the second regimen is to use hydroxyzine in a dose of 25 to 50 mg 1 hour before bedtime. This evening regimen seems to cause less drowsiness the next day and avoids the drowsiness associated with daytime use of the drug. If the patient does not respond to hydroxyzine or has used it previously without success, then I use one of the other H_1 antihistamines in comparable doses. The *recent* introduction of terfenadine has provided an antihistamine with only minimal sedative side effects; the recommended dosage is 60 mg twice daily. The concurrent use of the H_2 antihistamine cimetidine with an H_1 blocker may be helpful in some cases, but this combination in my experience has been rather disappointing. Combinations of the various H_1 antihistamines are sometimes useful in patients with chronic pruritus. I try to avoid the use of systemic corticosteroids except in acute dermatoses such as allergic contact dermatitis.

INPATIENT THERAPY IN SKIN DISEASE

MARIE-LOUISE JOHNSON, M.D., Ph.D.

Emergency room assessment of skin disease can be challenging. The overwhelming cutaneous disruption of widespread poison ivy may threaten the diagnostic confidence of the physician, but the problem can be readily and competently handled at home. By contrast, the weeping disruption of blistering diseases such as toxic epidermal necrolysis and pemphigus threaten life and demand admission, even when the presenting cutaneous change is fairly limited. Edema about the mouth of a young man may manifest a mild allergic response to cheese or may be the first sign of the hereditary fatal angioedema.

Which cutaneous problems, then, should be considered for emergency care and inpatient treatment? Generally, these may be divided into chronic problems that would benefit from intensive care, acute and subacute problems perhaps presently contained but in danger of exacerbating, and a third group in which skin change is an associated marker of serious underlying disease.

CHRONIC DISEASE

Chronic dermatological problems are easiest to consider at the outset, because the diagnosis is usually known and the differential diagnosis not a challenge. Occasionally the patient's recognition of his diagnosis or admission of chronicity will be withheld, not so much to test the examiner as to ensure hospital admission.

Atopic Dermatitis

The atopic diathesis may present in either the skin or the respiratory system or both. There may be a history of urticaria as well as eczematous change of the skin, which is characteristically weeping in children and drier and lichenified in adults, with an intensification in the flexural areas, behind the ears, and about the eyes. Reactions to airborne contact irritants may mimic atopic dermatitis in appearance, but a lifelong history of intermittent rash beginning at 2 to 3 months of age, combined with a his-

With appropriate therapy, most skin diseases respond quickly and with gratifying results. Appropriate care and referral in the emergency department can contribute to better care and faster recovery.

tory of seasonal rhinitis or family history of the atopic diathesis, should confirm the clinical impression.

Acute atopic dermatitis in the *child* is best managed by open wet dressings with Burow's solution, 1 to 3 hours a day, divided into four time intervals; a light cotton pajama wet with solution can keep a dressing applied to an active 2-year-old. An oil-in-water lubricant such as cetaphil (containing 0.25 percent menthol if pruritus is severe) overcomes dryness without being occlusive. Heavier lubricants retain heat and aggravate the pruritus. Intermediate-strength topical steroids in a similar cream base, applied twice daily under the light lubricant and at bedtime when itching is worse, reduce the erythematous response. Diphenhydramine hydrochloride as elixir or capsules is useful. If this is too soporific (as in 25 percent of patients) or too stimulating (as in 10 percent of patients), other antihistamines may be tried, such as dexchlorpheniramine maleate (Polaramine), the dextrorotatory form of chlorpheniramine maleate (Chlor-Trimeton), which is well tolerated, or Chlor-Trimeton itself, tripelennamine (Pyribenzamine), or hydroxyzine (Atarax).

Although steroids in low dosage may be needed eventually to bring the problem under control, a trial of 24 to 48 hours of intense topical care in the protective environment of the hospital is essential for adequate assessment of severity and complications.

Threatening infections, such as herpes simplex, must always be considered if the erythema or vesiculation seems excessive. A Tzanck smear of a vesicle (Table 2) shows multinucleated giant cells if the vesicle is viral. Superimposed pyodermas are also possible. However, bacterial cultures of eczematous skin may reveal opportunistic pathogens that are growing in a favorable environment without infecting the skin. Erythema, tenderness, and lymphatic response give clues as to whether there is active infection. If infection is not clinically apparent, restoring the skin to its normal state permits natural barriers to over-

TABLE 1 Open Wet Dressings

Immerse a soft, closely woven cloth such as cotton sheeting in tepid water, wring thoroughly, and apply one layer to the area to be treated. In 15 minutes or so, depending on the ambient temperature and humidity, the cloth should be removed and reimmersed. Repeat the process over an interval of at least 1 hour, 4 times a day.

To enhance the therapeutic effects of the wet dressing, aluminum acetate may be added—1 Domeboro powder pack or tablet to 1 pint of water (full-strength Burow's solution).

come the pathogens. When there is doubt, broad-spectrum antibiotics such as erythromycin or cephalexin (Keflex) may be started pending the outcome of appropriate cultures.

Atopic dermatitis in the *adult* patient, with extensive, chronic eczematous change in the skin present intermittently over a lifetime, is an infrequent problem but one best managed by someone familiar with the disease and its manifestations. There is a time to hospitalize such patients and a time to use a small dose of systemic steroid, but such times are infrequent.

When intensive topical outpatient therapy has failed and the patient's function is compromised, hospitalization is in order. As with the child, open wet dressings, light mentholated lotions, and systemic antihistamines should be begun with a view to resuming the hardening effect of ultraviolet light with or without tar. Attention to stress and the host response to stress, whether psychic or physical, is important.

Psoriasis

Afflicting no more than 1 percent of the population and ignored or suffered patiently by many, psoriasis can present in such a generalized way that the body is encased in scale, with function severely limited by tense fissured skin, hyperkeratotic palms and soles, and associated arthritis. Pruritus may be present and so intense that the skin is scratched raw. Patients in such cases benefit from the intense therapy possible only in a supervised, assisted environment. Without such therapy there is risk of extending to an exfoliative erythroderma, which in the older patient may become a chronic exfoliative dermatitis with consequent protein loss and debility.

Therapy begins with quieting the reactive process. Open wet dressings may be useful if erythema and pruritus are major components. Soothing tub baths with cautious use of tar, 1 to 2 capfuls of a tar emulsion per bath, and topical steroid applied 2 or 3 times daily in a nonocclusive base (e.g., triamcinolone acetonide cream 0.1 percent) reduce the reactivity of the skin and permit more aggressive therapy with ultraviolet light.

Scalp Psoriasis

Scalp psoriasis (seborrheic dermatitis in the extreme) can present as a helmet of scale with an erythematous base impossible to treat until the scale is softened with occlusive warm oil, washed away with keratolytic shampoos such as Sebulex, and treated with topical steroid lotion (Table 3).

TABLE 2 Tzanck Smear

Unroof a vesicle with a scalpel. Using the blunt side of the scalpel, gently curette the vesicle base. Smear the accumulated cells on a clean slide. Wright's or Giemsa stain demonstrates the cellular morphology to show the multinucleated epidermal giant cells of a viral infection or the acantholytic cells of certain blistering diseases.

TABLE 3 Triple "8" Regimen

Apply warm olive oil to scalp, cover with a shower cap or plastic-wrap turban, and leave for 8 hours; then shampoo with Sebulex or Sebutone.

Next, apply Baker's P&S liquid to scalp and leave undisturbed for 8 hours, followed by another (optional) shampoo.

Finally, apply steroid lotion (Valisone lotion 0.1%) to scalp (but avoid wasting on hair). Use twice in the next 8-hour interval.

Repeat this 24-hour regimen once or twice.

Pustular Psoriasis

Usually chronic and indolent, psoriasis may present as a life-threatening problem in a generalized pustular form. An acute eruption of superficial sterile pustules that coalesce into lakes of pus may appear on normal skin or previous psoriatic plaques. The superficial pustules become denuded, leaving raw eroded areas; circinate lesions may appear on the oral mucosa. Dehydration and electrolyte imbalance are common; septicemia may be a complication. The differential diagnosis includes pustulation due to bacterial infection. Smears of pus in search of bacteria and appropriate cultures of skin and blood must be taken.

Immediate therapy includes hydration and the correction of electrolyte imbalance, with every effort to quiet the reactive process in the skin through wet dressings and sedation. No specific psoriatic therapy should be undertaken until the pustulation has ceased and the systemic manifestations have abated.

The generalized pustular eruption of pregnancy is probably a form of pustular psoriasis. It portends distress for mother and fetus, leading occasionally to abortion or stillbirth or even to maternal death secondary to cardiac and renal failure. Hospitalization and obstetric consultation are urgent.

Localized groups of pustules may appear on plaques of psoriasis, often as a reaction to the primary irritation of topical therapy. No significant signs are associated, and cautious outpatient management is safe. Pustules may also appear on normal skin of the palms and soles with plaque psoriasis elsewhere, a form of psoriasis frequently associated with arthropathy of the distal interphalangeal joints. Hospitalization is not indicated.

Other Pustular Conditions

Similar pustules occurring without psoriatic plaques elsewhere may or may not be a manifestation of psoriasis. When arthritis is associated with such pustules, Reiter's syndrome is difficult to rule out; if there is urethritis preceding or concomitant with the pustular lesions, or if the arthritis involves larger joints, the diagnosis is probably Reiter's syndrome. Signs and symptoms include mild to crippling arthritis with fever, polymorphonuclear leukocytes, and elevated erythrocyte sedimentation rate, plus systemic manifestations warranting hospitalization for bed rest and protection of the inflamed joints. Aspirin in an adequate dosage to produce a blood level of 20 mg per deciliter, steroidal and other nonsteroidal anti-inflammatory agents, and even the antimetabolite methotrexate have been used. The nonspecific urethritis tends to be unresponsive to antibiotics.

More common than Reiter's syndrome is dyshidrotic eczema, which presents as extensive vesicles of the feet or hands. With secondary bacterial infection these may be confused with pustular psoriasis or Reiter's syndrome or with fungal infection. Open wet dressings with Burow's solution, or 0.125 percent silver nitrate solution if the organisms warrant it, cleanse and calm the eruption as topical steroids bring it under control.

ACUTE CONDITIONS

Acute dermatologic problems with no antecedent history of cutaneous disruption present more of a challenge. Some are so devastating and the systemic effects so severe that there is no question about hospitalization. Others with an adequate supporting environment might fare as well without hospitalized care. These must be sorted out, and whether or not the patient is admitted to the hospital, intensive restorative therapy must be begun.

Contact Dermatitis

Acute extensive contact dermatitis may be an *allergic* contact dermatitis such as that evoked by the oleoresin of poison ivy or the chemical ingredients of a sun-protective lotion; it may be a *primary irritant* contact dermatitis, as can be seen with the chemicals of a pesticide; or it may be a *photoallergic* contact dermatitis that for its expression requires cutaneous contact with a chemical, such as the salicylanilides, plus exposure to ultraviolet light.

All of the above produce an eczematous cutaneous reaction that varies with the extent of the exposure and host response. Here the history usually helps (e.g., if the patient has been working in the garden or using new chemicals or old soaps). Pruritus is a clue to the underlying pathogenesis, and distribution, such as a clothing pattern or brush streaking as from plants, indicates possible etiology.

If the cutaneous distribution is extensive, if the skin is blistered and weeping, if the patient is debilitated, or if there is obvious secondary infection, hospitalization may be necessary to maintain electrolyte balance and treat opportunistic infection. However, most acute contact dermatitis can be managed on an outpatient basis.

Whether the patient is hospitalized or not, good therapy mandates drying and cleansing of the skin, readily achieved with immersion tub baths using inert powder as obtained from oatmeal (Aveeno), corn (starch), or soy (Soyaloid), one-half cup per tubful of water. Open wet dressings with Burow's solution should also be used 2 to 3 hours a day over the entire involved area of skin. Dividing the areas to be treated so that no more than one-quarter of the skin is wet-dressed at any one time, and ensuring

protection from drafts by cradle-supported covers, avoids uncomfortable chilling and hypothermia. If the eruption is extensive, *systemic steroids* should be used (30 to 40 mg of prednisone in a once-daily dose, with tapering withheld until there is reduction in erythema and no evidence of extension). If there is a history of hypertension, diabetes, peptic ulcer, tuberculosis, osteoporosis, malignancy, or even psoriasis, one should pause long and thoughtfully before initiating even a short course of steroids. However, with close monitoring, even the patient at greatest risk can be given a short course of systemic steroids. Although the young healthy adult is the ideal risk for short-term steroids, the older patient may need them to thwart an exfoliative erythroderma. Once an extensive eczematous dermatitis extends to exfoliation, it is always difficult to manage, and in the elderly it takes months or more to clear. Along with systemic steroids, *antihistamines* should be used in full dosage, such as 250 mg of diphenhydramine daily.

Topical steroids are of little value added to high systemic doses of steroids, but they should be used as the systemic steroids are tapered, always in a cream base to avoid occlusion. An intermediate-strength steroid such as triamcinolone acetonide 0.1 percent in a cream base is useful for lesions other than on the face, where using a less potent hydrocortisone cream, 1 percent or 2.5 percent reduces the risk of atrophic effects on facial skin. Overlayering the steroids with a mentholated lotion is an important added antipruritic maneuver and also provides lubrication without occlusion.

Photosensitivity, whether induced topically by cutaneous contact or systemically by drugs, usually does not warrant admission. However, associated leukopenia, fever, albuminuria, or friction rub should bring the diagnosis of lupus erythematosus to mind and warrant concern for worsening of the autoimmune disease because of the photosensitive response.

Angioedema and Urticaria

Angioedema and acute urticaria frequently present in an emergency fashion. *Anaphylaxis*, beginning as a sensation of warmth, pruritus, or burning, may lead to death within minutes. (See the chapter on *Anaphylaxis and Serum Sickness*.) After stabilizing treatment, the patient should be admitted for observation, because the antigen load may escape control. Death from anaphylaxis has been known to occur after 4 days.

Angioedema represents a mild form of localized tissue swelling of and about the eyelids, lips, tongue, and even the pharynx, without extending to anaphylaxis. It may involve an extremity. Lesions arise suddenly, rarely persist beyond a day or two, and may recur. Such change about the head and neck must always suggest the possibility of anaphylaxis. Without a history of sting or injection, perhaps with a history of previous angioedema, anaphylaxis is less likely. Nonetheless, those with angioedema, especially complement-mediated angioedema (both inherited and acquired), can have involvement of the skin, mucous membranes, and respiratory and gastrointestinal tracts. They can die from anaphylaxis. Treat them as for urticaria, but be prepared for anaphylaxis.

Urticaria, erythematous and pruritic wheals with edema in the superficial portions of the dermis, presenting without angioedema, is a more common problem. IgE-dependent *allergic urticaria* can be seen in the atopic diathesis, with specific antigen sensitivities, and as a response to cold, light, pressure, or heat (cholinergic). This must be distinguished from *complement-mediated urticaria*, which may be part of hereditary or acquired angioedema, necrotizing vasculitis, serum sickness, or reactions to blood products. It must also be distinguished from reaction to substances that provoke urticaria directly by *anaphylactoid responses* through the stimulation of mast cells (e.g., opiates, polymyxin B, curare, and radiologic contrast media). Aspirin, nonsteroidal anti-inflammatory agents, azo dyes, and benzoates (presumably through altering the metabolism of arachidonic acid) are known to cause urticaria and anaphylactoid responses, but many cases are idiopathic.

The patient who presents with acute urticaria should be treated with subcutaneous epinephrine 0.3 ml of 1:1,000 concentration, plus antihistamines such as intramuscular diphenhydramine, 100 mg, and observed. A careful history should be taken for previous allergic responses, for a familial predisposition to such responses, and for a recent exposure that may be the precipitating event.

Blisters and Bullae

Vesicles and bullae without background erythema (not a thermal burn and not an eczematous process such as atopic dermatitis or acute contact dermatitis) may be infectious (viral or bacterial), allergic (drug induced), or one of the blistering diseases such as pemphigus.

Viral blisters, discrete in a dermatome distribution, are recognized as herpes zoster. If the patient is elderly and without pain, or if there are scattered blisters outside the primary dermatome, the diagnosis may be challenged. A Tzanck smear (see Table 2) confirms the process as viral. Some 20 percent of immunologically competent individuals have lesions at a distant site. Should the patient be immunologically compromised, there is risk of dissemination and death. Only such compromised patients should be admitted. Acyclovir should be begun at once in an intravenous dosage of 250 mg per m² every 8 hours in patients with normal renal function. Open wet dressings with Burow's solution cleanse and dry the denuded dermatome. Erythromycin (Ilotycin) or Polysporin ointment reduces the risk of secondary bacterial infection; topical viscous lidocaine (Xylocaine) provides some anesthesia if pain is a problem.

Grouped vesicles in an extensive, nondermatome distribution about the face or genital area, associated with fever and pain, probably represent primary herpes simplex. Again, the positive Tzanck smear proves the viral etiology of the vesicle. Unless the individual has the atopic

diathesis or is pregnant and close to term, there is no need for hospitalization, but viral cultures should be taken to confirm herpes simplex infection, wet dressings should be instituted, and oral acyclovir should be begun, 200 mg every 4 hours.

Bullae on a slightly erythematous base in a localized or random distribution without Nikolsky's sign (separation of skin layers when pressure is applied) are probably *bacterial or bullous impetigo*. Bacterial cultures and sensitivities should be obtained from the blister, and wet dressings should be begun with topical antibiotic solution applied (erythromycin, tetracycline, or clindamycin in an alcohol base). If the lesions are extensive, oral antibiotic therapy is required (erythromycin cephalexin, or Keflex, 1.5 g in the first 24 hours, then 1 g per day, or for children the pediatric equivalent).

In infants, children, and occasionally adults, infection with phage group 2 staphylococci, usually phage type 71 staphylococci, may begin as bullous impetigo with Nikolsky's sign, spreading to become the *staphylococcal scalded skin syndrome* (SSSS), with large flaccid bullae around body orifices extending to denude the integument, a phenomenon attributed to an exotoxin elaborated by the staphylococcus. The prompt initiation of therapy with penicillinase-resistant penicillin is mandatory. Hospitalization is needed to replace the water, colloid, and electrolytes lost through the denuded integument. Even with such measures, the risk of fatal outcome is still 2 to 3 percent.

Distinct from SSSS is *toxic epidermal necrolysis*, (TEN), characterized by the explosive appearance of widespread skin erythema and then denudation. It affects adults more than children, is unassociated with bacterial infection, and frequently has an antecedent drug history. The mucous membranes and conjunctivae are often severely involved. The diagnosis is best made by examining a denuded sheet of skin in which there is necrolysis beginning in the basal layer with only necrotic epidermal cells, polymorphonuclear leukocytes, and debris, in contrast to SSSS, in which the cells appear normal, although acantholytic.

Current therapy for TEN is corticosteroids in high dosage: 150 to 250 mg of prednisone daily. Fluid and electrolytes must be maintained as in a burn patient, and eye care is important to reduce ocular damage. A fatal outcome can be expected in some 30 percent of cases.

Because toxic shock syndrome (TSS) can also present explosively with diffuse erythema, it must be considered in the differential diagnosis of TEN and ruled out. Both TEN and TSS may have multiple system involvement with high fever plus conjunctival, oropharyngeal, and vaginal hyperemia. However, systemic steroids, lifesaving for the patient with TEN, might have disastrous effects if used as the only therapy in TSS. Cutaneous histopathology of TSS fails to show subepidermal vesiculation, intracellular edema, or confluent epidermal necrosis.

The patient with pemphigus, although a candidate for totally denuded skin, does not have such an explosive course and usually has no history of erythema or burning of the skin. Rather innocuous blisters with Nikolsky's sign appear on normal skin, often asymptomatically. Lesions of the oral mucosa are common and may be painful, compromising nutrition.

The patient with pemphigus requires admission for assessment, immunofluorescent studies of serum and skin, and institution of specific therapy (high-dose corticosteroid therapy, the equivalent of 80 to 120 g of prednisone a day with antimetabolites such as azathioprine 100 mg for its steroid-sparing effect). Wet dressings to denuded areas and topical antimicrobial and drying agents such as Castellani's paint are useful.

Other bullous problems, bullous pemphigoid and bullous drug eruptions, are characterized by tense bullae but not Nikolsky's sign and are often associated with pruritus. If extensive, the denuded surfaces permit loss of electrolytes and risk of infection.

Immediate therapy is to remove the cause if a drug is suspected and, depending on the extent of the eruption, to initiate corticosteroids, 40 to 80 mg a day of prednisone or equivalent, if needed. With bullous pemphigoid, prolonged steroid therapy may be required for control, and in such cases antimetabolites may be useful.

Erythema multiforme, which must also be considered as a bullous disease, has a spectrum from scattered target lesions to profound systemic symptoms with severe mucocutaneous involvement (Stevens-Johnson syndrome). The appearance is sudden and often recurrent, but the problem is usually self-limited, although blindness and death can occur. The condition is a reaction pattern associated with infections, ingestants, physical factors, and even malignancy, but often is of unknown etiology. Therapy relates to symptoms and the disruption of the integument. Mild cases need little treatment. In the more severe cases, compresses and appropriate antimicrobial and supportive therapy are indicated. Systemic steroids are often used because of the severity of the systemic involvement but are probably not helpful and may be contraindicated.

DERMATOLOGIC SIGNS ASSOCIATED WITH UNDERLYING DISEASE

There are patients with certain skin changes that alert the examiner to link the presenting complaint with the cutaneous clue. Listed in Table 4 are some cutaneous markers of systemic disease associated with epistaxis and abdominal pain.

Vasculitis produces skin lesions and can affect any organ. Purpuric lesions on the skin can be the result of mechanical trauma or insect bites, but they may also represent damage to the blood vessels through immunologic mechanisms. In the skin, the vessels involved are almost always venules, and the necrotizing vasculitis is observed as *palpable purpura*. Among the more common chronic conditions underlying necrotizing vasculitis are rheumatoid arthritis, lupus erythematosus, and Sjögren's syndrome, but it is also seen with hypergammaglobulinemia, cryoglobulinemia, and lymphoproliferative disorders.

The *infectious agents* tending to provoke such cutaneous vasculitis are hepatitis B virus, group A hemolytic streptococci, *Staphylococcus aureus*, and in some populations *Mycobacterium leprae*.

Chronic *meningococcemia* produces tender papules having a dark blue hemorrhagic center. These may be scattered and have associated petechiae or ecchymoses; there may be pustules. Joint pain (especially of the temporomandibular joint) is common, and there may be splenomegaly. There will be a history of intermittent fever and shaking chills. Similar skin lesions are produced by gonococcemia, subacute bacterial endocarditis, rat-bite

TABLE 4 Cutaneous Markers of Systemic Disease Presenting as Abdominal Pain or Bleeding

Skin Sign	Diagnosis
Abdominal pain	
Brown/black macules on lips, face, buccal mucosa, dorsa of hands	Peutz-Jeghers syndrome
Nodules in groups along superficial arteries	Polyarteritis nodosa
Erythematous macules that become papules on limbs, buttocks, rarely face	Henoch-Schönlein purpura
Dark blue/purple macules that become nodules	Kaposi's sarcoma
Pink papules that become small white scars with peripheral telangiectasias on trunk	Degos's disease
Tender subcutaneous nodules on upper thighs and buttocks	Weber-Christian disease
Erysipelas-like erythema of feet and lower legs	Familial Mediterranean anemia
Pyoderma gangrenosum	Ulcerative colitis
Epistaxis	
Telangiectasias on upper half of body	Rendu-Osler-Weber syndrome
Fox-Fordyce disease of scrotum	Phlebectasia of oral cavity, jejunum, scrotum

fever, and rickettsial infection such as Rocky Mountain spotted fever.

Among the drugs predisposing a patient to vasculitis are the sulfonamides, the thiazides, and penicillin. In some 50 percent of patients, the cause of the vasculitis remains undiscovered. It is among this group that Henoch-Schönlein anaphylactoid purpura is found. A history of antecedent upper respiratory infection is sometimes elicited. Occurring more often in children, it frequently involves the skin, joints, gastrointestinal tract, and kidneys. When Henoch-Schönlein purpura occurs in the older individual, usually a woman, it presents with more urticarial lesions associated with arthralgias. This may be accompanied by abdominal pain, lymphadenopathy, and diffuse glomerulonephritis.

Erythema nodosum, a hypersensitivity vasculitis, presents as bilateral pretibial red nodules, occasionally with additional lesions of the extensor aspect of the arms. Leprosy, tuberculosis, or sarcoid may cause this lesion, as may streptococcal pharyngitis or primary atypical pneumonia. Less frequently it is seen in ulcerative colitis, regional enteritis, or even as a reaction to medications such as the iodides, bromides, sulfonamides, and oral contraceptives.

Sweet's syndrome (acute febrile neutrophilic dermatosis) produces painful nodules or even plaques, associated with high persistent fever, occurring asymmetrically over the extremities, face, and neck. It occurs mostly in middle-aged women and is associated with leukocytosis and an elevated erythrocyte sedimentation rate.

Pancreatitis can produce recurrent painful nodules, 0.5 to 5 cm, appearing on the legs or elsewhere, which soften and drain a viscous aseptic material, liquefied fat.

Erythema induratum produces nodular lesions occurring on the posterior aspect of the legs (rarely on the thighs) that are painful to pressure and apt to ulcerate. Classically these were associated with tuberculosis, but often there is no evidence of active mycobacterial infection. As in all patients with vasculitis, an underlying cause must be sought. The need for inpatient assessment and care depends on the severity of symptoms and activity of the underlying problem.

SUGGESTED READING

Fitzpatrick TB, Eisen AZ, Wolff K, Freedberg IM, Austen KF, eds. Dermatology in general medicine. 3nd ed. New York: McGraw-Hill, 1986.
Johnson ML. Skin diseases. In: Wyngaarden JB, Smith LH, eds. Cecil textbook of medicine. 17th ed. Philadelphia: WB Saunders, 1985.

CELLULITIS AND LYMPHADENITIS

J. STEPHAN STAPCZYNSKI, M.D.

CELLULITIS

Cellulitis is an inflammatory process of the deep dermis that occurs when bacteria breach the protective epithelium, gain access to the subcutaneous tissues, and produce the characteristic spreading infection. Although cellulitis can occur in areas of normal-appearing skin, prior trauma, ulcerations, venous or lymphatic stasis, and underlying immunodeficiencies are predisposing factors. The majority of cases of cellulitis have been documented to be caused by *Staphylococcus aureus* and group A streptococci, but other bacteria are found in high frequency in certain clinical circumstances (Table 1). The limited number of potential pathogens means that initial antibiotic therapy can be based on the patient's age, area of involvement, and underlying host factors. Additionally, many (probably most) cases of cellulitis are treated empirically without definitive microbiologic diagnosis and have a completely adequate response.

Cellulitis presents as a spreading inflammation with local warmth, erythema, and tenderness. If it is untreated, induration and suppuration can develop, and in severe cases, vesicles, bullae, and abscesses can occur. Lymphangitis and regional lymphadenopathy are common. In adults and most children with truncal or extremity cellulitis, fever and systemic toxicity are usually not prominent. In the preantibiotic era, cellulitis had up to a 25 percent mortality rate.

Because cellulitis due to *Haemophilus influenzae* can be associated with bacteremia and other disseminated infections, several studies sought out clinical clues that suggest the presence of this organism. These are (1) facial cellulitis, especially in a child less than 2 years old and without an obvious portal of entry; (2) extremity cellulitis in a child accompanied by fever and leukocytosis; (3) "violaceous hue" of the erythema; and (4) multiple separate areas of cellulitis. However, such clues are not found in all cases.

Erysipelas is a distinctive type of cellulitis involving the superficial dermis and is most often caused by group A streptococci. This disease is less common than simple cellulitis and is more often found in children and the elderly than in young and middle-aged adults. In the preantibiotic era, the face was most frequently involved, but the most recent report from Israel documents a preponderance of cases involving the legs, presumably owing to walking in sandals or barefoot. Erysipelas starts off as a small, raised, painful plaque that spreads with a dis-

TABLE 1 Clinical Syndromes of Cellulitis Associated With Bacteria Other Than Staphylococci and Streptococci

Clinical Syndrome	Causative Agent
Facial cellulitis in children, especially without a portal of entry	H. influenzae
Facial cellulitis with exterior trauma	S. aureus
Facial cellulitis from a dental abscess or intraoral laceration	Anaerobic mouth flora
Infants, especially with face or neck involvement	Group B streptococci
Cellulitis after a dog or cat bite	Pasteurella multocida

tinct advancing edge over several days to reach a maximal size, if untreated, of 10 to 15 cm in diameter. The involved area is typically elevated. As opposed to simple cellulitis, in erysipelas, high fever, systemic toxicity, leukocytosis, and bacteremia are common. During convalescence, desquamation of the involved skin occurs. In untreated cases of erysipelas, mortality can be as high as 40 percent, but antibiotics have rendered this disease benign.

Uncommon and Rare Forms of Cellulitis

Staphylococcus aureus and Group A streptococci are the cause of most cases of cellulitis, but other organisms are found depending on the clinical situation. Other streptococcal groups can cause cellulitis: Groups C, G, and B (especially in neonates). Pneumococcal cellulitis is rare, usually develops from a bacteremia, and looks similar to erysipelas.

Erysipeloid is a cellulitis that is due to *Erysipelothrix rhusiopathiae*. This bacteria is found in saltwater fish, shellfish, and occasionally in poultry, beef, and animal hides. The bacteria is usually innoculated though a break in the skin; most often on the hands. Within a week, a painful violaceous lesion develops that slowly spreads with distinct raised edges as the central portion clears. Erysipeloid responds well to penicillin.

"Seal finger" presents as a lesion similar to erysipeloid, but found in individuals who work with seals. The etiology is unknown. "Seal finger" is best treated with tetracycline.

Aeromonas hydrophila is a gram-negative rod found in freshwater lakes, rivers, and soil. An acute cellulitis may develop if this organism is innoculated into abraded or lacerated skin.

Various vibrio species (e.g., *V. vulnificus, V. alginolyticus*, and *V. parahaemolyticus*) may produce acute cellulitis if innoculated into a wound sustained while in salt water. The cellulitis may progress into bullous lesions, necrotic ulcers, and bacteremia which often require surgical debridement for treatment. These organisms are usually sensitive to chloramphenicol or tetracycline.

Sporothrix schenckii is a fungus found in plants and soil. If innoculated into a wound—most often on the hand—it slowly produces a small painless papule with some exudate. Secondary nodules develop along the path of ascending lymphatic channels, but regional lymphadenopathy is rare. Ulceration is common in the primary lesion and is sometimes seen in the secondary lymphangitic spread. This infection can be diagnosed by the clinical appearance, culture, lack of response to topical or the usual antibacterial agents, and response to topical or the usual antibacterial agents, and response to potassium iodide.

In immunocompromised individuals, a wide variety of bacteria (*Enterobacteriaceae, Pseudomonas*) and fungi (*Candida, Cryptococci*) may produce acute cellulitis.

Two major points must be remembered when evaluating a patient with cellulitis. First, although most patients with cellulitis are generally healthy, have limited involvement, and respond well to oral antibiotics, three high-risk situations indicate the need for more aggressive therapy; these are (1) cellulitis of the face, (2) cellulitis in the presence of venous or lymphatic edema, and (3) cellulitis in patients with asplenism, those on steroid therapy, alcoholics, and any others with depressed immune function. If the area around the eye is involved, it is important to differentiate between orbital and periorbital (preseptal) infection: in orbital cellulitis, globe mobility is usually impaired. Second, infections of the soft tissues may not be superficial and slowly spreading, but deeper and rapidly advancing along tissue planes. These necrotizing infections are usually caused by a polymicrobial mix of aerobic and anaerobic bacteria. A number of clinical syndromes have been described that usually have a distinctive picture in the pure state, but not all patients present with an easily recognizable pattern. Important clues to the presence of a deeper and rapidly spreading soft tissue infection are prominent systemic toxicity, high fever, gas formation in soft tissues (crepitus), overlying skin necrosis, foul-smelling discharge, and bleb or bullae formation. Patients with these deeper infections all need parenteral broad-spectrum antibiotics, admission to the hospital, and urgent surgical incision or drainage.

The microbial evaluation of patients with cellulitis can be done by a number of techniques; these are through swab cultures of open wounds or discharge, subcutaneous aspiration of the advancing edge, or blood cultures. Depending on the clinical presentation, these techniques isolate a pathogen between 10 and 90 percent of the time (Table 2).

Needle aspiration should be done through intact skin at the edge of the involved area. The skin should be first cleansed with a bacteriocidal agent (i.e., povidone iodine) and allowed to dry; this reduces the potential for surface organism contamination. Infiltrative anesthesia is to be avoided; the bacteriostatic additives may reduce culture yield. The skin surface is held steady and punctured with a 22 or 23 g needle attached to a 5 or 10 ml syringe; any available fluid or pus is then aspirated. If no fluid is obtained, then 1.0 ml of sterile, nonbacteriostatic saline is injected into the area and immediately aspirated. Any fluid obtained should be sent for Gram stain and culture.

As mentioned before, isolation of a pathogen often does not influence therapy, and most patients respond to empiric antibiotic selection. However, cultures should be done in the following patients: children and possibly adults with facial cellulitis, infants with cellulitis, patients with immunodeficiencies, patients with open wounds, and patients who do not respond to empiric therapy. Additionally, cultures are recommended in patients with erysipelas. Some authors also recommend that children suspected of *H. influenzae* cellulitis have a lumbar puncture done to exclude coexistent meningitis. Infants with cellulitis should have an aspiration culture of the involved area along with a generalized septic work-up and, thereafter,

be admitted for intravenous ampicillin and gentamicin treatment pending culture results.

Most cases of simple cellulitis can be managed on an outpatient basis with oral antibiotics (Table 3). The key is patient compliance with the therapeutic regimen and close follow-up. Conversely, the following patients should be admitted for intravenous antibiotic therapy: (1) children and adults with facial cellulitis, (2) children and adults with a high fever or significant systemic toxicity, (3) patients with immunodeficiencies or local host defense impairments, (4) patients with erysipelas, (5) patients suspected of having a deeper infection, and (6) infants with cellulitis.

Outpatient empiric therapy uses either an oral semisynthetic penicillinase-resistant penicillin, cephalosporin, erythromycin, or trimethoprim-sulfamethoxazole (Table 4). All are equally effective, and the antibiotic selection is usually determined by the patient's history of drug allergies and by cost. Treatment should continue for 7 to 10 days. Additionally, the patient should be instructed not to bear weight on the involved extremity, to keep the involved part rested or elevated, and to be rechecked in 2 days. The patient should also be instructed to come back sooner if symptoms worsen.

Inpatient empiric antibiotic therapy uses either a semisynthetic penicillinase-resistant penicillin or cephalosporin directed against gram-positive staphylcocci and streptococci (Tables 5 and 6). If *H. influenzae* is a possibility, the previous practice was to add both ampicillin and chloramphenicol, for a total of three antibiotics. Both ampicillin and chloramphenicol were used because of the incidence of ampicillin resistance that occurs in up to 20 to 25 percent of *H. influenzae* isolates in many communities. However, current experience with both second- and third-generation cephalosporins, which possess excellent activity against all three major pathogens (staphylococci, streptococci, and *H. influenzae*), has been that single-drug therapy with these agents produces as good a clinical response as previous triple-drug regimens. In addition to exposing the patient to only one drug and often having lower total cost, some agents need be given only once or twice per day. Intravenous therapy should continue until systemic toxicity and local inflammation have resolved (usually 4 to 6 days), and then the oral antibiotic should be started to complete a total of 10 days of treatment.

Patients with erysipelas should be admitted to the hospital for intravenous antibiotic therapy with penicillin

TABLE 2   Approximate Incidence of Pathogen Isolation In Previously Healthy Patients With Cellulitis

	Cultures	
Clinical Syndrome	Aspiration	Blood
Extremity or truncal cellulitis with intact skin	10–40%	< 5%
Extremity or truncal cellulitis with broken skin and purulence	80–90%	< 5%
Facial cellulitis in children	40%	40–80%

TABLE 3   Indications For Outpatient Treatment With Oral Antibiotics

Previously healthy
No host defense deficiencies (asplenism, steroids, alcoholism)
Truncal or extremity involvement
Little systemic toxicity

TABLE 4   Oral Antibiotics For Cellulitis

Antibiotic	Pediatric dosage	Adult dosage	Frequency
Penicillin V	25-50 mg/kg/day	1-2 g/day	q6h
Dicloxacillin	12.5-25 mg/kg/day	1-2 g/day	q6h
Cephalexin	25-50 mg/kg/day	1-2 g/day	q6-12h
Cephradine	25-50 mg/kg/day	1-2 g/day	q6h
Erythromycin	30-50 mg/kg/day	1-2 g/day	q6h
Trimethoprim-sulfamethoxazole	1 ml/kg/day suspension[*]	4 regular tabs/day[**]	q12h

* 1 ml = 8 mg trimethoprim (TMP) + 40 mg sulfamethoxozole (SMZ)
** 1 regular tablet = 80 mg TMP + 200 mg SMZ

**TABLE 5 Indications For Inpatient Treatment
With Intravenous Antibiotics**

Immunocompromised
Poor host defenses
Facial cellulitis
Marked systemic toxicity
Erysipelas
Suspicion of a deeper and more rapidly
spreading soft tissue infection

TABLE 6 Intravenous Antibiotics For Cellulitis

Antibiotic	Pediatric Dosage	Adult Dosage	Frequency
Penicillin G	20–40,000 U/kg/day	4–6 million U/day	q6h
Nafcillin or	25–50 mg/kg/day	2–4 g/day	q6h
Oxacillin	50–100 mg/kg/day	2–4 g/day	q6h
Cefazolin	25–50 mg/kg/day	3 g/day	q8h
Erythromycin	15–25 mg/kg/day	2–4 g/day	q6h
Ampicillin	100–200 mg/kg/day	4–8 g/day	q6h
Chloramphenicol	50–100 mg/kg/day	3–6 g/day	q6h
Cefuroxime	50–100 mg/kg/day	3–6 g/day	q8h
Cefotaxime	50–150 mg/kg/day	2–6 g/day	q6h
Ceftriaxone	50–75 mg/kg/day	1–2 g/day	q12–24h

G (40,000 to 80,000 units per kilogram per day in children and 4 to 8 million units per day in adults at 6-hour intervals). Alternatives to penicillin include cephalosporins and erythromycin. It is possible to treat selected patients with erysipelas involving an extremity as outpatients with oral antibiotics; the key is patient compliance.

Patients with simple cellulitis should respond rapidly to antibiotic therapy within a few days; if not, the patient should be investigated for a resistant pathogen or abnormal host defenses.

LYMPHADENITIS

Lymph node enlargement is a common physical finding, especially in children. This section discusses the evaluation of the patient with acute or subacute lymph node enlargement confined to a single region due to an infectious agent. Generalized lymphadenopathy and noninfectious causes of lymph node enlargement are not considered. Lymphadenitis commonly has the cardinal signs of inflammation, erythema, warmth, tenderness, and fluctuance, but these findings are not always present.

Cervical adenitis can be caused by almost any organism that can infect the head or neck area. To evaluate these patients properly, it helps to understand the areas drained by a particular group of lymph nodes. The posterior auricular nodes drain the scalp, posterior external ear, and external auditory canal. The anterior auricular nodes drain the eyes and temporal area of the scalp. The anterior cervical and submandibular nodes drain the teeth and pharynx. Most common causes of cervical adenitis are minor scalp infections, dental or pharyngeal infections, "primary" staphylococcal or streptococcal adenitis, and

mycobacterial infections. Patient history and physical examination are necessary to exclude minor skin or intraoral infections that may be causing cervical adenitis. Percutaneous needle aspiration can be done to isolate a pathogen, but is usually not required to begin empiric antibiotic therapy. An intradermal tuberculosis skin test is recommended, especially in children. Because the most common pathogen isolated from "primary" cervical adenitis is *S. aureus*, a penicillinase-resistant penicillin or cephalosporin is recommended as initial antibiotic treatment. Therapy is given for 10 to 14 days or until there is complete resolution of the swelling. Some patients form abscesses and eventually require surgical drainage, but most can be treated with antibiotics alone.

Supraclavicular adenopathy is always cause for suspicion of neoplasm, and early biopsy is strongly recommended.

The inguinal nodes drain the lower extremities and distal urethra, so a wide variety of soft tissue and venereal infections can cause inguinal node enlargement. For example, the following venereal infections have the indicated incidence of inguinal lymphadenitis: gonococcal urethritis, up to 40 percent; nonspecific urethritis, about 1 percent; primary syphilis, 50 to 70 percent; herpes, almost 100 percent; chancroid, 25 to 60 percent, and lymphogranuloma venereum, about 70 percent. It is important to examine both the legs and genitals for skin lesions and suppurative infections. Fluctuant nodes should be aspirated and, in addition to Gram stain and culture, also have a dark-field microscopic examination for spirochetes. Patients without associated skin lesions should receive a serologic test for lymphogranuloma venereum. Antibiotic treatment is guided by the associated leg or genital lesions, or if no portal of entry can be found and the node is obviously infected, then antistaphylococcal therapy is recommended. Regardless, all patients with inguinal adenopathy need follow-up within a week to assess regression in response to therapy.

It is important to remember that lymph node enlargement is only a physical finding, not a diagnosis. A course of antibiotics should not be considered curative. Follow-up is mandatory, and persistent enlargement requires an explanation.

SUGGESTED READING

Carter S, Feldman WE. Etiology and treatment of facial cellulitis in pediatric patients. Pediatr Infect Dis 1983; 2:222–224.

Fleisher G, Heeger P, Topf P. Hemophilus influenzae cellulitis. Am J Emerg Med 1983; 3:274–277.
Fleisher G, Ludwig S, Henretig F, Ruddy R, Henry W. Cellulitis: initial management. Ann Emerg Med 1981; 10:356–359.
Ginsberg MB. Cellulitis: analysis of 101 cases and review of the literature. South Med J 1981; 74:530–533.
Goldgeier MH. The microbial evaluation of acute cellulitis. Cutis 1983; 31:649–656.
Ho PWL, Pien FD, Hamburg D. Value of cultures in patients with acute cellulitis. South Med J 1979; 72:1402–1403.
Shimoni Z, Turgeman Y, Flatau E, Kohn D. Changing patterns of erysipelas. Isr J Med Sci 1984; 20:242–243.
Szilagyi A, Mendelson J, Portnoy J. Cellulitis of the skin: clinical observations of 50 cases. Can Fam Physician 1982; 28:1399–1402.

CUTANEOUS ABSCESS

HARVEY W. MEISLIN, M.D.

Cutaneous abscesses are one of the most common soft tissue infections encountered by emergency physicians. Approximately 1 to 2 percent of all patient visits are the result of abscesses or their complications.

The emergency physician must understand the extent of the soft tissue infection before simply labeling it an abscess. In general, abscesses tend to be localized and are rarely found in multiples. The physician, however, must realize that cutaneous abscesses may also be associated with deeper infections. A patient who has an abscess may also have an underlying necrotizing fasciitis or myositis. It is very important to recognize these deeper infections, since they can be life-threatening.

Cutaneous abscesses may also be manifestations of other systemic diseases. For example, it is estimated that between 25 and 50 percent of all patients with granulomatous inflammatory bowel disease will manifest a cutaneous abscess at some time. Cutaneous abscesses may be a manifestation of another process that may require different work-up and therapy, as is the case in a drug-induced abscess.

Abscesses tend to occur in all locations of the body, with most appearing in the head, neck, extremities, or the perineal region. Abscesses in the extremities tend to be associated with needle puncture wounds, cuts, abrasions, or minor trauma. Abscesses in the perineal region tend to be associated with bacterial spread that initially emanated from anal crypts. Vaginal abscesses tend to result from obstruction of Bartholin's glands. Abscesses in the head and neck region often result from the obstruction of sebaceous glands or from cystic acne. Abscesses in the axillae often manifest secondary to hidradenitis suppurativa in the adult. Abscesses in general tend to be isolated events, but certain entities predispose to recurrence, such as inflammatory bowel disease, hidradenitis suppurativa, and rectal fistula.

It may be difficult at times to determine the *cause* of a cutaneous abscess, but some clues may be helpful. A patient in the postpubescent population with recurrent abscesses in the axillae who, upon inspection of the axillary region, shows evidence of scarring and inflammation in various stages of healing most likely carries a diagnosis of hidradenitis suppurativa. This has a three to one female to male predominance. Abscesses of the extremity that tend to be associated with sclerotic veins and needle puncture wounds and that often occur in the left forearm tend to be associated with drug abuse and may even be sterile. Sterile abscesses are difficult to differentiate from abscesses due to other causes, except that they tend to occur very rapidly after injection of a foreign substance in the extremity of a young individual. Recurrent abscesses in the midline buttock crease are often associated with recurrent pilonidal sinuses. Recurrent perirectal abscesses are often an indication of fistula formation and may point to the presence of inflammatory bowel disease. Abscesses of the ear lobe, behind the ear, and of the posterior portion of the neck are often associated with infected sebaceous cysts.

CLINICAL PRESENTATION

Clinically the patient usually presents with a painful inflamed nodule that is often fluctuant, with surrounding granulation tissue. There may be associated localized cellulitis or even lymphangitis. Usually patients do not have toxic symptoms, and fever is rare. Not uncommonly, the patient has been squeezing the area or perhaps has attempted to drain it with a needle or knife.

PRE-HOSPITAL MANAGEMENT

Cutaneous abscesses are usually not a difficult problem to handle for paramedical personnel or in the prehospital environment. However, if paramedics have a patient with signs of toxicity or even in frank shock in addition to an abscess, the process cannot be considered localized. This patient should be treated with intravenous fluids with strict monitoring of vital signs and quickly transported to an emergency department, where a work-up can evaluate the extent of the soft tissue infection.

TREATMENT

The mainstay of treatment for cutaneous abscess is incision and drainage. One of the most common errors made by physicians is that if they do not see or feel pus, they put the patient on antibiotics and warm soaks with a return visit when the abscess either points or drains spontaneously. I have found this to result only in a delay in patient care, with the patient remaining in a painful state and often becoming septic. If an abscess is felt to be present, whether or not fluctuance can be truly demonstrated, then at the least purulence should be sought for by simple needle aspiration. Preferably incision and drainage should be carried out.

Incision and drainage are unavoidably painful processes. In the outpatient setting, we tend to use primarily local anesthetics to achieve adequate analgesia. However, local anesthetics do not perform adequately in areas of inflammation and infection, primarily because of decreased pH and an increased blood flow in the area. Also a significant portion of the pain of cutaneous abscess is caused by the pressure of the abscess cavity on surrounding tissue and cutaneous nerves. Instillation of additional volume into the abscess cavity will only worsen the pain.

It therefore may be advisable to use other forms of analgesia. Inhalation of nitrous oxide is useful, although in my experience, it does not suffice as the sole means of analgesia. Premedication of the patient with parenteral analgesics such as the use of meperidine, 50 to 100 mg IM, 20 to 30 minutes before incision, and diazepam, 5 to 10 mg slowly IV approximately 2 to 3 minutes before incision, can be most beneficial. The use of regional anesthesia is also a very effective way to achieve pain control. An intravenous Bier's block or axillary nerve block works well for the upper extremity. The physician must use his judgment in analgesic selection in certain patients because of age, preexisting medical condition, and location and extent of the abscess. Drainage in an inpatient or ambulatory surgical setting, using either general or spinal anesthesia, may be the most appropriate way to go.

Incision is best made with a number 11 scalpel. This is the only scalpel with a blade that can be used to both poke and incise in an upward direction. The incision should span the fluctuance and be deep enough to enter the cavity thoroughly. Abscesses may be under quite a bit of pressure and not uncommonly pus spurts out.

An abscess is not simply a hollow sphere but a series of granulation tissues with loculated areas of purulence. These loculations must all be removed in order to achieve adequate drainage. For incisions in which the overlying skin appears to be necrotic or very cellulitic, it may be advisable to cut an ellipse out of the roof of the abscess cavity. With Bartholin's abscesses, marsupialization is most appropriate.

Once the incision is made, all purulence must be removed. A small mosquito clamp is then inserted into the abscess cavity, breaking up all loculations. This must not be an aggressive process, but done gently so as not to instill bacteria in healthy adjacent tissue or produce bacteremia. The wound should then be irrigated, using a syringe and a plastic catheter, until all necrotic tissue and purulence are removed.

Packing can then be inserted into the cavity. The purpose of packing is twofold: (1) to provide a drainage route for any loculated areas of pus that have not drained or for any purulence that may form, and (2) to hold the surface open so that the drainage is complete before the epithelium closes.

The drain should be loosely placed, that is, installed in all the quadrants of the abscess cavity and exteriorized. It is not necessary to use antibiotic gauzes; plain one-quarter-inch or one-half-inch gauze will suffice. Excessive or tight packing impedes healing and only results in increased pain for the patient. Packing should be removed within 24 to 48 hours. In general, in cosmetically important areas such as the face, breasts, and inguinal area, I tend to remove the packing in 24 hours. In all other areas, I remove it in 48 hours. If purulence is still present, the wound should be reprobed, re-irrigated, and repacked.

It has been well documented for over a decade that antibiotics are not indicated in localized cutaneous abscesses in the patient with normal host defenses. If indeed antibiotics are not indicated, then there is no reason to culture the purulence or the abscess wall and a Gram stain is not necessary.

In patients with recurrent abscesses, in patients whose abscesses fail to respond to normal therapy, in patients who show signs of systemic toxicity, in patients who are immunocompromised, and in patients who have abscesses in areas such as the central triangle of the face that is drained into the cranial vault by the cavernous sinus, antibiotics may be considered. However, some logic must be used in selection. The flora of the abscess cavity tends to be reflective of the skin flora of the anatomic part involved. In the oral cavity, anaerobes outnumber aerobes by 10 to 1; in the perirectal area, anaerobes outnumber aerobes by 1,000 to 1; thus abscesses around the oral cavity and the perirectal area tend to show a predominance of anaerobes. Abscesses on the skin, extremities, and trunk tend to reflect the flora normally found on the skin. Obviously this may be altered in patients who are immunocompromised, those who have chronic abscesses, or those who have injected foreign substances subcutaneously.

If antibiotics are used to treat abscesses in the extremities, axilla, or head and neck region, an oral staphylococcal agent such as dicloxacillin, erythromycin, or cephaloridine is quite efficacious. Abscesses in the perineal region should be treated with drugs such as clindamycin or the new generation cephalosporin antibiotics, which are appropriate for both gram-negative enterics and fecal anaerobes.

The Gram stain can also be a very useful tool in predicting the flora present. It is useful in three circumstances:

1. The presence of gram-positive cocci in grape-like clusters probably indicates the presence of *Staphylococcus aureus,* which exists most of the time in pure culture.
2. The presence of gram-positive and gram-negative bacteria of various pleomorphic morphology is associated with anaerobic bacteria.
3. The presence of no bacteria and a significant number of white blood cells tends to be associated with sterile abscesses.

Odor may be somewhat helpful in that a feculent odor tends to be associated with anaerobes, although this is not a sensitive indicator.

SPECIFIC ABSCESS TYPES

Bartholin's cysts are abscesses that occur secondary to obstruction of Bartholin's duct. The patient presents with a painful mass in the lower outer margin of the vaginal opening. These abscesses should be drained through the mucosal (vaginal) side of the abscess. Marsupialization, a process in which the cyst wall is sutured to the mucosal surface, is recommended since these abscesses have a significant rate of recurrence after just simple incision and drainage. This process obliterates the cyst cavity. However, it does not need to be carried out at the time of initial treatment in the emergency department.

Hidradenitis suppurativa is a chronic inflammatory process of the apocrine glands. It has a three to one female to male predominance and only occurs after puberty, when these glands become active. Abscesses can occur in the axillary, inguinal, and perirectal regions. Although on an acute basis incision and drainage are indicated, for chronic recurring disease a more extensive inpatient surgical process should be performed and the apocrine glands or the hair-bearing surfaces of the area excised.

Perirectal abscesses originate within the anal crypts, burrow laterally to the ischiorectal space, and then penetrate to the skin surface in the perianal or perirectal area. A submucous abscess that presents as a tender mass protruding into the mucosa is picked up on rectal or anoscopic examination. High ischiorectal or supralevator abscesses do not point on the skin, and the patient presents with a tender rectal area without cutaneous fluctuance.

Abscesses that tend to point on the skin's surface often can be drained on an outpatient basis. Those abscesses that appear to be extensive, high up, or submucous need to be drained on an inpatient basis, usually in the operating room. Recurrent abscesses in the perirectal area and the lower abdominal area are often associated with either fistula formation or granulomatous bowel disease or both.

Pilonidal abscesses occur secondary to minor disruptions of the skin in the buttock cleft. They are often associated with prolonged sitting in hirsute and dark-skinned individuals. These skin disruptions tend to epithelialize over and often plug with hair or keratin, leading to infections and sinus formation. Unlike perirectal processes, culture of these abscesses demonstrates flora of the skin area rather than fecal flora. Thus while *Staphylococcus aureus* is rarely found in perirectal abscesses, it is found in pilonidal abscesses. These abscesses tend to be small and can be drained on an outpatient basis with a small midline incision, freeing the cavity of all purulence and hair-borne material. However, they may go on to form sinus tracts that may burrow toward the rectum. In this case an inpatient procedure must be performed, in which the soft tissue is excised down to the presacral fascia. In very extensive disease this may require a diverting colostomy and skin graft for closure.

DISPOSITION

All patients who have incision and drainage performed must be followed to ascertain that the purulent cavity is no longer draining and the patient is on the road to healing. Once the packing is removed, patients should be advised to use warm soaks and should be instructed concerning signs of infection or reoccurrence.

ADMISSION CRITERIA

Not all abscesses (even though they may be cutaneous and localized) can be drained in the emergency department or outpatient setting. In general, patients who have very large abscesses or abscesses that may be difficult to drain with local anesthesia (e.g., high ischiorectal abscesses) should have the procedure performed under general or spinal anesthesia in the operative suite. Patients who have systemic toxicity or are immunocompromised should be admitted to the hospital, parenteral antibiotics should be administered before incision and drainage, and the response to the procedures should be monitored on an inpatient basis. Occasionally, because of a patient's age or other underlying medical conditions, it is most appropriate to have the procedures performed on an inpatient basis.

In a patient with normal host defenses, abscesses primarily need incision and drainage. In patients with large abscesses, in immunocompromised patients, and in patients with abscesses in special locations, in addition to incision and drainage, a Gram stain and culture should be done of the exudate, the patient started on antibiotics, and hospital admission considered. Antibiotics should initially be chosen on the basis of the location and odor of the abscess and the results of a Gram stain. Appropriateness of choice should be confirmed by the results of cultures and sensitivity tests.

SUGGESTED READING

Brook I, Finegold SM. Aerobic and anaerobic bacteriology of cutaneous abscesses in children. Pediatrics 1980; 67:981–985.

Llera JL, Levy RC, Staneck JL. Cutaneous abscesses: Natural history and management in an outpatient facility. J Emerg Med 1984; 1:489–493.

Meislin HW, Lerner SA, Graves MH. Cutaneous abscesses. Anaerobic and aerobic bacteriology and outpatient management. Ann Int Med 1977; 87:145–149.

ECTOPARASITES

JAMES E. RASMUSSEN, M.D.

LICE

Head Lice

The head louse is a cylindrical, obligate human parasite 2 mm in length. This tan insect is found most commonly in the hair of children and young adults, but persons of any age may be affected. The primary symptom is pruritus; common physical manifestations include secondary infection, lymphadenopathy, and matted hair from scratching.

Any patient who complains of itching of the head, scalp, neck, or shoulders should be thoroughly examined for the presence of head lice. The organisms are usually few in number and difficult to see. Much more common are nits, which represent egg cases cemented to the sides of the shafts of hair. The eggs are normally laid close to the scalp (within 1 to 2 cm) and are gradually carried away from the scalp as the hair continues to grow. Consequently, nits more than 4 cm from the scalp (with none closer) usually represent old and inactive infections. Nits are most common and easy to find along the margin of the hair above the ears and around the back of the neck.

Treatment

General Therapy. All individuals who have personal contact with a patient infected with head lice should be treated regardless of whether they are symptomatic. Since the primary mode of transmission is either person-to-person or through fomites such as towels, caps, or coats, these items should be washed thoroughly in hot water. If this is not suitable, then dry cleaning or freezing will also suffice. Combs and personal toilet articles should be washed vigorously in hot, soapy water such as in the dishwasher. Nits should be removed with the use of a nit comb. These have recently been redesigned so that the spaces between the teeth have been greatly narrowed, allowing them to easily remove nits from hair. Many school districts have a "no nit" policy, i.e., children with nits in the scalp are not allowed to return to school until they are free of parasites.

Treatment involves destroying adult organisms, sterilizing unhatched nits, and removing their egg cases from the patient. There are several agents available that are effective for the treatment of head lice.

Specific Therapy. Kwell, 1 percent lindane shampoo, is a prescription medication that is very effective in eradicating adult organisms. The shampoo should be applied for 4 to 5 minutes and then thoroughly rinsed from the scalp. A repeat application should be given in 1 week, since lindane only destroys about 70 percent to 90 percent of unhatched nits. Daily shampoos are not indicated because of the problem of percutaneous absorption with repeated exposure. Lindane is safe to use on persons of all ages provided that the directions are followed explicitly. No significant toxic reactions have been reported from its proper use in the treatment of head lice. Although blood levels are detectable following its use, they are approximately one-tenth to one-twentieth those that occur when the product is used in the treatment of scabies. Parents with more than one child to treat should probably use gloves for each application to decrease percutaneous absorption.

Pyrethrin Products. Pyrethrins are extracts of a variety of chrysanthemum flower heads. They are usually combined with piperonyl butoxide, which enhances their insecticidal capacities. Pyrethrins are sold as a variety of over-the-counter (OTC) medications (Rid, A-200 Pyrinate and others), and most of them are contained in a petroleum-based vehicle. Many come with nit combs, and because of this, their OTC status, and their low cost, they are very useful in treating large groups of patients with head lice. The product is applied to the scalp according to directions (usually for 5 to 10 minutes) and then rinsed out. Repeat application is necessary in 1 week, since the drug is no more effective against nits than is 1 percent lindane. Pyrethrins are not known to have any appreciable toxicity for human beings, but their vehicle can be irritating if allowed to contact mucous membranes.

Crotamiton. Eurax, or 10 percent crotamiton, is an effective prescription pediculocide when applied for 12 to 24 hours. This long period of application time, compared with that of the pediculocides mentioned above, somewhat limits its utility. Its effect on nits is not known, but a second application a week after the first is usually prudent.

Prioderm or 0.5 Percent Malathion. This prescription item has recently been introduced into the United States market but it has subsequently been withdrawn. It is an effective pediculocide and also has a substantial effect on nits. Of all the commercially available agents, it alone has a nit kill rate of 95 percent or greater. The main disadvantage of the product is that it must be applied to the scalp for 8 hours. A shampoo preparation of malathion is currently widely used in Europe and probably will be marketed in the United States within 1 to 2 years. At that time, malathion shampoo will probably become the treatment of choice for patients with head lice.

Body Lice

Infestation with the body louse is usually limited to the poor, mentally ill, or substance-abusing patient. It is rarely seen in most parts of the United States. The predominant symptom is itching, with secondary excoriations and impetiginization. These signs are usually more prominent over the upper half of the body, particularly the shoulders, back, and chest. Unlike the head louse, the body louse does not spend much time on its human hosts, preferring the host's undergarments as a place to live and lay eggs. Consequently, a patient suspected of having body lice should have the seams of his or her clothing searched. Examinations with negative findings are often the result of patients changing clothes just before visiting the hospital in order to put on their "Sunday best."

Treatment of body lice involves a total body application of 1 percent lindane in either cream or shampoo form. All the patient's clothes should be disinfected, as should his or her home environment, if possible. All contacts should also be treated, since this is a contagious disease. Secondary infections should be treated with an appropriate antibiotic. It should be kept in mind that occasionally the human louse can transmit disease from person to person, in particular the *Rickettsia* responsible for typhus.

Pubic Lice

Infestation with the pubic louse (*Phthirus pubis*) is a common finding in young men and women in large urban populations. It is probably one of the more common venereal diseases. The main signs and symptoms are scratching and excoriations. The crab louse lays its eggs on pubic hair, and these nits serve as the hallmark of the diagnosis. Agents effective in the treatment of head lice are also effective against pubic lice.

Occasionally a patient will present with itching of the eyelashes and neck. This usually represents pubic lice of the eyelashes rather than an aberrant southward-bound head louse. Patients with lice of the eyelashes are usually prepubertal and consequently have no suitable locale for the pubic louse to set up housekeeping. All of the previously mentioned agents are too irritating or toxic to be used around mucous membranes such as the eye. Consequently, the treatment of choice for lice of the eyelashes is petrolatum (Vaseline), applied with a cotton swab or a finger to the eyelashes four to five times a day. This presumably suffocates the adult lice or it may make the hair so slippery that they fall to their death. Other potentially useful treatments include physostigmine, applied to the lashes not the conjunctiva, and fluorescein.

INSECT BITES

A variety of insects such as fleas, mosquitos, chiggers, and ticks can produce intensively irritating local reactions. They are most common on exposed body parts and are usually more apparent in spring, summer, and fall than in winter. Some (flea bites) may occur year-round because of the association with domestic animals. Local reactions to insect bites usually require nothing more than a soothing lotion such as calamine or an oral antihistamine. If the reaction is severe or truly allergic in nature (associated with hives or angioedema), systemic corticosteroids in a dose of 1 mg per kilogram per day for 7 to 10 days usually produce prompt resolution. Anaphylactic reactions to these insect bites are uncommon, usually occurring after encounters with stinging insects such as wasps and bees. For the patient who is chronically exposed and susceptible, insect repellents are most useful. Those containing DEET are widely sold under a variety of over-the-counter brand names (Cutter, 6-12, Deep Woods, Off). The concentration of DEET varies widely from product to product, and the patient should be encouraged to obtain one with the highest available concentration. A very high concentration of DEET may be associated with neurotoxicity.

SCABIES

Scabies is caused by a small (0.1 mm) eight-legged mite, *Sarcoptes scabiei* var *hominis*. The disease is most common in children or young adults, but it can affect patients of any age. The presenting manifestation is usually severe pruritus or the secondary infection that results from scratching. It is often stated that the itching of scabies is worse at night. While this is true, almost all diseases itch more at night, a fact that considerably detracts from the value of this often stated "diagnostic piece of history".

Any patient who complains of itching, particularly on the hands, waist, or genitalia, should be thoroughly examined for the lesions of scabies. The organism tends to cluster in certain body sites, which somewhat facilitates the diagnosis. Favored areas are the web spaces of the hands, belt area of the trunk, male genitalia, anterior and posterior axillary folds, and elbows. Only a few patients with established scabies infection have normal web spaces. Consequently it is most important to look here first for signs of the disease. The characteristic lesions range from small vesicles to burrows (irregularly "S"-shaped tracks) and nodules (particularly in the male genitalia and axillary folds). Frequently, more than one family member is affected, but this is not true in about 25 percent of patients. Once the diagnosis has been considered, a potassium hydroxide (KOH) scraping from the web spaces is most important. This is because many diseases that itch, such as atopic eczema, may superficially resemble scabies, including involvement of the web spaces. Most of the mites congregate on the hands and particularly in the interdigital spaces. Select a vesicle or a burrow from this site, moisten the skin with alcohol or water, and through scraping, remove the surface of the lesion with a round-bellied number 15 blade. Transfer the material to a slide and repeat the procedure at least four more times on separate lesions. Scraping a single lesion is usually not satisfactory, since the total number of mites on each patient is small, usually fewer than 12. After four or more lesions have been scraped, a drop of water or KOH is added to the slide, followed by a coverslip. The material is then examined under low-power microscopy for the presence of mites or eggs.

General Therapy It is most important that all exposed patients be treated, whether they are symptomatic or not. Treatment should be given from neck to toes, not just on visible cutaneous lesions. The patient's clothes, bedding, and towels should be washed thoroughly in hot water, but it is not necessary to disinfect the carpets, sofas, and mattresses, since the life span of the mite off the human host is very short and its degree of infectiousness is low.

Specific Therapy. Once the diagnosis has been established, 1 percent lindane remains the treatment of choice. The product should be applied in a cream or lotion vehicle and left on the patient for approximately 6 to 8 hours. Therapy should not be repeated within 1 week because of the dangers of convulsions associated with increased blood levels. Convulsions following a single application are exceptionally rare, with only a few instances having been reported in the United States from among millions of patient exposures. All family members and other close personal contacts should be treated simultaneously, even if they are not symptomatic. Failure to adhere to this rule will frequently result in a poor cure rate.

It is also important to realize that the signs and symptoms of scabies do not resolve promptly following treatment with lindane or any other scabicide. Patients may need to be treated with antihistamines and systemic antibiotics if infection is present. Intermediate to mild potency topical steroids (0.1 percent triamcinolone, 1 percent hydrocortisone) also decrease signs and symptoms. Large

nodular lesions on the genitalia or axillary folds respond slowly to therapy, often taking weeks to months to resolve.

Crotamiton is much less effective than 1 percent lindane in the treatment of scabies. Outpatient therapy of scabies with crotamiton produces about a 50 percent to 60 percent response rate, even when the drug is given for three to five daily applications. Current *Physicians Desk Reference* instructions suggest that crotamiton be used consecutively for 2 days. It is often used when the physician is concerned about the potential toxicity of lindane in a young child or pregnant mother. The reader should be aware that no study has documented the efficacy and safety of crotamiton in these situations. The drug has not been studied in pregnant women and cannot be assumed to be any more or less hazardous than 1 percent lindane.

SUGGESTED READING

Ginsburg CM, Lowry W, Reisch JS. Absorption of lindane (gamma benzene hexachloride) in infants and children. J Pediatr 1977;91:998–1000.
Rasmussen JE. Pediculosis and the pediatrician. Pediatr Dermatol 1984; 2:74–79.
Taplin D, Castillero PM, Spiegel J, et al. Malathion for treatment of *pediculus humanus* var *capitis* infestation. JAMA 1982; 247:3103–3105.

MUCOUS MEMBRANE DISEASE

THOMAS A. CHAPEL, M.D.

MUCOUS MEMBRANE

The differential diagnosis of mucous membrane dermatitis includes direct irritation, allergic reactions, erythema multiforme, pemphigus vulgaris, aphthous stomatitis, Behçet's syndrome, hand-foot-and-mouth disease, local trauma, herpes infection, and syphillis. The latter two are covered in separate chapters.

Mucous membranes are subject to two types of local reactions: primary irritation and allergic sensitization. Primary irritation of the oral mucosa is usually caused by heat or chemicals, while allergic stomatitis is most often caused by dentifrices and mouthwashes. Females may develop contact vulvitis after using douches, feminine hygiene deodorants, contraceptive foams and jellies, or contact with rubber products, and males may develop a contact balanitis from rubber condoms or products used by the sexual partner.

The subjective *symptoms of contact dermatitis* of the mucous membranes often are more prominent than the physical signs. Contact stomatitis frequently is associated with loss of taste and, in cases of allergic stomatitis,

coexisting cheilitis or circumoral dermatitis. Patients with inflamed mucosa also may complain of numbness, burning, soreness, and itch. Objective signs vary from barely visible erythema to intense redness with edema and vesicobullae that rupture, leaving shallow erosions. Contact reactions of the mucous membranes may be mistaken for candidiasis. However, mucosal candidiasis often manifests closely adherent cheesy deposits that leave an eroded bleeding site upon removal.

Treatment

Patients with painful thermal *burns or mild chemical injury of the mouth* should be given ice chips to suck or ice-cold glycerin to apply as needed to affected sites. If pain persists, lidocaine (Xylocaine), 2 percent viscous solution, is applied every 3 to 8 hours until the patient is comfortable. Thereafter, a small dab of triamcinolone acetonide in emollient dental paste (Kenalog in Orabase) is pressed to the lesion two to three times a day until it is healed.

Cure of allergic contact dermatitis of mucous membranes requires prompt removal of specific contact allergens. Allergic cheilitis and stomatitis with local swelling of the lips are treated with ice water compresses for 15 minutes three to four times a day, followed by application of fluocinolone acetonide (Synalar) ointment 0.025 percent. Painful erosions or ulcers of the oral mucosa are soothed by sucking ice chips and, if this is ineffective, by swishing 15 ml of undiluted lidocaine (Xylocaine), 2 percent viscous solution, or diphenhydramine hydrochloride (Benadryl) elixir around the mouth for 5 minutes every 3 to 4 hours and then expectorating. Later, Kenalog in Orabase can be patted on injured areas two to three times daily.

Mild contact *vulvitis or balanitis* usually responds to compresses with Burow's solution diluted 1:40 and applied for 15 to 30 minutes every 4 to 6 hours. After each compress, hydrocortisone 1 percent or 2.5 percent cream is gently massaged into the inflamed area.

Severe allergic dermatitis of mucous membranes producing great distress usually requires a single intramuscular injection of triamcinolone acetonide (Kenalog-40) suspension or triamcinolone diacetate (Aristocort) suspension in a dose of 40 mg for the average adult. After emergency care is rendered, patients requiring follow-up care should be referred to a dermatologist or an allergist.

ERYTHEMA MULTIFORME

Erythema multiforme (EM) is an acute, self-limited but occasionally relapsing eruption of the skin and mucous membranes. The clinical picture consists of macular-urticarial lesions, sometimes in pathognomonic "iris" or "target" configuration, and vesiculobullous lesions. Blistering of the mucous membranes occurs in approximately 25 percent of cases, and at times it represents the sole expression of the disease.

In severe EM, called *Stevens-Johnson syndrome*, the oropharynx is affected with extensive erosions, and the lips characteristically are covered with hemorrhagic crusts. Blisters also may develop on the bulbar conjunctivae, pharynx, external nares, larynx, esophagus, and genital surfaces. Bullous pemphigoid, pemphigus vulgaris, and mucocutaneous lymph node syndrome (Kawasaki's disease) may be confused with severe EM; however, the hemorrhagic crusted lips of patients with EM are not a feature of these other diseases.

EM is an immune-mediated hypersensitivity reaction precipitated by many antigens (Table 1). The physician should undertake studies to determine the underlying cause of EM, and the patient should stop taking all drugs of potential etiologic significance. Patients with limited cutaneous disease can be treated on an outpatient basis with triamcinolone (Aristocort, Kenalog) cream, 0.1 percent, applied three times daily. However, severe EM has substantial morbidity and a mortality rate of 5 to 10 percent. Patients with extensive mucous membrane involvement often require hospitalization with admission to a general medical floor under the care of an internist or dermatologist experienced in treating the condition.

Painful *stomatitis* may prevent oral intake, thereby requiring putting the patient on intravenous fluids for 2 or 3 days. Parenteral maintenance may be started in the emergency room by administering 1,000 ml of 10 percent dextrose in water with 20 mEq potassium chloride over the first 12 hours and 1,000 ml of .45 percent saline in 5 percent dextrose and water with 20 mEq potassium chloride over the second 12 hours of each day of maintenance therapy. Painful stomatitis can sometimes be relieved by treating the patient every 3 to 4 hours with 5 ml of diphenhydramine hydrochloride (Benadryl) elixir or lidocaine (Xylocaine) viscous 2 percent solution swished about the mouth for 3 to 5 minutes before expectorating.

A short course of *systemic corticosteroids* will provide symptomatic relief but is of unproven value in influencing the duration and outcome of the disease. Moreover, systemic corticosteroids are likely to lessen injury only when used early in the course of the disease. If corticosteroids are deemed necessary, the emergency physician can institute therapy using prednisone in a dosage of 1 to 2 mg per kilogram per day, given in three divided doses. The dosage is halved and given in two divided doses when the patient is afebrile, no new lesions have occurred for at least 72 hours, and old lesions are beginning to resolve. If there is no flare-up over another 72-hour period, then the dose is reduced to 5 mg per m of prednisone for a third 3-day period, and if no problems occur at this point, the drug is discontinued.

Denuded surfaces are susceptible to secondary bacterial infection, and such an occurrence requires appropriate antibiotics. Significant ocular sequelae occur in 10 to 15 percent of patients, and eye involvement requires ophthalmologic consultation. Respiratory failure secondary to mucosal sloughing, pneumonia, hematuria, renal tubular necrosis, and progressive renal failure occurs, but is rare. None the less, the physician should be alert to these possibilities and should monitor patients with appropriate tests.

PEMPHIGUS VULGARIS

Oral lesions of pemphigus vulgaris may precede cutaneous lesions by several months to several years, and unless the diagnosis of pemphigus is suspected, the condition is often misdiagnosed. Blisters on mucous mem-

TABLE 1 Some Recognized Causes of Erythema Multiforme

Infectious Agents and Diseases	Drugs	Other Factors
Herpes simplex virus	Sulfonamides	Radiotherapy
Epstein-Barr virus	Barbiturates	of malignancies
Mycoplasma pneumoniae	Penicillins	
Vaccinia	Phenylbutazone	
Mycobacterium Tuberculosis	Diphenylhydantoin	

branes rupture early, leaving ragged ulcerative lesions that may become so extensive and painful as to interfere with the intake of solid food. The mucous membranes of the pharynx, larynx, nose, vagina, and anus may also be involved, and accompanying cutaneous lesions present as flaccid, weeping blisters, that rupture, leaving large denuded areas of skin. Patients with pemphigus vulgaris have circulating antibodies of the IgG class to epithelial intercellular cement substance.

Pemphigus vulgaris has been mistaken for erythema multiforme and benign mucosal pemphigoid. Erythema multiforme has an abrupt onset of urticarial and blistering lesions, and if present, "iris" or "target" lesions are pathognomonic of the condition. Benign mucosal pemphigoid has a predilection for the conjunctivae and the oral mucosa, but unlike pemphigus vulgaris, the oral mucosa shows little edema, denuded areas cause less pain, and the vermilion border of the lips, a common site of lesions in pemphigus, is only rarely involved.

Physicians rendering emergency care should be familiar with the clinical expressions of pemphigus vulgaris, but both acute and long-term management are best handled by physicians skilled in treating the condition. Patients with limited lesions can be referred on an outpatient basis, while patients with pemphigus vulgaris and widespread lesions are best admitted to a general medical floor under the care of a dermatologist or internist experienced in diagnosing and treating the disorder.

APHTHOUS STOMATITIS

Aphthous stomatitis may present in one of three clinical patterns: (1) minor aphthous ulcers that recur in crops of one to five lesions, are less than 1 cm in diameter, and usually affect the lips, buccal mucosa, mucobuccal and mucolabial sulci, and tongue; (2) major aphthous ulcers that are larger than 1 cm in diameter, begin as solitary nodules, and subsequently destroy deeper tissue that may result in scarring; (3) herpetiform ulcers, which are recurrent, multiple, shallow, pinpoint lesions 1 to 2 mm in diameter that may affect any part of the mucosa.

Aphthous stomatitis is a disease of unknown cause. However, evidence shows that immunologic mechanisms of tissue injury are important in its pathogenesis.

Recurrent intraoral herpetic ulceration and oral lichen planus may mimic aphthous stomatitis. However, both conditions usually produce vesicles, and blister formation is not characteristic of recurrent aphthae. Aphthae are identical to the ulcers seen in Behçet's syndrome, but patients with Behçet's disease also have genital ulcers and ocular changes.

Patients with aphthous ulcers should be advised to reduce oral trauma by avoiding sharp-surfaced foods, such as peanuts, popcorn, potato chips, and tacos, and to brush carefully with a soft-bristled toothbrush. Citrus fruits, acidic foods, and spices may aggravate existing lesions and should be eliminated from the diet during flare-ups. Chocolate, nuts, and strong cheeses are suspected of inducing aphthae and should be avoided if recognized as precipitating factors.

The preferred therapy, if few lesions are present, is 0.1 percent triamcinolone acetonide in emollient dental paste (Kenalog in Orabase), gently pressed against the lesions twice each day. Patients with early lesions and a history of deep, painful ulcers often benefit from applications of escharotics, such as silver nitrate or negatol (Negatan) applied to each lesion by the physician. However, escharotics are not recommended for treating late lesions because excessive tissue necrosis retards healing. Severe pain sometimes associated with aphthous stomatitis can be treated with lidocaine (Xylocaine), 2 percent viscous solution, applied every 3 to 8 hours until the patient is comfortable.

Tetracycline oral suspension (Achromycin V oral suspension), 10 ml swished in the mouth for 2 minutes four times a day and then swallowed, is often helpful in controlling aphthous ulcers. A 2-week course of this syrup may be repeated as necessary to control recurrences. Patients with continuous or major types of aphthous stomatitis often require a prednisone equivalence of 40 mg orally for 7 days, followed by 20 mg orally for 7 days. Such patients should be referred to a dermatologist or primary care physician for follow-up care.

BEHÇET'S SYNDROME

Behçet's syndrome is characterized by recurrent ulcerations of the oral mucosa and external genitalia associated with a recurrent uveitis that is frequently complicated by hypopyon. The disease may begin at any one site and persevere for days to years before another location is affected. The diagnosis is generally made when two or more major sites are involved. The lesions should be thought of as only one phase of a widespread disorder that at times may include cutaneous, joint, pulmonary, intestinal, vascular, and central nervous system involvement. Behçet's syndrome with neuro-ocular involvement carries a more serious prognosis and a high mortality rate. The specific cause of Behçet's syndrome is unknown, but the evidence supports a delayed hypersensitivity reaction of a cell-mediated type in which immune complexes may be involved in the transition from focal ulceration to multitissue involvement.

The oral lesions of Behçet's syndrome are indistinguishable from those of recurrent aphthous stomatitis. They may be present on any oral site as small, superficial, single or multiple ulcers, and they tend to occur in crops lasting for 2 weeks or less. These lesions are treated symptomatically, as discussed under aphthous stomatitis. However, patients with Behçet's syndrome should be referred to an internist for long-term follow-up care. Patients with neuro-ocular presentation may need prompt referral or even general medical hospital admission.

VESICULAR STOMATITIS WITH EXANTHEM (HAND-FOOT-AND-MOUTH DISEASE)

Hand-foot-and-mouth disease is a disorder caused by an enterovirus, usually coxsackie A16, although coxsackie A5 and A10 also cause this symptom complex. The dis-

TABLE 2 Some Causes of Persistent Solitary Oral Ulcerations

	Clinical Characteristics	Diagnosis	Treatment and/or Disposition
Oral Cancer	Most occur on the lower lip or the posterior two-thirds and lateral borders of the tongue. Intraoral squamous cell carcinoma is an infiltrative, ulcerated or exophytic growth that may arise from preexisting velvety, red, granular thickenings. Early epidermoid carcinoma is rarely painful in contrast to similar-appearing inflammatory lesions.	All chronic ulcerative lesions that fail to heal within 2 to 3 weeks should be considered potentially malignant and must be biopsied for definitive diagnosis	Refer to oral surgeon or otolaryngologist for biopsy.
Traumatic ulcers	Occur any place on the oral mucosa. Dental structures and devices (carious teeth, irregular restorations, fractured or eroded teeth), bites, and penetration by foreign objects (e.g., toothbrush bristles, fish bones) are frequently responsible for ulcers in the vestibule. Ulcers are localized, discrete, and have red margins. If they are not secondarily infected, they will heal within 7 to 10 days after irritation is removed.	Identification of irritant.	Remove foreign body or refer to dentist for correction of offending dental structure or device.
Primary syphilis	Small papule that rapidly develops into larger, painless, indurated ulcer with unilateral lymphadenopathy. Most often seen on the lips, especially the upper; less common within the oral cavity.	Identification of *Treponema pallidum* on dark-field microscopic examination of exudate from lip lesion or, with intraoral chancres, aspirates from regional lymph node. Reactive Venereal Disease Research Laboratory or rapid plasma reagin test and reactive confirmatory test (fluorescent treponemal antibody absorption test or micro-hemagglutination-*Treponema pallidum*).	Benzathine penicillin G, 2.4 million units IM. Tetracycline hydrochloride or erythromycin, 500 mg by mouth 4 times a day for 15 days, for penicillin-allergic patients. Patients should be reported to the local or state health department for case tracing and to a dermatologist or primary care physician for follow-up visits, beginning 3 months after treatment.
Tuberculosis	Tuberculosis, either primary or secondary, occurs infrequently in the mouth; predilection for the gingiva, soft palate, and tonsils. Solitary irregular ulcer covered by a persistent exudate; ulcer has undermined, indurated border and is often quite tender.	Demonstration of acid-fast organisms in smears or biopsy from ulcer of draining lymph node. *Mycobacterium tuberculosis* can be identified on culture. Intradermal test to purified protein derivative reactive.	Refer to oral surgeon or otolaryngologist for biopsy for histopathology and culture.
Histoplasmosis	One of the more common fungal infections to involve the oral cavity. Lesions occur in any area of mouth, particularly the tongue, gingiva, or palate; single or multiple indurated ulcerative or vegetative erosions covered by a gray or pinkish membrane. Lesions are often painful; hoarseness and/or dysphagia may occur because of lesions on the larynx; usually associated with fever and malaise.	Biopsy using special stains (PAS or methenamine silver); culture of lesion on mycosel (Difco) or Sabouraud's agar with added chloramphenicol.	Refer to oral surgeon or otolaryngologist for biopsy for histopathology and culture.

ease may occur as an isolated phenomenon or in epidemic form. Infection usually begins with a brief prodrome of low-grade fever, malaise, and abdominal pain, followed by the appearance of vesicles on the margins of the palms and soles, dorsal surfaces of the hands and feet, and in the oral cavity. Oral blisters soon rupture, forming superficial erosions and ulcers. The disease usually runs its course in 7 to 10 days without disability, although a few cases of recurrent disease and single cases of fatal myocarditis and meningoencephalitis have been reported.

The diagnosis of hand-foot-and-mouth disease usually is evident from the clinical pattern, but in equivocal cases definitive diagnosis can be established by obtaining acute and convalescent sera for complement-fixing antibody testing or by culturing the virus from vesicle fluid or swabs from the mouth and anal canal. Occasionally hand-foot-and-mouth disease may be mistaken for herpes simplex gingivostomatitis. However, the latter is associated with greater toxicity, cervical lymphadenopathy, and vesicles that affect the entire buccal mucosa, but it is not associated with vesicles elsewhere on the skin.

Patients with hand-foot-and-mouth disease usually need no treatment, only reassurance as to the benign nature of their disease. Rarely, oral ulcers are painful, and in such cases symptomatic relief can be obtained by swishing 15 ml of undiluted diphenhydramine hydrochloride (Benadryl) elixir around the mouth for 5 minutes every 3 to 4 hours and then spitting it out. Follow-up care is rarely needed, but for cases of uncertain diagnosis or with particularly severe symptoms, referral to an infectious diseases specialist is appropriate.

PERSISTENT SOLITARY ULCERATIONS OF THE ORAL MUCOSA

Physicians rendering emergency care occasionally see patients with persistent, solitary ulcerations of the oral mucosa. Certain reactive or neoplastic processes should be considered in the differential diagnosis of such lesions, and the physician should take appropriate steps to establish a definitive diagnosis (Table 2).

SUGGESTED READING

Baker HW. Diagnosis of oral cancer. CA 1972; 22:31–39.
Berlin C. Behçet's disease as a multiple symptom complex. Arch Dermatol Syphilol 1960; 82:73–79.
Bickley HC. A concept of allergy with reference to oral disease. J Periodontal 1970; 41:302–312.
Cooper D, Penny R. Behçet's syndrome: Clinical, immunological, and therapeutic evaluation of 17 patients. Aust NZ J Med 1974; 4:585–596.
Crissey JT. Stomatitis, dermatitis, and denture materials. Arch Dermatol 1965; 95:45–48.
Francis TC. Recurrent aphthous stomatitis and Behçet's disease. A review. Oral Surg 1970; 30:476–487.
Lehner T. Progress report: Oral ulceration and Behçet's syndrome. Gut 1977; 18:491–511.
Lever WF. Pemphigus and pemphigoid. Am Acad Dermatol 1979; 1:2–31.
Lever WF, Schaumburg-Lever G. Immunosuppressants and prednisone in pemphigus vulgaris. Arch Dermatol 1977; 112:1236–1241.
Neiders ME. Early clinical diagnosis of oral cancer. Int Dent J 1972; 22:441–450.
Rasmussen JE. Erythema multiforme in children. Br J Dermatol 1976; 95:181–186.
Rogers RS III. Recurrent aphthous stomatitis: Clinical characteristics and evidence for an immunopathogenesis. J Invest Dermatol 1977; 69:499–509.
Schosser RH. The erythema multiforme spectrum: Diagnosis and treatment. Curr Concepts Skin Disorders 1985; 6:6–11.
Tucker HA, Mulherin JL. Extragenital chancres: Survey of 219 cases. Am J Syphilis, Gonorrhea, Vener Dis 1948; 32:345–364.
Turbiner S, et al. Orificial tuberculosis of the lip. J Oral Surg 1975; 33:443–447.
Turrell JJ. Allergy to denture materials—fallacy or reality? Br J Dermatol 1967; 79:331–338.
Young LL, et al. Oral manifestations of histoplasmosis. Oral Surg 1972; 33:191–204.

FUNGAL INFECTIONS OF THE SKIN

ALFRED D. HERNANDEZ, M.D.

DERMATOPHYTOSIS (RINGWORM OR TINEA INFECTIONS)

Dermatophytes, which are species in the genera *Trichophyton, Microsporum*, and *Epidermophyton*, infect the keratinous nonviable structures of the skin—stratum corneum, hair, and nails. Because the keratinous structures of the skin move outward until they are shed into the environment, a dermatophyte continues to infect a keratinous structure as long as it penetrates into the structure at a rate at least equal to the rate at which the keratinous structure moves outward.

Antifungal Agents Effective Against Dermatophytosis

Topical Agents. A variety of topical antifungal agents are available both by prescription and over the counter. Among the most effective of these are the imidazole derivatives, miconazole (Monistat-Derm), clotrimazole (Lotrimin, Mycelex), and econazole (Spectazole); they have a cure rate that exceeds 80 percent. These agents are effective against dermatophytes and yeast; but not dermatophytic infections of the hair or nails.

These agents should be applied twice daily to the affected areas for 2 to 8 weeks, depending on the type of infection being treated. In general, they are chosen to treat small areas of infection. Although extensive infections are commonly treated with systemic griseofulvin, a topical imidazole may be used as an alternative if the patient is either allergic to or has an underlying condition that prevents the use of a systemic antifungal agent.

A variety of other topical antifungal agents, including tolnaftate (Tinactin), haloprogin (Halotex), and undecylenic acid (Desenex) are available either by prescription or over the counter. These agents are only moderately effective against chronic noninflammatory infections. They may be used to speed the resolution of inflammatory infections that are generally self-limited whether they are treated or not.

Systemic Agents. Systemic antifungal agents effective against dermatophytes are usually reserved for stratum corneum infections that are either widespread or resistant to topical therapy. They are the only effective agents against hair and nail infections. Of the two systemic oral antidermatophytic agents on the market, only griseofulvin is currently approved by the Food and Drug Administration for treating dermatophytic infections. Ketoconazole, the other oral antifungal agent, is active against dermatophytes, but has been reported to cause idiosyncratic liver toxicity, which in some cases has led to death. Ketoconazole does not appear to be more effective than griseofulvin in eliminating infections or in preventing their recurrence. The risk-benefit ratio, therefore, does not favor its use.

Griseofulvin (Fulvicin, Grisactin, Gris-PEG): The dose of griseofulvin differs, depending on whether the micronized form (Fulvicin, Grisactin) or the ultrafine (Gris-PEG) form is used. The dose for the micronized form is 500 mg twice a day for adults, 750 mg daily in a divided dose for children weighing 50 to 90 lb, and 250 mg twice a day for children weighing 30 to 50 lb. The dose for the ultrafine form is one-half that of the micronized form of griseofulvin. The ultrafine form of this drug is more expensive and offers no therapeutic advantage over an equivalent dose of the micronized form.

Griseofulvin has relatively few side effects. The most frequently reported is headache. Skin eruptions and gastrointestinal disturbances also occur. Griseofulvin also increases the clearance of warfarin and may exacerbate symptoms of porphyria.

DERMATOPHYTIC INFECTION OF THE STRATUM CORNEUM

Tinea Corporis

Tinea corporis is a dermatophytic infection of glabrous skin, excluding the groin, palms, and soles. It typically produces a well-circumscribed, red, scaly, or vesiculopustular circinate patch accompanied by pruritus. In general, the more inflammatory the infection the shorter its duration, and even when not treated, it tends to be self-limiting. Noninflammatory infections tend to be chronic and more resistant to treatment.

The differential diagnosis includes the herald patch of pityriasis rubra, seborrheic dermatitis, allergic or irritant dermatitis, erythema annulare centrifugum, and other figurate erythemas. The diagnosis of tinea corporis is confirmed by demonstrating hyphal elements on potassium hydroxide (KOH) examination of scale removed from the lesion. However, a negative KOH examination does not necessarily rule out the diagnosis. Areas clinically suggestive of tinea corporis, but which have negative KOH examinations, should be cultured. Confirmation by culture may take up to 4 weeks. Patients may be started

presumptively on antifungal therapy while awaiting culture confirmation. Patients with tinea corporis who are initially misdiagnosed as having dermatitis and who are treated with a topical steroid will have some symptomatic improvement, but the infection will not totally clear. If after 2 weeks of topical steroids the patient still has an underlying rash, the lesions should be scraped again and examined for the presence of hyphae. Scales from these patients frequently show abundant hyphae after a course of topical steroids.

Treatment. The recommended therapy for most cases of localized tinea corporis is a topical imidazole derivative applied twice daily for 2 to 4 weeks. Although the topical imidazoles are also effective in treating widespread infections, patient compliance becomes a limiting factor. For widespread infections patient compliance is better when an oral agent, griseofulvin, is prescribed. Griseofulvin therapy should be continued for 4 weeks to avoid recurrence, even if the patient's infection appears to be cured prior to the end of the therapeutic course.

Tinea Cruris

Tinea cruris (jock itch) is a dermatophytic infection of the groin. The clinical manifestations are similar to those of tinea corporis. The most frequent area involved is the inner thigh. The penis and the scrotum are usually not infected.

The differential diagnosis of tinea cruris includes candidiasis, erythrasma, and local irritation or chafing. The diagnosis is confirmed by demonstrating hyphae on scales cleared with KOH and examined microscopically or by culturing the fungus. Candidiasis, unlike tinea cruris, frequently involves the scrotum and penis and often has satellite pustules adjacent to the scaly red lesions in the intracrural folds. The diagnosis of candidiasis can be confirmed by demonstrating budding yeast cells on KOH examination or Gram stain of pustules and by culturing the organism. When the KOH examination of crural scales fails to show hyphae, the affected area should be illuminated with a Wood's light. If the area fluoresces coral red, the patient has erythrasma and requires erythromycin to cure the infection.

Treatment. The treatment for tinea cruris is the same as that for tinea coporis. Because factors such as moisture, occlusion, and trauma increase susceptibility to infection, the patient should be advised to use powder and wear loose-fitting underwear in order to decrease moisture in the area. Wearing tight-fitting, nylon underwear or prolonged wearing of a wet bathing suit or working clothes should be discouraged.

Tinea Pedis

Tinea pedis is a dermatophytic infection of the plantar surface of the feet. There are three distinct clinical presentations. The most frequent form produces scales and redness between the toes. Depending on the amount of moisture and occlusion, the infected interdigital areas may also appear white and have small fissures. Other areas of the foot may or may not be concurrently infected. Patients with tinea pedis may also present with scales covering the entire plantar aspect of the foot. Itching with this type is usually minimal or absent, and there may be no signs of redness or active inflammation. Another form of tinea pedis may manifest with tense vesicles that leave a collarette of scale when they rupture. Occasionally this type of presentation will proceed from vesiculopustules to ulcerations, and it may produce sufficient amounts of pain to hamper walking.

The differential diagnosis for the interdigital form of tinea pedis includes candidiasis and erythrasma. The definitive diagnosis is made by demonstrating hyphae on KOH examination or by culturing the fungus. The scaly and the vesiculopustular form of tinea pedis must be differentiated from allergic dermatitis to shoes and gram-negative toe-web infection. In such infections culturing of the ulcers almost always fails to grow dermatophytes, but it does yield gram-negative bacteria. Tinea pedis is thought to be a predisposing factor. After being treated for the gram-negative bacterial infection, the patient should be treated prophylactically with topical antifungals in an attempt to prevent dermatophytic infection and thereby prevent recurrence.

Treatment. Tinea pedis is treated in the same manner as tinea corporis except that the duration of therapy is 4 to 8 weeks for topical agents and 4 to 6 weeks for griseofulvin.

DERMATOPHYTIC INFECTION OF THE HAIR

Tinea Capitis

Tinea capitis is a dermatophytic infection of scalp hair that is characterized by alopecia and by varying degrees of inflammation. The pustular component of inflammatory tinea capitis ranges from a mild folliculitis to fluctuant furuncle-like nodules called kerions. Severe inflammatory tinea capitis may be associated with fever, malaise, permanent hair loss, and regional lymphadenopathy. Noninflammatory tinea capitis is characterized by alopecia and scales. Instead of stubby hair within areas of alopecia (as in inflammatory tinea capitis), this infection usually has "black dots", follicles filled with infected hair that have broken before exiting the follicle. This form does not produce permanent hair loss, but tends to be chronic unless treated.

Inflammatory tinea capitis is most frequently confused with a bacterial infection of the scalp, particularly because it may be superficial colonized with *Staphylococcus aureus*. Children with pustules on their scalps should be considered to have tinea capitis until proven otherwise. The diagnosis may be confirmed by demonstrating spores either on the surface of or within infected hair examined with KOH, by growing a dermatophyte from culture seeded with scale and hair from affected areas, or by demonstrating hairs that fluoresce yellow-green when exposed to a Wood's light.

Noninflammatory tinea capitis may be misdiagnosed as trichotillomania, alopecia areata, or seborrhea (dandruff). The noninflammatory type organisms do not fluoresce when hair is exposed to a Wood's light. Diagnosis is limited to demonstrating fungal spores within infected hair or growing the fungus from infected hair. Scales are usually KOH- and culture-negative.

Treatment. Tinea capitis responds to orally administered griseofulvin, but not to topical antifungal agents. Although the optimal dose schedule is not known, the dose schedule used to treat tinea corporis is most commonly used. Most patients require 6 to 12 weeks of medication.

In patients with marked inflammation and kerions, 20 to 30 mg of prednisone given as a single dose in the morning for 1 week as an adjunct to griseofulvin therapy may help prevent permanent hair loss and scarring. Daily washing of the scalp may also be helpful. Topical antifungals and antibacterials are not effective.

Tinea Barbae

Tinea barbae is a dermatophytic infection of beard hair, commonly acquired from cattle. Inflammatory tinea barbae is most frequently misdiagnosed as bacterial folliculitis or herpes simplex infection when it occurs periorally. The diagnosis of tinea barbae is confirmed by demonstrating spores within or on the hair or by culturing the fungus from hair.

Treatment. The treatment of tinea barbae is griseofulvin. The dose schedule of griseofulvin is the same as that used in tinea capitis, for a period of 4 to 6 weeks. Topical agents are ineffective.

DERMATOPHYTIC INFECTION OF THE NAILS

Dermatophytic nail infections are of three types: distal subungual onychomycosis, proximal subungual onychomycosis, and white superficial onychomycosis.

In distal subungual onychomycosis, the most common form of dermatophytic infection of the nail, the fungus invades the keratinous material between the nail bed and the nail plate. A white to yellowish discoloration is observed at the distal portion of the nail; the infection progresses until the nail plate is lifted from the nail bed by induced hyperkeratosis and thickening. Because KOH examination cannot distinguish between the hyphae of dermatophytes and those of the many other fungi that frequently cause this infection, a positive culture should be obtained before prescribing long-term therapy with griseofulvin, which is only effective against dermatophytes. The differential diagnosis includes psoriasis and lichen planus.

In proximal subungual onychomycosis, white longitudinal bands traverse the width of the nail plate, but do not affect the surface contour of the nail. The differential diagnosis of this rare infection is leukonychia, which may be produced by trauma or phototoxic drug eruptions, such as those seen with Declomycin.

In white superfical onychomycosis the surface of the nail plate is infected, and a white to yellowish material extends over the surface of the nail. Scrapings of the material show hyphae on KOH examination.

Treatment. Griseofulvin is the treatment for the distal and proximal subungual types of nail infection. The dose schedule is the same as that used for tinea corporis, except that the duration of therapy is 3 to 4 months for fingernail infections and 6 to 10 months for toenail infections. The duration of treatment may be diminished by avulsing the entire infected nail plate. The cure rate for fingernail infection is higher than 90 percent whereas toenail infections have a much lower cure rate and frequently recur. No treatment is recommended for toenail infection because of the high failure rate, unless there is physical discomfort. The treatment for white superficial onychomycosis is paring away the fungal colony or killing it by applying dilute solutions of formaldehyde or glutaraldehyde onto the nail.

TINEA VERSICOLOR

Tinea versicolor is caused by *Malassezia furfur*, a lipophilic yeast that is a normal inhabitant of the skin. It begins as perifollicular hypopigmentation, then coalesces into well-circumscribed irregular areas covered with a fine scale. Less commonly the affected areas may be a pink or fawn color rather than hypopigmented. The patient with tinea versicolor is usually asymptomatic, but occasionally it produces mild itching. The differential diagnosis includes tinea corporis, pityriasis rosea when the lesions are pink, and vitiligo when they are hypopigmented. The diagnosis is made by demonstrating the organism on scales removed from the lesions. The scales typically show yeast forms and short, stubby hyphae whose appearance has been described as resembling "spaghetti and meatballs."

Treatment. The treatment of choice is selenium sulfide in a shampoo base (Selsun shampoo). The shampoo is used as a soap to lather the entire body, not just the involved areas; it is left in place for 10 minutes and then washed off. This is repeated every other day for 2 weeks. The shampoo should not be used daily because it dries the skin and may induce dermatitis. After the treatment, it may take several weeks (depending on the season) for the skin to regain its normal pigmentation. The patient is cured, when the hypopigmented areas will no longer be scaly. Although the cure rate is high, recurrences are frequent. Other therapeutic regimens include 20 percent sodium thiosulfate and both topical and systemic imidazoles. Oral ketoconazole for the treatment of tinea versicolor is strongly discouraged because of the high risk to benefit ratio.

TINEA NIGRA

Tinea nigra is a superficial infection caused by *Exophiala (Cladosporium) wernecki* that produces a well-circumscribed, irregularly shaped, tan- to black-colored macule without scales on the palms or soles. It most commonly occurs in children. It has been confused with stains, nevi, and malignant melanoma. The diagnosis is made by removing some of the overlying stratum corneum and examining it with KOH for the pigmented fungus.

Treatment. Because the fungus causing tinea nigra resides in the outermost layers of the stratum corneum, simply removing the layers cures the infection. This may be done manually with a blade, by repeatedly stripping the skin with tape, or by chemically removing the outer layers with keratolytic agents such as 4 percent salicylic acid. This infection does not respond to griseofulvin therapy.

CANDIDIASIS

Cutaneous Candidiasis

The most common cutaneous form of candidiasis occurs in intertrigenous areas of the body—the genitocrural folds, the gluteal folds, the inframammary folds, the axilla, and the interdigital area. It is characterized by a well-demarcated, red, errosive, or macerated area with scalloped borders. Pustules characteristically occur adjacent to the macerated areas. Depending on the age of the patient and the area involved, this type of infection may be confused with diaper rash, tinea cruris, or erythrasma. The diagnosis is made by smearing the contents of pustules or the material scraped from the macerated areas onto a microscope slide, treating it with KOH or Gram stain, and demonstrating budding yeast cells.

Treatment. Cutaneous candidiasis responds to treatment with topical nystatin or topical imidazoles (see *Topical Agents*). The addition of a topical corticosteroid to these antifungal agents helps to decrease the inflammatory component induced by *Candida* without decreasing the efficacy of the antifungal agent. These agents are usually applied two to four times a day for 2 to 3 weeks. The use of combination drugs that contain neomycin, ethylenediamine, and parabens should be avoided because of their potential for sensitizing the patient and inducing contact dermatitis. Because moisture and occlusion predispose to infection, patients should wear loose-fitting absorbent clothing and use powder in intertrigenous areas. Some patients with perineal candidiasis may require concurrent therapy with oral nystatin to control the gastrointestinal source.

Mucous Membrane Candidiasis

Candidiasis frequently affects the mucous membranes. In the mouth, the yeast produces white, curd like patches (thrush) on the tongue or buccal mucosa that may be painful. Candidiasis occurs under dentures and is a common cause of denture sore mouth. Patients who use steroid inhalers for pulmonary disease have an increased incidence of oral candidiasis, as do those with acquired immunodeficiency syndrome (AIDS). The diagnosis is made by scraping the involved areas and demonstrating hyphal elements. The finding of budding yeast cells by KOH examination or *Candida* on cultures taken from the mouth is not sufficient to make the diagnosis. The differential diagnosis of oral candidiasis includes lichen planus, white sponge nevus, and squamous cell carcinoma.

Another mucous membrane infected by *Candida* is the vagina. Vaginal candidiasis occurs frequently in conjunction with diabetes mellitus, antibiotic therapy, oral contraceptives, and pregnancy. The induced vaginitis is usually accompanied by a thick discharge and moderate to intense pruritus of the vulva. The vagina and labia are frequently red, and redness and erosions may extend to the perineum. The differential diagnosis includes vaginitis caused by other organisms.

Treatment. Oral candidiasis may be treated by having the patient swirl and swallow 4 to 6 ml of a nystatin suspension containing 100,000 U per milliliter four times a day. Nystatin vaginal tablets or clotrimazole troches sucked four times a day are also helpful in curing an oral infection. Vaginal infections respond well to the clotrimazoled troches inserted daily. The duration of therapy is usually 7 to 10 days.

Nail Candidiasis

Candida often causes paronychia in those who frequently have their hands immersed in water. If the infection persists, it may cause proximal nail ridging or nail loss. The diagnosis is made by culturing the organism or demonstrating it by KOH examination or Gram stain. The differential diagnosis includes bacterial infections and allergic contact dermatitis.

Treatment. The treatment for *Candida* paronychia is topical nystatin or one of the many topical imidazole preparations, applied to the affected area four times a day. The patient should be advised to dry the hands thoroughly after having them in water and to reapply the medica-

tion. The use of rubber gloves should be discouraged, since they tend to become colonized with the fungus and serve as a source for reinfection.

Candida also causes onycholysis of the nail; the yeast grows between the nail plate and the nail bed and causes them to separate, producing a whitish discoloration without surface changes. In women who do not respond to therapy, a thorough search for vaginal or gastrointestinal candidiasis should be conducted, and these areas should also be treated. The differential diagnosis includes psoriasis and trauma. *Pseudomonas* may also be isolated from onycholytic nails, but it usually turns the nail green. It is a secondary invader and is eradicated by treating the candidiasis.

Treatment. To successfully treat candidal onycholysis, the onycholytic portion of the nail plate should be cut off and a topical antifungal agent, either an imidazole or nystatin, should be applied four times a day under the remaining nail plate. The removal of the nail plate prevents trapping of moisture which favors the growth of *Candida*. The patient should be advised to dry the fingernails after having them in water and to reapply the medication. This therapy is continued until a normal nail plate has grown, usually 2 to 3 months. Failure to remove the nail plate before treating the infection may result in further extension of the infection.

SUGGESTED READING

Demis DJ, ed. Clinical dermatology. Philadelphia: Harper and Row, 1986.

Fitzpatrick TB, Eisen AZ, Wolff K, Freedburg IM, Austen KF, eds. Dermatology in general medicine. 2nd Ed. New York: McGraw Hill, 1979.

Mandell G, Douglas R, Bennett JE, eds. Principles and practice of infectious diseases. 2nd Ed. New York: Don Wiley and Sons, 1985.

MANAGEMENT OF NON-LOCALIZING INFECTIOUS DISEASE

ANTIBIOTIC SELECTION

THOMAS F. O'BRIEN, M.D.
KENNETH H. MAYER, M.D.

The ability of an antibiotic to kill a particular strain of bacteria depends on the antibiotic's specific target site, on its access to that target site through the walls and membranes of that type of bacteria, and on whether the infecting strain has acquired a resistance mechanism to inactivate the antibiotic. We can also now group the antibiotics by their actions on target sites, group the types of bacteria by their walls and membranes as reflected roughly in their shape and Gram stain color, and estimate the chances of a particular strain carrying a particular resistance mechanism by knowing when and where the patient got it.

We use these groupings to devise an overall scheme for selecting antibiotics for particular patients, and then we review exceptions. Even an imperfect scheme may be preferable to a catalog matching bacteria and antibiotics, because a scheme can be easier to remember and can be improved as our understanding of antibiotic actions, bacterial envelopes, and resistance mechanisms improves. A scheme also makes antibiotic selection look easier than it is. The clinician often has to guess at the most probable pathogen or pathogens from whatever clinical evidence is available, before any scheme can be used.

ACTIONS OF THE ANTIBIOTICS

Antibiotics inhibit specific steps in the life cycle of a bacterial cell to a greater degree than they inhibit the analogous steps in the life cycle of the patient's cell. The major steps and the antibiotics that inhibit them are reviewed in Figure 1.

The start of the life cycle may be viewed as the synthesis of the cell's genetic material, its deoxyribonucleic acid (DNA), which codes the amino acid sequence of all of the cell's proteins. Many chemicals inhibit this synthesis, but most do so in the cells of both bacteria and humans. Sulfonamides, trimethoprim, and nalidixic acid inhibit various parts of this process selectively in bacteria.

Rifampicin inhibits the synthesis of messenger RNA copies of the DNA.

The next major step in the life cycle of the bacterial cell, the synthesis on the ribosomes directed by the messenger RNA of all of the cell's proteins, is inhibited by two general groups of antibiotics. One of them consists essentially of tetracycline, chloramphenicol, erythromycin, and clindamycin. They tend to inhibit protein synthesis reversibly and so are bacteriostatic.

The other family of antibiotics inhibiting ribosomal synthesis of proteins are the aminoglycosides; streptomycin, neomycin, kanamycin, gentamicin, tobramycin, amikacin, and netilmycin. They inhibit irreversibly, and so tend to be bactericidal.

Among the structures then synthesized by the proteins is the bacterial cell membrane, which encloses the cell contents. Polymyxins disrupt this membrane, allowing the contents to leak out. Vancomycin and bacitracin inhibit the transport out through this membrane of the precursors needed for synthesis of the bacterial cell wall.

Outside of the bacterial cell membrane is the bacterial cell wall, a tough, durable structure that protects the cell from mechanical trauma and from osmotic rupture that would occur in the lower osmotic pressure of the patient's tissues if the wall were not there. The beta-lactam family of antibiotics, which includes all of the penicillins and cephalosporins, selectively blocks the synthesis of this cell wall and thus creates gaps through which the bacterial cell herniates and ruptures.

The patient has no structure analogous to the bacterial cell wall, and probably for this reason the beta-lactam antibiotics have remarkably little direct toxic effect on patient cells. This gives beta-lactam antibiotics some special advantages. Besides being bactericidal in very low concentrations for many major pathogens, beta-lactam antibiotics can often be given to patients in high concentrations. This added margin of security proves helpful in treating many kinds of infections and is one of the major determinants of the general scheme for antibiotic selection that follows.

GENERAL RULES

1. *Some penicillin or first-generation cephalosporin is the drug of choice for infections caused by gram-positive cocci or bacilli or gram-negative cocci.*

The above working rule applies to gram-positive and negative cocci and to gram-positive bacilli, and exempts

Bacterial Function	Antibacterial Action
1. *The bacterial chromosome, an extended single loop of double-stranded DNA, replicates for bacterial cell division.*	*Sulfonamides* and *trimethoprim* inhibit folic acid synthesis, hence nucleotide synthesis, hence DNA synthesis and chromosome replication, but reversibly so are bacteriostatic. *Nalidixic acid* also inhibits chromosome replication.
2. Messenger RNA copies nucleotide sequence of a portion (gene) of the chromosome, carries it to a ribosome.	*Rifampicin* inhibits synthesis messenger RNA.
3. Nucleotide sequence of messenger RNA threading through ribosomes determines sequence of amino acids being bonded onto growing polypeptide chains on each ribosome.	*Tetracycline* *Chloramphenicol* *Erythromycin* *Clindamycin* } inhibit ribosomal polypeptide growth reversibly, so are mostly bacteriostatic.
	Streptomycin *Neomycin* *Kanamycin* *Gentamicin* *Tobramycin* *Amikacin* } (Aminoglycoside family) disrupt ribosomal function irreversibly, so are bactericidal.
4. Proteins synthesized on ribosomes then synthesize other cell components, including cell membrane.	*Polymyxins* *Vancomycin* cause "detergent" disruption of bacterial cell membrane. stop membrane transport cell wall precursors.
5. Bacterial cell wall, a tough, durable, continuous network of cross-linked polysaccharide and polypeptide polymers, encases and protects the bacterial cell from osmotic rupture.	*Penicillins and Cephalosporins* (beta-lactam family) block final cross-linking (transpeptidation) of cell walls, cells herniate out through resulting gaps in cell wall, rupture, use bactericidial.

Figure 1 Steps in the life cycle of a bacterial cell and the antibiotics that inhibit them.

TABLE 1 Major Bacterial Pathogens

	Shape	
Gram Stain	Cocci	Bacilli
Positive	Streptococci Group A, B *viridans* enterococcus pneumococcus Staphylococci *aureus* *epidermidis*	*Clostridia* *Listeria* *Bacillus* *Corynebacteria*
Negative	*Neisseria* meningococci gonococci	Enterobacteriaceae *Escherichia coli* *Klebsiella* *Proteus* *Enterobacter* *Salmonella* *Serratia* *Hemophilus* Anaerobes *Bacteroides,* etc. Nonfermenters *Pseudomonas,* etc.

for separate consideration later only the gram-negative bacilli (Table 1, Fig. 2).

The gram-positive coccal pathogens include essentially five kinds of streptococci and two kinds of staphylococci. Group A beta-hemolytic streptococci cause pharyngitis, cellulitis, erysipelas, and occasional late sequelae, such as rheumatic fever and glomerulonephritis. Group B streptococci are a major cause of neonatal sepsis. *Streptococcus viridans* is the most common cause of bacterial endocarditis. The enterococcus is the second most common cause of endocarditis and also a cause of urinary tract infection. *Streptococcus pneumoniae* causes pneumococcal pneumonia, bacteremia, and meningitis.

These streptococci are susceptible to penicillin, and penicillin remains the drug of choice for infections caused by them. An aminoglycoside is added to increase the killing of enterococci that cause endocarditis. Penicillin-resistant pneumococci have been isolated in South Africa, but only extremely rarely in other parts of the world.

Staphyloccus aureus causes boils, abscesses, wound infections, osteomyelitis, septicemia, and acute bacterial endocarditis. *Staphylococcus epidermidis* usually causes infection only in or with an implanted foreign body, but the growing number of prosthetic joints and heart valves is increasing the opportunities for these. Most isolates of either produce a penicillinase that makes them resistant to penicillin, but most remain susceptible to the semisynthetic antistaphylococcal penicillins, such as methicil-

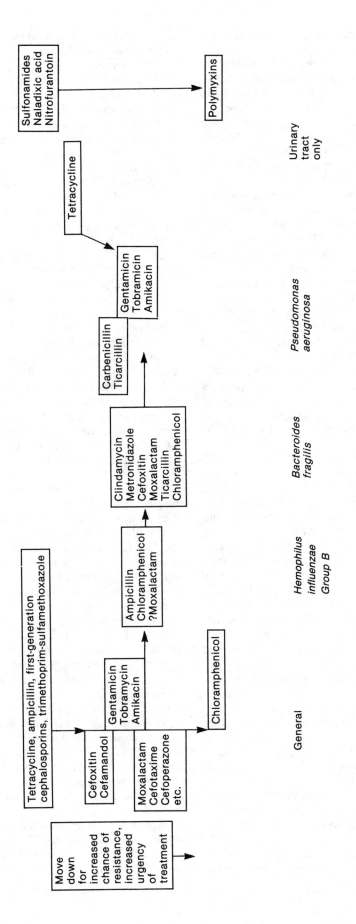

Figure 2 Treatment for infections caused by gram-negative bacilli

lin, oxacillin, cloxacillin, dicloxacillin, and nafcillin, and also to the cephalosporins.

A major exception to our working rule comes from the quarter or so of *S. epidermidis* isolates and the hospital isolates of *S. aureus* called methicillin-resistant staphylococci, which are increasing in number, but are still rare in the United States. Any staphylococcus that is resistant to methicillin (or oxacillin) should be considered resistant to *all* penicillins and cephalosporins, the individual susceptibility test results notwithstanding. These isolates should be treated with vancomycin.

Gram-positive bacilli include clostridia such as *Clostridium perfringens*, a common cause of gas gangrene, cellulitis, or septic abortion, for which penicillin has been the antibiotic therapy of choice, although surgical extirpation of the necrotic tissue is needed. They also include *Clostridium difficile*, which is a notable exception to our working rule. *C. difficile* overgrowth—now recognized as the cause of pseudomembranous colitis—far from being controlled by penicillins, may sometimes be induced by them. Treatment is oral vancomycin.

Also among the gram-positive bacilli is *Listera monocytogenes*, a frequent agent of bacteremia and meningitis in immunosuppressed patients, for which penicillin or ampicillin is the recommended therapy. The agents of anthrax and diphtheria are also penicillin-susceptible gram-positive bacilli, although tetracycline is often used for anthrax and antitoxin is the important part of diphtheria therapy.

The clinically significant gram-negative cocci is the meningococci, which cause meningitis, bacteremia, and pneumonia, and the gonococci, which may be isolated from urethra, cervix, rectum, pharynx, blood, or joints. Penicillin is the treatment of choice for infection with either, although minocycline, rifampicin, or sulfonamides (if isolate is susceptible) are used for eradication of pharyngeal carriage of meningococci. Also, the penicillinase producing *Neisseria gonorrhoeae*, still extremely rare in most parts of the United States, require treatment with other agents, such as spectinamycin or cefoxitin.

Patients with a history of penicillin allergy are an exception to the unqualified application of this rule. The seriousness of this exception has been diminished by the safe use of cephalosporins in many such patients, although some risk of cross allergy remains. Erythromycin, clindamycin, and tetracycline have also been used as alternative therapy in penicillin-allergic patients. For penicillin-allergic patients needing bactericidal therapy for severe gram-positive coccal infections, such as enterococcal endocarditis, vancomycin, with its previously mentioned bactericidal action on the bacterial cell wall, is an excellent choice of therapeutic agent.

2. Selection of an antibiotic for treatment of infection with gram-negative bacilli is determined by the urgency of treatment and by the probability that the bacilli are antibiotic-resistant.

Gram-negative bacilli are the most common cause of urinary tract and bowel-related infections, bacteremia, septic shock, and childhood meningitis, and a common cause of soft tissue infection.

The reason for the rule is that there are many relatively nontoxic, inexpensive antibiotics capable of treating successfully most infections due to gram-negative bacilli. We can identify some patients for whom therapy with these drugs would be more likely to fail, or for whom failure would be more serious, or both; and for these patients initial use of more expensive or more toxic antibiotics is justified.

Figure 2 diagrams these choices. The long box at the top of the diagram includes antibiotics such as tetracycline, ampicillin, first-generation cephalosporins, and trimethoprim-sulfamethoxazole, which are commonly used to treat less urgent infections caused by gram-negative bacilli less likely to be antibiotic-resistant. An example might be an infection of the lower urinary tract in a woman not previously hospitalized or treated with antibiotics. To the right is a box containing additional agents, such as sulfonamides, nalidixic acid, and nitrofurantoin, which are at the same level, but are exclusively for urinary tract infections.

To the left in Figure 2 is one major descending pathway for gram-negative bacilli generally, and to the right are separate blocks for each of three special gram-negative bacilli, *Hemophilus influenzae* group B, *Bacteroides fragilis*, and *Pseudomonas aeruginosa*, as well as the far-right pathway for urinary tract infections. The more urgent the patient's need for therapy and the more likely the isolate is to be resistant, the further down is the appropriate box for therapy.

Some boxes on the downward path are partly contiguous, to signify that one is not entirely higher or lower than the others, and also to indicate that synergy may be possible between agents from contiguous blocks, although the need for synergy seems to be infrequent and difficult to establish. Simultaneous treatment with more than one antibiotic is more often prompted by the need to treat more than one possible infecting agent, than by a demonstrated need for synergistic treatment of any one infecting agent.

Deciding where a patient fits on this decision tree is a matter of clinical judgment. For example, a patient who has been hospitalized and treated with antibiotics prior to developing gram-negative bacillemia would be far down on the diagram. Hospitalization and antibiotic therapy make it more likely that the infecting strain is antibiotic-resistant, and failure to treat promptly with an effective antibiotic increases the risk of death from bacillemia. The need to consider the block for *Pseudomonas* would be increased if *Pseudomonas* had been a nosocomial problem in that hospital, or the *Bacteroides* block if a bowel source of sepsis were suspected on clinical grounds.

The second box encountered in proceeding down the general pathway to the left contains the second-generation cephalosporins: cefoxitin and cefamandole. They kill all of the gram-negative bacilli that are killed by first-generation cephalosporins, and each kills some others in addition, which may be identified by susceptibility testing. This moderate increase in spectrum and their increased cost without increased toxicity determine their location on the diagram.

The third box down on the general pathway includes the currently used aminoglycosides: gentamicin, tobramycin, and amikacin. Their relatively narrow therapeutic ratio, potential nephrotoxicity, bactericidal efficacy, and wide spectrum put them here. When first introduced they killed nearly all gram-negative bacilli, but now something like 15 percent of *Pseudomonas* isolates everywhere and a similar proportion of other gram-negative bacilli (in some hospitals but not in others) are resistant to one or more of them. The experience of your own particular hospital is the deciding factor.

The fourth box down on the scheme for general treatment of gram-negative bacillary infection contains the third-generation cephalosporins: moxalactam, cefotaxime, cefoperazone, and others to come. Their present ability to kill nearly all gram-negative bacilli, perhaps excepting *Pseudomonas*, their high cost, and the desire to avoid development of resistance to them determine their position. The low concentrations of these agents needed to kill most bacilli and their moderate penetration of cerebrospinal fluid may prove to be useful for therapy of the rare, but otherwise difficult to treat, gram-negative bacillary meningitis.

A fifth box is added for chloramphenicol as a reminder that its wide spectrum occasionally makes it useful in treating sepsis severe enough to justify its low, but unpredictable, risk of bone marrow aplasia.

In the special categories to the right, *H. influenzae* group B gets a special box because it is a major cause of croup, pneumonia, bacteremia, and meningitis in childhood and because up to a fifth of its clinical isolates are now resistant to ampicillin. Treating it with chloramphenicol and ampicillin when it causes meningitis or other

major sepsis has been recommended until susceptibility tests can establish that ampicillin alone is adequate. This unfortunate need for chloramphenicol may be circumvented if agents such as moxalactam prove effective in clinical trials.

The next special category box is for *B. fragilis*. It is the most pathogenic of the anaerobic bacteria in the colon and thus is a cause of infection after leaks from the colon, such as appendiceal or diverticular abscesses or following trauma or bowel surgery. It is also usually resistant to tetracycline, penicillin, ampicillin, and first-generation cephalosporins, as well as having the resistance all anaerobes have to aminoglycosides. Most isolates are susceptable to clindamycin and metronidazole and virtually all isolates in the United States are susceptible to chloramphenicol. Most are killed by high concentrations of cefoxitin and many to high concentrations of ticarcillin or moxalactam.

A third special category box is given to *P. aeruginosa*. Carbenicillin or ticarcillin may be less toxic than the aminoglycosides, but a quarter or more of *P. aeruginosa* isolates may be resistant to either group, and some to both. For this reason, and in hope of some synergy, therapy including one of each is often used for severe sepsis due to *Pseudomonas*.

The tetracycline arrow angled from the urinary tract therapy box down to the *Pseudomonas* boxes represents the frequent ability of tetracyclines to suppress *Pseudomonas* infections of the urinary tract, presumably because of their high concentrations in urine. The box further down receiving arrows from both *Pseudomonas* and urinary tract boxes reminds us that polymyxins, such as Coly-Mycin, given systemically are effective in killing virtually any *Pseudomonas* in the urine although ineffective at any other site.

FEVER IN THE ADULT

STEPHEN E. FOLLANSBEE, M.D.

Fever is one of the most treated of symptoms, yet its pathogenesis and benefits are still only partially understood. Even in its most malignant form, fever is a byproduct of disease, and appropriate treatment requires some understanding of the underlying cause and pathophysiologic mechanism. Therefore, the practitioner must read this chapter in conjunction with one or more other chapters of this text when approaching fever in the adult patient.

PATHOPHYSIOLOGY

It is helpful to list the differential diagnosis of temperature elevation based on the pathophysiologic mechanism. A fever develops by resetting the hypothalamic thermoregulatory "set point." This most often occurs because of infection, but may be owing to malignant disease (through production of endogenous pyrogen), central nervous system bleeding (either intraventricular or hypothalamic), head trauma, collagen vascular disease, or drugs and medications (through hypersensitivity mechanisms). Hyperthermia develops despite a normal "set point" because of excessive heat production or defective heat dissipation. Excess heat production occurs in various metabolic or endocrinologic conditions (such as hyperthyroidism, primary adrenal insufficiency, or pheochromocytoma), salicylate overdose, drug overdose

(LSD, PCP), and malignant hyperthermia (an autosomally dominant inherited predisposition in the setting of anesthesia). Some infections such as tetanus produce fever by this mechanism owing to increased autonomic nervous system activity. Defective heat loss may occur in anticholinergic drug overdose, "overinsulation," excessive environmental temperature, and heat stroke and in autonomic dysfunction secondary to quadriplegia.

Fever itself is usually not harmful. It usually peaks spontaneously at about 40° C and causes no problems in the otherwise healthy adult. There are exceptions. Elevations greater than 41.1° C (106° F) in even previously healthy persons may be associated with severe dehydration and consequent metabolic disorders, delirium, and hepatic damage. Lower elevations (38.8 to 40° C) may be dangerous in children with febrile seizures (discussed in another chapter). The heart rate generally rises by 15 to 18 beats per minute per degree C (8 to 10 beats per minute per degree F), and metabolic demands increase 13 percent per degree C (7 percent per degree F). Fever in persons with cardiac disease and coronary artery insufficiency may lead to myocardial ischemia and infarction. Fever in those with severe lung disease may lead to hypoxia and then diffuse ischemia and infarction. Fever in patients with severe mental disorders may induce more severe psychosis. Brain edema may increase 40 percent with every 2 degree C increase in temperature; fever in patients with recent head trauma or neurosurgical procedures may precipitate coma. The fetus is unable to thermoregulate independent of the mother, and fever in pregnant women has been associated with congenital anomalies. Heat stroke produces hematologic sequelae, including disseminated intravascular coagulation.

DIAGNOSIS

The essentials of diagnosis are the history and physical examination (Table 1). Further evaluation will be dictated by critical findings, and reference is again made to other chapters, particularly those on bacterial infection,

TABLE 1 Essentials of Diagnosis of Fever in Adults

History of fever: duration, height, periodicity, associated complaints

Pertinent medical history: medications prescribed (phenytoin, antibiotics, Aldomet, phenothiazines, anticholinergics), recreational drugs (PCP, LSD, intravenous drug use), travel history, bites (insect, animal), recent trauma (surgical, nonsurgical, ?loss of consciousness), vaccinations (?tetanus), recent surgery and dental procedures, pregnancy, and menstrual history

Review of systems: skin rashes (rule out Rocky Mountain spotted fever, staphylococcus sepsis, meningococcemia), pulmonary disease, cardiac disease (including history of valvular heart disease or endocarditis), urinary tract symptoms, central nervous system (stiff neck, headache, photophobia, history of meningitis, loss of consciousness), gastrointestinal complaints

Physical examination: temperature (rectal), heart rate, respiratory rate, blood pressure, general perfusion and mentation; skin rashes; meningismus; pulmonary consolidation; heart murmur; abdominal tenderness; costovertebral angle tenderness; tenderness on rectovaginal examination; signs of autonomic activity; draining wounds or recent trauma

toxic shock, thyroid disorders, tetanus, heat injury, and hyperthermia.

The height of the fever is generally not helpful in distinguishing its cause, nor does a fever response to antipyretics distinguish bacterial from nonbacterial infection. A history of fever not confirmed on rectal measurement may be attributable to one of several causes, including recent antipyretics, oral temperature determination in a patient who is hyperventilating or unable to close his mouth, the fever pattern of certain conditions (e.g., malaria), and factitious fever history (in this case, the patient should be directly observed throughout the temperature-taking).

A "fever of unknown origin" is defined as a temperature elevation greater than 38.3° C (101.1° F) for more than 3 weeks, without documented cause after at least 1 week of intense medical evaluation. In general it is not a diagnosis established in the emergency department. However, the evaluation can be initiated in the emergency department upon referral to a family practitioner or internist.

MANAGEMENT

Therapy for temperature elevation is always undertaken in conjunction with treating the underlying cause. Recommendations for the choice of initial antibiotics, empiric treatment of many specific life-threatening infections, as well as treatment of other noninfectious causes of fever are found in other chapters. For conditions associated with a reset thermoregulatory "set point," therapy should include antipyretics. For conditions attributable to imbalance between heat generation and heat dissipation, antipyretics in general have no role. In some instances these may be contraindicated; e.g., aspirin may worsen acidosis. Table 2 summarizes some physical findings that may help distinguish these two categories of temperature elevation.

Therapy should initially be directed at correcting dehydration and metabolic disorders. Serum electrolyte and arterial blood gas levels should be obtained if there is question. Supplemental oxygen may be helpful for those with pulmonary and cardiac disease.

High fever, in addition to creating metabolic burdens on the cardiovascular system, generally contributes to patient discomfort and is thus worth treating. On the other hand, fever is a universal response to infection in mam-

TABLE 2 Physical Signs That May Distinguish an Elevated Thermoregulatory "Set Point" from True Hyperthermia

Elevated "set point" (fever)
  Shivering
  Curling into a ball
  Drinking hot liquids
  Vasoconstriction (cool, pale skin)

Imbalance between heat production and
heat dissipation (true hyperthermia)
  Sweating
  Lying straight out
  Drinking cool liquids
  Vasodilation (warm, flushed skin)

mals and has been shown to enhance the body's ability to kill bacteria; thus, eliminating it altogether may not be desirable.

Acetaminophen and aspirin are equally efficacious in adults for fever control in those with an elevated hypothalamic "set point." (Alternating 10 grains of each every 2 hours may be more effective.) There may be relative contraindications to acetaminophen in patients with underlying liver disease. Aspirin may be contraindicated in patients with bleeding disorders (hemophilia, anticoagulants), severe cirrhosis, gout, hyperuricemia, peptic ulcer disease, or aspirin-induced asthma. However, the potential danger of untreated temperature elevation may outweigh these relative contraindications in the case of extreme pyrexia. The patient's response to antipyretics does not distinguish those with bacteroid or viral infections.

Tepid sponging and cooling blankets help to rapidly decrease the body temperature in the patient when clothing is removed. Fans help move air and dissipate heat.

Iced bath emersion should be reserved for patients with severe hyperthermia (greater than 41.1° C). Iced gastric lavage and the use of cold intravenous fluids have not proven to be more effective than these other peripheral cooling methods. These more aggressive methods of cooling should be needed only in cases of hyperthermia, not ordinary fever.

In severe cases of hyperthermia, chlorpromazine may be useful in doses of 25 to 50 mg intramuscularly every 4 to 6 hours. It apparently is effective by blocking alpha-adrenergic mediated mechanisms of shivering and causing peripheral vasodilation. Phenothiazines should not be used in cases of pheochromocytoma and clearly not in patients taking phenothiazines with a history of environmen-

tal heat exposure. Nitroprusside has been used rarely (doses of 0.5 to 1 μg per kg per minute by constant intravenous infusion) to aid in vasodilation in refractory situations.

The only documented benefit of glucocorticoids in fever is for the treatment of primary or secondary adrenal insufficiency associated with (or without) fever. Their role in septic shock is addressed elsewhere.

DISPOSITION

Clearly any patient with severe hyperthermia (greater than 41.1° C) needs admission for management of fever as well as the underlying condition. A decision to admit a patient solely on the basis of fever less than this depends on the cause as well as potential sequelae of unmanaged or poorly controlled fever. Thus, the threshold for admitting a patient with coronary artery disease and fever is lower than in a patient with fever alone. Likewise, a pregnant women with mitral stenosis may need admission for temperature elevations considered trivial in other persons. Subspecialty referral likewise depends on the multitude of factors just discussed and cannot be simply delineated.

SUGGESTED READING

Done AK. Treatment of fever in 1982: a review. Aspirin Symposium. Am J Med, June 1983:27–35.
Simon HB. Extreme pyrexia. JAMA 1976; 236:2419–2421.
Simon HB, Daniels GH. Hormonal hyperthermia: endocrinologic causes of fever. Am J Med 1979; 66:257–263.

SEPSIS IN ADULTS

RICHARD A. JACOBS, M.D., Ph.D.

Bacteremic infections are a major cause of morbidity and mortality. It has been estimated that as many as 300,000 to 500,000 cases of gram-negative rod bacteremia occur yearly in the United States, and one-third to one-half end fatally. Early recognition of this disease and prompt institution of antimicrobial agents active against the causative organism are important elements in reduction of the mortality rates for this deadly disease.

The organisms most commonly associated with gram-negative sepsis include *Escherichia coli*, *Klebsiella* species, *Pseudomonas aeruginosa*, *Serrtia marcescens*, and *Enterobacter* species. Other organisms, such as *Proteus* species, *Bacteroides fragilis*, and other gram-positive and gram-negative anaerobes, can also invade the bloodstream, but do so less frequently.

The usual sites of origin for systemic gram-negative infections are the genitourinary tract, the gastrointestinal and biliary systems, and the lungs. Other less common sources include intravenous catheters (both peripheral and central), surgical wounds, surgical drains, and the skin (with cellulitis, decubitus ulcers, abscesses). The importance of localizing the source of bacteremia cannot be overemphasized—removing (catheters, drains) or draining (abscesses) the source of bacteremia greatly improves the outcome and makes a potentially fatal disease easily treatable.

CLINICAL DIAGNOSIS

A thorough physical examination looking for sources and manifestations of infection is critically important in the potentially septic patient. The physician should seek rashes, petechiae, splinter hemorrhages, retinal lesions (Roth's spots), and purpura on the skin as well as on the mucous membranes (mouth, vagina, conjunctiva). The entire body (including scalp, web spaces, perineum, and palms and soles) should be examined for abscesses, ulcers, or needle marks. Signs of meningeal irritation, heart murmurs, and abnormal lung sounds should be further investigated. All patients need a rectal examination (for abscess) and examination of all joints and the spine for arthritis or abscess, and all female patients should have a pelvic examination.

The clinical manifestations of sepsis are often nonspecific, and a high index of suspicion is required to make the diagnosis. Fever and chills are common, but not always present. Approximately 15 percent of patients are hypothermic (temperature $\leq 97.6\,°F$) at the onset of their bacteremia, and 5 percent will never develop a temperature above $99.6\,°F$ throughout the course of their illness. Thus, when present, fever and chills are helpful clues in making the diagnosis of sepsis, but their absence by no means excludes this disease. Other clinical manifestations that may be helpful in identifying the bacteremic patient are hypotension, shock [blood pressure (BP) $\leq 90/60$], and oliguria. Two important signs of sepsis are *hyperventilation* with a respiratory alkalosis, and changes in *mental status*. These findings are important because they occur very early in the course of illness, often before the onset of fevers, chills, or hypothermia. The changes in mental status may be very subtle, such as a slight change in personality or unusual behavior, or they may be more obvious, such as confusion, obtundation, or even coma.

Cutaneous lesions are also seen in sepsis. The one most commonly described, and seen primarily in *Pseudomonas aeruginosa* bacteremia, is ecthyma gangrenosum. This lesion is 1 to 5 cm in size and has a necrotic center surrounded by an indurated, erythematous halo. Although ecthyma gangrenosum is the best described skin lesion, a number of other cutaneous lesions can also be seen, including vesicles, bullae, petechiae, cellulitis, and even a diffuse erythematous reaction similar to that seen in scarlet fever. Thus, skin lesions can be quite varied and nonspecific and do not allow the physician to make a definitive diagnosis of sepsis, although their presence should certainly raise the suspicion that one is dealing with a bacteremic patient. If skin lesions are present in a patient with suspected sepsis, they should be scraped, Gram-stained, and sent for culturing. A positive Gram stain is confirmatory evidence of bacteremia and is very helpful in deciding which emperic antibiotics to initiate.

LABORATORY TESTS

Initial laboratory investigation may reveal a leukocytosis with immature forms, but a normal or even depressed white blood cell count can also be seen. Other laboratory abnormalities include thrombocytopenia (50 percent) and abnormal clotting parameters consistent with disseminated intravascular coagulation (10 percent), although only 2 to 3 percent of patients have clinical bleeding.

It is imperative that a careful and methodical search be made for an infection site in the patient thought to be septic. This includes a careful physical examination of all organ systems and of sputum, urine, and stool for evidence of bacteriologic infection. Specimens of cerebrospinal fluid (CSF) or ascitic fluid should also be examined where appropriate.

Although the clinical manifestations and examination of body fluids may suggest the diagnosis of sepsis, it is confirmed by obtaining a positive *blood culture*. Two frequently asked questions about blood cultures are (1) *how many* blood cultures should be obtained and (2) *how much* blood should be cultured? Because gram-negative rod bacteremia is intermittent, several cultures must be drawn to maximize results. There is a correlation between the number of blood cultures obtained and the likelihood of positivity: if one culture is drawn, there is an 80 percent chance that it will be positive; if two cultures are drawn, a 90 percent chance; and if three cultures are obtained, there is a 99 percent chance that one of them will be positive. Unfortunately, in the study cited above, cultures were obtained over a 24-hour period *before* antibiotics were administered. In patients suspected of being bacteremic, it is inappropriate to withhold therapy for 24 hours to maximize the results of blood culture. Instead, a single blood culture should be drawn and therapy initiated. When this course is followed, it is important to remember that there is a 20 percent chance that the culture will be falsely negative, i.e., the patient was bacteremic, but a single blood culture failed to detect the bacteremia.

Because gram-negative rod bacteremia is low grade, it has generally been recommended that 5 to 10 cc of blood be cultured. Recent information suggests that, if larger volumes of blood are cultured, the yield is higher. Culturing 30 cc of blood (placing 10 cc in each of three blood culture bottles) increases the rate of positive culture 65 percent over culturing only 10 cc of blood. Based on these data, a reasonable approach to the patient suspected of having bacteremia would be to obtain a single large volume of blood for culture and institute empiric antibiotic therapy immediately. This maximizes positive culture results and avoids the dangerous situation of delaying therapy to obtain blood cultures spaced over prolonged intervals.

TREATMENT

A major determinant of outcome of sepsis is the severity of the underlying disease of the patient. Patients with rapidly fatal underlying diseases (immunosuppression, leukemia) have a higher mortality rate than patients with ultimately fatal diseases (any disease likely to cause death in 5 years) and nonfatal diseases (or no underlying disease). If the underlying disease can be reversed (stopping or decreasing immunosuppressive drugs, or administering white blood cells to the leukopenic patient), survival will improve.

The importance of localizing the source of bacteremia and removing or draining it has been discussed. Therapy of disseminated intravascular coagulation and the use of fluids and pressors to treat shock are discussed elsewhere.

The early institution of at least one antibiotic active against the causative organism is the most important therapeutic maneuver in improving outcome of sepsis. From a careful history and physical examination, one can usually determine the organ system involved in the infection. A Gram stain of any fluid or secretions produced can be instrumental in selection of antibiotics. Urinary and respiratory infections severe enough to cause sepsis are usually associated with localizing symptoms and positive Gram stains.

If the Gram stain of a urinary sediment reveals gram-negative rods, an aminoglycoside such as gentamicin or tobramycin should be instituted (2 mg per kilogram loading dose followed by 1.8 mg per kilogram every 8 hours, adjusted for renal function). Gram-positive cocci in the urine usually represent *Streptococcus faecalis* and should be treated with an aminoglycoside plus ampicillin (6 to 12 g per day in divided doses every 4 hours) or vancomycin (8 to 10 mg per kilogram every 8 hours adjusted for renal function) if the patient is penicillin allergic. Rarely *Staphylococcus aureus* (gram-positive cocci in pairs and clusters) can cause urinary infections and should be treated with a beta-lactamase-resistant penicillin such as nafcillin (9 to 12 g per day in divided doses every 4 hours) or vancomycin in the penicillin-allergic patient.

An adequate sputum specimen (numerous polymorphonuclear leukocytes and few epithelial cells) will most commonly reveal gram-positive diplococci indicative of *Streptococcus pneumoniae* (penicillin 5 to 10 million units per day in divided doses every 4 hours), small gram-negative coccobacilli indicative of *Hemophilus influenzae* (ampicillin or in areas where ampicillin-resistant strains are prevalent, a third-generation cephalosporin), gram-negative rods indicative of enterobacteriaciae (gentamicin or tobramycin), or mixed gram-positive and gram-negative organisms suggesting aspiration (penicillin or clindamycin 600 mg every 6 to 8 hours).

Intra-abdominal infections and biliary tract infections are frequently polymicrobial, involving anaerobes (particularly *Bacteroides fragilis*), enteric gram-negative rods, and enterococci. Therapy usually involves ampicillin, gentamicin, or tobramycin and metronidazole (7.5 mg per kilogram every 6 to 8 hours).

Simple cellulitis is usually due to group A streptococci or *S. aureus* and can be treated with a first-generation cephalosporin (cefazolin 1 g every 8 hours). The bacteriology of decubitus and vascular ulcers is polymicrobial and requires therapy directed against *S. aureus*, anaerobes, and enteric gram-negative rods. In 25 percent of patients no source can be found for their bacteremia. Since the clinical manifestations of sepsis with gram-positive and gram-negative organisms are identical, initial therapy should include antibiotics active against both groups of organisms, i.e., nafcillin or cefazolin in combination with an aminoglycoside.

The initial therapy suggested is broad spectrum and frequently involves antibiotics with potential serious toxicities. Once an organism has been isolated and sensitivities are known, the antimicrobial agent that is least toxic and most efficacious can be substituted for the empiric regimen to complete the usual 10- to 14-day course of therapy.

The use of high-dose corticosteroids (3 mg per kilogram of dexamethasone or 30 mg per kilogram of methylprednisolone) remains controversial. A recent study indicated that the early use of steroids, before irreversible end-organ damage occurred, improved short-term survival (5 to 6 days) but had no effect on overall prognosis. Further studies to elucidate the role of steroids in sepsis are ongoing.

Similarly, the use of an opiate antagonist, naloxone, in the therapy of septic shock is controversial. Animal and human reports suggest that as little as 0.4 mg of naloxone can reverse the hypotension associated with gram-negative sepsis. The ultimate impact of this form of therapy on the outcome of sepsis requires further investigation.

The most exciting new form of therapy involves the use of J-5 antiserum. Most gram-negative organisms share a common constituent located in the outer membrane of the cell wall, termed lipid A. Lipid A has all of the properties of endotoxin and is thought to be the toxic moiety of gram-negative organisms. Using the J-5 mutant of *E. coli*, it has been possible to obtain J-5 antiserum that has antibody activity against the lipid A component. Clinical studies have indicated that administration of J-5 antiserum to patients with gram-negative bacteremia improves survival significantly. When administered prophylactically to patients at high risk for developing gram-negative infections, it significantly reduced the incidence of shock and shock-related deaths. Recently, a human monoclonal J-5 antibody with activity against lipid A was produced, providing hope that this biologic product may be available for widespread use in the near future.

SUGGESTED READING

Mandell GL et al, eds. Principles and practice of infectious diseases. 2nd ed. New York: Wiley Medical Publications, 1985:452.

Weinstein MP et al. The clinical significance of positive blood cultures: a comprehensive analysis of 500 episodes of bacteremia and fungemia in adults: I. Laboratory and epidemiologic observations. Rev Infect Dis 1983; 5:35–53.

Weinstein MP et al. The clinical significance of positive blood cultures: a comprehensive analysis of 500 episodes of bacteremia and fungemia in adults: II. Clinical observations, with special reference to factors influencing prognosis. Rev Infect Dis 1983; 5:54–70.

TOXIC SHOCK SYNDROME

ANN HARWOOD-NUSS, M.D.
DAVID S. SCHILLINGER, M.D.

In 1978, Todd and co-workers described a disease process in seven children characterized by high fever, hypotension, diarrhea, erythroderma, confusion, and acute renal failure; they labeled the disease toxic shock syndrome (TSS). In 1980, TSS was noted in menstruating women, and by 1981, an epidemic associated with tampon use was well recognized. Since 1978, the etiology and a proposed pathogenesis have been delineated, the clinical picture has been well described, and the epidemiology extensively studied.

ETIOLOGY AND PATHOGENESIS

It is well known that TSS is associated with infections caused by *Staphylococcus aureus*. Approximately two-thirds of the organisms are phage type I and 25 percent are nontypeable. In 1981, Schlievert demonstrated that pyrogenic toxin C was produced by 90 to 100 percent of the organisms isolated from patients with TSS; less than 25 percent of the control organisms produced the same toxin. Bergdoll identified an enterotoxin (enterotoxin F) in 91 percent of cases of toxic shock associated with cultures of *S. aureus* versus only 10 percent of cases caused by random strains. It is now thought that pyrogenic toxin C and enterotoxin F are probably the same protein and by some unknown mechanism mediate the disease. The toxin has been shown to enhance the effects of endotoxin and may directly damage cell membranes, thus activating the coagulation, the kinin, and the prostaglandin cascades. Furthermore, the immunologic status of the individual may play a role in the pathogenesis of the disease. Antistaphylococcal enterotoxin F antibody titers of 1:100 were seen in approximately 80 percent of control patients, whereas only 17 percent of patients with TSS had such titers.

EPIDEMIOLOGY

The vast majority of cases of TSS occur in white females. Ninety-two percent of cases in women occur during menstruation; 99 percent are associated with tampon usage, most notably the super-absorbant tampons. One percent of cases of toxic shock associated with menstruation have been associated with the use of sanitary napkins and sea sponges. Only 2 percent of menstruation-related TSS has occurred in the nonwhite population. Although an exact explanation has not been provided, the most plausible reason relates to racial preferences for sanitary protection during menstruation. *S. aureus* has been isolated from the vaginas of 98 percent of women with TSS, versus only an 8 to 10 percent vaginal carrier rate in the general female population.

Variant toxic shock (cases not related to menstruation) has been reported with a variety of staphylococcal infections (Table 1). In contrast to menstruation-related toxic shock, 13 percent of the patients are nonwhite, a figure more closely reflecting the racial distribution in the United States. However, 68 percent of variant TSS patients are female. This is partly attributable to the high number of cases related to postpartum and vaginal infections; these infections account for one quarter of all cases of variant TSS. Nasal packings ("nasal tampons") are also associated with a high incidence of TSS, since 20 to 40 percent of the adult population carry *S. aureus* on the anterior nasal vestibule. Nasal carrier rates are highest among hospital employees, intravenous drug abusers, hemodialysis patients, and insulin-dependent diabetics.

The overall incidence of TSS has decreased since 1980, but the percentage of variant TSS increased from 7 percent in 1980 to 29 percent in 1983. Mortality rates, originally reported to be between 5 and 10 percent, decreased to 2.5 percent in 1983. However, several opportunities for bias exist when discussing epidemiologic data on TSS. Many of the early reports were based on retrospective analyses and may have resulted in erroneously high mortality rates. Furthermore, the lack of a specific disease marker has made it necessary to adhere to a strict definition of the disease; therefore, milder forms of the disease often are not included in the statistical reports. Finally, physician bias exists: physicians tend to associate the syndrome only with menstruating women.

CLINICAL PRESENTATION

Toxic shock syndrome should be considered in any unexplained febrile illness associated with erythroderma, hypotension, and diffuse organ pathology, especially in menstruating women. The clinical criteria for the diagnosis of TSS are listed in Table 2. Patients with menstruation-associated TSS usually present between the third and fifth day of menses. The median time to onset of illness in postsurgical toxic shock is the second postoperative day.

Sudden onset of fever and chills occurs approximately 1 to 4 days prior to presentation. Diffuse myalgias—particularly in the proximal aspects of the extremities, abdomen, and back—are reported by virtally all patients;

TABLE 1 Clinical Settings Associated with Variant Toxic Shock Syndrome

Childbirth (vaginal or cesarian section)
Septic abortion
Mastitis
Nasal surgery with packing
Fasciitis
Osteomyelitis
Peritonsillar abscess
Subcutaneous abscess or lesion (furuncles, hydradenitis, insect bites, burns, abrasions)
Staphylococcal colonization of mucous membranes

TABLE 2   Criteria for Diagnosis of Toxic Shock Syndrome

Temperature 38.9 ° C (102 ° F)
Systolic BP 90 mm Hg, orthostatic decrease of systolic
  BP by 15 mm Hg, or syncope
Rash with subsequent desquamation, especially on palms
  or soles of feet
Involvement of 4 of the following organ systems
  clinically or by abnormal laboratory tests:
    Gastrointestinal: vomiting, profuse diarrhea
    Musculoskeletal: severe myalgias or 5-fold increase
      in CPK
    Renal: increase in BUN and creatinine 2 times
      normal; pyuria without evidence of infection
    Mucosal inflammation (vagina, conjunctiva,
      pharynx); hyperemia
    Hepatic involvement: hepatitis (increased bilirubin,
      SGOT, SGPT)
    Hematologic: thrombocytopenia (< 100,000
      platelets/mm³)
    CNS: disorientation without focal neurologic signs
    Pulmonary: ARDS
Negative serology for Rocky Mountain spotted fever,
  leptospirosis, measles, hepatitis B surface antigen,
  fluorescent antinuclear antibody, VDRL, monospot,
  and blood, urine and throat cultures

arthralgias are also common. Profuse, watery diarrhea and repeated vomiting are reported by 90 to 98 percent of patients. Patients also complain of sore throat, headache, paresthesias, and photophobia, as well as orthostatic dizziness or syncope.

Physical examination reveals hypotension or an orthostatic decrease in systolic pressure by 15 mm Hg in 100 percent of cases, since this is an inclusion criterion of the disease. Milder forms of the disease may not present with hypotension, however. The rash is classically a diffuse blanching erythroderma that fades within 3 days of its appearance and is followed by full-thickness desquamation, especially of the palms and soles. Variations include patchy erythroderma and localized maculopustular eruptions. One-half to three-quarters of patients have pharyngitis with a strawberry red tongue; conjunctival hyperemia and vaginitis are also seen. Tender, edematous external genitalia, diffuse vaginal hyperemia, scant purulent cervical discharge, and bilateral adnexal tenderness are seen in 25 to 35 percent of menstruation-related TSS. Approximately 75 percent of patients have nonfocal neurologic abnormalities without signs of meningeal irritation. Confusion, disorientation, agitation, hysteria. somnolence, and seizures have been reported, consistent with a toxic encephalopathy.

Numerous laboratory abnormalities indicative of multisystem involvement are common in TSS. Leukocytosis with an increase in immature forms is frequently seen; lymphocytopenia has also been reported. Azotemia and abnormal urinary sediments (sterile pyuria and red blood cell casts) are seen with the development of acute renal failure. Liver function abormalities and hyperbilirubinemia are seen in approximately half the patients. Despite increases in the prothrombin time, partial thromboplastin time, and fibrin split products in association with thrombocytopenia, only 3 percent of patients have clinical evidence of a coagulopathy. Electrolyte abnormalities

including hypocalcemia, hypophosphatemia, hyponatremia, and hypokalemia are common. Metabolic acidosis secondary to hypotension is also seen.

Acute renal failure secondary to acute tubular necrosis is a complication of TSS. Ventricular dysrhythmias, adult respiratory distress syndrome (ARDS), and refractory hypotension represent the ultimate end-organ damage secondary to TSS. Most patients recover without sequelae with appropriate treatment. However, numerous sequelae have been reported. Of these, the most common is the reversible loss of hair and nails, the late onset of a maculopapular rash, and prolonged fatigue and weakness. Neurologic sequelae have been fairly well documented. Memory deficits, difficulty remembering new information, and hyper-reflexia, associated with diffuse electroencephalographic abnormalities, are consistently seen in patients with neurologic sequelae. It is important to be aware that recurrence of the disease may occur in patients who are not treated with beta-lactamase stable antibiotics. However, recurrences tend to be less severe and seem to occur on the same day of the menses as the prior attack.

DIFFERENTIAL DIAGNOSIS

The patient with a fever, rash, watery diarrhea, myalgias, and multisystem involvement presents a true diagnostic dilemma to the emergency physician. Such protean manifestations require differentiating TSS from numerous other diseases (Table 3). The clinical picture of staphylococcal scarlet fever is so similar to TSS that only pathology specimens or serologic evidence of the exfoliative toxin can differentiate the two entities. However, streptococcal scarlet fever is rare after 10 years of age. Furthermore, the "sand paper" rash of scarlet fever is distinct from the macular rash of TSS. The staphylococcal scalded skin syndrome can be distinguished by rapid, superficial peeling in contrast to the full-thickness desquamation of TSS; in addition, the scalded skin syndrome usually occurs in children less than 5 years old. Mucocutaneous lymph node syndrome (Kawasaki disease) is generally limited to children less than 10 years old. Although the exanthems may be similar, Kawasaki disease may present with target lesions resembling erythema multiforme, and the bright red appearance of the vermillion border is not common in TSS. Finally, the rash of Rocky Mountain spotted fever may begin as a macular eruption and progress to a maculopapular rash and ecchymoses within a few days.

TABLE 3   Differential Diagnosis of TSS

Staphylococcal scarlet fever	Septic shock
Staphylococcal scalded skin syndrome	Rocky Mountain spotted fever
Streptococcal scarlet fever	Leptospirosis
Kawasaki disease	Reye's syndrome
Acute Rheumatic Fever	Gastroenteritis

TREATMENT

The pre-hospital management of patients with toxic shock syndrome is determined by the severity of the presentation. In the initial assessment, management of the circulatory status dominates, since hypotension is a common finding. Aggressive fluid resuscitation with crystalloid is the main therapeutic intervention initiated in the field.

In the emergency department, more extensive intervention may begin. Stabilization of vital signs is the priority. Aggressive fluid resuscitation is often required; some patients have required up to 20 liters of fluid in the first 24 hours of hospitalization. Patients with abnormal coagulation profiles and evidence of bleeding require colloid replacement; thrombocytopenia may require platelet transfusions. Fluid status should be monitored in the emergency department by assessing urine output, measuring central venous pressure, or, if feasible, measuring pulmonary capillary wedge pressure with a pulmonary artery catheter. In cases of refractory hypotension, vasopressors may be required to maintain adequate tissue perfusion. A dopamine infusion beginning at 5 to 10 μg per kilogram per minute may be used. The role of corticosteroids or nalaxone in TSS is not yet defined; preliminary evidence suggests that methylprednisolone, 30 mg per kilogram, may reduce the severity of the illness if administered within the first 2 to 3 days of onset of the illness. However, recent data has prompted the manufacturer to remove septic shock as a possible indication for methylprednisolone.

Electrolyte abnormalities are seen frequently in TSS. Hyponatremia may be corrected with normal saline infusion; potassium replacement may also be needed. Hypocalcemia is treated with intravenous calcium chloride or calcium gluconate. Electrolytes should be monitored closely during the phase of fluid resuscitation.

Following stabilization of the patient and correction of electrolyte abnormalities, a careful examination of the patient is required. In all patients with variant toxic shock, a focus of infection can be found and requires prompt attention. Women with tampon-related toxic shock should have the tampon removed; some authors recommend irrigation of the vagina with saline or povodone-iodine solution. Cultures of all potentially infected sites should be obtained, including blood cultures, before antibiotic therapy is initiated.

Antibiotic selection should include an antistaphylococcal penicillin or first-generation cephalosporin with beta-lactamase stability. Nafcillin or oxacillin, 1 to 2 g every 4 hours, provides adequate antimicrobial coverage. Cefazolin, 2 g every 6 hours, also provides adequate coverage, but the first-generation cephalosporins are less beta-lactamase stable than the antistaphylococcal penicillins. Vancomycin, trimethoprim-sulfamethoxazole, or rifampin may be used if methicillin-resistant strains are encountered. Data on the optimum duration of antimicrobial therapy are not available. It seems prudent to administer parenteral antibiotics for at least 3 days or until the patient improves clinically. Oral antistaphylococcal antibiotics (cloxacillin or dicloxacillin) should then be administered for an additional 10 days. Although prospective studies are lacking, the addition of rifampin to the oral regimen is suggested because of the unique ability of this drug to eradicate the carrier state. The precise role of antibiotics in treating the acute infection remains unclear; indeed, patients have recovered without antibiotic therapy and following therapy with beta-lactamase sensitive antibiotics. However, treatment with appropriate antibiotics does decrease the risk of recurrent infections.

Future prospects in the treatment of TSS may include methods to remove or neutralize the toxin. Pooled gamma globulin has high antibody titers to enterotoxin F (1:1,000 to 1:16,000), whereas patients with TSS usually have titers less than 1:5. However, the use of gamma globulin in TSS awaits further studies. In addition, the prospect of developing a specific horse antitoxin, analogous to the neutralizing antitoxin for botulism toxin, type E, also needs to be evaluated.

SUGGESTED READING

Wager G. Toxic shock syndrome: A review. Am J Obstet Gynecol 1983; 146:93–102.
Waldvogel F. *Staphylococcus aureus* (including toxic shock syndrome). In: Mandell G, Douglas R, Bennett J. Principles and practice of infectious diseases. New York: John Wiley and Sons, 1985, 1097.
The toxic shock syndrome. Ann Int Med 1982; 96 (part 2):831–996. (41 articles).

INFECTION IN THE PARENTERAL DRUG USER

HENRY F. CHAMBERS, M.D.

FEVER IN THE PARENTERAL DRUG USER

Fever and infection bring the parenteral drug user to the emergency department. Two-thirds or more of such patients have a documented infection as the cause of fever. The emergency physician is faced with finding the cause of the fever and determining whether or not the patient should be admitted to the hospital.

Perhaps most challenging are those patients who have fever, but no obvious infection, even after careful and complete physical and laboratory evaluation. Uncommonly, fever may be the only sign of a serious infection, such as endocarditis. Outpatient follow-up visits after blood cultures have been obtained may be reasonable in some of these patients. If there is doubt about the severity of the illness or the benign nature of the fever, because follow-up examination is often unsatisfactory and infections are so common, the patient should be admitted to the hospital for observation.

In order to manage these patients properly and to anticipate the type of infection, a history of parenteral drug use must be diligently pursued. All teenagers and young adults, in particular, should be asked direct questions about parenteral drug use. Persistence may be required, because the drug user may hide the habit or claim ''I used to do it, but quit.'' Practically speaking, any history of past or present parenteral drug use (even if only ''once'') should be considered positive and lead one to consider the infections discussed below.

SKIN AND SOFT-TISSUE INFECTIONS

These are the most common infections in parenteral drug users. Infection probably results from direct inoculation of bacteria. Consequently, besides staphylococci and streptococci, a significant proportion of infections are caused by anaerobes, gram-negative aerobes, or multiple organisms.

Because the list of potential pathogens is virtually limitless, specimens should be obtained for aerobic and anaerobic culture whenever possible. Areas of fluctuance and induration should be aspirated for pus and incised and drained, if necessary. The patient should be completely examined for signs of infection at other sites. If fever, chills, or other signs of systemic or metastatic infection are present, blood cultures and other appropriate studies (e.g., chest film, urinalysis, and other cultures) should be obtained.

Patients with uncomplicated infections, such as a localized cellulitis or focal subcutaneous abscess, often do not have fever and can be treated as outpatients. Follow-up of drug users is notoriously poor. If successful outcome depends largely upon patient compliance or if the severity of the infection is in question, hospitalization is advisable.

Indications for hospitalization are fever, lymphangitis, possible involvement of joints, fascia, muscle, blood vessels, or tendons, or extensive areas of infected soft tissue. Complicated infections, such as necrotizing fasciitis, myositis, and gas gangrene, involve structures beyond the skin and can be rapidly progressive and life-threatening. Emergency surgical exploration is mandatory to define the extent of the infection and for debridement and amputation, as indicated. Classically, streptococci, staphylococci, or *Clostridium* species cause these infections, but in drug users other organisms (e.g., *Bacteriodes,* gram-negative aerobes) can produce an identical clinical picture. Initial antimicrobial coverage should be broad until sufficient information is available to indicate a specific pathogen.

For outpatient therapy, any of several antimicrobials is effective, provided they are active against staphylococci and streptococci (Table 1). If gram-negative organisms are present in Gram-stained pus, then an oral cephalosporin might be preferred initially.

Cefazolin is very effective as a single agent for parenteral therapy of uncomplicated skin and soft-tissue infections. Either cefoxitin alone or clindamycin (with an aminoglycoside if gram-negative aerobes are suspected) provides suitable coverage for suspected anaerobic or mixed infections.

Coverage for extensive, complicated infections should be broad until the causative organism(s) is identified. Aqueous penicillin G is the drug of choice for clostridial infections and should be added to the regimen whenever this is suspected. For the penicillin-allergic patient, clindamycin or cefoxitin provides satisfactory coverage.

TABLE 1 Empiric Therapy of Cutaneous, Soft-tissue, and Musculoskeletal Infections in Parenteral Drug Users

Infection		Empiric Therapy*
Localized, often uncomplicated		
Cellulitis	Oral:	Dicloxacillin, 500 mg PO q.i.d.
Subcutaneous abscess		Erythromycin, 500 mg PO q.i.d.
		Cephalexin, 500 mg PO q.i.d.
	Parenteral:	Cefazolin, 1,000 mg IV/IM q8h
		Cefoxitin, 1,500 mg IV q6h
		Clindamycin †, 900 mg IV q8h
Complicated**		
Arthritis	Parenteral:	Nafcillin, 1.5 g IV q4h
Gangrene		Cefoxitin, 2.0 g IV q6h
Myositis		Clindamycin, 900 mg IV q8h
Necrotizing fasciitis		*plus*
Osteomyelitis		Gentamicin, 1.5 mg/kg IV q8h
Pyomyositis		

* Listing is according to order of preference; doses based upon normal renal function.
** For suspected clostridial infection, add aqueous penicillin G 4 million U IV q4h.
† For penicillin-allergic patients; add aminoglycoside for suspected mixed infection with gram-negative aerobes.

MUSCULOSKELETAL INFECTIONS

Pyomyositis is a primary muscle infection usually caused by *Staphylococcus (S.) aureus* and occasionally by other organisms. This infection often manifests as a tender muscle mass, with little or no involvement of overlying skin. Multiple abscesses may be present and can result from hematogenous spread during septicemia. Patients suspected of having this infection should be admitted to the hospital. Therapy requires surgical drainage and an antistaphylococcal antibiotic.

Acute osteomyelitis may be a primary infection or a sign of endocarditis; bacteremia is common in either case. *S. aureus* causes most of these infections, although *Pseudomonas*, other gram-negative aerobes, mycobacteria, and fungi have also been isolated. Vertebral bones are most often infected, but any site (clavicle, sternum, shoulder, wrist) can be involved. Patients with these infections present with focal pain and tenderness and sometimes with a mass over the involved bone.

Patients with suspected osteomyelitis should be admitted to the hospital for treatment and for bone biopsy for culture and sensitivity testing. It is neither necessary nor appropriate to begin therapy before cultures are obtained. Empiric therapy initiated before cultures only leads to confusion about drug selection and duration of therapy, if these cultures turn out to be negative. If bone biopsy is delayed or if the patient appears septic or has signs of endocarditis, then antimicrobials can be administered once blood cultures have been sent to the laboratory.

Infectious arthritis usually affects the knee or hip, but like osteomyelitis, any site may be infected. Bacteremia or endocarditis or both are commonly present. Otherwise unusual sites commonly associated with endocarditis are the acromioclavicular joint or the sacroiliac joint.

S. aureus, streptococci, and aerobic gram-negative organisms are the common pathogens. Because sexual promiscuity and prostitution are common among drug users, gonococcal arthritis is likely if blood and joint cultures prove negative.

Patients with septic arthritis should be admitted to the hospital. It is rarely necessary to initiate therapy before blood cultures have been obtained and the infected joint aspirated for Gram staining, culture, and sensitivity testing. Unless the hip is infected, open drainage of the joint is not required provided reaccumulated fluid can be removed by percutaneous needle aspiration.

PLEUROPULMONARY INFECTIONS

Depressed levels of consciousness, impaired clearance of secretions, and aspiration of oropharyngeal or gastric contents while under the influence of drugs contribute to the predisposition of drug users to pneumonia (Table 2).Thus, pneumococcal or aspiration pneumonia accounts for most cases, which can be treated with penicillin.

However, pneumonia may be secondary to bacteremia from associated endocarditis or septic thrombophlebitis in up to one-half of cases. This is particularly likely if signs of cavitation, multiple nodules, abscess, or effu-

TABLE 2 Differential Diagnosis of Pneumonia in Parenteral Drug Users

Pneumococcal or other bacterial pneumonia

Aspiration (anaerobic) pneumonia or lung abscess*

Tricuspid valve endocarditis*

Septic thrombophlebitis*

Foreign body aspiration

Heroin-associated pulmonary edema

Tuberculosis*

AIDS- associated opportunistic infection
(e.g., pneumocystis, cytomegalovirus)

* Commonly associated with signs of cavitation on chest films.

sion are present on chest films. Therefore, all intravenous drug users with suspected pneumonia should also be admitted to the hospital for observation until blood cultures are negative for at least 72 hours. After three blood cultures have been obtained, empiric therapy of either nafcillin, 1.5 g every 4 hours, or vancomycin, 500 mg every 6 hours (for the penicillin-allergic patient), plus an aminoglycoside, 1.5 mg per kilogram every 8 hours, is recommended. These regimens provide suitable coverage for most pneumonias as well as the likely causes of endocarditis. In regions where *Pseudomonas* species are a common cause of endocarditis, an antipseudomonal beta-lactam antibiotic (such as ticarcillin) should be added.

ENDOCARDITIS

Endocarditis is present in 10 to 20 percent of intravenous drug users who have fever and no skin infection. Although *S. aureus*, streptococci, *Pseudomonas,* and enterococci account for 90 percent of cases, virtually any organism can be responsible. Thus, endocarditis must be suspected whenever blood cultures are positive in an intravenous drug user (particularly in the absence of a source of infection).

S. aureus causes half or more of the cases of endocarditis, although unexplained regional variations occur and other species may be common in some areas. Approximately three-quarters of the staphylococcal infections involve the tricuspid valve only. In these cases a murmur may not be heard or may appear innocent. The chest film will reveal an infiltrate or some other abnormality in three-quarters of the patients with tricuspid valve involvement. Chest pain, hemoptysis, cough, and dyspnea may point to tricuspid valve infection. However, in a small number of patients, there are no localizing signs of infection.

Congestive heart failure, focal neurologic deficits, meningismus, metastatic foci of infection, embolic phenomena, stigmata of endocarditis (Janeway's lesions, Osler's nodes, petechiae), and murmurs of aortic or mitral valve origin are indicative of left-sided endocarditis. Besides *S. aureus*, other organisms, namely enterococci and viridans streptococci, and in some cities, *Pseudomonas*, assume a greater importance in left-sided as compared with right-sided endocarditis.

All patients who are suspected of having endocarditis should be admitted to the hospital for observation. At least three blood cultures and cultures of other potentially infected sites (e.g., pleural fluid, cerebrospinal fluid, septic joint) should be obtained prior to starting therapy. If there is a history of recent antimicrobial administration that may render cultures negative, then therapy can be safely withheld for 24 to 48 hours, during which time several additional cultures may be taken and the patient observed and evaluated for other signs of endocarditis. In the absence of prior therapy, particularly if the illness is acute and there are signs of left-sided involvement, empiric therapy should be initiated promptly. Therapy with a semisynthetic penicillin (e.g., nafcillin) or vancomycin (for the penicillin-allergic patient) plus gentamicin, in the doses listed above, is recommended until culture results are available. In medical centers or cities where endocarditis caused by *Pseudomonas* or enterococci is known to occur, then ticarcillin or penicillin, respectively, should be included in the empiric regimen.

Left-sided endocarditis in the drug user can be a rapidly progressive and lethal disease. Complications should be sought and identified as soon as possible. Patients should be carefully evaluated for evidence of central nervous system involvement (meningitis, brain abscess, mycotic aneurysm and hemorrhage, septic emboli and stroke), significant valvular insufficiency, hemodynamic compromise (owing to heart failure, pericarditis, hypovolemia, or sepsis), and renal insufficiency. Subspecialty consultation is recommended if complications are suspected in order to proceed with the necessary emergency studies (e.g., computed tomographic brain scan, arteriogram, echocardiogram).

OTHER VASCULAR INFECTIONS

Septic thrombophlebitis is a surprisingly uncommon infection in drug users. Localized infection of a thrombosed vein often can be managed on an outpatient basis by surgical incision, drainage, and oral antistaphylococcal antibiotics. This approach is recommended only if the infection has not progressed centrally and if the vein is superficial. Indication of more extensive disease are involvement of deep veins, tenderness or erythema centrally, or fever. Patients with these findings should be hospitalized, treated with parenteral antibiotics, and considered for vein resection.

Septic thrombophlebitis may resemble pneumonia and may be indistinguishable from tricuspid valve endocarditis. The veins of patients with these infections should be examined for evidence of thrombophlebitis as the source of infection.

Arterial mycotic aneurysms may or may not be associated with endocarditis. An aneurysm can be an occult source of bacteremia that is erroneously attributed to endocarditis. This distinction is important because aneurysms can cause serious bleeding, exert mass effects, and usually require surgical excision plus antibiotics for cure.

Any artery can be infected, but peripheral locations are more common in drug users (probably as a result of direct damage to or infection of the arterial wall during injection) than in other patients with mycotic aneurysms. The findings are tenderness or a pulsatile mass over the course of an artery or both. Abdominal aneurysms manifest as a palpable mass, unexplained abdominal pain, or occult or gross blood in the stool. The diagnosis is made by arteriography. All patients suspected of this complication should be admitted to the hospital for evaluation.

NEUROLOGIC DISORDERS

Meningitis, stroke syndromes, and epidural abscesses are the most common infectious complications of the central nervous system in drug users (Table 3). These often occur as a complication of staphylococcal endocarditis. Epidural abscess, however, may be the only site of infection and the source of bacteremia.

When purulent meningitis accompanies endocarditis, *S. aureus* is usually the cause. This complication is relatively rare. More commonly the patient has "aseptic" meningitis or meningoencephalitis (i.e., headache, wild alterations in mental status, meningismus, nonfocal results of a neurologic examination, cerebrospinal fluid pleocytosis, and negative cerebrospinal fluid cultures), which occurs in up to 10 percent of cases of endocarditis. Aseptic meningitis is probably an inflammatory response to bacteremia and microemboli; it occurs more often in left-sided as compared to right-sided endocarditis and requires no special therapy.

In addition to staphylococcal meningitis in association with endocarditis, pneumococci and meningococci also cause meningitis in intravenous drug users. Therefore, initial coverage for suspected meningitis should in-

TABLE 3 Infectious Neurologic Complications in Parenteral Drug Users

Bacterial meningitis
Aseptic meningitis or meningoencephalitis
Brain abscess
Epidural abscess
Mycotic aneurysm
Cerebral or spinal cord emboli
Stroke
Tetanus
Botulism

clude a penicillinase-resistant penicillin (such as nafcillin in doses of 12 to 16 g per day) and aqueous penicillin G, 24 million units a day. For penicillin-allergic patients, vancomycin plus chloramphenicol may be used, although a third-generation cephalosporin possessing significant antistaphylococcal activity, such as cefotaxime, may also be used.

Aseptic meningitis may also result from more serious complications of mycotic aneurysm, brain abscess, or parameningeal or epidural abscess. Cerebrospinal fluid pleocytosis in association with focal neurologic dificits or altered mental status or both is an indication for neurologic consultation and further special studies, such as computed tomographic brain scan and arteriography.

Bloody or xanthochromic cerebrospinal fluid is a sign of subarachnoid hemorrhage from a mycotic aneurysm. A few red blood cells may be the only sign of a leaking mycotic aneurysm. Although computed tomographic brain scan may disclose intracranial blood, arteriography is required to localize the aneurysm. Neurosurgical consultation should be obtained at the first suggestion that a patient may be bleeding from a mycotic aneurysm.

Brain abscess complicates 1 percent or less of endocarditis cases or may occur as a focal infection. The diagnosis is established by the typical findings on computed tomographic brain scan. Brain abscesses in association with endocarditis characteristically are small and multiple, so that surgical drainage is not necessary. If blood cultures are negative or the abscess is large, then surgical aspiration or resection is recommended for diagnosis and treatment.

Strokes in drug users are a sign of embolization from underlying aortic or mitral valve endocarditis or occasionally of brain abscess or mycotic aneurysm. Rapidly injected intravenous cocaine also may cause extreme elevation of blood pressure and stroke. Patients who present with a stroke should be elevated promptly by a neurologist or neurosurgeon and should undergo the appropriate studies to define the cause.

Spinal epidural abscess should be suspected in patients who complain of localized back pain, who have point tenderness over the spine, or who have signs and symptoms of spinal cord (sensory level, hyper-reflexia, incontinence of urine or feces, motor deficits) or nerve root irritation. The spine may be infected at any location, but the lumbar spine is the most common site. Epidural abscess may be the only focus of infection or may occur as a complication of vertebral osteomyelitis or endocarditis. Blood cultures frequently are positive for *S. aureus*. Computed tomographic scan of the spine with metrizamide contrast or standard myelography is a useful test to define these lesions. Neurosurgical consultation should be obtained if this complication is suspected.

Tetanus and botulism are rare complications of parenteral drug use. Both result from a toxin produced by clostridial organisms in an infected wound, which may be inapparent. Both cause neurologic syndromes in the absence of fever. Patients suspected of either should be admitted to an intensive care unit because symptoms may progress rapidly and result in death.

Tetanus should be suspected in patients who have trismus, muscle stiffness, or spasms. Treatment is debridement of wounds as indicated, high-dose parenteral penicillin (to eradicate residual organisms), and 10,000 U of human tetanus immune globulin intramuscularly. Intrathecal administration of 250 U of human tetanus immune globulin may be more effective than intramuscular injection of the higher dose. Clinical tetanus is not an immunizing experience, so once the patient has recovered, a full course of active immunization with tetanus toxoid should be given.

Botulism is characterized by ocular nerve palsies (ptosis, diploplia, blurred vision, dilated and fixed pupils), dry mouth and difficulty swallowing, postural hypotension, nausea and vomiting, and descending paralysis. The diagnosis is confirmed by detection of botulin in serum. Treatment is high-dose parenteral penicillin, drainage and debridement of any suspicious wounds, and antitoxin administered as one vial intravenously and one intramuscularly and repeated in 4 hours if symptoms persist. The antitoxin is prepared from horse serum, so appropriate precautions must be taken to determine hypersensitivity, with desensitization measures if necessary.

HEPATITIS

Hepatitis A, hepatitis B, non-A, non-B hepatitis, delta-agent infection, and chronic active hepatitis are more common in drug users than in the general population. Acute infections are associated with fever, sometimes arthralgias, and coexisting or ensuing jaundice. Patients with acute hepatitis and fever need not be admitted to the hospital unless there are signs of a concurrent bacterial infection or liver failure. Serum for hepatitis A IgM and hepatitis B surface antigen should be obtained for diagnosis, and the health department notified of suspected cases. Baseline liver function studies are also recommended, and the patient should be referred for follow-up examination.

ACQUIRED IMMUNODEFICIENCY SYNDROME

Parenteral drug users are at risk for acquired immunodeficiency syndrome (AIDS). Although most cases have been reported from the New York metropolitan area and Florida, up to 10 percent of drug users from other locations are seropositive for the AIDS-related virus. Patients who present with chronic illnesses, oral candidiasis, pulmonary infiltrates on chest film, and fever, but none of the usual bacterial infections, should be suspected of AIDS and evaluated for the presence of associated opportunistic infections.

SUGGESTED READING

Cherubin CE. The medical sequelae of narcotic addiction. Ann Intern Med 1967; 67:23–33.
Hussey HH, Katz S. Infections resulting from narcotic addiction. Report of 102 cases. Am J Med 1950; 9:186–193.
Reisberg BE. Infective endocarditis in the narcotic addict. Prog Cardiovasc Dis 1979; 22:193–204.
Webb D, Thadepalli H. Skin and soft tissue polymicrobial infections from intravenous drug users. West J Med 1979; 130:200–204.

ACQUIRED IMMUNODEFICIENCY SYNDROME

PAUL A. VOLBERDING, M.D.

Acquired immunodeficiency syndrome (AIDS) is a part of the spectrum of medical disorders caused by infection with a newly discovered, and probably newly evolved, human retrovirus called the human immunodeficiency virus or HIV. This virus, (initially termed HTLV-III, LAV, or ARV by various investigators) infects a variety of cells in the body, especially the subgroup of T-lymphocytes known as T-helper cells. In addition to these cells, there is evidence that HIV can infect other cells in the immune system and cells in the brain. Cases of acquired AIDS are being reported to the Centers for Disease Control in ever increasing numbers. Reports have now originated from all 50 states and from an increasing number of foreign countries as well.

There is a wide spectrum of clinical problems associated with HIV infection. These can range from subclinical infection to overt AIDS. At all phases of the infection, individuals are at risk of transmitting the virus to unprotected sexual partners, through transmission of blood products and organs, and by sharing of contaminated needles in the use of intravenous drugs.

The epidemiology of AIDS in the United States is relatively well understood. As has been true since the beginning of the epidemic, AIDS is primarily affecting homosexual men. This risk group represents over 70 percent of all reported cases to date. The next most common group affected by HIV infection are users of intravenous drugs who share contaminated needles and syringes with others. This group represents approximately 17 percent of all reported cases of AIDS. Additional risk groups include hemophiliacs, people from parts of the world where HIV infection is endemic, recipients of contaminated units of blood and blood products, and sexual partners of all the foregoing risk groups. Additionally, and perhaps most tragically, HIV infection is common in children born to women with an established HIV infection. (The risks of AIDS from blood products is discussed in the specific chapters on those products).

The stability of the relative proportion of AIDS cases in these risk groups over the past 5 years is encouraging and suggests that HIV infection is not spreading rapidly to other segments of the population. On the other hand, there is growing evidence that intravenous drug users constitute an increasing pool of infected individuals and may represent a slow but sure bridge of the AIDS virus infection to the broader population groups. Also, the implications of the large heterosexual epidemic of HIV infection in Central Africa in regard to populations in other parts of the world are not understood at the present time.

As the number of cases continues to increase, more and more medical providers and facilities are encountering patients with HIV infection or those who are concerned about the possibility of this infection. In many cases, these patients are being seen and cared for in an outpatient setting, especially hospital emergency departments. This and the concern for optimum patient management and occupation risk reduction make it imperative that emergency physicians and other staff understand the current status of HIV infection, its clinical spectrum, and current thinking about the transmissibility of this potentially lethal virus.

DIAGNOSIS

Several large patient groups can be expected to be encountered in the outpatient and emergency department setting. These include individuals who are not members of high risk groups, nor sexual contacts of risk group members, whose fears of infection are almost certainly not warranted, members of risk groups whose fear of infection is serious and who may well be infected, those with minimal symptoms, and those with fully established AIDS. With each group it is important for the emergency department staff to have a management plan established. In this way patient management can be optimized and stress on medical staff reduced.

An important function of emergency department personnel is to include the possibility of HIV-induced disease in their differential diagnoses. Here it is essential that the *risk group membership* of a patient be explicitly addressed. At present, if an individual is not a member of one of the known AIDS risk groups and is not a sexual partner of a risk group member, HIV-induced disease need not be seriously considered. If, on the other hand, the patient is in a risk group for this infection, the history and physical examination should be performed to include possible HIV-induced clinical manifestations. These can be broadly divided into those that are diagnostic for AIDS and those that are less immediately life-threatening, broadly called the AIDS-related complex or ARC.

The diagnosis of ARC is often difficult because the definition of this symptom complex is inprecise. In general, ARC is diagnosed when an individual suffers chronic symptoms of moderate immunodeficiency. These may include chronic fever, weight loss, diarrhea, lymphadenopathy, fatigue, and many other symptoms. To make the diagnosis of ARC, one must first establish the risk group status of the patient. In the emergency department setting it is not essential to perform immunologic or HIV antibody testing; this may be required at a later point in the patient's management. However, it is essential to confidently identify those complications of ARC that can be treated in an outpatient setting. These include moderate persistent diarrhea, cutaneous bacterial infections, and oral candidiasis. The management of each of these and other mild ARC-related infections is not different from that used when these infections are seen in other settings. Hospitalization in this situation is not indicated, but the individual should be referred to a physician comfortable with patients infected with HIV and aware of the complexities of this illness.

It is critical for the emergency department physician to recognize patients with *frank AIDS*. Many of these patients have life-threatening opportunistic infections that require immediate hospitalization and invasive testing and initiation of systemic treatment with antibiotics. The most common of these infections (termed opportunistic infections because of their nonpathogenecity for normal individuals) are *Pneumocystis carinii* pneumonia, cryptococcal meningitis, and toxoplasma brain abscess. Each of these AIDS-related opportunistic infections is likely to be encountered by the physician in the emergency setting, and each requires immediate diagnosis and treatment. In none of these, however, is it essential that the specific diagnosis be made in the emergency setting. Rather, they should be included in a differential diagnosis in appropriate patients, who should then be admitted for further testing. Because of the serious nature of each of these infections, they will be addressed separately.

Pneumocystis carinii pneumonia is a diffuse parasitic process that only affects patients whose host defense systems are seriously damaged. Typically, patients present with symptoms of cough, fever, and dyspnea on exertion are found on chest x-ray examination to have a mild diffuse interstitial pneumonitis. The symptoms, however, can be subtle, and the chest x-ray findings in many cases can be within normal limits. Arterial blood gas levels often show hypoxemia, but again the levels may be normal in early cases. In most cases, further invasive diagnostic testing is required after hospitalization. Therapy with specific antibiotics need not be initiated in the outpatient setting, but rather should follow appropriate diagnostic testing. (See *Pulmonary Problems in AIDS Patients*).

Cryptococcal meningitis often presents with complaints of fevers and severe persistent headaches. Physical examination may show nuchal rigidity, but this physical finding should not be relied on in considering this diagnosis. Lumbar puncture can be performed safely in patients with cryptococcal meningitis, but the results are atypical when this infection occurs in the setting of AIDS; pleocytosis and elevated protein level are less commonly found in patients with AIDS than in other patients with cryptococcal meningitis. For this reason it is recommended that specific diagnostic testing and antibiotic therapy for cryptococcal meningitis be deferred until the patient is hospitalized and evaluated by an infectious disease specialist.

Toxoplasma brain abscess is the third most common life-threatening infection seen in patients with AIDS. Patients with *Toxoplasma* brain abscess often present with neurologic deficits, including generalized seizure disorders. The clinical suspicion of *Toxoplasma* brain abscess should be confirmed by computed tomography (CT) or magnetic resonance imaging (MRI). Lumbar puncture should be deferred until this imaging is performed. Lumbar puncture is generally not helpful for *Toxoplasma* infection. The specific diagnosis requires brain biopsy, but this is rarely performed as the infection responds rapidly to antibiotic therapy, which must be initiated in a hospital setting.

In addition to these opportunistic infections, many patients with AIDS present to the emergency department with skin lesions of Kaposi's sarcoma. These skin lesions may be found in any body site including, it should be stressed, the oral cavity. They initially appear as red to purple, small subcutaneous nodules ranging in size from several millimeters to 2 or more centimeters in diameter. They are generally nonpainful and nonpruritic at the time of presentation. If typical lesions are seen in a patient who is a member of an AIDS risk group, especially a homosexual man, the patient should be referred to an appropriate specialist for a skin biopsy. This need not be performed in the outpatient or emergency setting, but the patient should be informed of the serious nature of the possible diagnosis and the need for rapid confirmation.

The role of laboratory testing in the initial management of a patient with or suspected of having clinical illness related to HIV infection is controversial. Some easily obtained laboratory tests can be helpful in increasing the suspicion of an HIV-related clinical problem. If, for example, anemia, leukopenia, thrombocytopenia, or an elevated erythrocyte sedimentation rate are seen, the suspicion of an AIDS-related problem is strengthened. There is, however, very little role for additional specific laboratory testing. Testing for the degree of immune competence or testing for HIV antibodies is to be strongly discouraged. While each of these laboratory procedures has a potential role in further management of a diagnosed patient, they are not required in the emergency setting.

INPATIENT VERSUS OUTPATIENT MANAGEMENT

When a probable clinical diagnosis of ARC or AIDS has been made in the emergency department, the next essential question is to decide whether hospital admission is required or whether the patient can safely be managed without hospitalization. This question is, of course, difficult to answer in the abstract. Two groups of patients should clearly be admitted to the hospital. The first are the patients with a probable AIDS opportunistic infection already discussed, which requires immediate diagnosis and prompt initiation of therapy. These patients again, especially those with *Pneumocystis* pneumonia, cryptococcal meningitis, or *Toxoplasma* brain abscess, should be treated as true medical emergencies in almost all cases. They should be hospitalized under the care of their own physician or, if possible, with a physician familiar and comfortable with the diagnosis and management of AIDS-related problems. As discussed, in most of these cases complex diagnostic procedures should be performed after hospitalization rather than in the emergency department.

The second group of patients who should be treated as inpatients are those with AIDS or ARC who are clinically symptomatic and unable to care for themselves properly at home. For example, some with chronic diarrhea and cachexia may benefit from a brief hospitalization to reassess palliative control of their symptoms and their need for specialized at-home nursing care or confinement to a more chronic care facility. Usually the patient himself is able to help guide the physician as to the need for hospitalization in this stage of the illness. It is essential for the emergency physician, however, to make specific inquiries as to the patient's social support structures, as some patients deny the existence of even very obvious living difficulties.

COUNSELING PATIENTS, FAMILIES, AND FRIENDS

Patients in groups at high risk for AIDS are often extremely aware of many features of the disease and often, in fact, have seen friends or close acquaintances die from AIDS. Because of this, anxiety in these groups is often very high when clinical symptoms appear. This can even be true when these symptoms are clearly not, to the physician's mind, related to HIV infection. It is important for all health care providers, including emergency department staff, to recognize this high baseline anxiety and to deal with it appropriately. To do this, it is imperative for the staff members to understand some of the medical and social realities of AIDS in order to provide consistent rational responses to questions. It is also important to acknowledge the very real nature of the fears patients have and understand that they cannot be ignored. The same concerns extend equally to the family, friends, and lovers of the ill patient. For homosexual men, their close friends or lovers may well be much closer emotionally than family members and therefore should be accorded the same privileges in a hospital setting usually reserved for next of kin. At all times the patient's confidentiality should be the first concern, and the patient should be consulted before any discussion of the possible diagnosis of HIV-related disease.

OCCUPATIONAL RISK OF AIDS AND ITS REDUCTION

Despite the devastation that can follow HIV infection, the virus itself is quite fragile, and transmission of the virus from person-to-person is very difficult. An extensive body of information has now been collected regarding the risk of acquiring AIDS in the medical setting. These studies have clearly established that the risk to health personnel of acquiring AIDS is, in fact, negligible. In a study of more than 305 medical employees at the San Francisco General Hospital, there has not been a single case of antibody conversion to HIV, despite years of repeated viral exposure, including, in some cases, repeated injuries by contaminated needles. Similarly, the risk of acquiring an AIDS-related opportunistic infection is nonexistent for normal hosts. For these reasons it should never be permissible for healthy employees to refuse to care for potential AIDS cases out of fear of becoming ill themselves. It is wise, however, for certain guidelines published by the Centers for Disease Control to be reviewed and followed by all medical staff. The essential recommendations are that hand washing be performed before and after each patient contact, that gloves be worn when exposure to blood or body secretions is anticipated, and that protective eye gear be worn when blood splashes of mucous membranes are possible. Although the risk of transmission is very low, saliva is a body secretion, and thus mouth to mouth resuscitation should be avoided whenever possible in favor of bag-valve-mask or pocket-mask ventilation. The HIV is easily killed, and instruments and surfaces can be disinfected by 5 to 10 minute exposure to fresh 3 percent hydrogen peroxide, a fresh 1:10 dilution of common household bleach (sodium hypochloride), or 70 percent ethanol or isopropanol. Masks, either for the patient or the health care provider, are almost never required, and excessive isolation precautions should be avoided because they are unnecessary and decrease the quality of care and efficiency of care that an emergency department can provide.

SUGGESTED READING

CDC. Recommendations for preventing possible transmission of human T-lymphotropic virus type III/lymphadenopathy-associated virus from tears. MMWR 1985; 34:533–534.

CDC. Update prospective evaluation of healthcare workers exposed via the parenteral or mucous-membrane route to blood or body fluids from patients with AIDS—United States. MMWR 1985; 34:101–103.

CDC. Update evaluation of human T-lymphotropic virus type III/lymphadenopathy-associated virus infection in health-care personnel—United States. MMWR 1985; 34:575–578.

Hirsch MS, et al. Risk of nosocomial infection with human T-cell lymphotropic virus-III (HTLV-III). N Engl J Med 1985; 312:1–4.

Kovacs JA, et al. Cryptococcosis in the acquired immunodeficiency syndrome. Ann Intern Med 1985; 103:533–538

Luft BJ, Brooks RG, Conley F, McCabe RE, Remington JS. Toxoplasmic encephalitis in patients with acquired immunodeficiency syndrome. JAMA 1984; 252:913–917.

Macher AM. Infection in the acquired immunodeficiency syndrome. In: Fauci AS (moderator, NIH Conference). Acquired immunodeficiency syndrome: epidemiologic, clinical, immunologic, and therapeutic considerations. Ann Intern Med 1984; 100:92–106.

Resnick L, Veren K, Salahuddin SZ, Tondreau S, Markham PD. Stability and inactivation of HTLV-III/LAV under clinical and laboratory environments. JAMA 1986; 255:1887–1891.

Sande M. Transmission of AIDS. The case against casual contagion. N Engl J Med 1986; 314:380–382.

Volberding P. Kaposi's sarcoma. In: Ebbesen P, Biggar RJ, Melbye M, eds. AIDS: a basic guide for clinicians. Copenhagen: Munksgaard, 1984.

Ziegler JL, Abrams DI. The AIDS-related complex. In: De Vita V Jr, et al, eds. AIDS etiology, diagnosis, treatment, and prevention. Philadelphia: JB Lippincott, 1985: 223.

PROPHYLAXIS FOR TRAVELERS

HERBERT L. DuPONT, M.D.

Persons who cross international boundaries may be exposed to infectious diseases not commonly found in their homelands. The regions putting the traveler at greatest risk to develop infection are tropical countries of Latin America, Africa, and southern Asia. The risk indirectly reflects the level of endemicity of the various infectious diseases in the local population.

Gastrointestinal infections represent particularly important health hazards to the international traveler to high-risk areas. Diarrheal diseases occur in about 40 percent of travelers to the high-risk areas mentioned above. The agents responsible for this illness show some regional differences. For example, *Vibrio parahaemolyticus* is particularly important in Japan as is *Aeromonas hydrophila* in Thailand, and rotavirus appears to occur with increased frequency among travelers to Mexico. The most important causative agents in the well-studied areas (e.g., Mexico) are enterotoxigenic *Escherichia coli* (40 percent); *Shigella* (15 percent); *Salmonella* (4 to 7 percent); *Campylobacter* (3 percent); *Rotavirus* (5 to 10 percent); and *Giardia lamblia* (less than 2 percent). *E. coli* possessing special enteroadherence properties may be found in as many as 10 percent of the cases. The fact that bacterial agents are responsible for about 80 percent of the disease explains the remarkable effect of antimicrobial agents in preventing and treating traveler's diarrhea. Another viral enteric infection causing morbidity among travelers to rural areas of the developing world is viral hepatitis type A.

Preventive medicine is of particular importance for the international traveler to disease-endemic areas. Pretravel planning can reduce the likelihood of developing an infectious disease. Obviously, travelers would benefit by knowing something about the specific infections endemic to the areas to be visited. Infections for which specific or nonspecific preventive measures are available include dengue, malaria, filariasis, trypanosomiasis (African and South American), schistosomiasis, tapeworm, flukes, hepatitis A, measles, poliomyelitis and the diarrheal diseases. For dengue, malaria, and filariasis a key to prevention is mosquito control in the form of using repellents; remaining indoors at night, and using insect netting during sleep. For prevention of African trypanosomiasis during travels to east Africa and northern Botswana, persons should wear long sleeves and trousers, avoid wearing brightly colored clothing, and use mosquito nets. For South American trypanosomiasis, persons traveling to rural Central and South America should stay in well-constructed housing without wall cracks and general debris. If it is necessary to live in poorly constructed housing, the traveler should use residual insecticides and mosquito nets during sleep.

VACCINES

A number of vaccines are available for certain travelers. Yellow fever and cholera vaccines are required by law for a few areas of the world. Yellow fever vaccine is a live vaccine and is given every 10 years to visitors traveling to the endemic regions of South and Central America, central Africa, and certain countries of Asia. Cholera vaccine may be required for travel to India, Bangladesh, or Pakistan or their border countries. The commercially available killed and parenterally administered typhoid fever vaccine is only partially effective and is associated with bothersome reactions. It is recommended only for the unusual traveler who will be living in very poor conditions in highly underdeveloped areas for periods of time exceeding 3 weeks. Persons traveling to tropical regions of the developing world who have not yet received polio virus vaccine should receive a complete vaccination series. Previously unvaccinated adults and those with diseases that affect their general immunity should receive inactivated vaccine to prevent vaccine-associated paralysis as a result of receiving the live vaccine. Recommendations for immunization for preventing hepatitis A and measles are given in Table 1.

PHARMACEUTICAL PROPHYLAXIS

Chemoprophylaxis is used for preventing malaria for all travelers to endemic areas. For malaria-endemic areas in which chloroquine-resistant *Plasmodium falciparum* is not present, 500 mg (300 mg base) chloroquine is given once weekly beginning the week of travel and continuing for 4 to 6 weeks after returning home. Primaquine is given in a dose of 15 mg once daily for 14 days after returning home if *Plasmodium vivax* or *Plasmodium ovale* is present in the area visited. When traveling to areas where chloroquine-resistant *P. falciparum* strains are endemic, chloroquine is given weekly as above. In addition, for short-term travel (3 weeks or less), febrile illnesses that occur while traveling are treated empirically with 75 mg pyrimethamine plus 1,500 mg sulfadoxine (Fansidar) as a single oral dose. For longer-term travel, in addition to the chloroquine prophylaxis detailed above, 25 mg pyrimethamine and 500 mg sulfadoxine (Fansidar) is taken weekly during travel and is continued for 4 to 6 weeks after returning home. Because of the changing distribution of drug-resistant malaria, it is necessary to review up-to-date information for the specific country and region to be visited from local health authorities or the Centers for Disease Control in Atlanta.

In preventing diarrhea and other intestinal infections among travelers to high-risk areas, good principles of food selection are critical. Safe foods are identified in Table 1. Items to be avoided include foods remaining at room temperature (buffet style), raw shellfish, rare meats, hot sauces that are left out on the table, desserts, tap water, and milk. Chemoprophylaxis is appropriate for selected travelers. Bismuth subsalicylate (BSS) (Pepto-Bismol) prevents 65 percent of cases of illness when taken in a dose of 2 tablets four times a day (2.1 g per day), with meals

TABLE 1   Preventive Measures to Minimize Infections During Travels to High-Risk Areas

Infectious Disease	Region Where Endemic	Precaution or Preventive Measure
Dengue	Most tropical and some subtropical areas where *Aedes* mosquitoes are present	Mosquito control: repellents; remaining indoors at night; using insect netting during sleep
Malaria	Where *Anopheles* mosquitoes and malaria are present in Central and South America, central and south Africa, southern Middle East, Asia, South Pacific	Same as dengue plus chemoprophylaxis (see text)
Chloroquine-resistant *P. falciparum*	Southern, eastern, and central Africa, southern and southeastern Asia, and the South Pacific	Same as dengue plus chemoprophylaxis (see text)
Schistosomiasis	Africa and Arabia, Middle East, South America, Caribbean, Japan, China, Philippines	Avoid swimming or bathing in fresh or salt water, lakes, irrigation channels, and questionably chlorinated swimming pools
Hepatitis A	All countries of the developing world (Latin America, Africa, southern Asia)	2 ml gamma globulin
Measles	Same as hepatitis A	Those born after 1956 and those who have not received vaccine or had clinical disease should receive vaccine
Diarrhea	Same as hepatitis A	Appropriate food selections: all that are steaming hot, citrus, bread, bottled liquids; and prophylaxis for selected travelers: bismuth subsalicylate, or antimicrobial agents (see text)

and at bedtime, for periods of time no greater than 3 weeks. The drug should be continued for 2 days after returning home. Common side effects of BSS are blackening of stools and tongues and mild tinnitus.

Other salicylate-containing drugs should be avoided during BSS prophylaxis. Trimethoprim–sulfamethoxazole (TMP–SMZ) is probably more effective when used to prevent the illness (160 mg TMP and 800 mg SMZ once a day) while traveling in areas where prevalent bacterial enteric strains are susceptible. As in BSS prophylaxis, TMP–SMZ should be continued for 2 days after returning home. The side effects are probably more important than those associated with BSS, however. These include skin rashes (3 percent), development of antimicrobial-resistant gut flora, and rarely more serious side effects (e.g., Stevens-Johnson syndrome, antibiotic-associated colitis). Antimicrobial prophylaxis is reserved for persons in whom the risk of side effects is outweighed by the advantage of remaining free of illness. These persons must understand the hazards of taking an antimicrobial agent.

SUGGESTED READING

Centers for Disease Control. Health Information for International Travel. Atlanta, U.S. Public Health Service.

INFECTIOUS DISEASE IN IMMIGRANTS AND TRAVELERS

ELAINE C. JONG, M.D.

Immigrants, refugees, and returned travelers are likely to seek emergency medical care for fever, diarrhea, worms, or skin lesions.

In trying to formulate a differential diagnosis for each of these problems, the American practitioner has to add exotic infectious disease possibilities to standard considerations when the patient has been abroad.

The risk of infection with agents causing exotic infectious diseases is somewhat determined by the location, duration, and conditions of exposure in the foreign country. Immigrants and refugees are likely to have had a more intensive exposure to endemic diseases in a given geographic location than Western tourists. Similarly, Peace Corps volunteers, students, and missionaries are likely to have had a more significant exposure than tourists and business travelers.

This chapter identifies a few of the infectious disease entities that should be considered in the sick patient who has immigrated or has traveled abroad.

MALARIA

The diagnosis and treatment of malaria are discussed in detail in an earlier section (see chapter on *Malaria*). A few therapeutic considerations for dealing with malaria in immigrants and refugees follow.

Malaria usually manifests as a flu-like illness with fever and chills, sometimes accompanied by headache, muscle aches, gastrointestinal discomfort, and general malaise. Malaria attacks commonly occur weeks to months after a person has been infected in an endemic area, but occasionally the first clinical attack occurs years after the person was originally infected.

Malaria must be considered in order to make the diagnosis. A history of mosquito bites in an area known to be endemic for malaria is the best indication in a febrile patient for ordering a thick and thin smear evaluation of the blood for malarial parasites. A history of the patient's having taken medication to prevent malaria should not dissuade the physician from considering the diagnosis, since the patient may have a resistant form of malaria or may not remember his or her pill-taking habits accurately.

The documentation of cyclical fevers and chills is less useful diagnostically, because in first attacks of malaria the fever spikes are often irregular and in recurrent attacks in natives from endemic areas the illness may be perceived by the patient as a set of subjective symptoms, in a nonquantitive context. Language barriers may also add to the difficulty of eliciting an accurate temporal history.

Another problem in dealing with malaria occurring in natives or travelers from endemic areas is that the patient may have partially or completely treated himself or herself with left-over medications after self-diagnosis and may present after the acute signs and symptoms are subsiding. In any case, blood smears should be examined for evidence of malarial parasites during and at the conclusion of antimalarial therapy. If parasitemia or symptoms did not improve during or following initial antimalarial therapy, the adequacy of that therapy would have to be reconsidered. In patients who respond to initial therapy with complete clearing of the parasitemia, blood smears should be reexamined 3 to 4 weeks after therapy for a test of cure.

If the species of *Plasmodium* cannot be identified from the blood smear, and if the patient is from an area where chloroquine-resistant and/or Fansidar-resistant *P. falciparum* malaria is known to occur, it may be appropriate to treat the patient for the worst-case diagnosis, that is, with quinine sulfate and tetracycline if the clinical status warrants immediate therapy. Most patients can be treated as outpatients if they can be relied upon to return for follow-up examination or worsening symptoms. Patients who are unable to take oral medications or who show a severely toxic reaction on presentation need prompt antimalarial therapy and supportive measures in the hospital.

DIARRHEA

Diarrhea is a common problem among immigrants, refugees, and returned travelers (see chapter on *Adult Infectious Diarrhea*). In addition to patient exposure to infectious agents by ingestion of contaminated food and water in foreign countries, food eaten en route to or from foreign destinations may also cause problems.

Toxigenic strains of *Escherichia coli* are thought to be responsible for over half of cases of traveler's diarrhea, a self-limited watery diarrhea lasting for 3 to 5 days that may be accompanied by gas, fatigue, nausea, and cramps. A smaller percentage of travel-acquired infectious diarrheas are caused by the bacteria traditionally considered enteric pathogens. Table 1 presents a list of common bacterial pathogens associated with infectious diarrheas and the drugs of choice for treatment. Rotavirus is recognized as a causative agent of watery diarrhea in some parts of the world, and in 10 to 35 percent of traveler's diarrheas, no pathogen is identified.

Patients usually seek emergency care when diarrhea and symptoms have persisted for a week or more, and thus work-up studies are directed toward identification of specific pathogens.

Clinical predictors of positive stool cultures include duration of diarrhea more than 24 hours, fever of higher than or equal to 37.8 ° C, blood in the stool, nausea or vomiting, abdominal pain, and a history of foreign travel within 60 days of the examination.

A general approach to the diagnosis of travel-associated or imported diarrhea follows:

1. Determine if blood is present in the stool.
2. Determine the presence or absence of fecal leukocytes.
3. Culture the stool for *Salmonella, Shigella,* and *Campylobacter*, up to two specimens cultured per episode of illness.
4. Ova and parasite examination of up to three stool specimens collected on 3 separate days, looking specifically for protozoan parasites such as *Giardia lamblia, Entamoeba histolytica,* and *Dientamoeba fragilis*.
5. Culture the stool for *Yersinia enterolitica* if fever, lymphadenopathy, or right lower quadrant pain is present.
6. Process the stool for culture of *Clostridium difficile* and detection of toxin if the patient has been on antimicrobials prior to the present occurrence of diarrhea.
7. Culture the stool for *Vibrio parahaemolyticus* and *Vibrio vulnificus* if a history of eating raw or undercooked seafood is obtained.
8. Request a *Cryptosporidium* stain if profuse watery diarrhea persists for longer than 5 to 7 days, and the routine ova and parasite examinations of the stool have been negative.
9. Do a "string test" if upper gastrointestinal symptoms are present, routine ova and parasite examinations are negative, and *Giardia* or *Strongyloides* is suspected. The string test is commercially available as the Enterotest (Hedeco Corp., California).
10. Consider sigmoidoscopy in the case of diarrhea with blood or fecal leukocytes or both present in the stool, and if the initial round of stool cultures and ova and parasite examinations was negative. Abnormal areas of intestinal mucosa should be swabbed and biopsied, and specimens examined as wet mounts and as histologic preparations. This is often the only way to make the diagnosis of amebiasis *(Entamoeba histolytica)*, or schistosomiasis *(Schistosoma mansoni* or *S. japonicum)* or to confirm the diagnosis of pseudomembranous enterocolitis caused by *C. difficile*.

TABLE 1 Common Bacterial Pathogens Causing Acute Diarrhea

Pathogen	Drug	Dosage For Adults	Dosage For Children
Enterotoxigenic *E. coli*	Bismuth subsalicylate (Pepto Bismol)	30 ml PO every 30 minutes for 8 doses	Not recommended (No specific treatment) (Oral rehydration important)
Shigella sp.	Trimethoprim-sulfamethoxazole (Bactrim, Septra)	160 mg + 800 mg PO every 12 hours for 3 to 5 days	10 mg + 50 mg/kg/day in 2 divided doses for 3 to 5 days
	or		
	Tetracycline	2.5 g PO in a single dose	Not recommended
	or		
	Ampicillin	0.5–1.0 g PO or 0.5–3.0 g IV every 6 hours for 5 days	100 mg/kg/day PO or IV in 4 divided doses for 5 days
	or		
	Nalidixic acid	0.5–0.75 g PO every 6 hours for 5 days	55 mg/kg/day PO in 4 divided doses for 5 days
Salmonella sp.	(Treat only severely toxic or life-threatening situations; no treatment recommended for routine gastroenteritis.)		
	Ampicillin	0.5–1.0 g PO or 0.5–3.0 g IV every 6 hours for 5 days	100 kg/day PO or IV in 4 divided doses for 5 days
	or		
	Chloramphenicol	0.5–1.0 g PO or IV every 6 hours for 5 days	50 mg/kg/day PO or IV in 4 divided doses for 5 days
Campylobacter	Erythromycin	500 mg PO every 6 hours for 5 days	50 mg/kg/day PO or IV in 4 divided doses for 5 days
	or		
	Tetracycline	500 mg PO every 6 hours for 5 days	Not recommended
Vibrio sp.	Tetracycline	500 mg PO every 6 hours for 5 days	Not recommended (Oral rehydration of greatest importance)
	or		
	Doxycycline	100 mg PO every 12 hours for 5 days	Not recommended
Clostridium difficile	Vancomycin	125 mg PO every 6 hours for 7–10 days	12.5 mg/kg/day PO in 4 divided doses for 5 days

Therapy is directed toward the specific pathogen when one is identified (Table 1). Often, however, the patient desires treatment prior to identification of specific pathogens or he or she may not be able to afford a full diagnostic work-up.

Broad-spectrum antimicrobials such as trimethoprim-sulfamethoxazole (Bactrim or Septra) or a tetracycline in therapeutic doses may be efficacious for presumptive therapy of traveler's diarrhea. Although identification of specific pathogens is ideal, a course of presumptive therapy with one of these antimicrobials may allow the patient a faster return to a comfortable status when no pathogen can be identified.

If the diarrhea is caused by a protozoan rather than a bacterial agent, the patient is likely to have a more prolonged course of diarrhea that is unresponsive to antibacterials. Unfortunately, diagnosis of protozoan pathogens in the stool is relatively time-consuming and expensive and may be missed under the best of circumstances. In addition, the commonly used antiprotozoan drugs, metronidazole (Flagyl), quinacrine (Atabrine), furazolidone (Furoxone), iodoquinol (Yodoxin), and tinidazole (Fasigyn) may cause unpleasant symptoms and have potentially serious adverse side effects, so that most physicians have a justifiable reluctance to use these drugs for presumptive therapy. Table 2 gives a list of common protozoan intestinal pathogens and drugs of choice.

WORMS

Passage of grossly visible worms is a common occurrence in rural populations all over the world, but is less commonly seen in the urban United States except among immigrants, refugees, and returned travelers. The worms are passed per rectum by themselves or with bowel movements. On rare occasions, roundworms are vomited up from the stomach.

In general, the presence of symptoms from intestinal worms is proportional to the worm burden or numbers of worms present within the body. Patients with light to moderate infections may be entirely asymptomatic or may have vague gastrointestinal discomfort. Heavy infections may predispose individuals, especially children, to complications such as intestinal obstruction, rectal prolapse, or ectopic migration of worms outside the intestinal lumen. Perforation or obstruction of a viscus may result from migrating *Ascaris lumbricoides*.

TABLE 2 Common Protozoan Intestinal Pathogens

Pathogen	Drug	Dosage for Adults	Dosage for Children
Giardia lamblia	Metronidazole*	500 mg PO 3 times a day for 7 to 10 days	15 mg/kg/day PO in 3 divided doses for 7 to 10 days
	or		
	Quinacrine	100 mg PO 3 times a day for 5 days	6–7 mg/kg/day PO in 3 divided doses for 5 days
	or		
	Furazolidone	100 mg PO 4 times a day for 7 to 10 days	5 mg/kg/day PO in 4 divided doses for 7 to 10 days
	Tinidazole†*	2.0 g PO as a single dose	
	or		
Entamoeba histolytica	Iodoquinol (for asymptomatic cyst passers)	650 mg PO 3 times a day for 20 days	30–40 mg/kg/day PO in 3 divided doses for 20 days
	plus		
	Metronidazole (for symptomatic intestinal disease or hepatic abscess)	750 mg PO 3 times a day for 5 to 10 days	35–50 mg/kg/day PO in 3 divided doses for 5 to 10 days
	or		
	Tinidazole*†	2.0 g PO as a single dose for 3 to 5 days	
Dientamoeba fragilis	Iodoquinol	650 mg PO 3 times a day for 20 days	30–40 mg/kg/day PO in 3 divided doses for 20 days
Balantidium coli	Tetracycline	500 mg PO 4 times a day for 10 days	10 mg/kg PO 4 times a day for 10 days (not recommended for children under 8 years)
Isospora belli	Trimethoprim-sulfamethoxazole*	160 mg + 800 mg PO 4 times a day for 10 days; then 2 times a day for 3 weeks	
Cryptosporidium	No specific drug has been found effective		

* Considered an investigational drug for this use by the FDA.
† Not available for purchase in the United States.

Table 3 lists common intestinal helminths or worms and the therapeutic drugs of choice. Most worms are acquired through the ingestion of microscopic parasite eggs in contaminated food or water. Two exceptions are hookworm and *Strongyloides*. Hookworm eggs hatch in the soil, and the larvae penetrate the skin during ground contact (usually through bare feet). *Strongyloides* eggs may hatch in the fecal stream of the host, releasing larvae that reach the infective stage by the time they are ready to exit from the body per rectum. The *Strongyloides* larvae then penetrate the skin in the perirectal area, buttocks, or upper thighs, causing an itchy rash and initiating a new cycle of infection. *Strongyloides* may thus increase the originally acquired worm burden through autoinfection. This parasite also has free-living stages in which larval stages passed in the feces survive in the environment and infect other hosts.

Common intestinal helminths take 4 to 6 weeks after infection by eggs or larvae to reach maturity and begin egg-laying. As mentioned earlier, most worm infections are asymptomatic, and thus newly acquired infections can be missed in diarrhea work-ups done shortly after patients arrive in the United States, despite the fact that three stool examinations for ova and parasites are performed in a reliable laboratory. In occasional patients, worm infections can be associated with chronic diarrhea.

The diagnosis of intestinal helminths can be made in the following ways:

1. Identification of gross parasite specimens (usually the case in *Ascaris [roundworm] or Taenia* [tapeworm] infections).
2. Identification of characteristic ova (eggs) or larval forms in stool specimens.
3. Identification of *Strongyloides* larvae from proximal jejunal aspirates or biopsies.
4. Serum antibody titers of greater than or equal to 1:128 against *Strongyloides*. This test is obtained through the State Health Department and will be performed upon request if the patient has a peripheral eosinophilia and three negative stool examinations for ova and parasites.
5. Identification of characteristic ova on a Scotch Tape test for *Enterobius* (pinworm) infections. (A piece of cellophane tape is pressed sticky side down onto the perianal skin folds and then is pressed sticky side down onto a clean glass microscope slide. The refractile eggs are visible at a magnification of 40× power. The specimen is best obtained first thing in the morning before a bowel movement.

Most patients with worm infections can be managed as outpatients after prescription of the appropriate oral

TABLE 3 Common Intestinal Helminths

Pathogen	Drug	Dosage for Adults (Children†)
Roundworms:		
Ascaris lumbricoides, Trichuris trichiura, Hookworm *Necator* and *Ancylostoma*	Mebendazole	100 mg PO 2 times a day for 3 days
Enterobius vermicularis	Mebendazole	100 mg PO; repeat dose in 14 days
Strongyloides stercoralis	Thiabendazole	25 mg/kg/day PO 2 times a day for 2 days (maximum dose is 3 g per day)
Tapeworms:		
Taenia saginata, T. solium, Diphyllobothrium latum, Dipylidium caninum	Niclosamide	A single dose of 2 g (4 tablets) chewed thoroughly‡
Hymenolepis nana	Niclosamide or Praziquantel*	A single dose of 2 g (4 tablets) chewed thoroughly for 7 days§ 25 mg/kg PO for a single dose
Flukes:		
Schistosoma haematobium, S. mansoni	Praziquantel	40 mg/kg PO for a single dose
Schistosoma japonicum, S. mekongi	Praziquantel	20 mg/kg PO for a total of 3 times in one day
Clonorchis/Opisthorchis, Fasciola, Fasciolopsis,Heterophyes, Metagonimus	Praziquantel*	25 mg/kg PO for a total of 3 times in one day
Paragonimus sp.	Praziquantel*	25 mg/kg PO 3 times a day for 2 days

* Considered an investigational drug for this use by the FDA.
† Doses given are appropriate for patients 2 years of age or older, unless otherwise indicated.
‡ Niclosamide pediatric dose: 11–34 kg: a single dose of 2 tablets (1 g); >34 kg: a single dose of 3 tablets (1.5 g)
§ The appropriate pediatric dose of niclosamide is taken daily for 5 days.

drug (see Table 3). Patients with *Ascaris* or *Taenia* infections need to be advised that grossly visible worm specimens may be passed in bowel movements for several days following medication and represent worms that are dead or dying. Occasionally, patients presenting with acute obstruction of a viscus (for example, acute bilary tract obstruction by ectopic *Ascaris* or by *Clonorchis-Opisthorchis*) need surgical intervention for definitive diagnosis and management. Acute bowel obstruction in children with heavy worm burdens of *Ascaris* may also require surgical management.

SKIN LESIONS

In addition to skin lesions such as superficial fungal infections, ectoparasites, and leprosy, which are discussed in chapters on *Fungal Infections of Skin* and *Ectoparasites*, patients who have originated or traveled abroad may present in emergency facilities with unusual skin lesions. Cutaneous myiasis and cutaneous larva migrans are two parasitic conditions that should be considered.

Cutaneous myiasis occurs when fly larvae burrow into the subcutaneous tissues and cause pustular lesions, ranging from pimple-sized to furuncle-sized, depending on the species.

The lesions are unsightly but rarely painful. Fly larvae penetrate the skin during bites with mosquitos or other biting insects previously innoculated during flight with eggs by flies (botflies) or from fly eggs laid on clothing worn next to the skin (tumbu flies) in tropical areas. After the eggs hatch, the newly released larvae burrow under the surface of the skin. Close inspection, preferably with a handlens, shows each papule to have a small central opening with some bristles or dark material or both visible through the hole. Removal of the larvae is best accomplished by occlusion of the air hole with Vaseline, occlusive tape, or even clear nail lacquer for several days. After death of the larvae, the remains are manually expressed. Large larvae may need to be delivered from their subcutaneous site through enlargement of the central air hole to a slit by surgical incision. Diagnosis is confirmed by identification of the larvae. The most serious complication of cutaneous myiasis is secondary bacterial infection, which must be diagnosed and treated appropriately.

Cutaneous larva migrans is a striking serpiginous, erythematous, and pruritic linear lesion that appears to advance a few millimeters each day. The lesion is commonly caused by a larva of dog hookworm, *Ancylostoma canis*. The parasite larva penetrates human skin and wanders around subcutaneously, for days to weeks, leaving a distinctive lesion following its path. Patients acquire this infestation by skin contact with wet sandy soil (such as at beaches) that is contaminated by dog excrement.

Diagnosis is best made by recognition of the peculiar lesion and eliciting an appropriate history of exposure. Biopsy of the advancing front of the lesion is rarely useful, since the actual larva is always in advance of the body's visible inflammatory reaction to its passage, and its route is unpredictable.

Treatment consists of thiabendazole (Mintezol), 25 mg per kilogram twice a day for 2 days. Symptomatic treatment with antihistamines may help to lessen the troublesome pruritus.

SUGGESTED READING

Barrett-Connor E. Latent and chronic infections imported from Southeast Asia. JAMA 1978; 239:1901–1906.
Blumenthal DS, Schultz MG. Incidence of intestinal obstruction in children infected with *Ascaris lumbricoides*. Am J Trop Med Hyg 1975; 24:801.

Cline BL. Current drug regimens for the treatment of intestinal helminth infections. Med Clin North Am 1982; 66:721–742.

Gorbach SL, Hoskins DW. Travelers' diarrhea. DM 1980; 27:1–44.

Jokipii L, Jokipii AMM. Single-dose metronidazole and tinidazole as therapy for giardiasis: success rates, side effects, and drug absorption and elimination. J Infect Dis 1979; 140:984–988.

Koplan JP, Fineberg HV, Ferraro MJB, et al. Value of stool cultures. Lancet 1980; 2:413–415.

Leksomboon U, Echeverria P, Suvongse C, et al. Viruses and bacteria in pediatric diarrhea in Thailand: a study of multiple antibiotic-resistant enteric pathogens. Am J Trop Med Hyg 1981; 30:1281–1290.

Ross TF. Health care problems of Southeast Asian refugees—Medical Staff Conferences, University of California, San Francisco. West J Med 1982; 136:35–43.

Welch JS, Powell BJ, Freeman C. Treatment of intestinal amoebiasis and giardiasis, efficacy of metronidazole and tinidazole compared. Med J Aust 1978; 1:469–471.

Wolfe MS. The treatment of intestinal protozoan infections. Med Clin North Am 1982; 66:707–720.

Wyler DJ. Malaria—resurgence, resistance, and research, Part I. N Engl J Med 1983; 308:875–879.

Wyler DJ. Malaria—resurgence, resistance, and research, Part II. N Engl J Med 1983; 308:934–940.

LYMPHADENOPATHY AND MALAISE

CHARLES E. HESS, M.D.

Few patients who present with lymphadenopathy and malaise require therapeutic intervention on an emergency basis. In many cases, no specific treatment is indicated if a diagnosis either is firmly established or is felt to be probable based on clinical and laboratory findings. As a result, the diagnostic approach is of utmost importance. Table 1 lists important diagnostic considerations that, if evaluated sequentially, should result in the prompt establishment of a diagnosis in the majority of patients with a minimal expenditure of resources.

As with any clinical manifestation, the *age of the patient* is diagnostically important. Lymphadenopathy, usually accompanied by malaise, fever, and skin rash, is a common occurrence in many viral illnesses in children

TABLE 1 Lymphadenopathy and Malaise: Diagnostic Considerations

Patient's age

Clinical history
  Mode of onset
  Nature of associated symptoms
  Drug exposure (e.g., Dilantin)
  Animal exposure
  Occupation

Physical examination
  Lymph node consistency
    Non-neoplastic: fat, relatively soft
    Neoplastic: round or irregular, hard
    Infections: tender, red, painful, hot, may be fluctuant
  Localized or generalized
  Presence or absence of hepatosplenomegaly, skin rash, or lesion in area of drainage of the enlarged lymph node or nodes

Laboratory studies
  CBC and careful inspection of a peripheral smear
  Monospot test

(e.g., measles). The lymphadenopathy may be generalized, but more frequently it is confined to the posterior and anterior cervical and posterior auricular areas. If a specific viral etiology is suspected from the clinical history (e.g., exposure to others with documented viral illnesses), follow-up care is all that is necessary. In young adults, malaise and lymphadenopathy are cardinal clinical manifestations of infectious mononucleosis and other mononucleosis-like syndromes (cytomegalovirus infection and toxoplasmosis). Again, the lymphadenopathy may be generalized, but is most often confined to lymph nodes in the neck. In the case of toxoplasmosis, it is frequently seen only in the posterior cervical lymph nodes. The diagnosis can be confirmed in the majority of cases by demonstrating a positive Monospot test. A careful examination of a peripheral blood smear for the presence of atypical lymphocytes is a simple, inexpensive, and valuable study to obtain in any patient suspected of having infectious mononucleosis or any viral illness. If such lymphocytes are present in significant numbers, even if a specific diagnosis cannot be made, the patient should be followed to determine if the course of the illness is self-limited.

From the clinical history there are several important considerations that often suggest a specific underlying etiology (see Table 1). In general, the infectious causes are of rather sudden onset, have a relatively rapid and progressive course, and in most instances resolve without specific treatment. In contrast, lymphadenopathy caused by malignant neoplasms often is characterized by a more indolent and not infrequently relatively asymptomatic course.

Certain *drugs* can produce lymphadenopathy and a serum sickness-type reaction. Dilantin is by far the most common one, but other drugs have been implicated. In any patient with unexplained lymphadenopathy and serum sickness-like symptoms, drugs should be considered as a possible cause and any that the patient is currently receiving should be discontinued before proceeding with expensive work-up studies. The lymphadenopathy usually subsides over a period of 1 to 3 weeks after discontinuance of the drug. A complete resolution of the lymphadenopathy should be documented, since an increased incidence of malignant lymphoma has been reported in patients who have developed lymphadenopathy while taking Dilantin.

A history of *animal exposure* also is an important factor. In most instances the lymphadenopathy is localized and associated with a demonstrable lesion at the entry site of the causative agent (e.g., ulceroglandular syndrome). In many cases, however, the entry site has healed by the time the lymphadenopathy occurs. The most common ulceroglandular syndromes seen in the United States are listed in Table 2.

Cat-scratch fever is by far the most common ulceroglandular syndrome. Some patients give a history of being scratched by a cat, usually a young healthy cat, but many do not recall a specific injury. A lymph node biopsy frequently is indicated to rule out other causes. Special stains to demonstrate a recently described pleomorphic gram-negative bacillus should be attempted if a lymph node is biopsied. Follow-up examination to document resolution is all that is indicated.

Rat-bite fever also is not an uncommon cause of the ulceroglandular syndrome, particularly in laboratory workers. Other ulceroglandular syndromes should be considered, depending on the specific nature of the exposure. In most instances the diagnosis can be made from serologic studies or cultures. Needle aspirations of lymph nodes for culture and cytologic study may be indicated. In some of these syndromes (e.g., tularemia, bubonic plague, and most of the rickettsial diseases), other clinical and laboratory manifestations (e.g., fever, pneumonia, skin rash) point to the systemic nature of the disorder. Specific treatment depends on the cause.

Toxoplasmosis is probably the most common infection transmitted through animal exposure. In most instances the infection occurs early in life and is not recognized as such. There are three recognized clinical syndromes: (1) lymphadenopathy that is frequently asymptomatic but that may be associated with malaise; (2) an infectious mononucleosis-like illness; and (3) reactivation infection (e.g., brain abscess) in immunocompromised hosts. Lymph node biopsy usually reveals characteristic (some feel diagnostic) histopathologic features. Pre- and convalescent serologic reactions should be obtained to confirm the diagnosis. Specific antimicrobial therapy usually is indicated only for reactivation infection in immunocompromised hosts.

A patient's *occupation* is often a helpful clue. Manual laborers frequently have easily palpable lymph nodes in the epitrochlear, axillary, femoral, and inguinal areas. If these lymph nodes are only moderately enlarged (1 to 1.5 cm in diameter) and not firm, they are frequently the result of recurrent trauma and are of no significance. Hilar and mediastinal lymphadenopathy also may be occupation-associated (pneumoconioses). The diagnosis, however, should be established in most patients by histopathologic examination of lung or lymph node tissue.

On the *physical examination*, there are several important factors (see Table 1). Non-neoplastic lymph nodes are often enlarged, flat, and relatively soft. Neoplastic lymph nodes usually are enlarged, irregular, and firm. Enlarged lymph nodes caused by infection demonstrate a variable degree of hardness, tenderness, redness, heat, and pain; they may also be fluctuant. Aspiration of fluctuant lymph nodes for culture and cytologic examination often is indicated and is diagnostically productive.

The presence of hepatosplenomegaly indicates a systemic process and frequently it is caused by a viral infection such as infectious mononucleosis or a malignant process (malignant lymphoma, chronic lymphocytic leukemia). The presence of a skin rash usually indicates either an allergic reaction or a systemic viral or rickettsial illness. The distribution and character of the rash are diagnostically important.

The anatomic location of isolated lymphadenopathy has diagnostic significance (Table 3). It should be emphasized, however, that other conditions can involve any of these areas. The reason that certain conditions involve

TABLE 2   The Ulceroglandular Syndromes

Syndrome	Vectors	Causative Agents
Cat-scratch disease	Cat	Gram-negative pleomorphic bacillus
Rat-bite fever	Rat	*Spirillum minus*
Tularemia	Several animals (e.g., rabbits, squirrels)	*Francisella tularensis*
Anthrax	Cattle, sheep	*Bacillus anthracis*
Erysipeloid	Several animals	*Erysipelothrix rhusiopathiae*
Bubonic plague	Rodents or rodent fleas	*Yersinia pestis*
Erythema chronicum migrans	Ticks	Unknown
Rickettsial diseases	Dog and rodent ticks and mites	Several
Orf	Lambs	Poxvirus

TABLE 3 Lymphadenopathy and Malaise: Diagnostic Significance of Anatomic Location of the Lymphadenopathy

Occipital—inflammatory scalp conditions
Posterior auricular—rubella
Anterior auricular—inflammatory eyelid and conjunctival conditions
Posterior cervical—toxoplasmosis
Anterior cervical—upper respiratory and oral cavity inflammatory conditions, mucocutaneous lymph node syndrome
Submental and submaxillary—oral cavity infections and neoplasms, sinus histiocytosis
Supraclavicular—malignant neoplasms, sarcoidosis
Axillary and epitrochlear—ulceroglandular syndromes, dermatopathic lymphadenopathy
Mediastinal—thymomas, malignant neoplasms, Castleman's disease
Hilar—sarcoidosis (bilateral), malignant neoplasms, pneumoconioses, pulmonary infections
Intra-abdominal—malignant neoplasms, nonspecific mesenteric adenitis
Inguinal and femoral—venereal diseases, dermatopathic lymphadenopathy

specific areas often relates to the entry site of the causative agent, but in some instances (e.g., posterior cervical lymphadenopathy in toxoplasmosis), the exact reason is not known.

A careful head and neck examination should be performed in any patient with unexplained lymphadenopathy involving any lymph node region in the neck. Supraclavicular lymphadenopathy almost always portends a serious underlying disease process, usually a malignant neoplasm, and warrants aspiration or biopsy in essentially every instance. In addition to a careful inspection of the upper extremities, a thorough examination of the breasts, including mammography, is recommended in any female patient with significant axillary lymphadenopathy.

In general, the etiology of mediastinal or hilar lymphadenopathy should be confirmed by needle aspiration or biopsy. However, in the diagnosis of *sarcoidosis*, many clinicians would accept the findings of bilateral hilar lymphadenopathy, with or without pulmonary infiltrates, with or without other characteristic clinical manifestations of the disease (e.g., erythema nodosum, uveitis, and polyarteritis), and with or without some of the characteristic laboratory signs (e.g., polyclonal gammopathy, hypercalciuria, hypercalcemia, and an elevated serum angiotensin-converting enzyme level) as confirmatory without obtaining histopathologic confirmation. If histopathologic confirmation is not obtained, very close follow-up examination is necessary to document the resolution of the symptoms and the lymphadenopathy, which occurs over a period of months to years in the majority of patients. Histopathologic confirmation should be obtained in all patients with atypical presentations. It is the author's opinion that histopathologic confirmation should be obtained in all patients. The choice of biopsy sites includes bronchial or transbronchial lung biopsy, minor salivary gland biopsy, percutaneous liver biopsy, a prescalene fat pad biopsy, or mediastinoscopy with biopsy, depending on the expertise available.

Specific treatment of sarcoidosis is not indicated in a majority of patients. Corticosteroids are indicated in patients with progressive pulmonary symptoms and with certain other extranodal involvement (e.g., uveitis, central nervous system, and cardiac involvement). Symptomatic relief and resolution of lymphadenopathy are usually dramatic, but evidence that corticosteroid therapy prevents progressive pulmonary fibrosis, which only occurs in a small percentage of patients, is lacking.

Techniques such as ultrasonography, lymphography, and computed tomographic (CT) scanning have revolutionized the ability to detect intra-abdominal lymphadenopathy. Malignant neoplasms are, by far, the most frequent causes. Needle aspiration under CT guidance should be the initial diagnostic test. If a positive diagnosis is not obtained, or if diagnosis cannot be established from a biopsy of a suspected primary lesion, laparotomy is indicated.

A thorough examination of the genitalia, perineum, and lower extremities should be conducted in patients with inguinal or femoral lymphadenopathy. Veneral diseases probably are the most common causes, and the causative agent usually can be identified with appropriate stains and cultures of the primary lesions.

Generalized lymphadenopathy is defined as involvement of two or more noncontiguous lymph node regions. Table 4 lists the most common causes of generalized lymphadenopathy. Autoimmune disorders such as rheumatoid arthritis and systemic lupus erythematosus often are not considered as causes of generalized lymphadenopathy. Biopsy is not indicated if appropriate serologic tests are positive (e.g., rheumatoid factor, antinuclear antibodies), unless other manifestations suggest the presence of another underlying disease process, or unless the lymphadenopathy progresses. Dermatopathic lymphadenopathy is most often the result of recurrent trauma in manual laborers, but the most dramatic cases are seen in patients with chronic skin conditions such as exfoliative dermatitis and mycosis fungoides.

Patients with the pre-acquired immune deficiency syndrome (AIDS) and AIDS frequently have generalized lymphadenopathy and malaise. The majority of cases in the United States occur in homosexual or bisexual men and drug abusers. An increased incidence also is seen in patients who require frequent transfusions of blood products (hemophiliacs, sickle cell anemia patients). Lymph node biopsy frequently is not indicated, since the diagnosis usually is established by other studies (see chapter on *Acquired Immunodeficiency Syndrome*).

An occasional patient has significant generalized lymphadenopathy for which no explanation can be found.

TABLE 4 Causes of Generalized Lymphadenopathy

Infections (e.g., measles, infectious mononucleosis)
Autoimmune disorders
Dermatopathic lymphadenopathy
Pre-AIDS and AIDS*
Malignant lymphomas
Chronic lymphocytic leukemia
Sarcoidosis
Metastatic carcinomas and sarcomas
Drug-induced (e.g., Dilantin)
Angioimmunoblastic lymphadenopathy
Idiopathic lymphadenopathy

* AIDS = acquired immunodeficiency syndrome

Such patients should be followed closely for the emergence of a definable underlying disorder.

The single most important *laboratory investigation* in patients with lymphadenopathy is a complete blood count and a careful inspection of the peripheral smear. A diagnosis of chronic lymphocytic leukemia usually can be made by obtaining a complete blood count and a differential. The diagnostic significance of finding atypical lymphocytes is referred to earlier. A Monospot test is indicated in any patient with unexplained lymphadenopathy. Appropriate cultures and specific pre- and convalescent serum titers should be obtained when the clinical history and physical examination indicate a possible underlying infectious etiology.

If a diagnosis cannot be made from a careful clinical history, physical examination, and inspection of a peripheral blood smear, a lymph node aspiration or biopsy or both are indicated. In general, a lymph node aspiration should be the initial procedure. In most instances a lymph node aspiration or biopsy does not need to be performed on an emergency basis, but there are situations in patients whose clinical course is rapidly progressing where these procedures are indicated prior to instituting empiric therapy.

SUGGESTED READING

Hess CE. Approach to patients with lymphadenopathy and splenomegaly. In: Thorup OA Jr, ed. Fundamentals of clinical hematology. Philadelphia: WB Saunders, 1987 (in press).

Jeghers H, Clark SL Jr, Templeton AC. Lymphadenopathy and disorders of the lymphatics. In: Blacklow RS, ed. MacBryde's signs and symptoms. JB Lippincott, 1983:467.

TETANUS

WESLEY FURSTE, M.D., F.A.C.S.
FERNANDO I. COLON-FIGUEROA, M.D.

Tetanus (lockjaw) is a severe and dreaded infection of wounds caused by the toxin-producing *Clostridium tetani*. This disease is characterized by tonic spasms of the voluntary muscles, by a tendency toward episodes of respiratory arrest, and, worldwide, by a mortality rate of approximately 50 percent.

Tetanus continues to occur as a complication of lacerations, open fractures, burns, abrasions, hypodermic injections, and (rarely in the United States) in operations on the gastrointestinal tract and after birth (infection of the umbilical stump in the newborn).

In contrast to gas gangrene (clostridial myonecrosis), which is a complication of the severe and sometimes neglected wound, tetanus occurs not only in severe, neglected, or old wounds, but may also occur in very minor and very superficial wounds, or in individuals without any demonstrable wound.

C. tetani is a large, gram-positive, actively motile bacillus, which, in its spore bearing form, has a characteristic "drumstick" appearance. Spores may develop at either end of the bacillus, giving it a "dumbbell" appearance. It is a strict anaerobe, and spores do not germinate in the presence of even the smallest amount of oxygen. The organism is ubiquitous.

DIAGNOSIS

In the generalized form of tetanus, the infection usually becomes evident 1 to 2 weeks after injury. The severity of the clinical picture and the mortality rate are roughly inversely proportional to the duration of the incubation period.

Some patients have prodromal symptoms of restlessness and headaches. In others, the first symptoms are those stemming from the developing muscle rigidity, with vague discomfort in the jaws, neck, or lumbar region. At an early stage, spasm of the muscles of mastication causes trismus and difficulty with chewing, i.e., lockjaw. Sustained contraction of the facial muscles produces a distorted grin (risus sardonicus). Spasm of the pharyngeal muscles makes swallowing difficult. Also, stiff neck and opisthotonos are among the early signs. Progressively, other muscle groups become involved, with tightness of the chest and rigidity of the abdominal wall, the back, and the limbs. Generalized tonic convulsions are frequent and exhausting. Any sudden jarring or sound, such as a hypodermic injection or the fall of an object onto the floor, will excite such generalized convulsions. In association with these convulsions, there sometimes is spasm of the laryngeal and respiratory muscles with possibly fatal acute asphyxia.

Cruelly, the patient is mentally clear throughout the course of the disease and suffers great pain from the muscle spasms. The pulse rate is elevated and there is profuse perspiration. Fever may or may not be present. Neurologic examination discloses hyperactive tendon reflexes, often with sustained clonus. There are no sensory changes.

If the patient survives, the intensity of the muscle contractions may begin to diminish slowly during about the second week. Complete recovery may take several months.

Occasionally, mild cases occur in which there is only moderate muscle rigidity without tetanus seizures. In a person who has not received tetanus toxoid prophylaxis prior to injury, the administration of toxoid may forestall the development of severe tetanus and may result in only mild tetanus or a local tetanus involving only the muscles around the site of the injury.

The diagnosis of tetanus must be based on the clinical picture, for laboratory examinations are of little assistance. The demonstration of *C. tetani* in a wound does not prove the diagnosis of tetanus; the failure to demonstrate the bacillus in a wound does not eliminate the possibility of tetanus. The urine is normal unless secondary urinary tract infection occurs. Tetanus itself produces a slight elevation in the leukocyte count, but secondary infection may produce greater elevation. Often, the cerebrospinal fluid is under increased pressure, but otherwise it is not remarkable.

There are two unusual forms of tetanus that may be missed. Localized tetanus presents with spasm only in a localized area, usually a limb; spasms in adjacent muscles may be seen. This form occurs in patients with partial immunity or very few *C. tetani* in their wounds. Cephalic tetanus results from infection of the head, neck, and eye or chronic otitis media; it presents with trismus and palsy of the cranial nerves in the affected region of the head. It is a form of localized tetanus and often progresses to generalized tetanus.

DIFFERENTIAL DIAGNOSIS

Early or mild tetanus may resemble certain other conditions, but severe tetanus is likely to be confused with few other diseases.

Careful history differentiates the tonic contractures of tetanus from the trismus and rigidity due to phenothiazine tranquilizer drugs, lead, and hepatic encephalopathy.

Meningitis and encephalitis must be differentiated from tetanus. Signs of meningeal irritation and of brain inflammation usually make this easy.

Rabies (hydrophobia) is exhibited by the patient's inability to swallow as an early symptom, drooling of saliva, and spasms of the muscles of deglutition. Later, in the course of the disease, it is characterized by fever, anxiety, excitement, delirium, hyperesthesia, and convulsions. Rabies particularly involves the muscles of respiration. A history of animal bite is usually obtainable.

The clinical picture of strychnine poisoning, with hyperexcitability of muscles, opisthotonos, risus sardonicus, and tonic convulsions, may mimic full-blown tetanus very closely, except that the muscles are relaxed between seizures in strychnine intoxication, whereas spasm tends to persist in tetanus. Moreover, in strychnine poisoning, the jaws and face are not particularly affected.

Acute psychoses may be difficult to differentiate from early or mild tetanus, and a thorough psychiatric evaluation and a test of time may be necessary to make an exact diagnosis.

Local tetanus may closely simulate the spasms of a localized group of voluntary muscles due to soft tissue or bone injuries.

Trismus—not due to tetanus—may occur with peritonsillar abscess and other local infections of the mouth and cervical regions, and with dentomandibular problems. Dysphagia, suggestive of tetanus, may actually be the result of upper respiratory infections.

In the newborn, neonatal tetanus may be confused with meningitis, hypocalcemic tetany, sepsis, and intracranial hemorrhage. Cerebrospinal fluid analyses, blood chemistry studies, wound and blood cultures, and neurosurgical evaluation may be necessary for a correct diagnosis.

Hypocalcemic tetany is less severe than tetanus, usually follows operations on the thyroid gland, and primarily affects the upper extremities. The muscle contractions of tetany are elicited by pressure on the nerves leading to the contracting muscles.

Formerly, before the availability of human tetanus immune globulin (TIG), a frequent diagnostic problem was differentiation of heterologous equine serum sickness from early tetanus, with approxmiately 5 to 30 percent of the patients subsequently developing serum sickness with temporomandibular arthralgia and trismus, arthralgia of other joints, urticaria, and generalized adenitis.

TREATMENT

The treatment of tetanus is complex, but can be successful. It requires devoted and exhausting attention by all echelons of health personnel. It is truly a team effort. The following recommendations for management are given in chronologic order of priority.

A complete medical history must be obtained and a complete physical examination performed, with particular inquiries about the date and circumstances of injury, the depth of the injury below the skin, and allergies. Such information forms a baseline for the recognition of complications, such as atelectasis, pneumonia, traumatic glossitis, fractures of the vertebrae, decubital ulcers, and fecal impaction. Basic laboratory work is also obtained (Table 1).

Intramuscular injection of tetanus immune globulin (TIG) is injected as soon as the diagnosis of tetanus is made; 500 to 6,000 units of TIG are given deeply intramuscularly. TIG is given in the proximal portion of the extremity in which the wound responsible for tetanus is located, or in the gluteal muscles when the wound is not in an extremity or when the causative wound cannot be found.

The exact effective dosage of TIG has not been clearly established. Since a serum tetanus antitoxin level of 0.01 units per milliliter prevents tetanus in the injured, a dosage of 10,000 units of TIG is more than adequate for severe

TABLE 1 Laboratory Evaluation in Tetanus

Complete blood cell count with differential white blood cell count	Arterial blood gases
	Chest roentgenogram
	Electrocardiogram
Urinalysis	Electroencephalogram
Serologic test for syphilis	Wound and—if the patient is febrile—blood cultures
Prothrombin time and partial thromboplastin time	If necessary for diagnoses,
Blood chemistry tests: urea nitrogen, creatinine, electrophoresis, bilirubin, calcium, glucose	cerebrospinal fluid for culture, smear, cells, and chemistry tests

tetanus. A dose of only 1,500 units may be therapeutic in less severe cases.

In the United States, there are no indications for the administration of heterologous equine and bovine antitoxins (rather than TIG), which have been responsible for serum sickness, myocardial infarction, peripheral neuritis, and anaphylactic shock with death. Moreover, in humans the life span of the heterologous antitoxins cannot be predicted with certainty.

Two hundred fifty units of TIG intramuscularly is proper for neonatal tetanus.

As soon as the diagnosis of tetanus is made, for all cases, give TIG intrathecally. For adult tetanus, the dose of TIG for the intrathecal route by lumbar puncture is 1,000 units; and for neonatal tetanus, 250 units of TIG is administered intrathecally.

Constant nursing care in an ICU is needed. A physician must be immediately available to treat complications, particularly respiratory arrest.

Administer analgesics in doses that relieve the pain associated with the tonic contractions of tetanus but that do not cause respiratory depression. Codeine, meperidine (Demerol), meperidine with promethazine (Phenergan), and morphine are suitable drugs.

Sedatives are needed to reduce the patient's threshold to external stimuli, with the hope of reducing the number and severity of seizures. In the mildest cases of tetanus the patient can be sedated adequately with phenobarbitol or paraldehyde, but more severe cases require thiopental sodium (Pentothal). Muscle relaxant drugs are difficult to administer because of the problems of overdosage or underdosage. Drugs more commonly suggested for use are diazepam (Valium), D-tubocurarine, succinylcholine (Anectine), pancuronium (Pavilon), atracurium (Tracrium), and vecuronium (Norcuron).

Meticulous surgical care of wounds must be carried out, with removal of all necrotic tissue and foreign bodies.

In vitro, penicillin and other antibiotics are effective against the tetanus bacillus. However, antibiotic therapy is disappointing because tetanus is a toxemia, not a bacteremia. In addition, necessary antibiotic concentrations within the wound may not be attained, because avascular conditions are frequently present. Nevertheless penicillin may be a useful adjunct to surgical wound care in that it may prevent or lessen the severity of wound infections other than tetanus. Penicillin does not prevent tetanus. If it is given, the route (oral, intramuscular, or intravenous) of penicillin administration and its dosage must be determined by the characteristics of the wound. Antibiotics are irreplaceable in the care of infectious complications of tetanus, especially in combating pneumonia or secondary invasive wound infections. The choice of most effective antibiotics for infectious complications should be determined by prior experience and by culture and sensitivity tests.

If adequate personnel and facilities, including adequate tracheostomy tubes and mechanical respiration units, are available, one performs a tracheostomy. Tracheostomy and controlled ventilation are not necessary for every patient, but patients with short incubation periods or those who manifest periods of respiratory arrest require long term respiratory control.

Infants with neonatal tetanus should be placed in an incubator in which the oxygen partial pressure, environmental temperature, and a nebulized atmosphere of distilled water can be monitored and maintained.

Roentgenograms may be needed for fractures associated with the initial injury, determination of pulmonary problems such as atelectasis and pneumonia, and fractures or avulsions of muscle insertions produced by the tonic muscle contractions of tetanus. Compression fractures of the vertebrae may be the result of the intense paroxysms that characterize the disease, and their diagnosis may be easily missed without roentgenograms.

Tetanus Prophylaxis in Wounds

As can be deduced from the lack of good specific therapy for tetanus and its high mortality rate, this is a disease in which prevention is of paramount importance. In the United States, routine tetanus immunization has made this previously commonplace disease rare. However, not all patients are adequately immunized, and the primary responsibility of the physician treating a patient with a wound is to ensure that the patient is adequately immunized. Accurate information about this is often lacking. Whenever in doubt, check the records, particularly in the case of persons from underdeveloped countries where childhood immunization is not routine. Many older patients are also not adequately immunized; over 50 percent of patients over age 60 have inadequate antibody titers to tetanus.

Patients who are not adequately immunized need immediate emergency department administration of tetanus toxoid (active immunization) and possibly tetanus immune globulin (passive immunization), as detailed in Table 2. Adults receive 0.5 cc of tetanus toxoid intramuscularly; this is ideally administered as tetanus-diphtheria (Td) toxoid, rather than just tetanus toxoid, because many adults no longer have adequate antibody titers to diphtheria and are potentially at risk for this disease. (The pertussis vaccine usually combined in DTP immunizations used in children under 7 years of age is not given because the disease is insignificant in adults, and reactions to the pertussis vaccine can be severe.) Patients who have never received initial immunizations and who have major or tetanus-prone wounds also need temporary passive protection from tetanus immune globulin, 250 mg administered intramuscularly in the other arm, and then a follow-up in 30 and 60 days to receive the remaining injections in the basic immunization series. Patients with particularly tetanus-prone wounds need 500 mg of TIG if TIG is indicated.

Meticulous surgical care of wounds is critically important as well in preventing tetanus. All the usual principles of wound care should be followed, with special emphasis on irrigation and debridement of crushed and devitalized tissue. Antibiotics cannot be relied upon to prevent tetanus, and should not be routinely administered.

TABLE 2 Guideline for Tetanus Immunization in Patients with Wounds

| Type of Wound | Patient Not Immunized or Partially Immunized | Patient Completely Immunized— Time Since Last Booster Dose | |
		5 to 10 years	>10 years
Clean—minor	Begin or complete immunization per schedule; tetanus toxoid, 0.5 ml	None	Tetanus toxoid, 0.5 ml
Clean—major or	In one arm: human tetanus immune globulin, 250 units[†] In other arm: tetanus toxoid, 0.5 ml complete immunization per schedule[†]	Tetanus toxoid, 0.5 ml	Tetanus toxoid, 0.5 ml
Tetanus-prone, delayed or incomplete debridement	In one arm: human tetanus immune globulin 250–500 units[†] In other arm: tetanus toxoid 0.5 ml, complete immunization per schedule thereafter,[†] antibiotic therapy	Tetanus toxoid, 0.5 ml; antibiotic therapy	Tetanus toxoid, 0.5 ml

[†] Use different syringes, needles, and injection sites.
NOTE: With different preparations of toxoid, the volume of a single booster dose should be modified as stated on the package label.

TABLE 3 Recommended Schedule for Active Immunization of Normal Infants and Children

Recommended Age*	Vaccine(s)	Comments
2 months	DTP-1§, OPV-1¶	Can be given earlier in areas of high endemicity
4 months	DTP-2, OPV-2	6-weeks–2-months interval desired between OPV doses to avoid interference
6 months	DTP-3	An additional dose of OPV at this time is optional for use in areas with a high risk of polio exposure
15 months**	MMR††	
18 months	DTP-4, OPV-3	Completion of primary series
4-6 years§§	DTP-5, OPV-4	Preferably at or before school entry
14-16 years	Td¶¶	Repeat every 10 years throughout life

* These recommended ages should not be construed as absolute, i.e., 2 months can be 6-10 weeks, etc.
§ DTP-Diphtheria and tetanus toxoids and pertussis vaccine.
¶ OPV-Oral, attenuated poliorirus vaccine contains poliovirus types 1, 2, and 3.
** Simultaneous administration of MMR, DTP, and OPV is appropriate for patients whose compliance with medical care recommendations cannot be assured.
†† MMR-Live measles, mumps, and rubella viruses in a combined vaccine
§§ Up to the seventh birthday.
¶¶ Td-Adult tetanus toxoid and diphtheria toxoid in combination, which contains the same dose of tetanus toxoid as DTP or DT and a reduced dose of diphtheria toxoid.
Source: CDC MMWR 32(1)11, 1983.

Immunization Precautions

The recommendations for routine immunization are summarized in Tables 3 and 4. Patients with wounds treated in the emergency department should receive immunization according to these guidelines.

Immunosuppressive therapies, including irradiation, antimetabolites, alkylating agents, cytotoxic drugs, and corticosteroids (used in higher than physiologic doses),

TABLE 4 Recommended Immunization Schedule for Persons 7 Years of Age or Older

Timing	Vaccine(s)	Comments
First visit	Td-1*, OPV-1[†] and MMR§	OPV not routinely administered to those ≥18 years old
2 months after first Td, OPV	Td-2, OPV-2	
6-12 months after second Td, OPV	Td-3, OPV-3	OPV-3 may be given as soon as 6 weeks after OPV-2
10 years after Td-3	Td	Repeat every 10 years throughout life

* Td-Tetanus and diphtheria toxoids (adult type) are used after the seventh birthday. The DTP doses given to children under 7 who remain incompletely immunized at age 7 or older should be counted as prior exposure to tetanus and diphtheria toxoids (e.g., a child who previously received 2 doses of DTP only needs 1 dose of Td to complete a primary series).
† OPV-Oral, attenuated poliovirus vaccine contains poliovirus types 1,2, and 3. When polio vaccine is to be given to individuals 18 years or older, IPV is preferred.
§ MMR-Live measles, mumps, and rubella viruses in a combined vaccine. Persons born before 1957 can generally be considered immune to measles and mumps and need not be immunized. Rubella vaccine may be given to persons of any age, particularly to women of childbearing age. MMR may be used since administration of vaccine to persons already immune is not deleterious.

may reduce the immune response to vaccines. Short term (less than 2 weeks) corticosteroid therapy or intra-articular, bursal, or tendon injections with corticosteroids should not be immunosuppressive. Although no specific studies with pertussis vaccine are available, if immunosuppressive therapy is to be discontinued shortly, it would be reasonable to defer immunization until therapy has been discontinued for one month; otherwise the patient should be vaccinated while still taking therapy.

When an infant or child returns for the next dose of DTP, the parent should be questioned about any adverse events occurring after the previous dose.

Tetanus toxoid reactions: mild local reactions, erythema, and induration are common after tetanus injections. Some patients with preexisting high antibody levels have a severe local Arthus-type hypersensitivity reaction of tenderness, redness, and swelling.

Special cautions must be observed in children under 7 years of age when administering DTP immunization (Table 3). Although pertussis is a significant disease of early childhood that warrants prevention, it is relatively rare, and there have been instances of severe neurologic complications (including encephalopathy and seizures) caused by pertussis vaccine. The current recommendation is that this vaccine not be given to those with a history of any untoward neurologic reaction within 3 days after receiving pertussis vaccine, or any history of seizures, or any neurologic condition characterized by changing developmental or neurologic findings (such as epilepsy, infantile spasm, or progressive encephalopathy). Stable conditions such as cerebral palsy and developmental delay are not a contraindication. Patients with stable and well-controlled seizures not related to vaccination may receive vaccine. When in any doubt, the emergency physician should contact the patient's primary physician for consultation before administering the DTP vaccine.

If any of the following adverse events occur after DTP or single antigen pertussis vaccination, further vaccination with a vaccine containing pertussis antigen is contraindicated:

1. Allergic hypersensitivity.
2. Fever of 40.5 ° C (105 ° F) or higher within 48 hours.
3. Collapse or shocklike state (hypotonic-hyporesponsive episode) within 48 hours.
4. Persisting, inconsolable crying lasting 3 hours or more or an unusual high-pitched cry occurring within 48 hours.
5. Convulsion(s) with or without fever occurring within 3 days (all children with convulsions, especially those with convulsions occurring within 4 to 7 days after receipt of DTP, should be fully evaluated to clarify their medical and neurologic status before a decision is made about initiating or continuing vaccination with DTP).
6. Encephalopathy occurring within 7 days. This includes severe alterations in consciousness with generalized or focal neurologic signs (a small but significantly increased risk of encephalopathy has been shown only within the 3-day period following DTP receipt; however, most authorities believe that an encephalopathy occurring within 7 days after DTP should be considered a contraindication to further doses of DTP).

SUGGESTED READING

Brand DA, et al. Adequacy of antitetanus prophylaxis in six hospital emergency rooms. N Engl J Med 1983; 309:636–640.

Centers for Disease Control, Public Health Service, U.S. Department of Health, Education, and Welfare. Recommendation of the Immunization Practices Advisory Committee (ACIP). Diphtheria, tetanus, and pertussis: guidelines for vaccine prophylaxis and other preventive measures. MMWR 1985 (July 12); 34(27):405–426.

Editorial. Tetanus immune globulin: the intrathecal route. Lancet 1980; 2:464.

Furste W. The sixth international conference on tetanus, Lyon, France, 1981. J Trauma 1982; 22:1032.

Furste W, Baird IM, Lobe TE. Tetanus. In: Simmons RL, Howard RJ, eds. Surgical infectious diseases. New York: Appleton-Century-Crofts, 1982:1089.

Furste W, Wheeler WL. Tetanus: a team disease. Curr Prob Surg 1972; 9:1–72.

MALARIA

PAUL B. BAKER, M.D.
STEVEN C. DRONEN, M.D.

Malaria is a blood-borne infection with protozoan parasites of the genus *Plasmodium*. Although it has been eradicated in the United States and Europe, the disease continues to be a major health hazard in most of the developing world. Because of increasing numbers of visitors and immigrants to and from these areas, physicians in this country should have a basic familiarity with the prevention, recognition, and treatment of malaria. Because of the often precipitous onset of symptoms, it is not uncommon for patients with acute malaria to first present to the emergency department.

ETIOLOGY

Malaria has a broad distribution in most tropical and subtropical regions of the world, including South and Central America, sub-Saharan Africa, Southeast Asia, the Eastern Pacific, and the Indian subcontinent (Fig.1). Of the more than 100 species of plasmodia, only four routinely cause clinical disease in humans—*P. vivax, P. ovale, P. falciparum,* and *P. malariae. P. ovale* is rare outside of West Africa, but the remaining three have nearly worldwide distribution.

The protozoan parasite is spread from one human host to another by an insect vector, the female Anopheles mosquito. Other modes of transmission include contaminated blood supplies, shared needles among intravenous drug users, and congenital malaria.

The life cycle of plasmodia in humans consists of both erythrocytic phases (within the red blood cell) and exoerythrocytic phases (usually within the liver) that vary, depending on the species. The maturation of the *P. fal-*

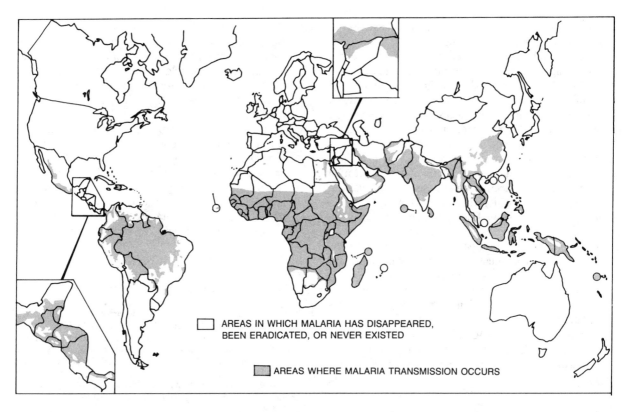

AREAS IN WHICH MALARIA HAS DISAPPEARED,
BEEN ERADICATED, OR NEVER EXISTED

AREAS WHERE MALARIA TRANSMISSION OCCURS

Figure 1 Epidemiologic assessment of status of malaria, 1982. (From MMWR 1984; 33:586.)

ciparum parasite occurs within the capillaries and sinusoids of visceral organs—the liver, the kidney, and the brain—and accounts for the greater morbidity and mortality of this strain. In addition, it must be emphasized that both *P. vivax* and *P. ovale* have prolonged exoerythrocytic forms in the liver that are capable of causing relapses weeks or months after the patient has left the malaria-endemic area. These forms of the parasite are resistant to most antimalarial drugs and may persist after a standard course of prophylactic therapy.

DIAGNOSIS

Although the clinical manifestations of malaria can be protean, certain features of the illness are easily recognized and common to all species. Symptoms coincide with rupture of the red blood cells and release of immature parasites into the circulation. Classic symptoms include chills, shivering, headache, and a paroxysmal rise in body temperature from 102 to 105° F (39 to 40.5° C). The attack ends after 4 to 12 hours with profuse sweating and defervescence, only to recur if the infection remains untreated. The characteristic fever patterns of tertian and quartan malaria may take several days to develop, and paroxysms may occur irregularly at the beginning or throughout the illness. Some degree of *hypotension* is not uncommon during the malarial paroxysm and usually responds promptly to fluid administration. Splenomegaly and jaundice are frequently noted in established infections, but are usually absent early in the course of the

disease. Anemia is usually mild initially, but may become profound in long-standing malaria or in fulminant infection and hemolysis with *P. falciparum*(blackwater fever). *Thrombocytopenia*, occasionally to levels less than 20,000 per cubic millimeter, is common, as is mild neutropenia. Coagulation abnormalities, such as elevation of the partial prothrombin time, are noted in many cases, although episodes of clinical bleeding are rare.

The severity of an acute attack of malaria depends on the immune status of the affected individual, with semi-immune individuals within endemic areas being subject to more benign chronic infections. Even in nonimmune patients, infection with *P. vivax*, *P. malariae*, or *P. ovale* usually results in a self-limited illness that is rarely fatal in the acute phase; much of the morbidity arises from the sequelae of long-term infection. However, infection with *P. falciparum* or malignant tertian malaria may have a case fatality rate of over 10 percent in some strains and must be identified early in its presentation to prevent unnecessary mortality. Because the *P. falciparum* parasite completes its maturation within the capillaries of various internal organs, infection with this strain may mimic a variety of pathologic conditions. Blockage of blood vessels by malarial parasites may cause symptoms suggesting acute appendicitis, cholecystitis, and even myocardial infarction. Other serious complications of falciparum malaria include cerebral hypoxia and coma, adrenal insufficiency (algid malaria), acute tubular necrosis, and pulmonary edema or adult respiratory distress syndrome.

TABLE 1 Areas Reporting Chloroquine-Resistant *Plasmodium falciparum*

Africa	*Asia*
Angola	Burma
Burundi	China (Hainan Island and
Central African Republic	southern provinces)
Comoros	Indonesia
Gabon	Kampuchea
Kenya	Laos
Madagascar	Malaysia
Malawi	Phillipines (Luzon, Basilan,
Mozambique	Mindoro, Palawan, and
Namibia	Mindanao Islands; Sulu
Rwanda	Archipelago)
Sudan (northern provinces)	Thailand
Tanzania	Vietnam
Uganda	
Zaire (northeastern)	
Zambia (northeastern)	
South America	*Oceania*
Bolivia	Papua, New Guinea
Brazil	Solomon Islands
Colombia	Vanuatu
Ecuador	
French Guiana	
Guyana	*Indian Subcontinent*
Panama (east of the Canal Zone,	Bangladesh (North and East)
including the San Bias Islands)	India
Peru (northern provinces)	Pakistan (Rawalpindi)
Surinam	
Venezuela	

From MMWR 1985; 34:186

The diagnosis of malaria can easily be missed by physicians in nonmalarious regions of the world who are unfamilar with the symptoms and presentation of the disease. The key to diagnosis is a high index of suspicion in patients returning from endemic areas of malaria transmission. A brief travel history is essential in the evaluation of any febrile illness that is without apparent source. Malaria can occur weeks to months after leaving an endemic region and after complete adherence to standard prophylactic therapy, either from drug-resistant strains of *P. falciparum* or from exoerythrocytic forms of *P. vivax* or *P. ovale*.

The most common erroneous diagnosis in such patients is to ascribe the symptoms of malaria to a nonspecific viral syndrome; the periodicity and recurrent nature of the malarial paroxysm usually lead to the correct diagnosis in time. Conversely, it is essential to rule out bacterial sepsis as the cause of any severe febrile illness before considering the diagnosis of malaria. Thorough physical examination and appropriate laboratory tests (appropriate cultures and blood smears) are indicated prior to treatment. In addition to the usual differential diagnosis of the febrile patient, consideration should be given to the diagnosis of viral hepatitis, dengue fever, typhoid fever, amebiasis, and other less common infections in such patients.

The standard method of confirming the diagnosis of malaria is the demonstration of the protozoan parasites on peripheral blood smears. In the majority of cases of acute malaria, the routine Wright or Giemsa stain of standard thin blood smears demonstrates plasmodia in various stages of development. Notification of the appropriate

clinical laboratory of the suspicion of malaria is vital, since lower levels of parasitemia may be overlooked by observers unfamiliar with the disease. Exact determination of malarial species may prove difficult and requires considerable experience, though a highly motivated novice can often make a crude distinction between the more virulent *P. falciparum* and the more benign species of *Plasmodium*. In cases in which clinical suspicion for malaria is high and routine thin smears are negative, special thick-blood smears may detect the parasite.

THERAPY

Pre-hospital Phase

Therapy for the patient with malaria at home or in the field is primarily supportive. Hyperpyrexia may be controlled with cool baths or compresses and antipyretics such as acetaminophen may prove useful. Aspirin is best avoided because of the frequency of thrombocytopenia in these patients. Many patients with malaria exhibit some degree of dehydration or volume depletion, and rehydration via oral or parenteral routes forms the mainstay of therapy. Transport to a physician's office or emergency facility is indicated in all but the mildest cases.

Emergency Department Phase

The most important part of the initial management is prompt consideration and recognition of the illness and

TABLE 2 Antimalarial Drugs

Agent	Brand Name	Dosage Forms	Indications	Precautions-Side Effects
Chloroquine phosphate	Aralen (Winthrop) Many generic forms available.	Oral Tablets of 500 mg and 250 mg of salt or 300 mg and 150 mg of base. Pediatric suspension unavailable in U.S.; dose should be calculated carefully using pulverized tablets.	Treatment and prophylaxis of erythrocytic forms of *P. vivax, ovale,* and *malariae.* Ineffective against exoerythrocytic forms of *vivax* and *ovale;* should be used in combination with primaquine phosphate to prevent relapse from liver parasites. Increasing levels of resistance of *P. falciparum* to this drug reported in many regions (see Table 1).	Usually well tolerated via oral route. Occasional GI upset, cutaneous reactions, transient ECG changes. Long-term therapy may be associated with neuromyopathy, corneal/retinal damage, and blood dyscrasias. Should be used with caution in pediatric age group, as toxicity may occur with relatively low doses.
Pyrimethamine-sulfadoxine	Fansidar (Roche)	Oral Tablets containing 25 mg 500 mg sulfadoxine. Pyrimethamine and 500 mg sulfadoxine.	Treatment and prophylaxis of chloroquine-resistant strains of *P. falciparum.* Should be used in conjunction with chloroquine to increase coverage of *P. vivax* and *ovale.* Strains of *P. falciparum* resistant to both pyrimethamine/sulfadoxine and chloroquine have now been reported.	Recent reports have implicated this agent in serious and even fatal cutaneous reactions (e.g., Stevens-Johnson syndrome) when used for *prophylaxis,* and its indications have been redefined by the CDC. As yet, this complication has not been reported when the drug is used as single-dose *treatment* for malaria.
Primaquine phosphate	Primaquine (Winthrop)	Oral Tablets containing 26.3 mg (15 mg base). Also available in combination form with chloroquine.	Treatment and prophylaxis of *P. vivax* and *ovale.* Will eradicate prolonged liver forms in these strains and prevent relapse. Should be used following treatment with standard agent such as chloroquine.	Can precipitate a hemolytic anemia in G-6-PD–deficient patients. Enzyme assay should be obtained prior to initiation of therapy. Enzyme-deficient patient may require alternative dosage schedule.
Quinine sulfate	Many generic forms available.	Oral Tablets and capsules containing 200 mg, 260 mg. 300 mg, and 325 mg.	Treatment of drug-resistant strains of *P. falciparum* or in severely ill patients with unidentified *Plasmodium species.* May be used in combination with pyrimethamine-sulfadoxine or tetracycline to increase effectiveness. Again no activity against exoerythrocytic forms.	Side effects include GI upset, cutaneous reactions, and hematologic disorders, in addition to hemolytic anemia in G-6-PD-deficient individuals.
Quinine dihydrochloride	Generic forms available. In U.S., CDC in Atlanta can assist in obtaining drug*	Intravenous Given as infusion of 600 to 500 ml of normal mg in 300 to 500 ml of normal saline over 2 to 4 hours.	Treatment of severely ill individuals unable to tolerate oral therapy. Should be switched to oral therapy as soon as possible.	Patients must be closely monitored for signs of hypotension or circulatory collapse. Arrhythmias and ECG changes have been reported.
Chloroquine hydrochloride	Aralen hydrochloride (Winthrop) Again, CDC can provide valuable assistance with therapy.	Intramuscular Ampules containing 250 mg salt or 200 mg base in 5 ml.	Treatment of individuals unable to tolerate oral therapy. Should be switched to oral therapy as soon as possible	Patients must be monitored closely for hypotension and arrhythmias. These reactions are more common in children, and agent should be used only in extreme cases.

* Consult Malaria Branch, Division of Parasitic Diseases, CDC, Atlanta: telephone (404) 452-4046 (days), (404) 329-2888 (nights).

TABLE 3 Treatment and Prophylactic Regimens for Antimalarial Agents

Treatment

Areas without chloroquine-resistant *P. falciparum*:

Oral treatment

Adults: Chloroquine phosphate 1,000 mg (600 mg base) initially, followed by 500 mg (300 mg base) at 6, 24, and 48 hours. If species is *P. vivax* or *P. ovale*, should be followed by primaquine phosphate 26.3 mg/day (15 mg base) for 14 days. G-6-PD activity must be determined prior to therapy.

Children: Chloroquine phosphate 10 mg/kg of *base* initially, followed by 5 mg/kg of *base* at 6, 24, and 48 hours. If species is *P. vivax* or *P. ovale*, should be followed by primaquine phosphate *base* 0.25 mg/kg/day for 14 days. G-6-PD activity should be determined prior to therapy. In no case should calculated doses for pediatric patients exceed the standard adult dose for either chloroquine or primaquine.

Parenteral treatment (for severely ill individuals unable to take oral medication)*

Adults: Quinine dihydrochloride 600 mg in 300 ml of normal saline given as an infusion over 2 to 4 hours every 8 to 12 hours until oral therapy with chloroquine can be instituted. Alternatively, chloroquine hydrochloride 250 mg (200 mg base) can be given intramuscularly every 6 hours until oral therapy with chloroquine phosphate can be started. With *P. vivax* or *P. ovale*, a course of primaquine phosphate is necessary to prevent relapse.

Children: Quinine dihydrochloride 10 mg/kg in 10 mg/kg of normal saline given as an infusion over 3 to 4 hours. May repeat 5 mg/kg dose every 8 to 12 hours until oral chloroquine can be tolerated. With *P. vivax* or *P. ovale*, therapy with primaquine phosphate is necessary to prevent relapse.

Areas with known or suspected chloroquine-resistant *P. falciparum*:

Oral treatment

Adults: Quinine sulfate 650 mg 3 times a day for 3 to 10 days. Most would use combination therapy with pyrimethamine/sulfadoxine 75 mg/1,500 mg (3 tablets) as a single dose on fourth day or tetracycline 250–500 mg 4 times a day for 7 to 10 days. Quinine may be given for a shorter course (3 to 5 days) if combination therapy is given.

Children: Quinine sulfate 10 mg/kg (not to exceed adult dose) given 3 times a day for 3 to 10 days. May combine with pyrimethamine/sulfadoxine 15 mg/500 mg tablet on fourth day using following schedule: 6 mo to 4 yr—½ tablet; 4 yr to 8 yr—1 tablet; 8 yr to 14 yr—2 tablets; 14 yr to adult—3 tablets. Tetracyclines may be used in older children, but should be avoided in children under 8 yr. Quinine may be given for shorter course if combination therapy is given.

Parenteral treatment (for severely ill individuals unable to tolerate oral therapy)*

Adults: Quinine dihydrochloride given as previously noted. Should be switched to oral quinine and second drug as soon as possible.

Children: Quinine dihydrochloride given as previously noted. Again, oral therapy should be initiated as soon as possible.

Prophylaxis

Areas without chloroquine-resistant *P. falciparum*:

Chloroquine phosphate 500 mg (300 mg base) once weekly beginning 1 week prior and 6 weeks after leaving malarious area. Pediatric dosage is 8.3 mg/kg (5 mg/kg base) on same schedule. Primaquine phosphate, 26.3 mg (15 mg base) per day for 14 days, may be indicated when exposure is long term and intense, but is rarely necessary in the average traveler. Pediatric dose is 0.25 mg/kg/day of base for 14 days.

Areas with known chloroquine-resistant *P. falciparum*:

Chloroquine phosphate, using previously detailed dosages, is indicated to protect against sensitive strains of *P. falciparum*, *vivax*, *ovale*, and *malariae*. In addition, prophylaxis with pyrimethamine/sulfadoxine should be considered if exposure is high risk (e.g., travel in rural areas of East Africa). Because of recent reports of severe and occasionally fatal cutaneous reactions, prophylactic therapy must be individualized, and consultation with state and federal health agencies is advised. Dosage of pyrimethamine/sulfadoxine in adults is one 15 mg/500 mg tablet once weekly beginning 1 week prior to entering a malarious area and continuing for 6 weeks after leaving. Medication must be discontinued at the first sign of skin or mucous membrane lesions. The pediatric dose of pyrimethamine/sulfadoxine is ¼ tablet weekly for those under 4 yr, ½ tablet weekly from 4 to 8 yr, and one tablet weekly from 8 to 14 yr.

---

* Early consultation with infectious disease specialists and state and federal health agencies is strongly recommended in such cases, both to optimize therapy and assist in obtaining parenteral antimalarial agents.

institution of appropriate therapy. The presentation of the patient with malaria may be quite dramatic, and those in the midst of a paroxysm appear acutely ill. The approach to such patients should follow standard emergency department protocol, with careful attention to airway integrity, maintenance of circulation, and establishment of intravenous access when indicated. Some degree of hypotension is not uncommon and will usually respond to fluid administration. Once the patient has been stabilized, the clinician must reliably exclude other more common causes of fever (e.g. bacterial or viral infection) before ascribing symptoms to malaria. A complete blood count with a peripheral smear, chest film, urinalysis, and appropriate cultures (blood, sputum, urine, and cerebrospinal fluid when indicated) should be obtained.

Once the diagnosis of malaria has been established by peripheral blood smears, treatment can be initiated in the emergency department, either on an inpatient or outpatient basis, depending on the clinical status of the patient. Using the travel history, initial clinical presentation, and examination of blood smears, the physician should attempt to differentiate cases of *falciparum* malaria from other less virulent types. The higher morbidity and mortality associated with this species and changing patterns of drug resistance require prompt recognition and vigorous therapy. Infectious disease consultants, state and local health departments, and the centers for disease control (CDC, Atlanta) can provide valuable expert assistance and should be contacted early on.

Infection with *P. vivax, ovale,* or *malariae* usually responds readily to standard oral therapy, and most authorities feel that such patients can safely be treated on an outpatient basis with close follow-up over the next 24 hours. Referral to a practitioner with interest and expertise in infectious diseases or malaria or both is indicated. Criteria for hospital admission and inpatient therapy include severe dehydration, inability to tolerate oral medications, central nervous system symptoms, preexisting severe medical illness, and cases in which the diagnosis or patient reliability is questionable. Consideration should be given to transferring severely ill patients with multiple organ system involvement to tertiary care facilities in the event that prolonged support (ventilatory or dialysis) or specialized therapy (exchange transfusions) is needed.

The chemotherapy of malaria has changed markedly over the past 20 years, owing to resistance of the parasites to standard antimalarial agents. Countries reporting chloroquine-resistant *P. falciparum* are shown in Table 1. Information regarding commonly used antimalarial drugs and current recommendations for therapy and prophylaxis are summarized in Tables 2 and 3, although it is advisable to check with the CDC for the most recent treatment regimens. Chloroquine remains the drug of choice for infections with *P. vivax, ovale,* and *malariae,* and resistance to this drug has yet to be reported with these species. Chloroquine and other schizonticidal agents are ineffective against exoerythrocytic forms of *P. vivax* and *P. ovale,* and therapy with primaquine phosphate is needed to prevent relapse after chloroquine therapy. Glucose-6-phosphate dehydrogenase (G-6-PD) activity must be determined prior to therapy with primaquine, and dosage must be modified in enzyme-deficient patients to prevent hemolytic crises.

Cases of falciparum malaria or severely ill individuals in whom the species is unknown are probably best treated with quinine, given the now widespread incidence of choroquine-resistant *P. falciparum.* Alternative therapy with pyrimethamine and or sulfadoxine (Fansidar—released in the United States in 1982) is possible in such cases, although scattered reports of resistance to this agent when used alone have already appeared. Therapy with primaquine is not necessary in confirmed cases of *P. falciparum* malaria given the absence of prolonged exoerythrocytic forms with this species. Both chloroquine and quinine can be given parenterally when the patient is unable to take oral medications, but careful monitoring is essential to prevent life-threatening hypotension or arrhythmias. When standard parenteral agents have been unavailable, therapy with intravenous quinidine has been used with reported success. Supportive therapy for the malaria patient includes maintenance of fluid balance, blood component therapy when indicated, exchange transfusion in overwhelming infection, and ventilatory or dialysis support in the event of respiratory or renal failure.

The most important phase of malaria control in this country is adequate prophylaxis. The physician who advises travelers must be acquainted with the various species causing malaria and drug resistance in the areas to be visited. Again, complete adherance to standard prophylaxis will not prevent infection with resistant strains of *P. falciparum* or relapse from exoerythrocytic forms of *P. vivax* or *P. ovale.*

In conclusion, the emergency physician must maintain a high index of suspicion for malarial infection in individuals arriving in the United States from endemic malaria regions. The travel history is an important part of the evaluation of fever without an apparent source and only takes a few moments. Malaria is an exotic though easily treated illness that may prove fatal if unrecognized.

SUGGESTED READING

Spencer HC, Strickland GT. Malaria. In: Strickland HC, ed. Hunter's tropical medicine. 6th ed. Philadelphia: WB Saunders 1984.
Stair T, Ricci R, et al. Malaria in the emergency department. Ann Emerg Med 1983; 12:422–425.
Wiley DJ. Malaria. In: Mandell GL, Douglas RG, Bennett JE, eds. Principles and practice of infectious disease. 2nd ed. New York: J Wiley & Sons, 1985.

HERPESVIRUS

GEORGE L. STERNBACH, M.D., F.A.C.E.P.

HERPES SIMPLEX

Manifestations

Infection with herpes simplex virus produces a variety of clinical syndromes. Among these, dermatitis involving either genital or nongenital areas, vulvovaginitis, and gingivostomatitis are most likely to be encountered by the emergency physician. Less common manifestations include eczema herpeticum, keratoconjunctivitis, meningoencephalitis, and disseminated visceral infection.

Eczema herpeticum is a diffuse form of cutaneous herpes simplex infection most commonly seen in children. Lesions of vesicular and crusting eruptions appear most consistently on eczematous skin, particularly on the face. Patients with atopic dermatitis are involved chiefly, but the condition may be seen in children with other skin disorders. Lesions may appear in areas of normal skin. High fever, restlessness, and irritability may accompany the eruption. The severity of the condition is variable, but it may be fatal. Secondary bacterial infection is common.

Disseminated herpes infection to the viscera and generalized cutaneous involvement may be seen in patients who are immunocompromised, including those with the acquired immunodeficiency syndrome (AIDS). Such infection is potentially fatal in these patients.

The hallmark of cutaneous herpesvirus infection is the presence of grouped vesicles on an erythematous base, usually localized in a nondermatome distribution. Prodromal symptoms occur from 3 to 7 days following exposure. Pain, hyperesthesia, burning, or paresthesias at the skin site may precede the appearance of lesions. Headache, fever, tender lymphadenopathy, and generalized aching may also be present. Prodromal symptoms tend to be absent or substantially less severe in recurrent infections. The disease is definitely transmissible whenever lesions are present, so patients should be advised to avoid sexual activity during this time. However, the virus may be shed even during times when skin lesions are absent.

The differential diagnosis of genital herpes simplex infection includes syphilis, lymphogranuloma venereum, granuloma inguinale, chancroid, herpes zoster, and erythema multiforme. Gingivostomatitis due to herpes may be confused with aphthous stomatitis, Vincent's angina, candidiasis, herpangina, and erythema multiforme. Pharyngeal involvement may produce a picture similar to that of streptococcal pharyngitis or infectious mononucleosis.

Viral culture may confirm a diagnosis suspected on clinical grounds. Virocult collection kits should be used to collect material from early active lesions. Results may be available 24 hours after incubation is initiated. The cost of herpes simplex viral culture is approximately $50.

The presence of multinucleated giant cells on Tzanck smear may affirm the presence of herpes infection. Tzanck preparation is performed by scraping the base of a previously intact vesicle with a No. 15 scalpel blade, and by applying the material onto a microscope slide, and staining with Giemsa, Wright's, or toluidine blue stain. Multinucleated giant cells may also be encountered in other viral vesicular diseases, such as herpes zoster and varicella. Although a positive Tzanck smear confirms the presence of herpetic infection (assuming a compatible clinical picture), a negative result does not exclude it.

Treatment

Application of the topical antiviral agent acyclovir (Zovirax) to lesions of initial episodes of genital herpes simplex infection reduces the duration of viral shedding, accelerates lesion healing, and shortens the duration of symptoms. However, such treatment does not prevent the development of recurrent infection and should not be considered curative. Five percent acyclovir ointment should be applied to lesions every 3 hours for 7 days. Alternatively, oral acyclovir, 200 mg 5 times per day for 5 to 10 days may be administered.

When applied to recurrent lesions, acyclovir may arrest their development and speed healing. Efforts have been made to prevent recurrent infection through the prophylactic administration of oral acyclovir. However, the effects of prolonged administration of the drug are unknown, and

such use should be considered investigative. There has been benefit found by some investigators in the topical application of acyclovir to lesions of recurrent herpes infection of the lips and perioral area, but this therapeutic efficacy has been disputed by others.

An intravenous form of acyclovir is available, which should be reserved for patients with eczema herpeticum and for immunocompromised patients with herpes simplex infection. The dosage of intravenous acyclovir is 5 mg per kilogram infused over 1 hour every 8 hours. Hospitalization of such patients is required.

Intravenous acyclovir may also be used for treatment of herpetic meningoencephalitis. This is the most common and lethal form of nonepidemic encephalitis in the United States. However, initiation of treatment should await definitive diagnosis, which requires hospitalization.

Herpetic keratoconjunctivitis may be treated with the topical application of idoxuridine (IDU). A drop of 0.1 percent solution should be instilled every 2 hours, day and night. Alternatively, IDU 5 percent ophthalmic ointment may be applied 5 times per day. Ophthalmologic consultation should be obtained in suspected cases of herpes simplex infections of the eyes. Oral acyclovir is not effective in this situation.

VARICELLA

Manifestations

Varicella, or chickenpox, is a common childhood infection that also occasionally affects adults. It is produced by the herpes zoster virus. The illness is self-limited and usually runs a benign course, especially in children. The hallmark of varicella is the appearance of skin lesions in various stages of development (papules, vesicles, crusted, and umbilicated lesions) in a single region of the body. Complications include encephalitis, pneumonia, and bacterial superinfection.

Treatment

There is no specific therapy for varicella. Aspirin may be administered for fever or myalgia. Oral antihistamines (diphenhydramine, 25 to 50 mg 3 to 4 times a day for adults, 5 mg per kilogram per day for children or hydroxyzine hydrochloride, 50 to 100 mg 4 times a day for adults, 50 mg a day in divided doses for children under 6 years) are helpful for controlling pruritus. Topical application of calamine lotion or baths in colloidal oatmeal (Aveeno) may likewise relieve itching.

Secondary bacterial skin or subcutaneous tissue infection should be treated with systemic antibiotics. Dicloxacillin, 250 mg every 6 hours for adults, 25 mg per kilogram per day for children, is recommended. Cephalexin (Keflex) may be used as an alternative, at the same dosage.

The treatment for varicella encephalitis is supportive. Similarly, there is no specific treatment for varicella pneumonia unless complicated by bacterial superinfection.

Children exposed to varicella who have a malignancy or who are immunocompromised should be given zoster

TABLE 1 Criteria for Administration of Zoster Immune Globulin

One of the following underlying illnesses or conditions:
  Leukemia or lymphoma
  Congenital or acquired immunodeficiency
  Under immunosuppressive medication
  Newly born of mother with varicella

One of the following types of exposure to varicella or zoster:
  Household contact
  Playmate contact (1 hour play indoors)
  Hospital contact (in same room or adjacent beds in a large ward)
  Newborn contact (mother contracted varicella from 4 days before to
    48 hours after delivery)

Negative or unknown prior disease history

Age younger than 15 years

Treatment initiated within 72 hours of exposure

immune globulin (ZIG). This product prevents varicella in normal children and has been found to reduce the morbidity and mortality of the disease among immunocompromised children. The criteria for administration of ZIG are listed in Table 1. Recommended dosage is 1.25 ml per 10 kilograms or fraction thereof, to a maximum of 5 ml, given by intramuscular injection.

HERPES ZOSTER

Manifestations

Herpes zoster, or shingles, is an acute infection in individuals who have previously been infected with chickenpox. Patients typically develop pain in a dermatomal distribution 1 to 10 days before the appearance of the rash. The eruption consists of grouped vesicles on an erythematous base involving one or several dermatomes. Thoracic or abdominal dermatomes are involved in the majority of cases. In instances in which the patient presents before the appearance of the rash, the clinical presentation may mimic that of other causes of chest or abdominal pain, such as angina pectoris, pericarditis, perforated peptic ulcer, appendicitis, and biliary of renal colic.

Herpes zoster has a very low mortality rate, even when disseminated. Complications include meningoencephalitis, myelitis, ophthalmic involvement, and postherpetic neuralgia. Herpes zoster that presents in several dermatomes or is disseminated should raise the suspicion of underlying immunocompromise, such as AIDS or occult malignancy.

Treatment

Treatment is rarely necessary. Analgesics containing codeine may be prescribed as necessary. Burow's solution compresses, 1:20 to 1:40 diluted in water, may be applied to hasten drying of lesions. Topical application of 5 percent acyclovir ointment may reduce pain and accelerate skin lesion healing. Although herpes zoster is not a specific indication for the use of oral acyclovir, this drug would be expected to reduce the duration and severity of infection.

Ocular complications occur in one-third to one-half of cases involving the ophthalmic division of the trigeminal nerve. Ophthalmologic consultation should be obtained in these cases. Treatment of herpetic keratitis with topical IDU and cytosine arabinoside has also been carried out.

Neuralgia that persists after the healing of skin lesions occurs more frequently in older (over 60 years) and immunosuppressed patients. Such pain may be prolonged and extremely severe. Although standard codeine-containing analgesics are commonly administered for this, the pain is frequently refractory to such treatment. There are those who favor the administration of corticosteroids to relieve pain of postherpetic neuralgia. The use of such medication is controversial, and steroids have not been shown to eradicate pain in all patients. Prednisone, 40 mg daily, may be administered for 10 days, with gradual tapering of the dosage carried out over 3 weeks. The use of other medications in treatment and prevention of postherpetic neuralgia is currently under investigation.

SUGGESTED READING

Corey L, Benedetti JK, Critchlow CW, et al. Double-blind controlled trial of topical acyclovir in genital herpes simplex virus infections. Am J Med 1982; 73:326–334.

Keczkes K, Basheer AM. Do corticosteroids prevent postherpetic neuralgia? Br J Dermatol 1980; 102:551–555.

Orenstein WA, Heymann DL, Ellis RF, et al. Prophylaxis of varicella in high-risk children: dose-response effect of zoster immune globulin. J Pediatr 1981; 98:368–373.

Straus SE, Rooney JF, Sever JL, et al. Herpes simplex virus infection: biology, treatment and prevention. Ann Intern Med 1985; 103:404–419.

RABIES

DANIEL B. FISHBEIN, M.D.

Rabies is an infection of the central nervous system caused by a number of antigenically related RNA viruses. Rabies viruses make up a species in the genus *Lyssavirus* of the family Rhabdoviridae. Clinical rabies has become extremely rare in the United States in the past 25 years, with an average of two cases reported each year. However, rabies should still be considered in the differential diagnosis of any patient with encephalitis of unknown etiology, even if no exposure is reported. Rabies, almost uniformly fatal after the onset of clinical illness, can be prevented by proper postexposure therapy during the incubation phase. Each year, approximately 25,000 persons in the United States receive rabies postexposure prophylaxis. Many more persons than this present to health care providers each year for evaluation of animal bites, and each evaluation should involve a decision as to whether postexposure prophylaxis is indicated.

THE DISEASE IN HUMANS

Human rabies is an almost invariably fatal disease that is rarely seen in the United States. Its division into five phases is useful in both understanding the pathophysiology of the disease and approaching the patient in whom the diagnosis of rabies is being considered. The *exposure* (introduction of the virus into the host) is followed by an *incubation phase*, during which there are no symptoms or signs of disease. During the incubation phase, which lasts from 9 days to 2 years (usually 1 to 3 months), the infection may terminate naturally or as a result of immunization. As the virus invades the central nervous system, a *prodromal phase* begins and is manifested by one or more nonspecific symptoms (fever, anorexia, headache, malaise). In about half of the cases there may also be a specific symptom, pain or paresthesias at the bite site. The *prodromal phase* lasts 2 to 10 days. It is followed by an *acute neurologic phase*, lasting 2 to 7 days. This phase is dominated by neurologic signs (hyperventilation, aphasia, incoordination, paresis, hydrophobia, pharyngeal spasms, confusion, delirium, hallucinations, hyperactivity). A *coma phase* follows, and usually begins abruptly with respiratory arrest. This phase almost always terminates within 14 days with death, but very rarely, a *recovery phase* may occur. Deviation from these phases is unusual and almost always indicates a diagnosis other than rabies. If clinical rabies is suspected, state health departments should be consulted immediately for assistance in diagnosis and institution of proper isolation measures.

DETERMINING THE NEED FOR RABIES PROPHYLAXIS

The decision whether to administer rabies postexposure prophylaxis can be based on an algorithmic analysis of the circumstances of the individual exposure (Fig. 1). Substantial savings result from administering postexposure prophylaxis (the cost of which ranges from $380 to $500) only when strictly indicated.

First, the physician must determine whether the patient has been exposed to the rabies virus. Exposures may occur in two ways. A *bite exposure* is a penetration of the skin by the teeth with the introduction of potentially infectious saliva into the wound. Bite exposures are the cause of nearly all human rabies cases. A nonbite exposure is a contamination of a scratch, abrasion, mucous membrane, or open wound (one that has been bleeding within the previous 24 hours) with potentially infectious material, such as saliva or central nervous tissue. Unusual nonbite exposures that have caused rabies include aerosol exposures in bat caves and rabies research laboratories and corneal transplants. Casual contact, such as petting a rabid animal, does not constitute an exposure. If no exposure has occurred, postexposure prophylaxis is not necessary, but many patients may require reassurance to allay the fear of rabies.

Once it has been determined that an exposure has occurred, the physician must then determine the risk of rabies in the animal species implicated and the geographic area involved. Carnivorous wild animals (especially skunks, raccoons, foxes, coyotes, and bobcats) and bats are the animals most commonly found infected with rabies and have caused most of the indigenous cases of human rabies in the United States since 1960. If the exposing animal is a dog or cat, every effort should be made to place the animal under observation. If the dog or cat remains healthy during a 10-day holding period, no treatment is necessary. If available, all other animals (wild and domestic) should be subjected to euthanasia and their brains examined for rabies virus antigen by trained personnel using direct fluorescent antibody techniques.

The geographic area in which the exposure occurred should be considered. In some parts of the United States, the risk of rabies in dogs, cats, and some terrestrial mammals is negligible, and postexposure treatments may be unnecessary. One state (Hawaii) and some countries of the world (e.g., Australia) are considered rabies free.

Finally, the circumstances of the bite (provoked or unprovoked) can be taken into consideration. In almost every state, local or state health officials provide 24-hour emergency consultation to health professionals. These consultants are best able to evaluate the exposure because they can take into account the exposing species, the circumstances of the bite, and the local rabies situation.

PROPHYLACTIC TREATMENT

The essential components of rabies postexposure prophylaxis are local treatment of the wound and immunization, including the administration, in most cases, of both human rabies immune globulin (RIG) and vaccine. Postexposure prophylaxis should be initiated as soon after the exposure as possible. In circumstances of low risk, treatment with RIG and vaccine may be delayed for up to 48 hours pending the outcome of a fluorescent anti-

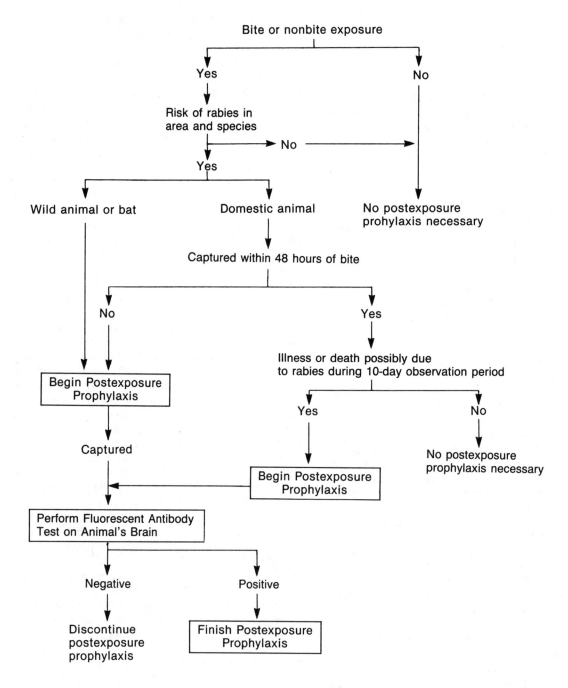

Figure 1 Algorithm for human rabies postexposure prophylaxis.

body examination of the animal brain. If there has been a long delay since the exposure, postexposure prophylaxis (with both RIG and vaccine) should still be instituted, unless clinical rabies has developed.

Local wound care is the first step in preventing rabies and should be administered as soon after the exposure as possible. Immediate and thorough washing of all bite wounds and scratches with soap and water is perhaps the most effective measure in preventing rabies and has been shown to reduce markedly the likelihood of rabies in experimental animals. Tetanus prophylaxis and measures to control bacterial infection should be administered as indicated.

After local wound care, at the time postexposure treatment is begun, RIG is administered once, in a dose of 20 IU per kilogram (9.1 IU per lb). If anatomically feasible, up to half of this dose should be infiltrated into the area of the wound. The rest should be administered intramuscularly in the gluteal area or lateral thigh (in divided doses if necessary). In small children and infants, the anterolateral aspect of the upper thigh is the preferred site for RIG. Human diploid cell rabies vaccine (HDCV) is the only type of rabies vaccine currently licensed in the United States. HDCV should be given intramuscularly in the deltoid muscle in adults and children and in the anterolateral aspect of the upper thigh in infants. The gluteal area should not be used. The first 1.0-ml dose of HDCV is administered at the same time as RIG at the beginning (day 0) of postexposure therapy. *HDCV should never be administered into the same anatomic location as RIG.* One additional 1.0-ml dose of HDCV should be given on each of days 3, 7, 14, and 28 for a total of five doses. The vaccine dosage is not modified for infants or children. Because the antibody response following the recommended vaccination regimen with HDCV has been so satisfactory, routine postvaccination serology is not recommended except in unusual circumstances (such as when the patient is known to be immunosuppressed). State health departments should be contacted in these circumstances.

Persons who either have previously received preexposure or postexposure immunization with HDCV or have a documented history of positive antibody response to a prior vaccination with any other type of rabies vaccine require only two doses of HDCV. They should receive one 1.0-ml dose intramuscularly on each of days 0 and 3.

If postexposure treatment is initiated outside the United States with locally produced biologics, it may be desirable to provide additional treatment when the patient reaches the United States. State health departments should be contacted for specific advice in such cases.

Preexposure Immunization

Preexposure immunization is offered to persons who are at high risk of an inapparent exposure to rabies and to persons whose postexposure therapy might be expected to be delayed. Preexposure immunization does not eliminate the need for prompt postexposure prophylaxis following an exposure, but it does eliminate the need for RIG and reduces the number of doses of vaccine needed from five to two. Preexposure prophylaxis consists of three 1.0-ml intramuscular doses or three 0.1-ml intradermal doses of HDCV, one on each of days 0, 7, and 28. The HDCV produced by Merieux Institute has been approved for preexposure immunization when administered with a specially designed syringe containing a single 0.1-ml dose of HDCV. The 1.0-ml vial currently available is not approved for intradermal preexposure immunization.

Adverse Reactions and Contraindications

Because the risk of rabies is always more serious than the risk of vaccination, postexposure prophylaxis is not contraindicated in pregnant women or in persons with history of an allergic reaction to HDCV. Reactions after vaccination with HDCV are less common than with previously available vaccines. Local reactions, such as pain, erythema, itching, and swelling at the injection site, are common. Mild systemic reactions are reported by up to 50 percent of recipients of postexposure prophylaxis with RIG and HDCV and may include headache, nausea, abdominal pain, muscle aches, and dizziness. Two cases of neurologic illness resembling Guillain-Barré syndrome that resolved without sequelae in 12 weeks, and a focal subacute central nervous system disorder temporarily associated with HDCV vaccine, have been reported. An "immune complex-like" allergic reaction has been noted in about 6 percent of persons who had received HDCV in the past and who subsequently received a booster dose of HDCV. The illness, which occurs 2 to 21 days after the booster dose, is characterized by a generalized pruritic rash or urticaria and may also include arthralgias, arthritis, angioedema, nausea, vomiting, fever, and malaise. In no vaccine recipient has the resulting illness been a threat to life. Symptoms are usually relieved by standard doses of antihistamines, but on rare occasions epinephrine and corticosteroids have been required. If a true rabies exposure has occurred and an allergic reaction develops during the course of vaccination, postexposure therapy should be continued in the proper medical setting.

SUGGESTED READING

Baer GM, ed. The natural history of rabies. New York: Academic Press, 1975.

Bernard KW, Hatwick MAW. Rabies virus. In: Mandell GM, Douglas F.G, Bennett JE, eds. Principles and practice of infectious disease. New York: John Wiley & Sons, 1984.

Centers for Disease Control. Rabies Prevention—United States, 1984. MMWR 1984; 33:393–402, 407–408.

RICKETTSIOSIS

THEODORE E. WOODWARD, M.D., D.Sc.(Hon)

Rickettsiae cause three major groups of illness: the spotted fevers (including Rocky Mountain spotted fever), the typhus group (including classic typhus and murine typhus), and Q (query) fever. Rash is a characteristic feature of all except Q fever. Table 1 outlines the salient features of the major rickettsial diseases. The following discussion focuses on the rickettsial diseases causing rash that are most common in the United States.

DIAGNOSIS

Differential Diagnosis

The suspicion of Rocky Mountain spotted fever (RMSF) should be raised for a patient with fever, prostration, headache, and a history of tick bite or tick exposure while engaged in work or recreation in a rural or wooded area of known endemicity. Early in the febrile illness before the rash has appeared, differentiation from other acute infections is confusing. The rickettsial rash is initially pink and macular, fades on pressure, and becomes petechial or ecchymotic more slowly over several days. This exanthem is not sensitive to palpation. Meningococcemia and measles are common misdiagnoses.

The rash of meningococcemia simulates RMSF and epidemic typhus in certain features because it may be macular, maculopapular, or petechial, in acute or subacute forms and either petechial, confluent, or ecchymotic in more acute types. Usually the hemorrhagic, purplish, necrotic exanthem develops rapidly in fulminant meningococcemia and is tender to palpation. Significant leukocytosis favors meningococcal infection. The features of gonococcemia resemble those of meningococcemia.

Measles, more often an autumn- and winter-occurring illness, is associated with coryza, cough, conjunctival injection and photophobia, and a characteristic cephalocaudal progression of the rash. It appears about 3 days after onset; first in the face and neck as pink macules, and soon becomes maculopapular and extends within a day or 2 to the trunk and extremities. Petechiae or ecchymoses may occur; Koplik's spots are distinctive. In rubella (German measles), the rash is frequently a flush, not unlike scarlet fever, which soon spreads from the face and neck to the trunk and extremities. It is less extensive and of shorter duration than measles with mild constitutional manifestations. Postauricular adenopathy and absence of Koplik's spots suggest rubella.

The initial lesions of varicella or variola are first exanthematous and later become vesicular. Rose spots in the typhoid fevers are usually on the upper abdomen and lower chest and remain delicate, without hemorrhagic characteristics. The macular lesions in RMSF, in contrast to those in typhoid, begin on the periphery of the body and later become petechial. The rash of infectious mononucleosis (uncommon except when associated with sensitivity to drugs) is usually morbilliform on the trunk and rarely becomes petechial. In pharyngitis, the presence of a whitish membrane, lymphadenopathy, and atypical lymphocytes in the blood are differentiating features.

Drug rashes, including that of erythema multiforme, often cause fever. Such patients are less toxic in their appearance than are those of RMSF, and the rash is frequently diffusely erythematous; the individual lesions are larger, raised, and vesicular.

Epidemic typhus frequently causes all of the pronounced clinical, physiologic, and anatomic alterations noted in cases of RMSF: hypotension, peripheral vascular failure, cyanosis, skin necrosis and gangrene of digits, renal failure with azotemia, and neurologic manifestations. However, the rash of classic typhus occurs initially in the axilla and on the trunk and later extends peripherally, rarely involving the palms, soles, and face. Classic or epidemic typhus occurs in the United States as Brill-Zinsser disease (recurrent epidemic typhus fever) and an endemic type associated with contact with flying squirrels. Each is usually milder than cases of classic typhus.

Murine typhus is a milder disease than RMSF and epidemic typhus, the rash is less extensive, nonpurpuric, and nonconfluent, and renal and vascular abnormalities are uncommon. Differentiation between these three major rickettsial diseases must often await the results of specific serologic tests.

An illness that simulates RMSF is caused by *Rickettsia canada*, a member of the typhus group. Rickettsialpox, caused by a member of the spotted fever group of organisms, is easily differentiated from RMSF by the initial lesion, the relative mildness of the illness, and early vesiculation of the maculopapular rash.

Q fever is the one rickettsial infection unassociated with a rash. Usually the illness is mild to moderate. It is manifested by fever for about a week to 10 days, severe headache, and pneumonitis in about 50 percent of cases. The roentgenographic findings are nonspecific and may resemble those of influenza or the atypical pneumonias. Occasionally, a dense infiltrate may suggest a neoplasm. An acute form of hepatitis, with or without jaundice, may progress to chronic granulomatous hepatitis. A chronic form of Q fever endocarditis is becoming clinically significant. In chronic hepatitis or endocarditis, antibodies to phase I antigens are present, which confirms the clinical diagnosis. The Weil-Felix reaction is negative.

Confirmatory Laboratory Diagnosis

In ordinary practice, the available serologic tests are adequate for laboratory confirmation of the rickettsioses provided two and preferably three serum samples are examined during the first, second, and fourth to sixth weeks, of illness. This allows demonstration of a rise in titer of specific antibody during convalescence. None of the tests is available in the emergency department and thus the initial diagnosis to treat with antibiotics is a clinical decision.

Weil-Felix Test

The Weil-Felix test, using *Proteus* strains of OX19, gives positive results in many patients with RMSF and epidemic and murine typhus and negative or nonspecific results in those with rickettsialpox, Q fever, and scrub typhus. A single convalescent serum titer of 160 to 320 is usually diagnostic, but demonstration of a rise in titer is of greater value. False-positive reactions may occur in urinary tract infections or bacteremia caused by *Proteus* organisms and in enteric, relapsing, and rat-bite fevers, leptospirosis, brucellosis, and tularemia.

Complement-Fixation Reaction

Group specific rickettsial antigens clearly differentiate the rickettsial disease group (the typhus fevers, spotted fevers, and Q fever). Complement-fixing antibodies appear during the second or third week in patients who receive no specific therapy and may be delayed when illness is shortened by vigorous antibiotic treatment initiated within several days after onset of fever.

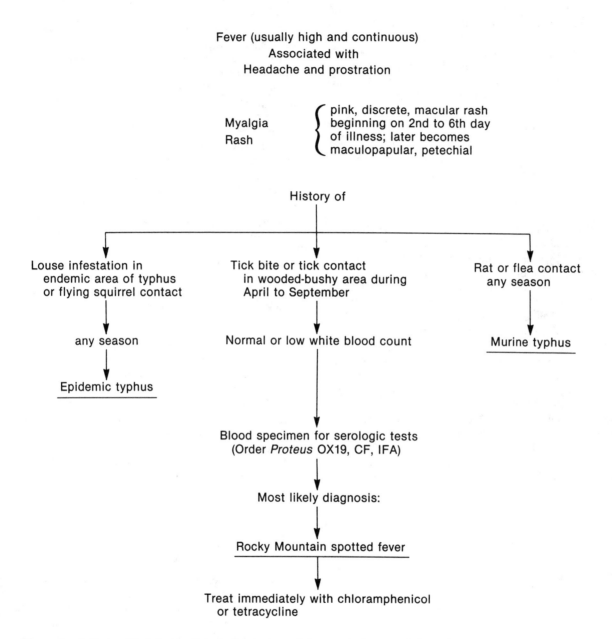

Figure 1. Salient epidemiologic, clinical, diagnostic, and therapeutic features of the major rickettsial disease. *Serology as for Rocky Mountain spotted fever.

Other Specific Serologic Tests

The following serologic tests are more reliable than the Weil-Felix or complement-fixation tests. Specific diagnoses of RMSF, other tick-borne rickettsioses, and the typhus fevers may be achieved by the rickettsial microagglutination and the indirect fluorescent antibody (or hemoagglutination) reactions.

Early Diagnosis by Identification of Rickettsiae in Tissues

Rickettsia rickettsii are identified by the indirect fluorescent antibody reaction in pink macular skin lesions obtained by biopsy as early as the third day or in ecchymotic lesions as late as the tenth day. The organisms show an identifiable morphology and staining properties. This technique may be used with formalized tissue.

THERAPY

There are important physicochemical changes that merit understanding in planning a therapeutic regimen for patients seriously ill with the spotted fever—typhus group of rickettsioses. Often there is circulatory collapse, oliguria, anuria, azotemia, anemia, hyponatremia, hypochloremia, hypoalbuminemia, edema, and coma. Management is much less complicated in mildly and moderately ill patients when these alterations are absent. The principles of treatment of all rickettsioses are specific chemotherapy and supportive care; most patients need hospital admission to the care of an internist or infectious disease specialist.

Specific Treatment

Chloramphenicol and the tetracyclines are specifically effective; they are rickettsiostatic and not rickettsicidal. When therapy is initiated during the early stages coincident with appearance of the rash, there is prompt alleviation of clinical signs. Response is less dramatic when therapy is delayed until the rash becomes hemorrhagic and diffuse.

Optimal antibiotic regimens are chloramphenicol, an initial oral dose of 50 mg per kilogram body weight, or tetracycline, 25 mg per kilogram body weight. Either is acceptable. Subsequent daily doses are calculated as the initial oral dose divided equally and given at 6- to 8-hour intervals. Antibiotic treatment is given until the patient improves and has been afebrile for about 24 hours. In patients too ill to take oral medication, intravenous preparations are employed for the loading and subsequent doses. All patients with rickettsioses respond promptly to antibiotic treatment when it is initiated early in illness, before serious tissue changes have occurred. Clinical improvement is obvious in 36 to 48 hours, with defervescence in 2 to 3 days. In scrub typhus, the response is even more dramatic.

Clinical improvement is slower and fever extends over longer periods in those patients first treated during the latter stages of illness. Large, single oral doses of chloramphenicol (50 mg per kilogram) have been effective in patients with RMSF and scrub typhus, although this regimen is not recommended. A single oral dose of 200 mg of doxycycline (a lipotropic tetracycline derivative that produces sustained high blood and tissue levels) has been shown in field trials to be practically effective for treatment of louse-borne typhus fever.

Tetracycline and chloramphenicol are quite effective for treatment of patients with the acute manifestations of Q fever. Recovery is usually prompt. Endocarditis is difficult to treat because the vegetations are rather large and the broad-spectrum antibiotics are rickettsiostatic and not rickettsicidal. Long-term treatment is necessary; this favors tetracycline as the antibiotic of choice. As a general rule, surgical intervention with valve replacement is necessary for cure. A few patients have recovered following extended antibiotic treatement.

Steroid Treatment

Large doses of adrenal cortical steroids (e.g., prednisone 1.0 mg per kilogram or solucortef 5.0 mg per kilogram) given for about 3 days in combination with specific antibiotics are recommended in patients critically ill with spotted fever or with typhus that is first observed late in the course of severe illness. Temperature abates more rapidly than usual, as do the toxic manifestations. Steroids are not recommended for mild or moderately ill patients.

SYPHILIS

F. MARC LaFORCE, M.D.

Syphilis is a systemic illness with protean manifestations caused by infection with a spirochete, *Treponema pallidum*. Except for rare cases, infections occur as a result of direct contact, usually sexual, with an infected person.

Syphilis can be divided clinically into various stages. The incubation period is usually about three weeks, and the disease is in its *primary stage* when a chancre, a painless shallow ulcer, is noted at the site of inoculation. Chancres heal spontaneously in 4 to 6 weeks, and from 2 weeks to 6 months later, the *secondary stage* becomes evident. This phase is characterized by mucocutaneous and systemic findings. The most commonly recognized lesions are discrete, nonpruritic macules commonly found on palms and soles. Highly infectious lesions may develop on mucous membranes. Other common manifestations of secondary syphilis include lymphadenopathy, anorexia, and a low-grade fever. Virtually any organ system can be involved, and aseptic meningitis, hepatitis, and nephrotic syndrome may result.

After the secondary stage, patients enter a phase of latency, and 10 or more years later about 10 to 20 percent of untreated patients develop central nervous or cardiovascular symptoms of *tertiary syphilis*. Classic neurologic syndromes include general paresis of the insane and tabes dorsalis. The Argyll Robertson pupil, an irregular pupil that does not react to light, but does accommodate, is virtually pathognomonic of tertiary syphilis. Cardiovascular syphilis is manifested by the development of a fusiform aortic aneurysm leading to aortic insufficiency.

Most new cases of syphilis are seen in 15- to 30-year olds, with a third of cases occurring in homosexual men. Because of the protean manifestations, the most prudent approach is to do serologic studies in any sexually active patient with findings consistent with syphilis or with any perplexing illness.

DIAGNOSIS

The clinical diagnosis of primary syphilis may be difficult. There are several other causes for ulcerative genital lesions: trauma, local infection, chancroid, or herpes. For the generalist, it is somewhat pointless to compare various lesions, since syphilitic chancres can range from a papule to a large ulcer, depending on the immune status of the patient and on the size of the inoculum. However, it is important to emphasize that a chancre will develop wherever the inoculation takes place. Therefore, the primary chancre may be found on oral, anal, cervical, or perineal sites. Any newly developed oral, anal, or genital lesion in a sexually active person requires that the diagnosis of syphilis be considered and appropriate darkfield or serologic tests done.

Secondary syphilis can have such a varied presentation that the differential diagnosis is virtually endless. Within the last year I have seen cases of secondary syphilis present as acute hepatitis, optic neuritis, and aseptic meningitis. Nonetheless, most patients have maculopapular skin lesions and lymphadenopathy. Furthermore, all patients with secondary syphilis have positive serologic tests, and thus establishing the diagnosis requires only that the disease be thought of and that serologic tests be obtained. *Any sexually active patient, particularly a male homosexual, with new skin lesions or constitutional symptoms or an undiagnosed illness* should have serologic tests to rule out syphilis.

A diagnosis of syphilis can be made with certainty only by identification of the organism by darkfield microscopy or by serologic tests. *Darkfield microscopy* is useful in examining exudates from chancres. *T. pallidum* can be identified as corkscrew-shaped organisms with a peculiar flexion type of motion at the center of the organism. For the most part, the darkfield technique is available only in venereal disease clinics. The most important *serologic tests* for the diagnosis of syphilis are the VDRL and the FTA-abs tests. The standard nontreponemal test is the Venereal Disease Research Laboratory (VDRL) test. An important modification of this test is the rapid plasmareagin card test (RPR), which can be done in an office or clinic setting. About 80 percent of patients with primary syphilis and virtually all patients with secondary syphilis have a positive VDRL test result. There are several causes of false-positive VDRL tests; however, the more specific FTA-abs test can be used to confirm the presence of syphilis. The most commonly used specific antitreponemal antibody test done today is the fluorescent treponemal antibody absorption (FTA-abs) test. The main use for this test is to verify the diagnosis of syphilis. Once positive it remains positive; therefore, while it is useful in making the initial diagnosis, the fluorescent test has limited value in following patients. The FTA-abs test has not been standardized for cerebrospinal fluid and is not recommended for spinal fluid specimens.

A suggested approach for the use of these tests is as follows:

1. Suspected primary syphilis: do darkfield examination if facilities are available. Draw VDRL specimen. If positive, do FTA-abs to confirm the diagnosis (positive VDRL and negative FTA-abs indicates a biologic false-positive and is not diagnostic of syphilis). If the VDRL is negative, have the patient return in one month to repeat it.
2. Suspected secondary syphilis: draw VDRL specimen. If positive, do FTA-abs to confirm the diagnosis. A negative VDRL rules out secondary syphilis.

TABLE 1 Treatment of Syphilis

Stage	Treatment	Alternative Therapy
Epidemiologic treatment*	Benzathine penicillin G, 2.4 million units IM	
Primary or secondary	Benzathine penicillin G, 2.4 million units IM	Tetracycline, 2 g per day for 15 days Erythromycin, 2 g per day for 15 days
Latent syphilis	Benzathine penicillin G, 2.4 million units IM weekly for 3 weeks	Tetracycline, 2 g per day for 30 days or Erythromycin, 2 g per day for 30 days
Tertiary syphilis	Aqueous penicillin G, 4 million units every 4 hours for 10 days followed by benzathine penicillin G, 2.4 million units IM weekly for 3 doses	

* These are individuals exposed to infectious syphilis (lues) who are felt to be at high risk of developing syphilis.

It must be reemphasized that FTA-abs will remain positive and is not helpful in following a patient who may become reinfected; rather, an increase in the VDRL titer is the important discriminating test.

The diagnosis of tertiary syphilis is made in patients with clinical findings characteristic of neurosyphilis or cardiovascular syphilis who have a positive serum VDRL and FTA-abs. A diagnosis of neurosyphilis should be confirmed with a spinal fluid VDRL. The FTA-abs test should not be done on spinal fluid; careful studies have shown an unacceptably high false-positive rate.

TREATMENT

Penicillin is the drug of choice for syphilis. Suggested treatment regimens are summarized in Table 1. Pregnant patients should receive penicillin according to the stage of the illness. Erythromycin is suggested for those who are sensitive to penicillin.

In treating cases of primary and secondary syphilis it is important that activity of the disease be followed by quantitative VDRL determinations taken on serum speci-mens drawn at 3-, 6-, and 12-month intervals. If treated early, patients with primary and secondary syphilis may become seronegative. Patients with latent or late syphilis may have a fixed VDRL, but usually not above 1:2 dilution. Retreatment should be considered when clinical signs and symptoms of syphilis recur or are sustained or when an increasing titer in VDRL tests is observed.

Treatment of primary and secondary syphilis with penicillin may bring on a systemic reaction called the Jarisch-Herxheimer reaction, characterized by chills, fever, myalgia, and headache about 1 to 2 hours later. Patients should be warned of the reaction and treated with bed rest and aspirin.

It is vital for disease control purposes that positive cases be reported to health authorities. This is important so that contacts may be tested and offered treatment. Several studies have shown that individuals exposed to persons with primary and secondary syphilis have a 20 to 30 percent chance of developing the disease. Thus, as soon as such individuals have been identified, prophylactic therapy is highly recommended along with screening studies.

MANAGEMENT OF THE MUSCULOSKELETAL SYSTEM

WOUND MANAGEMENT

JURIS BUNKIS, M.D., F.A.C.S.
ROBERT L. WALTON, M.D., F.A.C.S.

The phenomenon of healing is manifested by various cellular and intercellular events including epithelization, wound contraction, and collagen synthesis. Wounds heal at their maximum rate only when allowed to do so. An understanding of the basic principles of wound healing and management is necessary to allow the physician to make the right decisions in order to obtain a superior result. The practical management of wounds should be based on knowledge of the nature of the injury, functional anatomy, and the reparative process.

WOUND ASSESSMENT

A pertinent history and physical examination are essential. As with any injury, priorities are given to life-threatening conditions. Regardless of wound appearance, attention must first be directed toward establishing adequacy of airway, ventilation, and circulation. The history should be obtained from the patient or, if unattainable, from a reliable witness. The mechanism of injury should be determined to shed light on the nature and extent of the injury. Is the injury due to an automobile accident, a fall, a stab, or a gunshot wound? Was a pen knife or machine employed? Is the wound due to a bullet from a small-caliber, low-velocity handgun or to a powerful, short-range shotgun blast? Did the patient fall from 3 or 30 feet? Is the injury due to a relatively clean plate glass window or a barnyard pitchfork? How much time has elapsed since the injury? How much blood was lost at the scene? What symptoms—e.g., hemoptysis, dyspnea, hematuria, paresthesia—has the patient experienced?

Alterations in the body's capability to respond to injury may alter the healing process. Stress, diabetes mellitus, malnutrition, bleeding disorders, and immunotherapy or steroid therapy represent systemic factors that may impede wound healing. The presence of other local factors (e.g., peripheral vascular disease, prior radiation therapy, or cutaneous eruptions) that may affect the healing process should also be determined.

A thorough physical examination should be performed. Present comments are limited to examination of the wound, but one must remember to begin the examination with an overall assessment of the patient's nutritional status, vital signs, and other aspects of his general condition.

The examining physician must first ascertain the location of the injury. A stab to the neck, thorax, or abdomen presents a different set of potential problems than does a superficial laceration of the buttocks. Deep lacerations of the extremities also frequently involve important underlying structures. The evaluation and management of deep wounds of the head and neck, extremities, chest, and abdomen are discussed in separate chapters of this book.

The depth of injury—as determined by loss of function of the injured part as well as injury to underlying nerves, blood vessels, ducts, tendons, bones, and joints—should be noted. The location, extent, and cause of the wound indicate which laboratory or radiologic studies are needed.

Gross contamination of the wound or the presence of foreign bodies should be noted, as should the viability of tissues and the possibility of tissue loss.

Careful examination of the wound is imperative for proper diagnosis and management. Such examination is possible only in an appropriate facility equipped with adequate lighting and instrumentation. Frequently, this necessitates taking the patient to the operating room, but universal guidelines cannot be established owing to the variability of standards between different emergency departments. Except under conditions of significant vascular compromise, a tourniquet is helpful in providing a dry field for the controlled evaluation of extremity wounds. Needless to say, sterile technique and gentle handling of tissues are mandatory.

Definitive wound evaluation cannot be performed in an uncooperative patient. It may be necessary to consider restraints, sedation, general anesthesia, or even a delay of the evaluation until more favorable conditions (e.g., sobriety) can be obtained. If anesthesia is given for this purpose, a thorough functional (including neurologic) examination should be performed when possible, prior to administration of the anesthesia.

WOUND CLASSIFICATION

Tissue injury is caused by mechanical forces. Shear, tensile, and compressive forces, alone or in combination, produce predictable patterns of tissue injury. Knowledge of the nature and magnitude of wounding forces allows the prediction of the extent of tissue damage.

Lacerations result from shear forces applied to the skin by sharp objects. Relatively little energy is required to produce such lacerations, and a minimal amount of tissue is injured. Consequently, the general demands for wound healing are easily satisfied, and wound infections are relatively infrequent.

Tensile forces can produce tearing wounds. When tensile force exceeds the elastic yield of tissue, stretching and eventual separation of the parts occur. The extent of injury is greater than in simple lacerations because the amount of energy absorbed by the soft tissue is larger. Such injuries may produce intimal damage in surrounding blood vessels, with subsequent thrombosis and ischemia to the injured parts. The structural integrity of nerves, muscles, ligaments, and tendons may also be disrupted. Such an injury places a greater demand on the biologic process of repair, decreases wound defense mechanism, and enhances susceptibility to infection.

Soft tissue compression and crushing between two opposing forces results in the greatest amount of tissue damage. Hemorrhage occurs in the soft tissues, with subsequent ecchymosis and hematoma formation. Edema affects capillary blood flow and prolongs the inflammatory phase of wound healing. Intimal damage to blood vessels may result in thrombosis and tissue necrosis. If the forces of compression are of significant magnitude, actual separation of the skin and soft tissue can occur to produce a "bursting" or "degloving" injury. Such wounds are markedly impaired in their ability to heal.

Wounds can also be classified, according to the expected level of bacterial contamination, into the following categories: clean, potentially contaminated, or contaminated. A thyroidectomy incision produced under sterile operating room conditions represents an example of a clean wound. Potentially contaminated wounds include those in which a hollow viscus (e.g, gallbladder, trachea, ureter, appendix) has been entered, but gross spillage of infected contents has not occurred. Other examples of potentially contaminated wounds include stab wounds with a kitchen knife and lacerations with glass or other relatively clean objects. Contaminated wounds contain quantitative bacterial counts exceeding 10^5 bacteria per gram of tissue, and the high probability of wound infection exists if such wounds are closed primarily. A puncture wound made with a dirty pitchfork, human bites, and wounds that have sustained gross spillage of infected secretions fall into this category.

For therapeutic purposes, superficial wounds can be classified as being either tidy or untidy. Tidy wounds are caused by sharp objects, result in minimal tissue injury and contamination, and can usually be closed under favorable circumstances. Untidy wounds, however, are manifested by extensive soft tissue injury or contamination and require major intervention to allow satisfactory wound healing. Management of untidy wounds may be influenced by the extent and location of the injury. A physician may be able to surgically convert an untidy wound to a tidy one, and thus permit immediate closure.

ANESTHESIA

Satisfactory anesthesia often must be provided to ensure the patient's comfort while the wound is being assessed and treated. The age and mental status of the patient, as well as the extent of the wound, dictate whether a local, regional, or general anesthetic is preferable. Local or regional anesthesia requires the cooperation of patient, surgeon, and, if present, anesthesiologist.

Frequently, a supplemental tranquilizing agent may be beneficial in an anxious patient. Diazepam (Valium) provides good sedative and amnesic effects, but minimal respiratory and circulatory effects, at the usual dose of 5 to 10 mg. In addition, diazepam increases the threshold to lidocaine-induced seizures. It can be given orally or intravenously. If given intravenously, the injection site should be flushed with normal saline to avoid tissue irritation from the diazepam. Intramuscular administration, which frequently results in erratic absorption, should be avoided.

A "pediatric cocktail" containing meperidine (Demerol), 2 mg per kilogram, chlorpromazine (Thorazine), 1 mg per kilogram, and promethazine (Phenergan), 1 mg per kilogram, is a useful supplement for the pediatric population during suturing of lacerations or other potentially painful procedures. Such a "cocktail," however, should not replace a gentle, personal approach to the patient, and may result in prolonged and excessive sedation.

Local anesthesia is recommended for most minor wounds. The anesthetic agent may be infiltrated directly into the wound to reduce the discomfort associated with injection. Infiltration directly into the wound risks spreading potential infection and should be avoided in heavily contaminated wounds. The pain associated with cutaneous injection is due in part to the stretching of sensory nerve endings in the dermis. This can be minimized by using smaller, more concentrated volumes of anesthetic and slower infiltration rates. The least amount of anesthetic that provides adequate anesthesia should be employed to minimize distortion of important landmarks, particularly when dealing with facial lacerations. In certain critical situations (e.g., in approximating the vermilion border), the key anatomic structures may be approximated with a single 6-0 monofilament suture prior to instillation of any anesthetic solution. Alternatively, methylene blue tattoos can be placed at critical anatomic points prior to injection of the anesthetic agent to allow subsequent accurate alignment.

Hemostasis is frequently achieved following injury by vasospasm, platelet plugging, and fibrin clot formation. Lidocaine and similar anesthetic agents cause vasodilation, which may result in rebleeding. The addition of epinephrine to the local anesthetic solution will overcome this tendency. An epinephrine concentration of 1:80,000 provides as much vasoconstriction as a 1:200,000 solution, but more dilute solutions are virtually ineffective. A 1:200,000 solution is optimal, as it produces maximal vasoconstriction with minimal epinephrine-related side effects.

Epinephrine-containing solutions can severely compromise the local wound defense mechanisms by their vasoconstricting effects, and therefore should not be used in heavily contaminated wounds. Their use is also contraindicated in areas such as fingers and toes, which are supplied by terminal, segmental blood vessels. Epinephrine should also be avoided in patients with heart and peripheral vascular disease.

Signs of toxicity, which are remarkably similar among the different local anesthetic solutions, are always dose-related and include numbness, tingling, diplopia, mental confusion, and convulsions.

Allergy to the ester-linked local anesthetics (e.g., procaine, cocaine) is well documented, and cross-sensitivity exists between the ester-linked moieties. Allergy to the amide-linked local anesthetics (e.g., lidocaine, bupivacaine, mepivacaine) is virtually nonexistent, and most reported reactions are vasovagal in nature. No cross-sensitivity exists between the amide-linked and ester-linked local anesthetic agents.

Limiting the total dose of local anesthetic administered is the surest way to avoid systemic toxicity. The vasoconstrictive effect of epinephrine decreases the rate of anesthetic clearance from the wound, thus adding to the safety margin (Table 1). Should a toxic reaction occur, however, the physician must be prepared to oxygenate the patient and administer intravenous diazepam to increase the seizure threshold to the local anesthetic, and place the patient in the Trendelenburg position to ensure adequate cortical blood flow.

Certain wounds are particularly adapted to *regional anesthetic techniques*. Such techniques allow wider exploration and manipulation of deeper tissues than would be possible with local blocks. Regional techniques also avoid distortion of local tissues and allow precise alignment of injured parts. Regional anesthesia is especially applicable in extremity injuries (e.g., axillary block; isolated ulnar, median, or radial nerve blocks; digital nerve blocks; sciatic or femoral nerve blocks; spinal or epidural anesthesia; Bier blocks). Trigeminal nerve blocks are useful in providing segmental facial anesthesia.

Lidocaine and most other local anesthetics do not provide satisfactory local anesthesia in areas of established infection. Biochemical and physical mechanisms have been postulated for this clinical finding. Local anesthetics which are weak bases, are inactivated by the acidic environment (e.g., increased lactic acid production) found in areas of infection. In addition, diffusion of local anesthetic solution is hampered by loculations and other physical barriers present in infected wounds. If the wound cannot be adequately examined or treatment rendered with either local or regional nerve block techniques, general anesthesia may be indicated. After adequate anesthesia has been achieved, the wound may be examined and definitive management rendered.

WOUND PREPARATION

Hair Removal

Clinical data suggest that preoperative shaving is associated with increased wound infection rates. Depilatory use does not enhance the wound's susceptibility to infection. Although shaving may facilitate wound management, it may invite bacterial proliferation and wound infection if the infundibulum of the hair follicle is injured. This can be avoided by clipping the hair 1 or 2 mm above the skin or by using depilatory agents. Care should be taken to remove all shaved hair from the wound, as any hair left behind in the closed wound will act as a foreign body, in-

TABLE 1 Suggested Maximum Dosages of Local Anesthetics

Agent		mg/kg	Total Dose in Average 70-kg Patient
Lidocaine	With epinephrine	7	500 mg
	Without epinephrine	4	300 mg
Procaine	With epinephrine	14	1,000 mg
	Without epinephrine	8	500 mg
Cocaine		1	70 mg

0.5% = 5 mg/ml, 1% = 10 mg/ml, 2% = 20 mg/ml

viting infection and compromising the wound healing process.

Hair definitely should not be shaved if the laceration traverses the eyebrow or other hair-bearing area. The juncture between the hair-bearing and non-hair-bearing skin presents a critical landmark which allows accurate alignment of wound edges, thereby avoiding a step-off deformity, particularly in the brow line.

Skin Degerming

Although it is possible to sterilize surgical instruments, one cannot completely sterilize the skin of either the physician or the patient without damaging or destroying it. However, skin degerming techniques have been developed to decrease bacterial counts on the physician's hands, within the wound, and on the surrounding skin. A distinction must be made between techniques employed to decrease the resident bacteria on intact skin and those designed to decrease the bacterial contamination of the open wound. One must avoid placing anything into the wound that may cause further tissue injury or impede wound defense mechanisms. In the final analysis, one should avoid placing anything into the wound that one would not place into the conjunctival sac of the eye.

Initial cleansing of the skin surrounding the wound should be carried out by the physician or nurse employing soap, a nonirritating solution, or a fat solvent. Ionic soap and detergents (as found in Betadine Scrub) are satisfactory skin cleansers, but are extremely irritating to the open wound and, if allowed to bathe the wound, actually increases the potential for wound infection. After application to intact skin, the surgical scrub solutions should be removed by thorough rinsing with water. Such cleansing removes transient microflora, gross contaminants, and coagulated blood from the skin surrounding the wound.

A degerming agent should next be applied to the intact skin surrounding the wound. Commonly used solutions include iodine and iodine compounds, hexachlorophine, and alcohol solutions. Povidone-iodine (Betadine) solution, which is nonirritating to intact skin and has a rapid onset of action and a broad antimicrobial spectrum, is the most commonly used skin disinfectant. Such solutions reduce the number of resident and contaminating bacteria on the intact skin surface. If povidone-iodine gains access to an open wound, free iodine can be absorbed, leading to disturbingly high serum levels. When placed in an open wound, antiseptic solutions destroy not only bacteria, but also cells responsible for local defense and tissue repair, and may actually increase the incidence of wound infection. Therefore, such solutions should not be used in open wounds.

Necrotic tissue, exogenous debris, and bacteria promote the development of wound sepsis. A simple wash of the open wound with physiologic saline solution or a balanced salt solution may mechanically remove up to 90 percent of contaminating bacteria. However, normal saline (pH 5.0) may be irritating to the wound, particularly to the intima of blood vessels; lactated Ringer's solution (pH 6.7) is preferable to saline. Antibiotics may be added to the irrigating solution for heavily contaminated wounds.

The efficacy of wound irrigation is related to irrigation pressure. In heavily contaminated wounds, simple irrigation with an Asepto syringe does not adequately reduce the bacterial concentration. Pulsatile pressure delivered at 7 to 10 p.s.i., however, effectively removes debris, including bacteria, from the wound without disseminating microorganisms into the tissues. Irrigation with a 35-ml syringe through a 19-gauge needle produces irrigation pressures of 7 p.s.i., a useful technique in an emergency setting. Higher irrigation pressures are to be avoided, as tissue damage and increased potential for wound infection may result.

Mechanical cleansing of the wound by direct scrubbing techniques is effective for removal of particulate contamination and bacteria, but may further injure local tissues. If mechanical scrubbing is required, a highly porous sponge minimizes tissue trauma. Brushes and low-porosity sponges are apt to inflict further tissue injury in an open wound, but may be required to remove imbedded debris to avoid the persistence of abrasion tattoos. Soaps, detergents, and surgical scrub brushes should not be used in open wounds, as they inflict further tissue injury and decrease the wound's resistance to infection.

Surgical Debridement

Although conservative debridement is recommended for most wounds, it must be adequate. Necrotic wound edges must be debrided, regardless of the location or former importance of the devitalized tissue. Surgical debridement may also be required to remove severely contaminated tissues or wound edges that are so irregular as to make wound closure impractical. Closely parallel lacerations may be converted to a single wound by excising the intervening skin bridge.

The simplest method of debridement is total excision of the wound, creating a surgically clean one, but this should be limited to wounds that do not involve specialized structures. Complete excision of the wound is possible only in regions containing an abundance of soft tissues, such as the thigh or buttocks. Selective debridement of all grossly nonviable tissue is essential in wounds containing vital structures. Under special circumstances, tendons, fascia, or dura of questionable viability may be retained, but must be protected from further injury through desiccation. These structures may survive as free grafts if appropriate wound coverage is provided.

Guidelines for determining tissue viability must be based on careful examination of the wound and sound clinical judgement. A completely reliable test to predict tissue viability has not been perfected, although inspection of the wound with Wood's lamp for fluorescence following an intravenous fluorescein injection does provide a reflection of tissue perfusion at that moment. Especially with burn, crush, and blast injuries, the exact extent of tissue damage may be difficult to determine during the initial evaluation. The diffuseness of the tissue damage makes precise initial surgical debridement impossible. In such circumstances, grossly devitalized tissue should be debrided, but tissue of questionable viability may be initially preserved. The demarcated necrotic tissue can be debrided at a "second look" procedure in 24 to 48 hours.

Avulsed or amputated tissue will become necrotic unless the part can be converted to a graft or the blood supply reestablished. Unless cellular destruction has occurred, avulsed skin can frequently be debrided, defatted, and re-applied successfully as a free graft. Composite tissues rarely survive as free grafts, and microvascular revascularization should be considered if feasible.

Hemostasis

Thorough wound debridement and prevention of fluid collections are primary goals of good wound management. A blood clot acts as a foreign body and provides an excellent culture medium for bacteria within the wound. Hematoma is a common cause of skin graft loss, and its presence beneath a skin flap may compromise the flap's viability. Therefore, every effort must be made to obtain meticulous hemostasis before closing the wound. Even small clots within the deep recesses of a wound may led to fibrosis and palpable thickening in the postoperative period.

Spontaneous hemostasis may occur in an acute wound owing to vasospasm, fibrin deposition, and platelet plugging. If a known vessel traverses the wounded area, it should be examined for injury, regardless of the presence or absence of bleeding at the time of exploration.

Hemostasis can be achieved by the application of pressure or biologic solutions (e.g., crystalline collagen, thrombin solution) to the wound or by direct manipulation of injured vessels. Vessels may be suture ligated, clipped, or electrocoagulated. Vessels larger than 2 mm in diameter should be precisely clamped with as little adjacent tissue as possible and clipped or tied with the finest appropriate ligature to avoid necrosis of a large mass of tissue distal to the tie. Metal and synthetic absorbable (polydioxanone) ligature clips are commercially available. However, sutures and clips are foreign bodies and increase the wound's susceptibility to infection. Braided, nonabsorbable sutures have the highest propensity for infection in contaminated wounds and should be avoided. Quantitative bacterial studies have demonstrated that a single, buried silk suture enhances the possibility of infection by a factor of 10,000 times. Monofilament synthetic sutures are least reactive, but their low friction coefficient makes them unsuitable as ligatures, except in the repair of large vessels. For these reasons, absorbable sutures (e.g., polyglycolic acid, polyglactin, catgut) are recommended for use as suture ligatures in acute wounds.

Smaller vessels may be electrocoagulated. Vessels must be precisely clamped and the minimal amount of electrical energy necessary to provide hemostasism employed. Indiscriminate electrocoagulation results in significant amounts of charred, necrotic tissue within the wound, which increase the wound's susceptibility to infection.

Antibiotics

The reward for meticulous wound debridement and physiologic closure is timely healing without suppuration and rapid restoration of function. Fortunately, most civilian wounds are not heavily contaminated and contain less than 10^2 bacteria per gram of tissue at the time of presentation in the emergency department. Quantitative bacterial studies demonstrate that the critical factor in predicting wound sepsis is the number rather than the type of bacteria remaining in the wound at the time of closure. Infection predictably occurs if wounds containing more than 10^5 bacteria per gram of tissue are closed without adjunctive measures. The most important factor in preventing wound infection is adequate surgical debridement. If the likelihood of wound infection remains high, antibiotic prophylaxis is indicated.

Prophylactic antibiotics markedly decrease the risk of postoperative sepsis if the antibiotic can be delivered before the bacteria arrive in the tissues. For most clean outpatient wounds, prophylactic antibiotics have been proven to be of no benefit. If indicated, antibiotics should be administered promptly in the emergency department following wound evaluation. The effectiveness of antibiotics in preventing subsequent wound infection is markedly reduced by any delay in starting therapy and by delaying wound closure. Prophylactic antibiotics have a negligible beneficial effect if initial administration is delayed 4 hours following injury and bacterial contamination.

Assessment of Degree of Contamination

Wound quantitative bacterial counts give an accurate prediction of subsequent potential for wound infection. Properly managed wounds containing less than 10^5 bacteria per gram of tissue at the time of closure heal per primum without infection. The magnitude of bacterial contamination is provided by knowledge of the mechanism of injury and by the clinical appearance of the wound, but a more definitive assessment of the degree of contamination can be obtained by quantitative microbiologic assays. The "rapid slide technique" can provide the physician with this crucial information within 20 minutes (Table 2).

Clean acute lacerations rarely present with bacterial counts greater than 10^5 bacteria per gram of tissue. Following proper irrigation and debridement, such wounds can usually be closed primarily without risk of infection and do not require prophylactic antibiotic therapy. Wounds resulting from crush or blast injuries, on the other hand, frequently contain large quantities of devitalized tissue, foreign debris, bacteria, and blood clots. The level of bacterial contamination should be determined following irrigation and debridement. If counts greater than 10^5 organisms per gram of tissue persist, but the extent of tissue injury does not contraindicate wound closure, prophylactic antibiotics may allow uncomplicated primary wound closure and healing. A Gram stain from the wound helps to determine the appropriate antibiotics. However, antibiotics are effective in preventing wound infection only if the bacterial levels are less than 10^9 organisms per gram of tissue. If closed, wounds containing greater than 10^9 bacteria per gram of tissue following debridement suppurate regardless of the presence or absence of prophylactic antibiotics. Such grossly contaminated wounds (including those contaminated by feces, pus, or heterosaliva) should not be closed primarily. In such circumstances, the wound should be debrided and topical antimicrobials (e.g., silver sulfadiazine) added to the wound management regimen until bacterial counts drop below 10^5 bacteria per gram of tissue to allow delayed primary closure.

Any wound may provide the portal of entry for *Clostridium tetani*. Nail puncture wounds, splinter injuries, burns, and other traumatic wounds require tetanus prophylaxis (Table 3).

WOUND CLOSURE

Timing of Closure

Time elapsed since injury does not by itself represent a significant determinant for wound closure. The decision to close a wound is predicated on many factors, the most important of which is the level of contamination. The primary goal is to reduce the bacterial inoculum below the critical level of 10^5 organisms per gram of tissue prior to wound closure. However, a laboratory test must not replace sound clinical judgment. When faced with less than ideal circumstances (e.g., retained foreign body, necrotic tissue following debridement) or diminished wound defense mechanism (associated with systemic illness, malnutrition, impaired local blood supply, and so on), primary wound closure may produce disastrous results, regardless of the initial quantitative bacterial counts.

The timing of wound closure represents a compromise between the likelihood of infection and the ability to provide favorable conditions for closure. If appropriate, primary wound closure is clearly advantageous over other methods. An open wound invites fibrous tissue proliferation and contraction, both of which detract from final function and appearance. The wound should not be closed indiscriminately, as infection will defeat any possible gains from primary closure.

If left open, contaminated wounds gradually gain resistance to infection over a 4-day period. After initial debridement, the open wound may be dressed with sterile, fine-mesh gauze. A moist or greasy dressing prevents wound desiccation. The presence of wound debris, drainage, or fever dictates the frequency of dressing changes. On the fourth day, a quantitative bacterial assay helps to determine the appropriateness of wound closure. Following further debridement and antibiotic coverage as necessary, the wound may be closed using

sterile technique. If the wound is not located in a critical area and if it is small, it may be preferable to allow healing by second intention.

The most aesthetically pleasing scars and the most satisfactory return of function usually result from healing by first intention. Anything that interferes with primary healing may result in additional scarring and a less acceptable result. Proper wound debridement, closure, and postoperative management are prerequisites for satisfactory primary healing. Initial wound care has a significant influence on subsequent healing; surgical technique remains the most important determinant of successful wound closure. This includes gentle manipulation of injured tissues, precise sharp debridement, prudent use of electrocautery, avoidance of excessive or strangulating sutures, prevention of tissue desiccation, and diligent postoperative management.

Methods of Closure

The choice of method requires an understanding of the objectives of repair as well as the materials necessary to effect such a repair. The ultimate goal of any closure is to achieve precise tensionless alignment of the injured parts without further injury to adjacent structures. This allows prompt restoration of function and cosmetic appearance.

The choice of appropriate material for wound closure is based on its biologic and mechanical properties as well as characteristics of the tissues being approximated. Composition of the material, strength, knot efficiency, tissue response, and wound location should all be considered. The armamentarium includes a variety of suture materials, stainless steel staples, and surgical tapes. To a degree, however, the choice of material for surgical closure is less important than the surgical technique. Each suture must be properly placed and tied without excessive tension to minimize ischemia of the wound edges. The least reactive and the smallest size and amount of suture material that will adequately effect tissue approximation, particularly in contaminated wounds, should be employed.

The necessity to close individual layers of the wound is based on knowledge of local wound stresses, presence of dead space, and the necessity for accurate approximation of tissues. Dense *connective tissues* (e.g., dermis, fascia, ligaments, tendons) represent the strength layers of any wound closure. These tissues heal slowly, however, and the suture material chosen to approximate them should be capable of maintaining its strength until satisfactory union has occurred. Ideally, such a suture should incite a minimal amount of local tissue reaction. Synthetic, monofilament, nonabsorbable sutures are best suited for this purpose.

Muscle and adipose tissues do not hold sutures well. Closure of these layers is occasionally necessary in order to obliterate dead space. In the laboratory, dead space resulting from tissue loss has been shown to increase the likelihood of infection. However, obliteration of dead space with sutures, enhances the possibility of infection because the sutures act as foreign bodies in the wound. Suturing of the dead space is particularly contraindicated in the closure of contaminated wounds. When necessary, the dead space should be obliterated with a minimal number of loosely tied absorbable sutures.

Skin closure may be performed in layers or by full-thickness percutaneous sutures. Surgical tapes or staples may also be considered. The choice of method depends on the location of the wound, its direction, and local stress factors. Wounds that are oriented in the direction of skin wrinkles are subjected to less tension during healing, and consequently produce a more favorable scar. Examples include transverse lacerations involving the forehead or neck. Wounds that cross the lines of maximal stress are subjected to increased tension during healing and have a propensity to widen and hypertrophy with time. Examples include lacerations over the deltoid region or the cheek. In most situations, the acute wound should be debrided and closed without any attempt at reorientation of the direction of the scar. The scar should be allowed to mature before considering scar revision.

The degree of wound gaping prior to epidermal reapproximation reflects the potential width of the scar. Particularly in areas of high skin tension, layered wound closure is indicated to minimize the final width of the scar.

The dermis should be anatomically realigned with interrupted inverted sutures. A few well-placed 5-0 or 6-0 clear nylon sutures provide adequate reapproximation of the dermal layer until the wound has healed and the scar matured. Dermal nylon sutures, however, may remain palpable or visible through the skin. Catgut sutures, which are made from animal protein (available either in the plain or chromic form), are frequently employed for dermal closure. However, catgut sutures display erratic behavior in loss of strength, absorption, and tissue reaction. For these reasons, many surgeons prefer to use synthetic absorbable sutures (e.g., polyglycolic acid, polyglactin) for dermal reapproximation. Even though these sutures do have longer holding power than catgut, they too lose their holding power before wound maturation is complete. Recent studies with polydioxanone monofilament absorbable sutures have demonstrated prolonged breaking strength retention, a reliable absorption profile, and minimal tissue reaction. Experience with polydioxanone is still limited, but perhaps this suture will prove to be the most appropriate material for dermal approximation. Following closure of the dermis, the strength layer of the wound, the epidermal layer can be adjusted with fine, nonabsorbable, monofilament sutures—chosen for their low tissue reactivity—or surgical tape. If sutures are employed, they should be replaced before the fifth postoperative day with surgical tape to avoid unsightly cross-hatching of the final wound. This method of wound closure is designed to provide the least noticeable scar and is most appropriate for facial lacerations.

Percutaneous sutures that incorporate both the epidermis and dermis and a small amount of underlying subcutaneous tissue are frequently employed to close wounds elsewhere in the body. Such sutures are usually removed 7 to 14 days later. Without dermal support during the subsequent maturation phase, the scar tends to widen and hypertrophy. Here too, however, a layered closure and early replacement of the superficial sutures by surgical tape may minimize the subsequent scar.

Factors in obtaining a satisfactory scar include eversion of the wound edges to effect precise epidermal coaptation and proper suture tension to minimize ischemia of the wound margins. In order to obtain everted wound edges, the sutures must be placed so that the depth of each

TABLE 2 The "Rapid Slide" Bacterial Quantitative Assay

1. Clean the surface of the wound biopsy area with 70 percent isopropyl alcohol.
2. Obtain the biopsy specimen with a 3- or 4-mm dermal punch or with a scalpel. No anesthesia is required for an open wound.
3. After the tissue is weighed, flamed, and diluted 1:10 with thioglycollate (1 ml/g), it is homogenized.
4. Spread exactly 0.02 ml of the suspension with a 20-lambda Sahli-pipette on a glass slide. The inoculum is confined to an area 15 mm in diameter.
5. Oven-dry the slide for 15 minutes at 75 °C.
6. Stain the slide using either a Gram stain or the Brown and Brenn modification for tissue staining, to accentuate the gram-negative organisms.
7. Read the smear under 1.9 mm (magnification × 97) objective and examine all fields for the presence of bacteria.
8. The presence of even a single organism is evidence that the tissue contains a level of bacterial growth greater than 10^5 bacteria per gram of tissue.

TABLE 3 Tetanus Prophylaxis

Type of Wound	Patient Not Immunized or Partially Immunized	Patient Completely Immunized—Time Since Last Booster Dose	
		5 to 10 years	10 years*
Clean minor	Begin or complete immunization per schedule; tetanus toxoid 0.5 ml	None	Tetanus toxoid 0.5 ml
Tetanus prone	Human tetanus immune globulin, 250–500 units; tetanus toxoid, 0.5 ml, complete immunization per schedule; antibiotic therapy as indicated	Tetanus toxoid 0.5 ml; antibiotic therapy if indicated	Tetanus toxoid 0.5 ml; human tetanus immune globulin, 250–500 units; antibiotic therapy if indicated

* No prophylactic immunization is required if patient has had a booster within the previous five years.

bite exceeds its width. It has been clearly shown that the size of suture material employed is not so important as the tightness of the closure or the length of time that the sutures are left in situ. Sutures should be removed before the seventh day to avoid epithelization of the suture tracts with a resultant objectionable (railroad) appearance of the scar.

Monofilament, synthetic nonabsorbable sutures (e.g., nylon, polypropylene) are most frequently employed for percutaneous skin closure. Silk sutures, which are natural fibers, are significantly more reactive and have been shown to increase the incidence of wound infection. Silk should not be used in acute wounds, except occasionally for closure of intraoral mucosal laceration.

Stainless steel sutures, skin clips, and staples have been employed for years because of their presumed inertness. However, studies have suggested slightly increased infection rates, probably owing to the mechanical irritation because of their rigidity. This fact will be of little, if any, clinical significance if the staples are removed before the seventh postoperative day. A number of prepackaged skin staplers are now available. Most staplers are designed to produce an everted skin closure and can do so quickly. The main advantage of staplers is a significant reduction in wound closure time, particularly with extensive lacerations or in such specialized situations as securing multiple skin grafts.

Surgical tapes have the advantage of not requiring anesthesia or painful stimuli during wound closure. Such techniques are particularly attractive in the care of the pediatric population. Taped wounds also have the least propensity for infection. In certain situations, one may close the deeper layers of the wound (including the dermis) with sutures and close the epidermal layer with tape—thus avoiding the need to later remove skin sutures. Microporous, rayon reinforced wound tapes are widely used. Adherence is enhanced if all moisture is removed and the skin defatted with acetone before tapes are applied. Tincture of benzoin may initially enhance tape adherence but it is quickly solubilized by skin oils and loses its adherence capabilities, thus contraindicating its use. However, wound tapes do have significant disadvantages. It is difficult to obtain precise anatomic approximation of the skin edges with surgical tapes, particularly with irregular lacerations. It is impossible to obtain an everted closure solely with tape. Moreover, tape only approximates the superficial portion of the wound and leaves deeper layers vulnerable to biomechanical stresses, which may result in widening and a more prominent scar.

Wound Drains

Justification for drains has been stated to include obliteration of dead space and egress of material foreign or harmful to a particular location. Drains are rarely indicated in the closure of acute superficial wounds. Percutaneous drains constitute foreign bodies, enhance tissue necrosis, and serve as conduits for bacterial contamination. Contrary to popular opinion, drains do not prevent the formation of hematomas or seromas. If good surgical technique has been employed, it is unnecessary to drain most superficial wounds in the acute situation. If bleeding cannot be controlled at the time of operation, delayed primary wound closure should be considered. However, drains may be an important adjunctive measure in the treatment of superficial abscesses. The specific indications for drainage of body cavities and organs are discussed in separate chapters.

DRESSINGS

The physician's responsibilities do not end with wound closure. The physician must provide maximal support of the patient and a suitable environment for satisfactory wound healing, and he must direct the patient's rehabilitation.

Although wound healing may be considered a local phenomenon, the ideal milieu for the wound can only be provided by total patient care. Attention must be paid to associated injuries. In addition, nutrition, blood volume, and oxygenation must be maintained. A social worker may provide valuable assistance to a patient with a physically disabling injury. Likewise, a psychiatrist may help a patient to cope with an altered body image following a disfiguring injury.

The sutured wound should be protected from the environment with a dressing impervious to exogenous microbial contamination. Experimental studies have demonstrated that closed wounds can be infected by surface bacterial contamination within the first 2 or 3 days. Following this period, sutured wounds gain considerable resistance to infection, and dressings no longer serve a protective role. Taped wounds demonstrated superior resistance to infection, becoming resistant to surface contamination within 2 hours following wound closure.

A dressing may serve a number of functions that may contribute to healing. Ideally, a dressing should provide an atmosphere conducive to satisfactory wound healing. The dressing should keep the wound surface free of excess fluids to minimize maceration and bacterial proliferation while avoiding desiccation. The main functions of a dressing may be listed as follows: protection, immobilization, compression, absorption, debridement, medication, and cosmesis. As the wound heals, its needs may change and necessitate a different type of dressing.

Most dressings consist of a contact layer, an absorptive layer, and an outer wrap. Plastic-coated dressings (e.g., Telfa) or gauze impregnated with bismuth ointment (e.g., Xeroform) or petrolatum provides a satisfactory contact layer. A bulky intermediate layer should be applied to absorb wound exudate. A plaster or aluminum splint may be added to the dressing to enhance immobilization.

Dry gauze is frequently applied to a freshly closed wound. Such a dressing will adhere to the epithelium and vascular tissue of the wound and may result in interference with wound healing during dressing changes. Preferably, the contact layer should consist of nonadherent plastic-coated material or gauze impregnated with a bland ointment. This contact layer should be applied as a single sheet to allow continued egress of wound fluid through the contact layer. Fluffed gauze sponges, mechanics' waste, and bulk cotton may be added as an absorptive layer, to allow the dressing to conform to a desired shape, and to provide immobilization of the wounded part. Nonstretchable, firm, roller gauze bandage and adhesive tape complete the typical dressing, thus providing a compact and stable immobilizing influence.

Occlusive tapes limit vapor transmission, promoting tissue maceration and bacterial growth. Porous paper tapes are preferable as they allow moisture to be transmitted through the interstices of the tape, with resultant dry skin beneath the tape, which inhibits bacterial proliferation.

POST-TREATMENT WOUND CARE AND FOLLOW-UP

Certain wounds are not amenable to the satisfactory application of a dressing. It is frequently difficult to apply a conforming dressing to sutured facial lacerations. Meticulous suture line care may provide a reasonable alternative. This involves frequent cleansing with saline or dilute hydrogen peroxide solution to remove adherent coagulum, thus decreasing the likelihood of stitch abscess formation. Following cleansing, a thin layer of antibiotic ointment should be applied to the suture line.

Dressings may also be used to debride an open wound. The traditional wet-to-dry method utilizes avulsion of adherent tissues to provide the debridement. This method is effective if performed properly, but one must remember that the dressing does not discriminate between viable and nonviable tissues and tissue injury results with each dressing change. Moistening the dressing prior to removal defeats the purpose of such a dressing. A wet-to-dry dressing should not be employed in wounds containing viable periosteum, perichondrium, paratenon, or perineurium because such tissues desiccate during the "dry" phase, resulting in further tissue damage.

Enzymatic debridement provides an alternative to the wet-to-dry dressing. An enzyme produced by *B. subtilis* (Travase) is effective in removing particulate necrotic debris and coagulum without producing significant injury to viable tissues.

Medicated dressings are occasionally indicated. Topical antimicrobial agents, particularly silver sulfadiazine (Silvadene) and mafenide (Sulfamylon) are frequently employed to control surface contaminants in chronic granulating wounds. These agents are also useful in the management of partial-thickness injuries or wounds containing marginally viable tissues to decrease the potential for bacterial invasion with subsequent conversion to a full-thickness injury and necrosis. However, topical agents retard wound epithelization and should be discontinued as soon as their objectives have been reached (mainly bacterial counts less than 10^5 organisms per gram of tissue).

A physician should not discount the importance of a neat dressing. To the patient or casual observer, the sight of a wound may be abhorrent and incite fear or anxiety. A carefully applied dressing reassures the patient that the best possible wound care has been provided.

The timing of the first follow-up visit will be determined by multiple factors—the location and complexity of the wound, the potential for infection or other complications, and the ability of the patient to care for the wound and to follow instructions. Generally, patients should see a physician within 48 hours to re-evaluate the wound and answer questions. Subsequent frequency of visits will be determined by the progress of healing.

Immobilization may avert further tissue damage. Immobilization of the site of injury is essential in the management of contaminated wounds because lymphatic flow is thus reduced in the immobilized part, thereby minimizing the spread of wound microflora. Immobilization places the wound at rest, thus decreasing pain and metabolic demands of the tissues. In addition, immobilization may protect the newly formed capillaries from disruption, thus avoiding small clots and allowing the wound to heal more expeditiously. When combined with elevation and pressure, the transudation of fluid is minimized. Immobilization may be aided by bulky dressings, skin tapes, or splints. The length of immobilization varies according to the demands of local tissues and the status of the wound. However, prolonged immobilization may defeat its possible advantages.

One cannot overemphasize the advantage of elevating the injured part to minimize edema with its resultant deleterious effects. This is particularly applicable to extremity injuries. Edema, which has been stated to be "the mother of scar," slows down the machinery of repair and increases fibrous tissue proliferation. Elevation of the wounded part above the level of the heart is the simplest method of limiting the amount of edema. In certain situations, compression of the wound with bulky dressings may subserve the benefits of elevation. However, one must not apply tourniquet-like constriction to proximal parts or distal venous and lymphatic congestion could result. In extremity injuries, compression dressings should extend from the most distal point proximally, but access to the toes or fingertips should be maintained to allow assessment of the neurovascular status. Maximal wound edema occurs within the first 48 hours and gradually resolves over the next week. It may be necessary to adjust an extremity dressing during periods of fluctuating tissue edema.

A clean wound should have very little drainage and require few dressing changes. Unless clinical signs dictate otherwise, the initial dressing should be left intact over most sutured wounds for the first 48 hours. As mentioned previously, sealed wounds will be highly resistant to surface bacterial contamination by this time, and further dressings may be unnecessary. In most clinical situations, the patient with a well-healing wound may shower by the third day. However, wounds that continue to drain serous fluid require continued protection with an appropriate dressing.

LOCAL WOUND INFECTION

RICHARD L. LAMMERS, M.D., F.A.C.E.P.

Infection is a serious impediment to wound healing. Epithelialization is hindered by enzymes released from bacteria and from cells trying to destroy the bacteria. Infection occurs when the number of organisms contaminating a wound exceeds the ability of local and systemic defenses to destroy them. In immunologically healthy patients with simple wounds containing minimally traumatized tissue, wound infection occurs if after wound cleaning the remaining bacterial concentration is greater than or equal to 10^6 per gram of tissue. Impaired local tissue defenses may allow lower levels of bacteria to proliferate to that critical level.

ETIOLOGY AND PATHOGENESIS

Local and Regional Infections

The type of organism contaminating a wound and the depth of contamination determine the clinical characteristics of a wound infection. The majority of wound infections occur within the dermal and subcutaneous layers of skin. The spread of infection is limited vertically by fascia and horizontally by fascial adherence to bone and other prominences.

Introduction of bacteria into the epidermis and dermis may result in pyoderma or other types of impetigo, cellulitis, or erysipelas. Subcutaneous inoculation produces cellulitis and subcutaneous abscesses. Infections confined to the subcutaneous layer and adjacent to the wound are considered local wound infections.

There are many forms of regional infections. Lymphangitis is an inflammation of lymphatic channels (usually in the subcutaneous tissue) and appears as visible red streaks. If infection extends to the fascial cleft between superficial and deep fascia in a compromised host, a spreading, necrotizing fasciitis may develop. Myositis, myonecrosis, and osteomyelitis result from penetration into muscle and bone. Tenosynovitis, bursitis, and septic arthritis usually result from direct injury to these structures, but contiguous spread from a local wound infection is possible. Sepsis and hematogenous seeding of distant organs are rare complications of wound infections.

Microbiology of Wound Infection

The sources of bacteria causing wound infections include the patient's skin, the wounding agent, and the environment in which the wound occurred.

There are wide variations in concentrations of skin bacteria in different locations of the body. Bacterial counts vary depending upon individual hygiene, endocrine changes, exposure of the skin, and anatomic site. The lowest bacterial counts are located on exposed, cool, dry skin surfaces such as the arms and face. In areas with higher temperatures and relative humidities, such as in the mouth, anterior nares, axillae, perineum, and interdigital spaces, colonization by larger numbers of all types of bacteria is found. The scalp and forehead also have high bacterial counts; however, wound infection is less likely in these areas of high vascularity.

The resident flora of the skin consists mostly of diphtheroids and staphylococci. *Staphylococcus aureus* is the most frequent cause of soft-tissue and wound infections. Infections caused by this organism tend to be localized. Initial signs of inflammation are often followed by purulent drainage or abscess formation. Group A streptococcal infections are usually associated with cellulitis, lymphangitis, and lymphadenopathy. Abscess formation is unusual but possible. A thin, watery, purulent exudate is characteristic. Aerobic bacteria are the predominant infecting organisms in lesions on the trunk, axillae, and extremities. Anaerobic and mixed anaerobic and aerobic infections tend to occur in perineal regions. Other bacteria causing local wound infections are listed in Table 1.

Bite wounds and wounds occurring in certain environments may result in unusual types of local infections. There are large numbers and a wide variety of species of microorganisms found in the human mouth. The more common organisms include *Staphylococcus* and *Streptococcus* species, anaerobic micrococci, enterococci, peptostreptococci, *Veillonella alcalescens, Actinomyces israelii,* lactobacilli, enterobacteriaceae, *Bacteroides* and *Treponema* species, *Eikenella corrodens, Fusobacterium nucleatum, Candida albicans,* and *Streptococcus viridans.* All these organisms can be found in human bite infections.

Pasteurella multocida is an organism commonly found in the upper respiratory tracts of cats and less commonly in dogs. Infection with this organism produces inflammation, ulceration, and a small amount of gray, seropurulent drainage. This may progress to a rapidly spreading cellulitis with associated lymphangitis and lymphadenopathy, or it may result in local necrosis and abscess formation. This infection may manifest only as delayed healing.

Infections occurring in wounds exposed to a marine environment may involve the organisms listed in Tables 1 and 2.

The organism infecting a wound sometimes can be deduced from the mechanism of injury. Lymphangitis

TABLE 1 Bacteria Causing Local Wound Infection

Staphylococcus aureus	*Enterobacter*
Group A *Streptococcus*	*Pseudomonas aeruginosa*
Staphylococcus epidermidis	*Serratia*
Streptococcus faecalis	*Proteus mirabilis*
Streptococcus pneumoniae	*Klebsiella*
Peptostreptococci	*Bacteroides sp.*
Escherichia coli	*Clostridium sp.*

TABLE 2 Marine Bacteria Causing Wound Infection

Aeromonas hydrophila (fresh water)	*Vibrio sp.*
Providencia stuartii	*Acinetobacter*
Streptococcus sp.	*Mycobacterium marinum*
Pseudomonas putrefaciens	*Bacillus cereus*

resulting from a rodent bite may be evidence of rat-bite fever, an infection with *Spirillum minus* or *Streptobacillus moniliformis*. Painful, regional lymphadenitis 3 to 10 days after an injury, systemic signs, and a papule, vesicle, or small eschar at the site of inoculation are characteristic of cat-scratch fever, an uncommon infection usually following cat scratches or animal bites. Chronic lymphangitis following a minor wound infection on the extremity of a horticulturist, especially with painless ulcerating papules and nodules in a linear distribution, suggests sporotrichosis infection. Bite wounds resulting in suppurative granulomas and chronic wound infections with sinus tracts draining gram-positive sulfur granules are usually a result of actinomycosis. Persistent sinus tracts over an area of infection caused by common pyogenic bacteria suggest the presence of a retained foreign body or underlying osteomyelitis. A chronic wound infection following an injury sustained in a fish tank or in brackish water may be caused by *Mycobacterium marinum*. Nodules or ulcerations with superficial granulation tissue develop at the site of these wounds.

Erysipelothrix insidiosa is a gram-positive rod that lives in soil and decomposed organic matter. Skin infection can occur in patients who have handled dead animal matter, meat, fish or shells. Erysipeloid is an acute but slowly developing infection. A purplish-red, nonvesiculated nodule with an irregular, raised border is characteristic. The lesions itch and burn. Systemic spread is rare but may produce arthritis or endocarditis. Recent studies have demonstrated that *Pseudomonas aeruginosa* resides on the surface of feet. Patients with deep puncture wounds of the feet are particularly at risk for bone infections with this organism.

RISK FACTORS FOR WOUND INFECTION

The primary determinants of wound infection are the amount of bacteria and the amount of devitalized tissue remaining in the wound after cleaning and debridement. Other important factors include the nature of the contamination and the patient's local and systemic resistance to infection.

Devitalized Tissue

A critical number of bacteria must be present in a wound before an infection will develop. More bacteria are needed to produce infection in tidy lacerations that have sustained minimal tissue damage (i.e., 10^6 bacteria per gram of tissue) than in wounds with considerable crushed or devitalized tissue (i.e., 10^4 bacteria per gram of tissue). If the patient's immune system is intact, lesser amounts of bacterial contamination will be contained and infection prevented. Devitalized and necrotic tissue provides a culture medium for bacteria in the wound, hinders leukocyte phagocytosis, and creates an anaerobic environment favorable to certain species of bacteria. Leukocytes have a limit to their capacity to ingest and digest foreign material, devitalized tissue, and bacteria. Their ability to remove bacteria can be overwhelmed by the presence of large amounts of devitalized tissue.

Foreign Bodies

The presence of retained foreign bodies in sutured wounds commonly results in infection. The probability of infection is related to the reactivity of the foreign body. Inert foreign bodies (such as glass or bullet fragments) seldom produce infection by themselves, but they may carry contaminated or chemically reactive particles such as clothing, gun wadding, or soil into the wound. Soil types containing large amounts of infection-potentiating fractions (e.g., clay particles or organic matter) increase infection rates because of the chemical reactivity of these contaminants. In contrast, sand and road grease are relatively innocuous.

Immunologic Competence

Differences in regional blood supply affect infection rates. Ischemic extremities and areas of fibrosis are more prone to infection. Wounds on distal parts of extremities are more likely to become infected than proximal extremity, truncal or facial wounds. The vascularity of the scalp provides some degree of protection from the large numbers of bacteria endogenous to that area.

Factors reducing a patient's immunologic competence or impairing blood flow to the injured area increase the risk of wound infections. Patient age is important in host resistance—those individuals at the extremes of age are at greater risk. Infection rates are reportedly higher in patients with medical illnesses such as diabetes mellitus (particularly when associated with small vessel disease or with hyperglycemia), immunologic deficiencies, malnutrition, anemia, uremia, congestive heart failure, cirrhosis, malignancy, obesity, and in patients taking steroids or immunosuppressive drugs or those receiving radiation therapy. Shock, remote trauma, distant infection, bacteremia, and peripheral vascular disease also increase wound infection rates.

INITIAL WOUND MANAGEMENT

Cleaning and Debridement

Proper wound management can significantly reduce the risk of infection. A patient is at considerable risk of developing a wound infection from the bacteria transmitted by the hands and mouth of medical personnel. Hands should be washed for at least 15 seconds and gloves worn before examining, cleaning, or suturing any wound.

The use of vasoconstrictors in anesthetic solutions increases infection rates. Local infiltration may disseminate bacteria in heavily contaminated wounds; regional anesthesia techniques avoid this danger. Infection rate is higher in wounds that are shaved with a surgical prep razor that has a nonrecessed blade. Several studies have shown that scrubbing with coarse sponges, detergent solutions, and various antiseptics (povidone-iodine 5 to 10 percent solution, povidone-iodine surgical scrub, hexachlorophene, Hibiclens, quaternary ammonium compounds, hydrogen peroxide, acetic acid, sodium hypochlorite, ethyl alcohol, and green soap) destroys tissue and white blood cells, increases infection rates, and prolongs healing. Both Betadine 1 percent solution and Pluronic F-68 (Shur-Clens) are probably safe and effective agents for wound cleansing, although further studies are needed. Pluronic F-68 is nontoxic but nonmicrobiocidal and expensive.

High-pressure irrigation with normal saline delivered by a syringe through a 19-gauge needle or catheter has proved effective in reducing wound infections by removing particulate matter, bacteria, and loosely adherent devitalized tissue without damaging other tissue. Several investigators have added antibiotics to irrigation solutions, including ampicillin, tetracycline, penicillin, kanamycin, cephalothin, cephaloridine, a neomycin-bacitracin-polymyxin combination, and other combinations. In one study, irrigation with antibiotics achieved bactericidal concentrations that outlasted concentrations obtained with systemic adminstration. Complications to date have been unusual; however, aminoglycosides are absorbed from subcutaneous tissues and may cause ototoxic and nephrotoxic complications. Unless sensitization occurs, antibiotic solutions may prove to be less tissue-toxic and more effective in reducing infection in heavily contaminated wounds than dilute povidone-iodine solutions. An optimally bactericidal irrigation solution has not been found. The use of topical antibiotic solutions in clean wounds does not appear to be justified.

Debridement is of unquestionable importance in preventing infection in wounds. Devitalized tissue and tissue contaminated with bacteria or chemically reactive substances can be removed most effectively with this technique. Complete excision of grossly contaminated wounds allows primary closure of such wounds with no greater risk of infection than in relatively uncontaminated lacerations.

The configuration and size of wounds may affect incidence of infection. Bites resulting in puncture wounds are more likely to become infected than are extensive lacerations produced by the same mechanism. Punctures are more likely to penetrate several layers of tissue, depositing bacteria and debris into pockets inaccessible to effective cleansing.

Closure

Closure of contaminated wounds greatly increases the probability of wound infection. Sutured wounds are more likely to become infected than wounds closed with surgical tape, because sutures act as foreign bodies. Infection rates are directly proportional to the number and size of sutures placed in wounds. If stitches are placed too tightly, tissue is strangulated and necroses. The physician should choose the smallest suture that will hold the tissues in place and incorporate no more tissue in a skin stitch than is needed to coapt the wound edges with little or no tension. Absorbable or highly reactive sutures enhance infection more than nonabsorbable synthetic materials. Silk sutures provoke considerably more tissue reaction than absorbable and nonabsorbable synthetic sutures; therefore, silk should not be used as a wound closure material.

Skin and subcutaneous tissue that is handled roughly, stretched, twisted, or crushed by an instrument may also necrose. If tissue is manipulated gently and if skin hooks or toothed forceps are used to grasp subcutaneous tissue (and not skin surfaces), tissue damage will be minimized.

The presence of dead space in adipose tissue potentiates infection, but the closure of that dead space with sutures increases the risk of infection to a much greater degree. Dead space in deeper layers of traumatic wounds should be obliterated with the use of relaxing incisions or dressings that provide gentle surface pressure.

Persistent, uncontrolled bleeding resulting in a wound hematoma provides a substrate for the proliferation of bacteria. Hemostasis can be achieved by ligating actively bleeding arterioles, cauterization, compression, or apposition of wound edges. Although it is important to prevent the accumulation of blood within the wound, it is also important to minimize the amount of tissue strangulated by ligatures or destroyed by cauterization and the amount of suture material left in the wound. Approximation of wound surfaces controls most diffuse, capillary bleeding in traumatic wounds.

Drains do not prevent infection; they simply allow a path of drainage for any collection of purulence or blood that may develop. When no infection exists, they are more likely to produce infection than prevent it. Drains are not indicated in the repair of traumatic wounds and should not serve as substitutes for other methods of achieving hemostasis.

Delayed Primary Closure

Traumatized skin is most susceptible to infection during the first 3 days following the injury and increasingly resistant thereafter. Most wound infections occur during this time period. The technique of delayed primary closure is based on the observation that, after cleaning and debridement, heavily contaminated wounds left unsutured have a lower risk of infection during the first 3 to 4 days after injury than do closed wounds. In severe soft-tissue injuries, delayed closure also allows time for nonviable tissue to demarcate from uninjured tissue. Debridement can then be accomplished with maximal preservation of tissue.

In general, high-velocity missile or explosion wounds and other wounds with extensive tissue damage, wounds that have been contaminated with feces, purulence, or saliva, and wounds heavily contaminated with soil types known to potentiate infection should not be closed primarily. All infected wounds must be left to close by secondary intention.

Although it is clear that the infection rate in wounds increases in proportion to the time elapsed prior to definitive wound care, there is no precise maximum time period after injury that a wound may be safely closed without significant risk of infection. The "safe time" or "golden period" varies with amount and type of contamination, mechanism of injury, amount of tissue damage, location on the body, the patient's immunologic status, the physician's ability to clean and debride the wound satisfactorily, and other factors. Under optimal conditions, wounds located on distal parts of extremities, in the perineal region, or within the mouth should be considered for delayed primary closure if treatment is delayed more than approximately 6 to 8 hours. With the possible exception of clean, sharp facial lacerations, even wounds in highly vascular areas should not be closed primarily if they are older than about 24 hours. Contamination with large numbers of bacteria may shorten the safe period to less than a few minutes.

Open wound management consists of packing the wound with sterile, fine-mesh gauze and covering it with a sterile dressing. The dressing should not be removed during the first 3 days after injury unless the patient develops an unexplained fever. Unnecessary inspection risks contamination of the wound. On the fourth day, the wound is re-evaluated; if there is no evidence of infection, the wound may be closed, after additional debridement if necessary. Since the wound is closed prior to collagen formation, there is no delay in healing, and the results are indistinguishable from those of primary closure.

Wound Dressings

Among the many functions of wound dressings, one of the more important is the protection of the wound from exogenous bacteria. As long as the outer surface remains dry, a dressing serves as an effective barrier to bacteria. Sutured wounds are susceptible to infection from surface contamination during the first 1 to 2 postoperative days. Coagulum and superficial epithelialization seal the wound edges during this time. On the third day, the dressing may be removed for brief periods to allow gentle cleansing of the skin surface. However, if wound exudate saturates the dressing before this time or if the dressing becomes soiled or wet, it must be changed to prevent passage of

exogenous bacteria through the dressing and bacterial overgrowth beneath it. Dressings also absorb blood and exudate that might otherwise contribute to the formation of stitch abscesses.

It is unlikely that antibiotic ointments reduce the development of infections in wounds extending below the epidermis, but they are useful in minimizing the formation of a crust that covers and separates the edges of the wound.

Splints

Immobilized tissue is more resistant to infection than mobile tissue. When lymphatic flow is minimized by splinting, bacteria within the wound (especially an infected wound) are less likely to spread. In wounds of the extremities, edema enhances infection; splinting and more importantly elevation lessen the development of edema.

Prophylactic Antibiotics

Antibiotics are useful when (1) infection is already present, and (2) the risk of infection is considerable because the wound cannot be adequately cleaned or debrided. The risk of drug reactions and the potential for the emergence of resistant strains of bacteria outweigh the potential benefit of topical or systemic antibiotics in low-risk patients.

If the wound is so heavily contaminated that even the most skillful management is not likely to reduce bacterial concentrations below the infective level, it should not be closed primarily. Many careful studies have shown that prophylactic antibiotics have no effect on infection rates in simple, relatively uncontaminated wounds. When the wound is contaminated with exceedingly high numbers of organisms, such as are found in feces or pus, infection will develop despite antibiotic treatment.

However, the use of prophylactic antibiotics aimed at bacteria persisting within the wound is probable effective in a limited number of special circumstances. Imperfect studies suggest that patients with dog bites involving extremities and all cat bites should receive antibiotics. Although efficacy is not proved, it is common practice to give prophylactic antibiotics for human bites, bites of ungulates (hoofed mammals), sutured intraoral lacerations, wounds involving tendons, bones, or joint spaces, and wounds contaminated with feces, vaginal secretions, saliva, purulence, or soil containing large amounts of organic matter. Antibiotics should be considered for any puncture-type bite wound, as these have a higher incidence of infection (see chapter on *Human and Animal Bites*).

Studies indicate that systemic antibiotics are of no benefit more than 3 hours after injury unless the wound is thoroughly debrided. If antibiotics are considered necessary, they should be given intravenously or intramuscularly in the earliest stages of management. Broad-spectrum antibiotics should be used—cephalosporins, penicillinase-resistant penicillins, or if allergy or cost precludes the use of these two groups, erythromycin. Irrigation with solutions containing antibiotics may be of benefit in these types of wounds. In all cases, the use of antibiotics should be considered secondary treatment; careful cleaning and debridement are a much more effective means of minimizing the risk of infection.

DIFFERENTIAL DIAGNOSIS

The diagnosis of local wound infection is based primarily on the four classic signs of inflammation—redness, warmth, swelling and tenderness—or on the presence of purulent drainage. Uninfected wounds have little drainage after the first 24 hours. If the purulence has been completely absorbed by the overlying dressing, a malodor may provide a clue to the presence of infection.

Lymphangitis or lymphadenopathy proximal to the wound indicate spread of the infection beyond the borders of the wound. Fever without an obvious source requires removal of all dressings and a careful inspection of the wound. Fever usually indicates that the infection has become regional or systemic. The presence of bullae, blisters, unusual systemic toxicity and pain, and subcutaneous crepitus or rapidly advancing inflammation, suggests a necrotizing wound infection.   There are several noninfectious causes of inflammation. Combinations of redness, warmth, and swelling occur with contusions, wound hematomas, stitch abscesses, and dependent edema in an injured extremity. Fluctuant swelling indicates either an underlying abscess or a hematoma. Both can cause fluctuance, redness, warmth, mild tenderness, and mild fever. Hematomas are differentiated from wound abscesses by the withdrawal of liquified blood on needle aspiration. Stitch abscesses are microabscesses confined to the suture's point of entry in the skin. They resolve rapidly after the stitch is removed but result in a punctate scar. Dependent edema involves an area beyond the wound and is often pitting in nature. However, the tissues are pale and cool rather than red and warm. Extensive edema associated with warmth or tenderness may indicate cellulitis or a necrotizing wound infection. If signs of inflammation increase after the initial 12 to 24 hours, infection must be considered. Erythema and swelling with well-defined, elevated borders are characteristic of erysipelas, an infection caused by *Streptococcus*.

Pain associated with an uncomplicated wound is usually mild. Pain may be moderate to severe and throbbing in nature if the injured part is held in a dependent position. Significant tenderness that persists more than 12 to 24 hours after the injury is unusual and suggests infection. Of the four signs associated with inflammation, tenderness serves as the most specific sign of early infection.

Local tissue reaction caused by Hymenoptera envenomation is hard to distinguish from cellulitis. Redness, warmth, and swelling result from the local effects of the venom. The sting of Hymenoptera species that build mud nests (wasps, in particular) often results in cellulitis. The absence of tenderness in the area of the inflammation helps distinguish a toxic effect from a secondary infection.

Extensive ecchymosis not caused by blunt trauma may be a sign of an underlying gangrenous infection.

DIAGNOSTIC LABORATORY AND RADIOLOGIC STUDIES

Complete Blood Count

A complete blood count (CBC)is occasionally helpful in the evaluation of local wound infections, but should not be routinely done. When infection cannot be distinguished clinically from edema or soft-tissue contusion, a CBC with an elevated white blood cell count associated with an increase in band cells weighs in favor of infection.

Gram Stain

Gram stains of infected wound surfaces are seldom useful in the management of local infections. The Gram stain may not distinguish between contaminants and the infecting organism unless bacteria are present in large numbers (e.g., purulent drainage), and the results rarely alter therapy. However, a Gram stain of purulent drainage from a wound sustained in an atypical environment may be useful, since an uncommon organism is more likely to be responsible for the infection.

Staphylococcus aureus appear as gram-positive cocci in clusters, and the appearance of smaller gram-positive cocci in pairs or chains indicates infection with *Streptococcus*. A Gram stain with a mixture of bacilli and cocci suggests the presence of anaerobes with or without aerobes.

Wound Cultures

Cultures taken from the wound on initial presentation are not useful for predicting the likelihood of infection or the type of organism in subsequent infections. Wound cultures are not necessary in the management of uncomplicated, localized, minor wound infections. In vitro and in vivo antibiotic sensitivities often do not correlate well. Definite indications for cultures of infected wounds are (1) regional extension or systemic infection, (2) failure of initial treatment, (3) chronic infection, (4) prior use of prophylactic antibiotics, and (5) wounds contaminated with large number of species of bacteria (bites, fecal contamination) or sustained in unusual environments (e.g., ditch or pond water, aquariums, exposure to fresh meat or seafood).

Roentgenography

The indications for x-ray film evaluation of a wound infection include suspicion of (1) a foreign body, (2) osteomyelitis or infection near bone, or (3) infection caused by gas-forming organisms without obvious signs of subcutaneous emphysema.

THERAPY

Suture Removal, Debridement, Cleansing

Infected wounds should have sutures removed along the entire length of the infection, and devitalized tissue

TABLE 3 Oral Antibiotic Dosages* for Outpatient Treatment of Common Local Wound Infections

Antibiotic	Indications
Dicloxacillin	Initial therapy; *S. aureus* infections
Cloxacillin	Initial therapy; *S. aureus* infections
Cephalexin	Initial therapy; *S. aureus* infections
Cephradine	Initial therapy; *S. aureus* infections
Erythromycin	Initial therapy in patient allergic to penicillins and cephalosporins; erysipeloid
Penicillin VK	Streptococcal and anaerobic infections; initial therapy for intraoral infections; erysipeloid; *Pasteurella multicocida* infection; rat-bite fever; actinomycosis

* Dosage for each of these antibiotics is 250-500 mg (6.25–25 mg/kg) PO 4 times daily for 7 to 10 days; penicillin VK should be given in doses of 500 mg.

should be debrided. If a retained foreign body is suspected, the wound should be thoroughly explored and all foreign matter removed. Abscess cavities should be exposed completely by incision, drained, and irrigated with saline solution. All pus and necrotic tissue must be removed. The cavity is then loosely packed with fine-mesh gauze. If the infection is extensive or if lymphangitis, lymphadenitis, or septicemia is present, or if the patient has any immune suppression or cardiac valvular disease, antibiotics should be given prior to manipulation of the wound.

Wet Versus Dry Dressings

A small amount of viscous drainage that readily coagulates seals off the wound and thereby prevents inflammatory cells from reaching the infecting bacteria. A wet dressing helps remove thick secretions from an infected wound by diluting the exudate. Wounds that are draining large amounts of thin fluid are best managed with a dry, bulky dressing. A dry dressing absorbs more drainage than a wet one. Dressings have been used to debride an infected wound. Dry dressings become adherent to the wound, and when removed pull off loosely attached necrotic tissue. Wet dressings are relatively ineffective in cleaning the wound surface unless the dressing in contact with the wound is in place long enough to dry out. Other methods of debridement are preferable. Washing the wound seems to be more effective; debridement by surgical excision is more directed and controlled.

Various solutions have been used to wash or soak infected wounds. An acid pH seems to discourage growth of urea-splitting organisms. Salicylic acid and weak acetic acid solutions have been used to speed up enzymatic digestion and separation of necrotic dermis and fascia. These measures are probably less effective than washing and selective sharp excision.

The application of heat to infected wounds has two benefits. Moist heat applied to a wound increases the inflammatory response. A temporary benefit of heat application is improvement in the patient's comfort when wet to dry dressings are used; cold, wet dressings are uncomfortable.

TABLE 4 Continued Care of Infected Wounds: Patient Instructions

Take the antibiotics until all pills are gone.
Change dry dressings once a day, wet to dry dressings three times a day, and more often if the dressing is saturated with drainage.
Wash the wound with mild soap and water once daily.
Apply warm compresses (or soak wound in warm water) for 20 minutes 3 times a day.
Elevate the injured part as much as possible.
Observe for spread of infection.
Return for evaluation in 2–3 days.

Antibiotics

No single antibiotic can protect against all potential infecting organisms, even in uncomplicated local wound infections. The initial antibiotic chosen must be effective against the most common organisms found in wound infections, which includes the penicillin-resistant strains of *Staphylococcus aureus* (Table 3). When the infecting organism in a local wound infection is not known, a penicillinase-resistant penicillin or cephalosporin should be used. If the patient is allergic to those drugs or cost precludes their use, erythromycin may be used. Initial therapy can be adjusted on the basis of wound culture results, patient response, or both.

If a necrotizing infection is involved or a Gram stain shows a predominance of gram-negative rods and the patient requires hospitalization, an aminoglycoside in combination with clindamycin or chloramphenicol is the treatment of choice until the organism is identified.

Pasteurella multocida is an organism implicated in animal bite wound infections and is quite sensitive to penicillin. However, penicillin should not be given empirically to patients with these infections because multiple organisms are usually introduced into bite wounds, and penicillin-resistant *Staphylococcus aureus* is still the most common infecting organism. *Pasteurella* is sensitive to most antibiotics effective against *Staphylococcus* with the exception of erythromycin, and a penicillinase-resistant penicillin or a cephalosporin is a more reasonable choice. Penicillin-allergic patients with *Pasteurella* infection should be treated with tetracycline. Patients should receive verbal and written instructions on the further care of their wounds (Table 4).

Consultation and Hospitalization

There are several indications for consultation with a surgical or infectious disease specialist. A patient with a hand infection that fails to respond to initial therapy or that is the consequence of a human bite should be referred to a hand surgeon and probably admitted for parenteral therapy. Infection that has spread beyond the wound, such as deep space infection or tenosynovitis within the hand, necrotizing wound infection, fasciitis, osteomyelitis, and septic arthritis all require hospitalization, intravenous antibiotics, and in many cases, surgical debridement. Wound infections in critical areas, such as periorbital cellulitis or extensive scalp infections, usually require intravenous antibiotics and close observation for complications. Major systemic toxicity is an obvious indication for hospitalization. Wound infections in patients with major risk factors (e.g., major immune suppression, alcoholism, asplenism) are at risk for serious complications and, depending on the extent of the wound, may require aggressive treatment.

Antibiotic Treatment Failure

Initial antibiotic therapy may fail to control an infection. Several possibilities must be considered:

1. There may be a foreign body or excessive amounts of necrotic tissue present within the wound.
2. A subcutaneous abscess may be present, and incision and drainage are necessary in order for the infection to resolve.
3. Underlying structures, such as bones, joints, or bursae, may also be infected.
4. Inflammation on the skin surface may be a sign of a deep, necrotizing infection.

5. The organism may be resistant to the antibiotic being used; wound culture and sensitivity testing should be initiated. The antibiotic can be changed or another added for a synergistic effect.
6. The antibiotic is being given too infrequently, in too small a dose, or by an inappropriate route. The course of therapy may be too short or the patient may be metabolizing or excreting the drug too rapidly. (If penicillin is the antibiotic of choice, the excretion of this antibiotic can be delayed with the oral administration of 1 g of probenicid.)
7. The patient's immunologic defenses may be impaired.

SUGGESTED READING

Lammers RL. Principles of wound management. In: Roberts JR, Hedges JR, eds. Clinical procedures in emergency medicine. Philadelphia: WB Saunders, 1985:478.
Peacock EE. Wound repair. 3rd ed. Philadelphia: WB Saunders, 1984.
Simmons RL, Howard RJ, eds. Surgical infectious diseases. New York: Appleton-Century-Crofts, 1982:274–284, 291–295, 429–441, 449–472, 473–485, 507–583.

NECROTIZING WOUND INFECTION

H. HARLAN STONE, M.D.

The most serious of all wound infections are those associated with tissue necrosis; they uniformly threaten life or limb or both. Although antibiotics are useful in therapy, it is primarily early and aggressive surgery that determines the final outcome. Delay in initiating surgical care or timidity in its execution is consistently the cause of a poor result.

ETIOLOGY

In patients with relatively normal local and general host defense mechanisms, only the most virulent of bacteria can cause a necrotizing wound infection. Characteristically, any single pathogen capable of producing such an infection must be able to secrete potent proteolytic enzymes. Highly virulent strains of the hemolytic *Streptococcus* and *Staphylococcus aureus* are the commonly incriminated aerobic pathogens.

An impairment in local defenses against invasive infection, as in the contused or ischemic wound, permits single-species anaerobic growth and thereby the evolution of perhaps the most rapidly progressive of all necrotizing infections, *gas gangrene*. With a more generalized reduction in host defense effectiveness, especially whenever the humoral system (i.e., globulins and granulocytes) has been depressed, somewhat less virulent species with not as potent a set of proteolytic exotoxins can initiate an infectious gangrene. *Pseudomonas aeruginosa* and various fungi, such as *Aspergillus* and *Sporotrichosis,* are good examples.

By far the most frequent cause of necrotizing infection, however, is the microbial synergy created by the combination of aerobic and anaerobic bacterial species. In this symbiosis, the aerobic partner extracts most of the available oxygen from the local microenvironment so that conditions become suitable for anaerobic growth. The anaerobe component then secretes an array of relatively powerful proteolytic enzymes, which in turn destroy local host defenses, break down tissue barriers, and digest substrate for the nourishment of both sets of pathogens. One or more of the several enteric gram-negative rods generally function as the aerobic component, while a multitude of various anaerobic species are capable of providing the necessary anaerobe population.

PREDISPOSITION

Certain categories of patients are predisposed to developing a necrotizing infection. A severely contused or heavily contaminated fresh wound poses no problem if it is properly managed. Unfortunately, all too often debridement has been inadequate, wound cleansing has been incomplete, or a wound with a definite predilection for infection has been closed. Worse still, the patient with such a wound is discharged from the emergency area without steps being taken to obtain an early wound check, that is, scheduled returns on a daily basis for the next 4 to 6 days. For such patients, hospital admission may be required.

Another susceptible group is made up of those patients with altered host resistance. Diabetes mellitus, hypo- or dysgammaglobulinemia, advanced cancer with or without chemotherapy, diseases of the reticuloendothelial system, extremes of age, obesity, immunosuppression caused by organ transplantation, and major stress states are the more significant contributors to that immune impairment.

Finally, exposure of fresh wounds to the mixed microbial flora resident in the colon or wound contamination by highly virulent aerobic gram-positive cocci makes the outcome uncertain.

PRESENTATION

Whenever there is gangrenous tissue within an infected wound, the patient usually has an extremely toxic reaction. Fever is high, in the 39 to 40 °C range; often the patient is irrational. Leukocytosis is at the extreme, that is, either the peripheral white blood cell count exceeds 18,000 mm³ or there is the leukopenia of present or impending septic shock. In addition, hemolytic anemia may lead to jaundice, especially if sepsis is caused by gas gangrene or fulminating streptococcal infection. At more advanced stages, septic shock may already have become established, as reflected by hypotension, hypothermia, and a refractory oliguria.

On inspection of the wound, necrotic tissue is usually obvious. However, in some cases the area of gangrene lies well below the superficial fascia and can be missed unless the wound is more widely opened. Instead of normal-appearing pus, the wound discharges a fluid primarily derived from tissue autolysis, resembling dirty dishwater. This fluid should be cultured for both aerobes and anaerobes as well as smeared and stained to determine the presence of gram-positive cocci, gram-positive rods, or a polymicrobial mix.

The central area of infection is almost always anesthetic, even though the patient may complain bitterly of pain in that area. Gaseous crepitation is frequently noted on palpation and on x-ray evaluation of the involved tissues, regardless of the specific pathogen. Most characteristic of all, however, is the strong putrid odor emitted from the wound whenever anaerobes are involved.

Different pathogens create somewhat different clinical pictures. Accordingly, for clarification, the more common presentations are discussed individually.

Streptococcal Gangrene. The incubation period is quite short, being somewhere between 6 and 72 hours. Although deeper structures may be involved, the process is usually confined to the skin and subcutaneous tissues. Skin necrosis is patchy, with a central area of gangrene. Beyond is a halo of cutaneous hyperemia that is warm and exquisitely tender. Blister formation is common and may even suggest a partial-thickness burn (scalded skin syndrome). The wound discharge is pinkish and appears more like a serous exudate than in other forms of infectious gangrene. A smear of this fluid generally contains only gram-positive cocci. High fever and jaundice are characteristic.

Gas Gangrene. As with streptococcal necrotizing infections, the incubation period for gas gangrene is brief—12 hours to 5 days. The central area of dark, hemorrhagic discoloration rapidly advances, so that within as short a period of time as a single hour one may appreciate definite advancement of the infection. The wound is cool, often crepitant, and anesthetic. Nevertheless, the patient describes a continuous excruciating pain within the wound. High fever, jaundice, and irrational behavior are prominent within 12 hours of the onset of symptoms. Fluid obtained from the wound or its associated dark, hemorrhagic blisters contains gram-positive, club-shaped rods in only half the cases.

***Pseudomonas* Gangrene.** Patients with significant impairment in their host defense mechanisms are primarily the ones who develop *Pseudomonas* gangrene. Perianal necrotizing infection is commonly seen in patients with leukemia, lymphoma, and related malignancies of the reticuloendothelial system. Major deficiences in the humoral defense mechanism, such as hypogammaglobulinemia and agranulocytosis, are precipitating conditions. Deterioration of a wound into *Pseudomonas* gangrene is generally confined to patients with extensive losses of skin mantle, as with major thermal burn. In these cases, gangrene may be punctate (focal necrosis) or instead may involve somewhat broad areas of previously healthy granulation tissue (neoeschar formation). Both are referred to as pyoderma gangrenosa.

Fungal gangrene. With *Aspergillus* infection, there usually is focal necrosis within a large, already established surface defect, similar to what has been described for *Pseudomonas* gangrene. However, these areas of necrosis have a unique metallic gray color, and microscopic examination of an exudate smear demonstrates branching chains of yeast. Sporotrichosis, on the other hand, begins in a small skin wound, usually the result of a thorn or splinter puncture, and progresses slowly outward.

Synergistic gangrene. Necrotizing infections caused by the symbiosis between aerobic and anaerobic bacteria was first described by Meleney. This generally involves the skin and subcutaneous planes on an extremity, rarely penetrates the deep enveloping fascia, and progresses slowly over a period of days to weeks, somewhat resembling the pattern of a rodent ulcer. A smear of the necrotic tissue contains only gram-positive cocci.

Fusospirochetal infections tend to occur near mucocutaneous junctions, such as on the lip and along the gingival and buccal mucosa. Cancrum oris, an especially destructive lesion, is seen at the corner of the mouth and on the cheek of malnourished children. A smear of the exudate reveals spirochetes and a fusiform bacillus. Vibrio may occasionally be present as well.

Most common of all, however, are those necrotizing infections caused by one or more aerobic gram-negative rods and various anaerobes. These evolve in the immediate vicinity of the anus, the artificial anus as represented by a colostomy, or as an infectious complication following large bowel surgery. If the infection is located in the space between Scarpa's fascia and external oblique fascia, it is called necrotizing fasciitis. In this case, infection spreads along that plane, causing nutrient vessels to the overlying dermis to become thrombosed and thereby creating a rapidly progressive cutaneous gangrene. Necrotizing infection below the deep enveloping fascia is referred to as necrotizing cellulitis. By contrast, the skin may appear to be healthy and given no suggestion of the extensive gangrene beneath. The entire fascial compartment is routinely necrotic, yet vessels that pass through that same space remain patent, and distal pulses are equal to those on the opposite limb. Both necrotizing fasciitis and cellulitis may develop in a surgical incision on the abdominal wall or may specifically complicate an otherwise benign-appearing perianal or perirectal abscess. Differentiation is made by the fact that patients with infectious gangrene have exceedingly toxic symptoms such as high fevers and extreme degrees of leukocytosis. Instead of true pus being discharged from the wound, the characteristic odor and exudate of autolyzed tissue are noted on incision or aspiration.

If either necrotizing fasciitis or cellulitis develops in the external genitalia, then the process is usually called for Fournier's gangrene.

INITIAL MANAGEMENT

If the patient presents in septic shock, all initial efforts are directed toward resuscitation. These are standard and are detailed elsewhere. Nevertheless, it is important to obtain blood cultures for both aerobic and anaerobic bacteria as well as for fungi before any antimicrobial therapy is started. Otherwise, a septicemic process may be missed.

Likewise, after inspection of the wound, appropriate samples are taken of available exudate for culture. At the same time, smears for staining and microscopic inspection should be obtained.

Antimicrobials

Parenteral antimicrobial therapy must be started as soon as blood for cultures has been taken. Penicillin (aqueous penicillin G, 30,000 U per kilogram body weight every 4 hours) is administered intravenously for infectious gangrene clearly due to Clostridium. The dose is reduced to one-third (10,000 U per kilogram body weight every 4 hours) in cases of necrotizing infection caused by Streptococcus, Staphylococcus, and synergy due to the combination of streptococci and staphylococci (Meleney's gangrene) as well as the fusospirochetal combination. In patients with a history of penicillin allergy, tetracycline (20 mg per kilogram body weight every 6 hours) is an acceptable substitute.

For Pseudomonas gangrene, an aminoglycoside (tobramycin 1.5 mg per kilogram body weight every 8

hours) and carbenicillin (30 mg per kilogram body weight every 4 hours) are given intravenously. For fungal gangrene, amphotericin B (0.25 mg per kilogram body weight per day) is administered slowly by a constant intravenous infusion.

The majority of patients, however, have a polymicrobial synergy due to aerobic gram-negative rods and various anaerobes. Since there is compromised renal function and an anticipated need for prolonged antibiotic therapy, aminoglycosides should be avoided because of their predictable nephrotoxicity with high doses or extended therapy. Excellent results can be expected with a combination of third-generation cephalosporins (moxalactam, cefotaxime, or cefoperazone—20 mg per kilogram body weight every 8 hours) plus metronidazole (15 mg per kilogram body weight every 12 hours). It is important to give a dose of vitamin K (0.2 mg per kilogram body weight) initially and every fifth day while moxalactam and cefoperazone are being used to avoid bleeding problems from drug-induced hypoprothrombinemia.

Surgery

Antibiotics only temporize and aid in the control of the associated bacteremia. Absolutely crucial is surgical excision of all necrotic tissue. The wound must then be left open for delayed closure, usually by skin graft. Accordingly, efforts at surgical control of the process should be made within a very few hours of patient admission. No case can ever be managed on an outpatient basis. Each and every patient must be admitted for surgical care.

The responsible wound is excised as completely as possible. Topical antibiotic is applied (Neosporin aerosal), and the patient is returned to the operating room on a daily basis until the wound demonstrates no further progression of the gangrenous process. Initial measures are directed to this end: type and crossmatch for estimated volume of blood needed for transfusion, post for emergency operating room time, and perform preoperative anesthetic evaluation.

Hyperbaric Oxygen

With the exception of the treatment of gas gangrene, use of the hyperbaric oxygen chamber has never been shown to be of objective benefit. Even in the case of gas gangrene, reports are conflicting. Nevertheless, it is probably wise to transfer the patient to a facility equipped to give hyperbaric oxygen therapy if one is immediately available. Otherwise, therapy should be as outlined above.

SUGGESTED READING

Benjamin BI. Fournier's gangrene. Br J Urol 1979; 51:312–316.
Defore WW Jr, Mattox KL, Dang MH et al. Necrotizing fasciitis; a persistent surgical problem. JACEP 1977; 6:62–65.
Eckstein A. Noma. Am J Dis Child 1940; 59:219–237.
Giuliano A. Lewis F Jr, Hadley K, Balaisdell FW. Bacteriology of necrotizing fasciitis. Am J Surg 1977; 134:52–57.
Lee C, Oh C. Necrotizing fasciitis of the genitalia. Urology 1979; 13:604–606.

Meleney FL. Hemolytic Streptococcus gangrene. Arch Surg 1924; 9:317–364.

Stark S. Noma or gangrenous stomatitis. Oral Surg 1956; 9:1076–1079.

Stone HH, Martin JD Jr. Synergistic necrotizing cellulitis. Ann Surg 1972; 175:702–711.

LOW BACK PAIN AND DEGENERATIVE DISC DISEASE

FRANKLIN T. HOAGLUND, M.D.

The most common cause of low back pain is degenerative disease of the lumbar intervertebral discs. Symptoms may begin with a minor physical motion, such as bending, twisting, or lifting, or patients may even awaken with a backache. A preexisting degenerative process affecting the disc, the cause of which is unknown, disposes an individual to the problem. A symptomatic degenerative disc under mechanical stress produces symptoms across the low back region, in one or another lumbosacral angle, or is referred to the buttock, posterior thigh, or lower extremity (Fig. 1). If the disc protrudes, herniates, or dislodges a free fragment (sequestration) that causes local pressure on a nerve root, it produces radiculopathy. Pain in the distribution of the nerve root, which is most commonly at L5 or S1, may be intermittent or constant and depends on the size, severity, and location of the pressure; in some patients the extremity pain is present without noticeable back pain. Disc herniations can occur in the teenaged or elderly but have a peak incidence in the 30 to 40 year range. Chronic disc degeneration with associated facet hypertrophy, osteoarthritis, and thickening of the ligamentum flavum can result in a narrow spinal canal (spinal stenosis) and cause symptoms of neurogenic claudication.

PATHOPHYSIOLOGY

Pressure of the disc on the nerve root accounts for the lower extremity pain. When the pressure on the disc is at its greatest, as in sitting with abdominal muscles relaxed, there is presumably a greater protrusion to cause the nerve root pressure. Also, in certain positions, e.g., extension of the lumbar spine, or leaning backward, the space in the neural canal decreases and results in more nerve pressure and pain.

The actual mechanism of low back pain, when there is no direct pressure on a nerve root, is uncertain. Discs have nerve endings in the posterior annulus, so that injury, inflammation, or mechanical strain can produce symptoms. However, degenerative changes can be present for years before symptoms occur; many such patients never admit to a backache. Facet joints may be a source of such pain, but the pathologic findings in these structures are also present before and after a low back episode. Pressure on a disc is greatest when sitting; it is less when standing, and least when recumbent. Tightening of the abdominal muscles reduces the disc pressure and sometimes the symptoms, as does a lumbosacral corset that substitutes for the relaxed abdominal muscles.

DIFFERENTIAL DIAGNOSIS

Low back pain can be caused by any type of spinal pathologic process; also, many diseases affecting the abdominal organs or retroperitoneal areas may cause low back pain. It is mandatory to make a timely diagnosis of potentially life-threatening conditions. A leaking abdominal aneurysm, occlusion (acute or chronic) of the large vessels, renal tumors, infection, or a perforated abdominal viscus can all present as low back pain.

Other spinal conditions can resemble the pain attributable to degenerative disc disease. An acute intraspinal pyogenic or disc space infection may produce back or leg pain. Immunologically compromised individuals or intravenous drug users are at highest risk. Hematogenous inoculation can occur at any age. Disc space infection should be considered in the immediate postoperative postdiscectomy patient. The pain can be severe and is usually constant at rest. Other signs of infection supportive of the diagnosis are fever, chills, and general symptoms of illness. Plain lumbosacral x-ray views are usually negative during the acute phase.

Tuberculosis can involve any part of the spine. With disease in the upper lumbar spine, pain may be referred to the low back region. Bone destruction on both sides of the disc space is characteristic of tuberculosis and is usually evident when the patient presents.

Metastatic disease to the spine is more frequent in older individuals. Instability owing to pathologic fracture produces significant mechanical symptoms. Percussion tenderness of the spine, pain at rest, and the radiologic presence of a compression fracture, or fractures, in the absence of significant injury, indicate the need for a diagnostic bone scan. Compression fractures attributable to osteoporosis are common to the thoracic lumbar junction and may occur with minor trauma. Patients frequently experience pain in the low back region with tenderness over the involved vertebra.

Patients with ankylosing spondylitis may present with low back and leg pain. The costovertebral involvement from this disease limits rib excursion and, therefore, chest expansion to less than 1.5 inches at the nipple line and limited lumbar spine motion. Plain x-ray views show evidence of sacroileitis. The process frequently starts in the teen years and is most common in the male.

Herpes zoster, involving a lumbosacral root, is a rare cause of radiculitis, with diagnostic difficulty before the associated skin lesions are manifest.

ESSENTIALS OF DIAGNOSIS

Proper diagnosis depends upon suspecting and carrying out an appropriate physical examination in all patients with back pain. It is important to include historical questions concerning the genitourinary or gastrointestinal systems in order to consider these possibilities. A proper examination should include careful abdominal palpation for masses, evaluation of femoral and peripheral pulses, palpation for costovertebral angle tenderness, and a urinalysis. Pain in the upper lumbar region, costovertebral angle, flank, groin, testicular area, or iliac crest or associated abdominal pain may accompany low back pain, but usually suggests an etiology other than the lumbar discs.

Patients suffering from back pain only will have activity pain in the low lumbar region or midline or at the lumbosacral angle, S1 joint region, or medial buttock. The severity of this pain varies from inability to get up without assistance, to mild pain that does not interfere with most activities.

Physical examination reveals restricted lumbar spine motion when the patient is viewed from behind, with knees extended and then flexed forward to move in the direction of touching the toes. Restricted motion, such as the inability to reverse the normal lordosis, or spasm is apparent in any motion. Patients may flex forward and support themselves on the thighs, using this support to aid in returning to the upright position.

The straight leg raising maneuver, carried out in the recumbent position, may cause back pain. The straight leg raising maneuver is not specific for disc disease. When there is impingement on a nerve root from any cause (disc, tumor, or infection) and straight leg raising is carried out, the nerve root cannot move normally in its neural foramen. One of two things happens: when the maneuver is attempted, the patient guards against further elevation of the leg, or, during the maneuver, the nerve is stimulated by the pressure and produces pain in the distribution of the nerve root. A degenerative disc may only cause back pain, just from the motion over the currently painful disc. From a practical standpoint, however, straight leg raising positivity correlates with disc disease.

Plain film lumbar spine x-ray views may be needed to rule out other disease and may only show changes of disc space narrowing or marginal osteophytes associated with degenerative disc disease. Lumbosacral spine films are taken to rule out infection or tumor and to get a baseline for patients that do not get better initially. If the diagnosis of herniated disc or degenerative disc disease is made, there is some support for this diagnosis in the x-ray view that does not show other disease or perhaps shows a degenerative disc matching the level of radic-

ulopathy. In patients with short-term histories who have had previous x-ray examinations, there is no urgency in getting the films taken. In patients who get better quickly, there may not be an indication to obtain films on subsequent visits. Of course, if one suspects a pathologic fracture or infection (osteomyelitis, discitis) or if the patient has had more significant trauma, such as a fall, x-ray views are needed. When x-ray examination reveals spondylitis or spondylolisthesis, clinical interpretation of symptoms is necessary. Either finding may be present without symptoms or may be the cause of them.

In patients with radiculopathy, nerve root pressure or irritation may be constant or intermittent. Leg pain may occur in the absence of back pain, or pain may radiate only into the buttocks or posterior thigh (Table 1). However, pain in the lateral calf and dorsum of the foot is indicative of an L5 radiculopathy; pain in the posterior calf to the ankle or along the border of the foot is supportive of an S1 radiculopathy. Such patients may have sciatic scoliosis, e.g., involuntary muscle spasm in the upright position that causes tilt of the spine away from the involved nerve root but sometimes toward it. Patients avoid forward flexion in the upright position, and straight leg raising produces limitations. Usually patients guard the straight leg raising and do not allow elevation to the point where it aggravates the leg pain. Contralateral straight leg raising indicates a large disc protrusion, which will not improve on conservative treatment. Weakness of great toe dorsal flexion occurs with an L5 radiculopathy. Patients may have anterior tibial weakness and be unable to walk on the heels with the forefoot raised off the ground.

A difference in the Achilles tendon reflexes or any decrease or absence occurs with S1 root involvement. A decrease in the patellar tendon reflex is attributable to L4 radiculopathy, an L3–4 disc, or intraforaminal herniation of a lateral disc at L4–5. A decrease in sensation with pin prick or light touch occurs over the dorsal aspect of the great toe when an L5 radiculopathy is present and the lateral border of the foot or the heel with an S1 lesion. Plain film x-ray examination rules out other causes of back pain.

Patients with degenerative spinal stenosis have a characteristic history of back or leg pain with walking, but may get complete relief on sitting, with the back flexed (neurogenic claudication). Some patients, while standing, obtain pain relief by flexing one hip on a stair or chair.

Reflex changes and great toe extensor weakness, may be noted in various combinations. Plain film x-ray views show degenerative changes at one or more levels. The diagnosis is confirmed with a computed tomography (CT) scan showing encroachment on the neural canal because of disc protrusions, facet hypertrophy, or ligamentum flavum hypertrophy.

The cauda equina syndrome should be suspected in any patient with urinary retention or loss of anal tone. Such patients may have flaccid paralysis, bilateral leg symptoms, or saddle anesthesia.

TABLE 1 Common Nerve Root Compression Syndromes in the Lumbosacral Spine

Weakness	Reflexes	Sensory Deficit	Pain	Nerve Root	Disc
Quadriceps	Knee jerk decreased	Anterior-medial thigh, knee	Hip, posterior-lateral thigh, and anterior leg	L4	L3–4
Dorsiflexion of great toe, foot, and difficulty on heel walking	Usually absent	Lateral calf, first toe web	Lateral thigh and lateral calf	L5	L4–5
Plantarflexion of great toe, foot, and difficulty on toe walking	Ankle jerk decreased	Back of calf, lateral heel and foot, little toe	Posterolateral thigh, calf, and heel	S1	L5–S1
Bowel and bladder incontinence and/or variable paresis of legs	Ankle jerk decreased	Variable: perineum, legs, and feet (occasionally bilateral)	Same as sensory deficit	S1–5	Large lumbar herniation

THERAPY

The bed rest protocol is appropriate for patients with severe back pain only. In those who are able to walk and move without great difficulty, the prescription of a lumbosacral corset can be dramatically helpful. Such a corset provides immobilization and, more important, abdominal compression and thus reduces the force across the disc space. Outpatients can wear this corset when upright and remove it for bed rest. In those with low-grade back pain, Naprosyn (375 mg twice daily) or Motrin (800 mg 3 times daily) may be helpful; if there is no response to these drugs, other anti-inflammatory drugs (Tylenol No. 3 or Valium, 5 mg twice daily) may be tried.

Patients with disc protrusions and radiculopathy who are unable to stand because of back and leg pain require bed rest, lying recumbent in the semi-Fowler position, using three sofa cushion pillows beneath the knees, or lying on either side with the hips and knees flexed but avoiding the prone position. Such patients should use a bed pan or urinal for urination, but are generally more comfortable getting up to use a commode for bowel movements. Eating should be done while lying on either side.

When patients are sent home from the emergency department to bed rest, the administration of Demerol (75 to 100 mg) eases the discomfort of travel by automobile. Only rarely do some patients need hospitalization and bed rest for the management of pain.

On home bed rest, the treatment is Tylenol No. 3 or 4 (every 4 to 6 hours as needed), although Naprosyn, (375 mg twice daily after meals) can be tried and continued if helpful. Valium (2 to 5 mg twice daily) may be helpful for sedation and as a muscle relaxant.

Patients are specifically given instructions to avoid lying on the floor because of reinjury in getting up to use the commode. A plywood panel between the mattress and box spring can provide the needed bed stability. Higher beds are recommended because of the ease of getting up from them. Waterbeds are contraindicated. Patients are specifically instructed to call at once if there are any signs of sphincter weakness or bladder paralysis.

Most patients are improved with 1 week of bed rest; if so, they are encouraged to remain at bed rest for half-time for a second week, during which time walking is encouraged and sitting discouraged. During the third week, if the leg pain has resolved, patients are allowed to ambulate and be up as needed.

Patients are generally reexamined between 10 and 21 days, depending upon improvement. Persistent severe pain after 10 to 14 days calls for reexamination and readmission for a myelogram, computed tomography, and consideration of surgical decompression.

Return to work or activity after 3 weeks is dependent upon progess in pain relief as well as consideration of the occupation. Laborers or those who drive may be advised to stay off work for an additional 3 weeks or longer. A satisfactory response through this conservative regimen is indicated by the relief of symptoms; reflex changes and motor weakness also should be improved (or certainly not worsened). The degree of straight leg raising will diminish and indicates improvement; however, reflex changes may persist indefinitely.

In patients with mild backache and those with resolving radiculopathy, it is imperative that a permanent exercise and rehabilitation program be instituted to avoid back reinjury. This twice daily exercise provides abdominal strengthening by requiring 10 isometric abdominal contractions in the recumbent position, with hips and knees flexed. Patients are also instructed to do twice daily straight leg raising with the contralateral hip and knee flexed. They need to avoid sitting or driving for long periods, and should understand the proper body mechanics during weight lifting. Following an acute low back episode, these exercises are started gradually, with pain to be avoided.

Although heat, ultrasound, acupuncture, and massage have all been tried in patients with an acute low back pain, there is no evidence that recovery occurs any sooner with such treatments.

Patients with a suspected or definite cauda equina syndrome should be hospitalized immediately and a consultation sought with an experienced neurosurgeon or spine surgeon. A metrizamide myelogram is carried out promptly as well as a postmyelography CT scan, if available. Patients are managed with the insertion of a Foley catheter, strict bed rest in the semi-Fowler position, and appropriate analgesic medication. Morphine or Demerol may be necessary until posterior lumbar spine decompression can be accomplished. Spine fusion is usually not an initial consideration.

ACUTE BACK PAIN IN PHYSICALLY ACTIVE INDIVIDUALS

JAMES S. KEENE, M.D.
DENIS S. DRUMMOND, M.D.

Acute back pain often is experienced by physically active individuals, and usually is initially evaluated by primary care and emergency physicians. The cause of the back pain is best diagnosed by a thorough, well-conceived history and physical examination that uses time economically and enables the examiner to narrow down the diagnostic possibilities. To accomplish this, the examiner should begin the evaluation by determining whether the individual is suffering from mechanical or nonmechanical back pain. *Mechanical back pain* is caused by an injury or is the result of repetitive, subclinical injuries that occur in overuse syndromes. Spondylolysis is an example of an overuse injury that is caused by repetitive hyperextension of the spine. Mechanical back pain is aggravated by activities such as stooping, bending, walking, and lifting, and is improved by rest. Similarly, it may be relieved by activities that are opposite to those that aggravate the pain. For example, if extension of the spine aggravates the pain, often gentle flexion will ease it.

Nonmechanical back pain occurs spontaneously and is not associated with prior levels of physical activity. Rest is less likely to relieve the pain; in fact, rest pain is one of the hallmarks of nonmechanical back pain. An algorithm depicting the concept of mechanical and nonmechanical back pain is shown in Figure 1. Differential diagnosis within these categories is summarized in Table 1.

MUSCLE STRAINS AND ILIAC APOPHYSITIS

Muscle strains are the most common mechanical cause of acute back pain. A muscle strain is defined as a disruption of the muscle fibers, muscle-tendon junction, tendon, or either the bony or cartilaginous insertion of the muscle-tendon unit. Acute strains are the result of forces that exceed the strength or flexibility of the muscle-tendon unit. Individuals with this injury may feel "something tear" and experience acute pain, but more often the pain is most intense 24 to 48 hours after injury. Chronic strains are caused by repetitive forces that exceed the endurance capacity of the muscle-tendon unit. With this type of injury, the individual initially experiences pain after physical activity. Without treatment, the pain is experienced during strenuous activity, and ultimately the pain occurs with daily activities.

On physical examination, the pain is usually found to be localized to the insertion of the muscle at the iliac crest or within the muscle belly lateral to the spinous processes (area *B* in Fig. 2). Muscle spasm ranges from focal to generalized and causes a functional curvature of the spine (scoliosis) and limited motion of the spine.

Although muscle strains are experienced by all age groups, younger individuals with open iliac apophyses may have inflammation in the apophysis (iliac apophysitis) or separation of the apophysis rather than a chronic muscle strain. In these individuals, the pain is localized to the iliac crest (area *B* in Fig. 2), and anteroposterior roentgenograms of the pelvis may demonstrate a fracture and separation of the ilac apophysis. Treatment of acute strains is focused on limiting swelling, inflammation, and muscle spasm. Therefore, during the first 24 to 48 hours, ice is applied to the area of maximal tenderness for 10 to 15 minutes every 4 to 6 hours. This is effectively accomplished by using an ice "popsicle." The popsicle is made by freezing a paper cup filled with water and then tearing off the upper half of the cup. The area of maxi-

TABLE 1 Differential Diagnosis of Mechanical and Nonmechanical Causes of Acute Back Pain

Category	Cause	Diagnosis	Movement Causing Pain	Location of Pain (Fig. 2)	Special Tests (clinical)
Mechanical	Acute Injury	Muscle strain	Flexion	Areas *B* and *D*	None
		Iliac crest avulsion	Flexion, rotation	Area *B*	None
		Ligament sprain	Flexion	Area *C*	None
		Disc injuries	Hyperextension	Areas *C* and *E*	Straight-leg raising
		Compression fractures	Flexion	Area *A*	Post-void urine volume
	Repetitive trauma (overuse)	Kissing spines	Hyperextension	Area *C*	Hyperextension
		Leg-length inequality	Flexion	Area *E*	Leg measurements
		Spine instability	Flexion	Area *A*	Instability test
		Spondylolysis	Hyperextension	Area *D*	One-leg hyperextension
Nonmechanical	Infection	Discitis	Any direction	Area *A*	None
	Variable	Tumors	Variable	Variable	None

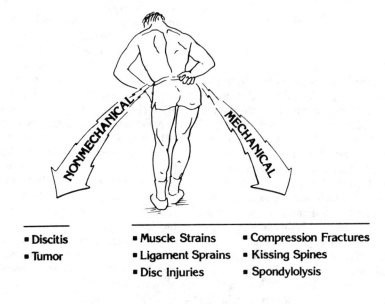

- Discitis
- Tumor

- Muscle Strains
- Ligament Sprains
- Disc Injuries

- Compression Fractures
- Kissing Spines
- Spondylolysis

Figure 1 An algorithm showing the most common mechanical and nonmechanical causes of acute back pain.

mum tenderness is then rubbed with a circular motion and the remainder of the cup is peeled as the ice melts. Oral nonsteroidal anti-inflammatory drugs should be included in the treatment regimen. However, oral corticosteroids should not be used because even a short course (up to 3 days) may cause avascular necrosis of the weight-bearing bones in both athletes and nonathletes.

After the muscle spasm has resolved, gentle stretching of the injured muscle is initiated. Local heat should be applied to the muscle for 15 to 20 minutes before stretching. The individual may return to physical activity only when he has regained full motion of the spine and has restored the strength, flexibility, and endurance of the injured muscle. The stretching modifies the inelastic scar tissue that forms as a result of the muscle strain and prevents future injury by enhancing the flexibility of the back musculature.

The young athlete with iliac apophysitis or an iliac apophysis avulsion should be withheld from any activities that cause pain at the site of this injury. The iliac apophysitis or avulsion heals with 4 to 6 weeks of rest.

After the pain has resolved, gentle stretching of the muscles that attach to this area of the iliac apophysis is initiated and performed as described for muscle strains.

ACUTE LIGAMENT SPRAINS AND INTERSPINOUS PROCESS BURSITIS

Back sprains are a second common mechanical cause of acute back pain. The term *sprain* denotes injury to one or more of the ligaments of the spine. The most common site of injury is the interspinous process ligaments. With this injury, a person experiences the acute onset of pain in the midline of the lower back (area *C* in Fig. 2). The pain is exacerbated by flexion of the lumbar spine. On physical examination, the tenderness is maximal over the interspinous ligament between the spinous processes, and there also may be compensatory paraspinous muscle spasm. Treatment of this condition is the same as that described for muscle strains.

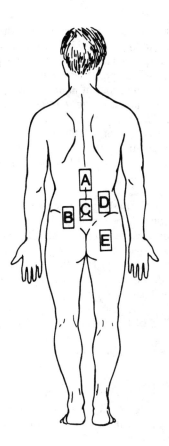

Figure 2 The locations of pain and tenderness with the following causes of mechanical and nonmechanical back pain: (*A*) compression fractures; (*B*) muscle strains and iliac crest avulsions; (*C*) ligament sprains, kissing spines, and disc injuries; (*D*) spondylolysis, articular facet fractures, and muscle strains; and (*E*) disc injuries and leg-length discrepancies.

Lumbar interspinous process bursitis (kissing spines) may have a more insidious onset and is caused by repetitive contact of the tips of the spinous processes. This condition, common in gymnasts and divers, is the result of repetitive hyperextension of the lumbar spine. In contrast to that of ligamentous sprains, the pain increases with hyperextension and decreases with flexion of the lumbar spine. The site of maximum tenderness is the same as that described for acute sprains. The most common level involved is between the spinous process of the fourth and fifth lumbar vertebrae (lower part of area *C* in Fig. 2). With both acute ligamentous sprains and interspinous process bursitis, roentgenograms of the lumbar spine usually do not reveal abnormalities of the spinous processes. Even if views in hyperextension do not demonstrate contact between the tips of the two adjacent spinous processes at the level of symptoms, the diagnosis can be made based on the results of the physical examination. The initial treatment of kissing spines is directed toward resolving the bursitis. This can be accomplished by short periods of restricted activity in conjunction with the use of oral nonsteroidal anti-inflammatory drugs. If the bursitis persists, the injection of dexamethasone (1 ml) and 1 percent lidocaine (2 to 3 ml) into the inflamed bursa between the spinous processes usually produces immediate and lasting relief.

LEG LENGTH AND EQUALITY

Minor differences in leg lengths occur commonly, but seldom result in significant back pain. However, in some persons, differences of only 1 cm can cause pain along the course of the sciatic nerve at the sciatic notch (area *E* in Fig. 2) on the side of the short extremity. Because leg-length discrepancies of up to 2.5 cm do not grossly affect an individual's gait, differences usually are not noticed. Thus, leg lengths should be determined during the initial examination of an individual with low back pain. This is accomplished by measuring both legs along the distance between the anterior superior iliac spine and the medial malleolus. The dull, aching pain caused by unequal leg length is usually aggravated by prolonged periods of standing. On physical examination, the pain can be reproduced by pressure over the sciatic nerve at the sciatic notch (area *E* in Fig. 2). Roentgenograms of the pelvis and the lumbar spine often demonstrate a curvature (scoliosis of the spine) and an elevation of the pelvis on the side of the longer extremity. However, long-term studies have shown that structural (fixed) curvatures or degenerative changes in the thoracic or lumbar spine do not occur.

Treatment of this condition, in skeletally mature individuals, consists of strengthening the abdominal musculature and leveling the pelvis. The pelvis is leveled with a heel lift applied to the shoe of the short extremity. The height of the lift should be equal to one-half of the difference between the lengths of the two extremities; greater height will give a person the sensation that he or she is tipping over to the long side. A heel-lift thickness of up to one-quarter inch will not cause the heel to be pushed out of the shoe. If additional height is needed, the outside of the shoe can be augmented. Leg-length equalization should be considered in individuals with open growth plates and discrepancies of 2.5 cm or more.

DISC INJURIES

Herniated nucleus pulposus (HNP) is not the most common cause of mechanical back pain seen in the adolescent or young athlete, but it is among the most disabling. The older the patient, the more the clinical presentation resembles the classic picture of the adult with an acute disc syndrome. In adult patients, low back pain and radiation of the pain along the sciatic nerve (sciatica) is characteristic of the syndrome (areas *C* and *E* in Fig. 2). In children and adolescents, the presentation often differs. Although 90 percent of the adolescents with HNP have sciatica, only 60 percent of them have back pain. Frequently the sciatica is associated with the stiff spine syndrome, which is characterized by a shuffling gait, severe paravertebral muscle spasm, reduced spinal movement, and tight hamstring muscles. The key to the diagnosis of the herniated disc in adolescents is the presence of sciatica. Although neurologic deficits are not commonly seen in the younger patient, they should be looked for, including competency of the anal sphincter. Initial treatment for HNP includes bed rest in a semi-Fowler's position (knees and hips flexed), analgesics, and nonsteroidal anti-inflammatory drugs. Recovery is marked by improvement in mobility of the spine as well as a diminution of the sciatic nerve irritability. Although HNP occurs less frequently in adolescents than adults, the prognosis is more guarded for successful recovery without surgery.

Fractures of the Vertebral Body and Posterior Elements of the Spine

Although uncommon, compression fractures of a vertebral body do occur in gymnasts, divers, and tobogganers. Symptoms include moderate paraspinal muscle spasm, limited motion of the spine, and pain in the midline directly over the spinous process of the fractured vertebra. The most common site of injury is the thoracolumbar junction (area A in Fig. 2), followed by the mid-lumbar spine (upper part of area C in Fig. 2). Most compression fractures heal without complications; however, genitourinary dysfunction and pain owing to chronic vertebral instability can occur and result in prolonged disability and numerous emergency visits.

Genitourinary dysfunction secondary to minor compression fractures of the lower thoracic and upper lumbar vertebrae has been documented in individuals with a normal neurologic examination. Specifically, they have normal sacral sensation and anal sphincter tone. For this reason, all individuals with vertebral fractures at the thoracolumbar junction should have two or more determinations of residual urine volume after voiding. If residual volume is more than 60 ml, the patient should be referred to a urologist.

Vertebral instability can be the result of fractures that appear benign, but are associated with ligamentous injuries of the thoracolumbar and the lumbar spine. Individuals with this condition present with midline back pain (area A in Fig. 2), that is aggravated by physical activity and relieved by rest. On clinical examination, these patients have a positive spine instability test. This test is performed with the patient prone on the examining table. The examiner applies ventral pressure to the spine at the level of the patient's symptoms. The patient is instructed to contract the paraspinous musculature, and the ventral pressure is then again applied to the level of the injury. The test is positive if the first step reproduces the patient's pain and the second step relieves it. The initial treatment includes strengthening of the abdominal and paraspinous musculature. If the pain does not abate after several months of nonoperative treatment, posterior spinal fusion is recommended.

Fractures of the posterior elements of the spine may be caused by acute or repetitive trauma. Acute fractures are usually the result of a direct blow to the back (e.g., in a football game) or excessive torsional loads applied to the lumbar spine. The inferior articular processes of the lumbar vertebrae are the structures most commonly fractured with these types of injuries. On clinical examination, the area lateral to the midline at the level of the fracture is tender to palpation (area D in Fig. 2). The pain is increased by rotation of the lumbar spine, and the patient has a positive spine instability test. These fractures usually heal with 8 to 12 weeks of immobilization and restricted activity.

Stress fractures of the posterior elements (spondylolysis) usually occur in the pars interarticularis and are the result of repetitive hyperextension forces that are not sufficient to produce an acute fracture. Although these fractures can occur with various types of physical activity, they are most commonly found in gymnasts and football linemen. With this injury, the patient presents with pain that is localized lateral to the midline at the belt level (area D in Fig. 2). The pain is aggravated by rotation and hyperextension of the lumbar spine. On clinical examination, the patient is found to have tight hamstrings, tenderness in the paravertebral muscles, and a positive one-leg lumbar hyperextension test. The test is performed by having the patient stand on one leg and then hyperextend his lumbar spine. The test is positive if this posturing reproduces his pain. In addition, the patient may have a positive result on the spine instability test. Results of the neurologic examination are normal.

Radiographic evaluation should include anteroposterior, lateral, and oblique views of the lumbar spine. The pars interarticularis is best visualized on oblique roentgenograms. However, the initial lumbar films, including oblique views, may appear normal in patients in whom a stress fracture of the pars interarticularis is developing. In these cases, the technetium (^{99m}Tc) polyphosphate scan is a valuable adjunct in early diagnosis of a pars defect. The scan demonstrates a stress fracture long before the injury may be confirmed radiographically. Stress fractures of the pars interarticularis should be treated symptomatically. This treatment involves restriction from activities that aggravate the pain, flexibility exercises to stretch the hamstrings, and hyperextension exercises to strengthen the paraspinous musculature. If the patient has pain during daily activities, he should be fitted with an antilordotic brace. This type of brace has proven effective for controlling the patient's symptoms to the extent that many of these individuals are able to remain active in sports. If bracing is not effective in controlling the pain or there is evidence of progressive anterior vertebral body displacement (spondylolisthesis), posterior spinal fusion may be indicated.

Disc Space Infection (Discitis)

Discitis is an infection that usually occurs spontaneously in the disc space and adjacent vertebral end-plate. Although it is not frequently seen in athletic individuals, it is the most common cause of nonmechanical back pain in the first and second decades of life. Therefore, the adolescent athlete who presents with severe back pain and muscle spasm without a clearly mechanical symptom pattern should be evaluated for discitis. The patient usually has severe muscle spasm, spinal deformity (scoliosis), and tight hamstrings. Systemic signs such as fever and leukocytosis are usually low grade, and blood cultures are frequently (55 percent) negative. Initial roentgenograms of the spine are normal. Abnormal film findings that include vertebral end-plate irregularities and disc space narrowing are not evident for many weeks. However, if a ^{99m}Tc bone scan is obtained after the third day of the illness, it usually demonstrates increased activity at the site of infection.

The most frequently involved disc spaces are L2–L3, L1–L2, and L3–L4, in that order (area C in Fig. 2). The most common infecting organism is *Staphylococcus aureus*.

Discitis usually responds well to bed rest and antistaphylococcal antibiotics. Intravenous antibiotics should not be used until blood cultures (positive in 45 percent of cases) have been obtained. The patient is mobilized and switched to oral antibiotics as soon as the symptoms begin to subside and the sedimentation rate starts to normalize. Mobilization usually can be accomplished without a cast or brace. Oral antibiotic therapy should be continued for 6 weeks.

SUGGESTED READING

DeOrior JK, Bianco AJ Jr. Lumbar disc excision in children and adolescents. J Bone Joint Surg 1982; 64-A:991–996.
Hazlett JW. Kissing spines. J Bone Joint Surg 1964; 46-A:1368–1369.
Jackson DW, Wiltse LL, Dingeman RD, Hayes M. Stress reactions involving the pars interarticularis in young athletes. Am J Sports Med 1981; 9:304–312.
Keene JS, Goletz TH, Benson RC. Undetected genito-urinary dysfunction in vertebral fractures. J Bone Joint Surg 1980; 62-A:997–999.
Papaionnou I, Stokes I, Kenweight J. Scoliosis associated with limb-length inequality. J Bone Joint Surg 1982; 64-A:59–62.

COMPARTMENT SYNDROME AND RHABDOMYOLYSIS

BARRY BRENNER, M.D.

Rhabdomyolysis occurs when an injury to skeletal muscle tissue causes the dissolution of the cells and the subsequent release of their contents into the circulation. Myoglobinuria often accompanies rhabdomyolysis and is responsible for the reddish brown discoloration of urine. This muscle damage subsequently can cause myoglobinuria, compartmental compression syndrome, hypocalcemia, hypoalbuminemia, hyperuricemia, hyperkalemia, hyperphosphatemia, and disseminated intravascular coagulation (Table 1). Myoglobinuria can lead to acute tubular necrosis. Early diagnosis and treatment are important to prevent acute renal failure or irreversible muscle tissue loss.

Compartment syndrome occurs when injured muscle tissue that is encased in a fascial sheath swells and causes secondary compression of any or all blood vessels and nerves that traverse the compartment. Compartment syndrome can lead to Volkmann's ischemic contracture, causing permanent loss of function.

There are nearly 100 specific diseases that can be grouped into five categories of causes of skeletal muscle injury (Table 2). These categories range from hereditary enzymatic defects, which cause inefficient energy production, to infectious diseases, such as Legionnaire's disease. Others include trauma, toxin-like snake venom, and hypoxia from carbon monoxide poisoning and arterial embolism.

DIAGNOSIS AND TREATMENT OF RHABDOMYOLYSIS

If awake, a patient with rhabdomyolysis presents with symptoms including weakness, myalgia, pain, and tenderness of the afflicted muscle or muscles. Passive or active movement may cause severe pain. The overlying skin may be erythematous and edema is common. If the disorder has been allowed to progress, deep tendon reflexes may be absent and irreversible muscle necrosis may have already taken place. Many patients, however, will be obtunded or unconscious owing to their precipitating disorder, such as stroke, hyperthermia, or overdose. The urine is frequently dark colored because of myoglobin.

There are many laboratory test results that confirm rhabdomyolysis and myoglobinuria. The most specific

TABLE 1 Progression of Compartment Syndrome and Muscle Injury

First stage:	Myoglobinuria CPK >10,000 IU/ml
Second stage:	Myoglobinuria Increased creatinine and BUN but normal urine output CPK >20,000 IU/ml Hypotension (from third space losses)
Third stage:	Oliguria Shock Metabolic acidosis Hyperkalemia Arrhythmias

TABLE 2 Causes of Skeletal Muscle Injury

Abnormalities of Energy Consumption	Hypoxia	Primary Muscle Injury	Infectious Diseases	Miscellaneous
Muscle overexertion (e.g., march myoglobinuria) Seizures	Generalized hypoxia	Crush injury	Infectious myositis	Hyperthermia
	Arterial embolism or injury	Trauma Fractures	Clostridia perfringens infection	Hypothermia Direct muscle injury by toxins (e.g., drugs, toluene)
Hereditary enzymatic defects (e.g., McArdle's syndrome)	Prolonged immobility causing ischemia: Drug overdose CVA Carbon monoxide	Electrical injury Burns Polymyositis	Legionnaire's disease Rocky Mountain spotted fever	Spider or snake bite

findings are myoglobin in the urine and elevated muscle enzyme activity in serum. Muscle aldolase activity levels as high as 100,000 IU per ml and CPK levels over 20,000 IU per ml are not unusual. In cases of lesser degrees of rhabdomyolysis, aldolase activity levels may range from 500 to 5,000 IU per ml, and a lower concentration of myoglobin in the urine may not be noted. A practical method for quickly differentiating rhabdomyolysis from hemolysis in patients with discolored urine is to look at the serum. Rhabdomyolysis does not discolor serum, whereas hemolysis turns it pink.

Hyperkalemia, hyperphosphatemia, hypocalcemia, hypoalbuminemia, and hyperuricemia are other findings. Hyperkalemia is potentially cardiotoxic. It should be anticipated in patients with severe rhabdomyolysis and should be prevented. Plasma calcium levels as low as 3.5 mg per deciliter have been reported, caused by the "dumping" of plasma calcium salts into the injured muscle tissue, where they are bound. Hypocalcemia usually corrects itself in several days and treatment is not required, although it may potentiate the cardiotoxicity of hyperkalemia. Calcium salts, however, may be used to treat hyperkalemia. Hyperuricemia with serum uric acid levels of 50 mg per deciliter may occur. Hypoalbuminemia may be present because of related capillary injury. Severe cases may occur even in previously healthy patients within the first few days. Albumin may be administered, but because it leaks from the capillaries and contributes to interstitial edema, the physician should watch for compartment compression syndrome. Disseminated intravascular coagulation can occur in major rhabdomyolysis, and fresh frozen plasma can be used, if severe hemorrhaging occurs, to replace coagulation proteins. Fibrin split products in serum or urine, thrombocytopenia, hypofibrinogenemia, and a prolonged prothrombin time are often found as well.

In patients with extensive rhabdomyolysis, one should keep the volume of fluid at an adequate level and maintain normal circulation to prevent acute tubular necrosis. Ten liters of normal saline in the first 12 to 24 hours may be needed to stabilize blood pressure and replace volume lost into muscle. Any ensuing edema, however, should be observed closely as a harbinger of the development of the compartment syndrome. In addition, the use of mannitol and furosemide dilutes the concentration of myoglobin in the urine, increases urine output, and reduces the renal toxicity of myoglobin.

DIAGNOSIS AND TREATMENT OF COMPARTMENT SYNDROME

The compartment syndrome is an important complication of rhabdomyolysis that should be detected and treated early. Skeletal muscle tissue comprises 40 percent of the body weight, and muscle injury is extremely common. Various groups of muscles are encased in fascial sheaths, which allow no room for swelling. In such a surrounding fascial sheath, any edema can cause secondary vascular compression of the traversing blood vessels. Muscle tissue more distal from the site of injury may become ischemic, and muscle necrosis with possible subsequent contracture may eventually result. The most common sites in the musculature where this may occur include the four fascial compartments in the leg—peroneal, anterior, deep posterior, and superficial posterior. Also included are the volar and dorsal compartments of the forearm and the interosseous muscles of the hand (Figure 1). The anterior compartment of the leg is the area most often afflicted by the compartment syndrome; if it is left untreated, the resultant muscle damage results in foot drop.

Early diagnosis is critical, since irreversible muscle damage occurs in four to six hours. A high index of suspicion is needed, particularly in unconscious or uncooperative patients. A complete neurologic and motor examination of the affected extremity is a must. Tenderness and pain during active or passive flexion are common signs. A sensitive and reliable early sign is heightened pain upon passive extension of the fingers or toes when the hand or foot is involved, but this is of use only when there has been no direct trauma that could also cause pain. An abnormal two point discrimination or light touch examination of a traversing nerve is a good early indicator of the compartment syndrome; this is often preceded by paresthesias. The affected area may also be indurated and erythematous, although this is a late sign.

Of particular importance is that capillary refill and distal pulse strength are helpful only when they are abnormal, suggesting reduced perfusion. However, both are

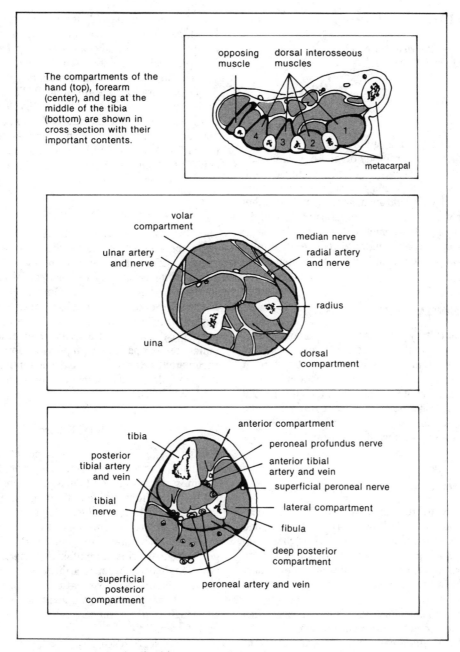

The compartments of the hand (top), forearm (center), and leg at the middle of the tibia (bottom) are shown in cross section with their important contents.

Figure 1 Three common compartments involved in compartment syndrome. (From In defense of limbs. Emerg Med 1981: 208.)

usually normal in patients with the compartment syndrome, and thus can never rule out this entity.

Suspicion of the compartment syndrome calls for immediate orthopedic consultation; if there is any doubt, the tissue pressures can be measured directly by inserting an 18 gauge needle into the compartment tissues and connecting to a manometer with saline-filled tubing. Tissue pressures of 0 to 8 mm Hg are normal; pressures over 30 mm can cause ischemia and are an indication for fasciotomy. Compression of a forearm or leg by the head or torso causes pressures of 30 to 50 mm, and the rib cage compressing the forearm causes a pressure of 180 mm Hg. Repeated serial observations are also mandatory if there is a suspicion of the compartment syndrome or if the patient is at high risk, e.g., the patient with severe fractures or trauma of the lower leg. Once the diagnosis is made, decompression by fasciotomy should be performed immediately to preclude further injury. Despite the presence of swelling, however, adequate hydration of the patient should continue to prevent acute renal failure attributable to myoglobinuria.

ARTHRITIS

DAVID B. HELLMANN, M.D.
MICHELLE PETRI, M.D.

The most important job of the emergency physician evaluating arthritis is to promptly diagnose patients having an infected joint. Diagnosing and treating crystal-induced arthritis (i.e., gout and pseudogout) are also important. The evaluation and management of most other arthritic and rheumatic conditions are the province of the consulting rheumatologist, internist, or orthopaedist.

The first step in evaluating arthritis is to determine whether the joint problem is inflammatory or noninflammatory.

NONINFLAMMATORY ARTHRITIS

In noninflammatory conditions (e.g., osteoarthritis), heat, soft-tissue swelling, redness, and systemic manifestations of inflammation are absent. Therefore, if a patient does not have at least one hot, swollen joint or systemic manifestation of inflammation, then that patient is unlikely to need emergency medical care and can be given aspirin, acetaminophen, or a nonsteroidal anti-inflammatory drug and referred to a primary care physician.

INFLAMMATORY (AND INFECTIOUS) ARTHRITIS

Inflammatory arthropathies are manifested by joint redness, heat, soft-tissue swelling, morning stiffness, and fatigue. In some inflammatory conditions, such as systemic lupus erythematosus, the degree of joint swelling is minimal or absent, but other manifestations of generalized inflammation (e.g., fever, pericarditis, pleuritis) are present.

Patients with inflammatory arthritis must undergo further evaluation to exclude the presence of infection. The duration of the arthritis greatly influences the differential diagnosis because, generally, inflammatory arthritis of more than 3 weeks' duration is rarely due to infection. Several exceptions to this rule are worth noting. For example, some chronic arthropathies such as rheumatoid arthritis are occasionally complicated by septic arthritis. Therefore, a patient with previously diagnosed rheumatoid arthritis who is having an atypical flare as indicated by fever or sudden increased swelling in only one joint, should be suspected of having a superimposed infection. In addition, patients with an undiagnosed arthropathy of more than 3 weeks' duration should be evaluated for the possibility of infection if the patient has fever or monoarthritis. Polyarthritis of more than 3 weeks' duration is rarely due to infection, although the polyarthritides of bacterial endocarditis and secondary syphilis are noteworthy exceptions. Patients having any of these risk factors

for infection must have their joint fluid aspirated and analyzed, as discussed later in this chapter. Otherwise, the patient with a chronic (longer than 3 weeks) arthritis is best referred to an internist or a rheumatologist.

For the patient with inflammatory arthritis of less than 3 weeks' duration, the differential diagnosis is usually limited to a few disorders. These are crystal-induced arthritis (i.e., gout and pseudogout), gonococcal arthritis, nongonococcal septic arthritis, and Reiter's syndrome (Table 1). A directed history and physical enable the diagnosis by focusing on host factors, the joint pattern, and the extra-articular manifestations.

Host Factors

Gonococcal arthritis and Reiter's syndrome nearly always occur in patients under the age of 40. Gonococcal arthritis predominates in women (and is especially common during pregnancy or menses), whereas gout and Reiter's predominate in men. Gout is rare before age 40. Diuretic use, obesity, alcoholism, renal disease, and low-dose aspirin use are other risk factors for gout. Nongonococcal septic arthritis can occur at any age and in either sex, but patients with previous joint disease (e.g., rheumatoid arthritis) or recurrent septicemia (e.g., intravenous drug abuse or valvular heart disease) are especially likely victims.

Joint Pattern

The pattern of joint involvement often provides additional clues about the correct diagnosis. Crystal disease is almost always monoarticular. Gout commonly attacks the great toe, foot, or knee. Pseudogout typically strikes the knee, wrist, or shoulder. Reiter's syndrome usually produces an oligoarthritis, chiefly involving the lower extremities. In contrast to gout or Reiter's syndrome, gonococcal arthritis more often affects the upper extremity. Nongonococcal septic arthritis is usually monoarticular and favors the lower extremity, especially the knee or hip. In intravenous drug abusers, however, unusual sites such as the sternoclavicular or sacroiliac joint can be infected.

The onset of disease is most rapid in the crystal diseases; usually the time from initial symptom to maximally intense pain is only a few hours. With septic arthritis and Reiter's syndrome the onset is slightly less rapid, taking 1 to several days before reaching maximal intensity. Gonococci often produce a migratory polyarthritis that evolves over several days into an oligoarthritis. The arthritis of Reiter's syndrome may be preceded by an episode of dysentery, nongonococcal urethritis, or conjunctivitis.

The exact form of the swelling may also be revealing. Tenosynovitis (swelling of the tendon sheaths), especially in the hand, is a classic feature of gonococcal arthritis. Sausage swelling of one entire digit (especially in the foot) is a hallmark of Reiter's syndrome, as is swelling of large tendons such as the Achilles tendon. In gout, surrounding sterile cellulitis is not uncommon.

TABLE 1 Major Causes of One Inflamed Joint

Cause	Risk Factors	Joint Pattern	Extra-articular Features	Laboratory Data
Crystal-induced				
Gout	Diuretic use Renal insufficiency Alcohol use Moonshine (lead) Low-dose aspirin Obesity	First MTP most common Also ankle-tarsal and knee May be polyarticular	Tophi	Negatively birefringent needle-shaped crystals in joint fluid
Pseudogout	Hyperparathyroidism Hemochromatosis	Knee, wrist, or shoulder	None	Postively birefringent rhomboidal crystals in joint fluid
Infection				
Gonococcal arthritis	Sexual exposure Onset during menstruation or pregnancy Late complement deficiency	Often migratory Rarely monoarticular Upper limb most common	Fever Skin lesions—pustules Tenosynovitis	Blood and joint cultures often negative Urethral, rectal, or pharyngeal culure may be positive
Other septic arthritides	Immunocompromised patient IV drug abuse Valvular heart disease Previous joint disease	May be an unusual joint such as sternoclavicular or sacroiliac usually monoarticular, especially knee or hip		Joint culture usually positive
Noninfectious				
Reiter's Syndrome	Young men Post-dysentery	Lower limb oligoarthritis May have sausage digit	Aphthous ulcers Conjunctivitis or iritis Urethritis Balanitis Keratoderma blennorrhagicum	Inflammatory joint fluid 90% HLA-B27 positive

Extra-articular Manifestations

The general physical examination can provide many important diagnostic clues. For example, the presence of small, erythematous, necrotic pustules distributed on the distal extremities indicates disseminated gonococcemia. Reiter's syndrome produces several mucocutaneous lesions including mild conjunctivitis, painless mouth ulcers, raw erythematous papules on the glans penis (circinate balanitis), and scaling of the palms or soles (keratoderma blennorrhagicum). Tophi, which are cutaneous urate deposits frequently found in the external ear, can suggest the diagnosis of gout.

Fever is not a very discriminating finding for the differential diagnosis under consideration. Some patients with acute gout have a raised temperature, whereas some patients with septic arthritis have no fever. Although the absence of fever is more common in patients with septic arthritis who are taking corticosteroids, fever may be absent even in otherwise normal individuals presenting with an infected joint. The risk of missing an infected joint in such a patient is especially high when the joint cannot be palpated, as with the hip. Therefore, a patient who has acute, unexplained hip pain (which is aggravated by moving the hip and unaffected by palpating the trochanteric bursa or sciatic notch) should be suspected of having an infection regardless of his temperature.

Laboratory Tests

The diagnosis suggested by the history and physical examination can be supported by judicious use of the laboratory. The most important test in any patient with the first episode of a hot joint is examination of the synovial fluid. The site of joint involvement and the training of the emergency physician determine whether aspiration can be done by that physician or whether an orthopaedist should be called.

The synovial fluid helps answer three questions: Is infection present? Is inflammation present? Are crystals present? Thus, the most important step is culturing the fluid and doing a Gram stain. The importance of the culture is emphasized by the fact that 20 to 50 percent of infected joint fluids may give a negative Gram stain. The next most important test is to examine the fluid for crystals. A microscope equipped with built-in polarizing lenses is ideal, but a less well-endowed microscope enhanced by a kit of polarizing lenses is adequate. Urate (gout) crystals are needle shaped and negatively birefringent, whereas calcium pyrophosphate dehydrate (pseudogout) crystals are rhomboidal and positively birefringent. Most crystals are small so that high dry or oil-immersion views are required. If there is sufficient fluid, some should be sent for cell count: more than 1,000 white blood cells suggest mild inflammation, more than 50,000 indicate more intense inflammation as is typical of gout, and more than 100,000 suggest infection. However, there is much overlap among these classifications. Infection cannot be excluded on the basis of cell count alone. Other synovial fluid tests such as glucose and protein are of limited value.

Patients with hot joints should have complete blood counts. Leukocytosis and increased immature polymorphonuclear leukocytes suggest infection but are also seen in inflammatory conditions such as gout. Patients suspected of having gout should have serum uric acid and baseline serum creatinine tests. X-ray films taken during the first several days of a joint infection rarely demonstrate bony changes, but do provide a helpful baseline. Patients suspected of having gonococcal arthritis should have cultures of the pharynx, rectum, and urethra because the joint fluid culture is frequently negative.

Management

If the synovial fluid Gram stain demonstrates organisms, then the patient has an infected joint and should be admitted. The only exception to this rule is in gonococcal arthritis; reliable patients who have a small effusion and do not appear toxic can be treated as outpatients with oral ampicillin, 3.5 g orally, plus 1 g of probenecid, followed by ampicillin, 0.5 g orally 4 times daily for 7 days. Such patients should be reevaluated by a primary care physician within 48 hours.

What should be done for the patient who has a picture consistent with an infected joint, but in whom the Gram stain is negative? Given that the outcome of septic arthritis is directly related to the speed of the correct diagnosis, the best course is to admit the patient. Usually the patient can be treated with empiric antibiotics while culture results are awaited. Additional tests, such as synovial biopsy and bone scan, may be needed.

If the patient is shown to have gout or pseudogout, then treatment with a nonsteroidal anti-inflammatory drug (e.g., indomethacin 25 to 50 mg orally 3 times a day with food) should be started. Colchicine is also effective for acute gout, but the diarrhea that usually complicates its use makes the nonsteroidal anti-inflammatory drugs preferable. The patient should be referred to an appropriate physician to determine the form of long-term treatment. Agents that abruptly lower the serum uric acid (e.g., allopurinol) have no place in the treatment of acute gout and, in fact, can aggravate the acute inflammation.

SUGGESTED READING

Goldenberg DL. Gonococcal arthritis. In: McCarthy DJ, ed. Arthritis and allied conditions. Philadelphia: Lea & Febiger, 1985: 1651.
Schmid FR. Approach to monoarticular arthritis. In: Kelley W, Harris ED, Ruddy S, Sledge CB, eds. Textbook of rheumatology. Philadelphia: WB Saunders, 1985: 391.
Simkin PA. Management of gout. Ann Intern Med 1979; 90:812–816.

HAND INFECTIONS

DAVID M. CONTRERAS, M.D.
LEONARD GORDON, M.D.

Although the majority of infections of the hand can be treated successfully in the emergency department, a small group of infections are serious and require hospitilization and more extensive treatment. Hand infections have the potential for prolonged disability, and they require accurate diagnosis and timely, effective treatment.

HISTORY

A careful history provides important information for proper diagnosis and treatment. Such factors as diabetes, steroid therapy, immunosuppressive therapy, and ischemic conditions are known to predispose a patient toward infection. While general malaise, fevers, and loss of sleep can be associated with established hand infections, a hand infection may, in turn, be a manifestation of a systemic problem, such as gonococcal infection. A careful history often differentiates infections from other inflammatory problems of the hand, such as arthritis, gout, pseudogout, and Reiter's syndrome.

Often, antibiotic treatment must be initiated even before a fluid specimen can be obtained for Gram stain and culture. In these situations, the choice of antibiotic is empiric, relying heavily on the patient's history (Table 1). Infection in an injury that is 24 to 48 hours old is often limited to a cellulitis, which can be controlled with antibiotics. Abscess formation involving the various spaces of the hand, or septic arthritis should be suspected when an injury is more than 48 hours old. These latter conditions usually require surgical intervention.

LABORATORY STUDIES

A complete blood count and differential leukocyte count should be performed for patients who have systemic signs or symptoms. The relevance of other tests is determined by the presence of predisposing conditions or other significant information revealed in the history. For example, in patients with a history of penetrating trauma, x-ray films of the hand may demonstrate a fracture or foreign body. A widened joint space or bone destruction in the x-ray film indicates septic arthritis or osteomyelitis. If fluid can be obtained, Gram stain can direct

TABLE 1   Hand Infection: Scheme for Initial Antibiotic Therapy based on Patient History

Situation	Organism	Antibiotic
Human bites	*Eichinella corrodens*, anaerobes, streptococci	Penicillin and cephalosporin
Animal bites	*Pasteurella multocida*	Penicillin
Aquatic environments	*Aeromonas hydrophila, Mycobacterium marinum*	Aminoglycosides (tetracycline)
Drug addicts	*Pseudomonas, Serratia*	Tobramycin, gentamicin
Dentists and nurses	Herpes simplex	No treatment available

TABLE 2   Hand Infection: Scheme for Initial Antibiotic Therapy Based on Gram Stain Results

Organism on Gram Stain	Approximate Incidence* (%)	Antibiotic		
		Oral	First IV	Second IV
Gram (+) cocci (*Staphylococcus*)	50	Dicloxacillin	Cephalosporin	Erythromycin
Gram (+) cocci (*Staphylococcus*)	30	Penicillin	Penicillin	Erythromycin
Gram (−) rod	20	—	Gentamicin	—
Mixed flora	55	Cephalosporin	Cephalosporin	Tetracycline

* Incidence varies widely in the literature and depends on geography and the particular patient population.

initial antibiotic therapy while awaiting culture results (Table 2).

CLASSIFICATION AND TREATMENT

The following are the three most common categories of hand infection seen in the emergency department: cellulitis, infections that occur on the dorsal surface of the hand, and infections that occur on the palmar surface of the hand.

Cellulitis

Cellulitis may result from a localized infection in the skin or be secondary to a deep-seated infection. A patient with cellulitis, fever, and leukocytosis should be hospitalized for parenteral antibiotic therapy and be evaluated by a hand specialist for a deep-seated abscess. Uncomplicated cellulitis usually presents within 24 to 48 hours of injury and is caused by group A streptococci. The drug of choice is penicillin, which is taken orally at a 500-mg dose 4 times daily; erythromycin at the same dosage should be used for penicillin-allergic patients. In addition to this specific treatment, a hand splint should be applied. Splints allow the inflamed part to rest, and they promote patient comfort during the acute phase of the infection.

Dorsal Surface Infections

Paronychia

Paronychia appears as a collection of pus in the nail fold, and is the most common infection of the hand (Fig. 1). If neglected, it may extend around the entire nail

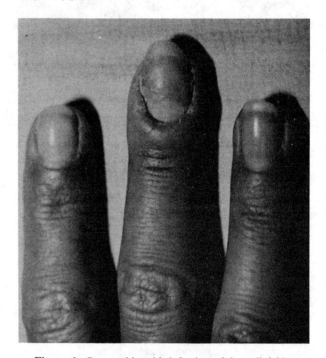

Figure 1   Paronychia with infection of the nail fold.

margin and cause a floating nail. Although the most common causative agent is *Staphylococcus aureus*, a variety of other bacterial and fungal organisms can also be responsible. Oral antibiotic therapy may be sufficient for early cases with cellulitis. The telltale symptoms of abscess formation are throbbing and pain that causes awakening from sleep at night. Treatment consists of incision and drainage of the nail fold and evacuation of accumulated pus. A digital block using xylocaine without epinephrine is usually

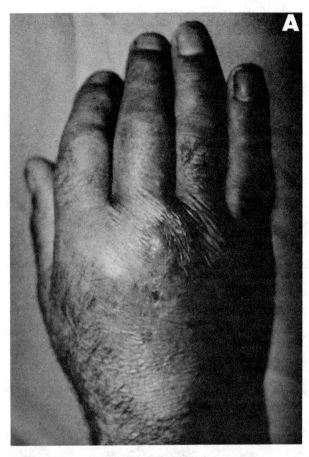

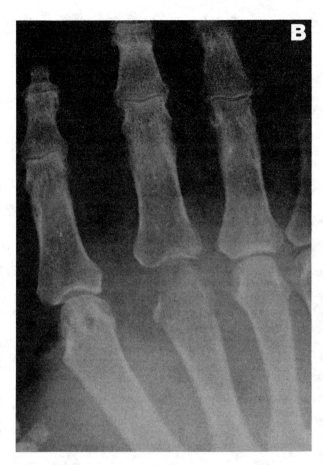

Figure 2 *A*, Several weeks after receiving a puncture wound from a tooth, this patient presented with septic arthritis of the second metacarpophalangeal joint. *B*, X-ray rilms show lytic change in the metacarpal head.

required. The wound is then loosely packed and the digit splinted and elevated. The packing is changed and the wound reexamined after 1 to 2 days.

Carbuncles and Boils

The dorsum of the hand has loose subcutaneous tissue. Local infection usually involves the hair follicles, which results in a boil or carbuncle. It is important to realize that swelling on the dorsum of the hand often occurs with deep palmar infections because of the loose subcutaneous layer dorsally. Treatment consists of local incision and drainage and loose packing of the wound. The hand is splinted and elevated, and the patient is told to return after 1 to 2 days for a dressing change and reexamination. Oral antibiotics are indicated if cellulitis or lymphangitis is present.

Septic Arthritis

The most common cause of septic arthritis in the hand is a bite from another human (Fig. 2A and 2B). Puncture wounds on the dorsum of the metacarpophalangeal joint often represent tooth marks received in an altercation. These human bites should be treated with exploration, operating room debridement, and parenteral antibiotics.

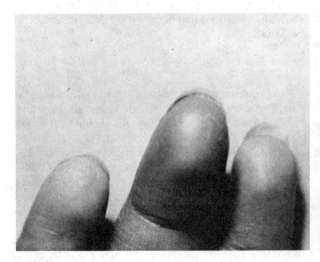

Figure 3 Felon; note the tense palmar pulp of the middle fingertip.

The seriousness of this kind of wound, and its potential for infective complication should not be underestimated. If joint swelling or a persistently draining wound is present, septic arthritis must be considered.

Palmar Surface Infections

Felon (Terminal Pulp Abscess)

A felon results from infection within the closed space of the digital pulp (Fig. 3). *S. aureus* is usually the causative agent. Treatment consists of incision and drainage at the point of maximal tenderness. A digital block using xylocaine without epinephrine provides appropriate anesthesia. The incision should be longitudinal over the mid-pulp area. The wound is loosely packed and the digit splinted and elevated. The patient should return in 1 to 2 days for removal of the packing and reexamination. Oral antibiotics should be administered.

Deep Space Infections: Web Space Infection, Deep Palmar Space Infection, and Thenar Infection

Web spaces are surrounded by several ligaments and the palmar fascia. When infected, they provide a closed compartment. Web space infections are characterized by a fixed, painful separation of the fingers. The deep palmar space lies deep to the palmar fascia. The thickness of the palmar fascia can mask severe infection and does not allow spontaneous drainage. Recognition of these infections is essential in order to prevent destruction of important hand structures. They require formal incision and drainage in the operating room.

Three simple rules of drainage should be applied in these situations:

1. Do not wait for fluctuant swelling.
2. Pus is likely, if the patient complains of throbbing pain or has lost a night's sleep because of the pain.
3. In the presence of pus, always incise over the area of maximal tenderness.

Tenosynovitis

Tendon sheaths represent a closed space that surrounds the flexor tendons in the index, long, and ring fingers. They extend from a point just beyond the distal digital crease to the midpalmar crease proximally. The sheaths of the small finger and thumb extend to the ulnar and radial bursae at the wrist. Tense infections in these closed spaces must be treated emergently, because the delicate vascularity to the tendon may be compromised with resultant tendon necrosis and serious long-term impairment of function.

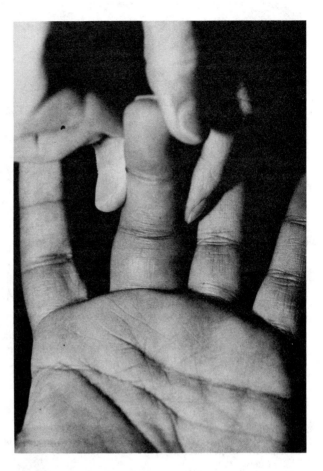

Figure 4 Flexor tenosynovitis, here being tested for pain with passive extension of the finger. Pressure on the palmar surface produces local pain and should therefore be avoided when performing this test.

Tendon sheath infections invariably show the following four classic signs described by Kanavel (Fig. 4):

1. Flexed position of the digit
2. Fusiform swelling and erythema
3. Intense pain on passive extension of the digit
4. Tenderness along the flexor sheath

Immediate hospitalization under the care of a hand specialist is required for open surgical drainage and parenteral antibiotic therapy.

SHOULDER PAIN

RENE CAILLIET, M.D.

Shoulder pain is usually a symptom of a localized orthopaedic problem that is the result of trauma or overuse. There are seven joints in the shoulder complex that may be the site of musculoskeletal pain and dysfunction (Figs. 1 and 2). Pain also may be referred to the shoulder from a distant visceral site.

In the differential diagnosis of shoulder pain, the conditions listed in Table 1 must be considered. In addition, visceral pain can be referred to the shoulder; two classic examples are myocardial infarction and diaphragmatic irritation due to blood or infection.

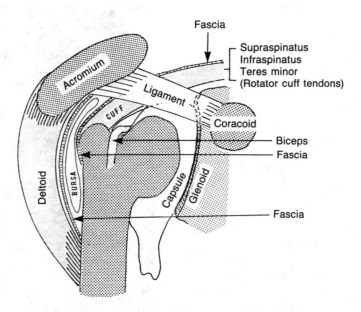

Figure 1 Anatomy of the shoulder. (From Goers HR, Hamaty D, Litton L. Calcific tendonitis and bursitis. Patient Care 1972, 6 (14):18–33.)

TABLE 1 Orthopaedic Causes of Shoulder Pain

Supraspinatus tendinitis
Subdeltoid bursitis
Rotator cuff tear—partial or complete
Acromioclavicular joint pain
   Degenerative arthritis
   Separation
Biceps tendinitis
Biceps tendon tear or dislocation
Referred pain from
   Cervical radiculitis
   Myocardial ischemia
Fracture-dislocation
Malignant disease—primary or metastatic

The history is of paramount importance. A direct fall or severe injury immediately alerts the examiner to fracture or dislocation. An insidious onset suggests more subtle and chronic causation; then examination and palpation are mandatory to isolate the exact tissue site of pain (Fig. 3). Certain movements may cause pain, as in the inability to brush the hair so typical of subdeltoid bursitis, or shoulder pain from cervical radiculitis that is elicited by turning the head.

The next step in evaluation is examination. The shoulder should be visually inspected and then palpated, noting localized tenderness in the structures in Figure 1. Active and passive range of motion should be tested and results noted on the chart for further reference. This includes an attempt at abduction, lifting the shoulder in as high an arc as possible. Finally, x-ray studies are obtained; routine are AP and lateral views. Weight-bearing views may be needed in cases of acromioclavicular separation. Special views are needed for dislocation.

The next important portion of the examination is attempted active motion, followed by passive motion.

ROTATOR CUFF TENDINITIS

Acute rotator cuff tendinitis causes painful movement of the shoulder. Abnormal overhead activity may be implicated, but it is surprising how often no history of trauma or abnormal activity can be elicited.

There is pain and tenderness of the shoulder with painful movement, usually forward flexion, abduction, or overhead elevation. A "painful arc" is often described, with less pain when the arm passes beyond that point (Fig. 4). Pain recurs at the same point in descent. External rotation may also be painful. There is tenderness at the greater tuberosity just lateral to the bicipital groove.

Inability to abduct the arm or externally rotate the humerus can indicate either an actively inflamed rotator cuff tendon or a rotator cuff tear. Passive and active abduction or forward flexion causes pain and incriminates an acutely inflamed rotator cuff tendon. If the patient can "hold" the arm abducted, this is an indication of absence of a complete rotator cuff tear. However, a positive test (failure to hold the arm abducted) does not always indicate a complete tear since pain alone may prevent one's holding the position.

Treatment usually is given on an outpatient basis and includes salicylates or one of the nonsteroidal anti-inflammatory agents taken three times a day with meals. Local measures such as an ice pack to the shoulder for 15 to 20 minutes three times a day for the first 24 to 48 hours are of value. An arm sling during the first day is soothing. Suprahumeral injection of 3 to 4 ml 1 percent lidocaine may be used if pain is severe, but usually can be delayed for 24 hours. Inclusion of steroids in the injection has no proven value.

ROTATOR CUFF TEAR

Rotator cuff tear presents with the same symptoms as rotator cuff tendinitis, but the patient cannot hold the

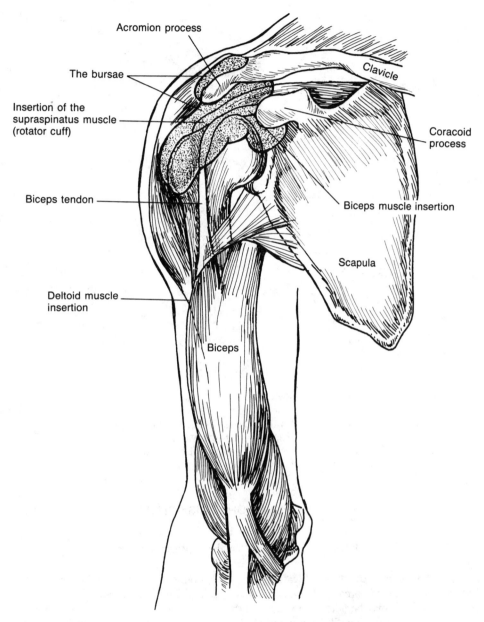

Figure 2 Anatomy of the shoulder. (From Goers HR, Hamaty D, Litton L. Calcific tendonitis and bursitis. Patient Care 1972, 6 (14):18–33.)

arm in the abducted position. Since the rotator cuff is also an external rotator, as well as an abductor, failure to externally rotate the arm or hold the arm in the extremely rotated position may be indicative of a complete tear.

Without severe trauma, a rotator cuff tear in the person under 40 years of age is rare; in older patients, a tear can occur with minimal trauma.

It is rarely necessary to accurately confirm the diagnosis of a completely torn rotator cuff on the first examination, but if it appears necessary, a suprahumeral injection of 3 to 5 ml 1 percent lidocaine relieves the pain sufficiently to allow the patient to actively attempt abduction or external rotation.

X-ray studies of the shoulder should be done routinely to rule out malignant disease, occult fracture, or disloca-

tion. Films of acute soft tissue disease are noncontributory and may be delayed.

If a suspected tear is clinically ascertained by failure to maintain abduction, an arthrogram should be obtained within a few days to ensure early surgical repair. A partial tear usually responds to conservative nonsurgical treatment as does the acute tendinitis. Arthroscopic examination currently is not an emergency procedure. Hospitalization is rarely indicated.

Partial Rotator Cuff Tear

A partial rotator cuff tear presents much the same symptoms as acute rotator cuff tendinitis, i.e., acute pain on active or passive movement, especially abduction, ex-

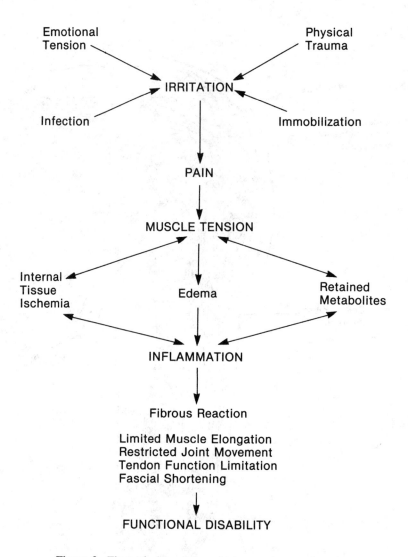

Figure 3 Theoretical causation of trigger point muscle pain.

ternal rotation, or attempted overhead elevation. There is usually tenderness over the area of the greater tuberosity. The "painful arc" may be noted as in acute tendinitis. As there are intact tendon fibers remaining, the patient *can* initiate abduction or external rotation and can hold the passively abducted arm.

The diagnosis and the treatment are the same as for acute tendinitis. Precise diagnosis depends on an arthrogram, but this is an elective procedure.

SUBDELTOID BURSITIS

The subdeltoid bursa lies under the acromion: its inner reflection is adherent to the humeral greater tuberosity, plus the outer layer of the supraspinatus tendon. The symptoms are the same as for rotator cuff tendinitis.

Although subdeltoid bursitis can occur as a primary disease, it is usually secondary to, or associated with, inflammation of the contiguous supraspinatus tendon and rotator cuff. Treatment consists of anti-inflammatory agents, local application of ice, and rest. Steroid injec-

tion is used only if pain is severe or disabling (see Rotator Cuff Tendinitis).

CALCIFIC TENDINITIS

Tendinitis even when recurrent, can exist without a calcific deposit, and a calcific deposit noted on the x-ray film may exist without pain or inflammation. Thus, x-ray findings of calcific deposits are not helpful. However, the deposit does confirm the presence of tendinitis, usually chronic and/or recurrent.

BICEPS TENDINITIS

The long tendon of the biceps passes within the biceps groove between the greater and the lesser humeral tuberosities, and hence is directly continuous with the supraspinatus tendon, infraspinatus tendon, and subdeltoid bursa. Inflammation of any of these structures can simultaneously inflame the biceps tendon, or the tendon can slip out of the bicipital groove. Tenderness can be elicited by palpating the tendon.

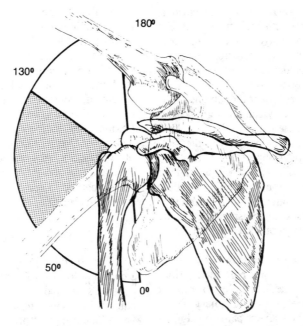

Figure 4 The painful arc caused by impairment on the bursa and rotator cuff from 50 to 130 degrees. (From Goers HR, Hamaty D, Litton L. Calcific tendonitis and bursitis. Patient Care 1972, 6 (14):18–33.)

The tendon is tested by having the patient flex the elbow. The wrist is then grasped to resist the biceps, and the arm is externally rotated. If the biceps tendon is unstable within the groove, it painfully pops out of the groove. If it is stable, there is no tendon slipping and no pain.

Treatment of biceps tendon subluxation or tendinitis is symptomatic pain relief with anti-inflammatory agents, local applications of ice, and avoidance of external rotation of the arm with flexed elbow. Orthopaedic consultation is advisable for subluxation.

BICEPS TENDON TEAR

The long head of the biceps tendon can tear at the bicipital groove with or without resultant shoulder pain. The pertinent findings are a bunching of the biceps muscle toward the antecubital fossa (a bulging "Popeye" biceps), a weakness or inability to supinate the forearm, a weakness of elbow flexion, and often a palpable defect of the entire upper portion of the arm.

Treatment consists of recognition of the problem and referral for orthopaedic consultation within 24 to 48 hours, so that repair, if indicated, is attempted before contracture of the biceps occurs.

ACROMIOCLAVICULAR JOINT

Direct trauma is usually responsible for pain in this joint. As the acromioclavicular joint is a synarthrosis, ligamentous strain is the major cause of painful dysfunction.

Pain and tenderness are found directly over the acromioclavicular joint. Shoulder scapular elevation, depression, and circumduction cause pain. Crepitation is palpable or audible through the stethoscope over the joint during active movement. Injection of several milliliters of lidocaine or procaine via a 25-gauge half-inch needle into the joint is diagnostic and temporarily therapeutic.

Plain films, taken with the arm weighted to distract the joint, can confirm the diagnosis and differentiate between separation and fracture. Treatment has recently become more conservative, and consists of fitting an arm-shoulder sling to prevent traction on the acromioclavicular joint by supporting the dependent arm. Oral anti-inflammatory, nonsteroidal medication given for 5 days, is recommended. Several injections of analgesic and soluble steroids into the joint given at 3 to 5 day intervals are also of value. Operation may be indicated if a severe separation occurs in a professional athlete or a heavy laborer whose professional future is involved; in this case, orthopaedic consultation should be obtained the same day.

CERVICAL RADICULOPATHY

Pain can be referred to the shoulder region from the cervical spine. The cervical lesion responsible may be an acute injury such as a hyperflexion-hyperextension injury (the so-called "whip-lash"), cervical degenerative disc disease, or postural cervical radiculopathy.

Most of these cervical problems involve the lower cervical segments (C5–C8, T1), with dermatomal referral into the shoulders. Injury to the upper cervical segment refers pain to the neck and the occiput (C1–C3). Shoulder pain that is thought to be referred is often muscular, due to the protective spasm of the trapezius or the scalenes.

When shoulder pain originates from the cervical spine, it should be reproducible with neck movement. Extension or rotation of the head narrows the foramina in the direction of the movement and reproduces the pain. Movement away from the shoulder region may cause pain from traction of the nerve roots.

When movement of the neck—*not* movement of the shoulder—causes the pain, a cervical etiology is suggested. Frequently there is muscle spasm of the neck, thus limiting active or passive motion. Palpation over the foramina may refer pain distally. A superficial neurologic examination of reflexes (triceps jerk, biceps jerk, and the brachioradialis reflex), a dermatomal mapping by light touch or pin scratch, and an evaluation of myotome involvement (biceps, C5, triceps, C7, supraspinatus, C5 and C6, wrist extensors, C6, and finger abductors, C8, T1) confirm the suspicion.

Treatment of the acute phase consists of cervical immobilization with a soft collar, oral pain medication, anti-inflammatory nonsteroidal medication, application of ice packs to the neck, and referral to the primary physician within 24 to 48 hours. Only severe pain and significant neurologic deficit justify admission to the hospital, where traction is instituted after orthopaedic or neurosurgical consultation. Otherwise, admission is to be avoided.

SUPRASCAPULAR NERVE TRACTION INJURY

A rare but painful shoulder condition is a traction injury of the suprascapular nerve, which usually follows acute and forceful movement of the arm across the chest wall. This distracts the scapula from the vertebral column (thoracic spine) and stretches the suprascapular nerve.

The suprascapular nerve supplies sensation over the deltoid muscle and motor function to the supra- and infraspinatus muscles, hence the external rotators become weak. Tenderness may be elicited over the supra- and infraspinatus muscles. Later atrophy is noted in the supra- and infraspinatus fossa, with weakness of arm external rotation. Within 21 days, the electromyogram (EMG) becomes diagnostic.

Treatment is supportive. Pain is relieved by the use of analgesics and anti-inflammatory nonsteroidal drugs. Hospitalization is not required, and referral to a neurologist should be the option of the primary physician.

SCAPULOCOSTAL MYALGIC PAIN

Pain in the interscapular region (trapezius muscles, levator scapulae, or rhomboids—the scapulocostal muscles), often termed myofascial pain, is rarely acute. Patients may come to the emergency room fearing "heart disease" or "lung disease". Its theoretic causes are summarized in Figure 2.

Finding localized deep muscle trigger points within tenderness of the involved muscles is suggestive. In a severe anxiety state, there may be restricted neck motion *in all directions* (flexion, extension, rotation, and lateral flexion), thus indicating muscle tension. Scapular movement may also be limited. Treatment consists primarily of explanation, reassurance, local applications of ice or heat, and oral anti-inflammatory medication. The "trigger areas" can be injected with 1 to 2 ml lidocaine through a 25-gauge needle.

ARTHRITIS

The shoulder joint does not bear weight and is not a common location for inflammatory arthritis. When it is, it is usually part of a repetitive pattern of polyarticular pain that responds to anti-inflammatory medications.

When a patient presents with what is thought to be new-onset arthritis of the shoulder joint, both bacterial and systemic causes must be ruled out, as in any other monoarticular arthritis. This is described in detail in the chapter on *Arthritis*.

VISCERAL CAUSES OF SHOULDER PAIN

Cardiac ischemia pain may be referred to the shoulder region; its management is discussed in the chapter on *Myocardial Infarction*.

Acute gallbladder disease, usually stones, may refer pain into the right shoulder. Albeit rare, it should be suspected in cases of right shoulder distress with no shoulder limitation and no cervical confirmatory signs.

SUGGESTED READING

Bateman JB. The diagnosis and treatment of the rotator cuff. Surg Clin N Amer 1963; 43:1523–1530.
Cailliet R. Shoulder pain. 2nd ed. Philadelphia: F.A. Davis Co., 1981.
Weviaser JS. Adhesive capsulitis of the shoulder a study of the pathological findings in periarthritis of the shoulder. J Bone Joint Surg 1945; 27:211–222.

DISORDERS OF THE HIP

JOSEPH F. WAECKERLE, M.D.

The hip joint—essential for an active, full life—is continuously under stress. In walking or running it can bear up to six times the body weight. Therefore, any disease process or trauma can adversely affect it, limiting the individual's existence. The diseases that affect the hip occur in the very young, the severely traumatized, and the elderly; a good prognosis depends on early diagnosis and treatment.

ANATOMY

The hip joint is a ball-and-socket joint made up of the acetabulum and femur. The functions of the hip are weight-bearing and movement. The hip moves in all planes. Because the shape of the hip joint is not symmetric, forces acting on it are not uniformly dispersed and may result in various patterns of injury. The fibrous capsule that surrounds the joint on all sides is exceedingly strong, but is weakest posteriorly. The vascular supply to the hip is threefold: (1) a vascular ring at the base of the neck derived from the circumflex arteries and gluteal arteries supplies intracapsular vessels; (2) two to three metaphyseal arteries supply the inferior lateral head; and (3) the ligamentum teres supplies a small area. The hip is surrounded by approximately 18 bursae, of which three are most important: the trochanteric, the iliopectineal, and the ischiogluteal.

THE PHYSICAL EXAMINATION

Examination of the hip begins with a detailed history and complete examination of the individual. The pelvis and hip are then carefully evaluated. The unclothed, erect patient is inspected for a list, asymmetry of the muscles, injuries, or scars. Gait should be tested, if possible.

If the patient is a trauma victim, after primary survey and initial stabilization the physician should observe the position of the extremities, looking for deformities, lacerations, or bruises. He should test for stability and range of motion. On palpation, the physician should feel for irregularities in movement at the iliac crest, pubic rami, and ischial rami. He should compress the pelvis lateral to medial through the iliac crest; anterior to posterior through the symphysis pubis; and anterior to posterior through each iliac crest, to elicit pain and tenderness. The physician should also compress the greater trochanters of the hips.

If no significant abnormalities are found, range of motion of the hips should be performed. If a hip or pelvic fracture or dislocation is identified in a trauma victim, the physician *must assume* that intra-abdominal, retroperitoneal, and urologic injuries have occurred as

well until it is proven otherwise. The physician should always perform a detailed neurovascular examination and a rectal examination to look for displacement of the prostate in the male patient.

X-RAY EVALUATION

Roentgenographic evaluation of the pelvis and hips is a must in all unconscious patients who have sustained multiple injuries. Lower-extremity long-bone fractures, as well as pelvic symptoms or signs, are also indications for these x-ray films. The x-ray evaluation should include a standard anteroposterior (AP) and lateral view of the pelvis. If further studies are needed, AP views of either hemipelvis, internal and external oblique views of the hemipelvis as described by Judet, or "inlet" and "tilt" views may be taken. In certain instances, such views allow better identification and detail of the acetabulum and femoral head and neck. The physician must always inspect not only the hip joint, but the femur and knee as well when evaluating hip disorders on x-ray films. Disorders of the knee and the femoral shaft can often occur with hip injuries.

The following discussion is divided into sections on traumatic conditions and nontraumatic conditions affecting the hip joint. Further subdivision includes intra-articular and extra-articular conditions affecting the joint. Intra-articular disorders of the hip are further categorized according to the age groups in which such conditions are presented to the physician.

TRAUMATIC DISORDERS OF THE HIP

Dislocations of the Hip

Dislocations of the hip are usually due to auto-pedestrian accidents. They are associated with other significant injuries, as well as local soft-tissue injuries. Numerous classifications have been utilized, but posterior, anterior, and central are used here.

Posterior Dislocations

Eighty to 90 percent of all dislocations are posterior. This type of dislocation is caused by force applied to a flexed knee with the hip in flexion, driving the femur posteriorly. If the femur assumes a more abducted position, posterosuperior acetabular fractures may occur in association with the dislocation.

Physical examination of the patient reveals a shortened, internally rotated, and adducted extremity with the muscles in spasm and pain, and deformity in the hip. Concomitant life-threatening injuries should always be excluded by careful examination. Once the primary survey and stabilization have been completed, the secondary survey may be performed and x-ray evaluation done. An anteroposterior view of the pelvis and hip reveals the dislocation, but further assessment of the acetabulum and femur should be conducted to rule out other fractures. The oblique views of Judet reveal such damage. Inlet and tilt views may be required as well.

The pre-hospital treatment of posterior dislocations of the hip should not be centered on the hip injury, since the real significance of hip dislocations is that the other, more severe injuries may have occurred. No attempt to reduce the hip in the field is recommended. It is much more appropriate that the patient be transported in the least painful position on a long spine board with the affected extremity splinted and stabilized as well as possible.

After evaluation and stabilization in the emergency department, treatment for the patient with a posterior dislocation is immediate closed reduction with general anesthesia. Because of the significant trauma, as well as the difficulty and skill required to reduce hip dislocations, orthopaedic consultation is recommended.

Although the gravity method of Stimson usually accomplishes the reduction with minimal trauma, the patient must be stable enough to assume the prone position. In most instances, the emergency physician cannot use this technique because the seriousness of the patient's condition or the lack of immediately available orthopaedic consultation requires that he attempt reduction in the emergency department without general anesthesia in a traumatized patient who is unable to assume the prone position. The Allis maneuver is recommended in this situation. Briefly, with the patient supine, an assistant stabilizes the pelvis. The knee is flexed and the hip is flexed after application of longitudinal traction in line with the femur. The physician then gently rotates the extremity internally and externally to obtain relocation.

Multiple attempts at reduction or forced maneuvers may produce more damage. In these instances, open reduction may be required. Postreduction evaluation and x-ray studies are important.

Early complications include sciatic nerve injury in 10 to 15 percent of patients, irreducibility, missed knee ligament injuries, missed femoral and pelvic fractures, and recurrent subluxation-dislocations due to instability of the joint. Late complications include myositis ossificans, recurrent dislocations, arthritis, and aseptic necrosis.

It has been demonstrated that the likelihood of aseptic necrosis, the most feared of all complications, is directly proportional to the length of time the hip is dislocated. In general, the prognosis of posterior hip dislocations is directly proportional to the degree of trauma the patient suffered during the injury.

Anterior Dislocations

Approximately 10 to 15 percent of all hip dislocations are anterior. A vast majority are secondary to auto accidents, but also occur as a result of falls or blows to the back while the individual is squatting. The mechanism of injury is usually forced abduction, causing the head to be levered out through the anterior capsule.

Inferoanterior dislocation is due to forced abduction with the hip in flexion. These patients present with the hip abducted, externally rotated, and flexed. Superoanterior dislocations are due to abduction of the hip while it is in extension. These patients present with the hip in abduction, external rotation, and extension. In superior dislocations the femoral head can sometimes be palpated near the anterior iliac spine or in the groin. Associated neurovascular damage should always be excluded. An AP pelvis x-ray study easily demonstrates the head to be dislocated. Other views or computed tomography may be required to assess the damage in certain instances.

The pre-hospital treatment of an anterior dislocation of the hip is similar to that of posterior dislocations. The focus should not be on the hip dislocation, but on properly evaluating the total patient because of the high-energy trauma sustained. Properly stabilizing and immobilizing the affected extremity in the position of least discomfort is appropriate. After the patient is completely evaluated and stabilized in the emergency department, immediate closed reduction, preferably under general anesthesia, is recommended; this usually requires orthopaedic consultation.

A modified Allis maneuver is recommended as the technique of reduction when an emergency physician must reduce an anterior dislocation. While an assistant stabilizes the pelvis, countertraction is applied in the groin. In superior dislocations, strong in-line traction pulls the head below the acetabulum, and the hip is then flexed and gently rotated internally. In inferior dislocations, continuous in-line traction along with hip flexion, gentle internal rotation, and adduction are carried out to reduce the hip. Postreduction evaluation and films are then done to rule out associated injuries and fractures not seen in the prereduction films.

The early complications associated with anterior hip dislocations are neurovascular injuries, irreducibility, and missed associated injuries such as femoral shaft injuries. Recurrent dislocations, arthritis, and aseptic necrosis may occur in later years. In general, the more severe the injury and the longer it takes to diagnose and treat, the worse the results are.

Central Acetabular Fracture-Dislocations

Central dislocations of the femoral head through acetabular fractures occur as a result of significant trauma. Usually the force is a lateral-to-medial blow to the greater trochanter. Rarely, such dislocations may be seen secondary to seizures or shock therapy.

The patient is evaluated by a primary survey and initially stabilized before a detailed examination of the hips is performed, because severe life-threatening injuries often occur in association with these dislocations. The patient presents with shortening of the affected extremity and severe pain. X-ray evaluation should include an anteroposterior view, and then the internal and external views of Judet, to properly assess the entire acetabulum.

The pre-hospital treatment of the patient with such an injury centers on proper assessment and immediate treatment for severe and life-threatening injuries associated with such dislocations. In some cases, pneumatic antishock garments are required because of associated pelvic fractures and severe hemorrhage. If a central acetabular fracture-dislocation is suspected and the patient is stable, immobilization in the position of least discomfort is recommended with careful attention to vital signs.

It is the goal of the emergency physician to restore the joint to as near normal anatomy as possible. Surgery is indicated if the difficult task of reduction of the femoral head and exact restoration of the displaced fractured acetabulum cannot be done quickly and safely by closed reduction with traction. Immediate orthopaedic consultation for the treatment in the emergency department is recommended.

Early complications include sciatic nerve injury, superior gluteal artery injuries, ileus, phlebitis, and infection. Late complications include myositis ossificans, infections, post-traumatic arthritis, and aseptic necrosis. There is a direct relationship between the severity of the injury and the prognosis, especially regarding arthritis and aseptic necrosis.

TRAUMATIC DISLOCATIONS IN CHILDREN

Hip dislocations in children are rare, but do occur more often than fractures. As with adults, posterior dislocations are more common, occurring in about 80 to 85 percent of cases. The mechanism of injury and clinical picture are similar to those in the adult. The majority of dislocations are simple hip dislocations, which can be easily seen on an anteroposterior view of the pelvis. Rarely, there is an associated fracture that usually occurs in older children and can be seen better on prereduction than on postreduction films.

The treatment for simple dislocations in children under 12 years of age is closed reduction after adequate relaxation. If the child is older than 12 or if the hip is irreducible after one or two attempts, then taking the child to the operating room and performing the reduction under general anesthesia is recommended. In either case, immediate orthopaedic consultation for treatment in the emergency department is recommended. Complications are identical to those seen in adults.

OPEN HIP INJURIES

Open wounds to the hip joint should be treated like any other open joint. An initial culture should be done and the wound cleaned by debridement and copious irrigation in the operating room. Primary wound care with secondary closure is suggested by most authorities. Tetanus prophylaxis is ensured by the administration of toxoid and immune globulin if indicated. Prophylactic antibiotics are recommended. Continuous irrigation of the hip may be indicated.

The other traumatic disorders that affect the hip are extra-articular and are discussed in the following sections.

BURSITIS

Approximately 18 bursa surround the hip joint. These are developmentally similar to synovium and tendon sheaths. As a result, they suffer from the same inflammatory afflictions that cause problems to the joint itself. Conditions that affect the bursa include traumatic inflammation, which is usually secondary to overuse or excessive pressure, infections, metabolic disorders such as gout, and benign and malignant growths.

Trochanteric Bursitis

Trochanteric bursitis is commonly divided into superficial and deep bursitis because of the presence of two layers of bursa. The deep bursa are located over the greater trochanter under the tensor fascia lata-gluteus maximus bipennate muscle mass. These patients present with pain on weight-bearing or sitting in a deep chair or car. Upon examination, local tenderness is found over the greater trochanter, especially posteriorly, as well as pain with range of motion, especially flexion and rotation. This pain may radiate into the thigh in these individuals. Vital signs and laboratory values are usually normal.

Superficial trochanteric bursitis is caused by bursa between the greater trochanter and the skin. These patients present with pain over the greater trochanter that is accentuated by range of motion, especially adduction.

The x-ray evaluation of patients with trochanteric bursitis usually reveals no significant findings. In some instances, soft-tissue shadows may be seen due to swelling overlying the greater trochanter.

Treatment consists of rest, application of ice, oral administration of anti-inflammatory medication, and occasionally intrabursal injections. Ultrasound physical therapy may help as well. The prognosis for such individuals is good as long as associated problems such as infection and low-back disc disease are ruled out. Mechanical problems, especially leg length discrepancies, must be sought and, if found, properly treated to prevent further trochanteric bursitis.

Iliopectineal or Iliopsoas Bursitis

This is the most constant and largest of the bursa that surround the hip joint. It is located between the iliopsoas muscle anteriorly and the iliopectineal eminence posteriorly over the hip capsule. The patient complains of pain over the lateral aspect of Scarpa's triangle (near the femoral triangle) and may present with some localized swelling in that area as well. The patient experiences tenderness with palpation in the anterior hip inferior to the midinguinal ligament. Inflammation in this area causes decreased range of motion secondary to the pain, especially adduction and external rotation. Iliopectineal bursitis may irritate the femoral nerve, causing pain with radiculopathy. The treatment is similar to the treatment for trochanteric bursitis.

Ischiogluteal Bursitis

This bursa is located superficial to the ischial tuberosity. Patients present with pain and local tenderness in this area. Occasionally the pain radiates down the back of the thigh along the course of the hamstring muscles. The mechanism of injury is usually sitting for prolonged periods and irritating this bursa by mechanical inflammation. The treatment is similar to the treatment for trochanteric bursitis.

TENDINITIS

The patient with hip pain due to tendinitis has the typical symptoms of inflammation. Usually the tendon of the gluteus medius lateral to the greater trochanter or the tendon of the gluteus minimus superior to the joint capsule is inflamed. The most common cause of inflammation is trauma and overuse, but rarely metabolic causes may precipitate the condition. The patient presents with pain and limited range of motion. The muscles may be in spasm and are locally tender. The patient attempts to put the muscle and tendon at rest by assuming a relaxed position. X-ray films may demonstrate a calcified tendon, but not always. Treatment is similar to that for tendinitis of the shoulder, consisting of moist heat and ice, ultrasonography, oral anti-inflammatory medications, and injections if needed.

STRAINS

Of the various muscles that surround the hip joint, any can be overused, causing strains in the belly or at the musculotendinous unit. The symptoms and signs are individualized, depending on which muscle has been strained. Of the various muscles reported to cause pain around the hip joint as a result of minor injuries, the most common are the iliopsoas, gluteus medius, sartorius, hamstrings, rectus femorus, and external or internal rotators of the hip.

The patient presents with pain when the muscle is put to use and assumes a position that relaxes the musculotendinous unit so that it does not cause further inflammation by contraction. Examination of the patient reveals local tenderness and pain with contraction of the muscle. Such examination obviously requires that the physician understand the origins, insertions, and major actions of the muscles listed above. The treatment approach is the same as that for tendinitis, except that special attention should be given to keeping the muscle at rest to facilitate the healing process.

VASCULAR PROBLEMS

Phlebitis of the femoral vein, or intermittent claudication of the terminal aorta, may cause ischemic-type pain, which can be referred to the hip. Such disorders need to be evaluated to ensure that they are not occurring when a patient presents with pain in the hip without obvious etiology. For further discussion of the diagnoses of these problems, refer to the appropriate sections in this chapter.

NONTRAUMATIC DISORDERS OF THE HIP

The differential diagnosis of nontraumatic hip problems is presented by age.

Congenital Hip Dislocations

The incidence of congenital hip dislocations is one in every 1,000 live births. Approximately 70 percent of these occur in the first baby of a family, and it is six times more common in females than in males.

The diagnosis of congenital hip dislocation in the newborn infant is made by examining the baby at birth and throughout the developmental period, if necessary. The examination should be made on the relaxed newborn, performed in proper sequence; it consists of the Ortolani and the Barlow examinations.

The Ortolani, or reduction, test is carried out to ascertain if the hip is subluxed or dislocated at the moment. Each thigh, examined individually, is grasped with the thumbs over the medial aspect and the middle fingers over the greater trochanter. The examiner gently lifts the thigh while simultaneously abducting it. This causes reduction of the femoral head, which is a palpable and sometimes audible "clunk."

The Barlow test is performed to demonstrate instability. It produces dislocation or subluxation if the hip is in place. The hand position is as described for the Ortolani test. The hip and knee are flexed to 90 degrees. The examiner then causes adduction with gentle downward pressure. If there is instability, the femoral head can slip out of the acetabulum as a result of these maneuvers.

In older babies, the muscles and ligaments tighten, limiting abduction. The thigh is found to be shorter on inspection because of the femoral head assuming a posterior position. This shortening causes "bunched-up" skin, which produces the asymmetric folds often mentioned as a sign of congenital hip dislocation. Moreover, the knees are not the same height when the hips and knees are flexed and the feet are placed on the table with the baby supine. The femur pistons during an examination as well.

In newborn infants, x-ray studies are not reliable because there is no visible bone to ascertain the femoral head position. When the infant is greater than 6 weeks old, x-ray films may be helpful, but they require very careful positioning and evaluation.

Orthopaedic consultation for further treatment is recommended in any child with a possible subluxation-dislocation of the hip. The orthopaedic surgeon attempts to restore the normal anatomy and maintain the restoration in order to reverse the pathologic changes. This requires reduction and positioning devices for periods of time.

With early diagnosis and treatment, the success rate of developing a normal hip joint is high—up to 96 percent. The complications of missed congenital hip disorders are poor hip development and, in some individuals, avascular necrosis.

Septic Arthritis

Septic arthritis is the most likely cause of painful hip joints in infants. About 70 percent of the time it occurs in children under the age of 4.

The septic hip is usually due to one of three causes: (1) hematogenous seeding, (2) metaphyseal spread to the joint (more common in the older child), or (3) direct contamination, such as a needle introduced into the hip while drawing arterial blood gases (ABGs). The most common organism causing septic arthritis of the hip is *Staphylococcus*, then *Hemophilus* and *Streptococcus pyogenes*. Hip destruction occurs by bacterial enzymes causing articular destruction and interruption of blood supply.

Symptoms and signs are consistent with most infective disorders in that the child is irritable, has fever, and shows a loss of appetite. The child presents with a flexed, abducted, and externally rotated hip. This position is assumed because it allows the most volume to be accommodated in the swollen hip joint. There is a decreased range of motion secondary to pain.

Laboratory examination reveals an increased white blood cell count and increased sedimentation rate. Blood cultures may be positive for the offending organism in 50 percent of cases. X-ray studies may be unremarkable or they may simulate other problems with capsular swelling secondary to accumulation of fluid. This may mimic a subluxation of the hip with a widened joint space.

The diagnosis of septic hip is made by aspiration of the hip joint. Such aspiration requires expertise and is usually best left to the orthopaedic or pediatric consultant rather than the emergency physician. Treatment of septic arthritis of the hip consists of immediate hospitalization with appropriate intravenous antibiotics and the possibility of surgical drainage to avoid the cartilage destruction.

Complications of the septic hip are caused by bacterial enzymatic destruction and decreased vascular supply because of the compression of the vascular supply by intra-articular joint swelling and septic thrombosis. These result in epiphyseal destruction with osteonecrosis and osteomyelitis in some instances.

The prognosis is very poor in the infant, but better in the child. The prognosis for both the infant and the child is directly proportional to the length of time that the destructive process continues without treatment.

Differential diagnosis includes any rheumatic disease, most notably transient synovitis. However, it is most important for the emergency physician to realize that *any* arthropathy, especially of the hips, is infectious until proven otherwise because of the rapid course and poor outcome without treatment.

Transient Synovitis

This is a common disorder most prevalent in males 2 1/2 to 10 years of age. It is usually unilateral, but can be bilateral. Although there is frequently no history of trauma, occasionally this condition occurs after minimal trauma or a low-grade febrile illness such as tonsillitis, allergic reaction, or any of the exanthems. It is a nonspecific, synovial inflammation of the hip joint.

The history is one of insidious onset. The patient may complain of pain radiating down the anterior, medial thigh into the knee. The patient walks with a limp or may not walk at all, simply holding the thigh in the flexed, abducted, and externally rotated position, which allows the

joint capsule to be relaxed. The anterior joint is tender on palpation, and in performing passive range of motion, significant hip irritability is found. Temperature may be normal or minimally increased.

Laboratory findings are commonly within normal limits. X-ray films usually demonstrate no abnormality. There may be some soft-tissue swelling, which overlies the interpelvic aspect of the acetabulum, forming a shadow known as the "obturator sign."

Differential diagnosis includes any arthritis, especially infection, slipped capital femoral epiphysis, or Legg-Perthes disease. The emergency physician must rule out a septic hip prior to making the diagnosis of transient synovitis, which is usually one of exclusion.

Treatment is bed rest, as transient synovitis is self-limiting and has a short course of only 3 to 4 days. In some patients, traction may help, requiring orthopaedic consultation and hospital admission.

Complications to transient synovitis usually do not develop, but in a small number of cases, Legg-Perthes disease may occur. Follow-up by the orthopaedic surgeon or pediatrician is recommended in all cases.

Legg-Calvé-Perthes Disease

The incidence of Legg-Perthes disease is not common. It is usually seen among 3- to 10-year-olds, especially in the 5- to 9-year-old age group, and more often in males. It may occur bilaterally in approximately 10 to 15 percent of cases. For some reason, it is more common in shorter children and is rare among the black population.

Legg-Perthes disease is an idiopathic avascular necrosis of the femoral head. It may be due to vascular interruption, causing necrosis of the head or of all or part of the epiphysis. It is usually self-limiting with new bone formation occurring within 2 to 3 years. Such new bone formation results in an abnormal joint—coxa plana.

The clinical picture is one of insidious onset with a prolonged course. The patient presents with a limp that is a constant, early sign. This progresses to decreased range of motion of the hip joint with muscle spasm. The patient may complain of pain with radiation into the thigh or knee, which worsens with activity. This condition is sometimes indistinguishable from transient synovitis. However, there is no spontaneous recovery within 2 to 3 days with Legg-Perthes disease. Laboratory results are not helpful because they are usually within normal limits.

X-ray films are often within normal limits early, or they may show a bulging of the capsule secondary to joint effusion with a lateral shift of the femoral head. In contrast, bone scan at an early stage may be helpful. If there is any suspicion of this disease occurring, a bone scan should be done quickly. As the disease progresses over 1 to 2 years, characteristic changes occur. In general, these include necrosis, reabsorption, and regeneration, which results in an imperfect joint.

Treatment of Legg-Calvé-Perthes disease is referral to the orthopaedic surgeon. The consultant attempts to maintain the femoral head anatomy by keeping it in the acetabulum with casts, braces, or surgical treatment. Early treatment may include bed rest with traction to decrease the pain and spasm and to regain full range of motion.

Differential diagnosis includes any joint disease, especially septic arthritis and transient synovitis. In certain individuals, it is difficult to distinguish early Legg-Perthes disease from transient synovitis. Therefore, Legg-Calvé-Perthes should be assumed and a bone scan ordered.

This disease may be limited, with some individuals undergoing spontaneous recovery. The prognosis is better if the femoral head is only partially involved, if there is no collapse of the femoral head, or if the patient is younger.

Slipped Capital Femoral Epiphysis

This condition usually occurs in adolescents and preadolescents between the ages of 10 and 16 years. It is five times more common in males than females and occurs bilaterally in 20 to 40 percent of cases. The cause is unknown.

The history is usually one of no predisposing injury or systemic disease and an insidious onset. Occasionally there may be an acute traumatic event associated with pain in the hip and decreased range of motion. Frequently, the obese male patient complains of hip and medial knee pain, walks with a limp, and has limited range of motion. Physical examination demonstrates pain over the joint and pain with guarding with abduction and rotation. There are no laboratory findings.

AP and lateral x-ray views may be within normal limits initially or may demonstrate widening of the epiphyseal line and joint space along with soft-tissue swelling. Later, a slip of the plate posteriorly can be seen most easily on the lateral view. Repeat x-ray evaluation is advised if initial films are negative and symptoms persist.

Treatment is centered on preventing further slipping. This is a semiemergent condition, and the emergency physician should ensure that any weight-bearing is eliminated immediately. The orthopaedic consultant usually hospitalizes the patient and may use traction and surgical fixation as well.

The prognosis is usually excellent in cases of minimal slips treated early; however, degenerative disease of the hip may occur in early to middle adult life. In more severe cases, attempts at reducing the epiphyseal segment may result in avascular necrosis, whereas accepting the position may result in malalignment of the femoral head and neck. In general, the prognosis depends on the degree of slip and time to diagnosis and treatment. The differential diagnosis is similar to that of the other conditions mentioned previously.

Avascular Necrosis of the Femoral Head

Avascular necrosis of the femoral head is a common complication of many hip disorders, which results from impaired blood supply to the head. It is not a disease process in itself but a consequence of many of the nontraumatic as well as traumatic disorders discussed in this chapter. In 30 percent of cases, however, the cause is unknown. In half the cases not due to trauma, bilateral involvement occurs.

The main blood supply to the hip is derived from the circumflex vessels. These vessels, which enter at the base of the femoral neck, send intracapsular vessels proximally toward the head. Because of this anatomic supply, they are very susceptible to disruption as in fractures of the neck of the femur and sepsis of the hip. This disruption causes avascularity of the femoral head resulting in subchondral bone cortical collapse with subsequent cartilage degeneration and ending in severe hip degeneration.

The physician must be suspicious of this condition, particularly in patients with predisposing factors such as alcohol use, liver disease, trauma, sickle cell disease and prolonged steroid use. The symptoms and signs are directly proportional to the cause and the patient's age. In the child, the patient presents with a limp, complains of thigh or knee pain, and experiences spasm of the thigh muscles. The adult patient also has a limp, complains of groin pain or pain in the thigh or knee worsened by weight-bearing, demonstrates decreased range of motion, especially rotation and abduction, and has atrophy of the thigh muscles.

X-ray studies in the early period of the condition are usually normal if no significant trauma has occurred. Later, various changes in proportion to the degree of vascular disruption will occur.

These changes are well-described in the standard radiology texts and are diagnostic. The orthopaedic surgeon bases treatment on the cause and the patient's age. Children may benefit from no weight-bearing to avoid collapse or may require operative measures. In certain adult cases, prosthetic replacement is required.

Rheumatic Disease

Like any other joint in the body, the hip joint is affected by various rheumatic diseases of diverse etiologies. Special efforts should be made to exclude the following disorders that can cause hip joint disease: rheumatoid arthritis, juvenile rheumatoid arthritis, infections including tuberculosis and viral hepatitis B, bacterial septic arthritis, crystal-induced hemoglobinopathies, primary and metastatic neoplastic disease, osteoporosis, Paget's disease, hemophilia, and drug-induced syndromes. For a complete discussion of rheumatic diseases, the reader is referred to the suggested readings.

SUGGESTED READING

Kelly WN, et al. Textbook of rheumatology. Vol 2. 2nd ed. Philadelphia: WB Saunders, 1985.

Resnick D, Niwayama G. Diagnosis of bone and joint disorders. Vol 3. Philadelphia: WB Saunders, 1981.

Rockwood CA, et al. Fractures in children. Vol 3. 2nd ed. Philadelphia: JB Lippincott, 1984.

Rockwood CA, Green DP. Fractures in adults. Vol 2. 2nd ed. Philadelphia: JB Lippincott, 1984.

Simon RR, Koenigsknecht SJ. Orthopaedics in emergency medicine. New York: Appleton-Century-Crofts, 1982.

Tachdjian MO. Pediatric orthopaedics. Philadelphia: WB Saunders, 1972.

Turek SR. Orthopaedics principles and their application. Vol 2. 4th ed. Philadelphia: JB Lippincott, 1984.

LIGAMENTOUS ANKLE INJURY

ROBERT R. SIMON, M.D.

ANATOMY

Eighty-five percent of all ligamentous injuries of the ankle involve the lateral side. Three ligaments compose the lateral ligament complex—the anterior talofibular ligament, the calcaneofibular ligament, and the posterior talofibular ligament (Fig. 1). On the medial side there is the deltoid ligament. The anterior inferior tibiofibular ligament joins the tibia and fibula anteriorly and is commonly injured in association with severe second and third degree injuries of the ankle.

ASSESSMENT

Lateral ligamentous injuries of the ankle normally occur when the ankle is plantar flexed and an inversion force is applied. In this position the first ligament to rupture is the anterior talofibular ligament. Thus, the anterior drawer sign of the ankle, which tests the anterior talofibular ligament, is the most reliable test to determine whether there is a complete rupture or instability in that ligament (Fig. 2).

To perform the anterior drawer sign of the ankle, one should cup the right hand around the heel and place the left hand along the anterior border of the tibia. While stabilizing the tibia, the heel is pulled forward, thus displacing the foot anteriorly out of the ankle mortis. If the patient has a rupture of the anterior talofibular ligament, the foot will come forward significantly as compared with the normal side.

If the anterior drawer sign is negative, one does not need to use the inversion stress test, which tests both the anterior talofibular ligament and the calcaneofibular ligament.

In performing the inversion stress test, the foot is inverted while the tibia is stabilized with the opposite hand. In order to assess this test adequately, one usually needs to take an anterior posterior x-ray view of the ankle while maintaining this inverted position. If the talus is displaced by more than a 20-degree angle as compared with the tibia, this usually indicates a positive test. However, the ideal method is to compare the normal with the abnormal side, and if there is more than a 10-degree difference, the test is positive, which means that the anterior talofibular ligament and the calcaneal fibular ligament are both ruptured.

The anterior drawer sign of the ankle can be performed regardless of the severity of the ligamentous injury and the pain the patient is in. If the anterior drawer sign is positive and the patient has some instability in the ankle, an inversion stress test with x-ray examination should be obtained. This determines whether both ligaments are completely ruptured, a finding that changes the prognosis and may change the therapy.

When a patient is suspected of having a ligamentous injury of the ankle, the most important initial care is to elevate the ankle in some type of splint, if this is possible. If not, elevation on a pillow is adequate. Ice packs should be applied around the ankle joint and the patient should be evaluated. During the evaluation the physician should attempt to determine whether the patient heard any

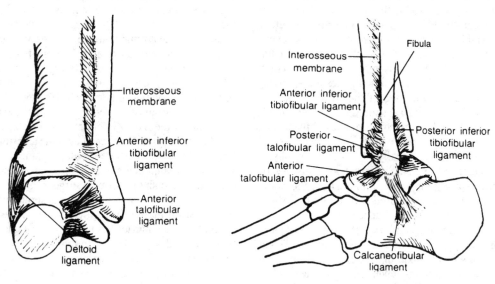

Posterior view

Lateral view

Figure 1 Ligaments of the ankle.

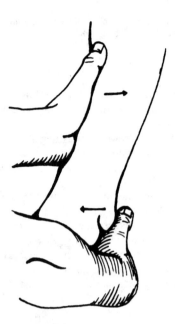

Figure 2 Testing for the anterior drawer sign.

audible pop or snap. This would indicate that there may be intra-articular or malleolar fracture, or a tendinous avulsion. An audible pop or snap may also occur with complete ruptures of the ligaments.

Radiographs should be obtained in all patients who present to the emergency department with ankle injuries in which the malleoli (rather than the ligaments below the malleoli) are tender to palpation. In addition, all patients who present with inability to bear weight should have an ankle x-ray examination. Patients presenting with an ankle sprain who are able to bear weight and have only moderate swelling do not necessarily require radiographic examination.

In examining the patient's ankle, one must be sure to examine the malleoli separately from the ligaments; if they are tender, this may indicate that there is a fracture of the malleolus. In addition, the anterior inferior tibiofibular ligament should be palpated to determine whether it is tender, as this indicates that there is usually a severe second or third degree injury of either the lateral or medial ligament complex. A commonly missed fracture, which occurs in association with inversion injuries to the ankle, is the Jones fracture at the base of the fifth metatarsal. The base of the fifth metatarsal should be palpated in all patients with suspected ligamentous injuries of the ankle. If this is tender, x-ray views of the foot as well as the ankle should be obtained. Finally, the examining physician should determine whether there was a history of weight bearing during the ankle injury. If so, the dome of the talus may have been injured and should be palpated for possible osteochondral fracture.

In children ligamentous injuries of the ankle are less common than epiphysial injuries of the malleoli. When a child presents with an ankle injury, one should palpate the malleoli carefully for any tenderness over the epiphysis. In addition, one should inform the parents that if any effusion occurs or a persistent pain in the ankle occurs, the patient should be re-examined because this may be

the only sign of a missed osteochondral fracture involving the dome of the talus or the malleoli.

TREATMENT

A great deal has been written in the past several years about the treatment of ankle sprains. In synthesizing all the recent literature, it appears that the following statements can be made: In first degree ankle injuries, which present with minimal or no swelling and in which the patient is able to bear weight without any pain, the treatment is early mobilization. The patient should be encouraged to bear weight as soon as it is comfortable to do so.

In second degree ankle injuries, one should divide these into severe or moderate sprains. In a severe second degree sprain, an anterior drawer sign will be slightly more positive than on the normal side. However, there is a firm end point. In this situation, the anterior talofibular ligament is partially ruptured, but there are some intact fibers. Usually these patients have marked swelling and tenderness. In this situation, the treatment of choice is to elevate the ankle for the first 2 days with ice applied periodically as the patient is able to do. This permits the swelling to decrease maximally. The patient should be discharged on crutches if necessary. A posterior splint can be applied so that the ankle is supported. If the patient has a moderate second degree sprain (able to bear weight but with pain), he can be discharged without a posterior splint and encouraged to use ice compresses and elevation. After the first 48 hours the patient should be placed in some type of commercially available ankle support. The ankle support should permit little inversion or eversion of the ankle, but a small amount of flexion and extension. Supports used in the past include the air cast, which is an inflatable support that fits around the ankle and can be worn in the shoe. In addition, the Futura ankle support is a good support, which can also be used with a shoe. This support should be worn and crutches used until the pain subsides with increasing weight bearing as the patient tolerates it. The patient should be encouraged to use peroneal strengthening exercises and exercises that strengthen the extensors and flexors of the ankle.

In third degree or complete ruptures of the anterior talofibular ligament, the treatment is similar to that of a severe second degree ankle sprain. However, it is not clear whether the prognosis may be worse in these patients, in that some of them may later develop instability in the ankle. In third degree ruptures of both the anterior talofibular ligament and the calcaneofibular ligament, the patient should be treated in a posterior splint, ice, and elevation, and referred to an orthopaedic surgeon. Some orthopaedic surgeons believe that young patients should undergo surgical repair if there is instability. Although cast immobilization for these injuries has recently come under disfavor, there are still a number of individuals who believe this to be the treatment of choice. Because there is controversy about the treatment of these injuries, it is best to refer these patients within the first 48 to 72 hours.

Unna boots and taping have been advocated for the treatment of second and third degree ankle sprains. There are a number of articles demonstrating that these are effective modalities of treatment. Both these modalities prevent some degree of inversion and eversion as well as flexion and extension of the ankle. Thus, they provide stability of the ankle while permitting the patient to bear weight and wear shoes, and are effective choices in treating second and some third degree injuries of the ankle. The important aspect in all these patients is early mobilization in a protective support of some type. This can be either an ankle support, which is commercially available and fits into the shoe, or an Unna boot or taping (which usually does not). The author prefers an ankle support that permits the patient to bear weight and wear his shoe.

In the athlete, protected early mobilization and peroneal strengthening exercises as well as exercises that strengthen the extensors and flexors of the ankle are vitally important in restoring the ankle to normal function. These should be commenced on early follow-up with the primary physician; they are too detailed for description here.

SUGGESTED READING

Hughes LH, Stetts DM. A comparison of ankle taping and semirigid support. Physician Sports Med 1983; 11:99–103.
Mack RP. Ankle injuries in athletes. Athletic Clinics—Sports Medicine. Philadelphia: WB Saunders, 1982, Vol. 1:71–84.
Sclafani S. Ligmentous injuries of the lower tibiofibular syndesmosis. Radiology 1985; 156:21–27.

LIGAMENTOUS KNEE INJURY

ROBERT R. SIMON, M.D.

ANATOMY

Ligamentous injuries of the knee are commonly seen in the emergency center. There are *four ligaments* that must be assessed when examining the knee joint—the medial collateral ligament, the lateral collateral ligament, the anterior cruciate ligament, and the posterior cruciate ligament (Fig. 1). In addition, the posterior capsule should be examined carefully.

ASSESSMENT

In examining the collateral ligaments, a valgus and varus stress test should be performed with the knee in 15 degrees of flexion. This makes possible the examination of the medial collateral ligament and lateral collateral ligament, respectively. In addition, the stress test should be repeated with the knee in full extension. One must com-

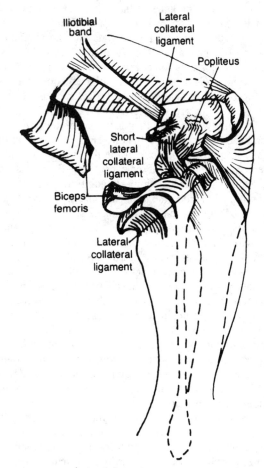

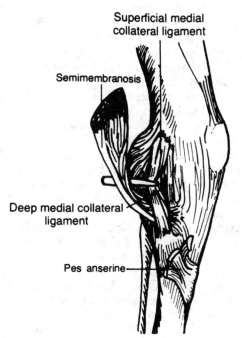

Figure 1 Ligaments of the knee.

pare opening of a joint on stress testing to the response on the normal side. A "positive" stress test may prove to be entirely normal for that patient when comparing opening of the joint to that on the normal side. If the valgus stress test is positive in flexion, but there is a firm end point, the patient has a partial tear of the medial collateral ligament. If the joint opens more than 1 cm as compared to the normal side and the end point is not clear, the patient has a rupture of both the medial collateral ligament and the anterior cruciate ligament. If the varus stress test is positive in flexion and the patient has opening of less than 1 cm with a firm end point, this means that the lateral collateral ligament is partially torn. If the patient has opening of the joint laterally on the varus stress test that is greater than 1 cm and there is not a clear end point, this is indicative of rupture of both the lateral collateral ligament and the anterior cruciate ligament.

The *anterior drawer test* is difficult to perform in a patient who has a ligamentous injury of the knee because it requires 90 degrees of flexion, which is often painful for the patient. In addition, the anterior drawer sign of the knee is unreliable in the acute injury. The best test to perform in determining the presence of acute ruptures of the anterior or posterior cruciate ligaments is the *Lachmann test*. The Lachmann test is done in 5 to 10 degrees of flexion, and the tibia is pulled forward and backward to determine whether there is opening.

In assessing the knee, if the stress test is positive in extension in either the valgus or varus position, the patient has rupture of both the cruciate and the respective collateral ligament as well as a tear in the capsule of the joint. These patients have very serious injury with instabilty and often present with no joint effusion. The examining physician should not be fooled by the fact that there is no joint effusion. Seventy-four percent of all patients with two or more ligaments completely ruptured in the knee have no joint effusion. The reason is that the effusion requires an intact capsule to be present, and if there is a severe rupture of the capsule and ligaments, the fluid leaks out of the knee joint. In addition, patients who have minimal to moderate joint pain may have significant ruptures of the ligaments of the knee. Well over 70 percent of the patients who present to the emergency center with two or more ligaments completely ruptured will have minimal to moderate pain. Partial tears of the ligaments with fibers that remain intact cause much more pain in association with stretching those fibers in performing a stress test than those ligaments with a complete rupture in which there is no intact neurovascular bundle to be stretched, causing pain. For this reason, third degree ruptures (complete ruptures) of two or more ligaments of the knee often are associated with very minimal pain. Thus, the patients who have the most serious knee ligament injuries have minimal or no effusion and minimal to moderate pain.

A patient who presents to the emergency center with an effusion of the knee occurring within two hours after injury usually has one of the four following: ligamentous rupture, peripheral meniscal tear, intra-articular fracture, or osteochondral fracture. If the patient has heard an audible pop or snap and presents to the emergency room with a traumatic effusion in the knee, there is a 60 percent chance that the anterior cruciate ligament has ruptured.

Roentgenography of the knee should be obtained whenever there is an effusion of the knee. This should be done prior to stress examination of the knee. In addition, roentgenographs should be obtained whenever there is a history of an axial load applied to the knee or a history of hearing an audible pop or snap. Finally, if the patient is unable to bear weight on arrival at the emergency center, x-ray views should be obtained prior to performing stress examinations.

Whenever a patient presents to the emergency department with a completely unstable knee on examination, one must always assume that the patient has had a dislocation of the knee that has spontaneously reduced. This is important because in many cases dislocations of the knee present to the emergency center having reduced spontaneously because of the severity of ligamentous rupture. The only positive finding for dislocation when the physician sees the patient is therefore complete instability of the knee in more than one direction. When a dislocation is suspected or seen, popliteal artery injury must be looked for. If a hematoma is noted in the popliteal fossa, one should have a high index of suspicion for popliteal artery injury. One should check distal pulses, but even if they are present, the patient should be treated with a splint and arteriography should be performed.

TREATMENT

The initial management of patients with knee ligament injuries involves splinting or supporting the knee in 20 to 30 degrees of flexion with ice compresses applied. The patient should be transported to the emergency department where an examination, as indicated above, is performed. The examination is the critical "treatment of choice" with regard to the emergency medicine specialist. If a partial tear is diagnosed in a collateral ligament and the patient has a stable knee joint otherwise, the treatment is to place the patient in a knee immobilizer, advocate ice compresses, and dispense crutches. The patient should be followed closely in 2 to 3 days to be certain that a complete rupture was not missed because of secondary spasm of the hamstrings, which may obscure the initial examination. If a complete rupture is diagnosed in either the collateral ligaments or the cruciates, an orthopedic surgeon should be consulted within 48 hours after injury and the patient again placed in a knee immobilizer or posterior splint and referred.

Tense effusions of the knee, which are traumatically induced, should be aspirated and drained. Blood under pressure in the knee joint causes articular cartilage to degenerate, and this may lead to early osteoarthritis. In addition, an adequate examination cannot be performed in a tensely swollen knee. After aspirating a hemarthrosis of the knee joint, 1 percent Xylocaine should be injected when there is significant pain in order to alleviate muscle spasm and permit a more adequate examination of the knee. Finally, if significant fat is found in the blood, this portends an intra-articular fracture or an osteochondral fracture. For these reasons blood should be aspirated out of the knee joint as soon as possible. If fat globules are seen in the fluid aspirated from the knee, but there is no fracture visualized, this usually indicates an impaction injury in which intra-articular fat has been compressed or rupture of one of the intra-articular ligaments of the knee, which also may release small amounts of fat globules. If a large amount of fat is seen, however, this usually indicates an intra-articular fracture, and one should carry out a careful assessment of the undersurface of the patella and the femoral condyles in order to be certain that there is no osteochondral fracture, which can be suspected by pinpoint tenderness over the articular surfaces of either the patellofemoral or femorotibial joints.

Arthroscopy is used increasingly in the evaluation of the injured knee, particularly in the athlete. If an athlete presents to the emergency center with an equivocal examination of the knee joint or hemarthrosis is present with negative stress tests, many orthopedic surgeons believe that arthroscopy should be done in all these patients. While this is not in the scope of the emergency medicine specialist, he should realize that, particularly in the athlete with an injured knee, arthroscopy should be done early and thus the patient should be referred, especially if there is an equivocal examination. Arthrograms, while still performed in many centers, have less importance with regard to emergency management or evaluation of injured knees.

SUGGESTED READING

Donaldson W, Warner R. A comparison of acute anterior cruciate ligament examinations. Am J Sports Med 1985; 13:5-10.
Houghotan JC, et al. Classification of knee ligament instabilities. J Bone Joint Surg 1976; 58: 159.
O'Donoghue DH. Treatment of injuries to athletes. 3rd ed. Philadelphia: WB Saunders 1976:71.

COMMON FOOT DISORDERS

FLAIR D. GOLDMAN, D.P.M., M.S.

Most foot pain is the result of a local abnormality. For this reason a working knowledge of the structure and function of the foot is helpful. There are, however, systemic disorders that result in local foot disorders. It is not the purpose of this chapter to review all the possible systemic causes of foot problems. However, the following must be kept in mind: vascular disease (Raynaud's disease, varicosities, lymphedema, and peripheral vascular disease), metabolic diseases (gout, diabetes mellitus, and hyperlipidemia), immunologic diseases (rheumatoid arthritis, Reiter's disease, ankylosing spondylitis, and psoriatic arthritis), and neurologic diseases (sciatica, Charcot-Marie-Tooth disease, and peripheral neuropathy).

When evaluating foot pain, it is best to divide the foot into three sections—the forefoot, including the toes and metatarsals; the midfoot, including the cuboid, navicular, and cuneiforms; and the hind foot, consisting of the talus and the calcaneus (Fig. 1).

PROBLEMS OF THE HIND FOOT

Sever's Disease (Calcaneal Apophysitis)

Sever's disease presents as pain in the area of the Achilles tendon in the adolescent. The condition is a form of aseptic necrosis of bone. It is believed to result from the strong pull of the posterior calf muscles on the calcaneal growth center. This is a self-limiting disease, most commonly found in athletically active adolescents.

Examination shows tenderness to palpation of the posterior calcaneus along the insertion of the Achilles tendon (Fig. 2). There is also pain with forced dorsiflexion of the foot. When symptomatic, the patient often walks with a short stride to avoid the need for excessive dorsiflexion. X-ray views may show fragmentation and condensation of the apophysis. X-ray examination, however, is helpful in ascertaining that the growth plate is indeed open and in ruling out other osseous disorders.

The treatment consists of rest, crutches, and a plantar flexed short leg cast if necessary. Reassurance should be given that once the growth plate is closed at about age 12 to 14 in girls, and 13 to 15 in boys, the symptoms will resolve. Until the growth plate is closed, symptoms may recur sporadically, and common sense and the avoidance of exertion are indicated.

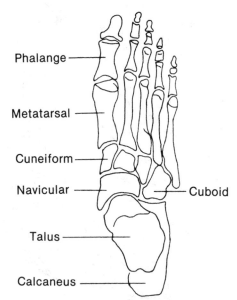

Figure 1 Bones of the foot

Achilles Tendinitis

Pain in the area of the Achilles tendon in adults is usually the result of tendinitis. Overuse and faulty mechanics are often to blame.

The symptoms may vary from a nagging pain with overexertion to the inability to walk. There is pain on palpation of the Achilles tendon itself. In severe cases there may be crepitus that is felt as the inflamed tendon rides through its sheath.

Treatment consists of rest and decreasing activity, as well as heel lifts and oral doses of nonsteroidal anti-inflammatory medicines. Ice applications are often helpful before and after activity.

Less common conditions that may mimic Achilles tendinitis include: partial rupture of the plantaris tendon or the Achilles tendon with resultant pain, swelling, and ecchymosis in the area (thick and painful tendons are the result of chronic microruptures of the tendon and subsequent healing with scarring); fatty deposition from hyperlipidemia; and Achilles bursitis, resulting from inflammation of the bursa between the calcaneus and the Achilles tendon.

Pump Bump

A pump bump is an exostosis (bony enlargement) of the posterior calcaneus. The exostosis results in irritation of the overlying skin as it rubs on the heel counter of the shoe. Often an adventitious bursa develops between the skin and bone, and irritation of this bursa may result. Causes include structural congenital anomaly of the posterior calcaneus, faulty shoe gear, and faulty foot mechanics causing excessive motion in the rear foot.

X-ray views are often not helpful in diagnosis, since standard lateral x-ray views often fail to show the bump, which is generally posterior and lateral on the calcaneus. The diagnosis is usually obvious as there is redness, irritation, blister formation, and occasionally callus tissue over the enlarged posterior lateral heel (Fig. 2).

Treatment consists of open heeled shoes, padding (including moleskin) to protect the skin, an arch support to control faulty foot motion, heel lifts, and if all else fails, surgical removal of the offending bone.

Plantar Heel Pain

The majority of cases involve the heel spur syndrome and bruising of the heel (Table 1). Other causes are rare, but should not be overlooked, especially in unresponsive cases.

Heel Spur Syndrome

The heel spur syndrome usually presents as a pain in the plantar or plantarmedial aspect of the calcaneus where the plantar fascia and intrinsic muscles of the foot insert into the calcaneus. The condition is caused by mechanical factors. As the foot pronates, the foot is lengthened and the plantar structures are put on a stretch.

TABLE 1 Causes of Plantar Heel Pain

Heel spur syndrome (periostitis, fasciitis)
Heel bruise
Stress fracture
Nerve entrapment (posterior tibial nerve, medial and lateral
  plantar nerves, sciatica)
Gout
Subtalar joint arthritis
Infection (especially in younger patients)
Tumor
Collagen vascular disease
Paget's disease
Calcium Pyrophosphate Dihydrate deposit disease

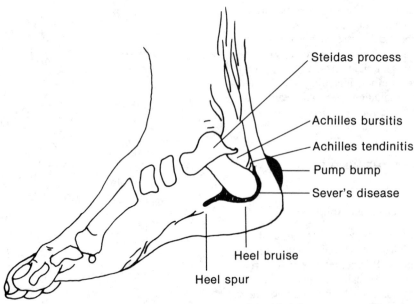

Figure 2 Disorders of the hind foot

There is pull at their origin on the calcaneus, resulting in a periosteal inflammation with pain and spur formation.

Examination shows pain on palpation of this area. If one is not sure of where to palpate, take a lateral non-weight bearing x-ray view and measure. X-ray finding of a spur is not pathognomonic of this condition, for many asymptomatic individuals have spurs, and in many symptomatic individuals this new bone has not yet been formed.

Treatment of the acute inflammatory process and correction of faulty mechanics are often necessary. The acute symptoms may be reduced with oral doses of anti-inflammatory medicines, a local injection of steroids, ice, ultrasound, and rest. Faulty foot mechanics can be corrected with foot supports. Weight reduction is also helpful. High heel shoes are often found to be more comfortable. In chronic cases, consider referral for surgical release.

Tarsal Tunnel Syndrome

The tarsal tunnel syndrome is an entrapment neuropathy of the posterior tibial nerve that occurs as it passes through the fibro-osseous tunnel created by the lacinate ligament as it crosses the calcaneus to the medial malleolus. Although this entrapment occurs in the rear part of the foot, the resultant symptoms from this entrapment may occur in the rearfoot, midfoot, or forefoot. Symptoms usually occur in the forefoot and include shooting and radiating pain from the medial malleolus to the plantar surface of the foot, which may be associated with anesthesia, paresthesia, or hypesthesia. The diagnosis is suspected whenever there is pain about the distribution of the medial or lateral plantar nerve, or when there is pain upon percussion of the region of the neurovascular bundle inferior to the medial malleolus (a positive Tinel's sign). If this diagnosis is strongly considered, it is advisable to order nerve conduction velocity measurements for confirmation. Since the posterior tibial nerve travels in this fibro-osseous tunnel with the tendons of the posterior leg muscles, one must also consider that tendinitis (overuse syndrome or collagen vascular disease) can put pressure on the nerve. Any condition that would result in peripheral edema must also be considered (varicosities, overuse, and hypothyroidism). Other causes of peripheral neuropathy make damage of this nerve more likely (commonly diabetes mellitus, and alcoholism).

Nonsurgical treatment consists of rest and anti-inflammatory medicines. Rest is accomplished by casting or taping the foot in a plantar flexed and inverted position to minimize tension on the nerve and relax the lacinate ligament. Surgical treatment consists of release of the lacinate ligament and decompression of the posterior tibial nerve.

PROBLEMS OF THE MIDFOOT
Pain in the Region of the Tarsal Navicula (Fig. 3)

Köhler's Disease

Köhler's disease (aseptic necrosis of the tarsal navicula) usually affects males between the ages of 5 and 10. The patient presents with a painful limp, swelling, and tenderness localized to the region of the tarsal navicular. X-ray examination shows a poorly developed ossification center with condensation and fragmentation. The treatment consists of rest and a below-the-knee cast if necessary. This is a self-limiting disease, and the child will outgrow it when this growth center reaches maturity.

Accessory Navicula

The accessory navicula represents a separate ossification center of the tarsal navicular medially that does not fuse to the main body of the navicular. X-ray views show an accessory ossicle.

Pain may occur in this region for several reasons. The enlarged navicular may simply become prominent and irritated by shoe gear. There can be motion between the accessory navicula and the true navicula, causing pain. The accessory navicula may cause an abnormal insertion of the posterior tibial tendon, giving rise to a painful flat foot. Conservative treatment is the same as that for posterior tibial tendinitis; in unresponsive cases, refer for possible surgical excision.

Posterior Tibial Tendinitis

The posterior tibial muscle is responsible for plantar flexing and inverting the foot and maintaining the medial arch of the foot. Arch collapse places an excessive burden on this muscle tendon unit.

The diagnosis is made by eliciting tenderness to palpation of the navicula at the insertion of the posterior tibial tendon, with pain when stressing the posterior tibial tendon. Stress the tendon by placing the foot in a position of plantar flexion and inversion and asking the patient to maintain this position against a force of dorsiflexion and eversion.

The treatment consists of rest, anti-inflammatory medications, and icing. Rest is effected by using crutches or by placing the foot in a below-the-knee cast slightly plantar flexed and inverted to take the tendon off stretch, or the use of arch supports.

Stress Fracture

When there is midfoot pain usually accompanied by swelling in the forefoot, a stress fracture of a metatarsal should be considered. Stress fractures were noted in new army recruits who were subjected to long forced marches; hence the alternate name, march fracture. Today these conditions arise when unconditioned people push their bones beyond their limits (e.g., long hikes, runs).

There are usually both pain and edema in the forefoot in variable degrees. Moving the affected metatarsal or palpation of the fracture is painful. The fractures are nondisplaced. As a rule, no fracture is noted on intitial x-ray views. Not until 2 to 3 weeks after injury are x-ray views helpful. X-ray views taken 2 to 3 weeks after injury show callus formation (bony healing) at the fracture site. (This bony proliferation, in the absence of a history of trauma, has been confused with an osteoblastic bone tumor.) The treatment is to decrease activity, elevate the

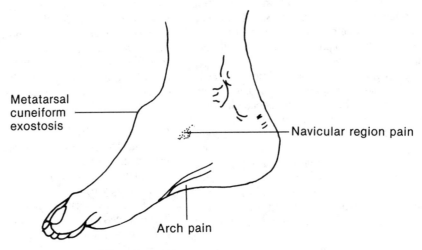

Metatarsal
cuneiform
exostosis

Navicular region pain

Arch pain

Figure 3 Problems of the midfoot

foot, and wear a stiff supportive shoe for 6 weeks; a short leg walking cast may also be used for comfort if necessary.

Pain on the Dorsum of the Midfoot

Metatarsal Cuneiform Exostosis

The metatarsal cuneiform exostosis is a bony enlargement on the dorsum of the foot in response to jamming of the dorsal metatarsal cuneiform joint (see Fig. 3). It may occur at any metatarsal cuneiform joint, but is most common at the first. Pain develops when the exostosis reaches a sufficient size to become a prominence on the dorsum of the foot. Structures such as skin, tendon, bursa, and nerve may then become pinched between this bump and the vamp of the shoe. There can be many associated conditions as follows:

1. Ganglion. Since the extensor tendons ride over this area, they may become irritated by the bony irregularity, and a cystic degeneration may occur in their sheath, thus giving rise to a ganglion.
2. Bursitis. A bursa may form between the skin and the bone as the result of pressure from the shoe. This bursa may then become inflamed.
3. Dorsal cutaneous nerve involvement. The dorsal cutaneous nerves may become entrapped in the fibrosis and scarring process and may become compressed between the exostosis and the shoe. The patient usually complains of numbness, tingling, and pain radiating from the point of the exostosis distally in the foot. Tapping in the area of the exostosis usually reproduces symptoms.
4. Arthritis. Longstanding changes may occur, giving rise to arthritis of the metatarsal cuneiform joint. X-ray views usually confirm a narrowed joint space, and moving the affected metatarsal plantarly and dorsally causes pain.

A simple metatarsal cuneiform exostosis, not complicated by any secondary changes, is best treated with accommodative padding and comfortable shoe gear. If bursitis is suspected, a cortisone and local anesthesia injection may be helpful. When ganglions are involved, aspiration of the ganglion with injection of cortisone and a compression dressing should be tried. Arthritis of the metatarsal cuneiform joint is managed by decreasing motion through a foot ortheosis, anti-inflammatory medicines, and, rarely, by fusion of the joint.

Arch Strain-Fasciitis

The long medial arch of the foot is made of three segments, two bony and one soft tissue (Fig. 3). The soft tissue segment is composed of intrinsic muscles of the foot and the plantar fascia. When the arch lowers, the foot is essentially lengthened and the soft tissue segment can be strained, causing fatigue, inflammation, and pain. The arch is also supported by muscles originating in the posterior leg, and flattening of the arch can be associated with posterior leg fatigue, pain, and cramps. To see whether the patient is flat footed, be sure to have him stand with his full weight on the feet, as many feet appear to have a good arch when the patient is not bearing weight.

Treatment is directed toward reducing acute pain and inflammation and correcting faulty biomechanics (flat footedness). Acute inflammation is best treated with rest (decrease activity, crutches) and oral doses of anti-inflammatory medication, or ultrasound. Once acute symptoms have resolved, and in chronic cases, orthotics (arch supports) are indicated.

FOREFOOT PAIN

Metatarsal Pain

Pain in the region of the metatarsals is usually located distally near the metatarsal heads (metatarsalgia), either under the metatarsal head or between them.

Intermetatarsal Neuroma

Intermetatarsal neuroma is a form of human mechanical neuropathy caused by compression and stretching of the common digital nerve (Fig. 4). Symptoms consist of a neuritic type of pain, burning, shooting and radiating pain, numbness, and tingling in the interspace of the affected nerve, sometimes radiating proximally, but most often distally into the adjacent sides of the toes. This condition most often affects females between the ages of 20 and 50 and is characterized by exacerbations and remissions.

Physical examination shows pain with dorsal-plantar compression using the thumb and index finger *between the metatarsal heads* of the affected interspace. While this maneuver is being carried out with one hand, the other hand compresses the forepart of the foot from medial to lateral. Occasionally the thickened nerve can be felt as it pops between the metatarsal heads. If this maneuver reproduces the symptoms the patient experiences during walking, neuroma must be considered. Referral to a podiatrist or orthopod is needed.

Intermetatarsal Bursitis

Intermetatarsal bursitis is often difficult to distinguish from intermetatarsal neuroma. Occasionally a large inflamed intermetatarsal bursa may act as a space occupying lesion, putting pressure on the intermetatarsal nerve and giving rise to a bursitis-neuritis combination. The treatment for suspected bursitis is similar to nonsurgical treatment of neuroma; cortisone injection and metatarsal pads.

Submetatarsal Head Pain

Care must be used in differentiating submetatarsal head pain from interspace pain. Submetatarsal head pain simply is pain to direct palpation of the plantar aspect of the metatarsal head.

Pain under the metatarsal head is usually the result of inflammation of the structures under the metatarsal head—the joint capsule, flexor tendons, subcutaneous tissue, skin, and on occasion the metatarsal head itself. Most cases are due to increased pressure under the metatarsal head. Chronic repetitive microtrauma from walking or running is usually to blame.

Tender or depressed metatarsal heads are best appreciated simply by looking for obvious bulges in the planter part of the foot and palpating the metatarsal heads in order, noticing whether one feels lower than the others. Plantar spurs and hypertrophied sesamoids are best demonstrated on oblique and axial metatarsal x-ray views and long metatarsals by anteroposterior x-ray views (weight bearing).

Treatment is aimed at decreasing the pressure under the affected metatarsal head. Conservative measures include flat shoes, which help keep the weight more posterior in the foot rather than on the ball of the foot. Shock absorbing material such as thick rubber soles shoes and cushiony innersoles are used as well as metatarsal pads

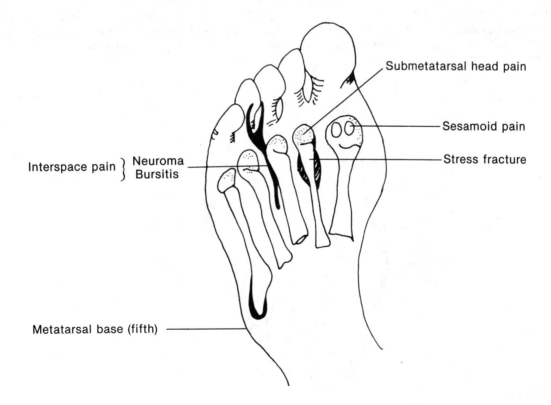

Figure 4 Sources of forefoot pain

to lift the metatarsal heads. Arch supports are also of value in transferring the weight off the ball of the foot.

Sesamoiditis

Sesamoiditis is an inflammation of the sesamoid and its surrounding structures. The tibial sesamoid is most frequently involved. Symptoms consist of plantar pain in the area of the first metatarsal head, with pain on palpation of the affected sesamoid. There is usually a limitation of range of motion, particularly dorsiflexion, at the first metatarsophalangeal joint, and there may be associated swelling. The treatment consists of decreased stress on the involved area, i.e., rest by means of padding or crutches, oral doses of anti-inflammatory medications, and local injection with steroids.

Fractured Sesamoid

One must consider a sesamoid fracture in cases of sesamoid pain that do not respond to conservative treatment, or when framk trauma is involved, or when palpation of the sesamoid is painful and there is surrounding edema. X-ray views should be ordered (anteroposterior, oblique, and axial sesamoid views). Interpretation of x-ray views is often complicated by the normal separation of some sesamoids (partism). When sesamoids are partite, they are usually in two pieces (bipartite). Approximately 20 percent of feet show partite sesamoids under the first metatarsal. The medial (tibial) sesamoid is partite five to ten times more often than the fibular.

Painful Callus on the Ball of the Foot

When examing a callus, one must note whether the callus has a nucleus (core). Calluses that have a nucleus are deep seated and are usually more painful than calluses that do not. If uncertainty exists, check for skin lines. In calluses that have a nucleus, the nucleus interrupts the skin lines. One must also be able to differentiate between a plantar wart and a callus. Warts are not on weight bearing surfaces as often as calluses are. Warts do show interruption of the skin lines. Calluses are generally tender to direct pressure (pushing) as compared with warts, which are more sensitive to lateral pressure (pinching). Warts, when pared, often exhibit pinpoint bleeding.

DIGITAL PROBLEMS

Toe Deformities

Hammer toes, mallet toes, and claw toes are deformities of the digits (Fig. 5). Hammer toes are the most common. These deformities are usually the result of muscle imbalance secondary to foot biomechanics and foot structure. Hammer toes contribute to submetatarsal head pain by depressing the metatarsal and displacing the fat pad on which it rests (Fig. 6). Also, when the toe is in a hammer position, it does not share its normal portion of weight, which is then taken by the metatarsal head.

In these digital deformities, bony prominences produce pressure points, which result in skin irritation, callus formation, and occasionally ulceration and infection. These toe deformities are easily identified on examination. Sometimes the patient must bear weight (standing) in order for the deformity to be appreciated.

Conservative treatment consists of routine shaving of the callus, protection of the bony prominence with pads (i.e., moleskin or store bought foam adhesive backed padding), and the wearing of shoes with a high toe box or custom made shoes.

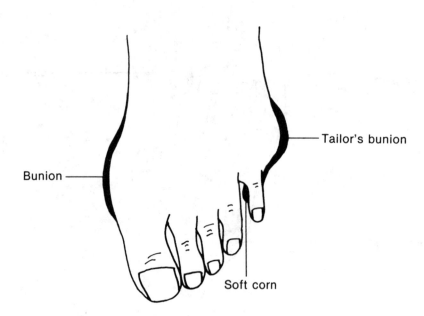

Figure 5 Digital problems

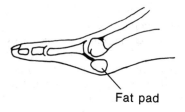

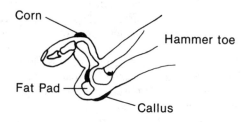

Figure 6 Hammer toe

Hallux Valgus Bunions

Hallux valgus is predominantly a bony deformity at the first metatarsophalangeal joint (See Fig. 5). Bunions become painful when the skin and soft tissue overlying the medial prominence become irritated from shoe pressure or when deviation of the big toe causes abnormal first metatarsophalangeal joint wear (DJD). Hallux valgus may also cause the big toe to hit the second toe and irritate the skin or nail, or cause a hammer toe when the second toe is pushed up by the underriding big toe.

In examination one looks for irritation of the skin over the bony prominence. Joints with a decreased range of motion, pain on motion, or crepitation indicate inflammation or degeneration of the joint. Pain only on palpation of the bony prominence medially with or without overlying skin irritation suggests only "bump" pain from shoe irritation.

Only if there is pain or functional limitation is treatment indicated. Conservative treatment consists of wide shoes, shoe stretching, soft leather shoes, pads, and molded shoes to accommodate for the deformity; oral doses of anti-inflammatory medicine is sometimes helpful if the joint is inflamed. If a bursa has developed between the skin and bony prominence, an injection of cortisone may be indicated.

Interdigital Corn (Soft Corns)

Interdigital corns form between the toes and cause toe bones from two adjacent toes to pinch the skin. This occurs mostly between the small toe (the fifth toe) and its neighbor, although any interdigital space may be involved (See Fig. 5). Patients usually present complaining of a painful growth between the toes. A history of recent change in shoes should be sought. Spread the toes and look for a corn. Since the interspaces are moist, the callused tissue is often macerated and appears white with a foul odor. Feel for any bony prominences. Examine for signs of cellulitis to rule out an infected corn. X-ray views may be necessary to determine which bones are involved.

A piece of metal (lesion marker) should be taped on the corn, the x-ray views should be weight-bearing views, and an anteroposterior view is most helpful.

Treatment in general involves removal of the excess callus tissue, and the involved toes should be separated with either foam pads or lamb's wool. Wide shoes should be recommended. If cellulitis is present, treatment with debridement, rest, elevation, warm soaks, and oral doses of antibiotics may be necessary.

Toenail Problems

Toenails can grow into the flesh of the toe at either nail border or at the end of the toe, resulting in pain from the pressure of the nail on the skin. If the nail punctures the skin, infection may follow. The common causes of ingrown toenails are congenitally deformed nails that incurvate at the borders, fungal infection, and trauma causing nail growth disturbances, and at times improper nail trimming. Patients usually complain of an acute pain localized to the toenail border. The nail groove may be inflamed or infected. The nail border may be hypertrophied from chronic irritation.

If there is infection, the offending portion of nail must be removed, followed by soaking in warm water with Epsom salts. This is accomplished by a digital block with local anesthesia. If the entire nail is to be removed, then lift the nail by inserting a straight clamp between the nailbed and nail. If only one border of the nail is to be removed, split the nail along the border to be removed and use the straight clamp to remove the involved nail border. Unless there is marked cellulitis, antibiotics are not indicated. Antibiotics alone without removal of the nail generally do not solve this problem in a timely fashion. Once the nail border is removed, antibiotics are rarely necessary.

When toenails are thick, crumbly, loose, and yellow, a fungal infection is often to blame. Once toenails become infected with a fungus, it is difficult, if not impossible, to get a normal looking, fungus-free nail. Treatments aimed at this are often doomed. Successful treatment of these nails consists of either routine debridement of the nail and at times topical application of antifungal medication, or permanent removal of the nail by removing the nail and destroying the entire nail growth center.

FLAT FEET

A flat foot condition refers to a low or absent medial longitudinal arch. Clinically there is turning in of the ankle, valgus (everted) heel, and an abducted forefoot. Many feet appear to have a good arch when examined with the patient sitting, but when the patient stands the arch collapses. Symptoms associated with flat feet include arch pains secondary to muscle ache or plantar fasciitis, tired feet and legs, heel pain, and posterior tibial tendinitis.

There are only a few flat foot conditions that are serious and need to be checked for. In general, any flat foot in a younger person that is rigid should be cause for concern and should result in referral to a specialist. Any patient who suddenly develops a unilateral flat foot should be examined for a rupture of the posterior tibial tendon. This is easily tested for and occurs only rarely.

DIABETIC FOOT INFECTION

More hospital days are spent treating diabetic foot infections than any other diabetic complication, and many such patients go on to major amputation.

The patient is examined to differentiate superficial infections of the skin and skin structures from deep space infections, and diabetics with intact circulation from dysvascular diabetic patients. The vascular evaluation includes femoral, popliteal, and pedal pulses and a Doppler examination when indicated. Gross sensory examination should be done to rule out neuropathy. Check the inguinal lymph nodes for adenopathy, and look for cellulitis and pointing abscesses. Unroof calluses, debride ulcers, and separate the toes to check for sinus tracts. Laboratory evaluation should include a complete blood count, sedimentation rate, random blood sugar, creatinine, Gram stain and culture, blood cultures, and arteriograms, as indicated. X-ray views are needed to rule out osteomyelitis, foreign body, gas, and Charcot joints.

In troublesome cases, *never hesitate to seek consultation*. If a deep space abscess is suspected because of frank sepsis, extending cellulitis, draining abscesses, and failure to respond to conservative treatment or if there is crepitus in the soft tissues, osteomyelitis, gas, or a foreign body present on x-ray views, a surgical consultation with a podiatric, orthopaedic or general surgeon is indicated. Dysvascular patients may benefit from a vascular surgeon's evaluation for bypass, endarterectomy, or balloon angioplasty once the infection has cleared.

Since most diabetic foot infections are mixed, broad spectrum antibiotic coverage is indicated initially and can be changed pending clinical progress and results of culture and sensitivity. I prefer the oral administration of cephalosporins for outpatient use in simple infections. When patients are hospitalized with more serious infections, I generally start using first generation cephalosporins intravenously unless anaerobes or gram-negative organisms are suspected to be of clinical significance. Then second or third generation cephalosporins may be indicated. Most often antibiotic treatment is combined with adequate surgical debridement, incision and drainage, or amputation. An alternate antibiotic coverage would be to use clindamycin for anaerobic coverage, ampicillin for coverage of enterococcus, and gentamicin or tobramycin with carbenicillin for gram-negative coverage.

Common pitfalls in the management of diabetic foot infections include failure to recognize deep space abscesses, osteomyelitis, or the patient's dysvascular status. Often patients are followed too long before consultation is obtained, and this at times can compromise limb salvage. Inadequate incision and drainage is often seen when small stab incisions are used rather than appropriate surgical techniques. Clinically, painless swollen feet are often misdiagnosed as infections when, in fact, Charcot joints are to blame. Likewise, radiographically Charcot joints are often misdiagnosed as osteomyelitis.

MUSCULOTENDINOUS CONTUSION AND RUPTURE

FREDERICK C. BALDUINI, M.D.

With all the time and paper devoted to ligamentous injuries of the knee, one might surmise that these are the most prevalent injuries in sports. Not so! It has been estimated that nearly 90 percent of all sport and recreational injuries are related to muscle contusion and strain.

The majority of muscle and tendon injuries are minor and rarely require medical attention. However, continued use of what may be a minimally traumatized structure can lead to a chronic disorder and the search for professional advice. In many instances simple reassurance that the injury is not severe and will respond to conservative measures is all the patient really wants to hear.

CONTUSIONS

By definition, contusions result from the impact of a blunt object on soft tissue, producing damage to skin, subcutaneous tissue, and underlying soft tissues (muscle, tendon, and neurovascular structures). The subsequent hemorrhage and severity of tissue damage are functions of the force of impact and may vary from a minimal "bump and bruise" to a severe thigh hematoma with up to 1,000 ml of blood loss.

The diagnosis of contusion is generally based on the history and findings of swelling and ecchymosis at the site of impact. One should be skeptical of patients presenting with signs disproportionate to the severity of trauma, for occasionally a patient with a previously unrecognized bone tumor may sustain a pathologic fracture with minimal trauma.

Contusions near or about joints warrant special attention. Frequently an athlete complains of medial knee joint pain believing he or she had sustained a contusion to the area, when in fact the impact was lateral, producing a medial meniscal or ligament tear and resultant medial pain. Any history of a periarticular contusion should suggest the possibility of ligamentous damage, and an examination to document ligament integrity should be performed. A patient demonstrating acute ligamentous laxity should be followed by an orthopaedist.

When patients present with progressive soft tissue swelling, the examiner should take serial measurements of limb circumference in an effort to assess continued hemorrhage. A one-inch difference in thigh circumference can represent a blood loss of 500 ml. Needles to say, a history of any bleeding disorder or therapeutic anticoagulation in a patient raises the possibility of coagulopathy, and levels of appropriate clotting factors must be measured.

There is little controversy concerning the early treatment of virtually any contusion. It is irrefutably accepted that ice application or other means of cooling the affected area along with application of a compressive dressing are the best means to control hemorrhage. It is my practice to apply crushed ice for a minimum of 20 minutes, following which a compressive dressing of bulky cotton and elastic wraps is loosely applied. The application of heat by any means is to be avoided for a minimum of 48 hours, or until the temperatures of the injured and normal limbs are similar.

Severe contusions of the thigh or upper arm deserve special attention, for these regions have an exceptional propensity for evolving into myositis ossificans. In the case of significant hemorrhage into these tissues, the respective part should be placed at rest (as well as receiving cold and compressive dressing). This is easily accomplished by the use of a sling for the arm or a knee immobilizer and crutches for the knee. The early goal of this type of management is directed at confining hemorrhage and preventing further soft-tissue damage.

Ice is frequently the only analgesic necessary. Aspirin and other nonsteroidal anti-inflammatory agents can potentially increase bleeding, and are therefore not recommended during the first 48 hours. If more analgesia is necessary, acetaminophen is usually adequate. Following the initial 48 hours, however, anti-inflammatory agents may facilitate the early mobilization and rehabilitation phase.

COMPARTMENT SYNDROME

One should always be cognizant of the potential development of an acute compartment syndrome with soft-tissue trauma. If unrecognized, this syndrome can result in permanent nerve and muscle damage. The criteria for establishment of this diagnosis are listed in Table 1. Pallor and pulselessness are late indicators, and their use as criteria could result in overlooking an impending compartment syndrome.

If one suspects or anticipates the possibility of this condition developing, the patient should be admitted and an orthopaedist or surgeon acquainted with compartment syndrome monitoring should be consulted. This condition is a potential surgical emergency and, as such, warrants prompt attention.

MUSCULOTENDINOUS STRAINS

Muscle strains can result from either acute or chronic trauma. Much like contusions, strains can vary in severity from minor (Grade I), with minimal fiber involvement,

TABLE 1 Clinical Criteria of Acute Compartment Syndrome

Tense tissues in compartment
Pain disproportionate to injury
Pain with passive stretch of muscle
Paresthesia

to severe (Grade III), with complete muscle or tendon rupture. Acute strains generally result from a rapid, asynchronous contraction of agonist and antagonist muscles and are frequently the consequence of an inadequate warm-up and stretching regimen prior to vigorous exercise.

Tendon ruptures in the lower extremity are frequently disabling injuries that can severely impair normal locomotion. Achilles tendon rupture is the most common of these injuries; patellar tendon, quadriceps, and biceps rupture are less common. Orthopaedic consultation should be sought with any of the lesions.

Achilles tendon rupture is frequently mistaken for an ankle sprain by both the patient and the inexperienced examiner. The patient frequently feels a "pop" near the ankle at the time of injury with diffuse pain and swelling. Physical examination may reveal ankle tenderness due to blood dissection within adjacent soft tissues, but there should be no pain in the "collateral" ligaments (deltoid and calcaneofibular) with stress. The examiner should always palpate the tendon itself for defects and tenderness. The sine qua non for Achilles rupture is the presence of a positive Thompson's test (Fig. 1). This test may remain negative with incomplete or partial ruptures. In these instances, active foot plantar flexion will be weak.

Radiographs may be helpful in making the diagnosis by demonstrating loss of the normal Achilles tendon shadow and disruption or obliteration of the radiolucent retrocalcaneal triangular fat pad (Kaygar's triangle).

Early treatment should include splinting of the lower extremity in a posterior plaster splint in passive equinus (the position the foot assumes when dependent). The patient should be instructed to keep the limb elevated and remain nonweight-bearing to prevent further extension of the rupture and retraction of torn ends. Immediate referral to an orthopaedist is advised.

A similar but less disabling injury has been seen with greater frequency recently with the increasing popularity of racquetball, squash, and handball. Partial rupture of the medial head of the gastrocnemius occurs at the musculotendinous junction, but continuity and function are maintained by the intact lateral head.

A characteristic feature of this injury is the searing pain that occurs in midcalf. Ambulation is difficult, and although Thompson's sign is negative, standing on tiptoe is difficult and painful. Soft-tissue swelling, erythema, and ecchymosis usually accompany this injury. The lesion must be differentiated from complete Achilles tendon rupture and venous thrombosis.

Treatment initially should be directed at immobilization with a posterior splint. Weight bearing should be protected with crutches. Ice, elevation, and oral anti-

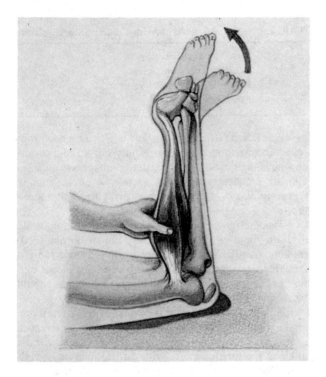 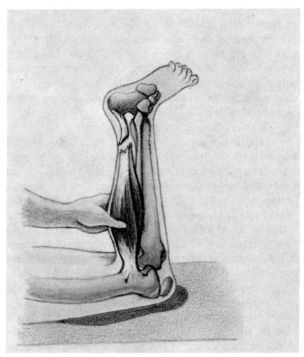

Normal   Abnormal

Figure 1 Positive Thompson's sign is indicated by failure of the foot to plantar flex against gravity with calf compression.

inflammatory agents diminish the swelling and discomfort. Weight-bearing can be started within a week with the use of bilateral heel lifts. Plantaris rupture presents with similar symptoms and findings, but fortunately treatment for this condition is similar; therefore it is not critical to differentiate these conditions.

Patellar tendon and quadriceps ruptures are serious injuries that inevitably require surgical repair for functional return. A history usually reveals the injury to be associated with jumping or coming to an abrupt stop.

Patients present with a swollen knee and complain of inability to extend the leg. With the instance of patellar tendon rupture, physical examination reveals an elevated or "high-riding" patella. With quadriceps rupture, the patella rides in its normal position but careful palpation proximal to the patella demonstrates a defect in the quadriceps mechanism. Attempted quadriceps contraction produces a mass in the anterior thigh. Radiographs should be included in the initial work-up to rule out patellar fracture or dislocation.

Treatment should again be directed at immobilizing the affected joint. Either a knee immobilizer or a bulky cotton dressing with plaster splints designed to hold the knee in extension is an effective means of accomplishing this goal. Pain and hemarthrosis can be quite severe with these injuries. Joint aspiration (from a lateral suprapatellar approach) can be of both diagnostic and therapeutic benefit and is recommended when the joint is distended.

Three other musculotendinous injuries are relatively common but of lesser severity and morbidity than those described above. Hamstring and groin pulls or strains are common injuries that are generally self-limited and respond well to the rest and gradual rehabilitation that common sense would dictate with any mild muscle strain. Biceps tendon rupture is a frightening occurrence to patients because of the resounding "snap" felt near the shoulder and the resulting mass that presents with attempted biceps contraction. Because of the anatomic duplication of the long and short heads of the biceps, there is rarely any permanent disability from this injury. Treatment is symptomatic for the initial 72 hours. The arm should be placed in a sling for that period, following which gradual mobilization should be encouraged. The patient needs to be reassured that the arm will function normally in spite of the cosmetic deformity.

The key to management of musculotendinous contusions and strains lies in a healthy respect for the hemorrhagic potential that exists in injuries to these tissues. Ice and compression remain the mainstays of therapy in that regard. Myositis ossificans and acute compartment syndrome are two significant complications associated with the hemorrhage accompanying muscle contusion and strain that have the potential for permanent disability. Appropriate early management is the best means by which these problems may be avoided. The astute emergency physician should always bear this in mind when evaluating trauma to the musculotendinous unit.

BURSITIS AND TENDINITIS

ROBERT W. BUCHOLZ, M.D.

Bursitis and tendinitis may involve any musculotendinous unit and its surrounding bursae. The nonspecific acute or chronic inflammation arises from overload or overuse of the extremity. Repetitive firing of the muscle leads to microtrauma of the tendinous fibers, often at their attachment to bony prominences. If the limb is not rested for sufficient time to allow for healing, an inflammatory reaction is initiated. Significant anatomic variations in osseous anatomy or extremity alignment occasionally may predispose individuals to particular forms of bursitis or tendinitis.

The following is a discussion of the three most common sites for this type of inflammatory condition.

BURSITIS AND TENDINITIS OF THE SHOULDER

Bursitis of the subacromial bursa, tendinitis of the rotator cuff or bicipital tendon, and supraspinatus syndrome represent variants of a syndrome with a common pathogenesis. Repetitive use of the shoulder in an elevated position results in impingement of the rotator cuff and bicipital tendon under the coracoacromial arch. The marginal vascular supply to the cuff at this location, along with the limited space available in the subacromial area, slows the healing process and predisposes this site to chronic inflammation. Direct trauma to the shoulder is a less common cause of bursitis.

Physical Examination

Physical examination reveals point tenderness over the greater tuberosity of the humerus at the supraspinatus insertion or over the bicipital tendon in its groove anteriorly. Diffuse tenderness over the deltoid muscle may also be present. Active abduction and flexion of the shoulder aggravates the discomfort. Impingement tests involving active resistive flexion or internal rotation of the shoulder at greater than 100 degrees elevation may be positive for bursitis and tendinitis as well as for supraspinatus syndrome. Chronic cases may demonstrate marked limitation of both active and passive shoulder motion along with crepitation and weakness.

Radiographic Examination

Radiographic examination is generally noncontributory unless there is extensive calcification within the tendon or bursa. Late radiographic changes may include cystic areas in the greater tuberosity and, if impingement is severe, sclerosis of the subchondral bone on the undersurface of the acromion.

Diagnosis

Differential diagnosis includes post-traumatic shoulder instability, glenohumeral and acromioclavicular degenerative arthritis, gout and other inflammatory conditions, septic arthritis, and cervical spondylosis. Localized signs to the subacromial region are usually sufficient to rule out these other entities. A major tear in the rotator cuff must be excluded. Such a tear may be the end result of chronic attrition of the cuff secondary to impingement. Loss of active initiation of shoulder abduction suggests a major disruption of the rotator cuff fibers.

Treatment

Treatment of shoulder tendinitis or bursitis centers around resting the joint. Cessation of the activity that incited the inflammatory reaction usually suffices in effecting a cure. Patients are often more comfortable resting in a sitting position so that the weight of the arm distracts the proximal humerus away from the acromium. The use of a sling for more severe cases should be limited to 5 to 7 days, minimizing the likelihood of shoulder stiffness. Mild analgesics, ice packs, and anti-inflammatories are most effective in acute cases. Chronic bursitis and tendinitis may necessitate steroid injections into the subacromial space. I prefer to use 40 to 80 mg of methylprednisolone mixed with an equal volume of 0.25 percent bupivacaine. The inflamed area is widely injected with this medication and then massaged to ensure dispersion of the steroid throughout the bursa and peritendinous tissues. If the correct area is injected, immediate relief of shoulder pain and improved range of motion should be evident.

If extensive calcific tendinitis is present, the needle can be used to morselize the calcific deposits. Barbotage of the material can be accomplished using sterile saline and a large-bore needle. Steroids are then injected into the subacromial space. The deleterious effects of steroids on collagen metabolism make it dangerous to perform more than two to three shoulder injections per year.

If there is not complete resolution of symptoms within several weeks, orthopaedic referral should be sought to assist in excluding other causes of the shoulder pain and in further managing the inflammatory condition.

TENDINITIS ABOUT THE ELBOW

Like the shoulder, the elbow is prone to overuse syndromes. Overload of the forearm extensor muscles results in lateral epicondylitis, or tennis elbow, and repeated microtrauma to the forearm flexor musculotendinous units leads to medial epicondylitis, or golfer's elbow. Weekend athletes, painters, maids, and other individuals who require repetitive wrist dorsiflexion and volar flexion are most susceptible to these types of elbow problems. Few clinical entities mimic these diseases, although golfer's elbow should not be confused with a subluxating ulnar nerve at the cubital tunnel. Radiographs are negative except in chronic cases with calcification of the degenerating tendon.

Tennis Elbow

Tennis elbow, the most common form of elbow tendinitis, is characterized by point tenderness 1 to 2 cm distal to the tendinous insertion of the extensors on the lateral epicondyle. The patient experiences pain in the elbow when he attempts active dorsiflexion of the wrist against resistance.

Treatment

Treatment revolves around modification of activity. Tennis players may need to change their backhand stroke or the grip circumference and string tension of their rackets. Forearm circumferential bands placed on the proximal forearm may aid in redistributing the impact loads on the muscle origins. Severe symptoms may require the temporary use of a cock-up splint to relieve the extended tendon from tension. Strengthening and stretching exercises for the forearm extensors should be instituted once the acute symptoms have subsided. Ice packs may be applied to the lateral aspect of the elbow following activity.

Refractory cases may necessitate steroid injections into the extensor tendons. Occasionally surgical release of the extensor mass from the lateral epicondyle is required.

TENDINITIS AROUND THE KNEE

Periarticular knee pain may be caused by a variety of different inflammatory conditions. Inflammations of the patellar tendon, the pes anserinus tendon, the iliotibial tract, and the prepatellar bursa are frequently encountered problems, especially in adolescents and athletes. Patellar tendinitis occurs mainly during the adolescent growth spurt. Inflammation of the pes anserinus bursa underlying the tendinous insertion of the gracilis, semitendinosus, and sartorius muscles is common in runners and cyclists.

Local swelling and tenderness usually identify which musculotendinous complex is inflamed. Prepatellar bursal swelling should be distinguished from a knee effusion. The prepatellar bursa is subcutaneous and located over the inferior aspect of the patella and the superior part of the patellar tendon. Radiographs are unremarkable except for soft-tissue swelling and occasional calcification of the insertion of the patellar tendon in cases of adolescent Osgood-Schlatter disease. Rarer causes of periarticular pain, including osteomyelitis, neoplasm, and septic bursitis, must be ruled out.

Treatment

As in the shoulder and elbow, most cases of knee bursitis and tendinitis respond well to rest, ice, and stretching exercises once the acute pain has diminished. Local steroid injections are helpful in refractory cases. Nonseptic prepatellar bursitis (housemaid's knee) is easily managed by aspiration of all bursal fluid, steroid injection in chronic cases, and application of a compressive dressing. It is critical that the patient abstain from kneeling directly on the patella during the recovery phase. Surgical excision of the bursa is the most effective treatment for chronic prepatellar bursitis.

Osgood-Schlatter disease may be symptomatic enough to warrant temporary immobilization of the knee in extension. Splints should be discontinued as early as possible. Weakening of the tibial tuberosity apophysis secondary to chronic Osgood-Schlatter disease may predispose the child to avulsion fracture of the tuberosity, especially during jumping sports. Most symptoms spontaneously resolve at the conclusion of the growth spurt.

OTHER SITES OF TENDINITIS AND BURSITIS

Acute or chronic inflammation may also commonly involve the calcaneal tendon, the retrocalcaneal bursa, the metatarsal bursae, the greater trochanteric bursa, the peroneal tendon sheaths, and the olecranon bursa. The basic management principles are identical to those already discussed for the shoulder, elbow, and knee.

SUGGESTED READING

Duthie R, Bentley G, eds. Mercer's orthopedic surgery. 8th ed. London: Edward, Arnold, 1983.
Turek S. Orthopaedics: principles and their applications. Philadelphia: JB Lippincott, 1977.

INJURIES IN RUNNERS

RICHARD C. LEHMAN, M.D.
JOSEPH S. TORG, M.D.

Running, jogging, and marathons are activities that have captured the attention of millions of Americans. From the novice to the elite, the overzealous runner pushes himself to ridiculous limits, and consequently injuries occur. Management of these problems includes accurate diagnosis, appropriate treatment, and rehabilitation.

HEAT INJURIES

Heat injuries are common in running sports and consist of heat cramps, heat exhaustion, and heat stroke.

Heat Cramps

Heat cramps are exceedingly common and occur mostly in the calf muscles. They are attributable to excessive sweating without replacement of water. This water deficiency results in muscle spasms, painful cramping, and an inability to use the affected extremity. Emergency management consists of stretching the involved muscles, replacement of fluids, and rest. Water is the fluid replacement of choice. It should be taken liberally before, during, and after practices and competition in hot humid weather.

Heat Exhaustion

The physician must differentiate the syndrome of heat exhaustion from heat stroke. Heat exhaustion occurs when the individual is exposed to excessive environmental temperatures and sweats profusely without adequate fluid replacement. The patient is volume-depleted and must be treated as such. The athlete experiencing heat exhaustion should be undressed and placed supine in a cool shaded area and oral fluid replacement should be instituted.

If the patient does not respond immediately, he should be transported to the nearest medical facility, where an intravenous line is placed and 2.5 percent dextrose in 0.2 sodium chloride (NaC1) is given as the replacement. Serum electrolytes and serum osmolality should be monitored in these athletes. If the serum sodium is monitored, the forumula:

$$\text{Change in body water} = 0.6 \times \text{body weight (kg) } (1\text{-}144/[\text{Na}])$$

is used to calculate the water loss in liters. If serum osmolality is used, Table 1 should be used to calculate the water deficit.

Once this deficit is determined, replacement is instituted in an attempt to replenish the deficit over 24 hours. The athlete's deficit plus insensible losses must be replace. An individual with normal renal function should receive a one-liter bolus over the first hour and then replace the rest of the deficit slowly. Vital signs, urine output, and clinical parameters are monitored.

Heat exhaustion is potentially fatal and must be treated as a medical emergency. The physician should become familiar with the signs and symptoms and employ aggressive management. Prevention of this potential catastrophe includes (1) acclimatization prior to competition; (2) adequate water intake before, during, and after an event; and (3) liberal use of table salt.

Heat Stroke

Heat stoke occurs in the unacclimatized individual who is exposed to strong sunlight and high temperatures. Failure of the thermoregulatory mechanism occurs, protective sweating stops, and the body temperature rises. The athlete presents with mental status change, rectal temperatures of 105 °F. or higher, cutaneous vasodilatation, and sometimes "the shakes." If the patient's temperature should rise above 107 °F, brain damage occurs and death may follow. The emphasis is on the lack of sweating. Emergency treatment consists of immediately placing the patient supine and packing him in ice. Transport the athlete to the hospital immediately and continue ice cooling.

Hospital treatment consists of (1) continuous cooling, (2) intravenous replacement fluids, (3) ECG monitoring and Foley catheterization, and (4) laboratory studies. Cooling with wet towels and immersion baths should be continued until the elevated temperature falls below 100 °F. Heat stroke may result in hepatocellular damage, diffuse intra-articular coagulation, or occult sepsis. Hospitalization of 48 hours is usually necessary, and follow-up after the injury is required (see also chapter on *Heat Illness*).

THE HIP

Hip pain occurring in runners should alert the emergency physician. Although most causes of hip pain are benign, the femoral neck stress fracture is an important exception. The athlete may present with hip or thigh pain that occurs while he or she is running. The pain decreases when the athlete stops running, and pain is directly related to activity. The athlete may also present with a limp and limited range of motion in the affected hip.

Anteroposterior (AP) and frog-leg lateral films are ordered. If the roentgenograms demonstrate a stress fracture involving only one cortex, non-weight-bearing locomotion is initiated on crutches. If the films demonstrate a complete fracture, this should be treated by operative closed femoral pinning. These fractures may go on to displace, increasing the risk of delayed union, nonunion, and avascular necrosis.

If the roentgenograms are negative, a bone scan is necessary to confirm the diagnosis. A runner with a posi-

TABLE 1 Clinical Laboratory Dehydration Criteria

Clinical Status	Serum Na	Serum OSM	HCT	H_2O Deficit (Liter)	% H_2O Loss
Normal	144	285	42		
Mild	149–151	294–298	42	1.5–2	3–4.5
Moderate	152–158	299–313	42.2	2–4	4.5–10
Severe	159–166	314–329	42.5	4–6	10–15
Lethal	>166	>330	>42.5	>6	>15

tive bone scan should stop running and rest the part. They should be kept non-weight-bearing as long as the hip is painful during routine daily activities.

THIGH AND GROIN

Pain in the thigh can be due to hamstring, groin, or quadriceps injuries. Hamstring injuries are commonly seen in sprinters, hurdlers, and athletes who fail to stretch before an event. The pain is usually disabling and may be associated with tenderness and sometimes ecchymosis. In the young athlete, if the complaints are referable to the ischium, roentgenograms may show an avulsion injury. The athlete is examined while prone, with the knee flexed at 90 degrees. Gentle resistance to knee flexion causes pain. Treatment consists of thigh wrap, ice, nonsteroidal anti-inflammatory drugs, and rest. Follow-up is important to institute stretching exercises and treatment with a high galvanic stimulator. Stretching is the most important exercise in the post-injury period.

Groin injuries in the runner can be separated into stress fracture of the pubis ramus, the sartorius syndrome, osteitis pubis, and adductor muscle strain. An AP view of the pelvis should be ordered. If the athlete has a stress fracture, a sclerotic line on the pubis ramus is seen on the roentgenogram. The treatment of a stress fracture of the pubis ramus is rest from athletic activities with continued weight-bearing. The sartorius syndrome can be diagnosed by tenderness at the insertion of the sartorius muscle in the area of the anterior superior iliac spine. Films may demonstrate a fleck of bone pulled off the pelvis at this anatomic site. Resisted flexion of the hip is painful. Treatment of the sartorius syndrome is rest, nonsteroidal anti-inflammatory drugs, and eventually stretching of the hip flexors. Osteitis pubis presents in the athlete with limited internal rotation of the hip, pain in the groin, and a positive roentgenogram showing obliteration of the cortical margin of the pubis. Treatment consists of rest and nonsteroidal medications. Osteitis pubis, in most cases, is refractory to treatment and may cause prolonged symptoms, but eventually resolves without sequelae.

THE KNEE

Knee injuries attributable to chronic overuse with an acute exacerbation may bring the runner to an emergency facility. These syndromes include overuse synovitis, lateral compression syndrome, chondromalacia, iliotibial band syndrome, patella, tendonitis, and bursitis. These injuries are treated by rest, ice, and nonsteroidal anti-inflammatory drugs. Patients with synovitis, and an effusion require knee aspiration to relieve discomfort. The aspirate is normal synovial fluid, and the effusions abate with cessation of running. Knee injuries that require acute attention include ligamentous disruption, patellar dislocations, and torn menisci. These are rare in runners, but do occur. Treatment of a ligamentous problem includes radiologic evaluation, stability testing, examination of tenderness, and aspiration. A knee immobilizer and

crutches are prescribed. Posterior splints exacerbate swelling and should not be used.

Injuries of the patella are separated into (1) direct trauma and (2) instability. If direct trauma has occurred, the athlete should be tested for active knee extension. If this is absent and the roentgenograms show a fracture, operative treatment may be indicated to repair the disrupted quadriceps mechanism. Place the patient in a knee immobilizer or cylinder cast and consult an orthopaedic surgeon for surgical repair.

Patellar instability may occur in the form of subluxation or dislocation due to a traumatic fall or twisting injury during events such as the hurdles and steeple chase. Most dislocations are reduced spontaneously. If the dislocated patella is noted on the patient's arrival, roentgenograms are obtained, and then the athlete is placed supine on the examination table. Gently reduce the patella by extending the knee and displacing the laterally dislocated patella medially. Apply a long-leg cylinder cast. Surgical treatment is rarely necessary for first-time dislocation without a concomitant fracture.

COMPARTMENT SYNDROME

Acute exertional compartment syndrome owing to overuse is not common, but catastrophic if missed. This injury can occur when the runner competes at distances to which he is unaccustomed. These athletes have severe pain over the compartment, and this pain can develop as late as 12 hours after the event. It may also develop during the run and is associated with numbness and weakness. The intensity of the pain increases, and the compartment feels tense. Stretching the involved muscle causes pain, and there is usually a sensory loss. The four P's associated with compartment syndrome are pulselessness, pallor, pain, and paresthesia. Compartment pressure measurements obtained by means of a wick catheter or a manometer confirm the diagnosis. All four leg compartments are tested. If compartment pressures are greater than 40 mm Hg and the aforementioned clinical features are present, four-quadrant surgical fasciotomy is done immediately.

Chronic exertional compartment syndrome occurs with exercise and presents as a dull ache or cramp. In most cases it is located in the anterior compartment. Rest after the activity decreases the pain, although the athlete may feel a fullness in the leg. The immediate treatment is rest acutely, but fasciotomy of the affected compartment may be necessary if the athlete chooses to continue running (see also the chapter on *Compartment Syndrome and Rhabdomyolysis*).

INJURIES TO THE LEG

Injuries in the leg include stress fractures of the tibia and fibula, posterior medial tibial syndrome, and "shin splints."

Stress fractures most commonly occur in the tibia and may be diaphyseal or metaphyseal. Antero-posterior, lateral, and oblique films should be ordered of the specific area that is injured. Tenderness and swelling identify the affected area. It should be noted that x-ray findings may be negative, and a bone scan may be necessary to identify a stress fracture.

Tibial diaphyseal stress fractures, which are diagnosed on plain films, are usually unicortical. Treatment for this fracture initially is rest, cessation of running, and nonsteroidal anti-inflammatory medications. Symptoms, in most cases, resolve with a decrease in activity. Follow-up examination and repeat films are performed to allow the physician to determine whether the athlete may return to running.

Metaphyseal stress fractures can also be diagnosed roentgenographically and may be subtle. A bone scan may be necessary to make the diagnosis. The athlete usually responds to a decrease in activity, and weight-bearing is tolerated. Since these fractures occur in cancellous bone, they are more likely to heal than the aforementioned diaphyseal fracture, which occurs in cortical bone. In both cases, follow-up, rehabilitative therapy, and a graduated increase in running when the athlete returns help to alleviate this problem.

Posterior medial tibial syndrome is characterized by tenderness along the posterior border of the medial tibia. The etiology is uncertain, but many people feel it is due to a periostitis at the muscular insertion of the posterior tibialis muscle. Pain may be acute after a long run and x-ray findings are usually normal. Rest, ice, nonsteroidal anti-inflammatory medication, and posterior tibial stretching relieve the symptoms. The hallmark of treatment is aggressive stretching of the posterior structures.

The etiology of "shin splints" is uncertain. Shin splints may occur in the anterior aspect of the tibia, which is felt to be due to overactivity in the unconditioned athlete. Shin splints in the posterior aspect of the tibia may be due to periostitis of the posterior tibial musculature, stress fracture, or overuse of the soft tissue structures in the posterior medial aspect of the tibia. Antero-posterior, lateral, and oblique films should be ordered specifically to rule out a stress fracture of the tibia. In patients with true shin splints, x-ray findings are normal. Rest, ice, nonsteroidal anti-inflammatory drugs, and, most important, stretching to relieve the symptoms are required. Low-dye strapping, a technique of taping to help support the medial arch and possibly orthotics may be appropriate if the symptoms are referrable to the posterior compartment. Rest and proper conditioning with appropriate stretching relieve symptoms in the anterior variety of shin splints.

ANKLE INJURIES

Ankle sprains commonly occur in athletes who run on uneven terrain, at night, or in events such as the high and low hurdles. Swelling and tenderness are noted on initial presentation. Examination of both the medial and lateral ligamentous structures is necessary to differentiate bimalleolar injuries from isolated lateral injuries. Ligamentous instability should be tested both medially and laterally, varus and valgus, and anteriorly and posteriorly. The proximal fibula must be palpated for tenderness to rule out a fracture with a concomitant injury to the del-

toid ligament. X-ray studies, including AP, lateral, and mortise views are ordered. In reviewing the films, a high index of suspicion is needed in searching for osteochondral fractures of the medial or lateral talus.

Treatment of simple ankle sprains includes ice, elevation, and crutch ambulation without weight-bearing. In cases of severe sprains, a short leg cast is excellent to decrease edema and allow comfort. Osteochondral fractures of the medial and lateral talus are treated either conservatively or with surgical intervention. Surgically, the fragment may be excised or replaced and may require cast immobilization after the procedure. Consultation with an orthopaedic surgeon is recommended.

PLANTAR FASCIITIS

Plantar fasciitis is common in runners. This is an overuse problem that occurs acutely if the unconditioned runner starts with high mileage. Tenderness occurs in the plantar fascia and its attachment posteromedial to the calcaneus. A heel spur may be seen on roentgenogram. These injuries are treated conservatively. Ice, rest, and nonsteroidal and anti-inflammatory drugs, as prescribed and taping of the medial arch of the foot (a low dye strap) is also helpful. After the acute episode, the athlete must stretch the posterior complex aggressively before running. If not treated appropriately, this injury may become chronic.

ACHILLES TENDINITIS

Achilles tendinitis is an overuse injury caused by increasing mileage too rapidly, change in surface, or a lack of conditioning and stretching. It also may be a recurrent injury that has not been allowed to completely recover. Pain occurs posteriorly in the Achilles area and is exacerbated by forced plantar flexion and toe standing. These injuries are treated conservatively with rest, ice, nonsteroidal anti-inflammatory drugs, and a heel lift. After the acute episode has resolved, adequate stretching and conditioning prevent recurrence.

ACHILLES TENDON RUPTURE

Complete rupture of the Achilles tendon is a severe injury that is often missed. The presenting complaint is sudden pain in the posterior aspect of the distal calf. The duration of the pain is short, and the athlete is unable to continue competing. The athlete presents with a swollen ecchymotic ankle that is only slightly tender. The athlete is able to actively plantar-flex his ankle using his or her toe flexors. Roentgenogram findings are normal, and many times the athlete is released with a diagnosis of acute ankle sprain. Do not be misled by active ankle plantar flexion. The proper test to determine a functioning tendo Achilles mechanism is performed with the athlete in the prone position with his feet hanging off of the table. The examiner squeezes the calf in the distal one-third and watches plantar flexion of the foot. Both legs should be examined. Asymmetry or loss of plantar flexion is diagnostic of a torn Achilles tendon.

Specific treatment of complete Achilles tendon rupture is somewhat controversial. Competitive athletes in our clinic are treated surgically with primary repair of the torn tendon. Conservative treatment consisting of cast immobilization is practiced by some orthopaedists and is left to the discretion of the consulting physician. Emergency management consists of non-weight-bearing crutch ambulation and referral. Follow-up should be immediate to improve results if surgical treatment is chosen.

COMPLICATIONS OF DISUSE AND IMMOBILIZATION

ROBERT SINE, M.D.

Most of the effects of disuse and immobilization develop slowly and should not—one might think—present in the emergency room. However, people judge the acuity of problems by the severity at first notice. Hence the conditions to be discussed may appear and require recognition.

The majority of the complications of immobility occur in patients with preexisting conditions that render them or a body part immobile. Among the most common such conditions are spinal cord injury, stroke, parkinsonism, and rheumatoid arthritis, but any condition producing enough motor or sensory loss, joint stiffness, chronic pain, or volitional paucity of movement to immobilize a person or extremity may produce these complications.

SYMPATHETIC REFLEX DYSTROPHY

Reflex sympathetic dystrophy is a series of changes in an extremity subjected to disuse, rather than a discrete syndrome. The early stages show the features of sympathetic activity from which the syndrome derives its name. The hand or foot is cool and wet. Frequently there is a history of trauma—often trivial—preceding the onset. There may be pain in the neighboring joint (shoulder-hand syndrome) and frequently pain and dysesthesias in the hand or foot itself.

As disuse persists, the joints initially show effusions and eventually go on to ankylosis. The sympathetic activity settles down, leaving an end stage of a warm, dry, boardlike hand with shiny, thin, atrophic skin and osteoporotic bones.

The early stages may develop rather quickly (over days) and appear rather dramatically in a patient's hand or foot. This stage is reversible with any treatment that reinstates use. Probably the most important treatment in the emergency department is reassurance, as the patient's anxiety itself heightens sympathetic activity. This dissuades the patient from using the hand or foot (to avoid pain and dysesthesia), thereby accelerating the cycle of disuse, leading to disuse phenomena, leading to more disuse. Exercises may start in a whirlpool bath or paraffin bath. I have had excellent results with "centripetal finger wrapping." The technique utilizes a string wrapped tightly and centripetally around a finger so as to milk fluid from the finger and provide an afferent sensory barrage. It is the same technique used to dislodge rings on swollen fingers and may be initiated in the emergency department.

The patient should then be referred to the physical medicine department for prompt vigorous treatment. The further the process evolves prior to treatment, the more difficult it is to reverse. Stellate ganglion block reportedly has been successful, but should await failure of more conservative measures and, when utilized, should be considered a means to the end of encouraging use.

AUTONOMIC HYPER-REFLEXIA

Although not caused by immobility, autonomic hyperreflexia is an emergency that presents among a visably immobile population—the high paraplegic or quadraplegic patient. The coexistence of immobility and a life threatening condition warrants its discussion here. The major features on presentation include hypertension and sweating, which are the direct effects of the overstimulated and unopposed sympathetic nervous system below the level of the spinal cord injury. Above the level of the injury, the secondarily activated parasympathetic nervous system may add the findings of bradycardia and conduction block with electrocardiographic abnormalities.

The hypertension is the focus of emergency attention because it commonly causes pounding headache and may cause hypertensive encephalopathy, confusion, visual disturbances, seizures, unconsciousness, hemorrhages, apnea, and cerebrovascular accident.

The originating hyperactivity of the sympathetic nervous system is usually triggered by a stimulus in the lower segmental distributions. The most common acute offenders are distention of the bladder or bowel. Less commonly, infections, cold, decubitus ulcers, or tight clothing may trigger the onset.

The diagnosis is complicated by the loss of sensation below the level of injury in the high level cord injured patient. Erroneous diagnoses can include essential or malignant hypertension, acute abdomen, cardiac disease, encephalopathy, or systemic infection. In short, a great deal of time may be spent on major work-ups of numerous systems if the syndrome is not recognized.

Initial measures include blood pressure monitoring at least every five minutes and elevation of the head of the bed. Abdominal palpation may reveal either a hard distended bladder or the unmistakable feel of feces—easily pitted—along the left abdomen. If neither is felt, the offending organ may still be the bladder, as bladder pressures may be high in a spastic bladder without high volumes. Free drainage should be assured by catheterization or a catheter change in the already catheterized patient. Catheters should be inserted slowly and lidocaine can be used with the lubrication. If bowel distention is the culprit, the situation is usually less acute, but may be tricky as disimpaction may trigger additional sympathetic activity. Awaiting lower blood pressures before proceeding and topical use of Nupercaine ointment is prudent prior to disimpaction. Clothes should be loosened and the skin inspected.

If all else fails, hydralazine (Apresoline) may be administered, 10 mg intravenously slowly.

If the episode dealt with is but one of recurrent episodes, the patient will require work-up to ascertain the nature of the offending stimulus and proper treatment. The patient will require education regarding the nature of the problem and self-care. A ganglion blocker may be required intermittently for control (Inversine, 2.5 to 5.0 mg twice daily).

Autonomic hyperreflexia is a potentially dangerous and initially perplexing syndrome, which, however, responds nicely to well considered therapy.

DECUBITUS ULCERS

If immobilization permits pressures exceeding capillary pressure to occur between a bony prominence and the external surface for a critical time, which may be as short as 20 minutes, infarction of the tissues may occur. The infarction includes all layers down to bone, though the skin portion will be most evident.

The lesion will present over a bony prominence, such as the sacrum, trochanters, or heels. Its first appearance will be as a reddened area. At this stage it is not possible to know whether infarction has occurred or whether there is simply a benign reversible hyperemia. If infarction has occurred, nothing will alter the situation, the area will whiten, demarcate, and eventually slough.

The patient and family should be counseled about the natural history of the lesion so that there is no undue alarm as the lesion appears to "worsen." Although a plethora of treatment regimes are utilized, the decubitus ulcer does not differ from other open wounds except for its mechanism of production by pressure. The general principles of good wound care hold, with the added caveat that reinjury by reintroduction of excessive pressures must be avoided.

Dressings are for the purpose of keeping the wound clean, reducing shear forces, avoiding maceration of adjoining skin, and soiling of clothes. To those ends they may be occlusive or nonocclusive, but should not be bulky, as such dressings are a source of increased pressure.

The laying down of new ground substance, collagen, and epithelium is an involved and delicate process, which should not be disturbed unnecessarily. Because the surface granulation tissue is resistant to infection, antisepsis should be restrained. Light cleansing will remove accumulated exudate. One percent hydrogen peroxide may be used. Powdered sugar sprinkled liberally into the wound produces a highly osmotic solution, which inhibits bacterial growth and is the least likely antisepsis to interfere with healing. Routine cultures are unnecessary. Infection is indicated by a malodorous colored exudate, which should be differentiated from necrotic sloughed material and is not common. In that case, a culture may be obtained and the organism treated appropriately. Debridement may be carried out when there is excessive loose necrotic tissue, but should be blunt and infrequent. An undermined wound should not be allowed to close over, leaving a potential space for infection, but should be lightly packed with gauze strips.

Finally, the patient should be made aware of the mechanism of production of the ulcer, the extent of the present one, and his role in treatment and prophylaxis.

CONSTIPATION

Inactivity per se can decrease bowel motility, leading to inspissated feces and eventually fecal impaction. Hence the impression of interns, that there is a generalized preoccupation with bowels among inactive hospitalized patients. When the condition is severe—as it can become in immobilized patients—it can present as a swollen, painful, tender belly and can be confused with conditions as diverse as peritonitis or ascites.

The usual symptoms are decreased stool and cramping pain. However, leakage around an impaction may elicit a report of diarrhea. The tenderness is generally more severe on the left along the descending colon. A pathognomonic sign may be present in patients without obesity. Firm digital pressure over the abdominal mass can produce an unmistakable "pitting" in the feces, which persists and can be repalpated.

If there has been no stool for 48 hours and there are active bowel sounds, treatment begins with a rectal check. If the finger finds hard inspissated stool filling the rectum, disimpaction is required or further efforts will simply meet the resistance of the fecal plug. Enemas should include a lubricant (oil, soap suds) as the stool is hard; laxatives should be of neurotropic type (senna, Dulcolax), as the already distended colon will respond poorly to laxatives, which depend on colonic distention to produce a purging reflex.

CONTRACTURES

The tissues across an immobile joint eventually assume the shortest resting length consistent with usual movement. Muscles and tendons shorten early and are the usual limiting structures. Spasticity seems to hasten the process. The condition is generally easily recognized. The patient may then be referred to the physical medicine department for slow stretching exercises. There is no urgency, but the patient and family should be counseled regarding the importance of maintaining range of motion.

SUGGESTED READING

Erickson RP. Autonomic hyper-reflexia: pathophysiology and medical management. Arch Phys Med Rehab 1980; 61:431–440.

Sine R. Identification and management of bowel problems. In: Base rehabilitation techniques. 2nd ed. Rockville, Maryland: Aspen Publishing, 1980:221.

Sine R. Pressure sores development, pathogenesis, prevention, and treatment. In: Basic rehabilitation techniques. 2nd ed. Rockville, Maryland: Aspen Publishing, 1980:237.

Steinbrocker O. The shoulder-hand syndrome: present perspective. Arch Phys Med Rehab 1968; 49:388–395.

FRACTURES NOT REQUIRING ORTHOPAEDIC CONSULTATION

RALPH J. DiLIBERO, M.D., F.A.A.O.S.

For most common fractures, the standard of care advocates that the emergency physician at least consult with an orthopaedic surgeon by phone, and for that reason the general topic of fracture treatment is not expounded on in this text. There are, however, certain fractures that an emergency physician, while recognizing certain parameters of precaution, can treat without initial orthopaedic consultation.

General complications of major fractures also apply to minor fractures. These include hematoma, infection, neurologic and vascular compromise, sympathetic dystrophy, pulmonary complications, ligamentous instability, and tendon avulsions and impalements. Errors in diagnosis include unrecognized pathologic fractures, epiphyseal plate injuries, and metabolic disturbances leading to fractures of nontraumatic etiology.

Late complications include avascular necrosis, malunion, bone growth stimulation or arrest, nonunion, associated joint loss of range of motion, angular and rotatory deformities, and bone shortening. Iatrogenic complications are also possible; usually these are produced by forceful manipulation. Skin avulsions in the elderly, secondary ligamentous and fracture injury, and crush injury to epiphyseal plates or neurovascular structures can be included in this grouping. Severe soft tissue swelling should also alert the emergency physician to look for hidden complications.

CLAVICLE FRACTURES

If a child sustains a bone shaft fracture, the most likely bone to be broken is the clavicle, and of all the clavicle fractures, half occur in children under 10 years of age. The closed shaft fractures are simple to manage and should be differentiated from those of the medial or outer end, which sometimes are difficult to maintain in acceptable reduction and require orthopaedic consultation if displaced or separated by soft tissue interposition.

An occasional complication of a clavicular shaft fracture is compression of the subclavian vein by an angulated fracture with a downward bow, for which management may include the use of a shoulder spica and bed rest. This complication occurs when there is encroachment of the space between the clavicle and the first rib, resulting in angulation or mechanical compression of the subclavian vessels, the brachial artery, or the carotid artery. *Brachial plexus compression* is also possible and should be differentiated from a stretching of the plexus by the history, physical examination, electromyogram, and strength-duration curves of involved muscles. *Vascular compression* can be identified by comparison testing of the radial pulses of both extremities while carrying out maneuvers that might constrict the artery, such as the Adson test, the costoclavicular maneuver, the attention test, the downward traction test, and the hyperabduction test. In Adson's test, the seated patient elevates his chin and points it toward the side on which the pulse is being palpated. In the costoclavicular maneuver, the examiner forces the seated patient's shoulders down and forward while an assistant checks the radial pulse. In the hyperabduction test, the seated patient places his hands behind his head, opening and closing his fist, while the radial pulse is palpated.

Fortunately, most shaft fractures do quite well, heal quickly and thus present no special complications. The aim of treatment is to prevent further displacement and angulation, not to reduce the fracture. A figure-eight bandage splint serves this function well. It is best applied with the child sitting with the hands raised over the head and the arms abducted to 90 degrees. Be sure that the bandage is not applied too tightly so that either axillary compression of vessels and nerves or pressure sores do not develop. The purpose of the splint is to provide comfort while healing with abundant fracture callus takes place. A perfect cosmetic result is not always expected.

RIB FRACTURES

The immediate aim in treatment of a fractured rib is relief of pain, so that a patient may breathe adequately. This is best accomplished by the use of intercostal nerve blocks of the fractured rib as well as the rib above and below the fracture with a long-acting anesthetic such as Marcaine. Various strapping and binding techniques to limit chest pain are not advised. They all tend to decrease ventilation and cause rather than correct problems.

It is most important to consider other possible associated respiratory complications when dealing with a simple fractured rib. Besides the obvious rule-outs such as pneumothorax and hemothorax, ventilation may be compromised by lung contusion, adult respiratory distress syndrome, and instability of the chest wall with paradoxical motion. Patients with these complications have suffered major trauma and need hospital admission and surgical consultation.

The patient with an uncomplicated rib fracture should be advised to take a slow deep breath every 15 minutes and should be given a surgical glove to blow up every half-hour as an incentive spirometer to prevent atelectasis. Elderly patients and those with severe pulmonary disease are more prone to complications; they should be carefully observed by a family member and occasionally admitted to the hospital.

FOOT FRACTURES

Fractures of the forefoot have probably been overprotected and overtreated in the past. Fractures of the phalanges require only sensible emergency care. Early ambulation and weight bearing in patients with minor foot fractures decreases rehabilitation time, time lost from work, the incidence of osteoporosis, and Sudeck's atrophy (sympathetic dystrophy).

Most people stub one of their toes from time to time, often while walking in a darkened room; this results in the *"night-walker" fracture of the proximal phalanx* of the toes. These injuries are usually self-treated and do well. The most common fracture of the forefoot is the fifth proximal phalanx, and occasionally a permanent deformity results, with the fifth toe angulating dorsally or the second, third, or fourth toe angulating to the plantar surface with a dorsal bump resembling a hammer toe. If not treated by initial closed reduction, these deformities may cause pain and problems with footwear, necessitating surgical correction. Since the most likely direction of future deformity is known, splinting should counter the deforming forces. Ice packs and elevation of the foot during the first few days should keep the patient quite comfortable. Symptomatic relief can be obtained by strapping adjoining toes together, after lining the intertriginous space with lamb's wool or cotton to prevent maceration of the skin. A shoe with an adequate toe box, a sandal, a stiff shoe with a cut-out toe, or, rarely, a short-leg walking cast with an expanded toe plate provides further comfort and protection.

Crush injury with resultant fracture of the toes, especially the distal phalanx of the great toe, is a common problem in industrial workers. Most of these fractures could be prevented simply by wearing shoes with reinforced metal plates over the toe portion. The treatment is usually directed to the soft-tissue component of the injury, since the fractures are adequately stabilized by the tense swollen toe. When the fracture is multiply comminuted, the transmitted force per unit area is usually more severe. The soft-tissue injury may include nerve and vessel injury leading to soft-tissue infection and necrosis. Metabolic disturbances, such as diabetes, and foreign body impalements can further aggravate the problems and may lead to eventual loss of the toe. Diabetics require special care, diligent follow-up, and especially avoidance of hot-water soaks. If there is a displaced intra-articular or compound fracture, an orthopaedic consultation is needed. I believe in prophylactic antibiotic coverage for even the slightest open wound, even though it often does not represent direct communication with bone or a "true" compound fracture.

A frequent and very painful fracture-related condition is traumatic avulsion of a toenail. Fortunately most injuries are quite minimal in extent, but if more than half the nail is involved or if the base is partially avulsed, the nail is usually lost. It is often necessary to remove the entire nail under local block anesthesia. After excision of the nail, the bleeding nail bed is best dressed with an anesthetic ointment and the dressing changed frequently over the next week. The great toenail takes approximately 4 to 9 months to completely regrow.

When a patient presents with a history of having turned the foot inward or of having stepped into a hole and experienced sudden pain and swelling on the lateral aspect of the foot, the most likely diagnosis is a fracture of the base of the fifth metatarsal, the most common of all metatarsal fractures. It is of key importance to ascertain that the base is fractured rather than the shaft of the fifth metatarsal, known also as a Jones fracture, which is sometimes difficult to treat and requires orthopaedic consultation. On reviewing the anteroposterior and oblique films of the foot, this fracture must be distinguished from the apophysis to which the peroneus brevis tendon attaches in a child or an accessory sesamoid bone, the *os vesalianum*, in an adult (Fig. 1). The fracture line in a child should be more transverse relative to the long axis of the metatarsal rather than oblique, as is the apophysis. The fractured fragment should be irregular in an adult rather than smooth, as is a sesamoid bone.

The aim of treatment is relief of pain and prevention of inversion for sufficient time to allow for fracture healing, usually 4 to 6 weeks. This can be accomplished by various methods, ranging from adhesive strapping to leather boots or a short-leg walking cast, depending on the severity of the symptoms.

STRESS FRACTURES

Paralleling the increased athletic participation of the American population is a concomitant increase in the incidence of stress fractures. These may occur in just about any part of the body, with the classic site being the "fatigue" or "march fracture" of the second metatarsal. This occurs because a common variation in foot symmetry is a second toe that protrudes beyond the first toe. This also produces a second metatarsal longer than the first and not able to absorb recurrent microtrauma, resulting in an increased incidence of stress fractures. Be sure to determine that the patient is not diabetic and developing the stress

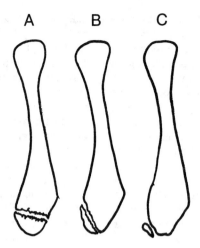

A B C

A. FRACTURE

B. APOPHYSIS (attachment of peroneus brevis tendon)

C. OSSICLE (accessory sesamoid bone)

Figure 1 Differential diagnosis of fractures of the base of the fifth metatarsal.

fracture as an early stage of an impending Charcot's foot. The patient's chief complaint will be pain, especially on weight bearing, and no definite history of trauma. Physical examination is usually unrevealing except for sharp pain in the area of the metatarsal head and shaft (on weight bearing or direct manipulative pressure) swelling, and increased local heat. In the early stages the fracture line is very fine and easily missed by x-ray examination for up to 6 weeks from onset. Eventually, the fracture line appears or the diagnosis is made by noting the formation of bony callus. Several metatarsals may be involved at the same time, with the second and third being the most common sites. Bone scans are occasionally necessary to diagnose early involvement. The aim of treatment is to avoid stress and microtrauma until the bone is healed. The degree of protection is titrated to the severity of the symptoms; thus treatment can range anywhere from avoidance of sports activity to plaster cast immobilization. It is also quite important to instigate a graded exercise program for muscle strengthening and flexibility before the patient is allowed to return to participation in sporting events.

SESAMOID FRACTURES

Sesamoid bones lie within a tendon to add leverage and thus mechanical advantage to a muscle's pulling force. Although uncommon, fractures of these bones do occur, especially of the medial sesamoid of the flexor tendon of the great toe. These should be differentiated from a bipartite or developmentally divided sesamoid. Treatment is symptomatic.

DISTAL PHALANX FRACTURES OF THE HAND

Finger-tip fractures are usually the result of crush injuries, traction, or direct trauma. Severe angulation trauma, flexion-extension, or sideways bending, can also cause fractures. Care is similar to the previously described crush injuries of the foot. It is important not only to recognize which of these can be treated with simple protective splinting of one's choice but also to select those that require a greater level of care. A *mallet finger* is caused by forceful flexion against resistance, rupturing the distal extensor mechanism. On examination the distal phalanx is partially flexed and cannot be actively extended. In an adult, there may or may not be a chip fracture of the dorsal articular surface. In a child, the fracture line runs through the epiphyseal plate, resulting in a Salter type 1 or type 3 fracture. Treatment of simple cases involves splinting the distal phalanx in extension and referring the patient for orthopaedic follow-up in a week. A mallet finger requires surgical repair when, after splinting in extension, there is subluxation of the distal interphalangeal joint. Occasionally the base of the nail is also avulsed, resulting in the Seymour injury. When the finger is forcefully hyperextended, there may be an *avulsion of the attachment of the profundus flexor tendon*, necessitating surgical repair. Always test flexion of the distal interphalangeal joint to rule out a rupture of the flexor digitorum profundus. Occasionally an x-ray film may show what appears to be a fracture through the growth plate of the fifth finger proximal phalanx, although the child has given no history of injury or symptoms. It is wise then to also observe an x-ray film of the finger of the opposite hand to rule out Kirner's developmental deformity, which is most often bilateral.

AVULSION FRACTURES

Strong forces exerted by the muscles of the thigh bone have the ability to pull off their tendinous origins on the pelvis, with accompanying attachment of bone. The displacement is ordinarily not severe, and these fractures can be treated conservatively utilizing ice, analgesics, and crutches or a cane for protected weight bearing. Two avulsion fractures that fit these criteria are avulsions of the sartorius muscle from the *anterosuperior iliac spine* and avulsions of the hamstrings from the *ischial tuberosity*. The diagnosis is made based on x-ray examination and physical examination findings of tenderness with palpation of the involved areas. Bone healing on x-ray evaluation and resolution of fracture site tenderness occur in approximately 6 weeks, which seems to be a time for many orthopaedic conditions to resolve.

SUGGESTED READING

Bateman JE. Foot science. Am Orth Foot Soc, Philadelphia: WB Saunders, 1976.

Howard FM, Shafer SJ. Injuries to the clavicle with neurovascular complications. J Bone Joint Surg 1965; 47A:1335.

HUMAN AND ANIMAL BITES

MICHAEL L. CALLAHAM, M.D.

Mammalian bites are an extremely common outpatient and emergency department problem. Accurate figures are only available for dog bites, but these number over 1.5 million per year in the United States alone, accounting for about 1 percent of typical emergency department visits. Worldwide, mammalian bites and injuries kill thousands of people; for example, an estimated 800 people a year are killed in Europe by domestic cattle, horses, and pigs alone. Deaths caused by large mammals are commonplace in much of Africa, India, and Asia, and even in the United States deaths attributable to attacks by dogs, bears, coyotes, and other large animals are a regular occurrence.

Nonbite injuries are not discussed in detail here, since their treatment does not differ from other types of trauma. The physician should always bear in mind, however, that anyone attacked by a relatively large or powerful animal often has fractures, contusions, and serious visceral injury, and such patients should be approached in the same fashion as victims of a motor vehicle accident.

On average, 75 to 90 percent of mammalian bite wounds needing medical treatment in the United States are inflicted by dogs; about 10 percent are inflicted by cats, and the remainder by a wide variety of species, including humans. There has been little scientific study of most of these injuries. Regardless of the inflicting species, all wounds should receive a certain basic assessment and care; certain wounds are selected for additional treatment on the basis of risk factors.

PRE-HOSPITAL CARE

In the field, wounds should be copiously irrigated with clean water and, if treatment cannot take place within an hour, they should be cleansed with plain white soap (which should then be rinsed from the wound). This will kill and remove many bacteria and, more importantly, the rabies virus. Dry, clean bandages should be applied and medical care sought. If the location is remote and medical care cannot be given for 6 hours or more, administration of prophylactic antibiotics in high-risk wounds is appropriate. If the animal is thought to be potentially rabid, an effort should be made to capture it and bring it back for examination, if this can be done without risk to others. The animal's brain should be preserved intact, preferably by refrigeration.

EMERGENCY DEPARTMENT ASSESSMENT AND TREATMENT OF WOUNDS

Once at the emergency department, the patient should again be assessed for possible major injuries, as in any other source of trauma. The wound should be carefully inspected for extent of injury and damage to deeper structures such as tendons, vessels, nerves, and joint capsule. This needs to be done with adequate local anesthetic and a proximal tourniquet to ensure a bloodless field. If there is thought to be a significant possibility of bone injury or of a foreign body, x-ray films should be obtained. A rapid initial assessment should be carried out for risk factors (Table 1) and if they are indicated, parenteral antibiotics should be given immediately. Prescription of oral antibiotics after several hours of waiting is essentially useless, since adequate blood and tissue levels of the drug will never be attained soon enough to be effective. Adequate tetanus prophylaxis should be assured (see chapter on *Tetanus*).

Wound toilet is critical. The common practice of soaking wounds in dilute povidone-iodine solution is completely unstudied and probably without benefit. Hair should be clipped from around the wound (never shaved), and the wound should be thoroughly irrigated with several hundred milliliters of 1 percent povidone-iodine solution (never povidone-iodine scrub) or saline using a 19-gauge needle and a 12-ml syringe or equivalent (this generates the 15 to 20 pounds per square inch (psi) necessary to dislodge bacteria and debris; lesser pressures such as are generated by bulb syringes and gravity drip methods are inadequate). Devitalized tissue should be debrided and the wound closed if appropriate. This wound toilet is far more important than any other treatment given; its omission cannot be overcome by any quantity of antibiotics.

TABLE 1 Risk Factors in Mammalian Bites

High Risk

Location:	Hand, wrist, or foot
	Scalp or face in infants (high risk of cranial perforation; skull x-ray studies mandatory)
Type of wound:	Punctures (impossible to irrigate)
	Tissue crushing that cannot be debrided (typical of injuries from herbivores such as cows, horses)
Patient:	Older than 50 years
	Asplenic
	Chronic alcoholic
	Altered immune status
	Diabetic
	Peripheral vascular insufficiency
	Chronic corticosteroid therapy
Species:	Cat
	Human (in hand wounds only)
	Primates (anecdotal evidence only)
	Pigs (anecdotal evidence only)

Low Risk

Location:	Face, scalp, and mouth (all facial wounds should be sutured)
Wound type:	Large clean lacerations that can be thoroughly cleansed; the larger the laceration, the lower the infection rate
Species:	Rodents

Uncomplicated low-risk wounds can be *sutured* and have an infection rate of about 10 percent, only slightly higher than that of nonbite lacerations in the same environment. The patient is done no favor if these low-risk wounds are left open to heal secondarily, since this produces not only a large scar but also a much longer period of disability. Moderate- to high-risk wounds are best treated by the method of *delayed primary closure*; they are left open initially, wet dressings are applied, and they are re-evaluated in 72 hours. If they are not infected then, they can be sutured with no increase in total wound healing time. This technique of delayed primary closure is well studied and very effective, but much underused. Allowing the wound to granulate by secondary intention should virtually never be necessary; this results in a large scar and is a very slow process that will unnecessarily delay return of function (and return to normal employment) for weeks. Although all wounds require meticulous basic wound toilet as described, fancy cosmetic repairs should not be attempted initially; these are usually not necessary. The small percentage of patients who ultimately need scar revision do much better if this is performed electively at a later date by a plastic surgeon.

If the risk of rabies is high (e.g., suspicious behavior or a bite from a high-risk species such as a bat, skunk, raccoon, or fox) (see chapter on *Rabies*), the wound should also receive a thorough *swabbing* with a cotton swab using 1 percent benzalkonium chloride solution (Zephiran). This is not an ideal agent, since it is irritating to tissue, but it is the only one proved effective against rabies virus experimentally. It should then be flushed from the wound with saline. Povidone-iodine is theoretically effective also since it is viricidal, but it has never been studied in relation to the rabies virus.

Initial *wound cultures* and *Gram's stains* are not cost-effective and are very poor predictors of subsequent in-

fection; most wounds are contaminated with any of a wide species of organisms (Table 2). The organism obtained on initial culture of a fresh wound does not correlate with the subsequent development of infection or with the infecting species. Cultures should be reserved for infected wounds in high-risk patients or those who have already failed to respond to initial treatment. Ordinary low-risk wounds do not need any prophylactic antibiotics; large, well-controlled studies have repeatedly shown them to be of no benefit.

RISK FACTORS

The *risk factors* that the physician must seek in every patient are listed in Table 1. Most are self-explanatory. Puncture wounds are a particular problem, since they are almost impossible to irrigate adequately, and it usually is not practical to debride or excise them (it results in too much tissue loss). However, these latter techniques should be considered in special high-risk circumstances or when cosmetic appearance is particularly important, since they convert this contaminated wound into a fresh, fairly clean one. Ironically, the bigger and worse-looking the animal-bite wound, the less likely infection is, usually because such wounds get proper respect (and subsequent wound toilet) and are easier to adequately irrigate and debride.

Alcoholics are particularly at risk for systemic sepsis, which is discussed below. This is important because the causative organisms are often unusual ones not normally thought of in sepsis.

Crush injuries are typically caused by the large herbivores (cows, horses), and such injury lowers the resistance of tissue to infection. If the skin is intact, the only treatment needed is prompt application of ice and a light pressure dressing to minimize the subsequent swelling, hematoma, and pain, all of which are often very se-

TABLE 2 Typical Pathogens Found in Animals' Mouths and as Infecting Agents in Bite Wounds

Aerobic Bacteria	Anaerobic Bacteria
Micrococcus sp.	*Bacteroides* sp.
Staphylococcus aureus	*Fusobacterium* sp.
Streptococcus	*Peptococcus*
Bacillis subtilis	*Veillonella* sp.
Corynebacterium sp.	*Propionibacterium*
Pseudomonas	*Eubacterium*
Brucella canis	*Leptothrix*
Bordetella sp.	
Neisseria sp.	*Rare pathogens*
Moraxella, sp.	Hepatitis
Acinetobacter	Versinia
Escherichia coli	Rat-bite fever *(spirillum, Streptobacillis)*
Enterobacter sp.	Tetanus
Serratia marcescens	*Leptospira*
Proteus mirabilis	Simian herpes
Aeromonas hydrophila	Herpesvirus
Pasteurella multocida	Rabies
Pasteurella sp.	Cat-scratch disease
Eikenella corrodens	Rio Bravo infection (virus)
Haemophilus aphrophilus	Sporotrichosis
Klebsiella	*Mycobacterium marinus*
	Vibrio sp.
	Erysipelothrix
IIJ	
EF-4	
M-5	

vere. If the skin is broken, debridement should be done where practical especially if the wound is considered high risk.

The most frequent bite injury dealt with by the physician is a *dog bite*; dogbites are low-risk wounds that need only good basic wound toilet, suturing, tetanus prophylaxis, and follow-up examination for wound infection in 3 to 5 days; without the need for cultures or antibiotics. Rabies prophylaxis for dog bite is virtually never indicated in the United States. Dog bites of the hand are discussed below.

Some risk situations deserve special mention. *Bites of the hand* are common and at risk because of the rapid spread of infection through the tendons and synovial sheaths, and the devastating and permanent consequences of inflammation and scarring in this part of the hand. Anything other than a trivial wound deserves x-ray evaluation and careful examination for fractures or violation of tendon sheaths or joint spaces; any of these mandates hospital admission. However, if these are not present, a fresh, well-irrigated hand wound can be treated well on an outpatient basis. Prophylactic antibiotics are traditional, although their value is unproved. Equally important is an immobilizing "mitten"-type dressing, elevation of the hand in a sling, and strict and total rest of the hand. Patients should be carefully re-examined the next day after treatment and then every few days for the first week. Patients with *established infections* of wounds in the hand always need consultation with a hand surgeon, and usually hospital admission for intravenous antibiotics or drainage or both.

Facial and scalp bites receive undue concern because of their cosmetic importance and the fear of periorbital

cellulitis (with subsequent cavernous sinus septic thrombosis), complications that in fact are exceedingly rare. These wounds heal extraordinarily well and are very low risk for infection. After good wound toilet, they should always be closed primarily (even if 12 to 24 hours old) for optimal cosmetic results. Prophylactic antibiotics are definitely not needed. However, a large animal's teeth can easily penetrate the cranium of infants (leading to meningitis or brain abscess) and skull x-ray studies are indicated in such cases. Any perforation of the cranium of course mandates hospital admission.

Human bites have a very bad reputation for developing infections, but most of that may be because of their high incidence of occurrence on the hand and the propensity for delayed presentation after infection is already present. Human bites other than those on the hand do not have a high infection rate, and few of the hundreds of species of bacteria in human mouths are unique to our species. Any laceration over the knuckles should be considered a human bite injury (inflicted by the fist's collision with an opponent's teeth) until proved otherwise. If infected, patients with such injuries need hospital admission, but if the wound is fresh and uninfected and otherwise uncomplicated, they can be treated very successfully as outpatients (see above for hand wounds). Such wounds should not be sutured primarily unless they are very small, but should receive delayed primary closure in 3 days.

Rats and other rodents conjure up horrible images, but in fact their bites almost never become infected and they are incapable of transmitting rabies.

Cats produce small puncture wounds, which are high risk, usually on the hand (also high risk), and they seem to have a higher incidence of transmitting *Pasteurella*; this is just as true of big cats such as tigers as it is of the household variety. Thus their wound infection rate is as high as 30 to 50 percent. Antibiotic treatment must be tailored to this bacterium as discussed above and prophylactic antibiotics are indicated in most cases.

Unusual species of biting animals (reptiles as well as mammals), especially marine dwellers, can carry seldom considered pathogens. Examples are infection with *Mycobacterium marinum* (which is clinically identical to sporotrichosis but must be treated on the basis of antibiotic sensitivities of the cultured organism) after dolphin and seal bites. *Aeromonas hydrophila*, a common organism in all fresh water, has caused infection after alligator bite (and more frequently after trauma occurring in lakes, rivers, and ponds). It is of significance because it can cause fatal sepsis and because it is typically resistant to penicillin and its derivatives requiring tetracycline as initial outpatient treatment and aminoglycosides for inpatient treatment. Various *Vibrio* species are found universally in sea water, mollusks, and shark's teeth; these can cause either local wound infection or sepsis, particularly in alcoholic patients. Initial treatment is with tetracycline, as is true for infection with most marine bacterial species.

ADDITIONAL TREATMENT

If risk factors are present, *prophylactic antibiotics* may be needed, although their effectiveness has not been well proved. Antibiotics are useless and inappropriate in ordinary low-risk bite wounds. Such prophylaxis, to be effective, must be given as early in the patient's treatment as possible—preferably parenterally, while still at the emergency department triage desk. Handing the patient a pill or prescription at the end of the emergency department treatment is useless. Oral treatment should be continued for 5 to 7 days with either a cephalosporin such as cephalexin (50 to 100 mg per kilogram per day in four divided doses in children or 500 mg by mouth four times a day in adults) or dicloxacillin (in the same dose). Both of these are effective against about 95 percent of potential infecting organisms; there is no one antibiotic that can span the entire spectrum. If the patient is penicillin-allergic, erythromycin should be used (30 to 50 mg per kilogram per day in four divided doses in children, 500 mg four times a day in adults).

Cat bites have a high incidence of infection with *Pasteurella multocida*; this infection can become symptomatic within 12 hours of inoculation and spread rapidly. If the wound is from a cat bite, or is suspected or known to be infected with *Pasteurella multocida*, penicillin V in the same doses should be used. If the patient is penicillin-allergic, tetracycline (500 mg four times a day in adults), not erythromycin, must be used. Unfortunately no one drug provides effective coverage against *Staphylococcus aureus* and *Pasteurella*, both of which are commonly found in the oral flora of most species and both of which cause about 10 to 20 percent of wound infections.

COMPLICATIONS OF BITE WOUNDS

Far and away the most common complication of a bite wound is local wound infection; it is prevented and treated as discussed above.

Sepsis is a very rare complication that may occur after animal bite, usually in asplenic or alcoholic patients. A variety of organisms have been reported, including such unusual strains as DF-2, II-J, and *Aeromonas*. Such patients should have thorough aerobic and anaerobic cultures of blood and material available from all infection sites, and antibiotic coverage should address the widest range of unusual pathogens possible.

Cat-scratch disease usually manifests as a regional lymphadenitis of an extremity 14 days (range, 3 to 50 days) after a cat scratch (although dog and monkey bites, splinters, fishhooks, porcupine quills, and thorns have also been reported). There is usually a raised, erythematous, slightly tender, nonpruritic papule with a small central pustule or eschar (often mistaken for an insect bite) at the site of inoculation. Two-thirds of patients experience mild constitutional symptoms of fever, malaise, and nausea. Evanescent morbilliform and pleomorphic rashes have been reported. Some patients develop Parinaud's oculoglandular syndrome of granulomatous conjunctivitis and an ipsilateral, tender, enlarged preauricular lymph node. Serious complications are rare. The only specific diagnostic test is the CSD (cat-scratch disease) skin test. Recently the etiologic agent has been identified as a small, gram-negative pleomorphic bacterium, as yet unnamed. These can be identified in biopsy sections of the inoculation site and lymph nodes; at present this procedure is done chiefly by the Armed Forces Institute of Pathology in Washington, D.C. The chief diagnostic dilemma is usually to differentiate the lymphadenopathy from other causes of regional adenopathy such as tuberculosis, tularemia, lymphogranuloma venereum, lymphoma, brucellosis, and sporotrichosis. There is no specific treatment of the disease; various antibiotics have been tried in the past without success. No doubt the recent discovery of the bacterium will soon lead to an effective antibiotic agent.

Rat-bite fever is an uncommon infection with either *Streptobacillus moniliformis* or *Spirillum minus* transmitted by bites from rats or carnivores that have preyed on rats and mice. The streptobacillary variety, an occasional hazard to laboratory workers, manifests as fever, chills, cough, malaise, headache, and sometimes lymphadenitis, followed by a nonpruritic morbilliform or petechial rash that frequently involves the palms and soles. Migratory polyarthritis is also common. Twenty-five percent of victims develop a false-positive VDRL test; the diagnosis is made by agglutinating antibodies to *Streptobacillus* or by culture. The differential diagnosis includes viral and rickettsial infection. The mortality rate for untreated cases is 10 percent, owing mostly to pneumonia and endocarditis; the treatment is procaine penicillin 8,000 to 16,000 IU per kilogram per day, in two divided doses parenterally. Endocarditis should be treated with high-dose intravenous penicillin G. Patients allergic to penicillin may be treated with tetracycline, 30 mg per kilogram per day orally in four divided doses, or streptomycin, 15 mg per kilogram per day intramuscularly in two divided doses. Admission to the hospital depends on the clinical status of the patient.

The spirillar form of rat-bite fever is similar to the streptobacillary form, except that the rash is a dark red macular one, myalgias are common, but arthritis is absent. The disease is episodic, with a 24- to 72-hour cycle. The diagnosis must be made by darkfield microscopic demonstration of the *Spirillum* organism. The incidence and mortality of this disease are much lower than that of the streptobacillary form, and the antibiotic treatment is the same.

Other Diseases Transmitted by Mammals

This topic is not expanded here, but there are a number of significant diseases that are transmitted by contact with mammals, although not precisely by animal bite. In the United States, significant examples are rabies, tularemia, leptospirosis, brucellosis, and plague; the last is seldom considered but is endemic in the western United States. An exceedingly rare example is the transmission of Creutzfeldt-Jakob disease (a progressive, untreatable fatal encephalopathy caused by a slow virus) caused by eating the brains of wild goat or squirrel, a common custom in certain areas of the United States. The reader is referred to any infectious disease text or the first suggested reading for details.

SUGGESTED READING

Callaham M. Domestic and feral mammalian bites. In: Auerbach PS, Geehr EC, eds. Management of wilderness and environmental emergencies. New York: Macmillan Publishing, 1983:310.
Clarke J. Man is the prey. London: Andre Deutsch, Ltd, 1969.
Hanson PG, Standridge J, Jarrett F, et al. Freshwater wound infection due to Aeromonas hydrophila. JAMA 1977; 238:1053–1054.
Johnston JM, Becker SF, McFarland LM. Vibrio vulnificus: Man and the sea. JAMA 1985; 253:2850–2853.
Margileth A, Wear DJ, Hadfield TL, et al. Cat-scratch disease: Bacteria in skin at primary inoculation site. JAMA 1984; 252:928–931.
Ordog GJ, Balasubraminium S, Wasserberger J. Rat bites: Fifty cases. Ann Emerg Med 1985; 14:126–130.
Weber DJ, Wolfson JS, Wartz MN, et al. Pasteurella multocida infections: Report of 34 cases and review of the literature. Medicine 1984; 63:133–154.

ENVIRONMENTAL HAZARDS

NEAR-DROWNING

JEROME H. MODELL, M.D.

PRE-HOSPITAL CARE

Drowning is defined as suffocation by submersion, especially in water; *near-drowning* implies that the patient has survived a submersion episode, at least at the time the diagnosis is made. The patient who suffers cardiac arrest during this process would be drowned unless resuscitation were successful, in which case the term near-drowned would be applicable.

Approximately 10 to 12 percent of patients who suffer a severe submersion episode do not aspirate water and, if the patient responds promptly to cardiopulmonary resuscitation (CPR) before irreversible cerebral hypoxia has occurred, complete recovery is likely without further therapy. The patient who does aspirate water, however, presents a far more complex problem. Since the degree of hypoxia increases with the duration of apnea, the victim should receive artificial ventilation as soon as possible. Preferably, this should be done in the water by performing mouth-to-mouth or mouth-to-nose respiration, provided that the rescuer does not place himself at risk. Most frequently, both clinically and experimentally, apnea precedes circulatory arrest in victims of submersion. Therefore, early institution of effective mouth-to-mouth ventilation may avert a frank cardiac arrest. If airway obstruction is present and is not relieved by manipulation of the mandible, a foreign body may be lodged in the larynx; in such cases, an abdominal thrust may help to dislodge the obstruction.

As soon as the victim is brought to land or any reasonably stable platform, adequacy of circulation should be evaluated. Near-drowning victims frequently suffer intense vasoconstriction and, although the heart may be pumping, cardiac output and cardiac rate may be extremely low. When mechanical ventilation improves arterial oxygenation, cardiac output frequently increases and mechanical measures to support circulation are not necessary. However, if there is any question as to whether an effective heart beat is present or whether the cardiac output is adequate, closed-chest cardiac massage should be instituted in conjunction with artificial ventilation.

When the patient aspirates water, a significant intrapulmonary physiologic shunt occurs; the shunt and the accompanying arterial hypoxemia persist even after spontaneous ventilation, circulation, and consciousness are restored. Therefore, supplemental oxygen should be administered to all such patients as soon as it is available, and they should be transported to a hospital for further evaluation and therapy.

Lactated Ringer's solution should be infused intravenously through a large-bore cannula. Early literature emphasized that when dogs were drowned in fresh-water, there was marked dilution of serum sodium and chloride, whereas with sea-water there was marked concentration. In humans, usually enough water to significantly disturb serum electrolyte concentrations is not aspirated, and absorbed fluid is redistributed rapidly; therefore, lactated Ringer's solution is the initial solution of choice.

Patients who are awake and breathing adequately should receive supplemental oxygen by mask. Comatose patients or those who remain apneic should have an endotracheal tube placed and should be ventilated mechanically. After sea-water aspiration, the pulmonary defect is fluid-filled, but perfused alveoli. After fresh-water aspiration, alterations in the surface tension properties of pulmonary surfactant lead to alveolar instability and collapse. In either case, adequate ventilation should be ensured and continuous positive airway pressure (CPAP), if available, of at least 5 cm H_2O, but not to exceed 10 cm H_2O, should be applied during transport to the hospital. More precise adjustment of the level of CPAP should take high priority when the patient arrives at the hospital and pulmonary status can be evaluated. Pulmonary edema occurs frequently and is best treated by CPAP. Replacement of intravascular fluid that is lost as pulmonary edema fluid may be necessary to maintain cardiac output and oxygen delivery.

HOSPITAL CARE

As soon as the patient reaches the emergency department, arterial blood should be drawn for analysis of oxygen (PaO_2) and carbon dioxide ($PaCO_2$) tensions and pH, and bicarbonate should be calculated. The degree of mechanical ventilation provided should ensure that hypercarbia does not occur. CPAP should be applied incrementally until the intrapulmonary physiologic shunt is reduced to low levels or has returned to normal. Several methods have been proposed for evaluating the effectiveness of CPAP therapy clinically. These include titration of shunt, compliance, carbon dioxide gradient, and PaO_2. The fraction of inspired oxygen may be decreased as CPAP is applied and adequate oxygenation obtained. Respiratory acidosis should be treated by more effective elimination of carbon dioxide, whereas metabolic acidosis causing a pH of less than 7.3 should be treated by the administration of sodium bicarbonate. The formula I recommend is sodium bicarbonate (mEq) = patient's weight (kg) × base deficit × 0.2.

Blood should be analyzed for PaO_2, $PaCO_2$, and pHa as often as necessary to guide therapy. In patients with severe pulmonary dysfunction or those who have cardiovascular instability, a Swan-Ganz catheter should be inserted. Use of a triple-lumen catheter permits evaluation of pulmonary artery occlusion pressure and cardiac output, and the third port can be used for infusion. Intravenous fluid therapy should be guided in these cases by the filling pressures, cardiac output, systemic blood pressure, and renal output. While a pulmonary artery catheter is not always required, I recommend its use when there is cardiovascular instability or when the amount of CPAP required to treat the pulmonary insufficiency exceeds 15 cm H_2O.

Renal output should be monitored carefully. In addition to obtaining blood to monitor PaO_2, $PaCO_2$, and pHa, a hemogram and electrolyte profile should also be obtained. While changes in serum electrolyte concentrations needing therapy usually do not occur, on rare occasions an adjustment of intravenous fluid may be required to treat a specific problem; or, if marked hemolysis occurs secondary to absorption of fresh-water, blood replacement and forced diuresis should be considered.

In treating near-drowned victims, the most consistent problems that require therapy are respiratory distress and hypoxemia. Pulmonary status must be evaluated frequently, and the level of mechanical ventilatory support adjusted accordingly. The goal of such therapy is to reduce the intrapulmonary shunt to normal as quickly as possible and, during therapy, to try to ensure adequate arterial oxygenation without excessively high inspired oxygen concentrations. As the patient improves, the level of CPAP and the rate of mechanical ventilation can be reduced accordingly. However, arterial oxygenation not only needs to be improved, but oxygen must also be delivered to the tissues. Therefore, cardiac output may have to be supported because relatively high levels of intrapleural pressure may result during mechanical ventilatory support and may interfere with venous return and cardiac output. Experimental studies have shown that in near-drowned animals cardiac output can be supported more effectively by fluid administration than by inotropic agents. Thus, it may be necessary to infuse more intravenous fluid when the cardiac output is low, even in the face of pulmonary edema. It is important to point out that the pulmonary edema of near-drowning is predominantly one of altered permeability in the lungs rather than a failing myocardium.

In the last few years, considerable emphasis has been placed on cerebral salvage after near-drowning. Patients who are awake and alert or obtunded but not comatose when they arrive at the emergency department have an excellent chance of survival when pulmonary, cardiovascular, and renal problems are adequately addressed. For those patients who are comatose on arrival, however, consideration should be given to whether specific treatment is indicated for cerebral salvage. Protocols consisting of dehydration, hyperventilation, deliberate hypothermia, muscle paralysis with mechanical ventilation, barbiturate coma, and corticosteroids have been recommended by some authors for all patients assumed to have increased intracranial pressure (ICP) or severe cerebral dysfunction. To date, there are no well-controlled studies demonstrating that this regimen of therapy improves the rate of normal survival. Many aspects of this therapy, particularly hypothermia, corticosteroids, and barbiturate coma, may result in severe complications in and of themselves.

This author recommends that whenever a near-drowned comatose victim does not respond immediately in the emergency department to adequate oxygenation, carbon dioxide removal, and restoration of acid-base balance, hyperventilation should be instituted because it decreases cerebral blood flow and thereby also decreases ICP and cerebral edema. A monitor should then be placed to measure ICP directly. If it is elevated, fluid restriction and barbiturate-induced coma are indicated to reduce ICP. The exact dose of barbiturate varies from patient to patient and the degree of fluid restriction also must be individualized. The goal of therapy is to decrease ICP below 20 cm H_2O and to keep it below that level. This therapy should be continued until it can be withdrawn without an increase in ICP. Once ICP stabilizes, barbiturates can be discontinued, ventilation can be readjusted to produce normocarbia, and fluid restriction can be discontinued.

In the past, parenteral corticosteroids and prophylactic antibiotics were recommended for all near-drowned victims. Neither of these is currently advocated. While corticosteroids are thought to lessen the initial inflammatory response to water aspiration, they interfere with normal healing mechanisms and may make the lung more susceptible to secondary infection and abscess formation. Antibiotics should be withheld unless there is evidence of secondary infection, in which case antibiotics specific to the invading organism should be administered.

If aggressive therapy, particularly aimed at the pulmonary lesion, is instituted quickly, near-drowned victims can make a remarkably rapid recovery. Many, however, require prolonged therapy; these patients should be admitted to an intensive care unit and, whenever possible, placed under the care of a physician who specializes in critical care medicine. The long-term therapy of patients with refractory pulmonary lesions or of those who remain comatose beyond the first several hours is beyond the scope of this chapter. The suggested readings deal more extensively with those problems.

SUGGESTED READING

Barnes PA, Modell JH. The near-drowned victim. In: Cherniack RM, ed. Current therapy of respiratory disease, 1984–1985. Philadelphia: BC Decker, 1984:150.

Modell JH. Drowning. In: Staub NC, Taylor AE, eds. Edema. New York: Raven Press, 1984:679.
Modell JH, Boysen PG. Drowning and near-drowning. In: Shoemaker WC, Thompson WL, Holbrook PR, eds. Textbook of critical care. Philadelphia: WB Saunders, 1984:39.

SCUBA DIVING ACCIDENTS

KENNETH W. KIZER, M.D., M.P.H., F.A.C.E.P., F.A.C.P.M.

The popularity of scuba diving has markedly increased in recent years. There are now about three million recreational scuba divers in the United Sates, and over 300,000 new sport divers are trained each year. In addition, scuba diving has become an integral part of many occupations.

Commensurate with the rise in its popularity there also has been an increased frequency of scuba diving accidents in recent years. Instead of occurring at only a selected few coastal areas, these accidents are now being seen throughout the country because of the increased popularity of diving in lakes, rivers, abandoned quarries, and underwater caves and because of the tremendous growth of the dive-travel vacation industry. As an outgrowth of the latter, scuba diving accident victims may present to emergency departments hundreds or even thousands of miles away from their dive site within hours after their last dive.

Diving medical problems are attributable to the intrinsic hazards of the aquatic environment and the breathing of air at increased pressure. Not surprisingly, an array of medical problems are associated with scuba diving (Table 1). Because of space constraints, this section will focus only on some of those pressure related syndromes that are largely unique to diving.

PRESSURE

When a scuba diver submerges under water the ambient pressure increases because of the increased weight of the water. Since water is much more dense than air, pressure changes substantially with even small changes in depth. Among the physical environmental conditions that are encountered under water, it is increased atmospheric pressure that, either directly or indirectly, causes the greatest proportion of diving maladies.

Pressure related diving problems can be categorized into problems caused simply by the mechanical effects of pressure (e.g., barotrauma) and those caused by breathing compressed air (e.g., decompression sickness and nitrogen narcosis).

BAROTRAUMA

The air pressure within gas filled spaces of the body is normally in equilibrium with the environment. However, if anything obstructs the free passage of air into and out of these spaces when ambient pressure changes, pressure disequilibrium will develop. If the space cannot expand or contract to accommodate the change in gas volume, injury will result. Such injuries are collectively

TABLE 1   Medical Problems of Divers*

Environmental exposure problems
Motion sickness
Near drowning and other immersion syndromes
Hypothermia
Heat illness
Sunburn
Phototoxic and photoallergic reactions
Irritant and other dermatitides
Physical Trauma
Dysbarism
Barotrauma
Dysbaric air embolism
Decompression sickness
Dysbaric osteonecrosis
Hyperbaric cephalgia
Breathing gas-related problems
Nitrogen or other inert gas narcosis
Hypoxia
Oxygen toxicity
Hypercapnia
Carbon monoxide poisoning
Nitrogen oxide toxicity
High pressure nervous syndrome
Lipoid pneumonitis
Hazardous marine life
Envenomations
Animals that bite
Toxic ingestions
Infectious diseases
Miscellaneous
Hyperventilation
Hearing loss
Carotogenic blackout
Panic
Claustrophobia

* Adapted from Kizer KW. Diving medicine. Emerg Med Clin N Am 1984; 2:513–530.

known as barotrauma and, overall, are the most common notable affliction of scuba divers.

Barotrauma of Descent

Barotrauma of descent, or "squeeze," as it is known in common diver's parlance, results from the compression of gas in enclosed spaces as atmospheric pressure increases with descent under water. The ears and sinuses are most often affected. More than one type of barotrauma may be present at the same time.

Aural barotrauma affects essentially all divers at one time or another and is the most frequent type of barotrauma. Although the external ear canal can be affected, this is unusual, and when it does occur, it is treated essentially the same way as other types of external otitis.

Much more common is middle ear squeeze, or barotitis media, which results when the diver fails to equalize pressure in the middle ear because of occlusion or dysfunction of the eustachian tube, e.g., as a consequence of upper respiratory infection or allergy.

Divers usually notice a sense of fullness, followed by increasingly severe pain, when middle ear volume is reduced by 20 percent or more (i.e., at a pressure disequilibrium of 100 to 150 mm Hg or greater). Examination usually reveals hypomobility and inward bulging of the tympanic membrane, along with erythema, gross hemorrhage, or perforation, depending on the severity of the injury.

The treatment of uncomplicated middle ear squeeze consists of the use of decongestants and analgesics and abstinence from diving or other pressure exposures until the condition resolves, which usually occurs in a few days. Antihistamines should be used if the eustachian tube dysfunction has an allergic etiology. A combination of an orally administered decongestant and a long-acting nasal spray, at least for the first couple of days, is most effective.

Although less common, inner ear barotrauma causing a perilymph fistula, owing to round or oval window rupture, is much more serious than middle ear barotrauma. The perilymph fistula is caused by the sudden development of markedly different pressures between the middle and inner ear, such as may occur from an overly forceful Valsalva maneuver intended to equalize the pressure in the middle ear or an exceptionally rapid descent in which middle ear pressure is not equalized.

The classic triad of symptoms indicating inner ear barotrauma is roaring tinnitus, vertigo, and deafness. A feeling of fullness or "blockage" of the affected ear, nausea, vomiting, nystagmus, pallor, diaphoresis, disorientation, or ataxia may also be present. The onset of these symptoms may occur soon after the injury or may be delayed many hours, depending on the size of the fistula and the diver's activities during and after the dive. Findings on physical examination may be normal or may reveal signs of middle ear barotrauma or vestibular dysfunction. Audiometry demonstrates a sensorineural hearing loss.

This condition is a true emergency, that results in permanent hearing loss if not properly treated. Obviously, recompression treatment is contraindicated because of the potential for worsening the condition with further pressure exposure, and all divers suspected of suffering inner ear barotrauma should have a complete otologic evaluation as soon as possible. These patients need to be hospitalized and placed at bed rest, with the head of the bed elevated, and anything that increases cerebrospinal fluid pressure should be avoided. Vertigo, nausea, and similar manifestations should be treated symptomatically with hydroxyzine, meclizine, or similar medications, but there is no role for vasodilators or anticoagulants. Controversy still exists as to when surgical exploration and repair are indicated, although it is the author's opinion that early surgical intervention is preferred. No further diving should be done after a perilymph fistula develops.

Just as with the ears, the paranasal sinuses may also fail to equalize pressure during descent, thus resulting in sinus squeeze. The frontal and maxillary sinuses are most often affected.

Sinus squeeze usually causes pain in the affected sinus, and the diver may notice bleeding from the nose or the mouth. Examination may be unremarkable or may elicit tenderness to percussion over the affected sinus. Roentgenograms may demonstrate cloudiness or air-fluid levels.

Treatment of sinus squeeze is similar to that for middle ear squeeze and consists of the use of decongestants, antihistamines, and analgesics and abstinence from diving until the condition is resolved. Antibiotics (e.g., ampicillin) are usually indicated in cases of frontal sinus squeeze because of concerns about complications resulting from frontal sinusitis.

Rarely lung squeeze may occur in breathholding divers who dive deeper than the depth at which the total lung volume is compressed to less than the residual volume (usually at depths in excess of 120 to 130 feet of sea water). As a result, the underventilated portions of the lung fill with fluid and blood. Chest pain, cough, hemoptysis, dyspnea, and other manifestations of pulmonary edema characterize this disorder. The treatment is similar to that for other types of noncardiac pulmonary edema, although positive pressure breathing should be avoided if at all possible because the lung injury increases the risk of further dysbaric injury—especially systemic arterial air embolism.

Barotrauma of Ascent

Although it is much less common than squeezes, scuba divers may also suffer barotrauma of ascent, which is the reverse process of what happens in the squeeze syndromes. Indeed the only type of barotrauma of ascent that occurs with any real frequency is the *pulmonary overpressurization syndrome* (POPS).

The POPS, a dramatic clinical demonstration of Boyle's law, results from the expansion of entrapped air in the lungs. Air entrapment may occur because of breath-holding during ascent (e.g., because of running out of air at depth or because of panic); less commonly it may result from focally increased elastic recoil. Whatever the case, the net effect leads to alveolar rupture and extravasation of air into extra-alveolar locations, thereby resulting in pneumomediastinum, subcutaneous emphysema, pneumopericardium, pneumothorax, pneumoperitoneum, or systemic arterial air embolism.

Mediastinal emphysema is the most common form of the POPS and usually presents with gradually increasing substernal chest pain, hoarseness, and neck fullness several hours after diving. In severe cases there may be more generalized chest pain, dyspnea, and dysphagia. Subcutaneous emphysema may be present. Roentgenograms may demonstrate the specific locations and extent of extra-alveolar air.

The treatment of mediastinal emphysema usually consists only of observation and abstinence from further diving for 4 to 6 weeks after the condition has resolved. In severe cases, or with unreliable patients, hospitalization may be necessary. Administration of supplemental oxygen may hasten resolution of the condition. An important point, except in exceedingly rare situations in which the volume of extra-alveolar air compromises the patient's airway or central venous return, is that recompression is contraindicated because of the fear of causing further pulmonary barotrauma and systemic arterial air embolism.

Pneumothorax is an infrequent manifestation of the POPS and is treated with needle aspiration or tube thoracostomy, as when it occurs in other situations. Pneumopericardium and the other manifestations of the POPS are treated in essentially the same fashion as dysbaric pneumomediastinum.

AIR EMBOLISM

The most serious complication of pulmonary barotrauma and, indeed, the most dramatic and serious medical emergency associated with scuba diving is dysbaric air embolism (DAE). Next to drowning, cerebral air embolism is the leading cause of death in sport scuba divers and accounts for 25 to 30 percent of recreational scuba diving fatalities and for about 35 percent of the cases treated at active diving accident treatment centers in the United States.

DAE typically presents immediately upon surfacing from a scuba dive, at which time the diver exhales and relieves the high intrapulmonic pressure that has resulted from lung overexpansion; this allows bubble-laden pulmonary venous blood to return to the left side of the heart. It is axiomatic that symptoms of DAE occur within 10 minutes after surfacing from a dive, although the majority of cases present almost immediately on surfacing.

Manifestations of DAE are myriad, depending on the exact location of the arterial occlusion(s), the volume of gas released into the systemic circulation, and the rate at which air leaves the left ventricle, but they tend to be dramatic, the brain being affected most often. Loss of consciousness, convulsions, blindness or other visual disturbances, aphasia, confusion, dizziness, vertigo, headache, focal weakness or asymmetric multiplegi, and various sensory disturbances are the most common manifestations. Sudden loss of consciousness in a scuba diver immediately upon surfacing should always be considered to be attributable to cerebral air embolism until proved otherwise. Less frequent manifestations include cardiac arrest attributable to coronary artery occlusion and abdominal pain owing to visceral ischemia.

Both the symptoms and physical findings of DAE are extremely variable and depend on the specific site(s) of vascular occlusion. Also because of the random and diffuse distribution of air bubbles in the cerebral circulation, the clinical findings may not fit with expected anatomic patterns of central nervous system injuries. Indeed, the clinical picture may be quite bizarre.

All patients suspected of suffering an air embolism must be referred for recompression (i.e., hyperbaric oxygen treatment) as rapidly as possible. This is the primary and essential treatment. Discussion of the specific hyperbaric regimens employed is beyond the scope of this section.

The majority of DAE patients have definite signs and symptoms of neurologic injury when first evaluated. However, a significant number manifest spontaneous recovery, at least initially. Nonetheless they must still be referred for recompression treatment, since it is impossible to fully exclude neuropsychologic impairment in the acute care setting, and many of these patients deteriorate over the ensuing hours, often to a worse condition than originally.

As soon as possible, all DAE patients should be given high flow supplemental oxygen, and other supportive measures should be instituted according to the patient's specific clinical condition. If endotracheal intubation is necessary, make sure to fill the balloon with normal saline and not air, since the air volume decreases during recompression and may result in the patient's inadvertently becoming extubated.

In the field or during transport, the patient should be placed in the Trendelenburg or Durant (head down and on the left side) positions, since these positions decrease the chance of any additional air emboli traveling to the brain. As well, they may cause cerebral vasodilation and consequent opening of arteriovenous shunts, both of which should facilitate passage of entrapped air bubbles back to the venous circulation. However, leaving patients in a head-down position for longer than 30 to 60 minutes may cause or worsen cerebral edema.

Manifestations of the POPS may or may not be present, but they must be carefully looked for. Pneumothorax, if present, should be decompressed prior to recompression, since it may progress to tension pneumothorax during recompression treatment.

High dose parenteral corticosteroids are probably of benefit in these patients, and should be given early in their treatment, although most of the evidence supporting their efficacy is anecdotal.

DECOMPRESSION SICKNESS

Decompression sickness (DCS), or, as it is more often called, the bends, is a multisystem disorder that develops when atmospheric pressure is decreased, thus causing the liberation of inert gas (nitrogen in compressed air scuba divers) from solution and, consequently, the formation of bubbles in blood and other tissues.

Bubbles cause mechanical effects (e.g., vascular occlusion), and they initiate a series of biophysical reactions at the blood-bubble interface, most notably the activation of Hageman factor and other components in the clotting cascade. The overall effect is to decrease tissue perfusion and cause ischemic injury.

The clinical manifestations of DCS are protean, with the central nervous and musculoskeletal systems being most often affected. Periarticular joint pain is the single most common symptom of DCS, and occurs in about three-fourths of the patients. In scuba divers the joints most often affected are the shoulders and elbows, although any joint may be affected. The pain is usually described as dull and is usually localized deep in the joint. Movement of the joint worsens the pain.

Neurologic manifestations of DCS are less common—occurring in 20 to 60 percent of patients, depending on the population in question. Because of the random manner in which bubbles may affect the central nervous system, essentially any symptom is compatible with neurologic DCS. Nonetheless the lower thoracic, lumbar, and sacral portions of the spinal cord are most often affected, and consequently paraplegia or paraparesis, lower extremity paresthesias, and bladder or bowel dysfunction are the most common symptoms of neurologic DCS. (Unlike arterial air embolism, the pathophysiology of DCS involves the evolution of bubbles in the venous circulation.)

Infrequently in scuba divers, lymphatic, inner ear, brain, pulmonary, and cardiovascular forms of DCS may be seen, each with its own peculiar clinical characteristics, which are beyond the scope of this section. However, anyone who manifests symptoms after a scuba dive that cannot be adequately explained by other conditions should be presumed to have decompression sickness until proved otherwise. Such a patient should be referred for recompression treatment without delay.

All patients suspected of having DCS should be started on high flow supplemental oxygen as soon as possible, and other life support measures should be given according to the patient's specific condition. Again, parenteral corticosteroids are probably beneficial and should be administered early. Because of the often profound loss of intravascular fluids and the impairment of microvascular circulation, which typically occurs in DCS, substantial quantities of isotonic intravenous fluids may be needed to resuscitate serious DCS cases. Indeed, in Hawaii, where many DCS cases are treated, it is not unusual to see patients with hematocrit levels in the 50s or 60s.

As with air embolism, discussion of the various hyperbaric treatment regimens that may be used to treat DCS are beyond the scope of this brief review. If the physician is unsure about either the need for recompression or the location of the nearest hyperbaric treatment facility, consultation may be obtained at any time through the *National Divers Alert Network* at Duke University (919:684-8111) in North Carolina.

In both DAE and DCS, patients should be transported to the recompression chamber in the most expeditious manner possible. In some cases this means aeromedical evacuation. In such situations the patient should be subjected to the least possible pressure reduction so as not to cause further bubble formation or expansion of existing bubbles. Depending on the specific circumstances (e.g., weather, geography, transport distance, available aircraft), either helicopters or fixed-wing aircraft may be used if they can be safely flown at less than a 1,000 foot altitude. Alternatively, aircraft capable of maintaining sea level cabin pressure may be utilized; this includes the Learjet, Cessna Citation, Hercules C-130, DC-9, and most commercial aircraft.

SUGGESTED READING

Edmonds C, Lowry C, Pennefather J, eds. Diving and subaquatic medicine. 2nd ed. Mosman, N.S.W., Australia: Diving Medical Centre, 1981.

Hallenbeck JM, Bove AA, Elliott DH. Mechanisms underlying spinal cord damage in decompression sickness. Neurology 1975; 25:308–316.

Kizer KW. Delayed treatment of dysbarism—a retrospective review of 50 cases. JAMA 1982; 247:2555–2558.

Kizer KW. Diving medicine. Emerg Med Clin North Am 1984; 2:513–530.

Shilling CW, Carlston CB, Mathias RA, eds. The physician's guide to diving medicine. New York: Plenum Press, 1984.

MARINE ENVENOMATION

PAUL S. AUERBACH, M.D.

In the aquatic environment, humans may encounter hazardous wildlife that feeds or defends itself by using a stinging mechanism. The organisms range from primitive invertebrates to highly evolved vertebrates, and they may inflict injury with a weapon as simple as a nematocyst or as sophisticated as a venom-filled lance. Although most envenomations occur in the temperate or tropical seas of the Indo-Pacific region, creatures with such mechanisms for inflicting injury can be found in virtually all waters.

SPONGES

More than 4,000 species of sponges are found worldwide, each composed of an elastic skeleton with tiny spicules of calcium carbonate or silica embedded in the connective tissue interstices.

Two syndromes may be induced upon contact with certain sponges. The first is an allergic inflammatory reaction akin to irritant plant dermatitis. The dermatopathic toxin is probably introduced into the skin from spicule-induced abrasions. A common offender is the yellow-orange-vermilion "fire sponge" (*Tedania ignis*), frequently found in Hawaiian and Floridian coastal waters. The reaction is largely one of itching and burning, which may progress to swelling of the joints, particularly of the hands. Severe involvement may resemble erythema multiforme with or without an anaphylactoid component. Immediate therapy is topical application of a 5 percent acetic acid soak; isopropyl alcohol is less effective as a topical agent. Steroid lotions are useless for initial decontamination. Severe reactions with vesiculation, pain, and swelling should be managed with a 10 to 14 day tapered dose of prednisone, beginning with 50 mg. It is not unusual for the surface epithelium to desquamate painlessly after a delay of 10 days to 2 months.

The second syndrome associated with sponge contact is an irritant dermatitis caused by the penetration of calcium carbonate or silica spicules into the skin. Largely a noninflammatory pruritic reaction, this may be managed by removing the spicules with adhesive tape, followed by an acetic acid soak. Because it is frequently difficult to differentiate between sponge spicule dermatitis and toxin-induced inflammation, it is usually necessary to treat all victims initially with adhesive tape and vinegar.

COELENTERATES

Coelenterates are a group of over 9,000 species that may be encountered in the ocean. Those that carry venom-inducing stinging cells, or nematocysts, are called cnidaria. The cnidaria are divided into the hydrozoans (e.g., fire coral, Portuguese man-of-war), scyphozoans (e.g., box-jellyfish), and anthozoans (e.g., anemones). In all cases, the stinging organelles are found near the mouth or on the outer surface of the tentacles. Each nematocyst contains a hollow, coiled, and sharply pointed thread tube of 200 to 400 μm in length, which floats in the liquid venom. The severity of envenomation is related to the toxicity of the venom, number of nematocysts discharged, and physical condition of the victim.

Fire corals are not true corals but rather sessile tropical ocean bottom creatures often mistaken for seaweed in their attachments to rocks, shells, coral, pilings, or shipwrecks. They often grow to 2 meters in height and have a razor-sharp lime carbonate exoskeleton, from which protrude thousands of tiny nematocyst-bearing tentacles.

The Portuguese man-of-war (Atlantic *Physalia physalis* and Pacific *Physalia utriculus*) is a pelagic animal widely distributed throughout the tropical oceans. Nematocyst-bearing tentacles of up to 100 feet in length are suspended from the nitrogen-and carbon monoxide-filled sail. If the animal encounters a foreign object, the nematocysts are discharged. A single man-of-war envenomation may involve several hundred thousand nematocysts. Detached tentacle fragments retain their potency for months and may envenom the unwary beachcomber. In the Chesapeake Bay, the sea nettle (*Chrysaora quinquecirrha*) poses a similar hazard.

The scyphozoan *Chironex fleckeri* (box-jellyfish) is reputed to be the most venomous sea creature, capable of inducing death within 1 minute after a significant sting. It is found predominantly in the quiet protected waters off the coast of northern Queensland, Australia.

Sea anemones are colorful flower-like bottom-dwellers that are often found in tidal pools. The finger-like projections are covered with modifications of the nematocyst, called sporocysts. In general, with the exception of *Actinodendron plumosum* (Hell's Fire sea anemone), the sting of most anemones is minor to moderate in severity.

Coelenterate envenomation ranges in severity from irritant dermatitis to excruciating pain, respiratory depression, and life-threatening cardiovascular collapse. A milder envenomation is characterized by stinging, paresthesias, pruritus, and pathognomonic reddish-brown linear wheals or "tentacle prints." A more severe inoculation of venom causes local edema, desquamation, and skin hemorrhages, with subsequent necrosis, ulceration, and secondary infection. If a potent venom or a large body surface area is involved, systemic symptoms include the rapid onset of nausea, vomiting, abdominal pain, myalgias, arthralgias, headache, aphonia, vertigo, ataxia, paralysis, seizures, arrhythmias, hemolysis, bronchospasm, pulmonary edema, coma, hypotension, and respiratory arrest.

The dermatitis should be managed as follows:

1. Immediately rinse the wound with seawater. Do not use freshwater or abrasion, as these will activate dormant nematocysts. Tourniquets are not recommended. Pressure or immobilization dressing techniques are not recommended and theoretically may worsen the envenomation.
2. Apply acetic acid (5 percent) solution in a copious irrigation. If vinegar is not available, less effective remedies include isopropyl alcohol, a baking soda slurry, dilute household ammonia, or a paste of unseasoned meat tenderizer (papain). There is continuing controversy in the laboratory and among clinicians as to the mechanism of action and efficacy of a variety of decontaminants. Pending a definitive evaluation of these different substances, acetic acid is the solution of choice. Topical lidocaine and ice packs are minimally efficacious for pain relief.
3. Remove visible tentacle fragments with forceps. Avoid self-contamination.
4. To remove invisible nematocysts, apply a lather of shaving cream and gently shave the affected area with a razor edge.

5. Reapply acetic acid or alcohol until pain is largely alleviated.
6. If the skin is inflamed, apply hydrocortisone (1 percent) cream or lotion.

A victim who is very young or elderly should be observed in the hospital for at least 6 hours for signs of systemic illness. If significant pain, vomiting, or any degree of hypotension is evident, intravenous access should be obtained for fluid replacement and analgesic administration.

Envenomation by *Chironex fleckeri* that results in respiratory distress, hypotension, intractable pain, or a severe skin reaction may necessitate the administration of antivenin (prepared from the hyperimmunization of sheep), available from Commonwealth Serum Laboratories in Melbourne, Australia. This is initiated with a primary dose of 20,000 U (1 ampule) intravenously, (IV), with appropriate premedication (diphenhydramine, 1 mg per kilogram IV, and methylprednisolone sodium succinate, 1 to 2 mg per kilogram) for the management of hypersensitivity to the animal product. The antivenin should be diluted 1:10 in normal saline or lactated Ringer's solution prior to administration. An instruction leaflet accompanies each ampule of antivenin. Repeat doses of antivenin are titrated to recurrent clinical decompensation. Tapered systemic administration of corticosteroid preparations is directed at the amelioration of the primary inflammatory response and against the development of delayed serum sickness. Delayed hypersensitivity reactions distant to the site of the initial envenomation have been attributed to the sting of *Physalia physalis*.

SEA URCHINS

Sea urchins are sedentary bottom- and crevice-dwellers covered with spines and delicate triple-jawed seizing organs called globiferous pedicellariae. The spines may or may not bear venom. The sharp tips are often broken off into the skin of the unwary diver or tidepooler. The pedicellariae use their venom-coated terminal pincer jaws to attach to the victim and will be torn from the shell rather than release their grasp.

The most common envenomation occurs when a spine penetrates the skin. This causes immediate burning pain and local myalgias, which may progress to paralysis, bronchospasm, hypotension, and collapse if numerous puncture wounds are present. Pain may disappear after the first few hours, with residual paralysis for 4 to 6 hours.

Immediate therapy is immersion in hot water to tolerance (110 °F or 43.5 °C) for 30 to 90 minutes to provide pain relief. Detached pedicellariae should be removed from the skin. Embedded spines are often difficult to extract, since they are brittle and easily broken. If left undisturbed, some delicate spines may be absorbed; however, heavier spines, those that have entered into joints, or those that are closely aligned to neurovascular structures should be removed. This should be accomplished in an operating room using surgical magnifica-

tion. In no case should a physician probe blindly into a wound in an attempt to fish out a spine. Because of the wide spectrum of microorganisms present in the aquatic environment, wounds that show evidence of minor infection should be cultured for *Vibrio* species and may initially be managed with oral trimethoprim-sulfamethoxazole (160/800 mg). Severe wound infections should be managed initially with an intravenous aminoglycoside (gentamicin 1 to 1.5 mg per kilogram every 8 hours) in combination with a third-generation cephalosporin(cefotaxime, 1 g every 8 hours, or moxalactam, 2 g every 8 hours), pending culture results. *Vibrio vulnificus* may invade the immunocompromised host and rapidly induce necrotizing myositis and septicemia.

SEA CUCUMBERS

Sea cucumbers are free-living sausage-shaped animals that live on the ocean floor. They produce a visceral liquid toxin, holothurin, that is excreted anally when the animal initiates a defense. This cantharidin-like substance may induce contact dermatitis and intense corneal inflammation. Because cucumbers occasionally feed on coelenterates, holothurin may be accompanied by excreted nematocyst venom. The initial treatment of cucumber dermatitis is therefore the application of acetic acid or isopropyl alcohol. If the cornea is involved, therapy is initiated with copious saline irrigation. The corneal abrasion is managed in standard fashion with cycloplegic, mydriatic, and antibiotic medications, taking care not to patch the eye closed if there is any chance of residual debris being adherent to the cornea.

STINGRAYS

In the warmer latitudes, stingrays are the most frequently incriminated group of coastal fishes with respect to human envenomations. At least 1,500 injuries per year are reported in the United States. The venom organ is composed of from one to four stings arranged on the dorsum of the whiplike tail. The sting is a bilaterally retroserrate dentinal dorsal tail spine, with an integumentary sheath that overlies the venom glands. When an unwary person surprises the creature, the tail lashes up, thrusting the spine into the victim. The foot and leg are most frequently involved, but penetrating fatal injuries to the thorax and abdomen have been reported.

Local venom effects include hemorrhage, intense inflammation with vasculitis, and necrosis. In animal models, stingray venom is capable of inducing local vasoconstriction, bradyarrhythmias, atrioventricular conduction abnormalities, subendocardial ischemia, respiratory depression, seizures, and death. The clinical wound is traumatic and envenomating. A severe laceration may be accompanied by secondary bacterial infection with ulceration. The envenomation causes immediate intense pain, local bleeding, and persistent edema. Systemic symptoms include abdominal pain, vomiting, diarrhea, diaphoresis, weakness, myalgias, headache, vertigo, arrhythmias, hypotension, and death.

Therapy is directed to life support, alleviation of pain, inactivation of venom, and prevention of infection. The wound should immediately be irrigated copiously with normal saline or fresh water. If medical aid is more than 1 hour distant and if the envenomation appears to be life-threatening, a proximal, loose lymphatic-occlusive tourniquet may be applied, although this is somewhat controversial. As soon as possible, the wound should be immersed in hot water to tolerance (110° F or 43.5° C) in order to inactivate the venom. If necessary, a local anesthetic without epinephrine may be injected into the wound or a regional nerve block may be performed. With early pain relief, the wound should be superficially explored to remove any retained fragments of the sting and integumentary sheath. Cryotherapy is absolutely contraindicated. After the soaking procedure, the wound must be thoroughly explored in the operating theater and debrided to the obvious margins of necrosis. All wounds should be closed loosely around drains or packed open for secondary closure, to minimize subsequent infection. The use of prophylactic antibiotics is currently under investigation. Infected wounds should be cultured for *Vibrio* species, aerobes, and anaerobes. Pending identification of organisms, patients should be treated with gentamicin or tobramycin and a third-generation cephalosporin. Proper antitetanus prophylaxis is mandatory.

SCORPION FISH

In the United States, scorpion fish (family Scorpaenidae) are most commonly found off the Florida Keys and Gulf of Mexico and along the coastlines of California and Hawaii. The most dangerous stonefish species are inhabitants of Indo-Pacific waters and the tanks of amateur aquarists. Scorpion fish are divided into three genera—*Pterois* (zebra fish), *Scorpaena* (scorpion fish), and *Synanceja* (stonefish)—on the basis of venom organ structure. Venom varies in toxicity according to the species and season, with that of the stonefish being the most potent.

The wound and surrounding area may rapidly become ischemic and cyanotic, painful to a degree sufficient to cause delirium. Local edema and erythema often spread to involve the entire extremity. Delayed necrosis and an indolent tissue reaction are common. Systemic symptoms include skin rash, abdominal pain, vomiting, diarrhea, restlessness, paralysis, arthralgias, fever, hypotension, bronchospasm, arrhythmias, congestive heart failure, and death. Wounds frequently become infected.

The therapy is similar to that for stingray envenomation. Stonefish antivenin is available from Commonwealth Serum Laboratories, Melbourne, Australia. It is recommended for serious stonefish stings and can be used for other varieties of scorpion fish, with the benefits obtained weighed against the risk of anaphylaxis and serum sickness. Instructions for use accompany the antivenin. Neither intravenous calcium chloride nor calcium gluconate have been effective in the alleviation of muscle cramps caused by Scorpaenidae envenomation.

SEA SNAKES

Sea snakes are distributed in the tropical and temperate Pacific and Indian Oceans. They are not found in the Atlantic Ocean or in the Caribbean Sea.

The venom apparatus of the sea snake is composed of two to four hollow maxillary fangs, associated with a pair of venom glands. The fangs are short and easily dislodged, which spares many victims from envenomation. The venom is generally considered to be more toxic than terrestrial snake venom and contains neurotoxic, hemolytic, and myotoxic components. Bites are incurred most frequently by native fishermen or the unwary snake handler. Diagnosis of a sea snake bite is contingent upon the following:

1. Location. Sea snake bites do not occur on land, with the rare exception of snakes that migrate briefly into mangrove-infested areas during tidal changes.
2. Absence of pain at the bite site.
3. Fang marks. These are minute puncture wounds, which usually number from one to four, but may number up to 20.
4. Identification of the snake.
5. Development of characteristic signs and symptoms. These include myoglobinuria, restlessness, malaise, euphoria, myalgias, extremity paralysis, trismus, and ptosis. If symptoms are not present by 6 to 8 hours, the envenomation is not significant.

The onset of symptoms may be within 5 minutes or delayed by 6 to 8 hours, depending on the nature of the venom, the site of envenomation, and the underlying condition of the victim. In a serious envenomation, the victim develops flaccid or spastic paralysis, dysphasgia, vomiting, aphonia, and cranial nerve dysfunction. Patients may lose vision, suffer respiratory distress, have seizures, and become comatose. Myoglobinuria is pathognomonic and manifested 3 to 6 hours after the bite. The victim often deteriorates in hours to days under the burdens of central respiratory paralysis, bulbar dysfunction, electrolyte aberrations, renal failure, and cardiotoxicity.

The therapy is similar to that for terrestrial snake bite. Incision and suction are of no value if not initiated within 3 to 5 minutes after the bite. The affected limb should be immobilized and kept in a dependent position. The pressure-immobilization technique may effectively retard the absorption of venom. A lymphatic-occlusive tourniquet should only be used if the victim is more than 1 hour away from definitive care and pressure-immobilization is impractical. Cryotherapy is not recommended. At the first sign of envenomation, the victim should be rushed to a medical facility, where polyvalent sea snake antivenin (Commonwealth Serum Laboratories) or tiger snake antivenin can be administered according to the instructions that accompany the product. Antivenin is specific and absolutely indicated in all severe cases of envenomation, as supportive therapy is frequently inadequate to rescue the victim. In general, the initial dose of polyvalent sea snake antivenin is 1,000 to 2,000 U diluted in 500 to 1,000 ml of normal saline.

SUGGESTED READING

Auerbach PS, Halstead BW. Hazardous marine life. In: Auerbach PS, Geehr EC, eds. Management of wilderness and environmental emergencies. New York: Macmillan, 1983:213.

Barss P. Wound necrosis caused by the venom of stingrays. Med J Aust 1984; 141:854–855.

Kizer KW, McKinney HE, Auerbach PS. Scorpaenidae envenomation. JAMA 1985; 253:807–810.

Williamson JA, LeRay LE, Wohlfahrt M, Fenner PJ. Acute management of serious envenomation by box-jellyfish (*Chironex fleckeri*). Med J Aust 1984; 141:851–853.

FROSTBITE AND LOCAL COLD INJURY

LINDA G. PHILLIPS, M.D.
JOHN P. HEGGERS, Ph.D.
MARTIN C. ROBSON, M.D.

Historically, localized cold injury was divided into many clinical syndromes such as chilblain, trench foot, and frostbite. However, based on the pathophysiology, it is better to regard all local cold injury as a continuum and discuss it under one heading—frostbite.

Frostbite occurs as a consequence of exposure to cold. The skin first becomes blanched, and a stinging or burning sensation is felt. The exposed part rapidly becomes numb and feels clumsy. Later, the part becomes firm and tense and is, indeed, frozen. Upon thawing or partial thawing, edema becomes manifest, with swelling and blister formation. This is accompanied by severe aching pain. If the injury is severe, the blisters progress to further injury with eventual gangrene. Without proper treatment, repeated episodes of partial thawing and refreezing result in a much more severe injury than the original local injury and are the cause of the requirement for major amputations so common in the past.

PATHOPHYSIOLOGY

Understanding the pathophysiology of frostbite allows comprehension of the rationale for treatment and of why treatment regimens attempted in the past were not successful. The pathophysiology can be divided into two distinct phases: the *immediate phase*, secondary to the formation of ice crystals in the tissue, and the delayed phase, which results in progressive dermal ischemia and tissue loss. When ice crystals form in tissue, water is drawn out of the cells into the extravascular spaces. These crystals expand and cause a mechanical destruction of cells. The intracellular electrolyte concentration increases drastically, further causing or initiating cellular destruction. Damage may occur to the blood vessels, particularly the endothelial cells, causing a loss of vascular tubular

integrity and leading to local edema and loss of distal nutritive flow. Actually, the initial formation of ice crystals in the tissue is not the most damaging; the partial thawing and refreezing cause the most severe injury. In addition, cold produces arteriolar vasoconstriction and tissue ischemia. With thawing, the arterioles reopen and blood flow is re-established with a reactive hyperemia. After a mild cold injury, this initial vasoconstriction followed by a flare-type hyperemia may be all that occurs. However, after a more severe injury or after repeated thaw-freeze cycles, a progressive thrombotic phase occurs.

The *progressive phase* is attributable to a progressive dermal ischemia very much like that following a thermal burn. The vascular injury discussed above, which occurs immediately, damages the endothelium and each dermal cell. This type of injury to the cell can give rise to the production of prostanoid derivatives such as prostaglandin E_2, prostaglandin $F_{2\alpha}$, and, more importantly, thromboxane. Thromboxane is a strong vasoconstrictor, platelet aggregator, and leukocyte-sticking agent. This results in deterioration of the microvasculature. The authors have shown both experimentally and clinically that thromboxane is the mediator of progressive dermal necrosis in frostbite injury. The longer the tissue is exposed to the lower temperature environment, the more serious the injury will be.

PREDISPOSING FACTORS TO LOCAL COLD INJURY

If cold exposure is the key to frostbite, there are other predisposing factors. The most important of these are environmental: humidity and wind. An increase in humidity or in the wind velocity can further increase the damage potential of the absolute temperature. This is why the wind-chill index is so important in predicting weather that may cause cold injuries. Patient factors may cause a predisposition to frostbite. Anything that decreases local tissue perfusion, such as atherosclerosis, tobacco smoking, or tight constrictive clothing, has been implicated. In addition, anything that causes vasodilatation, such as drugs or alcohol, can increase the rate of heat loss and result in more rapid and profound cooling. Since heat loss is what causes the body to become cold, it is important to wear clothes that maintain heat. Stocking caps, neck mufflers, and mittens (not gloves) are the most effective at preventing heat loss.

CLINICAL DIAGNOSIS

Local cold injury is easy to diagnose if a high index of clinical suspicion is maintained. Whenever the weather is conducive to injury, either with high humidity or a significant wind-chill index, anyone who presents with unprotected bodily parts should be presumed to have frostbite. Frostbite can be divided into first-, second-, and third-degree injury. If a firm white plaque is the only manifestation, this is considered first-degree frostbite. For the other two degrees, blisters are usually present. Blister fluid color can be used to assess the severity of frostbite injury. The blister fluid that is clear or white reflects a frostbite of short duration and second-degree injury. The hemorrhagic type of blister reflects a structural damage to the subdermal plexus and is an injury of longer duration. Purple hemorrhagic blisters are diagnostic of third-degree injury. Occasionally the third-degree injury appears as a deep purple firm part with no blister; this is the pregangrenous part, the most severe form of injury.

PRE-HOSPITAL THERAPY

There is very little role for pre-hospital management of the patient with frostbite. Certainly most of the treatments previously advocated have no place and are, indeed, contraindicated. Snow or ice should not be applied, since this will only worsen the injury. Partial slow warming with blankets is also injurious. Blisters should not be broken or damaged in any way prior to hospitalization. Do not mistake the clear or white blisters on a frostbitten hand for burn blisters. An appropriate or adequate history should be taken at the time the patient is picked up. All exposed parts, particularly extremities, should be kept elevated until arrival at an appropriate treatment facility.

EMERGENCY DEPARTMENT THERAPY

Rapid rewarming is the single totally agreed-upon treatment for frostbite of all degrees. This should be performed in a 40 °C (104 °F) waterbath. Usually 30 minutes is required. Active motion during rewarming is helpful. Intravenous analgesia in the form of small repeated doses of morphine or meperidine may be necessary during the rewarming process.

This rapid rewarming therapy reverses the ice crystal formation in the tissue. However, it does nothing for the progressive phase of injury. Therefore, additional treatment is necessary to prevent progressive dermal ischemia and tissue loss. This consists of topical and systemic agents to minimize the production of thromboxane by the injured cells. Therefore, the clear or white blisters should be debrided because they have been shown to contain thromboxane. The deeper hemorrhagic blisters should be aspirated but not debrided. The preferred continuing therapeutic regimen should include elevation of the extremity; tetanus prophylaxis; analgesics, either intravenous or intramuscular morphine or meperidine as indicated, unless contraindicated by medical history; aspi-

rin, 325 mg by mouth every 6 hours for adults and 125 mg by mouth every 6 hours for children; penicillin, 500,000 U every 6 hours for adults until the edema resolves and approximately 50,000 U per kilogram per day for children, given in four divided doses. All wound areas should be covered with a topical treatment of Dermaide aloe every 6 hours until disposition. Dermaide aloe is an inhibitor of thromboxane A_2, which has been identified as a major mediator of progressive dermal ischemia. In this manner, the progressive dermal ischemia is limited by use of a systemic, nonsteroidal anti-inflammatory agent (aspirin) and a topical, nonsteroidal anti-inflammatory agent (Dermaide). Dermaide aloe can be purchased from Dermaide Research Corporation, P.O. Box 562, Palos Heights, Illinois 60463, telephone (312) 448-9180.

DISPOSITION

Patients with all but the most minor localized cold injuries should be admitted to the hospital. Even those with minor injuries should be admitted after rewarming if a warm environment cannot be assured for them. The patient should not be discharged from an emergency department into subfreezing weather. If a warm car is waiting, the patient should only be allowed to leave after proper clothing has been obtained (stocking cap, wool mittens, and wool socks).

Any patient with suspected or confirmed frostbite injuries requires admission to the hospital. The antithromboxane treatment needs to be continued for approximately 96 hours. The antistreptococcal therapy begun in the emergency department also must be continued during the edema phase of the injury, which often lasts for 48 to 72 hours. Since frostbite generally involves injuries to the upper or lower extremities, appropriate physical therapy and occupational therapy should be recommended. Daily hydrotherapy for active and passive range of motion exercises has proved to be of extreme value in preservation of function. Finally, if the frostbite is so severe or the treatment is delayed, the therapeutic measures outlined may not prevent the progressive injury, and gangrene may result. This may require local treatment to the part in the form of a penetrating antibacterial cream such as Sulfamylon, while evaluating the need for amputation.

SUGGESTED READING

Heggers JP, Robson MC. Prostaglandins and thromboxanes. In: Ninemann J, ed. Traumatic injury—infection and other immunologic sequelae. Baltimore: University Park Press, 1983.

McCauley RL, Hing DN, Robson MC, Heggers JP. Frostbite injuries: A rational approach based on the pathophysiology. J Trauma. 1983; 23:143–147.

Robson MC, Krizek TJ, Wray RC Jr. Care of the thermally injured patient. In: Ballinger WF, Rutherford RB, Zuidema GD, eds. The management of trauma. Philadelphia: WB Saunders, 1979.

HYPOTHERMIA

J. DOUGLAS WHITE, M.D.

Hypothermia, defined as a core temperature of less than 35 °C, is both a sign of disease and a disease entity per se. This temperature has physiologic significance, as it indicates the patient is no longer able to maintain thermogenesis. The patient essentially becomes poikilothermic, and the core temperature continues to drop until it attains that of the ambient environment (usually air but often water, as in cases of immersion-associated hypothermia). Theoretically, then, patients may become hypothermic in exposure circumstances that are decidedly warm (i.e., ambient temperatures below 35 °C or 95 °F). Body temperatures in this range must be treated specifically in addition to making efforts to diagnose any underlying, predisposing illness.

ETIOLOGY

Simple exposure is the most common etiology for hypothermia. This usually takes place during cold weather when the patient's clothing, shelter, metabolism, or medical state is inadequate to cope with climatic conditions. Also, hypothermia can occur surprisingly rapidly when high wind velocities and immersion occur because of tremendous augmentation of convective and conductive heat loss. Severe medical illnesses, particularly involving metabolism and cardiovascular status, also predispose patients to hypothermia. Finally, extremes in age are often associated with hypothermia because of immature or aged thermoregulatory systems that are less sensitive and effective.

Hypothermia is also frequently associated with drug ingestions (both chronic and acute), and even therapeutic levels of sedatives or modest intoxication can contribute substantially to its development. Head and spinal trauma, strokes, and sepsis are also common causes of hypothermia. Uncommon endocrine-metabolic abnormalities (hypoglycemia, myxedema, Addison's disease, and hypopituitarism) often are accompanied by hypothermia. Finally, loss of skin thermal integrity as a result of burns or erythroderma poses a substantial risk of hypothermia.

DIAGNOSIS

By definition, the diagnosis is made by a temperature reading. The *most common diagnostic error* is a casual approach to vital signs. By definition, hypothermia will be disclosed if core temperatures are taken. Lapses usually occur when other primary diagnoses seem obvious (sepsis, stroke) or the physician is understandably distracted by other more serious conditions (e.g., cardiac arrest, trauma resuscitation). The vigilant physician who employs thermometers capable of accurately registering temperatures below 35 °C rarely misses this diagnosis, even in the most unusual circumstances. Given the undifferentiated nature of emergency patients, it is sound practice to obtain temperature readings on all patients and to obtain core temperatures on all patients with subnormal oral readings.

Clinically, hypothermic patients follow a progression of signs and symptoms outlined in Table 1. Electrocardiogram (ECG) changes are common, including shivering artifact, atrial fibrillation, bradycardia, and the characteristic J wave (Fig. 1). However, these changes are not present in every case.

THERAPY

Pre-hospital Management

Prolonged therapy in the field is to be condemned, and conventional cardiopulmonary resuscitation (CPR)

TABLE 1 Signs and Symptoms of Hypothermia

Temperature (°C)	(°F)	Findings
37	(98.6)	Normal oral temperature
35	(95.0)	Shivering, increased metabolic rate
34	(93.0)	Early mental status changes: poor judgment, slurred speech, ataxia
33	(91.4)	Approximate temperature to which patient must be rewarmed before CPR can be declared unsuccessful
32	(89.6)	Stupor
31	(87.9)	Shivering (and increased heat generation) stops, unable to generate heat
30	(86.0)	Cardiac dysrhythmia (especially atrial fibrillation), bradycardia, insulin becomes ineffective
29	(85.2)	Pupils dilated, comatose
		Decreased pulse, blood pressure, respiration
28	(83.0)	Decreased ventricular fibrillation threshold
27	(80.6)	Reflexes absent, no response to pain
24	(75.2)	Marked hypotension
22	(71.6)	Maximal risk of ventricular fibrillation
20	(68.0)	Lowest temperature at which cardiac resuscitation possible
19	(66.2)	ECG flat, asystole
16	(61.0)	Lowest recorded survival from accidental hypothermia

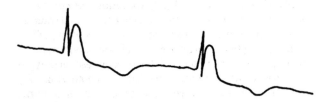

Figure 1 Classic J or Osborne wave of hypothermia.

and ACLS medications are customarily useless until the patient's temperature approaches euthermic levels. Rapid transport to the hospital for definitive rewarming is essential in all hypothermic patients.

Pre-hospital care should emphasize prevention of further heat loss and cardiac arrest rhythms (asystole, ventricular fibrillation). These patients often have spontaneous respirations and nonarrest rhythms (atrial, junctional, and bradycardic) and should be handled gently without excessive manipulation, chest compressions, or intubation for fear of precipitating refractory and usually fatal ventricular fibrillation. It is acceptable and even prudent to place a protective cervical collar in any situation where head and neck trauma cannot be excluded.

Patients with spontaneous respirations, even as low as 4 per minute, should only receive oxygen by mask, while patients without spontaneous respirations should be intubated and ventilated with warm humidified oxygen. Ventilatory rates should be modest (8 to 12 per minute) to avoid excessive alkalosis in a patient with a precarious myocardial status.

An attempt should be made to insert a peripheral intravenous line to infuse glucose, naloxone, and thiamine; however these attempts should be gentle and quickly abandoned if unsuccessful (quite probable in a rigid, poorly perfused limb).

A core temperature (usually rectal) should be obtained with thermometers capable of reading below 28 °C, and the patient's ECG monitored. If a comatose patient's core temperature is above 28 °C, pre-hospital CPR protocols, with the emphasis on rapid transport for definitive rewarming and resuscitation, should apply. If the patient is not comatose, he or she should be rapidly transported to the nearest emergency facility with minimal movement and manipulation.

For patients with a core temperature below 28 °C, bretylium tosylate, 5 mg per kilogram intravenously (IV), should be given as ventricular fibrillation prophylaxis. If the ECG reveals an arrested rhythm (asystole, ventricular fibrillation), CPR with chest compressions should begin and cardioversion attempted. If the ECG reveals a nonarrest rhythm or no ECG is available, CPR should not be instituted. In any case, rapid transport for definitive resuscitation is mandatory. Field CPR on hypothermic cardiac arrest victims is rarely successful in restoring stable rhythms and hemodynamics.

Emergency Department Management

All hypothermic victims should receive the following measures in the emergency department if they have not been instituted in the field:

1. warm (less than 42 °C) humidified oxygen therapy,
2. continuous core temperature and ECG monitoring,
3. peripheral intravenous line with 5 percent dextrose in normal saline at maintenance infusion rates,
4. naloxone, 0.8 mg IV,
5. thiamine, 100 mg IV,
6. glucose, 50 ml of 50 percent solution intravenously,
7. arterial blood gas readings,
8. toxicology screen,
9. complete blood count and electrolyte, glucose, and amylase determinations,
10. bretylium, 5 mg per kilogram IV, if the core temperature is less than 28 °C.

If a blood pressure reading cannot be obtained by auscultation, an intra-arterial line (preferably femoral) should be inserted to monitor central arterial pressures. While central venous monitoring has value in these patients, right atrial catheters are best avoided because of their arrhythmogenic potential. It is still customary for most physicians to correct the pH, Pco_2, and Po_2 to core temperature (pH rises by 0.015 and PaO_2 and $PaCO_2$ decrease by 7.2 percent and 4.4 percent, respectively, per degree Celsius below 37 °C) and strive to avoid alkalosis and maintain adequate oxygenation. However, recent animal studies suggest that this may not be physiologic and that better results (particularly in terms of cardiac function) may be obtained by maintaining the usual physiologic values (especially for pH) in *uncorrected* arterial blood gases.

For patients with core temperatures above 28 °C, these measures should be sufficient. If the patient's temperature cannot be raised by more than 1 degree Celsius per hour, warm inhalation therapy should be augmented with peritoneal, colonic, or nasogastric lavage at 42 °C, with minimal dwell times and flow rates up to 12 liters per hour. If the physical examination or test results indicate the presence of an infection, this should be evaluated and treated in the same manner as for a euthermic patient. Prophylactic antibiotics and hormones, in the absence of any evidence of infection or endocrinologic disease, are not indicated. Conventional CPR protocols should be applied as necessary for patients whose core temperatures are above 28 °C; however, treating physicians should be aware that drugs and cardioversion may not be successful until core temperatures reach 32 °C. After several rounds of cardioversion and medication, therefore, more aggressive rewarming measures (see further on) should be instituted to raise core temperature above 32 °C as rapidly as possible.

Patients with core temperatures below 28 °C with nonarrest rhythms are at risk of developing spontaneous ventricular fibrillation, which, even in the emergency department setting, is refractory and usually fatal. All such patients should receive bretylium tosylate, 5 mg per kilogram IV, and it is incumbent on the treating physician to raise core temperature rapidly to 28 to 32 °C. This may be accomplished with a combination of the aforementioned central rewarming measures if the patient's initial temperature approaches 28 °C; however, femoral-femoral bypass should be considered in profoundly hypothermic victims (temperature under 25 °C).

Patients with core temperatures below 28 °C and arrested rhythms should be intubated and chest compressions begun immediately. The patient should be placed on a respirator delivering warm humidified oxygen. Femoral-femoral bypass should begin as soon as possible, with peritoneal, colonic, and nasogastric lavage in the interim. If these measures fail to raise the core temperature above 28 °C after 1 hour, open thoracotomy with warmed saline (42 °C) should be performed. CPR protocols may resume at 28 °C (including cardioversion), and chest compressions and rewarming measures should continue until the patient is hemodynamically stable or the patient's core temperature is 32 to 35 °C. Only when the patient's core temperature reaches this range can resuscitation efforts be deemed exhausted. Clinical experience indicates that efforts should be even more vigorous and prolonged in the near-drowning victim, and even heroic if a pediatric patient is hypothermic after an immersion accident. Physiologic responses to immersion and drowning can be protective in these situations of hypothermia.

DISPOSITION

All patients with presenting core temperatures below 30 °C should be admitted to an intensive care unit. All patients with presenting core temperatures below 35 °C should be considered for hospital admission or treated and held for observation until they become euthermic. The threshold for admitting patients should be commensurately lower in situations of age extremes, associated medical illness, drug overdose, or abnormal laboratory test results. Most moderately hypothermic alcoholics suffering exclusively from exposure, without evidence of associated illness or drug ingestion, usually respond well to warm, humidified inhalation and do not necessarily have to be admitted to the hospital.

SUGGESTED READING

Becker H, Vinten-Johnson J, Buckbery GD, et al. Myocardial damage caused by keeping pH 7.40 during systemic deep hypothermia. J Thorac Cardiovasc Surg 1900; 82:810–820.

Harnett RM, Pruitt JR, Sias FR. A review of the literature concerning resuscitation from hypothermia: Part 1—The problem and general approaches. Aviat Space Environ Med 1983; 54:425–434.

Harnett RM, Pruitt JR, Sias FR. A review of the literature concerning resuscitation from hypothermia: Part 2—Selected rewarming protocols. Aviat Space Environ Med 1983; 54:487–495.

Pozos RS, Wittmers LE, eds. The nature and treatment of hypothermia. Minneapolis: University of Minnesota Press, 1983.

White FN. A comparative physiological approach to hypothermia. J Thorac Cardiovasc Surg 1981; 82:821–831.

Zell SC, Kurtz KJ. Severe exposure hypothermia: A resuscitation protocol. Ann Emerg Med 1985; 14:335–338.

HEAT ILLNESS

JAMES P. KNOCHEL, M.D.

ACCLIMATIZATION

The term acclimatization to heat represents a constellation of physiologic adaptations that appear in a normal person as a result of repeated exposures to heat stress. The most important adaptations include retention of salt and water, expansion of the extracellular fluid volume, and slight hemodilution, which depends on the action of aldosterone produced in the adrenal cortex. When a person is exposed to heat, the body temperature rises and signals the hypothalamus to initiate reflexes that initiate cutaneous vasodilatation to deliver heated blood to the body surface. Heat can thereby be lost into the environmental air. Reflexes are also activated to initiate sweat formation. Upon repeated exposure to heat, the ability to sweat increases in terms of the maximal volume of sweat that can be produced. In addition, there is a progressive decline in the sodium concentration of sweat, owing to the action of aldosterone. A number of additional changes occur that depend on the status of physical training in that particular individual. For example, training increases the mass of mitochondria, hemoglobin, and myoglobin. An individual thereby improves biochemical efficiency to the point that heat production for a given amount of work is less than it was in an unacclimatized trained individual. Cardiovascular performance also increases; maximal cardiac output under conditions of work can increase to higher levels than before training. During hard work in the heat, normal untrained individuals show a virtual disappearance of glomerular filtration and renal plasma flow. However, following training and heat acclimatization, such drastic changes do not occur, and basal glomerular filtration rate even increases by about 25 percent.

When discussing heat acclimatization, one must carefully quantitate the term. For example, one person may be acclimatized to heat in the sense that he or she can perform sedentary activities in comfort and safety despite the heat. However, for an individual to run a 10,000 meter race or for a farmer to pitch bales of hay for 12 hours a day in the summer heat requires much higher degrees of acclimatization. The physiologic adaptations that we define as acclimatization appear within a few days after heat exposure and become about 90 percent complete after 2 weeks of repeated heat exposure, but require up to 6 weeks for their full development. Modest salt deprivation accelerates the process and a very high dietary salt intake delays development of acclimatization. Certain individuals, such as military recruits, football players during the two a day sessions in August, and joggers who run each day, or in general terms, individuals who produce voluminous quantities of sweat day after day, may become seriously potassium-deficient by means of losses in sweat as well as losses in their urine produced by the joint effects of aldosterone and excretion of sodium into the urine. It can be readily appreciated why lack of heat acclimatization is a common predisposing factor to the development of serious heat stroke.

MECHANISMS OF BODY COOLING

Heat is lost from the body by physical irradiation, conduction, and convection. Heat diffuses from blood through tissues to the air, and of most importance, during work in the heat, body heat is lost by vaporization of sweat from the body surface. Vaporization of 1 ml of sweat reduces the heat load by 1.7 Kcal. Vaporization sweat is dependent upon water saturation of the air (relative humidity), so that on dry days when the air humidity is low, vaporization occurs at a rapid rate, cooling is extremely efficient, and accordingly, the 'comfort index,' a lay term for heat stress, is high. On the other hand, when the air is nearly saturated with water, it is impossible for sweat to vaporize so that heat loss by vaporization of sweat becomes impossible. When environmental temperature matches body temperature, heat loss by means of vaporization of sweat becomes the only possible way of regulating temperature. As a consequence, hard work is virtually impossible when the weather is hot and the humidity is high. Such conditions characteristically favor development of heat stroke. Because of these important relationships, it is important to schedule activities at a favorable time of the day when acquisition of heat loads from the sun is less and when loss of heat from the body is also more likely to occur. Early morning and late evening are the best. However, on some days, events requiring expenditure of energy and endogenous production of heat, such as athletic events or work, should not be scheduled at all, since adequate body cooling becomes virtually impossible.

Three important forms of heat illness may be encountered by the emergency physician: heat cramps, heat exhaustion, and heat stroke. The majority of this chapter deals with heat stroke, since it is a potentially fatal condition and represents a true medical emergency.

HEAT CRAMPS

Heat cramps are characterized by exquisitely painful sustained muscular contractions that usually occur in muscles used during the day's work. They tend to occur toward the end of the day or after work has been finished, especially after a heavily used set of muscles has been rested or cooled down by a shower. While cramps most commonly involve the muscles in the lower extremities, any muscles in the body can be involved. Cramps of the rectus abdominis muscles may be so severe as to simulate an acute surgical abdomen. Patients with heat cramps tend to be highly trained, physically fit, and heat-acclimatized persons who give a history of profuse sweating while working in a hot environment. Such individuals characteristically replace sweat losses with water and inadequate salt. As a result, laboratory tests show hyponatremia and hypochloremia, reflecting salt depletion. Sweat is hypotonic because sweat glands extract sodium and chloride ions but not water from the precursor fluid. Heat-acclimatized, highly trained men have the ability to produce sweat voluminously as a physiologic adaptation to hot weather. When sweat is secreted at high rates, there is less time for reabsorption of sodium chloride. Consequently, such individuals can actually lose more salt than those who are not acclimatized to heat.

Replacement of sweat volume with water and no salt causes salt depletion and dilution of body fluids. Treatment of heat cramps is simple, consisting only of salt replacement. If vomiting is not present, salt may be replaced orally by means of lightly salted liquids or bouillon. If oral intake is not possible, intravenous normal saline administered in doses of 1 or 2 liters is usually satisfactory. Chemical evidence of mild rhabdomyolysis, specifically a slight or moderate rise in creatine phosphokinase enzymes in serum, is often observed in patients with heat cramps. There has been no evidence reported that rhabdomyolysis in heat cramps constitutes an important clinical problem.

HEAT EXHAUSTION

Heat exhaustion is a more serious condition resulting from losses of water or salt or both as the result of heat stress. Although heat exhaustion may be subclassified into that form mainly associated with dehydration or that form associated with salt depletion, most patients show findings of both. Heat exhaustion usually but not always occurs in unacclimatized individuals, in individuals who are unaccustomed to a high environmental temperature, and who have worked in the heat for several days. Presenting symptoms may include postural hypotension, orthostatic dizziness, palpitations, weakness, headache, intense thirst, depression, and confusion. Slight fever is common and in some individuals, a temperature up to 102° F may be observed. Such temperatures are more commonly seen in patients with primarily dehydration.

In some instances, myalgias, headache, nausea, vomiting, and diarrhea dominate the clinical picture, and in the presence of a mild fever, they may suggest a viral syndrome. Patients with heat exhaustion continue to sweat, accounting for the common clinical finding of cool, clammy skin despite a slight fever.

Heat exhaustion, especially the form dominated by dehydration, is a treacherous illness because if allowed to proceed, it may culminate in frank heat stroke.

Treatment of heat exhaustion consists of placing the patient in a cool, shaded area, fanning to promote evaporation of sweat, cooling the body surface with tepid water, and administering salt and water. If fluids must be administered intravenously, repair solutions should ideally be selected on the basis of laboratory measurements. If a laboratory profile shows hypernatremia, the patient should first receive 0.45 percent saline solution in 5 percent glucose in an amount sufficient to correct any disturbances in volume depletion, such as a drop in blood pressure on assuming the upright position, or until it has been shown that urine is being produced at a rate of 40 to 60 ml per hour. If an individual has sweated heavily day after day for a week or more, potassium deficiency may also exist. Thus it may also be necessary to replace potassium, depending upon laboratory measurements.

HEAT STROKE

Heat stroke is a life-threatening medical emergency. Its characteristic features include central nervous system dysfunction, hyperthermia (rectal temperature of 106° F or higher), and a hot, dry skin. These findings describe *classic heat stroke* that one might expect to find in an elderly person who has been confined to a hot room during a heat wave or a young child who is left in an enclosed automobile on a hot afternoon. *Exertional heat stroke*, on the other hand, usually occurs in men who have been performing work in a hot environment at such a pace that heat accumulates more rapidly in their body than it can be dissipated into the environment.

The central nervous system manifestations of heat stroke are variable. Some individuals simply present in frank coma, whereas others may show a period of bizarre, inappropriate behaviour or even frank psychosis before collapse. The range of body temperature in heat stroke is also variable. By definition, the minimum temperature is considered by most authorities to be between 105 or 106° F, and extreme temperatures of 116° F have been observed. Temperature should be recorded rectally using a probe thermistor device if possible, since misleadingly low temperatures can be recorded from the mouth or axilla. Sweating is nearly always absent in classic forms of heat stroke and thus accounts for the usual finding of hot and dry skin. Cutaneous flushing is a prominent finding because of extreme peripheral vasodilitation. In contrast, young men with exertional heat stroke, although usually showing a hot, flushed, and dry skin, may often present while still sweating, and because of intense catecholamine release they may show a relatively cool skin that appears blanched. The normal respiratory response

to heating is hyperventilation (like a panting dog) and respiratory alkalosis, and this is the usual finding in classic heat stroke. In contrast, young men with exertional heat stroke hyperventilate, and in addition, may have severe lactic acidosis. The latter occurs as a result of muscular exertion itself and of lactate accumulation secondary to hypoxia as a result of volume depletion. An important and consistent difference between classic and exertional heat stroke is the occurrence of significant rhabdomyolysis in the exertional variety. Rhabdomyolysis in itself contributes heavily to morbidity in this illness.

There are a number of well-recognized predisposing factors to exertional heat stroke. One of the most important is lack of heat acclimatization. Of equal importance are salt depletion, potassium deficiency, coexisting febrile illness, lack of sleep, the use of drugs that impair sweating (major tranquilizers, antihistamines, antiparkonsonian agents), drugs that interfere with cardiovascular performance (diuretics, antihypertensives, and beta-blockers), and finally drugs that add to the endogenous production of heat (amphetamines, neuroleptics, and possibly tricyclic antidepressants). Last but not least, many victims of exertional heat stroke have performed competetive events or physical work under hot and humid weather conditions that prevent adequate loss of generated heat.

Predisposing factors for development of classic heat stroke include any disease process that interferes with cardiovascular performance; fluid imbalance as may occur as the result of sweating, dehydration, or salt depletion; drugs that interfere with sweating; and chronic diseases such as diabetes mellitus and chronic alcoholism. Haloperidol appears to be implicated in some cases of heat stroke. In my experience, many elderly patients who are admitted to the hospital in the summertime with severe dehydration and hypernatremia have been medicated with haloperidol. This drug may reduce awareness or recognition of thirst and as such is potentially hazardous.

TREATMENT OF HEAT STROKE

Heat stroke is a dire medical emergency; if untreated, it almost invariably culminates in death. The most important factors that determine successful treatment of this condition are (1) anticipation, (2) prompt recognition, and (3) rapid cooling. When emergency medical personnel or triage nurses in hospitals appreciate those weather conditions in which heat stroke is likely to appear, preparation for such cases can result in treatment at such an early stage that there may be essentially no morbidity as a result of severe hyperthermia. In the city of Dallas, Texas, during sustained hot and humid weather, the Dallas Firemen Paramedics have supplies of ice readily available and have been well instructed in recognition of patients with heat stroke. Immediate treatment upon discovery often leads to prompt recovery from coma. In many cases, the patient has essentially recovered by the time he or she is delivered to a hospital emergency department because of prompt and effective treatment. On the other hand, if a patient is allowed to remain hyperthermic because the condition is not recognized or because facilities are not provided to effect rapid cooling, with every moment there is continued loss of vital function. It is of key importance to recognize that morbidity and mortality in this illness are directly related to the intensity and duration of hyperthermia.

The emergent problems that may exist in a patient with severe heat stroke are shown in Table 1. In light of these complications, one needs to have a predetermined course of action similar to that for managing any crisis situation, such as major trauma. Before initiation of cooling, and especially in people who are severely ill, there must be immediate access to the circulation, preferably with a large-bore central line. Second, in totally unresponsive patients, it is wise to quickly empty the stomach and instill a small amount of antacid, because vomiting and the possibility of aspiration are so common during the cooling phase. This type of patient should also be intubated both as a precaution against aspiration and because of the possibility of respiratory arrest during cooling. A core temperature device, such as a thermistor probe, should be inserted 15 to 20 cm into the rectum to record core temperature. Simple thermometers that measure anal temperature are totally unsatisfactory. It is helpful to draw baseline blood samples for measurement of arterial pH and blood gases, arterial lactate, a complete blood count, including platelets and standard clotting factors, serum electrolyte concentrations, creatine kinase activity, and creatinine or blood urea nitrogen and glucose concentrations.

Methods of Cooling

The conventional method of cooling comatose, hyperthermic patients is to immerse them in a tub of ice water while two attendants briskly rub the body surface to promote circulatory exchanges of heat. This maneuver is painful to the hands of the attendants and therefore several teams must be available to alternate this activity. Obviously, there must be a sufficiently large tub and ice available to effect such a procedure. While cooling the patient, one can anticipate the development of shivering, frank shaking, and in many cases convulsive seizures as the body temperature is being lowered. Defecation and vomiting are also common as body temperature is lowered. Because of such problems, it is much more convenient and equally effective to place the patient on a gurney and wet the body surface with plastic bags containing ice. If the attendants wear insulated gloves, they will not experience the usual pain associated with cooling. It is also helpful to employ a large, powerful fan to promote movement of air and enhance vaporization over the body surface. Using either the iced tub or the wet body surface fanning and ice massage technique, body temperature can effectively be lowered over the course of 30 to 60 minutes. Cooling measures should be stopped when core temperature falls to 102° F. At this point, even when additional cooling procedures are not used, the body temperature will continue to fall to the range of normal. If it rises again, such as may occur following a convulsive seizure, cooling methods should be reintroduced. Some have recommended the use of chlorpromazine, 50 mg intravenously, at the outset of treatment as a means to prevent muscular fasciculations, frank shaking, or convulsions that occur during the cooling phase. In elderly individuals, the use of chlorpromazine for this purpose has been associated with hypotension. On the other hand, chlorpromazine has been extremely effective in young individuals with exertional heat stroke. Whether small doses of diazepam have the same salutory effect has not been examined, but it would appear likely.

Cold peritoneal lavage, ice water enemas, and cooling mattresses or blankets have all been employed for the purpose of reducing body temperature in patients with heat stroke and have been uniformly unsuccessful.

TREATMENT OF SHOCK

A substantial number of patients with heat stroke, whether of the exertional or classic type, present with hypotension or frank shock. Although volume depletion could play a role, it is often not responsible. During the development of hyperthermia, there is a major translocation of blood volume to the vessels of the skin and an associated decline of the central circulatory volume. Because of the extreme tachycardia and decreased venous return, such patients may not be able to maintain a normal cardiac output or arterial pressure. In such patients, it is unwise to administer large amounts of intravenous fluids for the purpose of restoring central circulatory volume, since as soon as cooling is effected and the large volume of blood in the cutaneous vessels is shifted back to the central circulation, pulmonary edema may occur. For this reason, it is advisable to cool patients with hypotension first. In the majority of patients, the blood pressure will rise to a normal range by simple cooling. If it does not, then a small amount of normal saline should be administered, for example 500 ml in 15 minutes, to determine its effect on arterial pressure. Having cooled the patient, one should obtain an electrocardiogram. Many patients with acute heat stroke show nonspecific ST-T

TABLE 1 Emergent Problems in Heat Stroke

Hyperthermia	Pulmonary edema
Shock	Hyperkalemia
Convulsions	Lactic acidosis
Aspiration	Hypoglycemia
Myocardial injury	Rhabdomyolysis
Arrhythmias	Acute renal failure
Cardiorespiratory arrest	

changes and a variety of atrial or ventricular arrhythmias. Structural damage to the heart is common in heat stroke, although in most cases the damage is not extensive. On rare occasions, acute transmural myocardial infarction or widespread myocardial damage may explain circulatory instability. In such instances, one must be extremely cautious about fluid administration and employ the conventional cardioactive drugs indicated for arrhythmias or other complications. The use of norepinephrine has not been recommended to treat hypotension in patients with heat stroke because of its vasoconstrictor action on cutaneous vessels, which in turn reduces heat loss from the body. Substances with less intense action such as metaraminol or dopamine are more appropriate.

ACID-BASE DISTURBANCES

When a normal person experiences excessive body temperature, the rate and volume of ventilation increase, and respiratory alkalosis follows. Hyperventilation can be of such intensity that frank tetany may result, so-called 'heat tetany'. All such patients have associated symptoms of paresthesias about the face and mouth and tingling in the extremities. In classic heat stroke, respiratory alkalosis is a common early finding. In such patients, arterial lactate levels are ordinarily in the range of 2 or 3 mmol per liter, which is probably the result of acute alkalosis per se or increased diaphragmatic work. However, when patients with classic heat stroke have associated cardiovascular disease with circulatory insufficiency, the finding of an arterial lactate level of 5 mmol per liter or higher appears to be an ominous sign. In contrast to patients with classic heat stroke, nearly all patients with exertional heat stroke show arterial lactate levels above 5 mmol per liter and, in fact, levels of 25 or 30 mmol per liter may be seen. In nearly all instances, lactic acid has accumulated as a result of muscular work, volume depletion, and hypoxia. Such lactic acidosis is not an ominous sign in individuals with exertional heat stroke, since in nearly all cases it clears rapidly after adequate volume replacement and cooling. Indeed, the finding of lactic acidosis at the time such patients are admitted to the hospital serves as a strong indicator for fluid volume replacement.

In some patients with exertional heat stroke, lactic acidosis is relatively mild. For example, a patient may present with an arterial lactate level of 10 mmol per liter and an arterial pH of 7.30. In such individuals, especially those who are hypotensive at the same time, a rather sudden intensification of lactic acidosis may be seen early during the phase of fluid volume adminstration. Apparently such individuals have accumulated major quantities of lactic acid in poorly perfused skeletal muscle, which upon reperfusion as a result of circulatory stabilization, causes an intensification of lactic acidosis. At any rate, this seldom presents a serious problem because it also tends to correct itself spontaneously as the lactate is converted to glucose in the liver.

Hypoglycemia has been observed in about 20 percent of patients with exertional heat stroke. Its cause is unclear but it would seem to be the result of reduced hepatic perfusion attributable to shunting blood to the skin and the associated visceral ischemia. This is usually a transient finding and responds quickly to volume replacement and administration of glucose.

RHABDOMYOLYSIS

Measurements of serum creatine kinase (CK) activity and aldolase have shown that virtually all patients with exertional heat stroke have substantial degrees of rhabdomyolysis. In contrast, rhabdomyolysis of a significant degree is highly unusual in patients with classic heat stroke. In the exertional variety, CK levels ranging up to 1,500,000 IU per liter have been observed. When CK levels are above 20,000 IU per liter severe degrees of disseminated intravascular coagulation, acute renal failure, and potentially dangerous hyperkalemia are very likely to occur. Normal persons who subject themselves to strenuous physical exertion always show an elevated serum CK activity 12 to 24 hours after completing their exercise. If this exercise is conducted in hot weather, the CK release is exaggerated. In exertional heat stroke, since up to 5 percent of muscle CK might be the MB isoezyme it is difficult on the basis of CK isoenzyme analysis alone to determine whether the patient has only skeletal muscle damage or myocardial injury as well. Extensive skeletal muscle damage, with its associated lysosomal destruction, may be responsible for releasing destructive lysosomal enzymes into the circulation that in turn induce widespread capillary injury. Perhaps for this reason, patients with severe heat stroke who also have severe rhabdomyolysis are more apt to develop clinically important disseminated intravascular coagulation, with its associated depletion of coagulation factors and platelets and the danger of extensive hemorrhage. In addition, such patients are also much more likely to develop the acute respiratory distress syndrome with the potential danger of hypoxia. Acute renal tubular necrosis is also much more common. It is mandatory that careful observations of urine flow be made. Continued oliguria despite replacement of volume losses is an ominous sign. It is possible that acute renal failure may be prevented in such patients by early volume replacement in order to re-establish renal perfusion. Nevertheless, there is compelling evidence that certain cellular contents released into the circulation from damaged muscle, such as myoglobin or destructive enzymes or even vasoactive hormones, may all be implicated in acute renal failure. Some authorities advocate the use of a single dose of mannitol, 12.5 to 25 g given as a bolus, in conjunction with a single dose of furosemide, 200 mg intravenously, in an attempt to convert oliguric to a 'normal-output' acute renal failure or prevent its occurrence altogether. If a patient does indeed develop acute renal failure, the likelihood of hyperkalemia and hyperphosphatemia resulting from release of potassium and phosphates from injured skeletal muscle becomes especially important.

DELAYED COMPLICATIONS OF
ACUTE HEAT STROKE

A number of important complications may occur in patients with heat stroke. These are shown in Table 2. The central nervous system appears to be especially sensitive to the effects of hyperthermia, and clinical observations over many years have affirmed that the longer one remains hyperthermic, the more likely one is to develop permanent brain injury. Those areas that appear to be most susceptible to heat injury include the hypothalamus, with ongoing disturbances of thermal regulation, and the cerebellum, with the appearance of dyskinesia, dysmetria, nystagmus, and dysphonia. Such lesions may be compounded by the complicating effects of disseminated intravascular coagulation and bleeding resulting from thrombocytopenia.

Muscle and nerve entrapment are especially likely to occur in patients with exertional heat stroke who have extensive rhabdomyolysis. In severe cases, the existence of a capillary leak, often heralded by otherwise unexplainable hypoalbuminemia, predicts that a large amount of the saline administered during resuscitation will find its way to the interstitial space in skeletal muscle. Three muscle groups, namely, the anterior tibialis, the soleus as it inserts onto the posterior tibia, and the gluteus maximus, appear to be preferred sites for fascial entrapment syndromes. Muscle protein decomposes during the process of rhabdomyolysis in such areas, and because of its osmotic activity, it attracts inflowing water from arterial plasma. The muscle swelling within the enclosed compartment leads to such a rapid rise of compartmental pressure that arterial inflow is shut off. The muscle and any nerve coursing through that vicinity may thereby become damaged as a result of ischemia. In such instances, it is wise to measure tissue pressure and employ fasciotomy if the need exists.

Hypocalcemia of severe magnitude can be seen in patients who have widespread rhabdomyolysis. This apparently results from deposition of calcium salts as the phosphate or carbonate in injured skeletal muscle cells. Values as low as 3.2 mg per deciliter have been observed. Ordinarily, such patients do not demonstrate tetany, probably because the muscle cells are loaded with calcium. Although it is tempting to administer calcium salts to such individuals, they simply deposit in skeletal muscle cells. If the patient survives, calcium salts will be mobilized at a later date, and if excessive calcium salts have been administered, hypercalcemia at that time is a definite risk. It is currently recommended that calcium salts not be given for such hypocalemia. The only justification for giving calcium salts to such patients would be in the management of acute cardiotoxic hyperkalemia.

Hyperkalemia is most likely to occur on the second or third day following the development of acute exertional heat stroke. Acute renal failure in this subclass of heat stroke patients occurs in about 30 percent as compared with 5 percent of patients with classic heat stroke. Thus, hyperkalemia during the convalescent phase is much more common in exertional heat stroke. Because of its anticipation in such cases, it is wise to begin therapy with disodium polystyrene sulfonate early in the course of the illness. If hyperkalemia does occur, treatment with glucose-insulin mixtures or calcium salts may be warranted, especially to counteract the effects of cardiotoxicity. In many instances, hyperkalemia is of such severe magnitude that hemodialysis is required for its relief.

Disseminated intravascular coagulation occurs in virtually all patients with exertional heat stroke and in approximately 30 percent of those with classic heat stroke. In some instances, especially when tissue injury is widespread, it can be life-threatening. Fibrin split products in the blood are identifiable very early. Fibrinogen depletion and thrombocytopenia usually increase in severity during the first 36 to 48 hours. Thereafter, spontaneous improvement is the usual course. Whether treatment with heparin is advisable in patients with acute disseminated intravascular coagulation with heat stroke is a difficult question to answer. In most instances, recovery is spontaneous. However, in some cases in which it is especially severe, heparin treatment might be considered, but with the possibility in mind that further hemorrhage could occur in sites of tissue destruction and vascular damage that exist because of heat damage per se. Fibrinolysis has also been described as a rather unusual finding in patients with exertional heat stroke.

Pancreatitis, identified by elevations of pancreatic enzymes in serum, appears to be a common complication of severe heat stroke, especially the exertional variety. This can be an extremely severe complication. Liver injury in patients with exertional heat stroke may occur and usually becomes evident after several days. Elevation of serum transaminase activity could result from either muscle or liver damage. Complete recovery is the rule.

In general terms, management of patients with severe heat stroke requires good clinical judgment. The physician should be aware that some patients commonly require intensive dialysis therapy. Fluid management must be balanced with the knowledge that the cardiovascular system may be severely injured and as a result, tenuous in its ability to withstand fluid loads. In some parts of the world, there are advocates of plasmapheresis for such ex-

TABLE 2 Delayed Complications of Heat Stroke

Brain damage	Fibrinolysis
Muscle nerve entrapment	Pancreatitis
Hypocalcemia	Liver injury
Hypercalcemia	Oliguria, anuria
Disseminated intravascular coagulation	Acute respiratory distress syndrome

tensively injured patients, based on the experimental evidence that circulating destructive enzymes may be removable by such a procedure. At the present time, this is entirely experimental, and therefore it is not advocated as routine treatment.

Alternative methods to cool patients with heat stroke are under ongoing investigation. One method of treatment that appears to be promising but cumbersome is the use of the Mecca bed. This employs the theory that slow cooling with tepid water and forced air movement to promote vaporization over the body prevents catecholamine release that in turn could reduce the rate of body heat loss. Our experience with this device was that it was large, expensive, and time-consuming, but deserved further study. It cannot be recommended for general use at present.

SUGGESTED READING

Hart GR, Anderson RJ, Crumpler CP, et al. Epidemic classical heat stroke: Clinical characteristics and course of 28 patients. Medicine 1982; 61:189–197.

Knochel JP. Environmental heat illness: an eclectic review. Arch Intern Med 1974; 133:841.

Weiner JS, Khogai MA. Physiological body-cooling unit for treatment of heat stroke. Lancet 1980; 1:507.

BEE, WASP, AND SPIDER ENVENOMATION

PAUL S. AUERBACH, M.D.

Traditionally considered a hazard of field and forest, arthropod envenomations are equally prevalent in the urban environment. Stings by flying and crawling insects are the most common form of human envenomation in the United States, accounting for a predictable number of annual deaths from anaphylaxis. Pathognomonic local and systemic syndromes should alert the informed practitioner to an accurate diagnosis and appropriate current therapy.

HYMENOPTERA (BEES, WASPS, AND FIRE ANTS)

Bees, wasps, and ants are members of the order Hymenoptera. Venomous families that sting humans include the Apidae (honeybees), the Bombidae (bumblebees), the Vespidae (wasps, hornets, and yellowjackets), and the Formicidae (ants). In the United States, domesticated honeybees, feral bumblebees, paper wasps, yellowjackets, and fire ants are the most common attackers. Killer bees (*Apis mellifera adansoni*) are rarely identified in North America. Each of these insects uses a modification of the ovipositor located at the posterior end of the abdomen, which is composed of a stinger connected to a venom reservoir supplied by glands. The venoms are mixtures of protein or polypeptide toxins (e.g., mellitin), enzymes (e.g., hyaluronidase), and pharmacologically active low molecular weight compounds (e.g., histamine). Immune sensitivity is induced by various antigenic proteins.

Stings from bees, wasps, and hornets are generally single, unless an insect nest or swarm is encountered. The honeybee is usually disemboweled after it envenomates the victim and thus inflicts a single sting. Most persons are envenomated outdoors during the warm summer months. The most common site of the sting is the head and neck, followed by the extremities. Unusual locations for stings include the esophagus, cornea, and external ear canal.

A single sting in the unsensitized person causes immediate pain accompanied by erythema and edema. Mild sensitivity is marked by hives, wheezing, malaise, conjunctivitis, rhinitis, fever, and nausea. Severe sensitivity is marked by diffuse urticaria, profound facial swelling and laryngeal edema, bronchospasm, cyanosis, vomiting, abdominal pain, arrhythmias, and hypotension. The risk of a severe reaction is greatest following multiple stings. Persons who are under treatment with beta-adrenergic blocking agents may be at greater risk for more severe reactions, as $beta_1$-blockade interferes with compensatory cardiovascular responses during anaphylaxis and $beta_2$-blockade potentiates alpha-adrenergic activity and opposes $beta_2$-mediated bronchodilatation.

Fire ant (*Solenopsis invicta* and *S. richteri*) stings are often multiple and mark the path traveled by the ant. The insect attaches itself to the victim with its mandible, and then pivots about to attack the victim repeatedly with the 0.5 mm lancet shaped abdominal stinger. The sting is typically intensely painful, with immediate formation of a wheal and, in 18 to 24 hours, a sterile vesicle or pustule, surrounded by an erythematous halo. Delayed transient fibrotic nodules may develop at the vesicle sites.

Treatment

Appropriate first aid for a bee, wasp, or fire ant sting includes the application of a cold compress or ice pack. A topical paste of unseasoned meat tenderizer (papain) may denature elements of the protein bee or wasp venom and provide rapid pain relief. Baking soda is a harmless, but ineffective remedy. Stings or fragments retained in the skin should be scraped off, not removed with forceps. If the honeybee venom sac is grasped and squeezed, retained venom may be injected into the wound, worsening the reaction. The wound should be cleansed and tetanus prophylaxis completed.

Most severe allergic reactions occur within the first 15 to 30 minutes after envenomation, and nearly all occur within 6 hours. Fatalities are related to airway obstruction or hypotension in the majority of cases. Therefore, treatment must be prompt and decisive. At the first indication of serious hypersensitivity, aqueous epinephrine, 1:1000, should be administered subcutaneously. The dose is 0.3 to 0.5 ml in adults and 0.01 ml per kilogram in children. This dosage may be repeated every 20 to 30 minutes as necessary. Aqueous epinephrine by aerosol is not an adequate first aid measure to abort systemic anaphylaxis. In the event that the victim does not respond to subcutaneously administered epinephrine, as manifested by persistent hypotension or profound bronchospasm, the adult patient should receive a 0.1 mg (0.1 ml) bolus of 1:1000 aqueous epinephrine diluted in 10 ml of normal saline infused over 10 minutes (10 μg per min). A mixture for continuous infusion should be prepared by adding 1 mg (1 ml) of 1:1000 aqueous epinephrine to 250 ml of normal saline, to create a concentration of 4 μg per milliliter. This infusion should be started at a rate of 1 μg per minute and increased to 4 μg per minute if the clinical response is inadequate. In children and infants, a mixture for continuous infusion should be prepared by adding 0.5 mg (0.5 ml) of 1:1000 aqueous epinephrine to 100 ml of normal saline, to create a concentration of 5 μg per milliliter. This is followed by an intravenous infusion at a starting dose of 0.1 μg per kilogram per minute up to a maximum of 1.5 μg per kilogram per minute, noting that infusion rates in excess of 0.5 μg per kilogram per minute may be associated with cardiac ischemia and arrhythmias.

The airway should be maintained at all times, utilizing endotracheal intubation or cricothyroidotomy if necessary. High flow supplemental oxygen should be administered to all victims with bronchospasm. Hypotension may necessitate intravenous crystalloid fluid administration and mild dopaminergic pressor agents. In a critical situation, a brief augmentation of blood pressure may be achieved by judicious application of the Military Anti-Shock Trousers (MAST), which contribute to increased systemic vascular resistance.

Antihistamines are of little use in the acute severe reaction but are often useful in lesser envenomations. The dose of diphenhydramine is 50 to 100 mg intravenously, intramuscularly, or orally in an adult and 1 mg per kilogram in a child. In moderate or severe envenomations, an intravenous corticosteroid, such as hydrocortisone, 2 mg per kilogram, should be administered at the earliest opportunity, as the onset of action is delayed by 3 to 6 hours. A 5 to 10 day taper should be employed. If the patient can cooperate, inhalation of nebulized *metaproterenol* may diminish bronchospasm.

Disposition

Any person stung by more than 10 hornets or wasps, or by great numbers of other Hymenoptera species, should be observed in the hospital for 24 hours. This is necessary to identify early complications such as thrombocytopenia, rhabdomyolysis, recurrent hypotension, and acute renal failure. Other indications for admission include intractable vomiting and persistent facial swelling. Any patient who has suffered a severe reaction should be referred to an allergy specialist for consideration for venom desensitization.

SPIDERS

At least 20,000 species of spiders are found in the United States. Because nearly all spiders produce venom, those with fangs capable of human epidermal penetration may envenomate man. The two common species associated with envenomations in the United States are the black widow and brown recluse.

Black Widow Spider

The black widow spider (*Latrodectus mactans*) is found in both the temperate and tropical zones of North and South America. Other related widow spiders found in the United States include *L. hesperus*, *L. variolus*, *L. geometricus*, and *L. bishopi*. The hazardous adult female black widow is shiny and black, 12 to 18 mm long, with a red or yellow-orange hourglass marking on the ventral abdomen. The complex neurotropic venom has its greatest effects at the neuromuscular junction where it both stimulates the release and prevents the reuptake of neurotransmitter substances (acetylcholine and norepinephrine), interrupting normal neurotransmission. The nerve terminal may be directly injured.

Widow spiders are not aggressive unless actively disturbed. Men are bitten more commonly than women, perhaps because of their propensity for recreational outdoor activities. The initial bite is rarely painful and may go unnoticed. A small red puncture wound without tenderness or swelling is common. Ten to 60 minutes following the envenomation, the victim notes painful cramps and local muscle spasm, which in severe cases may centralize and become quite marked, with abdominal rigidity and thoracolumbar pain. Associated symptoms include localized or diffuse paresthesias, headache, dysphagia, hypersalivation, bronchorrhea, nausea, vomiting, fever, diaphoresis, facial edema, ptosis, tachypnea, priapism, seizures, and hypotension or hypertension. Small children and elderly victims most commonly suffer severe reactions. In the untreated patient and in the absence of a hypertensive or respiratory crisis, the symptoms will resolve over 24 to 96 hours.

Treatment

A victim who suffers a moderate or severe envenomation should be treated. Proper first aid includes cleansing the wound, applying an ice pack, and administering appropriate tetanus immunization. Muscle spasm may be controlled with a slow intravenous infusion of 5 to 10 ml (0.1 ml per kilogram in children) of calcium gluconate, repeated every 2 to 4 hours as necessary. An alternate therapy in adults is a slow intravenous infusion of methocarbamol, 1 gram no faster than 100 mg per minute. This does not appear to be as effective as calcium therapy. If calcium is ineffective, diazepam or narcotic agents may be used judiciously to control pain and muscle spasm. The use of dantrolene sodium is as yet anecdotal. Calcium administration generally helps to control hypertension and vomiting. Severe hypertension unresponsive to calcium infusion may require the administration of sodium nitroprusside, nifedipine, labetalol, hydralazine, or diazoxide. Nausea and vomiting unresponsive to calcium infusion should be managed with standard antiemetics (prochlorperazine or trimethobenzamide).

Latrodectus antivenin, an equine serum product, should be used only to manage severe envenomations complicated by uncontrolled hypertension or seizures. Other high risk groups include pregnant females, young children, and elderly victims. Prior to the administration of antivenin, skin testing should be performed to estimate the risk of an anaphylactic reaction. Antivenin is administered in a dose of one ampule (2.5 ml diluted in 10 to 50 ml of normal saline) in a slow intravenous infusion. It is unusual to require more than a single ampule. Patients who receive antivenin should be observed for delayed signs of serum sickness.

Disposition

A victim of a Latrodectus envenomation should be observed in the hospital for a minimum of 8 hours, as recurrent symptoms are common. All infants, children, pregnant women, senior citizens, and severely envenomated persons should be admitted to the hospital for a minimum of 24 hours.

Brown Recluse Spider

The brown recluse spider (*Loxosceles reclusa*) and related species (*L. unicolor, L. deserta, L. arizonica*, and *L. refescens*) reside mainly in the southern United States, with increasing presence in the western states. The brown recluse spider is 9 to 14 mm in body length, brown or reddish brown, with long slender legs and three pairs of eyes. A dark, violin shaped marking ("fiddleback") is present on the dorsal cephalothorax. Both males and females are venomous and dangerous. The venom contains multiple enzyme fractions, including hyaluronidase, cholinesterase, collagenase, desoxyribonuclease, ribonuclease, lipase, esterase, and a number of phospholipases and proteases. The phospholipase sphingomyelinase D binds to cell membranes and initiates an intense inflammatory response with microvascular thrombosis.

Symptoms

The shy spider bites its victim most often when trapped in clothing. The bite may or may not be initially painful. After 1 to 4 hours, a painful red blister develops at the inoculation site, surrounded by a pale ring, with or without a red halo (bull's eye lesion). At this early stage, systemic symptoms may include fever, chills, malaise, nausea, and a local scarlatiniform rash, a clinical picture easily confused with meningococcemia or other infectious emergencies. A severe systemic reaction with laryngospasm, respiratory distress, and hypotension is unusual. After 12 to 16 hours, the bite wound becomes vesiculated with marked edema and the appearance of cellulitis. Profound necrosis (necrotic arachnidism) may ensue over the next 2 to 6 days, accompanied by regional lymphadenitis and prostration. Untreated, the wound becomes an indolent ulcer that may require months to heal, leaving a large tissue defect. Pyoderma gangrenosum is a rare complication.

Children may suffer from intravascular hemolysis, marked by spherocytosis, hemoglobinuria, chills, headache, fever, jaundice, petechiae, and hypotension. Rare deaths are preceded by pulmonary edema, renal failure, and profound coagulopathy.

Treatment

The management of systemic symptoms is supportive. Treatment directed at the local wound has included intralesional injection of corticosteroids, surgical excision, hyperbaric or local oxygen treatment, systemic polymorphonuclear leukocyte inhibitor pharmacotherapy, and the administration of antivenin. The latter two currently appear to constitute the most efficacious early approach to therapy. 4-4-Diaminodiphenylsulfone (dapsone) therapy is recommended as early as possible following the envenomation. The victim should be screened for profound anemia (dapsone can cause bone marrow suppression) and glucose-6-phosphate dehydrogenase (G6PD) deficiency. The initial dose is 25 mg orally twice daily, up to 100 mg per day, until there is no sign of local inflammation (not to exceed 10 days). Side effects include hemolysis in the G6PD-deficient patient, diarrhea, and mild methemoglobinemia. Concomitant corticosteroid administration is of no benefit. Erythromycin or another lipophilic antibiotic should be administered orally for 7 to 10 days. A hyperimmune rabbit serum antivenin has been prepared at Vanderbilt University. The antivenin appears to inhibit the activity of sphingomyelinase D and is most efficacious when injected directly into the wound within 48 hours after the bite. Dapsone and antivenin appear to be more effective in combination.

Surgical wound management should minimize tissue loss. If in spite of dapsone or antivenin therapy the necrotic area attains a diameter of 1 cm, it should be debrided sharply using sterile technique. Daily wound care may include wet-to-dry dressings, hydrophilic beads, or enzymatic debridement. As soon as a healthy granulation tissue bed appears, split thickness skin grafts should be applied. In no case should heat therapy be applied to the lesion.

SUGGESTED READING

Barach EM, Nowak RM, Lee TG, Tomlanovich MC. Epinephrine for treatment of anaphylactic shock. JAMA 1984; 251:2118–2122.

Key GF. A comparison of calcium gluconate and methocarbamol (Robaxin) in the treatment of latrodectism (black widow spider envenomation). Am J Trop Med Hyg 1981; 30:273–277.

King LE Jr, Rees RS. Dapsone treatment of a brown recluse bite. JAMA 1983; 250:648.

King TP, Alagon AC, Kuan J, Sobotka AK, Lichtenstein LM. Immunochemical studies of yellowjacket venom proteins. Molec Immunol 1983; 20:297–308.

Minton SA. Arthropod envenomation. In: Auerbach PS, Geehr EC, eds. Management of wilderness and environmental emergencies. New York: Macmillan, 1983:270.

Rees RS, Altenbern BS, Lynch JB, King LE Jr. Brown recluse spider bites. A comparison of early surgical excision versus dapsone and delayed surgical excision. Ann Surg 1985; 202:659–663.

RADIATION EXPOSURE

HIROSHI NISHIYAMA, M.D.
EUGENE L. SAENGER, M.D.

A radiation accident is defined as an occurrence, either actual or suspected, involving exposure of or contamination on or within humans and the environment by ionizing radiation. Its occurrence is extremely infrequent compared to most types of accidents. The exposed victim is usually asymptomatic shortly after the actual episode. For these reasons, hospital personnel are unfamiliar with the clinical course of radiation injuries. The delay of the onset of symptoms and signs after exposure often is misleading in assessing the level of injury. Tables 2 and 3 serve as ready references for an emergency. Late radiation effects, either from high or low doses, are not discussed here.

TYPES OF RADIATION

Ionizing radiation can cause ionization in atoms or molecules by ejecting electrons from atoms, thereby producing ions. This ionization results in positively charged atoms and negatively charged electrons, which may themselves cause additional ionizations if they are sufficiently energetic. These processes disrupt molecular structures, resulting in cellular injury. Gamma rays and x-rays are forms of electromagnetic waves and are not easily stopped. Beta particles are fast-moving electrons and penetrate tissue up to a range of a few millimeters. Other particles that may be encountered include alphas and neutrons. Alpha particles have very weak penetration ability and are hazardous only when they enter body tissues. Neutrons are produced in abundance in nuclear reactors and around high-energy accelerators. Exposure to neutrons induces radioactivity within the body. The most common element made radioactive is stable sodium, which becomes radioactive sodium 24 with a half-life of 15 hours. This activity is not removable by decontamination measures and can be identified by measurements of half-life or by radioisotopic analysis of its energy.

The unit of absorbed radiation dose commonly used is the rads (radiation absorbed dose), defined as the absorption of 100 erg of energy per gram of matter. Other units are R (roentgen) and rem (roentgen equivalent in man). For most practical purposes in dealing with beta particles, x-rays, and gamma rays, values of exposure in R can be considered essentially and numerically equal to absorbed dose in rads and to dose equivalents in rems. (For the use of the newer SI units, see Addendum.)

In general, the following principles minimize radiation hazards: (1) the farther the distance from the radiation source, the smaller the radiation exposure; (2) the shorter the exposure time, the smaller the radiation exposure; and (3) the denser and thicker the shielding material, the smaller the radiation exposure.

RADIATION SOURCES AND MODES OF EXPOSURE

The identification of facilities where x-rays and radionuclides are either produced or used, the types of radiation sources, and the amounts of activity provide advanced information of what one can expect in the event of an accident. The most frequently encountered radiation sources are listed in Table 1. Group I is found most often in industrial and research facilities. Group II is encountered in both industrial and medical facilities. Sealed sources in Group III are widely used in industry and medicine. The accident most commonly experienced occurs in industrial radiography using sealed sources when the radiographer loses track of the location of the source or when the source becomes loose in open areas or ruptures. Group IV includes the largest number of facilities, but serious accidents are unlikely because of low levels of activity and the use of radionuclides with short half-lives.

There are two types of radiation exposure: (1) from sources external to the body, and (2) from sources incorporated inside the body (Table 1). In the case of external exposure, the radiation is usually distributed nonuniformly. The victim does not emit radiation except after neutron exposure.

Contamination or internal exposure results from radionuclide inhalation, ingestion, injection, or absorption through the skin or mucosa. Here the victim acts as an emitter of radiation. The deposition of radioactive material over the body surface or clothing is termed external contamination and almost always accompanies internal contamination.

BIOLOGIC RESPONSES TO RADIATION EXPOSURE

The degree of injury depends on the dose level, dose rate, type of radiation, sensitivity of the cell type, and the portion of the body and organ systems being exposed (Table 2). The severity of injury is greater when the whole body is exposed as compared to only a portion of the body. An absorbed radiation dose of about 350 to 400 rads is generally expected to result in the death of 50 percent of an untreated population. The LD_{50} can be increased to about 500 to 600 rads with adequate supportive treatment.

In the acute radiation syndrome, the prodromal phase may occur in minutes to a few hours after exposure and is characterized by anorexia, nausea, and vomiting. These symptoms then remit, leading to the relatively asymptomatic latent phase lasting 2 to 3 weeks. This is followed by the manifest illness phase. Clinical and laboratory evidence of hematopoietic damage can be seen after an exposure of about 100 to 1,000 rads. The circulating lymphocytes are one of the most radiosensitive cell lines, and a fall in the absolute lymphocyte count provides a good clue as to the level of radiation exposure in the early phase of observation. Signs and symptoms of marrow depression and immunologic dysfunction appear later, at about 3 weeks. Gastrointestinal injury is usually observed at doses in excess of 1,000 to 1,500 rads and accelerated prodromal and compressed latent phases may be followed by dysentery-like symptoms. The neurovascular injury syndrome occurs in exposures over several thousand rads and is characterized by the immediate onset of severe prodromata leading to vasomotor collapse and death within 1 to 2 days. There is no latent period.

Local radiation injury produced by high doses of gamma rays or x-rays or both produces signs and symptoms similar to those of a thermal burn and is usually not life-threatening (Tables 2 and 3). Clinical manifestations usually develop more slowly than after a thermal burn. Necrotic ulceration resulting from a few thousand rads may become complicated by infection. Epilation can occur when the scalp or other hairy bodily parts are exposed. It occurs at about 14 to 21 days and suggests a skin dose higher than about 300 rads. It also may indicate the direction and distribution of the radiation.

DIAGNOSIS

A careful history should inquire as to the possibility of radiation exposure, its source, and whether the ex-

TABLE 1 Radiation Source and Exposure Mode

Group	Source	External	Contamination	Mixed
I	Critical assembly	Yes	Yes	Yes
	Reactor	Yes	Yes	Yes
	Fuel element manufacture	Yes	Yes	Yes
	Radiopharmaceutical manufacture	Yes	Yes	Yes
II	Particle accelerator	Yes	*	*
	X-ray generator	Yes	No	No
III	Sealed source(intact)	Yes	No	No
	Sealed source (leaking)	Yes	Yes	Yes
IV	Nuclear medicine laboratory	Yes	Yes	Yes
	In vitro assay laboratory	Yes	Yes	Yes

* Neutrons may induce radioactivity within the body. See text.
Transportation accidents are the only ones in which the type of radiation exposure cannot be readily identified a priori.
Responsible authorities should be notified promptly.
The nuclear medicine physician should be notified promptly, as should the consulting radiation physicist.

TABLE 2 Cardinal Clinical Manifestation of Radiation Injury*

Procedure	Finding	Time of Onset	Minimum Exposure (rads)
History	Nausea, vomiting	Within 48 hrs	~100
Physical examination	Erythema	Within hours to days	~300
	Epilation	Within 2–3 weeks	~300
Blood count	Absolute lymphocyte count† <1,000 mm³	Within 24–48 hours	~100
Chromosome	Dicentrics, rings, fragments	Within hours‡	~10
Sperm	<20 million /ml	After 7 weeks	~15

* Adapted from Wald N. Diagnosis and therapy of radiation injuries. Bull NY Acad Med 1983; 59:1129–1138.
† Lymphocytes may decrease within hours. Obtain the baseline count as soon as possible and repeat the count.
‡ Requires 48–72 hours for analysis.

posure was external, internal, or a combination of both. It is safer and more cost-effective to proceed with radiation emergency measures when an accident is suspected rather than waiting for confirmation. All patients suspected of exposure should be surveyed for radioactivity. If found, measures are required to protect attendants and to minimize the spread of radionuclide contamination at the accident site, during transportation of patients, and at the medical facility (Tables 4 and 5). If local surface contamination is found, the proper decontamination measures are to be followed, as shown in Table 6. If there is no external contamination, the noncontaminated patient can be released.

When exposure to radiation is suggested or identified as a possible source of injury, if available, a local radiation physicist (health physicist) can be helpful in evaluating the situation. If one is not available, Table 7

lists major regional resources for consultation. The important information to be assembled includes the type of radiation source, length of exposure, environmental contamination, numbers of patients, and the parts of the body exposed. It is often difficult to determine the absorbed dose immediately following the event, and it is usually not essential for the initial management of the patient.

Treatment should be based on presenting symptoms, signs, and routine laboratory tests pending the availability of dose estimates (see Table 5). The initial symptoms and signs are not specific. Careful observation and repeated laboratory studies are the only means of evaluation until further information is gathered and clinical manifestations become apparent. The most useful single laboratory test to rule out severe injury within the first 48 hours is the absolute lymphocyte count (Fig. 1).

TREATMENT

Radiation exposure can be complicated by trauma. Although life-saving measures should be taken first, consideration should be given to the protection of the support team, so that its level of exposure to contamination does not produce acute radiation injury.

Decontamination

An initial and important consideration in the emergency department is to prevent the spread of radioactivity

TABLE 3   Clinical Manifestation of Local Radiation Injury*

Finding	Time of Onset
Irritation, tenderness, itching	Within 1–2 weeks
Restriction of motion, stiffness	Within 1–2 weeks
Erythema, edema, decreased sensation	Within 1–3 weeks
Bullae, ulcerations	Within 1–4 weeks

*These findings and times of onset may vary.

TABLE 4   Recommended Protective Measures for Treating Personnel

Attendant attire	Surgical cap, mask, gown, gloves, shoe covers and plastic apron. Duplicated gowns and gloves preferred. Tape edges of mask and gloves. Protective clothes for paramedic, i.e., coverall with hood, mask, and gloves.*
Room setting	Isolated room or room away from general emergency area. Turn off air circulation. Tub or table with drainage system. Containers for waste water and any contaminated materials. Plastic bags are useful.
Survey meter	Geiger-Mueller counter with beta and gamma detection capability usually suffices. Check working condition. A full scale meter deflection indicates a high exposure rate and a high range instrument (ion chamber) may be required. Survey about 1 inch away by moving no faster than 2 inches per second or back-and-forth movement.
Personal dosimeter	Film badge or thermoluminescent dosimeter. Attendant exposure should be limited to less than about 25 rads.

* Paramedic and ambulance should be surveyed for contamination before their release.

TABLE 5   Initial Patient Contamination Survey and Laboratory Test

	Recommendation
External contamination	Cotton swabs for skin, nostrils, ear canals, wound, or any contaminated object. Each swab should be placed in a labeled test tube for counting.
Internal contamination	Radionuclides may be in the blood or excreted in the feces or urine. Excreta in appropriate containers and blood sample in test tube for counting.
All exposed	Routine CBC with differential, absolute lymphocyte count, and platelet counts.
Other	For those who were heavily exposed or are suspected of heavy contamination, identify existing infection and organisms. Cultures from skin, nose, mouth, urine, vagina, and stool are considered.

Every specimen should have clearly written name, type of specimen, time obtained, and date.
Aseptic technique for venous puncture should be observed.

TABLE 6   Recommended Decontamination Procedure

External Contamination

Material	Lukewarm water, soap, or ordinary detergent, soft brush, sponges, plastic sheet, tape, towel, sheet, stable isotope if known and available, equipment and material for ordinary emergency care.
Procedural priority	Remove entire clothing and place in plastic bags. Life-saving measures first. Identify contaminated areas, mark clearly, and cover until decontamination measures take place. Start decontamination from the wound when present and move on to the highest contaminated area.
Wound	Irrigate the wound with normal saline repeatedly. Surgical debridement might be considered in some instances. Eyes and ears may be irrigated gently with isotonic saline solution.
Local	Cover uncontaminated area with plastic sheet and tape edges. Soak, gently scrub with soap, and rinse thoroughly. Repeat the cycle by noting activity changes. One cycle needs no longer than about 2–3 minutes. Avoid vigorous scrubbing. A stable isotope solution may facilitate the process.
Extensive	Shower for the patient who is not seriously injured. Bathing on the operating table or stretcher for the seriously injured patient. Soak-scrub-rinse cycle should also be observed.
End point	Radionuclide activity is no longer detectable or is not decreasing.
Preventive measure	Cover areas still contaminated with plastic sheet and tape edges. Gloves can be used for hands. Repeat washings after some rest to the skin.

Internal Contamination

Principle	Dilution, blocking, chelation, mobilization, and elimination of the contaminant.
Inhalation	Irrigate nasopharynx and mouth.
Ingestion	Cathartics for insoluble materials. Diuresis by forcing fluids for soluble contaminants.

Figure 1   Schematic relationships between absolute lymphocyte level and clinical injury as estimated in the first 2 days after exposure. (From Andrews GA, Auxier JA, Lushbaugh CC. The importance of dosimetry to the medical management of persons accidentally exposed to high levels of radiation. In: Personnel Dosimetry for Radiation Accidents. Vienna: International Atomic Energy Agency, 1965.)

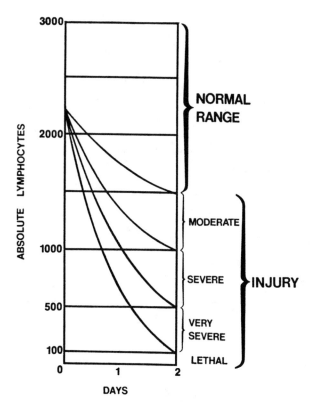

TABLE 7 Major Sources of Consultation in Radiation Emergencies

E. L. Saenger Radioisotope Laboratory
ML #577
University of Cincinnati Hospital
Cincinnati, Ohio 45267-0577
(513) 872-4282
Attn: Eugene L. Saenger, M.D.

University of Pittsburgh
Department of Radiation Health
Presbyterian-University Hospital
Pittsburgh, Pennsylvania 15261
(412) 647-3495
Attn: Niel Wald, M.D.

REAC/TS
Oak Ridge Associated Universities
P.O. Box 117
Oak Ridge, Tennessee 37830
(615) 576-3131
Attn: Robert Ricks, Ph.D.

Radiation Management Corporation
University City Science Center
3508 Market Street
Philadelphia, Pennsylvania 19104
(215) 243-2955
Attn: Roger E. Linnemann, M.D.

REMS Corporation
3004 La Mancha Street
Albuquerque, New Mexico 87104
(505)243-0236
Attn: Fred A. Mettler, M.D.

U.S. Nuclear Regulatory Commission Regional Offices

Region 1
(Maine, Vermont, New Hampshire, Massachusetts, Rhode Island, Connecticut, New York, Pennsylvania, New Jersey, Delaware, Maryland, District of Columbia)

631 Park Avenue
King of Prussia, Pennsylvania 19406
(215) 337-5000

Region 2
(West Virginia, Virginia, Kentucky, Tennessee, North Carolina, South Carolina, Georgia, Alabama, Mississippi, Florida)

101 Marietta Street
Suite 3100
Atlanta, Georgia 30303
(404) 221-4503

Region 3
(Ohio, Indiana, Michigan, Illinois, Wisconsin, Minnesota, Iowa, Missouri)

799 Roosevelt Road
Glen Ellyn, Illinois 60137
(312) 790-5500

Region 4
(North Dakota, South Dakota, Nebraska, Kansas, Oklahoma, Arkansas, Louisiana, Texas, Montana, Wyoming, Colorado, New Mexico, Idaho, Utah)

611 Ryan Plaza Drive
Suite 1000
Arlington, Texas 76012
(817) 334-2841

Region 5
(Washington, Oregon, California, Nevada, Arizona)

1990 North California Boulevard
Suite 202
Walnut Creek, California 94956
(415) 943-3700

U.S. Department of Energy Regional Coordinating Offices for Radiological Assistance

Region 1
(Maine, Vermont, New Hampshire, Massachusetts, New York, Rhode Island, Pennsylvania, Connecticut, New Jersey, Delaware, Maryland, District of Columbia)

Brookhaven Area Office
Upton, New York 11973
(516) 282-2200

Region 2
(West Virginia, Virginia, Kentucky, Tennessee, Missouri, Arkansas, Mississippi, Louisiana, Puerto Rico, Virgin Islands)

Oak Ridge Operations Office
P.O. Box E
Oak Ridge, Tennessee 37830
(615) 576-1005 or 525-7885

Region 3
(North Carolina, South Carolina, Georgia, Alabama, Florida, Panama Canal Zone)

Savannah River Operations Office
P.O. Box A
Aiken, South Carolina 29801
(803) 725-3333

Region 4
(Kansas, Oklahoma, Texas, New Mexico, Arizona)

Albuquerque Operations Office
P.O. Box 5400
Albuquerque, New Mexico 87115
(505) 844-4667

Region 5
(Ohio, Indiana, Michigan, Illinois, Wisconsin, Minnesota, Iowa, North Dakota, South Dakota, Nebraska)

Chicago Operations Office
9800 South Cass Avenue
Argonne, Illinois 60439
(312) 972-4800 (duty hours) or
972-5731 (off hours)

Region 6
(Montana, Wyoming, Colorado, Idaho, Utah)

Idaho Operations Office
P.O. Box 2108
Idaho Falls, Idaho 83401
(208) 526-1515

Region 7
(California, Nevada, Hawaii)

San Francisco Operations Office
1333 Broadway
Oakland, California 94612
(415) 273-4237

Region 8
(Washington, Oregon, Alaska)

Richland Operations Office
P.O. Box 550
Richland, Washington 99352
(509) 376-7381

and provide for appropriate decontamination (see Table 6). Prior notification of the arrival of a potentially contaminated patient is a great aid in preparation. If *wounds* are contaminated, decontamination should be carried out with repeated saline irrigation. Surgical debridement may be considered to remove embedded and highly hazardous contaminants. Absorption of the radionuclide, especially when in ionic or other soluble form, is very rapid when capillary networks are directly exposed. Similarly, abraded skin provides little protection from radionuclide absorption. Nasal and buccal mucosae are other ready entry points of radionuclides, and gentle nasal or oral irrigation with isotonic solutions may reduce the level of contamination and absorption.

The recommended procedure for *local surface contamination* is to cover the surrounding uncontaminated area with a plastic sheet, tape its edges, and then wash the area with soap or detergent. The contaminated surface should be blotted dry. After each rinsing of the exposed surface, the wash solution, and the sponges should be measured to determine the success of removal. The procedure should then be repeated. In practice, the initial two to three washings usually eliminate most of the contamination. Gentle scrubbing with soap or detergent followed by rinsing and repeat cycles is the most practical and effective approach. The recommended scrubbing time of 3 to 4 minutes and a thorough rinsing of 2 to 3 minutes are much too long. Abrasion of the skin by vigorous scrubbings or shaving should absolutely be avoided. An end point of the decontamination procedure is when the radionuclide activity is no longer detectable or no longer decreasing. Plunging the victim into a bathtub or sending him or her into the shower room as an initial measure is not recommended, since such steps spread contamination to clean areas. Note that fingertips, hair, nostrils, and ear canals are regions where decontamination is more difficult. Clipping nails facilitates the process, and cutting or shaving the hair may be considered when shampooings do not sufficiently remove the contaminant. Recommended measures of covering the still contaminated area with a plastic sheet with taped edges minimizes spread of contamination. Producing sweating in extremities by covering them with plastic or rubber gloves overnight may be helpful.

In the case of *ingestion*, mild cathartics shorten the intestinal passage time. Gastric lavage or emesis may also be considered. The bulk of solid foods are emptied from the stomach into the intestine by 2 hours, and clearance of liquid is much faster. Other drugs such as antacids, other cathartics, and chelating agents may be of value, as determined by the chemical form of the contaminant.

External Radiation

The severity of prodromal symptoms and signs is a function of the radiation dose. Patients in the emergency department who manifest nausea and vomiting should be treated symptomatically and should be followed based on daily blood counts. The victim who received only external radiation of less than 100 rads can be released if the dose estimate and laboratory tests (absolute lymphocyte count) seem appropriate. If doses higher than 100 to 150 rads are suspected, the patient should be observed carefully for potentially serious infection.

At this point in the course of the acute radiation syndrome, consideration should be given to the temporal sequence of events. Except in cases of massive exposure, more than 500 to 2,000 rads of total body exposure, the latent period of 2 to 3 weeks permits time to consider whether vigorous therapy is needed. Expert consultation can be obtained prior to the start of elaborate procedures. Cultures of regions of pre-existing infections should be carried out. Existing organisms from skin, nose, mouth, urine, vagina, and stool should be cultured and identified.

Later Consideration

It may be desirable to follow the patient in a facility where a sterile environment is available. At least reverse isolation should be provided. A room with laminar flow may be needed. Prophylactic antibiotics for bacterial and fungal infection should be considered when the granulocyte count falls below 1,500 per mm³. Cultures should be repeated. Scrupulous nursing care to maintain body cleanliness is recommended. Blood cultures should follow when a fever of over 101 °F develops. Since the care is directed at preventing the consequences of agranulocytosis and loss of immune competence, help from a hematologist or oncologist is valuable. Infusion of supplemental white blood cells and platelets can be considered for documented gram-negative sepsis in the presence of depressed bone marrow. White blood cells and platelets should not be used prophylactically. Sterile techniques are mandatory to avoid introduction of infection.

Addendum

These units are now being replaced by the SI (International System of Units) units used elsewhere in medicine and science. The rad now becomes the gray ($=100$ rads) and the rem becomes the sievert ($=100$ rems). The curie is replaced ty the becquerel ($=1$ disintegration per second).

Suggested Reading

NCRP Report No. 65. Management of persons accidentally contaminated with radionuclides. National Council on Radiation Protection and Measurements (NCRP), 7910 Woodmont Avenue, Bethesda, MD 20815, 1980.

Saenger EL, Andrews GA, Linneman RE, Wald N. Radiation accident preparedness—medical and managerial aspects. An audio-visual self-instruction course. New York: Science-Thru-Media, 1982.

Wald N. Diagnosis and therapy of radiation injuries. Bull NY Acad Med 1983; 59:1129–1138.

ELECTRICAL INJURY

MARY ANN COOPER, M.D., F.A.C.E.P

Electrical injuries account for between 800 and 1,000 deaths per year with nearly five times that number suffering injury. They account for 4 percent of burn unit admissions. Proper emergency department and pre-hospital care is essential to decrease the morbidity and mortality often associated with these injuries.

PATHOPHYSIOLOGY

Electrical injuries may be due to high voltage (greater than 1,000 volts) or low voltage (less than 1,000 volts). There are six factors that combine to determine the severity and character of the injury: type of circuit (alternating or direct current), duration of current exposure, voltage, amperage, resistance of the tissue through which the current passes, and the pathway of the current.

Alternating current is nearly three times more damaging than direct current of the same magnitude. This is partly because the 60 Hz current that is used in the United States is within the frequency range necessary to produce muscle tetany, which may lengthen the duration of exposure to the current if the hand, which is the most frequent entry point, is forced into a tetanic grip around an object that is in contact with the current. The longer the victim is in contact with the current, the worse the injury will be.

High-voltage injuries are almost always severe in nature, often leading to amputation of the digit or extremity. These injuries are often accompanied by cardiac arrest, severe burns, and myoglobinuria. Low-voltage injuries, particularly in the 110 to 220 volt range, seldom leave burns and may require little or no therapy after the initial screening for more serious accompanying problems such as cardiac arrhythmias.

The type of injury that can be expected varies with the resistance of the tissue through which the current passes (Table 1), with nerve tissue being the least and bone being the most resistant. Current passes most easily through nerves, blood, and muscle, often causing injury to these tissues, including destruction of nerves, permanent paresthesias, thrombosis of vessels, ischemia of tissue distal to the thrombotic vessel, and direct muscle damage with myoglobin release. Renal failure may occur owing to myoglobinuria unless proper fluid resuscitation is begun in the field and continued in the emergency department.

Resistance to the passage of electric current into the body is primarily provided by the skin. The amount of damage that is done to the skin and the underlying structures depends on the moisture content, cleanliness, and thickness of the skin. The thicker the skin or callus, the worse will be the burn, but the less energy will get into the deeper tissues, in general, as the energy of the current dissipates itself burning through the surface of the skin. When the skin is wet with sweat or bath water, the resistance of the skin is so lowered that no external burns may be present, but the patient may be dead from cardio-pulmonary arrest because all of the energy was delivered internally to such vulnerable structures as the heart or brain stem. The pathway that the energy takes is also important to the type of injury and complications that the physician may expect. If as little as 50 to 100 milliamperes is delivered to the heart, cardiac arrest may occur. Nearly every type of arrhythmia and block pattern has been reported with electrical injuries, as have S-T changes consistent with myocardial ischemia and damage. Respiratory arrest may also occur if the current passes through the respiratory center in the brain stem. Seizures can be expected if the current passes through the brain or as a result of hypoxia from an arrest. Electrical cataracts may occur if current passes anywhere above the shoulders of the patient.

DIFFERENTIAL DIAGNOSIS

High-voltage injuries are usually obvious from both appearance and history. However, occasionally low-voltage injuries may have no burns accompanying them and may be confused with cardiac arrhythmias from other causes, overdose, suffocation, or intracranial hemorrhage or trauma.

PRE-HOSPITAL TREATMENT

Pre-hospital therapy cannot be started until the victim is freed from the current source and the scene is secured so that none of the rescuers or bystanders becomes an additional victim. The best way to free a victim from the current is to *let the power company turn off the power.* Most of the ways touted to remove a victim from the current are not safe, particularly with higher voltages. One cannot tell the voltage of a line by where it is located or by how big it is, nor should one be fooled into thinking that the insulation on the wire is protection. The material coating electrical lines is used for protection of the line from environmental insults, not for protecting people.

After the victim and scene are both secure, the rescuers should assess the airway, breathing, and circulation (ABCs), initiating cardiopulmonary resuscitation (CPR), if indicated. Routine ACLS protocols are used, except that normal saline or Ringer's lactate is used as

TABLE 1   Resistance to Current Flow

Least resistant	Nerve
	Blood
	Muscle
	Skin
Most resistant	Tendon
	Fat
	Bone

the resuscitation fluid because of the shock that is so often present. Cardiac monitoring should be done, if possible, even in the apparently stable patient. In addition to assessing the ABCs, the rescuer must be aware that blunt injuries, including spinal and head trauma may be present. Treatment of burns should consist of fluid replacement, covering of the wounds with sterile dry sheets and dressings, and slight elevation of damaged extremities, if possible. The "Rule of Nines" cannot be used for evaluating the amount of fluid needed, because the external burn is often the only visible part of a much more extensive injury. Treatment of other life-threatening conditions, such as seizures, may be done in the routine fashion.

EMERGENCY DEPARTMENT ASSESSMENT

In the emergency department, the emergency physician should continue the therapy begun in the field and augment it with appropriate laboratory tests, drug therapy, and referral. The patient should be completely undressed and searched for signs of both burns and blunt injuries such as dislocations and fractures. Evaluation for spinal and head injuries should take a high priority. One must look for blunt injuries, because the victim may have fallen, been thrown by the force of the tetanic contraction, or had dislocations caused by the tetanic contraction of muscle around a joint. One must also look for exit burns in addition to entry burns, both of which may be multiple. The most common entry points are the hands and skull, and the most common exit points are the feet. The burns encountered with high-voltage electrical injuries are often very deep and severe and extend into the underlying tissues. In addition, the path of damage cannot be predicted from merely looking at the entry and exit points but may involve distant sites. Extensive debridement is often necessary. Between the burn edema and the thrombosis caused by damage to the walls of the vessels, distal ischemia and compartment syndromes are common with electrical injuries and are sometimes delayed from hours to days after the injury itself. Shock may be severe, from either cardiac arrest, burns, or release of toxic breakdown products into the bloodstream by the burned tissues.

An early baseline neurologic evaluation should be done in the emergency department because this is one of the areas that can change most rapidly and negatively for the patient. Normally the mental status of the victim continues to improve after the injury. If the level of central nervous system function deteriorates, a primary head injury or spinal injury should be ruled out with a computed tomography (CT) scan. Seizures are treated as any traumatic seizure would be.

The peripheral nervous system should be evaluated as well as the vascular status of the extremities, because this is a common area of deterioration as compartment syndromes, burn edema, and ischemia of tissues distal to thrombosed and damaged vessels develop. Fasciotomies may be needed to save as much tissue as possible in these cases. Carpal tunnel release is often indicated when the hand is involved.

A nasogastric tube should be placed in the severely burned individual. Burn ileus is common. However, if the ileus continues for more than 2 days, intra-abdominal injury should be suspected. Urinary catheterization is probably mandatory in the severely burned patient in order to monitor urinary output as well as the presence of myoglobinuria.

Eventually, an ophthalmologic evaluation should be done of those with injuries close to the face, because electrical cataracts are common; these may occur as late as 2 years after the accident.

Cases of electrical injuries almost always end up in court, either as a workman's compensation case or as a suit against a power company. Thus, clear, complete records often keep the physician from having to appear in court to document the injuries.

Laboratory tests should include an electrocardiogram, cardiac isoenzymes, complete blood count, baseline creatinine and blood urea nitrogen for later urinary function monitoring, urinalysis for myoglobin (which must be specifically requested), and other examinations as appropriate to the patient's injury severity including amylase, electrolytes, glucose, arterial blood gases (both to monitor the blood pH for use of bicarbonate therapy for myoglobinuria as well as for ventilatory status), and typing and crossmatching if extensive surgery and debridement are anticipated.

X-ray studies usually include cervical spine, chest, and other x-rays as indicated by the patient's areas of injury. As mentioned above, use of the CT scan may be indicated for the patient in whom intracranial injury is suspected. Monitoring should include cardiac monitoring for at least the first 24 hours in all but the most minor injuries, urine output for extensive burns or those with shock or myoglobinuria, central invasive monitoring for those patients in shock, and other monitoring as indicated by injuries (e.g., intracranial monitoring for those with intracranial injuries).

EMERGENCY DEPARTMENT TREATMENT

After initial assessment and stabilization, treatment of the burns includes cleansing, debridement of necrotic tissue, tetanus prophylaxis, and neurovascular checks of the extremities. Clostridial myositis is often seen with electrical injuries owing to the destruction of deep structures. Thus, tetanus prophylaxis should often include the use of human immune globulin or tetanus immune globulin (Hyper-Tet). Although silver sulfadiazine (Silvadene) is the drug most often chosen for most burns, mafenide, acetate (Sulfamylon) is preferred in most centers for electrical injuries because of its much deeper penetration of eschar. Use of prophylactic antibiotics varies with the institution and the extent of the burn. Most centers use at least penicillin initially. Repeated debridements over a period of several days may be necessary before viable graft sites may be obtained. The patient should be stabilized prior to any surgery, if possible. On rare occasions, especially when massive tissue damage has occurred, the release of toxic materials into the bloodstream may preclude stabilization until amputation or extensive debridement is performed.

The patient may be in profound shock from several causes, including major trauma and blunt injury, burn shock, release of toxic materials into the bloodstream from the burned tissue, and cardiac decompensation and hypoxia. Fluid resuscitation should be aggressive, both to combat the shock and to flush out the myoglobin released from the damaged muscles. If myoglobinuria is present, intravenous fluids should be run at levels sufficient to maintain a urine output of 1.0 to 1.5 cc per kilogram per hour. If myoglobinuria is not present, urine output should be maintained at 0.5 to 1.0 cc per kilogram per hour. A quick, presumptive test for myoglobinuria is to use a urine dipstick. If it is positive for blood but no red cells are seen when the urine is spun down, myoglobin can be presumed to be present. Of course, myoglobinuria is obvious when the urine is pigmented the typical wine or brown color. Myoglobin is cleared better if the urine is alkalinized. This is usually done by using one ampule of bicarbonate per liter of resuscitation fluid with careful monitoring of the blood pH to maintain it at 7.35 or above. Some institutions use mannitol or furosemide to enhance renal flow in the face of myoglobinuria.

For the victim with cardiac arrest CPR may be continued as judged feasible by the emergency physician. However, there is no evidence for the myth of "suspended animation" that is mentioned in some texts in discussing electrical injuries as a reason for prolonged CPR. Standard cardiac medications and dosages are used, as with an ordinary arrest, and standard therapy is established for the arrhythmias that any patient may suffer with electrical injuries. The only differences are that a resuscitation fluid of normal saline or Ringer's lactate is used to combat shock instead of dextrose and water.

ADMISSIONS, REFERRALS, AND DISCHARGE

Most patients with electrical injuries should be admitted. Most have severe burns, and they need cardiac monitoring for at least 24 hours because although most arrhythmias occur within the first few minutes of the injury, they have been reported as long as 24 hours after the injury. Many of these patients can be treated in the same manner as a rule-out myocardial infarction patient, using cardiac enzymes and cardiac monitoring. Their hospitalization should also include neurovascular checks of all extremities, including the ones that appear to be uninjured. If burns occur near the abdomen, intraabdominal injuries should be ruled out by frequent abdominal examinations.

The victim of a severe high-voltage electrical injury should have a trauma team approach with the management of the patient done on a long-term basis by a coordinated team. The victim should be referred to a burn center that is capable of providing not only the surgeons, the physical therapists, and other specialists that the patient will need, but also the psychological support and intervention that is necessary. These injuries can be extremely devastating, with the patient not only suffering major amputations but also changes in body image and self-image, loss of ability to continue his occupation, and major changes in family dynamics sometimes leading to divorce. Less severe burns may be handled by a surgeon (or hand surgeon if the case involves the hand, as is so often the case) on an outpatient basis if he is familiar with electrical burns and comfortable with the idea based on the history, physical examination, and the likelihood that the patient will follow up on his own care.

SPECIAL CASES

There are some special cases in which the patient may be treated differently from the typical patient with severe electrical injury. These include the victims of low voltage (up to 220 V) and children who have been chewing on electric cords. The patient with low-voltage injury may be treated as an outpatient, but only if he is completely oriented, is free of pain (especially chest pain), and has no external burns. Most of the time this therapy is enough if it includes cautioning the patient to return if he feels any palpitations or muscle pain or becomes disoriented. However, there are rare cases of arrhythmias occurring after apparently mild injury, so it is necessary to obtain a very good history and appropriate documentation, including an electrocardiogram, cardiac enzymes, and urinalysis for myoglobin.

The toddler who has been chewing on an electric cord has what appears to be severe burns about the mouth, but otherwise appear perfectly normal and alert. Usually child abuse or neglect is not a problem with this kind of patient, but the physcian should be alert to that possibility. Although these patients need the same evaluation as the patient with low-voltage injuries, the real danger is not in the first few days, but later when the eschar begins to separate and leaves the labial artery exposed, accounting for significant bleeding in about 10 percent of patients. Some centers prefer to admit such patients until the eschar separates. The other problem is long term, with scarring of the mouth, especially when the commissure is affected. These patients should be referred to an oral surgeon with experience with electrical burns so that appropriate debridement and splinting can be done. The splints, which are used to keep the scar from contracting the size of the mouth, are often worn continuously for 3 to 6 months and then only at night for another 3 to 6 months.

SUGGESTED READING

Artz CP, Moncrief JA. The treatment of burns. 2nd ed. Philadelphia: WB Saunders, 1969.
Butler ED, Grant TD. Electrical injuries with special reference to the upper extremity. Annals of Surg 1977; 134:95–101.
Hunt JL, Sato RM, Baxter CK. Acute electric burns. Arch Surg 1980; 115:434–438.
Larson TH. Splinting oral electrical burns in children. J Dent Child 1977; 44:382–384.

LIGHTNING INJURY

MARY ANN COOPER, M.D., F.A.C.E.P.

Lightning injuries account for nearly 1,000 injuries per year in the United States, of which 25 to 30 percent are fatal. Lightning injuries are markedly different than other forms of electrical injury and require different therapy. They occur most commonly in the South, along the Atlantic seaboard, and in the Midwest, and most frequently during the summer thunderstorm months when farmers, sportsmen, and campers are outside and susceptible to being struck.

ETIOLOGY AND PATHOPHYSIOLOGY

The same six factors that affect electrical injuries determine the kind of injury that a lightning victim suffers: type of circuit (alternating versus direct current), resistance of the tissues through which the current passes, voltage, amperage, duration of exposure, and pathway taken by the current.

However, these six factors interact in such a complicated way and their values are so different from those of electrical injuries that the type of injury normally found in lightning victims is unique. The type of circuit with lightning is, for all practical medical purposes, direct current, which is less dangerous than the alternating current most commonly found with high- and low-voltage electrical injuries. The resistance of the tissues is, of course, the same as with electrical injuries. The voltage and amperage found with lightning is tremendously higher than found with electrical injuries, but the two factors that make the most difference in the way that lightning affects the human victim are the last two: duration of exposure and pathway taken by the current. The duration of a lightning strike is normally 0.1 to 1 msec, so short that the current does not have time to burn through the skin and cause any significant internal flow of current. Thus, no significant burns are usually seen with the victim of lightning. In addition, because the duration is so short, very little energy actually gets delivered to the person, despite the incredibly high voltage and amperage. Because lightning does not break down the skin, the energy flashes over the outside of the person rather than going through the victim's core. Of course, a small amount of energy may leak internally, sometimes causing cardiac arrest and short-circuiting of the body's other electrical systems. This can result in temporary deafness, blindness, confusion, amnesia, loss of consciousness, vessel spasm, and so forth.

Because the pathway and duration are usually so different, victims of lightning seldom show the types of injuries found with high-voltage electrical injuries. Lightning deaths occur primarily from cardiac arrest or its sequelae and seldom from anything else.

DIFFERENTIAL DIAGNOSIS

The victim of lightning injury may be confused with victims of other etiologies, including cardiac arrhythmias, myocardial infarction, intracranial hemorrhage, seizure, heavy metal poisoning, and head and spinal cord injuries. The important differentiating factor is the history of a thunderstorm in the area, the report of witnesses, tympanic membrane rupture, or the destruction of the victim's clothing (the sweat or rainwater on the skin may turn to steam and blow the clothes apart).

PRE-HOSPITAL THERAPY

It is not uncommon to have multiple victims of a single lightning incident. In that case, the pre-hospital care personnel may be faced with serious triage decisions. Because the major cause of death is cardiac arrest, anyone who is moaning, rolling around, or showing other signs of life usually survives, often without permanent deficit, and may be quickly assessed and prevented from doing any further damage to himself. The sequence of events with the arrested victim seems to be that he suffers, in effect, a cosmic defibrillation, sending his heart into temporary standstill. Because these victims are often young and otherwise healthy, their hearts usually start up a rhythm again. However, the respiratory arrest is often not as quick to recover, leading to hypoxia and sometimes a second arrest. There is the potential that, if the rescuer can oxygenate the patient during this period, the secondary arrest may be averted.

Therapy of lightning victims in the pre-hospital care phase should include assessment of the airway, circulation, and breathing (ABCs) and initiation of cardiopulmonary resuscitation (CPR) or ACLS, if indicated. All patients should be placed on a cardiac monitor, have intravenous fluids started (usually dextrose and water unless there are other causes of shock present), and have any fractures or dislocations splinted. In some cases, the victim may have been thrown a distance, so spinal precautions should be taken. Blunt injuries seem to be rare. The rescuer should suspect that the patient may be hypothermic if he was exposed to a rainstorm. Transient hypertension and paralysis, especially of the lower extremities, from vascular instability, spasm, and sympathetic nervous system short-circuiting may be present but usually resolve without treatment.

EMERGENCY DEPARTMENT THERAPY

Cardiac monitoring and resuscitation should be continued at the emergency physician's discretion. *Examination* of the tympanic membranes is often overlooked, but it should always be done because over 50 percent of victims have at least one tympanic membrane ruptured. Cataracts may also occur with lightning injuries, so that a baseline look at the eyes is also a good idea.

Laboratory tests that should be done include electrocardiogram, cardiac isoenzymes, urinalysis for myoglobin, complete blood count, and baseline creatinine and blood urea nitrogen. X-ray studies should include the cervical spine as well as other spinal films as indicated by history or physical examination. To rule out intracranial trauma, the physician may want to get a computed tomography (CT) scan of the head if the patient does not seem to be recovering.

Treatment of lightning victims who have not undergone cardiac arrest is generally supportive, expectant, and based on common sense. Fluid loading is contraindicated if the patient does not have deep burns. Fasciotomies and escharotomies are rarely, if ever, needed.

Although a few cases of survival after prolonged resuscitation have been reported, there is no reason to believe in the myth of "suspended animation" occurring from lightning injuries that is sometimes mentioned in older texts. Standard ACLS and cardiac drug administration may be used unless the patient is found to be hypothermic, in which case hypothermia protocols should be followed. As mentioned before, the burns seen with high-voltage electrical injuries are seldom seen with lightning injuries. However, if they are present, they should be treated in the same fashion (see chapter on *Electrical Injury*). Tetanus prophylaxis is a must if the skin is broken. Myoglobinuria has rarely been reported but should be assessed. If it is present, fluid loading, alkalinization of the urine, and use of mannitol and furosemide may be indicated. Burns, when present, are generally very superficial and the result of the sweat and rainwater on the patient turning into steam. The resulting first- and second-degree burns occur along sweat lines or under metal objects such as jewelry or coins that are heated. Fine, lacy marks may appear transiently on the skin of some lightning victims but are not burns and do not seem to break the integrity of the skin.

Frequently the victim of lightning initially has transient hypertension, which need not be treated. He may also present with paralysis, particularly of the lower extremities, with blue, cold, mottled, pulseless legs or arms. This seems to be due to vascular spasm and sympathetic instability from the short-circuiting of the nervous system by the lightning strike, and it usually passes within a few hours. Almost all patients exhibit amnesia about the event, loss of short-term anterograde memory for several days, and confusion. Many have experienced loss of consciousness.

The patient should be monitored for arrhythmias for the first 24 hours, although they are rare. If the patient is in shock or recovering from an arrest, central monitoring may be indicated as well as monitoring of urine output. Intracranial pressure monitoring may be indicated if there is any evidence of increased intracranial pressure.

Admission, Referral, and Discharge

Most patients should be monitored for the first 24 hours. Referral is customarily made to a surgeon or internist. Other referrals should be made as indicated by the patient's other injuries (e.g., orthopaedic, tympanic membrane rupture).

SUGGESTED READING

Apfelberg et al. Pathophysiology and treatment of lightning injuries. J Trauma 1974; 14:453–460.
Bartholomew et al. Cutaneous manifestations of lightning injury. Arch Dermatol 1975; 111:1466–1468.
Bergstrom et al. The lightning damaged ear. Arch Otolaryngol 1974; 100:117–121.
Cooper MA. Prognostic signs for death in patients seriously injured by lightning. Ann Emerg Med 1980; 9:134–139.

HIGH-ALTITUDE ILLNESS

GARRETT FOULKE, M.D.

Many high-altitude visitors develop acute mountain sickness or other more severe forms of altitude-related illness (ARI). If they go untreated, the more severe conditions can be rapidly fatal. The most successful therapeutic efforts in ARI are preventive measures and prophylactic therapy. Once an altitude-related condition has developed, the key to successful therapy is rapid recognition. Table 1 summarizes high-altitude-related conditions.

The falling barometric pressure from increases in altitude produces *hypoxemia*. This hypoxemia caused by altitude is exacerbated by exercise or ventilatory depression during sleep. Arterial O_2 saturation falls sharply during exercise at high altitude. The normally mild fall in oxygen saturation with sleep at sea level is much more pronounced at high altitude. The periodic breathing (Cheyne-Stokes type respirations) that occurs with sleep at high altitude also worsens the oxygen desaturation. Increased ventilation stimulated by hypobaric hypoxia produces hypocarbia and respiratory alkalosis. The respiratory alkalosis initially inhibits maximal stimulation. During the first few days at high altitude, renal compensation partly corrects this alkalosis, resulting in increased ventilatory drive.

Hypoxia results in pulmonary vasoconstriction and increased pulmonary artery pressures. A hypoxic chemoreceptor reflex produces vasoconstriction in the skeletal muscle and splanchnic beds. Local hypoxic effects produce coronary and cerebral vasodilation. There is a distinct increase in cerebral blood flow at high altitude, which is attenuated by hypocarbia. The hypocarbia that occurs at high altitudes provides a "balancing" effect by acting as a stimulus to cerebral vasoconstriction. Additional physiologic alterations that occur at high altitude include an early tendency to intravascular volume loss (from increased ventilatory insensible loss as well as other forces) and increased renin production, with a tendency to fluid retention during more prolonged exposure. Fluid retention and peripheral edema often occur after several days to a week at high altitude and are most frequent when strenuous exercise is undertaken.

The stresses of the high altitude environment produce a number of *pathophysiologic conditions*. The most common conditions requiring therapy are acute mountain sickness, high-altitude cerebral edema, and high-altitude pulmonary edema. They represent a spectrum of disease, with the various conditions having considerable overlap in presenting features. The common symptoms are weakness, malaise, headache, and nausea. In the more severe conditions, these symptoms occur in concert with more specific signs such as the dyspnea and rales of high-altitude pulmonary edema. Individuals vary widely in adaptation to altitude and the severity of ARI they experience. Consequently, there are only very rough guidelines as to the specific altitude of onset or the severity of symptoms in ARI. In general, healthy persons are asymptomatic below 8,000 feet and symptomatic above 12,000 feet. High-altitude pulmonary edema and high-altitude cerebral edema most often occur with rapid ascent to higher than 12,000 feet. Elderly persons and patients with a variety of chronic medical illnesses may become symptomatic at levels near 6,000 feet. Children are also more predisposed to serious ARI (in particular, high-altitude pulmonary edema). It is also important to note that in addition to the directly altitude-related conditions covered in this chapter, there are numerous diseases such as coronary artery disease, congestive heart failure, chronic obstructive pulmonary disease, primary pulmonary hypertension, congenital cyanotic heart disease, and sickle cell anemia that are all worsened or precipitated by high altitude.

ACUTE MOUNTAIN SICKNESS

Acute mountain sickness (AMS) is the most common ARI. It is also the condition with the greatest individual variation in the severity of symptoms. Rapid ascent and vigorous exercise upon arrival appear to increase the incidence. Most symptoms appear after at least 6 to 8 hours of altitude exposure, achieve greatest severity within the first 24 hours, and remit untreated over the following 72 hours. Symptoms can sometimes require up to 5 days for full resolution. The usual symptoms are cerebral in nature and include a gradual onset of headache, nausea, vomiting, anorexia, lassitude, and insomnia. Daytime irritability and periodic breathing during sleep are also often noted. Further symptoms may include decreased concentration, poor judgment, and gait disturbances. When these latter symptoms become prominent, it is likely that frank high-altitude cerebral edema has ensued (most likely the two conditions are different ends of one disease spectrum). The differential diagnosis for AMS in its usual setting in-

cludes hypothermia, hypovolemia, and simple exhaustion. Victims complain of poor quality of sleep and routinely note the development of headache after the first night of sleep at high altitude. Many believe the pathogenesis of these symptoms to be an imbalance between the cerebral vasodilatation from hypoxia and the cerebral vasoconstriction stimulus from hypocarbia. The altitude-induced respiratory alkalosis and sleep-related relative hypoventilation produce peak CO_2 levels and the onset of symptoms. During the acclimatization process, renal compensation for respiratory alkalosis counteracts the relative hypoventilation. Symptoms resolve soon thereafter. The development of symptoms may be completely eliminated if the rate of ascent is geared to the rate of acclimatization.

Prevention

The best preventive measure is gradual ascent. Stopping for a day at less than 8,000 feet to allow acclimatization to occur is helpful. The subsequent rate of climb is best dictated by symptoms appearing in a member of the ascending party (ascending 1,000 feet per day can be used as a starting guideline). Visiting higher elevations during the daytime and sleeping at the lowest feasible elevation are also beneficial. Alcohol and sedative drugs can suppress ventilation with sleep and worsen symptoms and should be avoided. Prophylactic medication regimens are available but are best reserved for those with a repeated history of severe symptoms or emergency situations in which acclimatization is not feasible.

Acetazolamide has been shown to be an effective prophylactic agent in controlled trials. It acts to reverse respiratory alkalosis, increase ventilation, and increase oxygenation. These appear to be the important therapeutic actions, although the drug does have diuretic properties and a direct effect on cerebral blood flow, which may also be beneficial. An accepted regimen is 250 mg twice a day for 24 hours before and 3 days following ascent to high altitude. The regimen should not be interrupted, since severe symptoms have been reported when the drug was discontinued prematurely. Oral and peripheral paresthesias as well as altered visual acuity can be encountered with the use of this drug; these are usually avoided by its discontinuation in less than 5 days. If a physician is called upon to prescribe this regimen, it is important to stress to the patient the continued need for some restraint regarding rate of ascent. Acetazolamide does not have confirmed prophylactic value against high-altitude cerebral edema or high-altitude pulmonary edema. Acetazolamide every night at bedtime as an aid to sleep has also been recommended, but this regimen is less standard. Dexamethasone, 4 mg by mouth every 6 hours, has recently been reported to have prophylactic value. Further validating studies are pending.

Therapy

The treatment of severe AMS is descent from high altitude. Administration of oxygen partially relieves symptoms. Mild cases can be treated with bed rest while ac-

TABLE 1 Summary of High Altitude Conditions

	Acute Mountain Sickness	High–Altitude Cerebral Edema	High–Altitude Pulmonary Edema
Altitude	6,000–8,000 ft, uncommon 8,000–12,000 ft, common >12,000 ft, >50% have symptoms	Usually >12,000 ft	>8,000 ft
Frequency	Variable, most likely of all altitude-related illnesses	Rare	Mild (asymptomatic rales) 17–28% Overt 0.5–4%
Predisposing features*	Alcohol, sedatives, sleeping at high altitude	Same as AMS	Increased in the young; increased with vigorous exercise upon arrival, pulmonary artery atresia; increased in reascending high-altitude natives; increased in those with previous history of HAPE
Presentation	Onset after 6–8 hr of exposure (usually following first night's sleep), peak at 24 hr, resolution during next 72 hr	Onset: variable, 1–9 days Resolution: variable, several weeks	Onset 12–96 hr after arrival Resolution: variable
	Symptoms: headache, malaise, nausea/anorexia,vomiting, insomnia/ poor quality sleep, decreased concentration	Symptoms: symptoms of AMS, deteriorating concentration and mental faculties, hallucinations (rare)	Symptoms: nonproductive cough, increasing dyspnea, inappropriate fatigue; symptoms of AMS often occur as well, and may progress to severe respiratory distress and productive (edema fluid) cough
	Signs: periodic breathing with sleep, poor judgment, gait disturbance (suspect HACE).	Signs: ataxia, gait disturbances, deteriorating judgment seizures (rare), variety of motor and sensory deficits, obtundation, coma	Signs: rales, tachycardia, tachypnea, cyanosis, mild fever, stupor, coma, patchy infiltrates on x-ray films, right–sided heart strain on ECG
Prevention	Gradual ascent, acclimatization Sleep at lowest possible altitude Avoid alcohol or sedatives Acetazolamide 250 mg 24 hr before and first 3 days at high altitude ??Dexamethasone 4 mg q6h	Gradual ascent, acclimatization Sleep at lowest possible altitude Avoid sedatives	Gradual ascent, acclimatization Limit exertion on arrival Close observation if previous history
Treatment	Mild: Stop ascent and/or descent† Limit exertion/bed rest; maintain adequate fluid intake; acetaminophen for headache (codeine should be avoided if possible); ?? acetazolamide for sleep, 250 mg PO qhs	Descent O2 Supportive care ?? Dexamethasone	Descent (by litter if possible) Oxygen administration Bed rest Supportive care
	Moderate to severe: Descent; oxygen adiminstration; assistance with descent and observation for HAPE, HACE		

* AMS, HAPE, and HACE all are predisposed by rapid ascent, lack of acclimatization, and individual susceptibility.
† Indications for descent: severe headache unresolved by analgesia, protracted vomiting, impaired judgment, gait disturbances.

climatization occurs. Sedatives or analgesics with strong sedative properties should generally be avoided because of the ventilatory inhibition and subsequent symptom exacerbation they may produce. Furosemide, spironolactone, and ergotamine have all been reported to be useful in therapy. None has repeatedly proved to be of benefit or has been accepted as standard therapy. Sedative agents such as sleeping aids have been utilized on some mountaineering expeditions, but can produce significant adverse effects, as outlined above. Diazepam has been studied at high altitude and is reported to significantly decrease O_2 saturation.

HIGH-ALTITUDE CEREBRAL EDEMA

When several cerebral symptoms (impaired judgment, disorientation, and gait disturbances) are noted, the

diagnosis of high-altitude cerebral edema (HACE) should be suspected. This usually occurs above 12,000 feet, although there have been case reports at lower elevations. Fortunately, the condition is uncommon. Alterations in the cerebral vascular tone (as discussed under AMS) probably play a central role in HACE as well. Patients experience headaches, general malaise, and a truncal ataxia. Progression of the condition can cause severe gait disturbance, deteriorating judgment, obtundation, coma, and death. Papilledema, disorientation, and a variety of motor and sensory deficits have been reported.

Therapy

Adequate treatment requires rapid descent and high-flow oxygen administration. Dexamethasone administered in the same manner as it is used for brain injuries causing cerebral edema has been recommended. There is no definite proof of its therapeutic benefit in HACE. The guidelines of gradual ascent, acclimatization, avoidance of sedatives, and sleeping at the lowest possible elevation should all be followed as a routine precaution. There is no proven prophylactic drug regimen.

HIGH-ALTITUDE PULMONARY EDEMA

Rapid ascent without acclimatization results in overt high-altitude pulmonary edema (HAPE) in approximately 4 percent of individuals. Asymptomatic rales are present in a much larger percent of individuals (between 17 to 28 percent in various studies). Children have a much higher risk than adults (in some studies as much as a tenfold increase). Those who undertake vigorous exercise soon after arrival at high altitude are also at increased risk. There is a relatively high recurrence rate with repeated visits to altitude.

Symptoms usually develop between 12 to 96 hours after arrival at high altitude. Nonproductive cough, dyspnea, and fatigue are noted, along with headache and other nonspecific symptoms as experienced in AMS. Cyanosis and a cough producing edematous fluid develop in more severe cases. It remains unclear whether the release of some chemical mediator causing endothelial injury or alterations in the perfusion of the pulmonary vascular beds is the cause. The weight of evidence implicates altered capillary permeability pulmonary edema. Detailed examinations have revealed electrocardiographic evidence of right ventricular strain as well as radiographic evidence of the patchy interstitial and alveolar infiltrates seen in adult respiratory distress syndrome.

Therapy

High concentration oxygen is the best therapy known for HAPE. Rapid descent is also indicated and can often be life-saving. Descents of only 2,000 to 3,000 feet are often very helpful and usually the only therapy available in a wilderness environment. Bed rest is also recommended, because exercise exacerbates hypoxemia and worsens the already significant pulmonary hypertension. Seriously ill patients should thus be evacuated by litter if possible. Arranging this transportation should not delay the start of descent, however. Morphine sulfate, rotating tourniquets, and furosemide have all been recommended for treatment. Although such therapy may have advantages in reducing the pulmonary capillary pressure, this would seem to be outweighed in most instances by the potential disadvantage of hypovolemia, decreased cardiac output, and ventilatory depression that may be induced. Steroids, theophylline, digoxin, and isoproterenol are of no proven benefit. There have been two reports of patients with severe HAPE in whom mechanical ventilation and positive end expiratory pressure was effective.

OTHER CONDITIONS

Retinal hemorrhage occurs in altitude exposures above 14,000 feet. Strenuous exercise seems to be a major contributing factor to its appearance. The hemorrhages are generally asymptomatic and require no therapy. If visual disturbances occur at high altitude, descent is indicated. The visual deficits may persist and thus should not be allowed to worsen by the patient's remaining at high altitude. Deep venous thrombosis, pulmonary embolism, and cerebral thrombosis also have been reported at high altitude. It is unclear whether the incidence is increased over that of the general population. Dehydration and restricted activity during bad weather are likely to contribute. Gradual ascent is probably not preventive, but its prevention of AMS will allow maintenance of adequate activity and oral hydration.

SUGGESTED READING

Foulke GE. State of the art review: Altitude related illness. Am J Emerg Med 1985; 3:217–226.

Hackett PH, Rennie D. Rales, peripheral edema, retinal hemorrhage and acute mountain sickness. Am J Med 1979; 67:214–218.

Johnson TS, Rock PB, Fulco CS, et al. Prevention of acute mountain sickness by dexamethasone. N Engl J Med 1984; 310:683–686.

Meehan RT, Zavala DC. The pathophysiology of acute high-altitude illness. Am J Med 1982; 73:395–403.

Sutton JR, Houston CS, Mansell AL, et al. Effect of acetazolamide on hypoxia during sleep at high altitude. N Engl J Med 1979; 301:1329–1331.

EXPOSURE TO CHEMICALS AND HAZARDOUS MATERIALS

MICHAEL L. FISCHMAN, M.D., M.P.H.

The disastrous exposure in 1984 of residents of Bhopal, India, to methyl isocyanate leaking from a pesticide plant resulted in an estimated 1,700 deaths and focused considerable media attention on the problem of environmental and occupational exposure to toxic materials. The emergency physician will often be the first to examine the victim of a toxic exposure and to make decisions regarding further evaluation and treatment that may be critical to the patient's well-being. Such decisions must often be made without the benefit of precise information about the nature and severity of exposure.

This chapter provides an approach to the initial diagnosis and management of patients with acute chemical exposure and intoxication. It is obviously impossible to review the toxicologic properties of the 100,000 or more chemicals in regular use in this country. It is possible, however, to group these toxic agents into several general classes, with shared biologic and toxic effects. Recognition of these effects may assist in proper diagnosis and treatment. In addition, certain principles of management apply to virtually all cases.

ROUTES OF EXPOSURE

Unlike the more commonly encountered suicidal or accidental childhood ingestions of a drug or toxin, the route of exposure in most acute environmental poisonings is via inhalation or dermal absorption. The majority of air-borne materials, whether gases, vapors or aerosols, are easily absorbed from the vast surface area of the lung parenchyma. Here they may produce local effects on the respiratory mucosa or systemic effects after absorption. The skin acts as a barrier to the penetration of certain substances, but many other materials, such as some organic hydrocarbon solvents and organophosphate insecticides, are well absorbed through intact skin. Lethal intoxication from materials such as ethylene dibromide, a fumigant, and cyanide has resulted from primarily dermal exposure, without significant inhalation or ingestion. Dermal absorption is generally enhanced in areas of injured or abraded skin. The importance of the dermal route accounts for the need for adequate decontamination during first aid.

FIRST AID

The primary objective in the pre-hospital management of the patient with a chemical intoxication is removal from further exposure. With air-borne exposures, this requires removal to an uncontaminated atmosphere, usually outdoors. Such efforts often carry some risk for the rescue personnel, particularly when there is confined space entry. In order to avoid further casualties, no attempt should be made to enter a contaminated area without the use of proper *protective equipment*. Such protection usually includes an air-supplied respirator or self-contained breathing apparatus and impervious protective clothing. Fire department rescue teams should have access to this equipment, or it may be available at the industrial site. In addition, the contaminated area should be closed in order to restrict entry. An area for decontamination should be established to avoid further dispersion of the toxic material.

If the victim's skin or clothing has been contaminated with the chemical, the next step involves removal of all contaminated clothing and *cleansing of the skin*. Ideally, this should be done at the scene, while the rescuers are protected. All clothing should be placed in impervious plastic bags. The skin, as well as the hair and nails, should be washed thoroughly with soap and water, and an attempt made to collect the waste water for proper disposal. If decontamination first occurs at the hospital, care must be taken to avoid exposure of personnel and equipment. Use of surgical gloves, plastic sheeting, and gowns is generally sufficient, unless the material is extremely toxic on skin exposure.

If contact with acids, alkalis, or other corrosive materials is suspected, vigorous irrigation of the exposed skin is necessary as well. *Hydrofluoric acid* is unique in its propensity to cause severe soft tissue destruction and bone decalcification associated with severe pain, with manifestations that may be delayed for up to 8 hours. If the acid concentration is higher than 20 percent or there is exquisite pain, immediate irrigation should be followed by treatment with a 10 percent calcium gluconate injection. Following digital or regional block anesthesia, small quantities (about 0.5 ml per cm² of burned surface area) of calcium gluconate solution should be injected with a 30-gauge needle into the affected dermis and subcutaneous tissue and the immediately surrounding tissue. Injections should be performed as one would perform local anesthetic infiltration, without distending the tissues. Patients with extensive burns or burns requiring debridement should be hospitalized.

Eye contact with an irritant or corrosive material requires immediate irrigation with large quantities of water or normal saline. Alkali burns are particularly dangerous and require prolonged irrigation until the pH of eye secretions has returned to normal (7.0). The pH may be checked with litmus or other indicator paper. Such cases should generally be referred to an ophthalmologist for further treatment.

HAZARDOUS MATERIAL IDENTIFICATION

In the event of a transportation accident involving hazardous materials, an attempt can be made to identify the agent from shipping papers or placards on the transport vehicle. The United States Department of Transportation (DOT) requires that vehicles carrying hazardous materials must be placarded with diamond-shaped signs indicating the class of toxic material and an identification number (ID number), either on a placard or on an orange panel. The placards, some of which are illustrated here (see Fig. 1), indicate the general class of material, e.g., poison gas, corrosive, or flammable. Shipping papers are required to be visible in the cab of the vehicle and indicate the chemical name, classification, ID number, and weight of the material. The DOT issues an annual publication, *Emergency Response Guidebook for Hazardous Materials*, which contains a listing of the standard ID numbers with the corresponding chemical names and reference to enclosed guidelines for handling the material. The emergency response guides include information about the nature of the hazard, required protective equipment, and first aid. The *DOT Guidebook* is a useful publication that should be part of the emergency department library.

Once the agent has been identified, other resources are available to provide information and assistance. The Chemical Manufacturers Association has established an emergency hotline, CHEMTREC (Chemical Transportation Emergency Center), through which information regarding the handling and toxicity of hazardous materials is available 24 hours a day. Their telephone number (for emergencies only) is 1-800-424-9300. In addition, local or regional poison control centers may be able to

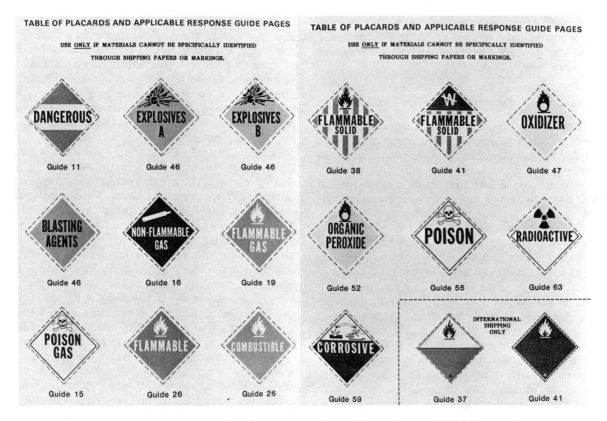

Figure 1 Illustration of placard designs to be posted on vehicles for various types of hazardous material. (From D.O.T. Emergency Response Guidebook for Hazardous Materials, United States Department of Transportation, 1983)

provide valuable information regarding the management of exposed patients.

CLASSES OF TOXIC AGENTS

Most toxins can be classified into one of several broad categories, based on their principal functional effects. This approach is useful because it provides a general framework for the diagnosis and management of exposures to a multitude of toxic materials. Particularly in the acute setting, when the identity of the toxin may not be known, a tentative treatment can still be established.

There are obvious limitations to this approach as well, because many toxins in any given class have unique biologic effects, not shared by other members of the group. Thus, benzene, an aromatic hydrocarbon solvent, falls into the category of central nervous system depressants, but has distinctive hematologic effects as well, including aplastic anemia and leukemia. Many of these unique effects are delayed in onset; thus they may not impact significantly on emergency management.

There are also overlaps in the classification scheme. Thus, xylene and styrene, both hydrocarbon solvents, are central nervous system (CNS) depressants and mild irritants to mucous membranes. Because of such overlap, certain nonspecific symptoms are quite common in many patients, even those who are only mildly intoxicated— headache, nausea, and eye, nose, or throat irritation.

Upper Respiratory Irritants

Exposure to air-borne mucous membrane irritants is commonly encountered. Symptoms and signs are as expected with air-borne contact: burning in the eyes, excessive lacrimation, rhinorrhea, and injection of the oropharyngeal, nasal, or conjunctival mucous membranes. Thus acetone, used as a cleaning solvent and in the dyeing and celluloid industries, particularly causes eye but also nose and throat irritation, with severity dependent upon concentration. Formaldehyde, used heavily in the pharmaceutical and chemical industries and present in particle board and plywood, generally produces mucous membrane irritation. However, in very high concentrations, reached when escape from a heavily contaminated area is prohibited, it may cause severe irritation and pulmonary edema. In low concentrations, many of the severe pulmonary irritants, such as ammonia and ethylene oxide, may produce only mucous membrane irritation. The major diagnostic challenge facing the emergency physician when the responsible agent has not been identified is to exclude the presence of significant lower respiratory involvement. This involves a thorough chest examination, as well as chest roentgenograms, arterial blood gas measurements, and spirometry in appropriate cases.

Treatment of upper respiratory irritation is symptomatic. Analgesics, gargles, and perhaps decongestant preparations should suffice in most cases. Reassurance in the mildly symptomatic patient is very important, in order to prevent undue concern. Of course, patients should be instructed to return if shortness of breath or other lower respiratory symptoms develop.

Pulmonary Irritants

Exposures to severe respiratory irritants pose the greatest danger with respect to the potential for mass poisoning of large populations. A large number of agents in various physical forms may, upon inhalation, cause severe inflammation of lower respiratory mucosa. Certain gases, liquids with high vapor pressure, aerosolized liquids, and fumes are capable of causing this type of reaction. Effects are dependent upon the concentration and duration of exposure, the solubility of the agent, and perhaps host susceptibility factors; they may be manifested as mild upper respiratory irritation, acute tracheobronchitis, acute laryngeal edema, noncardiogenic pulmonary edema, or some combination thereof. Acute tracheobronchitis may result in wheezing, chest tightness, blood-tinged sputum, or frank hemoptysis. The more soluble toxins, such as ammonia and hydrogen chloride, tend to cause immediate mucous membrane irritation, prompting the individual to leave the contaminated environment immediately; whereas relatively insoluble materials, such as nitrogen dioxide, do not have these warning properties.

Some important respiratory irritants are listed in Table 1. Some of these materials, such as chlorine and ammonia, which may be transported in large quantities in a pressurized liquid form in railroad cars or tank trucks, can pose a significant risk to large populations if an accidental leak occurs. A number of episodes have occurred with chlorine, resulting in mass poisoning of communities and significant morbidity and mortality. Phosgene, used as a chemical warfare gas during World War I, accounted for more than 80 percent of gas fatalities. Smoke inhalation during fires may result in severe respiratory irritation, probably from a variety of irritating agents, including aldehydes and oxides of nitrogen, depending on the nature of the combustible material. In addition, fires generate carbon monoxide and sometimes hydrogen cyanide, both chemical asphyxiants, to be discussed further on.

Evaluation of patients with suspected inhalation of severe respiratory irritants should include a thorough chest

TABLE 1 Common Pulmonary Irritants

Ammonia	Methyl isocyanate
Bromine	Nickel carbonyl
Cadmium oxide	Nitric acid
Chlorine	Nitrogen dioxide
Chromates	Ozone
Diazomethane	Phosgene
Epichlorhydrin	Phosphine
Ethylene oxide	Phosphorus trichloride
Fluorine	Sulfur dioxide
Hydrogen chloride	Sulfuric acid
Hydrogen fluoride	Toluene-2,4-diisocyanate
Methyl bromide	Zinc chloride fume

examination, with particular attention to auscultatory findings of wheezing or rales, and frequently a chest film, spirometry, and arterial blood gas measurements. In cases of noncardiogenic pulmonary edema, chest film findings vary from increased interstitial markings, to diffuse patchy infiltrates, to a "white-out" of the lung fields; they are usually bilateral. The film may be normal in patients with pure tracheobronchitis or early in the course of pulmonary edema. Spirometry may reveal reductions in 1 second forced expired volume (FEV_1) and FEV_1 percent, suggesting an obstructive defect in irritant bronchitis, or alternatively, a restrictive pattern with reduced forced vital capacity (FVC) in pulmonary edema. The decision to discharge the mildly symptomatic patient is complicated by the fact that many of these agents can produce a delayed pulmonary edema, up to 24 to 48 hours after exposure, and that usually there is little information as to the concentration and severity of exposure. Nevertheless, the findings on these studies and an assessment of the reliability of the patient and family assist in this decision.

Treatment of patients with significant lower respiratory injury is supportive in nature. Administration of supplemental oxygen is often necessary to treat hypoxemia. Good pulmonary toilet for removal of excess secretions is necessary. If hypoventilation occurs, endotracheal intubation with mechanical ventilation may be required. If hypoxemia persists despite high oxygen concentrations, mechanical ventilation with use of positive end expiratory pressure (PEEP) may be necessary, as in other forms of noncardiogenic pulmonary edema. Though their value is somewhat controversial, a short-term trial of high-dose corticosteroids is probably reasonable in chemically induced pulmonary edema. If acute laryngeal edema and obstruction occur, emergency cricothyrotomy or tracheostomy or both may be required.

When bronchospasm occurs as part of an acute tracheobronchitis, treatment measures are identical to those utilized in bronchial asthma. Aerosolized and parenteral beta-adrenergic bronchodilators, such as metaproterenol or terbutaline, and intravenous aminophylline are useful. If the response is inadequate, use of high-dose corticosteroids, e.g., 60 mg of methylprednisolone intravenously four times a day, with a rapid taper, is indicated.

Central Nervous System Depressants

Central nervous system (CNS) depressants constitute another large category of intoxicants. These agents are generally hydrocarbon solvents, although by producing cerebral hypoxia, other agents such as asphyxiant gases often cause CNS depression (Table 2). Exposure to solvents generally results from inhalation of vapors or direct skin contact. Some solvents are readily absorbed through intact skin. Because of their widespread use in both the home and the industrial environment—in degreasing, dry cleaning, chemical synthesis and extraction, painting, and myriad other applications—the potential for exposure is great.

In low concentrations, these solvents often produce mucous membrane irritation, mild headache, nausea, diz-

TABLE 2 Commonly Used Hydrocarbon Solvents	
Acetone	Petroleum distillates
Chloroform	(e.g., Stoddard solvent)
Freons	Toluene
Glycol ethers	Tetrachloroethylene
(e.g., methyl cellosolve)	(perchloroethylene)
Methylene chloride	1,1,1-Trichloroethane
Methyl ethyl ketone	Trichloroethylene
	Xylene

TABLE 3 Asphyxiants

Simple Asphyxiants	Chemical Asphyxiants
Acetylene	Acetonitrile
Argon, neon, helium	Acrylonitrile
Carbon dioxide	Carbon monoxide
Ethane	Cyanides (alkali)
Hydrogen	Hydrogen cyanide
Liquefied petroleum gas	Hydrogen sulfide
Methane (natural gas)	
Nitrogen	

ziness, and drowsiness. Such nonspecific symptoms may be confused with a variety of other entities, but the temporal correlation with exposure assists in the diagnosis. In higher concentrations, disorientation, abnormal behavior, and altered sensorium may occur, progressing to narcosis and coma. Heavy exposures tend to occur in poorly ventilated areas, usually indoors, and particularly when there is confined space entry. Confined space entry is responsible for many of the severe acute solvent intoxications, because minimal ventilation allows accumulation of high vapor concentrations, and small openings impair egress from the area after symptoms develop. Rescue efforts are also impaired, and multiple casualties may result if proper protective clothing is not worn.

Emergent evaluation requires thorough examination of mental and neurologic status as well as observation for complications such as respiratory depression that may require therapy. After removal from exposure and decontamination of skin, treatment is supportive in nature during the time the agent is being eliminated by metabolism and renal or respiratory excretion. With severe exposures, hypoventilation caused by respiratory center depression may require mechanical ventilation. Observe the patient for renal or hepatic dysfunction, as might occur from exposure to halogenated hydrocarbon solvents.

Simple Asphyxiants

Asphyxiants are gases which, by some mechanism, result in insufficient delivery of oxygen to the tissues. Simple asphyxiants are physiologically inert gases (such as nitrogen and carbon dioxide); in sufficient concentrations they displace oxygen from inspired air and thus cause tissue hypoxia. An oxygen-deficient atmosphere may also occur in an enclosed space where oxygen consumption takes place in the absence of adequate ventilation, for example, in sewer manholes. Table 3 lists a number of asphyxiants. Findings vary with the degree of oxygen deficiency, but may include tachypnea and tachycardia, emotional lability, nausea, vomiting, exertional dyspnea, fatigue, reduced level of consciousness, cyanosis, coma, and seizures. Treatment involves removal from exposure, administration of supplemental oxygen, and mechanical ventilation, if required.

Chemical Asphyxiants

In contrast, chemical asphyxiants interfere with cellular respiration or oxygen delivery by virtue of their chemical reactivity. The most common chemical asphyxiants are carbon monoxide, hydrogen cyanide and cyanide salts, and hydrogen sulfide (Table 3). Carbon monoxide results from the incomplete combustion of hydrocarbons. It is found in automobile exhaust, cigarette smoke, homes with defective furnaces and space heaters, fires, and a variety of other settings. Because of its greater affinity for hemoglobin, it displaces oxygen from hemoglobin and prevents adequate delivery of oxygen to tissues. Manifestations are dependent upon the duration of exposure, ambient concentration, and activity level (level of ventilation) and generally proceed through a spectrum of symptoms as the carboxyhemoglobin levels increase above 10 percent. Initial symptoms are usually headache and giddiness, followed by nausea, weakness, decreased alertness and sensorium, and, ultimately, collapse, coma, and death (see chapter on *Toxic Inhalation and Burns*).

Hydrogen cyanide and cyanide salts cause asphyxia by inhibition of cytochrome oxidase, preventing cellular oxygen utilization. Hydrogen cyanide is used as a fumigant and in chemical synthesis, while cyanide salts are commonly used in electroplating. Addition of acid to cyanide salts results in generation of hydrogen cyanide. Hydrogen cyanide may be in a gaseous or liquid form at room temperature. It may be absorbed via inhalation or skin contact. Sodium and potassium cyanide may be in a powder or granular (solid) form or in solution. These salts can be absorbed by skin or inhalant exposure, though less quickly than hydrogen cyanide. Symptoms depend on severity of exposure and vary from headache, dizziness, nausea, vomiting, and weakness to confusion, lethargy, dyspnea, convulsions, coma, and death. Initial tachypnea proceeds to respiratory depression, apnea, and cyanosis. Arterial and venous oxygen saturations remain high, until apnea ensues, but metabolic acidosis occurs early (see chapter on *Antidotes in Poisoning*).

Similarly, hydrogen sulfide inhibits cytochrome oxidase and causes tissue asphyxia. In addition, it is a severe respiratory irritant and may cause pulmonary edema. Hydrogen sulfide is present in a variety of industrial and environmental settings, including petroleum refineries, tanneries, mines, and in sewers and other areas where decay of organic material occurs. It tends to accumulate in low-lying areas because it is heavier than air. It has a characteristic "rotten-egg" odor, but rapidly occurring olfactory fatigue may confuse the individual into thinking the exposure has ceased. Exposure occurs via inhalation. Low-level exposures cause mucosal irritation, whereas at higher levels, headache, nausea, dizziness, decreased level of consciousness, progressing to coma, seizures, and pulmonary edema can occur. Evaluation should include thorough respiratory, mental status, and neurologic examinations and, frequently, chest x-ray films and measurement of arterial blood gases. Treatment is described in the chapter on *Toxic Inhalation and Burns*.

Acetylcholinesterase Inhibitors

Acetylcholinesterase inhibitors, the organophosphate and carbamate insecticides, result in accumulation of acetylcholine at nerve endings. These insecticides are widely used in home and agricultural settings. There are a multitude of active agents, including malathion, parathion, carbaryl, and diazinon, with even more trade names (Table 4). They are generally well absorbed from the skin, respiratory system, and gastrointestinal tract. Mild intoxication may cause headache, weakness, nausea, and vomiting without objective findings. Some symptoms may result from the vehicle for the pesticide, typically hydrocarbon solvents. Severe poisoning causes a classic picture of cholinergic excess (Table 5). Death after severe poisoning results from respiratory failure. Confirmation of a diagnosis may be made when the red blood cell ("true") acetylcholinesterase level is significantly depressed relative to the baseline, but results are generally not available before evaluation and presumptive therapy.

After thorough decontamination, the treatment of cholinesterase inhibitor poisoning varies, depending on the severity of intoxication. Mild symptoms may require immediate treatment with *atropine* in high doses, usually 2 mg intravenously repeated at 10-minute intervals until signs of atropinization occur (e.g., tachycardia, dry mouth, and flushing). The atropine blocks the effect of excess acetylcholine. Supportive treatment, e.g., oxygen administration, mechanical ventilation, suctioning of secretions, and perhaps anticonvulsants, may be required. Repeated administration of atropine is usually necessary because of the longer duration of action of the insecticides. Hospitalization for observation and further treatment is required for 24 to 48 hours. With the organophosphate insecticides, which cause irreversible inactivation of cholinesterase after a period of "aging," a

reactivator, *pralidoxime (2-PAM)*, is indicated, in addition to atropine. Pralidoxime is given in a dose of 1 g intravenously over 5 minutes and may be repeated several times over the succeeding 24 hours if needed. In carbamate poisoning, because the inhibition of cholinesterase is rapidly reversible, pralidoxime is *not* utilized.

Miscellaneous Agents

Inhalation or skin absorption of certain substances may result in *methemoglobinemia* and consequent hypoxia. For example, aniline, o-toluidine, and dinitrotoluene, used in dye and chemical synthesis, are potent methemoglobin formers. Headache and cyanosis, progressing to weakness, dizziness, dyspnea, and ultimately coma, occur with increasing methemoglobin concentrations. Treatment primarily involves thorough decontamination of skin, hair, and nails and oxygen administration. Only in severe intoxications, with CNS depression and methemoglobin concentrations above 60 percent, should use of methylene blue be considered. A 1 percent solution may be given over 5 minutes, in a dose of 1 to 2 mg per kilogram.

Several agents can cause significant *hemolysis*. After a delay of 2 to 24 hours, arsine (arsenous hydride, AsH_3), a gas used as a dopant in semiconductor wafer manufacture, can induce massive intravascular hemolysis, with abdominal pain, hematuria, jaundice, hemolytic anemia, oliguria, and renal failure. Stibine (antimony hybride, SbH_3) and phenylhydrazine, used in chemical and dye manufacture, are also capable of causing hemolysis, though probably less severe. Treatment of severe arsine poisoning involves exchange transfusion and, if renal failure occurs, hemodialysis.

Some chemicals that have received considerable media attention have negligible acute toxicity. In this situation, the emergency physician must provide more reassurance than treatment. The polychlorinated biphenyls (PCBs) fall into this category. Exposure frequently results from leaking capacitors or transformers in which PCBs are used as insulating fluids. Animal literature indicates that these compounds, given in high doses chronically, promote liver tumors. Demonstrated adverse effects in humans from heavy chronic industrial exposures, however, have been limited to chloracne, a unique acneiform eruption, and perhaps mild liver function test abnormalities. The PCBs do accumulate in tissues, particularly fatty tissue, and persist for prolonged peri-

TABLE 4   Some Common Cholinesterase Inhibitors (Insecticides)*

Aldicarb (Temik)
Azinphos-methyl (Guthion)
Carbaryl (Sevin)
Chlorpyrifos (Dursban)
Dichlorovos (DDVP, Vapona)
Dimethoate
Fenthion (Tiguvon, Baytex, Entex)
Malathion
Naled (Ortho-Dibrom)
Parathion
Ronnel
Tetraethyl pyrophosphate (TEPP)

* Trade names listed in parentheses

TABLE 5   Cholinergic Syndrome (from Acetylcholinesterase Inhibitors)

Excessive salivation
Involuntary urination and defecation
Diarrhea
Miosis
Hyperactive bowel sounds
Bronchospasm
Increased respiratory secretions
Respiratory distress and failure
Muscle weakness

ods in the environment. Fires involving PCBs may produce polychlorinated dibenzofurans (PCDFs) and dibenzodioxins (PCDDs). These materials may be more potent carcinogens. For these reasons, exposure to PCBs should be avoided. If skin contact occurs, thorough decontamination of the skin by washing and proper disposal of contaminated clothing should be performed. However, a single acute exposure is unlikely to cause any adverse effects and the patient should be adequately reassured.

SUGGESTED READING

Doull J, Klaassen C, Amdur M, eds. Casarett and Doull's toxicology: The basic science of poisons. 2nd ed. New York: MacMillan, 1980.

Gosselin R, Smith R, Hodge H. Clinical toxicology of commercial products. 5th ed. Baltimore: Williams & Wilkins, 1984.

Proctor N, Hughes J. Chemical hazards of the workplace. Philadelphia: Lippincott, 1978.

Rom W, ed. Environmental and occupational medicine. Boston: Little, Brown, 1983.

United States Department of Transportation. Emergency response guidebook for hazardous materials. DOT P 5800.3, 1984. (Available for a nominal fee from Labelmaster, 5724 N. Pulaski Road, Chicago, IL 60646.)

TOXICOLOGIC EMERGENCIES

In this section, the most common and most deadly forms of overdose (alcohol, opiates, and cyclic antidepressants) are discussed in detail. Poisonings for which there is a specific and immediate antidote are also discussed, as are the general principles of overdose management. However, no text can provide sufficiently up to date information about the tens of thousands of commercially available substances and potential toxins. Fortunately, up to the minute information about all these substances is available at any of the regional poison control centers, and a list of these with their phone numbers can be found in the final chapter of this section.

PREVENTION OF ABSORPTION IN OVERDOSE

ALAN H. HALL, M.D.
BARRY H. RUMACK, M.D.

Few drugs or poisons ingested in overdose have a specific antidote. Treatment therefore is directed at support of pulse, blood pressure, and respirations; enhancement of poison elimination; and prevention of further poison absorption. Currently accepted methods of preventing absorption of an ingested drug or poison are discussed below.

INDUCED EMESIS

Induction of emesis with syrup of ipecac is a standard procedure for many types of ingestions. Although it is frequently recommended, it has never actually been proved to be of benefit in terms of patient outcome. Syrup of ipecac is an effective emetic and produces good return of gastric contents. Older emetics such as apomorphine, copper sulfate, and salt solutions have been abandoned because of their deleterious side effects.

However, ipecac is not without its own potential toxicity. Mallory-Weiss tear of the esophagus, pneumomediastinum, retropneumoperitoneum, diaphragmatic rupture, aspiration pneumonitis, and possibly intracranial bleeding in the elderly have all been attributed to prolonged vomiting after administration of syrup of ipecac. There is also evidence that ipecac-induced vomiting delays the administration of activated charcoal.

Despite these cautions, ipecac is often used in the emergency department, particularly in accidental childhood ingestions. Syrup of ipecac oral doses are listed in Table 1. Contraindications to use of ipecac are listed in Table 2. In general, any patient with caustic ingestion should not have induced emesis, since this exposes the esophagus to the caustic substance twice and could produce further injury to the already injured mucosa and increase the potential for bleeding, perforation, and stricture formation. Patients with coma or seizures may aspirate gastric contents into the lungs with induced emesis. The procedure is contraindicated in these patients as

well as in patients ingesting poisons that may produce rapid coma or seizures, such as cyanide, strychnine, or camphor.

Ipecac acts both by local irritation of the gastric lining and by absorption and stimulation of the medullary vomiting center. Recent publications indicate that a substantial amount may be absorbed, and most authorities avoid using it in pregnant patients.

GASTRIC LAVAGE

Although numerous studies have attempted to compare the efficacy of gastric lavage with that of induced emesis, all were carried out using a small-bore nasogastric tube. Current practice is to utilize a large-bore (36–40 French) orogastric hose. This large tube should not be inserted through the nose, as it can damage the mucosa or turbinates and result in epistaxis. The most current study of gastric emptying procedures plus use of activated charcoal as opposed to activated charcoal alone showed that lavage with a large-bore orogastric hose within 1 hour of the overdose produced a significant difference in the clinical course in *obtunded* patients only.

When clinically indicated, gastric lavage should be performed with the patient in the Trendelenburg (head-

TABLE 1 Syrup of IPECAC Dose

Age	Dose (ml)
Less than 1 year	10
1 year to 12 years	15
Over 12 years	30

From Hall AH, et al. Management of acute poisoning and overdose. Denver, Co.: Rocky Mountain Poison and Drug Center, 1985.

TABLE 2 Contraindications to IPECAC-Induced Emesis

Coma
Convulsions
Ingestion of
  Alkali
  Acid
  Rapidly acting CNS depressants (i.e., cyanide)
  Rapidly acting CNS irritants (i.e., strychnine)
  Petroleum distillates (unless advised otherwise by
    a poison center)

From Hall AH, et al. Management of acute poisoning and overdose. Denver, Co.: Rocky Mountain Poison and Drug Center, 1985.

down) left lateral decubitus position to minimize the possibility of aspiration if emesis occurs. This precludes the need for endotracheal intubation prior to gastric lavage, unless it is indicated for central nervous system or respiratory depression.

Indications for gastric lavage are listed in Table 3.

Complications of gastric lavage include inadvertent intubation of the trachea, aspiration of gastric contents into the lungs, and perforation of the esophagus.

ACTIVATED CHARCOAL

Activated charcoal is an excellent adsorbent for the great majority of substances ingested in overdose. It is produced by burning organic materials and treating the residue with either steam or chemicals to remove impurities and increase surface area. Activated charcoal is not absorbed through the gastrointestinal mucosa and itself adsorbs large amounts of ingested poisons. Table 4 lists some agents that are not well adsorbed by activated charcoal. Since activated charcoal is a safe and effective treatment for most poisons, it should be administered to nearly all overdosed patients. The most recent studies indicate an equal or greater efficacy of activated charcoal when it is used alone than when it is used in conjuction with a gastric emptying procedure. Only in cases in which the overdose has occurred within 1 or 2 hours of the patient's presentation to the emergency department are gastric emptying procedures likely to decrease absorption. In cases in which there has been a longer delay between ingestion and presentation, administration of activated charcoal immediately after presentation is the treatment of choice. Activated charcoal may also bind drugs or poisons that are still unabsorbed in the proximal small bowel. Its administration should not be delayed for a likely futile gastric emptying procedure.

Contraindications to activated charcoal are caustic ingestions with potential esophageal injury, in which dilution with water or milk is the treatment of choice, and iron ingestion (see below). Although the other agents listed in Table 4 are poorly adsorbed, it does no harm to administer activated charcoal to patients ingesting them.

The usual dose of activated charcoal is 1 g per kilogram body weight (minimum adult dose is 30 g) as a slurry given either orally or by gastric tube. Providing nursing personnel with gloves and plastic aprons or raincoats to wear during administration may increase receptivity to the otherwise messy chore of instilling this valuable agent.

TABLE 3   Indications for Gastric Lavage

Poison recently ingested (1 hour or less)
Agent likely to slow gastric emptying
Patient is comatose, convulsing, or requires airway support
Ingested poison is rapidly absorbed (i.e., strychnine, cyanide) and induced emesis is too slow to be effective or too dangerous if the patient rapidly becomes obtunded and cannot protect the airway

From Hall AH, et al. Management of acute poisoning and overdose. Denver, Co.: Rocky Mountain Poison and Drug Center, 1985.

TABLE 4   Agents Not Well Adsorbed by Activated Charcoal

Acids
Alkalis
Cyanide
Ethanol
Ferrous Sulfate
Methanol
N-methylcarbamate

From Greensher J, et al. Activated charcoal update. Journal of the American College of Emergency Physicians 1979; 8:261–263.

Several investigators have found that drug excretion may also be enhanced by "pulsed" or multiple-dose oral activated charcoal. Phenobarbital, carbamazepine, phenylbutazone, and theophylline have been shown to have their elimination rates increased by multiple-dose oral activated charcoal. Anecdotal reports suggest that several other drugs, including tricyclic antidepressants, have decreased reabsorption in the gastrointestinal tract and therefore have increased gastrointestinal removal when multiple-dose charcoal is administered. Dosing regimens range from 20 g every 2 hours to 40 g every 4 hours with variable addition of cathartics. Children should receive one-quarter to one-fifth of the initial 1 g per kilogram dose every 2 to 4 hours.

CATHARTICS

Saline cathartics (magnesium sulfate, magnesium citrate, sodium sulfate) presumably act by presenting an osmotic load to the bowel, thereby increasing the volume of fluid in the gut and decreasing gastrointestinal transit time. They may be administered simultaneously with activated charcoal. The clinical effectiveness of saline cathartics is, however, unproved.

Sodium or magnesium sulfate is given in a dose of 250 mg per kilogram, or 15 to 20 g (adults) as a 10 percent solution, which may be repeated every 4 hours until charcoal stools appear. Magnesium citrate is given in a dose of 4 ml per kilogram or 4 to 8 oz (adults). Possible hazards include administration of significant magnesium loads to patients in renal failure or sodium loads to patients with heart failure. Documented toxicity from magnesium sulfate enemas and sodium phosphate (Fleet Phospha-Soda) in children should encourage physicians to use only appropriate doses of saline cathartics.

Sorbitol (70 percent premixed with 30 g of activated charcoal in a 150-ml solution) is an acceptable cathartic. Sorbitol may increase the palatability of activated charcoal, but it should be used with caution in young or dehydrated children or in multiple-dose oral activated charcoal regimens because of the potential for protracted diarrhea and fluid losses.

The potential for emesis and aspiration with resultant lipoid pneumonitis after administration of oil cathartics (i.e., castor oil) has caused them to be abandoned in treating poisoned patients.

SPECIAL CONSIDERATIONS

Iron (Ferrous Sulfate)

Ingestion of ferrous sulfate may be treated with either emesis or gastric lavage with an orogastric hose. Rather than activated charcoal and a cathartic, a dilute solution of sodium bicarbonate is instilled after the gastric emptying procedure. This 2 percent solution is made by diluting one ampule (44 to 50 mEq $NaHCO_3$) with normal saline or water to a total volume of 200 ml. Fifty to 100 ml are left in the stomach to permit partial conversion of ferrous sulfate to ferrous carbonate, which is much less well absorbed. Some authors alternately recommend lavaging the stomach with a deferoxamine solution until the return fluid loses its "vin rose" color, indicating that no further chelatable iron is present. This procedure has been abandoned by most poison experts because of expense and questionable efficacy. An x-ray film of the abdomen to evaluate residual iron should be obtained after completion of gastric emptying and instillation of the bicarbonate solution. In rare cases with large accretions of iron tablets in the stomach, surgical removal through a gastrotomy incision may be indicated.

Thallium

European authors routinely recommend the use of Prussian blue (ferric ferrocyanide) as an adsorbent of residual thallium in the gut and a chelator of any thallium in the enterohepatic or enteroenteral circulation. Although there is good evidence for its efficacy, Prussian blue is not routinely available in the United States and is not approved by the Food and Drug Administration. Activated charcoal is an acceptable alternative.

Paraquat

Fuller's earth has been recommended for years as the ideal adsorbent to prevent uptake of paraquat after ingestion of this highly lethal agent. A recent in vitro study showed equal efficacy of an activated charcoal-magnesium citrate mixture. As the latter agents are more readily available and familiar to clinicians, they should be administered immediately in patients with paraquat ingestions rather than delaying while making the attempt to find a source and protocol for the use of Fuller's earth.

Acetaminophen

When indicated, gastric emptying should be performed in cases of acetaminophen poisoning. At present, activated charcoal and a cathartic are not administered if the patient has ingested a potentially hepatotoxic amount (150 mg per kilogram or 7.5 g) or has a potentially hepatotoxic plasma acetaminophen level, unless the patient has also ingested another drug such as propoxyphene. There are some small studies suggesting that the antidote (N-acetylcysteine) is not well adsorbed by activated charcoal, but until further studies are reported it is best to avoid activated charcoal in cases in which the antidote may need to be administered. In mixed ingestions, activated charcoal and a cathartic should be given, with removal of residual activated charcoal by gastric lavage prior to the administration of N-acetylcysteine. In cases in which co-ingestants require administration of multiple-dose activated charcoal, the agents can be alternated every 2 hours, with removal of residual gastric activated charcoal just prior to administration of N-acetylcysteine.

SUGGESTED READING

Curtis RA, Barone J, Giacona N. Efficacy of ipecac and activated charcoal/cathartic: prevention of salicylate absorption in a simulated overdose. Arch Intern Med 1984;144:48–52.

Haddad LM. A general approach to the emergency management of poisoning. In: Haddad LM, Winchester JF, eds. Clinical management of poisoning and drug overdose. Philadelphia: WB Saunders, 1983:10.

Kulig K, Bar-Or D, Cantrill SV, et al. Management of acutely poisoned patients without gastric emptying. Ann Emerg Med 1985;14:562–567.

Rumack BH, ed. General or unknown, general toxicology information management. Englewood, CO: Poisindex Information System, Micromedex Publishers, 1974 through current year.

Wanke LA. Prevention of absorption: dilution, emesis, gastric lavage, adsorption, catharsis. In: Bayer MJ, Rumack BH, Wanke LA, eds. Toxicologic emergencies. Bowie, MD: Robert J. Brady Co. 1984:37.

TOXICOLOGY SCREENS AND ASYMPTOMATIC POISONING

KENT R. OLSON, M.D.

HOW TO APPROACH THE DIAGNOSIS OF POISONING

The toxicology laboratory can be helpful in diagnosing and managing poisoning or drug overdose, but should never replace a careful clinical examination. Over-reliance on the toxicology screen leads to unneeded expense, and may result in potentially tragic delay in providing life saving supportive care and specific antidotes or other interventions. Instead, the emergency physician can use simple clinical and laboratory tests to make a tentative diagnosis. This usually results in appropriate early management and also occasionally to selection of specific toxicology tests. The key question that should always be answered before any test is requested is this: How will the result of this test alter my approach to treatment?

The specimen for the *standard toxicology screen* available to most emergency departments (Table 1) has to be sent out to a reference laboratory and will not return for at least 6 to 8 hours, often over 24 hours. The screen employs several methods to test for perhaps 100 different drugs, and although it has reasonable positive predictive value (a positive result is probably true), it has poor sensitivity, and a negative result does not rule out intoxication. Many drugs, such as newer antidepressants, isoniazid, and ethylene glycol, are not specifically tested for on standard toxicology screens. In addition, even when a positive result is found, this is not proof that it is responsible for the state of intoxication. Quantitative blood levels of many drugs correlate poorly with the state of intoxication, and attempting to plan therapy on the basis of a drug level is often a waste of time and money.

Thus, the standard toxicology screen has limited usefulness. It may be used to confirm clinical impressions during the course of hospitalization, or it may provide medicolegal confirmation for the medical record. It should obviously be obtained whenever the diagnosis of brain death is being considered, in order to confirm the absence of common depressant drugs that might result in temporary absence of brain activity. Whenever possible, the physician should indicate on the laboratory slip the specific drugs or classes of drugs that are of concern. Tables 2 and 3 describe some of the drug classes associated with toxicologic syndromes and the types of screens (urine or blood) that are most likely to be positive. Tables 4 and 5 illustrate common causes of coma and metabolic acidosis which should be considered in the overdose patient.

TABLE 1 The Standard Toxicology Screen

Uses: Confirmation of clinical impression
Documentation for medical record or legal purposes
Rule out intoxication in suspected brain death cases

Problems: Low sensitivity ("rule-out" accuracy <30%)
Time consuming
Expensive

Common drugs screened for:

In the blood: acetaminophen, alcohols, barbiturates, benzodiazepines, carisoprodol, ethchlorvynol, glutethimide, meprobamate, methaqualone, phenytoin, salicylates

In the urine: acetaminophen, alcohols, barbiturates, chlorpheniramine, cocaine, codeine, dextromethorphan, diphenhydramine, ethchlorvynol, lidocaine, meperidine, meprobamate, methadone, methaprylon, morphine, pentazocine, phencyclidine, phenothiazines, propoxyphene, salicylates, tricyclic antidepressants

Note that generally the urine screen is more comprehensive, picking up drugs of abuse (opiates, stimulants) and antihistamines and in many cases also testing for drugs found in the serum.

TABLE 2 Common Drugs Causing Coma

Drug/Toxin	Best Specimen
Ethanol*	Serum (quantitative level)
Barbiturates	Serum (quantitative level)
Sedative-hypnotics	Serum, urine (qualitative)
Narcotics*	Urine (qualitative)
Antidepressants*	Urine (qualitative)
Phenothiazines*	Urine (qualitative)
Antihistamines*	Urine (qualitative)

* Simple clinical features; standard laboratory tests are usually sufficient to make the diagnosis.

TABLE 3 Common Drugs Causing Seizures

Drug/Toxin	Best Specimen
Antidepressants*	Urine (qualitative)
Theophylline	STAT serum level (quantitative)
Isoniazid	Blood (rarely done)
Cocaine, amphetamines*	Urine (qualitative)
Phencyclidine*	Urine (qualitative)
Phenothiazines*	Urine (qualitative)
Antihistamines*	Urine (qualitative)

* Simple clinical features; standard laboratory tests usually are sufficient to make the diagnosis.

TABLE 4 Important Considerations in Coma

A: Alcohol related problems—intoxication, withdrawal seizures, liver disease and encephalopathy

T: Trauma and CNS mass lesions—head trauma, intracranial bleeding

O: Overdose and poisoning

M: Metabolic problems—hypothermia or hyperthermia, hypoglycemia or hyperglycemia, hypoxia, hyponatremia or hypernatremia

I: Infections—meningitis, encephalitis, sepsis

C: Carbon monoxide poisoning

TABLE 5 Common Causes of Anion Gap*
Metabolic Acidosis

A.	Salicylates
A:	Alcohols (ethanol, methanol, ethylene glycol)
L:	Lactic acidosis:
	Shock, e.g., iron
	Hypoxia, e.g., carbon monoxide, cyanide
	Seizures, e.g., isoniazid
A:	Anuria
D:	Diabetic ketoacidosis

* Anion gap = Na—Cl—HCO_3 = 8–12 mEq/L

TABLE 6 Some Drugs and Toxins for Which Specific
Levels are Usually Readily Available and Results Will
Likely Alter Treatment or Disposition

Drug/Toxin	Intervention
Acetaminophen	Use of specific antidote N-acetylcysteine based on serum level
Carbon monoxide	High level of carboxyhemoglobin indicates need for 100% oxygen
Digitalis	Based on serum level and potassium, treatment with Fab antibody fragments may be indicated
Ethanol	Low serum level may suggest nonethanol cause for coma (e.g., trauma, other drugs, other alcohols); may also be used in monitoring ethanol therapy for methanol/ethylene glycol poisoning
Iron	High level may indicate need for chelation with deferoxamine
Lithium	Serum levels and calculated half-life can guide decision to hemodialyze
Methanol	Acidosis, high level, indicates need for hemodialysis, ethanol therapy
Methemoglobin	Methemoglobinemia can be treated with methylene blue intravenously
Salicylates	High level may indicate need for hemodialysis, alkaline diuresis
Theophylline	Immediate hemoperfusion may be indicated based on serum level

In contrast to the toxicology screen, specific levels of certain drugs along with some simple laboratory tests can provide enormous urgent help to the emergency physician treating the poisoning or drug overdose victim. Table 6 lists the common drugs for which most hospitals have rapid specific methodologies and for which specific action might be taken, depending on the result. Table 7 describes a recommended panel of commonly available laboratory tests that can assist in making a tentative diagnosis and that may be used in the initial evaluation of the intoxicated patient, and an algorithm to assist in ordering further specific toxicology tests. A description of the tests listed in Tables 6 and 7 follows.

USEFUL CLINICAL AND TOXICOLOGIC LABORATORY TESTS

Acetaminophen

Acetaminophen (APAP) overdose commonly accompanies ingestion of a variety of drugs. There are numerous prescription and over the counter preparations that contain acetaminophen. Most important, patients often do not recognize the seriousness of APAP overdose and do not volunteer such information in the history. Because there are no distinctive clinical or laboratory clues to the diagnosis early after ingestion, many clinicians routinely order a serum APAP level in every case of mixed or unknown drug ingestion. This is done to avoid missing an occult, but potentially severe overdose, and to allow early administration of the antidote, N-acetylcysteine. The best time for obtaining the level is about 4 to 6 hours after the ingestion.

Arterial Blood Gases

Arterial blood gas levels should be obtained to assess the adequacy of ventilation and to detect the presence of any underlying metabolic acidosis. Table 5 lists some common causes of anion gap metabolic acidosis. The presence of respiratory alkalosis and hyperpnea would suggest salicylate intoxication, which should be confirmed with a rapidly available specific assay.

Carboxyhemoglobin and Methemoglobin

Toxins that alter the capacity of hemoglobin to carry and deliver oxygen can result in significant cellular hypoxia and damage. Specific therapy exists for each of these conditions (100 percent oxygen for carbon monoxide and methylene blue for methemoglobin), and thus early diagnosis can have an impact on effective treatment. The routine arterial blood gas machine does not measure hemoglobin saturation. It measures the partial pressure of dissolved oxygen in the plasma and then calculates the saturation, assuming a normal hemoglobin. Therefore, when carbon monoxide poisoning or methemoglobinemia is suspected, specific determinations should be requested, and can be performed quickly on many of the newer generation blood gas machines. One clue to the presence of COHgb is the occasional observation of bright red color of the venous blood. Methemoglobinemia may be suspected when the blood appears a dark, chocolate brown color.

Digoxin

Serum digoxin levels may be useful in confirming toxicity, but are rarely used by themselves to determine treatment. Levels may be misleadingly high shortly after a massive single ingestion, before distribution of the drug into tissue sites. With acute ingestion (in contrast to chronic accidental overmedication) the serum potassium rises owing to inhibition of the sodium-potassium adenosinetriphosphatase (Na-K ATPase) pump and is a better predictor of digitalis toxic effect at the cell level (a chronic type of intoxication is usually associated with hypokalemia). Serious toxicity would indicate the need for pacemaker placement and/or digitalis specific antibodies.

**TABLE 7 Recommended Initial Laboratory Tests and
Strategy for Ordering Further Specific Tests**

Step 1. Order in all patients:

Arterial blood gas levels
electrolytes
CBC, glucose
Serum osmolality
Acetaminophen
ECG and abdominal x-ray examination

Step 2. Further test ordering strategy (refer to text for more details):

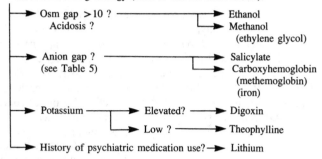

Tests in parentheses () are optional, indicated as suggested by the history and
clinical findings (see text).

Iron

Iron levels can be helpful in determining the need for admission and treatment with the chelating agent deferoxamine. Clues to the presence of iron poisoning include: the history of ingestion, especially if more than 60 mg per kg of elemental iron; vomiting and diarrhea, often bloody; and shock. In the asymptomatic person with a history of iron ingestion, additional support for the diagnosis of serious intoxication is the finding of an elevated blood glucose level (>150) or leukocytosis (>15,000).

Lithium

Patients with massive acute lithium ingestion may be asymptomatic shortly after the overdose, because the drug takes several hours to be distributed into the target tissues, especially the brain. During this time serum levels are high and the drug is easily accessible for hemodialysis. A serum level should be obtained whenever there are signs of intoxication (lethargy, slurred speech, muscle rigidity, or fasciculations) or whenever there is a likelihood of acute lithium ingestion (history of manic-depressive illness, psychosis, or if the patient is known to be taking lithium therapy). For acute single ingestions, serum levels of 4 mEq per liter or greater are considered significant (depending on the time after ingestion), while with chronic accidental intoxication serious toxicity may be seen with levels only slightly above 2 mEq per liter.

Serum Osmolality

The osmolality measures the concentration of molecules in solution and is generally well estimated by the calculation, Osm = 2(Na) + glucose/18 + BUN/2.8 = 290 mOsm per liter. This calculated osmolality agrees well with the result obtained by the laboratory measurement of osmolality using a freezing point depression device. When small, low molecular weight toxins such as alcohols or glycols are ingested, they may increase the measured osmolality, but they are not accounted for by the calculation. This results in an "osmolar gap" (in mOsm) between the measured and calculated results. The most common cause of an elevated osmolar gap is ethanol intoxication. For each mOsm of gap, the corresponding ethanol level is approximately 5 mg per deciliter. Thus, a person with a blood alcohol level of 100 mg per deciliter (0.10 percent), legally drunk in most states, would have a gap of 20 mOsm per liter. A specific serum ethanol level can also be obtained, and it should agree with the calculation. When a large gap is not explained by the specific ethanol result, one should immediately consider concomitant intoxication with methanol, ethylene glycol, or another alcohol substitute. With a large unexplained gap one might begin hemodialysis and other specific treatment for methanol or ethylene glycol without waiting for specific determinations of these toxins.

Salicylate

Salicylate intoxication should be suspected in the patient with hyperpnea, fever, and combined metabolic acidosis and respiratory alkalosis. The presentation is often subtle, especially in cases of chronic inadvertent repeated overmedication, such as the elderly patient with chronic arthritis who confuses her doses, or the young child overmedicated by well meaning, but over enthusiastic parents. In many of these patients the diagnosis is delayed for hours or days and recognized only when serious complications (pulmonary edema, cerebral edema, cardiovascular collapse) occur. It is wise to order a stat salicylate level in any patient with anion gap acidosis. A specific level will determine the need for hemodialysis.

Theophylline

This is one of the most important stat tests that an emergency physician should have available on a rapid turn-around basis. Acute massive theophylline overdose causes tremulousness, agitation, seizures, vomiting, tachycardia, hypotension, and profound hypokalemia. The serum potassium level is often less than 2.7 to 3 mEq per liter. Other laboratory abnormalities include hyperglycemia and metabolic acidosis. Hypokalemia and hypotension are not usually seen in patients with a chronic type of intoxication secondary to accidental repeated overmedication. A serum theophylline level greater than 90 to 100 mg per liter after acute ingestion, or over 40 to 60 mg per liter in a chronic case, would indicate the need for hemoperfusion.

ELECTROCARDIOGRAM AND X-RAY EXAMINATION

Electrocardiogram

The electrocardiogram can be a very useful test for the pharmacologic effects of several cardioactive drugs. Tricyclic antidepressants (TCAs) typically cause prolongation of the QT and QRS intervals, and a QRS duration greater than 0.12 seconds has traditionally been used to confirm significant TCA toxicity and determine the need for admission. QT and QRS prolongation may also be seen with phenothiazines, lithium intoxication, and type I antiarrhythmic agents (quinidine, procainamide, and disopyramide). However, it is important to recognize that serious ingestion may have occurred without any changes noted on the electrocardiogram, if for example, the drug is still in the stomach and not yet absorbed. Also, newer "noncardiotoxic" antidepressants such as amoxapine may cause serious poisoning (seizures, hyperthermia) without any associated electrocardiographic changes.

X-ray Examination

Standard x-ray views may reveal radiopaque pills or foreign bodies in an asymptomatic patient. Disc-shaped button batteries may be swallowed by infants and can become lodged in the esophagus. Within 24 hours these batteries can cause perforation and mediastinitis, exsanguination, and death. A chest x-ray view revealing a battery in the esophagus should be followed by early

TABLE 8   Some Radio-opaque Tablets

C:	Chloral hydrate
H:	Heavy metals
I:	Iron and iodides
P:	Psychotropics (antidepressants, phenothiazines)
S:	Sodium

Enteric coated tablets are most reliable of all

endoscopy for removal. Once in the stomach, these batteries usually pass into the stools without incident. A variety of pills may be seen on x-ray film of the stomach. Some radiopaque tablets are listed in Table 8. The most reliably positive of the tablets listed are the enteric coated products, which may remain intact for several hours. If a tablet bezoar or concretin is suspected, but is not seen on standard x-ray films, it may be outlined with oral contrast material.

Catastrophe can occur if a patient has ingested a serious toxin and this goes unrecognized or underestimated on initial evaluation. Some toxins produce few or no symptoms early after ingestion, only to become apparent after the victim has been discharged or transferred. For example, ingestion of acetaminophen, colchicine, or *Amanita phalloides* mushrooms causes no illness in the first few hours, but can result in death after several hours to days. A careful history may help to identify these ingestions. In addition, a serum acetaminophen level should be obtained as it is predictive of toxicity and may indicate the use of N-acetylcysteine.

Other toxins may normally produce prompt symptoms, but on occasion manifest delayed toxicity because of slow absorption. Any patient who ingests a sustained release or enteric coated preparation should be carefully monitored for several hours, and repeated serum levels should be obtained to rule out delayed absorption. Sustained release theophylline preparations taken in overdose typically cause a delay in reaching the peak serum level of 12 to 16 hours. Examples of drugs commonly prescribed in enteric coated or sustained release form include theophylline, aspirin, and lithium.

SUGGESTED READING

Hansen HJ, Caudill SP, Boone J. Crisis in drug testing—results of a CDC blind study. JAMA 1985; 253:2382–2387.

Ingelfinger JA, Isakson G, Shine D, et al. Reliability of the toxic screen in drug overdose. Clin Pharmacol Ther 1981; 29:570–575.

Rygnestad T, Berg KJ. Evaluation of benefits of drug analysis in the routine clinical management of acute self-poisoning. Clin Toxicol 1984; 22:51–61.

ANTIDOTES IN POISONING

CHRISTOPHER H. LINDEN, M.D.

Antidotes are specific agents capable of counteracting the effects of a poison. Mechanisms of action include chelation, competition for receptor sites, metabolic alterations, neutralization by antibodies, and physiologic antagonism. When used in conjunction with intensive supportive care and measures aimed at preventing poison absorption, antidotes can significantly reduce morbidity and mortality. Unfortunately, few poisons have antidotes. In addition, most antidotes are potential poisons and should not be used indiscriminantly. For this reason the indications, administration, and potential hazards of antidotal therapy are emphasized in the following pages.

PRE-HOSPITAL CARE

Supplemental oxygen, with assisted ventilation if necessary, should be considered a basic life support measure and given to all potentially poisoned patients, particularly those with abnormal vital signs, altered mental status, cyanosis, or dyspnea. Specific toxicologic indications include inhalation of simple pulmonary asphyxiants (methane, ethane, natural gas, volatile hydrocarbons, nitrogen, hydrogen, helium, carbon dioxide, and smoke), chemical-cellular asphyxiants (carbon monoxide, cyanide, and hydrogen sulfide), and pulmonary irritants (ammonia, chlorine, acid gases, metal and polymer fumes, isocyanates, nitrogen oxides, ozone, phosgene, sulfur dioxide, ethylene oxide, and smog). Although it should be used judiciously in patients with chronic obstructive pulmonary disease or paraquat poisoning, there are no contraindications to oxygen therapy.

Glucose and naloxone should also be given to any patient with abnormal vital signs or altered mental status, and particularly those with seizures. Details regarding the use of these antidotes are presented in the sections on hypoglycemia and narcotic overdose. When both agents are administered, they should be given sequentially, waiting several minutes for a response to one prior to giving the other. If possible, blood should be drawn (for later analysis) prior to glucose or naloxone administration. The practice of simultaneously administering a combination of glucose, narcan, and sometimes thiamine as a "coma cocktail" may lead to diagnostic confusion and should be discouraged. Although thiamine has no immediate effect even if the correct diagnosis is Wernicke's encephalopathy, it should be administered (100 mg, IV or IM) whenever glucose is given.

SPECIFIC INTOXICATIONS AND THEIR ANTIDOTES

Acetaminophen

Toxicity

Signs and symptoms: Day 1: Anorexia, nausea, vomiting, diaphoresis, pallor, malaise. Day 2: Right upper quadrant (RUQ) abdominal pain and tenderness, hepatic dysfunction; occasionally oliguria and renal failure. Days 3 to 4: Peak hepatotoxicity, anorexia, nausea, vomiting, malaise. Day 5 to 2 weeks: Fulminant liver failure or complete recovery.

Mechanism: An as yet identified intermediary metabolite, produced by the cytochrome P-450 mixed function oxidase pathway and normally detoxified by conjugation with glutathione, reacts with hepatocyte proteins, causing hepatic necrosis when glutathione stores are depleted by overdose.

Notes: Patient may be "asymptomatic" (early symptoms overlooked) until liver toxicity develops and it is too late for antidotal therapy. Acetaminophen should therefore be routinely included in drug screens.

Antidote

N-acetylcysteine (NAC, Mucomyst, Mead-Johnson).

Mechanism: Not completely understood. NAC is taken up by hepatocytes and metabolized to cysteine, a glutathione precursor.

Indications: Patient at risk for hepatotoxicity by Rumack-Matthew nomogram (Fig. 1). If plasma acetaminophen level cannot immediately be obtained, begin NAC treatment if amount ingested was more than 140 mg per kilogram (children) or 7.5 g (adults). NAC may be discontinued if level is subsequently found to be nontoxic.

Dose: 140 mg per kilogram orally followed by 70 mg per kilogram orally every 4 hours for a total of 18 doses. Dilute Mucomyst (20 percent NAC) with 3 parts juice or carbonated beverage prior to administration.

Notes: Treatment is most effective if started within 10 hours after ingestion, but may be effective up to 16 and possibly 24 hours of ingestion.

NAC smells and tastes like rotten eggs. Side effects (nausea, vomiting, and diarrhea) are frequent, but may be lessened by changing the diluent, increasing its amount, chilling the solution, giving it slowly or by nasogastric or duodenal tube. Dose must be repeated if vomiting occurs within an hour of administration.

NAC is adsorbed by large doses of activated charcoal. If charcoal has been given (e.g., mixed overdose or early presentation) options include waiting 1 to 2 hours or lavaging the stomach before giving NAC, giving a loading dose of 210 mg per kilogram of NAC, or repeating the NAC loading dose (140 mg per kilogram) at 4 hours. Intravenous NAC is preferred in Canada and Europe, but has not yet been approved for general use in the United States.

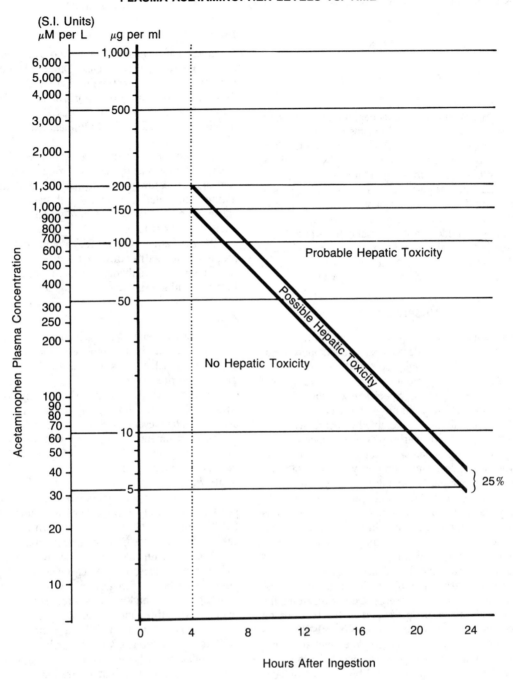

**SEMI-LOGARITHMIC PLOT OF
PLASMA ACETAMINOPHEN LEVELS VS. TIME**

Figure 1 Rumack-Matthew nomogram for acetaminophen poisoning.

Anticholinergic Agents

Toxicity

Signs and symptoms: Central nervous system: Anxiety, agitation, amnesia, aphasia, choreoathetoid movements, confusion, delirium, hallucinations, myoclonus, coma, seizures, respiratory depression, and circulatory collapse. Autonomic: Decreased gastrointestinal motility (decreased bowel sounds), dry skin and mucous membranes (thirst, dysphagia), fever, mydriasis, vasodilation (flushed skin), urinary retention, hypertension, tachycardia, and arrhythmias.

Mechanism: Action of acetylcholine in central and parasympathetic nervous systems is blocked by agents that compete for postsynaptic receptor sites.

Notes: Since central cholinergic pathways are both inhibitory and excitatory, blockade results in central nervous system excitation followed by depression. Drugs with anticholinergic properties include antihistamines, antiparkinson and antipsychotic agents, gastrointestinal and genitourinary antispasmodics, belladonna alkaloids, cyclic antidepressants, and topical mydriatics. Over-the-counter (OTC) analgesics, cold remedies, and hypnotics frequently contain anticholinergic agents. Mushrooms (e.g., *Amanita muscaria*) and plants (e.g., *Datura stromonium* or jimson weed) are additional sources of anticholinergic alkaloids.

Antidote

Physostigmine salicylate (Antilirium, O'Neal).

Mechanism: Reversibly inhibits central and peripheral acetylcholinesterase (the enzyme responsible for acetylcholine degradation), leading to increased cholinergic activity.

Indications: Severe agitation or hallucinations (patient dangerous to self or others), coma (diagnostic trial), extreme hypertension, incapacitating movement disorders, seizures, supraventricular tachycardia with hemodynamic instability, and ventricular arrhythmias unresponsive to standard therapy. Both central and peripheral anticholinergic findings must be present in order to ensure that a correct diagnosis has been made.

Contraindications: Gangrene, mechanical obstruction of gastrointestinal and genitourinary tracts, patients with active (symptomatic) asthma or cardiovascular disease, or those receiving cholinergic or depolarizing neuromuscular blocking drugs.

Dose: 0.5 mg (children) or 1 to 2 mg (adult) intravenously over no less than 2 minutes. May repeat dose every 10 to 20 minutes if necessary (incomplete response, severe or recurrent symptoms).

Notes: Hyponatremia, secondary to polydipsia induced by thirst and dry mouth, is common in patients taking anticholinergic medication and may cause similar clinical findings. Although reversal of symptoms by physostigmine has been said to confirm the diagnosis of anticholinergic poisoning, physostigmine has nonspecific analeptic properties and may arouse patients with coma of other etiologies. It should not be given merely to keep a comatose patient awake. The use of physostigmine in a cyclic antidepressant overdose is controversial and is recommended only after other measures have proven ineffective. Physostigmine induced cholinergic poisoning (see below) may be treated with atropine in a dose equal to one-half the amount of physostigmine given.

Anticoagulants (Oral)

Toxicity

Signs and symptoms: Spontaneous ecchymoses, hematomas, and hemorrhage (nose, gums, and gastrointestinal, respiratory, and urinary tracts).

Mechanism: Inhibition of vitamin K dependent epoxide reductase results in decreased synthesis of clotting factors II, VII, IX, and X with prolongation of the prothrombin and partial thromboplastin times (PT and PTT).

Notes: In contrast to chronic ingestions, single oral doses of most anticoagulants (e.g., anisindione, dicumerol, and warfarin) do not cause coagulation abnormalities even when ingested in massive amounts. However, some of the newer, more potent derivatives of 4-hydroxy-coumarin (e.g., brodifacoum, difenacoum, bromadiolone) and inandione (e.g., chlorphacinone, diphacinone, pindone) can produce severe and protracted anticoagulation in single doses of as little as 0.1 mg per kilogram. With these newer agents, inhibition of coagulation may develop within 24 hours and persist for as long as 8 months.

Antidote

Phytonadione (vitamin K_1; Mephyton-Aquamephyton, Merck, Sharp and Dohme; Konakion, Roche).

Mechanism: Inhibition of epoxide reductase is reversed by providing excess vitamin K.

Indications: Prolonged PT or PTT.

Dose: Excessive therapeutic anticoagulation or chronic accidental ingestion may be reversed with 10 to 50 mg (adult) or 0.2 to 0.6 mg per kilogram (children) of phytonadione orally, intramuscularly, or intravenously (diluted in normal saline and given no faster than 1 mg per minute) every 4 to 48 hours, depending on the clinical severity. Larger doses (100 to 125 mg per day for up to 8 months) may be required for the treatment of long-acting anticoagulant overdose.

Notes: Adverse reactions may occur with intravenous doses of phytonadione. Since it may take 6 to 12 hours for phytonadione to normalize the prothrombin time, active bleeding should be treated with fresh plasma or whole blood.

Arsenic-Mercury

Toxicity

Signs and symptoms: Nausea, vomiting, diarrhea, abdominal pain, gastrointestinal bleeding and perforation, mucosal burns and edema (pharynx, larynx), encephalopathy, peripheral neuropathy (delayed), shock, arrhythmias, myocardial depression, bone marrow suppression, hepatic dysfunction, and renal failure.

Mechanism: Mucosal corrosive. Metals bind to sulfhydryl groups of amino acids, resulting in inactivation of a variety of enzymes and inhibition of cellular metabolism.

Notes: Acute poisoning may occur rapidly following the inhalation of metallic (elemental) mercury vapors as well as the ingestion of inorganic arsenic and mercury salts (e.g., sodium arsenate, mercuric chloride), organic arsenicals (e.g., sodium methylarsonate), and arylated mercurials (e.g., phenylmercury compounds). Inhalation exposure may cause severe pulmonary damage (i.e., pneumonitis, necrotizing bronchiolitis, edema, and fibrosis) as well as systemic toxicity. Chronic poisoning may result from multiple inhalations, ingestions, or topical exposures to less concentrated formulations (including organic mercury salts). Ingested metallic mercury is nontoxic unless large quantities remain in the gut for prolonged periods (weeks).

Antidotes

Dimercaprol (British anti-lewisite (BAL) or BAL in Oil, Hynson, Westcott and Dunning); d-penicillamine (Cupramine, Merck, Sharp and Dohme).

Mechanism: Metals are chelated by (i.e., bind to) the sulfhydryl (thiol) groups of BAL and d-penicillamine, and the complex is excreted in the urine.

Indications: Symptomatic exposure to arsenic or mercury.

Contraindication: D-penicillamine (a metabolite of penicillin) should not be used in patients who are allergic to penicillin.

Dose: BAL: 3 to 6 mg per kilogram intramuscularly (gluteal) every 4 to 6 hours, depending on severity. D-penicillamine: 25 mg per kilogram up to 500 mg orally every 6 hours.

Notes: The persistence of radiodense material in the stomach following gastric decontamination procedures indicates the need for continued efforts such as repeat lavage, endoscopy, or gastrotomy to prevent absorption. Side effects of BAL (nausea, vomiting, pain, and sterile absess formation at the injection site, hypertension, tachycardia, headache, diaphoresis, anxiety, muscle cramps, seizures, coma, and urticaria) are usually transient and respond to supportive measures and decreased dosing. During chelation therapy with d-penicillamine, complete blood counts and renal function should be closely monitored.

Patients with severe symptoms should initially be treated for 10 days with both chelators. The dose of BAL may be tapered during this period. Since the d-penicillamine-metal complex can be absorbed from the intestine and may itself be toxic, it may be best to wait 12 to 24 hours following ingestion before beginning oral therapy. The endpoint of treatment is a urinary metal excretion of less than 50 μg per 24 hours and resolution of symptoms. Further courses of 5 to 10 days of d-penicillamine therapy with or without BAL (depending on severity), after withholding treatment for 3 to 5 days to allow redistribution of the metal, may be necessary in severe cases.

Asymptomatic patients exposed to arsenic or mercury may be given a 24 hour (4 dose) course of d-penicillamine as a mobilization test. If the 24 hour metal excretion is above 50 μg, a 5 to 10 day course(s) of chelation therapy with d-penicillamine is indicated.

Barium

Toxicity

Signs and symptoms: Nausea, vomiting, abdominal pain, diarrhea, muscle cramps, weakness, paralysis, severe hypokalemia, ventricular arrhythmias, renal failure.

Mechanism: Direct stimulation of smooth, striated, and cardiac muscle, intracellular shift of potassium, and precipitation of barium in renal tubules.

Notes: The onset of toxicity may be rapid. Only soluble salts (acetate, carbonate, hydroxide, nitrate, sulfide) are toxic. Barium sulfate is insoluble and nontoxic when ingested.

Antidote

Potassium chloride.

Mechanism: Reverses muscular and cardiac toxicity resulting from hypokalemia.

Indication: Laboratory or electrocardiographic evidence of hypokalemia.

Dose: Up to 75 mEq intravenously immediately and up to 40 mEq per hour for 24 hours, depending on severity.

Notes: Treatment should be started before the potassium level is known if malignant arrhythmias are present. Diuresis may also be helpful. Oral doses of magnesium (or sodium) sulfate will convert barium to its nonabsorbable salt within the gastrointestinal tract. The intravenous administration of magnesium sulfate may contribute to renal failure and is not recommended.

Beta-Adrenergic Antagonists

Toxicity

Signs and symptoms: Nausea, vomiting, diarrhea, confusion, lethargy, coma, seizures, respiratory depression, bronchospasm, pulmonary edema, hypoglycemia, hyperkalemia, bradyarrhythmias, cardiac conduction blocks, hypotension, and cardiogenic shock.

Mechanism: Blockade of beta-adrenergic receptors and direct effects (central nervous system and myocardial membrane depression). Decreased adenyl cyclase activity (decreased cyclic AMP synthesis) is the mechanism underlying adrenergic blockade (negative inotropic and chronotropic effects).

Notes: Although some beta-blockers (e.g., atenolol, metoprolol) are cardioselective (i.e., block only beta$_1$ receptors) at therapeutic doses, they are nonselective when taken in overdose. Drugs with high lipid solubility (e.g., alprenolol, metoprolol, oxprenolol, pindolol, practolol, propranolol) cause greater central nervous system effects than less soluble agents. Those with membrane depressant effects (e.g., acebutolol, alprenolol, oxprenolol, propranolol) are more likely to depress cardiac contractility and cause conduction disturbances. Agents with partial agonist or sympathomimetic activity (e.g., acebutolol, alprenolol, oxprenolol, pindolol, practolol, timolol) have less myocardial depressant effects and may even cause hypertension and tachycardia.

Antidotes

Atropine; beta-adrenergic agonists; glucagon.

Mechanism: Atropine: Increases heart rate by decreasing vagal tone. Beta-adrenergic agonists (e.g., dobutamine, dopamine, isoproterenol, norepinephrine): Stimulate beta-adrenergic receptors. Glucagon: Activates myocardial adenyl cyclase by stimulating a distinct (nonadrenergic) membrane receptor.

Indications: Hypotension or bradyarrhythmias causing hemodynamic instability.

Doses: Atropine, beta-agonists: Standard doses. Glucagon: 5 to 10 mg (adult) or 50 to 150 μg per kilogram (children) intravenously initially and then 1 to 5 mg per hour (adult) or 10 to 50 μg per kg per hour (children) as a continuous infusion.

Notes: Since the response to glucagon is often dramatic, this agent should be tried early in the course of overdose. Insertion of a pacemaker or Swan-Ganz catheter may be necessary in patients who are difficult to manage. Quinidine, pracainamide, and disopyramide should be avoided in the unlikely event that ventricular tachyarrhythmias develop.

Black Widow Spider Envenomation

See chapter entitled *Bee, Wasp, and Spider Envenomation*.

Brown Spider Envenomation

See chapter entitled *Bee, Wasp, and Spider Envenomation*.

Calcium Antagonists

Toxicity

Signs and symptoms: Nausea, vomiting, lethargy, confusion, seizures, hypotension, bradycardia, sinus arrest, heart block, asystole, nonspecific ST segment and T wave changes, and hyperglycemia.

Mechanism: Inhibition of transmembrane slow channel influx of extracellular calcium ions across myocardial and smooth muscle cell membranes leads to prolongation of the plateau phase (phase 2) of the action potential, vasodilation, cardiac conduction defects, and decreased contractility. Inhibition of insulin release causes hyperglycemia.

Notes: Verapamil depresses nodal conduction and myocardial contractility to a greater degree than diltiazem, nifedipine, and perhexilene.

Antidotes

Calcium gluconate; alpha- or beta-adrenergic agonists; atropine; glucagon.

Mechanism: Calcium: Increases flux of calcium ions. Adrenergic agents, glucagon: Stimulate their respective membrane receptors (see beta-adrenergic antagonist section). Atropine: Inhibits cholinergic receptors (decreases vagal tone).

Indications: Hypotension: Calcium, alpha-agonists (e.g., dopamine, norepinephine), glucagon. Symptomatic bradycardia, AV block, asystole: Calcium, atropine,

beta-agonists (e.g., dopamine, isoproterenol, epinephrine, norepinephrine), glucagon.

Dose: Calcium gluconate: 0.2 ml per kilogram (up to 10 ml) of a 10 percent solution intravenously over 5 to 10 minutes. May repeat as necessary provided that calcium levels are monitored. Glucagon: Same as for beta-blocker overdose. Alpha- and beta-agonists, atropine: Standard doses.

Notes: Cardiac pacing may be necessary for patients refractory to pharmacologic therapy. Seizures may respond to calcium or anticonvulsants. Calcium chloride (0.1 ml per kilogram up to 5 ml of a 10-percent solution over 5 to 10 minutes) may be used if the gluconate salt is not available.

Carbon Monoxide

Toxicity

Signs and symptoms: Same as hypoxia of any etiology (e.g., central nervous system depression, cardiac dysfunction, lactic acidosis) except for prominent headache, lack of cyanosis (unless respiratory depression supervenes), and occasionally cherry-red skin and retinal hemorrhages. Neuropsychiatric sequelae (e.g., blindness, deafness, extrapyramidal movement disorders, inability to concentrate, memory difficulty, personality changes, multiple sclerosis-like symptoms, and seizures) are common in patients who have been comatose.

Mechanisms: Carbon monoxide (CO) binds to hemoglobin (Hb), myoglobin, and the respiratory enzyme cytochrome oxidase A_3 more avidly than does oxygen. The oxygen carrying capacity of blood is reduced by carboxyhemoglobin (CO-Hb) formation, CO-Hb shifts the oxygen-Hb dissociation curve to the left (lower tissue Po_2 required for oxygen release), and oxygen delivery to muscle cells is reduced by carboxymyoglobin formation. Inhibition of cytochrome oxidase causes cellular asphyxia by blocking oxidative phosphorylation and ATP production. Myocardial depression may lead to ischemic hypoxia.

Notes: Carbon monoxide poisoning may result from the inhalation or ingestion of methylene chloride (in paint strippers and "bubbling" light bulbs) as well as the inhalation of CO (from incomplete combustion). "Normal" CO-Hb levels may be as high as 10 to 15 percent (of the total Hb) in heavy smokers. Since CO-Hb levels may not reflect tissue CO levels (duration of exposure) and often correlate poorly with symptoms, the neurologic status and degree of acidosis (pH) are more useful in assessing the severity of intoxication (effects of hypoxia). Arterial oxygen saturation is normal if calculated from the Po_2 (dissolved oxygen), but low if measured directly. The difference between the calculated and measured oxygen saturation, the oxygen "saturation gap," can be used to estimate the CO-Hb level when direct measurement capability is not immediately available.

Antidote

Oxygen.

Mechanism: Competes with carbon monoxide for binding sites on hemoglobin, myoglobin, and cytochrome oxidase.

Indications: 100 percent oxygen: Any patient with symptoms or CO-Hb level above 10 percent. Hyperbaric oxygen (HBO): Any patient who is or has been comatose (unresponsive to voice, unable to follow commands), infants and symptomatic children with levels above 30 percent, symptomatic adults with levels above 40 percent, and those with lower CO-Hb levels who remain symptomatic despite 100 percent oxygen therapy.

Dose: Awake patient: Nonrebreathing mask plus nasal cannula at 10 L per minute each (provides approximately 80 percent inspired oxygen concentration). Comatose patient: 100 percent by endotracheal tube followed by HBO. Therapy should be continued until patient is asymptomatic and Co-Hb level is less than 10 percent.

Notes: The half-life of CO-Hb due to inhalation of carbon monoxide is 4 to 6 hours in room air, 60 to 80 minutes when breathing 100 percent oxygen, and 20 to 30 minutes with HBO. In methylene chloride poisoning, the half-life is substantially longer.

Carbon monoxide binds to fetal Hb more tightly than to adult Hb, the normal fetal pO_2 is only 20 to 30 percent that of adults, and the developing nervous system is highly susceptible to the effects of carbon monoxide poisoning. Hence, infants, young children, and pregnant women should generally be admitted for prolonged treatment.

Although contraindicated in pregnancy, HBO is effective in the treatment of postanoxic cerebral edema and may reduce the incidence of permanent sequelae. Transfer of severely poisoned patients to a hyperbaric center is advisable whenever feasible.

Cholinergic Agents

Toxicity

Signs and symptoms: Muscarinic (parasympathetic): Nausea, vomiting, abdominal cramps, diarrhea, bronchospasm, increased tracheobronchial secretions, dyspnea, pulmonary edema, cyanosis, salivation, lacrimation, diaphoresis, blurred vision, miosis, urinary frequency, incontinence (stool and urine), bradycardia, and hypotension. Nicotinic (autonomic ganglia, neuromuscular junctions): Hypertension, tachycardia, vasoconstriction (pallor), hyporeflexia, fasciculations, twitching, tremors, weakness, and paralysis. Central nervous system: Anxiety, ataxia, confusion, headache, slurred speech, seizures, coma with cardiovascular and respiratory depression. Long-term sequelae include peripheral neuropathy and neuropsychiatric disorders.

Mechanism: Stimulation of muscarinic, nicotinic, and central nervous cholinergic receptors by agents that act directly or by inhibiting acetylcholinesterase (AChE) and hence the hydrolysis or acetylcholine.

Notes: Signs and symptoms of cholinergic poisoning are also known as the SLUDGE (Salivation, Lacrimation, Urination, Diaphoresis-Defecation, Gastrointestinal cramps, Emesis) syndrome. Direct acting cholinomimetic agents include choline esters (e.g., bethanechol, carbachol, and methacholine) and alkaloids (e.g., arecoline in betel nuts, muscarine in Boletus, Clitocybe and Inocybe mushroom species, and pilocarpine). Cholinesterase inhibitors include organophosphate and carbamate pesticides, and carbamate drugs, such as edrophonium, physostigmine, and other agents used in the treatment of myasthenia gravis (e.g., ambenonium, neostigmine, pyridostigmine).

Organophosphates inhibit AChE irreversibly, whereas other anticholinesterases reversibly bind to AChE. Low cholinesterase activity in red blood cell or plasma may confirm the diagnosis of organophosphate (and possibly severe carbamate) poisoning, but are not generally available as a stat test. In addition, cholinesterase levels do not correlate well with symptoms, are not helpful in guiding therapy, and vary widely among normal individuals (baseline level must be known for proper interpretation).

Antidotes

Atropine; pralidoxime (2-PAM; Protopam, Ayerst).

Mechanism: Atropine: Blocks muscarinic and central nervous system cholinergic receptors. Pralidoxime: Liberates (reactivates) AChE by competitively binding to organophosphates.

Indications: Atropine: Muscarinic–central nervous system symptoms. Pralidoxime: Nicotinic symptoms due to organophosphate poisoning.

Dose: Atropine: 0.5 to 1.0 mg (adults) or 0.01 mg per kilogram (children) intravenously over 1 to 2 minutes. Repeat or incremental doses may be given every 10 to 15 minutes until symptoms are relieved (i.e., secretions are decreased) or anticholinergic findings appear. Pralidoxime: 1 to 2 g (adults) or 25 to 50 mg per kilogram (children) in 50 to 250 ml saline intravenously over 15 to 30 minutes. Repeat doses (in 1 hour and every 8 to 12 hours) or a continuous infusion (0.5 g per hour for adults or 10 to 15 mg per kilogram per hour for children) for 24 to 48 hours may be necessary if symptoms persist or reappear. The reconstituted (but undiluted) 5 percent Protopam solution may be used in patients with pulmonary edema.

Notes: In severe poisonings, particularly those due to potent organophosphates, patients may have prolonged toxicity (up to 30 days) and may require large doses of atropine (several hundred milligrams per day).

Although pralidoxime is most effective in reversing nicotinic (neuromuscular) manifestations of organophosphate poisoning, it also acts (synergistically with atropine) at muscarinic and central nervous system sites. The use of pralidoxime in the treatment of carbamate intoxications is generally not necessary because of rapid, spontaneous reactivation of AChE and is contraindicated in carbaryl (Sevin) poisoning. Patients should be observed closely for 24 hours after treatment has been stopped because of potential rebound toxicity.

Cyanide

Toxicity

Signs and symptoms: Early: Agitation, anxiety, confusion, headache, dizziness, vertigo, nausea, vomiting, flushing, palpitations, weakness, dyspnea, tachypnea, hypertension with reflex bradycardia. Late: Hypotension, tachycardia, syncope, seizures, coma, rigidity, apnea, paralysis, pulmonary edema, arrhythmias, cardiac conduction block, terminal bradycardia, death.

Mechanism: Cyanide binds to the ferric (Fe^{+3}) ion of the respiratory enzyme cytochrome oxidase, thereby blocking oxidative phosphorylation and adenosine triphosphate (ATP) production.

Notes: Early symptoms are due to transient central nervous system and cardiovascular stimulation. Rapid onset, coma, intractible hypotension, and severe (lactic) acidosis are diagnostic clues. Many individuals cannot detect the classic "bitter almond" odor of cyanide. Inhibition of cytochrome oxidase prevents oxygen utilization, leading to an elevated venous Po_2 (greater than 40 mm Hg and approaching that of arterial blood) and equally red veins and arteries on funduscopic examination.

Antidotes

Oxygen; amyl nitrite, sodium nitrite, sodium thiosulfate (Cyanide Antidote Package, Lilly).

Mechanism: Incompletely understood. Oxygen displaces cyanide from cytochrome oxidase and enhances the efficacy of nitrate-thiosulfate therapy. Nitrites convert hemoglobin (Fe^{+2}) to methemoglobin (Fe^{+3}). Cyanide then binds to methemoglobin to form cyanomethemoglobin (liberating cytochrome oxidase). Cyanomethemoglobin slowly dissociates into cyanide and methemoglobin, and thiosulfate combines with free cyanide to form thiocyanate, which is excreted in the urine.

Indications: Altered mental status, abnormal vital signs or neurologic examination, and metabolic acidosis.

Dose: Oxygen: 100 percent by mask plus nasal canula or by endotracheal tube (see carbon monoxide section). Amyl nitrite: Place freshly broken pearl between two gauze pads and hold in front of patient's mouth for 15 out of every 30 seconds while continuing oxygen by canula, mask, or bag mask. Sodium nitrite (3 percent): 300 mg (10 ml or one ampule) for adults or 10 mg per kg (0.33 ml per kilogram) for children intravenously over 2 to 4 minutes. Sodium thiosulfate (25 percent): 12.5 g (50 ml) for adults or 1.65 ml per kilogram for children intravenously over 1 to 2 minutes.

Notes: Early central nervous system symptoms should not be used as the sole indication for antidotal therapy, since they are similar to those of anxiety reactions (which commonly follow cyanide exposures). Amyl nitrite should be used only as a temporizing measure until sodium nitrite can be prepared for injection. Sodium nitrite may cause hypotension if given rapidly. The pediatric dose of nitrite is designed to produce a methemoglobin level of 30 percent. Since a 30 kilogram child is given the full adult dose, it follows that a 70 kilogram individual may require more than the "standard" adult dose. Although the manufacturer recommends repeating half the original dose of sodium nitrite and sodium thiosulfate if the response is submaximal or signs of poisoning reappear, larger doses may be given provided methemoglobin levels are monitored and do not exceed 30 percent. Excessive methemoglobinemia should be treated by exchange transfusion rather than methylene blue, because methylene blue may cause cyanide to be released from the cyanomethemoglobin complex. Hyperbaric oxygn should be considered in patients who do not respond to antidotal therapy.

Digitalis

Toxicity

Signs and symptoms: Anorexia, nausea, vomiting, lethargy, weakness, disturbances of color vision, photophobia, scotoma, headache, parasthesias, confusion, hallucinations, cardiac arrhythmias, and conduction abnormalities.

Mechanism: Direct central nervous system effects, inhibition of the sodium-potassium-ATPase transport system, and increased vagal tone. Cardiac effects include increased contractility and excitability, decreased automaticity of the SA node with increased automaticity of other cardiac tissues, and slowed conduction (heart block) at the SA and AV nodes.

Notes: Although digoxin and digitoxin are the only digitalis preparations commonly used in clinical practice, many plants (e.g., foxglove, lilly of the valley, oleander) contain cardiac glycosides. Virtually any type or combination or arrhythmias and conduction abnormalities may be seen. Severe hyperkalemia is characteristic of acute poisoning, whereas hypokalemia is generally found in chronic poisoning.

Antidote

Digoxin-specific Fab fragments of sheep IgG antibodies (Dibibind, Burroughs-Wellcome).

Mechanism: Antibody fragments react with digoxin (and related glycosides), forming an inactive antigen-antibody complex, which is excreted in the urine.

Indications: Life-threatening cardic toxicity unresponsive to correction of electrolyte, calcium, and magnesium abnormalities, antiarrhythmic agents (e.g., lidocaine, phenytoin, magnesium, propranolol, and possibly bretylium), chronotropic agents (e.g., atropine, isoproterenol, glucagon), countershock, and pacemaker insertion.

Dose: The neutralizing dose of Fab, given intravenously over 15 to 30 minutes, is approximately 66 mg for each milligram of digoxin ingested or for each ng per milliliter of digoxin in serum. Lower doses may also be effective. Since digitoxin crossreacts weakly (about 7 percent) with digoxin-specific Fab fragments, a larger Fab dose may be needed for digitoxin intoxications.

Notes: Since distribution is limited and optimal doses are unknown, consult poison information center for nearest source of Fab and antibodies and package insert for latest dosing guidelines. For comments regarding antibody administration see the chapter *Bee, Wasp, and Spider Envenomation*.

Dystonic (Extrapyramidal) Reactions

Toxicity

Signs and symptoms: Involuntary, often sustained, muscle spasms of eyes and lids (oculogyric), tongue and face (buccolingual), neck (torticollic), back (opisthotonic), abdomen and pelvis (tortipelvic), or combinations thereof.

Mechanism: Appears to result from inhibition of central nervous system dopaminergic and cholinergic pathways, causing a relative excess of cholinergic activity.

Notes: Drugs known to cause dystonic reactions include antihistamines, antipsychotics (butyrophenones, phenothiazines, thioxanthenes), bromocriptine, cyclic antidepressants, carbamazepine, lithium, metoclopramide (Reglan), phenytoin, reserpine, and trimethobenzamide (Tigan).

Antidotes

Diphenhydramine (Benadryl, Parke-Davis); Benztropine mesylate (Cogentin, Merck, Sharp & Dohme).

Mechanism: Anticholinergic effects restore dopaminergic-cholinergic balance in the central nervous system.

Indication: Signs and symptoms as described above.

Dose: Diphenhydramine: 50 to 100 mg (adult) or 1 to 2 mg per kilogram (children) intravenously over 2 minutes followed by 50 mg (adult) or 1 to 2 mg per kilogram (children) orally 3 to 4 times a day for 2 to 3 days. Benztropine: 1 to 2 mg (adult) or 0.01 to 0.02 mg per kilogram (children) intravenously over 2 minutes followed by same dose orally twice a day for 2 to 3 days.

Notes: Benztropine should be used for dystonic reactions caused by diphenhydramine. The manufacturer states that benztropine is contraindicated in children under 3 years of age because of anticholinergic side effects. In this situation, however, this is precisely the intended effect. Alternative therapeutic agents include intravenous or oral doses of biperiden (Akineton) and oral doses of trihexyphenidyl (Artane). The response to treatment is immediate and dramatic except for reactions to metoclopramide (reactions are notoriously prolonged and resistant to treatment).

Ethylene Glycol

Toxicity

Signs and symptoms: Nausea, vomiting, ataxia, lethargy, nystagmus, slurred speech, hyporeflexia, metabolic acidosis (tachypnea), flank pain, renal insufficiency, hypocalcemia (hyperreflexia, myoclonus). Ophthalmoplegia, papilledema, coma, seizures, cerebral edema, cyanosis, pulmonary edema, cardiac failure, and oliguric renal failure may occur in severe cases.

Mechanisms: Direct central nervous system depression. Intermediary metabolites (e.g., glycoaldehyde and glycolic, glyoxylic, and oxalic acids) are responsible for metabolic, cardiopulmonary, and renal toxicity. Hypocalcemia results from formation of oxalic acid and precipitation of calcium oxalate crystals.

Notes: ethylene glycol is found in solvents, windshield de-icers, and radiator antifreeze. Ethanol-like inebriation, increased anion gap metabolic acidosis, increased serum osmolality (1 mOsm per kilogram water for each 5 mg per deciliter ethylene glycol), and an abnormal urinalysis (hematuria, proteinuria, calcium oxalate and hippuric acid crystals) are diagnostic clues. Renal insufficiency typically develops within 24 to 36 hours. Metabolic and renal toxicity may be delayed if ethanol is simultaneously ingested.

Antidote

Ethanol; pyridoxine; thiamine.

Mechanism: Ethanol competitively inhibits ethylene glycol metabolism by saturating alcohol dehydrogenase (the enzyme responsible for the first step in ethanol and ethylene glycol metabolism. Unmetabolized ethylene glycol is then excreted by the lungs and kidneys. Pyridoxal phosphate and thiamine pyrophosphate are cofactors in the pathways responsible for degrading glyoxylic acid (to nontoxic metabolites).

Indications: Symptoms of intoxication or ingestion of more than 120 mg per kilogram (0.11 ml per kilogram) of pure ethylene glycol (pending serum level); serum level greater than 20 mg per deciliter; acidosis or severe toxicity (regardless of serum level).

Dose: Ethanol: 10 ml per kilogram of 10 percent ethanol (in 5 or 10 percent dextrose) intravenously over 30 minutes followed by 1.5 ml per kilogram per hour of the same solution. Alternatively, 1 ml per kilogram 95 percent ethanol (with juice) followed by 0.1 ml per kilogram per hour may be given orally. Doses should be adjusted to achieve a steady state ethanol level of 100 to 150 mg per deciliter. Pyridoxine and Thiamine: 100 mg intravenously over 5 to 10 minutes initially and then once a day.

Notes: Sodium bicarbonate and calcium should be given to correct acidosis and hypocalcemia. Since ethanol may increase the ethylene glycol half-life from 2 to 4 hours to 15 to 20 hours, prolonged treatment is often necessary. Hemodialysis is recommended if the ethylene glycol level is above 50 mg per deciliter, acidosis persists despite ethanol and bicarbonate therapy, or symptoms are severe. The hourly dose of ethanol should be doubled during dialysis. Treatment may be stopped when symptoms and metabolic abnormalities have resolved and the ethylene glycol level is less than 10 mg per deciliter.

Fluorides

Toxicity

Signs and symptoms: Ingestion: Nausea, vomiting, diarrhea, abdominal pain, gastrointestinal bleeding, central nervous system depression, headache, paresthesias, weakness, paralysis, hypocalcemia (tetany, increased QT interval), hypomagnesemia, hypo- or hyperkalemia, coagulopathy, hematuria, arrhythmias, cardiac failure, and renal dysfunction. Dermal exposure (hydrofluoric acid): Burns, necrosis, ulceration. Inhalational exposure: Laryngeal and pulmonary edema.

Mechanism: Local corrosive effects. Absorbed fluoride ions form relatively insoluble complexes with calcium, magnesium, potassium, and zinc inhibit glycolytic (and other) enzymes, and cause direct neuromuscular toxicity.

Notes: Toxicity following ingestion or inhalation is often rapid in onset, whereas dermal injury after exposure to low concentrations of hydrofluoric acid (e.g., 20 percent) may be delayed up to 24 hours. The serum calcium level (both ionized and nonionized) may be profoundly depressed. In contrast to other acids, hydrofluoric acid causes liquefaction necrosis, resulting in deep tissue penetration, severe pain, and progressive burns. Ingestion of less than 5 mg per kilogram of free fluoride (as one of its salts) is unlikely to result in significant toxicity.

Antidotes

Calcium gluconate; magnesium sulfate.

Mechanism: Corrects hypocalcemia and hypomagnesemia. Calcium and magnesium bind free fluoride ions and precipitate as nontoxic salts (e.g., calcium fluoride).

Indications: Ingestion, inhalation: Hypocalcemia, hypomagnesemia, tetany, or symptomatic patient with arrhythmias or electrocardiographic evidence of hypocalcemia (i.e., increased QT interval) pending serum calcium and magnesium levels. Dermal exposure: Pain with or without objective evidence of burns.

Dose: Ingestion, inhalation: Calcium gluconate: Same as for calcium antagonist overdose. Repeat dose as indicated by serum calcium level, recurrence of tetany, or electrocardiogram evidence of hypocalcemia. Magnesium sulfate: 0.1 to 0.2 ml per kilogram of a 10-percent solution intravenously over 15 to 30 minutes. Repeat dose as indicated by serum magnesium level. Dermal exposure: 10 percent solution of magnesium sulfate or calcium gluconate, 0.5 ml per square centimeter of affected area and surrounding margin (0.5 cm), by subcutaneous infiltration using a 30-gauge needle. Repeat injection if pain recurs.

Notes: Diuresis may enhance the excretion of fluoride. Milk, antacids containing aluminum, calcium, or magnesium hydroxide, or calcium salts (e.g., chalk, lime water) may be given orally to bind ingested fluoride. Calcium or magnesium gels (2.5 to 10 percent) or iced solutions of magnesium sulfate (25 percent) or benzalkonium chloride may be applied to hydrofluoric acid burns as a first aid measure. If the subungual area is involved, the nail should be removed to permit local infiltration. Pain may be briefly worsened during infiltration, but should subside shortly thereafter. Since relief of pain is the endpoint of therapy, local anesthetics should be used only for surgical procedures such as nail removal. The intra-arterial (i.e., brachial) infusion of 10-percent calcium gluconate (10 ml in 50 ml 5-percent dextrose in water over 4 hours with repeat doses as necessary) has recently been shown to be highly effective alternative to local infiltration in the treatment of digital burns.

Hydrogen Sulfide

Toxicity

Signs and symptoms: Same as those of hypoxia of any etiology (e.g., central nervous system and cardiovascular dysfunction, lactic acidosis). Conjunctivitis, blepharospasm, blurred or halo vision, pruritis, skin erythema, seizures, and pulmonary edema may also be noted.

Mechanism: Inhibition of the respiratory enzyme cytochrome oxidase leads to cellular asphyxia by blocking oxidative phosphorylation and ATP production.

Notes: Hydrogen sulfide is a colorless gas, which smells like rotten eggs and is released from sulfur compounds by decomposition (e.g., sewers, liquid manure, and fish holding tanks) or the action of an acid (e.g., sulfuric acid, tanning). The rapid onset of coma, seizures, hypotension, and lactic acidosis is characteristic of exposure to high concentrations.

Antidotes

Oxygen; nitrites (Cyanide Antidote Package, Lilly).

Mechanism: Incompletely understood. Oxygen competes with hydrogen sulfide for binding sites on cytochrome oxidase. Nitrites convert hemoglobin to methemoglobin. Hydrogen sulfide then binds to methemoglobin (liberating cytochrome oxidase).

Indications: Severe clinical toxicity, metabolic acidosis, abnormal mental status, vital signs, or neurologic examination.

Dose: Oxygen: Same as for carbon monoxide poisoning. Nitrites: Same as for cyanide poisoning.

Notes: Nitrites should be reserved for severely intoxicated patients or those who do not improve with oxygen therapy. The sodium thiosulfate component of the cyanide antidote kit should not be given. Rescue personnel should wear self-containing breathing devices to avoid secondary casualties.

Hypoglycemia

Toxicity

Signs and symptoms: Anxiety, confusion, dizziness, headache, abnormal behavior, diaphoresis, tachycardia, tremors, coma, seizures.

Mechanisms: Underproduction of overutilization (i.e., hyperinsulinism) of glucose.

Notes: Symptoms are due to central nervous system dysfunction and adrenergic hyperactivity (epinephrine release). In addition to insulin and oral hypoglycemic drugs (i.e., sulfonylureas), agents known to cause hypoglycemia include acetone, alcohols (including alcoholic ketoacidosis), beta-adrenergic antagonists, ethylene dichloride, hepatotoxins, narcotics, and salicylates. Children appear to be more susceptible than adults.

Antidote

d-Glucose (Dextrose).

Indications: Abnormal vital signs or mental status.

Mechanism: Provides exogenous glucose.

Dose: 1 to 2 ml per kilogram of 50 percent dextrose (50 percent dextrose in water) intravenously over 2 minutes for adults or same volume of 10 to 20 percent dextrose for infants and children. Repeat dose if incomplete response or symptoms reappear.

Notes: Glucose may be given by mouth in awake patients or by nasogastric tube in comatose patients when venous access cannot be obtained. Glucose solutions are hypertonic and may cause severe tissue necrosis if extravasation of intravenous solutions occurs.

Iron

Toxicity

Signs and symptoms: Nausea, vomiting, diarrhea, gastrointestinal bleeding, fever, leukocytosis, hyperglycemia, acidosis, lethargy, confusion, coma, and shock. Hepatic and renal failure, pulmonary edema and hemorrhage, and bowel infarction may develop in severe cases. Intestinal stricture formation is a delayed complication.

Mechanism: Mucosal corrosive (gastrointestinal). Shock is secondary to gastrointestinal and intravascular fluid loss (capillary leak). Acidosis results from shock, conversion of ferrous iron to ferric hydroxide with concomitant release of hydrogen ions, and inhibition of the Krebs cycle, leading to anaerobic metabolism with lactic and citric acid accumulation. Hepatic toxicity is due to mitochondrial injury.

Notes: Gastrointestinal symptoms, leukocytosis (leukocyte count greater than 15,000 per cubic millimeter), hyperglycemia (serum glucose greater than 150 mg per deciliter), fever, and radiodense material in the stomach on kidney-ureter-bladder x-ray examination are risk factors that correlate with elevated iron levels. Patients with these findings or a history of ingesting more than 60 mg per kilogram of elemental iron should have serum iron (SI) and total iron binding capacity (TIBC) measured. Patients with lesser ingestions and no associated risk factors who remain asymptomatic during a 4 to 6 hour observation period may be discharged. Poisoned patients may show signs of apparent improvement 6 to 12 hours following ingestion, but subsequently relapse. Ferrous sulfate and ferrous gluconate tablets are the most common iron preparations and contain 20 percent and 12 percent elemental iron, respectively.

Antidote

Deferoxamine mesylate (DFO; Desferal, Ciba)

Mechanism: Free iron is chelated by DFO (8.5 mg iron per 100 mg), forming ferrioxamine (the iron-DFO complex), which is then excreted in the urine. Of importance in chronic iron overload is the fact that storage pool iron (hemosiderin and ferritin) is also chelated by DFO.

Indications: SI greater than TIBC, SI greater than 350 mg per deciliter if TIBC not available or, in presence of risk factors if neither SI or TIBC are available.

Dose: 15 mg per kilogram per hour intravenously in 5 percent dextrose or normal saline. May also be given intramuscularly (90 mg per kilogram up to 2 g every 8 hours) as a provocative (challenge) test or therapeutically in normotensive, mildly symptomatic patients.

Notes: DFO is more effective by the intravenous route. Although rapid intravenous administration of DFO may cause histamine release resulting in anaphylactoid reactions, doses as high as 35 mg per kilogram per hour have been used without adverse effects. Oral doses of DFO may lead to enhanced absorption of ferrioxamine, resulting in increased toxicity and should be avoided. Gastric lavage with 5 percent sodium bicarbonate (in addition to water or saline) may convert iron to the relatively insoluble carbonate salt and decrease its absorption. Ferrioxamine gives the urine a reddish ("vin rose") color. This color change is the criterion determining a positive chelation challenge test and the need for continued chelation. DFO may be stopped when the urine color returns to baseline (save a prechelation sample in a vacuum tube for comparison), the SI level drops below the TIBC level, and clinical toxicity resolves.

Isoniazid-Hydrazines

Toxicity

Signs and symptoms: Nausea, vomiting, confusion, dizziness, ataxis, slurred speech, hallucinations, hyperreflexia, coma, seizures, respiratory depression, hyperglycemia, hypotension, tachycardia, rash, and liver and kidney damage. Inhalation and topical exposure (hydrazines) may cause respiratory and skin irritation. Chronic isoniazid (INH) ingestion may cause optic and peripheral neuritis, psychosis, encephalopathy, seizures, and bone marrow suppression.

Mechanism: Inhibition of the coenzyme pyridoxal-5-phosphate results in decreased synthesis of the central nervous system neurotransmitter GABA (gamma-aminobutyric acid). Since GABA is mainly found in inhibitory neurons, decreased GABA levels result in central nervous system stimulation.

Notes: Hydrazines, used in chemical reactions and as rocket fuel, may also cause methemoglobinemia.

Monomethylhydrazine is the toxic principle in certain species of mushrooms (e.g., Gyromitra, Paxina). The onset of toxicity may be rapid and seizures may result in severe lactic acidosis.

Antidotes

Diazepam; pyridoxine.

Mechanism: Diazepam (and barbiturates) are GABA receptor agonists. Pyridoxine is converted to pyridoxal-5-phosphate, thus reversing the inhibition of this coenzyme.

Indications: Diazepam: Seizures. Pyridoxine: Acute ingestion of 80 mg per kilogram or more of INH or presence of symptoms.

Dose: Diazepam: 5 to 10 mg (adult) or 0.1 to 0.3 mg per kilogram (children) IV over 2 to 3 minutes. Repeat dose every 3 to 5 minutes until seizures cease. Pyridoxine: Same dose (in milligram) as estimated amount of INH or hydrazine ingested or 25 mg per kilogram in 5 percent dextrose in water as a 5 to 10 percent solution of pyridoxine over 5 to 30 minutes (depending on clinical severity) for topical or oral exposures in which the amount of toxin is unknown. Repeat dose if response is submaximal or symptoms recur.

Notes: The use of ample doses of diazepam and pyridoxine have essentially eliminated the need for barbiturates (e.g., amobarbital), paralyzing agents, general anesthesia, and hemodialysis in the management of acute INH-hydrazine poisoning. Although pyridoxine is generally considered relatively nontoxic, high doses have been reported to cause mild central nervous system depression, seizures, and peripheral (sensory) neuropathies.

Methanol

Toxicity

Signs and symptoms: Nausea, vomiting, abdominal pain, gastrointestinal bleeding, pancreatitis, transient liver function abnormalities, headache, dizziness, weakness, lethargy, confusion, photophobia, scotoma, blurred vision, tunnel vision, "white spots" or "snowfield" vision, and increased anion gap metabolic acidosis (tachypnea). Coma, seizures, shock, blindness, macula elevation, retinal edema, optic disk hyperemia, putamen infarction and persistent neurologic sequelae (e.g., Parkinson-like syndrome, spasticity, tremors) in severe cases.

Mechanism: Gastrointestinal irritation. Formation of toxic intermediary metabolite (formic acid).

Notes: Gastrointestinal symptoms, visual complaints, metabolic acidosis, and increased serum osmolality (1 mOsm per kilogram of water for each 2.6 mg per deciliter methanol) are diagnostic clues. Patients appear more sick than inebriated. Onset of symptoms may be delayed up to 18 hours after ingestion, particularly if alcohol was also ingested.

Antidotes

Ethanol; folate (folic acid).

Mechanism: Ethanol competitively inhibits methanol metabolism by starting alcohol dehydrogenase (the enzyme responsible for the first step in ethanol and methanol metabolism). Unmetabolized methanol is then excreted by the lungs and kidneys. Folic acid is a coenzyme in the metabolic conversion of formic acid to carbon dioxide and water.

Indications: Symptoms of intoxication or ingestion of more than 120 mg per kilogram (0.14 ml per kilogram) of pure methanol (pending serum level); peak methanol level of 20 mg per deciliter or greater; acidosis, visual symptoms, or severe toxicity (regardless of serum level).

Dose: Ethanol: Same as for ethylene glycol. Folate: 50 mg intravenously initially and then 50 mg intravenously every 4 hours.

Notes: Since ethanol may increase the half-life of methanol from 2 to 4 hours to more than 15 hours, prolonged treatment is often necessary. Hemodialysis is recommended if the methanol level is greater than 50 mg per deciliter, if acidosis persists despite ethanol and bicarbonate therapy, or if symptoms are severe or visual symptoms are present. The hourly dose of ethanol should be doubled during dialysis. Treatment may be stopped when symptoms and metabolic abnormalities have resolved and the methanol level is less than 10 mg per deciliter.

Methemoglobinemia

Toxicity

Signs and symptoms: Central nervous system and cardiovascular depression, seizures, nausea, vomiting, dyspnea, tachypnea, cyanosis, lactic acidosis, Heinz body formation, and hemolysis (delayed).

Mechanism: Oxidation of hemoglobin (Fe^{+2}) to methemoglobin (Fe^{+3}). Methemoglobin is unable to carry oxygen, and the oxygen-hemoglobin dissociation curve is shifted to the left (lower tissue Po_2 required for oxygen unloading). Further oxidation of methemoglobin causes Heinz body formation (precipitated hemoglobin), which makes erythrocytes more rigid and more susceptible to hemolysis.

Notes: Signs and symptoms are due to hypoxia. Cyanosis (violet, gray, or brown hues) becomes visible at methemoglobin levels of 15 to 20 percent (1.5 g), but symptoms do not usually develop until levels reach 30 percent. Cyanosis unresponsive to oxygen, a normal Po_2 level (and hence normal calculated oxygen saturation) with decreased measured (direct) oxygen saturation, and blood having a chocolate color when placed on filter paper next to a drop of normal (red) blood are diagnostic clues. If methemoglobin levels cannot be measured directly, the difference between the calculated and measured oxygen saturation, the "oxygen saturation gap," provides an estimate of the methemoglobin level. Agents capable of oxidizing hemoglobin include aniline and related aromatic amino-nitro-nitroso-compounds, antimalarial drugs (e.g., chloroquine), local anesthetics, chlorates, dapsone, nitrates and nitrites, phenacetin, phenazopyridine, phenols, quinones, and sulfonamides.

Antidote

Methylene blue.

Mechanism: Enhances enzymatic (NADPH-dependent methemoglobin reductase) conversion of methemoglobin to hemoglobin by acting as an electron donating cofactor (reducing agent).

Indications: Methemoglobin level of 30 percent or greater; lower levels in those with cardiovascular disease or symptoms that are not relieved by oxygen administration.

Dose: 1 to 2 mg per kilogram of a 1 percent solution (0.1 to 0.2 mg per kilogram) intravenously over 5 minutes. Repeat as necessary for persistent or recurrent methemoglobinemia.

Notes: Ascorbic acid (0.5 to 1 g intravenously or orally 4 times a day), another reducing agent, may be given in addition to methylene blue. Hyperbaric oxygen or exchange transfusion should be considered in patients unresponsive to methylene blue or those with methemoglobin levels above 60 percent. Side effects of methylene blue include headache, confusion, nausea, vomiting, diaphoresis, abdominal and chest pain, dysuria, repolarization changes on the electrocardiogram, blue-green saliva and urine, and hemolysis. Although high doses (7 mg per kilogram or greater) of methylene blue may induce methemoglobinemia, therapeutic doses have not been associated with this complication.

Narcotics

Toxicity

Signs and symptoms: Nausea, vomiting, ileus, diaphoresis, pinpoint pupils, central nervous system and respiratory depression, hallucinations, seizures, bradycardia, hypotension, noncardiogenic pulmonary edema.

Mechanism: Stimulation of opiate (endorphin-enkephalin) receptors in the central nervous system, increased vagal tone, vasodilation, and increased pulmonary vascular permeability.

Notes: Narcotic agents include opium and its derivatives (e.g., paregoric, morphine, codeine), morphine congeners (e.g., diphenoxylate, fentanyl), methadone and its congeners (e.g., propoxyphene), and synthetic agonist-antagonist compounds (e.g., butorphanol, nalbuphine, and pentazocine). Some agents (e.g., meperidine) have anticholinergic effects and may cause mydriasis. Following ingestion, symptoms may be delayed in onset and prolonged in duration. Pulmonary edema may develop up to 24 hours after recovery from coma.

Antidote

Naloxone hydrochloride (Narcan, DuPont).

Mechanism: Antagonizes effects of narcotics by competitively blocking opiate receptors.

Indications: Symptoms of narcotic overdose, especially central nervous system or respiratory depression and seizures.

Dose: 2 mg intravenously initially with repeat doses as often as necessary. Alternatively, a naloxone infusion (0.4 to 4 mg per hour) may be used to maintain narcotic reversal (e.g., adequate ventilation). If an intravenous line cannot be established, nalaxone may be given intramuscularly, by sublingual injection, or by the endotracheal route.

Notes: Larger doses of naxolone may be required to reverse intoxication due to methadone derivatives and agonist-antagonist agents. The diagnosis of narcotic overdose should not be excluded until a total dose of 10 mg of naloxone has been given. Although the manufacturer still recommends a pediatric naloxone dosage of 0.01 mg per kilogram followed by 0.1 mg per kilogram (if clinical response is less than optimal), the antidotal dose of naloxone should be the same for all patients (regardless of age and weight), since it depends on the amount of narcotic present and its affinity for opiate receptors (not the size of the patient). Since the pharmacologic half-life of naloxone (20 to 30 minutes) is short compared with that of narcotics, prolonged observation and repeat doses are often necessary. Hospital admission is mandatory for all toxic ingestions and any suggestion (by history) of narcotic ingestion in children because of delayed and prolonged toxicity. Narcotic withdrawal, the only side effect of naloxone administration, is short-lived and should not be treated with narcotics (except in neonates in whom withdrawal symptoms may be life-threatening). In known addicts, withdrawal may be prevented by giving smaller doses of naloxone (e.g., only enough to reverse respiratory depression). Naloxone may not reverse propoxyphene-induced hypotension and administration of a pressor agent may be necessary.

Snake Envenomation (Crotalidae)

Toxicity

Signs and symptoms: Local: Puncture wound(s), pain, swelling, erythema, ecchmyosis, paresthesias, bullae formation, necrosis, ulceration, and compartment syndromes. Systemic: Nausea, vomiting, diarrhea, gastrointestinal bleeding, diaphoresis, unusual taste sensations, salivation, perioral and scalp paresthesias, weakness, arrhythmias, cardiac ischemia, lethargy, coma, seizures, pulmonary edema, hemolysis, thrombocytopenia, coagulopathy, hematuria, proteinuria, and glycosuria.

Mechanism: Proteins and enzymes in venom cause local tissue necrosis and vascular damage (proteases, hyaluronidase), hemolysis (phospholipase), fibrinolysis (amino acid esterases), and neuromuscular dysfunction (cholinesterases, anticholinesterases).

Notes: Genera of the family Crotalidae include *Crotalus* (rattlesnakes), *Agkistrodon* (copperhead, cottonmouth), and *Sistrurus* (pigmy rattler and massasauga). The venom composition varies from species to species. The Mojave rattler (*C. scutulatus scutulatus*), found in southwestern states, may cause delayed neuromuscular paralysis with minimal local findings. Many bites do not result in envenomation. First aid measures include immobilization of the affected extremity and rapid transport to a hospital. Tourniquets (obstructing lymphatic, but not venous or arterial flow), incision (short, shallow, and perpendicular to line between fang marks), suction, and ice packs are unlikely to be of value unless utilized within 30 minutes after envenomation.

Antidote

Polyvalent Crotalidae antivenin (Wyeth)

Mechanism: Immune globulins in antivenin neutralize venom proteins by antigen-antibody reaction.

Indications: Local or systemic signs of envenomation.

Contraindications (relative): Allergy to horses or horse serum.

Dose: Mild envenomation (local reaction limited to hand or foot): 5 vials. Moderate envenomation (moderate or progressive local reaction with or without systemic symptoms and laboratory abnormalities): 10 vials. *Severe envenomation* (local reaction involving entire extremity, severe systemic symptoms or marked laboratory test abnormalities): 15 vials. Antivenin should be mixed with 20 ml per kilogram of normal saline and infused over 1 to 2 hours. Additional doses of antivenin may be necessary if symptoms or laboratory test abnormalities worsen or if systemic symptoms are not relieved by the initial dose.

Notes: The affected extremity should be immobilized in a horizontal position at heart level, and circumference measurements (at the bite site and several proximal locations) should be taken every 15 to 30 minutes to assess the progression of local reactions. Fasciotomy should be reserved for those with high intracompartmental pressures (i.e., greater than 40 mm Hg) documented by direct catheter measurement, since, despite severe edema, compartmental pressures are rarely elevated. See chapter, *Bee, Wasp, and Spider Envenomation* for notes on antivenin administration and serum sickness reactions. Patients with horse or horse serum allergies, or those previously treated with antivenin, may be pretreated with diphenhydramine, epinephrine, and corticosteroids.

Snake Envenomation (Elapidae)

Toxicity

Signs and symptoms: Local: Scratch, puncture wound(s),and minimal pain and swelling. Systemic: Nausea, vomiting, lethargy, salivation, headache, tremors, fasciculations, weakness, and paralysis (e.g., dysphagia, dysphonia, diplopia, ptosis, respiratory failure).

Mechanism: Venom proteins block neuronal transmission at neuromuscular junctions.

Notes: Elapidae indigenous to the southern United States include three *Micruris* species: the Eastern, Texas, and Arizona coral snakes. These small snakes are recognized by wide red and black bands separated by narrow yellow ones—("Red on yellow, kill a fellow. Red on black, venom lack.") Exotic elapidae (e.g., cobras, kraits) may be kept by zoos or amateur herpetologists.

Antidote

North American coral snake antivenin (Wyeth); exotic antivenins.

Mechanism: Immune globulins in antivenin neutralize venom proteins by an antigen-antibody reaction.

Indications: Symptoms of envenomation or unequivocal bite by a positively identified coral snake.

Contraindications(relative): Allergy to horses or horse serum.

Dose: Three to five vials initially with repeat doses if symptoms persist, reappear, or subsequently develop.

Notes: See discussions of black widow spider and crotadidae envenomation for notes about antivenin administration. Coral snake antivenin may be located by calling a local poison information center or Wyeth Laboratories in Philadelphia (215-688-4400). Exotic elapidae antivenin may be located by calling a local zoo, the Antivenin Index Center at the Oklahoma Zoo (405-424-3344), or the Oklahoma Poison Information Center (405-271-5454).

Thyroid Hormones

Toxicity

Signs and symptoms: Nausea, vomiting, diarrhea, abdominal pain, mydriasis, flushing, anxiety, agitation, hyperactivity, tremors, palpitations, tachycardia, fever, hypertension, diaphoresis, and hyperglycemia. Tachyarrhythmias, hypotension, cardiac failure, and seizures in severe cases.

Mechanism: Increased metabolic and sympathetic nervous system activity.

Notes: In contrast to the early onset of toxicity following a desiccated thyroid (T_3 and T_4) or liothyronine (T_3) overdose, toxicity due to levothyroxine (T_4) ingestion is typically delayed 12 hours to several days (until T_4 is metabolized to T_3, the more active hormone). Patients without symptoms during a 6 hour observation period may be discharged (with outpatient follow-up).

Antidotes

Propranolol (Inderal, Ayerst).

Mechanism: Counteracts adrenergic hyperactivity and inhibits conversion of T_4 to T_3.

Indications: Symptoms of metabolic or adrenergic hyperactivity.

Dose: 0.1 to 1 mg per kilogram orally every 6 hours. For rapid control of severe symptoms, 0.01 to 0.02 mg per kilogram intravenously every 5 to 10 minutes until symptoms abate.

Notes: Phenytoin, which also inhibits the conversion of T_4 to T_3, may be used (in addition to diazepam) for seizure control. Exchange transfusion, plasmapheresis, and the administration of antithyroid agents (e.g., propylthiouracil) have not been shown to be beneficial in treating exogenous thyroid hormone toxicity.

SUGGESTED READING

Goldfrank L, Cohen L, Flomenbann N, et al. Newer antidotes and controversies in antidotal therapy. In: Wolcott BW, Rund DA, eds. Emergency medicine annual. East Norwalk, Connecticut: Appleton-Century-Crofts, 1984: 221.

Haddad LM, Winchester JF, eds. Clinical management of poisoning and drug overdose. Philadelphia: W.B. Saunders, 1983.

Rumack BH, ed. Poisindex. Denver: Micromodex, 1985.

SEDATIVES AND OPIATES

TOBY LITOVITZ, M.D.

SEDATIVE-HYPNOTICS

In 1984, 19,325 reports to the American Association of Poison Control Centers National Data Collection System involved sedative-hypnotic agents. This represents an estimated 15 to 42 percent of the actual nationwide frequency of sedative-hypnotic overdoses. Table 1 presents the frequency distribution for the various drugs in this category, emphasizing the preponderance of benzodiazepines (63 percent), followed by barbiturates and over the counter sleep aids.

DIAGNOSIS

Except for minor clinical clues, diagnosis rests predominantly on ingestion history, labels on available prescription vials (often with pharmacy confirmation of the number dispensed), and toxicologic analysis of blood, urine, and gastric contents. Undifferentiated central nervous system (CNS) depression, variably accompanied by respiratory depression, hypotension, hypothermia, and pulmonary edema, is the common clinical denominator of all these agents. Additional unique clinical features associated with specific agents are delineated below and may allow more precise diagnosis.

Specific drug identification is generally a low priority. Its major utility is the exclusion of other agents that require more than supportive treatment. Determination of plasma drug concentrations rarely influences the management of the patient with a pure sedative-hypnotic overdose, but it is useful when alternative diagnoses are being considered and when extracorporeal drug elimination procedures are contemplated. Generally a poor correlation between blood levels and clinical manifestations is obtained in this pharmacologic group. However, a useful correlation of blood levels with clinical manifestations for uncomplicated single acute ingestions of short-acting barbiturates was devised by McCarron et al and is presented in Table 2. Patients with medical complications in addition to the acute intoxication or with multiple ingested substances would have significantly lower plasma levels at the same intoxication state; in contrast, patients with long-term sedative hypnotic use would be expected to have significantly higher levels.

Chloral hydrate is metabolized within just a few minutes to trichloroethanol, also an excellent hypnotic agent. Chloral hydrate mixtures with ethanol bear the street name "Mickey Finn," and ethanol has been demonstrated to cause an earlier and higher peak and more prolonged elevation of serum trichloroethanol levels. A unique feature of chloral hydrate intoxication is its corrosive action, frequently exhibited as gastritis with nausea and vomiting. Severe hemorrhagic gastritis, gastric necrosis, enteritis, and esophageal stricture formation have also been reported. Hepatic, renal, and cardiac toxicity less

TABLE 1 Frequency of Sedative-Hypnotic Overdoses Reported to AAPCC in 1984

Barbiturates	
Long-acting	2,391
Short- or intermediate-acting	1,014
Benzodiazepines	12,227
Chloral hydrate	186
Ethchlorvynol	247
Glutethimide	139
Meprobamate	383
Methaqualone	197
Sleep aids (OTC)	2,185
Other/unknown	356
Total	19,325

TABLE 2 Correlation of Intoxication State with Serum Barbiturate Concentration in Single-Drug Acute Intoxications of Short-Acting Barbiturates in Nonaddicted Patients without Medical Complications (McCarron et al, 1982)

Intoxication State	Mean Serum Level ($\mu g/ml$)
Alert	<6
Drowsy	8 (± 2)
Stuporous	14 (± 3)
Coma, grade 1	18 (± 2)
Coma, grade 2	22 (± 2)
Coma, grade 3	26 (± 2)
Coma, grade 4	34 (± 6)

frequently implicate a direct toxic effect of chloral hydrate, as jaundice, albuminuria, and cardiac arrhythmias have been reported.

Barbiturate toxicity is representative of the sedative-hypnotic group, manifested predominantly by CNS and cardiovascular depression. Reflexes are depressed and then eventually absent as CNS depression progresses. Miosis is typically noted early, although nonreactive mydriasis may be a later manifestation. Respiratory pattern variations eventually yield to respiratory depression, and pulmonary edema may develop. Hypotension may progress to shock, and hypothermia is frequent. Bullous skin lesions, once thought to be a unique feature of acute barbiturate overdose, more recently have been demonstrated with a wide variety of drug overdoses.

Benzodiazepines are considered to be relatively safe in oral overdose and pose mild symptoms when ingested alone. Concomitant drug or alcohol ingestions or intravenous dosing pose a more significant toxic hazard.

Ethchlorvynol overdose is marked by prolonged coma, up to 288 hours, with an average of 102 hours (Teehan et al, 1970).

Glutethimide overdose is complicated by profound and prolonged coma with cyclic fluctuations in the depth of coma and occasional focal neurologic deficits. Sudden deterioration, especially apnea, may occur despite apparent neurologic recovery. Anticholinergic manifestations are common, and a persistent hyperthermia, often following hypothermia, may last for many hours after consciousness returns. The clinical presentation is variable and generally considered to carry a higher fatality rate than most sedative-hypnotic overdoses.

Meprobamate overdose is more frequently characterized by severe and persistent hypotension, appearing with lesser degrees of CNS depression than is seen with other sedative-hypnotic agents.

Methaqualone overdose uniquely features increased deep tendon reflexes, muscular hypertonicity, myoclonus, generalized twitching, shivering, and occasionally seizures (which may also occur with other sedative-hypnotic agents). Neuromuscular paralyzing agents and mechanical ventilation may be required to control the muscular hyperactivity. Coma caused by methaqualone is less frequently accompanied by hypotension or respiratory depression than that caused by other sedative hypnotics. Excessive salivation and increased tracheobronchial secretions are commonly reported, resulting in more frequent aspiration pneumonia. Painful gross hematuria from a necrotizing cystitis has been reported in drug abusers ingesting illegally and improperly synthesized methaqualone contaminated with ortho-toluidine. Deaths frequently result from accidents or drownings while patients are intoxicated rather than a direct toxic effect of methaqualone.

Treatment

Therapy of sedative or hypnotic overdoses focuses on respiratory support. Less frequently, cardiovascular support is also required. Hypotension should be managed initially with fluids to restore central venous pressure; thereafter pressors may be required. As stabilization is achieved, pre-hospital rescue personnel are strongly urged to investigate the overdose site and gather any possibly implicated product or medication containers from the area, transporting these with the patient to the emergency department. A call should be placed to the regional poison center to assist in product ingredient identification and subsequent guidance of the patient's management. When the ingestion is limited to sedative or hypnotic agents, the thrust of therapy is supportive, since no specific antidotes are currently available in the United States, although a benzodiazepine antagonist (Ro 15-1788) has been employed experimentally in Europe.

Gastric decontamination and activated charcoal administration follow (or may be concurrent with) initial stabilization. In the alert patient without seizure activity or concomitant caustic ingestion, ipecac syrup is initially administered in a dose of 30 ml to adults, 15 ml to children aged 1 to 12 years, and 5 to 15 ml to children under 1 year. Where CNS depression has begun to develop and the patient is not sufficiently alert to protect the airway from aspiration, gastric lavage should be performed with a large-bore (No. 36 to 42) orogastric tube in the adult and the largest possible tube that can be inserted in the child. Activated charcoal administration (30 g in children, 60 to 100 g in adults) must follow gastric emptying promptly, since delayed administration has been demonstrated to decrease its efficacy. The palatability of activated charcoal may be improved by suspension in sorbitol, imparting a more viscous texture and sweet flavor. When the activated charcoal is administered per nasogastric or orogastric tube, mixing may alternately be accomplished in a slurry of water or magnesium citrate. Repeated dosing of activated charcoal (20 g every 4 to 6 hours) has been demonstrated to shorten the half-life and increase the clearance of both orally ingested (Pond et al, 1984) and intravenously administered phenobarbital (Berg et al, 1982). Though no data exist to support repetitive activated charcoal administration to enhance the elimination of other sedative-hypnotics, given the nontoxic nature of this therapy, its repetitive use for all sedative-hypnotic overdoses may be advisable.

Enhanced elimination may also be obtained with *alka-*

TABLE 3   Comparison of Various Extracorporeal Techniques That
Enhance Sedative-Hypnotic Elimination (Seyffart, 1977)

| | | | Clearance (ml/min) | |
	Peritoneal Dialysis	Hemodialysis	Hemoperfusion Charcoal	Resin
Chloral hydrate (trichloroethanol)		120–160	†	†
Ethchlorvynol	20	40–80	110–170	184–200
Glutethimide	10	29–109	70–200	up to 300*
Meprobamate	2.5–11	20–100	153–180	up to 300*
Methaqualone	7.5	29	55–230	100–20
Phenobarbital	9	45–80	up to 150	up to 300

* Corresponds to blood flow.
† Limited data, appears to be superior to hemodialysis.

line diuresis in the case of a phenobarbital or barbital overdose, but is ineffective for short-acting barbiturates. Alkalinization dramatically increases urinary excretion of phenobarbital by increasing the percentage of ionized drug. Phenobarbital diffuses across renal tubular cell membranes when nonionized and is therefore reabsorbed. In contrast, when ionized, phenobarbital is excreted in the urine, with renal clearances rising to 17 ml per minute. Alkalinization may be accomplished by adding 1 to 2 ampules (50 to 100 mEq) of sodium bicarbonate to a liter of 5 percent dextrose in water or 5 percent dextrose in half normal saline administered at a rate required to obtain a urine flow of 3 to 6 ml per kilogram per hour and a urine pH of 7 to 8. Both urine and blood pH should be monitored, and subsequent bicarbonate administration should be based on these results. Potassium administration may be required to obtain an alkaline urine.

Hemoperfusion is the preferred extracorporeal detoxification system, but is reserved for the few severely poisoned patients who fail to respond to routine supportive therapy. A comparison of the various extracorporeal techniques is presented in Table 3, based on available data. Although limited by availability, resin hemoperfusion is generally superior to charcoal hemoperfusion for the sedative-hypnotic drugs.

OPIATES

The opiate (plant-derived) and opioid analgesics produce similar effects through CNS opioid receptors. The terms are used interchangeably in the clinical discussion below. Their analgesic potency varies, and they possess psychotropic effects including euphoria and hallucinations, making users prone to addiction. Opiate overdose occurs most frequently with intravenous heroin in the drug abuser, generally resulting from inadvertent abuse of a more concentrated preparation. Other contributing causes are accidental pediatric ingestion of legally available opioids and suicide attempts. In overdose, fatal respiratory depression is the major concern.

The *clinical triad* of CNS depression, miosis, and respiratory depression is characteristic of the opioid overdose patient. Cardiovascular collapse (typically with hypotension or frank shock and less often with

bradycardia), hypothermia, pulmonary edema, and pneumonia are also common. Although pinpoint pupils are characteristic, severe hypoxia or mydriatic drugs may produce mydriasis instead. Noncardiogenic pulmonary edema is uniformly present in fatal cases. It follows opioid-induced hypoxia, generally developing early in the patient's course (within the first 24 hours). Dilution of street drugs with nonsterile potentially toxic substances and malnutrition, infection, and trauma occurring during intoxication are other major causes of morbidity and mortality in the opioid abuser.

Although routine airway maintenance procedures and mechanical ventilation may be necessary, the immediate focus of treatment of opiate overdose is the pure narcotic antagonist *naloxone*. This agent has been demonstrated to be extremely effective, reversing coma and hypotension induced by opioids and restoring ventilation. Naloxone is safe even when administered in very high doses and should be routinely incorporated in the initial approach to any comatose patient, along with dextrose and thiamine administration. As with dextrose, naloxone utilization is both therapeutic and diagnostic, producing immediate arousal and reversal of respiratory depression when administered in adequate doses to the opioid-poisoned patient.

The *recommended dose of naloxone* for the reversal of opioid-poisoning has recently been increased markedly after the observation of (1) occasional naloxone failure to reverse CNS or respiratory depression when given in small doses (0.4 to 0.8 mg intravenously) or when the patient has ingested "relatively refractory" drugs (propoxyphene, methadone, pentazocine, codeine), and (2) the remarkable safety of massive doses (Moore et al, 1980). This change in the naloxone dosing schedule follows documentation of failure to reverse coma with lower doses and subsequent prolonged requirements for ventilatory support, critical care, and extensive neurologic diagnostic studies. Current recommendations utilize naloxone doses of 2 to 4 mg as an initial intravenous bolus, with repeated dosing (an additional 2 mg every 3 to 5 minutes) up to 10 mg or more when opioid overdose is suspected, and the patient fails to respond clinically to the initial dose. An argument can be advanced to utilize the same doses in children as in adults, as it is not the weight of the child that is relevant to the need for the antagonist, but rather the amount of the opioid that was ingested.

In the patient whose coma or respiratory depression was reversed by naloxone boluses, a *naloxone infusion* should follow at a rate of 0.4 mg per hour. If relapses of CNS or respiratory depression occur, the infusion rate should be increased to 0.8 mg per hour (or more as necessary). Naloxone infusions should be continued for a minimum of 12 hours following demonstrated narcotic-induced CNS or respiratory depression. Most opioids have a longer half-life than naloxone; thus a recurrence of respiratory depression as the naloxone bolus wears off is likely, posing a potentially disastrous clinical scenario in the patient who is inappropriately discharged without an adequate observation period following naloxone bolus administration. In addition, the use of continuous infusions of naloxone following the initial bolus provides a safer inpatient management regimen, allowing slightly less meticulous patient observation and thereby freeing intensive care resources for utilization elsewhere.

Fear of precipitating withdrawal is not an indication to withhold naloxone. Because of its short elimination half-life (mean 65 minutes), the narcotic addict experiences transient discomfort (nausea, vomiting, diarrhea, abdominal cramping, sweating, anxiety, tachycardia, hypertension), which will resolve spontaneously if further naloxone dosing is withheld. It is important to realize that life-threatening complications of withdrawal do not develop in this setting. Naltrexone, a newly approved oral narcotic antagonist with a prolonged half-life, may precipitate protracted withdrawal. Therefore, naltrexone is not indicated for the emergency department management of opioid overdose in patients with known chronic use or evidence of possible opioid dependency.

Naloxone administration through the intravenous route is routine, but where intravenous access is difficult in the narcotic abuser with damaged peripheral veins or in the patient in shock, subcutaneous or intramuscular injection of naloxone has been advocated despite delayed and erratic absorption. *Endotracheal administration* of naloxone affords a superior, readily accessible route and allows rapid reversal of opioid depressant effects (Greenberg et al, 1980). Naloxone demonstrates very low oral potency (Bradberry et al, 1981), a factor that has been utilized to clinical advantage via the manufacturer's incorporation of 0.5 mg of naloxone in each 50-mg tablet of Talwin (pentazocine). Intravenous abusers of "Ts and Blues" (Talwin and tripelennamine) experience no narcotic-induced euphoria with this new formulation (and indeed, may actually experience withdrawal). In contrast, when ingested orally, the incorporated naloxone has no significant effect on analgesic potency.

Despite the remarkable safety record of naloxone, even when administered in high doses, sporadic reports of *adverse effects* have appeared in the medical literature.

These include cardiovascular complications (arrhythmias, pulmonary edema) in 7 to 10 reported cases, all of whom received the previously recommended low doses. The definitive implications for the use of naloxone are inconclusive, since all these patients had received general anesthesia and multiple drugs, and many had preexisting disease (including cardiac surgery in four cases). In addition, in most of these cases, symptoms of cardiorespiratory failure actually led to the naloxone administration; thus further deterioration after the drug was taken remains compatible with some other underlying problem.

Multiple additional uses of naloxone, including use for septic and hypovolemic shock, spinal injury, cerebrovascular accident, chronic obstructive pulmonary disease, obesity hypoventilation, neonatal apnea, sudden infant death, high-altitude pulmonary edema, schizophrenia, tardive dyskinesia, idiopathic constipation, and reversal of diazepam, ethanol, barbiturate, and non-narcotic anesthetic effects, are currently under investigation, but results are inconclusive (Milne, 1984). An interaction with endogenous opioids, endorphins, and enkephalins is implicated by proponents of these alternative uses.

The ready availability of a safe antidote for opioid overdose does not obviate the use of standard gastric decontamination procedures when the route of exposure is ingestion. Ipecac-induced emesis or gastric lavage, as outlined above for sedative-hypnotic overdose, is followed by activated charcoal administration. Forced diuresis or urinary pH manipulation are without significant effect, and extracorporeal elimination procedures have demonstrated little utility because of the availability of a safe and specific antidote.

SUGGESTED READING

1984 Annual Report of the American Association of Poison Control Centers National Data Collection System. Am J Emerg Med 1985;3:423–450.

Berg MJ, Berlinger WG, Goldberg MJ, et al. Acceleration of the body clearance of phenobarbital by oral activated charcoal. N Engl J Med 1982;307:642–644.

Bradberry JC, Raebel MA: Continuous infusion of naloxone in the treatment of narcotic overdose. Drug Intell Clin Pharm 1981;15:945–950.

Greenberg MI, Roberts JR, Baskin SI. Endotracheal naloxone reversal of morphine-induced respiratory depression in rabbits. Ann Emerg Med 1980;9:289–292.

McCarron MM, Schulze BW, Walberg CB, et al. Short-acting barbiturate overdosage: correlation of intoxication score with serum barbiturate concentration. JAMA 1982;248:55–61.

Milne B, Jhamandas K. Naloxone: new therapeutic roles. Can Anaesth Soc J 1984;31:272–278.

Moore RA, Rumack BH. Naloxone: underdosage after narcotic poisoning. Am J Dis Child 1980;134:156–158.

Pond SM, Olson KR, Osterloh JD, et al. Randomized study of the treatment of phenobarbital overdose with repeated doses of activated charcoal. JAMA 1984;251:3104–3108.

Seyffart G. Poison index: dialysis and haemoperfusion in poisonings. Bad Homburg: Fresenius Foundation, 1977.

Teehan BP, Maher JF, Carey JJH, et al. Acute ethchlorvynol (Placidyl) intoxication. Ann Intern Med 1970;72:875–882.

ALCOHOL INTOXICATION AND WITHDRAWAL

CHARLES G. BROWN, M.D., F.A.C.E.P.
RONALD B. TAYLOR, M.D.

ACUTE ETHANOL INTOXICATION

The diagnosis of acute ethanol intoxication is not difficult if clinical and laboratory assessment is used. The possibility of associated injuries, illnesses, and other intoxicants must always be considered especially when a patient presents with altered mental status. The patient's competency must also be considered. The physician is legally responsible to exercise reasonable prudence in preventing the intoxicated patient from harming himself or others. Most states allow for observing intoxicated patients until they are competent (sober).

The acute effects of ethanol depend not only on blood levels (Tables 1 and 2), but also on the amount consumed and the rate of consumption. These effects are caused by the release of cortical inhibitions and direct depression of cognitive, motor, associative, and judgment centers. Blood levels at which respiratory depression and death occur vary widely (350 to 750 mg per 100 milliliters). Patients with a high tolerance may be ambulatory at normally lethal levels. Generally, a dose of 3 g per kilogram body weight will be lethal in 50 percent of adults. This dose may be lower in various subgroups such as children, patients with Addison's disease, and patients taking drugs such as disulfiram (Antabuse), chlorpropamide, and ethacrynic acid (such drugs inhibit enzymatic degradation of ethanol).

The most common route of ethanol administration is intentional ingestion; however, accidental intoxication may occur. Transdermal absorption of toxic levels of isopropanol in children is well established. Many household products contain significant amounts of ethanol or related compounds. Mouthwashes, for example, may contain up to 27 percent ethanol and are packaged in sufficiently large quantities to supply a lethal dose in this age group. Ethanol is metabolized at a constant rate, 20 mg per 100 milliliters per hour (10 g per hour). In the average adult, about one drink is metabolized per hour. This rate may be increased in the chronic drinker.

Differential Diagnosis

A thorough physical examination and pertinent laboratory analysis generally allows the differentiation of ethanol intoxication from other causes of altered mental status (Tables 3 and 4). Historical information from the patient is often unreliable and should also be obtained from family members, police, or pre-hospital care personnel. This information should include a history of other potentially toxic ingestions. Over the counter medications and empty bottles found with the patient should be brought to the emergency department. Associated injuries and illnesses should always be sought and their effects on the intoxicated patient evaluated and treated. The suicide rate is high in the alcoholic population, and this risk should also be evaluated.

Evaluation of Metabolic Complications

Ethanol-induced metabolic abnormalities are common. Hypoglycemia, at times severe, may be seen. Ketoacidosis from starvation, ethanol, or both may occur. Pyruvate is more readily converted to lactate and a subsequent lactic acidosis may develop. Fluid imbalance may be present because of ethanol-induced diuresis (which occurs only while blood ethanol levels are rising), vomiting, poor nutritional status, diarrhea, or occult gastrointestinal blood loss. Vitamin K deficiency may also occur secondary to poor nutrition or hepatic disease. The most common electrolyte abnormalities are hypokalemia, hyponatremia, hypophosphatemia, hypomagnesemia, and hypocalcemia. Rhabdomyolysis may be present, resulting in myoglobinuria. Disulfiram (used to encourage abstinence from ethanol) may cause toxicity in the patient taking phenytoin secondary to inhibition of enzymatic degradation. Serum phenytoin levels should be obtained if toxicity is suspected. The ethanol-disulfiram reaction

TABLE 2 Blood Ethanol Levels Versus Effects

Blood Ethanol Level (mg/100 ml)	Effects
20 to 50	Dimished fine motor control
50 to 100	Impaired judgment and coordination
100 to 150	Difficulty with gait and balance
150 to 250	Lethargy; difficulty sitting upright without assistance
300	Coma in naive drinkers
400	Respiratory depression
>400	Death secondary to respiratory depression or aspiration

Notes: 1. 100 mg/100 ml is considered legally intoxicated in most states.
2. More than 50% of the adult population is intoxicated at a level of 150 mg/100 ml.

TABLE 1 Approximate Blood Alcohol Level (mg/100 ml)

	Weight (lbs)							
	100	120	140	160	180	200	220	240
Drinks								
1	40	30	30	20	20	20	20	20
2	80	60	50	50	40	40	30	30
3	110	90	80	70	60	60	50	50
4	150	120	110	90	80	80	70	60
5	190	160	130	120	110	90	90	80
6	230	190	160	140	130	110	100	90
7	260	220	190	160	150	130	120	110
8	300	250	210	190	170	150	140	130
9	340	280	240	210	190	170	150	140
10	380	310	270	230	210	190	170	160

Note: One drink contains approximately 12 ml of ethanol (about 10 g). This is equivalent to 1 oz of 80-proof liquor, one 12-oz beer, or one 5-oz glass of wine.

**TABLE 3 Differential Diagnosis of Altered
Mental Status in the Intoxicated Patient**

Focal/Lateralizing Neurologic Signs

  Epidural/subdural hematoma
  Brain abscess
  Cerebrovascular accident
  Tumor

Meningeal Irritation

  Subarachnoid hemorrhage—aneurysm, trauma
  Meningitis
  Encephalitis

No Focal/Lateralizing Neurologic Signs

  Intoxicants: ethanol, methanol, isopropanol, ethylene glycol
  Metabolic: diabetic ketoacidosis, alcohol ketoacidosis,
    hyperosmolar states, hepatic failure, uremia, hypoglycemia, hypoxia, hypercarbia
  Sepsis
  Shock
  Epilepsy—postictal state
  Environmental—hypothermia, hyperthermia, carbon monoxide
  Trauma—concussion

(flushing, hypotension, headache, and gastrointestinal distress) may occur from ingestion of ethanol or from exposure to ethanol-containing products (e.g., cologne). Supportive care and volume expansion are generally all that is required. Laboratory studies, as dictated by clinical evaluation (see Table 4), should include electrolyte readings, hemoglobin and hematocrit values, prothrombin time, calcium, magnesium, glucose, phosphorus, and blood urea nitrogen and creatinine (fluid status) determinations, serum ketones, and urinalysis (myoglobin). Appropriate cultures (cerebrospinal fluid, blood, urine, and sputum) should be obtained as clinically indicated.

Serum osmolality and osmolal gap cannot be used to accurately estimate serum ethanol levels. Other solutes (ethylene glycol, methanol) can affect the osmolality, and the freezing point depression method used by most laboratories to determine osmolality does not accurately correlate with the actual ethanol level. Serum ethanol levels should be measured directly. The serum sample must be drawn without the use of an alcohol prep pad (isopropanol), since erroneous levels may result. Most hospital laboratories report ethanol levels for diagnostic use only. Legal samples must be drawn and processed according to local law enforcement policies.

Treatment

The treatment of the acutely intoxicated patient is supportive. Naloxone is not useful as it has no specific ethanol receptors. The only agent known to significantly increase ethanol metabolism is fructose, and the adverse effects associated with its administration preclude any clinical benefit. Analeptic agents (doxapram, theophylline) have no value and can increase seizure activity, aggravate hypertension, and provoke cardiac dysrhythmias.

The foremost consideration is prevention of death from respiratory depression. Intubation and ventilatory support may be necessary. Alcoholic ketoacidosis usually responds to normal saline infusion. Severe acidosis (pH less than 7.10 or bicarbonate less than 8 mEq per liter) may require bicarbonate therapy. Usually 1 mEq per kilogram of bicarbonate is given initially and subsequent therapy administered as dictated by pH. Hypoglycemia is corrected by intravenous dextrose, 25 g (50 ml of a 50 percent solution). Thiamine (100 mg given intramuscularly or intravenously) is administered if dextrose is given or if any signs of Wernicke-Korsakoff syndrome are present (bilateral sixth nerve palsy, oculomotor paralysis, ataxia, dysarthria). Lavage and activated charcoal (30 to 60 g) are of little value in the acutely intoxicated patient unless given within 2 hours after ingestion or if a mixed ingestion is suspected. Activated charcoal should always be followed by a cathartic (250 mg per kilogram of magnesium citrate). Hyponatremia is corrected by infusing isotonic saline solutions. Hypokalemia is initially treated by administering 10 to 20 mEq of potassium chloride intravenously or by mouth. Hypocalcemia is treated with intravenous calcium chloride, 100 to 200 mg (10 to 20 ml of a 10 percent solution) over 10 to 15 minutes. Severe hypophosphatemia (less than 1.0 mg per 100 milliliters) is treated with an intravenous phosphate solution (2.5 to 5.0 mg per kilogram) over 6 to 8 hours. Hypomagnesemia is corrected with magnesium sulfate, 2 to 4 g intramuscularly (4 to 8 ml of a 50 percent solution), or intravenously as a 10 percent solution (infusion rates should not exceed 1.5 ml per minute). Potassium, magnesium, and phosphate repletion should be carefully monitored, especially if any renal impairment exists. If myoglobinuria occurs, mannitol and furosemide are indicated. Mannitol is given as a 20 percent solution in infusion rates titrated to maintain urine flow at 30 to 60 ml per hour (generally 2 to 4 g per hour). Furosemide is given intravenously in a dosage of 10 to 20 mg.

In general, the intoxicated patient should be observed and examined periodically in the emergency department until he or she is sober. Appropriate follow-up for detoxification or impending withdrawal and long-term rehabilitation (usually through social services programs) should be initiated.

TABLE 4 Clinical and Laboratory Evaluation
(Altered Mental Status)

Vital Signs	Diagnostic Considerations
Tachypnea	Metabolic acidosis, sepsis, hepatic failure
Fever	Sepsis, hyperthermia
Hypothermia	Sepsis, hypothermia
Bradycardia	CNS event, hypothermia

Clinical Signs

Skin	
burns	Carbon monoxide
jaundice	Hepatic failure
Head	
Battle's sign/raccoon's eyes	Basilar skull fracture
Ears	
hemotympanum	Basilar skull fracture
Eyes	
retinal edema	Ethylene glycol, methanol
nystagmus	Wernicke-Korsakoff syndrome, barbiturates, phenytoin
ophthalmoplegia	Wernicke-Korsakoff syndrome
Mouth	
fruity breath	Ketoacidosis, isopropanol
paraldehyde	Paraldehyde
Neck	
meningismus	Meningitis, subarachnoid hemorrhage, encephalitis
Neurologic examination	
focal findings	Epidural/subdural hematoma, brain abscess, cerebrovascular accident, tumor

Laboratory Evaluation

Arterial blood gases	Hypoxia, hypercarbia, acidosis
Carboxyhemoglobin level	Carbon monoxide poisoning
Glucose	Hypogleyemia, diabetic ketoacidosis
Ammonia	Hepatic failure
Urinalysis (oxylate crystals)	Ethylene glycol intoxication
Serum ketones	

	Acidosis	Ketonemia*	Osmolal Gap†
Ethylene glycol	+	0	up
Isopropanol	0	+	up
Methanol	+	0	up
Ethanol	+/−	+/−	up
Paraldehyde	+	+/−	−−

* Acetest method (only detects acetaldehyde/acetone. Beta-hydroxybutyrate is the principal ketone produced in ethanol-induced ketoacidosis).

† Serum osmolality may be measured and an "osmolal gap" calculated. The osmolal gap refers to the difference of measured versus calculated serum osmolality. Serum osmolality may be calculated as follows:

Serum Osm = (2Na) + BUN/3 + Glu/18 (normal = 280–295). An osmolal gap of greater than 10 suggests the presence of osmotically active agents such as ethanol, methanol, isopropanol, ethylene glycol, or mannitol. The osmolar contribution of ethanol may be taken into consideration by adding its activity to the above equation (mg/100 ml/4.6). If the osmolal gap remains elevated after taking into account ethanol's contribution, the presence of other osmotically active substances (e.g.,methanol from denatured ethyl alcohol) is suggested.

0 = generally absent; + = generally present; +/− = may be absent or present; up = elevated, i.e., >10

ALCOHOL WITHDRAWAL

Clinical experience has demonstrated that tolerance to ethanol develops with prolonged consumption. Compensatory physiologic mechanisms are initiated to counteract the depressant effects of ethanol during this time. This adaptation predisposes to withdrawal reactions. With a declining blood ethanol concentration, these compensatory mechanisms become unopposed and lead to the development of alcohol withdrawal reactions. Therefore, not only cessation, but also a reduction in ethanol intake may lead to the development of alcohol withdrawal. Although there is wide individual variation as to how severe any withdrawal reaction will be, in general it is dependent upon the amount and duration of ethanol consumption. A syndrome similar to alcohol withdrawal may also be seen in patients who consume smaller quantities of alcohol, but who concurrently take sedative-hypnotics (benzodiazepines, barbiturates). These agents are cross-tolerant with ethanol, and a reduction or cessation of their intake can induce a withdrawal syndrome.

The alcohol withdrawal syndrome is characterized by four stages (Table 5). Stage one is characterized by autonomic hyperactivity and begins 6 to 8 hours after the cessation or reduction of ethanol intake. This stage is often short-lived, with most symptoms resolving within 24 hours. Stage two is characterized by hallucinations. Although usually auditory, they can be visual, tactile, olfactory, or mixed. The hallucinations seen during this stage may be preceded by illusions. Stage three is characterized by grand mal seizures (''rum fits''), which may begin from 7 to 48 hours after the cessation or reduction of ethanol intake. From one to several brief seizures usually occur over a few hours, with more than half the patients having multiple seizures. Stage four (delirium tremens) is characterized by marked autonomic hyperactivity, hallucinations, and global confusion. It begins within 3 to 5 days after the discontinuation or decline in ethanol consumption. The development of seizures after the onset of delirium tremens is highly unusual.

Differential Diagnosis

The symptoms and signs seen in barbiturate and benzodiazepine withdrawal are similar to those seen in ethanol withdrawal. One distinguishing feature with short-acting barbiturate withdrawal is the occurrence of status epilepticus. With long-acting barbiturates and benzodiazepines, the symptoms progress more slowly than in ethanol withdrawal, and seizures may not become apparent for up to 7 days following cessation of the offending drug.

The tremor of alcohol withdrawal poses little diagnostic difficulty when other autonomic signs and symptoms exist and when given a history of recent ethanol cessation. The tremor of ethanol withdrawal is a postural tremor and is therefore maximal when the patient's arms are outstretched. Another postural tremor seen in this population is asterixis. This is seen with metabolic encephalopathies (e.g., hepatic failure) and is more intermittent and irregular than the tremor of alcohol withdrawal. Cerebellar tremors (intention tremor), which can be seen with alcoholic cerebellar degeneration or as part of Wernicke's syndrome, are made worse by movement and abate at rest.

Hallucinations seen during ethanol withdrawal often emerge from background noises. The patient's response to the hallucination is appropriate to its content (e.g., anxiety in response to hallucinatory threats). These hallucinations must be distinguished from those seen in schizophrenia, delirium, dementia, and the major affective syndromes, e.g., psychotic depression (Table 6).

The differentiation of idiopathic from withdrawal seizures may be difficult when not viewed within the context of the withdrawal syndrome. In patients with alcohol withdrawal seizures, the electroencephalogram (EEG) may show abnormalities during the seizure but returns to normal following it. In patients with underlying seizure disorders, an abnormal EEG is present both during and following the seizure. Most patients have two to six brief (less than 30 seconds) grand mal seizures over approximately an 8-hour time course. More frequent seizures, or seizures occurring past this time course, should alert the physician to seek other etiologies. Focal seizures seen during ethanol withdrawal should be fully evaluated to rule out space-occupying lesions (subdural-epidural hematoma), subdural empyema, brain abscess, intracerebral hemorrhage, cerebral infarction, tumor, or arteriovenous malformation. Status epilepticus seen during alcohol withdrawal is unusual and should suggest short-acting barbiturate withdrawal or central nervous system infections (e.g., meningitis).

Patients presenting in delirium from ethanol withdrawal must be differentiated from those with central nervous system or systemic infections, barbiturate and benzodiazepine withdrawal, and metabolic etiologies, including hypoglycemia and thyrotoxicosis.

Therapy

The goals of therapy are (1) to allay symptoms, (2) to diagnose and initiate treatment of underlying disord-

TABLE 5 Stages of Alcohol Withdrawal

Stage	Onset	Symptoms and Signs
1	6–8 hours	Tremulousness, anxiety, tachycardia, hypertension, hyper-reflexia
2	24 hours	Hallucinations
3	7–48 hours	Grand mal seizures
4	3-5 days	Autonomic hyperactivity, hallucinations, global confusion

TABLE 6 Major Diagnostic Features (Mental Status Examination) of Patients Presenting with Hallucinations

	Alcohol Withdrawal	Schizophrenia	Delirium	Dementia	Major Affective Syndromes
Mood		Inappropriate, bland			Predominant disturbance
Thought process		Loose, tangential			
Thought content		Feelings of influence, reference			
Perceptions	Auditory hallucinations often emerge from background noises	Hallucinations often bizarre and symbolic	No distinguishing feature of hallucination		
Cognitive function	Usually remain well oriented	Usually remain well oriented	Disoriented	May be disoriented, significant intellectual decline	Not a diagnostic feature

ers, and (3) to prevent progression of the syndrome to the more serious later stages of withdrawal, which carry a mortality rate up to 25 percent. Several clinical series have suggested that treatment of patients during early withdrawal with drugs that are cross-tolerant with ethanol decreases the incidence of seizures and delirium tremens.

In the pre-hospital setting, no therapy is indicated for the early stages of withdrawal. Patients presenting with withdrawal seizures or delirium are managed with standard supportive care. This includes protection from injury (for the patient with seizures), airway management (maintenance of a patent airway, oxygen, prevention of aspiration by suction or transport in left lateral decubitus position), treatment of shock, and treatment of reversible metabolic causes of seizures and delirium (e.g., hypoglycemia).

In the emergency department, therapy is best organized according to the presenting stage of withdrawal. To allay the symptoms seen during stages one and two and to abate progression of the withdrawal syndrome, initiation of therapy with drugs that are cross-tolerant with ethanol is most effective. Although self-treatment with ethanol is a widely employed therapeutic modality, this is discouraged. Ethanol has a short duration of action, a narrow therapeutic window, and numerous metabolic disturbances result from its consumption. More effective therapy is initiated with paraldehyde or one of several benzodiazepines.

Paraldehyde, 10 ml by mouth every 2 to 3 hours, is an effective therapy. It cannot be administered intramuscularly since sterile abscesses may occur or given rectally because of the risk of regional proctitis. Although its odor has been considered a detracting factor, this may significantly reduce its abuse potential. Treatment with benzodiazepines may be preferred if outpatient treatment is decided upon. Diazepam (Valium), 5 to 20 mg by mouth every 6 hours, chlordiazepoxide (Librium), 25 to 100 mg by mouth every 6 hours, or oxazepam (Serax), 15 to 30 mg by mouth every 6 hours, are alternative therapeutic regimens. The dose should be titrated individually so as to achieve a calm state without inducing central nervous system depression. Therapy should be continued over the high-risk period (about 5 days) for the development of severe withdrawal reactions. In patients with hypoproteinemia or hepatic disease, diazepam and chlordiazepoxide must be administered cautiously. These drugs are metabolized by the liver to pharmacologically active metabolites that are protein bound. This may produce a cumulative toxic effect. Oxazepam does not pose this problem since it is metabolized to an inactive form. Intramuscular administration of diazepam and chlordiazepoxide should be avoided because of their erratic absorption by this route. Antihistamine therapy (e.g., hydroxyzine) and phenothiazine therapy should be avoided. Their anticholinergic effects can cause tachycardia, hallucinations, and delirium, whereas phenothiazines lower the seizure threshold.

All patients should be monitored during these early stages for progression to the more serious stages of ethanol withdrawal. This may be done at home if there is a supportive environment. Patients who previously have had serious withdrawal reactions are probably at greater risk for recurrence, and hospitalization should be considered. Once the acute abstinence syndrome has been treated, plans for rehabilitation should be initiated through the patient's private physician or through alcoholism or social services programs.

The following recommendations are outlined for the management of alcohol withdrawal seizures. In patients who present in alcohol withdrawal, but also have an underlying seizure disorder, the most likely explanation for the occurrence of seizures is noncompliance with their antiseizure medication. Pending results of serum determinations, patients should be reloaded and maintained on their antiseizure drug regimen. Benzodiazepine or paraldehyde therapy as outlined above should also be instituted to allay symptoms and halt progression of the withdrawal syndrome. Those patients in early withdrawal who have not had seizures and who have no history of an underlying seizure disorder or of ethanol withdrawal seizures should be considered at low risk for the development of withdrawal seizures. Prophylactic anticonvulsant therapy is not indicated. In those patients who have not had seizures, but who have a history of ethanol withdrawal seizures, prophylactic therapy with chlordiazepoxide (up to 400 mg by mouth per day) and phenytoin (100 mg by mouth three times a day) for 5 days may be effective in preventing the development of withdrawal seizures. (Although unusual in its omission of the usual 500 to 1,000 mg loading dose, this regimen was very effective in a study in which both drugs were used. Studies of phenytoin alone have never been done.) In those patients who present with seizures and who have a history of withdrawal seizures, prophylactic anticonvulsant therapy is not indicated. Paraldehyde or benzodiazepine therapy should be withheld during an initial observation period of 6 to 8 hours. Patients with alcohol withdrawal seizures should only have several brief seizures over this time course, and if protected from injury and aspiration, they rarely suffer any sequelae. This observation period allows the physician to characterize the type of seizures.

As noted previously, focal seizures, status epilepticus, and frequent or prolonged seizures require further diagnostic evaluation. Similarly, the initial presentation of patients with "alcohol withdrawal seizures" should be completely evaluated. The emergency physician should initially evaluate for structural lesions (focal neurologic signs), intracranial infections (meningeal signs), and reversible metabolic and electrolyte disturbances. If the initial evaluation is negative, and an outpatient work-up is decided upon (computed tomographic scan, electroencephalogram, cerebrospinal fluid examination), patients should still be observed in the emergency department for 6 to 8 hours, as noted above. Following this period, paraldehyde or benzodiazepine should be initiated as previously outlined.

Patients presenting with delirium tremens frequently have underlying pulmonary disease, electrolyte and fluid disorders, and are also at risk for seriously injuring themselves. To evaluate, manage, and prevent injury in these patients, sedation with intravenous diazepam is indicated. Initially 10 mg can be given, followed by 5 mg every 5 minutes until a calm state is achieved. Physical restraints may also be necessary during this initial phase of management. Maintenance therapy is then initiated with oral diazepam, 5 to 20 mg every 6 hours.

Underlying medical and surgical problems (head trauma, central nervous system and pulmonary infections, pancreatitis, hepatic disease, or gastrointestinal hemorrhage) may lead to cessation of alcohol intake and thus precipitate withdrawal. In addition, hypokalemia and hypomagnesemia (for treatment, see previous section) are frequently observed during alcohol withdrawal and are factors in the pathogenesis of seizures and delirium. Fever and hypertension are also frequently noted. Hypertension

usually resolves over several days and does not require specific therapy unless the patient is symptomatic or has preexisting cardiac, renal, or vascular disease. Whenever fever appears, underlying causes should be sought, including pneumonia and dehydration. Finally, all patients in withdrawal should receive thiamine 100 mg intramuscularly or intravenously and multivitamin therapy.

SUGGESTED READING

Brown CG. The alcohol withdrawal syndrome. Ann Emerg Med 1982;11:276–280.
Sellers EM, Kalant H. Alcohol intoxication and withdrawal.N Engl J Med 1976;294:757–762.

CYCLIC ANTIDEPRESSANT OVERDOSE

MICHAEL L. CALLAHAM, M.D.

The cyclic antidepressants (chiefly the tricyclic antidepressants) are the pharmacologic therapy of choice for the treatment of major depression and were the third most common cause of drug-related death in the United States in 1982. This combined with their unpredictable clinical course and their cardiovascular toxicity makes them major management problems for the emergency physician.

PHARMACOLOGY AND NEW ANTIDEPRESSANTS

The cyclic antidepressants (CA) are a group of closely related cyclic compounds, analogs of the phenothiazines, which share to different degrees the anticholinergic and amine pump blocking properties of the phenothiazines. Classically the original agents in this group were all tricyclic, but newer agents are unicyclic, bycyclic, and tetracyclic as well (Table 1).

No major differences have been shown to exist among the older CAs in terms of toxicity. Thus the treatment of toxic reactions is the same for all of them. New cyclic antidepressants are continually coming on the market, with claims of decresed toxicity in overdose. Such claims for older CAs have not been sustained. However, four recent new CAs are of significance and warrant brief discussion. Maprotiline (Ludiomil) is a tetracyclic antidepressant that causes an increase in seizures in overdose, but possibly fewer (but not nonexistent) cardiovascular side effects. Not enough cases have been reported to draw conclusions. Amoxapine (Asendin) is a metabolite of loxapine, which has few cardiovascular side effects in overdose but a

dramatically higher incidence of seizures (36 percent) and death (15 percent) as compared to 5 to 10 percent and less than 1 percent, respectively, for all tricyclic antidepressants (TCA) combined. Trazadone (Desyrel) is a triazolopyridine compound unrelated to the TCA, which has equal clinical efficacy and virtually no cardiac and few central nervous system effects in overdose. The few overdose cases reported so far have followed a benign course comparable to that of benzodiazepine overdose. The fourth drug is fluoxetine, not yet released in this country. It is clinically as effective as older CAs, but since it is a pure serotonin blocker with little muscarinic, histaminic, or adrenergic activity, it has virtually no cardiovascular toxicity. Nine human overdoses have been reported; all were relatively benign, although one patient had seizures. These new drugs, if their early promise endures, may offer the solution to the dilemma of dangerous, hard to treat drug overdoses in the hands of depressed patients.

PREDICTORS OF OUTCOME

Accurate plasma CA levels are measurable by gas chromatography and are clinically important for monitoring therapy, but are considerably less useful in overdose. First, very few laboratories do the tests on a stat basis, usually returning results after 24 hours, long after the worst toxicity has been dealt with. (However, the new EMIT assay can be done in minutes and detects all levels higher than 200 ng per milliliter.) Second, plasma levels are not predictive; a low level does not mean that the level will not be toxic (and the patient moribund) in 30 minutes.

Plasma levels do correlate in a general way with toxicity and outcome. Levels of 1,000 ng per milliliter or more are associated with coma, seizures, respiratory depression, conduction blocks, arrhythmias, and death. However, plasma levels fail to accurately predict seizures or dysrhythmias in individual patients, and both plasma

TABLE 1 Common Cyclic Antidepressants*

Generic name	Trade name	Type	Outpatient Daily Dose (mg)	Mg/kg Dose of 2-Week Supply
Amitriptyline	Elavil Endep Amitril Amitid Etrafon (with perphenazine) Triavil (with perphenazine) Limbitrol (with chlordiazepoxide)	Tertiary TCA	125	25
Amoxapine	Asendin	Dibenzoxazepine (TCA derivative)	300	60
Desipramine	Norpramin Pertofrane	Secondary TCA	200	40
Doxepin	Sinequan Adapin	Tricyclic	125	25
Imipramine	Tofranil Janimine Presamine Imavate SK-Pramine	Tertiary TCA	150	30
Maprotiline	Ludiomil	Tetracyclic	150	30
Nortriptyline	Aventyl Pamelon	Secondary TCA	100	20
Protriptyline	Vivactil	Secondary TCA	40	8
Trazodone	Desyrel	Triazolopyridine (not related to TCA)	400	80 (Animal LD$_{50}$ =500 mg/kg)
Trimipramine	Surmontil	Tertiary TCA	150	30

*Estimated LD$_{50}$ is 35 mg/kg; ingestions of 14 mg/kg or less are usually minor.

TABLE 2 Central Nervous System Signs of CA Toxicity (in Approximate Order of Appearance)

Disorientation
Agitation
Hallucinations
Myoclonic jerks
Coma
Pyramidal signs—clonus, Babinski present, hyperreflexia
Seizures

TABLE 3 Peripheral Signs of CA Toxicity (Peripheral Anticholinergic Syndrome) in Approximate Order of Appearance

Tachycardia*
Hypertension
Fever
Mydriasis
Dry red skin
Decreased bowel sounds
Urinary retention
Respiratory depression

* In a quietly resting patient, a pulse of 90 per minute or more is suspicious.

TABLE 4 ECG Abnormalities in CA Overdose (in Approximate Order of Appearance)

ST and T wave changes
Prolonged Q-T interval
Prolonged P-R interval
QRS greater than 100 milliseconds*
Bundle branch block (especially RBBB)
Atrioventricular conduction blocks (1st, 2nd, or 3rd degree)
Dysrhythmias
    Sinus tachycardia
    Premature ventricular contractions
    Aberrantly conducted beats
    Ventricular tachycardia
    Sinus arrest
    Slow idioventricular rhythm
    Electromechanical dissociation

* Correlated with high plasma levels and major complications.

levels and clinical signs can change within minutes for better or worse.

By contrast, a QRS duration of 100 msec or more is useful, since most patients with seizures or dysrhythmias have this degree of QRS prolongation. It is thus best to rely on a high index of suspicion and good preventive care. Treatment should never be delayed until plasma level values are returned from the laboratory.

Just as plasma levels are not sensitive predictors of outcome, neither are ingested dose levels, even in the rare case when this is accurately known. There are huge individual differences in sensitivity and metabolism. Owing to the unpredictable variations in response, it is wise to treat the patient on the basis of his clinical condition, not the amount or type of drug ingested. For purposes of initial evaluation at least, any CA ingestion is significant.

CLINICAL SIGNS AND SYMPTOMS

The symptoms and signs of CA overdose are those of central nervous system depression, anticholinergic tox-

TABLE 5   Clinical Signs in CA Overdose

	All Published Cases Since 1967	Petit (ref.20)*
Total number of patients	1815	40
Coma	35%	47%
Conduction block	20%	65%
Supraventricular dysrhythmias	17%	30%
Ventricular dysrhythmias	11%	17%
Hypotension	14%	15%
Seizures	10%	20%
Death	2.6%	5%

* This study is listed because all patients had plasma levels of drug drawn and the correlation with clinical signs and outcome was determined.

icity, and depression of cardiac conduction and contractility. These are listed in Tables 2 through 5 in approximate order of appearance. Generally tachycardia, slurred speech, and lethargy are the earliest signs of toxicity, but these cannot be relied upon as warning signs, since 17 percent of fatal CA overdose cases presented to the emergency department awake and alert, and 45 percent had a normal sinus rhythm.

The major *central nervous system signs* are those of coma (with respiratory depression prominent even in only partially obtunded patients) and seizures. Coma lasts for an average of 24 hours. Twitching, jerking myoclonic movements are seen in 40 percent, are commonly confused with seizures, and do not respond to phenytoin. Grand mal seizures are seen in 10 to 20 percent of the cases and contribute greatly to hypoxia and acidosis, which directly worsen cardiac complications.

CA *cardiovascular toxicity* is probably the most feared. Continuous intravenous infusion of CA causes the electrocardiographic effects listed in Table 4. Arrhythmias such as ventricular tachycardia and frequent aberrant and premature ventricular beats occur after there is significant intraventricular conduction block (with a widened QRS) and before bradycardia; by the time these arrhythmias occur, cardiac contractility is only a small fraction of normal (see Table 3). Although most of the literature dealing with humans has focused on these ventricular dysrhythmias, in the laboratory they do not seem to be an important mechanism of mortality, often being virtually absent. Myocardial depression is much more significant. Most patients who die suffer from hypotension, conduction blocks, and tachycardia, not ventricular dysrhythmias.

The interplay of these cardiotoxic effects in the patient is exceedingly complex and poorly understood. Hypoxia, seizures, acidosis, intubation, and any sympathetic nervous system stimulation may further alter the balance and can trigger or alter dysrhythmias or induce cardiac arrest. Any patient may skip one or several stages, stay in one phase a long time, or move quickly back and forth between different phases of toxicity.

PRE-HOSPITAL CONSIDERATIONS

There is little effective pre-hospital treatment for the major toxicity of CA overdose, and rapid transport should be instituted. In 25 percent of the fatal cases the patients were alert and awake, and 75 percent had normal sinus rhythm when pre-hospital personnel first encountered them in one series. Thus all patients giving a history of CA ingestion should be placed on a monitor, have an intravenous line started, and be under constant observation while being transported to an emergency department. Ipecac is not recommended since patients may easily become obtunded by the time vomiting begins. Activated charcoal, 50 to 100 g should be given if the patient has an active gag reflex; this is particularly important owing to the time consumed in transport and the difficulty of removing these drugs once absorbed. Any patient who is obtunded should be given assisted ventilation and oxygen supplementation. Treatment of other complications is as described for the emergency department, but stabilization of the toxic patient is unlikely under field conditions.

ASSESSMENT AND STABILIZATION IN THE HOSPITAL

The mainstays of treatment in cases of CA overdose are prevention of absorption of the drug and good respiratory support. Once absorbed, the drug is highly tissue bound; thus even efficient methods of removal, such as charcoal hemoperfusion, have little impact since the size of the tissue-bound drug pool makes the effort akin to draining Lake Erie through a garden hose.

MANDATORY PREVENTIVE CARE

Any patient who presents to medical care with any history of ingestion of CA must be immediately placed on a cardiac monitor, have an intravenous line established, and have the stomach emptied. Patients should never be allowed to "wait their turn"; fatal cases can present to the emergency department with only trivial signs of poisoning and develop major toxicity and life-threatening complications in a very short period of time.

Emptying the stomach is a must. Owing to the possibility of precipitous deterioration, an argument can be made for using lavage instead of ipecac. Ipecac may produce results just as the patient loses his gag reflex, and it delays administration of activated charcoal by at least an hour. Putting charcoal down the lavage tube before lavage may further limit the amount of drug absorbed.

Activated charcoal effectively binds CA and can decrease plasma levels 58 percent as compared with controls. Multiple doses of charcoal every two hours are even more effective, presumably binding CA secreted later in the biliary and gastric juices. Such multiple doses reduce the drug half-life from the usual 36 hours to a mere 4 hours; 100 g will bind about 4 g of amitriptyline and should be the minimum initial dose.

Cathartics such as sodium and magnesium sulfate (250 mg per kilogram) are routinely recommended to speed drug removal from the gastrointestinal tract. No clinical study has demonstrated the effectiveness of this technique with CAs. Nonetheless it seems theoretically sound and is without major side effects. There may be no cathartic effect or passage of stool until the patient begins to awaken from coma, since the CAs have anticholinergic properties that inhibit peristalsis.

Ventilatory support and careful monitoring of the acid-base status is even more important than for most other overdoses, because of the many cardiovascular complications of CAs that are directly pH dependent and triggered by acidosis. Patients with CA overdose who are only lightly obtunded and judged by experienced clinicians to be ventilating adequately nonetheless have low minute volumes, hypoxia, and metabolic acidosis. Any CA overdose patient with even a minimal decrease in the level of consciousness should have arterial blood gas levels determined and ventilatory assistance as needed to maintain optimal blood gas levels. Any acidosis (pH less than 7.40) should be immediately corrected, and all patients should have a high normal Po_2 maintained at all times with oxygen administration.

An electrocardiogram should be obtained as soon as the patient arrives, seeking telltale signs such as tachycardia and QRS prolongation. A QRS duration of 100 msec or less puts the patient in a relatively low risk group according to one recent study, whereas a level of 100 msec or more is associated with a 34 percent incidence of seizures and a level of 160 msec or more with a 14 percent incidence of dysrhythmias. However, changes in condition are very unpredictable, and the patient should remain on a cardiac monitor at all times.

Drug removal from the body cannot be achieved by peritoneal dialysis or forced diuresis. Hemoperfusion with activated charcoal removes the drug very efficiently from the blood, but the total dose removed is very small and no reliable effect on clinical outcome has been shown in various studies. Nonetheless minor fluctuations of plasma CA levels may have great clinical impact, and this technique may be worth a try in the critically ill patient in whom all simpler and more proven measures (such as

alkalinization, fluid loading, and pressors) have been tried and failed.

Patients who are admitted to the hospital must of course receive constant cardiac monitoring. Routine blood work should be carried out, including electrolyte levels and liver function tests. Drugs such as diazepam may slow hepatic clearance of the drug and should be avoided if possible.

TREATMENT OF SPECIFIC COMPLICATIONS

Despite an abundance of literature, information about proven and effective treatment for CA complications does not exist. The preventive measures already mentioned are far more important. The currently recommended therapy is summarized in Table 6, and only a few key points are emphasized in the following text. Our understanding of the pharmacology of CA overdose is in fact very poor, despite the tidy explanations in review articles, and the relative importance of the various effects is a matter of debate. Similarly, treatments based on these pharmacologic mechanisms (such as the use of physostigmine or beta blockers) have not been either successful or safe.

Physostigmine, 2 mg intravenously over 2 minutes, and repeated every 20 to 30 minutes, or 2 mg intramuscularly every 2 hours, has enjoyed periodic popularity. Physostigmine is a cholinergic drug, which reverses the anticholinergic effects of the CA. Unfortunately physostigmine is a nonspecific analeptic and will waken patients obtunded for a wide variety of reasons. It also has a very narrow therapeutic toxic ratio. In one large study, although the intravenous administration of physostigmine rapidly and dramatically awoke CA overdose patients, 10 percent had grand mal seizures attributed to the physostigmine and another 10 percent had cholinergic crisis (excessive salivation, bronchial secretions, vomiting, diarrhea, and bradycardia). Physostigmine can also worsen conduction blocks and produce cardiac arrest and asystole. Although it can reverse seizures in CA overdose, it is short acting and itself causes seizures, which usually occur within 20 minutes after administration. The use of physostigmine should be avoided whenever possible.

Alkalinization of the blood to a pH of 7.5 is probably the best treatment available for most forms of cardiovascular CA toxicity; this can narrow the QRS, abolish arrhythmias, and improve perfusion in minutes. Alkalinization can be accomplished by either hyperventilation or the intravenous administration of sodium bicarbonate, 1 to 3 mEq per kilogram or titrated to pH. A number of human case reports and large animal studies over the years show that hyperventilation can be dramatically effective. Hyperventilation offers the advantage of being administered immediately, of being completely reversible, of not adding a sodium load to the patient, and of not causing paradoxical intracellular acidosis as does bicarbonate. It is a good initial choice and can be later followed with bicarbonate, which some believe to have a more potent effect.

TABLE 6 Summary of Treatment of Specific CA Complications (in Order of Preference and Effectiveness)

Coma:	Arterial blood gas monitoring and respiratory support
Seizures:	Respiratory support and alkalinization for all patients
	Diazepam
	Phenytoin (not effective for myoclonic jerks)
	Phenobarbital
	Physostigmine
	General anesthesia and paralysis
Tachycardia:	Alkalinization
	No other treatment unless hypotensive
Conduction blocks and ventricular dysrhythmias:	Alkalinization
	Phenytoin (unproven; may worsen ventricular tachycardia) hypotension)
	Only if hypotensive: bretyllium, lidocaine (cautiously); all other antiarrhythmics significantly worsen myocardial depression
Hypotension:	Alkalinization
	Fluid loading
	Pressors with predominant alpha-adrenergic effect:
	Epinephrine
	Norepinephrine
	High dose dopamine
	Phenylephrine
	Digitalis (experimental)
	Physostigmine (in extremis only)
	Charcoal or resin hemoperfusion
	Cardiopulmonary bypass
Contraindicated drugs:	Absolute: Procainamide
	Quinidine
	Any type I antiarrhythmic
	Beta—blockers
	Relative: Corticosteroids
	Metaraminol
	Mephentermine
	Isoproterenol, dobutamine, low dose dopamine (may worsen hypotension and arrhythmias)

Phenytoin is theoretically a logical treatment, since it may improve cardiac conduction and has little cardiodepressant activity. However, phenytoin has never been studied in any large series of human CA overdose patients. Phenytoin can cause hypotension itself if given rapidly, and it would not be expected to improve cardiac contractility, which may be a more important cause of cardiac arrest than conduction defects. Recent experiments in our laboratory demonstrated that "prophylactic" phenytoin in dogs provided no benefit in morbidity or mortality and, in fact, doubled the frequency and duration of hypoperfusing ventricular tachycardia. Therefore it may be rational in an individual case, but its widespread use for "prophylaxis" in cases of CA overdose is not supported by published evidence at this time. It is a rational treatment for seizures but is not effective against myoclonic jerks.

Hypotension is present in 14 percent of CA overdose cases, but significant depression of cardiac contractility is present long before it appears. Usually accompanied by conduction blocks and apparent ventricular arrhythmias, it progresses to cardiac arrest and death in 2.6 percent. (Since the myocardium of the younger patient is usually healthy, prolonged CPR or cardiopulmonary bypass can result in complete recovery once the immediate drug toxicity is past, unlike the situation with cardiac arrest in older patients due to ischemic heart disease.)

Alkalinization has been shown effective in hypotension, and it is safe. Intravenous fluid loading is also useful. If these two methods fail, catecholamine pressors are a rational choice. Drugs with potent vasoconstricting properties, such as epinephrine, norepinephrine, and phenylephrine, are desirable, since CAs produce strong alpha-adrenergic blockade and deplete endogenous norepinephrine. Use of isoproterenol may worsen hypotension and cardiac irritability through an unopposed beta-adrenergic effect. All vasopressors may increase the risk of arrhythmias. Dopamine has not been studied in humans; it would be logical at high doses but low doses carry the same risks as isoproterenol. Dobutamine, a predominantly beta-adrenergic drug, would be contraindicated. Indirect acting sympathomimetics, such as metaraminol and mephentermine, are not logical choices, since the CAs block their uptake into the adrenergic neuron, and they act by releasing endogenous norepinephrine, which may already be depleted.

The list of noncatechol inotropic agents is short. Glucagon has not been studied. Digitalis has been used

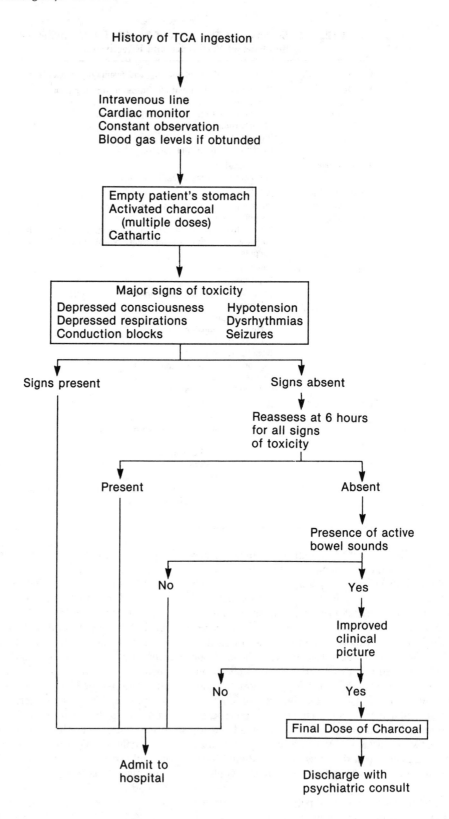

Figure 1 Initial management of TCA ingestion.

clinically with and without conduction blocks. In overdosed dogs without dysrhythmias, ouabain completely reversed the myocardial depression of desipramine, even with 66 to 100 percent depression of contractile force. Digitalis increases cardiac irritability and increases AV block, although in dogs there was no effect on the already increased PR and QRS duration. Some conduction block may occur secondary to poor perfusion and could actually be improved with digitalis. The literature suggests that digitalis must be used with caution in patients with significant block or ectopy, but it may be useful as a last resort.

Physostigmine has been recommended for hypotension, but it can worsen hypotension and block and cause asystole. Many of the anecdotal beneficial effects of physostigmine may have been due to its analeptic property of increasing wakefulness and stimulating respiration in patients who are not receiving ventilatory assistance. It should be regarded as a last-resort drug.

Hemoperfusion with activated charcoal or resin has already been discussed. Although the impact is minor, it may tip the scales in critical cases and should be considered when simpler methods are failing.

DISPOSITION AND ADMISSION CRITERIA

The patient should receive the initial assessment and treatment already described and be observed for at least 6 hours. If at any time during this period he develops major signs of poisoning (decreased level of consciousness, respiratory depression, seizures, hypotension, dysrhythmia, or conduction block), he should be admitted to hospital. If after 6 hours of observation none of these major signs has developed, he should receive a final dose of charcoal and may be discharged to psychiatric evaluation. A patient who after 6 hours demonstrates only minor signs, such as tachycardia less than 120 or slightly slurred speech, may be discharged if the presence of active bowel sounds suggests that both the ingested CA and the administered charcoal and cathartic are progressing on their way out of the gastrointestinal tract, and if signs of poisoning are decreasing rather than increasing. If bowel sounds are absent or markedly decreased, peristalsis may be inhibited by the anticholinergic effects of the CA and delayed absorption is more likely. In this case, admission for further monitoring and observation is prudent.

Management by the algorithm shown in Figure 1 should allow prompt identification and treatment of seriously poisoned patients. At the same time the high incidence of hospitalization and unnecessary costs for trivial ingestions will be lowered while still providing an adequate margin of safety for borderline cases.

DELAYED COMPLICATIONS

In the 1960s a few cases were reported in which dysrhythmias occurred days after ingestion. Tachycardia commonly persists for several days. Such prolonged effects are easily explained by the long and varied half-life of CAs in overdose, which ranges from 25 to 81 hours. This raised justifiable concern about sudden death late in the course of CA ingestion and led to recommendations for prolonged monitoring. However, more recent studies of hospitalized inpatients have allayed fears of serious delayed complications. In a series of 129 patients, all who developed cardiovascular or central nervous system complications did so within an hour of admission. No patient who had normal electrocardiographic findings for an hour developed a subsequent dysrhythmia. Two other studies documented that all severe cardiac complications were initially manifested in the first 24 hours. Another recent study found that in 48 of 49 patients the electrocardiogram taken in the emergency department showed the maximal QRS prolongation during the hospitalization, and that all patients who had major complications developed them within the first six hours after hospitalization. A study of fatal cases found that 75 percent of the deaths occurred within the first six hours and 100 percent within 24 hours; the mean time from arrival to the development of the first major sign of poisoning was only 58 minutes. In every fatal case major signs developed within two hours after arrival.

Thus, the first 24 hours are critical. After this time, continued monitoring is needed only for patients manifesting major signs of toxicity—which should be very few. Monitoring patients for six hours after all cardiovascular toxicity (including any electrocardiographic abnormalities) disappears should allow a generous margin for error.

SUGGESTED READING

Boehnert M, Lovejoy F. Value of the QRS duration versus the serum drug level in predicting seizures and ventricular arrhythmias after an acute overdose of TCA. NEJM 1985; 313:474–479.

Callaham M. Antidepressant toxicity. Ann Emerg Med, 1986; 15:1036–1038.

Callaham M. TCA poisoning. J Emerg Med 1984; 1:453–457.

Callaham M. Tricyclic antidepressant overdose: a collective review. JACEP 1979; 8:413–425.

Callaham M, Kassel D. Epidemiology of fatal TCA ingestion: implications for management. Ann Emerg Med 1985; 14:1–9.

Litovitz TL, Troutman WG. Amoxapine overdose: seizure and fatalities. JAMA 1983; 250:1069–1071.

SNAKEBITE

JOHN B. SULLIVAN Jr., M.D.

Snake venom poisoning is an uncommon medical emergency that many physicians may feel uncomfortable in managing. Consultation on management of snake envenomations can be obtained through local or regional poison centers, and this consultation should be sought if the physician remains uncomfortable in caring for the patient.

The venomous snakes indigenous to the United States are the pit vipers (Crotalidae) and coral snakes (Elapidae). The majority of bites and envenomations are inflicted by pit vipers (rattlesnakes, cotton mouths, and copperheads). Most contacts with these snakes occur in warm months; however, because some people keep these snakes as pets, envenomations also occur during winter months. The pit viper has a unique infrared thermoreceptor organ ("pit") on each side of the head that allows the snake to seek out warm-blooded prey.

DIAGNOSIS OF ENVENOMATION

The diagnosis of snake venom poisoning is usually not difficult. In some cases however, the snake may not be seen or found, or the patient may be a small child incapable of giving accurate history. In these instances the diagnosis may be delayed or missed (Table 1). The patient may have a history of being in an environment where snakes may be found or of handling snakes; the snake may not be seen or found. The majority of rattlesnakes do not give warning rattles before striking. Fang marks may be seen at the bite site; these may appear as tiny puncture wounds or as scratches. There may be one, two, or more marks, depending on the number of strikes.

Venom is composed of a variety of proteins that produce many toxic effects on blood and other tissues. Proteolytic enzymes produce tissue destruction and edema and pain (within minutes), local tissue necrosis and ecchymosis, and coagulopathy.

These pathophysiologic findings may not be present in all envenomatins, and 20 percent of bites do not result in envenomation. Diagnosing the envenomation also means grading the severity that affects therapy. Grading envenomatins is a clinical interpretation and falls into one of the categories noted in Table 2.

The treating physician should remember that envenomation grades change with time. A mild envenomation can become severe over a matter of hours. Venom, like

TABLE 1 Degrees of Envenomation

No envenomation (dry bite)

Mild envenomation (local edema and pain only)

Moderate envenomation (pain, edema beyond bite site accompanied by other systemic manifestations, such as nausea, vomiting, orthostasis)

Severe envenomation (shock, severe coagulopathy massive edema)

TABLE 2 Common Errors in Diagnosis

Not considering snake venom poisoning in the case of an edematous, ecchymotic extremity in a child who was playing in an area where snakes may be found

Not looking for fang marks at the site of pain

Not considering that an envenomation grade can change with time and thus that the clinical status of the patient may worsen over a period

Not checking initial coagulation studies and repeating these at a later time

Not considering the diagnosis of envenomation because a snake was not seen

any drug or toxin, has absorption, distribution, and elimination characteristics. Also a snake has control over the amount of venom it wishes to deposit. Thus, multiple bites usually result in more venom being deposited. The venom will leave this deposition site and circulate throughout the body. Venon proteins may be eliminated slowly and can be found after a week following an envenomation in the urine and plasma of patients.

THERAPY OF SNAKE VENOM POISONING

Prehospital Care

This is a controversial area. Once the diagnosis of actual envenomation has been made, there is time to proceed to an emergency department in an orderly manner. However, if the patient is hemodynamically unstable, emergent care is necessary. The bitten extremity can be splinted and the person kept at rest. The use of a lymphatic-venous constriction band can help retard the systemic spread of venom. However, this should not be very tight and should not be kept on longer than 30 minutes. In the early phase of the envenomation, the majority of victims experience some pain and manifest edema at the bite site.

Vital signs should be assessed and, if necessary, an intravenous line started in an uninvolved extremity. If a patient is hypotensive in the field, the main treatment is the intravenous administration of crystalloid. A vasopressor may also be necessary. Antivenin administration in the field is not recommended. In fact, antivenin is not an emergent mode of therapy for snake venom poisoning.

Newer prehospital care methods for removal of venom are being developed. One such method involves a suction device (Extractor, Sawyer Products) that is applied over the fang marks. This device has been demonstrated to remove a mean of 23 percent of injected venom after only a three minute suction period. The extractor device does not require incision and removes venom by creating a negative suction of one atmosphere. There is no evidence that incision of the wound and suction are any more effective, and vital structures can be damaged by the inexperienced or hasty incision. There is no need for application of ice or for excision of the bite site; both do more harm than good. The patient should be transported to the hospital as soon as possible.

Hospital Management

Upon arrival in the emergency department, vital signs should be assessed, any constriction band removed, and

978

the envenomation graded as mild, moderate, or severe. At this time the most crucial decision is whether to use *antivenin*.

Not every envenomated patient should receive antivenin. Antivenin is equine in source and is obtained from horses hyperimmunized with particular snake venoms. There are many potential problems. Some patients may be allergic to horse serum. Antivenin also contains other horse proteins besides neutralizing antibodies. The incidence of serum sickness varies between 50 to 75 percent following its use. Patients with a history of allergies to horse serum or with mild envenomations can be managed with antivenin.

A patient who sustains a mild envenomation should be observed for signs and symptoms of changing envenomation grade. Antivenin is indicated for moderate and severe envenomations.

Before antivenin is administered in any case, *skin testing* should be undertaken with the dilute horse serum present in the kit or with dilute antiven (Table 3). Antiven is approximately 10 times more concentrated than the horse serum in the kit.

The appropriate method for skin testing is administration of 0.1 ml of the 1:10 dilution of horse serum intradermally. The serum should not be given subcutaneously. A proper skin test will raise a small skin bleb. Skin testing should not be performed with the antivenin itself unless it is diluted at least to 1:100. Antivenin is much more concentrated than the normal horse serum and contains the same proteins present in horse serum.

HOW TO ADMINISTER ANTIVENIN

Each vial of antivenin contains approximately 1.5 g of processed, freeze dried horse hyperimmune serum. Dilute the antivenin volume to be given to at least 1:2 or 1:4 with the accompanying dilutant. Foaming indicates denaturing of the protein. Make sure it is all dissolved by gently shaking; this may require 20 minutes. Administer the antivenin intravenously, starting the administration slowly at first to avoid hypotension and urticaria caused by a rapid bolus of foreign protein. If hypotension or urticaria occurs, stop the antivenin and administer diphenhydramine intravenously. The infusion can be started back slowly. If hypotension occurs again, consider terminating the antivenin administration and managing the patient conservatively. Antivenin can be given as rapidly as the patient can tolerate it. Full doses should be ad-

TABLE 3 Skin Testing for Antivenin Sensitivity

Administer dilute horse serum or very dilute antivenin intradermally (not subcutaneously).

Wait at least 30 minutes before determining a negative skin test.

A positive skin test is an erythematous reaction.

Always be prepared to treat anaphylaxis during skin testing.

Do not skin test if antivenin is not going to be given.

A negative skin test does not insure that anaphylaxis will not occur upon administering antivenin.

TABLE 4 Important Points to Remember Concerning Anaphylaxis

Anaphylaxis may occur up to two hours following exposure to foreign protein.

If a patient is taking beta-adrenoceptive blocking agents such as propranolol, anaphylaxis may be more prolonged and severe.

Fluid administration along with epinephrine is the mainstay of therapy for anaphylaxis.

Diphenhydramine intravenously is also helpful in moderating anaphylaxis.

Corticosteroids have no role in the acute management of anaphylaxis. The onset of action requires 4–6 hours.

ministered early in the course. Points to remember about anaphylaxis are summarized in Table 4.

Determining the amount of antiven required depends on the grade of envenomation. Mild envenomation should not be treated with antivenin. Moderate envenomations may require 10 to 15 vials of antivenin. Severe envenomation may require 15 or more vials of antivenin. Clinical judgment must be used as well as patient monitoring to titrate the appropriate amount of antivenin to prevent further complications.

Coagulopathy is caused by some venins and may present with thrombocytopenia, prolongation of prothrombin time and partial thromboplastin time, decrease in fibrinogen, and elevation of levels of fibrin degradation products. Management of coagulopathy includes the administration of antivenin and the judicious use of either fresh frozen plasma or cryoprecipitate. In a patient with allergies or allergy to horse serum, severe coagulopathy can be managed conservatively without antivenin as long as the patient is not showing signs of clinical bleeding.

Response to antivenin therapy will be manifested by a termination in the progression of edema, relief of pain, and reversal of coagulopathy. Antivenin will not reverse edema once it is present. Also the platelet count may not return to normal quickly. This may require a few days even with antivenin therapy. Therapy can be monitored by observing for further edema spread, progression of coagulopathy, or a worsening clinical picture. Antivenin should be titrated against these pathophysiologic changes. Some edema spread may continue to occur after antivenin therapy. This may simply be dependent edema in an extremity and may occur hours following therapy.

Serum sickness may occur at any time 7 days to 3 weeks after antivenin therapy. The treatment of serum sickness consists of the administration of antihistamines and corticosteroids on an outpatient basis.

DISPOSITION OF THE PATIENT

A patient with a mild envenomation can be observed for a few hours. If signs and symptoms do not progress and coagulopathy is not present, the patient can be sent home and rechecked the following day. Make sure the patient has an up to date tetanus immunization status. Snakes harbor gram negative bacteria and Clostridium species in their mouths; in an envenomated extremity it is very difficult to document infection. A patient with moderate or severe envenomation should be admitted to the hospital. A moderately envenomated patient can be admitted to a ward bed. A severely envenomated patient usually requires intensive care. The average patient who is treated with antivenin requires hospitalization for up to 3 days. Sequelae of envenomation include lymphangitis and lymphadenopathy.

THE CONTROVERSY CONCERNING SURGERY

There is absolutely no need for surgical intervention in an envenomated patient unless a compartmental syndrome can be demonstrated by intracompartmental pressure monitoring. Tissue necrosis can occur, but is rare. It is difficult to clinically assess the presence of a compartmental syndrome in an envenomated extremity, since pain, edema, and ecchymosis are present. Even with a large amount of edema, the majority of envenomated extremities do well and can be easily managed by elevation of the extremity along with the administration of Mannitol. Drastic surgical remedies previously recommended do more harm than good. Application of ice is of no benefit and can particularly harm tissue if applied too long; it is not recommended. Surgical management of envenomated extremities can be disfiguring and result in unnecessary hospitalization.

MANAGEMENT WITHOUT ANTIVENIN

Patients who have allergies to horse serum or who have experienced anaphylaxis on skin testing or when an-

tivenin is administered are a management dilemma. In some cases, treatment with intravenous diphenhydramine, 50 mg, will allow further antivenin administration. However, in other cases, the patient can be conservatively managed by observation and judicious administration of blood products as needed. Generally, these patients are hospitalized for up to 10 days before coagulopathy and edema reverse. Expert consultation should be sought in these cases.

EXPERT CONSULTATION

Most poison centers have access to clinical toxicology consultants to advise about the management of snake venom poisoning. These poison centers are open 24 hours a day and have consultants available at all times. Information on treatment and antivenin for exotic species can be obtained from the Arizona Poison Center (602) 626-6016.

REFERENCES

Dart R, Sullivan J, Troutman W. Management of severely envonomated patients without antivenin. (Abstract) Veterinary and Human Toxicology 1986; 28(5):485.

Russell FE. Snake venom poisoning. Great Neck, New York: Scholium International, Inc, 1983.

Sullivan JB: Crotalidae envenomation. In: Edlich R, Spyker D, eds. Current emergency therapy. Appleton Century Crofts, 1985.

Wingert WA, Sullivan JB. Snakebite management—which approach to use. Emerg Med Rep 1984; 5:37–44.

DIRECTORY OF POISON CONTROL CENTERS

The clinician is advised to institute all the basic initial measures for toxicologic management discussed in the previous chapters and then call the nearest poison control center for more specific information.

AMERICAN ASSOCIATION OF POISON CONTROL CENTERS

ALABAMA

Alabama Poison Center
Tuscaloosa, AL 35401
800-462-0800 (AL)
205-345-0600

Children's Hospital of Alabama Poison Center
Birmingham, AL 35233
205-933-4050
800-292-6678
205-939-9201

ARIZONA

Arizona Poison and Drug Information Center
University of Arizona
Tucson, AZ 85724
800-362-0101 (AZ)
602-626-6016

Central Arizona Reg. Poison Management
  Center
St. Lukes Hospital
Phoenix, AZ 85006
602-251-8186

ARKANSAS

Arkansas Poison and Drug Information Center
Little Rock, AR 72205
501-666-5532

CALIFORNIA

Central Valley Poison Control Center
Fresno, CA 93715
209-442-1222

Lacma Reg. Poison Information Center
Los Angeles, CA 90057
213-484-5151

San Diego Regional Poison Center
San Diego, CA 92103
619-294-3666
619-294-6000

San Francisco Bay Area Reg. Poison Control
  Center
San Francisco, CA 95404
415-666-2845

Sonoma Country Poison Control Center
Santa Rosa, CA 95404
707-527-7177

U.C. Davis Medical Center
Sacramento, CA 95817

U.C. Irvine Medical Center
Irvine, CA
714-634-5988

COLORADO

Rocky Mountain Poison Center
Denver, CO 80204
303-629-1123

CONNECTICUT

University of Connecticut Poison Control
  Health Center
Farmington, CT 06032
203-674-3456

DISTRICT OF COLUMBIA

Georgetown University Hospital
Washington, DC 20007
202-625-3333

FLORIDA

St. Vincents Medical Center
Jacksonville, FL 32203
904-387-7500

Tampa General Hospital
Tampa, FL 33679
813-251-6995

Winterhaven Hospital
Winterhaven, FL 33880
813-299-9701

GEORGIA

Grady Memorial Hospital
Atlanta, GA 30335
404-589-4400

Poison Center, Memorial Med.
Savannah, GA 31403
912-355-5228

IDAHO

Pocatello Regional Medical Center
Pocatello, ID 83201
800-632-9490 (ID)
208-234-0777 X5019

ILLINOIS

Brokaw Hospital Poison Center
Normal, IL 61761
309-454-1400

Chicago and N.E. Illinois
Regional Poison Control Center
Chicago, IL 60612
800-942-5969 (IN, IL)
312-942-5969

St. Francis Medical Center
Peoria, IL 61637
309-672-2662
309-672-2334

St. Johns Hospital Regional Central and
  Southern Illinois Poison Resource Center
Springfield, IL 62769
800-252-2022

INDIANA

Indiana Poison Center
Indianapolis, IN 46202
800-382-9097
317-630-7351

IOWA

Iowa Methodist Medical Center
Des Moines, IA 50308
512-283-6408

Marian Health Center, Poison Center
Sioux City, IA 51103
712-279-2066

St. Lukes Poison Center
Sioux City, IA 51104
800-352-2222 (IA)
800-831-1111 (NE.SD)

University of Iowa Hospital and Clinic
Iowa City, IA 52242
319-356-2922

KANSAS

Stormont-Vail Regional Medical Center
Topeka, KS 66606
913-354-6100

University of Kansas Medical Center
Kansas City, KS 66103
913-588-6633

KENTUCKY

Kosair Children's Hospital
Louisville, KY 40232
800-722-5725 (KY)
502-589-8222

Northern Kentucky Poison Information Center
FT. Thomas, KY 41075
800-352-9900
606-572-3215

LOUISIANNA

Louisianna Regional Poison Center
Shreveport, LA 90057
800-535-0525 (LA)
318-425-1524

MAINE

Maine Medical Center
Portland, ME 04102
800-442-6305 (ME)

MARYLAND

Maryland Poison Center
Baltimore, MD 21201
800-492-2414 (MD)
301-528-7701

MASSACHUSETTS

Massachusetts Poison Control System
Boston, MA 02115
800-682-9211 (MA)
617-232-2120 (Other)

MICHIGAN

Blodgett Regional Poison Center
Grand Rapids, MI 49506
800-442-4571 (MI AC 616)
800-632-2727 (MI Other)
Borgess Medical Center
Kalamazoo, MI 49001
800-632-4177
616-383-7070
Bronson Methodist Hospital
Kalamazoo, MI 49007
800-442-4112 (AC 616)
616-383-6409
Children's Hospital of Michigan
Detroit, MI 48201
313-494-5711
Saginaw Reg. Poison Center
Saginaw, MI 49602
517-755-1111
Univeristy of Michigan Hospital
Ann Arbor, MI 48109
313-764-7667

MINNESOTA

Hennepin Poison Center
Minneapolis, MN 55415
612-347-3141
St. Marys Hospital
Rochester, MN 55902
507-285-5123
St. Paul Ramsey Medical Center
St. Paul, MN 55101
800-222-1222 (MN)
612-221-2113

MISSISSIPPI

U.M.C. Poison Services
University of Mississippi Medical Center
Jackson, MS 39216
601-354-7660

MISSOURI

Cardinal Glennon Children's Hospital
St. Louis, MO 63104
800-392-9111 (MO)
314-772-5200

Children's Mercy Hospital
Kansas City, MO 64108
816-234-3000

NEBRASKA

Children's Memorial Hospital
Omaha, NE 68114
800-642-9999 (NE)
800-228-9515 (Sur states)
402-390-5400

NEVADA

St. Marys Hospital Poison Control Center
Reno, NV 89520
702-789-3013

NEW HAMPSHIRE

Dartmouth-Hitchcock Medical Center
Hanover, NH 03756
603-646-5000

NEW JERSEY

Middlesex General University Hospital
New Brunswick, NJ 08901
201-937-8583
New Jersey Poison Information
800-962-1253 (NJ)
201-926-8005
Warren Hospital
Phillipsburg, NJ 08865
201-859-6767
West Jersey Health System
Berlin, NJ 08009
800-962-1253

NEW MEXICO

University of New Mexico
Albuquerque, NM 87131
800-432-6866
505-843-2551

NEW YORK

Childrens's Hospital of Buffalo
Buffalo, NY 14222
716-878-7654

Life Line Finger Lakes
Regional Poison Control Center
Rochester, NY 14607
716-275-5151
Nyack Hospital
Nyack, NY 10960
914-353-1000
New York Poison Control Center
New York, NY 10016
212-340-4494
Southern Tier Poison Center
Binghamtom, NY 13760
607-723-8929

NORTH CAROLINA

Duke Poison Control Center,
Duke Medical Center
Durham, NC 27710
800-672-1697 (NC)
919-684-8111
Mercy Hospital
Charlotte, NC 28207
704-379-5827
Moses Cone Hospital
Greensboro, NC 27401
919-379-4105

NORTH DAKOTA

St. Lukes Hospital
Fargo, ND 58122
701-280-5575

OHIO

Central Ohio Poison Center
Columbus, OH 43205
614-228-1323
Children's Hospital Medical Center
Akron, OH 44308
216-379-8562
Children's Medical Center
Dayton, OH 45404
800-762-0727
513-226-8352
Greater Cleveland Poison Control Center
Cleveland, OH, 44106
216-844-1573
St. Elizabeth Hospital Medical Center
Youngstown, OH 44501
216-746-2222
University of Cincinatti
Cincinnati, OH 45267
800-872-5111 (SW OH)
513-872-5111

OREGON

Oregon Poison Control Center and
    Information Center
Portland, OR 97201
800-452-7165 (OR)
503-225-8968

PENNSYLVANIA

Allentown Hospital
Allentown, PA 18102
215-433-2311
Capital Area Poison Center
717-534-6111
Children's Hospital of Pittsburg
Pittsburgh, PA 15213
412-681-6669
Mamot Medical Center
Erie, PA 16550
814-452-4242
Mercy Hospital
Altoona, PA 16603
814-946-3711
Philadelphia Poison Information Center
Philadelphia, PA 19104
215-WA2-5523
St. Vincents Health Center
Erie, PA 16544
814-452-3232

RHODE ISLAND

Rhode Island Poison Center
Providence, RI 02906
401-277-5727

SOUTH DAKOTA

McKennan Poison Center
Sioux Falls, SD 57101
800-952-0123 (SD)
800-843-0505 (IA, MN, NE)
Rapid City Reg. Poison Center
Rapid City, SD 57709
605-341-3333

TENNESSEE

Johnson City Medical Center
Johnson City, TN 37601
615-461-6572
Southern Poison Center
Memphis, TN 38103
901-528-6048

TEXAS

East Texas Poison Center
Tyler, TX 75711
915-533-1244

TEXAS

El Paso Poison Control Center
El Paso, TX 79905
915-533-1244
Medical Center Hospital
Conroe, TX 77305
409-539-7700
North Central Texas Poison Center
Dallas, TX 75235
214-920-2400

Texas State Poison Center
Galveston, TX 77550
409-765-1420

UTAH

Humana Hospital Davis Nth
Layton, UT 84041
801-825-825-4357
Intermountain Reg Poison Control Center
Salt Lake City, UT 84123
800-662-0062 (UT)
801-581-2151

VERMONT

Medical Hospital of Vermont
Burlington, VT 05401
802-658-3456

VIRGINIA

Central Virginia Poison Center
Richmond, VA 23298
804-786-9123
Depaul Hospital
Norfolk, VA 23505
800-552-6337
804-489-5288
Hampton General Hospital
Hampton, VA 23669
804-727-7195
Roanoke Memorial Hospital
Roanoke, VA 24033
703-981-7336
University of Virginia Medical Center
Charlottesville, VA 22908
804-924-5543

WASHINGTON

Deaconess Medical Center
Spokane, WA 99210
800-572-5842 (WA)
800-541-5624 (Other)
Seattle Poison Center
800-732-6985 (WA)
206-526-2121
Yakima Valley Memorial Hospital

Yakima, WA 98902
800-572-9176 (WA)
509-248-4400 (Other)

WEST VIRGINIA

West Virginia University Medical Center
Charleston, WV 25304
304-348-4211

WISCONSIN

Luther Hospital
Eau Claire, WI 54702
715-835-1515
Milwaukee Children's Hospital
Milwaukee, WI 53233
414-931-4114
St. Francis Medical Center
Lacrosse, WI 54601
608-784-3971
St. Vincent Hospital
Green Bay, WI 54307
414-433-8100
University of Wisconsin Hospital
Madison, WI 53792
608-262-3702

WYOMING

Wyoming Poison Center
Cheyenne, WY 82001

PUERTO RICO

University of Puerto Rico
San Juan, PR 00936
809-753-4849
809-763-0196

JAPAN

Japan Poison Center
Sakura-Mura, Niihari-Gun
Japan 305
0298-51-9999

PEDIATRIC EMERGENCIES

FEVER IN THE CHILD

CAROL D. BERKOWITZ, M.D., F.A.A.P.

Fever, a frequent presenting complaint of children in the emergency department, is noted in one-third of all pediatric emergency department visits. Fever is not a disease but rather a nonspecific symptom of some underlying process involving inflammation or infection. The physician must be aware of the characteristic signs and symptoms of these processes, differentiate the seriously ill from the mildly ill child, and institute appropriate therapy.

ETIOLOGY

Fever is caused by a rise in core body temperature that follows a resetting of the body's thermostat. This thermostat is located in the preoptic region of the anterior hypothalamus. Resetting the thermostat occurs in response to endogenous pyrogens (fever-inducing agents that are released from leukocytes, alveolar macrophages, and Kupffer cells in the liver) that in turn are responding to exogenous pyrogens such as bacterial antibodies, antigens and viruses.

Resetting the body's thermostat leads to a number of physiologic and behavioral changes. The first sign of fever in the affected individual is a sensation of being cold or chilled. This occurs because the body temperature is lower than the central thermostat setting. Behaviorally, the individual responds to the feeling of being chilled by putting on additional clothes, climbing under the covers, and drinking hot beverages. Physiologically, there is peripheral vasoconstriction and central pooling of blood. The individual starts to shiver. Body temperature then rises until it equals the temperature of the thermoregulatory center.

For many years, the term fever has been synonymous with disease; many diseases include the word fever in their name, e.g., thyroid fever, scarlet fever, rheumatic fever. But fever is not a disease, but rather a symptom of some underlying disorder.

DIAGNOSTIC EVALUATION

All children should be evaluated with a medical history. The duration and the severity of the fever may be clues to the etiology. The presence of associated symptoms, such as rhinorrhea, cough, respiratory distress, vomiting, diarrhea, anorexia, lethargy, irritability, or changes in mental status, may point to specific organ system involvement. Any other changes from the normal state of the child should be noted. It is useful to inquire about exposure to communicable diseases or the presence of illness in other family members. In children with prolonged fevers, history of foreign travel, drug (including antibiotic) ingestion, or contact with animals should be elicited.

A complete physical examination should be performed on any febrile child, even if the history suggests a disorder of one organ system. Children with otitis media frequently present with gastrointestinal symptoms; the correct diagnosis would go unrecognized if a complete examination were not performed. The overall well-being of the child should be determined. A child with a toxic reaction, regardless of age, does not interact appropriately with the examiner. The child should be observed for spontaneous movements, eye contact, consolability, and negative reactions (e.g., crying) to aversive stimuli. Absence of these activities suggests a seriously ill child. Vital signs should be measured. The heart rate increases by 10 beats per minute for each degree of temperature elevation (°F) above normal. Tachycardia disproportionate to the degree of fever suggests sepsis or dehydration. Tachypnea is seen with metabolic acidosis (as in sepsis or shock) or respiratory tract infection. It may be the only clue to the latter. Other signs of respiratory tract infection are rales, rhonchi, wheezing, or stridor. The fontanelle should be palpated; a depressed fontanelle is seen in dehydration and a bulging fontanelle in central nervous system infection or congestive heart failure. A careful assessment of the ears, including pneumatic otoscopy, often reveals the source of the fever, especially in children under the age of 5 years. Tonsillitis secondary to infection with group A hemolytic streptococci is a common cause of fever in children between 5 and 10 years. Other disorders that may be apparent from the physical examination include exanthems, which suggest viral infection, or localized areas of pain or swelling or both, which are seen with cellulitis, osteomyelitis, or septic arthritis. Nuchal rigidity and a positive Kernig's or Brudzinski's sign may be noted in the older child with meningitis but are frequently absent in the infant under 2 years of age. The physician must maintain a high index of suspicion for meningitis when evaluating such young infants.

Two other groups that require special attention are febrile infants under the age of 2 months and infants under 2 years of age with no focus of infection.

INFANTS UNDER 2 MONTHS

Febrile infants under 2 months of age present a diagnostic dilemma for the emergency department physician. Such young infants lack the interpersonal skills noted previously (e.g., eye contact), and it is more difficult to clinically assess their well-being. Some investigators have noted that these infants are at particularly high risk for serious infections, such as bacterial meningitis, bacteremia, and aseptic meningitis. Because the history may not provide specific clues to the diagnosis and the physical examination may be equally unrevealing, these infants deserve a comprehensive laboratory work-up, including complete blood count, differential analysis, chest x-ray study, lumbar puncture, urinalysis and culture, and blood culture. Hospitalization is recommended if any of these studies is abnormal, if the infant appears ill, or if follow-up care is uncertain.

INFANTS LESS THAN 2 YEARS WITHOUT A FOCUS OF INFECTION

There has been much interest in the febrile infant between 3 and 24 months who has no focus of infection. Numerous studies have shown that these infants may be bacteremic. The most common organisms implicated are *Streptococcus pneumoniae* (65 percent) and *Haemophilus influenzae* (25 percent). Certain characteristics distinguish this group. Infants generally have fever higher than 39 °C, white blood counts higher than 15,000 per cubic millimeter, and/or an erythrocyte sedimentation rate of greater than 30 mm per hour. The incidence of bacteremia in this group is approximately 12 to 15 percent. The presence of pneumonia on chest roentgenogram increases the incidence of bacteremia in this age group to about 25 percent.

The risk of meningitis in bacteremic infants is about 6 to 8 percent. It is uncertain whether this figure is influenced by the institution of antibiotics at the initial visit. In general, institution of antibiotics at the initial visit is associated with a good outcome, and particularly with resolution of the bacteremia.

The approach to the febrile infant between 3 and 24 months should be guided by the clinical assessment noted above. A blood culture is useful in infants with high fevers and elevated white blood cell counts who have no focus of infection.

THERAPY

Fever Control

Therapeutic intervention is twofold: controlling the fever and treating the infection causing the fever. Prehospital care is limited to fever control. There is no evidence that fever per se is harmful, and numerous studies in animals suggest that fever may have beneficial effects. In 1666 Sydenham said that "Fever is a mighty engine that nature brings into the world for the conquest of her enemies." Many parents are fearful of fever and are concerned about the risk of febrile seizures or brain damage. They should be reassured that the fever may be helping their child fight off the infection.

In spite of the possible beneficial effects of the fever, many children do not feel comfortable while they are febrile, and so fever-reducing measures may be instituted to assure patient comfort. Simple measures to assist with fever reduction include unbundling, sponging with tepid water, or bathing with tepid water. Ice-water baths should be discouraged because of the degree of patient discomfort, and alcohol baths should also be discouraged because of reported episodes of alcohol intoxications through inhalation. Such intoxication is associated with seizures and hypoglycemia. Antipyretics such as aspirin or acetaminophen may also be given at a dosage of 10 to 15 mg per kilogram per dose every 4 hours. Because of the association with Reye's syndrome, aspirin should be avoided in any child with chickenpox, influenza, or an influenza-like illness. The response of the fever to antipyretics does not distinguish between bacterial and other infections.

Hospitalization

The decision to hospitalize versus manage as an outpatient must be determined on the basis of the age of the child, the severity of the illness, and the reliability of follow-up care. In general, infants under the age of 2 to 3 months with fever should be evaluated with a full septic work-up as outlined and should be admitted to the hospital. All children with bacterial infections requiring systemic antibiotics (meningitis, omphalitis) should also be admitted. Infants under the age of 1 year with aseptic meningitis should also be admitted to assure adequate hydration and follow-up. These infants are at high risk for subsequent hearing and learning disabilities.

Antibiotic Management

Antibiotic therapy should be initiated in any child with a suspected bacterial infection. Mildly ill children such as those with otitis media, pharyngitis, pneumonia, or urinary tract infection may be managed as outpatients. Antibiotics should be selected to cover the suspected organisms. In general, ampicillin, at a dose of 50 to 100 mg per kilogram per day in four divided doses, covers the usual pathogens implicated in outpatient infections. Viral illnesses do not require antibiotic therapy.

Children with suspected bacterial infections who are admitted to the hospital should be managed with systemic antibiotics. Antibiotics should be selected to cover the pathogens usually implicated in the specific illness. These are somewhat different in different age groups. Infants under the age of 3 weeks who have been discharged from the nursery and are now patients are at risk for infection with gram-negative organisms, group B *Streptococcus*, *Listeria monocytogenes*, and occasionally *Haemophilus influenzae*. The antibiotics recommended for suspected bacterial meningitis in this age group are ampicillin, 300 mg per kilogram per day in four divided doses, and gentamicin, 2.5 mg per kilogram per dose every 12 hours for infants under 1 week of age, and every 8 hours for infants over 1 week of age. If sepsis but not meningitis is suspected, the choice of antibiotics is the same, but the dosage of ampicillin is only 100 mg per kilogram per day in four divided doses. Older infants between 3 weeks and 2 months of age are at risk for the same group of organisms, but the risk of *Haemophilus influenzae* is somewhat higher. As a result, more definitive coverage of possible ampicillin-resistant *H. influenzae* infection must be instituted. Because of the potential danger of toxicity from chloramphenicol in this age group, recommended antibiotics include ampicillin at the same dosage as noted and cefotaxime at 100 mg per kilogram per day in four divided doses. Infants over the age of 2 months with suspected bacterial meningitis should be managed with ampicillin at 200 mg to 300 mg per kilogram per day in four divided doses and chloramphenicol at 100 mg per kilogram per day in four divided doses. The dosage of chloramphenicol should be lowered to 50 mg to 70 mg per kilogram after the initial few days of therapy, or if meningitis is not suspected.

Children with specific infections (e.g., osteomyelitis, omphalitis, mastitis) associated with other organisms (e.g., *Staphylococcus aureus*) should have additional antibiotics. Antistaphylococcal coverage is best accomplished with a semisynthetic penicillin, such as oxacillin, 100 mg to 200 mg per kilogram per day in four divided doses, or nafcillin, 20 mg per kilogram per day in two divided doses in neonates and 50 mg per kilogram per day in two divided doses in older infants and children, or a cephalosporin, such as cefazolin (for infants older than 1 month) 25 to 100 mg per kilogram per day in three or four doses. Other antibiotics may be instituted if culture and sensitivity testing reveal other organisms with different sensitivities.

Other therapeutic measures should be instituted as deemed necessary. Infants with respiratory distress may benefit from oxygen, and dehydrated infants require rehydration.

Follow-up Care

Infants who are bacteremic and are sent home must be recalled for repeat evaluation. Children treated with antibiotics at the initial visit will have cleared their bacteremia in about 80 percent of cases. If the child has not received antibiotics, but is afebrile and doing well, there is no need to institute antibiotic therapy. If, on the other hand, the infant returns febrile, anorectic, lethargic, or doing poorly, regardless of whether he is receiving antibiotics, he should be completely reassessed. A repeat complete blood count, differential analysis, lumbar puncture, urinalysis and urine culture, and chest x-ray film should be obtained. All bacteremic infants who are febrile or symptomatic should be admitted to the hospital and treated with parenteral antibiotics pending the outcome of the repeat cultures.

SUGGESTED READING

Dershewitz RA, Wigder HN, Wigder CM, Nadelman DH. A comparative study of the prevalence, outcome, and prediction of bacteremia in children. J Pediatr 1983; 103:352.

Dinarello CA, Wolff SM. Pathogenesis of fever in man. New Engl J Med 1978; 293:607.

McCarthy PL. Controversies in pediatrics: what tests are indicated for the child under 2 with fever? Pediatr Rev 1979; 1:51.

Soman M. Diagnostic work-up of febrile children under 24 months of age: a clinical review. West J Med 1982; 137:1.

COMMON PEDIATRIC RASHES WITHOUT SYSTEMIC ILLNESS

ILONA J. FRIEDEN, M.D.

ATOPIC DERMATITIS

Atopic dermatitis is an extremely common skin disorder of childhood. Its precise etiology is not known, but there is often a positive family history of allergic rhinitis, asthma, or atopic dermatitis. The skin of individuals with atopic dermatitis is more easily irritated, itchier, drier, lichenifies more readily, and is more susceptible to certain bacterial and viral infections than is the skin of individuals without atopic dermatitis. The presence of cutaneous infection with *Staphylococcus aureus* or sudden changes in the weather often precede exacerbations of atopic dermatitis, but frequently no precipitating factor can be found.

The differential diagnosis of atopic dermatitis includes scabies, contact dermatitis, and psoriasis. The duration of scabies is usually less than two months. The rash is often more papular and less lichenified than that of atopic dermatitis. The presence of papules, vesicles, and pustules on the hands and feet and extensive axillary involvement may help differentiate scabies from atopic dermatitis. Contact dermatitis may be difficult to differentiate, but the distribution of the rash together with a history of a likely irritant may be helpful. Contrary to popular belief, laundry detergents are rarely a cause of contact dermatitis if clothing is adequately rinsed. Psoriasis is usually more sharply marginated, with a denser, micaceous scale, and is most commonly located in the scalp and on the extensor elbows and knees. It usually does not itch as severely as atopic dermatitis.

The skin lesions of atopic dermatitis are usually lichenified, scaly plaques with some degree of erythema. The erythema may be difficult to appreciate in darker skinned individuals. Distribution may vary, depending on the age of the child. Typically, young infants have involvement of the cheeks and extensor surfaces of the arms and legs, while toddlers and older children have more involvement of the flexural creases, such as the antecubital and popliteal fossae. Areas of oozing, honey-colored crusts, or the prescence of small pustules should alert the clinician to the possibility of superinfection with *S. aureus*. The presence of multiple, 1- to 2-mm vesicles or shallow ulcerations, either individually or in groups, may indicate cutaneous infection with herpes simplex virus, so-called "eczema herpeticum." The diagnosis may be confirmed by a Tzanck preparation, direct immunofluorescence, or viral culture.

The treatment of atopic dermatitis requires a concerted approach, using a dry skin care regimen, topical corticosteroids, oral antihistamines, and oral antibiotics when indicated. One useful dry skin regimen consists of brief showers or baths in tepid water followed by the application of corticosteroid creams or ointments to affected areas of skin. An emollient, such as Nutraderm, Moisturel, Eucerin Cream, or petrolatum is then applied over the entire body. The choice of emollient depends on patient preference and the degree of skin dryness. Most patients can tolerate a mild soap such as Dove or Purpose. Ivory should *not* be used, because it is very drying. For patients who cannot tolerate soap, Cetaphil lotion may be used as a soap substitute. Without using any water, the patient applies the lotion all over and then wipes it off with a soft cloth.

Corticosteroids are the mainstay of atopic dermatitis therapy (Table 1). The choice of corticosteroid potency depends on both the severity of the rash and its location. Potent fluorinated steroids should generally be avoided on the face and in intertriginous areas. The choice of the vehicle used depends on the location and the morphology of the eruption. If lesions are extremely inflamed and oozing, a corticosteroid cream or lotion is preferable to an ointment. Such lesions may also be helped by the use of aluminum acetate (Domeboro, Bluboro) compresses diluted to a 1:40 concentration (1 packet or tablet per pint of water) or oilated colloidal oatmeal baths (Aveeno). This should be followed by the appliction of a thin coat of a corticosteroid cream or lotion, such as triamcinolone

acetonide (TAC), 0.1 percent. Lesions that are heavily lichenified generally respond better to ointments than to creams. Scalp lesions should be treated with corticosteroid solutions or lotions, such as Synalar, 0.01 percent solution, or TAC, 0.1 percent lotion. Oral corticosteroids are rarely necessary in the treatment of atopic dermatitis in childhood.

Anithistamines should be used in oral dosages sufficient to stop severe pruritus and to allow patients and their families to sleep at night. This may require dosages that are substantially higher than the usual dosage recommendations for age and weight. Their usage is particularly important at night, since many children do most of their scratching at this time. In infants, diphenhydramine elixir or hydroxyzine hydrochloride syrup may be used, beginning with one-half to 1 tsp at bedtime and increasing the dosage as needed. Older children may require as much as 50 to 100 mg of diphenhydramine or 25 to 50 mg of hydroxyzine to adequately control pruritus, but it is better to start with a slightly lower dose and increase as needed.

The treatment of exacerbations of atopic dermatitis should include a one-week course of oral antibiotics with coverage for *S. aureus*. Erythromycin, 25 to 50 mg per kilogram per day up to a total of 1 g per day is usually effective unless significant *S. aureus* resistance to erythromycin is present in the community. In this case, dicloxacillin, 12.5 to 25 mg per kilogram per day divided into 4 doses or cephradine, 25 to 50 mg per kilogram per day divided into 4 doses may be given. Erythromycin should also be avoided in patients taking theophyllin derivatives, since it may increase the serum theophyllin level and could lead to toxic drug levels.

Patients with severe atopic dermatitis may improve rapidly with 2 or 3 days of inpatient hospitalization. This should be considered in children with widespread unremittent atopic dermatitis, despite adequate therapy, when areas of frank cellulitis or widespread superficial infection are present, or when parental compliance is likely to be poor.

Many patients with eczema herpeticum require hospitalization and intravenous treatment with acyclovir, but patients who are afebrile and look well may be followed closely as outpatients taking oral doses of acyclovir. Although the oral dosage levels for this condition are not well established, 200 mg every 4 hours would probably be a reasonable starting dose for children older than 3 years of age. Younger children should probably be hospitalized for observation and treatment.

DIAPER DERMATITIS

Diaper dermatitis, while rarely life-threatening, can be an uncomfortable condition for both infants and parents. The eruption may be itchy or even painful, especially if erosions are present. Parents often blame themselves for the presence of a diaper dermatitis, and feel that its presence may be taken as a sign of parental neglect. In fact, it is the wearing of diapers per se that is the underlying cause of most cases of diaper dermatitis.

TABLE 1 Treatment of Atopic Dermatitis

Mild	Moderate	Severe
Dry skin regimen	Dry skin regimen	Dry skin regimen
Hydrocortisone cream, or ointment 1 to 2.5%	Face: hydrocortisone cream or ointment, 1 to 2.5%	Face: Desonide, 0.05%, cream or ointment
	Body: triamcinolone acetonide cream or ointment, 0.025 to 0.1%	Body: triamcinolone acetonide, 0.1%, cream or ointment or Cyclocort, Maxiflor, or Lidex cream or ointment
	Antihistamines as needed	Antihistamines as needed
	Antibiotics with infection or exacerbation	Antibiotics with coverage for *S.aureus*
		Hospitalization as indicated

Five common forms of diaper dermatitis and their respective treatments are described in Table 2. These five conditions can usually be distinguished from one another by their morphology, distribution, and the presence or absence of other cutaneous findings. Together they account for over 90 percent of all cases of diaper dermatitis.

Mycolog cream (or its generic equivalent) has been used as a panacea for diaper dermatitis. This is an unfortunate practice, since in addition to containing two common contact sensitizers, neomycin and ethylenediamine, Mycolog also contains triamcinolone acetonide, 0.1 percent. This is an inappropriately strong corticosteroid for use in the diaper area, especially since it is being occluded by the diaper with its plastic wrap, thus further enhancing its cutaneous absorption. A more reasonable approach to the treatment of diaper dermatitis that does not fit into the catagories described in Table 2 is to use a combination of mystatin ointment and hydrocortisone ointment, 1 percent. This is an adequate treatment for most cases of diaper dermatitis.

Several conditions not mentioned in Table 2 may also present, although less commonly, as a diaper dermatitis. Scabies may be characterized by prominent groin involvement, but characteristic papules, vesicles, and occasional burrows are usually found on the feet and hands. Rare metabolic disorders such as acrodermatitis enterophathica and biotin-multiple carboxylase deficiency may present with a severe diaper dermatitis. Perioral dermatitis, diarrhea, and metabolic acidosis may also be present. Letterer-Siwe disease, a form of histiocytosis X, may also present with a severe diaper dermatitis. These conditions are extremely rare, but do point out the importance of taking a good history to ascertain that the infant is healthy, feeding well, and generally thriving. Recalcitrant cases of diaper dermatitis should be referred to a pediatrician or dermatologist for further evaluation.

WARTS AND MOLLUSCUM CONTAGIOSUM

Warts and molluscum contagiosum, common viral infections of the skin, are not generally considered to be emergencies, but pain, bleeding, or the sudden onset of a blister-like eruption may cause patients to seek emergency medical care. Warts usually become painful because of trauma or because repeated pressure causes warts to become endophytic, thereby impinging on nerves and other vital structures. This occurs most commonly with warts on the weight-bearing surfaces of the foot, so-called plantar warts, but may also occur with warts on the palm or other locations where repeated pressure is exerted. Treatment should be aimed at relieving the pressure by paring down the thickened areas of hyperkeratosis as much as possible. The patient (or parents) should then be instructed to use a 40 percent salicylic acid plaster cut to the size of the wart and secured in place with waterproof tape for 24 to 48 hours. The area should then be soaked in water, and any excess keratin can again be scraped off with a pumice stone, emery board, or dull paring knife. This process should be continued as often as is necessary to relieve the pressure.

TABLE 2 Diaper Dermatitis

Diagnosis	Distribution	Morphology	Treatment	Remarks
Irritant diaper dermatitis	Convex surfaces; "tide-water marks," located on waist and thighs at diaper's edges; spares folds	Erythema; variable scale; skin may look chapped; superficial erosions may be present	Increase diaper changes; use paper diapers or diaper service; hydrocortisone oint., 1% b.i.d.-t.i.d.; Desitin or A&D ointment after rash is improved	May occur at any age as long as child is still in diapers
Seborrheic diaper dermatitis	Sharply demarcated +/− involvement of folds	Scaly erythema without satellite pustules; occasionally greasy scale is present	Hydrocortisone oint., 1% t.i.d.; if severe, or if present more than 72 hours, add miconazole cream or nystatin oint. t.i.d.	Seborrheic dermatitis of scalp or face is usually present
Candida diaper dermatitis	Involves both convex surfaces and folds; may also be perianal	Beefy red with whitish scale; satellite papules and vesicopustules are present	Nystatin cream or oint. *or* miconazole cream; if marked erythema, add hydrocortisone ointment, 1%; use oral nystatin if oral thrush is present or if rash is recurrent	Frequently follows oral antibiotics; KOH prep. of satellite pustule may show hyphae
Napkin dermatitis with psoriasiform id reaction	Extensive diaper dermatitis involving folds with multiple papulosquamous plaques located on torso, face, and scalp	Erythema and scale in diaper area; psoriasiform lesions elsewhere	Combine miconazole cream and hydrocortisone ointment, 2.5% in diaper area t.i.d.-q.i.d.; use triamcinolone oint., 0.025%, in other affected areas	Dramatic eruption, but usually self-limited; may indicate predisposition toward atopic dermatitis or psoriasis in a minority of cases
Bullous impetigo in diaper area	Often spread from umbilicus downward, +/− folds	Varies from tiny vesicopustules to large tense bullae; lesions are discrete, without underlying erythema; usually multiple	Dicloxacillin, 12.5-25 mg/kg/day divided q.i.d., *or* erythromycin, 25-50 mg/kg/day divided q.i.d.	Usually occurs in newborns, after the umbilicus is colonized with *S. aureus*; culture or Gram stain will confirm diagnosis

Warts are nourished by a rich blood supply, and minor trauma may cause them to bleed. No treatment other than direct pressure is necessary if this occurs, but the patient should be reassured that this is not a sign that the wart has become malignant.

Molluscum contagiosum is a common cutaneous eruption caused by a pox virus. Although lesions generally present as flesh colored or pink umbilicated papules, they may look vesicular or pustular. They are usually multiple and may occur on any part of the skin. A useful diagnostic test to distinguish molluscum from true vesicular disorders consists of puncturing the center of a lesion with a small needle. If fluid is present, the lesion is a true vesicle. A white curd-like material, which can be expressed from lesions of molluscum contagiosum, may be examined for the presence of "molluscum bod-ies," large intracytoplasmic inclusions, which may be easily seen with a light microscope. Molloscum contagiosum is a self-limited disorder, but infection can persist for months to years and may spread to other individuals. Treatment with Cantharone, a blister-causing agent, liquid nitrogen, or curretage may require multiple visits and need not be initiated in the emergency room.

SUGGESTED READING

Hurwitz S. Clinical pediatric dermatology. Philadelphia: WB Saunders Company, 1981.

Tunnessen WW. Cutaneous infections. Pediatr Clin North Am 1983; 30:515–532.

Weston W, et al. Diaper dermatitis: current concepts. Pediatrics 1980; 66:532–536.

PEDIATRIC GASTROINTESTINAL PROBLEMS

DON K. NAKAYAMA, M.D.
HARRY C. BISHOP, M.D.

Evaluation and treatment of abdominal emergencies in infancy and childhood offer unique clinical challenges. Particularly in small infants, a series of blood tests may produce hypovolemia or anemia; the use of micromethods in the clinical laboratory can significantly reduce the volume of blood necessary for a test. Transport incubators or heating lamps protect infants from prolonged exposure to cold, particularly during radiologic tests.

Children with possible surgical conditions should be given nothing by mouth. Fluid should be administered at a rate calculated to meet maintenance requirements (4 ml per kilogram per hour for the first 10 kg; 2 ml per kilogram per hour for the second 10 kg; 1 ml per kilogram for each kilogram thereafter) and to correct pre-existing deficits. Since deficits are rarely more than 10 percent of body weight, an additional 2 to 4 ml per kilogram per hour usually suffice if depletion is present. The requirement for blood is estimated by the child's hemoglobin concentration. If needed, blood is generally administered in increments of 10 ml per kilogram, over 2 to 3 hours, but rapid transfusion of 20 ml per kilogram is tolerated if necessary. Prophylactic antibiotic therapy is usually used for infants who require major surgery. Ampicillin (100 to 200 mg per kilogram per day in four divided intravenous doses) and gentamicin (7.5 mg per kilogram per day in three divided intravenous doses) should be started before operation.

Narcotics are generally not used in infants under 6 months of age because the respiratory depressant effects of opiates and bartiturates are unpredictable and often pronounced.

Surgical conditions of infancy and childhood fall under broad categories based upon symptoms and age. Pediatric abdominal emergencies requiring surgical treatment are discussed as part of the differential diagnosis of the following presenting symptoms: vomiting, abdominal distention, abdominal pain, and gastrointestinal bleeding. Conditions that are primarily seen in the newborn period are not discussed here.

VOMITING

The etiology of vomiting, a very common symptom in childhood, includes most of the major disease categories in pediatrics (Table 1). A thorough search for extra-abdominal causes of vomiting should include examinations of the neck (nuchal rigidity may suggest meningitis), eyegrounds (for papilledema), ears (for otitis media),

TABLE 1 Nonsurgical Causes of Vomiting Beyond the Neonatal Period

Infection	Toxic
Gastroenteritis	Ingestions
Otitis	Medication
Meningitis	Radiation
Pneumonia	
Urinary tract infection	
Exanthematous diseases	
Metabolic	Gastroesophageal
Congenital adrenal hyperplasia	Reflux
Renal failure	Overfeeding
Hypoglycemia	
Diabetic ketoacidosis	
Adrenal insufficiency	
Hypothyroidism	
Central Nervous System	
Tumors	
Infection	

chest (for pneumonia), and flanks (for urinary tract infections). Laboratory studies reveal glucose abnormalities (diabetes), azotemia (renal failure), and leukocytosis (sepsis). Electrolyte concentrations not only guide fluid resuscitation of children with dehydration caused by vomiting, but may suggest its cause (e.g., adrenal insufficiency, adrenogenital syndrome, hypocalcemia, hypokalemia). Specific questions about possible ingestions or accidental poisoning, always a possibility in the young, are necessary parts of the history. An apparently trivial fall can cause significant trauma in infants and children, with vomiting resulting from pancreatitis, duodenal hematoma, or ileus from hemoperitoneum.

Surgical causes of vomiting are often more obvious to a surgeon, and early consultation may expedite the evaluation (Table 2). Bilious vomiting suggests intestinal obstruction and demands urgent attention, including further radiologic study. An abdominal mass may be present (intussusception, pyloric stenosis, periappendiceal abscess). An abdominal scar from a previous laparotomy makes the diagnosis of small bowel obstruction caused by postoperative adhesions more likely. The inguinal regions must be carefully examined for incarcerated hernia. Testicular torsion can cause reflex vomiting.

Left lateral decubitus views of the abdomen are the most sensitive for free air in the abdominal cavity, because they display the air against the liver's edge. Normal plain films of the abdomen show gas-filled bowel loops of uniform size and distribution. It usually is not possible to distinguish the colon from the small bowel in young children. Bowel loops that are markedly dilated are abnormal, as are those that have fluid levels.

Infants and young children with vomiting rapidly become dehydrated. Resuscitation with crystalloid (10 ml per kilogram over 20 minutes) may be necessary if dehydration is severe, followed by infusion of crystalloid at one and a half to two times the maintenance rate. Electrolytes are also lost in vomiting. Special attention must be paid to serum electrolyte concentrations, which may vary widely, depending on the level of obstruction (e.g., metabolic alkalosis in pyloric stenosis) and what the child was given to drink and was able to retain (causing hyponatremia or hypernatremia).

TABLE 2 Surgical Causes of Vomiting Beyond the Neonatal Period

Nonbilious, No Abdominal Distention

  Pyloric stenosis
  Gastroesophageal reflux

Bilious, No Abdominal Distention

  Malrotation
  Annular pancreas
  High small bowel obstruction from adhesions

Bilious, Abdominal Distention

  Malrotation with volvulus
  Internal hernia (mesenteric defect, omphalomesenteric
    duct remnants)
  Incarcerated inguinal hernia
  Low small bowel obstruction from adhesions
  Hirschsprung's disease

Passage of a nasogastric tube is necessary to decompress the stomach and prevent aspiration. Because the duodenum decompresses easily into the stomach, long intestinal tubes are seldom needed in pediatric patients.

ABDOMINAL DISTENTION

A distended abdomen is always abnormal and requires a diagnostic work-up. Generalized distention of bowel loops appearing on abdominal plain film can be caused by partial or complete bowel obstruction, gastroenteritis, chronic constipation, or Hirschsprung's disease. A prone, cross-table lateral view is useful to detect the presence of air in the rectosigmoid in infants.

Fluid-filled and solid *masses* often reach enormous size before the child is brought to medical attention. Leukemia, lymphoma, and portal hypertension are common causes of hepatic enlargement and splenomegaly in childhood. Retroperitoneal masses frequently arise from the kidney or adrenal gland. Roughly half are neoplasms (Wilms' tumor and neuroblastoma) and half are benign (hydronephrosis owing to ureteral or urethral obstruction, and multicystic kidney). Less than 10 percent of abdominal masses are intracoelomic in origin (hydrometrocolpos, enteric duplications, ovarian neoplasms or cysts). Infants under 3 months of age have masses that are predominantly benign renal anomalies. Neuroblastoma and Wilms' tumor become more frequent in later infancy, and malignant neoplasms account for more than half of abdominal masses in children older than 1 year.

Because of the possiblity of malignancy and obstructive uropathy, urgent evaluation of all children with abdominal masses is required. This may include laboratory evaluation of liver enzymes, bilirubin, alpha-fetoprotein, and human chorionogonadotropin levels. Urine studies include 24-hour collections for vanillylmandelic acid (VMA) and catecholamines when neuroblastoma is suspected. Chest films are routine, as are intravenous urograms and ultrasonographic examination of the liver, spleen, retroperitoneum, and pelvis. Bone marrow examination, bone scan, and computed tomographic (CT) scan may be indicated.

ABDOMINAL PAIN

Abdominal pain is also a common presenting symptom in childhood and has a varied etiology (Table 3). Pain is subjective, so in young children it is hard to evaluate unless it is severe. Young children just learning how to talk cannot describe their symptoms with accuracy and often are frightened and communicate poorly.

Certain conditions that occur outside the gastrointestinal tract should be specifically sought. Despite the presence of abdominal pain, suspicions of pneumonia, urinary tract infection, and meningitis can lead to the correct diagnosis. A recent skin rash or sore throat may suggest rheumatic fever. Purpuric skin rash and arthralgia suggest Henoch-Schönlein's purpura, but may follow the onset of abdominal pain. An abdominal sickle cell crisis is a possibility in black children. A high index of sus-

TABLE 3 Causes of Abdominal Pain Beyond the Neonatal Period

Infection	Gastrointestinal
Pneumonia	Appendicitis
Urinary tract infection	Intussusception
Gastroenteritis	Volvulus
Salmonella enteritis	Cholecystitis
Shigella enteritis	Meckel's diverticulitis
Amebiasis	Hemolytic-uremic syndrome
Meningitis	Perforation
	Obstruction
Toxins	Gynecologic
Bites (snake, insect)	Ovarian cyst or teratoma
Lead poisoning	Ectopic pregnancy
Food poisoning	Hematocolpos
Inflammatory	Urologic
Pancreatitis	Obstruction
Inflammatory bowel disease	Tumor
Peptic ulcer	Stones
Miscellaneous	Retroperitoneal tumors
Henoch-Schönlein's purpura	Very rate
Rheumatic fever	Trauma
Constipation	
Diabetic ketoacidosis	
Sickle cell crisis	
Porphyria	
Hemophilia	

picion under appropriate circumstances may help make the diagnosis of lead poisoning in a child from an impoverished home, of snake or insect bites, of hemophilia, or of diabetes with ketoacidosis. Pediatric solid tumors occasionally cause pain, either from invasion or from acute necrosis or hemorrhage within the tumor. Trauma is always a possibility in children.

Many causes of abdominal pain can be diagnosed, however, on the basis of the history and observations obtained from the parents. Take time to engage the child with gentle small talk without touching him. Parents' observations have particular diagnostic importance in infants and young children who cannot communicate. Is the child eating normally? Does he appear "sick", and is he avoiding activity? An infant may be so irritable that examination is difficult and, at times, unreliable. Mild sedation may allow adequate examination. Narcotics should be avoided until the diagnosis is established, and narcotics should not be given routinely to infants under 6 months of age because of the risk of respiratory depression.

Simple observations may suggest the presence of significant abdominal pathology. A youngster lying still, on his side, with his legs drawn up, is more likely to have significant peritoneal irritation than one who is playing in the examination room. The best way to localize tenderness is to begin with gentle palpation, then proceed with more vigorous maneuvers until abdominal pain is produced. Too vigorous a stimulus may make the entire abdomen hurt and prevent any further examination. Does changing position or coughing cause pain? Does gentle shaking of the examination table or of the patient's hips produce pain? Finally, the abdomen is gently palpated, starting at the point farthest from where pain was produced or where the child indicated the pain was located. Once the painful area is reached, a useful maneuver is to have the child hold the examiner's fingers as palpation is first light and then progressively deepened to assess rigidity. This allows the patient to protect himself and increases trust during examination. Never suddenly press down on the abdomen and release suddenly in a child with abdominal pain. This maneuver produces excruciating pain in a child with true peritonitis.

Once nonintestinal causes of abdominal pain are ruled out, the main clinical problem is distinguishing surgical conditions—for the most part, intussusception in the older infant to toddler age group, and appendicitis in children and adolescents—from gastroenteritis. In older girls, gynecologic problems must be considered. Early surgical consultation may avoid unnecessary delays in diagnosis and treatment. Children admitted to the hospital for the evaluation of abdominal pain should receive nothing by mouth. Those with vomiting should have nasogastric tube decompression. Again, vigorous intravenous fluid resuscitation is indicated for children who require an operation.

GASTROINTESTINAL BLEEDING

Gastrointestinal bleeding in a child is an alarming symptom; a calm assessment must include answers to basic questions that are frequently overlooked. First, is it really blood? Red dye from candy, soft drinks, or beets may give stool the appearance of blood. Second, is there a bleeding disorder? A consistent family history or unexplained bruising or bleeding may suggest an inherited disorder. Check for medication such as aspirin, steroids, or anticoagulants, or for recent disease (e.g., cancer chemotherapy). Coagulation studies (prothrombin time, partial thromboplastin time; and platelet count) should be obtained. Third, is bleeding from the gastrointestinal tract? Careful inspection of the nose, pharynx, and gums excludes swallowed blood as a cause. Blood in the diaper or toilet may also be from the urethra, vagina, or foreign bodies inserted into a perineal orifice by the child or caretaker.

Hematemesis usually indicates that the source of bleeding is proximal to the ligament of Treitz. If the child has not vomited and bleeding is suspected, a nasogastric tube is passed and the stomach is lavaged with saline; if the saline is bloody, an upper gastrointestinal source is confirmed. (The appearance of vomitus and stools suggests the rate of bleeding and its source.) Peptic ulcers and esophageal varices can produce massive hematemesis. Meckel's diverticulum, communicating duplications, and hemangiomas can bleed heavily from the rectum. Patients with bleeding from an upper gastrointestinal source usually pass tarry stools, but if the bleeding is active, bright red blood may pass from the rectum. Intussusception produces small amounts of blood mixed with mucus (i.e., "currant jelly"). Colonic polyps rarely bleed profusely, and rectal polyps and anal fissures streak normal stool with red blood.

Three major *age groups* categorize the etiology of gastrointestinal bleeding in infants and young children (Table 4): younger than 6 months, 6 months to 3 years, and older than 3 years. Older children and adolescents exhibit adult causes of bleeding, particularly from peptic ulcer, esophageal varices, and inflammatory bowel disease.

Initial management is based on how much blood the child has lost and the rate of ongoing losses. Children can maintain a nearly normal blood pressure with vasoconstriction in the face of severe blood loss, making it an insensitive measure of shock. More sensitive are the skin temperature (because shock results in cool extremities) and an elevated heart rate for age (an initial compensatory response to volume loss). Normal values for vital signs and hematologic values vary significantly with age (Table 5). A decreased urinary output of less than 1 ml per kilogram per hour or a urine specific gravity of greater than 1.020 suggests hypovolemia. Serial measurements of hemoglobin (Hgb) concentration provide an objective means of following the rate of bleeding, but 4 to 8 hours are required for equilibration of Hgb to a lower level. Orthostatic changes in vital signs occur late and indicate severe volume depletion. Admission to an intensive care area is mandatory for any child with significant bleeding.

PYLORIC STENOSIS

Hypertrophy of the muscle fibers of the distal antrum and pyloris results in pyloric stenosis. This condition predominantly affects male infants (4 to 1 sex ratio).

Symptoms from gastric outlet obstruction usually begin 2 to 3 weeks after birth, although less frequently within a week or as much as 4 months later. The infant regurgitates a few feedings at first, but over several days vomits more frequently. The vomitus contains undigested food and no bile. Blood from gastric irritation and stasis is present in 5 percent of cases. Vomiting is usually projectile, but frequently effortless regurgitation occurs, particularly in chronically starved, premature infants. Shortly after vomiting the infants act starved and will eat again. Weight loss results from starvation and dehydration, but if the diagnosis is made early, the infant may appear fat and healthy.

Between bouts of vomiting, a distended stomach may distend the epigastrium and left hypochondrium. Gastric peristalsis can often be seen moving from left to right. The enlarged pylorus can be palpated in the majority of cases, which makes x-ray studies and sonography unnecessary. Palpating the "olive" is best done with the examiner on the infant's left; the patient's lower extremities are gently lifted with the examiner's left hand to relax the abdomen. The right hand palpates the upper

TABLE 4 Causes of Gastrointestinal Bleeding in Children

Younger than 6 Months	*6 Months–3 Years*	*3 Years or Older*
Upper Tract		
Swallowed maternal blood (neonate)	Nasogastric tube irritation	Gastritis
Nasopharyngeal bleeding	Esophageal varices	Peptic ulcer
Peptic ulcer	Peptic ulcer	Medications
Necrotizing enterocolitis	Esophageal foreign body	Mallory-Weiss syndrome
Esophagitis due to reflux	Medications	
Hemorrhagic disease of newborn		
Lower Tract		
Anal fissure	Anal fissure	Anal fissure
Necrotizing enterocolitis	Meckel's diverticulum	Polyps
Midgut volvulus	Intussusception	Intussusception
Intussusception	Polyps	Hemolytic-uremic syndrome
Meckel's diverticulum	Infectious diarrhea	Inflammatory bowel disease
Hemangiomas	Henoch-Schönlein's purpura	Henoch-Schönlein's purpura
Duplications	Duplications	Trauma
Ingested maternal blood	Hemolytic-uremic syndrome	Duplication
	Hemangioma	Hemangioma

TABLE 5 Normal Vital Signs for Age

	Respirations	*Heart Rate*	*Blood Pressure*	*Urine Output**[*]*
1 yr	40/min	120	80/40	10 ml/hr
1 yr–5 yr	30/min	100	110/60	20 ml/hr
6 yr–12 yr	20/min	80	120/80	30 ml/hr

[*] Another criterion is 1 ml/kg/hr.

abdomen from above. The pyloric "olive" is firm, mobile, and about a fingertip in size. It is deep to the liver edge, generally in the epigastrium or to the right of the midline. Abdominal relaxation is often obtained by feeding the baby a small amount of sugar water; the examination should be repeated in a half-hour if it is initially negative. A distended stomach obscures the pylorus, so emptying of the stomach contents through a nasogastric tube is frequently necessary.

A *gastrointestinal series* is indicated only in the 10 percent of cases in which a pyloric tumor cannot be palpated. Ultrasonographic examination of the pylorus measures the width and length of the pyloric muscle. Barium swallow has an advantage over ultrasonography in that gastroesophageal reflux, antral web, and malrotation, important causes of vomiting in infancy, can be detected if pyloric stenosis is absent.

Preoperative treatment is directed toward correcting dehydration and hypokalemic, hypochloremic metabolic alkalosis. Nasogastric decompression is necessary to empty the stomach of feedings and barium if an upper gastrointestinal study was done. Surgery should be delayed until fluid and electrolyte deficits have been corrected. Pyloromyotomy is curative.

DUODENAL OBSTRUCTION CAUSED BY MALROTATION

Congenital duodenal obstruction caused by duodenal atresia and most cases of duodenal stenosis and annular pancreas are detected shortly after birth. Malrotation, a dangerous cause of upper gastrointestinal tract obstruction, may cause symptoms later in infancy. When normal intestinal rotation fails to occur in fetal life, normal fixation of the small bowel mesentery to the retroperitoneum is absent. Adhesive bands are usually present; commonly the cecum lies in an abnormal position high in the right upper quadrant, and adhesive bands between the cecum and the right posterior abdominal wall compress or obstruct the underlying duodenum. This predisposes to volvulus, with clockwise twisting of the bowel around the superior mesenteric vessels. Midgut ischemia and infarction may follow, making the diagnosis of malrotation an urgent priority in any child with bilious vomiting.

Abdominal distention may be absent if obstruction is produced by bands, and plain films may appear normal. Volvulus and gaseous distention of closed loops of twisted bowel cause massive abdominal distention. Bowel ischemia and infarction cause bloody stool and peritonitis, with a metabolic acidosis that resists correction by intravenous bicarbonate infusion.

Once this diagnosis is suspected, an immediate upper gastrointestinal series is indicated. The diagnostic goal is to verify the position of the ligament of Treitz to the left of the vertebral column in the upper abdomen. Any other position means that malrotation is present. Urgent laparotomy is indicated.

INTUSSUSCEPTION

Intussusception, the telescoping of a segment of bowel into the adjacent segment, is a common cause of intestinal obstruction in children under age 2 and creates a risk of ischemia and gangrene. Ileocolic intussusception is most common, but ileoileal, ileoileocolic, jejunojejunal, and colocolic intussusceptions do occur. A seasonal variation is noted, with cases clustering in midsummer and midwinter, apparently associated with adenovirus infections. In older children, structural lesions and anomalies such as inverted Meckel's diverticulum, polyps, intramural duplications, lymphoma, and intramural hematoma from Henoch-Schönlein's purpura account for an increasing number of cases.

The child with intussusception suddenly doubles up and cries, experiencing crampy, abdominal pain. The bouts last a minute or so and are separated by symptom-free intervals. Reflex vomiting may occur. As strangulation of the intussusceptum occurs, blood and mucus may be passed as a "currant-jelly" stool. Small infants may appear withdrawn and may not exhibit the characteristic colicky behavior. Vomiting is the most common symptom, with pallor and sweating occuring during colic. The intussusceptum is occasionally palpable on rectal examination and may even prolapse through the anus.

Plain *films* of the abdomen may show evidence of intestinal obstruction with dilated loop with fluid levels and a soft-tissue mass. The process may leave the right lower quadrant devoid of bowel gas on x-ray film, which may be noticeable on physical examination. A barium enema establishes the diagnosis.

Intravenous access and fluid resuscitation are the initial priorities. Contrast enema reduction with a surgeon present is successful in more than 50 percent of cases. The radiologic maneuvers require experienced judgment to recognize failure and to avoid perforation of the intussuscipiens. Prompt laparotomy is indicated if enema reduction has failed.

MECKEL'S DIVERTICULUM

Meckel's diverticulum, the most common form of omphalomesenteric duct remnant anomalies, is found in about 2 percent of the population. Located in the ileum, it may contain small bowel, colonic, or gastric mucosa and aberrant pancreatic tissue. It usually produces no symptoms, and the patient is unaware of its presence. When symptoms occur, there may be gastrointestinal bleeding in 40 percent of cases, a lead point for intussusception in 20 percent and, very rarely, perforation of the diverticulum in 15 percent.

Rectal bleeding caused by a Meckel's diverticulum results from peptic ulceration of the small bowel mucosa adjacent to the ectopic gastric mucosa. Most patients are 2 years or less. Bleeding is usually brisk, resulting in bright red rectal bleeding. Young patients may exsanguinate. Melena and occult bleeding are unusual. Forty percent of patients have a history of a previous episode of bleeding.

Contrast studies seldom diagnose a Meckel's diverticulum. Technetium-99m pertechnetate localizes gastric mucosa and may identify a Meckel's diverticulum with heterotopic mucosa as the source of gastrointestinal blood loss. After restoration of blood volume, treatment of symptomatic Meckel's diverticulum is resection.

HIRSCHSPRUNG'S DISEASE

Hirschsprung's disease, an absence of cephalocaudal growth of myenteric nerve cells into the rectum, lower colon, and rarely the entire colon or entire colon and the small bowel, produces a functional lower gastrointestinal bowel obstruction. Symptoms almost always occur shortly after birth. The newborn produces little or no meconium within 24 hours of birth, abdominal distention occurs, and surgery is necessary.

However, some cases are not diagnosed until later in infancy or childhood. The infant may have chronic constipation, with infrequent passage of large amounts of flatus with stool and occasionally foul-smelling diarrhea. Progressive abdominal distention, vomiting, poor feeding, listlessness, irritability, and poor growth may occur. Foul-smelling diarrhea and abdominal distention in infancy should be considered signs of Hirschsprung's disease until proved otherwise. Older children exhibit chronic constipation and abdominal distention.

Certain features distinguish Hirschsprung's disease from chronic functional constipation. In Hirschsprung's disease symptoms begin in early infancy, stools are small in caliber, and encopresis occurs rarely. The rectum is small and empty in children with Hirschsprung's disease, and impacted feces are often palpable higher in the abdomen. Children with functional constipation usually have symptoms beginning later in childhood, around the time of toilet training. The stools are normal in caliber, and fecal soiling is frequent because of stretching of the anus. The rectal ampulla is full of stool, within reach of the examining finger, and there may be liquid stool around the large rectal bolus of stool.

Barium enema supports the diagnosis of Hirschsprung's disease. Do not give a cleansing enema or attempt to disimpact the child, since these maneuvers decompress the dilated colon and obscure diagnostic roentgenologic signs. Follow-up films 24 to 48 hours after study show retained barium. Definitive diagnosis may require biopsy.

Fever, toxicity, abdominal distention, and foul-smelling diarrhea indicate enterocolitis, a rapidly lethal complication of untreated Hirschsprung's disease. Immediate volume resuscitation is indicated, and broad-spectrum antibiotics are administered (ampicillin, 200 mg per kilogram per day in four divided doses, and gentamicin, 7.5 mg per kilogram in three divided doses). Saline irrigation through a large rectal tube may relieve enterocolitis temporarily, but frequently a colostomy must be performed as an urgent procedure.

INGUINAL HERNIA

Persistence of the patent processus vaginalis after birth is the explanation for congenital indirect inguinal hernias in infants and children. This condition is particularly common in premature infants, and these hernias are the most common congenital anomaly. Occasionally fluid is entrapped in the tunica vaginalis and is found at the time of birth. This is a physiologic hydrocele and will absorb during the first month of life. However, there can be an opening of the processus vaginalis with a localized narrowing just at the top of the tunica vaginalis and accumulation of hydrocele fluid distally. This represents a communicating hydrocele that needs surgical repair because of its hernial component. Occasionally a hydrocele forms along the spermatic cord; this can occur only if there is an opening back to the abdominal cavity, where there is a fluid reservoir. If this hydrocele occurs high along the spermatic cord, it may be difficult to differentiate from an incarcerated inguinal hernia, and occasionally infants need to be operated on immediately to rule out the possibility of an incarcerated hernia.

A straightforward empty hernial sac usually bulges intermittently with small bowel loops that enter it. This becomes tense during increased intra-abdominal pressure from crying, but most of the time the bowel spontaneously reduces. These hernias are operated on soon after they are discovered to avoid the complication of incarceration with the potential for strangulation and gangrene of the entrapped bowel.

If the infant or child has an incarcerated hernia, an effort is made to reduce this by placing him in a head-down position and applying an ice bag to the area. Manual reduction should be attempted if this is unsuccessful. This is best done by compressing the internal ring area and then gradually pushing from the bottom up, so that the bowel loop will slip back into the intra-abdominal cavity. If an incarcerated hernia cannot be reduced, emergency surgery is necessary. After reduction of an incarcerated hernia, we admit the child to the hospital for observation. Clear liquids are given, and the edema of the sac is allowed to subside for 24 to 48 hours before elective repair is done.

SUGGESTED READING

Raffensberger JG. Swenson's pediatric surgery. 4th ed. New York: Appleton-Century-Crofts, 1980.

Sheldon CA, Martin LW. Pediatric surgery. Surg Clin North Am, 1985; 65:1059–1687.

Welch KJ, Randolph JG, Ravitch MM, O'Neill JA Jr, Rowe MI. Pediatric surgery. 4th ed. Chicago: Year Book Medical Publishers, 1986.

THE PEDIATRIC TRAUMA PATIENT

PAUL M. COLOMBANI, M.D.
J. ALEX HALLER Jr., M.D.

In the pediatric population under age 15, injuries constitute more than 50 percent of deaths, numbering approximately 30,000 per year. Beyond the neonatal period, deaths from injuries in children outnumber the combined total from congenital malformations, cancer, and infectious disease. More than a million children are hospitalized for injuries each year with significant morbidity. While injury control and prevention may appear to be the best method to lower these statistics, a systematic approach to the expeditious transport, evaluation, and treatment of an injured child must be implemented to prevent significant mortality and morbidity following injury. These measures must be implemented most often in the field and in community hospital emergency departments. As a result, the most critical period of initial resuscitation and evaluation of the majority of these patients is the responsibility of field care providers, emergency physicians, and pediatricians.

PATTERNS OF INJURY

Knowledge of the common mechanisms of injury and of patterns of injury in pediatric trauma is essential. In a recent series of our pediatric trauma patients constituting a mixed urban, suburban, and rural population, the majority of injured children were boys (75 percent) with blunt injuries (more than 90 percent). Motor vehicle accidents were the most common mechanism of injury (54 percent), with 75 percent of these injuries being pedestrian motor vehicle accidents. Falls were the second most common injury, and 15 percent of these were bicycle injuries. Other miscellaneous injuries included sports injuries, farming injuries, and assaults. The preponderance of motor vehicle accidents and falls contributes to the high incidence of blunt multisystem injuries seen in children. The most common single organ system involved is the craniocervical, usually associated with skeletal and ab-

dominal injuries. In our own series, the presence of head injury was the most important factor in determining morbidity and mortality. Injuries that are out of proportion to the purported mechanism of injury as well as evidence of old injuries or a history of previous injuries should alert the emergency physician to possible child abuse.

PRE-HOSPITAL CARE

As with any injured patient, the goals of pre-hospital care of the injured pediatric patient should be to ensure an adequate airway and ventilation, treat shock, and prevent further deterioration or injury in an efficient and rapid fashion. Bag and mask ventilation with humidified oxygen may be required. Endotracheal intubation may be necessary and can be utilized if personnel are adequately trained. Needle cricothyroidotomy is rarely indicated. A frequent problem encountered in the pediatric patient is gastric distention with the potential for vomiting and aspiration. A nasogastric tube should be placed in any patient requiring ventilatory assistance and transport. Remember that cervical spine injury cannot be excluded by physical examination, and in-line cervical immobilization is required when manipulating the airway.

Shock treatment should include direct control of bleeding, placement of military anti-shock trousers (MAST), and insertion of a large-bore intravenous line for administration of lactated Ringer's solution. MAST trousers should be inflated in patients with systolic blood pressures less than or equal to 60 mm Hg or with signs of shock. They are also useful in field management of pelvic fractures, abdominal or retroperitoneal bleeding, lower extremity soft tissue bleeding, and fractures. Fluid administration should be determined by evidence of shock and calculated on patient weight (estimated blood volume). Normal blood pressure in children is 80 plus twice the age in years (mm Hg), and normal blood volume is 80 ml per kilogram. Patients should receive 20 ml per kilogram of lactated Ringer's solution if there is evidence of shock but normal blood pressure. Patients with hypotension should receive a rapid infusion of 40 ml per kilogram of lactated Ringer's. To prevent further deterioration, a number of principles should be observed: prevent hypothermia; frequently assess neurologic status; maintain oxygenation; check ventilation and perfusion pressure; maintain cervical spine immobilization with in-line traction, backboards, and rigid cervical collar; and splint potential extremity fractures. Prompt transport should be made to the appropriate trauma facility. The patient should be monitored during transport, and personnel should have direct access to the patient so that they can assess his or her condition and continue resuscitation.

EMERGENCY DEPARTMENT CARE

Initial assessment of the pediatric trauma patient in the emergency department follows the general guidelines for any trauma patient. The physicians evaluating the patient must have an organized approach. Resuscitative efforts to stabilize the patient must be implemented to prevent immediate life-threatening problems while a complete physical examination, history, x-ray films, and laboratory examinations are completed.

A primary survey must be performed to ensure an adequate airway, ventilation, and circulation as well as to assess the patient's neurologic status. The child's clothing must be completely removed to facilitate a complete physical examination. Hypothermia, however, should be avoided by external warming. Electrocardiogram monitoring leads should be applied.

The airway is secured by chin lift or jaw thrust. If an adequate airway cannot be secured in this way, then oral endotracheal intubation should be performed. In-line cervical traction should be used to prevent cervical spine injury during intubation. The pediatric larynx is more anterior and superficial than in adult patients. Endotracheal tube size may be estimated by using the formula:

$$\frac{16 + \text{age in years}}{4} = \text{ETT I.D.}$$

Patients should always have bag and mask ventilation with 100 percent oxygen prior to intubation. Muscle relaxants may be required to ensure atraumatic intubation.

Following intubation, ventilation should be assessed. Inability to ventilate the patient after the airway is secured may indicate tension pneumothorax, massive hemothorax, or flail chest. Measures to alleviate these problems should be instituted immediately.

Circulation should next be assessed by gauging the quality, rate, and regularity of the pulse, peripheral perfusion (capillary refill), and blood pressure. Blood pressure is an unreliable guide for judging blood volume status in the pediatric age group because extensive vasoconstriction may keep the blood pressure in a low normal range in spite of major blood loss. Staff should also be familiar with blood pressure norms for the pediatric age groups. A rule of thumb for blood pressure is 80 plus twice the patient's age in years (mm Hg); for maximal normal pulse rate, 140 beats per minute for infants, 120 for toddlers, and 100 for school-age children. Shock, defined as an inadequate circulating blood volume, most commonly occurs secondary to external or internal blood losses (thoracic, abdominal, or retroperitoneal) in the pediatric population. Occasionally, tension pneumothorax or cardi-

ac tamponade may be the cause of the shock state. Rarely, a patient with cervical cord transection presents with signs and symptoms of shock secondary to profound vasomotor collapse.

Vascular access should be obtained during this initial period. Two large-bore intravenous catheters should be placed. If no vein is readily accessible, a saphenous vein cutdown should be made at the ankle. Blood for laboratory studies and cross-matching should be drawn at this time. The emergency department is *not* the setting for percutaneous subclavian access in the pediatric patient.

Initial fluid resuscitation should begin with lactated Ringer's solution at a rate dependent on estimated blood loss as determined by circulatory assessment. Patients with mild blood losses (less than 15 percent) as evidenced by a slight increase in pulse, normal blood pressure, and a mild decrease in capillary refill, should receive a 20 ml per kilogram fluid bolus. Moderate blood losses (20 to 30 percent) evidenced by tachycardia, tachypnea, decreased blood pressure, and poor capillary refill should be treated initially with a 40 ml per kilogram bolus of lactated Ringer's solution. Patients with evidence of severe blood loss (more than 35 percent) should be managed with lactated Ringer's and packed red blood cells initially. At any level, patients who do not improve after initial fluid replacement challenges should be considered to be at the next higher level of blood loss, i.e., patients with mild losses with no improvement should receive an additional 20 ml per kilogram fluid bolus and patients with moderate losses with no improvement should receive packed red blood cells. In general, one-half of major blood losses should be replaced with packed red blood cells, and the remainder is replaced with lactated Ringer's according to the 3:1 rule (3 ml lactated Ringer's solution for each 1 ml of blood loss).

The MAST trousers should be inflated for any child presenting with a blood pressure less than two-thirds of normal systolic and evidence of decreased circulatory blood volume (shock). MAST trousers should be left inflated until the patient is stabilized, then gradually deflated (abdominal compartment deflated first), and the patient's status should be checked frequently for deterioration prior to deflating the extremity compartments.

A mini-neurologic examination should be performed during this initial phase. The Glascow coma scale for the patient should be recorded, scoring eye opening, best verbal, and best motor responses. For children under age 2, responsive crying indicates a full verbal response. Pupillary reactions and spontaneous movements should also be noted.

Following this primary survey and initiation of resuscitative efforts, a complete head-to-toe secondary survey should be performed to assess the patient for additional injuries that are not immediately life-threatening, as well as for concurrent or preexisting medical conditions. Up to 15 percent of pediatric trauma patients have concurrent infections (otitis media, asymptomatic urinary tract infection) or a chronic medical condition (seizure disorder, asthma, congenital heart disease) that may not have been previously diagnosed or is under current treatment.

All patients should receive a lateral cervical spine, supine chest, and supine abdominal x-ray study, including the pelvis. Additional x-ray films of the cervical spine, chest (upright), and abdomen (lateral decubitus) can be performed when indicated. Other x-ray examinations (skull, extremities) are also ordered when indicated. Urinalysis, including microscopic examination, should be performed on all patients. Severely injured children should have a urinary drainage catheter placed. Nasogastric or orogastric tubes should be placed in pediatric patients (especially patients with altered levels of consciousness) to prevent vomiting, or aspiration, or both because of the high frequency of gastric distention and reflex ileus.

Significant head injury is present in up to 75 percent of pediatric patients. Skull fractures are less common. Increased intracranial pressure in most patients is secondary to cerebral edema and not to space-occupying hematomata. Maxillofacial injuries are uncommon in children (approximately 10 percent). Knowledge of the normal development of aeration of the nasal sinuses is useful in this evaluation. Cervical spine fractures are uncommon (5 percent). The most common "abnormality" seen on cervical spine x-ray study is the subluxation of C2 on C3, which is a normal variant if less than 5 mm. Thoracic injuries constitute approximately 15 percent of childhood injuries. Rib fractures are less common, but pulmonary contusion is more likely present in the absence of overt chest wall injury. Injuries to the thoracic aorta are also uncommon because of the mode of injury (pedestrian) and a relatively mobile mediastinum in this patient group. Occult abdominal injuries are common in the pediatric patient with blunt injury. The most common injuries are to the spleen, liver, and kidneys. Pancreaticoduodenal and intestinal injuries are less common. The most common cause of abdominal pain and tenderness, however, is acute gastric dilatation, and effective treatment is insertion of a nasogastric tube.

In addition to plain abdominal x-ray films, a number of auxillary diagnostic tests can be utilized to assess for abdominal injury. Abdominal computed tomography and liver and spleen radionuclide scans can be used to diagnose intra-abdominal injuries. The majority (up to 90 percent) of injuries to the liver and spleen can be managed nonoperatively. This approach is best utilized in trauma referral centers, where there is intensive monitoring and 24-hour availability of surgical personnel. Peritoneal lavage and operative exploration for positive intra-abdominal bleeding are the best approaches in a community hospital setting. Genitourinary injuries evidenced by hematuria or abnormalities noted on examination of the rectum and external genitalia should be evaluated by intravenous pyelogram combined with retrograde urethrocystography when indicated. Extremity fractures are common (30 percent), but may not be immediately obvious in the emergency department, especially greenstick fractures.

After the secondary survey, a detailed history can be obtained from the family to include past illness, allergies, current illness, or medications. The paramedics at the scene are also a good resource for obtaining details of the time and mechanism of injury. A list of the patient's injuries should be made, and priorities of management outlined. Once the airway, ventilation, and circulating blood volume are ensured, head injury and cervical spine injury are the next priorities. Adequate oxygenation and hyperventilation to lower arterial PCO_2 and fluid restriction are basic ingredients of head trauma management. Steroids and osmotic diuretics should be administered only after consultation with the neurosurgical team. The cervical spine must be stabilized early. Abdominal and thoracic injuries take the next priority. Extremity, facial, and soft-tissue injuries take last priorities in management.

Remember that the levels of anxiety and fear are very high for both the children and their families. The treating physician should approach the patient in a calm and reassuring manner. The child, if alert, should be informed of what procedures are to be performed before they occur, such as intravenous access, blood drawing, or x-ray studies. The patient's family must also be handled in a calm, direct, and sensitive manner.

DISPOSITION

Patients with potentially significant head, chest, or abdominal injuries that may not be apparent in the emergency department should be admitted for observation. Patients suspected of being victims of child abuse or patients whose family dynamics may preclude adequate follow-up visits or prompt return for problems should also be admitted. Patients with serious injuries should be transferred to a major trauma center, preferably a pediatric one. Patients with the following spectrum of injuries should be transferred: complicated head injury, serious injury to more than one organ system, shock, complicated or multiple extremity fractures, suspected spinal cord injuries or axial skeletal fractures, and patients requiring ventilatory support. Any patient whom the treating physician thinks would benefit from transport to a children's trauma center should be stabilized as much as is practical and then sent urgently to that center.

SUGGESTED READING

Colombani PM, Buck JR, Dudgeon DL, et al. One year experience in a regional pediatric trauma center. J Pediatr Surg 1985; 20:8–13.
Haller JA, Buck JR. Trauma in the child: regional pediatric centers for life-threatening injuries. Prog Crit Care Med 1984; 1:208–217.
Mayer TA, ed. Emergency management of pediatric trauma. Philadelphia: W.B. Saunders, 1985.

ORTHOPAEDIC INJURY IN CHILDREN

ALVIN H. CRAWFORD, M.D., F.A.C.S.

GROWTH PLATE INJURY

Our major concerns in a child have to do with the basic differences between children and adults, namely, growth plates. Trauma in the child more frequently injures the growth plate rather than a ligament or the metaphysis of a long bone. Therefore, when an injury occurs, one has to determine whether the child has fractured a bone, torn a ligament, or injured the growth plate. The ramifications of growth plate injuries are significant because, depending upon the type of injury, the limb may show continued normal growth, shortening or delay followed by normal growth, or an angular deformity caused by the formation of a bony bridge connecting the metaphysis to the epiphysis on one side. It is therefore important that the examiner be familiar with the types of growth plate injuries.

Several types of growth plate injuries have been described based on their radiographic interpretations, but the more commonly used classification is that of Salter and Harris (Fig. 1). The type I injury occurs through the line dividing the growth cartilage and the proximal portion of the metaphysis of a long bone. This is usually a benign injury; rarely is there displacement and they tend to heal with minimal, if any, residual deformity. The type II injury occurs through the growth plate, but extends into the metaphysis usually carrying a small bone fragment or chip called a "Thurston-Holland" sign. This injury in young children has a benign prognosis and tends to heal well. The fracture is easily reducible, because the periosteal sleeve on the side of the metaphyseal fragment remains intact and overcorrection cannot usually be performed. Except for the open Salter II injury of the distal radius and the distal femur in the adolescent, the majority of these injuries respond well with no residual. Shortening of the distal radius may result from this injury when associated with either compounding or significant soft tissue damage. The femoral Salter II injury, especially when associated with high intensity trauma such as a clipping injury from American football, has about a 33 percent incidence of either growth discrepancy or angular problems following the injury. The Salter III fracture is one that occurs through the bony epiphysis, transgresses the epiphyseal line, and exits through the periosteum. It usually occurs in and about the distal lateral tibia where is is called the juvenile fracture of Tilleaux; it occasionally occurs through the distal femoral epiphysis. This is an intra-articular injury in which an anatomic reduction is mandatory. The type IV injury occurs through the bony epiphysis and the epiphyseal plate and exits through the metaphysis. This injury occurs most frequently in the area of the lateral condyle of the humerus. It is both an intra-articular and metaphyseal injury as a result requires an anatomic reduction to prevent nonunion, delayed union, or angular deformities associated with malreduction. The injury also occurs at the distal medial tibia or ankle joint and is associated with a high incidence of angular deformity and partial growth arrest. For those reasons, anatomic reduction of this injury to within 2 mm of its normal alignment is mandatory. The type V Salter injury occurs through the growth plate itself with no metaphyseal involvement. The injury usually crushes the germinal cell layer of the growth plate itself, thus destroying the most active area of growth. It cannot be distinguished radiographically from a type I injury. The resultant deformity might be significant shortening, a delay in growth followed by normal growth, or an angular deformity.

INJURY NEEDING IMMEDIATE TREATMENT

When an injured child is first seen, it may not be appreciated whether he has a sprain, strain, or fracture. Certain orthopaedic injuries require immediate definitive care, and orthopaedic consultation as soon as possible.

1. *Open fractures* should be handled directly by an orthopaedic surgeon. They may temporarily be managed with warm saline dressings over extruded bone. Culture and sensitivity tests should be performed as soon as possible and tetanus prophylaxis carried out if immunization is not current.

2. *Traumatic dislocations* occur in children most frequently at the elbow, hip, and ankle. The hip in a child may be dislocated with no evidence of fracture (although occasionally there are osteocartilaginous or cartilaginous fractures that cannot be appreciated on plain x-ray films). Because of the high incidence of avascular necrosis associated with traumatic dislocations of the hip, efforts should be made to reduce the dislocation as soon as possible. An anteroposterior x-ray view of the pelvis is mandatory prior to performing a reduction. The hip is most commonly dislocated posteriorly. The limb is flexed and adducted at the hip. One method of reduction is sustained traction. The patient is given a muscle relaxant, after which longitudinal traction is applied to the femur with the knee flexed. An assistant applies countertraction and direct pressure over the greater trochanter. Once reduction has been accomplished, the hip should be placed through a range of motion to determine stability and rule out the presence of intra-articular osteochondral fragments. Careful assessment of the sciatic nerve is carried out immediately. Traumatic dislocations of the ankle do occur, but usually with accompanying fractures and tend to reduce fairly easily, although, again, osteocartilaginous fractures may involve the joint.

Traumatic dislocations about the elbow secondary to falling on the outstretched hand do not involve the associated problems of avascular necrosis of the humerus, although they are associated with a high incidence of fracture of the medial epicondyle. X-ray views should be taken after reduction, but before cast application, to determine

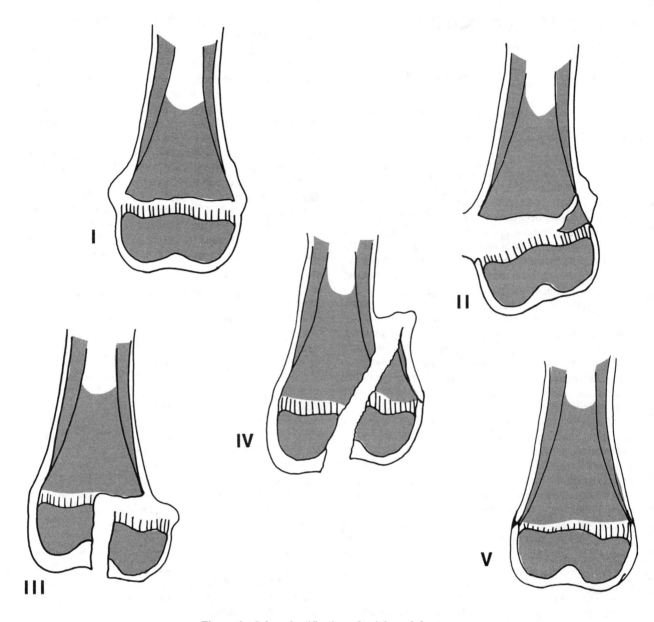

Figure 1 Salter classification of epiphyseal fractures.

whether there are bone fragments (usually the medial epicondyle) entrapped in the elbow joint. It may be necessary to obtain an x-ray view of the opposite elbow if there is uncertainty. A careful evaluation of the ulnar nerve is then carried out. Because of the possibility of ulnar nerve entrapment, local anesthesia is discouraged.

Dislocations of the shoulder are rare in young children, but in older adolescents they do occur frequently. The dislocation is most often anterior and is usually associated with abduction and external rotation of the arm. Unfortunately, even when treated quite well initially, the result may be a chronic recurrent dislocation.

Traumatic dislocation of the knee is extremely rare in children. Fracture through the distal femoral or proximal tibial epiphysis is more common. X-ray views are necessary to confirm the diagnosis. For a knee dislocation to occur, most of the ligaments have to be torn, with

significant trauma to the neurovascular structures. The emergency treatment should be directed toward obtaining full extension of the joint and monitoring distal pulses.

3. *A pulseless extremity* is a cause for grave concern. This may represent a laceration of an artery due to a fracture or a contusion, or secondary spasm of an artery due to blunt trauma. Immediate steps should be taken toward re-establishing either the pulse or perfusion of the extremity: Volkmann's ischemia or a compartment syndrome can occur within hours, resulting in devastating muscle destruction. This requires direct surgical release or repair of the vessel.

4. *Injuries to the pelvis and spine* are somewhat uncommon in children. With a pelvic fracture one is concerned with the possibility of urethral damage as well as neurologic damage. Injuries to the spine are also uncommon in children. Several common associations have to

be remembered, such as after a fall from a height. Even though there might be a fractured calcaneus, one has to also investigate even minor back pain lest one misses a lumbar spine flexion-compression fracture. Because of the lack of ossification of the epiphyseal rings of the vertebrae in children, one might miss a fracture of the epiphysis with displacement which, even though it does not show up on x-ray examination, can cause significant neurologic damage. The combination of computed tomography (CT) scan and CT myelography has allowed this diagnosis to be made much earlier.

For the spine fracture, a careful neurologic examination, including an anal wink test for spinal cord continuity, should be performed, as well as the insertion of a nasogastric tube because of the possibility of paralyticileus. A nasogastric tube should also be passed in case of pelvic fracture, as well as a urethral catheter to determine whether the urethra is intact and to assess the possibility of urinary tract injury.

5. *Child abuse* should be considered whenever the child presents with injuries encountered unless less than normal circumstances of trauma. All too often the child who presents with a femoral shaft fracture after "falling off the studio couch" or "slipping out of the babysitter's lap" is subject for investigation of child battering. When one appreciates the magnitude of a femoral shaft fracture in a small child, the resulting trauma should in accord with the history. A recent review of hospital incident reports of children falling from the height of a hospital bed revealed that less than 1 percent sustained a fracture of a long bone, with less than 1 percent being injuries to the femur.

Management of orthopaedic injuries are secondary to management of life threatening problems. The ABC investigations (airway, breathing, and circulatory status) are to be undertaken first, even though the fractured shaft of a bone emerging from the skin might draw more attention. Life saving procedures such as establishing an airway and the control of hemorrhage are more important than attention to the damaged extremity.

RADIOLOGIC EXAMINATION

The unconscious and preverbal child is not able to give a history and may present only with a limb deformity. If there is swelling or pain in the area of deformity, an x-ray examination should be carried out prior to attempting to evaluate further. Place a splint on the extremity and send the child to the x-ray department.

The initial radiographic assessment of patients with orthopaedic injuries should include anteroposterior and lateral views of the extremity and comparison with the normal limb when there is doubt regarding the diagnosis. The presence of the emerging secondary centers of ossification (bony epiphysis)—around the elbow especially—creates much confusion.

Except for frank dislocation, one should exercise care in correcting the position of an extremity prior to obtaining x-ray views because of the possibility of aggravating a pre-existing condition.

Bone Abnormality. This is sometimes seen after trauma. This does not mean that trauma caused the condition, but that an intrinsic problem of the bone causes it to be weaker so that pathologic fracture occurs.

Bone cyst. The most frequent bone cyst is the simple or unicameral cyst. It looks like a clear hole in the bone as opposed to fibrous dysplasia, which has a ground glass appearance. The unicameral bone cyst is seen most commonly in the proximal humerus. There may be multiple small loculations and a ballooning expansive contour of the bone. (If so, aneurysmal bone cyst would have to be ruled out.) The unicameral bone cyst causes pain secondary to a pathologic fracture. The treatment initially is application of a sling and rest of the extremity. The definitive treatment is saline irrigation and injection of steroids.

Osteomyelitis. This condition most frequently mimics a tumor. If there is a history of acute fever and swelling, (tumor, rubor, dolor, calor), the diagnosis is simple. It is chronic osteomyelitis with persistent swelling and sclerotic bone changes (increased density) that is difficult for the emergency physician. A sedimentation rate should be obtained whenever extremity pain presents with such x-ray view changes.

Rickets. This condition presents as swelling of the joint region (metaphyses) and pain. The x-ray views are diagnostic. The emergency physician needs to be aware that conditions other than classic nutritional deficiencies may cause the problems, e.g., selective nondairy diets, commune dwellers, and religious sects. Patients taking anticonvulsant medications may also present with rickets. The emergency treatment consists of immobilization. The child with renal rickets invariably has a prolonged history of illness or progressive dehabilitation. A retrospective history can be obtained once the x-ray films are reviewed.

Fatigue Fractures. This is somewhat rare in children. The young child under 5 years old may present with a limp of 2 to 3 weeks duration. Early x-ray views are most frequently normal. X-ray views taken after 2 to 3 weeks most often show increased density in the distal third of the fibula. A bone scan in these children allows the diagnosis to be confirmed much earlier, but should not be overused. Adolescents present with pain in the proximal tibia, usually in the child who has not been athletic, but decides to become a long distance runner or sprinter. The x-ray changes have frequently been interpreted as being indicative of osteogenic sarcoma. Even though the x-ray picture is characteristic, if not diagnostic, a bone scan, CT scan, or MRI should be performed prior to considering a biopsy.

Osteogenesis Imperfecta. This is an intrinsic bone deformity (fragilitas ossium, brittle bones) that causes the bones to fracture with less than usual trauma. The vera form usually has a history presenting from birth; however, the tarda form may present as multiple sprains or fractures. The x-ray views of the vera form are diagnostic (thin, gracile bone, remodeling of previous fractures). The tarda form may present more difficulty with the first injury.

Tumor. Tumors such as osteogenic sarcoma and Ewing's sarcoma are rare. The osteogenic sarcomas occur at the areas of most rapid growth, i.e., distal femur, proximal tibia, and proximal humerus. X-ray views may show blastic, lytic, or mixed configuration. These patients require comprehensive work-up, staging, and biopsy prior to selection of a treatment. Ewing's sarcoma tends to occur in the flat bones (pelvis) and long bone diaphyses. It tends to mimic an infection. Staging and biopsy are important. The tumor most frequently encountered in children is the benign osteochondroma. This lesion is seen most frequently at the knee and is pedunculated. Multiple exostosis usually carries a family history and involves multiple lesions. They are usually benign; however, those appearing in the axial skeleton are at greatest risk of malignant degeneration.

GENERAL PRINCIPLES

1. Remove all clothing surrounding the fracture or dislocation.
2. Cover all wounds with sterile dressings before splint applications.
3. Avoid pushing bone fragments back beneath the skin in compount (open) fractures when the bone extrudes through the skin.
4. Pad the splint to prevent excessive pressure.
5. In a fracture-dislocation use the splint to immobilize the joint above and below the site of injury.
6. Straighten severely angulated fractures with general traction so that the limb can be incorporated into a splint. Pay careful attention to the pulse with any change in position; if the pulse is lost when the patient assumes the new position, revert to the previous position.
7. Dislocation or obvious fracture with deformity near a joint can be a serious injury because of possible damage to adjacent nerves and blood vessels. In general, the deformity may be straightened with steady, general traction, if the maneuver does not significantly increase pain for the patient and if no resistance to correction is encountered.

COMMON ERRORS

One of the more common erroneous diagnoses in children is that of a sprain or strain, especially about the ankle. More often than not, this represents a lateral malleolar fracture of the distal fibular epiphysis.

The treatment of sprains should initially be ICE (*ice, compression, and elevation*). Elevation and ice application should be initiated as soon after the injury as possible. The definitive management of an injury is usually carried out in the hospital.

Not enough can be said about the need for attention to the neurovascular status of the extremity distal to a fracture or dislocation. The four ''Ps'' (*p*ulselessness, *p*ain, *p*allor, and *p*aralysis) denote loss of vascular integrity and should be thoroughly investigated.

TYPES OF INJURY

Forearm Fractures

Forearm fractures constitute the most common fracture in children. They most frequently occur at the wrist and account for 15 to 20 percent of the total number of fractures in children. They usually result from a F.O.O.S.H., or fall-on-the-outstretched-hand. When a fracture is noted in the forearm, an x-ray view of the entire extremity should be obtained to preclude the possibility of an unrecognized injury at either one of the ends, such as a dislocation of the wrist or elbow. The fracture should be casted or splinted into the neutral position with careful attention paid to pulse and circulation. If there is significant swelling, elevation, and compression, application of ice should be carried out early. Most angular deformities resolve in the child under 10 years of age. The major residual deformity following reduction of a forearm injury tends to be a slight loss of rotation. An anatomic reduction is not usually required in a child under 10 years of age. One can accept approximately 30 to 35 degrees of angulation and expect complete remodeling if the child is less than 10 years of age, but only 15 to 20 degrees of angulation if the child is older than 10 years of age.

Once an adequate reduction has been accomplished in a forearm fracture, the child should usually be comfortable, if not pain free, within 3 to 4 hours. If there is continued irritability and discomfort, the possibility of a compartment syndrome should be recognized. Clinically, the compartment syndrome can be evaluated by passive stretching of the deep finger flexors. The test is performed by placing the metacarpophalangeal joints in full extension and passively extending the fingers. If passive finger extension causes disproportionate pain in the volar forearm or deep flexor compartments, the test is positive for ischemia. One can also use a commercial wick device to measure forearm compartment pressure if the pain is continuous and there is no capillary refill to circulation distally.

Last, but not least, one has to make the parent aware of the possibility of a growth discrepancy whenever an epiphyseal injury occurs, regardless of how mild the x-ray characteristic appears to be. Remember that it is impossible to distinguish a type I (benign) injury to the growth plate from a type V (severe) injury by x-ray characteristics alone. If the parents are aware of the possibility of the complication of growth arrest, which occurs at the time of injury and has nothing to do with the treatment and follow-up, the management of the injury becomes much easier.

Elbow Injury

Injury around the elbow in children is the second most common injury of the upper extremities. A problem occurs when there is a question as to whether there is a chip fracture around the elbow or an emerging ossific center. One method of evaluating a bone density relative to an ossific center or a fracture is simply to obtain x-ray views of the opposite elbow for comparison. A mnemonic for memorizing the chronologic appearance of the ossific centers is CRITOE (*capitellum, radial head, internal humeral condyle or medial epicondyle, trochlear, olecranon, external humeral condyle or lateral epicondyle*). The position of the radius in relation to the capitellum or lateral condyle following injury to the elbow should always be observed. A line drawn through the radius under normal circumstances always points to the capitellar epiphysis of the lateral condyle. This provides an excellent landmark to determine whether a dislocation of the elbow has occurred, which is the case if a line drawn through the radial shaft does not intersect the capitellum.

The presence of a displaced, bulging, periarticular fat pad (an area of radiolucency seen on a lateral x-ray view of the elbow just above the olecranon process posteriorly or above the radial head anteriorly) indicates an effusion of the radiohumeral joint. This could be due to a nondisplaced fracture of the supracondylar region, radial head, capitellum, trochlear, olecranon, or coronoid process. It is nonspecific, but causes the examiner to take a closer look at the elbow joint when it is present and the patient is clinically symptomatic. The appearance of a posterior fat pad sign is of greater importance than an anterior fat pad sign.

The supracondylar humeral fracture is the most common injury to the elbow. Because of the neurovascular structure surrounding the elbow joint, i.e., the brachial artery and median, ulnar, and radial nerves, one must be meticulous in evaluating the distal extremity for the four Ps (pain, pallor, pulselessness, and paralysis), which may be indicative of ischemia. Following reduction of a supracondylar fracture, one should check carefully for possible compromise of the anterior interosseous nerve. This can be evaluated by having the patient make a perfect O sign with the index finger and thumb. This determines whether there has been neuromuscular damage to the flexor digitorum profundus to the index finger and the flexor pollicis longus. If the child cannot make a perfect O, but pinches the thumb to the side of the interphalangeal joint of the index finger, there is a strong possibility that there is injury to this nerve. Also after reduction of a dislocation of the elbow, one should carefully evaluate the ulnar, nerve to rule out entrapment. A general rule is that a neurocirculatory evaluation of the distal extremity should be carried out following the reduction of all elbow injuries.

Transcondylar Fractures

Fractures through the distal humeral epiphysis tend to occur most often during infancy. In children under 5 years of age, a supracondylar fracture through the distal humeral epiphyseal plate may imitate an elbow dislocation; the forearm is displaced medially as opposed to the lateral displacement seen with true elbow dislocations; also a line drawn through the radius points to the capitellar epiphysis, which does not occur with a dislocation. There is a significant association of child battering with this injury, and this possibility should be ruled out.

So-called Y or T condylar fractures of the distal humerus are uncommon in young children, but occur most frequently in adolescents. The treatment is reduction by either closed overhead traction or open reduction and pin fixation.

Radial Head Fractures

Radial head fractures may result from the valgus strain mechanism after a fall on the outstretched hand that causes a dislocation of the elbow. Occasionally there is a nondisplaced crack in the radial head or the neck that is not visible on x-ray examination, but presents only as pain and a positive anterior or posterior fat pad sign. Patients under 12 years old can best be treated by splintage. In those over 12, the effusion is enough that aspiration of the joint with injection of Marcaine is necessary to relieve the pain.

Monteggia Injury

This is a fracture of the proximal ulna with dislocation of the radial head. The ulna fracture is almost always identified, but the radial head dislocation may frequently be missed. X-ray films should include both the wrist and elbow when there is a single bone forearm fracture, especially the ulna. Again, a line drawn through the radius should point to the capitellar epiphysis on all views. If this is not the case and there is a fracture of the ulna, one has to consider a Monteggia injury. One also has to be concerned about neuropraxia of the median or radial nerve following a Monteggia injury.

Unicameral Bone Cyst

Pathologic fractures do occur to the upper extremity. The most common cause is a unicameral bone cyst of the proximal third of the humerus. There may be no displacement or deformity beyond simple swelling. The x-ray view is characteristic. Because the x-ray findings are almost 99 percent diagnostic of unicameral bone cyst when a cystic lesion occurs within 1 inch of the humeral proximal epiphysis, treatment can be carried out directly by an orthopaedist. Our current treatment is multiple aspirations of the cyst, with pressure forced saline irrigation and instillation of methylprednisolone acetate.

Nursemaid's Elbow

This is a common injury to the elbow in a very young child who is subjected to forceful extension of the elbow joint. Another term is "nanny yank." It most often occurs when one is walking along holding a child by the arm or hand who then steps off a curb, thereby leaving him or her suspended by the arm. Most often there is subluxation of the radial head from its orbicular ligament. The child presents with a refusal to flex the elbow and significant irritation. Reduction is most often accomplished through supination and flexion or may occur spontaneously. We most often see reduction carried out by the x-ray technologist who forces the child into a flexion and extension of the elbow for a scout film to determine whether there is any bone injury. This usually resolves the problem by the time the child returns to the office. The injury can usually be treated by a sling or collar and cuff for 3 to 4 days. If the patient has had repeated subluxation, he should be treated in a long arm cast for approximately 3 weeks in the 90 degree flexed position. Recurrent subluxations are quite uncommon.

Shoulder Injuries

Dislocation of the Shoulder. This is rare prior to skeletal maturity. The arm is usually in forced abduction and external rotation when dislocation occurs. The treatment, following reduction of the initial dislocation involves strapping the arm in adduction and internal rotation. The shoulder is immobilized for approximately 6 weeks, after which physical therapy and rehabilitation are carried out. Most dislocations are anterior subglenoid with a defect sustained in the posterolateral aspect of the humeral head. This defect is called the Hill-Sachs lesion. The presence of this defect causes ease of redislocation during abduction and external rotation motions.

Acromioclavicular Separation. This is unusual in a child and occurs infrequently prior to skeletal maturity. The philosophy of treatment of this injury varies considerably. In the skeletally mature adolescent, fixation of the clavicle to the coronoid process by a Bosworth screw is carried out. For the younger child, strapping of the shoulder is the preferred method of treatment.

Clavicle Fracture. This is a common injury in a child usually caused by a direct fall on the shoulder. The treatment of this injury by a figure-of-eight bandage is tradition bound, although occasionally exceedingly uncomfortable for the patient. If there is minimal displacement, I recommend the collar and cuff or a sling and swath. The displacement is rarely significant enough to require open reduction. Considerable spontaneous remodeling can be expected.

Hand and Wrist Injury

The sprain of the wrist is uncommon in both the child and the adult. In the adult most often there is an injury to the carpal navicular bone. In the child most often there is a nondisplaced fracture of the distal radius. Most of the sprains of the wrist can be treated with a prefabricated splint or plaster volar splint. Only rarely does a carpal navicular fracture occur in a child. However, when it does occur, it has to be treated by anatomic reduction and a thumb spica cast; otherwise it is subject to nonunion and avascular necrosis.

Fractures of the metacarpals are usually the result of direct trauma from an object falling on the hand or someone stepping on the hand during team sports activity. The boxer's fracture of the fifth metacarpal is usually the result of indirect trauma, either from striking someone's jaw or, in the pediatric age group, striking a wall, a locker, or other fixed object after a frustrating game or ego deflating practice situation. This fracture is also somewhat overtreated, and except for angular deformities in excess of 50 to 60 degrees in a child over 12 years of age, one can expect considerable remodeling and minimal functional

loss. Manipulative reduction can be carried out under local anesthesia, and a bulky dressing or an ulnar gutter splint is all that is required for treatment.

The other metacarpals are rarely injured except for direct trauma. Most heal with minimal difficulty and angular deformities will remodel. One has to be concerned about rotational alignment. Most often they can be managed by "buddy taping" the fingers to the adjacent fingers to effect alignment and rotation. Splintage is necessary only to relieve initial discomfort. Rarely is more aggressive treatment required for a child.

Metacarpophalangeal Injury

Dislocation of the metacarpophalangeal joint, especially the thumb metacarpal and index metacarpal, is not infrequent in children. The thumb metacarpophalangeal joint and some finger metacarpophalangeal joints may be reducible by closed means. Most often the index finger metacarpophalangeal joint dislocation has to be treated operatively because of the interposition of the volar plate between the metacarpophalangeal joint. The finger flexors and supporting ligaments tend to trap the volar plate, preventing reduction. Once reduction has been obtained and prior to application of a cast, x-ray films should be obtained to rule out persistent displacement or entrapped osteochondral fractures.

Finger Fractures

Most commonly, finger fractures in children occur at the base of the proximal phalanx of the fourth and fifth fingers, usually a Salter type II epiphyseal injury. The metaphyseal fragment may be either frankly displaced or buckled. The injury has been called the "pencil fracture" because it can be treated by placing a regular lead pencil in the web space and approximating a deviated finger until they touch. There is occasionally an audible snap, which usually results in anatomic reduction. The fingers can then be "buddy taped" together with good results. Definitive healing usually occurs within 3 weeks.

Hip Injury

Femoral neck fractures are unusual in children. These fractures are usually the result of a significant amount of trauma, such as a fall from a height or vehicular-pedestrian accident. There are various classifications of these injuries that have to do with the anatomic location, e.g., through the epiphyseal plate, through the neck, through the trochanter, and subtrochanteric. Avascular necrosis is not uncommon in injuries that occur through the epiphysis and through the neck of the femur. These may, of course, lead to growth problems, and the parents should be informed of this.

Dislocation of the hip joint may occur following the same types of trauma that cause a fracture of the hip. Because of the strong potential for injury to the blood supply to the femoral head, all hip dislocations should be reduced immediately. Once reduction has been accomplished, the hip joint should be placed through a full range of motion. If there is any crepitus, pain, or limitation in range of motion, polytomography or computed tomography should be carried out to rule out any osteochondral fragments in the joint. In hips that have been dislocated in excess of 12 hours, avascular necrosis is the rule rather than the exception. A bone scan can be performed to determine whether avascular necrosis has occurred. Orthopaedic consultation is always needed after reduction.

Slipped capital femoral epiphysis can be considered a fracture through the epiphyseal plate, but is most often an insidious, progressive injury rather than an acute break. The child usually complains of knee pain for several weeks to months and has a limp. The characteristic body type is that of a eunuchoid male or somewhat plump female. There invariably is an externally rotated limb on the involved side. The x-ray films are usually diagnostic. Both anterior and posterior pelvis films showing both hips and frog-leg pelvis film should be taken. It is not unusual for a minimal slip not to be seen on the anteroposterior films, but should be obvious on the frog-leg lateral films.

To diagnose the minimally slipped femoral epiphysis, one needs to project a line tangential to the neck of the femur. On each view this line should intersect into the head. If the line does not intersect to the head, the head has slipped, thus identifying a minimal slip. The patient should be referred to an orthopod.

Avulsion Injury

Avulsion injuries frequently occur around the pelvis and may initially mimic hip injuries. These injuries result from strong contracture against resistance. They usually occur during athletic events in adolescents and come under the heading of "overuse syndromes." They occasionally present problems in diagnosis when seen on x-ray films. The two most common injuries are avulsion of the anterior superior iliac spine and ischial tuberosity. Avulsions of the greater and lesser tuberosities of the femur are far less common.

Anterior Superior Iliac Spine. This is most frequently avulsed in track and field events. The patient complains of a sharp pain at the anterior pelvis just above the hip. There may be localized swelling and inability to bear weight. The x-ray view is diagnostic, with the appearance of a sliver of bone off the anterior superior iliac spine. Rest is important. The patient should not return to participation until he is pain free and there is evidence of the fragment healing.

Ischial Tuberosity Apophysis. This is most frequently avulsed in hurdlers. They usually feel a pop and hear a tear during participation. There is pain and localized swelling. Occasionally the condition is chronic, in which case the patient is aware of a "pull" in the ischial region. X-ray views during this time usually show abundant new bone in the area of the ischium of a suspicious character that could be confused with a tumor and suggests the diagnosis of "pseudotumro ischia." The bone scan is invariably "hot" early, and a biopsy reveals aggressive repair of bone, which could be considered sarcomatous. The history is most important. The acute injury presents as a sliver of bone off the ischium and is easy to identify. Rest and early healing prior to return to participation constitute the treatment of choice.

Trochanteric Avulsions. Trochanteric avulsions are relatively rare and are treated by compression, ice, and rest. The child should not be allowed to return to participation until he is pain free and rehabilitation has been achieved.

Femoral Shaft Fracture

A significant amount of trauma (such as a vehicular-pedestrian accident) is required to break the femur in a child. Profound blood loss and shock may result, especially in infants. The child must be admitted to the hospital for evaluation. One must always be alert for possible child abuse when young children present with femoral shaft fractures.

Growth plate injuries to the distal femur may result in shortening or angular deformities. Whenever one evaluates an injury to the adolescent distal femoral metaphysis with soft tissue swelling, especially if it appears to be somewhat older with an increase in sclerosis and new bone formation in and about the area, one must consider this possibly to have been a pathologic fracture, with osteogenic sarcoma high on the list of possible diagnoses. Benign pathologic fractures of the femoral shaft are usually proximal and caused by unicameral bone cysts, except for those found in individuals with known metabolic disorders, such as osteogenesis imperfecta and fibrous dysplasia.

Knee Injury

The ligaments of the knee in a child are stronger than the epiphyseal plates. If there is an apparent effusion and no evidence of fracture, the possibility of an epiphyseal plate injury must be considered. The parents must be made aware that 65 percent of lower extremity growth occurs around the knee, with a 39 percent contribution from the distal femoral growth plate and a 26 percent contribution from the proximal tibial growth plate.

When plain films are normal and there is an effusion, stress x-ray views are indicated. The varus-valgus stress x-ray view can be obtained by placing the child supine and pressing against the outside of the knee (valgus stress) or against the inside of the knee (varus stress). If the knee joint tends to open up on either side, the injury is primarily ligamentous, whereas if the epiphyseal line opens, a growth plate fracture is diagnosed.

If there is an effusion of the knee, the joint should be aspirated and examined for fat droplets to rule out the possibility of an unrecognized tibial spine fracture or some other intra-articular injury. Tibial spine fractures are more common when the injury is noted to have been a fall from a bicycle. If there is a tibial spine fracture and it is non-displaced, it can be treated initially with a compression dressing followed by a cylinder cast. Displaced fractures require open reduction and internal fixation.

If the stress view does not open at the growth plates, but at the knee joint, arthroscopic examination is indicated. The results of operative repair of the major knee ligaments in children and nonoperative results remain controversial.

Dislocations of the knee are rare, but when they do occur, there is great concern for neurovascular injuries. With any massively swollen or injured knee, a possible spontaneously reduced dislocation must be suspected. With any history of dislocation of the knee, admission to the hospital and careful observation for 48 hours are necessary.

Patella Fractures

These fractures are unusual in children and usually result from direct trauma. The presence of bipartite patella must be ruled out. Bipartite lesions are usually peripheral with smooth edges as opposed to the irregular edge seen with fractures. When there is less than 2 to 3 mm of displacement of fragments, the injury can be treated by aspiration of joint effusion and placing the child in a long leg cast. If effusion is significant, a compression dressing might be applied for 5 to 7 days, followed by a formal cylinder or long leg cast.

Fractures of the patella sustained in dashboard injuries are frequently associated with dislocation of the hip on the same side. If the patient was rendered unconscious and has hip pain, an x-ray view of the pelvis should be taken.

The most frequent injury to the patella in a child, especially young females, is the dislocation-subluxation rather than a fracture of the patella. The patella usually dislocates laterally and may cause an osteochondral fracture of the lateral femoral condyle or the medial facet of the patella. Comprehensive x-ray views should be taken to rule out a fracture with a dislocation. Reduction is carried out by extension of the knee to relax the quadriceps and gentle pressure on the lateral border of the patella. The treatment is aspiration of the effusion and a compression dressing. Many orthopaedists now perform arthroscopy following acute patellar dislocation to rule out osteochondral fractures, and thus consultation is recommended.

Tibial Fractures

These fractures are usually the result of motor vehicular trauma. There is the occasional pathologic fracture through a benign cyst of the tibia. Stress fractures may also be seen in the proximal posteromedial tibial metaphysis. They most often follow significant change of physical activity, such as track and cross country training in the spring. The x-ray views may occasionally be alarming and may appear to represent tumor. One should refrain from early biopsy of these lesions lest they be mistakenly diagnosed as osteogenic sarcoma.

The parents should be informed that all fractures of the lower extremity long bones potentially may cause growth problems. These may include growth inhibition and shortening; growth stimulation; and progressive angulation following fracture of the proximal medial tibial metaphysis.

Nondisplaced tibial fractures can be maintained in a long leg cast. Displaced fractures or open fractures require operative treatment. It is rarely necessary to fix a child's fracture with threaded pins or a plate. Healing is usually uneventful.

Fibular injuries are rare and usually aproblematic. The most common fibular diaphyseal fracture is the distal third stress fracture. It may not be seen initially on radiograph, but shows periosteal new bone at 7 to 10 days. Supportive and symptomatic treatment with a short walking cast is occasionally necessary. Most often the healing process is well on its way at the time of diagnosis.

Proximal fibular fractures are benign, but may be associated with peroneal nerve neuropraxia.

Lower-Extremity Injuries

The most common injury of the lower extremity in children is an ankle sprain. A common sprain that results in injury to the anterior talofibular ligament in adults is usually an epiphyseal injury of the distal fibula in a child. The epiphyseal plate is the weak link in the chain, as all ligaments attach distal to it. The fracture is usually a Salter type I epiphyseal injury and cannot be appreciated on the initial x-ray views. There is usually swelling in and around the anterolateral aspect of the ankle. The treatment is a compression dressing using Webril and an ACE bandage initially, if there is significant swelling. This is supplemented by plaster splinting. The patient must not bear weight. This dressing is usually replaced by a cast in approximately 1 week; it takes about 3 weeks for the injury to heal.

Repeated ankle sprains and strains should stimulate investigation of a subtalar *tarsal coalition*. Special views including CT scans are often required to identify the abnormal osteochondral formations. The most common coalition is the calcaneonavicular.

The medial aspect of the ankle is rarely strained or sprained, and the injury most often results in a fracture through the medial malleolus. This tends to be a Salter-Harris type IV fracture through the distal aspect of the articular weight-bearing surface. It has be anatomically reduced, as it can result in angular deformities of the ankle joint secondary to partial growth plate arrest or closure.

Foot Injuries

Fractures of the foot in children are most often due to direct trauma, such as an object falling on it from a height. The calcaneus is rarely injured, but is the most common tarsal bone injury. The treatment consists of compression initially, followed by application of a short leg walking cast.

Metatarsal fractures are usually nondisplaced and can be managed by early compression dressing followed by application of a short leg walking cast. It is common in the Midwest to see a number of lawnmower injuries in the spring that result in significant loss of bone. Treatment is supportive and directed toward the individual injury.

Phalangeal injuries are unusual in children and usually can be treated by a hard soled shoe or short leg cast if swelling is significant.

Rang M. Children's fractures, 2nd ed. Philadelphia: JB Lippincott, 1983.
Rockwood CA, Wilkens KE, King RE. Fractures in children. Philadelphia: JB Lippincott, 1984.

SUGGESTED READING

Crawford AH. Pediatric orthopaedic surgery. Burbank, CA: Sci Image Communicat 1981.

PEDIATRIC BRONCHIOLITIS AND ASTHMA

CHRISTOPHER J. L. NEWTH, M.B., F.R.C.P.(C.)

PEDIATRIC BRONCHIOLITIS

Bronchiolitis is an inflammatory disease of the respiratory tract that predominantly affects the peripheral airways. The inflammation can result from infection, which is most commonly viral; chemical factors, such as hydrocarbons; or physical factors, such as cigarette smoke. In this article the discussion is limited to acute viral bronchiolitis.

Bronchiolitis is clinically characterized by an upper respiratory tract infection followed in 2 to 3 days by cough, tachypnea, wheezing, and a temperature that is usually less than 39.5 °C. Apnea can occur in younger infants, especially those who were premature at birth. The usual course of illness is clinical improvement within 3 days, although some wheezing can occur for 1 to 2 weeks.

Although bronchiolitis occurs at all ages, infants suffer the most severe clinical illness. Children under 1 year of age have the highest incidence of disease, with more males than females requiring hospitalization. The peak incidence of hospitalization occurs in infants aged 2 months. In children under 2 years of age in whom the virus is isolated, respiratory syncytial virus (RSV) accounts for 45 percent of the cases. The radiographic findings in bronchiolitis are nonspecific, ranging from a normal appearance to hyperinflation and sometimes extensive patchy atelectasis. Mild to moderate hypoxemia is always present, but significant arterial carbon dioxide retention reflecting respiratory failure is uncommon. The major differential diagnoses are given in Table 1.

Pre-hospital Treatment

During the transport of the infant to hospital, therapy should be directed at two areas.

Support of the Infant

Oxygen administration is helpful in correcting the hypoxemia present in all infants suffering from moderate or severe clinical illness. An inspired oxygen concentration of 30 to 40 percent is usually adequate. The oxygen should be humidified and delivered by head hood (or by mask, if tolerated).

Handling should be minimal, to provide the maximum of observation without increasing the infant's restlessness and hence oxygen comsumption.

Detection of Complications

Continuous clinical observation should be instituted for apnea and cyanosis. A portable sensor for skin surface (transcutaneous) oxygen and carbon dioxide can be used if available to monitor gas exchange.

Initial Hospital Treatment

Support of the infant

Oxygen, humidified and at a concentration of 30 to 40 percent should be administered. (Oxygen that has not been humidified is irritating and contraindicated.)

An oxygen tent can deliver 40 percent oxygen at best. This is seldom achieved, because access to the infant requires opening and closing the tent, which mixes the oxygenated air with room air. Another disadvantage is that the humidification causes mist, which "rains out" on the inside of the tent, making it difficult to observe the infant. In addition, the mist can cause excessive cooling of the baby. The infant head hood gives better control over oxygen concentration and allows access to the baby, but some infants do not tolerate these hoods well. If a tent is not available, humidified oxygen at 40 percent can be blown in the child's face, or a pediatric nasal cannula can be run at 2 to 3 liters per minute.

Nursing should be undertaken in a thermoneutral environment, to reduce oxygen consumption. For the same reason, acetaminophen should be given to decrease the body temperature.

Fluids. Infants with bronchiolitis need fluids to prevent the dehydration that results from poor fluid intake prior to admission and the increased respiratory losses secondary to tachypnea. Excess fluid may be harmful, however; fluid intake and body weight must be carefully monitored.

Detection of Complications

Apnea is commonly associated with bronchiolitis, particularly in infants born prematurely. Continuous respiratory and heart rate monitoring should be undertaken to detect apnea and subsequent bradycardia.

Gas exchange. The state of oxygenation can be monitored either by clinical observation of cyanosis (a late feature), by the use of finger or ear oximetry, or by skin surface oxygen electrodes. The latter are often inaccurate, but a significant decrease in oxygen tension measured by this device should alert the clinician to be wary. Skin sur-

TABLE 1 Differential Diagnosis of Acute Viral
Bronchiolitis in Infants

Infantile asthma
Aspiration syndromes
Foreign body inhalation
Cardiac disease with pulmonary edema
Cystic fibrosis

---

face carbon dioxide sensors can be used for measurement of adequate alveolar ventilation and are generally accurate. An initial arterial blood gas determination is required (usually drawn from the radial or dorsalis pedis artery) for correlation with the skin surface electrodes and also for detection of metabolic acidosis. Subsequently arterial blood gas determination should be performed when indicated by changes in clinical condition.

Bacterial superinfection. Antibiotics are not indicated in the treatment of bronchiolitis. If the diagnosis is in doubt, however, and the respiratory distress may be secondary to bacterial infection, it is prudent to start antibiotic therapy. Ampicillin (100 mg per kilogram per day divided into doses given every six hours) and gentamicin (5 mg per kilogram per day divided into doses given every eight hours) intravenously are the usual choices. If the subsequent clinical course, cultures, and radiologic findings then confirm the diagnosis of acute viral bronchiolitis, the antibiotics can be discontinued.

Nasopharyngeal aspirates can be taken for rapid immunofluorescent confirmation of respiratory syncytial virus (RSV). It is advisable to check the capabilities of your own laboratory in this respect.

Association with *patent ductus arteriosus* (PDA). Rarely, but particularly in the baby who was born prematurely, the ductus arteriosus can reopen in response to the hypoxemia of severe bronchiolitis. The presence of a cardiac gallop rhythm, a large liver, and radiographic evidence of an enlarged heart and pulmonary edema should alert one to this possibility. The PDA murmur is often difficult to hear in this clinical situation. If a PDA is suspected, an electrocardiogram and appropriate two dimensional echocardiographic studies should be done and a pediatric cardiologist consulted.

Protection of Others

All staff should be aware of the potential hazard of nosocomial transmission of RSV. The infection is highly contagious and is spread by infectious secretions through direct inoculation of large droplets or contaminated hands. Thus, careful hand washing should be stressed.

Pharmacologic Agents (See Table 2)

Studies of the effects of pharmacologic agents and bronchiolitis have been limited by the lack of objective methods for assessing pulmonary function in infants and young children. Thus, the efficacy of beta-adrenergic drugs and atropine-like drugs is controversial. Clearly some infants respond clinically to beta-adrenergic drugs, and it is recommended that every infant with bronchiolitis, irrespective of age, receive a 24 hour trial of therapy with inhaled metaproterenol or subcutaneous epinephrine. Clinical trials of theophylline and steroid therapy have demonstrated no benefits in bronchiolitis, unlike asthma.

Antiviral Agents

When RSV can be documented as the cause of the acute viral bronchiolitis, the antiviral agent ribavirin can be delivered by aerosol. Theoretically the sooner this is given the better. It has been found efficacious when administered for as little as 12 hours each day and should be continued for 3 to 6 days.

Management and Disposition

With careful observation and a minimum of handling, most children with acute bronchiolitis have an uncomplicated course if the therapy just outlined is instituted. Children with mild disease can be managed as outpatients. If there is any question as to the adequacy of ventilation, arterial blood gases should be obtained. Infants with respiratory distress, exhaustion, difficulty in feeding, or an episode of apnea all need hospital admission. A small group of patients will proceed to acute respiratory failure and require intubation and mechanical ventilation. The principles of such intervention are summarized in the section on pediatric asthma, and tube sizes are recommended in Table 3. Their management should be carried out in a pediatric intensive care unit.

PEDIATRIC ASTHMA

Asthma is a disease characterized by increased responsiveness of the trachea and bronchi to various stimuli. It is manifested by a narrowing of the airways that can change in severity either spontaneously or as a result of therapy. Any infant with recurrent (three or more) episodes of wheezing, which have no other specific cause identified, should be considered to have asthma; this is regardless of age of onset, evidence of atopy, apparent precipitating factors, or frequency of wheezing.

At least 5 to 10 percent of infants younger than the age of 2 years suffer from asthma; boys have a higher incidence than girls. The majority of childhood asthmatics develop their first symptoms before the age of 3 years. The most common precipitant of wheezing is a viral infection of the respiratory tract. Conversely, bacterial infection is a rare precipitant of wheezing.

Infants and young children with acute asthma often present with tachypnea, cough, and evidence of dyspnea. Hypoxemia is always present, and the most obvious radiologic finding is air trapping, which is usually bilateral and symmetrical. Patches of atelectasis varying in size from a segment to a lobe are not unusual. Signs of pulmonary edema are sometimes evident.

Pre-hospital Treatment

As with bronchiolitis, support of the child involves administration of humidified oxygen at a concentration of 35 percent, delivered by head hood or face mask, to relieve hypoxemia. To provide the maximum of observation without increasing the child's restlessness and anxiety, and hence oxygen consumption handling should be minimal.

Initial assessment is fundamental to useful serial clinical observation of improvement or deterioration. The following baseline observations should be recorded: restlessness, fatigue, respiratory and heart rates, use of accessory muscle of respiration, pulses paradoxus (greater than

TABLE 2 Pharmacologic Agents in Bronchiolitis and Asthma

Agent	Parenteral Administration	Oral Administration	Aerosol Administration
Sympathomimetics			
Epinephrine (adrenaline)	Subcutaneous: 1:1,000, 0.01 ml/kg, can be repeated twice at 20 min intervals		
Isoproterenol (Isuprel)	Intravenous: 0.1 µg/kg/min; can be raised in increments of 0.1 µg/kg per 15 min to a maximum of 1.0 µg/kg/min	Not recommended because of poor oral absorption	0.5% (1:200) respirator solution, 0.25 ml diluted to 2 ml, up to 4 times daily
Metaproterenol (Alupent)		10 mg per 5 ml syrup, 0.5 mg/kg/dose, 3 to 4 times daily	5% respirator solution, 0.015–0.02 ml/kg to a maximum of 1.0 ml diluted with saline up to 2 ml, up to 1 hourly
Methylxanthines			
Theophylline preparations (anhydrous preparations 100% bioavailable)	Loading dose: aminophylline 6 mg/kg IV diluted in saline run over 15 min. Maintenance: (a) 1.0 mg/kg/hour, begun 30 min after loading dose finished, or (b) intermittent bolus every 4 to 6 hours to a maximum of 24 mg/kg/day	16-24 mg/kg/24 hours. Immediate release: divided 6 hourly. Sustained released: divided 8 or 12 hourly	

Note: Serial serum theophylline concentrations should be monitored. Intravenous drug is aminophylline; 100 mg of this is equivalent to 80 mg of theophylline.

Steroids			
Hydrocortisone	Loading dose: 5 to 7 mg/kg IV. Maintenance: 0.5 to 1 mg/kg/hour IV		
Prednisolone		2 mg/kg to start; reduce dose to minimum possible over 5 days	

10 mm Hg drop in systolic pressure with inspiration), and cyanosis.

Initial Hospital Treatment

Support of the Child

Oxygenation and nursing are the same as for bronchiolitis. The serial observations already mentioned should be continued. Measurements of peak expiratory flow rate before and after bronchodilator therapy should be carried out (in children old enough to cooperate, i.e., 6 years or older). Not all asthma patients in the emergency department need ABGs, but any patient who is thought to be in respiratory failure or who is not improving despite aggressive therapy should receive them. In patients who meet these criteria, serial arterial blood gas levels are mandatory, until the patient has improved.

Detection of Complications

Pneumothorax is an uncommon complication, but unless there is the sudden appearance of subcutaneous emphysema, it can be difficult to detect. A decrease in breath sounds on the affected side, which is the earliest warning, is unfortunately common in asthma secondary to mucus plugging of airways. After stabilization, a chest film should be taken in all moderate to severe asthmatics. A lack of improvement in air entry to the affected lung following bronchodilator therapy should alert the clini-

cian to the possibilty of pneumothorax or massive atelectasis.

Bacterial superinfection is infrequent, and antibiotics are not usually indicated.

Establish an intravenous line early, using a conventional hypotonic replacement solution in order to administer drugs and to correct dehydration and electrolyte imbalance.

TABLE 3 Size of Endotracheal Tubes

Approximate Age of Patient	Internal Diameter (mm)	Length (cm)* Oral	Length (cm)* Nasal
Premature	2.5 to 3.0	11	13.5
Newborn	3.0 to 3.5	12	14
6 Months	3.5	12.5	14.5
1 Year	4.0	13	15
2 Year	4.5	14	16
4 Year	5.0	15	17
6 Year	5.5	17	19
8 Year	6.0	19	21
10 Year	6.5	20	22
12 Year	7.0	21	22
14 Year	7.5	22	23
16 Year	8.0	23	24

* The length referred to here is that to which the ETT should be "precut" to allow adequate room for immobilization of the tube connection to the ventilator. For patients above 1 year of age, the following formula is convenient:

$$\frac{\text{Age of patient (yr)} + 16}{4} = \text{Tube size (in mm ID)}$$

Beta-adrenergic drugs work poorly if the pH is less than 7.25. Thus, *acidosis* of this degree, irrespective of metabolic or respiratory origin, should be corrected with sodium bicarbonate as soon as possible. The intravenous dose of bicarbonate in mEq is $0.3 \times$ body weight (in kilograms) $\times$ base deficit.

Protection of Others

In many of these infants and young children asthmatic attacks are precipitated by viral infections. Therefore vigorous hand washing by staff and avoidance of infant-to-infant contact should be undertaken.

Pharmacologic Agents

A beta-adrenergic bronchodilator is the first treatment of choice; this can be metaproterenol (Alupent), isoproterenol (Isuprel) respiratory solution given by nebulizer, or epinephrine (1:1,000) given subcutaneously. Inhaled metaproterenol generally works extremely well in infants and young children. The actual dose of the inhaled drug is initially limited by the (low) tidal volumes. Provided there is good clinical observation and continuous electronic cardiac monitoring, inhalations can be given continuously until the bronchospasm decreases and secretions are mobilized. In very severe cases, intravenous administration of isoproterenol may be required.

Although theophylline is used widely in the United States for the management of asthma, it is not a good bronchodilator in the acute situation. At best it is adjuvant therapy to beta-adrenergic agents, but it should never be used alone in the management of acute asthma. If the child is not vomiting, the oral route can be safely substituted for the intravenous one to provide the loading dose of 5 mg per kilogram. However, an immediate release or liquid (not sustained release) preparation must be used.

Theophylline is contraindicated if the patient has a known theophylline idiosyncrasy. Heart failure, liver disease, and erythromycin alter metabolism and may produce toxic levels with conventional theophylline doses. The loading dose should be reduced to 3.5 mg per kilogram if the patient has used theophylline products in the previous 12 hours (serum levels cannot be accurately predicted).

In the uncomplicated acute asthmatic attack, corticosteroids (Table 2) have been shown to have no benefit in children. However, if the child has been on long-term systemic steroid treatment within the previous 2 years or the clinical history indicates that the present hospitalization is due to an acute attack superimposed on chronic symptoms (weeks), corticosteroids should be used. Dosages for these pharmacologic agents are given in Table 2.

Assisted Ventilation

Once it has been decided that artificial ventilation is necessary, full control over the patient's airway and ventilation must be achieved as rapidly as possible if unnecessary hypoxia is to be avoided. The patient should be preoxygenated with 100 percent oxygen by face mask for 1 to 2 minutes (using hand ventilation if necessary). Then a large dose of pancuronium (0.15 mg per kilogram) is injected intravenously, an orotracheal tube is passed, and intermittent positive pressure ventilation is started by hand. Secretions are aspirated through the endotracheal tube and sent for culture and immunofluorescence studies.

The choice of tube size is important. Uncuffed tubes are generally used in children (see Table 3). Too large a tube compresses the subglottic mucous membrane and may lead to subglottic edema or stenosis. Too small a tube allows an excessive leak of gas from the larynx and, in view of the high inflating pressures required, makes it difficult to achieve adequate alveolar ventilation. Ideally there should be a slight leak of gas from the larynx when the lungs are inflated, but if a tube allows a large leak and the size larger is occlusive, the larger tube should be used or a cuffed tube substituted. Further ventilatory management should only be undertaken by a pediatric intensivist.

Disposition

With adequate and aggressive bronchodilator therapy and oxygen, most children with asthma do well. If they respond quickly and adequately, they can often be sent home from the emergency department provided a suitable beta-adrenergic drug (preferably inhaled) is made available with appropriate instructions for use. Albuterol and metaproterenol metered dose inhalers can be used in a dose of 2 puffs every 4 hours in children old enough to cooperate (i.e., about 6 years of age). These same agents can be used in younger children and even infants when an inhalation aid (such as Aerochamber or Inspirease) is attached to the inhaler. In this latter case, the dose should be increased up to double the amount.

Failure of management is manifested by worsening clinical signs, progressive hypoxemia, and a rising arterial carbon dioxide tension. This may indicate the need for hospital admission and intravenous, administration of isoproterenol (see Table 2) or assisted ventilation.

SUGGESTED READING: PEDIATRIC BRONCHIOLITIS

Hall CB, McBride JT, Gala CL, Hildreth SW, Schnabel KC. Ribavirin treatment of respiratory syncytial infection in infants with underlying cardiopulmonary disease. JAMA 1985; 254:3047–3051.

Levison H, Tabachnik E, Newth CJL. Wheezing in infancy, croup, and epiglottitis. In: Gluck L, ed. Current problems in pediatrics. Chicago: Year Book Medical Publishers, 1982:22.

Wohl MEB, Chernick V. Bronchiolitis—state of the art. Am Rev Resp Dis 1978; 118:759–781.

Soto ME, Sly PD, Uren E, Taussig LM, Landau LI. Bronchodilator response during acute viral bronchiolitis in infancy. Pediatr Pulmonol 1985; 2:85–90.

SUGGESTED READING: PEDIATRIC ASTHMA

Gurwitz D, Levison H, Mindorff C, Reilly P, Worsley G. Assessment of a new device (Aerochamber) for use with aerosol drugs in asthmatic children. Ann Allergy 1983; 50:166–170.

Simpson H, Mitchell I, Inglis JM, Grubb DJ. Severe ventilatory failure and asthma in children. Arch Dis Child 1978; 53:714–721.

Speight ANP, Lee DA, Hey EN. Underdiagnosis and undertreatment of asthma in childhood. Brit Med J 1983; 36:1253–1256.

CONGESTIVE HEART FAILURE IN INFANTS AND CHILDREN

GERARD R. MARTIN, M.D.
SCOTT J. SOIFER, M.D.

Congestive heart failure (CHF) is a symptom complex in which the heart is unable to meet the metabolic requirements of the body, including those for growth. In its most severe form, cardiovascular collapse with metabolic acidosis and death may occur. CHF may result from a variety of cardiac and noncardiac causes. The age at which a pediatric patient develops CHF may be helpful in determining the specific etiology and in choosing a treatment regimen. In this chapter we will review the symptoms of CHF, discuss the various causes, and present an overview for treatment.

RECOGNITION OF CONGESTIVE HEART FAILURE

The most common signs and symptoms of CHF are poor feeding, failure to thrive, dyspnea, diaphoresis, pallor, and irritability (Table 1). These symptoms may result from inadequate systemic output, pulmonary congestion, or from the body's compensatory mechanism (increased adrenergic tone). Tachypnea and tachycardia are almost always present. Rales, heart murmurs, gallop rhythm, hepatomegaly, and peripheral edema may be present on physical examination. Cardiomegaly, increased pulmonary blood flow, or interstitial edema may be present on chest x-ray films.

ETIOLOGY

The causes of congestive heart failure vary with age (Table 2). *Newborns* who develop congestive heart failure require prompt evaluation and treatment, because they may rapidly develop metabolic acidosis and cardiovas-

cular collapse. Congenital heart malformations producing obstruction to left ventricular output (hypoplastic left heart syndrome, coarctation of the aorta, interrupted aortic arch, and aortic stenosis) are the most common causes of CHF during the first week of life. In these infants, systemic blood flow is dependent on the patency of the ductus arteriosus, which directs right ventricular output from the pulmonary artery to the descending aorta. As the ductus arteriosus closes after birth, systemic blood flow decreases and metabolic acidosis develops. The peripheral pulses are diminished and may completely disappear when the ductus arteriosus closes. There is also increased pulmonary blood flow with pulmonary overcirculation, resulting in dyspnea, tachypnea, and poor feeding.

Newborns are dependent on a normal heart rate to maintain an adequate cardiac output. Heart rates greater than 200 beats per minute (supraventricular tachycardia) or less than 60 beats per minute (complete heart block) decrease cardiac output and produce CHF. Myocardial dysfunction and CHF may also be produced by a variety of noncardiac conditions, including hypoglycemia, hypocalcemia, birth asphyxia, severe anemia, or polycythemia. Sepsis should always be considered in any newborn with CHF.

In *older infants*, CHF develops slowly. These infants often present with poor weight gain and failure to thrive. Cardiovascular collapse is rare. Congenital heart malformations producing ventricular volume overload (ventricular septal defect, atrioventricular canal defects, and anomalous pulmonary venous return) are common causes of CHF in this age group. As pulmonary vascular resistance falls normally over the first months of life, left-to-right shunting of blood and pulmonary blood flow in-

TABLE 1 Signs and Symptoms of Congestive Heart Failure

Decreased Systemic Output

Pallor
Peripheral edema
Decreased urine output
Hepatomegaly

Pulmonary Congestion

Poor feeding
Tachypnea
Dyspnea
Rales

Increased Adrenergic Tone

Diaphoresis
Tachycardia
Irritability

TABLE 2 Causes of Congestive Heart Failure by Age

Newborn

Hypoplastic left heart syndrome
Severe coarctation of the aorta
Interruption of the aortic arch
Severe aortic stenosis
Supraventricular tachycardia
Complete heart block
Other: hyperviscosity, hypoglycemia, hypocalcemia, birth asphyxia, severe anemia, sepsis

Infant (1–12 months)

Ventricular septal defects
Atrioventricular canal defect
Anomalous pulmonary venous connection
Coarctation of the aorta
Aortic stenosis
Supraventricular tachycardia
Endocardial fibroelastosis
Other: severe anemia, trauma, sepsis

Children

Infections: myocarditis, endocarditis, rheumatic heart disease
Cardiomyopathies: idiopathic, metabolic
Hypertension
Cardiac dysrhythmias
Ischemia: congenital coronary artery malformation, coronary arteritis, Kawasaki disease
Other: severe anemia, trauma, sepsis

crease, resulting in ventricular volume overload and CHF. Obstruction to left ventricular output and cardiac dysrhythmias may also produce CHF in these infants. Endocardial fibroelastosis and other cardiomyopathies are rare causes of CHF in older infants.

In *children*, congenital heart malformations are rare causes of CHF, while acquired heart diseases (myocarditis, endocarditis, pericarditis, and rheumatic heart disease) are more common. Idiopathic cardiomyopathies, inherited metabolic disorders, acute hypertensive crises, and drug-induced myocardial dysfunction may also produce CHF. Myocardial ischemia and myocardial infarction secondary to congenital coronary artery malformations (anomalous origin of the left coronary artery from the pulmonary artery) or from the coronary arteritis of Kawasaki disease produce CHF. Though the causes of congestive heart failure in infants and children are numerous, a rational approach to evaluation and treatment is based on improving the ability of the myocardium to meet the metabolic needs of the patient.

EVALUATION

An accurate history and physical examination of an infant or child with CHF help make the appropriate diagnosis and determine specific therapy. A rapid assessment of the respiratory status of the patient is mandatory. The cardiovascular system can be rapidly evaluated by checking the arterial pulse quality and rate. Blood pressures should be obtained in both the upper and lower extremities using the appropriate size blood pressure cuffs. Increased cardiac activity is determined by observation and palpation of the precordium. Auscultation of the heart and lungs determines whether heart murmurs are present. Auscultation of the skull and abdomen can reveal bruits that would suggest an arteriovenous malformation. Initial laboratory tests should include arterial blood gases, blood glucose level, serum electrolytes (calcium, blood urea nitrogen, and creatinine), and a hematocrit reading. A chest x-ray study to evaluate heart size and pulmonary parenchymal changes and an electrocardiogram to evaluate ventricular hypertrophy, myocardial ischemia, or cardiac dysrhythmias should be obtained.

TREATMENT

For infants and children with severe CHF, prompt intervention is necessary. Respiratory insufficiency or severe dyspnea produced by pulmonary interstitial edema should be treated by the administration of supplemental oxygen and, when necessary, endotracheal intubation and assisted ventilation with positive end expiratory pressure. Correction of hypoxemia or hypoventilation alone may improve CHF. Metabolic acidosis should be corrected by the administration of sodium bicarbonate (1 to 2 mEq per kilogram per dose given intravenously). In newborns with CHF and weak or absent femoral pulses, an intravenous infusion of prostaglandin E_1 should be started. This metabolite of arachidonic acid dilates the ductus arteriosus and maintains systemic blood flow in congenital heart

malformations with severe obstruction to left ventricular output. The starting dose is 0.05 μg per kilogram per minute. If there is no improvement, the dose should be increased to a maximum of 0.15 μg per kilogram per minute. The side effects of prostaglandin E_1 include apnea, hyperthermia, jitteriness, and seizures. Caution should be used when administering oxygen to newborns, since the marked increase in arterial P_{O_2} may actually constrict the ductus arteriosus, further decreasing systemic blood flow and increasing the metabolic acidosis. Newborn infants with CHF should be given supplemental oxygen to maintain an arterial P_{O_2} in the normal range (60 to 100 mm Hg).

All newborns and other infants with CHF should be treated with intravenous *antibiotics* even if the appropriate bacterial cultures have not been obtained. The choice and doses of antibiotics are age-dependent. Hypoglycemia may occur because of decreased oral intake and increased utilization of glucose secondary to anaerobic tissue metabolism. Fifty percent dextrose (1 g per kilogram) should be given until the serum glucose is in the normal range. Hypocalcemia can also impair myocardial function. Treatment with calcium chloride (10 mg per kilogram per dose) may lessen the symptoms of CHF. Severe anemia in association with CHF leads to inadequate oxygen delivery to the tissues and worsens metabolic acidosis. The hematocrit in patients with congestive heart failure should be maintained at greater than 30 percent. All newborn and young infants with CHF should be referred to a tertiary care center with diagnostic and surgical capabilities as soon as stabilization has occurred.

Older infants and children are less likely to present with cardiovascular collapse. If CHF is mild, then an adequate history, thorough physical examination, and chest x-ray study are sufficient. Respiratory and metabolic abnormalities should be rapidly corrected. If the symptoms are moderate in severity, then additional therapy may be of benefit regardless of age.

Infants and children with CHF have increased extracellular volume secondary to decreased renal excretion of sodium and water retention. There is decreased glomerular filtration and increased aldosterone and vasoactive peptide secretion, which enhance sodium reabsorption. The excess interstitial fluid may cause pulmonary and dependent edema. Fluid restriction is necessary in all patients with CHF. Diuretics are given to increase the excretion of excess sodium and water and to prevent their reaccumulation when fluid restriction is lessened.

Furosemide is a potent diuretic having a rapid onset of action when given intravenously. For the acutely ill patient, it is the diuretic of choice (Table 3). It can be given intramuscularly or orally. Because furosemide may result in marked potassium and calcium losses, the electrolyte levels should be routinely monitored in patients on this drug. Hypochloremic metabolic alkalosis, auditory nerve damage, and renal calculi may occur. When furosemide is given chronically, potassium supplementation should also be given. Chlorothiazide and spironolactone are less potent diuretics that are useful for long-term therapy. These agents are slower acting than furosemide

TABLE 3 Drug Dosages of Diuretics

Drug	Dosage	Route
Furosemide	1–3 mg/kg/dose 1–4 times/day	IV, IM, PO
Chlorothiazide	25–50 mg/kg/day q8–12h	PO
Spironolactone	1–3 mg/kg/day q8h–q12h	PO

and should not be used when rapid diuresis is indicated.

Inotropic agents improve myocardial contractility. They are used to treat myocardial dysfunction and in ventricular volume overload states. *Digitalis* is the most commonly used inotropic agent in the pediatric age group. Digitalis improves myocardial contractility, prolongs atrioventricular conduction, and slows the heart rate. Digoxin is the most frequently used frug preparation. Since it has a long half-life (T½ = 36 hours), a loading or total digitalizing dose (TDD) should be given (Table 4). The TDD varies with age and is usually given orally. In infants or children who are unable to take oral medications or who require a rapid response, the TDD is given intravenously. The TDD is decreased by 20 percent for intramuscular or intravenous administration. It is divided into three doses given every 8 hours. Because ST-T wave changes occur following digitalis administration, a 14-lead electrocardiogram should be obtained prior to starting digoxin. A lead II rhythm strip should be obtained prior to each dose to determine heart rate and the duration of the P-R interval. If bradycardia or marked first-degree heart block develops, digoxin should be stopped. The maintenance dose of digoxin is one-fourth of the TDD. It is divided into two doses and given every 12 hours. The first maintenance dose is given 12 hours after the last digitalizing dose. Digoxin is excreted by the kidneys. Patients with impaired renal function should receive a full digitalizing dose, but require a decreased maintenance digoxin dose.

Digoxin toxicity may occur in infants and children because of accidental ingestion or from overdosage. Digoxin toxicity is exaggerated by electrolyte disorders (hypokalemia, hypomagnesemia, or intravenous calcium administration). Bradycardia, P-R interval prolongation (greater than 50 percent of pretreatment), second- or third-degree heart block, ventricular tachycardia, or ventricular fibrillation all may occur. When digoxin toxicity is suspected; (1) discontinue digoxin, (2) draw blood for digoxin level and serum electrolyte levels, (3) induce vomiting and give activated charcoal to impair drug absorption, (4) correct electrolyte disorders, and (5) monitor cardiac rhythm. For the treatment of bradycardia, atropine (0.01 mg per kilogram per dose intravenously) or the insertion of a temporary transvenous pacemaker may be necessary. Phenytoin (5 mg per kilogram per dose) is the drug of choice for ventricular arrhythmias caused by digoxin toxicity. Recently, antibodies to digoxin have been created that when infused accelerate the removal of free digoxin from the body.

In critically ill infants and children who need rapid inotropic support, *intravenous catecholamines* may be used. Dopamine, isoproterenol, dobutamine, norepinephrine, and epinephrine have been used with varying effects. Dopamine has beta$_1$, and beta$_2$ adrenergic, and dopaminergic effects at low doses. The beta adrenergic effects tend to increase cardiac output primarily by increasing myocardial contractility, but also by increasing heart rate. The dopaminergic effects increase renal blood flow and may improve renal function. Heart rate increases frequently with dopamine infusions. The renal effect of dopamine occurs at doses of 1 to 3 μg per kilogram per minute. Doses of 5 to 10 μg per kilogram per minute are used for increasing cardiac output. Doses of higher than 15 μg per kilogram per minute have strong alpha adrenergic effects; the renal effect is lost, and tachycardia occurs.

Isoproterenol has pure beta-adrenergic effects. It increases heart rate and myocardial contractility, resulting in increased cardiac output and elevation of systolic blood pressure. The diastolic blood pressure usually decreases,

TABLE 4 Drug Dosages of Digoxin

Age	Digitalization	Maintenance
Premature	20–25 μg/kg PO TDD ½, ¼, ¼ q8h or	5–8 μg/kg/day q12h PO
	15–20 μg/kg IV TDD same schedule	4–6 μg/kg/day q12h IV
Full-term newborns and infants	40–50 μg/kg PO TDD same schedule or	10–12 μg/kg/day q12h PO
	30–40 μg/kg IV TDD same schedule	8–10 μg/kg/day q12h IV
Children	20–40 μg/kg PO TDD same schedule maximum TDD 1.0 mg IV or 15–30 mg/kg IV TDD	8 μg/kg/day q12h PO maximum dose 0.25 mg/day

TABLE 5 Drug Dosages of Vasodilators

Drug	Dosage	Route	Site of Effect
Nitroglycerin	0.5–20 μg/kg/min (maximum 60 μg/kg/min)	IV	Venous
Hydralazine	0.1–0.8 mg/kg/dose q4–6h over 30 min	IV	Arterial
	0.15 mg/kg/dose q6–8h (maximum 7 mg/kg/day)	PO	
Captopril	0.1–1.0 mg/kg/dose q6h	PO	Arterial
Nitroprusside	0.5–8.0 μg/kg/min	IV	Combined
Prazosin	5–25 μg/kg/dose q6h	PO	Combined

resulting in a wide pulse pressure. In patients with CHF produced by bradycardia, isoproterenol is the drug of choice. Side effects include tachycardia, arrhythmias, and myocardial ischemia. The starting dose is 0.05 to 0.10 μg per kilogram per minute.

Dobutamine is an analogue of isoproterenol. It has beta$_1$ selectivity and little effect on heart rate. It may also have myocardial alpha-adrenergic effects. Dobutamine primarily increases contractilit, stroke volume, and cardiac output. There is no direct effect on renal blood flow. The starting dose is 2 μg per kilogram per minute (maximum 40 μg per kilogram per minute).

Norepinephrine has potent alpha-adrenergic and myocardial beta$_1$-adrenergic effects, which produce elevation of systolic blood pressure. The starting dose is 0.05 μg per kilogram per minute and may be increased to 1.0 μg per kilogram per minute. Epinephrine has dose-dependent effects. At low doses, beta$_1$ myocardial effects and beta$_2$ peripheral vascular adrenergic effects predominate, resulting in increased cardiac output and widening of the pulse pressure. At higher doses, alpha-adrenergic effect occurs, producing elevation of the systolic and diastolic blood pressure. The starting dose is 0.05 μg per kilogram per minute and may be increased to 1.0 μg per kilogram per minute. Norepinephrine and epinephrine are useful in maintaining cardiac output and blood pressure in patients who are unresponsive to dopamine.

The use of *vasodilators* to decrease the afterload of the myocardium is the most recent addition to the treatment of CHF in infants and children. The primary goal is to lower systemic vascular resistance and augment myocardial function by decreasing the resistance to left ventricular ejection. These drugs are helpful in the management of mitral or aortic regurgitation, systemic hypertension, cardiomyopathy, or myocardial ischemia. Nitrates are venodilators. Hydralazine and captopril are arterial dilators, while nitroprusside and prazosin are both arterial and venodilators (Table 5).

Supraventricular tachycardia (SVT) and complete heart block can cause CHF in newborns and young infants. The treatment of choice for SVT with CHF is syn-chronized cardioversion (1 to 2 joules per kilogram). Cardioversion is followed by the administration of digitalis to prevent recurrences of SVT. In young patients without CHF, vagal maneuvers, including carotid massage, rectal stimulation, or placing an icebag over the face for 30 seconds (diving reflex) are sometimes effective. If vagal maneuvers fail, drug therapy is indicated. Verapamil (0.1 mg per kilogram intravenously given over 30 seconds), a calcium-channel blocker, is usually effective in terminating SVT. Hypotension can occur and is treated by the administration of calcium chloride (10 mg per kilogram). Pretreatment with calcium chloride may prevent hypotension. Verapamil is contraindicated in infants under 12 months of age. Digoxin is frequently used in the treatment of SVT but takes several hours to take effect (see Table 4). Propranolol (0.01 mg per kilogram per dose) is effective in terminating SVT. Sinus bradycardia and myocardial dysfunction may occur. Propranolol should not be used with verapamil because severe hypotension and cardiovascular collapse may occur. Phenylephrine (0.02 mg per kilogram intravenously slowly) and edrophonium chloride (Tensilon)(2.0 mg intravenously for infants, or 5.0 mg intravenously for children) may also terminate episodes of SVT.

If *complete heart block or bradycardia* is causing CHF, then atropine (0.01 mg per kilogram per dose) or isoproterenol may increase heart rate and decrease the signs and symptoms of CHF. The insertion of a temporary transvenous pacemaker should be considered if drug therapy does not increase the heart rate. Other types of cardiac dysrhythmias are uncommon in infants and children.

SUGGESTED READING

Friedman WF, George BL. New concepts and drugs in the treatment of congestive heart failure. Pediatr Clin North AM 1984; 31:1197–1227.

Hoffman JIE, Stanger P. Congestive heart failure. In: Rudolph AM, ed. Pediatrics. 17th ed. Norwalk, Conn: Appleton-Century-Crofts, 1982;1352.

Talner NS. Heart failure. In: Adams FH, Emmanouilides GC, eds. Heart disease in infants, children, and adolescents. 3rd ed. Baltimore: Williams and Wilkins, 1983;708.

PEDIATRIC DYSRHYTHMIA AND OTHER CARDIAC EMERGENCIES

PAUL C. GILLETTE, M.D., F.A.C.C.

Many emergency situations in children are due to cardiovascular abnormalities. These may be either primary or secondary. When treating noncardiac emergencies the effects on the heart should always be considered. This chapter focuses on primary cardiovascular emergencies, discussing clinical situations as they would present to the clinician. Children do not always have the same disease etiologies or responses to treatment as do adults, so adult treatment guidelines cannot be indiscriminately applied.

The history and phsyical examination should be carried out as soon as possible, i.e., as soon as the patient is stabilized or by one physician while the patient is being stabilized by a second physician. Virtually all pediatric cardiac emergencies need immediate pediatric consultation and admission to the hospital.

CARDIOVASCULAR COLLAPSE

Cardiovascular collapse may be attributable to one of several etiologies. When confronted with this situation one should begin cardiac (and if appropriate pulmonary) resuscitation according to the American Heart Association guidelines. The electrocardiogram (ECG) immediately differentiates electromechanical dissociation from asystole, a tachyarrhythmia, or ventricular fibrillation. Each of these rhythms may present as essentially absent pulse and blood pressure. Each is obviously treated differently. In the rare case in which an ECG is not available but a defibrillator is, defibrillation is indicated with 1 watt-sec per pound. This may convert a tachydysrhythmia and does not cause further harm in the presence of hypovolemia or bradycardia.

BRADYCARDIA OR ASYSTOLE

If the diagnosis of severe symptomatic bradycardia is made by ECG or by the presence of a slow but full pulse, then atropine 0.04 mg per kilogram intravenously (IV) should be given. This often improves atrioventricular conduction or increases sinus rate in children. Intravenous isoproterenol (Table 1) 0.1 microgram per kilogram per minute often increases atrioventricular (AV) conduction or sinus bradycardia, but it may also cause premature ventricular contractions (PVCs) hypotension, or more serious ventricular arrhythmias. Temporary pacing may be carried out noninvasively if one of the new external transcutaneous pacemakers is available or by the transthoracic route. Transvenous pacing takes longer but is useful in less acute situations.

VENTRICULAR FIBRILLATION

Ventricular fibrillation (VF) is an ECG diagnosis. Once it is made the treatment is defibrillation using 1 watt-sec per pound. If VF is not converted, higher doses may be used. If it is converted and recurs, there is no need for a higher dose. Xylocaine 1 mg per kilogram IV (Table 2) should be given before the next defibrillation. If VF recurs again, bretylium tosylate 5 mg per kilogram IV should be given; this is successful even in the face of digitalis toxicity.

WIDE QRS TACHYCARDIA

A wide QRS tachycardia is always a true medical emergency. In a pediatric patient it should be assumed to be ventricular, although in a few it may be due to Wolff-Parkinson-White syndrome. Virtually no pediatric supraventricular tachycardias are continuously aberrant. Verapamil and digitalis are very dangerous in ventricular tachycardia, so great precautions must be taken to avoid giving them. Instead, the wide QRS tachycardia should be treated by synchronized direct current (DC) cardioversion using 1 watt-sec per pound. Synchronization is important to avoid inducing VF. Intravenous lidocaine may work in some cases, but it is not as reliable as cardioversion. Recurrences may be treated with repeat cardioversion after lidocaine 1 mg per kilogram or procainamide 15 mg per kilogram IV over 30 to 60 minutes. Intravenous phenytoin 15 mg per kilogram over 60 minutes is useful in some ventricular tachycardias, especially in postoperative patients and in digitalis toxicity. Propranolol is also sometimes useful if there is not an underlying cardiomyopamy.

TABLE 1 Intravenous Iontropic Drugs

Drug	Dosage
Isoproterenol	0.05–0.4 μg/kg/min
Dobutamine	2–20 μg/kg/min
Dopamine	2–20 μg/kg/min
Amrinone	0.5–1 mg/kg
Calcium chloride	100–200 mg

TABLE 2 Intravenous Doses of Antiarrhythmic Drugs

Drug	Dosage
Verapamil	0.15 mg/kg over 3 minutes
Lidocaine	1 mg/kg
Bretylium	5 mg/kg
Phenytoin	15 mg/kg over 60 minutes
Procainamide	15 mg/kg over 60 minutes
Propranolol	0.1 mg/kg over 10 minutes

IRREGULAR WIDE QRS TACHYCARDIA

An irregular wide QRS tachycardia is rare in pediatrics, but it is usually due to atrial fibrillation in a patient with Wolff-Parkinson-White syndrome. It should be treated with synchronized DC cardioversion. Intravenous digitalis or verapamil often leads to VF.

NARROW (NORMAL) QRS TACHYCARDIA

Narrow QRS tachycardia is often, but not always, an emergency. It depends on the heart rate and clinical status of the patient and how well he maintains cardiac output under these conditions. One particular narrow QRS tachycardia is particularly dangerous. A narrow QRS tachycardia with AV dissociation, with junctional rate faster than atrial, is virtually always due to an automatic focus in the bundle of His. It will not respond to cardioversion or other usual measures, and verapamil often worsens it. Hemodynamic support should be given with digitalis. The addition of oral propranolol or amiodarone often slows the rate, but 50 percent die in the next year anyway. The patient should be admitted so that the bundle of His can be destroyed and a pacemaker implanted.

Ninety percent of narrow QRS tachycardias with AV association are due to reentry, usually at least partially involving the AV node. They may, therefore, respond to vagal maneuvers such as the diving reflex or carotid sinus massage. The diving reflex (reflex bradycardia and vagal stimulation) is provoked by placing the patient's face in cold (ice) water and having him hold his breath for 15 to 30 seconds. Increases in effective vagal tone by Neo-Synephrine (0.01 to 0.1 mg per kilogram) to elevate the blood pressure or Tensilon 0.1 mg per kilogram may also be effective. In the emergent patient, synchronized DC cardioversion is the treatment of choice using 0.25 watt-sec per pound. In less sick patients, intravenous verapamil 0.15 mg per kilogram IV over 3 minutes is safe and effective in children over 1 year of age who do not have sick sinus syndrome or cardiomyopathy. Atropine and calcium chloride should be immediately available to treat bradycardia or hypotension. Verapamil in infants younger than 1 year causes an unacceptable incidence of cardiovascular collapse. Overdrive pacing, through either a right atrial catheter or a transesophageal electrode, may convert a supraventricular tachycardia, but special equipment is necessary, limiting its usefulness.

THE CYANOTIC NEWBORN

The management of the cyanotic newborn has improved markedly in the past 5 years. We now recognize that the anatomic diagnosis of the heart defect is not immediately necessary. The differentiation of heart and lung disease can often be made by history and physical. The hyperoxygenation test with 100 percent oxygen is also useful. If the PaO_2 is increased to over 110, a significant cyanotic congenital heart defect is very unlikely. If the PaO_2 after 100 percent O_2 is under 100, prostaglandins should be begun at 0.1 microgram per kilogram per minute to stimulate ductus arteriosus opening and the infant should be transferred to a cardiac center. Precautions against apnea must be taken during transfer either by intubating and ventilating the patient or by sending a professional capable of doing this on the transport. The exact anatomic diagnosis is made in an essentially well infant at the cardiac center, and further treatment carried out. In the patient in whom 100 percent FIO_2 does not appreciably increase PaO_2, then room air should be used.

THE PULSELESS INFANT

Many infants with severe congestive heart failure have weak pulses, but the truly pulseless infant usually has severe obstruction to left ventricular outflow. Many of these infants can be salvaged. In addition to supportive measures such as intubation, ventilation, digitalis, and diuretics, prostaglandins often allow the right ventricle to perfuse the body.

HYPERCYANOTIC SPELLS

Hypercyanotic spells can occur in infants and children with cyanotic congenital heart disease. They are characterized by irritability, hyperventilation, and increased cyanosis. Because pulmonary blood flow is very decreased, it matters little what the FIO_2 is. If giving the child O_2 causes him to be more irritable, it should not be done. The knee-chest position is very helpful, as is anything that calms the child. Morphine sulfate 0.01 mg per kilogram subcutaneously often aborts the spell. Intravenous Neo-Synephrine 0.01 to 0.1 mg per kilogram IV increases systemic resistance and, therefore, pulmonary blood flow. Intravenous propranolol 0.1 mg per kilogram may also help hypercyanotic spells.

SEIZURES IN CHILDREN

RONALD DIECKMANN, M.D., M.P.H., F.A.A.P., F.A.C.E.P.

EPIDEMIOLOGY

The childhood seizure is a common problem in the emergency department. About 5 percent of all children have one or more seizures before they are 16 years of age. Of those who have any seizures during life, 75 percent experience their first event before age 20. Epilepsy, a chronic condition of recurrent seizures, fortunately develops in only a small proportion of patients.

Usually, the seizure has occurred prior to arrival in the emergency department and has lasted less than 10 minutes. A "prolonged seizure" is one of longer than 10 minutes' duration. "Convulsion" refers to a seizure with primarily motor manifestations. "Status epilepticus" is continuous seizure activity, or recurrent seizures without intervening return of consciousness, for more than 30 minutes.

CLASSIFICATION

Seizures may be generalized or focal. Generalized forms include grand mal, petit mal (absence seizures), or myoclonic seizures (infantile spasms). Focal or "partial seizures" include motor, sensory, or complex (psychomotor)seizures. An acute focal seizure may evolve into a generalized seizure.

Status epilepticus may be either generalized grand mal or generalized petit mal. It may also present as a continuous focal seizure, with consciousness preserved.

The emergency physician is most often called upon to treat the grand mal convulsion, since it is dramatic and unmistakable and usually prompts an urgent quest for medical assistance. Also, it is convulsive grand mal status epilepticus that is most dangerous and demands the most skillful medical intervention.

CAUSES

The causes of seizures in children are multiple (see Table 1). The most frequent causes are (1) fever; (2) drug noncompliance in a child with known epilepsy; (3) head trauma; (4) intracranial infection; (5) metabolic disturbance; and (6) poisoning. In the neonatal period, hypoxia or hemorrhage from birth injuries, metabolic disorders, and infections represent the most important causes.

A disciplined approach to seizure management minimizes sequelae from the acute electrical and metabolic derangements and averts iatrogenic complications. Emergency treatment must focus first on stopping the seizure and reversing the metabolic imbalance, then on establishing cause. Later, long-term prophylactic anticonvulsant therapy and appropriate neurologic follow-up examinations are considered.

MANAGEMENT OF THE ACTIVE SEIZURE

A child in seizure on arrival in the emergency department is usually in status epilepticus. Hypoxia, acidosis, increased intracranial pressure, hypoglycemia, and hyperthermia may be present and, together with the disordered electrical activity, pose a major neurologic emergency.If status epilepticus is not stopped, Hypotension eventually ensues, with cardiovascular, respiratory, and renal failure. Mortality may reach 10 to 12 percent, and brain injury is almost universal after 60 minutes.

The first response is to *open and secure the patient's airway*. Gentle hyperextension of the neck, with chin thrust or jaw lift, permits placement of a mechanical airway device. The head should be held or otherwise softly restrained during the acute convulsive period.

Next, *assist breathing*, after careful suctioning of the airway to remove blood, secretions, and foreign objects. Tight-fitting clothing should be loosened. Administer 100 percent oxygen by nasal cannula. Bag-mask, mouth-to-mouth, or mouth-to-nose-and-mouth ventilation may be indicated if the child remains cyanotic. However, hypoventilation with hypercapnia and hypoxemia, along with metabolic acidosis, is expected. These derangements will typically correct themselves with cessation of the convulsion and with general supportive measures. Intubation, for airway protection or mechanical ventilation or both, is rarely necessary and should usually be withheld until the patient fails to respond to initial medical management. A cardiac monitor discloses significant rate, rhythm, or conduction abnormalities.

Once airway and breathing are established, *obtain vascular access*, draw blood, and begin pharmacologic therapy. We administer 50 percent dextrose in water at 1 ml per kilogram in the older child, or 25 percent dextrose in water at 2 ml per kilogram in the infant. Naloxone may be given at 0.01 mg per kilogram. If active seizure activity continues, *diazepam*, 0.3 mg per kilogram, is immediately infused by slow intravenous injection, at 1 mg per minute. The maximum doses are 3 to 5 mg in children under 5 years, and 5 to 10 mg in those over 5 years.

Gaining venous access is often the limiting step in emergency control of the child with seizures. Peripheral veins are usually present in the scalp, neck, or extremities. Sometimes, however, an intravenous route cannot be readily secured, or a peripheral line is inadvertently lost. Saphenous vein cutdown, although often difficult in the young child, is one recourse for the experienced clinician. Other routes for rapid access are either *intraosseous* or *endotracheal*. Deep-vein cannulation of the internal jugular or subclavian veins in the child in seizure is fraught with hazards and should not ordinarily be performed in the emergency department.

The *intraosseous route* is a safe and effective method of drug administration in children. We prefer either the

TABLE 1 Common Causes of Seizures in Childhood

Acute:
  Fever
  Noncompliance with anticonvulsants
  Head trauma
  Intracranial infection
  Metabolic problems
    Hypoglycemia
    Hyponatremia
    Hypocalcemia
    Pyridoxine deficiency
    Phenylketonuria
    Pertussis vaccine
  Poisoning
    Lead
    Sympathomimetics (phencyclidine, cocaine, LSD, amphetamine)
    Aspirin
    Isoniazid
    Theophylline
    Hydrocarbons
    Antidepressants
    Phenothiazines
  Hypertensive encephalopathy
  Renal failure
  Hepatic failure and Reye's syndrome
  Brain tumor
  Brain hemorrhage

Chronic
  Posthypoxic
  Posthemorrhagic
  Postinfectious
  Post-traumatic
  Degenerative disease
  Developmental defects
  Idiopathic

midline distal femur (2 cm above the patella) or a midline proximal tibial site. Once the area is prepared, an 18- or 20-gauge spinal needle with stylet is inserted at a 60-degree angle to the bone axis, into the marrow cavity. A bolus of 10 ml of normal saline is injected to assure proper catheter placement (by low resistance to injection). The needle is then carefully secured to the overlying skin. Diazepam may then be slowly infused into the intraosseous space.

The intraosseous route offers an effective conduit for administration of other essential drugs and fluids. Additional anticonvulsants may be given, as well as sodium bicarbonate, calcium, dextrose, dopamine and other inotropic drips, or blood products. Multiple intraosseous lines may be useful in emergency circumstances requiring several infusion sites. Cumulative experience at our institution and elsewhere indicates a complication rate of less than 1 percent with this procedure. Complications have included osteomyelitis, abscesses, and stress fractures.

When vascular access is impossible, a route of last resort for diazepam administration, is the *endotracheal* tube. Intubation of the child with a seizure is quite hazardous; airway trauma, aspiration, and gastric intubation are not uncommon sequelae. However, if no intravenous or intraosseous line is available, endotracheal intubation becomes necessary. Diazepam is injected directly into the trachea through an infant feeding tube inserted past the distal tip of the endotracheal tube, after dilution to 3 ml with distilled water or normal saline. Bag ventilation disperses the drug distally for rapid absorption into the tracheobronchial tree.

Most children stop seizing within minutes of receiving diazepam. Its pharmacologic activity, however, is 15 minutes or less. Multiple administrations of diazepam in the emergency department should be avoided because of the potential for unpredictable and sudden respiratory depression and hypotension. These effects are potentiated in a patient who is already being treated with phenobarbital. Therefore, after the first diazepam dose, a second anticonvulsant with longer duration of action is given.

Our pharmacologic approach to status epilepticus is outlined in Table 2. Oxygen, dextrose, and naloxone are given, followed by diazepam. The child under 12 months should receive 100 mg of pyridoxine. The patient is then loaded with 20 mg per kilogram of *phenytoin*. The drug is infused in normal saline at 1 mg per kilogram per minute, (20 mg per minute maximum) with the patient on a cardiac monitor. The infusion is stopped for blood pressure drops of more than 10 mm, for second- or third-degree heart block, or for bradycardia.

If the seizure continues 30 minutes after administration of both diazepam and phenytoin, or if the child is below 1 month of age, give *phenobarbital*, 20 mg per kilogram, at 1 to 2 mg per kilogram per minute. (In the neonate, reverse the order, so that phenobarbital is administered first, phenytoin second.) The child should be monitored closely for hypotension and respiratory depression. Capability for emergency intubation should be readily available.

Rarely, status epilepticus continues after maximum doses of diazepam, phenytoin, and phenobarbital. Paraldehyde or lidocaine is the next choice of drug. Paraldehyde is administered at 0.3 ml per kilogram diluted 1:2 in mineral oil, high in the rectum. The buttocks are then taped. Lidocaine may also be useful; it is given at a 1 mg per kilogram bolus, then 20 to 50 μg per kilogram per minute. If paraldehyde or lidocaine is unsuccessful within 20 minutes, pentobarbital coma is indicated. Pentobarbital doses are 5 mg per kilogram each hour for 2 hours, then 1 to 2 mg per kilogram per hour thereafter; the patient must be intubated and carefully monitored in an intensive care area.

SEARCH FOR THE CAUSE

Once the seizure has stopped, the practitioner must search for a specific etiology. A history obtained from the parents or supervising adult is essential, beginning with a precise description of the seizure itself. Breath-holding spells, syncope, and night terrors must be distinguished. Noncompliance with anticonvulsant therapy in an epileptic patient is frequent. A history of head trauma, fever, infection, alcohol consumption, or drug use (including aspirin, acetaminophen, and isoniazid) may provide a likely etiology. Consider poisoning with drugs (e.g., phencyclidine, cocaine, amphetamines) or other household

TABLE 2 Pharmacologic Management of Status Epilepticus

Drug	Dose	Route	Rate	Complications
First Line Agents				
Oxygen	100%	Nasal cannula, Mask, endotracheal	Maximum	None with brief use
Dextrose	D50W at 1 ml/kg D25W at 2 ml/kg (Infants)	IV, intraosseous	Bolus	Hyperosmolality
Naloxone	0.01 mg/kg	IV, IM, intraosseous, endotracheal	Bolus	None
Diazepam	0.3 mg/kg	IV, intraosseous, endotrachal	1 mg/min	Respiratory arrest, hypotension
Pyridoxine	100 mg (Infants)	IV	Bolus	None
Phenytoin	20 mg/kg	IV, intraosseous	1 mg/kg/min (0.5 mg/kg/min in infants)	Heart block, bradycardia hypotension
Second Line Agents				
Phenobarbital	20 mg/kg	IV, IM, intraosseous	1-2 mg/kg/min	Respiratory arrest, hypotension
Last Line Agents				
Paraldehyde	0.3 ml/kg	Per rectum, diluted 1:2 in mineral oil	Bolus	Pulmonary edema, coma, hypotension
Lidocaine	1 mg/kg	IV, intraosseous	Bolus, then 20–50 μg/kg/min	Respiratory depression, bradycardia, hypotension
Pentobarbital	5 mg/kg/hr for 2hrs	IV, IM	Bolus, then 1–2 mg/kg/hr	Respiratory arrest, hypotension

products (e.g., insecticides, hydrocarbons). Document both a developmental history and family history of epilepsy.

Attention to age-adjusted vital signs is next. Abnormalities of heart rate or rhythm may suggest poisoning (e.g., tricyclics, theophylline). Reduced blood pressure may indicate hemodynamic insult (e.g., trauma, sepsis). Persistent temperature elevation suggests a febrile seizure, meningitis, or encephalitis.

Physical examination should especially exclude head trauma, bulging fontanel, papilledema, meningitis, focal neurologic signs, cutaneous lesions, evidence of systemic disease, or developmental lags.

Laboratory tests include arterial blood gases, complete blood count, glucose level, electrolyte determinations, lead level, calcium and magnesium levels, liver function tests, renal function tests, urinalysis, ammonia, toxicology screen, and pertinent drug levels. A urine spot test for amino acids is indicated for infants. Patients on anticonvulsants should have specific serum levels tested.

Spinal fluid analysis is necessary in selected seizure patients who present with *fever* and *any* of the following additional characteristics: (1) age less than 18 months; (2) meningeal irritation on physical examination; (3) prolonged seizure or status epilepticus; (4) focal seizure or focal neurologic examination; and (5) high fever over 24 hours' duration (makes febrile seizure unlikely).

A computerized tomographic (CT) brain scan may be invaluable, especially in the patient with an *afebrile* seizure. This study may be useful in several patient groups: (1) the older child, with or without fever, with focal neurologic examination results or a history of a focal seizure (CT should precede lumbar puncture in this group); (2) afebrile patients with findings of increased intracranial pressure; (3) children with alterations of consciousness, persisting after the expected postictal period; and (4) those experiencing an early post-traumatic seizure (less than 24 hours after trauma).

Indications for CT in childhood seizures, however, are fewer in the young *febrile* child. Meningitis in children under two years of age may manifest with focal abnormalities and prolonged postictal confusion. Lumbar puncture and immediate antibiotic administration should not be delayed for CT when clinical suspicion is strong for central nervous system infection.

Skull x-ray films and electroencephalograms, both useful ancillary tests in work-ups for some types of seizures, are usually not indicated in the emergency department.

CRITERIA FOR HOSPITAL ADMISSION

Occurrence of a seizure in a child may require hospital admission for neurologic monitoring, further search for etiology, or specific treatment. A frequent management dilemma is the febrile seizure. Patients between the ages of 18 months and 6 years who do not have signs of meningeal irritation can usually be discharged to stable home environments. Parent education concerning temperature reduction with antipyretics and tepid bathing should be part of the general reassurance of the benign nature of the simple febrile seizure. Only 2 to 3 percent of children with a single or recurrent simple febrile seizure develop epilepsy. Therefore, no anticonvulsant therapy is needed. If the cause of the fever is bacterial infection, antibiotics are, of course, also part of outpatient therapy of this group.

While the simple febrile seizure is usually benign, a small subgroup of children with febrile seizures is at high risk for recurrent *afebrile* seizures. This subgroup requires hospitalization and anticonvulsant therapy. (Phenobarbital is the agent of choice.) High risk is defined by the presence of two or more of the following characteristics: (1) age less than 18 months; (2) *complex* first seizure: focal onset, postictal neurologic abnormalities, or more than 15 minutes' duration; (3) prior neurologic or developmental abnormalities; (4) history of epilepsy in the nuclear family.

Other seizure patients requiring hospitalization include those presenting in status epilepticus; those with first seizures that are not simple febrile seizures; noncompliant epileptics with unstable home situations; and epileptics with changing seizure patterns that are not controlled on current anticonvulsants.

LONG-TERM MANAGEMENT

For the treated epileptic who is presenting with a new seizure, management is based on serum anticonvulsant levels. If levels are subtherapeutic, the physician is alerted to possible noncompliance or drug underdosing. If levels are adequate, the physician is directed toward careful search for precipitating systemic or central nervous system insults. Modification of the drug regimen is often required.

Generally, consideration for long-term anticonvulsant therapy should be coordinated with the child's pediatrician or primary care physician. Successful outpatient management of the epileptic is premised on a consistent physician-patient relationship. Committing a child to long-term anticonvulsant drug therapy is not ordinarily the responsibility of the emergency physician.

SUGGESTED READINGS

Aicardi J, Chevrie JJ. Convulsive status epilepticus in infants and children: A study of 239 cases. Epilepsia 1970; 11:187-197.
Fishman M. Febrile seizures: The treatment controversy. J Pediatr 1979; 94:177-184.
Livingston S. Comprehensive management of epilepsy in infancy, childhood and adolescence. Springfield, Illinois: Thomas Press, 1972.
Rothner AD, Erenberg G. Status Epilepticus. Pediatr Clin North Am 1980; 27:593-602.
Simon RP. Management of status epilepticus. In: Pedley TA Meldrum BS, eds. Recent advances in epilepsy. Edinburgh: Churchill Livingstone Press, 1985:137.

SEPSIS IN CHILDREN

MARK W. KLINE, M.D.
SHELDON L. KAPLAN, M.D.

The term *septicemia* refers to systemic disease caused by the presence of bacteria in the blood stream. *Bacteremia* is the preferred term when bacteria are recovered from the blood of a patient who does not appear seriously ill. A substantial percentage of febrile children without signs of localized infection or with trivial illnesses such as pharyngitis or otitis media have positive blood cultures, even though they may look well enough to be treated on an outpatient basis. This condition has been referred to as occult bacteremia. Although bacteremia can be transient and self-limited, its presence calls for an organized diagnostic and therapeutic approach aimed at eliminating infection and correcting or preventing its sequelae.

The bacteremic or septicemic child may present in a variety of ways, determined in part by age. In the young infant, symptoms and signs of septicemia are frequently subtle and nonspecific. Temperature imbalance with hyperthermia or hypothermia, tachypnea, tachycardia, apnea, lethargy, vomiting, a change in feeding pattern, or refusal to eat may be noted. The septicemic infant is frequently inattentive to the environment, irritable, and difficult to console. Jaundice, petechiae, or seizures may be the only observed findings in some young infants. Shock and disseminated intravascular coagulation (DIC) are late and ominous findings. The incidence of septicemia in otherwise normal newborns up to 1 month of age is about 1 per 1,000 live births. The incidence is increased by a number of perinatal factors, such as maternal abruptio placentae, placenta praevia, toxemia, prolonged rupture of the membranes, and chorioamnionitis. Infants born prematurely are at greater risk for infection. Any microorganism may cause septicemia in the newborn, and acquisition of the organism may follow vertical transmission from the mother or occur via environmental or nosocomial sources. Up to 1 month of age, the most common bacterial pathogens are the group B streptococcus and *Escherichia coli*. Other streptococci and gram-negative enteric organsims such as *Klebsiella pneumoniae* are less prevalent, but are serious causes of infection in this age group. *Listeria monocytogenes*, a gram-positive coccobacillus, has a well-known predilection for causing septicemia and meningitis in the young infant.

The older infant or child with bacteremia or septicemia may present with a spectrum of findings, ranging from fever alone to lethargy, irritability, or shock. The history and physical examination may reveal a focus of infection and heighten the suspicion of blood stream invasion. In the immunologically normal child between 1 month and several years of age, the most prevalent pathogens are *Haemophilus influenzae* type b, *Streptococcus pneumoniae,* and *Neisseria meningitidis.* The presence of generalized petechiae is particularly suggestive of septicemia caused by *N. meningitidis.* Septicemia in a patient with impetiginous lesions or a history of recent trauma may be due to *Staphylococcus aureus* or *Streptococcus pyogenes.* The child with hemoglobinopathy (especially sickle cell disease) or with anatomic or functional asplenia is predisposed to overwhelming infection with *Streptococcus pneumoniae* or *H. influenzae* type b and also has an increased risk of septicemia produced by *Salmonella.* In the older child and adolescent, *H. influenzae* type b assumes less prominence as a pathogen, while *Streptococcus pneumoniae* and *N. meningitidis* remain important causes of septicemia.

A diagnosis of presumptive septicemia is made on the basis of the history and physical examination. A high index of suspicion is warranted, particularly in the young infant. Any newborn or young infant manifesting one of the aforementioned subtle signs of septicemia at home should be transported expeditiously to a clinic or emergency department for evaluation. Usually, this is accomplished safely by the parents' own means of transportation. On occasion, infants with unstable vital signs, apnea, or seizures need to be transported from the home to the clinic or from one medical facility to another by ambulance. Ideally, such infants should have a secure intravenous line in place prior to transport. Endotracheal intubation may be indicated in the newborn who is experiencing severe apnea or respiratory distress. The child in shock must be stabilized, and empiric antibiotic therapy should be initiated, if feasible, before transfer.

In the emergency department, the infant or child with presumed septicemia is evaluated first for adequacy of the airway and stability of vital signs. Then a diagnostic work-up is initiated. A complete blood count with differential white cell count and preferably two blood cultures should be obtained from every child. Urine is collected for analysis and culture. In an infant, this is best accomplished by either catheterization or suprapubic aspiration of urine. Countercurrent immune electrophoresis (CIE) or latex particle agglutination may be performed on urine, serum, or cerebrospinal fluid for the rapid detection of several of the prevalent pathogens (e.g., *H. influenzae* type b, *Streptococcus pneumoniae, N. meningitidis,* or group B *Streptococcus*). A lumbar puncture should be performed on any child with meningeal signs or other findings suspicious for meningitis. Infants less than 6 to 9 months of age frequently fail to manifest meningeal signs even in the face of documented bacterial meningitis, so patients in that age group with presumed septicemia should probably have a lumber puncture as a matter of routine. Since pneumonia is difficult to diagnose clinically in infants and young children, a chest roentgenogram should be obtained.

Oxygen by mask or hood is begun on any child with signs of shock. If severe respiratory distress or periods of apnea are noted, endotracheal intubation may be indicated. A 3.0- to 3.5-mm uncuffed endotracheal tube suffices in most newborn infants. A secure intravenous line is established. Generally, we empirically administer 5 percent dextrose in 0.2 percent sodium chloride at a maintenance rate of 1,600 ml per square meter body surface area every 24 hours initially, and adjust the composition and rate of administration based on the level of hydration, clinical setting, and initial laboratory data. If volume expansion is necessary for support of perfusion or blood pressure, we administer either normal saline or 5 percent albuminized saline. A 10 ml per kilogram bolus is given initially and is repeated if necessary. Caution should be exercised in the child with cardiac disease. Sympathomimetic amines may be necessary for additional support of perfusion and blood pressure. A combination of dopamine and dobutamine, each at an infusion rate of 5 to 10 μg per kilogram per minute is effective therapy for most patients with shock due to septicemic complications. The use of corticosteroids in septicemia patients with shock is controversial. We would administer either methylprednisolone, in a dose of 30 mg per kilogram, or dexamethasone, in a dose of 2 mg per kilogram initially, and repeat the dose once 4 to 6 hours later. DIC is a frequent concomitant to the shock state and should be documented and treated. Routine laboratory studies, as described for the stable patient with presumed septicemia, should be obtained as the clinical condition permits.

Our recommendations for initial antibiotic therapy in the patient with presumed septicemia are shown in Table 1. These are guidelines only. Specific clinical situations may necessitate deviation from this routine. Any systemically ill-appearing child with presumed septicemia should be admitted to the hospital for initiation of intravenous antibiotic therapy. If the clinical condition appears unstable in any way (e.g., changes in vital signs or perfusion, respiratory distress, or apnea), admission should be to an intensive care unit. We avoid chloramphenicol in the patient with shock because of its altered hepatic metabolism in that setting, and its cardiac depressant effects at toxic levels. We prefer cefotaxime over chloramphenicol in the 1- to 2-month old child with septicemia because of uncertainties about dosing and erratic serum levels of chloramphenicol in that age group. Although cefotaxime generally achieves adequate levels in cerebrospinal fluid for the treatment of meningitis due to susceptible organisms, we still prefer the combination of ampicillin and chloramphenicol for the older infant or child who has meningitis without signs of shock. The choice of antibiotics is reevaluated when culture results become available. The necessary duration of intravenous antibiotic therapy varies with the clinical situation and may range from 7 days in the patient with blood stream infection alone to a minimum of 10 days in the patient with meningitis and septicemia.

The *child with bacteremia* (i.e., bloodstream infec-

TABLE 1 Guidelines for Antibiotic Use in Children with Presumed Septicemia*

Category	Recommended Regimen	Precautions
Less than 1 month old with or without shock, no meningitis	Ampicillin 150 mg/kg/day in 4 divided doses, plus gentamicin 7.5 mg/kg/day in 3 divided doses	Follow renal function tests and urine output. Renal failure may necessitate dosing modification
Less than 1 month old, meningitis known or suspected	Ampicillin 300 mg/kg/day in 4 divided doses (after 100 mg/kg loading dose), plus gentamicin 7.5 mg/kg/day in 3 divided doses	A loading dose of aminoglycosides is not necessary
One to 2 months old with or without shock, no meningitis	Ampicillin 150 mg/kg/day in 6 divided doses, plus cefotaxime 100–150 mg/kg/day in 4 divided doses	
One to 2 months old, with or without shock, meningitis known or suspected	Ampicillin 300 mg/kg/day in 6 divided doses (after 100 mg/kg loading dose), plus cefotaxime 200 mg/kg/day in 4 divided doses	
Over 2 months old, without shock or meningitis	Ampicillin 150 mg/kg/day in 6 divided doses, plus chloramphenicol 50–75 mg/kg per day in 4 divided doses	Hepatic dysfunction may necessitate chloramphenicol modification
Over 2 months old, without shock, meningitis known or suspected	Ampicillin 300 mg/kg/day in 6 divided doses (after 100 mg/kg loading dose), plus chloramphenicol 75 mg/kg/day (age 2–6 months) or 100 mg/kg/day (>6 months) in 4 divided doses	Never give a loading dose of chloramphenicol
Over 2 months old, with shock, with or without meningitis	Ampicillin 300 mg/kg/day in 6 divided doses(after 100 mg/kg loading dose), plus cefotaxime 200 mg/kg/day in 4 divided doses. Cefuroxime 200 mg/kg/day in 4 divided doses can be used in place of ampicillin and cefotaxime for children over 3 months of age	

* If staphylococcal disease is suspected clinically, nafcillin or methicillin may be substituted for ampicillin at a similar dosage and interval.

tion without evident systemic illness) may be managed somewhat differently. We would admit to the hospital any child with suspected bacteremia who is under 6 months of age and we would initiate intravenous antibiotic therapy. A syndrome of occult bacteremia has been described in children between 6 and 24 months of age. These children do not appear seriously ill, generally have rectal temperatures higher than 38.9° C (102 °F), and usually have total white blood cell counts of 15,000 per cubic millimeter or higher. Toxic granulation or Döhle's bodies may be evident on peripheral blood smears from these patients. About two-thirds of patients with occult bacteremia are infected with *Streptococcus pneumoniae*; most of the remainder have *H. influenzae* type b infection. In general, a child with the findings of occult bacteremia may be managed on an ambulatory basis with oral or intramuscular antibiotic therapy. If a positive blood culture is obtained, the patient should be reexamined carefully for signs of systemic illness or focal infection and the blood culture should be repeated. Hospital admission and initiation of intravenous antibiotics are indicated for the child who has failed to respond or deteriorated on outpatient management. This appears to occur more often in patients with infections caused by *H. influenzae* type b than in those with *Streptococcus pneumoniae* bacteremia.

SUGGESTED READING

Grossman M. Septicemia and septic shock. In: Rudolph AM, eds. Pediatrics. Norwalk: Appleton Century Crofts, 1982:509.

Klein JO, Marcy SM. Bacterial sepsis and meningitis. In: Remington JS, Klein JO, eds. Infectious diseases of the fetus and newborn infant. Philadelphia: WB Saunders, 1985:679.

Teele DW, Marshall R, Klein JO. Unsuspected bacteremia in young children. Pediatr Clin North AM 1979; 26:773–784.

REYE'S SYNDROME

DAVID B. SWEDLOW, M.D.
MARK S. SCHREINER, M.D.

EPIDEMIOLOGY, PATHOGENESIS, AND DIAGNOSIS

Reye's syndrome (RS) is an illness of unknown etiology that is characterized by diffuse fatty infiltration of the viscera with widespread impairment of mitochondrial function. The major clinical features include a viral prodrome followed by lethargy, vomiting, confusion, and agitation, with frequent progression to coma and death. RS is a disease of infancy and childhood, with only rare cases reported over age 18. There is no sex predilection. A prodromal viral illness is reported in most patients, with nonspecific upper respiratory tract infections accounting for 60 to 75 percent of cases, varicella for 20 to 30 percent, and gastroenteritis the remainder. RS following upper respiratory tract infections is largely attributable to influenza B infection, and to a lesser extent influenza A infection. Most cases occur in the winter months, and the total number of cases reflects the severity of the yearly influenza season.

RS is largely a disease of rural and suburban children with few cases occurring in urban areas. Less than 10 percent of cases occur in children less than one year, and more than 90 percent occur in children less than 15 years of age. Although only 5 to 6 percent of all cases occur in blacks, nearly half of all infant cases occur in black infants. The mortality rate has dropped from a high of 42 percent in 1977 to 22 percent in 1980. Part of the improvement in prognosis is represented by recognition of milder cases, which may be more common than previously thought.

RS is characterized by fatty infiltration of the viscera without evidence of inflammation. The pathologic findings in the liver are reversible. Patients who succumb usually die secondary to cerebral swelling. The etiology of the encephalopathy remains unknown.

The manifestations of hepatic dysfunction present as hypoglycemia, elevated serum transaminase concentrations, an elevated prothrombin time, and hyperammonemia.

Environmental and genetic factors may predispose individuals to RS in the setting of a viral illness, starvation, dehydration, fever, and possibly toxins. Of all the proposed toxins, *salicylates* have received the most attention. The Surgeon General of the United States has cautioned against the use of aspirin and other salicylate containing compounds in the treatment of children with flulike illnesses or with varicella. The American Academy of Pediatrics has recommended that "aspirin should not be prescribed under usual circumstances for children with varicella or those suspected of having influenza on the basis of clinical or epidemiologic evidence." The epidemiologic studies upon which these recommendations were based show a strong association with RS and aspirin usage, but a direct causal relationship has not yet been established. Although recent reviews detail some of the inherent difficulties with the studies implicating aspirin usage and RS, a conservative approach avoiding salicylates seems reasonable until additional data are available.

The fatal lesion in RS is *cerebral swelling*, which is probably attributable to a combination of cerebral hyperemia and edema. The cerebral swelling results in an elevation in intracranial pressure (ICP), which may result in local or global ischemia or frank herniation of cerebral contents from one intracranial compartment to another. Herniation results in compression of the arterial supply and ischemia.

DIAGNOSIS

The clinical history in an older child with RS is stereotypical. The child develops a viral illness, usually mild in severity. At first, the child appears to recover, but 3 to 8 days after the onset of the prodromal illness, the child becomes lethargic and mildly obtunded. If the illness progresses, the child develops persistent vomiting unrelieved by typical measures. (Antiemetics should not be used as they tend to be ineffective in controlling the persistent vomiting and merely cloud the clinical picture, with the result that diagnosis is delayed.)

The next step in the evolution of the illness is agitated delirium, with kicking, biting, and screaming very common. An adolescent may appear to have developed an acute psychosis or to have ingested a toxic drug. He may be violent and injure himself and others. With further progression, coma develops with posturing and brain stem abnormalities. Lastly, flaccidity, apnea, and death from cerebral swelling and herniation supervene. The progression of the illness is so typical that the National Institutes of Health has adopted standard staging criteria for the syndrome (shown in Table 1) based on the system proposed by Lovejoy in 1974.

The infant with RS usually presents with a different history from that in the older child. Vomiting is uncommon. Hyperpnea or apnea is often a part of the initial presentation as are seizures and coma. Black infants are represented disproportionately, account for nearly 50 percent of all cases in infancy, and constitute the majority of cases in the first 5 months of life. After 6 months of age, white patients predominate.

To make the diagnosis of Reye's syndrome, most of the diagnostic criteria shown in Table 2 should be met.

If a patient presents with a history consistent with the diagnosis, the *work-up* should begin in the emergency department to confirm the diagnosis and to exclude other possible causes of acute encephalopathy. A screen for toxins, including heavy metals, salicylates, phenothiazines, and street drugs, on blood, gastric contents, and urine should be obtained. Metabolic screening of urine will detect most urea cycle defects, which can present in the same fashion. Liver function studies should include transaminases, ammonia, PT, PTT, and bilirubin. The ammonia concentration is of diagnostic and prognostic significance. Serum levels greater than 300 μg per deciliter (normal, less than 48 μg per deciliter) are associated with an increased mortality. Blood chemistries help-

TABLE 1 Clinical Staging System Adopted by NIH

Stage 1 Precoma

The child presents with vomiting, lethargy, and indifference, but will obey commands. He does not lapse into sleep when undisturbed. There is laboratory evidence of liver dysfunction, including positive biopsy.

Stage II Precoma

The child demonstrates disorientation, delirium, and combativeness when aroused. Hyperventilation and hyperactive reflexes may be present. The child lapses into sleep when left undisturbed. He may be postictal. He usually responds appropriately to noxious stimuli.

Stage III Coma

The child is comatose with no verbalization or response to commands. There is no appropriate motor response to pain, but there may be generalized nonspecific responses including decorticate or decerebrate posturing or rigidity. Pupillary light reflexes are preserved, although dilated pupils may be seen. Oculovestibular and doll's eyes reflexes are intact.

Stage IV Coma

There is deepening coma with decerebrate posturing and rigidity. The oculocephalic and oculovestibular reflexes may be lost or dysconjugate. Large "fixed" pupils or hippus may be present. Other brain stem reflexes may be lost.

Stage V Coma

There is flaccidity, irregular or agonal respiration, fixed dilated pupils, and signs of herniation (asymmetrical pupils). There is loss of deep tendon reflexes and absence of brain stem reflexes. Spinal reflexes may be present.

ful for management include serum sodium, potassium, uric acid, phosphate, blood urea nitrogen, creatinine, and osmolarity. Many patients are dehydrated as a result of poor oral intake and persistent vomiting. A blood glucose level is essential to screen for hypoglycemia, especially in infants. A complete blood count should be obtained and blood for typing and cross-matching should be sent. Coagulopathies are common and often need to be corrected with fresh frozen plasma.

To rule out encephalitis or meningitis, a *lumbar puncture* should be performed. There is a potential risk of herniation in patients who may have an incresed intracranial pressure. However, the benefit of finding a treatable disease such as meningitis outweighs the potential risks in our view. We use a 22 or 25 gauge needle to minimize the extent of cerebrospinal fluid leakage.

TREATMENT

Because nearly 50 percent of all patients continue to progress after hospital admission from the presenting stage to a deeper clinical stage, we strongly urge that any child with stage II or more advanced RS be transferred to a tertiary care center experienced in the care of children with RS.

We direct therapy in RS to the reduction of elevated intracranial pressure, with the view that its successful con-

trol reduces the probability and severity of secondary damage.

Central to the goal of aggressive intracranial pressure reduction is the need to *monitor the intracranial pressure*. This technology requires experience and special equipment and should be performed at tertiary care centers experienced in the treatment of elevated intracranial pressure. Rises in intracranial pressure may occur suddenly and without clinical warning and may be of sufficient magnitude to compromise either local or global cerebral blood flow. If one waits for a clinical finding such as fixed and dilated pupils or hemiparesis before treating an elevated intracranial pressure, the patient will have suffered potentially irreversible damage. Many therapies used to control intracranial pressure have serious side effects. It seems prudent to titrate such therapy against a reliable measurement of intracranial pressure so that excessive therapy is not employed on the basis of the subjective clinical findings, but rather on the basis of reproducible measurements.

Establishment of a Secure Airway

The child with acute brain swelling secondary to RS cannot tolerate even transient episodes of hypoxia or hypercarbia resulting from airway obstruction or hypoventilation. Therefore, the first priority for emergency

TABLE 2 Reye's Syndrome: Diagnostic Criteria

1. Clinical history consistent with the diagnosis
2. No other obvious, reasonable explanation or diagnosis, including toxins, encephalitis, meningitis, or trauma
3. A threefold rise in SGOT, SGPT, or serum ammonia levels
4. Serum bilirubin concentration less than 3.0 mg per liter
5. Liver biopsy showing diffuse fatty infiltrate, with no necrosis or inflammation

management should be to secure the airway. In the noncomatose child, evaluation of the airway usually confirms that the child's natural airway is functioning well and that there is no need to intervene. In the comatose child, however, the normal airway protective reflexes are often absent or compromised. In this case an artificial airway should be established quickly via intubation. Management of the airway in the child with diminished intracranial compliance and a potential "full stomach" is best done by an anesthesiologist, using a modified rapid sequence induction of anesthesia and tracheal intubation. In this technique, the child is preoxygenated with 100 percent oxygen using a reservoir bag and mask device. A large dose of pancuronium (0.15 to 0.20 mg per kilogram) is rapidly administered intravenously, followed closely by a dose of thiopental (2 to 6 mg per kilogram, depending on the cardiovascular status) to quickly reduce brain swelling, ablate the hypertensive response to tracheal intubation, and lower the intracranial pressure. An assistant presses on the cricoid cartilage (Selick's maneuver) to occlude the esophagus and reduce the risk of regurgitation and aspiration of gastric contents. The patient is then hyperventilated for 1 to 2 minutes until full paralysis is established. Many clinicians also administer lidocaine, 1 to 1.5 mg per kilogram intravenously, to further minimize airway responsiveness. The trachea is then gently intubated with a tube of appropriate size according to the formula: internal diameter (ID) = (age in years + 16) ÷ 4. Hyperventilation is then continued.

Electrolyte Therapy

Hypokalemia may be a problem if there is persistent vomiting in the prodromal stage of the disease. Hypophosphatemia during RS is common. Patients frequently present upon admission with serum phosphate concentrations of 1.5 to 2 mg per deciliter. We recommend administering phosphate as its potassium salt up to a total 3 mEq per kilogram per day. Hypophosphatemia is not usually a major clinical problem when it is recognized and treated early.

Glucose

Hypoglycemia is often seen in RS with young children. Hypoglycemia may precipitate seizures if not treated promptly. Hypertonic glucose should be administered to maintain a blood glucose concentration between 200 and 300 mg per deciliter. This usually can be accomplished with the infusion of 10 percent dextrose in a balanced electrolyte solution, although in unusual cases the concentration of dextrose may need to be increased. When more than 10 percent dextrose is required to maintain hyperglycemia, access to the central circulation is desirable.

Euvolemic Dehydration

Administration of excessive free water to patients with cerebral swelling results in an increase in cerebral edema and intracranial pressure, often with disastrous results. Electrolyte free solutions, such as 5 percent dextrose in water, should be avoided. Instead, *balanced electrolyte solutions* should be administered to provide solute along with free water. While it is obvious that administration of excess free water will exacerbate cerebral edema, it is not obvious that restriction of free water will prevent or reduce existing cerebral edema. Nevertheless, a large body of anecdotal experience suggests that *restriction of free water* and the maintenance of a dehydrated state may benefit the patient. Simultaneous with establishing a deficit of free water in relation to solute (i.e., dehydration), the normal circulating blood volume must be maintained. This combination results in a condition known as euvolemic dehydration. The simplest means by which euvolemic dehydration may be established is to provide volume expansion with colloid or blood products while maintaining a deficit of free water by restriction of crystalloid and electrolyte containing fluids to two-thirds or three-fourths of the normal maintenance rates.

Head Position

Any impediment to free venous drainage of blood from the head will raise jugular venous pressure and with it the intracranial pressure. The patient should be nursed in a 30 degree head-up tilt with the head oriented such that there is no rotation of the neck. The head should be slightly extended to avoid compression or kinking of the jugular veins. Sandbags placed on either side of the patient's head or soft blankets rolled up will provide adequate stability to keep the head from turning from side to side and compressing the jugular veins.

Hyperventilation

The mainstay of intracranial pressure (ICP) oriented neurointensive care is the manipulation of cerebral blood volume and ICP via manipulation of the systemic carbon dioxide level. The cerebral blood volume in the normal brain is very responsive to changes in the $PaCO_2$. Over the physiologic range of $PaCO_2$ between 20 and 80 mm Hg, there is a nearly linear change in cerebral blood flow with a change in the $PaCO_2$. We usually try to keep the $PaCO_2$ at or below the values seen in the patient before intubation.

Oxygenation

Hyperoxia has little effect on cerebral blood flow (CBF) until the PaO_2 rises above 600 mm Hg, at which point the CBF falls slightly. As the PaO_2 falls to 50 or 60 mm Hg, however, there is a dramatic rise in the CBF in response to the hypoxemia. Maintenance of a secure airway is crucial to insure adequate alveolar ventilation and oxygenation in the patient with cerebral damage. Airway obstruction with hypercarbia and hypoxemia can result in a devastating rise in the CBF and ICP.

Neuromuscular Blockade

The use of neuromuscular blockade in comatose patients with RS is controversial. The advocates of blockade cite the facilitation of passive hyperventilation, the lack of coughing, bucking, and straining attendant to endotracheal tube suctioning, and the decrease in venous tone that accompanies muscle paralysis. Those who oppose the use of neuromuscular blockade cite the loss of the neurologic examination for following the clinical course of the patient and the risk of interruption in ventilation in the event of an accidental disconnection of the endotracheal tube from the ventilator delivery tubing. There is a large body of clinical experience, (but no controlled studies), attesting to the intracranial pressure lowering effect of neuromuscular blockade. The usual drug employed for this purpose is pancuronium bromide in doses of 0.1 mg per kilogram as an intravenous bolus followed by a continuous infusion of 0.05 to 0.1 mg per kilogram per hour.

Sedation

The use of sedation in comatose children is also controversial. Advocates point to their experience with sedation in lowering the intracranial pressure, while opponents feel that sedation makes no sense in a comatose patient and that the drugs only serve to lower the blood pressure in an uncontrolled fashion. It is our practice *not* to use sedation until the recovery phase of the acute illness, when the patient manifests a reaction to stimulation. If sedation is to be used, we prefer morphine sulfate, 0.1 mg per kilogram intravenously; although diazepam, 0.15 mg per kilogram intravenously may also be used.

Osmolar Therapy

Mannitol is typically administered as a 20 or 25 percent intravenous solution over 5 to 15 minutes. It is hypertonic compared with plasma and rapidly draws water out of the intracellular and interstitial spaces into the intravascular space. There appears to be no difference in the speed, maximum value, and duration of intracranial pressure reduction in brain injured adults treated with 0.25 g per kilogram, 0.5 g per kilogram, and 1.0 g per kilogram. Our current practice is to treat elevations in intracranial pressure that are uncontrollable using hyperventilation with 0.25 g per kilogram intravenously over 5 to 10 minutes and to double the dose in 15 to 20 minutes if the first dose is unsuccessful. A problem with large doses of mannitol is that fluid and electrolyte wasting becomes severe as the dose of mannitol increases. We therefore use the lowest dose of mannitol effective in lowering the intracranial pressure. As the plasma osmolarity approaches 340 mosm per liter, renal failure due to reversible mannitol crystalization in the tubules begins to occur.

Extraordinary Therapy: Barbiturates and Hypothermia

There appears to be no evidence now favoring the prophylactic use of high dose infusion of barbiturate to protect the brain from intracranial swelling and elevated intracranial pressure. Barbiturates definitely reduce brain swelling quickly and will lower an elevated intracranial pressure. Their use is dangerous, however, and should optimally be left to a tertiary care center experienced in advanced cardiovascular monitoring and support. The same is true of total body hypothermia.

SUGGESTED READING

Center for Disease Control: Surgeon General's advisory on the use of salicylates and Reye syndrome. MMWR 1982; 31:289.

Center for Disease Control: National Reye syndrome surveillance—United States, 1982 and 1983. MMWR 1984; 33:41.

Daniels SR, Greenberg RS, Ibrahim MA. Scientific uncertainties in the studies of salicylate use and Reye's syndrome. JAMA 1983; 249:1311.

Fisher DM, Frewen T, Swedlow D. Increase in intracranial pressure during suctioning—stimulation vs. rise in PaCO$_2$. Anesthesiology 1982; 57:416–417.

Shaywitz B, Rothstein P, Venes JL. Monitoring and management of increased intracranial pressure in Reye syndrome: results in 29 children. Pediatrics 1980; 66:198.

Shaywitz SE, Cohen PM, Cohen DJ, et al. Long-term consequences of Reye syndrome: a sibling-matched, controlled study of neurologic, cognitive, academic and psychiatric function. J Pediatr 1982; 100:41.

PEDIATRIC DIARRHEA

ALFRED V. BARTLETT III, M.D.
LARRY K. PICKERING, M.D.

Physicians treating infants and children with acute diarrhea should consider several basic areas: (1) recognition and management of fluid and electrolyte abnormalities, (2) determination of the need for specific diagnosis and therapy, and (3) assessment of associated symptoms requiring therapy. Acute diarrhea in children is often infectious and includes a wide range of symptom complexes produced by a variety of enteropathogens. In almost all episodes, fluid loss is the most important determinant of morbidity and mortality. All patients with diarrhea require some degree of fluid and electrolyte therapy. Some need other nonspecific support, and others benefit from specific antimicrobial therapy.

ETIOLOGY

Common causes of acute infectious diarrhea in the United States are shown in Table 1. *Rotavirus* is the most

TABLE 1 Important Causes of Acute Infectious Diarrhea in Children

Etiology	Common Age Group	Characteristics	Epidemiologic Considerations	Means of Diagnosis	Therapy
Viruses*					
Rotavirus Enteric adenovirus	3 mo–2 yr	Acute watery diarrhea; vomiting and dehydration; often low-grade fever, occasionally to 39 °C	Common in colder months	ELISA or latex agglutination commercial kits available for rotavirus only	Supportive
Bacteria					
Campylobacter	Any	Watery diarrhea or dysentery; sometimes with fever	Animal or food exposure	Stool culture	Erythromycin
Shigella	1–5 yr	Watery diarrhea or dysentery; fever with leukocytosis common; convulsions	Exposure to an infected person	Stool culture	Trimethoprim-sulfamethoxazole
Salmonella	1 yr	Watery diarrhea or dysentery; may have sepsis or meningitis	Travel or exposure to contaminated food	Stool culture; blood culture; CSF analysis as indicated	Treat invasive disease only: ampicillin or trimethoprim-sulfamethoxazole or chloramphenicol.
Clostridium difficile (antimicrobial-associated colitis)	Any	Watery diarrhea or dysentery	Exposure to antimicrobial agents	Anaerobic stool culture; toxin assay sigmoidoscopy	Vancomycin or metronidazole
Bacterial toxins (food poisoning)	Any	Vomiting; short incubation from ingestion of food; others who ingested food also ill	Exposure to contaminated food	Culture stools and food; detection of toxins	Supportive
Parasites					
Entamoeba histolytica	Adults	Often chronic; severe colitis or dysentery or milder disease	Travel; contaminated food	Ova and parasite examination of stool	Carrier: iodoquinol or paromomycin Tissue invasion: metronidazole or dehydroemetine plus iodoquinol
Giardia lamblia	Any	Acute watery or chronic, relapsing diarrhea	Travel; contaminated water; day care	Ova and parasite examination of stool	Furazolidone or metronidazole or quinacrine
Cryptosporidium	Any	Acute watery or chronic diarrhea	Animal exposure; immune deficiency; day care	Weak acid-fast stain of stool	None

* Norwalk virus affects all age groups, mostly as a cause of water- or food-borne disease.

common cause of acute dehydrating diarrhea in young children. The exact significance of *enteric adenovirus* and Norwalk virus in children in the United States is unknown. Bacterial diarrhea usually is caused by *Campylobacter* and *Shigella* and less commonly by *Salmonella* and various disease-causing strains of *Escherichia (E.) coli*. Pseudomembranous or antimicrobial-associated colitis (AAC) should be suspected in a child with fecal leukocyte-positive diarrhea occurring after a course of antibiotics, generally ampicillin, a cephalosporin, or clindamycin. Noncholera vibrios and *Vibrio (V.) parahemolyticus* may cause diarrhea in those with a history of raw seafood consumption. The clinical spectrum of bacterial diarrhea extends from watery diarrhea indistinguishable from viral disease to severe dysentery with fever plus blood, mucus, and leukocytes in stool. Watery diarrhea with low-grade fever is caused by bacteria that produce enterotoxins (*E. coli, V.*

cholerae, Campylobacter, and occasionally *Shigella* and *Yersinia (Y.) enterocolitica*), whereas organisms that invade the gastrointestinal tract or produce cytotoxins (*Shigella, Salmonella, Campylobacter*, invasive *E. coli, Clostridium (C.) difficile, Y. enterocolitica*, and *V. parahemolyticus*) cause diarrhea that contains blood, mucus, and fecal leukocytes. Patients who have infections with invasive organisms often complain of tenesmus and have fever. Septicemia or meningitis associated with *Salmonella* infections should be suspected in infants with diarrhea plus fever, toxic appearance, marked irritability, or symptoms of meningitis. Those who have ingested foods with preformed enterotoxins produced by staphylococci, *Bacillus cereus*, or *Clostridium perfringens* may experience severe diarrhea, often associated with vomiting or abdominal pain; these illnesses are self-limited, and treatment is supportive.

Diarrhea caused by parasites tends to be chronic or relapsing, but may be acute. *Entamoeba histolytica* is uncommon in the United States, but should be suspected in patients with relapsing diarrhea or colitis-like illness. In some parts of the United States, *Giardia lamblia* is a common cause of diarrhea in older infants and toddlers; however, it also may be an incidental finding unrelated to the acute episode. *Cryptosporidium* diarrhea is common among immunocompromised hosts and has been increasingly recognized among normal hosts.

In children, mild diarrhea often accompanies *infection outside the gastrointestinal tract*, such as otitis media or pneumonia. Usually the principal symptoms are referable to the site of infection. In addition, patients with noninfectious conditions may present with acute diarrhea. Diseases such as congenital adrenal hyperplasia or congenital metabolic abnormalities should be considered in infants with severe dehydration, acidosis, and electrolyte abnormalities who respond poorly to therapy. Children with intoxication with aspirin, organophosphates, poisonous plants, and heavy metals occasionally may present with acute diarrhea.

Not all episodes of diarrhea in children require diagnostic studies. Appropriate investigations for etiology should be undertaken in those admitted to a hospital as well as those with severe dehydration, high fever, or toxic appearance, blood, mucus, or leukocytes in the stool, or a history of exposure to an enteropathogen. Regardless of etiology, enteric precautions should be observed in handling children with acute diarrhea, since nosocomial transmission of these agents commonly occurs.

ASSESSMENT

The initial assessment of a child with acute diarrhea should revolve around a general evaluation, which may provide clues as to the cause of the episode, and an evaluation of the fluid and electrolyte status. A rapid but thorough medical history, including information about epidemiologic factors, a physical examination, and a knowledge of the pathophysiology of various enteropathogens are critical.

General Assessment. A brief history should determine

1. onset of illness,
2. quantity, frequency, and character of stool, including presence of blood or mucus,
3. changes in activity level and neurologic status,
4. amount of urine output,
5. presence and degree of fever,
6. occurrence of convulsions, severe abdominal pain, or other major symptoms,
7. quantity and type of foods and fluids administered since onset of diarrhea,
8. medication or other therapies given,
9. possible exposures, including common source (multiple patients with simultaneous illness), household, daycare, or other exposure to gastrointestinal illness, and possible ingestion of toxins.

Fluid and Electrolyte Status. Whether the child is first seen in an outpatient setting or in a hospital emergency department, the assessment of hydration status and institution of appropriate therapy are the most important parts of the clinical evaluation. The initial physical examination should include vital signs and a baseline weight. The clinical criteria for evaluating degree of dehydration are presented in Table 2. Infants and young children develop significant dehydration more rapidly than older children and adults.

Several specific circumstances should be considered in an evaluation of hydration status. A comparison of the ill child's *weight* to a recent "well" weight can be used to quantitate dehydration. Because of variability among scales and inadequacies of recall, careful clinical evaluation should take priority over an apparently contradictory weight. Hypernatremia can mask several signs of dehydration, including decrease of skin turgor, depression of the anterior fontanelle, and sunken eyes. Children with hypernatremic dehydration may have "doughy" skin; mucous membranes will be dry and urine output decreased with high specific gravity. Persistent thirst in the absence of decreased skin turgor may be a clue to hypernatremic dehydration. Such dehydration requires special care in fluid repletion. Children who have been consuming hypotonic fluids or those with severe malnutrition may pass relatively large volumes of dilute urine while experiencing significant dehydration.

TREATMENT

In caring for patients with acute diarrhea and dehydration, therapy should be considered under several major headings: (1) need for hospitalization, (2) fluid and electrolyte therapy, (3) nonspecific therapy with antidiarrheal compounds, and (4) specific therapy with antimicrobial agents.

Hospitalization. When a patient develops moderate to severe diarrhea, a decision should be made regarding hospitalization. The following children should be considered for hospitalization: (1) those with severe dehydration or high rates of fluid and electrolyte loss through stools, especially when associated with vomiting, (2) children (especially infants and young toddlers) who appear toxic or have high temperatures, (3) children with grossly bloody stools, (4) children who are immunocompromised, and (5) dehydrated children whose home situations do not ensure adequate treatment. Once this decision has been made, appropriate diagnostic procedures and therapy can be instituted.

Fluid and Electrolyte Therapy. Fluid and electrolyte therapy should be instituted as soon as the initial evaluation is completed. Treatment of dehydration is divided into rehydration and maintenance phases. The oral method of rehydration with appropriate solutions is generally the treatment of choice for infants and children with diarrheal dehydration. Intravenous therapy is indicated in the following circumstances: severe dehydration or shock, depressed state of consciousness or other abnormality preventing adequate oral intake, nonavailability of ap-

TABLE 2 Signs and Symptoms Associated with Degree of Dehydration in Acute Pediatric Diarrheal Illness

| Signs/Symptoms | Dehydration | | |
	Mild	Moderate	Severe
Weight loss (%)	3–5	6–9	≥10
General condition:			
infants and young children	Thirsty, alert, restless	Thirsty, restless or lethargic, irritable on stimulation	Drowsy or apathetic; extremities limp, cold, sweaty, cyanotic; possibly comatose
older children	Thirsty, alert, restless	Thirsty, alert, light-headed with postural changes	May be unconscious or apprehensive; extremities cold, sweaty, cyanotic; possibly muscle cramps
Pulse	Normal rate, full	Rapid and weak, orthostatic changes	Rapid, feeble, sometimes not palpable
Respirations	Normal rate and volume	Deep, possibly rapid	Deep, rapid
Systolic blood pressure	Normal	Normal to low, orthostatic changes	Low, possibly unmeasurable
Anterior fontanelle	Normal	Sunken	Deeply sunken
Skin turgor	Normal (pinch retracts immediately)	Decreased (pinch retracts slowly)	Markedly decreased (pinch retracts in >2 seconds)
Eyes	Normal	Sunken	Deeply sunken
Tears	Present	Absent	Absent
Mucous membranes	Moist	Dry	Dry
Urine output	Normal	Reduced, dark	None for several hours, bladder empty
Urine specific gravity	Normal to mildly increased	High	Very high
Estimated fluid deficit	30–50 ml/kg	60–90 ml/kg	100–110 ml/kg

Adapted from A manual for the treatment of acute diarrhoea. Geneva: World Health Organization, 1984.

propriate oral rehydration solution, and nonavailability of parent or nursing personnel to administer an oral solution. Vomiting is usually not a contraindication to oral rehydration. Vomiting frequently accompanies pediatric diarrheal illness; in most cases, oral rehydration is successfully accomplished by administering the required volume in frequent, small amounts. Oral rehydration solutions do not reduce stool output; however, they accomplish rehydration despite continuation of diarrhea.

Solutions appropriate for *oral rehydration* include those specifically designated for this purpose. Such solutions contain 75 to 90 mEq per liter of sodium, with approximately 2 percent glucose, 20 mEq per liter of potassium, and 30 mEq per liter of base (bicarbonate or citrate). Since the transport of sodium from the gastrointestinal tract is linked to glucose transport, the glucose concentration of these solutions is as important as the electrolyte content. Available rehydration and maintenance solutions are listed in Table 3. Initial therapy of fluid and electrolytes should be administered as shown in Table 4. During therapy, signs of dehydration should be monitored frequently. Rate of fluid administration should be increased if stool output is high or if the child fails to improve. If failure to rehydrate persists or if there is progression to signs of severe dehydration, intravenous therapy should be initiated (Table 4).

Once rehydration has been accomplished, fluid therapy should provide maintenance hydration. Maintenance therapy should be instituted in children with diarrhea who are not dehydrated. Maintenance includes two compo-

nents: replacement of ongoing abnormal fluid and electrolyte losses in diarrhea and vomitus, and provision of normal daily fluid and electrolyte requirements.

Stool and vomitus losses can be quantitated by weighing soiled pads and diapers. These losses also can be effectively estimated by assessing severity of diarrhea. Children with mild to moderate diarrhea (less than one stool every 2 hours or less than 5 ml per kilogram per hour stool volume) should be given 5 ml per kilogram per hour of fluid to balance stool losses. More severe diarrhea with higher stool volume should be treated in a medical facility until stool output shows a sustained decrease. Children with severe diarrhea should receive 10 to 15 ml per kilogram per hour as replacement for ongoing stool losses. In the United States, most infectious diarrhea is nonsecretory and results in a volume of less than 10 ml per kilogram per hour. The electrolyte content of this stool is roughly 50 mEq per liter sodium, 45 mEq per liter potassium, and 30 to 50 mEq per liter bicarbonate. In developing countries secretory diarrheas, including cholera and diarrhea caused by enterotoxigenic E. coli, are more common and can result in up to 20 ml per kilogram per hour stool volumes with higher electrolyte content.

In addition to replacement of abnormal fluid losses, normal metabolic requirements must be met to maintain hydration. Normal fluid requirements are approximately 100 ml per kilogram per day for children under age 1 year, 80 ml per kilogram per day for children ages 1 through 5 years, and 60 ml per kilogram per day for children ages

TABLE 3 Composition of Available Oral Rehydration and Maintenance Solutions

	Sodium (mEq/l)	Potassium (mEq/l)	Chloride (mEq/l)	Base (mEq/l)	Glucose (g/dl)
Rehydration					
WHO solution	90	20	80	30	2.0
Pedialyte RS	75	20	65	30	2.5
Maintenance					
Infalyte	50	20	40	30	2.0
Lytren	50	25	45	30	2.0
Pedialyte	45	20	35	30	2.5

TABLE 4 Initial Fluid Therapy According to Degree of Dehydration

Degree of Dehydration	Fluid	Amount	Route	Planned time to Administer
Mild	Oral rehydration solution	Calculated deficit or 50 ml/kg	Oral	4 hours
Moderate	Oral rehydration solution	Calculated deficit or 100 ml/kg	Oral	4 hours
Severe or shock				
Infant	Ringer's lactate	30 ml/kg	IV	1 hour then,
	Ringer's lactate	40 ml/kg	IV	2 hours then,
	Oral rehydration	40 ml/kg	Oral	2 hours
Older child	Ringer's lactate	110 ml/kg	IV	Initiate rapid infusion until adequate blood pressure is restored; remainder over 4 hours, then
	Oral rehydration solution		Oral	2 hours

Adapted from A manual for the treatment of acute diarrhoea. Geneva: World Health Organization, 1984.

6 through 10 years. Maintenance fluids should contain approximately 3 mEq per kilogram per day of sodium and 2 mEq per kilogram per day of potassium.

Choice of Fluids for Maintenance. Oral rehydration solutions provide the extra potassium and bicarbonate lost in stools, but contain too much sodium to be used for all maintenance therapy. One suitable approach is to replace ongoing stool and vomitus fluid losses with rehydration solution and simultaneously provide normal daily requirements with clear liquids, breast milk, or one-half strength formula, progressing to full-strength formula within 12 to 24 hours. In practice, this balance can usually be achieved by providing two-thirds of *total* maintenance needs (stool losses plus daily requirements) as rehydration solution and one-third as milk or other fluids. Oral maintenance solutions (50 mEq sodium per liter, Table 3) may be used during the maintenance phase. However, feeding of breast milk or formula also should be begun shortly after rehydration. In all children, nutrition should be provided beginning within the first 12 hours of therapy.

Electrolyte Abnormalities. Most children with significant diarrhea experience net losses of sodium, potassium, and bicarbonate. If serum electrolytes are measured, mild hypokalemia, moderately increased base deficit, and elevated blood urea nitrogen are likely to be found. The amounts of electrolytes in the fluid therapy described generally are adequate to repair these abnormalities. Significant abnormalities of sodium are less common in acute diarrhea, but are more likely to be of clinical consequence. Sodium passes the blood-brain barrier less readily than water, allowing for relative shifts in these components and resulting in edema or irritability of the central nervous system. Management of these disorders requires special care. Electrolytes should be measured in children with severe diarrhea, severe dehydration, substantial lethargy or irritability, convulsions, low urine specific gravity in the presence of dehydration, or physical findings of hypernatremia. Correct use of oral rehydration solutions in the management of dehydration accompanied by hypo- or hypernatremia is not associated with rates of complications significantly different from those with intravenous therapy.

Hypernatremic Dehydration. High concentrations of sodium can result in vascular thrombosis, and if water losses are replaced too rapidly, central nervous system edema can occur. Rehydration volume should be administered over 12 to 24 hours, with ongoing stool losses replaced volume for volume with oral rehydration solution. Use of orally administered fluids results in seizures significantly less often than administration of fluid intravenously. Hypernatremia may be accompanied by other metabolic derangements. Hyperglycemia is common and can be corrected with oral rehydration solution, and hypocalcemia is sometimes encountered. Significant hypocalcemia with hypernatremia requires intravenous correction.

Intravenous therapy may be required in hypernatremia accompanied by severe dehydration, shock, or abnormal mental status. To avoid rapid osmotic shifts in the central nervous system, total correction should be accomplished over 48 hours. If shock is present, initial therapy should be with lactated Ringer's solution or colloid (e.g., 5 percent albumin), with rapid infusion of 20 ml per kilogram over the first half-hour. Otherwise 5 to 10 ml of Ringer's lactate per kilogram should be given over 1 hour. In either case, therapy is continued with Ringer's lactate with 5 percent dextrose, 10 ml per kilogram plus estimated stool losses, over 4 to 6 hours. Serum electrolytes, glucose and calcium levels, and osmolality should be monitored at 4 hours; if sodium concentration has fallen more than 5 mEq per liter, the rate of infusion should be slowed. Thereafter, infusion should be continued with intravenous solution containing approximately 40 mEq per liter of sodium; one-fourth of the sodium can be bicarbonate if acidosis is still present. If urine flow is adequate, 40 mEq per liter of potassium should be added; this higher concentration of potassium is often required to replace losses associated with hypernatremia. Fluids also should contain 5 percent glucose, whether or not hyperglycemia is present; hyperglycemia is usually corrected as volume status corrects, and excess glucose provides an osmotic buffer, since it freely equilibrates with the central nervous system compartment. Volume should be calculated to replace normal daily losses, excess ongoing losses in stool and vomitus, and one-half of the volume deficit each day. If neurologic status is normal and serum sodium is corrected to less than 150 mEq per liter, oral rehydration may be substituted for continuing intravenous therapy. Emergency peritoneal dialysis may be required for patients with sodium concentrations above 180 mEq per liter.

Hyponatremic Dehydration. Hyponatremic dehydration may occur if stool losses are replaced with fluids having a low electrolyte content. Hyponatremia exacerbates symptoms of dehydration. However, children often have no symptoms attributable to the electrolyte abnormality despite serum sodium concentrations below 125 mEq per liter. Asymptomatic hyponatremia above 115 mEq per liter may be corrected by oral or intravenous therapy in the same volume and route as indicated for the same degree of isotonic dehydration. Serum sodium levels below 115 mEq per liter, or associated with marked irritability or seizures, should initially be corrected with 3 percent saline solution intravenously. If significant acidosis is present, 1.5 ml of sodium bicarbonate ($NaHCO_3$ 1.0 mEq per milliliter) may be added to every 10 ml of 3 percent saline (yielding 0.57 mEq of sodium per mil-

liliter in final solution). Correction should be administered at a rate of 5 mEq sodium per kilogram per hour until serum sodium reaches 125 mEq per liter; time for the correction can be calculated by [(125-measured serum Na) × body weight (kg) × 0.65] ÷ (mEq Na per hour infused). Once sodium is above 125 mEq per liter, rehydration can proceed as appropriate to the state of dehydration.

Nonspecific Therapy. A large number of antidiarrheal compounds are available for the symptomatic treatment of patients with diarrhea. These over the counter and prescription preparations are reported to act by decreasing the volume of diarrhea by increasing absorption of water and electrolytes, decreasing intestinal secretion, or decreasing intestinal motility. The majority of these compounds are not effective in children with acute infectious diarrhea or have significant side effects and should not be used.

Specific Therapy with Antimicrobial Agents. Antimicrobial therapy is administered to selected patients with acute infectious diarrhea to abbreviate the clinical course or decrease excretion of the causative organisms or both. Table 1 shows recommended therapy for patients with acute infectious gastroenteritis owing to known causes. The finding of fecal leukocytes significantly increases the likelihood of a bacterial etiology, but does not distinguish between *Shigella, Campylobacter, Salmonella*, and the other less common invasive bacterial enteropathogens. Isolation of *Campylobacter* from stool does not imply the need for antimicrobial therapy. The decision should be made on clinical grounds, but therapy with erythromycin probably should be given to patients with high temperatures, bloody diarrhea, or severe diarrhea. In children with known ampicillin-susceptible strains of *Shigella*, ampicillin eradicates clinical symptoms and fecal shedding. Amoxicillin is not as effective as ampicillin in the treatment of shigellosis and should not be used. The treatment of choice for shigellosis when susceptibility is unknown is trimethoprim plus sulfamethoxazole. The type of syndrome produced by *Salmonella* influences the selection and duration of antimicrobial therapy. Antimicrobial agents are not indicated in the treatment of persons who are nontyphoid *Salmonella* carriers or in most patients with mild gastroenteritis. Antimicrobial treatment of patients with *Salmonella* infection is restricted to those with (1) typhoid fever, (2) bacteremia caused by nontyphoidal strains, and (3) dissemination with localized suppuration. Antimicrobial agents should be considered in patients with *Salmonella* enterocolitis if the disease appears to be evolving into one of the systemic syndromes and in patients with a major disease or condition that impairs host resistance to infection, such as young infants and those with hemoglobinopathies or malignancies. Ampicillin, trimethoprim-sulfamethoxazole, and chloramphenicol are the current drugs of choice. In toxic-appearing children with high fevers, diarrhea, and other findings suggestive of disease owing to *Shigella, Salmonella*, or invasive *E. coli* (fecal leukocytes, guaiac-positive stools, leukocytosis), empiric therapy with trimethoprim-sulfamethoxazole pending culture results may be appropriate. Antimicrobial-associated pseudomembranous colitis (AAC) is treated by removing the offending antimicrobial agent and treating the patient according to the extent of symptoms. Mild cases generally require no additional treatment. Moderately severe illness is best treated with oral vancomycin. Metronidazole is an alternate therapy for AAC. In treating patients with amebiasis, iodoquinol is the best luminal amebicide currently available commercially in the United States. This drug is effective against both cysts and trophozoites in the lumen of the gut, but is ineffective against tissue forms of the disease. Invasive amebiasis of the intestine, liver, or other organs necessitates the additional use of a tissue amebicide such as metronidazole. Quinacrine hydrochloride, metronidazole, and furazolidone are effective in treating patients with infections caused by *Giardia lamblia*; only furazolidone is available in liquid form. Optimal therapy of patients with cryptosporidiosis is not known.

Associated Symptoms Requiring Management. High fever may accompany infectious diarrhea; *Shigella* infection often produces temperatures over 39 °C. Significant dehydration also can produce high fever, especially in infants. High doses of antipyretics should be avoided, since dehydration may contribute to development of toxic drug levels. Fever in diarrheal dehydration is best managed by rehydration, cool soaks or baths, and low doses of antipyretics. Seizures associated with diarrhea may represent electrolyte abnormalities, febrile convulsions, *Shigella* neurotoxin–mediated central nervous system irritability, or meningitis. Electrolyte, calcium, and glucose concentrations should be determined. Lumbar puncture for analysis and culture of cerebrospinal fluid is generally indicated. Loading doses of phenobarbital should be given to children with seizures, followed by maintenance doses during the acute illness.

SUGGESTED READING

A manual for the treatment of acute diarrhoea. Geneva: Publication WHO/CDD/SER/80.2, World Health Organization, 1984.

Pickering LK, Cleary TG. Approach to patients with gastrointestinal infections and food poisoning. In: Feigin RD, Cherry JD, eds. Textbook of pediatric infectious disease. 2nd ed. Philadelphia; W.B. Saunders, 1986.

Pickering LK. Evaluation of patients with acute infectious diarrhea. Pediatr Infect Dis 1985;4:S13–S19.

Santosham M, Daum RS, Dillman L, et al. Oral rehydration therapy of infantile diarrhea: A controlled study of well-nourished children hospitalized in the United States and Panama. N Engl J Med 1982;306:1070.

CHILDHOOD AND ADOLESCENT GYNECOLOGIC PROBLEMS

ALBERT ALTCHEK, M.D., F.A.C.S., F.A.C.O.G.

VULVOVAGINITIS IN THE INFANT AND CHILD

Vulvovaginitis is the most common gynecologic problem of the child because the vulvar skin is thin and easily irritated, the vulva lacks the protection of the adult labial fat pads and hair, the vaginal mucosa is atrophic owing to lack of estrogen (and thus has a neutral pH), and the hygiene of the child is often poor. Some believe that at one time or another every child will experience vulvovaginitis. Bacterial culture is usually nonspecific.

For severe, weeping, vesicular, pruritic, painful, *acute vulvar dermatitis*, wet compresses with Burow's solution (aluminum acetate) 1–40 one packet or tablet of Domeboro dissolved in 1 pint of water) may be used as well as 0.9 percent physiologic saline (1 level teaspoonful of salt mixed in a large glass of water), or plain water. The solution is prepared at room temperature just before each treatment. Two to four layers of muslin cotton or well-laundered handkerchief linen are soaked, rung out, and applied in a smooth layer. Evaporation of the water cools the skin. After 5 to 10 minutes, the compress will be dry. Do not pour more solution on the dry compress, because this will increase the solute concentration. Instead, remove the dressing, rinse and rewring it, and reapply. Wet compress dressings are used for 20 to 30 minutes and may be repeated at 2- to 6-hour intervals. After each treatment, the skin is carefully patted dry, and if desired, a bland, nonspecific topical water-based medication may be applied. Powders are not used because of caking. No plastic wrappings or coverings are used over the compresses. With small children it is imperative not to use cold water or wet compresses on more than one-quarter of the body to avoid excessive cooling. A wet compress also makes it difficult to keep the bed dry.

An alternative to wet compresses is a tepid sitz bath for 15 to 30 minutes with plain water, colloidal oatmeal, baking soda, saline, starch, or skim milk. If needed, a cotton ball with vegetable oil may be used for cleansing. In the acute phase, soap is avoided, since it aggravates the inflammation.

After 2 or 3 days the acute vulvar dermatitis should subside, and if not the child's condition should be re-evaluated. Failure to respond may be caused by a reaction to topical specific therapy or to topical anesthetics (neither of which should be used in the acute phase); secondary infection (which requires oral systemic rather than topical antibiotics); irritation from soap, bubble bath, perfume, or hot water; or irritation from clothing heat, friction, dye, residual detergent, or wool or synthetic fabrics.

In the *subacute phase of vulvitis*, a shake lotion of a powder in a liquid (calamine lotion) may be painted on the skin, avoiding oozing and hairy areas. Later use antipruritic lotion with menthol (0.124 or 0.25 percent); or an emollient cream or lotion; or 1 percent hydrocortisone; or iodochlorhydroxyquin cream. Do not use ointments or pastes, because they occlude the skin.

Specific medication is used after the acute phase has

been reduced to the subacute one. For *candidiasis* of the vulva (one of the most frequent offenders), nystatin, miconazole, or clotrimazole creams are applied twice daily for 1 to 2 weeks. Nystatin is not as efficacious as the others but has less tendency to irritate. Vaginal candidiasis is more difficult to treat because of the problem of getting medication into the child's vagina, which can be done by instilling nystatin oral suspension with a dropper. Nystatin cream can be squirted into the vagina through a narrow tube nozzle (pediatric adaptor) or through a cut segment of urethral catheter.

Another frequent vaginal infection is caused by betahemolytic *Streptococcus* group A. It is treated like a traditional strep throat with oral penicillin for 10 days.

Pinworms are treated with a single dose of Vermox (mebendazole) as a 100-mg chewable tablet. This infestation has not been studied extensively in children under 2 years of age. Usually the entire household is treated simultaneously. Hygienic practices are also important: wash hands after bowel movements and before eating, avoid scratching the anal area, and wear underpants at night. Vermox is not prescribed for pregnant patients.

Gonorrheal vulvovaginitis is treated by aqueous procaine penicillin G (APPG), 100,000 units (U) per kilogram of body weight intramuscularly (IM), preceded by oral probenecid 25 mg per kilogram. If the child weighs 48 kg or more, she is given the adult dose of 4.8 million U IM in two separate sites with 1 g of probenecid. An alternative oral medication is a single dose of amoxicillin 50 mg per kilogram (maximum dose 3 g) with probenecid. If the child is allergic to penicillin and is under age 6, then a course of erythromycin, 40 mg per kilogram per day, may be used. Over the ages of 6 to 8 years, oral tetracycline may be used as 25 mg per kilogram initially, followed by 50 mg per kilogram per day in four divided doses for 1 week. Spectinomycin is the choice for penicillinase-producing gonorrhea (PPNG) and may also be used for the penicillin-sensitive child. The dose is 40 mg per kilogram intramuscularly into the buttock or anterior thigh. If more than 3 ml are given, two injection sites are used. Unlike APPG, spectinomycin does not cure incubating syphilis. Like APPG, it does not affect *Chlamydia*, which may coexist and continue to cause vaginitis. It is not effective in pharyngeal gonorrhea. It is not recommended for the newborn pending toxicity studies.

Disposable diapers are the leading cause of *diaper rash* in the infant. Although advertising claims that the infant's skin is protected and kept dry, in fact, the outer plastic covering (to keep the mother dry) is a heat and humidity shield. This causes a build-up of hot, steamy urine. To treat diaper rash, the mother should use cloth diapers without an outer plastic diaper covering and change the diaper the moment it is soiled. The diaper should be washed completely, rinsed twice, and sterilized if feasible. Whenever possible, diapers should not be used at all. At night, leave the area uncovered, and place diapers under the infant. The acute diaper rash may be treated with wet compresses of water, saline, or Burow's solution. Topical nystatin cream or powder is used for

candidal infections. Oral nystatin may be prescribed for primary or secondary candidal diaper area infections.

Recurrent vulvovaginitis may be caused by repeated vaginal infections from pharyngeal infections, a foreign body in the vagina, chronic vulvar dermatitis, allergic-irritant reactions, sexual abuse, ectopic ureter, pinworm infestation, diabetes mellitus, ectopic anus, draining pelvic abscess, and infrequent specific infections caused by *trichomonads, Haemophilus (Gardnerella) vaginalis*, and *Shigella*. Vaginoscopy or expert consultation or both are indicated for persistent or recurrent vulvovaginitis, vaginal bleeding, and suspicion of foreign body, neoplasm, or congenital anomaly.

VAGINAL BLEEDING

Vaginal bleeding in the child may be produced by trauma, severe vaginitis, foreign body, vulvar skin disease, clear cell adenocarcinoma of the vagina or cervix, or both, rhabdomyosarcoma (sarcoma botryoides) of the vagina and cervix, precocious puberty, unwitting exposure to exogenous estrogen, functional ovarian neoplasm, and a prolapsed urethra.

The most common cause is trauma, usually from an accident, less often from sexual abuse. Usually there is a vulvar or perineal laceration. Bleeding is managed initially by a cold compress. If the bleeding stops, usually no surgery is needed. Have the child void to be certain that the bladder is intact, and do a vaginoscopy and rectal examination. The abdominal and renal areas are carefully palpated and vital signs checked. If significant vaginal bleeding persists or if there is a tear of the rectal sphincter, or the suspicion of a tear of the posterior vaginal fornix or a recto- or vesicovaginal tear, then the child should be taken to the operating room, given general anesthesia, and completely examined.

Vaginal bleeding in the adolescent may be caused by spontaneous or induced incomplete abortion, in which case a gentle uterine curettage is done to remove necrotic placental tissue.

Rhabdomyosarcoma is a rare but very malignant tumor, usually of the upper vagina and cervix. It manifests itself as protrusion of a smooth mass, deceptively benign in appearance, resembling clusters of small translucent seedless grapes, together with small amounts of bleeding. Otherwise, these children look perfectly well. Ruling out this condition is the main reason for performing vaginoscopy for vaginal bleeding. This tumor is not palpable by rectal examination in its early stages, and superficial biopsy may show only benign vaginal mucosa. Previously this tumor resulted in a 90 percent fatality rate, but today as high as an 85 percent cure rate is expected with chemotherapy and local excision; however, this depends on early diagnosis and treatment.

Precocious puberty occurs more often in girls than in boys. Usually it is true idiopathic precocious puberty caused by premature activation of the hypothalamus and anterior pituitary. The sequence of normal puberty occurs but at an earlier age, that is breast buds, genital and axillary hair, height spurt, and menstruation. In very young children, vaginal bleeding may occur early. Such patients should be referred to a specialist promptly.

IMPERFORATE HYMEN

Imperforate hymen is usually not diagnosed until puberty, when it presents as primary amenorrhea. Unfortunately, newborns are not carefully examined and the area often is also overlooked at well-child examinations. If the open hymen cannot be visualized at birth, the area should be gently probed with a urethral catheter or medicine dropper. The differential diagnosis includes congenital absence of the vagina, vaginal septum, and feminized male pseudohermaphroditism (androgen insensitivity).

It is now recognized that even if the child with imperforate hymen is asymptomatic during childhood, the vagina may distend with mucus from endocervical gland secretion. Therefore these children should be examined vaginally, at not less than yearly intervals to look for bulging of the hymen; rectal examination should be done at the same time. If the vagina distends, surgery is indicated.

URINARY HYDROCOLPOS

Occasionally an acute situation arises in the newborn created by imperforate hymen, profuse fetal endocervical secretion owing to maternal estrogen, and massive *hydrocolpos*. The ureters are compressed laterally, which causes hydroureter and hydronephrosis; the urethera is compressed with dilatation of the bladder; the intestines are pushed into the upper abdomen; and there may be cardiovascular embarrassment. This requires immediate management by a surgeon.

URINARY TRACT OBSTRUCTION

Secondary *urinary tract obstruction* may occur from congenital anomalies such as female hypospadias, with the urethra exiting into the upper vagina with a distal vaginal stenosis; hydrocolpos with the distended vagina compressing the urethra; prolapse of a ureterocele into the urethra; or an atonic neurologic bladder. Urinary tract obstruction may also result from neoplasms such as a sarcoma botryoides. Often after a temper tantrum, a prolapse of the urethra may occur that obstructs or causes pain and thereby prevents voiding. Painful herpetic periurethral vulval ulcers may have the same effect.

A frequent cause of distortion of the urinary voiding stream and sometimes of urinary infection and partial obstruction is severe agglutination of the labia minora. The urethra cannot be visualized because the labia minora come together in the midline in a vertical white tinted line. The most efficacious treatment is the daily application of an estrogenic vaginal cream (Premarin). Within 2 weeks, a spontaneous opening of the labia occurs. Although the package insert states that estrogens may cause cancer of the uterus, cancer has not been documented for this use. As an alternative, the labia may be gently pulled apart

daily, combined with meticulous hygiene and if desired the use of 0.50 or 1 percent hydrocortisone cream.

PREGNANCY COMPLICATIONS IN THE ADOLESCENT

The diagnosis of pregnancy and its complications is difficult because we do not often associate it with the adolescent, because the adolescent often has irregular menses, and because the patient generally denies the possibility, either consciously or unconsciously.

With *spontaneous abortion* (miscarriage), characteristically there is one or more missed menses, severe midline lower abdominal cramps, and heavy bleeding with clots ("liver slices") and sometimes tissue (gray color). The diagnosis is confirmed by pelvic examination, with the findings of a dilated cervix with tissue passing and a tender, enlarged uterus (from borderline enlarged to up to 12 weeks' size). There are no adnexal (tube or ovary) masses. The proper treatment is uterine evacuation. Depending on the severity of the bleeding, the amount of tissue, the risk of anesthesia, the degree of dilation of the cervix, and the state of the patient, the evacuation may be done in an emergency department or gynecologic examining room with a polyp forceps, gentle sharp curettage, gentle dull curettage, and a uterine suction tube.

If the adolescent with spontaneous abortion has a *fever* or *peritonitis* or both, the process may have been going on for several days, or perhaps the patient has had an unprofessional induced incomplete abortion. (Since the legalization of abortion, this situation is unusual). Septic shock should be anticipated. Prompt, rapid intravenous fluids and antibiotics (to cover a broad spectrum, including *Escherichia coli*, aerobic streptococci, and anaerobes) are administered, and uterine evacuation is carried out. The vital signs and urine output are monitored. If necessary, a central venous pressure line or Swan-Ganz vascular catheter is placed to guide fluid intake. Steroids are given if necessary. If a septic course continues, the patient may have abscesses in the myometrium (which may require hysterectomy), tubo-ovarian abscesses (which may require salpingo-oophorectomy), or septic pelvic thrombophlebitis (which may require heparin anticoagulation).

Since government funds for abortion are very restricted, some economically disadvantaged women who want to have their pregnancies terminated may resort to *illegal abortion*. Such abortions are very dangerous. Illegal abortions are done with abortifacient, irritant chemicals that can cause vaginal bleeding ulcerations (potassium permanganate), by introducing chemicals into the uterus that may cause infections and disseminated intravascular coagulation, or by introducing a urethral catheter into the uterus. Characteristically, the patient experiences cramps, bleeding, shaking chills, fever, and pelvic peritonitis.

With the increase in sexual activity in adolescents, there is an increase in *ectopic tubal pregnancies*. Unfortunately, we do not normally consider this in the differential diagnosis of lower abdominal pain or abnormal bleeding or both. Characteristically, one or two periods are missed, and a small amount of vaginal bleeding and left or right unilateral pain occur, followed by generalized abdominal and shoulder pain and fainting. The last three symptoms are associated with rupture of the ectopic tubal pregnancy. A quantitative beta subunit human chorionic gonadotropin (hCG) blood pregnancy test should be ordered. A negative test almost always rules out ectopic pregnancy. If the hCG titer is 6,500 mIU per milliliter or higher and there is a normal intrauterine pregnancy, a pelvic sonogram will show a gestational sac. Absence of this sac suggests ectopic pregnancy. With a normal intrauterine pregnancy, the hCG titer doubles every 2.4 days early in pregnancy, and failure to do this suggests ectopic pregnancy or threatened intrauterine abortion. Next to the beta subunit hCG test, laparoscopy is the most important method of detecting an unruptured ectopic pregnancy. The optimal approach is to diagnose ectopic pregnancy before it ruptures, not only to avoid life-threatening rupture and hemorrhage, but also for the possibility of preserving the involved tube. After the hCG test and sonogram, schedule the patient for dilatation and curettage (if she does not wish to continue an intrauterine pregnancy) to rule out intrauterine pregnancy (combined intrauterine and tubal pregnancy is rare), laparoscopy, and possible laparotomy.

Rarely, the ectopic pregnancy is located in the part of the fallopian tube that goes through the uterine wall and develops in the cornual angle. This is a deadly variety, since the tubal fetus may develop to 12 to 16 weeks without symptoms and suddenly the tube ruptures. The patient then goes into hemorrhagic shock, and immediate laparotomy is necessary.

VULVOVAGINITIS

It is not unusual to have more than one cause of vulvovaginitis in the sexually active adolescent. In fact, finding one sexually transmitted disease should alert the clinician to look for others.

The most common ulcerative vulvitis in the female, and in some series the most common vulvovaginitis in the adolescent who first begins sexual activity, is caused by herpes virus. A cluster of small papules develops on the vulva on an erythematous base. In a day or two they rupture to become painful, soft, superficial ulcerations. With the first attack, the ulcers may persist for 2 to 4 weeks and there may be regional inguinal swollen and tender nodes, malaise, and low-grade fever. Ulcers near the urethra may cause dysuria and inability to void. About half the cases continue to have recurrences, and over the following few years the recurrences become shorter and milder. There is often a resultant and emotional depression caused by interpretation of the infection as a punishment for premarital sex, knowledge of the lack of true cure, the possible need for a cesarean section delivery if the patient wishes to have children later on, fear of later cancer of the cervix, or fear of spreading the infection to other sexual partners.

The standard treatment is the topical application of acyclovir ointment 5 percent (Zovirax) every 3 hours six times daily. Sexual relations are eschewed until 1 week after the ulcers clear in order to avoid pain and spread

of the disease. Recently, acyclovir has become available in oral tablet form. It may be taken as 1 tablet five times daily for acute, severe infections and three times daily to prevent recurrences if they are frequent. Use of a condom during sexual intercourse is a wise precaution to prevent spread, since there may be mild recurrences without ulceration. Emotional support for the patient may also be helpful.

Haemophilus vaginitis is also called nonspecific vaginitis and *Gardnerella vaginitis*. It is the most common vaginitis in the adult and is characterized by a stale fish odor and a watery gray, sometimes frothy discharge. There is usually very little pruritus. A vaginal smear shows "clue cells" or vaginal epithelial cells covered with myriads of short bacilli, giving a stippled appearance. The surrounding area is clear, that is, with no or few white blood cells or lactobacilli. Current theory is that it is an anaerobic infection associated with *Haemophilus*, which is difficult to culture. In the past, therapy entailed use of a sulfa cream, but the present treatment is metronidazole. The single 2-g oral dose for trichomonads may not work as well as the 1-week dose, 500 mg by mouth twice a day for 1 week. It is taken with food to avoid nausea; consumption of alcohol precipitates vomiting. If there are recurrences, consider treating the male partner with a similar dose. Although metronidazole is used in pregnant patients in England, in the United States, usually it is avoided during the first trimester, and some clinicians do not use it in pregnancy at all. Occasionally, there is a *Candida* overgrowth, and sometimes anticandidal vaginal medication is prescribed simultaneously. Previous fears that metronidazole causes cancer or chromosome damage have not been substantiated.

Candida albicans has a wide spectrum of activity. It may be resident in the vagina without causing symptoms; or it may cause a vaginitis with erythema and a lumpy, white, cottage-cheese–like vaginal discharge; or it may cause a vulvitis with mild to intense, burning, agonizing pruritus. The condition of the vulva may vary from mild erythema of the posterior fourchette to an extensive, symmetric, raw beefy, weeping, exudative, raised vulvitis with satellite, red, pustular, elevated lesions. The predisposing factors are antibiotics, pregnancy, diabetes mellitus, and immunodeficiency. In recent years, it is not unusual to see frequent recurrences of candidiasis, without apparent reason. Sometimes there may be a chronic vulvar skin disease—seborrheic dermatitis—which predisposes to fissures and maceration, and this provides fertile ground for candidiasis. The diagnosis is confirmed by a wet microscopic smear that shows hyphae filaments and spores.

For the agonizing acute case of *candida* vulvitis, first reduce the inflammation with sitz baths (plain tepid water, saline, bicarbonate of soda, corn starch, colloidal oatmeal baths) and mild hydrocortisone cream (1 percent). Avoid hot water and soap. Keep the vulva cool and dry. After 1 to 2 days or for the subacute phase, specific therapy is used. I usually use miconazole nitrate 2 percent (Monistat 7) vaginal cream or vaginal suppositories nightly for 1 week. Monistat 3 vaginal suppositories may be used for a shorter, 3-day course.

Clotrimazole (Gyne-Lotrimin vaginal cream or tablet suppositories; or Mycelex-G 1 percent vaginal cream) may also be used. The shortest treatment schedule is one Mycelex-G 500-mg vaginal tablet for the unreliable patient. It maintains a therapeutic vaginal level for 3 days. Although miconazole and clotrimazole are effective, there is a small chance of an irritant reaction. A less efficacious medication but one without an irritant reaction is nystatin vaginal tablets or cream for the vulva (Mycostatin) daily for 2 weeks.

In cases of recurrences, which are usually premenstrual, prescribe prophylactic medication monthly for several months before menses. In addition, oral nystatin tablets (Mycostatin) may be taken, 1 tablet three times daily for 2 to 3 weeks, to reduce intestinal colonization and therefore perhaps reduce recurrence. This drug is not absorbed systemically.

SUGGESTED READING

Altchek A. Chapter 2. In: Nichols DH, Evrard JR, eds. Pediatric and adolescent gynecology. New York: Harper & Row, 1985:20–62.

Altchek A. Psychological aspects of adolescent obstetric and gynecologic conditions. In: Heacock DR, ed. A psychodynamic approach to adolescent psychiatry. New York: Marcel Dekker, 1980:239–278.

Altchek A. Recognizing and controlling vulvovaginitis in children. Contemp Pediatr 1985; 2(5):59.

Altchek A. Vulvovaginitis, valvar skin disease and pelvic inflammatory disease. Pediatr Clin North Am, 1981; 28:397.

Huffman JW, Dewhurst CJ, Capraro VJ. The gynecology of childhood and adolescence. 2nd ed. Philadelphia: WB Saunders, 1981.

MANAGEMENT OF THE EMERGENCY DEPARTMENT

DIAGNOSTIC IMAGING IN THE EMERGENCY CENTER

MARK G. STEIN, M.B., B.Ch., B.Sc.
ROBERT C. BRASCH, M.D.

Diagnostic imaging examinations, including plain film radiography, computed tomography (CT), ultrasonography, and possibly in the future, magnetic resonance imaging (MRI), may contribute essential information for the treatment of the acutely ill patient. However, imaging evaluations by their very nature cause delays in therapy and should be undertaken only after obtaining a pertinent history and performing a careful physical examination to avoid wasting time on unnecessary examinations. Certain principles should be followed in ordering any emergency radiological study:

1. *Patients should be stabilized* prior to transportation to the radiology department. For critically ill patients, call ahead to the radiology department to expedite the examination. Never leave critically ill or injured patients unattended in radiology; a nurse or someone on the medical team should be with the patient at all times.

2. *Minimize movement of the traumatized patient*, particularly if there exists a possibility of spinal cord injury. Be aware of the amount of movement required for the examinations that have been ordered, and order those examinations less likely to involve unnecessary movement for the patient.

3. Decide for yourself the information required for the care of the patient, and *prioritize the examinations* to obtain the most urgent information first. Discuss the problem with the radiologist, giving him the pertinent history and physical findings, and decide in consultation with the radiologist which examinations should be performed and their order. The emergency setting does not justify lack of communication with the radiologic consultant.

Examples:

A. In severe abdominal trauma an abdominal CT examination may be more useful to assess hematuria than an excretory urogram; CT will simultaneously image the other abdominal viscera, e.g., liver, spleen, and pancreas. An initial urogram will potentially impede subsequent CT with an intravenous contrast medium (essential to evaluate liver and spleen) due to the contrast load.

B. All urographic procedures must precede barium studies.

C. With a fractured pelvis, retrograde urethrograms should be performed prior to the placement of a bladder catheter to prevent further trauma to a possibly already traumatized urethra. One may convert an incomplete tear of the urethra to a complete tear during attempted passage of a urethral catheter.

4. *Location*: Decide whether the radiologic procedures can be performed in the emergency department(as a portable examination), in the emergency x-ray department, or necessarily in the main radiology department.

Examples:

A. Emergency pelvic ultrasonography may be performed portably in the emergency department where the patient can be more easily monitored and will require no transportation.

B. CT examinations can often only be performed in the main x-ray department. CT may be used to evaluate abdominal trauma with only one move of the patient, as opposed to transporting the patient to nuclear medicine (for liver spleen scan) and to radiology for the excretory urogram. CT may also take a fraction of the time if both these examinations are required.

C. Chest radiography can be obtained portably in the emergency room and although not optimal may give more than adequate information for a particular emergency situation. If small abnormalities are suspected, an examination in the x-ray department should be obtained.

D. Portable skeletal x-ray views will only show gross fractures; subtle fractures, such as nondisplaced hip fractures, may be missed.

5. *Avoid unnecessary radiographic examinations.* This minimizes costs and, more important, time. Review, rather than repeat, examinations from outside facilities. Decide whether a procedure is really necessary or whether it merely satisfies one's intellectual curiosity or is performed for potential medicolegal liability. Plan procedures in advance so that all necessary procedures are performed at one time rather than moving the patient back and forth from the emergency department to the x-ray department.

TABLE 1 Guidelines for Diagnostic Imaging

Situation	Examination	What To Look For
Resuscitation and Trauma		
Cardiopulmonary arrest	Chest roentgenogram	Location of tubes and drains, pneumomediastinum, pneumothorax, subcutaneous emphysema, lung consolidation and edema, contusion, fractures
Assisted ventilation	Chest roentgenogram	Endotracheal tube location, pneumothorax, pneumomediastinum, stomach distention, atelectasis-consolidation
Airway obstruction	Chest and neck roentgenogram	Foreign body, mass, tracheal caliber, epiglottis size, pulmonary hyperinflation or consolidation
Head trauma		
Severe head injury (with loss of consciousness, neurologic abnormality, or strongly suspected bone injury)	Skull roentgenogram	Fracture, sphenoid sinus fluid level, pineal shift, pneumocephalus, cervical integrity
	Head CT (usually without intravenous contrast medium)	Mass; bleed-epidural, subdural, subarachnoid, parenchymal; fracture; sphenoid sinus fluid level; pneumocephalus
Basilar skull fracture	CT scan (without intravenous contrast medium)	Fracture (best seen on thin sections), bleed (as above), mass (as above), mastoid opacification, sphenoid sinus fluid level
	Thin-section CT of petrous bone	Fracture, ossicle dislocation, sphenoid sinus fluid level, mastoid opacification
Eye emergencies	Orbital CT	Foreign body, fracture, size of optic nerve, orbital content
	Orbital-facial roentgenograms	Fracture-dislocation, foreign body, sinus opacification
Facial fracture	Orbital-facial roentgenograms (horizontal beam)	Fracture, maxillary sinus fluid level, soft tissue swelling
ENT emergencies	Depends on signs and symptoms: sinus and pharyngeal roentgenography	Foreign body, opacification, mass, fracture
Dental emergencies	Roentgenography of maxilla, mandible, temporomandibular joints	Fracture, foreign body, bone destruction, teeth
Mandible fracture	Mandible and temporomandibular joint roentgenograms	Fracture, dislocation of temporomandibular joint, fracture of neck of mandible
Mandible dislocation	Open and closed mouth temporomandibular roentgenograms	Dislocation of mandibular head on closed mouth view, fracture of neck of mandible
Foreign bodies	Depends on site: if possible a roentgenogram of foreign body identical in composition to that being sought helps to determine degree of radiopacity	Foreign body, abnormal air collection, soft tissue swelling
Airway obstruction	Neck roentgenography (lateral in slight extension)	Mass including epiglottis, soft tissue swelling, tracheal caliber, tracheal deviation, retropharyngeal abscess
	Chest roentgenography including expiratory view (bilateral decubitus views in infants)	Air trapping, tracheal caliber, pulmonary consolidation, masses
Neck trauma		
Laryngeal fracture	Frontal and lateral neck	Subcutaneous air, soft tissue swelling
	CT	Fracture of thyroid cartilage, arytenoid dislocation
Cervical spine trauma	Initial cross table lateral followed by full cervical spine series if cross table is normal	Abnormal soft tissue swelling, bony alignment, disk space narrowing, facet joint alignment, subluxed or locked facets, foreign body
	CT spine (with or without metrizamide)	Fracture, spinal cord swelling, soft tissue swelling
Chest trauma		
Closed or open chest trauma	Chest roentgenogram	Pneumothorax, lung contusion, lung consolidation from aspiration, bone fractures, mediastinal widening, displacement of nasogastric tube
	Chest CT (with intravenous	Aortic laceration, mediastinal hemorrhage, lung consolida-

TABLE 1 Guidelines for Diagnostic Imaging (continued)

	contrast medium)	tion, pneumothorax, pneumomediastinum
	Aortic angiography (indicated for wide mediastinum or suspected aortic laceration)	Traumatic aneurysm, internal flap of aorta, extravasation, pleural effusion, apical cap
Rib fracture	Rib series (use markers at site of point tenderness)	Cortical break, pleural based mass, pneumothorax, pleural effusion
Pneumothorax	Expiratory chest roentgenogram with horizontal beam	Pleural line of collapsed lung, air-fluid level in pleural space
Abdominal trauma		
Penetrating abdominal trauma	Abdominal series (including supine, erect, or left lateral decubitus films)	Free intraperitoneal air or fluid foreign body, mass
	Excretory urogram	Presence of both kidneys, extravasation of contrast medium, renal outline
Blunt abdominal trauma	Abdominal series and chest roentgenogram	Free intraperitoneal air, loss of psoas line
	CT scan (with oral and intravenous contrast medium)	Liver laceration, splenic laceration, renal contusion-laceration, renal function bilaterally, presence of both kidneys, pancreatic mass, pancreatic rupture, free intraperitoneal air, pneumothorax on higher sections
Pelvic trauma		
Pelvic fracture	Pelvic roentgenogram	Fracture, intraperitoneal fluid
	Retrograde urethrogram	Extravasation, stretching of urethra, urethral tear
	Cystogram	Extravasation, extrinsic mass
	Water-soluble contrast enema	Sacral fracture, displacement of rectum by extraluminal mass, extravasation of contrast medium
	CT scan with intravenous, oral, and rectal contrast media	Fracture, extravasation, organ integrity including bladder, hip fractures
	Angiography	Bleeding sites, therapeutic (embolization of bleeders)
Extremities		
Fractures	Plain roentgenograms and special views of area of interest	Cortical breaks, must include joint above and below areas of interest
	Bone scan (if fracture is suspected but not visualized on plain film)	Abnormal uptake of radionuclide
	Tomography	Cortical break not seen on plain film
	CT (if all else fails and one still suspects a fracture)	Cortical breaks

Medical Emergencies

Head, neck, and upper airway		
Sinusitis	Sinus series	Opacification, fluid levels, bone destruction
Epiglottitis	Lateral neck	Swelling of epiglottis, thickening of aryepiglottic folds
Swallowed fish bone	Frontal and lateral neck	The bone itself, soft tissue swelling, air in prevertebral space
	Xerogram of neck	Bone itself
	Esophagram with water soluble contrast agent	Leak of contrast agent, coating of foreign body
Central nervous system		
Coma	Cranial CT (noncontrast, possibly with contrast enhancement)	Mass effect—cerebral swelling, intracranial hemorrhage (subarachnoid, subependymal, subdural, or intraventricular) abnormal brain density, calcifications, ventriculomegaly
	Skull roentgenography	Fracture, sutural diastasis, enlarged sella turcica, pineal displacement

TABLE 1 Guidelines for Diagnostic Imaging *(continued)*

	Chest roentgenography	Pulmonary consolidation or edema
	Cerebral arteriography	Vascular injury or malformation, contrast extravasation
Convulsions	Cranial CT (without contrast initially)	Mass lesion, intracranial hemorrhage, ventriculomegaly, abnormal brain density including calcification, metallic deposition, and demyelinization
	Skull roentgenography	Increased pressure (sellar erosion, sutural diastasis), focal or diffuse bone abnormality, mass effect
	Chest roentgenography	Pulmonary consolidation or edema, pleural effusion, cardiomegaly, mediastinal mass adenopathy
	Abdominal roentgenography (pediatrics)	Abnormal bowel gas pattern, focal mass effect—fluid collection, organomegaly, calcification
	Others depending upon physical findings	Osteomyelitis, soft tissue swelling
Acute toxic encephalopathy	Cranial CT	Mass lesion-brain edema, abnormal brain density, intracranial hemorrhage, ventriculomegaly
Cerebrovascular accident	Cranial CT (initially without contrast medium)	Normal scan may equal acute CVA, mass lesion, hemorrhage (intraparenchymal, subarachnoid, subdural)
	MRI	Not usually done in acute phase
Metastatic disease	Contrast CT (possibly with and without contrast as an initial study)	Mass lesions-effect, enhancement, bone lesions
Spinal and sensory motor levels	Spine roentgenograms	Lytic lesion, alignment abnormalities
	Myelogram (with or without follow-up CT)	Masses, cord displacement
	MRI	Mass lesions and cord displacement (may become imaging examination of choice)
Psychiatric		
Psychiatric emergencies	Cranial CT depending on circumstances	(See *Coma* and *Behavioral Emergencies*)
Uncomplicated asthma	None	
Drug abuse	Chest roentgenography depending on circumstances	Pulmonary consolidation (aspiration, pneumonia, hemorrhage), atelectasis
Pulmonary system		
Pneumonia	Chest roentgenography	Areas of consolidation, pleural effusions
Status asthmaticus	Chest roentgenography	Pulmonary consolidation, peribronchial cuffing, atelectasis, extra-alveolar air, heart size, pneumomediastinum-pneumothorax
Pulmonary embolus	Chest roentgenography	Normal chest x-ray, film consolidation, pulmonary edema, pleural effusion, areas of hypoperfusion
	Ventilation-perfusion scintigraphy	Areas of decreased perfusion associated with normal ventilation (high probability lung scan)
Heart		
Arrhythmias	Chest roentgenography	Heart size, pulmonary edema, pleural effusion
Cardiac tamponade	Chest roentgenography	Pulmonary edema, cardiomegaly, large azygos vein, pericardial effusion on lateral view, pericardial calcification
Myocardial infarct	Portable chest roentgenogram	Vascular redistribution, pulmonary edema, cardiomegaly
Congestive heart failure	Chest roentgenography	Pulmonary edema, pleural effusion, upper lobe redistribution, Kerley B lines, Kerley A lines
Aortic dissection	Chest roentgenography	Widening of superior mediastinum, pleural effusion, apical cap, cardiomegaly, medial displacement of aortic calcification
	CT scan of chest with intravenous contrast medium	Pleural effusion, "flap" within aorta
	Angiography	"Flap" within aorta

TABLE 1 Guidelines for Diagnostic Imaging (continued)

Ischemic bowel	Abdominal series	Dilated bowel loops, "thumb printing," air in bowel wall, free intraperitoneal air, portal venous air
Deep venous thrombosis	Venogram	Intraluminal filling defects
Genitourinary system		
Renal failure	Chest roentgenography	Cardiomegaly, pulmonary consolidation (edema, hemorrhage), pleural fluid
	Abdominal radiography	Mass, renal size, renal calcification, foreign body ingestion
Hematuria	Abdomen	Renal or ureteric calcification, bladder calcification, abdominal mass
	Voiding cystourethrogram	Bladder tumor, prostatic enlargement, reflux
	Excretory urogram	Ureteric obstruction, tumor (kidney, ureters, bladder), papillary necrosis
Pyelonephritis	Excretory urogram	Renal abscess, hydronephrosis, decreased opacification of infected kidney
	Voiding cystourethrogram (especially in pediatrics)	Ureteral reflux, urethral valves, strictures of urethra, large diverticula
Acute urinary retention	Abdominal roentgenography or ultrasonography	Bladder size, sacral anomaly (children), mass
	Excretory urography and voiding cystourethrogram (depending on circumstances)	Renal function, site of obstruction
Torsion of testis	Scrotal ultrasonography	Fluid collections, size of vas deferens and epididymis
	Testicular flow study (nuclear medicine)	Decreased perfusion of affected testis
Epididymo-orchitis	Scrotal ultrasonography	Fluid collections, evidence of abscess
	Testicular flow study	Increase uptake in affected site
Abdomen and genitourinary system		
Acute abdomen	Abdominal series	Free air, dilated small bowel loops, hernias, air in bowel wall or extraluminal gas in abscess
	Water-soluble contrast upper gastrointestinal series	Extravasation of contrast medium, bowel obstruction, ulcer
Right upper quadrant pain	Abdominal series	Gallstones, renal stones, free air, air within liver from abscess, air in gallbladder wall
	Ultrasonography	Gallstones, tenderness of gallbladder and thickened gallbladder wall, dilated bile ducts, hydronephrosis, evidence of liver mass or abscess
	Biliary scintigraphy (HIDA)	Nonvisualization of gallbladder (patency of cystic duct), bowel activity indicating patency of common bile duct
	Excretory urogram	Ureteric stone, hydronephrosis
Perforated ulcer	Abdominal series	Free intraperitoneal air
	Water-soluble upper gastrointestinal series	Extravasation of contrast material, evidence of ulceration
Pancreatitis	Abdominal series	Calcification, sentinel loop
	Abdominal ultrasonography	Fluid collection within enlargement of pancreas, pseudocyst, gallstones, enlargement of liver, bile duct dilatation
Jaundice	Abdominal ultrasonography	Dilatation of bile duct, mass in pancreas, gallstones, common bile duct stones
	Abdominal CT scan	Pancreatic mass, dilatated bile duct, tumors within liver
Bowel obstruction	Abdominal series	Bowel distention, bowel wall thickening, air in bowel wall
Ileus	Abdominal series (including upright or left lateral decubitus film)	Dilatation of both large and small bowel, fluid levels within both large and small bowel
Gastrointestinal bleeding	Abdominal series	Abnormal calcification, enlargement of liver, enlargement of spleen

TABLE 1 **Guidelines for Diagnostic Imaging** *(continued)*

	Upper gastrointestinal series	Ulcers, varices, tumors
	Barium enema	Tumor, diverticula
	Nuclear medicine gastrointestinal bleeding study	Persistent area of abnormal isotope collection, which moves along bowel with time
	Angiography	Extravasation of contrast medium, tumors, study may be used for treatment (e.g., local infusion of pitressin or embolization of a bleeding site)
Acute appendix	Abdominal series	Appendicolith, abnormal air collection within abscess
	Barium enema	Filling of appendix, evidence of cecal mass
Abdominal abscess	Abdominal series	Abnormal gas collection, displacement of bowel gas by mass
	Ultrasonography	Abnormal masses
	Abdominal CT scan (oral and intravenous contrast media)	Abnormal air fluid collection
Diverticulitis	Water-soluble contrast enema	Extravasation of contrast medium, mass effect on colon
Rectal foreign body	Pelvic x-ray film	Foreign body, free intraperitoneal air, retroperitoneal air
	Water-soluble contrast enema	Extravasation
Obstetrics and gynecology		
Threatened abortion	Pelvic ultrasonography	Fetal heart activity, fetal size, clot within uterine cavity
Prepartum hemorrhage	Pelvic ultrasonography	Fetal maturity, placental maturity, fetal motion, fetal heart, placental placement, abruptio placentae
Ectopic pregnancy	Pelvic ultrasonography	Intrauterine gestational sac, free fluid within cul de sac, adnexal mass, fetal heart within adnexa
Pelvic inflammatory disease	Pelvic ultrasonography	Free fluid in cul de sac, adnexal mass, complex cystic mass within adnexa
Intrauterine contraceptive device	Pelvic ultrasonography	IUD in uterus
	Abdominal roentgenography	Only if IUD is not seen in uterus; if IUD is seen elsewhere, it must have perforated
Endocrine system		
Diabetic ketoacidosis	None	
Disseminated intravascular coagulation	Depends upon circumstances	
Bleeding disorders	Depends upon circumstances	
Sickle cell crisis	Chest roentgenography	Heart size, pulmonary consolidation, spleen size
	Possibly abdomen or extremity roentgenography	
Hypovolemic shock	Dependent upon cause	Identify sites of internal blood loss
Anaphylaxis	None	
Central venous line	Chest roentgenogram	Location of CVP catheter
Acid-base disorders	Depends upon circumstances	
Acute dehydration	Depends upon circumstances	
Hypernatremia	Depends upon circumstances	
Hyponatremia	Depends upon circumstances	
Infectious diseases (nonlocalizing)		
Meningococcemia	Possible cranial CT	Impending brain herniation with compromise of subarachnoid space
Meningitis	Cranial CT (with contrast)	Dural plaques, fluid collections, brain edema or calcifications
Diphtheria	Neck and chest roentgenography	Mass, inflammation, tracheal caliber, sinus opacification
Botulism	None	
Gas gangrene	Site of involvement	Gas in soft tissues, soft tissue swelling, focal bony destruction

TABLE 1 Guidelines for Diagnostic Imaging (continued)

Tetanus	Site of infection	Soft tissue abnormality, osteomyelitis
Rabies	Possible injury site	
AIDS	Depends on symptoms	
Musculoskeletal system		
Joint pain	Depends on symptoms	
Osteomyelitis	Bone roentgenography	Periosteal reaction, bone destruction, soft tissue swelling
	Bone scan	Hot spot in region of interest
Environmental hazards		
Smoke inhalation	Chest roentgenography	Consolidation, pulmonary edema, atelectasis
Carbon monoxide poisoning	Cranial CT (without contrast)	Abnormal low density of basal ganglia
Drowning	Chest roentgenography	Pulmonary edema, consolidation
Burns	Depends upon circumstances	
Radiation injury	None acutely	
Sunburn	None	
Heatstroke	None	
Frostbite	None acutely	
Bites and stings	None	
Poisoning	Depends upon circumstances	Radiopaque tablet or substance in bowel, pulmonary edema, aspiration pneumonia
Specific pediatric emergencies		
Battered child syndrome	Skull, chest, abdomen, and extremity roentgenography (possible cranial CT)	Fracture dislocation, soft tissue swelling, organomegaly, pleural fluid
	Bone scintigraphy	Occult bony injury
Sudden infant death syndrome	Possibly chest roentgenography	
Sexually molested child	None unless foreign body suspected	
Emergencies in newborn	Depends upon circumstances	
Croup-epiglottitis	Lateral and frontal soft tissue neckviews	Subglottic narrowing

6. Review all x-ray films under *optimal viewing conditions*—good lighting and view boxes. Check the x-ray film thoroughly; do not rush! Important, often crucial, information may be missed by hasty review. Review all parts of the film, not only the area of interest. This will avoid missing unsuspected abnormalities, e.g., pneumoperitoneum on a chest x-ray view or rib fractures in a suspected myocardial infarct. If possible, review all films with the radiologist. Correlate all abnormal findings with appropriate history to obtain the maximum information from each examination.

7. An appropriate concentration of *water soluble contrast agent* should be used instead of barium for studies when extravasation of contrast medium is possible. Do not use hypertonic ionic contrast material when the patient may aspirate it, as this will result in pulmonary edema. Newly available nonionic contrast media (e.g., iohexol or iopamidol), useful for contrast examinations in isotonic concentrations, may be utilized in situations of potential aspiration or perforation.

8. *Interventional radiology* is now a function of many diagnostic radiology departments. In appropriate settings, therapy may be initiated in the radiology department, e.g., with embolization of bleeding sites, or drainage of abscesses.

Examples:

A. Pelvic trauma with massive bleeding is often managed by angiography and embolization of the bleeding vessels, thus saving patients major surgery.

B. Abscess drainage under CT or ultrasound guidance is routinely performed under local anesthesia, decreasing the length of the hospital stay and saving the patient general anesthesia.

The situations in Table 1 are arranged by and large in the order by which they appear in the text. For some situations, there may be a choice of imaging studies that may depend on the availability of modalities and the level of diagnostic suspicion based on the findings from the physical examination and the severity of symptoms. The list of examinations may need to be adapted for individual patients and specific situations. The list is not intended to be exhaustive, but to provide a general guide to many of the more common emergency situations.

SUGGESTED READING

Harris JH. The radiology of acute cervical spine trauma. Baltimore: Williams & Wilkins, 1978.
Harris JH, Harris WH. Radiology of emergency medicine. 2nd ed. Baltimore: Williams & Wilkins, 1981.
Keats TE. Atlas of normal roentgen variants that may simulate disease. 3rd ed. Chicago: Year Book Medical Publishers, 1984.
Keats TE, Smith TH. An atlas of normal developmental roentgen anatomy. Chicago: Year Book Medical Publishers, 1977.

RESPONSE TO DISASTER

JACEK BRONISLAW FRANASZEK, M.D., F.A.C.E.P.

The emergency department constitutes the major locus of activities in any hospital's response to a disaster. This is so because it is the main area to which patients arrive from a mass casualty incident and because of its traditional orientation to victims of precipitous injury. The ongoing interaction of the emergency department with prehospital care providers in the community's emergency medical services system, and particularly the provision of medical control, makes the transition to the disaster response a natural one. Moreover, the orientation and experience of the emergency staff are very well suited to an adequate disaster response, which involves rapid deployment of resources, crisp decision making on the part of health care providers, and establishing priorities with respect to patient care.

The best disaster response is achieved when details of expected behavior on the part of staff have been outlined in an emergency department plan, that is well integrated with the hospital-wide plan and the community-wide plan and that has been rehearsed so as to familiarize staff with anticipated courses of action in the event of a disaster. Such activities are in fact mandated by the Joint Commission on Accreditation of Hospitals (Table 1). By definition, a "disaster" occurs when the influx of patients exceeds immediately available resources of personnel and materials. In some instances, prior notification of the emergency department to anticipate a large number of victims allows recruitment of appropriate resources to forestall a disaster taking place.

This notification and continuing information from the site are functions of the Emergency Medical Services (EMS) system. Such communication is vital to the success of managing disasters outside the hospital and should be rehearsed in conjunction with hospital disaster drills. Patients must be triaged in appropriate numbers to hospitals with appropriate areas of expertise (e.g., trauma, burn, spinal cord injury).

Generally speaking, most disasters are not like the one that occurred in Bhopal, India, which involved thousands of patients. Instead they might involve a dozen or less. Different resources are needed for these much more frequent "minidisasters." In our institution, there are two plans, one of which calls for a "minidisaster" response. Only emergency department personnel are recalled, and the next shift are asked to arrive earlier and the current one to stay later, thereby allowing some additional personnel and equipment to be brought to the emergency department in order to be able to treat a relatively small number of critical patients. If the anticipated case load exceeds this number of patients, a full-scale disaster plan or "maxidisaster" plan is invoked, which involves a more elaborate recruitment of resources and mobilization of the hospital as a whole. A graded response is desirable, so as to avoid being overwhelmed, but not to incur costly manpower and supplies when they are not needed.

It is important to rehearse the disaster plan on all three shifts so that every employee has a sense of his or her duties in the course of the disaster response. Often, drills in emergency departments are only coordinated during the daytime, and personnel working the evening or nighttime shifts fail to understand the plan. Off-hours personnel and new personnel should be apprised of the disaster plan by staging disaster drills throughout the year. Action cards, or brief descriptions of expected behaviors, may be utilized as checklists, or reminders, for expected courses of action for any given type of staff. The plan or its synopsis may be added to the universally available telephone directory.

Coordination of the emergency department response through the hospital disaster committee and with various community agencies assures proper mobilization of resources and facilitates communication during a disaster.

TABLE 1 Summary of 1986 JCAH Guidelines for Disaster Planning

Emergency preparedness program must be in place.

The program is adaptable to a variety of disasters, concise, and documented.

The plan addresses hospital resources utilization, staff prepardness, and community plan integration.

Hospital personnel are provided with training.

The plan addresses patient management issues (discharge; relocation).

The program is implemented, evaluated, and documented semiannually.

Staff performance will be better if it has been discussed in advance, and the performance of individuals will be better if they are called upon to do what they already do on a regular basis, operating with familiar equipment in familiar surroundings. The emergency department response plan should be flexible and kept as simple as possible.

Initial notification should be subject to corroboration and should initiate a cascade of events that prepares the emergency department and the hospital. The more information that can be gleaned from the scene regarding the number and nature of casualties, the better prepared the hospital and the emergency department will be to handle the incoming cases. The preliminary preparation should include clearance of nonemergency patients from the area securing the area, (including routes of access to the emergency department), asking visitors to stay in alternative areas, and rapid disposition of any other patients who are present in the emergency department. If the anticipated number of victims is large, the emergency department and the hospital have to prepare what our institution has termed the "critical capacity inventory." This includes an assessment of number of available beds, number of available intensive care unit beds, operating theater capability, and blood bank capability. Usually the emergency department personnel initiate this critical capacity inventory. Notification from the disaster site should precede the actual arrival of casualties, allowing this preparation phase.

It is important to have a mechanism for recruiting additional staff in order to be able to handle a large number of incoming patients. Thus, one person is assigned the responsibility of augmenting the physician, nursing, technician, and clerical staff within the emergency department proper or re-deploying in-house personnel to the emergency department. In our emergency department, this task is given to a member of the clerical staff. Contacted individuals are asked to contact other members of the staff so as to hasten the rapidity with which personnel can be recruited. Staff is asked to identify themselves appropriately so as to be given access to the emergency department on arrival, since it will otherwise have been secured to traffic.

One other clerk is designated as a communications clerk within the department in an effort to handle most of the telephone traffic. The hospital switchboard should be notified to divert all routine calls away from the emergency department. It is prudent to have alternative forms of communication available, such as intercoms throughout the emergency department connected with other areas of the hospital or walkie-talkie radios to circumvent an already overloaded telephone system.

Since additional supplies may be necessary, these should be obtained from a central area. We use a disaster cart that is already made up and present in the area; some supplies are periodically removed and utilized before they become outdated. Other previously prepared disaster carts and supplies are available in the central supply area of the hospital and may be requisitioned by emergency department personnel when the need arises. Internal preparation should be made to be able to handle power, food, and water shortages. Supplies are more readily available than personnel; therefore, the initial thrust should be to recruit additional personnel to the department.

It is important to establish a chain of command within the emergency department proper and to clearly distinguish between treatment and administrative functions. In our institution, a disaster command center is established that is somewhat removed from the emergency area. This command center is staffed by leading administrative physicians and nursing personnel who receive information from all departments, including the emergency department, and who are able to deploy resources, facilitate patient discharges, analyze needs, and organize the entire institution's disaster response based on information that is made available. A link with the emergency department is crucial. The disaster command center becomes the hub of all operations in the hospital disaster plan and the administrative center of the disaster response. The emergency department serves to provide the initial treatment area for incoming casualties and serves less of an administrative role.

In our institution, it is the emergency department director or emergency physician who assumes command over the emergency department area. Triage is performed by the emergency physician. The chairman of the surgical department assumes responsibility for the operating theaters, and the trauma surgeon on call assumes responsibility for the care of the critically injured. The nursing director assumes responsibility for nursing care and supplies, and the departmental administrator assumes responsibility for clerical and logistical functions. In their absence, the most senior personnel assume the roles of the directors. Those assuming control of the area are identified to the staff. The emergency department assumes responsibility for notification of other departments in the hospital—the various medical departments, administration, nursing supervisors, admitting office, dietary, engineering, housekeeping, laboratory, medical records, radiology, pharmacy, security, and social service—all of which are expected to provide support to the patients who will be coming through the emergency department. Employees from nonclinical departments report to the administrator stationed in the emergency department; additional nursing personnel report to the emergency department nursing director; and physicians and surgeons report to the emergency department director or trauma surgeon responsible for the handling of casualties. Admitting personnel station themselves close to the entry point of patients and utilize preexisting medical records kept on hand for disaster patients. Records are kept with the patients as much as possible. Other departments, such as public relations, have their own discrete area in which to operate, but may send representatives to the emergency department in order to acquire enough information to be able to assist families who may arrive or call regarding their relatives as well as representatives of the media who are investigating the incident.

It is important to designate different areas in which different kinds of patients can be treated.

Most patients arriving from a disaster have been sorted at the scene and are already tagged according to the severity of their injury. Upon arrival, a reassessment of the extent of injury should be made. In our institution, this is done by an emergency physician and an emergency nurse acting in concert. The triage area should be designated very close to the entry to the emergency department. The role of the emergency physician responsible for triage is to designate the next appropriate area to which a patient will be deployed and where treatment will be initiated. All patients should enter through a common triage area. Security personnel should be expected to provide access to this triage area and to maintain traffic flow. Triage categories established in the emergency department mimic those established in the field. These categories are

1. High priority (red tag). This type of patient has very serious injuries but is salvageable (e.g., shock, compromised airway). Immediate attention is required.
2. Middle priority (yellow tag). This type of patient needs urgent care and may have serious injury, but his or her life is not immediately threatened (e.g., multiple fractures or a serious burn).
3. Low priority (green tag). This type of patient is ambulatory and has minor injuries.
4. No priority (black tag). This type of patient is dead or will be imminently.

Area designation facilitates team response and care of patients. Patients with red tags are deployed to a resuscitation area or trauma room. Patients with yellow tags are deployed to bays in the emergency department proper. Patients with green tags are deployed to a clinic area or to the vacated waiting room. Patients with black tags are deployed to the morgue. Staffing in these areas should reflect these needs. Patients who are seriously ill or injured should be managed in the emergency department by emergency physicians, surgeons, and nursing teams; patients with relatively less severe injuries may wait or be dealt with by additionally recruited medical personnel; and patients with trivial injuries may be asked to wait until all other patients have been reviewed and treated. It is helpful to have a discrete area for patients with acute psychiatric illness so they may be cared for in a less hectic environment by incoming social service or psychiatric personnel.

If a large number of victims is anticipated, it is appropriate for the disaster command center to cancel all elective surgeries and to recruit personnel for the operating theaters and recovery rooms as well as critical care units. It is equally important to prioritize the order in which patients are operated on.

A family waiting and discharge area must be established away from the emergency department, and a person should be stationed there to inform families of the status of their relatives. Communications from this area to the emergency department or operating theaters may be facilitated by a walkie-talkie; in our experience, a member of the social service department or chaplain functions well in this capacity. Similarly, public relations activities are less obtrusive if representatives from the media are handled in a designated area that is not in the emergency department. Immediate caregivers should not participate in media interviews; rather, a person provided with information from a number of hospital sources should interact with the press.

It should be kept in mind that the therapeutic goals of patient care are to stabilize life-threatening illnesses and not to provide exhaustive management for every patient until the majority have been sufficiently stabilized to prevent loss of life. A large number of patients must be evaluated and treated rapidly; therefore, it is appropriate that diagnosis and treatment take place as rapidly as possible. Unnecessary or cosmetic procedures must wait until the area has been cleared.

Following the episode, a staff debriefing should always take place in order to approve the response to subsequently occurring disasters. Not only should the hospital as a whole conduct a critique, but also the emergency department should review its own performance. It should be kept in mind that both the victim of a disaster and the rescue worker in a disaster incur a significant psychological burden that must be resolved following the acute incident.

SUGGESTED READING

American College of Emergency Physicians.Disaster management and planning for emergency physicians. Emmitsburg, Maryland: Federal Emergency Management Agency, 1983.
Mitchell GW. Emergency disaster management. In: Topics in emergency medicine. Vol. 7, No. 4. Aspen Systems, 1986 (January).

QUALITY ASSESSMENT OF EMERGENCY CARE

JANE G. MURPHY, Ph.D.

Quality assessment (QA) of emergency services has become a subject of increasing concern to all emergency physicians. This concern stems largely from the professional goal of providing the highest quality care possible to all patients. In addition, the influx of governmental funds into emergency services during the past 20 years has been accompanied by regulations requiring emergency departments to develop QA programs.

For the most part, emergency departments meet their own needs and the new regulations by establishing QA committees, with physician members and with support from medical record technicians, to audit medical records for form and process. However, the Joint Commission on Accreditation of Hospitals does recommend the use of "potentially useful sources" of data in addition to medical records. In particular, they suggest that QA programs include "specific process-oriented and outcome-oriented studies" and solicit "patient surveys or comments." Some departments act on these recommendations and take the relatively time-consuming and expensive step of "auditing" patients' health outcomes.

Alternate methods of conducting both process and outcome audits exist. These methods and the advantages and disadvantages associated with each are reviewed here. The major issues to be addressed are summarized in Table 1.

QUALITY ASSESSMENT OF THE PROCESS OF EMERGENCY CARE

The two most frequently used methods of assessing the quality of the process of emergency care are observation and medical records review.

Observation

Observation is touted by many as the ideal method of assessing the quality of emergency care. The method is prospective and reflects actual events rather than a record of events. In addition, observation is flexible since the observer can respond to changes in patients' needs at the same time that physicians respond.

The major disadvantage of observation as a QA method is its expense. Data recording forms must be developed or adapted. Such forms must be complex and detailed to allow information concerning a wide range of

patient's conditions and medical procedures to be summarized. As a result, extensive training of observers is needed to ensure the validity and reliability of data recorded. Given the large amount of data available, automated processing is required.

An additional problem associated with observation is the "Hawthorn effect." It is impossible to know how—if at all—the very presence of an observer changes the behavior of physicians and other medical personnel. Without such information, the validity of the method in any given situation is questionable.

Medical Records Review

By far the most common method of QA is the medical records review. Clinical conditions are selected for review. The method is most useful when conditions are chosen whose audit can be expected to yield important results—e.g., chest pain or abdominal pain as opposed to urinary tract infections. Medical records usually are reviewed by physicians from a variety of disciplines who serve as members of a QA committee and who set standards for care. Each record is rated on how closely it conforms to the standards established. Since physicians are not compensated for their committee activities and since the limited amount of data generated can be analyzed manually, the method is relatively inexpensive. Moreover, because medical staff generally do not know which records will be selected for review, it is unlikely that either patient care or the recording of such care will be changed in response to a planned audit.

A major advantage of medical records review is the understanding that is generated among medical disciplines, particularly when significant clinical problems are selected

TABLE 1 Methods of Assessing the Quality of Emergency Care

Aspect of Care	Method	Advantages	Disadvantages
PROCESS	Observation	Prospective Reflects actual events Flexible	Expensive "Hawthorne effect"
	Medical record review	Relatively inexpensive "Hawthorne effect" unlikely Increases understanding among disciplines	Retrospective Reflects recording of events rather than actual events Relatively inflexible
OUTCOMES	Re-examination of patients	Prospective Can alter treatment regimen Reflects objective and subjective health Compliance assessed via pill counts Understanding and satisfaction can be determined	Patient compliance with request to return variable Expensive
	Telephone interviews	Prospective Understanding and satisfaction can be determined. Less expensive than re-examination Generates good will and research	Not all patients have telephones Reflects subjective, not objective, health Relies on patients' reports of compliance
	Mailed questionnaires	Prospective or retrospective Understanding and satisfaction can be determined Relatively inexpensive	Often has low return rate Reflects subjective, not objective, health Relies on patients' reports of compliance

for review. The multidisciplinary nature of committees means that a variety of points of view and areas of expertise are brought to each clinical problem. Emergency medical staff can make valuable changes in programs and approaches to patient care based on suggestions from other specialists. By the same token, physicians practicing in other areas learn the principles of emergency medicine and come to understand the challenges unique to emergency care.

There are significant disadvantages in relying entirely on medical records reviews to ensure the quality of emergency care. The method is retrospective. The results reflects the recording of events rather than actual events. It is very difficult to determine in any given case the extent to which the information recorded in the medical record gives an accurate and complete picture of care rendered.

Finally, reviewing medical records to evaluate the process of medical care tends to be inflexible. Standards for the care of conditions can be structured to include decision-making algorithms. However, the more usual practice involves simply setting criteria and applying these to each case in a checklist fashion. The individual needs of patients are not well reflected in this rigid approach to quality assessment.

QUALITY ASSESSMENT OF THE OUTCOMES OF EMERGENCY CARE

The outcomes of emergency care provided to patients requiring hospital admission can be determined from in-hospital follow-up. It is more difficult to evaluate the outcomes of patients discharged. The three most frequently used methods of assessing the quality of the outcomes of emergency care provided to discharged patients are reexamination of patients, telephone interviews, and mailed questionnaires.

Reexamination of Patients

The ideal method of assessing the outcomes of emergency care generally is agreed to be the prospective reexamination of patients. Each patient selected is instructed to return to the emergency department at a time appropriate to his or her condition. A physician or nurse practitioner reexamines the patient and assesses his or her objective health status outcome. The patient's subjective assessment of health can also be elicited, and the treatment regimen can be altered if required. Compliance with medication regimens can be evaluated on the basis of pill counts. Questions concerning the patient's understanding of treatment and follow-up instructions and satisfaction with care can be posed.

However, the method has two major disadvantages. First, patient compliance with requests to return for reexamination is highly variable. Patients who are still symptomatic when reexamination is scheduled are likely to return, whereas those who are asymptomatic are not. Second, the method is expensive. Patients must be seen by a physician or a nurse practitioner. Health insurance plans rarely cover return visits to emergency settings, leaving the cost to be borne by the patient or by the emergency department.

Telephone Interviews

An alternative to reexamination of patients to determine outcomes is telephone follow-up. Selected patients are contacted by telephone at a time appropriate to their physical complaints. Each patient's subjective assessment of symptomatic relief can be determined, and patients with significant complaints can be advised to seek additional medical treatment. Questions concerning understanding of and compliance with the treatment regimen and satisfaction with emergency care may be asked.

This prospective method of quality assessment of patients' outcomes is significantly less expensive than reexamination. Its cost-effectiveness derives primarily from the fact that a secretary or research assistant can be trained to administer the questionnaire. Although automated data processing is preferable, most data can be analyzed manually.

Two additional characteristics contribute to the method's cost-effectiveness. First, telephone interviews with patients generate enormous goodwill for an emergency department—an advantage not to be taken lightly in this time of competition for patients. Second, the large amounts of information generated provide a rich source for clinical and social science research.

However, the method has disadvantages as well. Not all patients have telephones and not all patients with phones are easy to contact. An average of two to three attempts per patient contacted is common. In addition, only subjective health status can be evaluated, and patients' reports of compliance with treatment regimens often overstate actual compliance.

Mailed Questionnaires

The least expensive method of assessing the quality of patients' outcome is to mail questionnaires to selected patients. Selection of patients can be prospective or a retrospective sample can be chosen. Questions regarding subjective health, the understanding of and compliance with the treatment regimen, and the satisfaction with care can be included.

A low rate of return is the major problem with mailed questionnaires. Returns of between 5 percent and 10 percent are not uncommon. Analyses of data are not useful unless at least 25 percent of questionnaires distributed are completed.

The method also shares two of the disadvantages of telephone interviews. First, only subjective health status can be evaluated, and second, patients' reports of compliance with treatment regimens often overstate actual compliance.

Perhaps a broad-based group of emergency physicians will soon begin to work together to develop and promulgate workable question and answer formats. These criteria also should take into account the effect of pre-hospital care on patients' emergency department outcomes and, perhaps, should allow for the dependent evaluation of the quality of pre-hospital care.

In the interim, an ongoing program to assess the quality of care should be an integral part of all emergency departments. No method of assessment is ideal. QA programs that combine several methods of evaluating the process and outcomes of care are best able to meet the professional needs of physicians and the health care needs of patients.

SUGGESTED READING

Accreditation manual for hospitals. Chicago: Joint Commission on Accreditation of Hospitals, 1981.

Anderson GV, Ashutosh R, Looney GL, et al. A unique approach to evaluation of emergency care. JACEP 1977; 6:254–258.

Brook RN. Quality of care assessment: a comparison of five methods of peer review. Department of Health, Education, and Welfare Publication No. HRA–74–3100, Rockville, MD, 1973.

Hulka BS, Romm RJ, Parkerson GR, et al. Peer review in ambulatory care: use of explicit criteria and implicit judgement. Med Care 1979; 17:1–73.

McAuliffe WE. Studies of process-outcome correlations in medical care evaluations: a critique. Med Care 1978; 16:907–930.

Murphy JG, Jacobson S. Assessing the quality of emergency care: the medical record versus patient outcome. Ann Emerg Med 1984; 13:158–164.

Payne BC. The medical record as the basis of assessing physician competence. Ann Intern Med 1979; 91:623–629.

Roy A, Looney GL, Anderson GV. Prospective vs. restrospective data for evaluating emergency care: a research methodology. JACEP 1979; 8:142–146.

AVOIDANCE OF MALPRACTICE

JOSEPH J. TRAUTLEIN, M.D., F.A.C.P., F.A.A.I., F.A.C.A., F.C.P., F.A.C.U.R.P.
ROBERT LAMBERT, M.D., F.A.C.C.P.

Under the "holding forth doctrine," the existence of an emergency sign is an implied endorsement of the people who work within its wall. The four D's of culpability are slightly modified in this setting. The four D's are *duty* to perform a service, *dereliction* in the performance of that service, *damages* as a result of that dereliction, and *direct* causation attributable to the agent. In a practice setting, the choice by physician or patient to accept or reject treatment or management and establish a doctor–patient relationship is subject to certain limitation. In a nonemergent setting, during the initial contact, a physician and a patient have the option of whether to establish the doctor–patient relationship. For any of many reasons they may part ways without necessarily engendering an obligation on the part of the physician to treat or manage, as long as the desires are explicitly documented in the record. In an emergency setting, the patient (who may present in a state of diminished mental and legal competence) is not in a position to choose, nor is the emergency physician, who cannot refuse treatment if the patient is unpleasant or there are already too many patients in the department.

Allegations of malpractice are common events in the emergency department. One major insurance carrier, for example, finds that fully one-fifth of its allegations of malpractice stem from the emergency department*. Risk management in the emergency department can be defined in two broad categories: those areas that are common to lawsuits whenever physicians and patients interact, and specific areas where the emergency department, because of its unique role in patient care, is particularly susceptible.

---

* Pennsylvania Hospital Insurance Company

In the first category, bad outcome, high costs, and negative interpersonal relationships lead the list of reasons for suing. Paradoxically, the ability to do much more for a patient *in extremis* than in the past has caused a revolution of high expectations on the part of the consumer. Movies, television, and the popular press have painted a picture of high-tech professionals poised and ready to offer the full spectrum of modern medicine to every victim who appears. Ability to provide the most sophisticated diagnostic and therapeutic interventions in a timely manner is expected; when a less than ideal outcome occurs there is potential for litigation. Cost plays a significant role. In urban areas, in particular, the emergency department is frequently used as a walk-in clinic by the medically indigent, by transients and by other medically unsophisticated consumers. Although urgent care centers are making some inroads with this clientele, there still exists substantial traffic in those who are reluctant to pay their share of the high amortization costs of a 24-hour-a-day, 7-day-a-week hospital-based facility.

The breakdown in doctor-patient communication is a third contributing cause. No one who has worked in an emergency department has not encountered the belligerent, hostile, demanding, and even abusive patient who requires extreme patience to be handled with marginal civility. The physician himself is subject to the human lapses of fatigue, irritability, annoyance, stress, and overwork that might be interpreted as callousness, indifference, or cursoriness.

The only cure for the problem of "bad" outcome is staffing of emergency departments with personnel who are knowledgeable, competent, and demonstrably skilled in advanced life-support techniques and the management of life-threatening emergencies as set forth elsewhere in this book. The hospital that puts this first triage responsibility on the shoulders of a junior staff person or worse yet, a moonlighting resident, does so at its peril. The financial cost issue can best be dealt with by full disclosure in advance of treatment. Eye-level signs should indicate the changes for registration and intake clerks should be well versed in the details of various insurance coverages.

When an individual shows up in the emergency department he has self-identified a situation that he perceives to be threatening to health or life. That perception must be dealt with in a compassionate, cool, and timely manner. Performing any part of the physical examination necessary for including or excluding the most critical disorders and considering the differential diagnosis of the chief complaint, as well as any laboratory tests deemed appropriate according to reasonable standards of care, is the best approach. In the current day, not only do many patients present to the emergency department with no funds, but many also have insurance (usually with special conditions of financial coverage) that cannot be verified on evenings or weekends, or belong to Health Maintenance Organizations or Preferred Provider Organizations (PPO) with elaborate and varying restrictions and definitions of an emergency. The physician and hospital thus often fear partial or no reimbursement, but the emergency department must accept all patients. The physician must be sure that the usual standard of care is met in such patients, that they receive a thorough and fully documented examination, and that they receive whatever laboratory tests or x-ray examinations are essential (Table 1). If they are to be transferred to another institution for primarily financial reasons, it is particularly essential that the evaluation be thorough enough to ensure stability during transport.

The emergency physician is working under an additional burden. Physicians who have a long term relationship with a patient get to know him, his complaints, and any associated diseases and the patient's handling of these interrelationships, and thus has a chance to build a bonding and trusting relationship over time. Physicians who have more impersonal or episodic exposure to patients, especially if they are dealing in a crisis situation, have no such back-ground of residual trust to engender compliance.

TABLE 1 Essential Elements for Avoiding Malpractice

Conduct and document a thorough and appropriate examination in all cases, regardless of patient finances, personality, or emergency department case load.

Document not only the patient's history and examination, but also any complications and changes during the emergency department stay.

Obtain needed laboratory tests, x-ray examinations, and ECGs regardless of patient's financial status.

Obtain expert consultation when unable to rule out serious conditions.

Be particularly thorough in evaluation and stabilization of patients for transfer.

Deal with all patients and families in a sympathetic and professional manner.

Ensure immediate critical value reporting for laboratory tests, x-ray examinations, and ECGs.

Avoid controversial or "experimental" procedures and uses of drugs.

Carry out regular quality assurance audits to identify high-risk diagnoses, situations, and personnel.

Provide understandable and detailed follow-up instructions.

Explain in advance the purpose and possible complications of any procedure performed.

A law suit has been defined as the ultimate breakdown in the doctor–patient relationship. Any interaction between two human beings is an interaction between personalities. If a physician is perceived as being abrupt, abrasive, uncaring, superficial, or cavalier, the stage is set for subsequent legal activity, if there is a bad outcome or an expensive encounter. (Most patients do not sue over a bad outcome alone; a negative relationship with the physician is usually a motivating factor.) The patient who is obstreperous, demanding, insinuating, or hostile does not always bring out the best in us. Physicians should keep in mind that an emergency department encounter with such a patient does not have the same social implications as say; a battle of wits at a cocktail party. Behavior of all emergency personnel should always be professional. Particular care should be taken to ensure that the behavior of difficult patients is not due to head trauma, hypoxia, shock, hypoglycemia, or some other true emergency, even if alcohol, drugs, or psychiatric problems appear at first glance to be the culprit.

As a rule of thumb, approximately 40 percent of all potentially compensable events are rendered indefensible because of *poor documentation*. It is particularly difficult to defend a case when a ward clerk or triage nurse's documentation of the patient's complaint varies considerably from the physical examination, or the differential diagnosis considered by the physician who actually treats the patient.

In this era of cost containment and outpatient management; it is chilling to note that in one series the basis of the malpractice suit in almost half of cases was the failure to admit a patient whom the courts decided a prudent physician would have admitted for close physiologic monitoring. Failure to perform and document a baseline physical examination of the body part relating to the chief complaint was the most common single reason for suit. A close second was the failure to order proper diagnostic studies or properly read x-ray films or properly interpret diagnostic studies that were performed. About half (155) of these instances resulted in deaths; 45 later at home, 35 in the emergency department, 68 in the hospital, and several at other locations. The causes of death in those cases were myocardial infarction, arterial bleeding, septicemia, meningitis, ruptured aortic aneurysm, pulmonary embolus, ruptured appendix, and suicide. The consensus of impartial reviewing experts was that three fourths of these deaths were preventable. What is especially ironic is that more than half of all the cases that resulted in suit in this series pertained to patients who had visited the emergency department with the same complaint or illness twice or more.

In reviewing actual cases that have engendered legal acitivity, it is clear that there are certain *high-risk* diseases, conditions and circumstances peculiar to the emergency department that are susceptibel to preventive risk management. In most series the most commonly identified error is the failure to recognize a fracture or dislocation on x-ray examination. This is a necessary skill for the emergency physician, as is the interpretation of electrocardiograms (ECGs), and deficits in this area should be corrected promptly with study and formal courses. Ruptured appendix, missed fractures, sepsis, retained foreign bodies in wounds, undiagnosed nerve injuries, and missed tendon lacerations are also high on the list. Less common but more catastrophic are hypoxic brain damage, missed myocardial infarction (often misdiagnosed as "indigestion" or "costochondritis"), ectopic pregnancy, and testicular torsion. Knowledge of this list of problems should cause the emergency physician to develop the habit of being particularly alert to them and carefully seeking them out. In addition, it should emphasize the need to know one's own limitations and to seek competent consultation in appropriate cases.

Another area that causes problems is that of *follow-up and patient instructions*. All patients should be given detailed instructions for care and follow-up, and these should be documented in writing. The commonly employed mimeographed instruction sheet is of little value for legal protection because the patient can easily state that he never received it or did not understand it; written documentation on the chart is ideal. Instructions for care should be in simple lay language and should include all complications that might arise, so that the patient will know to seek medical care immediately should they occur. Follow-up for continuing care should be recommended also; no specific physician need be recommended, but the need to see a particular type of physician within a particular time period is important. Instructions are not of any use if the patient is incapable of understanding them or carrying them out; so it is important that emergency staff determine that the patient's condition is sufficient for self-care, or that sufficient resources exist at home to care for the patient without risk. If these support systems do not exist, alternative support should be arranged or the patient should be admitted to the hospital. Follow-up phone calls to patients a day or two later not only determine the patient's condition and compliance, but also serve as a teaching tool and are part of building a trusting and caring relationship with patients that diminishes feelings of alienation and thus the likelihood of suit.

The risk factors for malpractice suits described previously can all be substanially lessened by active *quality assurance audit*. In one series of 362 emergency department malpractice cases, the most likely litigant was a man between the ages of 30 and 45 with a general surgical problem, and more than half of these patients were managed by house officers or moonlighters acting beyond the scope of their knowledge without appropriate concurrent audit or consultation. A key element of quality assurance is a *critical value reporting system*, which is set up to ensure that the emergency department is promptly notified of critical abnormalities in laboratory tests, x-ray examinations, and ECGs. This is particularly important in small hospitals, where the latter may not be officially interpreted for days. On-line telephone interpretation of ECGs is one method of ensuring that such abnormalities are not missed when less experienced or less well-trained personnel must work in the emergency department. Such values must be immediately reported to the emergency department and personnel must immediately follow-up to ensure that the patient was appropriately treated. It is wise to track individual physicians in this regard and identify those who are consistently in error in their interpretations. Chart review and other forms of audits of care are a requirement of the Joint Commission on the Accreditation of Hospitals, and they allow the department to monitor the quality of care and identify problem areas and personnel. Such review can be conducted on a random basis, but malpractice experience suggests that particular scrutiny should be paid to diagnoses known to be high risk.

SUGGESTED READING

Informed Consent. Quality Review Bulletin 1981; 7(5):9–13.

Legal precedence in American law for patient education. Patient Counselling Health Education 1979; 1(4):135–141.

Malpractice session. Emergence Medicine Clinic North American 1985; 3(3):437–446.

Malpractice in the emergency department, a review of 200 cases. Ann Intern Med 1984; 13:709–711.

INDEX